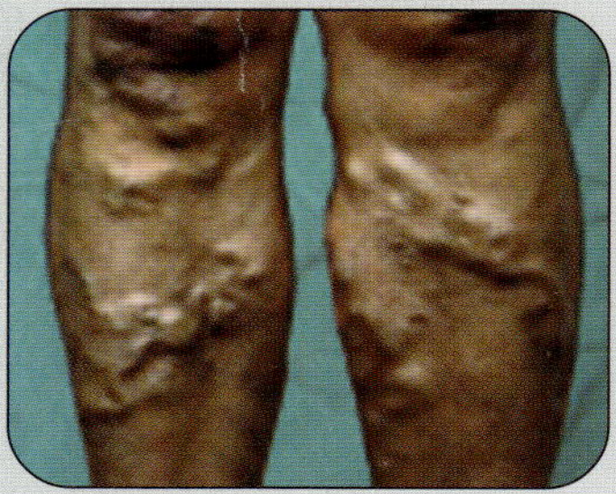 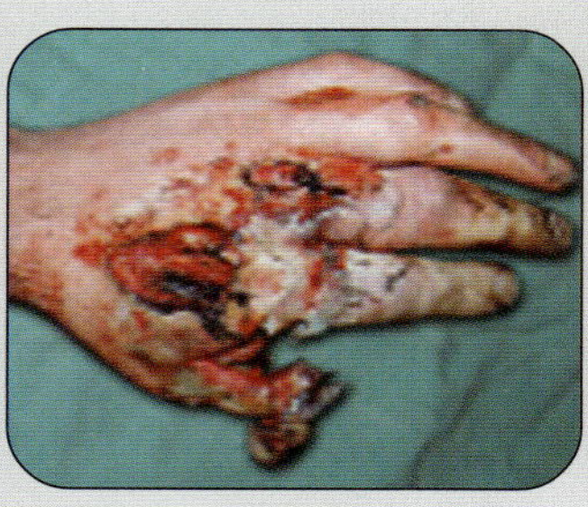 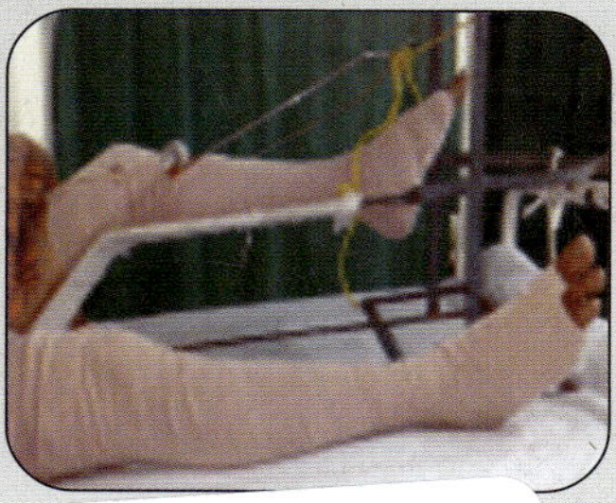 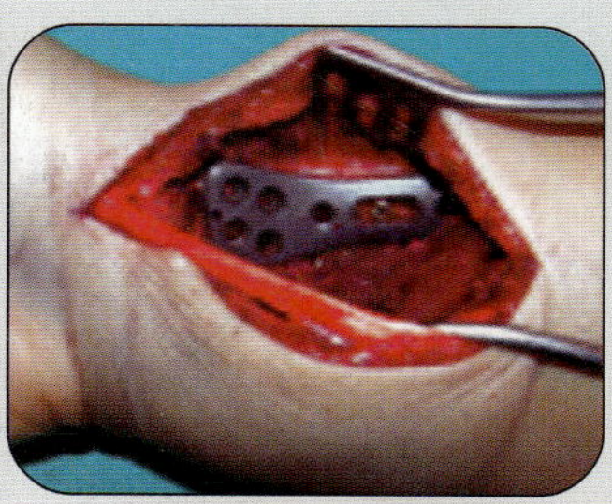

ORTHOPEDICS

(A Postgraduate Companion)

ORTHOPEDICS

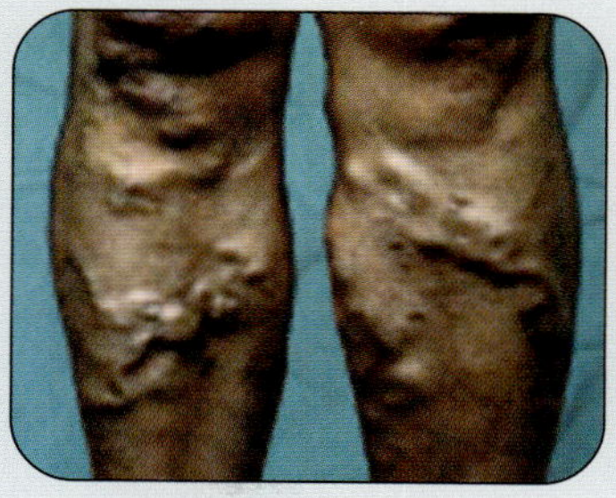
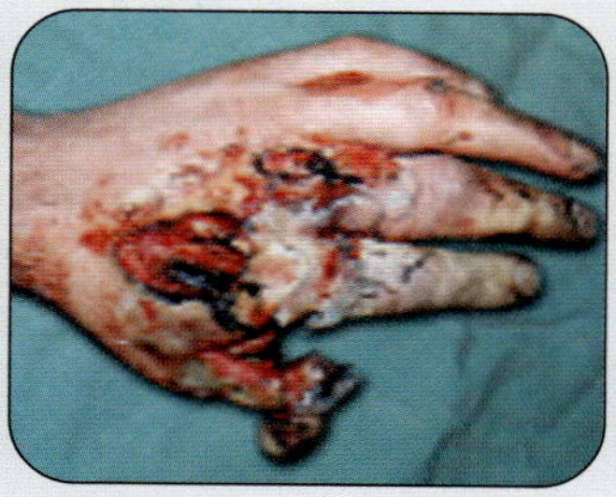
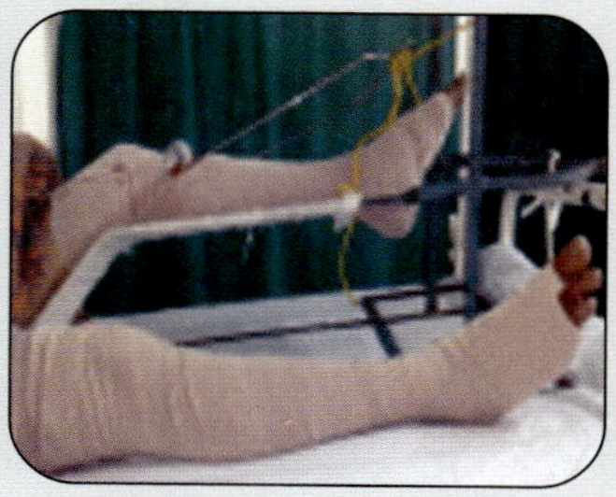
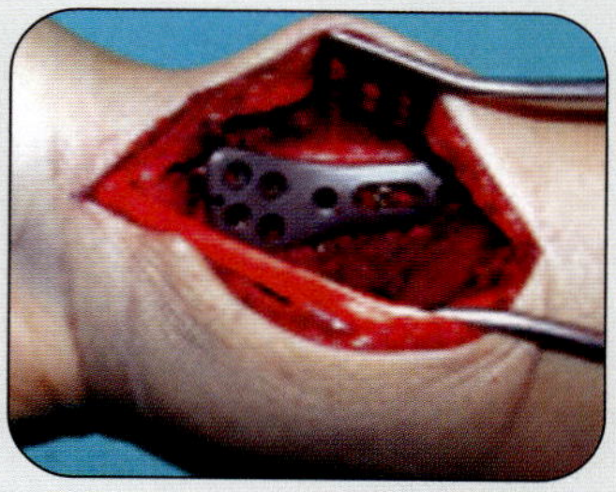

ORTHOPEDICS

(A Postgraduate Companion)

Dr (Col) Samar Kumar Biswas MS
General Surgery, Orthopedics
Foot and Ankle Institute of San Francisco (FAISF)
Professor and Head
Department of Orthopedics
Padmashree Dr DY Patil Medical College
Hospital and Research Centre
Pune, Maharashtra, India

Foreword

KH Sancheti

JAYPEE BROTHERS MEDICAL PUBLISHERS (P) LTD

New Delhi • Panama City • London • Philadelphia (USA)

Jaypee Brothers Medical Publishers (P) Ltd

Headquarters

Jaypee Brothers Medical Publishers (P) Ltd
4838/24, Ansari Road, Daryaganj
New Delhi 110 002, India
Phone: +91-11-43574357
Fax: +91-11-43574314
Email: jaypee@jaypeebrothers.com

Overseas Offices

J.P. Medical Ltd
83, Victoria Street, London
SW1H 0HW (UK)
Phone: +44-2031708910
Fax: +02-03-0086180
Email: info@jpmedpub.com

Jaypee-Highlights Medical Publishers Inc.
City of Knowledge, Bld. 237, Clayton
Panama City, Panama
Phone: +507-301-0496
Fax: +507-301-0499
Email: cservice@jphmedical.com

Jaypee Brothers Medical Publishers, Ltd
The Bourse
111 South Independence Mall East
Suite 835, Philadelphia, PA 19106, USA
Phone: + 267-519-9789
Email: joe.rusko@jaypeebrothers.com

Jaypee Brothers Medical Publishers (P) Ltd
17/1-B Babar Road, Block-B, Shaymali
Mohammadpur, Dhaka-1207
Bangladesh
Mobile: +08801912003485
Email: jaypeedhaka@gmail.com

Jaypee Brothers Medical Publishers (P) Ltd
Shorakhute, Kathmandu
Nepal
Phone: +00977-9841528578
Email: jaypee.nepal@gmail.com

Website: www.jaypeebrothers.com
Website: www.jaypeedigital.com

Inquiries for bulk sales may be solicited at: jaypee@jaypeebrothers.com

Orthopedics (A Postgraduate Companion)

First Edition: **2013**

ISBN: 978-93-5025-279-6

Printed at Replika Press Pvt. Ltd.

Dedicated to

My parents

My teachers

My family, and

My beloved PG students

Best Wishes

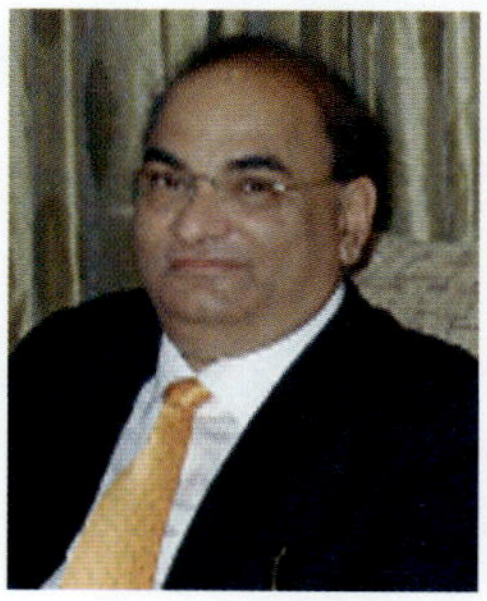

It gives me immense pleasure to pen a few lines of greetings and good wishes to Dr (Col) Samar Kumar Biswas for this book.

I know Dr Biswas over the last eight years, when he joined as a Professor and Head, Department of Orthopedics in Padmashree Dr DY Patil Medical College, Hospital and Research Centre, Pune, Maharashtra, India. In a short span of time, he became a popular Professor amongst undergraduate as well as postgraduate students for his excellent teaching practices. The classes and clinics of Dr Biswas were well attended and appreciated by the students. Even students from other institutions, in and around Pune, were also interested in attending his lectures. He has been honoured with 'Best Teacher Award'.

Dr Biswas has a dynamic personality. He has good relations with his colleagues, who revere him for his vast knowledge and pleasant personality.

As Albert Einstein aptly said, 'The only source of knowledge is experience.' Dr Biswas has put his vast teaching experience in this book to share his knowledge for the betterment of the postgraduate students. I am sure that his book will also become as popular amongst the students as were his teachings.

I congratulate Dr Biswas for this book and wish him all the success in future endeavor.

Dr PD Patil
Honourable President
Dr DY Patil Vidyapeeth
Pune, Maharashtra, India

Foreword

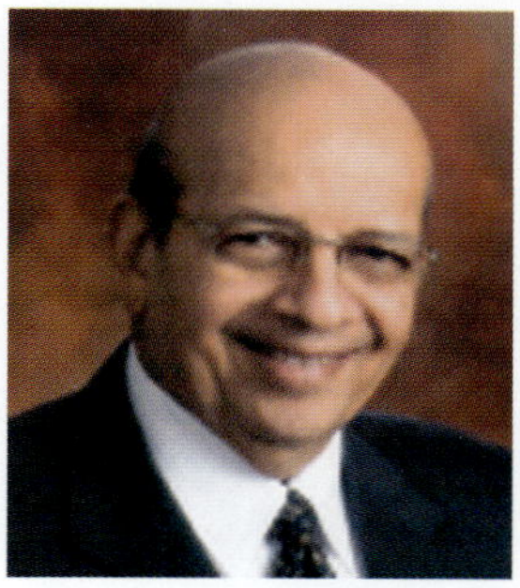

As a student, whenever I found information on any topic to be scattered and incomplete, I often had to refer to many books to get a complete picture. Nowadays, information available on any subject is enormous. A book that is comprehensive and covers every topic from A to Z was deeply needed to make the life of the postgraduate students easier. I think Dr (Col) Samar Kumar Biswas has been successful in accomplishing this feat.

I have gone through his book and I found that each region is adequately covered, from anatomy to the latest advances in surgical management. There is a lot of emphasis on basic principles and clinical examination, both of which are very close to my heart. This book eliminates the need to refer to a separate book on clinical skills. He has addressed controversies without bias and the sections on 'Recent Advances' is updated with current literature. The sections on 'Congenital Anomalies and Trauma' are a pleasure to go through. All recent classifications have been included and topics, like 'Scaphocapitate Fracture Syndrome,' have been explained in a lucid and clear manner.

A section on 'General Surgery' is given which would rival any general surgery textbook, means a student has to deal with one less book. The information is with special reference to the orthopedic students, so that this extra nonetheless essential knowledge is easy to grasp.

The real surprise, however, is the chapter on the Spine. Dr Biswas has truly done justice to this complicated and difficult topic.

I would encourage every postgraduate student to take advantage of this wonderful book. I have already decided to keep copies of this book in our institute's library.

I congratulate Dr Biswas for his vision and his tireless efforts to convert it into a reality.

Padma Vibhushan **Dr KH Sancheti**
MS, PhD (Ortho), FRCS (Edinburgh) FICS, FACS (USA)
Sancheti Institute for Orthopedics and Rehabilitation
Pune, Maharashtra, India

Preface

I got inspired to write a book, mainly for the postgraduate students, while teaching them and examining the postgraduate candidates during examinations of various universities, as a postgraduate teacher and examiner over the last fifteen years. I felt the necessity of a book describing regions, like hip, knee, elbow, etc. right from the anatomy and development of the regions to trauma, tumors, infections and even reconstruction or replacement of the part in one chapter. There is lack of such a book, as a guide for postgraduate students in market today. Orthopedics today is not just a crude way of treating with plasters, screws and plates, it is advancing day-by-day with new techniques and concepts of management from noninvasive to minimally invasive. This has been possible also from early diagnosis for proper institution of appropriate treatment, to join the patients back to their jobs early. Keeping the above, I have prepared the seminar topics accordingly, for my postgraduate students and guided them in making the seminars. I have also included the recent advances and concepts on the subjects, even by consulting the Internet. I have given special emphasis on the clinical methods of examination in detail, as during most of the examinations, postgraduate students are asked to demonstrate the clinical tests and signs.

Hence, by taking the name of Lord Ganesha, I made a fair attempt to prepare this book, describing the topics region-wise, encompassing from the very basics to most recent advances in that particular subject.

I will consider my attempt to be successful only when this book will be welcomed by the postgraduate students, as a constant companion while preparing their tough subject and will help them in becoming a successful orthopedic clinician.

Dr (Col) Samar Kumar Biswas

Acknowledgments

At the outset, I want to acknowledge my family members, my wife Mrs Smriti Biswas, my daughter Snigdha Dutta and my son Somnath Biswas, for their constant inspiration and selfless encouragement and cooperation, without these, I would not have been able to complete this impossible work, of writing this book.

I want to acknowledge the continuous help from my beloved postgraduate students, specially Dr Tanveer Singh Bhutani, Dr Mahendra Kumar Reddy, Dr Praful Kilaru, Dr Ganesh Kumar Reddy, Dr Dhyan Patel and Dr Shalin Maheswari, in preparing and editing the manuscript of this book.

My special thanks to my students, my colleagues, Assistant Professor, Dr Rahul Salunkhe; Dr Samir Deshmukh and Dr Abhijit Shroff. My thanks also goes for some of my favorite students, my colleagues, Professor, Dr Suahs Kamble; Associate Professor, Dr Amit Swamy; Professor, Dr Anil Salgia; Dr Subhash Puri for their continuous inspiration in writing this book for postgraduate students.

I will be failing in my duty, if I do not remember our Honourable President Dr PD Patil, without his blessings and best wishes I could not have completed this work.

My special acknowledgments go for Dr (Brig) Amarjit Singh, Vice Chancellor and Dr BS Mane, Registrar of our prestigious university Padmashree Dr DY Patil, Medical College and Vidyapeeth, Pune, Maharashtra, India.

My special gratitude goes for our artist Mr Pomaji, who has taken pain-taking task of making beautiful illustrations for this book.

I take this opportunity to thank Jaypee Brothers Medical Publishers (P) Ltd, New Delhi, India, who took keen interest in publishing this book.

Contents

SECTION 1: GENERAL ORTHOPEDICS

SECTION 2: GENERAL SURGERY RELATED TO ORTHOPEDICS

SECTION 3: REGIONAL ORTHOPEDICS

SECTION 4: RECENT ADVANCEMENTS IN ORTHOPEDICS

Section 1

General Orthopedics

1 History of Orthopedics

- Important Figures in Orthopedics
- Total Joint Replacement

■ Introduction

Orthopedics, like many specialties has developed through a necessity. A necessity to correct deformity, restore function and alleviate pain. Orthopedic surgeons have developed an ability to prevent major losses of bodily functions and indeed they can prevent an otherwise inevitable death. They seek perfection of their art, by ensuring that the patient reaches optimal condition in the shortest period of time by the safest possible method.

■ History

Ancient Egypt

- Splints have been found on mummies and they were made of bamboo, reeds, wood or bark, padded with linen
- There is also evidence of the use of crutches, with the earliest known record of the use of a crutch coming from a carving made in 2830 BC on the entrance of a portal on Hirkouf's tomb
- In the Papyrus (a book), the examination of peripheral limbs was described
- In this Papyrus, injuries were classified according to their prognosis into three categories:
  1. An ailment, which they would treat
  2. An ailment that they would contend
  3. An ailment, which they would not treat
- The Papyrus also mentioned many cases and the treatment involved.

Ancient Greece

- Many principles behind conditions and their treatment have been attributed to the ancient Greecs
- They could be regarded as the first to use a scientific approach
- They were also the first to document in detail their history and developments
- Hegetor of Alexandria (100 BC), described in detail the anatomical relations of the hip joint and was the first to record a description of the ligamentum teres
- In Corpus Hippocrates (it is named after Hippocrates, who is known as the Father of Medicine), dislocation of the shoulder was described together with the various methods used in reduction and correction of club foot
- Hippocrates had a thorough understanding of fractures. He knew the principles of traction and counter traction. He developed special splints for fractures of the tibia, similar to external fixation.

Roman Era

- Another respected roman figure of Greec origin by the name of Galen (129 to 199 BC) "Father of Sports Medicine"
- He gave a good account of the skeleton and the muscles that move it
- He first recorded a case of cervical ribs
- He described bone destruction, sequestration and regeneration in osteomyelitis and sometimes performed resection in such cases
- During this Greeco-Roman period, there were also attempts to provide artificial prosthesis
- It is said that both linen and catgut sutures were used for the procedures, during this period
- Various drills, saws and chisels were also developed during this period.

Arab Era

- Although, the Arab practices were regarded as an extension of those of the Greecs, the use of plaster of Paris in the tenth century was significant
- With the addition of water to a powder of anhydrous calcium sulfate, a hard crystalline material was produced
- It was not until the l2th century that Europe began to awake gradually from its dark ages

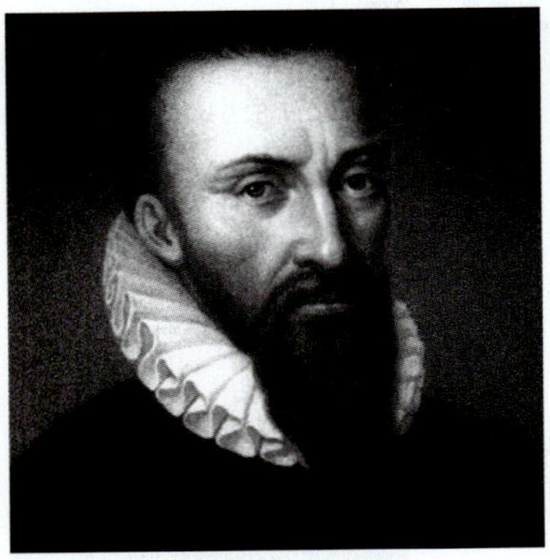

Fig. 1.1: Ambroise Paré

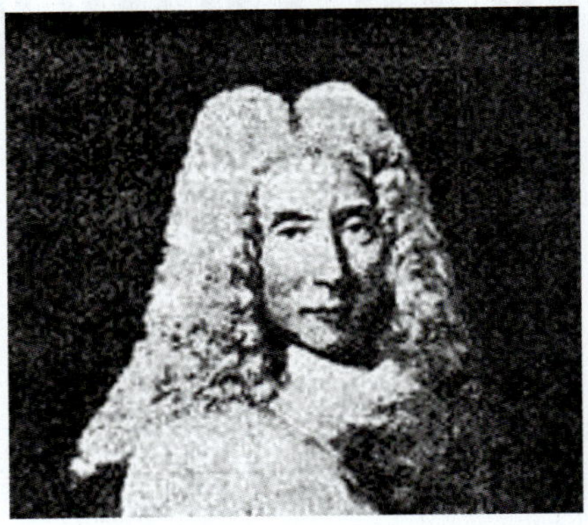

Fig. 1.2: Nicholas Andry

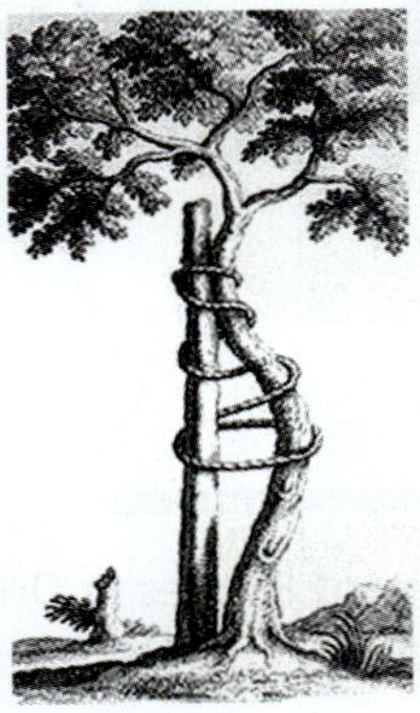

Fig. 1.3: Andry Tree—A symbol for orthopedics

- Until the 16th century, all developments remained within the shadow casted by Hippocrates.

Important Figures in Orthopedics

Ambroise Paré (1510–1590) (Fig. 1.1)

- Most famous surgical figure of the 16th century and the Father of French Surgery
- Used ligature, for large vessels in amputations
- Used a tourniquet in his amputations
- Paré, designed scoliosis corset and clubfoot boot.

Nicholas Andry (1658–1742) (Fig. 1.2)

- Father of Orthopedics
- He coined the term, "Orthopedics" (Greec word *Orthos*, means straight and *Paed*, means child) in 1741
- He published, a famous book called "Orthopedia" or the "Art of Correcting and Preventing Deformities in Children"
- He gave the symbol "Andry Tree" (Fig. 1.3), which has been adopted worldwide, as the symbol for orthopedics.

Percival Pott (1714–1788)

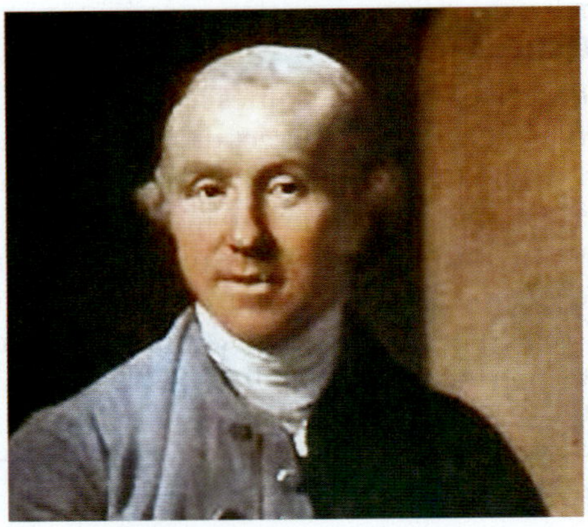

Fig. 1.4: Percival Pott

- Percival Pott (Fig. 1.4), was born in the Threadneedle Street of Cockney
- He obtained grand diploma of Barber Surgeon's Company in 1736 from St Bartholomew's Hospital and was soon appointed to the staff of the same hospital eight years later
- He is best known for the fracture that bears his name, Pott's fracture, as he was the first to give a good description of this ankle fracture
- In 1756, Pott sustained a broken leg after fall from his horse. It is often assumed that his injury was the same one that later came to be known as Pott's fracture, but in reality Pott's broken leg was much more serious compound fracture of femur
- As he lay in the mud, he sent a servant to buy a door from nearby and had himself placed on the door. Surgeons cleaned the wound and discussed amputation, but Pott insisted to splint the leg and recovered completely
- In 1775, Pott found an association between exposure to soot and high incidence of scrotal cancer. This was the first occupational link to cancer
- Pott was the first person, to demonstrate that malignancy could be caused by environmental carcinogen
- Pott's most famous work is on the paraplegia of spinal tuberculosis, where he stressed that the condition was not related to spinal cord compression, but associated with strumous disorders in the lungs. This is known as Pott's paraplegia. His account of tuberculosis paraplegia was first published in 1779.

John Hunter (1728–1793)

- John Hunter's (Fig. 1.5) saying "Do not think, try the experiment", has inspired generations of modern surgeons
- He described how to assess power in a weak muscle

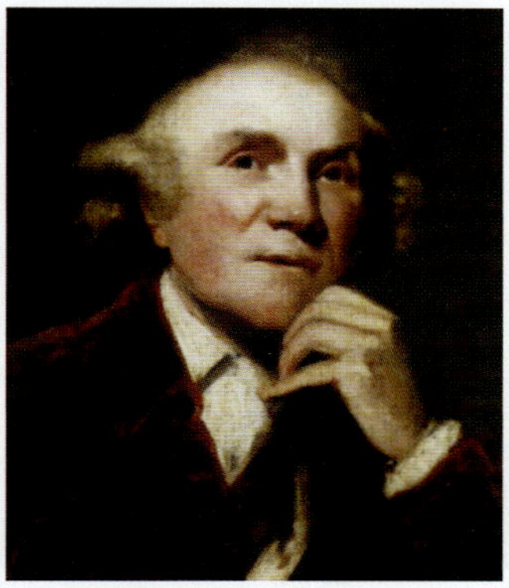

Fig. 1.5: John Hunter

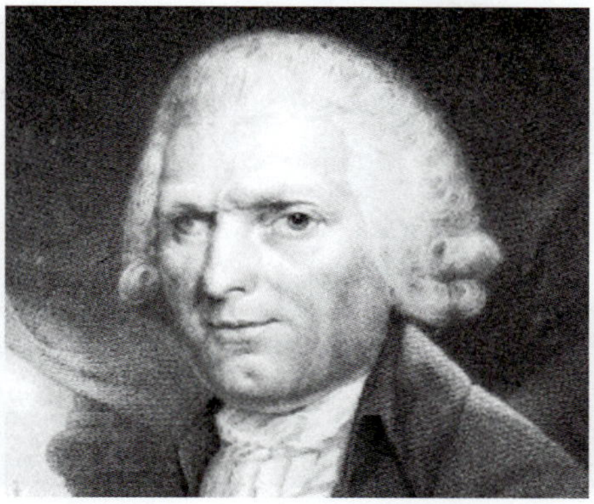

Fig. 1.6: William Hey

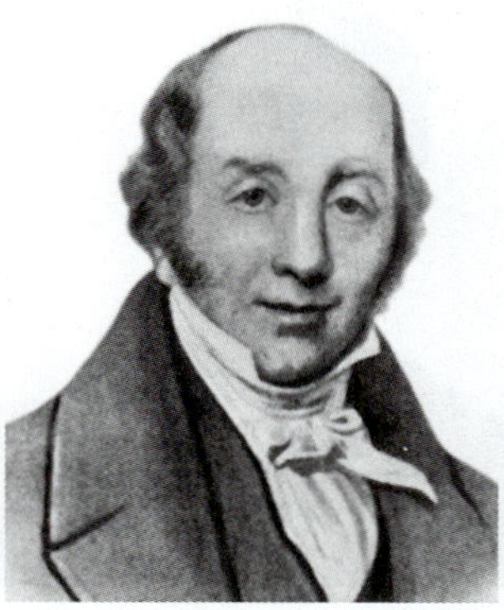

Fig. 1.7: Abraham Colles

- He believed that healing depends on the body innate power and that the surgeon's task was to aid this
- He studied loose bodies in joints, pseudoarthroses and fracture healing.

William Hey (1736–1819)

- Subacute osteomyelitis of the tibia, was described by him and he advocated deroofing of the lesion
- In 1773, Hey (Fig. 1.6), banged his knee getting out of the bath and many attribute his subsequent interest in the knee to this
- He coined the phrase "Internal Derangement of the Knee", and described meniscal injuries
- Hey, described loose bodies and introduced tarsometatarsal amputation.

Abraham Colles (1773–1843)

- Abraham Colles (Fig. 1.7), was responsible for much of the early scientific development of surgery in Ireland and was the leading Irish surgeon of his time
- On January 4, 1802, when only 29 years of age, he was elected as president of the Royal College of Surgeons in Ireland
- He was the first to tie the first stage of the right subclavian artery for a large axillary aneurism in 1811
- Best known for his description of Colles' fracture in 1814.

Colles' Fracture

In his classical paper, "On Fracture of the Carpal Extremity of the Radius" in 1814, when no X-rays were available, he had described accurately the classical deformity following the fracture of lower end of radius, which is known as "Colles' fracture" after him.

Colles' Fascia

In the perineum, the middle fascia of the urogenital triangle, the attachments of which served to confine within strict limits extravasation of urine from a ruptured urethra is known as Colle's fascia.

Colles' Ligament

It is the name sometimes given to the small triangular fascia that springs from the pubic crest and iliopectineal line and passes upwards and inwards towards the linea alba, under cover of the internal pillar of the external abdominal ring.

Colles' Law

- In 1837, Colles published a book entitled "Practical Observations", on the venereal disease and on the use of mercury. In a chapter, dealing with syphilis in infants, he made an observation that later became known as Colles' law, which can be stated as, "a child born of a mother, who is without any obvious venereal symptoms and which, without being exposed to any infection subsequent to its birth, shows this disease. When it is a few weeks old, this child will infect the most healthy nurse, whether she suckle it or merely handle and dress it and yet this child is never known to infect its mother, even though she suckle it, while it has venereal ulcers on the lips and tongue"
- He clearly observed the apparent immunity of the mother, but could not have guessed that she already had the disease in a mild form. It was nearly 70 years later, that the *Fritz Schaudinn,* discovered *Spirochaeta pallida* and the serological test devised by Wassermann
- This work on venereal disease was his last important contribution.

Antonius Mathijsen (1805–1878)

Antonius Mathijsen (Fig. 1.8), was a Dutch military surgeon, who in 1851 invented the Plaster of Paris (POP) bandage, which has become so important in orthopedic practice.

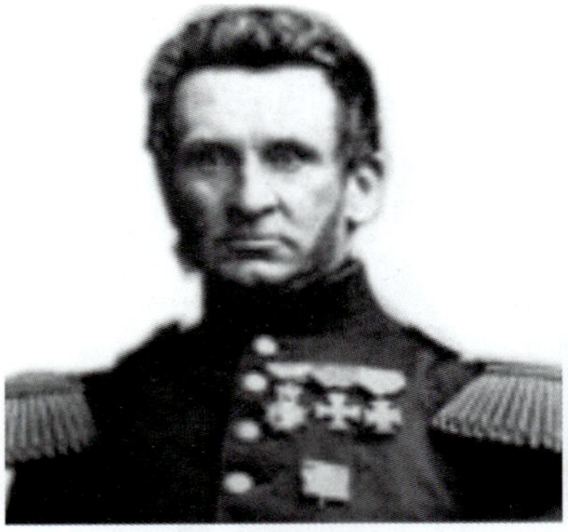

Fig. 1.8: Antonius Mathijsen

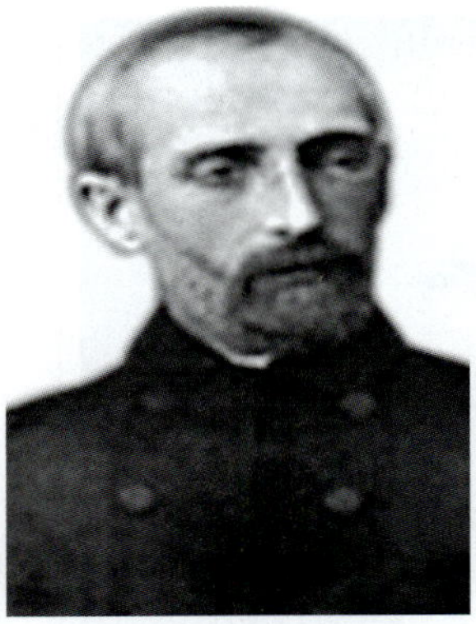

Fig. 1.9: Hugh Owen Thomas

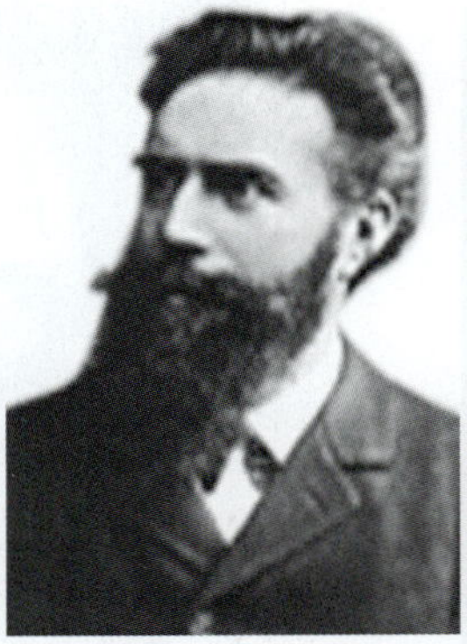

Fig. 1.10: William Conrad Roentgen

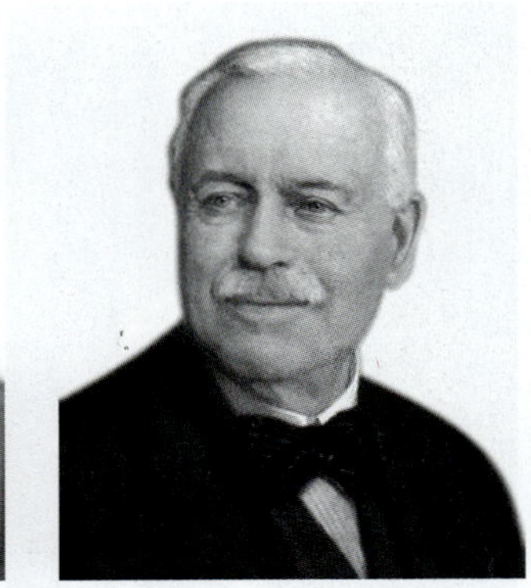

Fig. 1.11: Sir Robert Jones

Hugh Owen Thomas (1834–1891)

- Hugh Owen Thomas (Fig. 1.9), is known as Father of British Orthopedics
- He was the eldest of five sons born to a well known bonesetter at that time
- He could not even work with his father and never held a hospital appointment
- He treated all his patients at home
- His practice was so busy that he started his rounds at five or six in the morning and never left his home for other than professional purposes. Thomas would designate sunday, as his free day and hundreds of patients from the country would surround his house in order to be treated
- The people of Liverpool knew Thomas, as a short and quick man. A man who always wore a black coat buttoned up to the neck and a sailor's cap pulled over a damaged eye. A cigarette was also seen constantly in his mouth
- Thomas contributions include:
  - Thomas splint
  - Thomas wrench
  - Cervical collar
  - Metatarsal bar
  - Heel wedge
  - Knee splint
- Many of these are still in use, such as the Thomas splint
- He was the first to demonstrate concealed flexion of the hip joint and a way of unmasking this, by performing the "Thomas test".

The Modern Era (20th Century Orthopedics)

The discovery of the X-ray almost marked 1900 and orthopedics was only now being seen, as a true specialty of its own.

William Conrad Roentgen (1845–1923)

- Roentgen (Fig. 1.10), was a professor of physics at Wurzburg, his discovery of X-rays (Roentgen rays) and their use has been a huge contribution to orthopedics
- The first radiography that Roentgen took was of his wife's hand on December 22nd 1895. This was allegedly her christmas present
- Roentgen received the nobel prize for his discovery in 1901.

Sir Robert Jones (1857–1933)

- Jones (Fig. 1.11) was a nephew of the great Hugh Owen Thomas and became one of his apprentices in Liverpool
- In 1896, Jones published the first report of the clinical use of an X-ray, to locate a bullet in a wrist
- His textbook "Orthopedic Surgery", is said to be the first to have dealt systematically with the diagnosis and treatment of fresh fractures
- In World War I, Jones headed the orthopedic section of the british forces
- Jones was an advocate of:
  - Tendon transplantation
  - Bone grafting
  - Other conservative and restorative procedures.

World War I

- It must be noted that war has played an important part in orthopedic history
- Many of our greatest contributors were military surgeons
- It is interesting to note that many of the achievements during and after World War I, were not related directly to traumatic injuries received at war
- Orthopedics was definitely seen as a separate speciality, after World War I and that this was the first major war, where aseptic techniques were saving many more lives than in the past wars.

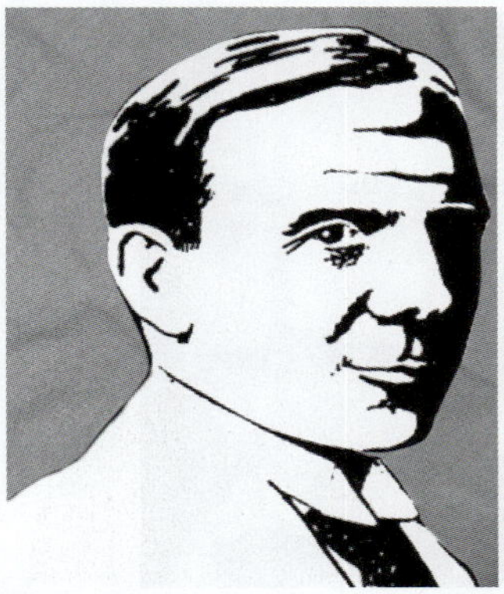

Fig. 1.12: Thomas Porter McMurray

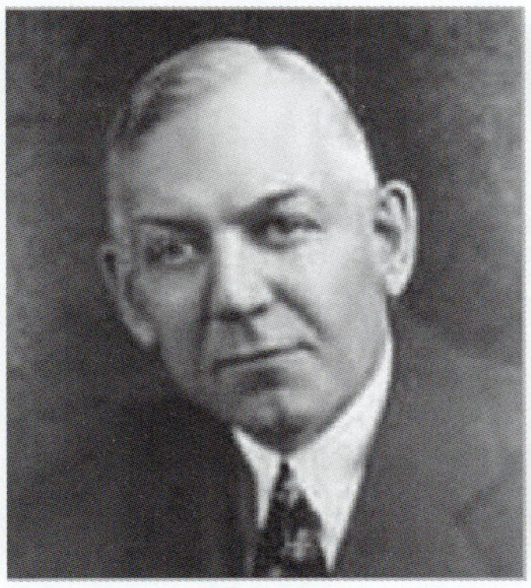

Fig. 1.13: Willis Campbell

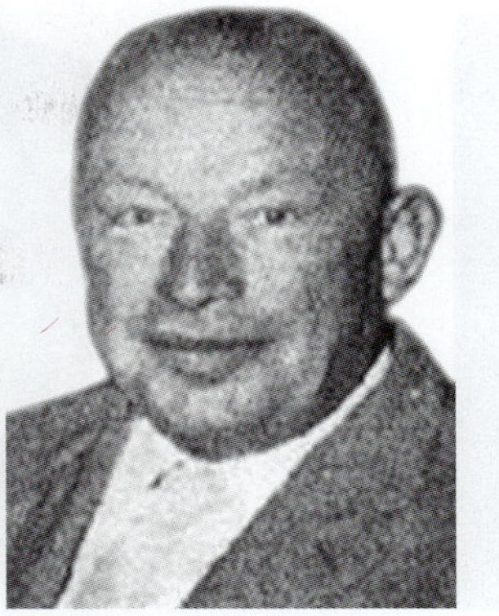

Fig. 1.14: Gerhard Kuntscher

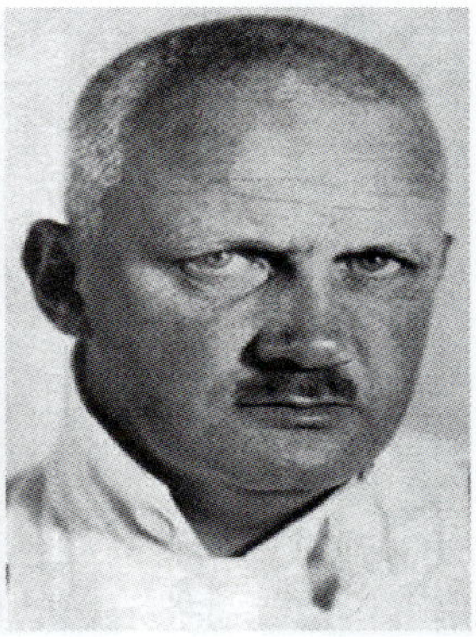

Fig. 1.15: Martin Kirschner

Thomas Porter McMurray (1888–1949)

- In the chain of great surgeons that followed Hugh Owen Thomas, came Thomas Porter McMurray (Fig. 1.12), who worked for Robert Jones
- His operative dexterity was renowned, for he could remove an entire meniscus in five minutes and disarticulate a hip in ten minutes
- He introduced his sign for a torn meniscus, McMurray's sign.

McMurray's Osteotomy

An operation was also named after him, as McMurray was the first to perform a displacement osteotomy, for ununited fractures of the femoral neck and arthrosis of the hip.

World War II

- The knowledge learnt in fighting World War I, helped in treating the casualties of World War II
- In World War II, there were less amputations performed, less gangrene and better measures for fixation of fractures
- We must not forget the importance of penicillin (whose effects were discovered by Sir Alexander Fleming, in 1928)
- The Germans needed quick measures, to restore their fighters to optimal fighting potential and developed a number of nailing procedures, during this period
- Together with this, the Americans were now making more contributions than ever before.

Willis Campbell (1880–1941)

- Campbell (Fig. 1.13) was the main advocate of interpositional arthroplasty at that time
- Campbell used a free autogenous transplant of fascia lata
- Campbell was also a key figure in bone grafting and performed inlay full thickness grafts, for nonunion bones fixed with screws of beef bone
- He published three volumes:
  - A monograph, "Orthopedics of Childhood", 1927
  - A textbook, "Orthopedic Surgery", 1930
  - His last publication was "Operative Orthopedics", in 1939.

Gerhard Kuntscher (1900–1972)

- Gerhard Kuntscher (Fig. 1.14), served in the German army, during the World War II and published his revolutionary procedure in the opening months of the war
- His work was concerned with the intramedullary nailing of fractures of the shafts of long bones and his name is associated with the nail.

Martin Kirschner (1879–1942) (Fig. 1.15)

- Known for his methods of fixation, in particular for the Kirschner or K-wire
- He also performed the first successful pulmonary embolectomy.

Sir Reginald Watson-Jones (1902–1972)

- Watson Jones (Fig. 1.16) was born in Brighton, England on March 1902
- He acquired an interest in the field of medicine after about with typhoid fever
- He was graduated form the University of Liverpool in 1922
- He decided to pursue orthopedics, following an operation to remove hemangioma from his leg
- During World War II, he was among the leading teachers in fracture therapy
- He was responsible for and was the first editor of the British volume of the Journal of Bone and Joint Surgery (JBJS) and retained the post through four decades
- He was the orthopedic surgeon for England's King and Queen
- Watson-Jones published, "Fractures and Joint Injuries" in 1940, which remained a standard reference

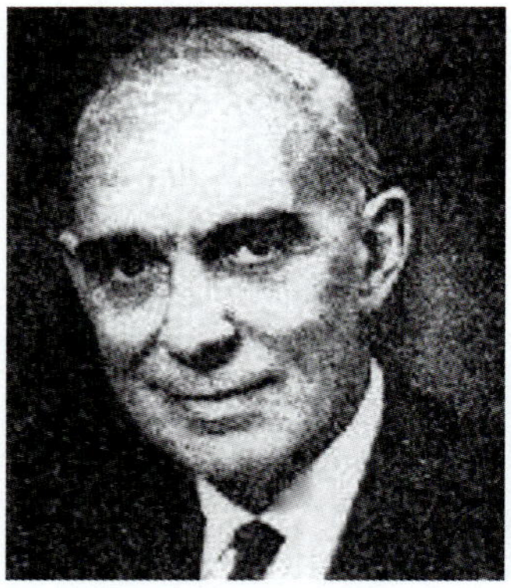

Fig. 1.16: Sir Reginald Watson-Jones

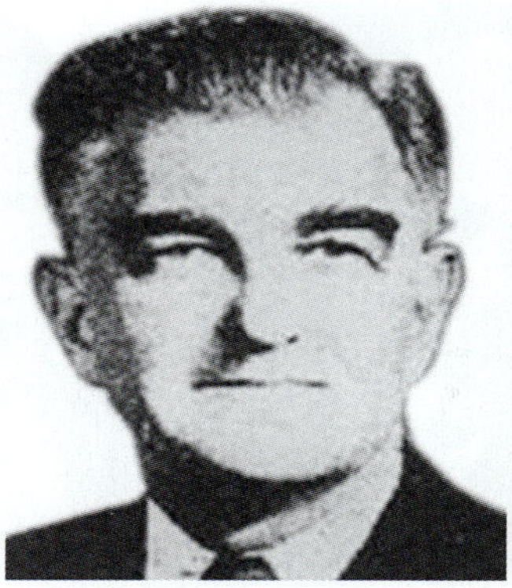

Fig. 1.17: Austin T Moore

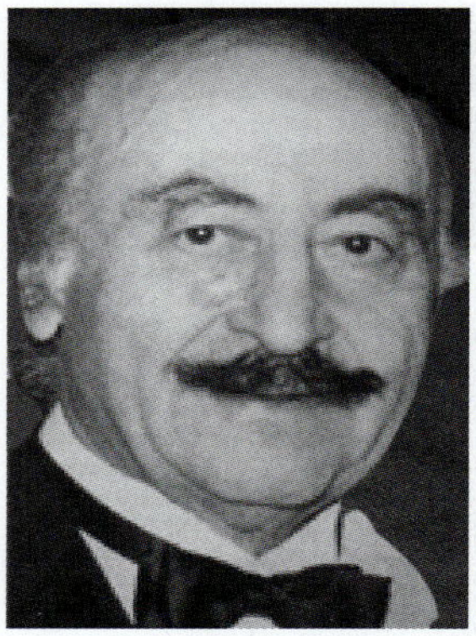

Fig. 1.18: Gavriil A Ilizarov

for several decades and was considered as a bible of the fracture and joint injuries. It was translated into many languages.

Austin T Moore (1899–1963)

- Moore (Fig. 1.17) performed the first metallic hip replacement. He had replaced for the first time, the entire upper portion of the femur with a vitallium prosthesis
- Over the years, the design of the prosthesis and the procedure improved. Consequently, there is one type of prosthesis called the Austin-Moore, which is still used today.

Gavriil A Ilizarov (1921–1992)

- G Ilizarov (Fig. 1.18) was born in the Caucasian Mountains and did not attend school until he was 12 years old, because his family had no money for shoes
- He graduated from Simferopol Medical School, which had been moved during the war to the Soviet near east
- During World War II, he was evacuated to Dolgovka, near Kurgan and ran a hospital single handed, where working conditions were primitive with no antibiotics and inadequate equipments. The operating room was heated by a wood fire
- Injured Russian soldiers, came through the village and this is when he started developing his famous apparatus, circular frame for distraction osteogenesis
- His theory that bone would grow, if gradually distracted and his external fixator of circular steel haloes connected by rods and bone-fixating wires, produced dramatic results not seen before in orthopedics
- His work was the beginning of a new medical paradigm, the conservation and exploitation of the unlimited natural plasticity of bone
- Although Dr Ilizarov's results were astonishing, his theory was contrary to orthodox views on bone regeneration
- His reputation remained confined to Siberia, until 1967, when he successfully treated the Russian olympic highjumper, Valery Brumel, who after a motorcycle accident, had chronically infected nonunited fractures of both legs, even after 14 operations, by the best surgeons in Moscow. After treatment by Ilizarov, he completely healed and went onto jump again in competition
- From then, his reputation soared into national and international prominence and by 1984, he presided over a new 1,000 bed, Scientific Center for Reconstructive Orthopedics and Traumatology, with over 350 surgeons, 1,500 nurses, 60 doctorate researchers and 24 operating rooms
- By 1986, North American orthopedic surgeons had learned the Ilizarov techniques from Europeans, who had worked directly with him and were performing Ilizarov limb-saving operations
- The use of his methods is widespread. The North American Association for the Study and Application of the Methods of Ilizarov (ASAMI), now includes over 200 surgeons.

After the Wars

- In the years following the war, orthopedic surgeons sought to perfect their treatment of fractures, in particular with the use of metallic pins and wires for fixation
- With the introduction of alloys, that could be used effectively, there was also a new wave of prosthesis, which are developing for treatment of arthritis as well as problematic fractures
- Antibiotics have greatly improved and so have our diagnostic devices.

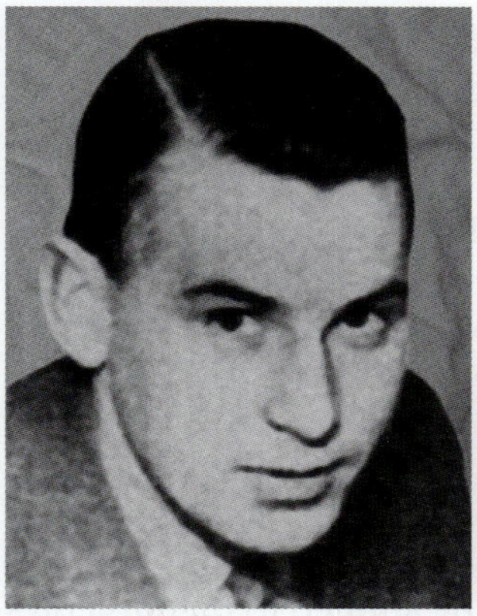

Fig. 1.19: H Lowry Rush

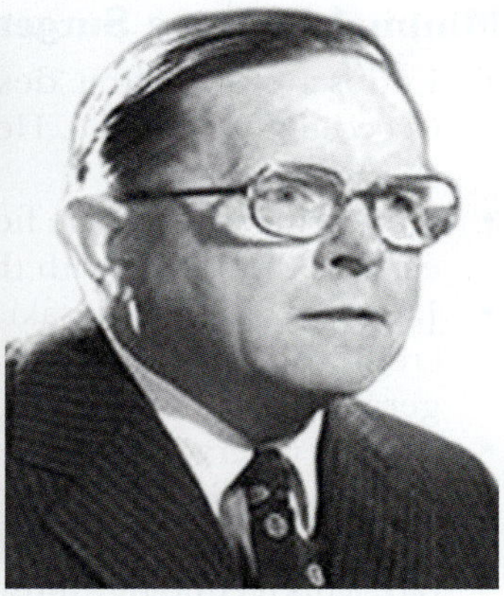

Fig. 1.20: Sir John Charnley

H Lowry Rush (1879–1965) (Fig. 1.19)

Used pins made of especially hardened stainless steel, for treating long bone fractures.

Sir John Charnley (1911–1982)

- Sir John Charnley (Fig. 1.20) wrote a classic book on the nonoperative approach to fractures, "Closed Treatment of Common Fractures"
- Sir Charnley is however renowned, as the effective innovator of the total hip replacement and development of a self-curing acrylic bone cement
- Many of the total hip replacements, that he performed in the 1960's are still sound and serving their patients effectively.

■ Total Joint Replacement

Hip

- In 1925, a surgeon in Boston, Massachusetts, MN Smith Petersen MD, molded a piece of glass into the shape of a hollow hemisphere, which could fit over the ball of the hip joint and provide a new smooth surface for movement. While proving biocompatible, the glass could not withstand the stress of walking and quickly failed
- Frederick R Thompson of New York and Austin T Moore of South Carolina, separately developed replacements for the entire ball of the hip. This type of hip replacement, called hemiarthroplasty, only addressed the problem of the arthritic femoral head (the ball). The diseased acetabulum (hip socket) was not replaced. While very popular in the 1950's, results remained unpredictable and arthritic destruction of the socket persisted
- As early as 1938, Dr Jean Judet and his brother, Dr Robert Judet of Paris, attempted to use an acrylic material, to replace arthritic hip surfaces. This acrylic provided a smooth surface, but unfortunately tended to come loose
- In 1950's, Charnley devised effective methods of replacing both the femoral head and acetabulum of the hip. He first used teflon implant for acetabular component, but when it failed, he tried polyethylene, which worked wonderfully well. In order to obtain fixation of this polyethylene socket as well as the femoral implant to the bone, Charnley borrowed polymethyl methacrylate from the dentists. This substance, known as bone cement was mixed during the operation then used as a strong grouting agent, to firmly secure the artificial joint to the bone. Truly this was the birth of "total hip replacement"
- In the last 10 years, there had been considerable effort and research done, in trying to improve the methods of fixation. Occasionally, it has been found that cement fixation breaks down over time. Due to this, implants with textured surfaces, which allow bone to grow into them have been developed. These have been used experimentally in animals and are now being used in humans. The results of these cementless joints look very promising, when utilized in the correct circumstances.

Knee

- The first attempt at total knee arthroplasty was a prosthesis, which was really a hinge fixed to the bones with stems into the medullary canals (the hollow marrow cavity). These hinges provided good short-term pain relief, but function was not always great due to the limitations of motion and were abandoned
- McKeever (1957) and Macintosh (1958, 1964) tried to treat arthritis of the knee with a metal spacer, which was placed between the bones of the knee to eliminate the rubbing of irregular surfaces on each other. These implants achieved some success, but were not predictable and many patients continued with significant symptoms
- Surgeons at Massachusetts General Hospital, made a prosthesis in the shape of the femoral half of the knee joint. This mold type arthroplasty, helped in relieving symptoms but was not predictable nor were the results always lasting
- During the late 1960s, a Canadian orthopedist, Frank Gunston from Sir John Charnley's Hip Center, developed a metal on plastic knee replacement, which secured to the bone with cement. This was really the first metal and plastic knee and the first with cement fixation (1968). Hence, the era of total knee arthroplasty, had begun

- In 1972, another englishman living in New York City, John Insall, MD, designed what has become the prototype for current total knee replacements. This was prosthesis, made of three components, which would resurface all three surfaces of the knee, i.e. the femur, tibia and patella (knee cap). They were all fixed with bone cement and the results were outstanding. This was the first total knee complete with specific instrumentation, to help with accurate bone cutting and implantation
- Since then, by reviewing the cases of patients, who have had total knee replacements, further significant improvements have been introduced. Today with metal backing of the plastic components, an increased inventory of appropriate sizes of implants and markedly better instruments, to perform the procedure, knee replacement results have equaled or surpassed those of hip replacement
- Cementless fixation, using prosthesis with a textured and porous surface, into which bone can grow, may provide biologic fixation. That is, the bone grows into the prosthesis and holds it in place. This may be more durable than cement used in the past. Cementless total knee arthroplasty is currently being used in patients and the results look very promising
- The most recent significant change has been the development and use of total knee implants, that are gender specific developed by Dr Bertin.

Minimal Invasive Surgery (MIS)

- Endoscopy was first described by Hippocrates in Greece (460–375 BC). He made reference to a rectal speculum
- Pioneering work in the field of arthroscopy began, as early as the 1920s, with the work of Eugen Bircher
- Japanese surgeon Masaki Watanabe, receives primary credit for using arthroscopy, for interventional surgery
- History is very important to any surgeon, particularly an orthopedic surgeon. An orthopedic surgeon has once again been presented with advancing technology. This technology must be applied to the surgeon's practice, but it is best applied only when the surgeon has an underlying knowledge of the history of his art. He must be aware of the way surgeons in the past have contributed to orthopedics and more importantly, of the mistakes that they have made in the process. A surgeon, who makes same mistake that was made by someone before him, is surely seen as poorly educated. So is he, who states that he has developed a technique that no one has thought of before, as chances are, that it has been thought of in the past
- For orthopedics to advance in an optimal manner, it is clear that attention must be paid to it's history. Past is our foundation for future developments, we must build upon it, so that we too can act as a stable foundation for future generations.

2 Bone

- Bone Structure
- Fracture
- Bone Grafting

BONE STRUCTURE

Introduction

Mammalian bones (including humans) are constructed of two types of grossly recognizable bones termed "cortical" and "cancellous" respectively.

Cortical Bone

Cortical bone (Fig. 2.1) is a dense, solid and grossly resembles ivory. In the arch typical long bone, the cortical type bone forms the cortex, which is a solid tubular structure that comprises the outer shell of the bone.

Cancellous Bone

Cancellous bone (Fig. 2.2) describes the bone structure that is found within the center of the long bones.

Cortical bone has tremendous strength approximating that of tempered steel. Its main function is to provide a rigid structure, which can provides a platform for the attachment of skeletal muscles. Due to its rigidity, cortical bone allows vertical posture. Cortical bone has a low surface to volume ratio, a fact that is important regarding its role in skeletal remodeling and calcium ion homeostasis.

Cancellous bone, demonstrates a tremendously high surface to volume ratio and grossly, it resembles the porous structure of a sponge. This accounts for the alternative designation of cancellous bone as "spongy bone". Cancellous bone is found within the marrow cavities of long and flat bones. It is principally concerned with transmitting the forces, directed across synovial joints from the articulating surface to the adjacent metaphyseal and diaphyseal cortical bone. Since the surface to volume ratio of cancellous bone is large, so it has an important role to play in calcium ion homeostasis (the importance of cancellous bone in calcium homeostasis is exemplified by the fact, that 99 percent of the total body calcium is stored within the skeleton).

The terms cortical and cancellous, describe the gross arrangement of bone tissue. Microscopically, bone is composed of cells and extracellular matrix. Bone is unique among all human tissues, due to its calcified matrix. This is formed by the crystallization of calcium

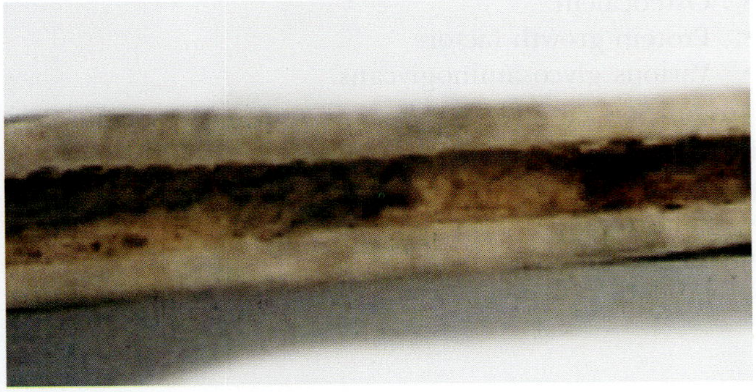

Fig. 2.1: Normal cortex

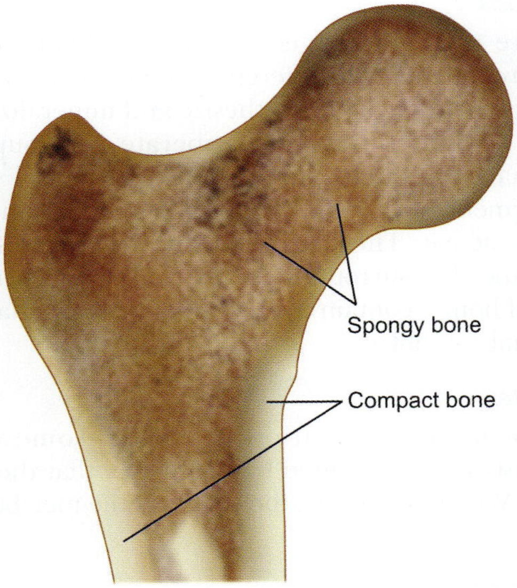

Fig. 2.2: Cancellous bone in the femoral head

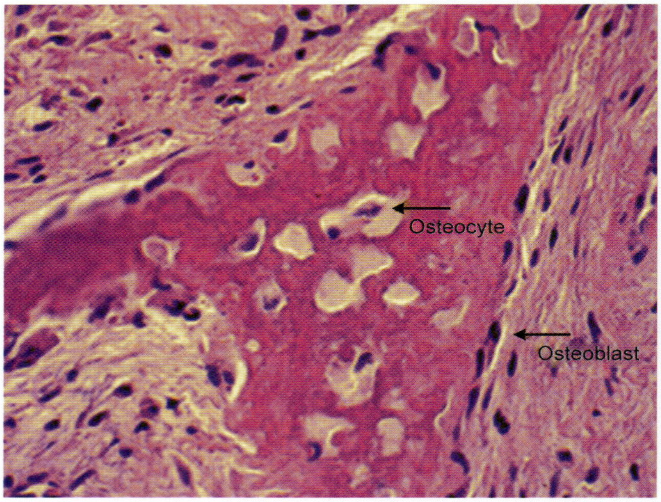

Fig. 2.3: Normal cells of bone

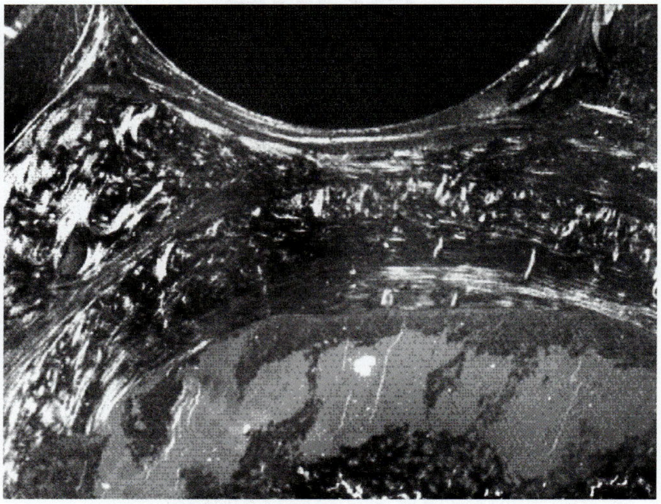

Fig. 2.4: Woven and lamellar bone

hydroxapatite crystals [$Ca_{10}(PO_4)_6(OH)_2$] within the extracellular matrix that surrounds the bone cells.

Functionally, there are four types of bone matrix cells, as shown in Figure 2.3.

Osteoclasts

They are syncytial multinucleated cells of monocyte origin. These cells reabsorb calcified bone matrix. They perform this function, while attached to mineralized bone within a concave depression called a Howship's lacuna. Osteoclasts are able to reabsorb bone, by selectively producing an extremely low pH within the immediate microenvironment of their action (the Howship's lacuna). The acidification of the extracellular space, results from the intracellular production of H^+ ions, by carbonic anhydrase II.

Osteoblasts

They are mononuclear cells of mesenchymal origin. These are the uniquely differentiated mesenchymal cells, that have the capacity to synthesize and mineralize bone matrix. Osteoblasts typically operate in groups and functionally are often arranged on the external surface of a segment of cortical or cancellous bone, on which they are active. The periosteum, which is the fibrous membrane that surrounds the external nonarticulating aspect of bones, contains cells that may differentiate into functional osteoblasts.

Osteocytes

As bone matrix formation proceeds, some of the osteoblasts get surrounded by the matrix that they have formed. When this occurs, the cells become metabolically less active and assume an inactive appearance. They are termed as osteocytes. The osteocytes are the same cells, as the osteoblasts, they merely change their appearance and function.

Osteoprogenitor Cells

These are functionally undifferentiated mesenchymal cells, that morphologically do not appear to be differentiated (they microscopically resemble the least differentiated mesenchymal cell, the fibroblast). Under the appropriate stimulation, these cells may differentiate into functional osteoblasts. Many of the cells that reside within the periosteum of adults (a nonactive structure under normal circumstances) are osteoprogenitor cells, although these cells are found throughout the bones.

Bone Matrix*

It is composed of an inorganic phase (calcium hydroxyapatite) and an organic phase. The organic phase, consists predominantly of type I collagen, however there are numerous additional protein and proteoglycan structural components of bone matrix. These include:

- Osteonectin
- Osteocalcin
- Protein growth factors
- Various glycosaminoglycans.

The structural strength (and therefore its mechanical function) of any bone is determined by the following parameters:

- The volume of bone matrix
- The type of bone matrix (woven or lamellar, as shown in Figure 2.4)

* Bone matrix (for the purposes of this section the word bone refers to microscopic tissue, i.e. cells and extracellular matrix)

- The degree of mineralization of the matrix
- The structural arrangement of the matrix.

Alterations in any of these parameters, will result in a potentially mechanically dysfunctional skeleton.

Types of Bone Matrix

- *Woven bone:* It is bone in which the collagen fibrils, which have been manufactured by osteoblasts, are distributed within the matrix in a haphazard arrangement. This type of bone matrix is rapidly formed however, it is mechanically weak. Woven bone is the first bone matrix formed in enchondral and intramembranous bone formation, during skeletal growth and development. Woven bone is always abnormal in the context of the mature skeleton, suggesting an abnormal pattern of bone formation. The finding of woven bone in the mature skeleton, while abnormal, is completely nonspecific.
- *Lamellar bone:* It is a bone, in which the collagen fibrils, that are manufactured and secreted into the extracellular space, by the osteoblasts, having an orderly arrangement in "curving linear arrays." This is mechanically, more sound matrix. It is the type of bone found in the mature skeleton. Within the cortex, the lamellar bone is functionally arranged as virtually solid tubes, centered upon a capillary in the cortex. These tubular structures are termed haversian systems or osteons. Within the marrow cavity, the lamellar bone forms linear anastomosing trabeculae (cancellous or trabecular bone).

Bone Remodeling

- The change in size, composition and arrangement of the components of the skeleton that occur in embryological development and growth is called "bone modeling." During this time, it is obvious that the skeleton is active, by virtue of the striking changes in size and shape of its components. When skeletal maturity is reached (i.e. when growth ceases), there is an apparent cessation of its activity. This apparent inactivity is erroneous. The skeleton remains one of the most active of the body's organs (do not be fooled, simply because the skeleton fails to alter its shape or manufacture some noxious liquid, gas or solid, like many of the other viscera). In fact, the activity of osteoclasts and osteoblasts persist throughout life. This activity, within the mature skeleton is termed "bone remodeling"
- The functional unit of bone remodeling is formed by the sequential coordinated activities of osteoclasts, osteoprogenitor cells, osteoblasts and finally osteocytes
- A group of osteoclasts commences bone resorption, by attaching to a mineralized bone surface. Each individual cell acidifies the local extracellular space and secretes active lysozomal enzymes, which enzymatically breaking down the bone matrix. These enzymes include serine proteases, collagenases and tartrate resistant acid phosphatase (the latter can be measured within serum and its level crudely reflects osteoclastic activity). The enzymatic destruction of the bone matrix releases various proteins, including growth factors, previously stored during bone formation. These, in addition to cytokines, manufactured the osteoclasts themselves and other cells, recruit adjacent ostoprogenitor cells to become osteoblasts. In general, osteoclasts function as groups that resorb cones of bone termed cutting cones (Fig. 2.5)

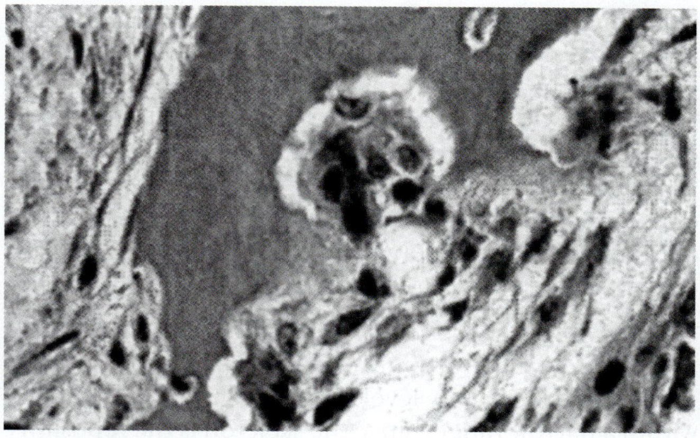

Fig. 2.5: Cutting cone

- The osteoblasts, which typically function in groups, enter the resorption defect created by the osteoclasts and manufacture new bone matrix of either woven or lamellar type. As the cells become entrapped within the bone matrix, they are transformed to osteocytes
- This sequential activity of osteoclast resorption, followed by osteoblastic bone formation is constantly occurring within the skeleton at all times. Since the surface to volume ratio of cancellous bone, is so much greater than that of cortical bone, this presents a greater area for bone remodeling. In fact, studies have estimated that up to 25 percent of the cancellous bone of humans may be remodeled each year, under normal circumstances. In comparison, three percent of cortical bone is remodeled annually. Under normal circumstances, the net effect of these sequences of bone resorption and formation resulted in, as such no overall change in skeletal mass. This process, whereby the degree of new bone formation is linked to the preceding bone resorption, is termed "coupling".

Factors Affecting Bone Remodeling

There are three broad categories of conditions that result in altered bone remodeling. These can be classified as:

Metabolic activity of the relevant cells: In practice, inborn metabolic dysfunction of cells, involved in bone remodeling is extremely rare and in addition to affecting "remodeling", these disorders typically have profound effects on growth and development (skeletal modeling). In contrast, acquired metabolic abnormalities of these cells are relatively common and account for the commonest of all metabolic bone diseases, such as osteoporosis.

Calcium homeostasis and nutritional status: Calcium ions are required for numerous intracellular enzymatic reactions. Extracellular calcium levels are stringently maintained within a narrow range. Since the skeleton is the repository of 99 percent of the body's calcium, it is clear that circumstances affecting calcium homeostasis, can have major effects on remodeling activities too. In this regard, the level of hormones "parathyroid hormone" and "vitamin D", may have major effects on the skeleton. In general terms, parathyroid hormone, stimulates osteoclastic activity and recruitment of osteoclast precursors (monocytes) to become osteoclasts, producing a net increase of osteoclastic function.

Physical stress: Bone is not unique in its ability to react to altered physical stress (the myocardium reacts by hypertrophy of cells, when it faces altered systolic pressures), however the extent and precision of the skeletal reaction, to physical stress is unique among all viscera. "Wolff's law", states that bone (an individual bone or group of bones) remodels itself, based upon the physical stresses placed upon it. The denser bones that are present within the dominant arms of professional tennis players, best exemplify this. Conversely, bones that lose their physical stressors for any reason, typically become more lucent reflecting a net resorptive state.

Regardless of which of the above factors pertain in any circumstance, the osteoclasts, osteoprogenitor cells, osteoblasts and osteocytes, always mediate remodeling activities within the skeleton. It has become increasingly clear that cytokines, manufactured by these cells, acting in a paracrine and autocrine fashion, actually mediate the activities of all these cells. The interleukin family of cytokines appears particularly important in this regard, especially regarding the function of osteoclasts.

FRACTURE

■ Introduction

A fracture may be defined as any break in continuity of a bone's structure. Fractures are virtually always associated with soft tissue injury and the healing process, which occurs with fracture repair, inevitably will have major effects on these structures. However, for the purposes of this discussion, comments will be confined to the sequence of events, which occur at the time of bone injury and subsequently with bone healing.

The following is a brief glossary of terms pertaining to fractures:

- *Closed fracture*: In this, the skin overlying the fracture bone is intact
- *Complete fracture*: In this, a full thickness break of the affected bone
- *Comminuted fracture*: It is a fracture that results in multiple separated bone fragments
- *Compound fracture*: It is a fracture in which the skin overlying the fracture is broken
- *Avulsion fracture*: It is a fracture due to pulling of a tendon or ligament at its insertion site
- *Greenstick fracture*: It is an incomplete fracture of the shaft of a long bone in the immature skeleton
- *Pathologic fracture*: It is a fracture occurring in abnormal bone (for any reason). In clinical practice, this is often used to describe fractures through bone tumors
- *Stress fracture*: It is an undisplaced fracture, usually involving a part of the cortex of bone that occurs due to excess loading. Stress fractures are sometimes referred to as "fatigue fractures".

Fracture Healing

A fracture occurs, when the continuity of a bone is broken and local blood supply is interrupted. If the overlying soft tissues are also injured, fracture healing may be delayed or disrupted, particularly in anatomic regions with decreased vascular networks, such as the tibial diaphysis. Bone is unique in its ability, to regenerate itself. Healing occurs, via reactivation of embryologic processes, resulting in the formation of bone not scar. Fracture healing can be described in three conceptual stages. An understanding of the timing and mechanisms associated with each stage is important in planning fracture treatment. The stages are:

Inflammation

This begins immediately after bone injury, with the formation of a local hematoma or fibrin clot. There is local cell death, where vessel disruption has resulted in ischemia, usually at the very ends of the fractured bone. Over the course of the next few days, this area becomes infiltrated by inflammatory cells and is characterized by local swelling and warmth. The inflammatory cells release lysozomal enzymes and other mediators that attract pluripotent cells to the area. They also act to remove necrotic tissue. Fibroblasts, mesenchymal cells and osteoprogenitor cells appear and may transform nearby tissues. The fracture is tender and may be grossly mobile to physical examination at this stage. Inflammation is at its peak, after 48 hours following a fracture.

Repair

The reparative phase begins a few days after the injury, with the arrival of mesenchymal cells, which are able to differentiate into fibroblasts, chondroblasts and osteoblasts. The repair phase persists for several months. It can be divided into two distinct phases, i.e. soft and hard callus formation.

Soft Callus Formation

It lasts for approximately six weeks from the time of injury. During this preliminary stage of repair, pain and swelling subside and bony fragments become united by fibrous and cartilaginous tissue and woven bone is formed. While this creates some stability, the fracture may still angulate at this stage if not held with stable external support, such as a cast or external fixator or internal support provided by plates, screws or intramedullary devices.

Hard Callus Formation

During this second stage of repair, woven bone is transformed into lamellar bone and this takes, approximately three months.

Remodeling

Remodeling is the process, by which bone is removed in tiny increments and then replaced by new bone. After a fracture, remodeling may continue for months or even years. The adult human skeleton continuously replaces itself at rate of 10 to 18 percent per year. The rate of remodeling is accelerated in children and during fracture repair. In addition to being an essential part of fracture healing, remodeling plays an important role in calcium homeostasis. During the remodeling phase, the woven bone is converted to lamellar bone and the medullary canal is reconstituted. During this phase, bone responds to loading characteristics, according to Wolff's law. Some angular deformities may correct during this stage, in children with sufficient growth remaining (up to 5° per year of growth remaining).

The efficiency of bone healing is determined by the following parameters:

- The general health of the patient, in particular the patient's nutritional status
- The presence or absence of pre-existing skeletal conditions, either localized or generalized
- The number of fragments in the fracture
- The alignment of the fracture fragments
- The presence and extent of adjacent soft tissue injury
- The presence of intervening soft tissue between the bone fragments
- The presence or absence of infection at the fracture site.

Systemic Factors Affecting Bone Healing

Various local and systemic factors affect the duration and effectiveness of the healing process. Abnormalities in any of these areas may lead to abnormally slow healing (delayed union) or failure to heal (nonunion). These factors include:

Age

Young patients heal rapidly and have a remarkable ability to remodel and correct angulation deformities. These abilities decrease, once skeletal maturity is reached.

Nutrition

A substantial amount of energy is needed for fracture healing to occur. An adequate metabolic stage with sufficient carbohydrates and protein is necessary.

Systemic Diseases

Diseases like osteoporosis, diabetes and those causing an immunocompromised state will likely delay healing. Illnesses, like Marfan's syndrome and Ehlers-Danlos syndrome, cause abnormal musculoskeletal healing.

Hormones

Thyroid hormone, growth hormone, calcitonin, parathyroid hormone (PTH) and others play significant roles in bone healing. Corticosteroids impede healing through many mechanisms:

- *Thyroid hormones:* They affect bone growth and maturation. Maturation of skeleton is mainly dependent on thyroid hormone. The growth action of growth hormone is potentiated by T_4. Thyroid hormone promotes the release of calcium from bone. Hyperthyroidism causes bone resorption, leading to osteopenia, hypercalcemia and hyperphosphaturia, etc. The rates of calcium deposition and resorption in bone is increased by several folds and returned to normal with treatment of hyperthyroidism. However, resorption always exceeds formation. In hypothyroidism, a state of secondary hyperparathyroidism develops and renal tubular resorption of phosphate is decreased. There is increased urinary excretion of hydroxyproline due to collagen breakdown, as a result of bone destruction
- *Calcitonin:* It is released from C cells of thyroid. Its function is to inhibit bone resorption and to reduce tubular resorption of calcium. It is therapeutically used in conditions of excessive bone resorption, like osteoporosis, Paget's disease and renal osteodystrophy
- *Parathyroid hormone* (PTH): The hormone carried out following functions:
  - Maintains blood calcium levels, by resorption of bone, promoting tubular resorption of calcium and

acting with vitamin D, to promote intestinal absorption of calcium
  - Encourages glomerular filtration of calcium and phosphate ions
  - Stimulates osteoclasis
  - Lowers serum phosphorus levels, by inhibiting tubular rebsorption of phosphate from glomerular filtrate
  - Directly effects dissolution of bone
  - Increases solubility of calcium and phosphate
  - Inhibits mineralizing effect of vitamin D.
- *Growth hormone*: Proliferation and hypertrophy of chondrocytes, in the epiphyseal growth plate are controlled by growth hormone. An abnormal increase in growth hormone, leads to proliferation of cartilage cells in the epiphyseal plate. It may continue even beyond the usual time of skeletal maturation and epiphyseal closure. Also subperiosteal ossification is increased, resulting in increased cortical thickness
- *Estrogen*: Estrogen is thought to stimulate calcium absorption and to protect bone from unrestrained action of PTH. Estrogen withdrawal, leads to bone depletion and osteoporosis
- *Androgen*: It affects anabolic proteins, which is exerted on muscles, skeleton, sex organs and other structures. When testosterone is administered to a child, it results in early growth spurt, but skeletal maturation is accelerated, leading to premature epiphyseal fusion, resulting in shortened stature
- *Adrenal corticosteroids*: In excess, they can cause pernicious type of osteoporosis, due to combination of increased bone resorption, diminished bone formation, decreased intestinal calcium absorption from intestine and increased calcium excretion. Collagen synthesis may also be defective.

Drugs

Nonsteroidal anti-inflammatory drugs (e.g. ibuprofen) and antibiotics (ciprofloxacin), depress healing.

Smoking

Found to decrease the process of bone healing.

Local Factors Affecting Fracture Healing

Type of Bone

Cancellous (spongy) bone fractures are usually more stable, involve greater surface areas and have a better blood supply than the cortical (compact) bone fractures. Cancellous bone, heals faster than the cortical bone.

Degree of Trauma

The more extensive the injury to bone and surrounding soft tissues, the poorer the outcome. Mild contusions with local bone trauma will heal easily, whereas severely comminuted injuries with extensive soft tissue, damage heal poorly.

Vascular Injury

Inadequate blood supply impairs healing. Especially, vulnerable areas are the femoral head, talus and scaphoid bones.

Degree of Immobilization

The fracture site must be immobilized for vascular ingrowth and bone healing to occur. Repeated disruptions of repair tissue, especially to areas with marginal blood supply or heavy soft tissue damage will impair healing.

Intra-articular Fractures

These fractures communicate with synovial fluid, which contains collagenases that retard bone healing. Joint movement will cause the fracture fragments to move, further impairing union. When intra-articular fractures are comminuted, the fragments tend to float apart, owing to loss of soft tissue support.

Separation of Bone Ends

Normal apposition of fracture fragments is needed for union to occur. Inadequate reduction, excessive traction or interposition of soft tissue, will prevent healing.

Infection

Infections cause necrosis and edema, take away energy from the healing process and may increase mobility of the fracture site.

Local Pathology

Any disease process that weakens the musculoskeletal tissues, like osteoporosis or osteomalacia, may impair union.

Primary Bone Healing

- In this kind of healing, callus is not formed at all and requires rigid stabilization, with or without compression of the bone ends
- Rigid stabilization suppresses the formation of callus, in either cancellous or cortical bone
- Primary bone healing can be divided into gap healing and contact healing. Union occurs in both the types.

Gap Healing

Gap healing occurs in two stages. These are:

- Firstly, the width of the gap is filled by direct bone formation. An initial scaffold of a woven bone is laid down, followed by formation of a lamellar bone as support. The orientation of the new bone formed in this first stage is transverse, to that of the original lamellar bone orientation

- In the second stage, which happens after several weeks, longitudinal haversian remodeling, reconstructs the necrotic fracture ends and leads the newly formed bone, to replace the woven bone with osteons of the original orientation. In the end, the normal bone structure results.

Contact Healing

- Contact healing occurs, where fragments are in direct apposition and osteons can grow across the fracture site, parallel to the longitudinal axis of the bone
- When fracture fragments are in contact, osteoclasts on one side of the fracture, undergo a tunneling resorptive response, forming cutting cones that cross the fracture line
- This tunneling, allows the penetration of capillaries and eventually the formation of new Haversian systems. These blood vessels are then accompanied by endothelial cells and osteoprogenitor cells for osteoblasts, leading to the production of osteons across the fracture line, eventually leading to regeneration of the normal bone architecture.

Secondary Bone Healing

It occurs, when there is no rigid fixation of the fractured bone ends, which leads to the development of a fracture callus. It includes, an inflammatory phase, a reparative phase and a remodeling phase.

Complications During Fracture Healing

Early Complications

Local

- *Vascular injury:* This can cause external or internal hemorrhage
- *Visceral injury:* This can cause damage to vital organs, like kidneys, intestine or bladder
- Neural damage
- Injury to surrounding tissue
- *Hemarthrosis:* There is blood in the joint
- *Compartment syndrome:* Due to bleeding, the blood gets accumulated in the closed compartment, formed by fascia and bone. When this accumulation is too much, with increase in intracompartmental pressure in closed compartment, which does not expand, pressure is produced, on the surrounding tissues, leading to ischemia or lack of oxygen, following a poor blood supply.
- Wound contamination, that could lead to infection.

Systemic

- Fat embolism
- Shock
- Thromboembolism
- Acute respiratory distress.

Late Complications

Local

- *Delayed union:* The bone takes more time to heal than the normal limit. Union occurs, eventually with or without augmentation procedure.
- *Nonunion:* There occurs a complete cessation of fracture healing process, clinically and radiologically, beyond the stipulated optimum time for healing, for that particular bone, site of fracture, type of fracture and age. In this case, fracture would not heal without any intervention (surgical), like open reduction and internal fixation augmentation procedure, like bone grafting.

  Nonunion as defined by FDA panel (1986) is as follows: A fracture is said to be nonunited, when at least nine months have passed since injury and when the last three months have elapsed, without progress in healing, clinically and radiologically. Exception, e.g. fracture neck femur, three months, since injury (and not 9 months). Local causes of nonunion are illustrated in the Table 2.1 and types on nonunion are expianed in the Table 2.2.
- *Malunion:* The fracture unites with fragments in unacceptable position, leading to deformity and other potential problems of malalignment.
- Joint stiffness.
- *Contractures of soft tissue:* This may include tendon, ligaments, joint capsule and skin
- *Myositis ossificans:* This is a term used for abnormal ossification of soft tissues. If present around joint, it may limit the range of motion.
- Avascular necrosis
- *Algodystrophy or Sudeck's atrophy (refer to chapter on CRPS in wrist and hand):* It is neurovascular disturbance following abnormal behavior of sympathetic nervous system
- *Osteomyelitis (refer to chapter on osteomyelitis):* It is infection of bone and medulla
- Growth disturbance or deformity, leading to limb length discrepancy

Table 2.1: Different causes of nonunion
Essential local causes of nonunion (DISCO)
Distraction
Especially, by gravity or excessive traction. For nonunion of tibia, additional reasons can be delayed weight-bearing and distal third fracture
Infection
Inadequate fixation, ill advised operation and insufficient immobilization
Segmental fractures
Soft tissue interposition, severe soft tissue damage
Comminuted fractures
Open fractures

Table 2.2: Showing different types of nonunion

Types of nonunion
Hypertrophic type • *Due to mechanical failure*: Vascularity not compromised. They are rich in callus. They result from insecure fixation, inadequate immobilization and premature weight-bearing • *Elephant foot nonunion*: Hypertrophic and rich in callus • *Horse hoof nonunion*: Mildly hypertrophic and poor in callus. They result from unstable fixation with plates and screws
Oligotrophic nonunion • Callus is absent. They occur after major displacement of fracture or distraction of fragment
Atrophic type • *Due to biological failure*: Vascularity is compromised • *Torsion wedge nonunion*: It is characterized by presence of an intermediate fragment, in which the blood supply is decreased or absent. The intermediate fragment has united to one main fragment and not to other • *Comminuted nonunion*: It is characterized by presence of one or more intermediate fragments • *Defect nonunion*: It is characterized by loss of a fragment of the diaphysis of a bone. Ends of the fragments are viable, but union across the defect is impossible and end in becoming atrophic

- Pressure ulcers, following cast
- Pin tract infection
- Volkmann's ischemia and ischemic contracture (refer to chapter on VIC in elbow).

Systemic

- *Gangrene:* It may occur due to vascular injury, failed vascular repair or as a complication of a plaster cast.
- *Tetanus:* This may occur, as a result of contamination by tetanus spores, at the time of injury.
- Septicemia.

BONE GRAFTING

Introduction

A bone graft is a transfer of living bone tissue.

Mechanism

Three biological mechanisms are involved in bone grafting, these are:

Osteogenesis

It is the production of a new bone, by proliferation, osteoid production and mineralization.

Osteoconduction

It is the production of new bone and migration of local osteocompetent cells, along a conduit, e.g. fibrin, blood vessel or even certain alloplast material, like hydroxyapatite. New bone originates from the endostium or residual periostium of the host bone.

Osteoinduction

It is the formation of bone, by stem cells transforming into osteocompetent cells by bone morphogenetic protein (BMP). It inducts the recipient tissue cells, to form periostium and endostium.

Indications

- Delayed unions, nonunions, osteotomies and arthrodeses
- Replacement of lost cortical segments
- Cavities or defects, secondary to cysts or neoplasia.

Types of Grafts

Autograft

- Taken from same individual
- Allows for osteogenesis, osteoinduction and osteoconduction
- Free (10%) or vascularized (90%).

Isograft

Taken from same family.

Allograft

From same species.

Xenograft

From different species.

Sources of Grafts

Cancellous Bone

- Taken from metaphyseal regions
- Has increased surface area
- Has 80 percent porosity.

Cortical Bone

- Increased mechanical strength
- Has 10 percent porosity
- Frequently corticocancellous grafts are used.

Osteochondral

Cartilage attached to parent bone.

Composite Bone Graft

A composite bone graft is made up of hydroxyapatite (HA) crystals, tricalcium phosphate (TCP) and bone marrow.

Vascularized Grafts (Corticocancellous)

- Increased cell survival
- Increased patient morbidity
- Generally for large bony defects.

Sites for Graft Collection

- Cancellous bone metaphyses, e.g. olecranon, distal tibia, etc.
- Cortical bone graft, e.g. ribs, fibula, iliac crest, tibia, etc.

Techniques for Graft Collection

- Aseptic collection
- Avoid oscillating equipment
- Place directly onto the host bone, as air kills the cells
- Place into blood soaked sponge, as saline kills cells
- Be generous
- Implant in stable and sterile environment
- Can regraft in eight weeks.

Process of Graft Healing

- *Inflammation*
- *Revascularization:* Takes more time for cortical grafts because of less porosity
- *Osteoinduction*: Decreased with cortical grafts
- *Osteoconduction:* Decreased with cortical grafts
- *Remodeling*.

Healing of Allografts

- "Creeping substitution"
- Basic bone remodeling, at graft host interface
- Bone resorption is followed by bone production
- May take years.

Harvesting Grafts from Different Bones

Ribs

- Indicated for costochondral graft, to restore pseudoarticulation of the temperomandibular joint (TMJ) or to replace a missing part of the anterior mandible, to reconstruct a functional articulation
- The rib is usually, fifth or sixth, the typical one
- The sixth rib has the distal origin of the pectoralis major muscle and dissection transect the muscle minimally
- Right rib is always preferred because:
  - It could be contoured to fit either side of the mandible or facial bones
  - Postoperative pain is less likely to be confused with cardiogenic pain.

Surgical Access

- Incision is placed in the inframammary crease, to hide the scar
- Sharp dissection is carried through full thickness of skin, subcutaneous tissues and the muscle, to expose the rib periostium and chest wall cortex
- The periosteum is incised from 1 cm onto the rib cartilage, to the full desired length, the anterior border of the latissimus dorsi muscle, about 12 cm
- Reflected carefully from the chest wall cortex, around the inferior and superior rib edges to the pleural cortex periostium, using a maxillofacial surgery periosteal elevator, rather than Doyen rib stripper
- This is to avoid creating pleural tear because of the irregularities and bony projections, to which periostium and lung pleura are firmly attached, leading to pneumothorax
- A releasing incision made at right angle to the rib incision, carried to the rib edges, help in reflecting the perichondrium and gaining access to the cartilage
- The cartilage is separated first, by scalpel blade and the proximal part is cut with a saw or rib cutter, after lifting the rib and carefully separating any adherent periosteal membrane from the pleural cortex
- The closure is layered as periostium, subcutaneous tissue, dermis and lastly skin
- Drain is not necessary
- The length of the cartilage is related to the growth of the graft, not to the prevention of bony ankylosis.

Disadvantages

- Longer length, creates a longer lever arm, promoting separation (2–3 mm)
- Associated with overgrowth
- Incorporation of the perichondrium or periostium sleeve, in the graft does not enhance survival or stability of the graft
- In children, the cartilage is easily separated from bone sleeve, thereby reducing the chance of separation
- In adult the cartilage is firmly incorporated to the bone
- Increases the probability of pneumothorax
- It is recommended that a 2 to 3 mm of cartilage length, without adherent periostium or perichondrium for both costochondral growth grafts in children and articulation graft in adult.

Iliac Crest

- The lateral approach to the anterior ilium, gives most effect on the gait
- The medial anterior approach involves the large iliacus muscle, which is not necessary for normal gait, but large medial hematoma might produce gait disturbances.

Surgical Access

- Incision should be placed 1 cm posterior to the antero-superior iliac spine and extend to the iliac tubercle
- It should be placed lateral to the bony prominence, to prevent irritation by tight cloths or belt

- Proceed down to bone medial to the muscles, tensor fascia lata and gluteus medius and lateral to the iliacus and the external abdominal muscles
- Cancellous bone is available in the anterior ilium within the upper 2 to 3 cm, between the tubercle and the anterosuperior iliac spine
- "Trap door" is one of the most common osteotomy used for anterior ilium harvest
- During closure, strict attention should be followed in order to reorient and reposition the muscles in their original positions
- A drain is required because of the dead space and should be placed within the bony cavity.

Tibia

- The extensive subcutaneous surface of the tibia makes it an accessible donor site for bone grafts
- The tibial plateau is an excellent reservoir for cancellous bone
- It can provide up to 40 cc of bone, without affecting the structural support of the tibia.

Bone Harvesting

Indications

Small bony defects, include:

- Nonunion
- Osteotomy defects
- Dentoalveolar defects
- Sinus lift procedure.

Surgical Access

- Could be done under local anesthesia
- Incision over the lateral tubercle, best accomplished by flexing the leg at the knee joint
- It is 6 to 10 mm, from the skin and dissection is made through the thin subcutaneous tissue
- Sharp dissection is done, to reflect the tensor fascia lata band and make 1 cm opening into the cortex. The cancellous bone could be harvested, lateral and inferior to the midline, to avoid damage to the knee.

Bone Graft Substitutes

- Demineralized bone matrix
- Porus calcium phosphorus ceramics
- Collografts
- Orthografts
- Hydroxyapatite cement
- Platelet gel
- Bone marrow cells
- Bone morphogenic protein
- Composite bone graft.

Properties of Bone Graft Substitutes

- Should be osteoconductive
- Should have load bearing capacity
- Should allow attachment, spreading, division and differentiation of cells, to produce lamellar bone on its mineral surface.

Demineralized Bone Matrix

It is produced by acid extraction of bone and has a variable amount of bone morphogenic protein. It is available as paste, powder and gel, with no intrinsic strength (allomatrix).

Porus Calcium Phosphate Ceramics

- Hydroxyapatite [Ca_{10} $(PO_4)_6$ $(OH)_2$]
- Tricalcium phosphate [Ca_3 $(PO_4)_2$]

Collografts

- These are granular composites of hydroxyapatite and tricalcium phosphate, with added dermal collagen
- Used with autogenous bone marrow, aspirate to have both osteoconductive and osteoinductive agents.

Orthografts

- They are made of pure tricalcium phosphate
- It is resorbed by dissolution.

Hydroxyapatite Cement

- It is a mixture of inorganic calcium phosphate and water. Setting time is 10 to 20 minutes
- It can be contoured, to fill any bony defect before setting
- It bears minimal load
- It is replaced by host bone at the rate of 3 to 4 mm in 6 to 8 months, by cell mediated response
- It gives no adverse effects on bone remodeling.

Autologus Platelet Concentrate (Platelet Gel)

This product is harvested from blood. It has multiple growth factors (osteoinductive) and may be combined with matrix, to enhance bone formation.

Ceramics

- These are derived from marine corals, that is porus and brittle, have variable resorption and is often used for augmentation of fractures
- It is highly crystalline hydroxyapatite porous material, which mimics human cancellous bone in appearance and architecture
- Bone regenerates into the pores
- Preparation is done by hydrothermal conversion reaction, where organic material is washed out
- *Advantages:* Biocompatible, with no inflammatory reaction

- *Disadvantages:* Weak, brittle, unable to bear cyclical loading and fixation required with grafting.

Bone Morphogenic Protein

- It was discovered by Dr Marshall Urist
- It is osteoconductive in nature
- Bone morphogenic protein (BMP) can be produced, concentrated and placed in the body, where bone formation is needed
- They stimulate regular cells, into bone forming cells
- It can be used for:
  - Intractable nonunion
  - Large bone defects
  - Massive trauma
  - Old infection
  - Excision of tumors
  - Congenital malformations.

Composite Bone Graft

- Composite bone graft is made up of hydroxyapatite (HA) crystals, tricalcium phosphate (TCP) and bone marrow
- Composite bone grafting consists of combination of osteoconductive matrix and bioactive agents, that provides osteoinductive and osteogenic properties
- Thus, the osteoconductive substrates, becomes a delivery system for bioactive agents, requiring less chemotaxis and less migration of osteoblasts progenitor cells to graft site
- The composite bone graft is nonantigenic, noncarcinomatous and noninfective
- Advantages include:
  - It is useful, when large quantities of bone are required to bridge a bone defect
  - Useful in pediatric and geriatric age groups
  - Have good osteoinductive and osteoconductive properties
  - No donor site morbidity, in contrast to autograft
  - Healing time of fracture and consolidation of bone was almost same as autograft
  - Easy availability of composite bone grafts in all sizes and shapes, facilitate better and more compact packing of bone defect.

3 Anomalies Related to Development of Bones

- Classification of Developmental Disorders
- Limb Anomalies
- Osteogenesis Imperfecta
- Achondroplasia
- Hypochondroplasia
- Metaphyseal Chondrodysplasia (Dysostosis)
- Osteopetrosis (Marble Bones, Albers-Schonberg Disease)

CLASSIFICATION OF DEVELOPMENTAL DISORDERS

The grouping used here, is a convenient way of dividing, the various clinical syndromes.

Disorders of Cartilage and Bone Growth

- *Dysplasias with predominantly physeal and metaphyseal changes*
  - Hereditary multiple exostosis
  - Achondroplasia
  - Hypochondroplasia
  - Metaphyseal chondrodysplasia
  - Dyschondroplasia (enchondromatosis, Ollier's disease)
- *Dysplasias with predominantly epiphyseal changes*
  - Multiple epiphyseal dysplasia
  - Spondyloepiphyseal dysplasia
  - Dysplasia epiphysealis hemimelia
  - Chondrodysplasia punctata (stippled epiphysis)
- *Dysplasias with predominantly metaphyseal and diaphyseal changes*
  - Metaphyseal dysplasia (Pyle's disease)
  - Craniometaphyseal dysplasia
  - Diaphyseal dysplasia
  - Craniodiaphyseal dysplasia
  - Osteopetrosis
  - Pyknodysostosis
  - Candle bones spotted bones and striped bones
- *Combined and mixed dysplasias*
  - Spondylometaphyseal dysplasia
  - Pseudoachondroplasia
  - Diastrophic dysplasia
  - Cleidocranial dysplasia
  - Nail-patella syndrome
  - Craniofacial dysplasia.

Connective Tissue Disorders

- *Generalized joint laxity*
- *Ehlers-Danlos syndrome*
- *Osteogenesis imperfecta (brittle bones)*
  - Mild
  - Lethal
  - Severe
  - Moderate
  - Fibrodysplasia ossificans progressiva

Storage Disorder and Metabolic Defects

- Mucopolysaccharidoses
- Hurler's syndrome
- Hunter's syndrome
- Morquio-Bralisford syndrome
- Gaucher's disease
- Homocystinuria
- Alkaptonuria
- Congenital hyperuricemia.

Chromosome Disorders

- Down's syndrome
- Thoracospinal anomalies
- Elevation of the scapula
- Limb anomalies.

LIMB ANOMALIES

■ Introduction

Localized malformations of limbs include extra bones, absent bones, hypoplastic bones and fusions. Complete absence of bones is called "amelia", almost complete absence (a mere stub remaining) "phocomelia" and partial absence "ectromelia". Defects may be transverse or axial. In the hands and feet brachydactyly, syndactyly, polydactyly and symphalangism, are among the many possibilities.

The embryonal limb buds, appear at about 26th day of gestation. By the 30th day, upper limb starts differentiating into its three segments (upper arm, forearm and hand) and in the lower limb, the same process occurs shortly afterwards. By the end of the 6th week, the embryo acquires a recognizable human form. The upper limb is fully formed by 12 weeks and the lower limb by 14 weeks. During this period, the muscles and nerves also develop and by the 20th week joint movement becomes possible.

Most of the malformations, involving limb reductions are due to embryonal insult, between the fourth and sixth week of gestation. Some are genetically determined and these usually have an autosomal dominant pattern of inheritance.

Classification

Various classifications of limb deficiencies have been proposed, but none is completely satisfactory. Some veer towards the purely descriptive, others go into almost obsessive detail, based on topographical and morphological features. Their usefulness lies in the elaboration of an agreed terminology, which will aid communication and permit sensible auditing of the results of various forms of treatment.

Some of the important disorders are referred to below and further details appear in the section on Regional Orthopedics.

Clinical Features

Radial Deficiency

Absence or hypoplasia of the radius may occur alone or in association with visceral anomalies or (more rarely) certain blood dyscrasias. Sometimes, the thumb is missing too and the elbow is often abnormal. In about half the cases, the condition is bilateral.

The forearm is short and bowed and the hand is underdeveloped and markedly deviated towards the radial side (radial club hand). In some cases the thumb is absent.

The clinical deformity may look bizarre, but children often acquire excellent function. If these seem unlikely, operative reconstruction may be advisable.

Ulnar Deficiency

Hypoplasia of the distal end of the ulna is usually seen as a part of generalized dysplasia, but occasionally it occurs alone. The radius is bowed (as if growth is tethered on ulnar side) and the radial head may dislocate and along with wrist, deviated medially. If the function is severely disturbed, only then the wrist stabilization, should be advised.

Congenital absence of the ulna is extremely rare. The forearm deformity is not as marked as in radial deficiency, but overall function is severely restricted. Operative reconstruction may provide some improvement.

Transverse Deficiency of the Arm

Transverse deficiency of the distal part of the arm will leave a stump below a normal elbow. This can be managed, by fitting prosthesis, with a mechanical facility for grasp.

Femoral Deficiency (Congenital Short Femur)

In its most benign form, femoral dysplasia consists merely of shortening of the bone, with a normal hip and knee. This can be dealt with, by limb lengthening procedures, if shortening is very marked, then by adding a distal orthosis.

Dysplasia of the Distal Third

Although uncommon, sometimes occurs with synostosis of the knee. Since the hip permits normal weight-bearing, so this condition can be managed by limb lengthening operations.

In most cases, it is the proximal third, which is under developed or absent. This results in a two fold problem of shortening of the limb and defective weight-bearing, at the hip.

Various grades of proximal femoral dysplasia are encountered. There may be coxa vara with moderate shortening of the shaft. This can be dealt with, by corrective osteotomy and limb lengthening. Severe degrees of coxa vara, sometimes associated with pseudoarthrosis of the neck, may result in marked shortening of the femur. In the worst set of cases, most of the femoral shaft is missing, the knee is situated at thigh level and the foot hangs, where the knee is normally expected to be. If the deformity is bilateral and symmetrical, walking is possible and some individuals acquire remarkable agility. However, they may still seek treatment, to overcome the severe cosmetic problem. Unilateral deformities are not only unsightly, but also very disabling. Effective limb lengthening is out of the question and fitting prosthesis to a short limb, with flexion deformities of hip and knee with a foot jutting forwards, where the knee hinge of the prosthesis will lie is a daunting prospect. In the past, there was some enthusiasm for the Van Nes operation, i.e. fusion of the knee and 180° rotational osteotomy of the leg bones, to get the foot facing back to front and the ankle substituting for the knee, followed by fitting an "above knee" prosthesis. However, the trick is easier and looks better in drawings, than in real life and the procedure is seldom done nowadays. One alternative is to fuse the knee in a functional position, amputate the foot and fit a suitable prosthesis. The earlier this is done, the better the outcome.

Tibial Deficiency

Congenital absence of the tibia is extremely rare. When it occurs, it is usually associated with other anomalies of the limbs. The ankle is non-existent and the foot is in varus. It is quite possible to construct a functioning one bone leg, by transposing the fibula and fusing it to the center of the femoral articular surface. Once the fusion is achieved, a Syme's amputation can be performed. This should be done as soon as the fibula has developed sufficiently, to permit fusion at the knee. If the procedure fails or if the associated abnormalities turn out to be more severe than expected, proximal amputation can be undertaken at a later stage.

Fibular Deficiency

Mild fibular dysplasia causes little shortening or deformity. However, complete absence of the fibula, leads to considerable shortening of the leg, bowing of the tibia and valgus deformity of the unsupported ankle. There may also be absence of the fourth and fifth rays of the foot and underdevelopment of the entire limb. Sometimes, if only the distal fibula is absent, there is a fibrous band in its place. Excision of this remnant may permit correction of the valgus deformity. If the overall limb length is markedly affected and the foot deformity intractable, distal amputation of the leg may be needed.

Congenital Pseudoarthrosis of the Tibia

This rare condition is usually diagnosed in early infancy. The child may be born with a fractured tibia or the bone may be attenuated and then get fractured some months later. In either cases, the fracture fails to unite or heals very poorly, only to get fractured again, shortly afterwards. By the age of two years, the leg is noticeably short and bowed anteriorly. By then, it has become obvious, that this is an intractable condition, which will not yield to ordinary forms of fracture treatment. X-ray shows a gap or marked thinning of the tibial shaft. Sometimes, the fibula also is affected.

Biopsy of the abnormal segment may show histological features of neurofibromatosis and other stigmata of this condition are present in about half of those affected.

Treatment is likely to be prolonged. Simple immobilization will certainly fail and internal fixation, with bone grafting succeeds occasionally. Better results have been achieved, by correcting the deformity, bone grafting the fracture and immobilizing the tibial fragments in a circular external fixator (the Ilizarov technique). Success has been claimed for extension of the abnormal segment and replacement by a vascularized fibular graft (Weiland et al. 1990).

Congenital Tibial Bowing

Congenital tibial bowing, compromises a spectrum of disorders, with significant differences in both etiology and prognosis for the different types (Crawford and Schorry, 1999).

Posteromedial tibial bowing is a relatively benign condition, which resolves spontaneously as the child grows. However, the leg may end up shorter than normal, requiring epiphysiodesis on the opposite side, to counteract the limb length inequality.

Anteromedial bowing is almost always associated with fibular deficiency and congenital defects of the foot or some type of femoral dysplasia. Treatment depends on the presence or absence (and severity) of the associated disorders and varies from reconstructive procedures of the ankle to (in the worst cases) amputation.

Anterolateral tibial bowing, with failure of normal tubularization may be the forerunner of localized osteolysis and eventual fracture, with persistent nonunion and pseudoarthrosis of the tibia. Corrective osteotomy, should be avoided because of the high risk of nonunion. When the bone is intact, treatment consists of bracing, until the bone matures. If a fracture occurs, treatment is same, as for congenital pseudoarthrosis.

Pseudoarthrosis of the Clavicle

A child sometimes presents with a painless lump over the clavicle and X-rays confirm the presence of a nonunited fracture or pseudoarthrosis. The condition is not really comparable to pseudoarthrosis of the tibia and is thought to be due to pressure by the subclavian artery, on the developing bone. In every reported universal case, the right side has been affected, except in the presence of dextrocardia. Treatment, if required is by excision and grafting.

Synostosis

The various types of interosseous fusion (radioulnar, tibiofibular, carpal or tarsal) are discussed in the relevant chapters. They rarely cause significant disability, except tarsal synostosis (which may be associated with spastic flat foot) or radioulnar fusion, which limits forearm supination (a considerable disability, if both forearms are affected). In spastic flat foot, division or removal of the bony bridge, may improve symptoms. Radioulnar fusion resists any form of operative mobilization because of the associated soft tissue involvement. However, the bones can be osteotomized and rotated to leave the hand in a more functional position.

Digital Anomalies

There are numerous digital anomalies, e.g. missing digits, extra digits or split deformities of the hand or foot, which may occur in isolation, in combination with each other or as part of a generalized dysplasia. Short digits seldom require any form of treatment. Extra digits, if simply hanging by a neck of skin, can be amputated at any time. The more complex anomalies, which involve not only bone, but also the associated muscles and neurovascular structures, may be treated by operative reconstruction, when the child is 3 to 4 years old, but only after painstaking assessment and by someone experienced in this branch of surgery.

■ Mucopolysaccharidoses

Introduction

The polysaccharide glycosaminoglycans (GAGs), form the side chains of macromolecular proteoglycans, a major component of the matrix in bone, cartilage, intervertebral disks, synovium and other connective tissues. Defunct proteoglycans are degraded, by lysosomal enzymes. Deficiency of any of these enzymes causes a hold up on the degradative pathways. Partially degraded GAGs, accumulate in the lysosomes in the liver, spleen, bones and other tissues and spill over in the blood and urine, where they can be detected by suitable biochemical tests. Confirmation of the enzyme lack can be obtained, by tests on cultured fibroblasts or leukocytes.

Clinical Features

Depending on the specific enzyme deficiency and the type of GAG storage, a number of different clinical syndromes have been defined. All except, Hunter's syndrome (an X-linked recessive disorder) are transmitted as autosomal recessive. As a group they have certain recognizable features, such as excessively short stature with vertebral deformity, coarse facies, hepatosplenomegaly and (in some cases) mental retardation. X-rays show bone dysplasia, affecting the vertebral bodies, epiphyses and metaphyses. Typically the bones have a spatulate appearance.

There is superficial similarity to spondyloepiphyseal dysplasia (SED) and spondylometaphyseal dysplasia. However, careful observation reveals several points of difference and the diagnosis can be confirmed, by testing for abnormal GAG excretion or demonstrating the enzyme deficiency in blood cells or cultured fibroblasts.

At least ten different disorders are recognized, here only the three important conditions will be described:

Hurler's Syndrome (MPS 1)

Infants look normal at birth, but over the next 2 to 3 years, they gradually develop a typical appearance. They are undersized, with increasing kyphosis, hepatosplenomegaly, coarse facies, protruding tongue, defective hearing and mental retardation. Speech is very poor, joints are stiff and walking is delayed. There may be corneal opacities, respiratory difficulty and cardiac anomalies. X-rays usually show unmistakable features, such as hypoplastic epiphyses and vertebral bodies, poorly modelled metaphyses, short but wide metacarpals, underdeveloped mandible, spatulate ribs and clavicles, flared iliac blades, shallow acetabuli and coxa valga. Cardiac or respiratory complications usually cause death in later childhood.

Hunter's Syndrome (MPS II)

This is also a recessive disorder, but X-linked, so all patients are male. Clinical features are similar to those of Hurler's syndrome, but are less severe. Suspicious features usually appear at about three years, cardiorespiratory complications gradually become more severe and death usually occurs in middle or late teens.

Morquio-Brailsford Syndrome (MPS IV)

Development seems normal for the first year or two, although walking may be delayed. Thereafter, the child begins to look dwarf, with a moderate kyphosis, short neck and protuberant sternum. There is marked joint laxity and progressive genu valgum. Suitable tests will reveal a conductive hearing loss. However, the face is unaffected and intelligence is normal. X-rays of the spine, show the typical ovoid, hypoplastic vertebral bodies, which end up abnormally flat (platyspondyly) and peculiarly pointed, anteriorly. Odontoid hypoplasia is usual. A marked manubriosternal angle (almost 90°) is pathognomonic. By the age of five years, the femoral head epiphyses are underdeveloped and flat, along with abnormally shallow acetabula. The long bones are of normal width, but the metacarpals may be short and broad, having pointed proximal ends.

Management

- There is yet no specific treatment for the mucopolysaccharide disorder. However, enzyme replacement and gene manipulation are possible in the future
- Hurler's syndrome has very poor prognosis, but the complications (e.g. respiratory infection) may need treatment
- Morquio's syndrome presents, several orthopedic problems. Genu valgum may need correction, by femoral osteotomy, though this should be delayed till growth has ceased. Coxa valga and subluxation of the hips, if symmetrical, may need femoral or acetabular osteotomy. Atlantoaxial instability may threaten the cord and require occipitocervical fusion. All the spondylodysplasias carry a risk of atlantoaxial subluxation, during anesthesia. Intubation and special precautions are needed during operation.

OSTEOGENESIS IMPERFECTA

■ Introduction

Also termed as, fragilitas ossium, idiopathic osteopsathyrosis or periosteal dysplasia. It is a hereditary condition and is characterized by:

- Fragility of bones, with tendency to fractures and bowing
- Deafness

- Blueness of sclerae
- Laxity of joints
- Tendency to improve with age.

Etiology

- The pattern of inheritance is autosomal dominant in postnatal cases and autosomal recessive in prenatal cases
- Each and every child of an affected parent has a 50 percent chance of inheriting the faulty gene and of having osteogenesis imperfecta
- However, this can also be a result of spontaneous genetic mutation.

Pathogenesis and Pathology

- Primary defect is the failure of osteoblasts formation
- Very few osteoblasts appear and osteoid formation is minimal
- Some of calcified cartilage may undergo direct metaplasia to bone.

Features of Bones

Features of bones are shown in Figure 3.1. These are described as follows:

- Periosteum is thick, but cambium layer is thin
- Bone is short and thin
- Epiphysis is bulbous
- Cortex is thin and medullary contents are fatty and fibrous
- Deformity results from fractures and bending
- Callus formation is abundant, except in severe cases.

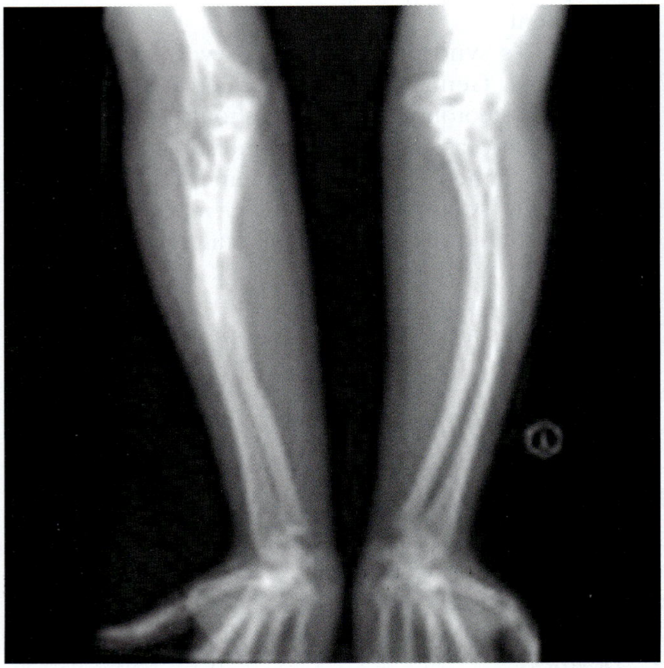

Fig. 3.1: X-ray, showing features of bones

Table 3.1: Types of osteogenesis imperfecta

Type	*Description*
Fetal/prenatal/congenital form (Osteogenesis imperfecta gravis)	• Multiple fractures present at birth • In severe forms, infant may be stillborn or die in first few weeks • Skull feels like membranous bag of bones
Infantile form	• Less severe • Skull is thin and globular-like hydrocephalic • Multiple fractures • If child survives first few years, prognosis is good • Child is normal at birth
Adolescent form (Osteogenesis imperfecta tarda)	• Fractures due to trivial trauma in childhood • Later, tendency to fracture is lost • Prognosis is good

Classification

Types of osteogenesis imperfecta (Table 3.1).

Sillence and Danks Classification

Sillence and Danks classification is depicted in Table 3.2.

Shapiro's Classification

Shapiro's classification is depicted in Table 3.3.

Falvo's Classification of Osteogenesis Imperfecta

Type 1: Osteogenesis Imperfecta Tarda

Presence of bowing of long bones (Fig. 3.1).

Type 2: Osteogenesis Imperfecta Tarda

- No bowing of long bones
- Fractures may be present in both types, but less in type 2.

Clinical Features

- Condition may vary from mild to severe
- Onset occurs from anytime before birth, to late adolescence and rarely in adults
- Patients present, with blue sclera and blue line on gums, dentinogenesis imperfecta and generalized osteoporosis (Fig. 3.2)
- Osteoporosis gives rise to bowing of bones and multiple
- *Spontaneous fractures:* Seen in severe cases
  - Healing occurs readily, with deformity
  - Abundant callus formation is seen
  - Tendency to fractures, lessens with age
- *Deafness:* Hearing decreased in 80 percent patients by third decade of life. Can be caused by otosclerosis

Table 3.2: Sillence and Danks classification of osteogenesis imperfecta

Type	*Inference*	*Description*
1 A	Autosomal dominant	Without dentinogenesis imperfecta; blue sclerae
1 B	Autosomal dominant	With dentinogenesis imperfecta; blue sclerae
2 (Osteogenesis imperfecta gravis)	Autosomal recessive	Lethal type; blue sclerae and blue line on gums severe crumpled bones; marked absence of ossification; perinatal death
3	Autosomal recessive	Severe bone fragility; multiple fractures; severe growth retardation, sclerae change from blue to white with age
4 A	Autosomal dominant	Without dentinogenesis imperfecta; variable severity to fractures and deformity more severe than type 1
4 B	Autosomal dominant	With dentinogenesis imperfecta; variable severity of fractures and deformity more severe than type 1

Table 3.3: Shapiro's classification

Type	*Description*	*Deaths*
Osteogenesis imperfecta Congenita A	*In utero*/birth fractures, short, broad, crumpled femora and ribs	94%
Osteogenesis imperfecta Congenita B	*In utero*/birth fractures, normal long bone contours, no chest deformity	8%
Osteogenesis imperfecta Tarda A	Fractures after birth, but before walking	0%
Osteogenesis imperfecta Tarda B	Fractures after walking	0%

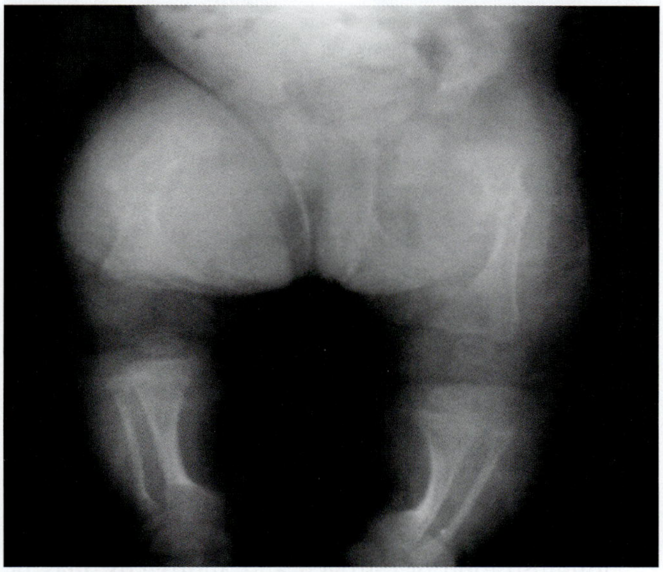

Fig. 3.2: X-ray, showing generalized osteoporosis in osteogenesis imperfecta

- *Laxity of joints:* Increased tendency to strains and dislocations
- Blue sclerae (Figs 3.3A and B) is present in 92 percent cases. A fairly deep indigo color is seen
- Dentinogenesis imperfecta, with characteristic blue line along the gums, more pronounced on the lower gums (Fig. 3.4)
- Feeble musculature
- *Dwarfing:* Due to deformities of lower limbs and spine
- *Broad skull:* Parietal and occipital bones are prominent and is called "Crâne-à-rebord"
- *Poorly calcified decidous teeth:* Permanent teeth are normal
- Normal blood chemistry
- X-ray findings
  - Skeleton is osteoporotic
  - Long bones appear thin and elongated, with thinned cortices and bulbous epiphyses (Fig. 3.5)

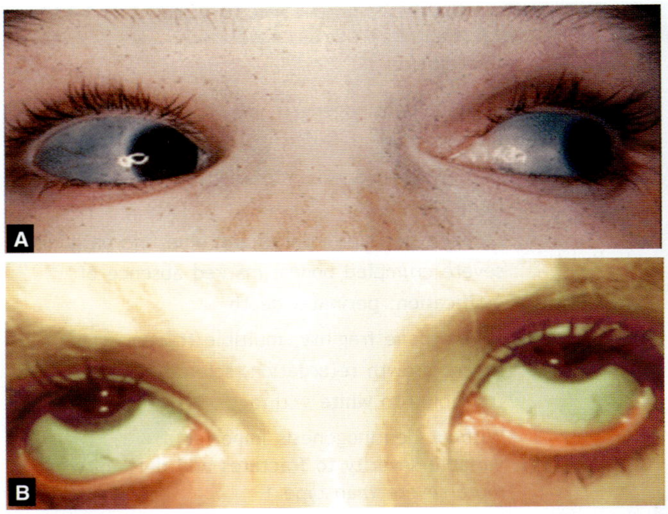

Figs 3.3A and B: Deep indigo color of sclerae or blue sclerae, is one of the clinical feature, associated with osteogenesis imperfecta

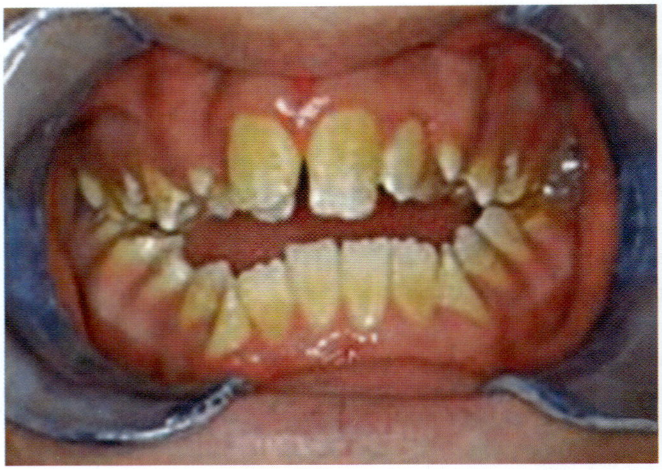

Fig. 3.4: Dentinogenesis imperfecta with blue line on gums

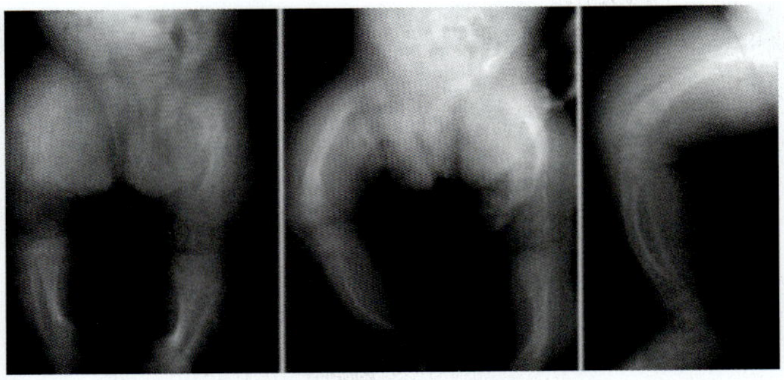

Fig. 3.5: X-ray findings, in patients with osteogenesis imperfecta

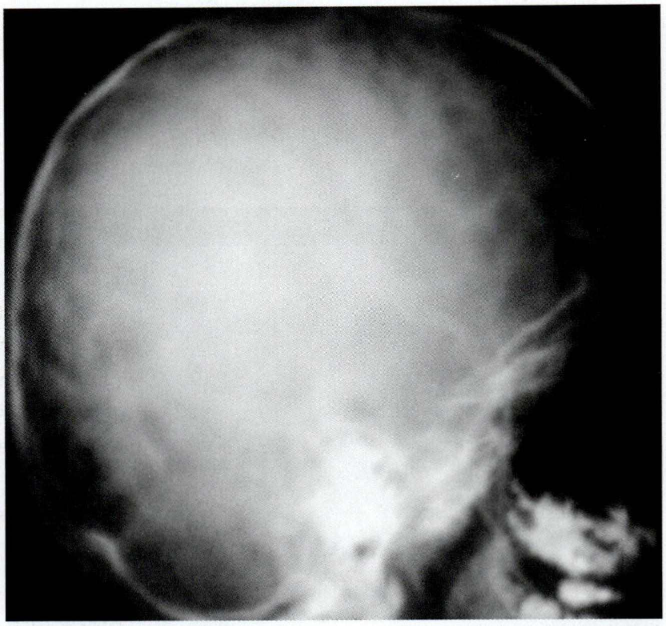

Fig. 3.6: X-ray, showing thin skull

- Skull is very thin, wormian bones may be present (Fig. 3.6)
- Vertebral bodies are translucent, shallow and biconcave, but disks are biconvex
- Severe cases show numerous fractures, especially in ribs
- Major long bones may be short, broad and thick.

Prenatal Diagnosis

- Probability of osteogenesis imperfecta in fetus can be confirmed, by amniocentesis and measurement of inorganic pyrophosphate
- The compound is consistently elevated 3 to 4 times, the normal value for gestational age. Normal values of inorganic pyrophosphate are shown in Table. 3.4

Table 3.4: Normal value of inorganic pyrophosphate

0-14 weeks	6 µg/dl
15-24 weeks	18 µg/dl
25 weeks to term	13 µg/dl

Treatment

- Protection of child, until tendency for fractures decreases
- Adequate vitamin intake for deposition
- Guard against overdosage of vitamin D, which leads to decalcification
- Administration of estrogen and androgens, may be helpful

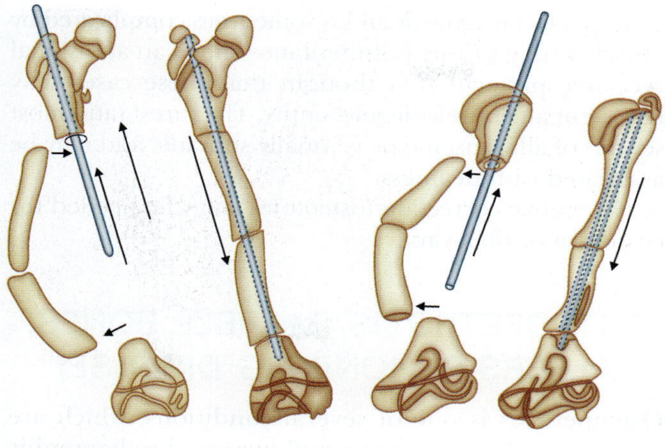

Fig. 3.7: Bailey and Buboy's method

- Severe deformities of long bones may be corrected, by multiple osteotomies through the metaphyses as well as through shaft of the bone and threading the fragments on an intramedullary rod
- *Bailey and Buboy's method (Fig. 3.7):* Telescoping medullary rod is used, which elongates as growth occurs
- *William's method:* Retrograde nailing is done, by fixing an extension to distal end of rod and driving the nail through the heel.

ACHONDROPLASIA

Introduction

This is the commonest form of abnormally short stature. Adult height is usually around 122 cm (48 inches). Severe, disproportionate shortening of the limb bones is diagnozed by X-ray before birth.

Pathology

This is an abnormality of endochondral longitudinal growth. The physes show, diminished and less regular cell proliferation, which accounts for the bone formation, is unaffected hence the normal growth of the skull vault and the periosteal contribution to bone width.

Clinical Features

The abnormality is obvious in the childhood, as growth is severely stunted, the limbs (particularly the proximal segments) are disproportionately short and the skull is quite large, with prominent forehead and saddle shaped nose. The finger appear stubby and somewhat splayed (trident hands). Joint laxity is common. Many infants have a thoracolumbar kyphosis, but this almost always disappears in a year or two. Mental development is normal.

By early childhood, the trunk is obviously disportionately long in comparison to the limbs. The standing posture is typical, i.e. the back is excessively lordotic, the buttocks are prominent, the hip flexed, the legs bowed and elbows are bent.

During adulthood, shortening of the vertebral pedicles may lead to lumbar spinal stenosis and disc prolapse, which is quite common and has exceptionally severe effects. Cervical spine stenosis, may cause typical features of cord compression.

X-ray

The tubular bones are short, the metaphyses wide and the physeal lines somewhat irregular, however the epiphyses are usually normal. Although the proximal limb bones are disproportionately affected (rhizomelia), changes are also seen in wrists and hands, where the metaphyses are broad and cup-shaped. The pelvic cavity is small (too small for a normal delivery) and the iliac wings are flared, producing an almost horizontal acetabular roof. The skull vault is large, but the base is rather short and the forearms magnum smaller than usual. The pelvic cavity is small (too small for normal delivery) and the iliac wings are flared, producing an almost horizontal acetabular roof. The skull vault is large, but the spinal cord is reduced in size. These features are clearly defined on computed tomography (CT) or magnetic resonance imaging (MRI).

Diagnosis

Achondroplasia should not be confused with any other types of short limbed dwarfism. In some (e.g. Morquio's disease) the shortening affects distal segments more than proximal and there may be widespread associated abnormalties. Others (e.g. pseudoachondroplasia and the epiphyseal dysplasias) are distinguished by the fact that the head and face are quite normal, whereas the epiphyses show characteristic changes on X-ray examination.

Genetics

Achondroplasia occurs, in about one in 25,000 births. There is autosomal dominant inheritance, however because few achondroplastic people have children, over 80 percent cases are sporadic. The fault has been shown to be point mutation in the gene coding for fibroblasts growth factor receptor three, which apparently plays a role in endochondral cartilage growth.

During childhood, operative treatment may be needed for lower limb deformities (usually genu varum). Occasionally, the thoracolumbar kyphosis fails to correct itself. If there is significant deformity (angulation of more than 40°), by the age of five years, there is a risk of cord compression and operative correction, may be needed.

During adulthood, spinal stenosis may require decompression. Intervertebral disk prolapse, superimposed on a narrow spinal canal, should be treated as an emergency.

Advances in the method of external fixation has made leg lengthening a feasible option. This is best achieved, by chondrodiatasis of the physis or callotis of the shaft. However, there are drawbacks, like complications, including nonunion, infection and nerve palsy, which may be disastrous and the cosmetic effect of long legs and short arms, may be less pleasing than anticipated. It is essential that the details of the operation, its aims, limitations and the patient (and where appropriate with the parents) should be carefully discussed and prioritized, as anesthesia carries a greater than usual risk and requires expert supervision.

HYPOCHONDROPLASIA

This has been described, as a very mild form of achondroplasia. However, apart from shortness of stature (with the emphasis on proximal limb segments) and noticeable lumbar lordosis, there is little to suggest any abnormality, the head and face are not affected and many of those with hypochondroplasia pass for normal stocky individuals. X-rays may show, slight pelvic flattening and thickening of long bones. The condition is transmitted, as autosomal dominant. Those affected, sometimes ask for limb lengthening and after careful discussion, this may be done, with a considerable chance of success.

METAPHYSEAL CHONDRODYSPLASIA (DYSOSTOSIS)

■ Introduction

This term, describes a type of short limbed dwarfism, in which the bony abnormality is virtually confined to the metaphyses. The epiphyses are unaffected, but the metaphyseal segments adjacent to the growth plates are broadened and mildly scalloped, somewhat resembling rickets. There may be bilateral coxa vara and bowed legs, as patients tend to walk with a waddling gait. Apart from the lordotic posture, the spine is normal. The main deformities are around the hips and knees.

There are several forms of metaphyseal chondrodysplasia. The best known, Schmid type has the classic features described above, with autosomal dominant inheritance. Another group (McKusick type) is associated with sparse hair growth and is sometimes complicated by Hirschsprung's disease. Inheritance shows an autosomal recessive pattern. It is thought that these cases may represent an entirely distinct entity. The rarest (and most severe) of all, Jansen type is usually sporadic and may be associated with deafness.

Operative correction (osteotomy) may be needed for coxa vara or tibia vara.

OSTEOPETROSIS (MARBLE BONES, ALBERS-SCHONBERG DISEASE)

Osteopetrosis is one of several conditions, which are characterized by thickening and increased radiographic density of the bone, differences in the pattern of inheritance, the age of presentation and the distribution of the clinical and X-ray changes, shows that they are genetically distinct conditions.

Osteopetrosis Tarda

The common form of osteopetrosis is a fairly benign, autosomal dominant disorder that seldom causes symptoms and may only be discovered in the adolescence or adulthood, after the pathological fracture or when an X-ray is taken for other reasons, hence the designation tarda. Appearance and function are unimpaired, unless there are complications, like pathological fracture or cranial nerve compression, due to bone encroachment or foramina. Sufferers are also prone to bone infections, particularly of the mandible, after tooth extraction.

X-rays show increased density of all the bones, such as cortices are widened, leaving narrow medullary canals, sclerotic vertebral end plates produce a striped appearance (Rugger jersey spine), the skull is thickened and the base density is sclerotic. Treatment is required, only if complications occurs.

Osteopetrosis Congenita

This rare, autosomal recessive form of osteopetrosis, present at birth and causes severe disability. Bone encroachment on marrow results in pancytopenia, hemolysis, anemia and hepatosplenomegaly. Foraminal occlusion may cause optic or facial nerve palsy. Repeated hemorrhage or infection, usually leads to the death in early childhood.

Treatment, in recent years has focused on the methods of enhancing bone resorption. This has been achieved by transplanting marrow from normal donors, suggesting that the condition is due to lack of marrow cells that control osteoclastic activity.

4 Genetic Disorders

- Introduction to Genetics
- Patterns of Inheritance
- Gene Mapping and Genetic Markers
- Prenatal Diagnosis
- Childhood Diagnosis
- Management of Genetic Disorders
- Down's Syndrome (Trisomy-21)
- Marfan's Syndrome
- Turner's Syndrome
- Ehlers-Danlos Syndrome

INTRODUCTION TO GENETICS

■ History of Genetics

People have known about inheritance for a long time, as evident from following facts:

- Children resemble their parents
- Domestication of animals and plants, selective breeding for good characteristics
- Sumerian horse breeding records
- Bible and hemophilia.

Old Ideas

Despite knowing about inheritance in general, a number of incorrect ideas had to be generated and overcome before modern genetics could arise. All lives come from other lives. Living organisms are not spontaneously generated from nonliving material. Big exception though is origin of life itself.

Species concept: Offspring arise only when two members of the same species mate. Monstrous hybrids do not exist. Organisms develop by expressing information carried in their hereditary material. As opposed to "preformation" the idea that in each sperm (or egg) is a tiny, fully-formed human that merely grows in size. Male and female parents contribute equally to the offspring. Ancient greec idea, male plants a "seed" in the female "garden".

Mid 1800's Discoveries

Three major events in the mid 1800 directly led to the development of modern genetics. Some of the major related discoveries are:

1859: Charles Darwin publishes *The Origin of Species*, which describes the theory of evolution by natural selection. This theory requires heredity to work.

1866: Gregor Mendel publishes his experiments in plant hybridization, which lays out the basic theory of genetics. It is widely ignored until 1900.

1871: Friedrich Miescher isolates "nucleic acid" from pus cells.

1900: Rediscovery of Mendel's work by Robert Correns, Hugo de Vries and Erich von Tschermak.

Major Events in the 20th Century

1902: A Garrod discovers that alkaptonuria, a human disease, has a genetic basis.

1904: G Bateson discovers linkage between genes. He also coins the word "genetics".

1910: Thomas Hunt Morgan proves that genes are located on the chromosomes (using Drosophila).

1944: Oswald Avery, Colin MacLeod and Maclyn McCarty, show that DNA can transform bacteria, demonstrating that DNA is the hereditary material.

1953: James Watson and Francis Crick determine the structure of the DNA molecule, which leads directly to knowledge of how it replicates.

1966: Marshall Nirenberg solves the genetic code, showing that three DNA bases code for one amino acid.

2001: Sequence of the entire human genome is announced.

"Blending" Theory of Inheritance

Before Mendel's work, the most popular theory of inheritance stated that the qualities of the parents blended to form the qualities of the child. Under this theory, one tall parent and one short parent would produce a child of medium height. Most ordinary observations seemed to support this hypothesis, which rejected the notion of discrete units of inheritance (i.e. genes). However, this theory was poorly equipped to deal with such phenomena, as two brown-eyed parents giving birth to a blue-eyed baby.

Early Genetics

The study of genetics began with observations made by Gregor Mendel. After noticing that the flowers of his pea plants were either violet or white, Mendel began to study the segregation of heritable traits.

Because the principles established by Mendel form the basis for genetics, the science is often referred to as Mendelian genetics. It is also called classical genetics to distinguish it from another branch of biology known as molecular genetics.

Mendel devised two fundamental principles of inheritance:

1. *Mendel's principle of segregation:* The factors of inheritance (genes) normally are paired, but are separated or segregated in the formation of gametes (eggs and sperm).
2. *Mendel's principle of independent assortment:* Each factors distribution in the gametes is not related to the distribution of any other factor (This principle is not strictly true due to the organization of genes on chromosomes).

Mendel's Observations

- Mendel made numerous important observations in his exhaustive study of pea plants characteristics. He elaborated an important distinction between dominant and recessive traits through his work with pea plants
- By studying the characteristics of pea plants, such as their height, seed shape, seed color, flower position and other traits
- This discussion will use height as a primary example. Mendel first crossbred one tall, true-breeding plant with one short, true-breeding plant. Contrary to the blending theory, all the offspring were tall. In terms of genotype, the original tall plant was "TT" (two dominant alleles; homozygous), the short plant was "tt" (two recessive alleles; homozygous) and the second generation plants were "Tt" (one dominant and one recessive allele; heterozygous)
- When Mendel next time allowed these plants to self-fertilize, he found that the short trait reappeared in the third generation. The ratio of tall to short plants was almost exactly 3:1. Their genotypes were in ratio of 1:2:1 [one short (tt), two tall (Tt) and one tall (TT)].

Limitations of the Mendelian System

The simple system of Mendelian genetics is very powerful and serves to explain the inheritance patterns of numerous traits. However, many traits are controlled by many genes acting in tandem, and thus do not obey strict Mendelian patterns (although their constituent genes may). Furthermore, many human traits are strongly influenced by the environment as well, therefore their phenotypes cannot be said to be Mendelian (though the genetic components may be). In sum, Mendelian patterns are important, but cannot be applied universally. Individual traits must be researched to find out, if they obey typical Mendelian patterns.

What is Gene?

A gene is an information entity. It is a sequence of DNA that codes for a single genetic instruction. Usually, this instruction is the sequence of a protein, but a gene may also serve to activate or deactivate other genes, in a cell or in neighboring cells. Every aspect of our species is constructed based on information encoded in genes. The genes themselves do very little, they are information storage molecules. It is the cytological machinery of our cells, passed from one generation to the next, that translate these instructions into a living organism. The effects of every gene depend both upon other genes and on the environment.

What is an Allele?

An allele is one variant of a gene. Many genes have two, several, or many different variants of the same basic genetic information. Some alleles are minor differences that to not significantly affect the organism, while others cause profound changes.

Example: Nucleotide substitutions in the third codon position often produces no change at all, because they code for the same transfer RNA and thus the same protein is produced:

- In humans CCU, CCA does not cause a change, both triplets code for proline. Other substitutions may produce profound effects
- Sickle cell anemia is caused by a single nucleotide substitution, GAG to GUG changes normal hemoglobin to hemoglobin, that "sickles" under.
- In humans, a cell's nucleus contains 46 individual chromosomes or 23 pairs of chromosomes. Half of the chromosomes come from one parent and half come from the other parent
- Chromosomal DNA contains other things besides genes:
  - Centromere (where the mitotic spindle attaches)
  - Telomeres (special structures on the ends of chromosomes)
  - Origins of replication (where copying of DNA starts)
  - Pseudogenes (nonfunctional, mutated copies of genes)

- Transposable elements AKA transposons (intranuclear parasites)
- Genes that make small RNAs and not proteins.

- The set of all genes that specify an organisms traits is known as the organism's genome. The genome for a human cell consists of about 100,000 genes. The gene composition of a living organism is its genotype. For a person's earlobe shape, the genotype may consist of two genes for attached earlobes or two genes for free earlobes or one gene for attached and one gene for free earlobes. The physical expression of the genes is referred to as the phenotype of a living thing. If a person has attached earlobes, the phenotype is "attached earlobes." If the person has free earlobes, the phenotype is "free earlobes." Even though three genotypes for earlobe shape are possible only two phenotypes (attached earlobes and free earlobes) are possible
- As you remember, diploid organisms have two sets of redundant genetic information and two copies of every gene
  - An individual is homozygous at a locus, if they have two alleles for a gene and heterozygous at that locus, if they have different copies
- Dominant alleles mask the effect of a recessive allele at that locus they are expressed in the homozygous or the heterozygous state
- Recessive alleles are only expressed in the homozygous state
- *Example:* Alleles for albino coloration in many animals result from recessive alleles. Thus, for albino coat color in mice, individuals with either one or two copies A (dominant) allele have brown fur. Therefore, "AA" and "Aa" have brown fur. Note that "Aa" individuals can pass on the allele, even though they do not express it themselves, they are carriers. Individuals with two copies of the albino allele, "aa" have white fur
- Some alleles of medical interest, when rare, recessive alleles are usually in the heterozygous state and not subject to natural selection, human populations harbor quite a few harmful, recessive alleles at low frequencies
- For instance, a rare, autosomal recessive allele on chromosome 7 disrupts the normal migration of neurons, leading to an abnormally thick and smooth cerebral cortex and reduced cerebellum, hippocampus and brainstem causing a condition called lissencephaly. It is typical of these conditions for an affected individual to be born to normal parents
- Dominant alleles, by contrast are generally manifested in the parents. For instance, ectrodactyly a condition, where the affected individual has severely deformed digits is caused by a dominant allele. It runs in families, conspicuously
- *Codominance* (sometimes called incomplete dominance) is the allelic interaction, where in the heterozygous state, both alleles are expressed (for attributes) or the heterozygote is in between the phenotypes of the homozygous individuals for those alleles (in the case of measurable characters). Thus, the heterozygote has a unique phenotype. For example, in chickens, black feather color is codominant with white feather color. Heterozygous chickens have black and white feathers in a checkered pattern.
- *Mitosis:* Mitosis, the duplication of the genetic material within a eukaryote cell, is worth mentioning here because of what it IS and what it IS NOT. A cell gives rise to two, smaller but genetically identical copies of itself. It is a duplication of the genetic complement of a eukaryote cell. Since it is usually followed by cell division, it can lead to growth, in a multicellular organism, or asexual reproduction, in a single-celled organism. It is not a means of producing gametes. In sexual organisms, mitosis is peripheral to sexual reproduction, it serves to give rise to cell types which ultimately "kill themselves off" by splitting and splitting again, into four, very different, cells.
- *Meiosis:* Meiosis is that process, by which a single diploid cell gives rise to four genetically different, haploid cells. It works like this (forget the phases):
  - The diploid progenitor duplicates its genetic material, thus every chromosome is composed of two identical, chromatids joined at the centromere (this happens before meiosis starts)
  - Each chromosome finds its match, to form "matching pairs" of homologous chromosomes. This process, which occurs during the first of the two meiotic divisions is unique to meiosis, it does not occur during mitosis
  - Four strands (two homologous chromosomes, composed of two identical strands each) cluster in structures sometimes called tetrads, along a plane in the center of the dividing cell. A process called "crossing over" may occur at this time
  - First division, homologous chromosomes separate
  - Spindle fibers drag them to opposite poles of the cell. The cell then divides. Where chromosome ends up, is completely random and is not influenced by the fate of the other chromosomes around it. The cell then divides
  - Second division, chromatids separate
  - Spindle fibers drag them to opposite poles of the cell. The cell then divides. This gives you four, genetically different, daughter cells from a single parent.
- *Errors in meiosis:* Errors in meiosis have the potential to produce unusual phenotypes in the offspring

- The most common meiotic error is nondisjunction, where an entire homologous pair of chromosomes migrates to the pole of a cell, without splitting
- If this happens to a single pair, it causes either a trisomy or a monosomy in the resulting offspring
- If it happens to the entire genome, it can produce triploid or even tetraploid offspring
- The human condition of Down's syndrome results from a trisomy at chromosome 23, a trisomy at chromosome 18, 13, or the sex chromosomes, is also survivable. In humans, trisomies for other chromosomes are not usually viable
- In other organisms, triploids and tetraploids may be viable.

PATTERNS OF INHERITANCE

■ What is Inheritance?

Inheritance is the transfer of characteristics from parents to their offspring, e.g. hair, eye and skin color.

■ What is Inheritance Patterns?

Inheritance patterns trace the transmission of genetically encoded traits, conditions or diseases to offspring.

Modes of Inheritance

- Single gene or Mendelian
- Multifactorial
- Mitochondrial.

Single Gene or Mendelian Inheritance

- Genetic conditions caused by a mutation in a single gene follow predictable patterns of inheritance within families
- Single gene inheritance is also referred to as Mendelian inheritance, as they follow transmission patterns that he observed in his research on peas
- There are four types of Mendelian inheritance pattern:
  - Autosomal dominant
  - Autosomal recessive
  - X-linked dominant
  - X-linked recessive
- *Autosomal:* The gene responsible for the phenotype is located on one of the 22 pairs of autosomes (non-sex determining chromosomes)
- *X-linked:* The gene that encodes for the trait is located on the X chromosome
- *Dominant:* Conditions that are manifest in heterozygotes (individuals with just one copy of the mutant allele)

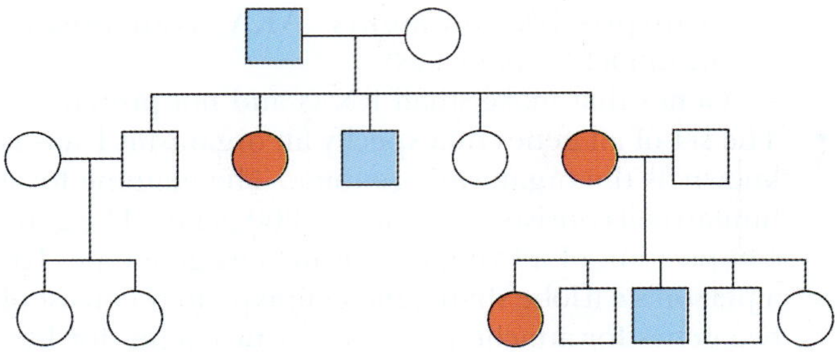

Fig. 4.1: Pedigree chart, showing the transfer of the mutant genes to offsprings

- *Recessive:* Conditions are only manifest in individuals who have two copies of the mutant allele (are homozygous).

Autosomal Dominant

- Dominant conditions are expressed in individuals, who have just one copy of the mutant allele
- Affected males and females have an equal probability of passing on the trait to offspring
- Affected individual's have one normal copy of the gene and one mutant copy of the gene, thus each offspring has a 50 percent chance on inheriting the mutant allele
- As shown in this pedigree (Fig. 4.1), approximately half of the children of affected parents inherit the condition and half do not
- *Autosomal dominant diseases:* The most common diseases are:
  - Achondroplasia
  - Marfan's syndrome
  - Brachydactyly
  - Ehlers-Danlos syndrome
  - Osteogenesis imperfecta
  - Neurofibromatosis.

Autosomal Recessive

- Recessive conditions are clinically manifest only when an individual has two copies of the mutant allele
- When just one copy of the mutant allele is present, an individual is a carrier of the mutation, but does not develop the condition
- Females and males are affected equally by traits transmitted by autosomal recessive inheritance
- When two carriers mate, each child has a 25 percent chance of being homozygous wild-type (unaffected), a 25 percent chance of being homozygous mutant (affected) or a 50 percent chance of being heterozygous (unaffected carrier) (Fig. 4.2)
- *Autosomal recessive diseases:* Most common diseases are:
  - Chondrodystrophia calcificans
  - Hurler's syndrome

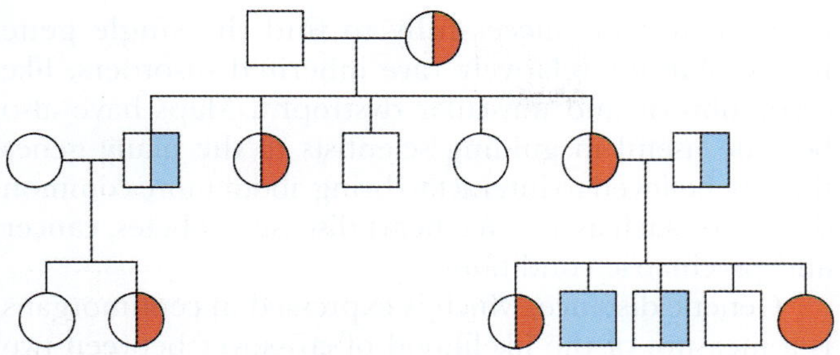

Fig. 4.2: Pedigree chart showing, each child has a 25 percent chance of being homozygous wild-type (unaffected); a 25 percent chance of being homozygous mutant (affected); a 50 percent chance of being heterozygous (unaffected carrier)

- Tay-Sachs disease
- Phenylketonuria
- Cystic fibrosis

X-linked Recessive

- X-linked recessive traits are not clinically manifest, when there is a normal copy of the gene
- All X-linked recessive traits are fully evident in males because they only have one copy of the X chromosome, thus do not have a normal copy of the gene to compensate for the mutant copy
- For that same reason, women are rarely affected by X-linked recessive diseases, however they are affected, when they have two copies of the mutant allele
- As the gene is on the X chromosome, there is no father to son transmission, but there is father to daughter and mother to daughter and son transmission. If a man is affected with an X-linked recessive condition, all his daughters will inherit one copy of the mutant allele from him
- *X-linked recessive diseases (Fig. 4.3):* Some of these diseases are:
- Duchenne dystrophy
- Fragile X syndrome
- Hemophilia A.

X-linked Dominant

- As the gene is located on the X chromosome, there is no transmission from father to son, but there can be transmission from father to daughter
- All daughters of an affected male will be affected, since the father has only one X chromosome to transmit
- Children of an affected woman have a 50 percent chance of inheriting the X chromosome with the mutant allele
- X-linked dominant disorders are clinically manifest when only one copy of the mutant allele is present

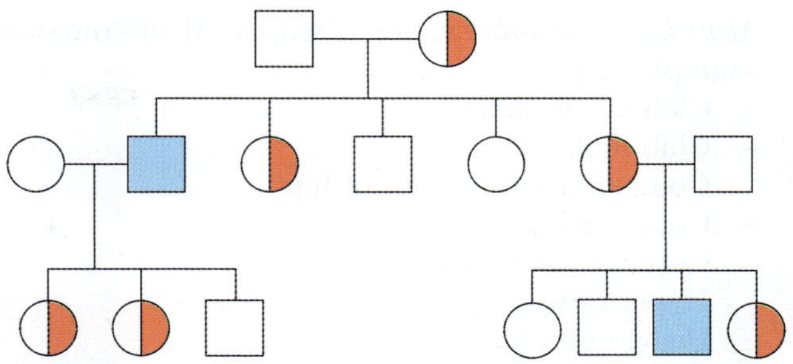

Fig. 4.3: Pedigree chart for X-linked recessive gene transmission

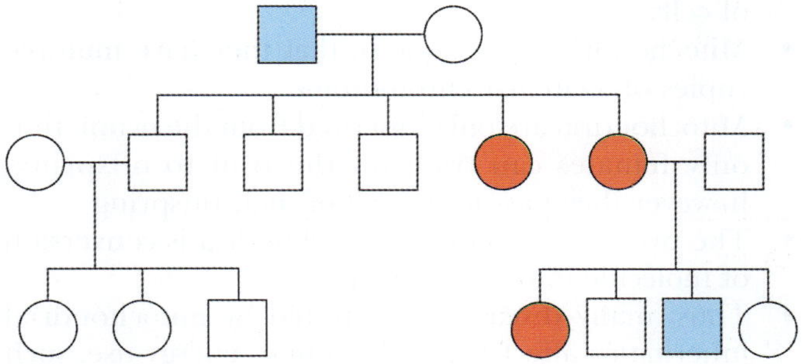

Fig. 4.4: Pedigree chart for X-linked dominant transmission of genes

- *X-linked dominant diseases (Fig. 4.4):* Most common diseases are:
  - Chondrodysplasia punctata
  - Hypophosphatemic rickets
  - Vitamin D resistant rickets
  - Morquio's osteochondrodystrophy.

Multifactorial Inheritance

- Most diseases have multifactorial inheritance patterns. As the name implies, multifactorial conditions are not caused by a single gene, but rather are a result of interplay between genetic factors and environmental factors
- Diseases with multifactorial inheritance are not genetically determined, but rather a genetic mutation may predispose an individual to a disease
- Other genetic and environmental factors contribute to whether or not the disease develops
- Numerous genetic alterations may predispose individuals to the same disease (genetic heterogeneity). For instance coronary heart disease risk factors include high blood pressure, diabetes and hyperlipidemia. All of those risk factors have their own genetic and environmental components
- Thus, multifactorial inheritance is far more complex than Mendelian inheritance and is more difficult to trace through pedigrees

- *Multifactorial inheritance diseases:* Most common examples are:
  - Cleft lip or palate
  - Club foot
  - Congenital dislocation of hip
  - Congenital heart disease
  - Coronary artery disease
  - Hypertension
  - Diabetes mellitus
  - Schizophrenia.

Mitochondrial Inheritance

- Mitochondria are organelles found in the cytoplasm of cells
- Mitochondria are unique in that they have multiple copies of a circular chromosome
- Mitochondria are only inherited from the ovum, thus only females can transmit the trait to offspring, however they pass it onto all of their offspring
- The primary function of mitochondria is conversion of molecule into usable energy
- Thus, many diseases transmitted by mitochondrial inheritance affect organs with high-energy use, such as the heart, skeletal muscle, liver, and kidneys
- *Mitochondrial inheritance disease:* Maternally inherited diabetes and deafness (MIDD) is a disorder with this type of inheritance pattern.

GENE MAPPING AND GENETIC MARKERS

■ Gene Mapping

Gene mapping is an intensively developing area of modern genetics that is highly relevant to studies of the organization of the human genomes. Its narrow scope is building of genetic maps, providing a basis for medical and human genetics. Its broader scope is to open up new possibilities to a better understanding of the anatomy of the genome and its organization principles.

Comparative gene mapping has offered new prospects for the research of the patterns, produced by evolving linkage groups, chromosomes and single gene associations that brought closer to examination of a fundamental biological problem that "Do genes combine randomly or not into linkage groups?" and for the research of, may be the role of natural selection in their combination.

Genetic mapping, also called linkage mapping, can offer firm evidence that a disease transmitted from parent to child is linked to one or more genes. It also provides clues about which chromosome contains the gene and precisely where it lies on that chromosome. Genetic maps have been used successfully to find the single gene responsible for relatively rare inherited disorders, like cystic fibrosis and muscular dystrophy. Maps have also become useful in guiding scientists to the many genes that are believed to interact to bring about more common disorders, such as asthma, heart disease, diabetes, cancer and psychiatric conditions.

Genetic distance, which is expressed in centimorgans is a measure of the likelihood of crossover between two loci. Two loci are 1 cm apart, if there is a 1 percent probability of crossover during meiosis in males and perhaps twice as many during meiosis in females. Feasibility of human linkage analysis was revolutionized by demonstration of genetic variation in the size of fragments generated, by digestion of normal human DNA with restriction endonuclease. Restriction fragment length polymorphisms (RFLPs) are the consequences of DNA sequence polymorphisms and inherited according to Mendelian principles.

Restriction enzyme digestion and southern blotting, makes it possible to utilize these polymorphisms as genetic markers for sites within genomes. If one of the base pairs in the recognition sequence for restriction enzyme differs between individual copies of the genome or if there is a length variation in DNA, then there will variation in the size of DNA fragments generated by restriction enzyme digestion. Genetic linkage can be assesed between any group of markers, one of which genes may represent a mutation that causes a diseases of phenotype.

For autosomal gene, each individual inherits one copy of each chromosome from each parent. Based on the following methods:

- Chromosomal and regional assignments of genes were made
- Genes were ordered on physical and genetic maps (Fig. 4.5).

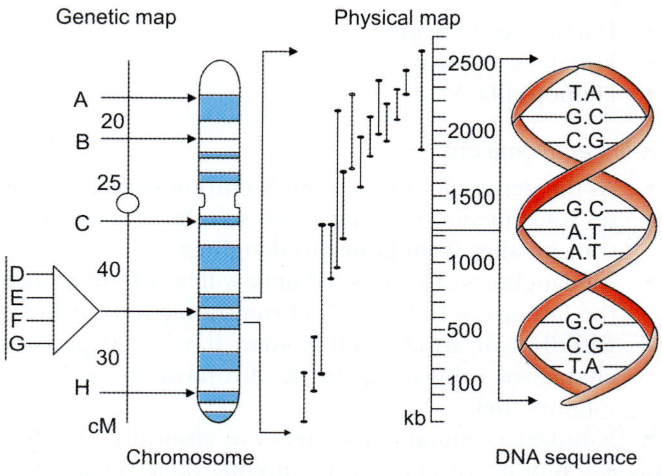

Fig. 4.5: Genes order, as shown on genetic and physical maps

RFLP Process

- Blood sample extracted
- It is digested by restriction enzyme and seprated by gel electrophoresis
- Double stranded DNA is denatured and is converted to single stranded
- Then blotted on solid membrane (southern transfer) and hybridized with radio probe
- On X-ray exposure specific DNA fragment can be seen (Fig. 4.6).

Variable number of tandem repeat (VNTR) polymorphisms (Fig. 4.7)

- Restriction enzymes cleave DNA on two different chromosomes, on either sides of the tandem repeat sequence
- Radioactive probes hybridized to the DNA
- They undergo complementary base pairing
- Autoradiography reveals fragments of different length.

Western blot method for proteins (Fig. 4.8).

Northern blot method for RNA (Fig. 4.9)

Southern blot method for DNA (Fig. 4.10)

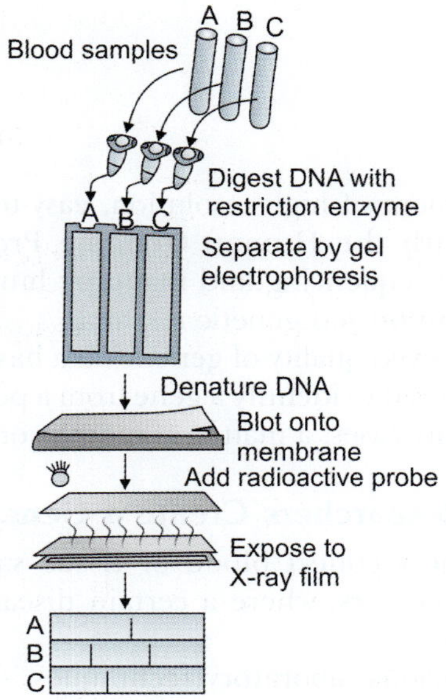

Fig. 4.6: Showing steps of RFLP process

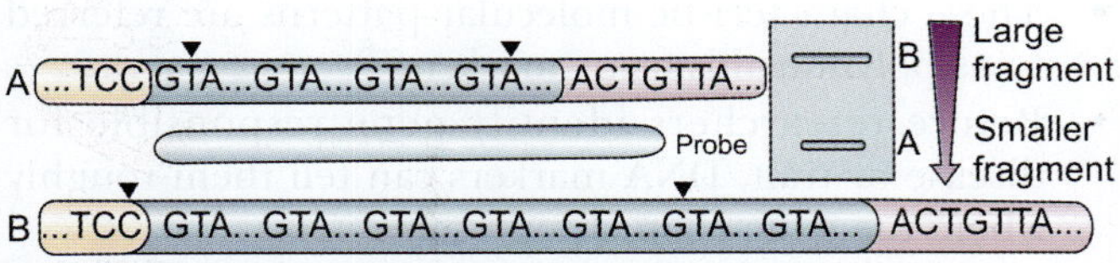

Fig. 4.7: VNTR polymorphisms: Restriction enzyme cleave DNA on two different chromosomes—(A) Smaller chromosomal segment; (B) Larger segment

- DNA is applied to gel
- Electrophoresis is done
- DNA is blotted with the help of salt solution by capillary action
- DNA is transferred to filter
- It is then hybridize with unique nuleic acid probe
- Then unbound probe is removed
- Exposure to X-ray produces the desired autoradiogam.

Approaches used to Build Genetic Maps

- Interspecific cell hybridization
- Radiation hybridization
- *In situ* hybridization

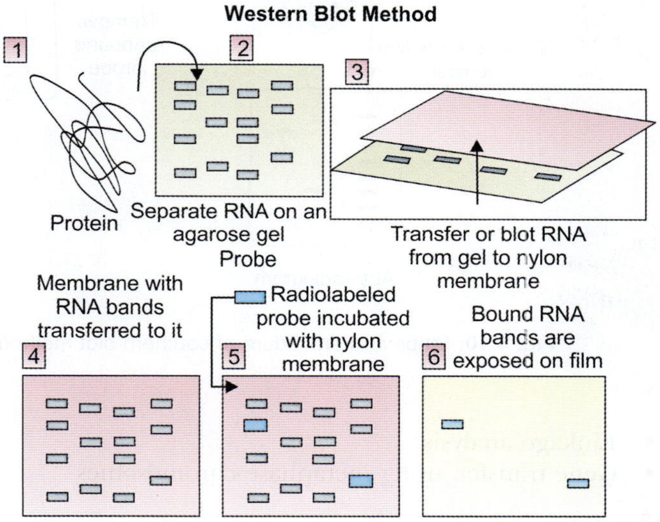

Fig. 4.8: Steps and procedure of western blot method for proteins

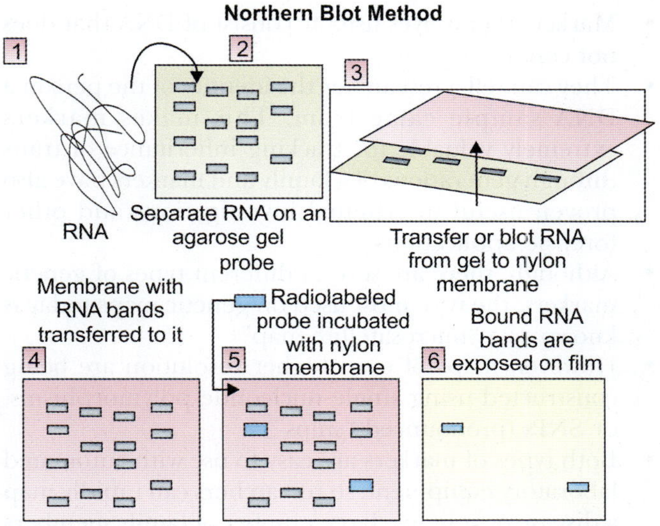

Fig. 4.9: Steps and procedure of northern blot method for RNA

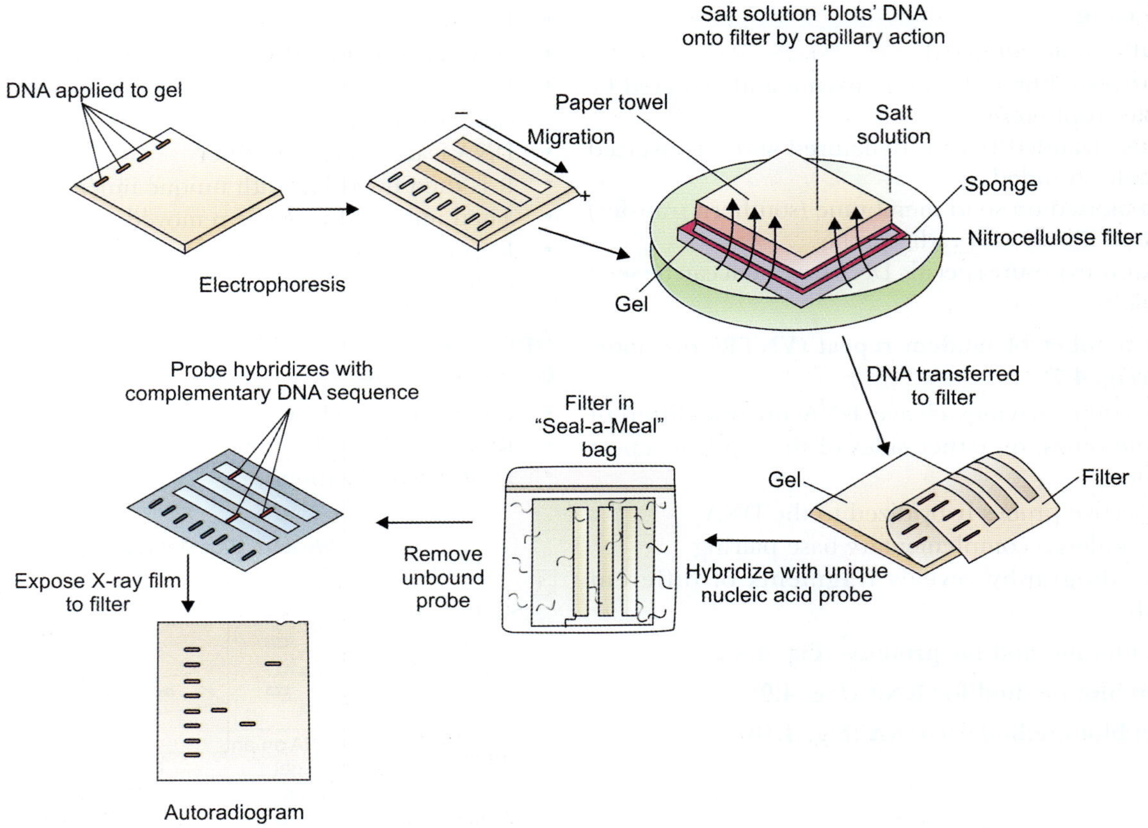

Fig. 4.10: Steps and procedure of southern blot method for DNA

- Linkage analysis
- Gene transfer, using metaphase chromosomes

Genetic Markers

What are Genetic Markers?

- Markers themselves usually consist of DNA that does not contain a gene
- They can tell a researcher the identity of the person a DNA sample came from. This makes markers extremely valuable for tracking inheritance of traits through generations of a family and markers have also proven useful in criminal investigations and other forensic applications
- Although, there are several different types of genetic markers, the type most used on genetic maps today is known as a "microsatellite map"
- However, maps of even higher resolution are being constructed using single-nucleotide polymorphisms, or SNPs (pronounced "snips")
- Both types of markers are easy to use with automated laboratory equipment, so researchers can rapidly map a disease or trait in a large number of family members
- Development of high-resolution, easy-to-use genetic maps, with the Human Genome Project (HGP) successful sequencing and mapping human genome has revolutionized genetic research
- The improved quality of genetic data has reduced the time required to identify a gene from a period of years to, in many cases, a matter of months or even weeks.

How Do Researchers Create a Genetic Map?

- Researchers collect blood or tissue samples from family members, where a certain disease or trait is prevalent
- Using various laboratory techniques, the scientists isolate DNA from these samples
- Then it is examined for unique patterns of bases, seen only in family members who have the disease or trait
- These characteristic molecular patterns are referred to as polymorphisms or markers
- Before researchers identify gene responsible for disease or trait, DNA markers can tell them roughly where the gene is on chromosome
- This is possible because of a genetic process known as recombination

- As eggs or sperm develop within a person's body, the 23 pairs of chromosomes within those cells exchange or recombine genetic material
- If a particular gene is close to DNA marker, the gene and marker will likely to stay together during the recombination process and passed on together from parent to child
- If each family member with a particular disease or trait also inherits a particular DNA marker, chances are high that gene responsible for the disease lies near that marker
- The more DNA markers on a genetic map, the more likely that one will be closely linked to a disease gene and the easier it will be for researchers to zero-in on that gene
- One of the first major achievements was to develop dense maps of markers spaced evenly across the entire collection of human DNA.

Clinical Relevance (Table 4.1)

Table 4.1: Genetic diseases, type of chromosomal aberration and the genes or chromosomes involved

Diseases	*Aberration*	*Chromosome*
Ewing's sarcoma	Translocation	11q24 and 22q12
Germ cell tumor	Isochromosome	12p
Sarcoma, synovial	Translocation	Xp11 and 18q11

PRENATAL DIAGNOSIS

■ Introduction

Many genetic disorders can be diagnosed before birth, thus improving the chances of treatment or at worst, giving the parents the choice of selective abortion. Ultrasound imaging is harmless and is being done almost routinely. On the other hand test that involve amniocentesis or chronic villous sampling, carry a risk of injury to fetus and are therefore used only when there is reason to suspect some abnormality. Indications are:

- Maternal age over 35 years or an unduly high paternal age
- A previous history of chromosome abnormalities or genetic abnormalities amenable to biochemical diagnosis
- To confirm noninvasive test, suggesting an abnormality.

Maternal Screening

Fetal neural tube defect is associated with increased level of alpha-fetoproteins in amniotic fluid and to lesser extent in maternal blood. Women with positive blood test may be given the option of further investigation by amniocentesis. It has also been noted that abnormally low level of AFP are associated with Down's syndrome.

Amniocentesis

Under local anesthesia a small amount (200 ml) of fluid is drawn from amniotic sac with a needle and syringe. The procedure is usually carried out between 14th and 18th weeks of pregnancy. The fluid can be directly examined for AFP and desquamated fetal cells can be collected and cultured for chromosomal studies and biochemical tests for enzymes disorders.

Chronic Villous Sampling

Under ultrasound screening, a fine needle catheter is passed through cervix and a small sample of chorionic is sucked out. This is usually done between 8th and 10th weeks of pregnancy. Mesenchymal fibroblast can be cultured and can be used for chromosomal studies, biochemical test and DNA analysis. Rapid advances in DNA technologies have made it possible to diagnose sickle cell anemia and hemophilia during early pregnancy.

Fetal Imaging

By the 18th week of pregnancy, high resolution ultrasonography may show anatomical abnormalities, such as open neural tube defect and short limb. In late pregnancy X-ray examination will reveal any marked change in bone density and multiple fractures.

CHILDHOOD DIAGNOSIS

■ Introduction

It is a difficult task for a physician to determine whether the disease with which the patient is afflicted, is genetic in origin. Towards the end, accurate diagnostic steps become imperative. Retarded growth, disproportionate length of the upper or lower trunk, childhood deformity and any malformations are the most commonly encountered conditions in childhood, which need to be corrected in the pediatric age group itself, to avoid any disability in the adulthood.

Predisposing Factors

- An abnormal fetus detected in intrauterine life by ultrasonography (USG)
- A child with mental retardation or delayed physical and mental milestones
- An infant with single or multiple malformations
- When it is suspected that the disease is either an inherited metabolic disorder, a single-gene disorder or a chromosomal disorder

- Consanguinity marriage
- History of multiple miscarriages
- Exposure to teratogens.

History

- A thorough detailed history and physical examination are essential
- A detailed history about the individual's prenatal period, labor, delivery and documentation of family relationships, i.e. charting the pedigree are useful
- In pedigree charting, gender of each individual and the relationship between individuals should be indicated using standard pedigree symbols
- In patients with X-linked recessive disorders, the history of the male relatives on the mother's side of the family is important, the age should be recorded along with the history of the presence or absence of any disease.

Examination

- In the clinical examination, attention should be paid to physical variations or minor abnormalities, which can provide clues to diagnosis
- Following physical examination, relevant routine laboratory tests, such as blood examination, ECG, imaging studies, special molecular cytogenic studies, molecular biochemical tests, etc. are carried out
- Routine tests usually enable recording of physical features, such as cardiac anomalies or musculoskeletal deformities
- Chromosomal analysis helps to establish diagnosis in cases, such as failure to thrive, developmental delay, multiple malformations, sexual dysmorphism, mental retardation, etc.
- Specific recombinant DNA tests enable the detection of mutation and establish diagnosis.

Prenatal Diagnosis

- Prenatal diagnosis includes both screening and diagnostic tests
- A popular screening test used for prenatal diagnosis is an assay of maternal serum alpha-fetoprotein (AFP), at 15 weeks of gestation
- The diagnostis tests can be used for two purposes:
  - Analysis of fetal tissues, e.g. aminocentesis, chorionic villus sampling (CVS), cordocentesis and in *in vitro* fertilization (IVF) diagnosis
  - Visualization of the fetus, e.g. USG.

Clinical Features

- Retarded growth and shortness of stature
- Disproportionate length of trunk and limbs
- Localized malformations (dysmorphism)
- Soft-tissue contracture
- All the skeletal dysplasis affect growth, although this may not be obvious at birth
- Children should be measured at regular intervals and a record kept of height and length of lower segment (pubic symphysis to heel) and upper segment (pubis to cranium), head circumference and chest circumference
- Failure to reach the expected height for the local population group should be noted and marked shortness of stature is highly suspicious
- The normal upper segment ratio changes gradually from about 1.5:1, at the end of the first year to about 1:1 at puberty
- Shortness of the stature with normal proportions is not necessarily abnormal, but it is also seen in endocrine disorders, which affect the different parts of the skeleton more or less equally
- By contrast, small stature with disapropriate shortness of the limbs is characteristic of skeletal dysplasia, the long bones being more markedly affected than the axial skeleton
- The different segments of the limbs also may be disproportionately affected
- The subtleties of:
  - Rhizomelia proximal segments (humeri and femora)
  - *Mesomelia:* Short middle segments (forearms and legs)
  - *Acromelia:* Stubby hands and feets
- Dysmorphism (a misshapen part of the body) is the most obvious in the face and hands
- There is a remarkable consistency about these changes, which makes for a disturbing similarity of appearance in members of a particular group
- Local deformities, such as kyphosis, valgus or varus knees, bowed forearms and ulnar deviated wrists result from disturbed bone growth.

Radiological Findings

- Presence of any above features calls for a limited radiograph survey. Anteroposterior views of the skull and thoracolumbar spine
- Fractures, deformity in bones, tumors, etc.
- Epiphyseal dysplasia and spinal deformaties may be obvious, especially in the older child
- Sometimes a complete survery is needed and it is important to know, which portion of the long bone (epiphysis, metaphysis or diaphysis) is affected
- With severe and varied changes in the metaphyses, periosteal new bone formation or epiphyseal separation always consider the possibility of non-accidental fractures. The battered baby syndrome.

Special Investigations

- In most cases, the diagnosis can be made without laboratory tests
- Routine blood and urine is helpful in excluding metabolic and endocrine disorders, such as rickets and pituitary or thyroid dysfunction
- Special tests are also available to identify specific excretory metabolites in the storage disorders, and specific enzyme activity can be measured in the serum, blood cells or cultured fibroblasts.

MANAGEMENT OF GENETIC DISORDERS

Genetic Consultation

Definition or Purpose

- To relay information on diagnoses, prognoses, risk, implication, options, test, therapy, services and mode of inheritance for genetic disorder
- To maintain confidentiality
- For accurate diagnosis
- To relieve anxiety
- To provide management.

Reasons for Reference

- Advanced maternal age (AMA)
- Previous family history
- Single gene defect
- Chromosomal anomalies
- Multifactorial disorders
- Cancer history
- Repeated miscarriages
- Infertility
- Abnormal prenatal diagnosis
- Teratogen exposure.

Ideal Consultation Schedule

Session 1

- Obtain family and medical history
- Available options and test
- Cost of test
- Collection of samples
- Schedule next session.

Session 2

- Discussed test results
- Explain mode of inheritance
- Explain risk to future childrens and other family members.

Counseling

- *Achondrogenesis*: The recurrence risk for siblings for type 1B is one in four, whereas for type 2 it is much lower
- *Achondroplasia*: Counseling is for autosomal dominant inheritance. When both parents have this disease, there is one chance in four that each of their children will be affected homozygotes, almost all such infants die before or after birth
- *Heriditary multiple exostosis:* Counseling is on the basis of autosomal dominant inheritance with variable expression
- *Osteogenesis imperfecta:* Counseling is for autosomal dominant inheritance for type 2
- *Osteopetrosis:* Measuring the level of carbonic anhydrase activity in erythrocytes, counseling for autosomal dominant and recessive inheritance
- Similarly, the other genetic disorders are counseled based on their inheritance pattern.

Treatment and Therapy

- Fetal surgery
  - Open fetal surgery
  - Laser treatment
- Prenatal stem cell and gene therapy.

Fetal Surgery

Fetal surgery is a unique field in maternal-fetal medicine, detecting birth defects prenatally has allowed physicians to provide better perinatal care, but many of these babies were already too sick to treat them successfully after they were born. This dilemma led to the development of fetal surgery.

Open Fetal Surgery

- Repairing birth defects in the womb:
- Open fetal surgery involves cutting into the mother's abdomen and uterus in order to operate on the fetus, to remove abnormal masses or patch an opening
- Fetal surgery places special demands on care givers, to ensure safety for two patients, the mother and the fetus
- Adzick in his first article, described fetal surgeries for two life-threatening defects:
  - Lung masses, which may compress the developing heart, leading to heart failure
  - Sacrococcygeal teratomas, which can lead to heart failure or a fatal hemorrhage before birth
- Adzick in his second article, described fetal surgery for myelomeningocele. To repair a myelomeningocele, fetal surgeons shield the developing spinal cord by closing the defect with the fetus's own tissue.

Laser Treatment

- Another application of fetal surgery is for twin-twin transfusion syndrome, occurring in 10 to 15 percent of identical twins
- In this condition, one fetus grows at the expense of its twin because of abnormal blood vessel connections in their shared placenta.

Procedure: Selective Laser Photocoagulation

In this procedure, using a viewing instrument called a fetoscope, the fetal surgeon employs a laser to seal off the blood vessels that carry hazardous blood flow between the two fetuses, thus shutting off dangerous twin-to-twin connection.

Prenatal Stem Cell and Gene Therapy

- The greatest future impact of fetal treatments probably lies in nonsurgical approaches—prenatal stem cell therapy and gene therapy
- In contrast to the relatively rare anatomical defects addressed in fetal surgery, cell and gene therapy offer the possibility of treating many genetic diseases before birth, including sickle cell anemia, immune deficiency disorders and some types of muscular dystrophy.

In Utero Hematopoietic Stem Cell Transplantation (IUHCT)

- It focuses on stem cells that develop into all the types of cells found in the blood
- The keystone of this approach is the fetal immune system's unique tolerance of transplanted cells
- Flake's strategy involves, using prenatal stem cell transplants to achieve tolerance of foreign cells, which are incorporated into the fetal circulation
- This sets the stage for postnatal transplant of therapeutic blood cells from the same donor that will not be rejected by the infant's immune system
- The specific characteristics of severe combined immunodeficiency (SCID) make this disease uniquely amenable to a prenatal stem cell approach
- At present, research in animal models is progressing toward using IUHCT, to treat other immune deficiency diseases, the hemoglobin disorders sickle cell anemia and thalassemia, and lysosomal storage diseases (genetic disorders in which the lack of an enzyme causes metabolic chemicals to accumulate to toxic levels in cells)
- Some diseases that progress to irreversible organ damage may offer targets for prenatal gene therapy, in which physicians deliver therapeutic DNA to correct a genetic defect
- Proof-of-principle studies in animals have produced preclinical successes for prenatal gene therapy in cystic fibrosis, Duchenne's muscular dystrophy, Pompe disease and the lysosomal storage disease, Sly syndrome
- There have also been promising animal studies in types of hemophilia
- As with postnatal gene therapy, important safety issues remain to be solved before prenatal gene therapy can be offered in the clinic
- Fetal gene therapy is still in the early experimental stage, said Flake, while noting great progress in this field.

Ex Utero Intrapartum Therapy (EXIT)

- The EXIT procedure is a partial delivery, in which the fetus is partially removed from the uterus, but remains attached to the circulation carried by the umbilical cord and placenta, so that surgeons can correct airway blockages before performing a full delivery
- It is a partial delivery, which buys time for fetal surgery eventually
- Clinicians at Children's Hospital of Philadelphia, USA have the world's most extensive experience in performing the EXIT procedure.

Set-Up

In order to carry out these procedures, there should be a multidisciplinary team and sophisticated imaging technologies, used to assess patients referred to the center and the facilities should include a "special delivery unit" for mothers carrying babies, with known birth defects.

DOWN'S SYNDROME (TRISOMY-21)

Introduction

- It is a chromosomal disorder caused by the presence of all or part of an extra 21st chromosome
- It is named after John Langdon Down, the British physician who described the syndrome in 1866
- The disorder was identified as a chromosome 21 trisomy, by Jerome Lejeune in 1959
- The condition is characterized by a combination of major and minor differences in structure.

Incidence

- The incidence of Down syndrome is estimated as 1 per 800 to 1,000 births
- Although, it is statistically much more common with elderly females.

Genetics

- Trisomy-21 (47 and +21), frequency of occurrence is about 94 percent. The frequency of trisomy increases with increasing maternal age (Figs 4.11 and 4.12)

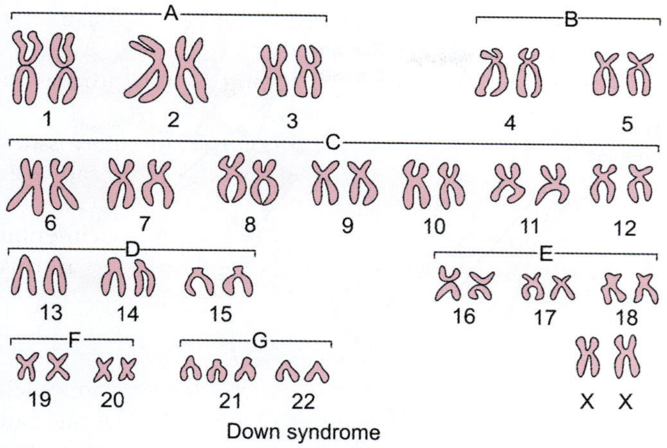

Fig. 4.11: Presentation of different chromosomal pattern in Down's syndrome (21st chromosome showing trisomy)

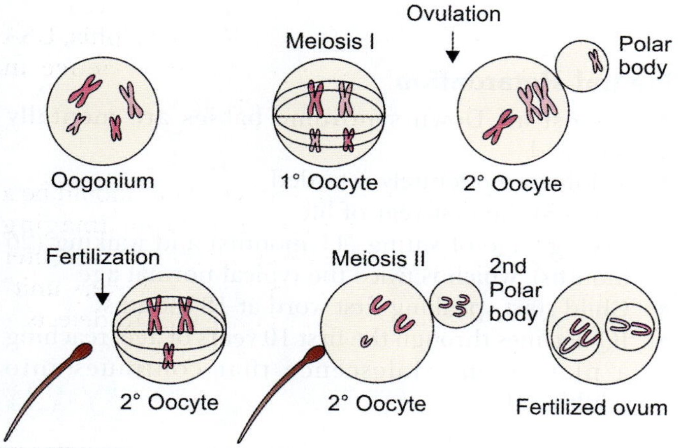

Fig. 4.12: Chromosomal nondisjunction in meiosis I, resulted in trisomy

- Robertsonian translocation, involving chromosome 21, approximately 3 to 4 percent, not related to maternal age (Figs 4.13A and B)
- Trisomy-21 mosaicism: 2 to 3 percent cases.

Clinical Features (Fig. 4.14)

- Brachycephaly
- Up-slanting palpebral fissures
- Epicanthal folds
- Brushfield spots (Figs 4.15A and B)
- Flat nasal bridge
- Folded or dysplastic ears
  - Open mouth
  - Protruding tongue
  - Short neck
  - Excessive skin at the nape of neck
  - Extremities

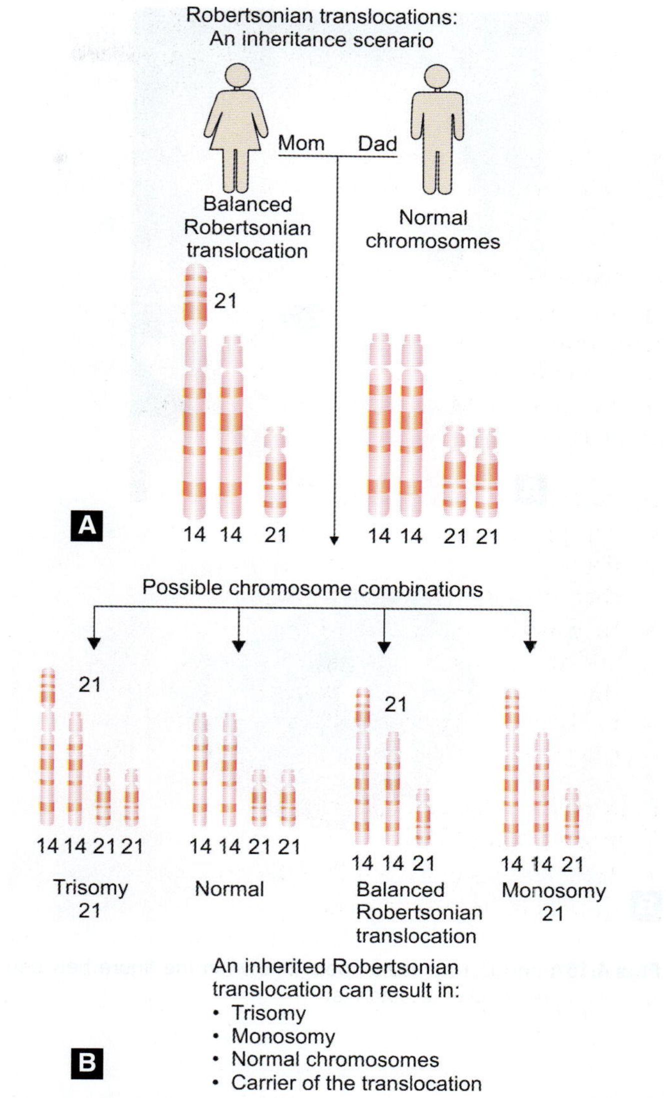

Figs 4.13A and B: Robertsonian translocation—(A) Showing an inheritance scenario; (B) Possible chromosomal combinations

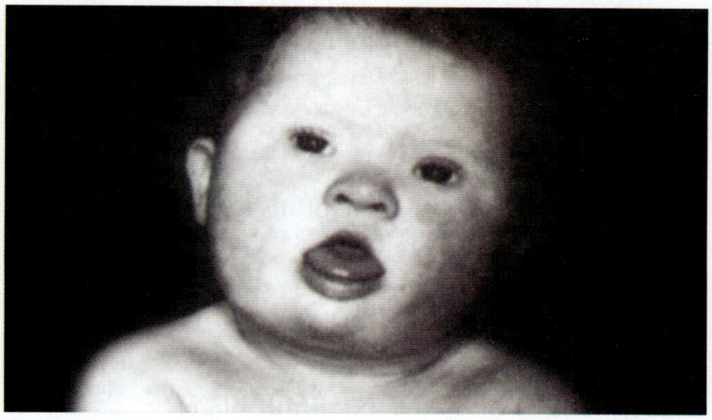

Fig. 4.14: A child suffering from Down's syndrome, with protruding tongue, open mouth and other presentable clinical features of Down's syndrome

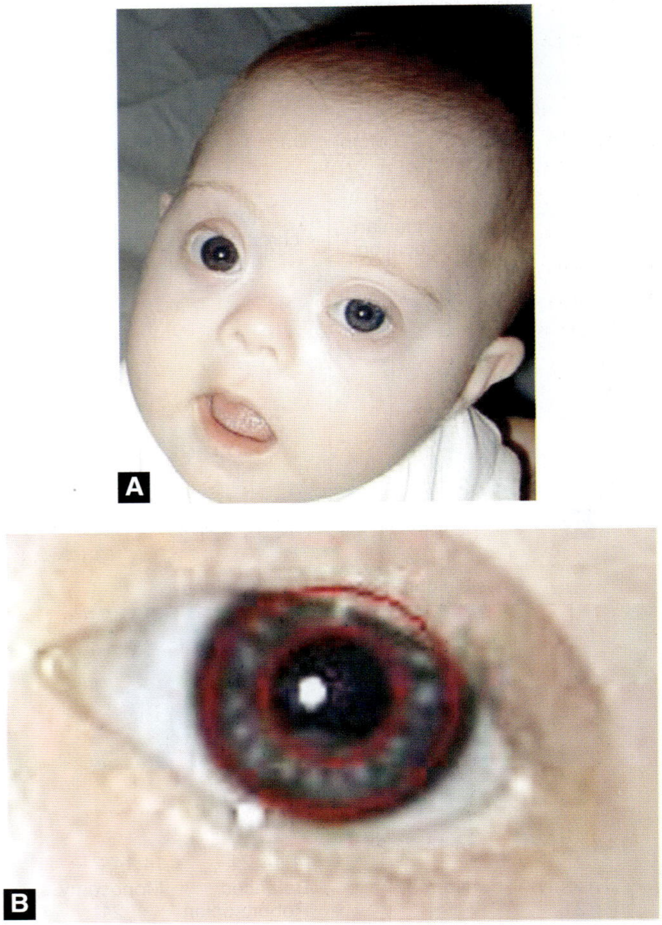

Figs 4.15A and B: Brushfield spots (shown in the figure between red circles around iris)

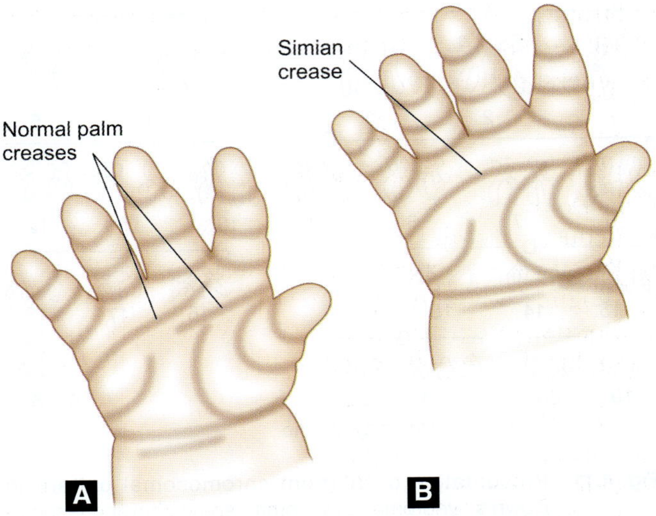

Figs 4.16A and B: Transverse palmar crease, a typical neonatal feature of Down's syndrome

- Short broad hands
- Short fifth finger
- Incurved fifth finger
- Transverse palmar crease
- Space between first and second toe
- Hyper flexibility of joints.

Neonatal Features

- Flat facial profile
- Poor moro reflex
- Excessive skin at the nape of neck
- Slanted palpebral fissures
- Hypotonia
- Hyper flexibility of joints
- Dysplasia of pelvis
- Anomalous ears
- Dysplasia of midphalanx of fifth finger
- Transverse palmar crease (Figs 4.16A and B)

Mental Retardation

- Almost all Down syndrome babies are mentally retarded
- Mildly to moderately retarded
- Starts in the first year of life
- Average age of sitting (11 months) and walking (26 months), which is twice the typical normal age
- Child start speaking first word at 18 months
- IQ declines through the first 10 years of age, reaching a plateau in adolescence that continues into adulthood.

Heart Diseases

Fifty percent of Down syndrome patients have heart disease, most common defects include:

- Atrioventricular septal defect
- Ventricular septal defect
- Secundum atrial septal defect
- Patent ductus arteriosus
- Tetrology of fallot
- Mitral valve prolapse
- Aortic regurgitation and mitral regurgitation.

Gastrointestinal (GI) Abnormalities

- Only in five percent of cases
- Duodenal atresia or stenosis, sometimes associated with annular pancreas in 2.5 percent of cases
- Imperforate anus
- Esophageal atresia, with tracheoesophageal fistula is less common
- Hirschsprung's disease

- Strong associated with celiac disease between 5 and 16 percent, 5 to 16 fold increase as compared to general population.

Growth

- Body weight, length and head circumference are less in Down syndrome
- Reduced growth rate
- Prevalence of obesity is greater in Down syndrome
- Weight is less than expected for length in infants with Down syndrome and then increases disproportionally, so that they are obese by the age of 3 to 4 years.

Eye Problems

Most common disorders are:

- Refractory error (35-76%)
- Strabismus (25-57%)
- Nystagmus (18-22%)
- Cataract occur in 5 percent of newborns
- Frequency increases with age.

Hearing Loss

- Unilateral or bilateral
- Conductive, sensorineural or mixed
- Otitis media is a frequent problem.

Hematologic Disorders

- The risk of leukemia is 1 to 1.5 percent
- Sixty-five percent of newborn have polycythemia, resulting in hypoglycemia
- Risk of acute myeloid leukemia and acute lymphocytic leukemia is also much higher than the general population
- Transient leukemia, exclusively affects newborn. It is asymptomatic with spontaneous resolution in 2 to 3 months
- Vesiculopustular skin eruptions are common and resolve with disorder.

Endocrine Disorder

- *Thyroid disease:* Hypothyroidism occurs more frequently than hyperthyroidism
- *Diabetes:* The risk of type 1 diabetes is three times greater than that of the general population.

Reproduction

- Women with Down syndrome are fertile and may become pregnant
- Nearly all males with Down syndrome are infertile. The mechanism is impairment of spermatogenesis

Atlantoaxial Instability

- Excessive mobility of atlas (C1) and the axis (C2), may lead to subluxation of the cervical spine
- Diagnosis made by lateral neck radiograph
- Patients are advised, to avoid contact sports.

Sleep Apnea

Obstructive sleep apnea is more common.

Skin Disorder

- Palmoplantar hyperkeratosis
- Seborrheic dermatitis
- Fissured tongue
- Cutis marmorata
- Geographical tongue
- Xerosis.

Mortality

- Median age of death for Down syndrome patients was 25 years in 1983 and with the advancement of medicine field the survival age has been increasing at the rate of 1.7 years per year
- Improved survival is because of increased placements of infants in homes and changes in treatment for common causes of death
- Most likely cause of death is congenital heart disease, dementia, hypothyroidism and leukemia
- Survival is better for males and blacks.

Counseling

- May begin, when a prenatal diagnosis is made
- Discuss the wide range of variability in manifestation and prognosis
- Medical and educational treatments and interventions should be discussed
- Initial referrals for early intervention, informative publications, parent groups and advocacy group.

Diagnosis

- Prenatal screening
- Genetic testing, such as amniocentesis, chorionic villus sampling (CVS) or percutaneous umbilical cord blood sampling (PUBS)
- *If no screening:* It is recognized from the characteristic phenotypic features, confirmed by karyotype.

Examination at Birth

- Particular attention to physical signs
- Evaluation of the red reflex can help identify congenital cataracts. Movement of the eyes should be observed to identify strabismus
- Constipation should raise concerns for Hirschsprung's disease and feeding problems should prompt intense education, to ensure adequate input and nutrition
- Ultrasound of the heart (echocardiogram) should be done immediately

- Complete blood count should be done in order to identify pre-existing leukemia immediately, in order to identify congenital heart disease.

Investigation

- *Growth based:* Measurements should be plotted on the appropriate growth chart for children with Down Syndrome. This will help in prevention of obesity and early diagnosis of celiac disease and hypothyroidism
- *Cardiac disease:* All newborns should be evaluated by cardiac echo for congenital heart disease in consultation with pediatric cardiologist
- *Hearing:* Brainstem auditory evoked responses (BAERs) testing is to be done in the newborn periodically in every 6 months until 3 years of age and then annually
- *Eye disorders:* An eye exam should be performed in the newborn period or at least before 6 months of age, to detect strabismus, nystagmus and cataracts
- *Thyroid function:* Normal values in newborn v/s values in Down syndrome should be done in newborn period and should be repeated at six and 12 months and then annually
- *Celiac disease:* Screening should begin at 2 years. Repeat screening, if signs/symptoms develop
- *Hematology:* Complete blood count with differential at birth, to evaluate for polycythemia as well as WBC
- *Atlantoaxial instability:* X-ray for evidence of atlanto-axial instability or subluxation at 3 to 5 years of age
- *Alzheimer's disease:* Adult with a Down syndrome has earlier onset of symptoms. When diagnosis is considered, thyroid disease and possible depression should be excluded.

Management

- Treatment of individuals with Down syndrome depends on the particular manifestations of the disorder
- For instance, individuals with congenital heart disease may need to undergo major corrective surgery soon after birth
- Other individuals may have relatively minor health problems requiring no therapy.

Plastic Surgery

- It has sometimes been advocated and performed on children with Down syndrome, based on the assumption that surgery can reduce the facial features associated with Down syndrome, therefore decreasing social stigma and leading to a better quality of life
- *For example:* Facial reconstruction and glossectomy (tongue reduction).

Cognitive Development

- Individuals with Down syndrome differ considerably in their language and communication skills
- Low gain hearing aids other amplification devices can be useful for language and learning
- Individualized speech therapy can target specific speech errors, increase speech intelligibility and in some cases encourage advanced language and literacy
- Augmentative and alternative communication (AAC) methods, such as pointing, body language, objects or graphics are often used to aid communication.

Follow-up

- As children with Down syndrome grow, their progress should be plotted on a growth chart, in order to detect deviations from expected growth. Special growth charts are available so that children with Down syndrome can be compared with other children with Down syndrome
- Thyroid function testing should be performed at 6 months and 12 months of age as well as yearly, thereafter
- Evaluation of the ears for infection as well as objective hearing tests should be performed at every visit
- Formal evaluation for refractive errors requiring glasses should be performed at least every two years with subjective vision assessments with each visit
- After the age of three, an X-ray of the neck should be obtained to screen for atlantoaxial instability
- As the child ages, yearly symptom screening for obstructive sleep apnea should be performed.

MARFAN'S SYNDROME

■ Introduction

- Marfan syndrome is an inherited connective-tissue disorder, transmitted as an autosomal dominant trait (Figs 4.17A and B)
- It is noteworthy for its worldwide distribution, relatively high prevalence, clinical variability and pleiotropic manifestations, some of which are life-threatening
- Cardinal features of the disorder include tall stature, ectopia lentis, mitral valve prolapse, aortic root dilatation and aortic dissection
- About three quarters of patients have an affected parent and new mutations account for the remainder.

Pathophysiology

- Marfan syndrome results from mutations in the Fibrillin-1 (FBN1) gene on chromosome 15, which encodes for the glycoprotein fibrillin

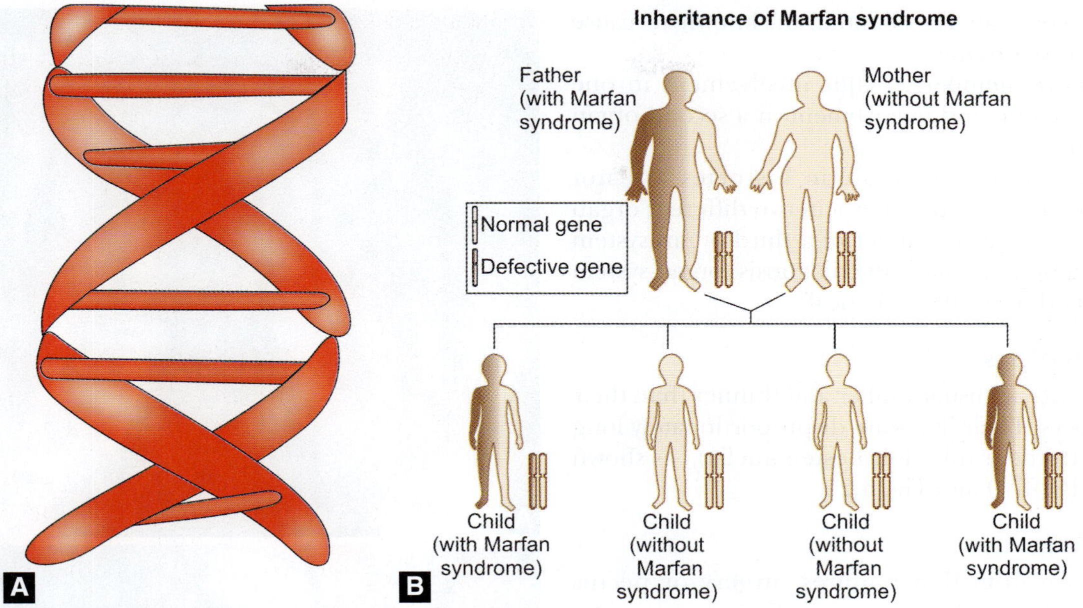

Figs 4.17A and B: Inheritance of Marfan's syndrome or transfer as autosomal dominant trait

- Fibrillin is a major building block of microfibrils, which constitute the structural components of the suspensory ligament of the lens and serve as substrates for elastin in the aorta and other connective tissues
- Abnormalities involving microfibrils weaken the aortic wall. Progressive aortic dilatation and eventual aortic dissection occurs
- Likewise, deficient fibrillin deposition leads to reduced structural integrity of the lens zonules, ligaments, lung airways and spinal dura
- Recent studies have suggested that abnormalities in the transforming growth factor-beta (TGF β)-signaling pathway may also involve in the development of the Marfan's phenotype. The gene defect ultimately leads to decreased and disordered incorporation of fibrillin into the connective tissue matrix
- *Frequency:* Marfan syndrome is one of the most common single-gene malformation syndromes with incidence of about 1 in 10,000 individuals
- No geographic predilection is known
- *Race:* Marfan syndrome is panethnic
- *Sex:* No sex predilection is known
- *Age:* Marfan syndrome may be diagnozed prenatally, at birth or well into adulthood. Neonatal presentation is associated with, a more severe course than that associated with other presentations
- Most clinical features are specific to age and some features may not manifest, until relatively late in life. This feature may make diagnosis in a child difficult
- *Mortality and morbidity:* Cardiovascular disease (aortic dilatation and dissection) is the major cause of morbidity and mortality. Progression from mitral valve prolapse to mitral regurgitation, often in conjunction with tricuspid prolapse and regurgitation is the most common cause of infant morbidity. If untreated, Marfan's syndrome is highly lethal. The average age at death is 30 to 40 years
- Death after infancy usually involves ascending aortic dissection and chronic aortic regurgitation. Dissection generally occurs at the aortic root and is uncommon in childhood and adolescence.

Clinical History

- Marfan syndrome is currently diagnozed using criteria based on an evaluation of the family history, molecular data and six organ systems
- The diagnosis cannot be based on molecular analysis alone because molecular diagnosis is not generally available, mutation detection is imperfect and not all FBN1 mutations, are associated with Marfan's syndrome
- Due to this Berlin criteria is used for diagnosis of Marfan
- In 1995, a group of the world's leading clinicians and investigators in Marfan's syndrome proposed revised diagnostic criteria, which is known as the Ghent criteria, they identify major and minor diagnostic findings
- The major criteria include the following:
  - A first-degree relative (parent, child or sibling), who independently meets the diagnostic criteria

- Presence of an FBN1 mutation known to cause Marfan syndrome
- In family members, major involvement in one organ system and involvement in a second organ system
- If the family and genetic histories are not contributory, major criteria in two different organ systems and involvement of a third organ system are required, to make the diagnosis (organ system criteria described in physical).

Skeletal Findings

Affected patients are usually taller and thinner than their family members. Their limbs are disproportionately long compared with the trunk (dolichostenomelia), as shown in Figures 4.18, 4.19 and Fig. 4.21.

Major Criteria

- Pectus excavatum that requires surgery or pectus carinatum (Fig. 4.20)
- *Pectus excavatum of moderate severity:* Reduced upper-to-lower body segment ratio (0.85 vs 0.93) or arm span-to-height ratio greater than 1.05. Arms and legs may be unusually long in proportion to the torso
- *Positive wrist (walker) and thumb (Steinberg) signs (Figs 4.22 to 4.24):* Two simple maneuvers may help demonstrate arachnodactyly. First, the thumb sign is positive if the thumb, when completely opposed within the clenched hand, projects beyond the ulnar border. Second, the wrist sign is positive if the distal phalanges of the first and fifth digits of one hand overlap when wrapped around the opposite wrist

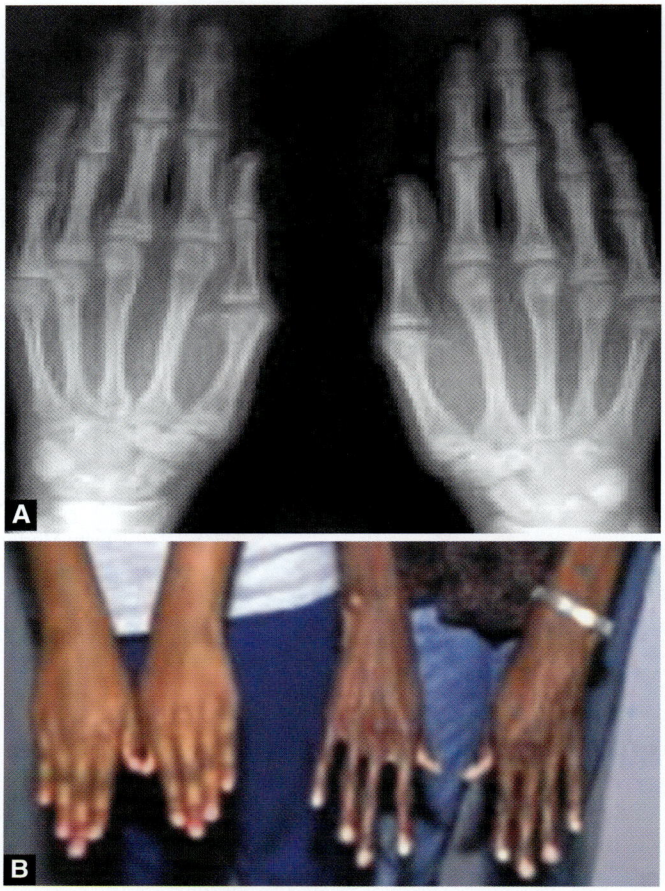

Figs 4.19A and B: Arachnodactyly in Marfan's syndrome—(A) X-ray findings; (B) Comparison of normal hands with the Marfan's syndrome patient

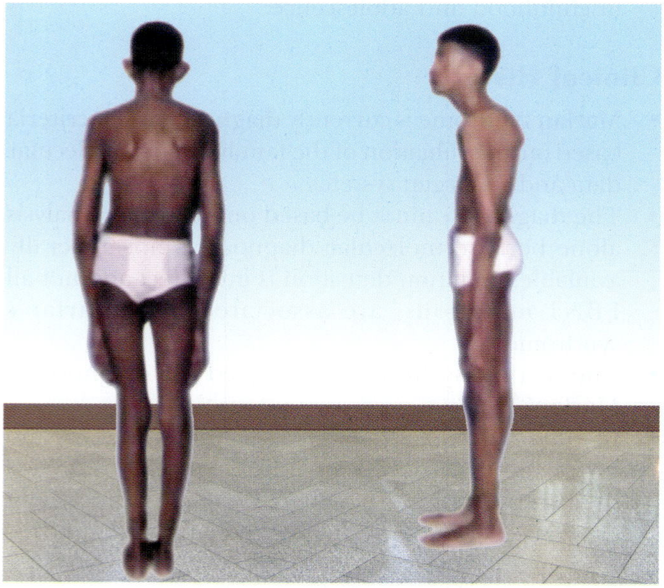

Fig. 4.18: Skeletal findings in Marfan's syndrome, Note tall and thin build, disproportionately long arms and legs and kyphoscoliosis

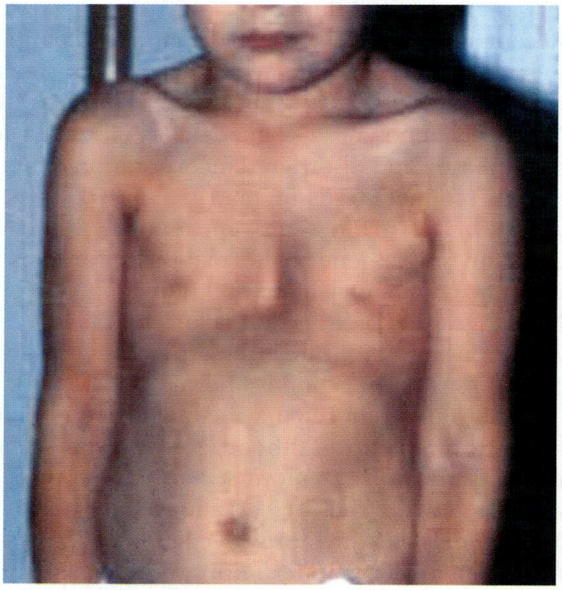

Fig. 4.20: Pectus excavatum

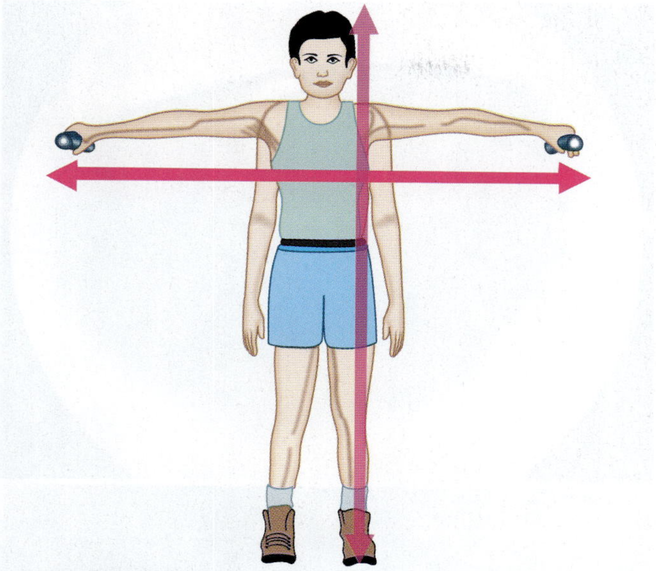

Fig. 4.21: This person in the figure with Marfan's syndrome is tall and thin and has an arm span that exceeds his height

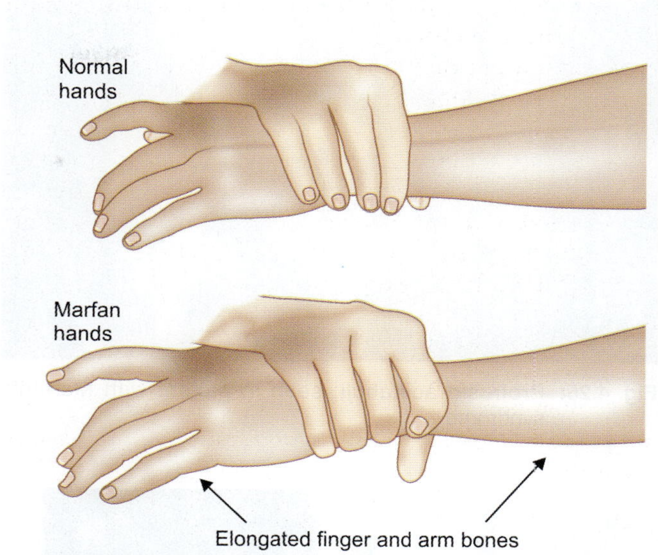

Fig. 4.23: Elongated arm and fingers in patient with Marfan's syndrome, compared to normal hands

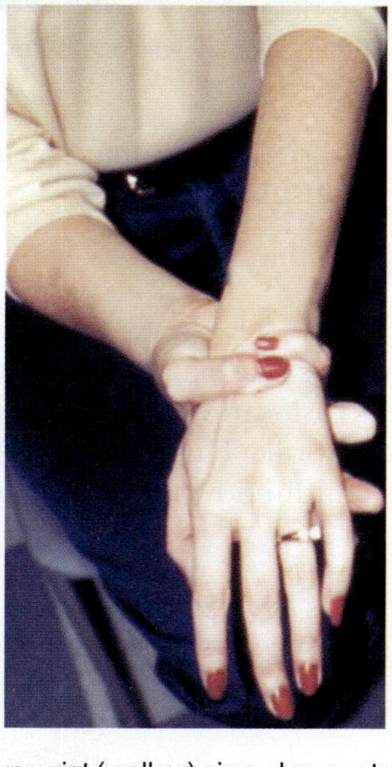

Fig. 4.22: Positive wrist (walker) sign, demonstrate arachnodactyly

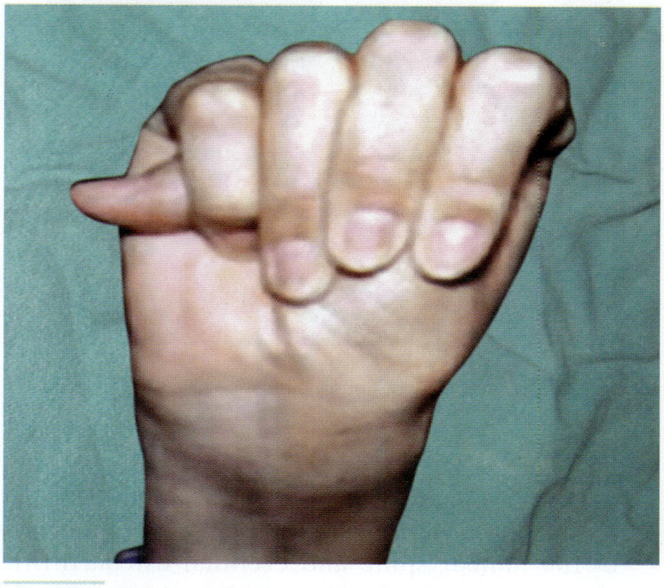

Fig. 4.24: Steinberg sign or positive thumb sign

- *Scoliosis greater than 20°:* More than 60 percent of patients have scoliosis. Progression is most likely with curvature of more than 20° in growing patients
- Reduced extension of the elbows (less than 170°)
- Medial displacement of the medial malleolus, resulting in pes planus. Pes planus is best diagnosed by examining the foot from behind. A valgus deviation of the hindfoot indicates pes planus
- *Protrusio acetabuli of any degree:* This is a deformity of the hip joint, in which the medial wall of the acetabulum invades the pelvic cavity with associated medial displacement of the femoral head and is ascertained using radiography. Protrusio acetabuli affects 31 to 100 percent of patients to varying degrees (Fig. 4.25)
- Clinical manifestations include hip joint stiffness and progressive limitation in activity related to joint pain,

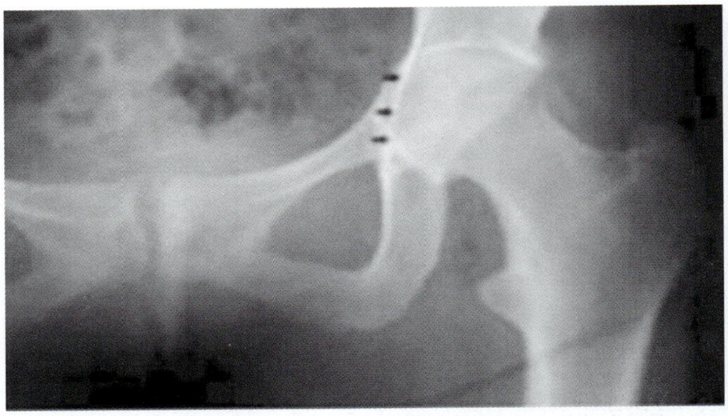

Fig. 4.25: Protrusio acetabuli, seen in patient with Marfan's syndrome

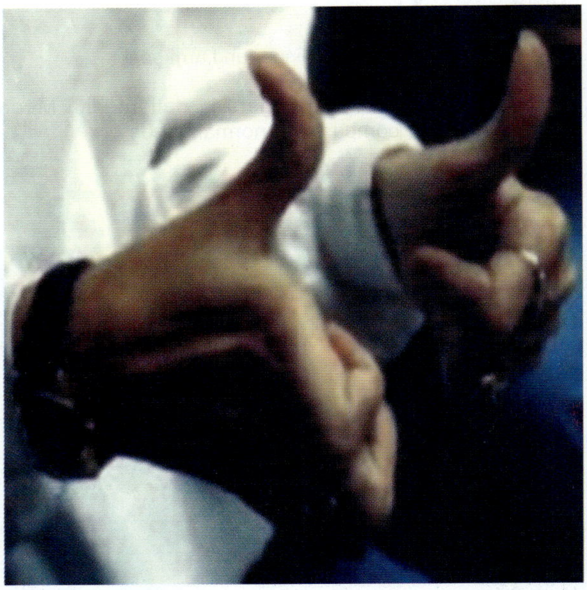

Fig. 4.26: Hypermobility of finger joints

a waddling gait, limited range of motion, flexion contracture, a pelvic tilt, with a resulting hyperlordosis of the lumbar spine and eventual osteoarthritic changes. Local progressive protrusion can lead to early hip pain and osteoarthritis.

Minor Criteria

- Pectus excavatum of moderate severity
- Scoliosis less than 20°
- Thoracic lordosis
- Joint hypermobility (Fig. 4.26)
- Highly arched palate
- Dental crowding
- Typical facies (malar hypoplasia, enophthalmos, retrognathia, down-slanting palpebral fissures)
- For the skeletal system to be involved

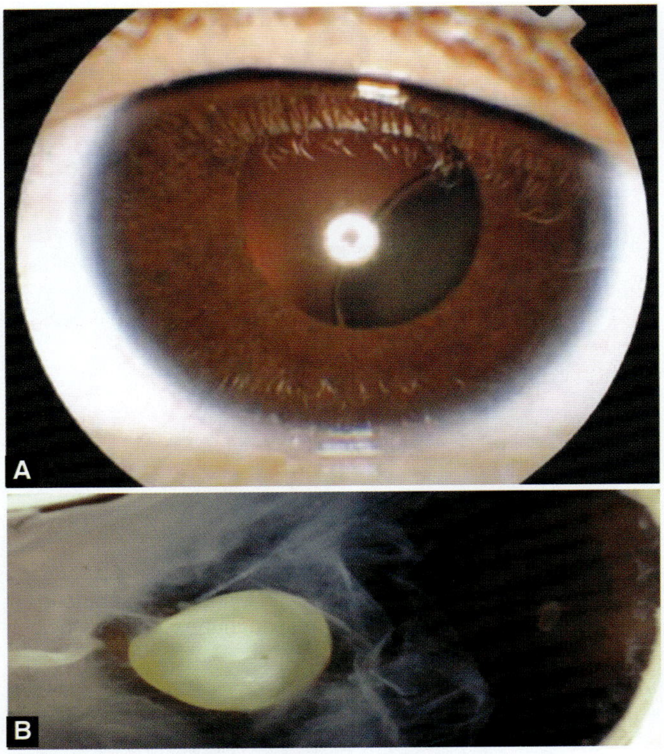

Figs 4.27A and B: Ectopia lentis—dislocated eye lens

- At least 2 major criteria or 1 major criterion plus two minor criteria must be present.

Ocular Findings

Major Criteria

The major criterion is ectopia lentis. About 50 percent of patients have lens dislocation. The dislocation is usually superior and temporal. This may present at birth or develop during childhood or adolescence (Figs 4.27A and B).

Minor Criteria

- Flat cornea (measured by keratometry)
- Increased axial length of the globe (measured by ultrasound)
- Cataract in patients younger than 50 years
- Hypoplastic iris or hypoplastic ciliary muscle that causes decreased miosis
- Nearsightedness regardless of whether the lens is in place the most common refraction error is myopia due to elongated globe
- Glaucoma (patients less than 50 years)
- Retinal detachment
- At least 2 minor criteria should be present.

Cardiovascular Findings

Cardiovascular involvement is the most serious problem associated with Marfan's syndrome.

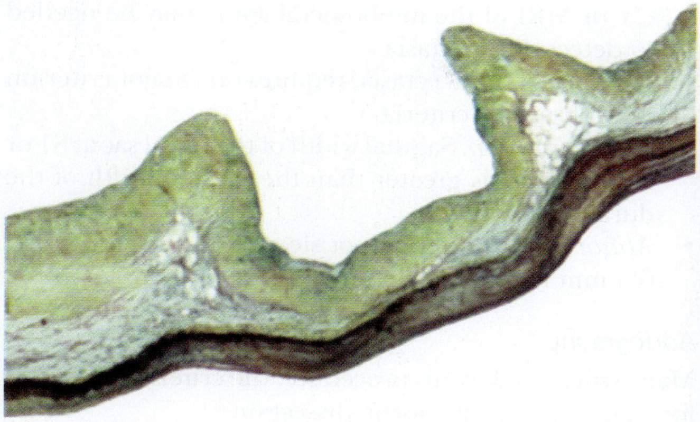

Fig. 4.28: Manifestation of Marfan syndrome—myxomatous degeneration of the aortic valve

Major Criteria

- Aortic root dilatation involving the sinuses of Valsalva. Its prevalence in Marfan's syndrome is 70 to 80 percent
- Aortic dissections involving the ascending aorta.

Minor Criteria

- *Mitral valve prolapse (55-69%):* Midsystolic clicks
- Dilatation of proximal main pulmonary artery in the absence of peripheral pulmonic stenosis or other cause
- Calcification of mitral annulus (patients less than 40 years)
- Dilatation of abdominal or descending thoracic aorta (patients less than 50 years)
- For the cardiovascular system to be involved, a major and a minor criterion must be present
- Micrograph demonstrating myxomatous degeneration of the aortic valve, is common (Fig. 4.28).

Lungs

- Marfan's syndrome is a risk factor for spontaneous pneumothorax
- The lung becomes partially compressed or collapsed. This can cause pain, shortness of breath, cyanosis, and, if not treated, death
- Marfan's syndrome has also been associated with sleep apnea and idiopathic obstructive lung disease.

Central Nervous System

- Another condition that can reduce the quality of life for an individual, though not life-threatening is dural ectasia, the weakening of the connective tissue of the dural sac, the membrane that encases the spinal cord
- Symptoms that can occur are lower back pain, leg pain, abdominal pain and other neurological symptoms in the lower extremities or headaches. Such symptoms usually diminish when the individual lies flat on his or her back

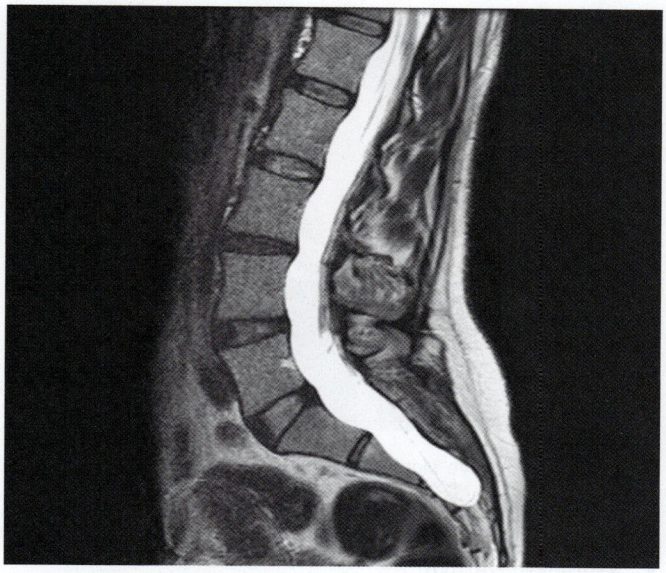

Fig. 4.29: Dural ectasia in the lumbosacral region

- Other spinal issues associated with Marfan include, degenerative disk disease and spinal cysts
- *Dural findings:* For the dura, only one major criterion is defined, "dural ectasia" must be present and confirmed using CT or MRI
- Dural ectasia is a common feature of Marfan's syndrome. The prevalence of dural ectasia among patients with Marfan's syndrome is 65 to 92 percent
- Dural ectasia is defined as a ballooning or widening of the dural sac, often associated with herniation of the nerve root sleeves out of the associated foramina. Dural ectasia most frequently occurs in the lumbosacral spine (Fig. 4.29).

Skin and Integumentary Findings

- For skin and integument, only minor criteria are noted
- Minor criteria include the following:
  - Striae atrophicae in the absence of marked weight changes, pregnancy or repetitive stress. Stretch marks are usually found on the shoulder, mid back and thighs
  - Excessive skin elasticity (Fig. 4.30)
  - Stretch marks (striae atrophicae) in the lower back
  - Recurrent or incisional hernia

Differential Diagnoses

- Ehlers-Danlos syndrome
- Fragile X syndrome
- Gigantism and acromegaly
- Hyperpituitarism

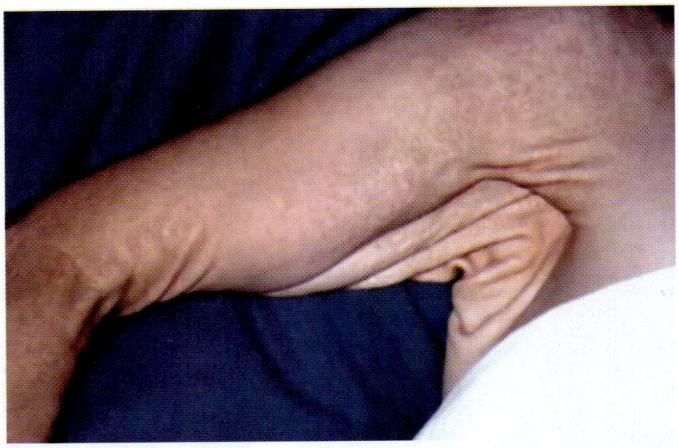

Fig. 4.30: Excessive skin elasticity, seen in Marfan's syndrome

- Hyperthyroidism
- Klinefelter syndrome.

Laboratory Studies

- As no common mutations have been identified, genetic testing includes screening the entire FBN1 gene
- DNA testing cannot exclude a diagnosis of Marfan's syndrome
- By 1998, 137 FBN1 mutations had been characterized in patients with Marfan's syndrome. Mutations are distributed throughout the FBN1 gene.

Imaging Studies

Radiography

- Chest radiography should be focused on apical blebs. Chest radiographs may also be of value in detecting a thoracic aortic dissection, by demonstrating enlargement of the aortic and cardiac silhouette
- Pelvic radiography is required only if a positive finding of protrusio acetabula is needed for the diagnosis.

Echocardiography

- Cross-sectional echocardiography is a common tool in the diagnosis and management of aortic root dilatation
- Standard echocardiography is valuable in assessing mitral valve prolapse, left ventricular size and function, function of the tricuspid valve and left atrial size.

CT and MRI

- MRI is the best choice for assessing chronic dissection of any region of the aorta. It should be performed in any patient at any age who has an aortic root dimension of more than 150 percent of the mean for their body surface area
- CT or MRI of the lumbosacral spine may be needed to detect dural ectasia
- Presence of dural ectasia, requires one major criterion or both minor criteria
- *Major criterion:* Sagittal width of the dural sac at S1 or below, which is greater than the sagittal width of the dural sac above L4
- *Minor criteria:* Nerve root sleeve at L5 of more than 6.5 mm in diameter or at S1 of more than 3.5 mm.

Aortography

Many still consider this procedure, the criterion standard for diagnosing acute aortic dissection.

Other Tests

Histologic Findings

- Immunohistologic evaluation of the skin for abnormal fibrillin has been reported, but is not widely available
- This is partly due to the high incidence of false-positive, results in patients with other connective-tissue disorders
- Electron microscopy of fibrillin from cultured fibroblasts has shown a substantial increase in fraying of microfibrils in patients with Marfan's syndrome.

Treatment

Medical Care

- Moderate restriction of physical activity
- Cardiac care in the form of, endocarditis prophylaxis
- Echocardiography at annual intervals
- Beta-blocker therapy should be considered at any age, if the aorta is dilated, but prophylactic treatment may be more effective in those with an aortic diameter of less than 4 cm
- At least annual evaluation should be offered and should include clinical history, examination and echocardiography
- In children, serial echocardiography at 6 month to 12 month intervals is recommended and the frequency depends on the aortic diameter (in relation to body surface area) and the rate of increase
- Prophylactic aortic root surgery should be considered, when the aortic diameter at the sinus of Valsalva is more than 5 cm
- Counseling for pregnancy 50 percent risk of transmitting the disease to offsprings.

Other Therapy

- Anticoagulant medications, such as warfarin are needed after artificial heart-valve placement
- Progesterone and estrogen therapy have been used to induce puberty and reduce the patient's ultimate height, if hormonal treatment is begun before puberty,

but no conclusive data are yet available to show whether this therapy reduces scoliosis
- Conservative treatment of protrusio acetabuli mostly involves physiotherapy, by forcible stretching (stress fractures of the femoral neck due to stretching are documented), weight extension on an abduction frame, local heating and re-education concerning daily activities
- Myopia is treatable with refraction
- Patients with flat feet may wear shoes with adequate arch support
- Psychological counseling is helpful for families coping with feelings of denial, anger, blame, depression or guilt.

Future Therapeutic Strategy

TGF β antagonism is a general strategy against aneurysm progression in patients with Marfan's syndrome and other disorders of the TGF β, signaling network.

Scoliosis Surgery

- Severe scoliosis requires surgery. Bracing has a limited role in treating the most severe form of infantile scoliosis
- Surgery should not be performed on a child younger than 4 years because many patients with large curves before this age spontaneously die of cardiac complications. Results of spinal fusion are better in children older than 5 years
- Indications for surgery in adults, include pain, neurologic signs and thoracic curves greater than 45°, which can cause restrictive lung disease.

Protrusio Acetabuli Surgery

This is directed at arresting progression, relieving pain and restoring the function of the hip through hip replacement with bone grafting of the medial acetabular cavity, in older patients and closure of the triradiate cartilage in a child or adolescent.

Pectus Repair

The shape of the front of the thorax becomes stable and established by mid adolescence. Therefore, repair of pectus excavatum to improve respiratory mechanics should be delayed, until then to lessen the risk of recurrence. Pectus carinatum repair is mainly performed for cosmetic reasons.

Pneumothorax Therapy

Chest tube is an appropriate initial therapy. After one recurrence, a more aggressive approach involving bleb resection and pleurodesis is recommended.

Diet

No special diet is needed.

Activity

- In general, patients can remain fully active unless their symptoms limit them. Patients should be discouraged from participating in demanding sports because several Marfan's syndrome patients have suddenly died from ruptured aortic aneurysm
- To protect against pneumothorax, patients should avoid the rapid decompression associated with quick ascents in elevators, scuba diving and flying in unpressurized aircraft
- Patients should avoid activities involving isometric work, such as weightlifting, climbing steep inclines, participating in gymnastics and performing pull-ups
- No strenuous activities and sports.

Complications

- Complications that affect the aorta are the primary cause of death
- Aortic dissection
- Mitral valve prolapse may be the most common cause of death with Marfan's syndrome
- Bacterial endocarditis
- Severe pectus excavatum can compromise cardiac and pulmonary function
- Rarely, the retina may detach.

Prognosis

- The patient's prognosis depends on the severity of cardiovascular complications and is mainly determined by progressive dilation of the aorta, which potentially leads to aortic dissection and death at a young age
- Improved detection, timely and improved surgical techniques and the prophylactic use of beta-blockers, all are helping to prolong survival. The average lifespan is now about 70 years.

TURNER'S SYNDROME

Turner's syndrome or congenital female hypogonadism is a rare abnormality caused by a defect in one of the X chromosomes. Those affected are phenotypically females, with a normal vagina and uterus, but the ovaries are markedly hypoplastic or absent.

■ Clinical Features

- Short stature
- Webbing of the neck
- Barrel chest
- Increased carrying angle of the elbows
- Cardiovascular and renal abnormalities are common, they have primary amenorrhea and hypogonadism leads to early onset osteoporosis.

■ Treatment

Estrogen replacement from puberty onwards.

EHLERS-DANLOS SYNDROME

■ Introduction

The syndrome is named after two doctors, Edverd Ehlers of Denmark and Henri Alexander Danlos of France. Ehlers-Danlos syndrome (EDS) is characterized by hyperelasticity of the skin and hypermobility of joints.

Epidemiology

Incidence: 1 in 5000 births

Race: Higher incidence in blacks

Sex: Affects both males and females of all racial and ethnic backgrounds

Types: The most commonly occurring type is the hypermobility type, followed by classical type. The others types of EDS are very rare (Table 4.2).

Etiology

- EDS is group of inheritable connective tissue disorder. There are problems of collagen formation and affect the musculoskeletal system, either by bone weakness (osteogenesis imperfecta) or soft tissue weakness (Marfan's, homocystinuria, EDS, etc.)

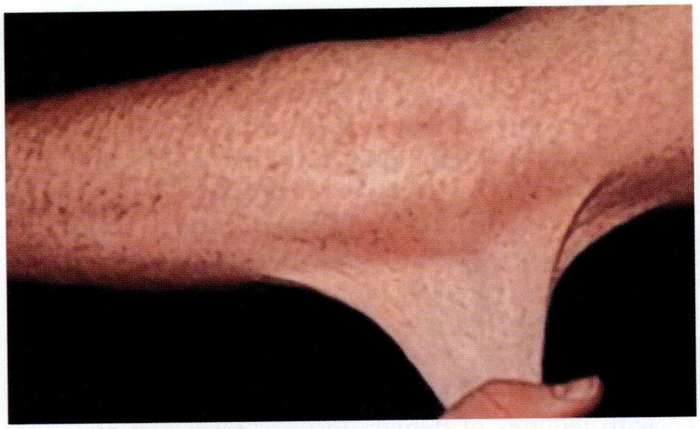

Fig. 4.31: Rubber man syndrome, with dramatically hyperextensible skin

- In EDS, there appear to be disorganization of the cross linkages due to reduction of the enzymes lysyl hydroxylase.

Clinical Features

- *Skin:* Skin changes vary from thin and velvety to skin, that is either dramatically hyperextensible, e.g. "rubber man syndrome" (Fig. 4.31) or easily torn or scared. Patients with classical EDS develop characteristic "cigarette paper scars" (Fig. 4.32)
- *Ligaments and joint changes:* Laxity and hypermobility of joints vary from mild to unreducible dislocations

Table 4.2: Different types of EDS, their clinical features and associated defects

Type	*Typical features*	*Inheritance*	*Gene defect*	*Protein defect*
Classic (EDS1-Severe and EDS2-MILD)	Skin hyperextensibility and fragility, joint hypermobility tissue fragility manifested by widened atrophic scarring	AD AR	COL5A1 COL5A2 COL1A1 COL1A2	Collagen 5
Hypermobile (EDS3)	Joint hypermobility moderate skin involvement, absence of tissue fragility	AD	TNX	Tenascin
Vascular (EDS4)	Marked reduced life span due to spontaneous rupture of internal organs such as arteries and intestines	AD	COL3A1	Collagen 3
X-linked (EDS5)	Similar to classic type 2	XR	Unknown	Unknown
Ocular-scoliotic (EDS6)	Severe muscular hypotonia after birth, progressive kyphoscoliosis, rupture of eye globe and arteries	AR	PLOD1	Def. of procollagen lysine 5 dioxygenase activity
Arthrochalasic (EDS7)	Cong. b/l dislocation of hip, hypermobile joints, osteopenia	AD	COL1A1 COL1A2	Mutation that prevent cleavage of N pro-peptides
Periodontotic (EDS8)	Premature loss of permanent teeth	AD	Unknown	Unknown

[Note: AD: Autosomal dominant; AR: Autosomal recessive; XR: X-linked recessive]

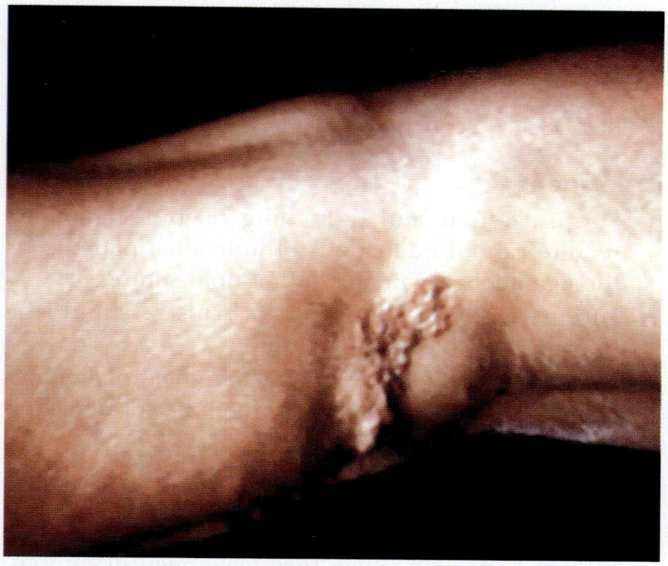

Fig. 4.32: Cigarette paper scars, as seen in patients with EDS

of hip and other large joints. In mild forms, patients learn to reduce dislocations by limiting physical activity (Figs 4.33A to C).

Other Features

- Flat feet
- High and narrow palate, resulting in dental crowding
- Fragile blood vessels, resulting from cystic medial necrosis with tendency towards aneurysm
- Abnormal wound healing and scar formation
- Early onset of osteoarthritis
- Low muscle tones and muscle weakness
- Cardiac effects, like dysautonomia accompanied by valvular heart diseases, such as mitral valve prolapse
- Myalgia and arthralgia
- Osteopenia
- Congenital talipes equinovarus (CTEV), especially in the vascular type
- Deformities of the spine, such as scoliosis, kyphosis, occipitoatlantoaxial hypermobility, etc.

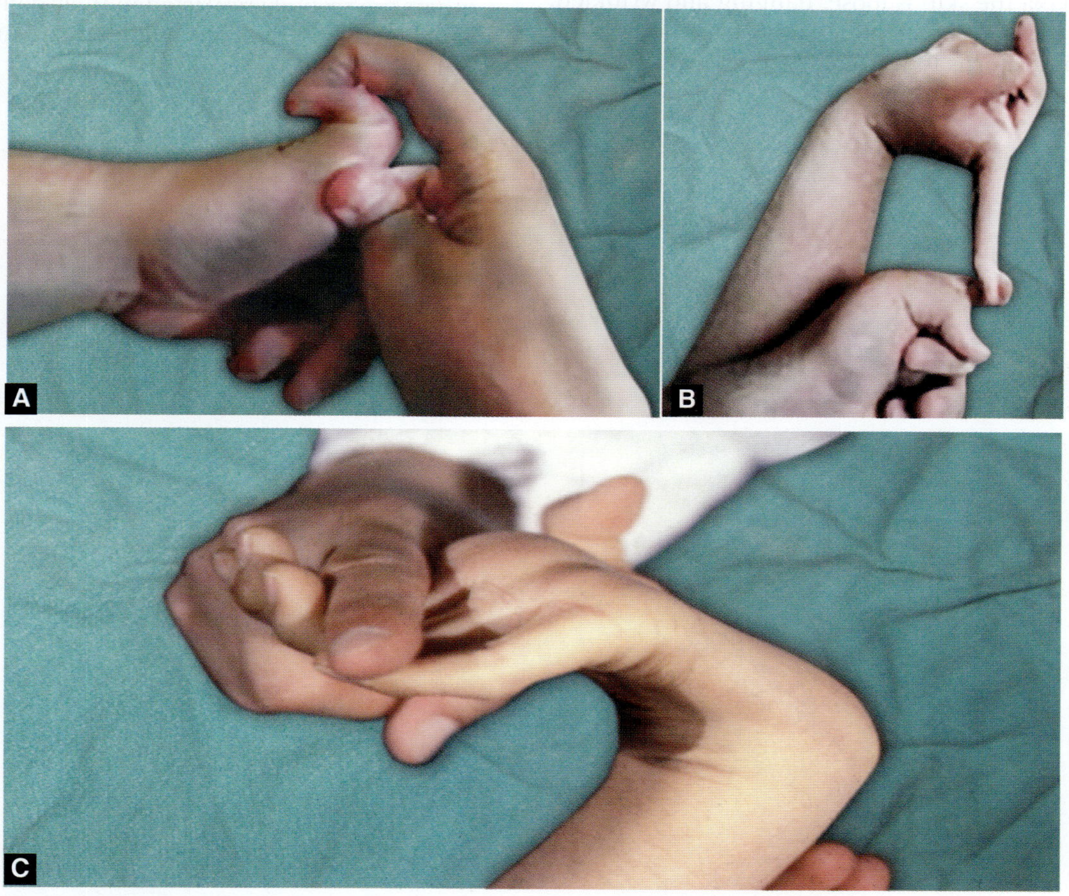

Figs 4.33A to C: Excessive laxity and hypermobility of joints, seen in patients with EDS

- Nerve compression disorders, e.g. carpel tunnel syndrome (CTS), acroparesthesia, neuropathy, etc.
- Raynaud's phenomenon
- Otosclerosis
- Functional bowel disorders
- Delayed development of motor skills, such as sitting, walking and standing.

Diagnosis

- Based on clinical criteria, both DNA and biochemical studies can be used to help identify affected individual. In some cases, a skin biopsy has been found to be useful in confirming a diagnosis. Unfortunately, these tests are not sensitive enough to identify all individual with EDS
- If there are multiple affected individual in family, it may be possible to perform prenatal diagnosis using a DNA information technique known as linkage study.

Differential Diagnosis

There are several disorders that have some of characteristic of EDS:

- In cutis laxa the skin is loose, hanging and wrinkled. In EDS, the skin can be pulled away from body, but is elastic and returns to normal when let go
- In Marfan's syndrome, the joints are very mobile but skin elasticity not seen. In the past, Menkes disease a copper metabolism disorder, was thought to be a form of EDS.

Treatment

- Surgical repair and tightening of joint ligaments require careful evaluations of individual patients, as the ligaments frequently do not hold sutures
- Patients with easily prone to bruises, should be evaluated for bleeding disorders
- Patients with type 4 EDS and members of families should be evaluated at regular intervals for detection of aneurysm.

Prognosis

- The outlook of individuals with EDS depends on the type of EDS, with which they have been diagnosed. Symptoms vary in severity, even within one subtype and the frequency of complications changes on individual basis
- Some individuals have negligible symptoms, while others are severely restricted in their daily life. Those with blood vessels involvement have an increased risk of fatal complications.

5 Metabolic Disorders

- Osteoporosis
- Scurvy
- Rickets
- Renal Rickets
- Osteomalacia
- Ochronosis (Alkaptonuric Arthritis)
- Fluorosis
- Mucopolysaccharidoses
- Gaucher's Disease

OSTEOPOROSIS

Introduction

Osteoporosis is a bone disease, in which bone tissue is normally mineralized, but the amount of bone is decreased. The structural integrity of trabecular bone is impaired and cortical bone becomes more porous and thinner.

WHO Definition

It is a reduction in bone mass density, beyond a standard deviations value of "2" from the mean, for a given age, sex and given site of the bone. It indicates weak bones, prone for getting fractured.

Risk Factors

Nonmodifiable

- Female sex
- Advanced age
- History of fractures
- Dementia.

Modifiable

- Smoking
- Alcoholism
- Low body weight
- Low calcium
- Estrogen deficiency
- Decreased physical activity.

Classification of Nordin (1964)

Generalized

- Primary
- Secondary.

Classification of Riggs and Melton (1988)

Primary Osteoporosis

Type 1

- Postmenopausal 51 to 70 years
- Sex ratio of female: Male= 5:2
- Mainly trabecular bone
- Vertebral fractures are more common
- Parathyroid hormone (PTH) decreased
- Calcium absorption decreased
- Cause is related to menopause

Type 2

- Senile
- *Age:* Greater than 70 years
- *Sex ratio:* Female to male ratio is 2:1
- Both cortical and trabecular bone
- Mainly fracture of neck of femur and intertrochanteric fractures
- PTH increased
- Calcium absorption decreased
- Cause related to aging.

Secondary Osteoporosis

Hormonal

- Hypogonadism
- Hyperadrenocorticism
- Thyrotoxicosis
- Hyperprolactinemia
- Diabetes mellitus

Nutritional

- Calcium deficiency
- Malabsorption
- Malnutrition
- Alcoholism
- Scurvy
- Liver disease
- Vitamin D deficiency

Drugs
- Glucocorticoids
- Thyroxine excess
- Anticonvulsants
- Heparin
- Cytotoxic drugs
- Alcohol
- Lithium.

Metabolic diseases
- Osteogenesis imperfecta
- Ehlers-Danlos syndrome
- Homocystinuria
- Marfan's syndrome.

Other causes
- Multiple myeloma
- Rheumatoid arthritis
- Mastocytosis
- Thalassemia
- Pregnancy.

Localized Osteoporosis

- Disuse osteoporosis
- Sudecks osteodystrophy
- Transient osteoporosis
- Regional migratory osteoporosis
- Idiopathic chondrolysis of hip.

Clinical Features

- Low backache, usually mild
- Loss of height
- Thoracic kyphosis
- Fractures.

Chronic pain in osteoporosis is due to:
- Vertebral fracture
- Kyphosis and scoliosis, with stretching of ligaments
- Iliocoastal friction syndrome.

Physical Examination

- Careful measurement of height
- Detection of kyphosis
- Blue sclera, thin skin
- Hepatosplenomegaly (Systemic disease)
- Skin pigmentation (Cushing's syndrome).

Differential Diagnosis

Differential diagnosis is shown in Table 5.1
- Hyperparathyroidism
- Paget's disease
- Osteomalacia
- Osteogenesis imperfecta
- Multiple myeloma
- Secondary tumors.

Table 5.1: Differential diagnosis of secondary osteoporosis

	Ca	*PO_4*	*ALP*
Osteoporosis	N	N/decreased	N
Hyperparathyroidism	Increased	Decreased	Increased
Paget's	N/increased	N/decreased	Increased
Osteomalacia	N/decreased	Decreased	Increased
Osteogenesis imperfecta	N	N	N/increased
Multiple myeloma	N/increased	N/decreased	N

[N: Normal; ALP: Alkaline phosphatase; Ca: Calcium; PO_4: Phosphate]

Laboratory Investigations

- Blood routine examination
- Serum calcium
- Serum phosphorous
- 24 hours urine calcium
- Alkaline phosphatase
- Increased serum calcium
  - Hyperparathyroidism
  - Malignancy
- Decreased serum calcium
  - Malnutrition
  - Osteomalacia
- If calcium level is increased, test PTH levels
- If increased, it indicates hyperparathyroidism
- If decreased, it indicates malignancy
- Increased levels of parathyroid hormone related protein (PTHP), leads to malignancy
- *Urine calcium:* If low, i.e. less than 50 mg/24 hours, causes osteomalacia, malnutrition and malabsorption
- *High urine calcium:* Greater than 300 mg/24 hours.

Causes

- Increased renal calcium leak
  - Males with osteoporosis
- Absorptive hypercalciuria
  - Idiopathic
  - Granulomatous disease
- Malignancy and diseases, with increased bone turnover
- Thyroid stimulating hormone (TSH): To rule out hyperthyroidism
- Urinary free cortisol, e.g. Cushing's disease
- Urine, Bence Jones proteins (myeloma).

Biochemical Markers

Bone Formation Markers

- Serum bone specific ALP
- Serum osteocalcin
- Serum probe peptide of type I procollagen

Bone Resorption Markers
- Urine hydroxyprolene
- Serum tranexamic acid phosphatase
- Serum bone sialoprotein
- Urine and serum cross-linked biochemical markers
- Immunoassay of pyridinoline.

Uses of Biochemical Markers
- Monitoring response to treatment
- Resorption marker is used
- Measure 4 to 6 months prior and after starting the treatment.

X-ray
- Postmenopausal osteoporosis
- Trabecular resorption and cortical resorption
- Senile osteoporosis
- Endosteal resorption
- Hyperparathyroidism
- Subperiosteal resorption
- Osteoporosis produces, increased radiolucency of vertebral bone
- Approximately 30 to 80 percent of bone tissue must be lost, before a recognizable abnormality can be detected on spinal radiographs
- Lesions less than 2 cm, may escape detection.

Vertebral Osteoporosis (Fig. 5.1)
- Cod fish vertebra
- Kyphosis
- Fractures
- Kleer Koper score:
  - Grade 0: Normal
  - Grade I: Biconcave deformity
  - Grade II: Wedge deformity
  - Grade III: Compression deformity
- Assessed from lateral view of spine T4 to L5.

Bone Mass Density (BMD)

Indications
- Estrogen deficient women are at risk of osteoporosis
- Vertebral abnormalities on X-ray
- Steroid treatment, greater than 3 mg and greater than 7.5 mg of prednisone
- Primary hyperparathyroidism
- Monitoring response to treatment.

Histological Method

It is given by Beck and Nordin
- Sample is taken from iliac crest biopsy
- Scoring is based on amount of bone present per unit area of biopsy sample. This is illustrated in Table 5.2.

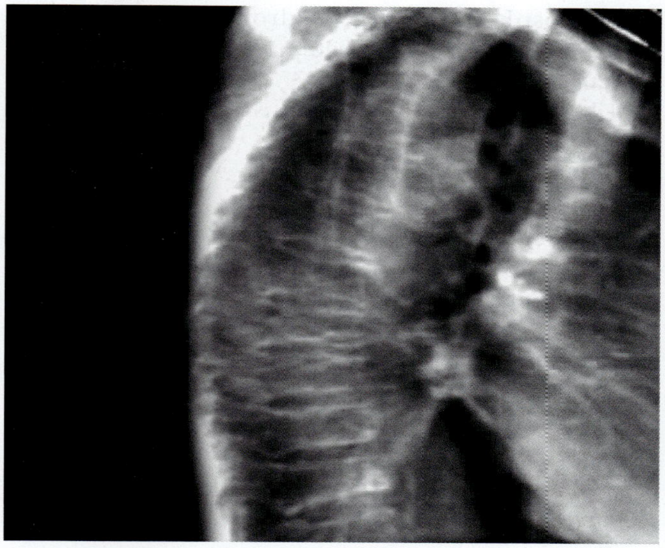

Fig. 5.1: X-ray, showing vertebral osteoporosis

Table 5.2: Histological scoring (Beck and Nordin), based on the amount of bone present per unit area of bone biopsy sample

Score assigned	*Bone percentage per unit area of biopsy sample*
Score 1	6%
Score 2	9%
Score 3	12%
Score 4	14%
Score 5	16%
Score 6	18%
Score 7	21%
Score 8	24%
Score 9	27%

[Normally score >5]

Management

Prophylaxis
- Calcium: 1 to 1.5 g/day
- Vitamin D: 400 to 800 IU/day
- Weight-bearing and gravity resistant exercises
- Avoid alcohol, cigarette
- Moderate phosphate intake
- Prophylactic agents
  - Alendronate (5 mg)
  - Raloxifine (60 mg).

Antiresorptive Agents
- *Hormone replacement therapy (HRT):* Estrogen and progesteron

- Biphosphonates, e.g. etidronate, alendronate, pamidronate, zolendronate, etc.
- Calcitonin
- Tibolone

Hormone Replacement Therapy

- *Dose:* 0.625 mg/day
- *Duration:* At least 5 years, to reduce risk of fractures
- *Timing:* Start HRT at perimenopause, for at least 5 years and start at late 60's.

Biphosphonate

Mechanism of Action

They binds to the surface of hydroxyapatite crystals and inhibits its resorption and digestion of bone by osteoclast.

Example: Alendronate

- *Dose:* 10 mg/day
- *Side effects*
  - Gastrointestinal intolerance
  - Esophagitis
  - Bone pain.

Selective Estrogen Receptor Modulators

Raloxifene

- *Dose:* 60 mg/day
- Reduces the occurrence of vertebral fracture by 30 to 50 percent
- Not associated with increasing risk of uterine cancer or benign uterine disease.

Tamoxifene

Calcitonin

- *Dose:* Nasal spray, containing 200 IU/day
- Not for prevention of osteoporosis
- Analgesic affect on bone pain
- *Mechanism of action:* Inhibit osteoclast activity by direct action on osteoclast calcitonine receptor
- Action on cortical bone is doubtful.

Orthopedic Management

Prophylactic Measures

- Avoid lifting heavy weight
- Avoid lifting weight in forward bending position
- Pectoral stretching, deep breathing and back extension exercises
- Avoid kyphotic posturing
- Low healed soft shoes and walking aids.

Rehabilitation in Established Osteoporosis

- Improve posture
- Relieve pain
- Activity and ambulation
- Low self esteem and depression have to be treated.

Treatment

- Improve posturing
- Superficial heat, like infrared therapy
- If pain persists, penetrating heat, like ultrasound or shortwave diathermy
- If pain still persists, rule out malignancy
- Back strengthening extension exercises.

Types of Osteoporosis

Steroid Induced Osteoporosis

- Most common cause, therapeutic dose
- Depends on dose and duration of treatment
- Bone loss is more, during early months of treatment
- Trabecular bone severely involved.

Mechanism of Action

- Inhibit osteoblast
- Increase resorption
- Decrease calcium absorption from GIT
- Increase urinary calcium dose.

Prevention

- Use low dose
- Prefer topical and inhaled route
- Risk factor reduction

Treatment

Biphosphonates.

Idiopathic Osteoporosis

- Idiopathic juvenile osteoporosis, between 8 and 14 years, abrupt appearance of bone pain, fracture after minimal trauma
- *Causes*
  - Malabsorption of calcium
  - High urinary calcium loss
- Vertebrae on X-ray
  - Regular biconcavity, with large disk space
- Usually self limited
- No response to vitamin D or calcium therapy.

Transient (Regional) Osteoporosis

- Rare
- Affects large joint
- Femoral head, most common site
- Young to middle age
- Male more than female
- In female
  - Left hip, most common site
  - In third trimester of pregnancy
- Resolve spontaneously in 4 to 6 months.

Regional Migratory Osteoporosis

- Mainly knee, ankle, foot are involved
- Males, affected more than females
- Between 30 and 50 years
- Involvement of each joint lasts 9 months
- Recurrence in other joints occur successively or be separated by 2 years or more.

Indices of Osteoporosis

Bone Mineral Density

- Bone mineral density (BMD), a measure of bone density, reflecting the strength of bones, as represented by calcium content
- Bone mineral density (BMD) is scored by two measures:
  - T-score
  - Z-score.

T-score

The T-score is a comparison of a patient's BMD, to that of a healthy 30 years-old, of the same sex and ethnicity. This value is used in postmenopausal women and men over aged 50 because it better predicts, risk of future fracture. The criteria of the WHO are:

- *Normal:* A T-score of 1.0 or higher
- *Osteopenic:* Less than 1.0 and greater than 2.5
- *Osteoporotic:* 2.5 or lower, meaning a bone density that is two and a half standard deviations below the mean of a thirty year old woman.

Z-score

The Z-score is the number of standard deviations, a patient's BMD differs from the average BMD of their age, sex and ethnicity. This value is used in premenopausal women, men under the age of 50 and in children.

Spinal Deformity Index

- The spinal deformity index (SDI), described by Minne et al. and Genant et al. is an assessment tool that integrates both number and severity of fractures, by summing the vertebral fracture grades along the spine from T4 to L4
- Lateral radiographs of the spine should be taken
- Assessment of each vertebra from T4 to L4 should be performed
- Grading scale is as follows:
  - Grade 0: Normal
  - Grade I: Mild (a decrease in a height of a vertebra of 20–25%)
  - Grade II: Moderate (a decrease of 25–40%)
  - Grade III: Severe (a decrease of 40% or more) fracture.
- A spinal deformity index (SDI) is calculated, by adding the grade of each vertebra from T4 to L4
- The SDI value, can vary between zero (no fracture) to 39 (all the assessed vertebrae are grade 3)
- SDI is a good predictor of incident vertebral fractures
- Patients with highest SDI, should receive highest priority to treatment.

Strength Index (SI)

- Reflection of both bone mass and structural architecture
- Calculated as section modulus × bone mineral, apparent density
- Section modulus is an estimate of the ability of distal radius to withstand bending forces
- Bone mineral (BM) apparent density is tissue mineral content or cortical area
- Low calculated SI and section modulus is a more accurate predictor of fracture risk than BMD
- SI, which reflects both bone density and bone size, appears to predict the risk of future fragility-related fractures (at distal radius)
- Femur strength index (FSI), predicts hip fracture, independent of bone density and hip axis length
- Femur strength index (FSI), calculated as the ratio of estimated compressive yield strength of the femoral neck to the expected compressive stress of a fall, on the greater trochanter.

Hip Axis Length (Fig. 5.2)

- Hip axis length (HAL) has been reported to be an independent predictor of hip fracture
- Hip axis lengh (HAL) provides the length of hip axis and the variance from the expected values, based on that patient's height. Every standard deviation (SD) above the average length or expected length represents a 1.8 fold higher risk for hip fracture.

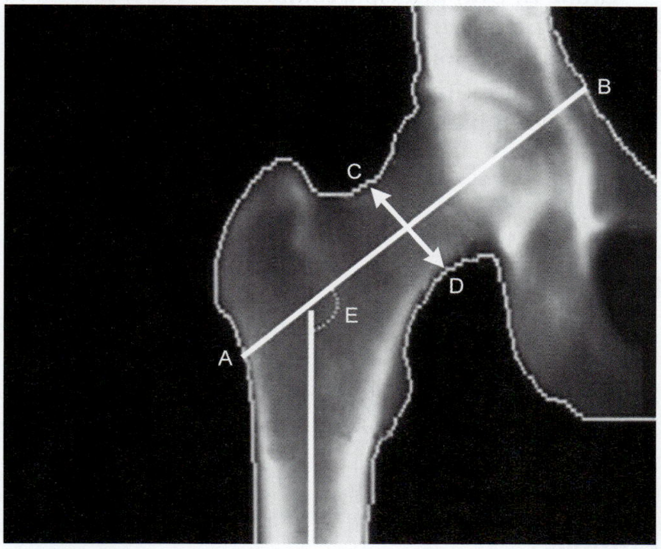

Fig. 5.2: Line AB, represents the HAL (see the text), line CD represents femoral neck diameter, and E is the neck-shaft angle

Table 5.3: Stiffness index values and its interpretations

Value of SI	*Interpretation*
<57%	High risk of having osteoporosis
57-77%	Moderate risk of having osteoporosis
>78%	Low risk of having osteoporosis

Stiffness Index (SI)

- Ultrasonographic stiffness index of calcaneum, is a noninvasive indicator of osteoporosis
- Different SI values and risk of accompanied osteoporosis are illustrated in Table 5.3.
- *Stiffness index is calculated using the following formula:* Stiffness index=broadband ultrasound attenuation (BUA)+speed of sound (SOS).

Singh Index

- The Singh index, which describes trabecular patterns in the proximal femur, has been used as a predictor for hip fractures and as an indicator of osteopenia
- *Grading*
  Grade VI: All normal trabecular groups are visible. Upper end of femur, seems to be completely occupied by cancellous bone.
  Grade V: Principal tensile and principal compressive trabeculae is accentuated. Ward's triangle, appears prominent.
  Grade IV: Principal tensile trabeculae are markedly reduced, but can still be traced from lateral cortex to upper part of the femoral neck.
  Grade III: There is a break in the continuity of the principal tensile trabeculae, opposite the greater trochanter. This grade indicates definite osteoporosis.
  Grade II: Only principal compressive trabeculae stand out prominently, remaining trabeculae have been essentially absorbed.
  Grade I: Principal compressive trabeculae are markedly reduced in number and are no longer prominent.

SCURVY

■ Definition

It is a nutritional disorder, caused by deficiency of vitamin C (ascorbic acid) and is characterized clinically, by a generalized hemorrhagic tendency

Daily recommended intake:
- 0 to 1 year: 35 mg
- 1 year to adults: 40 mg.

Etiology

- Most frequent between 5 and 10 months, in artificially fed children
- Vitamin C deficient diet (especially in old age, with restricted diet)
- When seen with rickets, it is called Barton's disease.

Pathology

- Inability to form normal intercellular collagen and organic bone matrix
- Hemorrhagic tendency due to fragility of capillary walls due to poor intercellular cement substance
- *Sites include*
  - Extra skeletal sites are gums, intestine, conjunctiva, skin, bladder and kidney
  - Skeletal sites are subperiosteal and marrow bleeding, particularly in metaphysis and especially, adjacent to actively growing epiphysis
  - Within bone, subperiosteal hemorrhage is characteristic, with ballooning of periostium resembling tumor
- *Later it can get*
  - Completely resorbed
  - Replaced by fibrous tissue
  - Ossified, forming fine periosteal trabeculations.
- Hemorrhage, within metaphysis near metaphysio-epiphyseal junction, can interfere with in-growth of osteoblasts into calcified cartilage, resulting in failure of conversion of calcified cartilage into ossified bone
- So excess of calcified cartilage accumulates and appears as a characteristic dense line on X-ray known as "White Line of Fraenkel"
- Metaphysis in response to hemorrhage, undergoes hyperemia causing increased resorption of bone, forming dark zone of radiolucency (*Scurvy line*), adjacent to Fraenkel's line
- In epiphysis, a zone of calcified cartilage is formed, encircling the bony centrum, which is known as "Wimberger's line"
- Weakening of epiphysiometaphyseal junction can occur, which can lead to fractures and complete/incomplete epiphyseal separation
- Hemorrhage in medullary cavity, undergoes fibrous organization and replacement of hematopoietic tissue. This causes secondary anemia
- Fractures can easily occur, through metaphysis in children and diaphysis in adults
- Osteoporosis of alveolar bone can cause loosening of teeth.

Clinical Features

Infants

- Irritable, restless, night cries, pale and febrile
- Extremities are held immobile, due to muscular spasm (pseudoparalysis). Any attempt to move the limbs, causes the child to cry

- Subperiosteal hemorrhages are caused, forming palpable and soft, extremely tender swelling, fixed to bone
- Gum are bluish, swollen, tender and bleeds on touch
- Petechial or ecchymosis hemorrhage in skin and mucous membrane
- Hematemesis or hemoptysis may develop
- Epiphyseal separation in lower end of femur, upper end of tibia and upper humerus
- *Scorbutic rosary:* Due to costochondral separation
- Severe cases, show anorexia, weight loss, anemia, hyperpyrexia, pneumonia and even death.

Adults

- Petechiae in skin and conjunctiva
- Bleeding gums, with bluish discoloration
- Alveolar loose teeth
- Anorexia and weight loss
- Pain and tenderness, over bony structures
- A fracture, with minimal trauma is suggestive.

Diagnosis

Laboratory

Serum ascorbic acid level, less than 0.5 mg/dl (Normal 0.7 to 1.2 mg/dl).

Radiologically

- White line of Fraenkel
- Scurvy line (also called Trummerfeld's zone of rarefaction)
- *Pelkan spur:* A small bony spur, protruding from lateral or medial border of epiphysiometaphysis junction
- Ground glass translucency of bones, due to generalized osteoporosis
- *Pencilling of cortex:* Cortex is thinned out, leaving out a mere pencil streak
- *Wimberger's line:* Epiphysis is outlined, as a rim standing out against a rarefied body, with pencilling
- Epiphyseal separation or fracture
- Ribs, show subluxation at costochondral junction (scorbutic rosary)
- Large subperiosteal hematomas, produce regional increase in soft tissue density. Calcification of hematoma occurs later, appearing as a shell enveloping the shaft
- Fissuring and fracture above calcified cartilage, in the metaphysis is common. Diaphyseal fractures are less common.

Differential Diagnosis

- Rickets
- Osteomalacia
- Acute osteomyelitis
- Osteogenesis imperfecta
- Septic arthritis
- Pseudoparalysis, may resemble poliomyelitis
- Other bleeding disorders.

Treatment

- Ascorbic acid tablets 500 to 1000 mg, daily for 1 week
- Vitamin C rich foods (citrus fruits, e.g. orange, lemon, etc.)
- Immobilization of fracture and painful joints with plaster splints.

RICKETS

Introduction

It is a metabolic disease of childhood, in which the osteoid, the organic matrix of bone fails to mineralize, due to interference with calcification mechanism. It commonly occurs between 6 months and 2 years.

Causes

Four main causes are:

- Vitamin D deficiency
- Reduced dietary intake
- Reduced amount of sunlight
- Pigmented skin

Other Causes are Malabsorption

It occurs due to:

- Celiac disease
- Hepatic osteodystrophy

Renal disease

- Glomerular failure
- Renal osteodystrophy

Antiepileptic drugs

They favor the formation of hepatic enzyme, which prevents conversion of calciferol.

Types of Rickets

Fetal Rickets

Children born to osteomalacic mother.

Infantile Rickets (Nutritional Rickets)

Most common form seen between 6 months and 3 years. Rarely seen before 6 months of age.

Late Rickets or Rachitic Tarda

Late onset rickets, familial, vitamin D resistant rickets.

Clinical Features

Symptoms

- Complains of bone pain during rest.
- Excessive perspiration in upper half of the body

- Weakness of proximal muscle of the lower limb produces waddling gait
- Irritability of CNS produces convulsion, laryngismus, spasmophilia, Chovsteck's sign, opisthotonos, etc.

Signs

Different body parts show following signs:

Skull

- Broadened forehead
- Skull square (caput quadratum)
- Frontal and parietal bossing
- Craniotabes is ping pong sensation on compressing the membranous bone of the skull.

Chest

- Pigeon chest due to prominent sternum
- Narrow chest
- Rickety rosary (enlargement of costocondral junction)
- Harrison's sulcus due to diaphragmatic pull on the soft ribs.

Abdomen

Protrubent abdomen (pot belly), develops due to weakness and hypotonia of muscles.

Spine

When the child starts sitting, he may develop kyphosis in thorax and lumbar spine scoliosis. Lordotic deformity, may develop when child starts walking.

Pelvis

Pelvic deformity with retardation of growth. Pelvic inlet is narrowed, by forward projection of promontory. Pelvic outlet is narrowed, by forward projection of caudal part of sacrum and coccyx. Changes become permanent in females, leading to obstetric problems.

Muscles: Lacking tone.

Extremities

- Epiphyseal enlargement of wrist and ankle
- Enlarged epiphysis can be seen or palpated, but cannot be seen on X-ray, as it consists of cartilage and uncalcified osteoid tissue
- Softened bones are vulnerable to bend and causes deformity like knock-knee or bow leg
- Decreased stature, giving rise to rachitic dwarfism.

Other Features

Delayed dentition, deficient dental enamel and secondary anemia, etc.

Laboratory Findings

- Calcium level is normal or deceased (due to compensatory hyperparathyroidism)
- Serum phosphorous is low
- Alkaline phosphates is normal
- Urinary calcium is low
- Serum 25-hydroxycholecalciferol is decreased.

Differential Diagnosis

- Acute poliomyelitis
- Congenital syphilis
- Septic arthritis
- Infantile scurvy.

Treatment

Prevention

- Adequate exposure of sunlight and consumption of milk and cheese
- Daily requirement of vitamin D is 10 mcg (400 IU).

Active Treatment

- Oral or parental administration of vitamin D is preferred, as follows:
  - *In active stage:* 15,000 mcg (600,000 IU)
  - *In milder cases:* 50 to 150 mcg (2000 to 6000 IU)
- Adequate intake of calcium is ensured
- It takes 2 to 4 weeks for X-ray healing.

RENAL RICKETS

■ Renal Osteodystrophy

This is the term given to the bone changes, which accompany chronic renal failure. The changes are due to a combination of hyperparathyroidism and osteitis fibrosa, osteomalacia, osteoscelerosis, periosteal new bone formation, osteoporosis and growth disturbances in children.

Clinical Features

- Children are always stunted in growth, often to a degree not equaled, by any other form of infantilism
- Less body weight
- May show infantilism and dwarfism
- Bone pain
- Muscle weakness
- Softening of bone causes skeletal deformity, like thoracic kyphosis and lumbar scoliosis
- Pruritis in skin, due to extraskeletal calcification
- Interstitial keratitis and conjunctivitis in eye.

Pathophysiology

Normal vitamin D metabolism is shown in Flow chart 5.1 of vitamin D metabolism.

Flow chart 5.1: Vitamin D metabolism

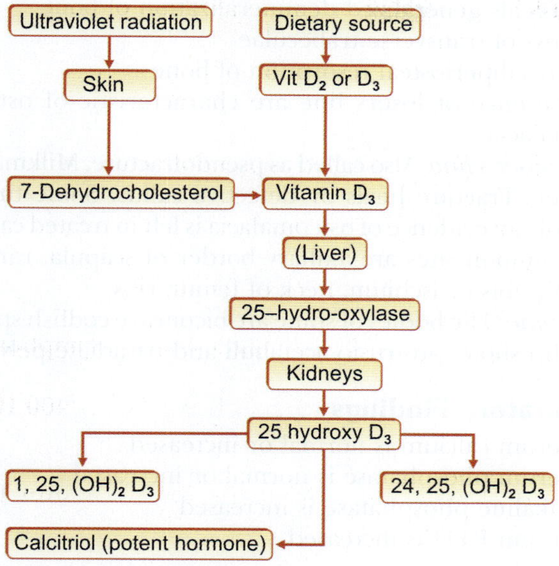

Abnormal Vitamin D Metabolism

- The major active metabolites of vitamin D is 1, $25(OH)_2D_3$ (calcitriol) which is produced by 1α-hydroxylation within the kidney
- Serum level of calcitriol is decreased when the glomerular filtration rate drops below 40 ml/min and is very low in end stage renal failure
- Lack of calcitriol leads to diminished intestinal calcium absorption, retardation of skeletal growth and defective mineralization
- A further vitamin D metabolite, 1-alpha, $25(OH)_2D_3$ and $24R,25(OH)_2D_3$ is also produced by the kidney. Low levels of this compound in renal failure may contribute to abnormalities of bone homeostasis.

Abnormal Calcium and Phosphate Metabolism

- In chronic renal failure (CRF), due to loss of renal tissue, the ability of body to excrete phosphate is diminished
- Increased phosphate lowers the ionized serum calcium and tends to cause extraskeletal calcification, by raising the calcium and phosphate product.

Abnormal Parathyroid Hormone (PTH) Metabolism

- Pure hyperparathyroidism or fibro-osteoclasis is still the most common form of renal bone disease
- Excretion of PTH degradation products is reduced in renal impairment.

Aluminium Toxicity

- Patients on dialysis accumulate a number of trace elements from the dialysis fluid
- Aluminium has been shown to be important in the pathogenesis of osteomalacia.

Pathological Changes in Kidneys

Kidney Leisons

- Kidney lesions occur, due to total renal insufficiency, as found in chronic glomerulonephritis, focal nephritis and congenital cystic disease, where there is reduced glomerular function, with failure to excrete phosphorus, as well as general uremia and acidosis
- The main skeletal change is an osteitis fibrosa, with little osteoid formation, either as rickets or as osteomalacia.

Tubular Insufficiency

- The resorption of phosphorus, amino acids, glucose, electrolytes and water is impaired, particularly from the proximal convoluted tubules
- If there is disease of the distal tubules, there is disturbance of potassium and creatinine secretion in the urine
- There is marked disturbance in the general acid-base regulation of the body, by alteration in bicarbonate, ammonium and hydrogen ions concentrations.

Syndromes Related to Rena Rickets

Snapper and Nathan (1957), reviewed the renal lesions and gave rise to the following syndromes:

Lignac-Fanconi Syndrome

- In this syndrome, there is proximal tubular deficiency, with polydipsia, polyuria, anorexia and vomiting
- The children exhibits rickets and dwarfism and usually die before puberty
- Hyperphosphaturia, with a low serum phosphate level, but normal calcium level
- Massive dosage of vitamin D, may improve skeletal disorder.

Renal or Hyperchloremic Acidosis

- Primary defect is in the distal tubules, which fails to resorb water and to secrete ammonium
- Excrete large amount of sodium, potassium and calcium
- Marked disturbances in acid-base mechanism
- Skeletal changes of either osteitis fibrosa or rickets are caused by excessive mobilization of calcium, from bone
- Condition can be improved, by administering excessive alkalizing salts, ammonium or calcium chlorides and vitamin D.

Characteristics of Different Types of Rickets

Various characteristics of different types of rickets are illustrated in Table 5.4.

Table 5.4: Characteristic features of different types of rickets

Vitamin-D	Renal deficiency	Renal tubular	Renal glomerula
Family history	-	+	-
Myopathy	+	-	+
Growth defect	±	++	++
Serum			
Ca	↓	N	↓
P	↓	↓	↑
Aik. Phos	↑	↑	↑
Urine			
Ca	↓	↓	↓
P	↑	↑	↑
Osteitis fibrosa	±	+	++
Other	Dietary deficiency or malabsorption	Aminoaciduria	Renal failure anemia

Treatment

- Ingested phosphate load is reduced by administration of oral phosphate binding compounds
- *Active treatment:* Oral or parental administration of Vitamin D is preferred
  - *In active stage:* 15,000 mcg (600,000 IU)
  - *In milder cases:* 50–150 mcg (2,000 to 6,000 IU)
- Adequate intake of calcium is ensured
- Parathyroidectomy
- Renal transplantation.

OSTEOMALACIA

Introduction

Definition

It is an adult counterpart of rickets characterized by failure of mineralization and an excess of osteoid due to interference of calcium metabolism.

Etiology

- Decreased vitamin D absorption from intestine
- Derangement of vitamin D and phosphorous metabolism.

Clinical Features

- Generalized skeletal pain and muscle weakness
- Acute pain due to fracture
- Other symptoms may be related to causative factor like GIT, renal, dietary
- Deformities like scoliosis, khyphosis, coxa vara, protrusion of acetabula, pelvis is trifoil, knock knee, etc. are encountered.

Radiological Features

- Reveals generalized demineralization of bone
- Loss of transverse trabeculae
- No subperiosteal resorption of bone
- Presence of losers line are characteristic of osteomalacia
  Looser's line: Also called as pseudofracture, Milkman's line. Fracture heals by defective callus. Some times only an evidence of osteomalacia is left in treated cases.
- Common sites are axillary border of scapula, ramus of pubis or ischium, neck of femur, ribs
- *Spine:* The bodies of spine are biconcave codfish spine
- Hip shows protrusio acetabuli and triradiate pelvis.

Laboratory Findings

- Serum calcium is normal or increased
- Serum phosphatase is normal or increased
- Alkaline phosphatase is increased
- Serum PTH is increased.

Treatment

- Calcium is given at 0.5 to 3 gm/day
- Vitamin D 10,000 IU/day
- High protein diet.

OCHRONOSIS (ALKAPTONURIC ARTHRITIS)

- Homogentisic acid is an aromatic acid, formed from incomplete breakdown of the amino acids tyrosine and phenylanine in the body
- It has affinity for certain tissues, particularly cartilages, which becomes brittle and disintegrates
- Secondary degenerative arthritis ensues.

Etiology

- Congenital and inherited, as a Mendelian recessive tract
- Occurs in the offsprings of consanguineous parents.

Pathology

- Homogentisic acid is a strong reducing agent, which when oxidized is converted to a dark pigment
- Tissues in which it is deposited are sclera, ligaments, tendons and cartilages of ears, nose, joints and intervertebral disk
- Cartilage loses its elasticity, becomes brittle and has poor resistance to mechanical strain
- Cracks easily and is worn away by friction and compression
- Exposed bony surfaces, undergo sclerosis and formation of marginal exsotoses, which are the changes, typical of degenerative arthritis

- Intervertebral disks, particularly in lumbar area, degenerate and calcify
- Disk space decreases and opposing surface of vertebral bodies become irregular sclerotic.

Clinical Feature

First Phase: Simple Alkaptonuria

Child passes urine which on exposure to air turns black.

Second Phase: Ochronosis

Deposit of ochre. Colored deposits in bone, cartilage, tendon sheath, pinna of ear. Sclera slate colored patches.

Third Phase

Alkaptonuric arthritis patient develops, generalized pain and stiffening of spine, peripheral joints, like hip and knee. Perspirations stain the clothing.

X-ray Findings

- Disks appear eliptical, thin and calcified wafer like
- Opposing vertebral bodies are sclerotic and spurred
- Evidence of degenerative arthritis is seen in large joints.

Laboratory Findings

- Homogentisic acid is a strong reducing agent that is oxidized on exposure to air and turns the urine black
- Heating or addition of alkali, fasten the reaction
- Cooper solution (Benedict's or Fehling's) is reduced
- Fermentation tests are negative
- Diagnostic test is the bluish green coloration, produced by the addition of a drop of dilute ferric chloride solution to urine.

Treatment

Reduction of intake of food, containing tyrosine and phenylalanine plus administration of high dosage of vitamin C will reduce excretion of homogentisic acid, but have no effect on progression of the disease.

FLUOROSIS

Fluorine in very low concentration, 1 part per million (ppm) or less, has been used to reduce the incidence of dental caries. At slightly higher levels (2–4 ppm) it may produce mottling of the teeth. It is a condition, which is fairly common in those parts of the world, where fluorine appears in the soil and drinking water. In some areas, notably parts of India and Africa, where fluorine concentrations in the drinking water may be above 10 ppm, chronic fluorine intoxication (fluorosis) is endemic and widespread skeletal abnormalities are occasionally encountered in the affected population. Mild bone changes are also sometimes seen in patients, treated with sodium fluoride for osteoporosis.

Fluorine directly stimulates osteoblastic activity, fluoroapatite crystals are laid down in bone and these are unusually resistant to osteoclastic resorption. Other effects are thought to be due to calcium retention, impaired mineralization and secondary hyperparathyroidism. The characteristic pathological features in severe cases are subperiosteal new bone accretion and osteosclerosis, most marked in the vertebrae, ribs, pelvis and the forearm and leg bones, together with hyperostosis at the bony attachments of ligaments, tendons and fascia in these areas. Despite the apparent thickening and density of the skeleton, tensile strength is reduced and the bones fractures occur more easily, under bending and twisting loads.

Patients complain of backache, bone pain and joint stiffness. Examination may show thickening of the tubular bones. Sometimes, the first clinical manifestation is a stress fracture. In the worst cases, there may be deformities of the spine and lower limbs, hyperostosis can lead to vertebral canal encroachment and resultant neurological defects.

The typical X-ray features are osteosclerosis, osteophytosis and ossification of ligamentous and fascial attachments. Changes are most marked in the spine and pelvis, where the bones become densely opaque.

In full blown cases, the diagnosis should be obvious, but the rarity of the condition leads to it being overlooked. X-ray features at individual sites can be mistaken for those of Paget's disease, idiopathic skeletal hyperostosis, renal osteodystrophy or osteopetrosis.

There is no specific treatment for this condition. After exposure ceases, it still takes years for bone fluoride to be excreted. If there is evidence of osteomalacia and secondary hyperparathyroidism, this can be treated with calcium and vitamin D.

MUCOPOLYSACCHARIDOSES

Introduction

- Mucopolysaccharidoses are a group of metabolic disorders, caused by an absence or malfunctioning of lysosomal enzymes, needed to breakdown molecules called glycosaminoglycans, long chains of sugar carbohydrates, in each of our cells, that help to build bone, cartilage, tendons, corneas, skin and connective tissues. Glycosaminoglycans (formerly called mucopolysaccharides) are also found in the fluid that lubricates our joints
- People with a mucopolysaccharidosis disease, either do not produce enough of one of the eleven enzymes, required to break down these sugar chains into simpler molecules or they produce enzymes that do not work properly
- Over time, these glycosaminoglycans collect in the cells, blood and connective tissues. The result is

permanent, progressive cellular damage, which affects appearance, physical abilities, organ and system functioning and in most cases, mental development
- The mucopolysaccharidoses are part of the lysosomal storage disease family
- Affects 1 in 25,000 babies
- It is an autosomal recessive disorder, except mucopolysaccharidosis (MPS II), which shows X-linked recessive inheritance.

Clinical Features

- The clinical features may not be apparent at birth, but may appear later, as storage of glycosaminoglycans affects bone, skeletal structure, connective tissues and organs
- Neurological complications may include damage to neurons, as well as pain and impaired motor function, resulting from compression of nerves or nerve roots in the spinal cord or in the peripheral nervous system
- Depending on the mucopolysaccharidosis subtype, affected individuals may have normal intellect or profoundly retarded, may experience developmental delay or may have severe behavioral problems
- Many individuals have hearing loss, either conductive, neurosensitive or both
- Communicating hydrocephalus is common in some of the mucopolysaccharidoses
- The cornea, often becomes cloudy from intracellular storage and glaucoma, along with degeneration of the retina, which also may affect the patient's vision
- Physical symptoms generally include:
  - Coarse or rough facial features (including a flat nasal bridge, thick lips and enlarged mouth and tongue)
  - Short stature with disproportionately short trunk (dwarfism), dysplasia (abnormal bone size and/or shape) and other skeletal irregularities
  - Thickened skin
  - Enlarged organs, such as liver (hepatomegaly) or spleen (splenomegaly)
  - Hernias
  - Excessive body hair growth
  - Short and often claw-like hands
  - Progressive joint stiffness
  - Carpal tunnel syndrome
- Recurring respiratory infections are common
- Many affected individuals also have heart disease
- Another lysozomal storage disease, often confused with the mucopolysaccharidoses is mucolipidosis. In this disorder, excessive amounts of fatty materials (lipids) are stored, in addition to sugars. Persons with mucolipidosis, may share some of the clinical features, associated with the mucopolysaccharidoses (certain facial features, bony structure abnormalities and damage to the brain) and increased amounts of the enzymes, needed to break down the lipids are found in the blood.

Types

- There are seven distinct clinical types and numerous subtypes of the mucopolysaccharidoses that have been identified and are shown in Table 5.5
- Although each mucopolysaccharidosis (MPS) differs clinically (Table 5.5), most patients generally experience a period of normal development, followed by a decline in physical and or mental function.

MPS I

- MPS I is divided into three subtypes, based on severity of symptoms:
  - MPS I H
  - MPS I S
  - MPS I H-S
- All three types, result from an absence of or insufficient levels of the enzyme, α-L-iduronidase
- Children born to an MPS I parent, carry the defective genes.

MPS I H

- Also called Hurler's syndrome or α-L-iduronidase deficiency
- It is the most severe of the MPS I subtypes
- Developmental delay is evident, by the end of the first year and patients usually stop developing between age of 2 to 4 years
- This is followed by progressive mental decline and loss of physical skills
- Language may be limited, due to hearing loss and an enlarged tongue
- In time, the cornea became clouded and retina may begin to degenerate
- Carpal tunnel syndrome and restricted joint movement are common
- Affected children may be quite large at birth and appear normal, but may have inguinal or umbilical hernias
- Many children develop, a short body trunk and a maximum stature of less than 4 feet
- Distinct facial features (including flat face, depressed nasal bridge and bulging forehead) become more evident in the second year
- By age of 2 years, the ribs have widened and are oar-shaped
- The liver, spleen and heart are often enlarged
- Children may experience noisy breathing and recurring upper respiratory tract and ear infections
- Feeding may be difficult for some children and many experience periodic bowel problems

Table 5.5: Types of mucopolysaccharides and associated symptoms

Type	*Main disease*	*Deficient enzyme*	*Accumulated products*	*Symptoms*
MPS I	Hurler syndrome	α-L-iduronidase	Heparan sulfate Dermatan sulfate	Mental retardation Micrognathia Coarse facies Macroglossia Retinal degeneration Corneal clouding Cardiomyopathy
MPS II	Hunter syndrome	Iduronate sulfatase	Heparan sulfate Dermatan sulfate	Mental retardation (similar, but milder, symptoms to Hurler syndrome is also X-linked recessive, as opposed to autosomal recessive)
MPS III	Sanfilippo syndrome A Sanfilippo syndrome B Sanfilippo syndrome C Sanfilippo syndrome D	Heparan sulfamidase N-acetylglucosaminidase Acetyl-CoA:alpha-glucosaminide acetyltransferase N-acetylglucosamine 6-sulfatase	Heparan sulfate	Developmental delay Severe hyperactivity Spasticity Motor dysfunction Death by the second decade
MPS IV	Morquio syndrome A Morquio syndrome B	Galactose-6-sulfate sulfatase β-galactosidase	Keratan sulfate Chondroitin 6-sulfate Keratan sulfate	Severe skeletal dysplasia Short stature, motor dysfunction
MPS VI	Maroteaux-Lamy syndrome	N-acetylgalactosamine-4-sulfatase	Dermatan sulfate	Severe skeletal dysplasia Short stature Motor dysfunction Kyphosis Heart defects
MPS VII	Sly syndrome	β-glucuronidase	β-glucuronidase	Hepatomegaly Skeletal dysplasia Short stature Corneal clouding Developmental delay
MPS IX	Natowicz syndrome	Hyaluronidase	Hyaluronic acid	Nodular soft-tissue masses around joints Episodes of painful swelling of the masses Short-term pain Mild facial changes Short stature Normal joint movement Normal intelligence

- Children with Hurler's syndrome, often die before 10 years of age from obstructive airway disease, respiratory infections and cardiac complications.

MPS I S (Scheie Syndrome)

- It is the mildest form of MPS I
- Symptoms, generally begin to appear after 5 years, with diagnosis most commonly made after age of 10 years
- Children with Scheie syndrome have normal intelligence or may have mild learning disabilities, some may have psychiatric problems
- Glaucoma, retinal degeneration and clouded corneas may significantly lead to impaired vision.
- Other problems, include Carpal tunnel syndrome or other nerve compression, stiff joints, claw hands and deformed feet, a short neck and aortic valve disease
- Some affected individuals also have obstructive airway disease and sleep apnea. Persons with Scheie syndrome can live into adulthood.

MPS I H-S (Hurler-Scheie Syndrome)

- It is less severe than Hurler's syndrome alone
- Symptoms generally begin between 3 and 8 years
- Children may have moderate mental retardation and learning difficulties
- Skeletal and systemic irregularities include short stature, marked smallness in the jaws, progressive joint stiffness, compressed spinal cord, clouded corneas, hearing loss, heart disease, coarse facial features and umbilical hernia
- Respiratory problems, sleep apnea and heart disease may develop in adolescence

- Some persons with MPS I H-S, need continuous positive airway pressure during sleep, to ease breathing
- Life expectancy is generally into the late teens or early twenties.

MPS II

- MPS II, Hunter' Syndrome or iduronate sulfatase deficiency, is caused by lack of the enzyme iduronate sulfatase
- Hunter syndrome has two clinical subtypes and (since, it shows X-linked recessive inheritance) is the only one of the mucopolysaccharidoses, in which the mother alone can pass the defective gene to a son
- The incidence of Hunter's syndrome, is estimated to be 1 in 100,000 to 150,000 male births.

MPS II A

- It is more severe form of Hunter's syndrome
- Children share many of the same clinical features associated with Hurler syndrome (MPS I H), but with milder symptoms
- Onset of the disease is usually between 2 and 4 years of age
- Developmental decline, is usually noticed between the ages of 18 to 36 months, followed by progressive loss of skills
- Other clinical features include, coarse facial features, skeletal irregularities, obstructive airway and respiratory complications, short stature, joint stiffness, retinal degeneration (but no corneal clouding), communicating hydrocephalus, chronic diarrhea, enlarged liver and spleen and progressive hearing loss
- Whitish skin lesions, may be found on the upper arms, back and upper legs
- Death from upper airway disease or cardiovascular failure, usually occurs by age of 15 years.

MPS II B

- Physical characteristics of MPS II B are less obvious and progress at a much slower rate
- Diagnosis is often made in the second decade of life
- Intellect and social development are not affected
- Skeletal problems may be less severe, but Carpal tunnel syndrome and joint stiffness can restrict movement and height is somewhat less than normal
- Other clinical symptoms, include hearing loss, poor peripheral vision, diarrhea and sleep apnea, although respiratory and cardiac complications, can contribute to premature death
- Persons with MPS II B, may live into their 50's or beyond.

MPS III

- MPS III, Sanfilippo syndrome, is marked by severe neurological symptoms
- These include progressive dementia, aggressive behavior, hyperactivity, seizures, some deafness and loss of vision, with an inability to sleep for more than a few hours at a time
- This disorder tends to have three main stages:
  - During the first stage, early mental and motor skill development may be somewhat delayed. Affected children show a marked decline in learning between 2 and 6 years, followed by eventual loss of language skills and loss of some or all hearing. Some children may never learn to speak.
  - In the second stage, aggressive behavior, hyperactivity, profound dementia and irregular sleep, may make children difficult to manage, particularly those who retain normal physical strength.
  - In the last stage, children become increasingly unsteady on their feet and most are unable to walk by age of 10 years.
- Thickened skin and mild changes in facial features, bone and skeletal structures become noticeable with age
- Growth in height, usually stops by age of 10 years
- Other problems may include, narrowing of the airway passage in the throat and enlargement of the tonsils and adenoids, making it difficult to eat or swallow. Recurring respiratory infections are common
- There are four distinct types of Sanfilippo syndrome, each caused by alteration of a different enzyme, needed to completely breakdown the heparan sulfate sugar chain
- Different types of MPS III syndromes are:
  - *Sanfilippo A:* It is the most severe of the MPS III disorders and is caused by the missing or altered enzyme heparan N-sulfatase. Children with Sanfilippo A, have the shortest survival rate among those, with the MPS III disorders
  - *Sanfilippo B:* Caused by the missing or deficient enzyme, alpha-N-acetylglucosaminidase
  - *Sanfilippo C:* Results from the missing or altered enzyme acetyl-Ca alpha-glucosaminide acetyltransferase
  - *Sanfilippo D:* This is caused by the missing or deficient enzyme, N-acetylglucosamine 6-sulfatase.
- Little clinical difference exists between these four types, but symptoms appear most severe and seem to progress more quickly in children with type A. The average duration of Sanfilippo syndrome is 8 to 10 years, following onset of symptoms. Most persons with MPS III live into their teenage years and some live even longer

- The incidence of Sanfilippo syndrome (for all four types combined) is about one in 70,000 births.

MPS IV

- MPS IV, Morquio syndrome, is estimated to occur in 1 in 700,000 births
- Its two subtypes, result from the missing or deficient enzymes, N-acetylgalactosamine 6-sulfatase (Type A) or beta-galactosidase (Type B) needed to break down the keratan sulfate sugar chain
- Clinical features are similar in both types, but appear milder in Morquio type B
- Onset is between age of 1 and 3 years
- Neurological complications, include spinal nerve and nerve root compression, resulting from extreme, progressive skeletal changes, particularly in the ribs and chest, conductive and or neurosensitive loss of hearing and clouded corneas
- Intelligence is normal, unless hydrocephalus develops and is not treated
- Physical growth slows and often stops between 4 and 8 years
- Skeletal abnormalities include a bell-shaped chest, a flattening or curvature of the spine, shortened long bones, along with dysplasia of the hips, knees, ankles and wrists
- The bones that stabilize the connection between the head and neck can be malformed (odontoid hypoplasia), in these cases, a surgical procedure called spinal cervical bone fusion, can be life saving
- Restricted breathing, joint stiffness and heart diseases are also common
- Children with more severe form of Morquio syndrome, may not live beyond their twenties or thirties.

MPS VI

- Children with MPS VI, Maroteaux-Lamy syndrome, usually have normal intellectual development, but share many of the physical symptoms found in Hurler's syndrome
- It is caused by the deficient enzyme N-acetylgalactosamine 4-sulfatase and Maroteaux-Lamy syndrome, has a variable spectrum of severe symptoms
- Neurological complications, include clouded corneas, deafness, thickening of the dura and pain caused by compressed or traumatized nerves and nerve roots
- Growth is normal at first, but stops suddenly around 8 years
- By age of 10 years, children have developed a shortened trunk, crouched stance and restricted joint movement
- In more severe cases, children also develop a protruding abdomen and forward curving spine
- Skeletal changes (particularly in the pelvic region) are progressive and limit movement
- Many children also have umbilical or inguinal hernias
- Nearly all children have some form of heart disease, usually involving valve dysfunction
- An enzyme replacement therapy was tested on patients with MPS VI and was successful in, that it improved growth and joint movement.

MPS VII

- MPS VII, Sly syndrome, one of the least common forms of the mucopolysaccharidoses, is estimated to occur in less than 1 in 250,000 births
- The disorder is caused by deficiency of the enzyme beta-glucuronidase
- In its rarest form, Sly syndrome causes children to be born with hydrops fetalis, in which extreme amounts of fluid are retained in the body
- Survival is usually a few months or less
- Most children, with Sly syndrome are less severely affected
- Neurological symptoms may include mild to moderate mental retardation by 3 years of age, communicating hydrocephalus, nerve entrapment, corneal clouding and some loss of peripheral and night vision
- Other symptoms, include short stature, some skeletal irregularities, joint stiffness and restricted movement, with umbilical and/or inguinal hernias
- Some patients may have repeated bouts of pneumonia during their first years of life
- Most children with Sly syndrome, live into the teenage or young adult years.

MPS IX

- As of 2001, only one case of MPS IX, Natowicz syndrome or online mendelian inheritance in man (OMIM)), had been reported
- The disorder results from hyaluronidase deficiency
- Symptoms include, nodular soft tissue masses located around joints, with episodes of painful swelling of the masses and pain that ended spontaneously within 3 days
- Pelvic radiography, showed multiple soft tissue masses and some bone erosion. Other traits included mild facial changes, acquired short stature, as seen in other MPS disorders and normal joint movement and intelligence.

Diagnosis

- By clinical examination
- Urine tests (excess mucopolysaccharides are excreted in the urine)
- Enzyme assays
- Prenatal diagnosis, using amniocentesis and chorionic villus sampling, can verify if a fetus either carries a

copy of the defective gene or is affected with the disorder
- Genetic counseling can help parents, who have a family history of the mucopolysaccharidoses, determine if they are carrying the mutated gene that causes the disorders.

Treatment

- Currently, there is no cure for these disorders
- Medical care is directed at treating systemic conditions and improving the person's life quality
- Physical therapy and daily exercise may delay joint problems and improve the ability to move
- Changes to the diet will not prevent disease progression, but limiting milk, sugar and dairy products, has helped some individuals experiencing excessive mucus
- Surgery to remove tonsils and adenoids may improve breathing among affected individuals, with obstructive airway disorders and sleep apnea. Some patients may require surgical insertion of an endotrachial tube to aid breathing
- Surgery can also correct hernias, help to drain excessive cerebrospinal fluid from the brain and free nerves and nerve roots compressed by skeletal and other abnormalities
- Corneal transplants may improve vision among patients, with significant corneal clouding
- Enzyme replacement therapy (ERT) is currently being tested. Enzyme replacement therapy has proven useful, in reducing non-neurological symptoms and pain
- Bone marrow transplantation (BMT) and umbilical cord blood transplantation (UCBT) have had limited success in treating the mucopolysaccharidoses. Abnormal physical characteristics, except for those affecting the skeleton and eyes, may be improved, but neurological outcomes have varied. BMT and UCBT are high-risk procedures and are usually performed only after family members receive extensive evaluation and counseling.

GAUCHER'S DISEASE

The genetic disorder, first described by Gaucher over 100 years ago is now known to be caused by lack of a specific enzyme, which is responsible for the breakdown and the excretion of the cell membrane products from defunct cells. This is a classical example of a lipid storage disease, for which the pathogenesis has been painstakingly worked out, leading to the development of an effective treatment.

Each time one of the cells in the body dies, a glucocerebroside is released from the cell membrane. Before it can be excreted, the glucoside bond holding the glucose molecule, has to be split by a specific enzyme, glucosylceramide beta-glucosidase. If this enzyme is lacking, the glucocerebroside cannot be excreted and instead is stored in the lysosomal bodies of macrophage of reticuloendothelial system, notably in the marrow, spleen and liver. Accumulation of these abnormal macrophage leads to enlargement of the spleen and liver, along with secondary changes in the marrow and bone.

Most patients suffer from a chronic form of disorder, with changes predominantly in the marrow, bone and spleen and varying degree of pancytopenia (Type 1). A rare form of the disease affecting central nervous system (Type II), appears in infancy and usually causes death within a year. Type III is a subacute disorder, characterized by the appearance of hepatosplenomegaly in childhood and skeletal and neurological abnormalities during adolescence.

Like other storage disorders, Gaucher's disease is transmitted as an autosomal recessive trait. Males and females are affected equally with relative high incidence in Jewish people of Ashkenazi descent. The phenotype is associated with a large number of different gene defects, five of which appear in the majority of cases.

Clinical Features

In the commonest form of disease (Type 1), patients present in the childhood or adult life with anemia, thrombocytopenia, hepatosplenomegaly or bone pain, about two-thirds of affected people develop skeletal abnormalities. Older patients may develop back pain due to vertebral osteopenia and compression fractures. Femur neck fractures also are not uncommon, however diaphyseal fractures are rare. The hematocrit and platelet counts are usually diminished. A suggestive finding (when positive) is elevation of serum acid phosphatase level. The diagnosis can be confirmed by demonstrating low glucocerebrosidase activity in blood or by identifying abnormal gene mutations in DNA tests.

A common complication is osteonecrosis, usually of femoral head, but sometimes in the femoral condyles, the proximal head of humerus or the bones around the ankle. The patients (usually a child or adolescent) may present with an acute bone crisis, with unrelenting pain, local tenderness and restriction of movement, accompanied by pyrexia, leukocytosis and elevated erythrocyte sedimentation rate (ESR). The clinical features resemble, those of osteomyelitis or septic arthritis, indeed Gaucher's disease predisposes to bone infection and this may be a source of confusion.

Imaging

X-rays show a variable pattern of radiolucency or patchy density, more marked in cancellous bone. The distal end of femur may be expanded, producing Erlenmeyer flask appearance. A skeletal survey, may lead to reversal of osteonecrosis of femoral head, femoral condyles, talus or humeral head.

A radioisotope bone scan may help to distinguish a crisis episode from infection, the former is usually "Cold" and the later is "Hot". MRI is the most reliable way of defining marrow involvement.

Treatment

Bone pain may need symptomatic treatment. For the acute crisis analgesic medication and bed rest are followed by nonweight-bearing walking with crutches. Specific therapy, is now available (albeit costly) in the form of replacement enzyme, alglucerase. This has been shown to reverse the blood changes and reduce the size of the liver and the spleen. The bone complications also are diminished.

Osteonecrosis of the femoral head, usually result in progressive deformity of the hip. However, most patients manage quite well with symptomatic treatment and surgery should be deferred for as long as possible.

6 Endocrine Disorders

- Hypothyroidism
- Hyperparathyroidism
- Hypopituitarism
- Hyperpituitarism
- Hypervitaminosis

HYPOTHYROIDISM

Hypothyroidism takes various form, depending on the age of onset. These are explained below, with associated clinical features.

Congenital Hypothyroidism (Cretinism)

- It may be caused by developmental abnormalities of thyroid, but it also occurs in endemic form in areas of iodine deficiency
- Unless the condition is treated immediately (diagnosis at birth is not easy), the child becomes severely dwarfed and mentally retarded
- X-ray may show irregular epiphyseal ossification
- Treatment with thyroid hormone is essential.

Juvenile Hypothyroidism

- It is usually less severe than congenital type
- Growth and sexual development are retarded and the child may be mentally subnormal
- X-rays show the typical epiphyseal "fragmentation" appearance
- Treatment with thyroid hormone, may reverse these changes.

Adult Hypothyroidism (Myxedema)

- It may result from some primary disorder of thyroid function (including Hashimoto's disease) or from iatrogenic suppression, following treatment for hyperthyroidism
- The onset is slow and there may be long period of nonspecific symptoms, such as weight increase, a general lack of energy and depression
- Later complications, include deafness, thinning of hair, muscle weakness, nerve entrapment syndromes and joint pain, sometimes associated with calcium pyrophosphate dehydrate crystal deposition
- Treatment with thyroxine is effective and will have to be continued for life.

HYPERPARATHYROIDISM

Introduction

Excessive secretion of parathyroid hormone (PTH), may be primary (usually due to an adenoma or hyperplasia), secondary (due to persistent hypocalcemia) or tertiary (when secondary hyperplasia leads to autonomous over activity).

Pathology

Overproduction of PTH enhances calcium conservation, by stimulating tubular absorption, intestinal absorption and bone resorption. The resulting hypercalcemia, leads to an increase in glomerular filtration of calcium, so there is hypercalciuria, despite the augmented tubular resorption. Urinary phosphate also is increased due to suppressed tubular resorption. The main effects of these changes are seen in the kidney, as calcinosis, stone formation, recurrent infection and impaired function. There may also be calcification of soft tissues.

There is a general loss of bone substance. In more severe cases, osteoclastic hyperactivity produces subperiosteal erosions, endosteal cavitation and replacement of the marrow spaces, by vascular granulations and fibrous tissue (osteitis fibrosa cystica). Hemorrhage and giant cell reaction within the fibrous stroma, may give rise to brownish, tumor-like masses, whose liquefaction leads to fluid-filled cysts.

■ Primary Hyperparathyroidism

Primary hyperparathyroidism is quite common, the usual cause is a solitary adenoma in one of the small glands.

Patients are middle-aged (40–65 years) and women are affected, twice as often as men. Many remain asymptomatic and are diagnosed only because routine biochemistry tests unexpectedly reveal a raised serum calcium level.

Clinical Features

They are mainly due to hypercalcemia, anorexia, nausea, abdominal pain, depression, fatigue and muscle weakness. They may develop polyuria, kidney stones or nephrocalcinosis due to chronic hypercalciuria. Some complaint of joint symptoms, due to chondrocalcinosis. Only a minority (probably less than 10%) present, with bone disease and this is usually generalized osteoporosis rather than the classic features of osteitis fibrosa, bone cysts and pathological fractures.

X-rays show signs of osteoporosis (sometimes including vertebral collapse) and areas of cortical erosion. Hyperparathyroid "Brown Tumors", should be considered in the differential diagnosis of atypical cyst-like lesions of long bones. However, the classic and almost pathognomonic feature, which should always be sought, is subperiosteal cortical resorption of the middle phalanges. Nonspecific features of hypercalcemia are renal calculi, nephrocalcinosis and chondrocalcinosis.

Biochemical tests show hypercalcemia, hypophosphatemia and a raised serum PTH concentration. Serum alkaline phosphatase is raised with osteitis fibrosa. Diagnosis involves the exclusion of other causes of hypercalcemia (multiple myeloma, metastatic disease, sarcoidosis), in which PTH levels are usually depressed. Hyperparathyroidism also comes into the differential diagnosis of all types of osteoporosis and osteomalacia.

Treatment is usually conservative and includes adequate hydration and decreased calcium intake. The indications for parathyroidectomy are marked and unremitting hypercalcemia, recurrent renal calculi, progressive nephrocalcinosis and severe osteoporosis. Postoperatively, there is a danger of severe hypocalcemia due to brisk formation of new bone (the "Hungry bone syndrome"). This must be treated promptly, with one of the fast acting vitamin D metabolites.

■ Secondary Hyperparathyroidism

Parathyroid over secretion is a predictable response to chronic hypocalcemia. Secondary hyperparathyroidism is seen, therefore, in various types of rickets and osteomalacia and accounts for some of the radiological features in these disorders. Treatment is directed at the primary condition.

HYPOPITUITARISM

■ Pituitary Dysfunction

The posterior lobe of the pituitary gland has no influence on the musculoskeletal system. The anterior lobe is responsible for the secretion of pituitary growth hormone, as well as the thyrotropic, gonadotropic and adrenocorticotropic hormones. Abnormalities may affect the production of some of these hormones and not others, thus there is no single picture of pituitary deficiency or pituitary excess. Moreover, the clinical effects are determined in part, by the stage in skeletal maturation, at which the abnormality occurs.

■ Hypopituitarism—Etiology

Anterior pituitary hyposecretion, may be caused by intrinsic disorders, such as infarction or hemorrhage in the pituitary, infection and intrapituitary tumors or by extrinsic lesions (such as a craniopharyngioma), which press on the anterior lobe of the pituitary. In some cases, there may also be features, due to posterior lobe dysfunction (e.g. diabetes insipidus) and space occupying lesions, are likely to have other intracranial pressure effects, such as headache or visual field defects. In childhood and adolescence, two distinct clinical disorders are encountered.

Childhood

In the Lorain syndrome, the predominant effect is on growth. The body proportions are normal, but the child fails to grow (proportionate dwarfism). Sexual development may be unaffected. The condition must be distinguished from other causes of short stature, i.e. hereditary or constitutional shortness, which is not as marked as childhood illness or malnutrition rickets and the various bone dysplasias, which generally result in disproportionate dwarfism.

In Fröhlich's adiposogenital syndrome, the effects include those of gonadal hormone deficiency. There is delayed skeletal maturation, associated with adiposity and immaturity of the secondary sexual characteristics. Weakness of the physes combined with disproportionate adiposity, may result in epiphyseal displacement (epiphysiolysis or slipped epiphysis) at the hip or knee.

Adults

Panhypopituitarism causes a variety of symptoms and signs, including those of cortisol and sex hormone deficiency. The only important skeletal effect is premature osteoporosis.

Investigations

These should include direct assays and tests for hormone function.

X-rays

X-rays of the skull may show expansion of the pituitary fossa and erosion of the adjacent bone. CT and MRI may reveal the tumor.

Treatment

Treatment will depend on the cause and the degree of dwarfism. If a tumor is identified, it can be removed or ablated. A word of warning, the sudden reactivation of pituitary function, after removal of a tumor may result in slipping of the proximal femoral epiphysis. Awareness of this risk, will make for early diagnosis and if necessary, surgical treatment of the epiphysiolysis. Growth hormone deficiency has been successfully treated, by the administration of biosynthetic growth hormone (somatotropin). The response should be checked, by serial plots on the growth chart.

HYPERPITUITARISM

Over secretion of pituitary growth hormone, is usually due to an acidophillic adenoma. However, there are rare cases of growth hormone secretion, by pancreatic (and other) tumors. The effects vary according to the age of onset.

■ Gigantism

Over secreation of growth hormone in childhood and adolescence, causes excessive growth of entire skeleton. The condition may be suspected quite early and it is important to track the child's development, by regular clinical and X-ray examinations. In addition to being excessively tall, patients may develop deformity of the hip, due to epiphyseal displacement (epiphysiolysis). There may be mental retardation and sexual immaturity. Treatment is directed at early removal of the pituitary tumor.

■ Acromegaly

Over secretion of pituitary growth hormone in adulthood causes, enlargement of the bones and soft tissues, but without the very marked elongation, which is seen in gigantism. The bones are thickened, rather than lengthened. Due to appositional growth, there is also hypertrophy of articular cartilage, which leads to enlargement of the joints. Bones, such as the mandible, clavicle, ribs, sternum and scapulae, which develop secondary growth centers in late adolescence or early adulthood, may go on growing longer than usual. Thickening of the skull, prominence of the orbital margins, overgrowth of the jaw and enlargement of the nose, lips and the tongue produce the characteristic facies of acromegaly. The chest is broad and barrel-shaped and the hands and feet are large. Thickening of the bone ends may causes secondary osteoarthritis. About 10 percent of acromegalics develop diabetes and cardiovascular disease more commonly than usual.

Treatment

The indications for operation are the presence of a tumor in childhood and cranial nerve pressure symptoms at any age. Transsphenoidal surgery has a high rate of success, provided the diagnosis is made reasonably early and the tumor is not too large.

Mild cases of acromegaly can be treated by administering growth hormone suppressants (a somatostatin analogue or bromocriptine, a dopamine agonist).

HYPERVITAMINOSIS

■ Hypervitaminosis A

- Occurs in children, following excessive dosage
- In adults, it seldom occurs except in explorers, who eat Polar bear's liver
- There may be bone pain and headache and vomiting, due to raised intracranial pressure
- X-ray shows increased density in the metaphyseal region and subperiosteal calcification.

■ Hypervitaminosis D

- Occurs, if too much vitamin D is given
- It exerts a PTH like effect and so as in the underlying rickets, calcium is withdrawn from bones, but metastatic calcification occurs
- In treatment, the dose of vitamin D must be properly regulated and the infant should be given a low calcium diet, but plentiful fluids.

7 Blood Disorders

- Hemophilia in Orthopedics

HEMOPHILIA IN ORTHOPEDICS

Definition

It is characterized by a bleeding diasthesis, due to the defect in the clotting mechanism of the blood.

Coagulation Factors of Blood

- Factor I: Fibrinogen
- Factor II: Prothrombin
- Factor III: Tissue thromboplastin (tissue factor)
- Factor IV: Ionized calcium (Ca^{2+})
- Factor V: Labile factor or proaccelerin
- Factor VI: Unassigned
- Factor VII: Stable factor or proconvertin
- Factor VIII: Antihemophilic factor
- Factor IX: Plasma thromboplastin component, Christmas factor
- Factor X: Stuart-prower factor
- Factor XI: Plasma thromboplastin antecedent
- Factor XII: Hageman factor
- Factor XIII: Fibrin-stabilizing factor

Types of Hemophilia

Hemophilia A:	Due to the deficiency of factor VIII (Antihemophilia factor)
Hemophilia B:	Due to deficiency of factor IX (Christmas factor)
Hemophilia C:	Due to deficiency of factor XI (Plasma thromboplastin antecedent)
von Willebrand's: disease	When both Factor VIII and platelet are deficient.

Clinical Features

The common orthopedic manifestations are:
- Hemorrhage into the following structure
  - Joints
  - Muscles
  - Peripheral nerves
- Hemophilic cyst (Fig. 7.1)

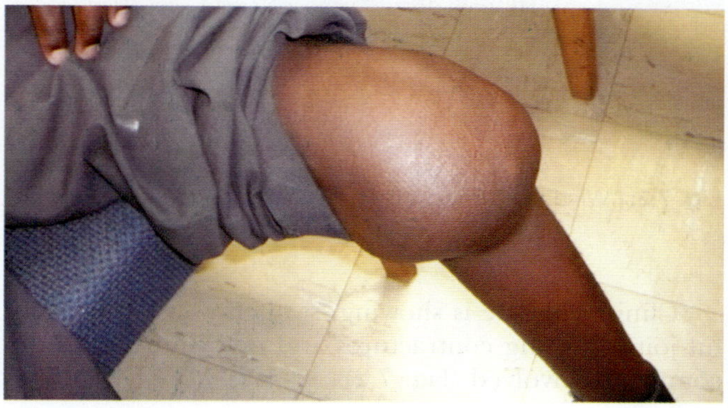

Fig. 7.1: Hemorrhage into the joint (knee)

Hemorrhages into Joint

There is a sudden attack of hemarthosis in joint, following minimal trauma. The bleeding occurs not only inside the synovial cavity of joint, but also intraosseous hemorrhages from subchondral bone. In later stage, destruction of cartilage, takes place with fibrous ankylosis and deformity. Knee, elbow, ankle and hip are commonly involved.

Hemorrhages into Muscle

Bleeding into iliacus, results in lump in iliac fossa and flexion deformity of hip, due to spasm of muscles. In calf, it gives rise to equinus deformity. In forearm produces Volkmann ischemic contracture (VIC) occasionally.

Hemorrhages into Nerves

Nerve lesion occurs, due to intraneural hemorrhages.

Hemophilic Cyst

The bleeding, form cysts in various planes of muscles, fasciae or in bones (pseudotumor).

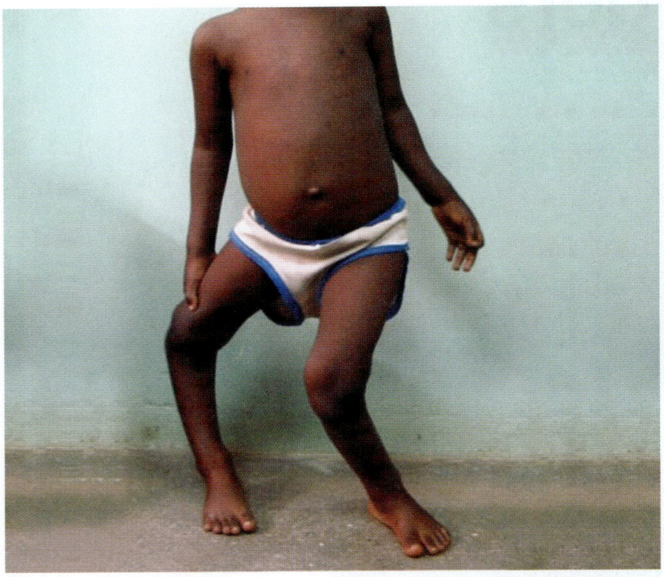

Fig. 7.2: "Wind swept deformity" of knee joint

Clinical picture is showing, swollen, warm and painful joint, causing contractures and deformities. Knee is commonly involved (Fig. 7.2).

Stages of Joint Involvement

Stage I

Trauma to joint, hemarthrosis, with mild to severe effusion.

Stage II

- Articular damage is present, with, widening of intercondylar notch
- Due to subchondral cysts, joint space is reduced and squaring of patella, is present
- Patient may have subluxation of tibia and lateral rotation.

Stage III

- Patient is bed ridden, with joint severely deformed and ankylosed
- Late arthritic changes, with subluxation of tibia.

Laboratory Findings

- Bleeding time and prothrombin time are normal
- Deficiency of factor VIII, IX
- Plasma thromboplastin time is elevated
- Blood HIV should be tested in hemophilia, as transfusion related AIDS is a well recognized complication of hemophilia.

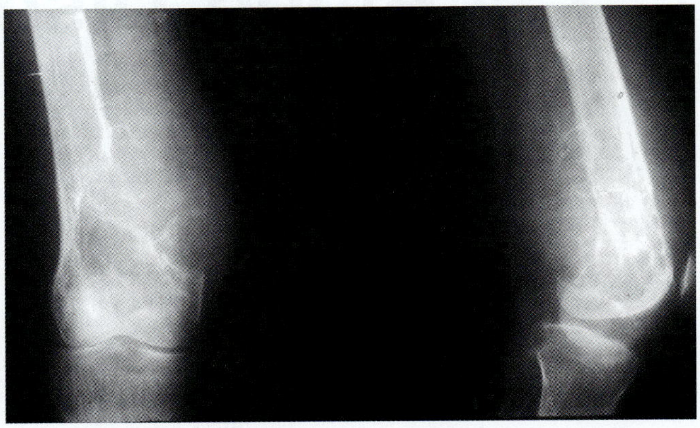

Fig. 7.3: X-ray showing, pseudotumor in a joint, as cystic, expansile and lucent, soft tissue swellings, eroding the cortex

Radiological Findings

Early Stage

Distended synovium, no para-articular skeletal deformity.

Intermediate Stage

Persistent boggy swelling and osteoporosis, with subchondral cyst are present. Squaring of patella is present and intercondylar notch of femur, along with trochlear notch is widened.

End Stage

- Joint is disorganized. Subchondral cysts are large and fibrous ankylosis is present
- Pseudotumor is seen as cystic, expansile and lucent, soft tissue swellings, eroding the cortex (Fig. 7.3).

Management

This varies according to stage.

Acute Stage

- Factor VIII is replaced
- Joint aspiration is done
- Immobilized with splint.

Late Cases

- Prolonged immobilization, with caliper or splint is recommended
- Trial aspiration.

Surgical Methods

- Fresh frozen plasma and blood transfusion
- Synovectomy
- Osteotomy, for severe flexion contracture
- Arthrodesis

- Lengthening or release, for contractures
- Joint replacement.

Surgical Approach

Principal of Surgery in Hemophilia

- HIV and inhibitors of factor VIII (antibodies) must be assayed in serum preoperatively
- Factors VIII replacement, must be started 45 minutes to 1 hour before surgery and continue till suture removal
- Factor VIII levels in serum must be maintained at 100 percent for the first week, following surgery and at 50 to 75 percent during the second weeks
- Tourniquet should be used, wherever possible
- Sharp dissection is preferred, blunt dissection should be avoided
- Drains should not be used
- Bulky dressing should be used
- Physiotherapy should be continued, under the coverage of factor VIII.

8 Gouty Arthritis

- Pseudogout (Chondrocalcinosis)
- Hydroxyapatite Crystals Deposition Disease

Introduction

Gout is a hereditary condition of disturbed uric acid metabolism, in which sodium urate salts are deposited in articular, periarticular and subcutaneous tissues. It is characterized, by recurring attacks of acute arthritis, with intervals of freedom from pain.

Etiology

Actual cause is unknown. Predisposing causes are:

Hereditary (Heredity)

Occurs in families.

Sex

Males predominantly affected and in females, usually occur at menopause.

Age

Second to fourth decade. Common at about 40 years.

Adrenal Cortex Activity

An adequate amount of cortical steroids counteracts gouty attack.

Vascular Changes

Extremity involved by acute gouty arthritis, displays increased blood flow and amplitude, suggesting vascular disturbance, as the cause of extreme pain.

Disturbed Electrolyte Equilibrium

Marked diuresis, that precedes acute attacks of gout.

Decreased Urinary 17-Ketosteroids

Formed from metabolism of adrenocortical and testicular androgens. Reduction below 3 mg/24 hours is a constant finding in gout.

Pathology

- Sodium urate crystals are deposited on the surface of and replacing articular cartilage
- Articular cartilage is eroded, the subchondral bone is replaced in well circumscribed punched out areas, by crystalline deposits
- Pannus of granulation tissue, grows over the articular surface, invades and replaces the cartilage and may bridge the joint to opposite articular surface, producing fibrous ankylosis
- Irregularity of joint surfaces, leads to secondary degenerative arthritis
- Urate crystals are deposited in the synovial membrane, periarticular soft tissues and subcutaneous tissues
- Microscopically, deposits are surrounded by an inflammatory reaction, fibrous tissues and giant cells
- Urate salts are found in articular cartilage, bone marrow, synovial membrane, joint capsules, ligaments, periosteum, tendons, bursae, subcutaneous and intramuscular tissues
- Metatarsophalangeal joint of big toe is predisposed
- Next affected parts are intertarsal joints, ankles, fingers and the wrist
- Cause of death is usually cerebral or coronary disease or nephrosclerosis with uremia.

Clinical Features

- Serum urate level, exceeds 6 mg/dl
- Initial attack is acute and may be precipitated by trauma, dietary indiscretions (high fat diet), drugs (liver extract), surgical operations, exposure to cold and withdrawal of adrenocorticotropic hormone (ACTH)
- *Attack:* Sudden onset, frequently at night
- *Joint:* Swollen, red and tender. May mimic cellulitis. Pain is excruciating
- Inflammation may involve a nonarticular urate deposit, such as a subcuatenous tophus or in a bursa
- *Constitutional symptoms:* Fever, tachycardia and headache
- Attacks last from a few days to several weeks before it subsides, with complete restoration of function of the joint

- Desquamation is involved up to final stage
- Intervals between attacks, may vary in length, they tend to become progressively shorter and the intensity of succeeding attacks, become progressively severe
- Small deposits of urate salts, in subcutaneous tissues are seen as a pearly white appearance. Characteristic location for these deposits is about ears
- Tophi may increase in size and assume large globular shapes, distending the overlying skin and rupturing it, to form a chronically discharging sinus, exuding milky white material
- Main complication is due to deposits of urate crystals in the kidneys. Impairment of renal function, due to chronic glomerulonephritis and interstitial nephritis, leads to uremia and death.

Diagnosis

Main diagnostic factors include:

- Family history of gouty arthritis
- Repeated attacks, with intervals of freedom from pain
- Renal disturbance
- Hyperuricemia
- Satisfactory response to adequate dose of colchicines.

Laboratory Findings

- *Blood:* Leukocytosis, increased erythrocyte sedimentation rate (ESR)
- Increased concentration of sodium urate. Normal level is less than 5 mg/dl
- Microscopic examination of joint fluid include:
  - Sodium biurate crystals, found in joint aspirates
  - Needle shaped crystals, show strong negative birefringence, when viewed under polarizing microscope digested by uricase
  - It helps in differentiating from pseudogout, in which rhombic calcium phosphate crystals are seen, showing positive but weak birefringence, not digested by uricase
  - *Murexide test:* Few drops of nitric acid are added to a suspected substance. Mixture is evaporated to dryness and is then moistened with ammonium hydroxide. If uric acid is present, a purple color (due to murexide) comes.

X-ray Findings

- Earlier, joint appears normal
- Later, replacement of bony structure by urate crystals, gives the characteristic punched out appearance
- Cartilage is destroyed, joint becomes narrowed
- Degenerative arthritic changes are seen.

Factors Influencing Uric Acid Levels

- Endogenous uric acid, arises from destroyed nuclei, particularly extruded nuclei of normoblasts, during process of maturation of erythrocytes
- Certain diseases such as polycythemia and drugs, such as liver extract, can precipitate arthritis
- High fat diet decreases its excretion
- Uric acid is an end product of purine metabolism.

Treatment

Prophylaxis demands, avoiding provocative factors.

Acute Attack

- Absolute bed rest
- Affected extremity immobilized in a splint
- Ice pack reduces the pain
- Colchicine (colchicum) specific for gout, acts as both analgesic and diuretic
- Salicylates, also valuable for their uricosuric effect
- High carbohydrate diet
- Phenylbutazone given, as enteric coated tablets (200 mg three times a day) and oral predinosolone (20 mg to 40 mg /day) is effective
- Since colchicines have no uricosuric effect, it should be combined with allopurinol
- Allopurinol is an inhibitor of the enzyme xanthine oxidase, thereby preventing final step in production of uric acid
- Principal side effects of allopurinol are gastrointestinal irritation and dermatitis
- Fever, blood dyscrasia and hepatic damage can occur rarely
- 300 mg/day is the starting dose of allopurinol.

Surgical Procedure

- During acute attack, immobilization of affected joint will lessen the degree of joint destruction
- A bursa may become distended by urate deposits and the overlying skin is thinned and penetrated or the tendon may be invaded
- A fusiform, nodular enlargement develops within the tendon, which interferes with tendon motion and may predispose to tendon rupture
- Invasion of joint, destroys articular cartilage and capsular structures
- Severe disintegration of joint structure, leads to fibrous ankylosis, which ultimately leads to bony ankylosis
- Surgical stabilization of the joint, in functional position is indicated
- Large bony lesion adjacent to a joint, removal of focus may preserve joint function
- Surgery of gouty lesions, demands observance of following principles:
  - Avoid local anesthesia, as it might impair local blood supply
  - Incision should be made parallel, with course of blood vessels

- Sharp dissection
- Loose suturing, to allow escape of liquified deposits
- Pressure dressing
- Avoidance of prolonged splinting, which encourages ankylosis.

PSEUDOGOUT (CHONDROCALCINOSIS)

- Pseudogout arthritis, occurs due to deposition of crystals of calcium pyrophosphate dihydrate deposits (CPPD) in synovium or articular cartilage or menisci
- Clinically it resembles gout, but serum uric acid is normal
- Most commonly affected joint is knee.

Investigation

X-ray

Calcified spots in menisci and articular cartilage.

Synovial Fluid Analysis

Rhomboid shaped crystals, under microscope.

Treatment

Respond to indomethacin.

HYDROXYAPATITE CRYSTALS DEPOSITION DISEASE

Clinical Presentation

- It may present, as primary crystal induced arthopathy or secondary to trauma or degenerative joint disease
- Hydroxyapatite crystals are deposited in soft tissue of joint space, rotator cuff tendons or bursa
- Shoulder and knee are commonly involved
- Hydroxyapatite crystals are non-birefringent
- Radiologically, the disease appears as radio opaque calcification, in a local tumor mass like fashion.

Treatment

- Treatment is with nonsteroidal anti-inflammatory drugs (NSAIDs), colchicine and oral and intra-articular corticosteroids and physiotherapy
- Large tumor mass-like deposits, may some time need excision.

9 Degenerative and Inflammatory Disorders

- Osteoarthritis
- Rheumatoid Arthritis
- Seronegative Arthropathies

OSTEOARTHRITIS

Introduction

It is characterized by degenerative changes in articular cartilage of diarthrodial joints and subsequent new bone formation at the articular margins.

Incidence

- By the age of 40 years, about 40 percent of population have radiological sign of osteoarthritis of major weight-bearing joints (knee, hip)
- Fifty percent of these will be symptomatic.

Types of Osteoarthritis

Predisposing Factors

- Trauma
- Metabolic disorders
- Infection
- Hemophilia
- Congenital and developing disorders, rheumatoid arthritis, etc.

Etiology

Age

Process begins in second decade of life and by that age 80 percent have radiological evidence of disease.

Sex

Females, affected more than males.

Hereditary

Articular expression of generalized constitutional condition from inherited metabolic abnormalities.

Obesity

Is prevalent in obese.

Biomechanical Factors

- Structural abnormalities, like articular, dislocation, acetabular dysplasia, slipped epiphysis and Perthe's disease, will cause abnormally high pressure over the articular surfaces and predispose it for early degeneration
- Similarly malalignment of joints, like genu varum, genu valgum and menisceal tears, leads to abnormal stresses, predisposing the joint to early degeneration.

Hormonal Effects

- Acromegaly notably effects articular cartilage
- Diabetics are often prone for degenerative arthritis.

Chemical Injury

Corticosteroids injected in joint or given systemically, are known to reduce synthesis and loss of prostaglandins (PG).

Repeated Intrasynovial Hemorrhage

Iron and blood pigments, alters physical and chemical properties of cartilage, causing early degeneration, e.g. hemophilic arthritis.

Areas of Involvement

- Varies from person to person and from joint to joint
- In females, distal interphalangeal (DIP) and first metacarpophalangeal (MCP) joints are most commonly involved
- In males, hips are most commonly involved
- In females, knees are most commonly involved
- Any synovial joint may be affected, but those under compression are more prone
- Inflammatory process, like rheumatoid arthritis destroys articular cartilage
- Metabolic disorders, like gouty deposits of urates and alkaptonuric ochronosis deposits, makes cartilage susceptible to destruction.

Changes with Age (Primary Osteoarthritis)

Fibrillation of articular cartilage is age related and is peculiar to certain locations (e.g. hip, inferiomedial to fovea and beneath femoral head; patellar medial facet), can lead to osteoarthritis.

Cellular Changes

- In growing epiphyseal cartilage mitotic activity is present, but in adults there is no change in cell count in superficial zone of cartilage, but increased cellularity is evident in transitional zone, marking the beginning of osteoarthritis
- *Collagen ageing*: With increasing maturity of collagen fibers
- *Protein and glycosaminoglycan synthesis*: Balance between rate of synthesis and rate of degradation is altered with ageing
- *Chemical composition*: Chondrotin-6-sulphate forms the principal GAG, which with advancing age decreases to the level of less than 5 percent in elderly.

Physical Alterations

- Permeability of articular cartilage decrease, with advancing age up to 40 years, then a variable increase in permeability takes place
- Elastic properties of articular cartilage also suffers, with advancing age
- Tensile stiffness of cartilage refers to forces parallel to articular surface, produced as a secondary effect of compression and ability to resist such force is the function of articular cartilage, which decreases with advancing age.

Pathophysiology

- Degeneration of hyaline cartilage is the first lesion
- Spotty degeneration of hyaline cartilage exposing subchondral bone, with healthy areas intervening
- Normal areas of cartilage at periphery along with perichondrium, stimulates to overcome losses
- As a result nonarticular area elevates above remainder and projects circumferentially known as "lipping".

Formation of Osteophytes

- The cartilaginous outgrowths are ossified, to form osteophytes
- Local periosteal new bone formation, particularly around capsular attachment, also leads to osteophyte formation.

Synovitis and Capsulitis

- Detached cartilaginous flakes lies freely in joint. Cavity readily absorbs the synovial membrane and leads to synovitis, followed by fibrosis
- Proteoglycans leaks from damaged articular cartilage, leads to irritation of synovial membrane and capsule, which undergoes hyperplasia.

Subchondral Sclerosis

- Proliferation of blood vessels along subchondral bone leads to osteoporosis initially, followed by invasion of larger blood vessels, leading to subchondral sclerosis
- Formation of subchondral cyst
- Edema of subchodral bone marrow, followed by formation of mucinous fatty marrow, with dilatation of surrounding sinusoids leads to cyst formation, which increases in size by osteoclastic activity and finally sclerosis around margins of cyst appears due to osteoblastic activity
- Another theory regarding formation of cyst, is from herniation of synovial fluid through denuded subchondral bone
- An osteoarthritic joint rarely gets completely ankylosed, but gross proliferation with presence of osteophytes out growths and dense capsular fibrosis, may impede free movement of joint, which may simulate some degree of fusion, which in fact does not exist.

Formation of Loose Bodies

Cartilaginous tags occasionally get detached and form loose bodies.

Eburnation

- Exposed bone ends of articular surface are subjected to considerable friction, which leads to bone trabeculae in immediate neighborhood fracture, leading to obliterated marrow spaces
- Changes involved in only a thin layer abutting on joint and this layer gradually becomes more smooth and polished, as a result of continuous rubbing. This process is known as eburnation.

Stages of Osteoarthritis (As Seen Under Light Microscopy)

Early Stage

- Surface irregularities or fibrillation with small clefts not extending beyond superficial zone
- Slight hypercellularity
- Minimal loss of mucopolysaccharides.

Moderately Advanced

- More extensive loss of surface
- Clefts extending into middle zone and occasionally into calcified zone
- Loss of mucopolysaccharides, extending into middle zone
- Hypercellularity in clusters of cells or chondrocyte clones.

Advanced Changes

- Thickness of cartilage is reduced
- Clefts may extend down to subchondral bone
- Mucopolysaccharides, markedly reduced through entire thickness of cartilage
- In some areas, complete loss of cartilage with exposure of thick, eburnated subchondral bone.

Clinical Features

Joint Involvement

- Primary generalized osteoarthrosis
- DIP joints of hand with Heberden's nodes
- More or less symmetrical involvement of other joints, like knee, MP joints of foot, posterior spinal joints and elbow joint.

Primary Osteoarthritis

Most commonly affected joints are:

- Knee joint
- Hip joint
- CP joint of thumb
- MP joint of great toe
- Posterior spinal joint
- Elbow joint.

Radiological Appearance

Stage I

Hyperemia with periarticular osteoporosis.

Stage II

Reduction in joint space.

Stage III

Osteophytes formation with subchondral sclerocystic changes.

Stage IV

Complete loss of joint space with or without subluxation.

Signs and Symptoms

Joint Pain

- Stiffness
- Difficulty in movement.

Deformities (Fig. 9.1)

Investigations

- Routine investigations in primary OA, are usually in normal limits
- Other investigations are dependent upon the predisposing factors, if present.

Management

Conservative

- Rest
- Range of motion exercises
- Abstinence from weight-bearing
- Vertical load reduction
- Traction
- Physical therapy
- Orthotics

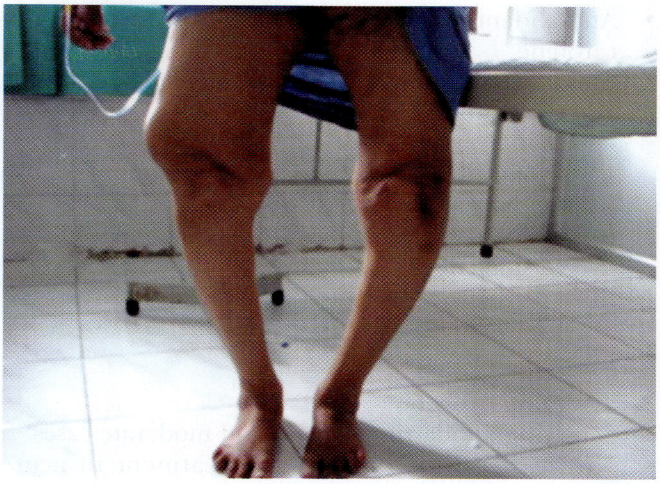

Fig. 9.1: Deformity of limb present in osteoarthritis

- Heat therapy
- Graduated exercise.

Drug Therapy

- NSAIDs, such as diclofenac and aceclofenac, produces their anti-inflammatory and analgesic effect, by inhibiting cyclo-oxygenace and thus preventing production of prostaglandins from arachidonic acid
- In addition, acelofenac has shown some stimulatory effects on cartilage matrix synthesis, that may be linked to ability of drug, to inhibit IL-1 activity
- Chondro synthesis drugs, i.e. glucasamine and amino monosaccharide
- Contains component of all human connective tissue
- Used in body to synthesize GAGS and glycoproteins
- Proteoglycan and HA synthesis
- Imparts high electronegativity in cartilage resulting in water retentions
- Maintains viscosity of synovial fluid—hyaluronate formation
- Anti-inflammatory property
- Active principle, e.g. chondroitin 4 and 6 sulfate
- Chondroitin
- Nonspecific slow acting chondro-protective, but helps in chondro synthesis
- Supplement action of glucosamine
- Inhibits proinflammatory prostaglandin/leukotrienes
- Inhibit hyaluronidase enzyme
- Breakdown HA molecule
- Viscosity of synovial fluid
- Chondroprotective and disease modifying drugs
- Inhibit pain, by inhibiting synthesis of cytokines
- Improves mobility, by stimulating the production of collagen II and proteoglycan
- Reduces stiffness, by stimulating the production of hyaluronic acid

- Antioxidant vitamins, e.g. vitamins C, E and beta-carotene
- Antioxidant minerals are selenium, manganese, zinc and their properties are:
  - Chondroprotective
  - Given with glucosamine and chondroitin
  - Building blocks in GAGS synthesis
  - *Efficacy:* Well tested
  - No side effects.

Semi-invasive Treatment Corticosteroids

Intra-articular Cortisone

- Temporary relief
- Satisfying and lasting in mild and moderate cases
- No response to conservative treatment in acute inflammatory phase
- Severe OA.

Local Steroid

Shows good result, for pain in pericapsular site (outside joint), e.g. Pes anserinus and biceps (Repeated long acting depot preparation)

- Risk of joint infection
- Hypo-pigmentation
- Subcutaneous atrophy
- Osteonecrosis.

Repeated Long Acting Depot Preparation

Intra-articular injection of hyaluronic acid or visco-supplementation therapy

- Safe and effective
- Pain, improves joints function for months
- Five injections, weekly
- Shock absorber. Joint capable of withstanding mechanical stress
- Molecular weight
- Greater viscoelasticity
- Better response.

Other Methods of Treatment

- Surgery
- Synovectomy
- Arthrodesis
- Osteotomies
- Arthroscopic lavage with debridement
- Arthroplasties.

Osteotomies

Features of Osteotomies

- Correction of mechanical malalignment
- Brings into contact nondamaged articular surface, hence reducing friction and pain

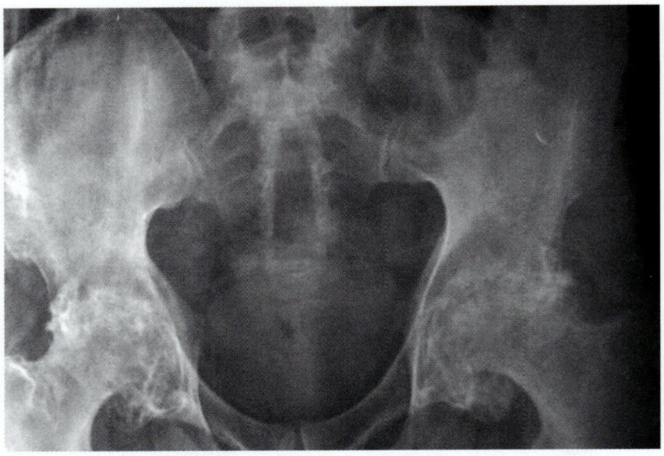

Fig. 9.2: X-ray, showing hip osteoarthritis

- Alters weight-bearing and joint reaction forces
- Decongests venous stasis and venous hypertension in metaphyseal trabecular bone.

Hip Osteoarthritis (Fig. 9.2)

Valgus Osteotomy (Figs 9.3A to C)

Varus Osteotomy (Figs 9.4A to D)

Total Hip Replacement (Figs 9.5 to 9.6)

Osteoarthritis of Knee

High Tibial Osteotomy (Figs 9.7 to 9.8)

Total Knee Replacement (Fig. 9.9)

OA Elbow (Figs 9.10A and B)

RHEUMATOID ARTHRITIS

Introduction

It is a systemic disease of young and middle aged adults, characterized by:

- Proliferation and destructive changes in synovial membrane
- Periarticular structure
- Skeletal muscles and perineural sheaths
- Eventually, the joints are fused and ankylosed.

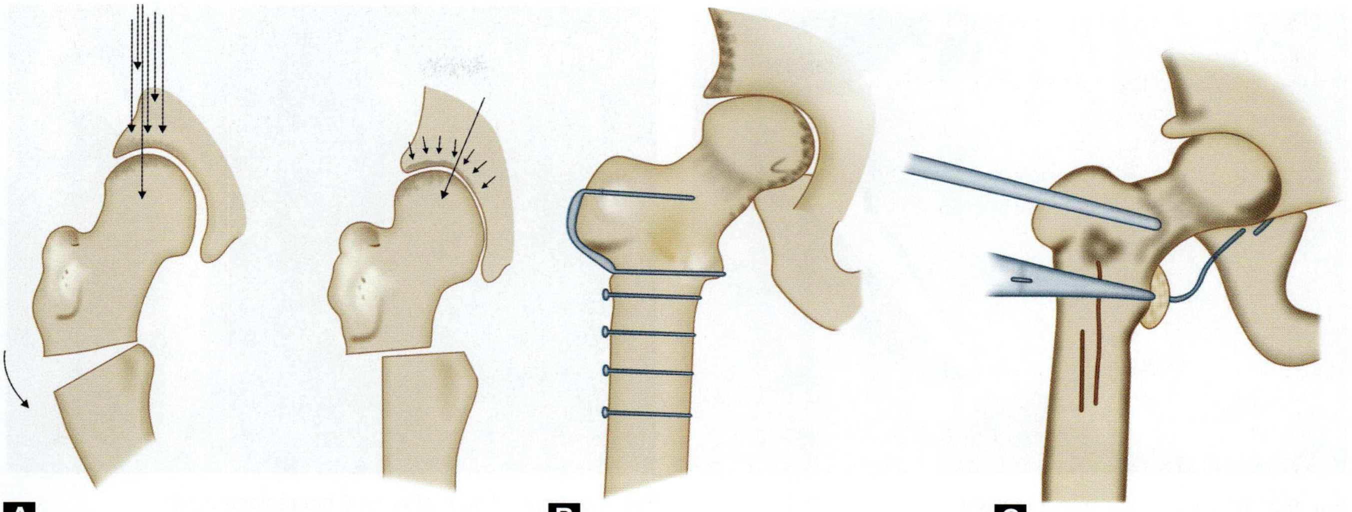

A B C

Figs 9.3A to C: Valgus osteotomy

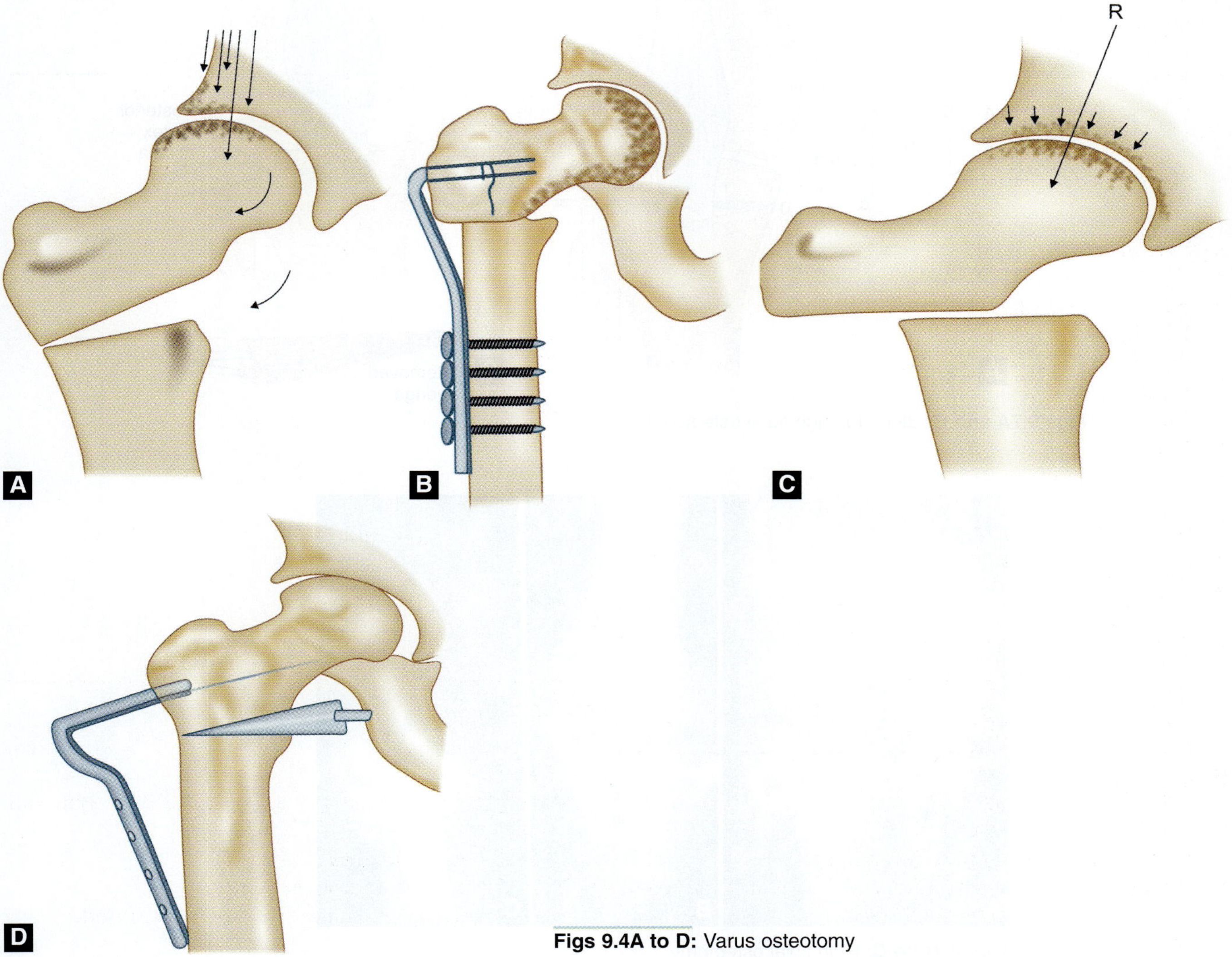

A B C D

Figs 9.4A to D: Varus osteotomy

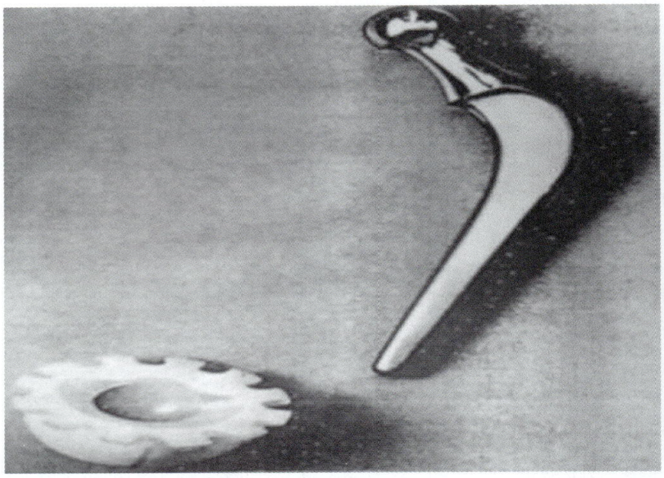

Fig. 9.5: Total hip replacement implant

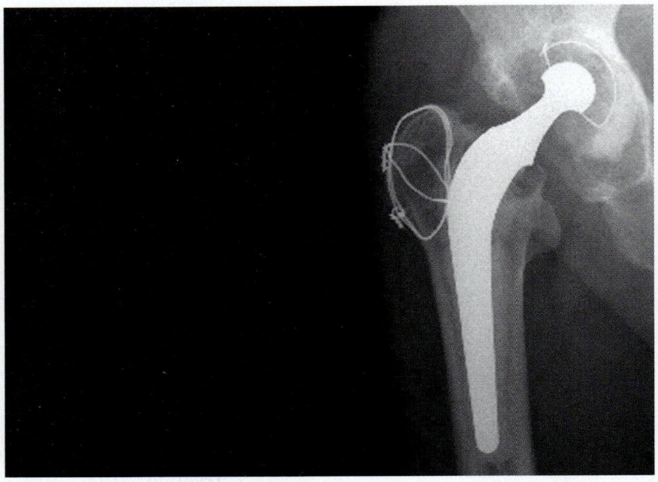

Fig. 9.6: Image taken after total hip replacement

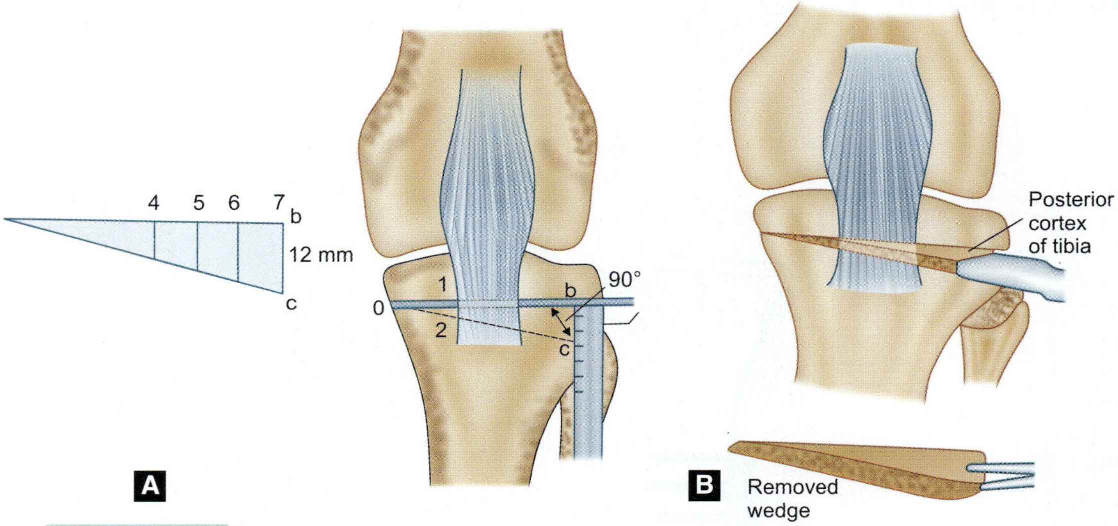

Figs 9.7A and B: Steps for high tibial osteotomy

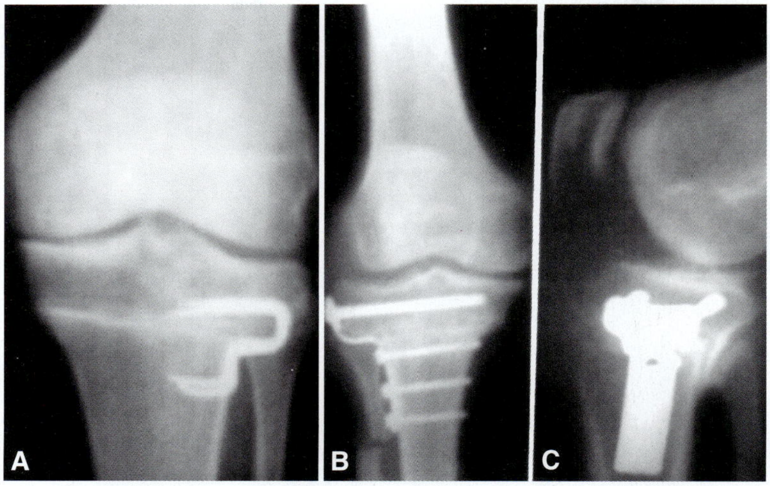

Figs 9.8A to C: High tibial osteotomy

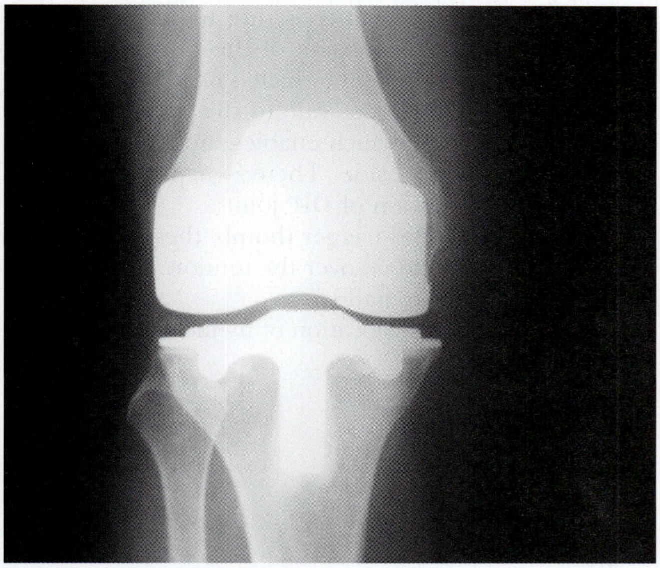

Fig. 9.9: Total knee replacement

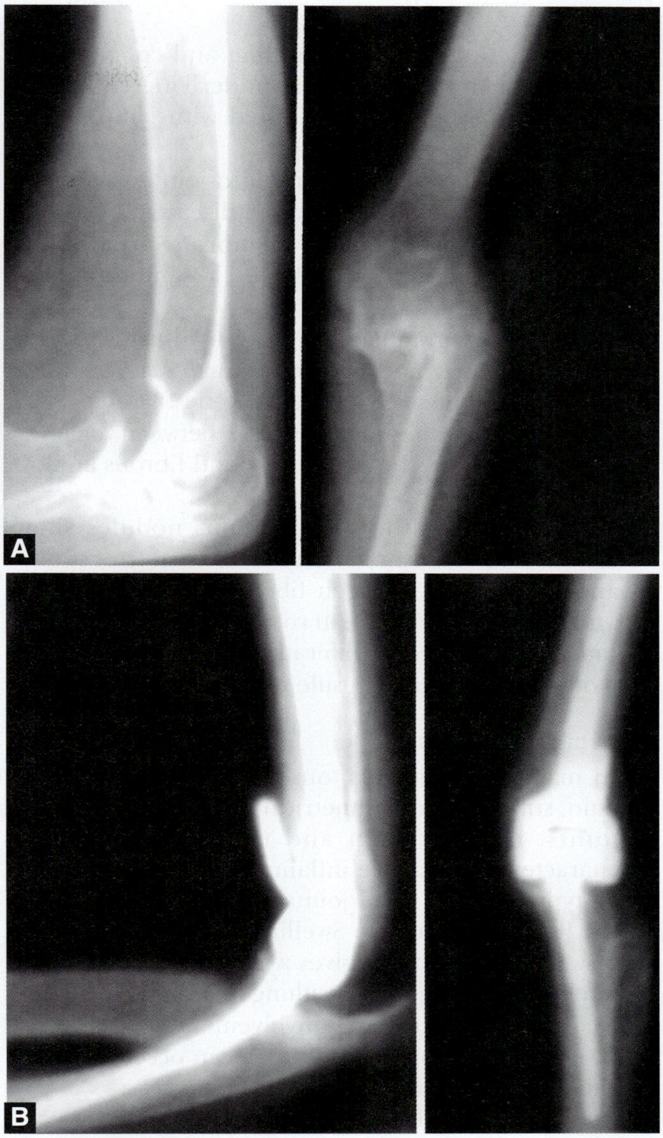

Figs 9.10A and B: X-ray film, showing OA elbow

Etiology

- *Sex:* Eighty percent affected are women, male to female ratio is 1:3
- *Age:* No age is exempted, mean age is 40 years
- The exact cause is unknown, theoretical causes include the following:
  - *Infectious:* Hemolytic and non-hemolytic types of streptococci, had been isolated from joint and regional lymph nodes
  - *Endocrines:* This is suggested by response to adrenocortical steroids
  - *Allergic:* Rheumatoid arthritis, frequently exhibits various allergic manifestations, eosinophilia is frequently present
  - *Genetic influence:* Increasing evidence, which suggest that the disease is triggered by T-lymphocytes activation in a genetically predisposed individual, with defined HLA-class II haplotypes (HLA DR4, HLA DR1)
  - *Immune over reactivity:* RA is characterized by persistent cellular activation, autoimmunity and the presence of immune complexes, at site of articular and extra-articular lesions.

Pathogenesis

- Most accepted theory is of immunogenic response, taking place in the synovium
- An unknown exogenous antigen encounters the defender cells, the lymphocytes, which are transformed into plasma cells
- The plasma cells manufactures antibodies
- Antibodies, antigen and complement combine to form complex
- Scavenger phagocytic cell, engulf the complex, as these phagocytes contain small enzyme sac (lysosomes), that destroys the complex
- Some of the lysozomes, escapes the phagocyte cells and their protease attack the cartilage and synovium
- Destruction of tissue produces debris, that calls for more phagocyte activity to remove the debris
- Consequently, more phagocyte activity cell pour out more enzymes, which create more destruction and further inflammation and the arthritic changes become self perpetuating
- The inflammed synovium forms pannus, a granulomatous mass, that grows over the destroyed cartilage, tendon and ligaments.

Pathology

- The earliest changes are swelling and congestion of synovial membrane and the underlying connective tissue, which becomes infiltrated with lymphocytes, plasma cells and macrophages
- Effusion of the synovial fluid into joint space, takes place during active phase of the disease
- Hypertrophy of synovial membrane occurs with formation of lymphoid follicles, resembling active lymph node changes
- Inflammatory granulation tissue (pannus) is formed, spreading over and under the articular cartilage, which is progressively eroded and destroyed
- Later, fibrous adhesion takes place between the layers of pannus across the joint space and fibrous anklosis may occur
- Microscopically, the subcutaneous nodules shows central area of fibrinoid necrosis, consisting of swollen and fragmented collagen fibers, fibrinous exudates and cellular debris, surrounded by palisade of radically arranged proliferating mononuclear cells
- Nodules have loose capsule of fibrous tissues.

Clinical Features

- In majority of patients, onset is insidious with joint pain, stiffness and symmetrical swelling of peripheral joints, but rest pain and morning stiffness is characteristic of active inflammatory arthritis
- In typical cases, small joints of fingers and toes are the first to be affected. Swelling of proximal, but not distal joints of fingers gives a spindled appearance
- Swelling of MTP joints, resulting in broadening of toes
- As the disease progresses, involvement of elbow, wrist, shoulder, knee, ankle joints, etc. can occurs
- The hip joint is involved late in the disease
- Cervical spine affection is common
- As the disease progresses muscle atrophy, tendon sheath and joint destruction, results in limitation of joint motion, joint instability occurs
- Characteristic deformities, like flexion contracture of small joints of hand and feet, besides other joints, i.e. knee, hip and elbow occurs.

Deformities

Rheumatoid Hand

The following are some of the common deformities seen in the hand:

- Symmetrical peripheral joint swelling of metacarpophalangeal and interphalangeal joints
- Ulnar deviation of the hand is due to rupture of the collateral ligaments at the metacarpophalangeal joints, which enable the extensor tendons to slip from their grooves towards the ulnar side
- Boutonniere's deformity is due to the rupture of central extensor expansion of the fingers, resulting in flexion at the PIP joint, which is nearest the knuckle
- Swan neck deformity is due to the rupture of volar plate of PIP joint, which enables the tendons to slip towards the dorsal side. There is hyperextension of PIP joint and flexion of DIP joint
- Trigger fingers and trigger thumb, these deformities are due to the nodule over the tendon
- Z-deformity of the hand
- Subluxation and dislocation of metacarpophalangeal joints.

Rheumatoid Foot

- Callosity under PIP joint
- Plantar callosity
- Claw toes
- Hammer toe
- Rheumatoid nodules
- Flattening of longitudinal arch
- Hallus valgus.

Other Joints

In knee, initially there is gross swelling due to synovitis, but in later stages patient may develop fibrous ankylosis or bony ankylosis, due to destruction of cartilage by pannus. Similarly other joints are involved and frequency of joints involvement is shown in Table 9.1.

Extra-articular Features

Two or more features are present in 75 percent of cases:

- Subcutaneous nodules
- Widespread vasculitis
- Keratoconjunctivitis sicca or scleritis
- Heart affection like arrhythmias and heart block.

Investigations

- Hemoglobin is low
- WBC is decreased
- ESR raised
- Increased C-reactive protein
- Increased alkaline phosphatase.

Table 9.1: Frequency of involvement of joints

MCP/MTP/PIP joints	90%
Knee, ankle, wrist	80%
Shoulder	60%
Hip, acromion process and elbow joint	50%
Cervical spine	40%
Temporomandibular joint and sternomastoid joint	30%
Cricoarytenoid joint	10%

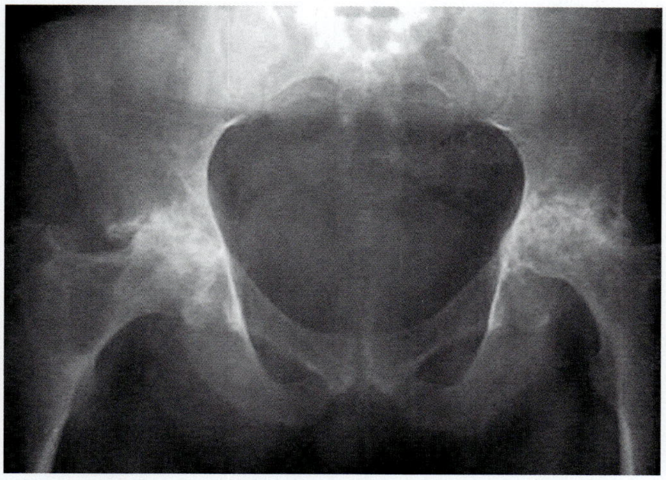

Fig. 9.11: X-ray showing RA

- Increased platelets
- Decreased serum albumin
- Synovial fluid analysis
- Serological tests
  - Latex fixation test
  - Inhibition test.

X-ray (Fig. 9.11)

- Juxta-articular osteoporosis
- Erosion of joint margin
- Joint space is decreased
- Deformities of joints
- Subcondral erosion and cyst formation
- Fibrous and bony ankylosis, develop in late stages.

Criteria for Diagnosis

- Morning stiffness
- Pain on motion or tenderness in at least one joint
- Swelling (soft tissue thickening or fluid, not bony outgrowth alone) in at least one joint continuously for not less than 6 weeks
- Symmetrical joint swelling
- Subcutaneous nodules
- X-ray changes, typical of rheumatoid arthritis
- Positive latex fixation test
- Poor mucin clot
- Characteristic histological changes in synovial membrane
- Characteristic histological changes in nodules.

Classic case of RA: Any seven criteria for at least 6 weeks

Definite case of RA: Any five criteria for at least 6 weeks

Probable case of RA: Any three criteria for at least 4 weeks.

Table 9.2: ACR clinical classification criteria for rheumatoid arthritis

Morning stiffness ≥ 1 hour
Arthritis of 3 or more of the following joints: right or left PIP, MCP, wrist, elbow, knee, ankle, and MTP joints
Arthritis of wrist, MCP, or PIP joint
Symmetric involvement of joints
Rheumatoid nodules over bony prominences, or extensor surfaces, or in juxta-articular regions
Positive serum rheumatoid factor
Radiographic changes including erosions or bony decalcification localized in or adjacent to the involved joints

American College of Rheumatoid, Clinical Classification Criteria for Rheumatoid Arthritis

American college of rheumatoid (ACR) clinical classification criteria for rheumatoid arthritis, using findings of history, physical examination, laboratory and radiographic findings is described in Table 9.2 and Flow chart 9.1. For making the diagnosis of rheumatoid arthritis, four of the below enumerated criteria must be present out of which at least one must be present for a minimum of 6 weeks.

ACR Classification Criteria for Determining Progression of Rheumatoid Arthritis

It is shown in Table 9.3.

Flow chart 9.1: ACR clinical classification criteria for rheumatoid arthritis

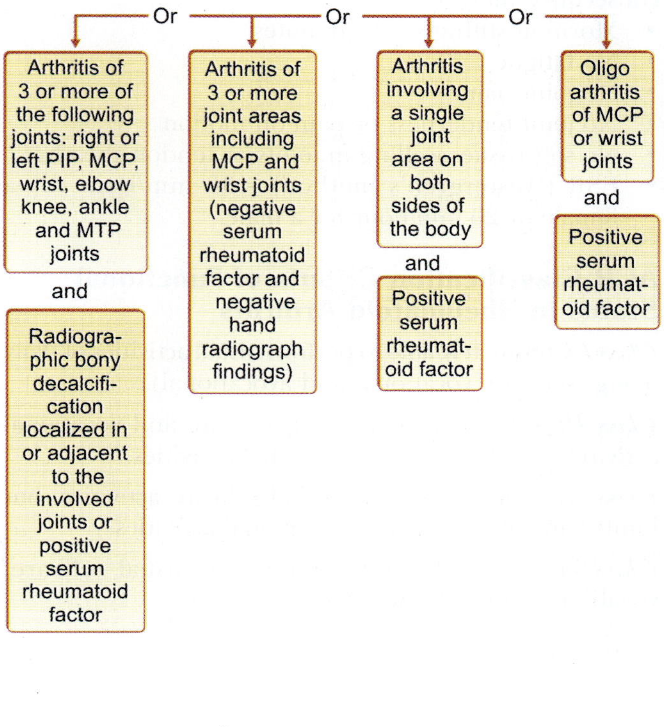

Table 9.3: ACR Classification criteria for determining progression of RA

Stage I	**Early**
	• No destructive changes on roentgenographic examination • Radiographic evidence of osteoporosis may be present
Stage II	**Moderate**
	• Radiographic evidence of osteoporosis, with or without slight slub • No joint deformities; slight cartilage destruction may be present • Adjacent muscle atrophy • Extra-articular soft tissue lesions, such as nodules and tenosynovitis may be present
Stage III	**Severe**
	• Radiographic evidence of cartilage and bone destruction, in addition to osteoporosis • Joint deformity, such as subluxation, ulnar deviation, or hyperextension, without fibrous or bony ankylosis • Extensive muscle atrophy • Extra-articular soft tissue lesions, such as nodules and tenosynovitis may be present
Stage IV	**Terminal**
	• Fibrous or bony ankylosis • Stage III criteria

ACR Classification Criteria for Determining Clinical Remission in Rheumatoid Arthritis

Five or more of the following are present for at least two consecutive months

- Morning stiffness <15 minutes
- No fatigue
- No joint pain
- No joint tenderness or pain on motion
- No soft tissue swelling in joints or tendon sheaths
- ESR (Westergren's method) <30 mm/hour for a female or 20 mm/hour for a male.

ACR Classification Criteria of Functional Status in Rheumatoid Arthritis

Class I: Completely able to perform usual activities of daily living (selfcare, vocational and avocational).

Class II: Able to perform usual selfcare and vocational activities, but limited in avocational activities.

Class III: Able to perform usual selfcare activities, but limited in vocational and avocational activities.

Class IV: Limited ability to perform usual selfcare, vocational and avocational activities.

Management

Aims of Treatment

- To keep inflammatory treatment to minimum
- To keep constitutional symptoms to minimum
- Appropriate splinting to prevent deformities
- Surgical measures to correct deformity.

Drug Therapy

- *Analgesics and anti-inflammatory:* NSAIDs, e.g. aspirin, ibuprofen, diclofenac sodium
- *Disease modifying antirheumatic drugs (DMARDs):* Injectable gold and oral gold (sodium aurothiomalate), penicillamine, sulphasalazine, antimalarials (dapsone and levamisole).

Surgery Methods

- Synovectomy
- Osteotomy
- Arthrodesis
- Arthoplasty.

SERONEGATIVE ARTHROPATHIES

Introduction

Seronegative arthropathies can be defined as an acute or chronic condition with characteristic involvement of axial joints, absence of RA factor and with HLA abnormality.

Clinical Entities

- Ankylosing spondylitis
- Reiter's disease
- Psoriatic arthritis
- Enteropathic arthritis
- Ulcerative colitis
- Crohn's disease
- Whipples disease
- Behcet's syndrome

Etiology

- Exact pathological mechanism is not known
- Genetic factors play an important role (the most complete evidence for familial aggregation is that for ankylosing spondylitis, children of a person with HLA-B27 have 50 percent chance of carrying the same antigen)
- *Salmonella, Shigella, Chlamydia, Yersinia* play an important role in the pathogenesis of this group of arthritis
- Virus.

Signs and Symptoms

Articular Features

- Low backache
- Morning stiffness
- Decreasing lumbar lordosis
- Diffuse swelling of fingers and toes
- Enthesopathy.

Common Features of Spondyloarthropathies

- Familial clustering
- Association with HLA-B27
- Axial joint involvement
- Asymmetrical peripheral joint involvement
- Enthesitis
- Extra-articular signs
- Negative rheumatoid factor
- Diagnosis of spondyloarthropathies is shown in Table 9.1

Extra-articular Features

- *Skin lesions:* These include
  - Psoriasis
  - Pitting of nails
  - Penile ulcer
- *Eye lesions*
  - Conjunctivitis
- Bowel disorders and GIT disturbance
- Dysuria
- Urethral discharge.

Diagnosis

Radiological Diagnosis

- Affected joint will show punched out areas, exceeding deep into subchondral bone
- CT scan is indicated, when plane X-ray is normal. Used to see early changes of bone erosion and sclerosis.

Hematological Diagnosis

- HLA-B27 positive in 16 to 100 percent
- RA factor negative.

Reactive Arthritis (Reiter's Arthritis)

Introduction

- Fifteen to thirty percent patients progress from acute to chronic arthritis
- Acute arthritis occur after genitourinary *(Chlamydia)* or gastrointestinal *(Shigella, Campylobacter, Salmonella, Yersinia)* infection
- It is a clinical triad of urethritis, arthritis and conjunctivitis.

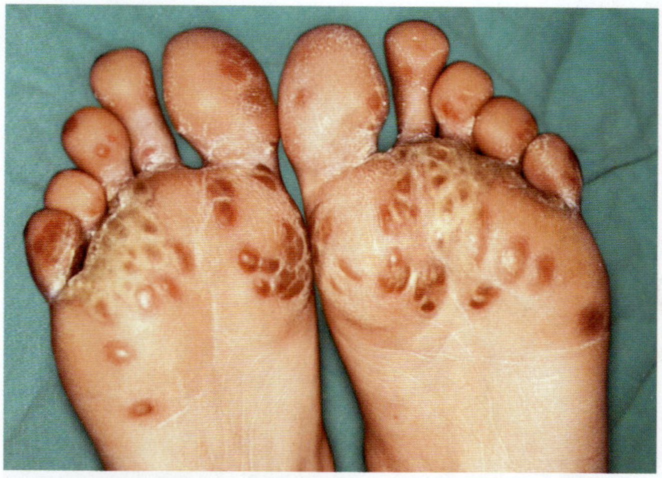

Fig. 9.12: Keratoderma blennorrhagica in Reiter's syndrome—keratoderma blennorrhagica on the soles of a patient with Reiter's syndrome. These lesions, which are indistinguishable from pustular psoriasis, begin as clear vesicles on erythematous bases and progress to macules, papules and nodules

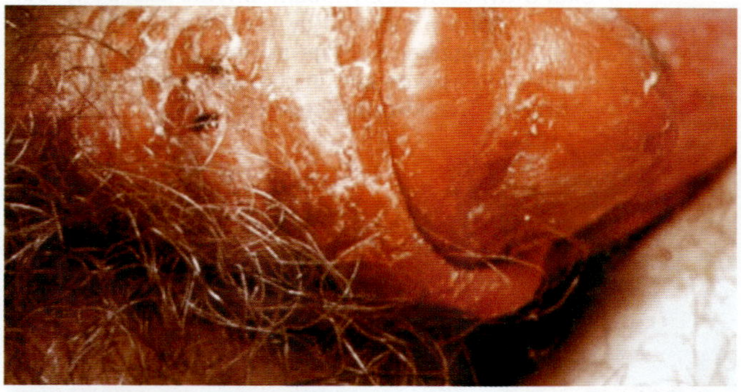

Fig. 9.13: Circinate balanitis in Reiter's syndrome—circinate balanitis characterized by shallow ulcers on the glans penis and the shaft of the penis. The lesions are generally asymptomatic

Clinical Features

- Mono/oligoarthritis
- Conjunctivitis
- Urethritis
- Keratodermititis (Fig. 9.12)
- Balanitis (Fig. 9.13)
- Enthesitis (Fig. 9.14)
- Circinate balanitis
- Dactylitis
- Recurrent attacks common in *Chlamydia*-induced arthritis (Figs 9.12 to 9.15)
- Prognostic signs for chronicity
  - Hip/heel pain
  - High ESR
  - Family history and HLA-B27 positive.

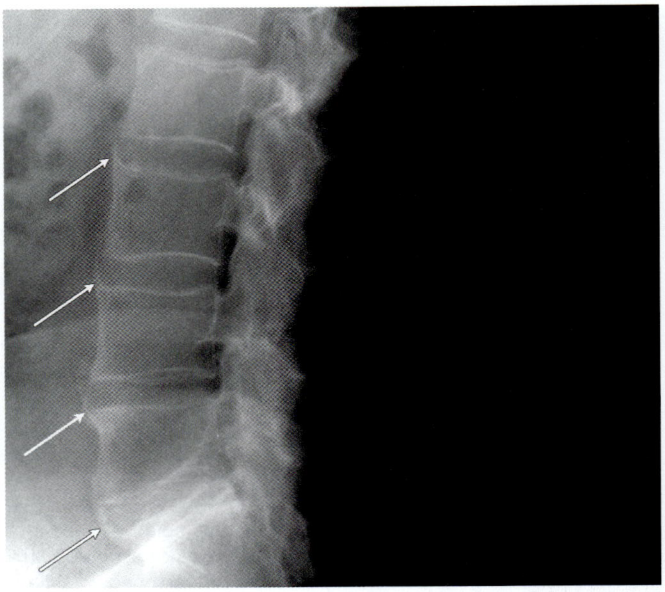

Fig. 9.14: Syndesmophytes in Reiter's syndrome—anterior syndesmophytes of the spine (arrows) in a patient with Reiter's syndrome. Syndesmophytes are bony outgrowths that are induced by an enthesopathy of the spine. The syndesmophytes in Reiter's syndrome and psoriasis are asymmetric, in contrast to their symmetric occurrence in ankylosing spondylitis

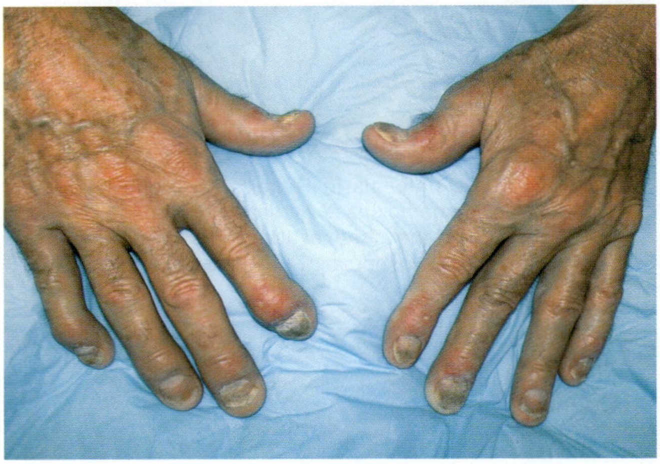

Fig. 9.15: Distal interphalangeal joint involvement in psoriatic arthritis—psoriatic arthritis with distal joint involvement in the third and fifth digits. Onycholysis is also seen in most of the fingernails.

Therapy for Reactive Arthritis

Acute

- NSAID
- Joint injection (if infection excluded)
- Tetracycline for 3 months in *Chlamydia* infection.

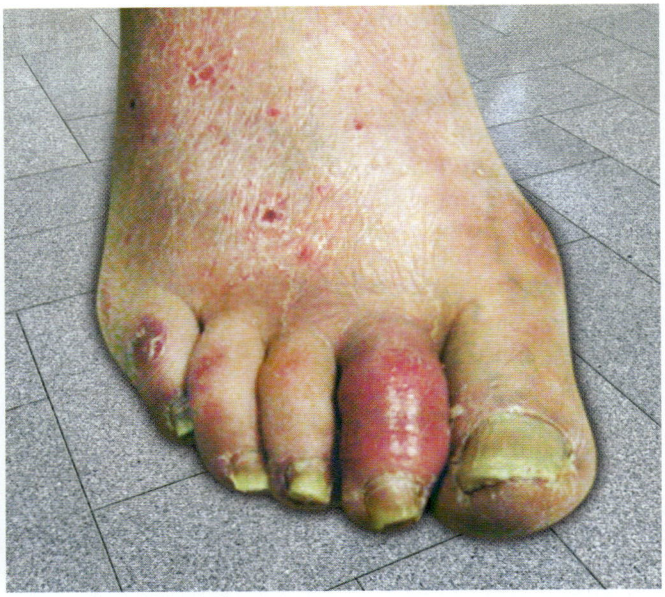

Fig. 9.16: Psoriatic arthritis—this photograph of the foot of a patient with psoriatic arthritis shows an early separation of the nails (onycholysis), swelling of the entire second toe (dactylitis) and some psoriatic skin lesions

Chronic

- NSAID
- DMARD (e.g. sulfasalazine, methotrexate).

Psoriatic Arthritis

Clinical patterns may include one or more of:

- Symmetrical inflammatory arthritis
- Distal interphalangeal involvement
- Axial disease (often involving cervical spine)
- Monoarthritis
- Oligoarthritis
- Skin lesions.

Other features (Figs 9.15 to 9.17)

- Dactylitis, enthesistis, nail pitting
- *Psoriasis:* It may be very mild or extensive and it precedes joint disease (Fig. 9.18)
- Colitis related arthritis.

Pathogenesis

It is an immune mediated disease, with inflamed synovium and infiltrated with T-cells, B-cells and macrophages. Synovium produces cytokines.

Arthritis Mutilans

Widespread shortening of digits (telescoping) occur along with co-existing ankylosis and contractures in other digits. This typical pencil-in-cup position is called "opera glass hand".

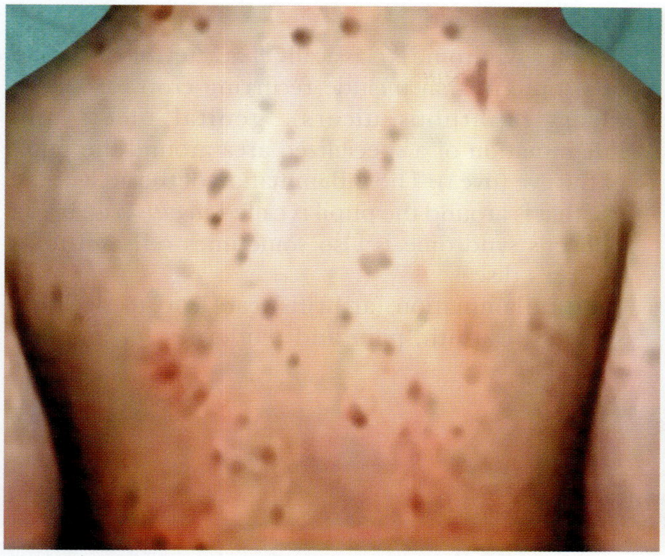

Fig. 9.17: Skin lesions, seen in psoriatic arthritis

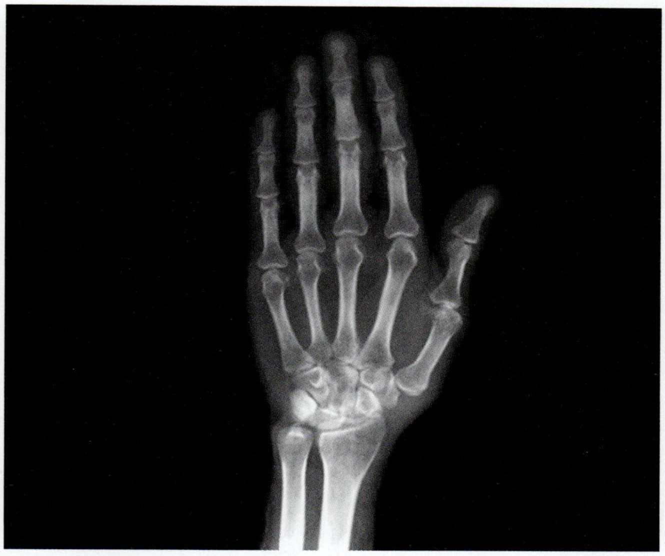

Fig. 9.19: X-ray, showing periostitis of bones

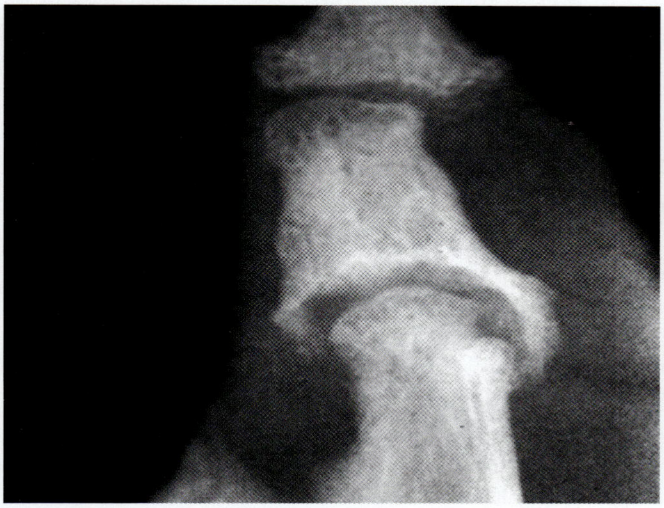

Fig. 9.18: X-ray, showing telescoping of phalanges

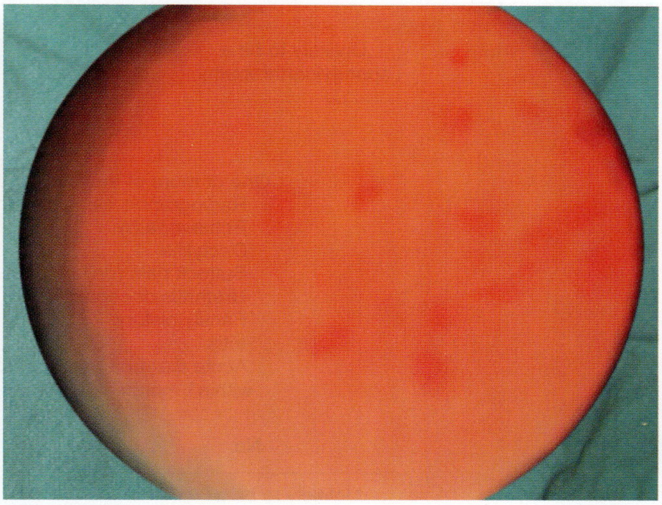

Fig. 9.20: Uveitis

Investigations

- ESR and CRP often elevated
- Mostly seronegative
- Uric acid may be elevated in presence of extensive psoriasis
- HLA-B 27 positive in 50 to 70 percent, with axial involvement. Positive in less than 15 to 20 percent with peripheral joint involvement.

X-ray (Peripheral)

DIP joint involvement with pencil-in-cup deformity. Marginal erosion with adjacent bony proliferation (whiskering), small joint ankylosis is seen with osteolysis of phalanges and metacarpals and telescoping of digits, periostitis of bones (Figs 9.18 and 9.19).

Colitis Related Arthritis

- Can occur in association with Crohn's or ulcerative colitis
- Peripheral arthritis (often a mono or oligoarthritis) improves with colectomy, axial disease does not improve
- Sulfasalazine is helpful.

Differential Diagnosis

- Septic arthritis
- Gout
- Acute onset of other seronegative spondyloarthritis

Investigations

- Raised ESR/CRP
- Aspirate joint to exclude infection/crystals
- Urethral swab, stool culture
- Contact tracing if necessary (Flow chart 9.2).

Behcet's Disease

- Behcet's syndrome is classically characterized as a triad of symptoms that include recurring crops of mouth ulcers (aphthous ulcers), genital ulcers and inflammation of a specialized area around the pupil of the eye (uvea). The inflammation of the area of the eye that is around the pupil is called *uveitis* (Fig. 9.20). Behcet's syndrome is also sometimes referred to as Behcet's disease
- Joint inflammation (arthritis) can lead to swelling, stiffness, warmth, pain and tenderness of joints in

Flow chart 9.2: Diagnosis of spondyloarthropathies

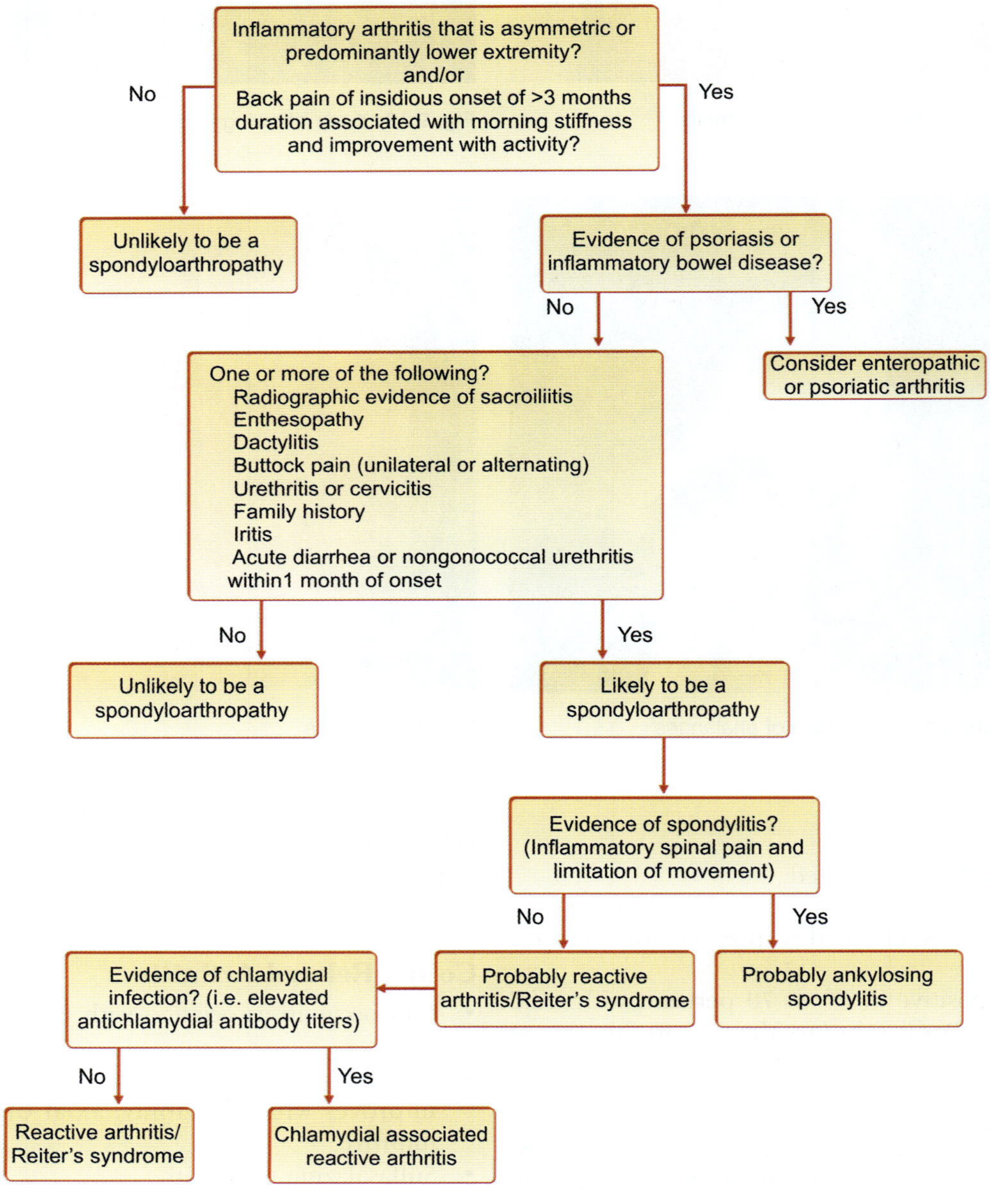

patients with Behcet's syndrome. This occurs in about half of patients with Behcet's syndrome at sometime during their lives. Knees, wrists, ankles and elbows are the most common joints affected

- The symptoms of Behcet's syndrome depend on the area of the body affected. Behcet's syndrome can involve inflammation of many areas of the body. These areas include the arteries that supply blood to the body's tissues. Behcet's syndrome can also affect the veins that take the blood back to the lungs to replenish the oxygen content. Other areas of body that can be affected by the inflammation of Behcet's syndrome include the back of the eyes (retina), brain, joints, skin and bowels.

Marie Stumpell Disease/Bekhterev Disease (Ankylosing Spondylitis)

Definition

It is a chronic progressive inflammatory disease of the sacroiliac joint and the axial skeleton.

For ankylosing spondylitis, please refer to spine section.

10 Infections in Orthopedics

- Pyogenic Osteomyelitis
- Septic Arthritis
- Tuberculosis of Musculoskeletal System
- Tuberculosis of Spine
- Skeletal Tuberculosis of Hip, Knee, Shoulder, Ankle, Elbow and Wrist
- Actinomycosis
- Mycetoma (Maduromycosis)

Introduction

The term indicates inflammation of bone caused by infective organisms.

Common Causative Organisms

- Nonspecific pyogenic organisms, like *Staphylococcus, Streptococcus*
- Specific organisms, like syphilis, tuberculous, typhoid, paratyphoid, causing organism
- Mycetomal (fungal) organisms
- Parasitic infection, e.g. hydatid cyst.

History

- Recognized as an old disease in Egyptian mummies
- Nelaton (1844): Coined the term osteomyelitis
- Hartmann (1855): Hypothesis of thrombosis of main trunk of nutrient artery
- Lennelongue (1879): Metaphyseal infection
- Rodet(1884): Experimental production of acute hematogenous osteomyelitis (AHOM) in animals following IV injection of *Staphylococcus*
- Lexer (1894): Suppuration at the site of trauma, produced experimentally shortly after injecting IV measured dose of cultured *S. aureus* in animals
- Starr (1922): Infection is carried by blood stream till they reach inner capillaries of juxta-epiphyseal region of long bone, lowering the undermined general resistance of patient.

PYOGENIC OSTEOMYELITIS

Following are the routes, through which infection may occur:

- *Hematogenous*: Through blood stream from focus of infection elsewhere
- Direct invasion from atmospheric air, e.g. open fractures
- Spread from neighboring focus of infection, e.g. mastoiditis from middle ear infection and osteomyelitis of mandible from dental root infection
- Osteomyelitis associated with vascular insufficiency, mostly involving lower extremity, as in diabetic neuropathy.

Etiology

Patient Dependent Factor

- Nutritional status of the patient
- Immunological status.

Surgeon Dependent Factor

- Skin preparation
- Operating room environment
- Prophylactic antibiotic therapy.

Skillful Surgery

- Proper dissection
- Proper homeostasis
- Proper tissue handling
- Avoid prolonged surgery.

Clinical Features

- Antecedent infection is usually present
- Irritability, restlessness, headache, vomiting, convulsion, chills, fever, etc.
- Pain and swelling
- Local increase of temperature
- Overlying skin becomes shiny, red and edematous
- Discharging sinus may be present
- Sympathetic synovitis of adjacent joint.

Investigations

- *Laboratory studies:* Complete blood count, including differential blood count and erythrocyte sedimentation rate or C-reactive protein
- Synovial fluid analysis
- Plain X-rays
- CT scan
- MRI
- Bone scan
- Leukocyte scanning technique
- Blood culture study
- Pus culture sensitivity
- Ultrasonography
- Polymerase chain reaction (PCR).

Treatment

- Appropriate antibiotic
- Surgical debridement, incision and drainage
- Polymethylmethacrylate (PMMA) beads
- Closed suction irrigation
- Splinting and rest to the affected area.

Clinical Types

- Acute hematogenous osteomyelitis (Eary acute, late acute)
- Subacute osteomyelitis
- Chronic osteomyelitis

Acute Hematogenous Osteomyelitis

Definition

It is defined as a suppurative process of the bone, caused by pyogenic organisms or simply a pyogenic infection of the cancellous portion of bone.

Etiology

Agent factors

Following myriad of incriminating organisms are responsible for its causation:

- "S" series organism are *S. aureus* (60–85%) and it is most commonly found. *S. haemolyticus* (8–10%), *Salmonella, etc.*
- "P"series organism: *Pseudomonas, Pnemococcus,* etc.
- "C"series: *Clostridium welchii, Coliforms (E. coli),* etc.

Host factors

- *Age:* In children the incidence is 88 percent and in adults 12 percent
- Low socioeconomic groups are more susceptible
- General factors.

Other factors

- Anemia
- Debility
- Infection
- Poor nutrition
- Poor immune status
- Trauma

Local factors

- Hair pin bend vessels
- Metaphyseal hemorrhage
- Defective phagocytosis
- Rapid growth at metaphysis
- Necrotic tissue act as culture media
- Anoxia
- Vasospasm.

Pathophysiology

- Osteomyelitis is initiated from introduction of bacteria from wound or hematogenous spread from pre-existing focus
- Infective embolus enters the nutrient artery and trapped in vessel of small caliber and blocks it
- Small areas of bones become necrotic
- Active hyperemia develops and polymorphonuclear leukocytes are poured out as exudates, to combat the invader
- Hyperemia causes decalcification of surrounding bone
- Proteolytic ferments formed by leukocytes, destroys bacteria, necrotic bone and medullary elements Spread of pus takes place along the medullary canal (Fig. 10.1)
- Along the Harvesian and Volkmann's canal superiolaterally, to form subperiosteal abscess, pus penetrates the periosteum and in the soft tissues
- In the joint, if capsular attachment is up to metaphyseal region, growth plate is resistant to spread of pus, e.g. hip.

Clinical Features

Symptoms

- Fever (95%)
- Sweating

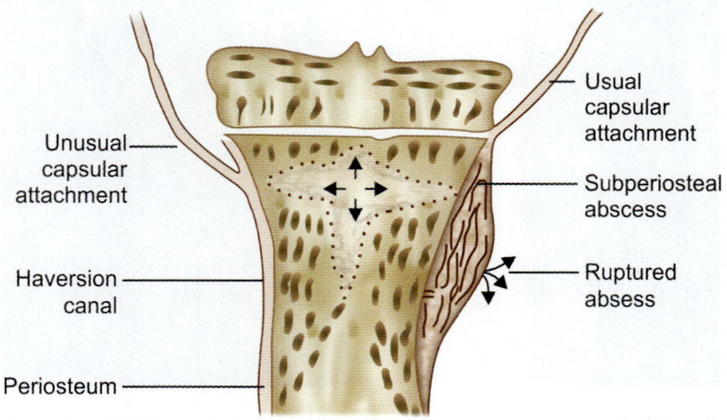

Fig. 10.1: Showing spread of pus through various channels

- Chills and rigors
- Local swelling
- Limitation of movement, due to muscle spasm and pain
- Patient may be in shock.

Signs

- Increased temperature
- Increased pulse rate
- Signs of dehydration
- Tenderness
- Local erythema
- Raised temperature
- Joint effusion
- Decreased movement.

Laboratory Investigations

- Hemoglobin is normal or increased
- ESR, can be normal or increased
- WBC, neutrophil increased
- Films are negative within the first week or 10 days
- Localized area of bone destruction is observed in metaphysic, surrounded by a wide zone of decalcified bone
- Later, within next few weeks the periosteal shadow is elevated and multiple lamination of bone deposition is present parallel to shaft
- Eventually more spongy trabeculae are destroyed giving a moth-eaten appearance, extending for varying degree in the diaphysis in 10 to 20 days (Fig. 10.2)
- The external and internal surface of cortex may display multiple scalloped lesion.

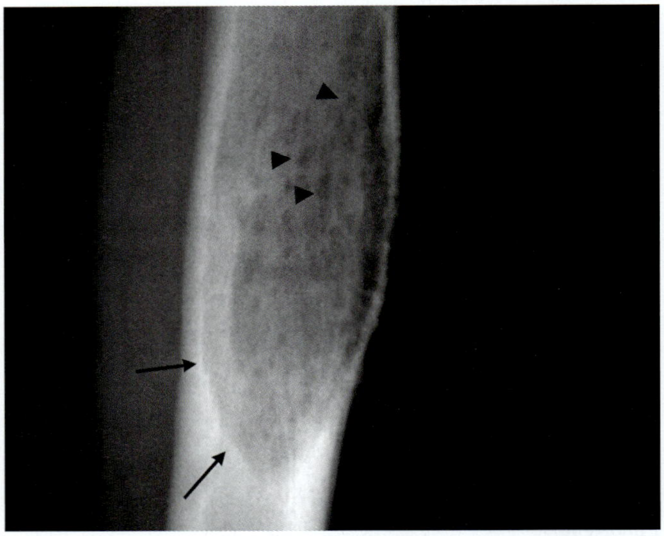

Fig. 10.2: Trabeculae showing moth-eaten appearance (arrow heads) in X-ray film

Bone Scan

- Confirms diagnosis in 24 to 48 hours, after the onset in 90 to 95 percent of cases
- Focal area of uptake.

Blood Culture

- It is positive in 60 percent of cases
- Pus culture demonstrates the bacteria.

Ultrasound

- Soft tissue swelling or subperiosteal abscess
- *Leukergy test:* Leukergy is phenomenon, in which WBC agglomerates in the peripheral vessel. This is a sensitive test.

Management

- Easy to remember as "RESTS"
- Rest in bed, protect the affected part with splint, to alleviate pain and spasm
- Elevation of part, warm and moist packs, to reduce swelling
- *Systemic treatment:* Blood transfusion and intravenous fluid, to correct shock and hypovolemia
- Treatment with antibiotics
- Surgery.

Treatment

Nade's Principle of Treatment of Acute Osteomyelitis

- An appropriate antibiotic is effective before pus formation
- Antibiotics will not sterilize avascular tissue and purulent material that must be removed surgically
- If such removal is effective, then antibiotics should prevent their reformation and therefore primary wound closure should be safe
- Surgery should not damage already ischemic bone and soft tissue
- Antibiotics should be continued after surgery.

Antibiotics

- Penicillins
- β-lactamase inhibitor
- Cephalosporins
- Ciprofloxacin
- Parental antibiotic for 2 weeks
- Oral antibiotic for 4 weeks
- *Local antibiotics:* Antibiotics impregnated with cemented beads, provide high dose of antibiotics locally.

Surgical Treatment

- *Aspiration:* It helps in decompression and the material so obtained may be used to identify the organism and also check for antibiotic sensitivity

- *Incision and drainage:* To drain the subcutaneous abscess
- Multiple drill holes
- Small bone window.

Subacute Osteomyelitis

Features

- Primary infection of bone
- More insidious onset
- Slow in progress
- Less severe symptoms
- Less virulent organism
- Difficult to diagnose.

Types

- Brodie's abscess
- Salmonella osteomyelitis (Typhoid osteomyelitis)
- Sclerosing osteomyelitis garre.

Brodie's Abscess

- In medulla of bone
- Low grade infection, by *Staphylococcus*
- Common-metaphyseal area, proximal end
- End of tibia or distal end femur.

Clinical Features

- Intermittent attacks of pain and swelling
- Local tenderness.

Radiological Findings

X-ray shows osteolytic area in the bone with a ring of diffuse sclerosis.

Treatment

Deroofing and curettage.

Salmonella Osteomyelitis

- Ulna, rib and vertebra are commonly affected
- Occurs after some months or years of typhoid or paratyphoid fever attack
- *Infection:* Hematogenous spread from persistent focus of infection in gallbladder
- Also occurs as a complication of sickle cell anemia.

Causative Factors

- Local bony tenderness
- Moderate signs of inflammation
- Typhoid spine often mimics caries spine.

Investigations

- *X-ray:* Central or cortical area of rarefication with periosteal reaction
- *Blood:* Widal test
- *Treatment:* Surgery always required along with curettage and local application of chloramphenicol/ciplox.

Sclerosing Osteomyelitis of Garre

- Abscesses and sequestra absent
- Affects children and young adults
- Cause unknown, possibly anaerobic bacteria:

Clinical Features

- Intermittent pain of moderate intensity
- Swelling and tenderness over affected bone.

Investigations

- X-ray, shows expanded bone with generalized sclerosis (Fig. 10.3)
- ESR is increased
- *Treatment:* Fenestration of sclerotic bone and antibiotic.

Classification Modified from Roberts

- *Type 1:* Central metaphyseal lesion
- *Type 2:* Eccentric metaphyseal lesion, with cortical erosion
- *Type 3:* Diaphyseal cortical lesion
- *Type 4:* Diaphyseal lesion with periosteal new bone
- *Type 5:* Primary subacute epiphyseal osteomyelitis
- *Type 6:* Subacute osteomyelitis, crosssing physis, to involve both metaphysis and diaphysis.

Chronic Osteomyelitis

Any osteomyelitis lasting for more than 3 weeks is termed as chronic osteomyelitis.

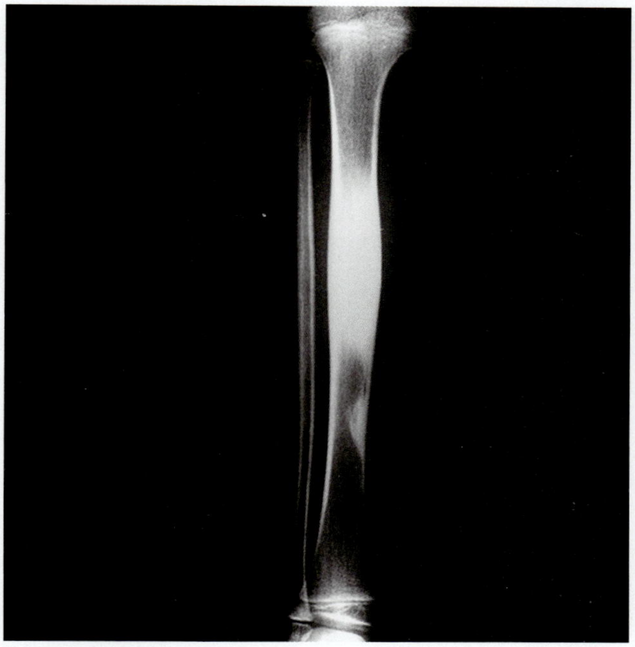

Fig. 10.3: Thickened and distended bone

Etiology

Chronic osteomyelitis, can arise from any one of the following:

- Sequel of acute osteomyelitis (5–10%)
- Following compound fractures
- Following surgery in bone and joints
- Chronic from the beginning (e.g. tuberculosis, syphilis, brodies abscess, etc.)
- Anaerobic organisms (sclerosing OM of Garre)
- Fungal osteomyelitis.

Cierny and Mader Classification

It is based on anatomic and physiologic criteria.

Anatomic Criteria

- Intramedullary (Fig. 10.4)
- Superficial (Fig. 10.5)
- Local (Fig. 10.6)
- Diffuse with segmental bone loss (Fig. 10.7).

Physiologic Criteria

- Normal immune system and adequate soft tissue envelop

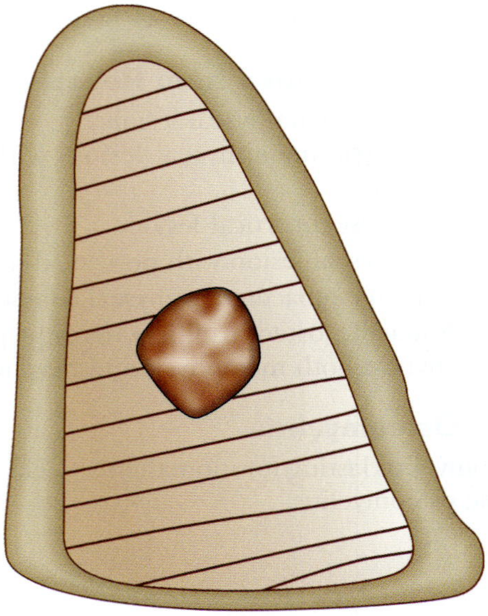

Fig. 10.4: Intramedullary osteomyelitis

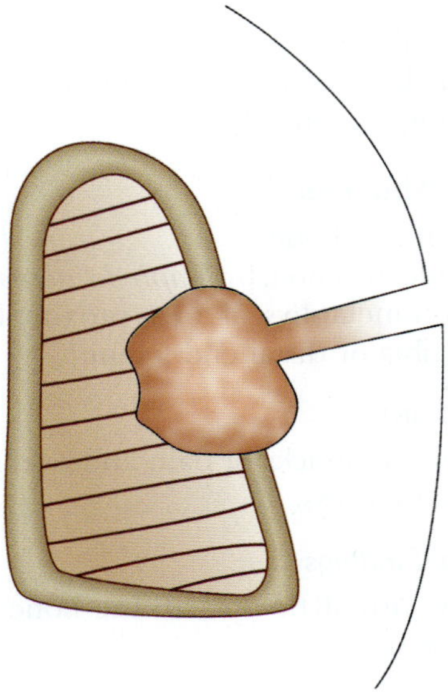

Fig. 10.6: Local osteomyelitis

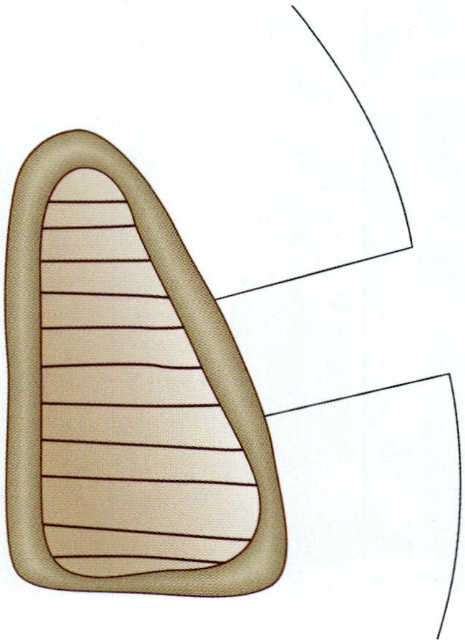

Fig. 10.5: Superficial osteomyelitis

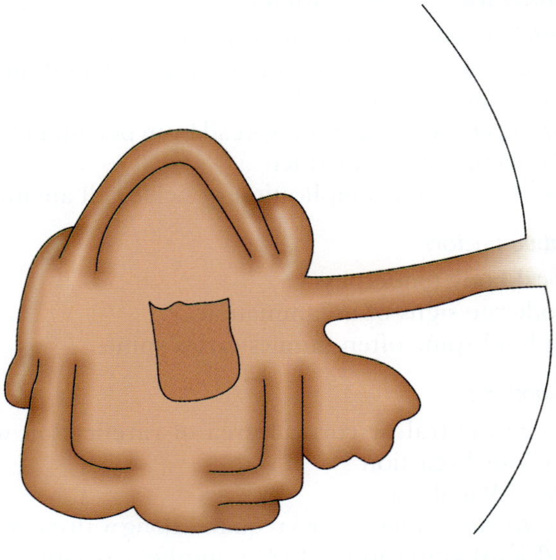

Fig. 10.7: Diffuse osteomyelitis with segmental bone loss

- Local, systemic or both compromised patients
- Immunoincompetent (requires immunosuppressive therapy).

Prognosis

- Type I, II, III and A: Good prognosis
- Type I, II, III and B: Guarded
- Type I, II, III, IV and C: Poor prognosis.

The conventional way of classifying these lesion

- Chronic post-traumatic osteomyelitis, without bone injury
- Chronic post-traumatic osteomyelitis, after open fracture
- Chronic post-traumatic osteomyelitis, after osteosynthesis (postsurgical).

Pathogenesis

- In any infection, if any attempt to repair remains incomplete, then it results in chronicity
- This repair is accomplished by hyperemia of surrounding tissue, which causes decalcification of bone
- Granulation tissue forms and carries osteoclasts and osteoblasts activity
- Necrotic cancellous tissue is readily absorbed and new bone is formed
- Dead bone is gradually absorbed and is detached from living bone to form sequestrum
- Due to loss of blood supply, sequestrum appears dense than the surrounding tissue
- After complete sequestration, the dead fragment lies free within the cavity and is absorbed slowly
- The surrounding living bone attempt to wall off infection by forming a thick, dense wall, called involucrum. It has multiple openings the cloaca, through which exudates debris, sequestra pass through sinus tract to the surface
- Constant destruction of soft tissue leads to cicatrix formation and skin becomes thin and distorted
- The skin epithelium grows inward and line sinus tract. Later forms epithelioma of sinus tract. After sequestrum is discharged, the sinus tract closes and cavity may feel with new bone
- In adults the cavity may persist and harbors organism and may not correlate with cultures of bone biopsy.

What is Sequestrum?

- It is a piece of dead bone, separated from healthy bone. It has no periosteal covering and outer surface is smooth and shiny. Inner surface is rough and edges are serrated because of osteoclastic absorption
- Radiologically, sequestrum appears as a dense irregular piece of bone, surrounded by radiolucent area.

Formation of Sequestrum

Formation of sequestrum is shown in Figure 10.8.

Types

- Feathery sequestrum, e.g. pyogenic infection (Fig. 10.9)
- Coarse sandy sequestrum, e.g. tuberculosis
- Dense ivory, e.g. syphilis
- Colored sequestrum (black), e.g. ulna and tibia OM
- Ring sequestrum, e.g. amputation stump
- Bombay sequestrum, e.g. phalanx and traumatic amputation
- Coralliform sequestrum, e.g. pyogenic infection
- Button hole, e.g. pin tract infection.

Clinical Features

- *Symptoms*: Fever, pain and swelling are seen in acute exacerbation of chronic osteomyelitis
- *Signs*: Irregular thickening develops due to unequal pace of destruction and new bone formation

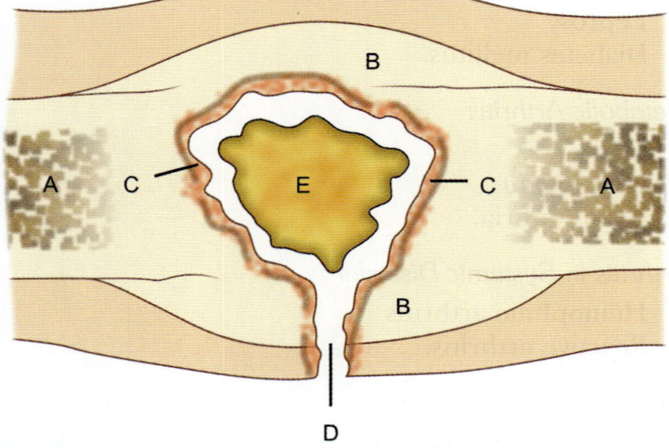

Fig. 10.8: Formation of sequestrum—A. Sound bone; B. New bone; C. Granulations, lining involucrum; D. Cloaca; E. Sequestrum

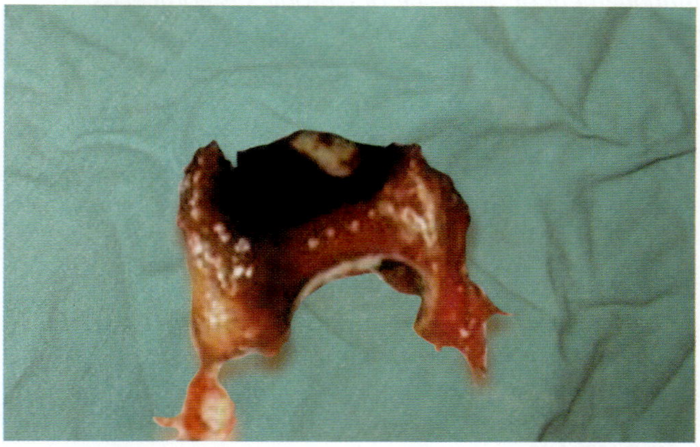

Fig. 10.9: Isolated sequestrum

- Multiple sinuses develop and their presence indicates unabsorbed sequestra, with presence of secondary infection
- Scars and muscle contracture develops
- Shortening or lengthening of bone develops
- Deformities and decreased movements
- Pathological fractures.

Investigations

X-ray Findings

- Early stage-moth-eaten appearance
- Elevation of periosteum and subperiosteal new bone formation
- Sharply delineated areas of dense bone with surrounding decalcification
- Gradually necrotic dense bone area is surrounded by white ring of involucrum.

Treatment

- Sequestrectomy and saucerization
- Open bone grafting (papineau technique) is done in three stages:
  - *Stage I:* Excision of infected tissue, sinus tract and sequestrum is done. After 4 to 5 days, daily dressing is done and next stage is delayed until signs of infection are absent and healthy granulation tissue is present
  - *Stage II:* Autogenous cancellous bone grafting is done
  - *Stage III:* Some cases show spontaneous epithelization, otherwise skin grafting, myocutaneous flap and muscle pedicle flap can be done by either of the following methods:
    - Gentamycin PMMA beads/antibiotic impregnated rod
    - Closed suction drain
    - Soft tissue transfer

Management of Sequelae of Chronic Osteomyelitis

This is done by Ilizarov's technique. Various sequelae of chronic osteomyelitis can be grouped as follows:

- *Group A:* Acute onset, but ends up as chronic osteomyelitis, with persistent infection
- *Group B:* Post-traumatic chronic osteomyelitis, associated with fractures either united or with nonunion
- *Group C:* Postoperative iatrogenic osteomyelitis.

Main line of treatment for chronic OM sequelae are:

- Removal of hardware and as per groups A and B
- Hyperbaric oxygen therapy
- Amputation and prosthesis

Complications

- Growth disturbances
- Pathological fractures
- Muscle contractures
- Secondary septicemia
- Epithelioma
- Joint stiffness
- Amyloidosis

■ Diseases of Joints (Arthritis)

Definition

It is an inflammation of joints. It is characterized by pain, swelling and limitation of movement and arthralgia is termed for pain in joints, without inflammation.

Classification

Infectious Arthritis

Acute infection: These include following arthritis:

- Acute pyogenic arthritis
- Acute gonococcal arthritis
- Acute rheumatic arthritis
- Smallpox arthritis.

Chronic infection

- *Nonspecific:* Pyogenic arthritis
- *Specific:* Tuberculous arthritis, syphilitic arthritis, gonococcal arthritis, etc.
- *Parasitic:* Guinea worm arthritis
- *Rheumatoid arthritis:* Rheumatoid arthritis, juvenile rheumatoid arthritis, etc.
- *Seronegative spondyloarthropathy:* Ankylosing spondylolitis, Reiter's disease, psoriatic arthritis, enteropathic arthritis, etc.

Degenerative Arthritis

- Primary osteoarthritis
- Secondary osteoarthritis.

Neuropathic Arthopathy

- Charcot's arthopathy
- Syringomyelia
- Leprosy
- Diabetes mellitus.

Metabolic Arthritis

- Gout
- Pseudogout
- Alkaptonuria.

Arthritis in Systemic Disorder

- Hemophilic arthritis
- Reactive arthritis.

Miscellaneous Condition

- Villonodular synovitis
- Synovial chondromatosis.

SEPTIC ARTHRITIS

Definition

It is defined as a bacterial infection of the joints, which causes an intense inflammatory reaction with migration of polymorphonuclear leukocytes and subsequent release of proteolytic enzymes, causing destruction of articular cartilage and later the joint.

Causative Organisms

Most common organisms are:
- *Staphylococcus aureus* (50%)
- *Streptococcus* (20%)
- *Pneumococcus* (10%)
- *Gonococcus*
- *E. coli*
- *H. influenzae* is common in children less than 2 years of age.

Predisposing Factors

- Trauma
- Diabetes
- Steroid therapy
- Malignancy
- HIV

Routes of Entry

These includes five P's:
1. Primary focus is in respiratory system, GIT, urinary system, etc.
2. Pyogenic osteomyelitis
3. Punctured wound
4. Pneumonia, typhoid, etc.
5. Primary focus in joint.

Sites of Involvement of the Joints

In adults
- Knee (53%)
- Hip (20%)
- Elbow (17%)
- Shoulder (10%).

In children
- Knee (32%)
- Hip (39%).

Pathogenesis

- The presence of bacteria in the joint, incites an intense local reaction
- The synovial membrane becomes hyperemic, edematous and proliferates, producing purulent fluid containing markedly increased leukocytes
- As a result, the synovial sac is greatly distended by large amount of fluid
- The condition is designated as serous arthritis or when precipitation of fibrin is excessive, it is called serofibrinous arthritis
- Areas of vascular thrombosis and focal necrosis occur
- Proteolytic enzymes originating from polymorphonuclear leukocytes, dissolve the articular cartilage and may even erode the bone
- The intense intra-articular pressure, causes necrosis and destruction of intra-articular soft tissue and capsule
- The exudates erupts into the surrounding soft tissue and into the skin, forming multiple sinuses
- This is typical of purulent arthritis characteristic of *Staphylococcus* infection
- Hemolytic infection is fulminating and quickly destructive
- The synovial inflammatory signs are intense; vascular thrombosis and necrosis are extreme
- The exudation in the joint is bloody serous typical of serosanguinous arthritis, the danger of septicemia is greatest
- In mild cases, healing takes place by resolution
- In severe cases, healing takes place by resorption of purulent exudates and repair by granulation tissue, which bridges the joint forming fibrous ankylosis
- The capsule becomes fibrotic, thickened and inelastic. Loss of articular cartilage, exposes the bone to mechanical trauma, resulting in degenerative arthritis.

Clinical Features

Septic arthritis is usually present as monoarticular feature in (90%) and polyarticular in (10%) of cases.

Symptoms
- Constitutional symptoms are chills, fever, sweats, malaise, anorexia and in infants nausea, vomiting, etc.
- Pain gradually increases in intensity over several hours and becomes excruciating
- Pain accentuates on movement of joints and thus limits the movement
- Swelling
- The patient holds the limb in position of maximum capacity to reduce the intra-articular pressure and thus minimizes pain
- *The position of maximum intra-articular volume are:*
  - *Hip:* 60° flexion, 15° abduction and 15° of external rotation
  - *Knee:* 30 to 60° flexion
  - *Ankle:* 15° plantar flexion
  - *Shoulder:* 30 to 60° abduction
  - *Elbow:* 30 to 60° flexion
  - *Wrist:* Neutral

Signs

- The joint is swollen, red, warm and tender throughout
- Patient holds the limb in position of maximum relief
- Local temperature is increased
- Muscle spasm is seen
- Reduced range of motion
- In case of knee, due to distention of joint, patellar tap is positive due to floating patella.

Laboratory Investigations

- WBC's (polymorphs) are raised to 50,000 to 100,000 (80%)
- ESR is raised more than 20 mm/hour (50%)
- Hemoglobin is decreased
- Blood culture is positive in 35 to 50 percent of cases
- CRP is positive, it should be done 24 hours before presentation. Note, if CRP is less than 10 mg/dl, the probability that the patient does not have septic arthritis is 87 percent
- *Joint fluid aspirate and synovial fluid aspirate:* It is critical for diagnosing and treatment of septic arthritis. Diagnosis of septic arthritis, is based on the results of analysis of synovial fluid is shown in Table 10.1.

Radiological Findings

- Films are generally negative in beginning
- Ballooning of synovial sac may be seen from rounded soft tissue swelling
- If infection persists, osteoporosis of adjacent bone is seen

Table 10.1: Diagnosis of septic arthritis, based on the results of synovial fluid analysis

Analysis	*Nonseptic arthritis*	*Septic arthritis*
Gross appearance		
Color	Straw or clear yellow	Serosanguinous or purulent
Volume	0.13 ml to 0.5 ml	Increased
Clarity	Clear	Turbid
Viscosity and mucin		
Clot viscosity	High	Very low
Mucin clot	Good	Poor
Microscopic examination		
Leukocytes	<300	>50,000
Neutrophils	<25%	>80%
Bacteria	Negative	Positive
Biochemistry		
Serum/synovial fluid glucose ratio	0.8 to 1.0	Low
Protein	2g/dl	<8 d/dl
Culture	Negative	Positive

- Destruction of cartilage and narrowing of joint space
- Degenerative arthritis supervenes
- In late cases, fibrous ankylosis and bony ankylosis is seen.

Treatment

- *Arthotomy or joint drainage:* The joint is aspirated first, if pus is present
- Arthroscopic drainage
- Antibiotics are given in adequate amount. Cephalosporins or penicillin, which combat gram-positive organisms and aminoglycosides, which combat gram-negative organism are started in combination
- Broad spectrum antibiotics, like chlortetracycline and oxytetracycline can be given. Appropriate antibiotics can be started after culture sensitivity
- *Immobilization:* It is done by plaster of Paris. Splint in functional position reduces pain.

TUBERCULOSIS OF MUSCULOSKELETAL SYSTEM

■ Introduction

- Though ubiquitous in distribution, tuberculosis (TB) has firmly entrenched itself with the third world. The main causes are illiteracy, poverty, poor hygienic condition and other favorable factors
- Tuberculosis bacilli have lived in symbiosis with mankind, since time immemorial
- In India *Rigveda, Atharvaveda, Charaka Samhita* and *Sushruta,* have mentioned the disease by the name *Yakshma* in all its form
- TB is the oldest disease affecting mankind. It has been found in egyptian mummies, dating back to 3400 BC
- Hippocrates (460–370 BC) was the first to suggest relationship between pulmonary and spinal deformity
- Percival Pott (1714–1788), described the Gibbus deformity and its sequelae
- Laennec (1781–1826) described the basic microscopic lesion the tubercle
- Drugs streptomycin was first introduced in 1947, para aminosalicylic acid (PAS) in 1949 and isoniazid (INH) in 1952
  - India is infamous of for hosting nearly one fifth of the 30 million people, suffering from tuberculosis throughout the world
  - There are 6 million radiologically proven cases of tuberculosis in India and perhaps a quarter of these are sputum positive
  - Skeletal tuberculosis is always secondary, the primary foci being the lungs, lymph nodes and gastrointestinal tract

– Of all the patients, suffering from tuberculosis, nearly 1 to 3 percent show, skeletal system involvement
– Vertebral tuberculosis is the commonest form and it constitutes 50 percent of skeletal tuberculosis
– The major area of predilection are spine, hip, knee, foot, elbow, hand, shoulder and others.

Causative Organisms

- *Mycobacterium* tubercle is the main causative organism. In 1882, Robert Koch discovered the tubercle bacillus. Most of the skeletal TB is caused by typical *Mycobacterium*. *Mycobacterium* tubercle bacilli, varies in size about 3 × 0.3 μm
- They are acid fast bacilli, aerobic and grow at temperatures varying from 30 to 40°C and can be grown on Lowenstein-Jensen medium
- They are killed by heat at 60°C in 15 to 20 minutes and survive for many weeks in moist conditions.

Predisposing Factors

- Malnutrition
- Poor sanitation
- Living in crowded area
- Close contact with TB patient
- Repeated pregnancies
- Exanthematous fever
- Immuno-deficiency status.

Pathology and Pathogenesis

- A minimum period of 2 to 3 years is required between the primary and secondary TB
- Primary focus, may be active or quiescent (lungs, tonsils, mediastinum, mesentery, etc.)
- *Bacillemia:* Through the arteries and veins (e.g. Batson's plexuses in spine) reach the skeletal system, tubercle develops.

What is Tubercle?

The tubercle is a microscopic pathological lesion with a central necrosis, surrounded by epitheloid cells, Langerhan's giant cells and round cells.

The future course of tubercle varies.

- *It may resolve completely:* The disease may heal completely with varying degrees of residual deformities and/or loss of function. The lesion may be completely walled off and the caseous tissue may be calcified. A low grade chronic fibromatous granulating and caseating lesion, may persist with a grumbling activity
- The infection may spread locally by contiguity and systemically by blood stream, as seen in immuno-compromised patients.

Clinical Features

- The disease may be insidious in onset
- Monoarticular and mono-osseous involvement
- Other visceral lesions
- *Constitutional symptoms:* Low grade fever, especially in evening, anorexia, weight loss, night sweats, night cries tachycardia and anemia
- *Local symptoms and signs:* Swelling, synovial involvement, pain, tenderness, muscle spasm, night cries, stiffness and later actual limitation of movements, due to fibrous ankylosis, limp and muscle atrophy.

Types

Granular: Mild, nondestructive and fibrosing
Caseous and exudative: Destructive abscess forming.

Laboratory Findings

- HMG with ESR is raised
- TLC and DLC
- Culture sensitivity
- ZN staining
- Sputum for AFB
- Guinea pig inoculation
- Mantoux test
- X-rays
- Biopsy of draining lymph nodes
- CT scan
- MRI.

Treatment

General Treatment

This includes rich protein diet, rest, immobilization and braces, hematinics, adequate exposure to sunshine, etc. The aim is to improve the immunity.

Chemotherapy

Drugs used for the treatment of tuberculosis are grouped as follows:

First line of drugs

P: Pyrazinamide
R: Rifampicin
I: INH
S: Streptomycin
E: Ethambutol

Second line of drugs

C: Capreomycin/ciprofloxacin/ofloxacin
A: Amikacin
K: Kanamycin
E: Ethionamide
C: Cycloserine
A: Para aminosalicylic acid (PAS)

Drugs useful for chemotherapy in skeletal system are shown in Table 10.2.

Chemotherapy Regime

- *Nine months regime:* Nine months of rifampicin and INH are effective in all forms of disease.
- *Six months regime:* First 2 months INH, rifampicin and pyrazinamide
- Next four months INH and rifampicin. When primary resistance to INH is high, therapy is usually initiated with four first line drugs.
- *Eighteen months regime:* Four drug therapy is done by rifampicin, INH, pyrazinamide and ethambutol for 3 months. Ethambutol is withdrawn and three drugs are continued for 9 months. Later, rifampicin and INH is continued for 6 months
- *Tuli's sixteen months regime:* Rifampicin, INH and ethambutol for first 4 months
  Pyrazinamide replaces rifampicin in second 4 months.
  In next 4 months, rifampicin is given with INH
  In last 4 months, INH is only drug given.

Local Treatment

Aim is to prevent, correct or decrease the deformities. If the disease is osseous, aim at ankylosis in functional position by immobilization. If the disease is synovial, aim at mobility with traction.

Operative Treatment

- Synovectomy
- Curettage
- Osteotomies
- Arthrodesis
- Drainage of abscess

Recent Advancements in Management of Skeletal TB

- Lab investigations
- Imaging modalities
- Treatment

Lab Investigations

Routine

- Complete blood count
  - Hemoglobin decreased
  - *TLC:* Increased
  - *DLC:* Increased lymphocytes
  - *Lymphocyte:* Monocyte ratio normally is 5:1. If less than 5:1, bad prognosis
  - Blood culture
  - Pus culture
  - *Sputum:* AFB
  - Tissue biopsy
  - FNAC
  - RFT
  - LFT
  - Blood sugar
  - *Skin test:* Mantoux test
  - HIV
  - HBsAg

Table 10.2: Chemotherapeutic drugs in skeletal system

S. No.	*Drugs*	*Daily adult dose*	*Drug toxicity*
1.	Streptomycin (injection)	20-35 mg/kg	Vestibular damage, deafness, fever, rashes, contact dermatitis, nephrotoxicity
2.	INH	300-400 mg (5 mg/kg of body wt in adult, 10-20 mg/kg of body wt in children	Peripheral neuropathy, behavior disorders, convulsions, hepatitis, hypersensitivity
3.	Ethambutol	15-25 mg/kg in single or divided doses (not used in children <5 yrs)	Retrobulbar neuritis with loss of vision and color blindness
4.	Para-aminosalicylic acid	12 gm in single or divided doses	Gastrointestinal disturbances, rashes, fever, lymphadenopathy, hepatotoxicity
5.	Thiacetazone	150 gm in single dose	Anorexia, nausea, vomiting, liver damage, marrow depression
6.	Ethionamide	250 mg/BD, 15-20 mg/kg	GIT upsets, abnormal liver test, peripheral neuritis, convulsion
7.	Pyrazinamide	40 mg/kg in single or two divided doses	Hepatotoxicity
8.	Cycloserine	15-20 mg/kg	CNS toxicity
9.	Capreomycin	15-30 mg/kg single dose	Nephrotoxicity
10.	Kanamycin	15 mg/kg single dose	Ototoxicity
11.	Amikacin	15 mg/kg/day	Ototoxicity, nephrotoxicity

Recent

- Twenty-four hours urine for AFB, TB-PCR
- *Blood TB-PCR:* Here amplification of the nucleic acid is done enzymatically, by polymerase chain reaction and identified, by using nucleic acid probes. It is very beneficial
- *TB-ELISA:* IgG, IgM assessment by A60 Ag. It has 60 to 80 percent specificity
- *ELISPOT (T-spot ELISA):* It measures the T-cell interferon γ (secreted by the T-lymphocytes of the affected person)
- *BACTEC:* It is a rapid culturing method. BACTEC radiometric cultural assay, can detect *Mycobacterium tuberculi,* as early as 7 days on the basis of release of radio labelled CO_2, from growth of *Mycobacterium* in a selective liquid medium containing C-14 labeled isotopes. It has 95 percent sensitivity
- *HPLC (High performance liquid chromatography):* It measures the mycolic acid, which is present in the cell of *Mycobacterium* TB. It helps in differentiating various acid fast bacilli
- *GLC (Gas liquid chromatography):* Mycobacteria are identified on the basis of secretion of cellular fatty acid, by gas liquid chromatography
- *QTB (Quantiferin gold TB):* It measures the T-lymphocytes secreting γ-interferons, when the whole blood is attached by antigen. It can be measured by blood sample. Results come in 3 to 5 days and are not affected by previous BCG vaccination
- *FTB (Fast plaque TB):* It can be done on anybody fluid, like aspirate, pus, sputum, blood. It gives results in 48 to 72 hours. It can also infer about the effectiveness of the drug
- Nucleic acid probe (Radioactive labeled DNA probes)
- Molecular typing.

Imaging

Routine

- *X-ray chest:* PA view
- *X-ray spine (cervical, D-L, L-S):* AP and lateral views
- USG
- Myelography
- CT myelography
- MRI.

Recent

- *Abreugraphy:* It is also called as miniature chest radiography and is helpful in detection of TB and its differentiation from other respiratory diseases. It is cheaper, comparative to other techniques and is used for mass screening.
- *Contrast MRI:* It gives accurate idea about intraosseous abscess, ligamentous involvement and dural involvement. It helps in postoperative imaging add in doing follow-ups of cases. It can be done in patients with titanium implants
- *Bone scan:* Technetium 99m, ciprofloxacin scintigraphy is more sensitive. It can be done in patients with stainless steel implants
- *PET scan:* It gives early diagnosis
- *MP CT:* Multiplanar CT
- *3D CT:* Reconstructive CT.

Treatment

- Conservative
- Surgical.

Conservative Treatment

- Anti-tubercular drugs
- High protein diet
- *Braces:* Somi, for cervical spine, Taylor's brace for dorsolumbar spine, etc.
- Early mobilization and rehabilitation
- Adequate exposure to sunlight and fresh air
- Improve hygiene.

Anti-tubercular Drugs Therapy

First line drugs

- Isoniazid – 5 mg/kg body wt
- Rifampicin – 10 mg/kg
- Pyrazinamide – 25 mg/kg
- Ethambutol – 15 mg/kg
- Streptomycin – 15 mg/kg

Second line drugs

- Para aminosalicylic acid (PAS)
- Thiacetazone
- Ethionamide
- Capreomycin
- Ethambutol
- Kanamycin
- Amikacin
- Ciprofloxacin

Recent drugs

- *Rifamycin:* Rifabutin, rifapentin
- Clofazimine
- *Beta lactams:* Augmentin
- *Macrolides:* Azithromycin, clarithromycin

Future drugs

- Immunomodulators
- Gamma interferons
- Interleukins - 2 and 12
- Alfa TNF.

Recent Treatment Regimen According to Revised National TB Control Program (RNTCP)

Category I (Table 10.3)

- New (untreated) smear positive pulmonary TB
- New smear negative pulmonary TB with extensive parenchymal involvement
- New cases of severe forms of extrapulmonary TB like meningitis, miliary, pericarditis, peritonitis, bilateral or extensive pleural effusion, spinal, intestinal, genitourinary TB.

Category II (Table 10.4)

- Smear positive failure cases
- Relapse cases
- Interrupted treatment cases.

Category III (Table 10.5)

New cases of smear negative pulmonary TB with limited parenchymal involvement or less severe forms of extrapulmonary TB, e.g. lymph node, unilateral pleural effusion, bone (excluding spine), peripheral joint or skin TB. This is shown in Table 10.5.

Category IV

- Multidrug resistant (MDR) TB cases
- Second-line of drugs are used.

Table 10.3: Category I of recent treatment regimen, according to RNTCP

Category	*Initial phase*	*Continuation phase*	*Total duration in months*
I	2HRZE	4HR/$4H_3R_3$ or 6HE	6 8

Table 10.4: Category II of recent treatment regimen, according to RNTCP

Category	*Initial phase*	*Continuation phase*	*Total duration in months*
II	2HRZES + 1HRZE	5HRE or $5H_3R_3E_3$	8 8

Table 10.5: Category III of recent treatment regimen, according to RNTCP

Category	*Initial phase*	*Continuation phase*	*Total duration in months*
III	2HRZ	4HR/$4H_3R_3$ or 6HE	6 8

Surgical Treatment

Indications in patients with no neurological deficit:

- No recovery after treatment
- First-line drug resistance or irregular treatment
- To prevent deformity
  - *In adults:* If vertebral height loss (collapse) in dorso-lumbar spine is greater than 0.75 and in lumbar spine greater than 1
  - *In children:* If kyphosis is greater than 30°
- Children with "spine at risk signs", explained in Table 10.6
- Each sign is allocated one point, to create a spinal instability score:
  - If score is greater than 2, need surgery and spinal fixation
  - If score is less than 2, no need of fixation, observe following:
    - If CT guided biopsy study is inconclusive
    - If cervical spine abscess is causing compression and difficulties in swallowing
    - If abscess is not healed
- Indication for patients with neurological deficit:
  - Neurological deficit develops, while patient is under treatment
  - No recovery after 4 weeks of chemotherapy
  - Exaggeration of deficit, while under treatment
  - Recurrence after correction
  - Advanced stage of deficit (bladder involvement, etc).

Surgical Options

- Drainage of abscess
- Costotransversectomy
- Anterolateral decompression
- Anterior decompression with interbody fixation
  - By using cage with bone graft: It can be expandable or nonexpandable
  - Using local graft
- Posterior decompression
- Posterior decompression with fixation (instrumentation)
  - Use of transpedicular screws, e.g. stainless steel, titanium, etc.
  - *Use of Mosmiami system:* Unidirectional or polydirectional screws
  - Titanium implants are generally used because postoperative MRI, can be done for evaluation, follow-up MRI can be done
  - *Global fixation:* Anterior spinal fusion, posterior spinal fusion, interbody fusion, intertransverse fusion and instrumentation
  - Recently, endoscopic spine surgery
- Surgery should be done under ATT (Antitubercular treatment) cover.

Table 10.6: Spinal instability scores

S.No.	Radiological signs of instability	Score
1.	Separation of facets	1
2.	Posterior retropulsion	1
3.	Lateral translation on AP view	1
4.	Toppling (sign) of superior vertebra	1

Table 10.7: Prognosis of TB

	Good	Bad
Age	Younger	Older
Onset	Early	Late
Duration	Shorter	Longer
Kyphosis	<60°	>60°
Stage	Active	Healed

Prognosis (Table 10.7)

"Middle Path Regime", by Tuli

- Bed rest on hard bed or plaster shell
  Drug regime: Total duration is 16 months (H: Isoniazid, R: Rifampicin, E: Ethambutol, Z: Pyrazinamide, S: Streptomycin)
  - 4 months: HRE
  - 4 months: HZE
  - 4 months: HR
  - 4 months: H
- Supportive treatment with vitamins, antioxidants
- X-ray at 3 to 6 months
- Drainage of abscess
- Decompression
- Fusion for unstable spine
- Postoperative care

Note: Implants can be used in TB, under ATT cover as no biofilm is produced.

TUBERCULOSIS OF SPINE

■ Introduction

- It is the most common type of skeletal TB, constituting of 50 percent of all cases
- Regional distribution of TB are
  - *Cervical:* 12 percent
  - *Cervicodorsal:* 5 percent
  - *Dorsal:* 42 percent
  - *Dorsolumbar:* 12 percent
  - *Lumbar:* 26 percent
  - *Lumbosacral:* 3 percent
  - Thus, lower thoracic and lower lumbar accounting for about 80 percent of all cases.
- The reason for this area of predilection are
  - Large amount of spongy tissues within the vertebral body
  - Degree of weight-bearing, which is comparatively more
  - More vertebral mobility is seen here.

Sites of Involvement within the Vertebra

Spinal TB can start in any part of vertebrae, but there are mainly four sites, as shown in Figure 10.10

- Paradiscal
- Central
- Anterior
- Appendical (involving pedicles, laminae, spinous process or transverse process)
  - Ninty-five percent: Anterior element
  - Five percent: Posterior element.

Pathogenesis

- Primary foci in lung, lymph nodes or abdomen. Bacillemia develops and the organism reach the spine through the Batson's plexus
- Tuberculosis endarteritis, which develops following the infection, results in marrow devitalizations. Later on, the tubercular follicle develops. Lamellae are destroyed due to hyperemia, causing osteoporosis. As a result the vertebral body gets easily compressed
- In thoracic vertebrae because of normal kyphotic curve, anterior wedging is common. In lordotic, cervical and lumbar vertebra, wedging is minimal
- Two types of vertebral reactions, commonly encountered in skeletal TB are shown in Table 10.8

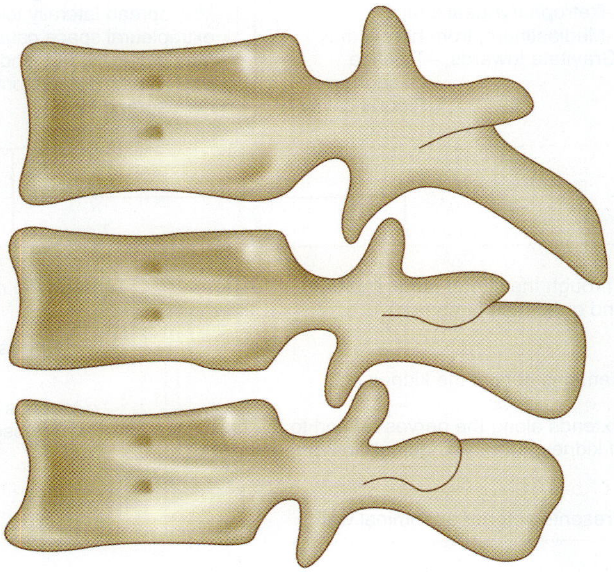

Fig. 10.10: Major sites of vertebral TB

Table 10.8: Two types of vertebral reactions commonly encountered in skeletal TB

Exudative reaction	*Caseative reaction*
• Common	• Rarer
• Sever hyperic reaction severe osteoporosis	• Mechanism of formation and spread is similar to exudative type but is slower
• Rapid spread	
• Abscess is formed frequently	
• Constitutional symptoms are more pronounced	

Abscess Formation

- It is most common complication about 20 percent
- At first, abscess collects under the anterior longitudinal ligament in front of the vertebral bodies and then it further disseminate along one or several courses
- It may pass backward and invade the vertebral canal, a serious complication and causes pressure on the spinal cord
- It may track forwards and become diverted by various anatomical structures, such as blood vessels, nerves or muscles (Flow chart 10.1).

Clinical Features

- Constitutional symptoms includes weakness, anorexia, weight loss, night sweats and evening rise of temperature, etc.
- Patient gives a history of backache
- Slight pain and stiffness are earliest complaints
- Pain is initially localized, dull aching, brought down by jarring or movement of spine
- Later on, it is referred pain depending on the nerve root involvement, e.g. cervical lesion causing pain over occiput, ear, jaw, upper limb; upper thoracic, intercostals neuralgia, thoracolumbar girdle pain or epigastric pain and lumbar to hips and legs
- Patient gives history of night cries
- Pressure symptoms due to cold abscess
- Paraplegia
- *Attitude:* It is characteristic of disease in different regions of spine
- *Cervical spine:* There is obliteration of cervical lordosis, position of head is similar to that of in "Wry neck", but face is not rotated
- *Lower cervical:* Head is thrown backward to one side and may be supported by hand

Flow chart 10.1: Showing spreading of abscess, from different vertebral sections to different anatomical body parts

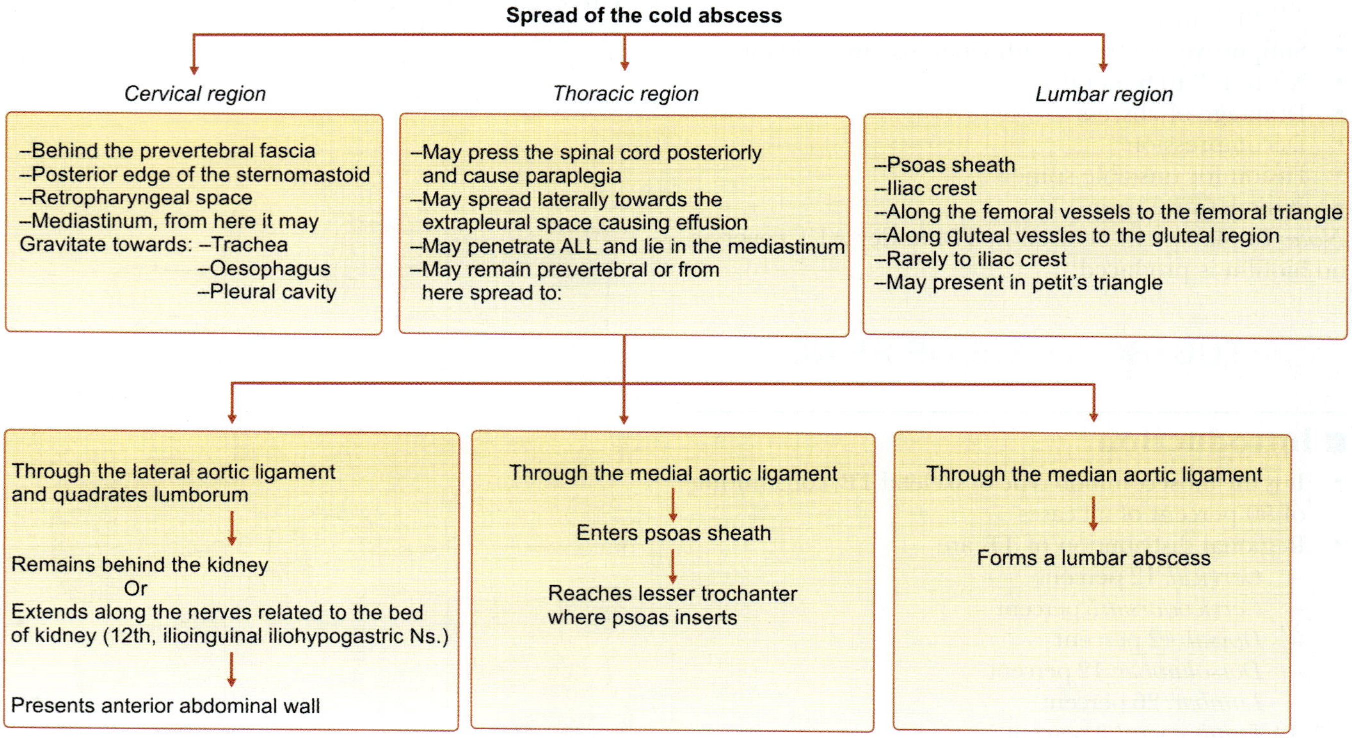

- *Upper thoracic:* Head appears shrunken, due to shortening of neck
- *Mid thoracic:* AP diameter appears increased, due to shortening of stature (Fig. 10.11)
- *Lower lumbar:* Pronounced lordosis
- *Gait:* Patient is very cautious and avoids jarring of spine and walks with legs apart and waddles, so called "Alderman's gait"
- Muscle spasm
- Angular type of kyphosis or gibbus is present
- Tenderness is present over the vertebrae
- Movement of spine are restricted
- Formation of cold abscesses and spread.

Radiological Findings

Earliest Changes (Fig. 10.12)

- Consists of disc space narrowing. Subsequent loss of disc space is common
- *Paradiscal lesion:* The bones look rarified and osteopenic.

Late Changes

It includes the following (Fig. 10.13):

- This includes anterior wedge compression in anterior vertebral involvement
- Central vertebral body collapse also called as "concertina collapse" in central involvement
- Destruction of the posterior elements in the posterior affection
- Soft tissue swelling and its calcification are highly predictable of tuberculosis
- In healing stage, the vertebral body and posterior elements may appear more dense due to sclerosis paravertebral shadow, which indicates cold abcesses
- *Cervical region:* Retropharangeal
- *Upper thoracic:* V-shaped shadow and widened mediastinum
- *Below fourth thoracic vertebra:* Fusiform or birdnest appearance
- Bilaterally widened psoas shadow, in lumbar region.

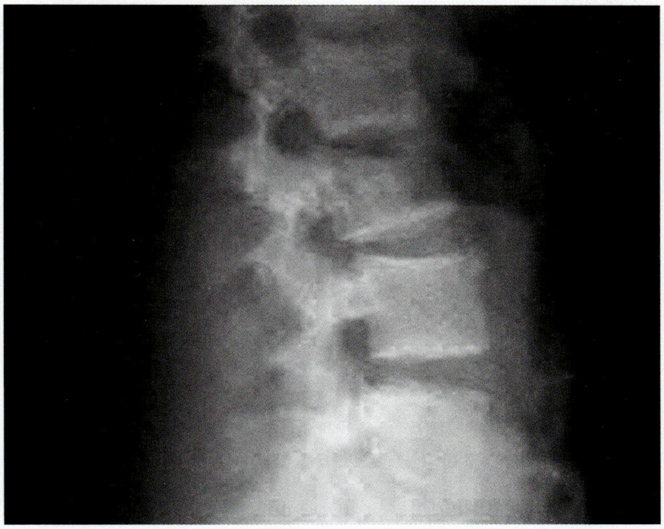

Fig. 10.12: X-ray film, showing earliest changes in the vertebrae

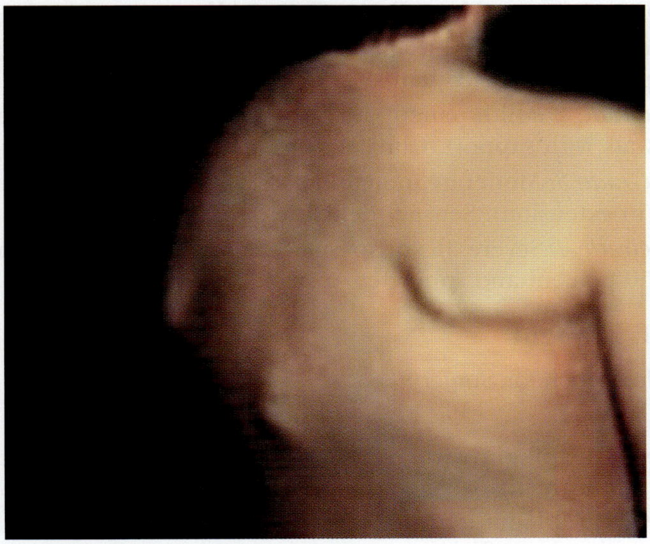

Fig. 10.11: Mid thoracic, AP diameter increases due to shortening of stature

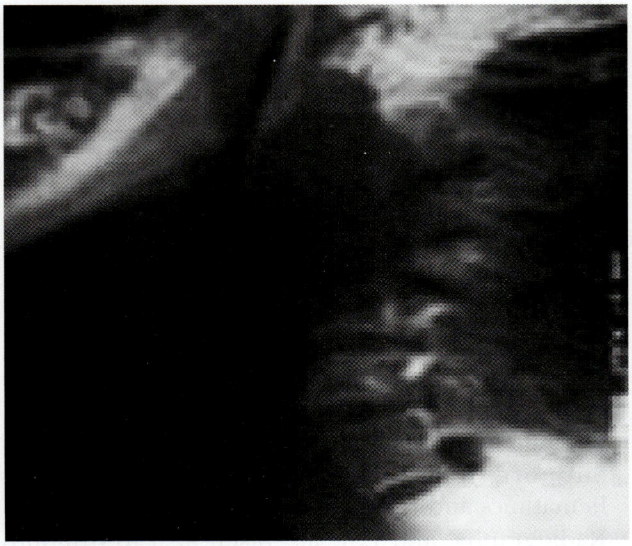

Fig. 10.13: Late changes

Investigations

- *Hemoglobin:* Reduced hemoglobin. High lymphocytes and low monocytes count, suggest good resistance
- If ratio is 5:1, it is favorable ratio. If it is less than 5:1, then it is poor prognosis
- ESR raised
- Mantoux test positive
- Sputum for AFB
- Biopsy and aspiration of abscesses
- CT scan
- MRI
- Bone scan
- Sonography
- Twenty-four hours urine for PCR and AFB.

Treatment

General treatment: Rest, well balanced diet and hygienic surroundings are essential with chemotherapy.

Antitubercular Drugs

- *INH:* 5 to 10 mg/kg up to 300 mg
- *Rifampicin:* 10 mg/kg up to 600 mg
- *Streptomycin:* 15 to 20 mg/kg up to 0.75 g
- *Pyrazinamide:* 20 to 35 mg/kg up to 2.09 g
- *Ethambutol:* 15 mg/kg
- *PAS:* 150 to 300 mg/kg up to10 g

Drug Recommendation for Tuberculosis of Bones and Joints

Intensive phase

- SM/EMB
- INH
- Rifampicin daily for 2 months
- Pyrazinamide

Continuation phase

- INH
- RMP daily for 7 months.

Tuli's Middle Path Regime

- Rest in hard bed or plaster of Paris bed
- Antitubercular drugs for 16 months
- INH and rifampicin for first 4 months
- INH and pyrazinamide for second 4 months
- INH and rifampicin for next 4 months
- INH alone for last 4 months
- Support should be given, with multivitamins, hematinics and high protein diet
- Radiographic and ESR are taken at 3 to 6 months interval
- Gradual mobilization
- Abscesses are aspirated, as they cause pressure effect and complications
- Sinus excision
- Decompression
- Operative debridement.

Complications

- Paraplegia
- Cold abscess
- Sinuses
- Secondary infection
- Amyloid disease.

Pott's Paraplegia

Incidence of this complication is 10 percent of all cases.

Causes of Paraplegia

Inflammatory: Edema, TB granulation tissue, TB abscesses, TB caseous tissue, etc.

Mechanical: Tubercular debris, sequestra from vertebral body, constriction of vertebral body due to stenosis of vertebral body and localized pressure due to internal gibbus.

Intrinsic: Prolonged stretching of cord over a severe deformity, infective thrombosis, pathological dislocation, tuberculous meningomyelitis, spinal tumor syndrome, etc.

Classification

Depending on the Onset and Duration of Disease (Griffiths and Seddon)

Group A: Early onset paraplegia.
Group B: Late onset paraplegia.

Depending on Motor Power (Tuli and Kumar)

Grade 1: Negligible, patient unaware of neural deficit, physician detects plantar extensor and/or ankle clonus

Grade 2: Mild, patient aware of deficit, but manages to walk with support. Clinical signs of spastic paresis

Grade 3: Moderate, nonambulatory because of paralysis (in extension). Sensory deficit less than 50 percent

Grade 4: Severe, flexor spasm, sensory deficit more than 50 percent and sphincter involved.

Treatment

Indication for Surgery

Absolute

- Paraplegia with onset during usual conservative treatment
- Paraplegia getting worse or remaining stationary, despite sufficient conservative treatment
- Complete loss of motor power for 1 month despite sufficient conservative treatment

- Paraplegia accompanied by uncontrolled spasticity
- Severe paraplegia of rapid onset
- Any severe paraplegia.

Relative

- Recurrent paraplegia
- Paraplegia with onset in old age
- Painful paraplegia
- Complication such as UTI and renal stones.

Rare indication

- Posterior spinal disease
- Spinal tumor syndrome
- Severe cauda equina paralysis.

Surgery

- Costotransversectomy
- Anterior decompression
- Laminectomy
- Posterior spinal fusion.

Note: Please also refer TB spine in spine Chapter.

SKELETAL TUBERCULOSIS OF HIP, KNEE, SHOULDER, ANKLE, ELBOW AND WRIST

Tuberculosis of Hip

Please refer to Hip section regional orthopedics chapter 24.

Tuberculosis of Knee

Introduction

- Knee is the third most common site and accounts for 10 percent of skeletal involvement
- Knee involvement more in adults. Tubercles may remain dormant for years
- It is always secondary and may start in any of the following sites:
  - Synovium (common)
  - Subchondral bone (of lower end of femur, upper end of tibia or patella)
  - Juxta-articular osseous foci.

Pathology

- Typical granular infection, starting in synovial membrane is of two types:
  1. Low grade (hematogenous; more common)
  2. High grade (osseous).

Low Grade Infection

- Synovial membrane becomes congested, edematous and studded with tubercle
- Caseative destruction is not a common tendency towards resorption of tubercles or healing by fibrosis
- Pannus formation at synovial reflection
- Articular damage with subchondral bone erosion
- Synovial fluid is thin, watery, opalescent, increased in quantity contains flakes of fibrin and mononuclear cells.

High Grade Infection

- Tuberculous granulation tissue, like pannus erodes the articular margins, destroys the bones and involves periarticular tissues, capsule and ligaments
- Nutrition is thus interfered and articular cartilage looses its smooth glistening appearance, becoming rough, pitted and soft
- Caseating destruction, with marked synovial swelling, sinus formation, effusion and tuberculous abscess in subchondral bone, epiphyseal or metaphyseal bone
- Muscles atrophy of thigh and calf occurs rapidly
- Knee flexion with posterior subluxation, abduction and external rotation of knee, due to contracture of biceps femoris and iliotibial band (triple deformity).

Clinical Features

Early Stage

- Joint effusion and evidence of synovial hypertrophy
- Skin may be stretched and blanched, giving an appearance of a white swelling (tumor alba) and is edematous
- Tenderness along the joint line and synovial reflection.

Middle Stage of Arthritis

- Joint movements are grossly restricted, with painful spasms (particularly of hamstrings)
- Quadriceps atrophy
- Lymphadenopathy
- In growing child, transient limb lengthening may be seen due to juxtaepiphyseal hyperemia.

Advanced Stage

Triple deformity (actually is a quadruple deformity): It is characterized as:

- Flexion (to accommodate for increased swelling and is the position of ease as well as maximum capacity)
- External rotation (from the hip) posterior and lateral subluxation (due to action of biceps femoris and ITB contracture)
- Abduction of tibia (above deforming forces further pull the leg into valgus).

Radiology

- Osteoporosis of juxta-articular structure
- Ballooning of capsule
- Enlarged ossification center
- Loss of definition of articular cortex with extreme thinning
- Posterior subluxation and valgus deformity

Treatment

Synovitis

- Chemotherapy
- Traction
- Joint aspiration.

When Active Symptoms Decrease?

- Active and assisted exercise
- Crutch walking for 6 to 12 months
- Protected weight-bearing for 18 to 24 months
- If disease is not responding favorably, arthotomy and synovectomy should be done.

Early Arthritis

- Synovectomy
- Joint debridement
- Curettage of juxta-articular foci.

Postoperative Regimen

- Drug therapy
- Traction
- Exercise
- Suitable braces

Advanced Arthritis

Arthrodesis.

■ Tuberculosis of Shoulder

Introduction

This is very rare constituting nearly 1 to 2 percent of skeletal tuberculosis and can start in any of the following sites:

- Synovium (rarely)
- Glenoid
- Head of humerus.

Clinical Features

Earlier Stage

- Painful limitation of abduction and external rotation occur early
- Marked wasting of the deltoid, supraspinatus and other muscles
- Common variety is dry type and is called "caries sicca", since there is no effusion in the joint
- Cold abscess formed could present at:
  - Supraspinous fossa
  - Deltoid
  - Biceps

Late Stage

- Destruction of the upper end of the humerus and glenoid cavity
- Fibrous ankylosis is the end result.

Radiology

- Generalized rarefaction (Fig. 10.14)
- Articular cartilage erosion
- Cavities in the head of humerus
- Periosteal reaction (Fig. 10.15)

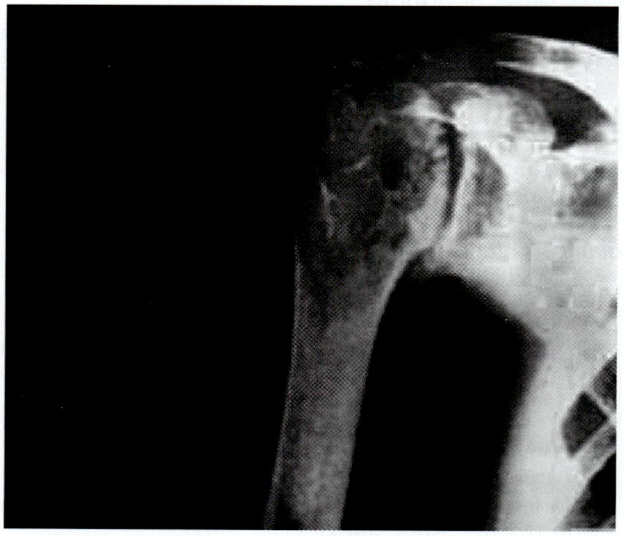

Fig. 10.14: Generalized rarefaction

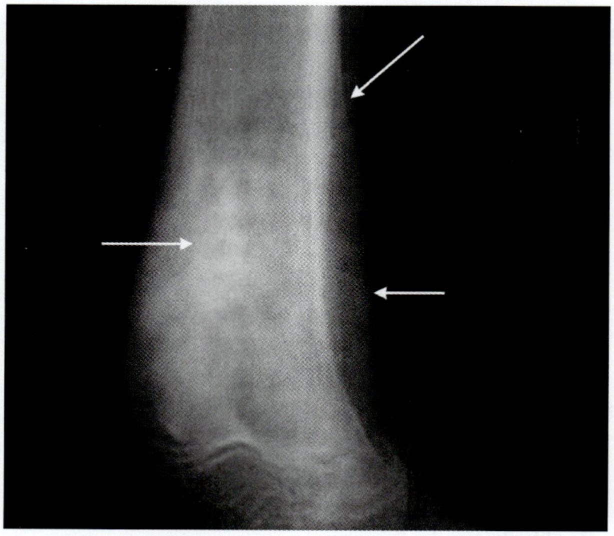

Fig. 10.15: Periosteal reaction

Treatment

- Chemotherapy is the mainstay of the treatment
- Shoulder immobilization by plaster shoulder spica in 70° to 90° of abduction, 30° of forward flexion and about 30° of internal rotation (saluting position), to encourage ankylosis in functional position, for 3 months
- Arthrodesis in painful ankylosis, recurrence, etc.

■ Tuberculosis of Ankle

This is very uncommon and the incidence is only 5 percent. Sites of involvement could be:

- Synovium
- Distal end of tibia
- Malleoli
- Talus
- Calcaneum (rarely).

Clinical Features

Early Stage

- Pain
- Limp
- Swelling
- Ankle is held in plantar flexion.

Late Stage

- Pathological anterior dislocation of the ankle
- Limitation of movements
- Wasting of calf muscles
- Sinus formation.

Radiology

- Marked osteoporosis (Fig. 10.16)
- Destruction of ankle joint (Fig. 10.17)

Treatment

- Chemotherapy is the mainstay of the treatment
- Below knee plaster cast for 8 to 12 weeks
- Synovectomy and joint debridement, during earlier stages
- Arthrodesis for advanced and persistence disease.

■ Tuberculosis of Elbow

Introduction

Tuberculosis of the elbow is rare and constitutes nearly 2 to 5 percent of all skeletal tuberculosis. The sites are:

- Olecranon
- Lower end of humerus
- Synovium
- Upper end of radius.

Clinical Features

- Pain
- Swelling
- Limitation of movements
- Wasting of arm and forearm muscles
- Lymphadenopathy
- Sinus.

Radiology (Figs 10.18 and 10.19)

- Destruction commonly in olecranon or left at the end of humerus
- Generalized demineralization and fuzziness of joint margins
- Subperiosteal new bone formation on the upper end of ulna resembling (spina ventosa) or lower end of humerus
- Pathological posterior dislocation

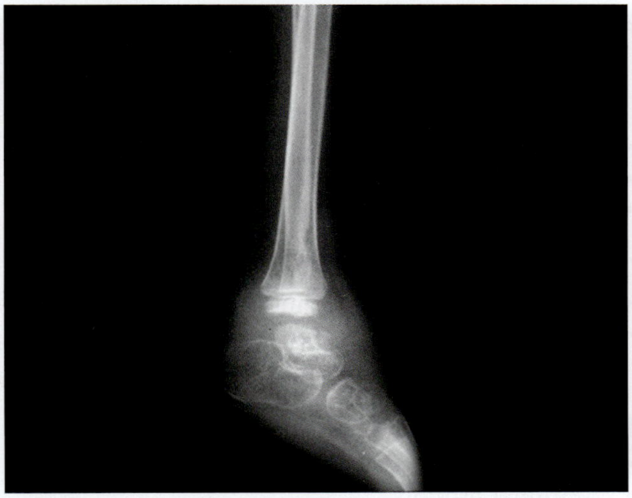

Fig. 10.16: Marked osteoporosis

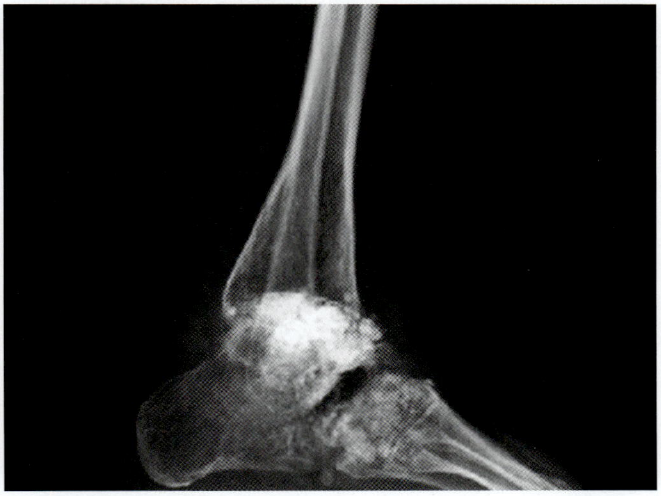

Fig. 10.17: Destruction of ankle joint

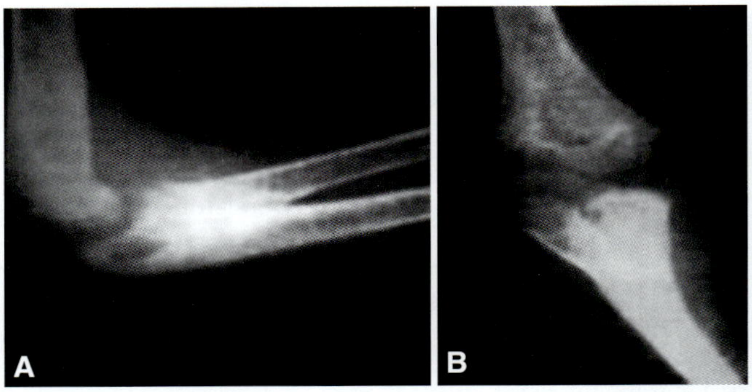

Figs 10.18A and B: X-ray, showing tuberculosis of the elbow

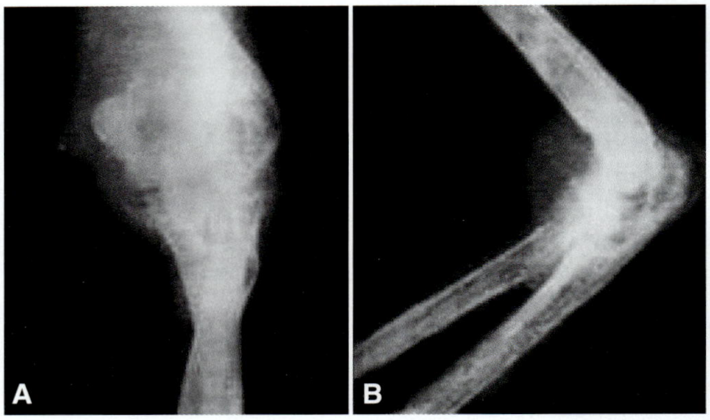

Figs 10.19A and B: Pathological posterior dislocation, due to TB of elbow joint

Treatment

- Chemotherapy is the mainstay of treatment
- Plaster in 90° of flexion and midprone position of the forearm is advisable
- As pain reliefs, splint is advisable for 6 to 9 months
- Synovectomy
- Excision arthroplasty in advanced arthritis/ankylosis
- Rarely arthrodesis of elbow is justified for heavy manual work.

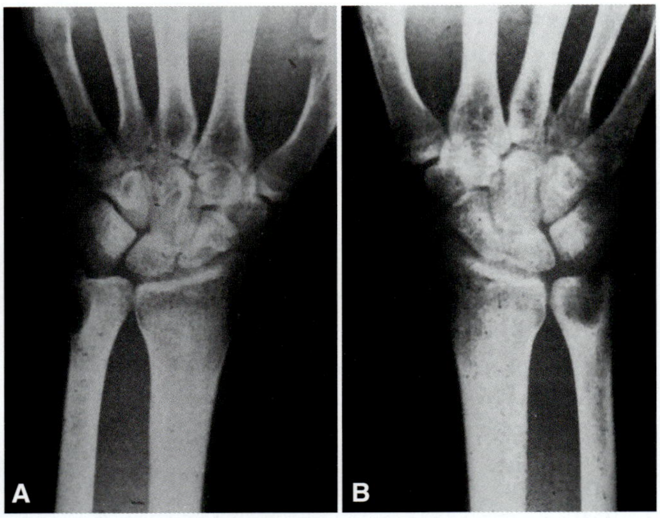

Figs 10.20A and B: X-ray, showing TB of wrist

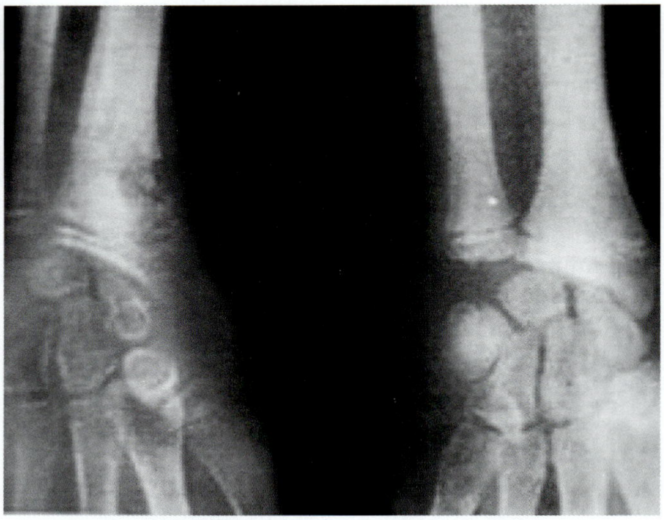

Fig. 10.21: Slight diminuation of joint space

■ Tuberculosis of Wrist

Introduction

It is very rare, localized and more frequent in adults. The sites are:

- Synovium
- Whole carpus
- Dorsal end of radius
- Neighboring extensors/flexors tendons.

Clinical Features

Early Stage

- Pain
- Swelling
- Lymphadenopathy
- Limitation of movements
- Palmar flexion deformity.

Late Stage

- Limitation of pronation and supination
- Anterior subluxation/dislocation at the radiocarpal articulation.

Radiology (Figs 10.20A and B)

- Demineralization
- Marginal erosion
- Slight diminuation of joint space (Fig. 10.21).

Treatment

- Chemotherapy is the mainstay of treatment
- Splinting of wrist in 10° to 15° of dorsiflexion and forearm in midprone position for 12 to 18 months in between exercises
- Synovectomy and curettage
- Arthrodesis in severe ankylosis.

ACTINOMYCOSIS

Introduction

- The disease is a chronic granulomatous infection, occurring in human beings and animals. It is characterized by the development of indurated swellings, mainly in the connective tissue, suppuration and discharge of sulfur granules (Figs 10.22 and 10.23)
- The lesion often points towards the skin, leading to multiple sinuses (Fig. 10.23)
- Actinomycosis in human beings is an endogenous infection
- The *Actinomyces* species are normally present in the mouth, intestine and vagina
- Trauma, foreign bodies or poor oral hygiene may favor tissue invasion
- *Actinomyces israelii* is the most common causative agent
- Actinomycosis is usually a cooperative disease, the *Actinomyces* being accompanied by other associated bacteria, which may enhance the pathogenic effect
- Actinomycosis in human beings occurs in four main clinical forms:
  1. *Cervicofacial:* With indurated lesions on the cheek and submaxillary regions.
  2. *Thoracic:* With lesions in the lung that may involve the pleura and pericardium and spread outwards through the chest wall.
  3. *Abdominal:* Where the lesion is usually around the cecum, with involvement of the neighboring tissues and the abdominal wall. Sometimes, the infection spreads to the liver via portal vein.
  4. *Pelvic:* Many cases of pelvic actinomycosis have been reported in association with the use of intrauterine devices.
- *Actinomyces* has been incriminated in inflammatory diseases of the gums (gingivitis and periodontitis) and with sublingual plaques, leading to root surface caries
- Actinomycosis may also present as mycetoma.

Laboratory Diagnosis

- The diagnosis is made by demonstrating actinomycetes in the lesion, by microscopy and by isolation in culture (Figs 10.24 and 10.25)
- The specimen to be collected is pus
- In pulmonary disease, sputum is collected
- Sulfur granules may be demonstrated in pus, by shaking it up in a test tube with some saline (Fig. 10.26)
- On standing, the granules sediment and may be withdrawn with a capillary pipette
- Granules may also be obtained by applying gauze pads over the discharging sinuses
- The granules are white or yellowish and ranges in size from minute specks to about 5 mm
- They are crushed between slides and stained by gram stain and examined
- The granules are in fact, bacterial colonies and will be found to consist of dense network of thin gram-positive filaments, surrounded by peripheral zone of

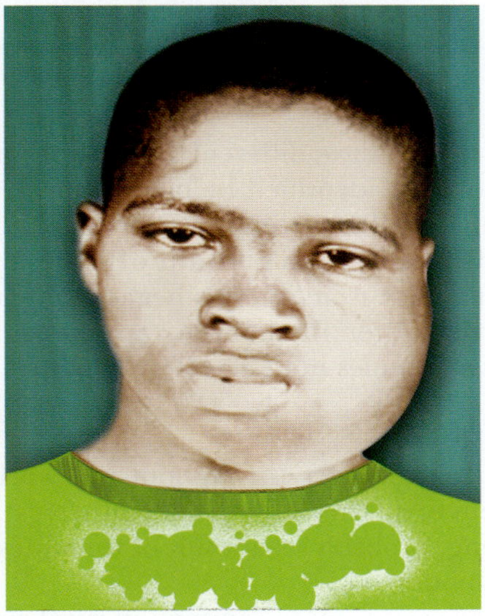

Fig. 10.22: Actinomycosis of jaw

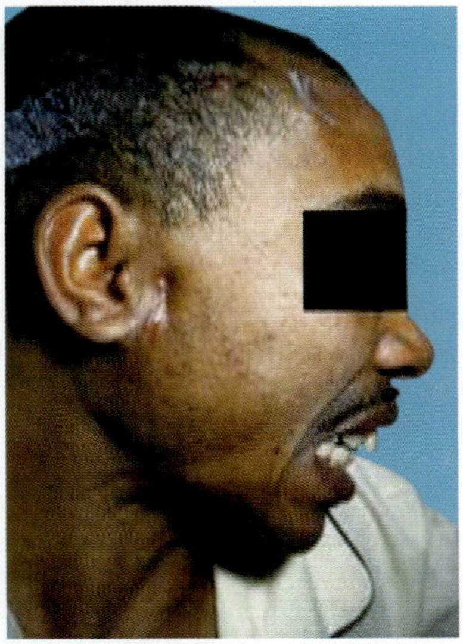

Fig. 10.23: Actinomycosis, with multiple sinuses in the skin

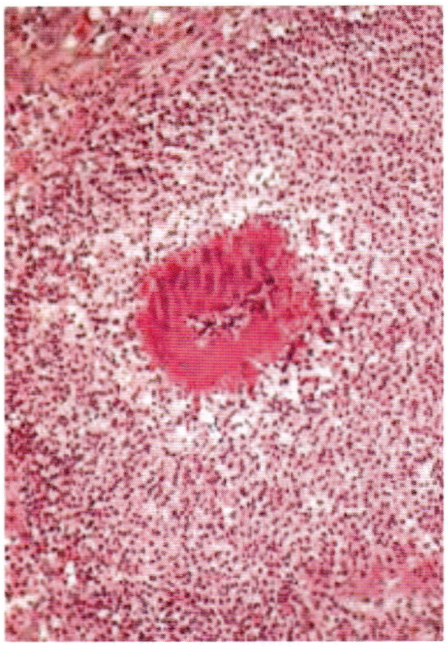

Fig. 10.24: Demonstration of actinomycetes (Low power)

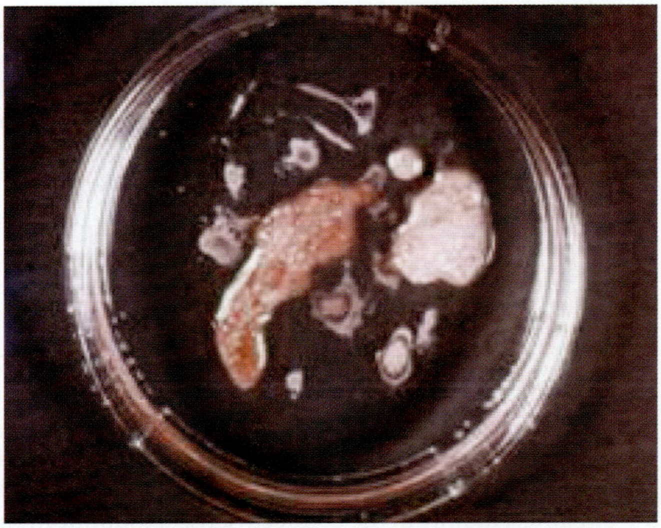

Fig. 10.26: Demonstration of sulfur granules in pus, by shaking in test tube

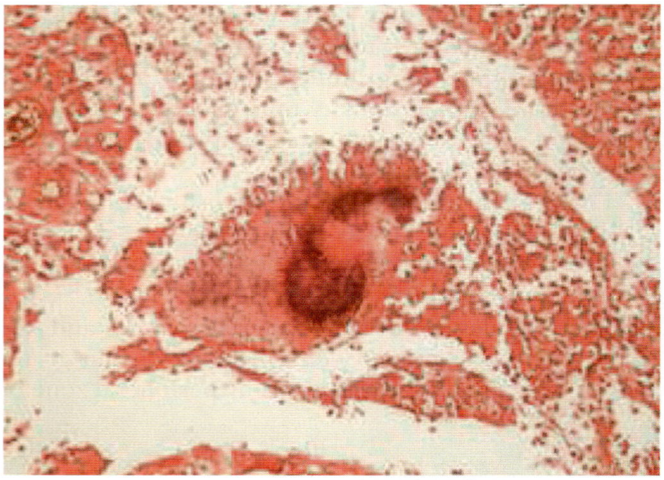

Fig. 10.25: Demonstration of actinomycetes (High power)

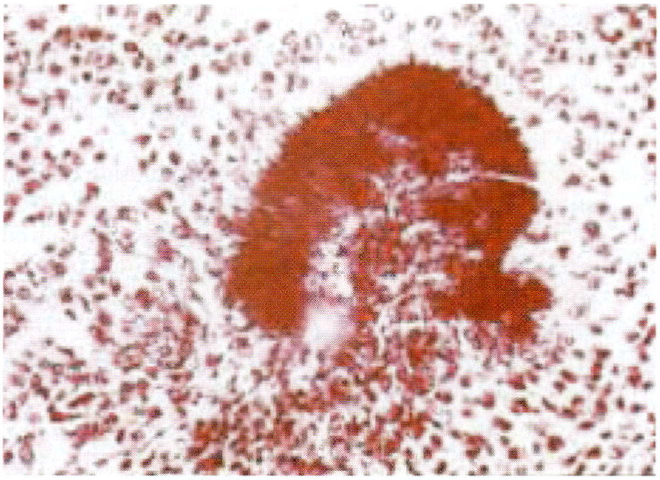

Fig. 10.27: Granules presenting a sun-ray appearance

swollen radiating club shaped structures, presenting a sun ray appearance (Fig. 10.27)

- The clubs are believed to be antigen-antibody complexes
- Sulfur granules or pus containing *Actinomyces* are washed and inoculated into thioglycollate liquid medium or streaked on brain-heart infusion agar and incubated anaerobically at 37°C
- In thioglycollate, *A. bovis* produces general turbidity, whereas *A. israelii* grows as fluffy balls at the bottom of the tube
- On solid media, *A. israelli* produces small spidery colonies in 48 to 72 hours that become heaped up, white and irregular or smooth, large colonies in 10 days
- Other species have different types of colonies
- The isolate is identified by microscopy, biochemical reactions and fluorescent antibody methods
- Gel diffusion and immunofluorescence can differentiate *A. israelii* from other actinomycete species and from other filamentous anaerobes that may produce granules in tissues (Fig. 10.28).

Epidemiology

- The disease occurs throughout the world, but its incidence in the advanced countries has been declining, probably as a result of the widespread use of antibiotics
- Actinomycosis is more common in rural areas and in agricultural workers

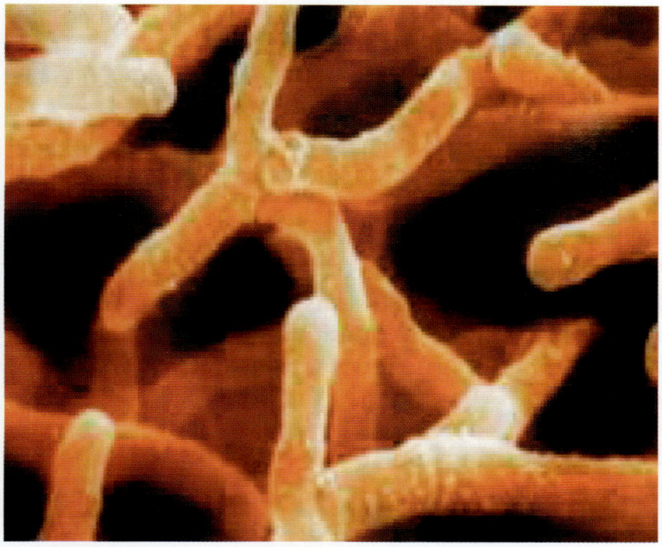

Fig. 10.28: Differentiating *A. israelii* from other actinomycetes

- Young male patients are most commonly affected
- The reason for this predisposition is not known
- About 60 percent cases are cervicofascial and 20 percent are abdominal.
- Pelvic actinomycosis is seen mainly in women, using intrauterine devices.

Treatment

- The bacterial infection is mostly treated with antibiotics, such as penicillin, usually given through a vein in the first instance, followed up by tablets. Depending on the seriousness of the infection, it may be necessary to continue antibiotics for 6 to 12 months, to prevent relapse
- In some cases, surgery may also be necessary to drain deep abscesses and to remove the sinuses. Surgery can also be used to remove the large infected lumps and to seal off any sinuses, which have moved into the bone structure
- *Actinomyces* bacteria can also be treated with other medications, including chloramphenicol, erythromycin, tetracyclines and clindamycin. However, they almost always respond to the combination of antibiotics and surgery.

MYCETOMA (MADUROMYCOSIS)

Introduction

Mycetoma or maduromycosis, is a slow growing bacterial or fungal infection, focused in one area of the body, usually the foot. For this reason and because the first medical reports were from doctors in Madura India, an alternate name for the disease is Madura foot. The infection is characterized by an abnormal tissue mass beneath the skin, formation of cavities within the mass and a fluid discharge. As the infection progresses, it affects the muscles and bones and at this advanced stage, disability may result.

Description

Although the bacteria and fungi that cause mycetoma are found in soil worldwide, the disease occurs mainly in tropical areas in India, Africa, South America, Central America and South-east Asia. Mycetoma is an uncommon disease, affecting an unknown number of people annually.

There are more than 30 species of bacteria and fungi that can cause mycetoma. Bacteria or fungi can be introduced into the body, through a relatively minor skin wound. The disease advances slowly over months or years, typically with minimal pain. When pain is experienced, it is usually due to secondary infections or bone involvement. Although it is rarely fatal, mycetoma causes deformities and potential disability at its advanced stage.

Source of Infection

Thorn trees contain the organisms, when it injures the skin and open the wound, it inoculates the organisms into subcutaneous tissues. When conditions are suitable, they grow and form grains and granuloma will be formed around the grain as a part of the host response to the organisms. The granuloma is firm, but can be cystic or soft. As the grains grow upwards, they attach to the skin and through it the sinus opens and discharges pus. The color and consistency of the pus depends on the etiological agent.

They may spread downwards affecting muscles and bones. Mycetoma affects many sites of body, but more commonly the foot (Madura foot). It can also infect upper limb, chest, abdomen, perineum, head and neck. Infection of head and neck is the most serious condition, as it compresses the cranium and causes abnormal neurological signs and symptoms.

Classification

Eumycete or True Fungi

It is a fungal infection:
- *Madurella mycetomatis*: Form big black grains
- *Madurella grisea*: Form black grains
- *Curvularia lunata*: Also cause black grain
- *Aspergillus nidulans*: Form white soft grains.

Actinomycetoma

It is a bacterial infection:
- *Streptomyces somaliensis*: Causes dirty yellow grains like sand
- *Actinomadura madurae*: Cause white soft grains
- *A. pelletierii*: Small red soft grains

- *Nocardia brasilienses*: Form very small creamy white or orange colored grains
- *Pseudallescheria boydii (Scedosporium apiospermum)*

History

- The earliest sign of mycetoma is a painless subcutaneous swelling. Some patients have a history of a penetrating injury at that site
- Several years later, a painless subcutaneous nodule is observed. After some years, massive swelling of the area occurs, with induration, skin rupture and sinus tract formation
- As the infection spreads to contiguous body parts, old sinuses close and new ones open
- Nearly 20 percent of patients with mycetoma experience associated pain, usually due to secondary bacterial infection or less commonly due to bone invasion
- Constitutional symptoms and signs of mycetoma are rare
- Patients may report a deep itching sensation.

Clinical Features

- Irrespective of the causative agent, the appearance of the mycetoma lesion is consistent as follows:
  - Initially, subcutaneous swelling is present
  - In a later phase, a subcutaneous nodule develops
  - Eventually, massive swelling with induration, rupture of the skin and formation of sinus tracts occur (Fig. 10.29)
- A chronic, slowly progressing bacterial or fungal infection, usually of the foot or leg, characterized by nodules that discharge an oily pus. Also called "Madura boil"

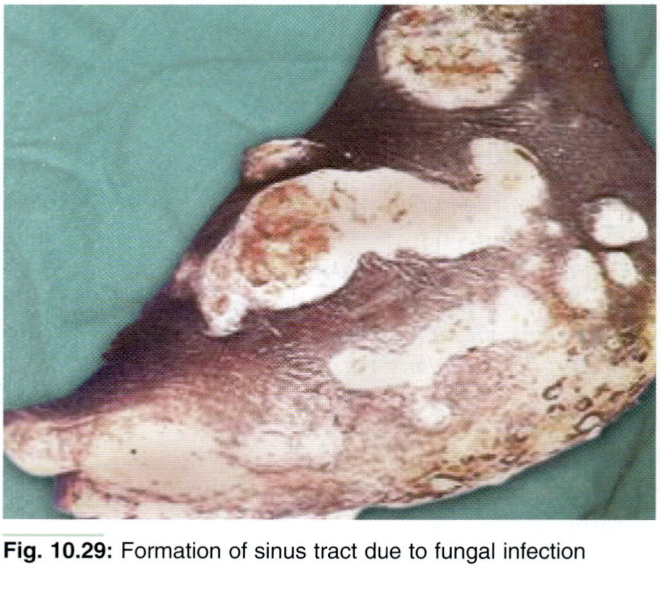

Fig. 10.29: Formation of sinus tract due to fungal infection

- In general, eumycetoma is more circumscribed and progresses slower than actinomycetoma
- Regional lymphatic obstruction and fibrosis can cause *lymphedema* and *erythema*
- Pulmonary mycetoma has been found to develop and progress more rapidly in individuals infected with HIV.

Primary Osseous Mycetoma

This results from direct inoculation of the organisms into bones, causing bone lesions especially in tibia and calcaneous bones. The condition is presented with pain and can be diagnozed by radiology or surgical exploration.

Spread of Infection

The organisms spread from one site of body to another sites by fascia and less commonly by lymphatics. Hematogenous spread is unknown to occur in individuals except in immunocompromised patients.

Microscopic Features (Figs 10.30 and 10.31)

Treatment

Actinomycetoma

- It is a bacterial infection that can respond to antibiotics if treatment is administered early in the course of the disease
- A combination of two drugs in 5 weeks cycles is used. If needed, the cycles can be repeated once or twice
- The following agents have been used in combination:
  - Trimethoprim-sulfamethoxazole (TMP-SMZ)
  - Dapsone (diaminodiphenyl sulfone)
  - Streptomycin sulfate
- Amikacin can be substituted for streptomycin, but is usually kept as a second-line drug because of its cost
- Rifampin has been used as a second-line drug in resistant cases
- An effective and convenient regimen combining a short course of intravenous gentamicin with a 6 months oral course of cotrimoxazole and doxycycline has recently been described.

Eumycetoma

- It may respond partially to antifungal agents, although surgical therapy is preferred for localized disease
- *Madurella mycetomatis,* mycetoma may respond to ketoconazole (200 mg bid)
- *P. boydii (S. apiospermum)* mycetoma should be treated primarily with voriconazole, although it may also respond to itraconazole
- Other agents that cause eumycetoma, may respond intermittently to itraconazole (200 mg bid) or amphotericin B
- The minimum treatment duration is 10 months

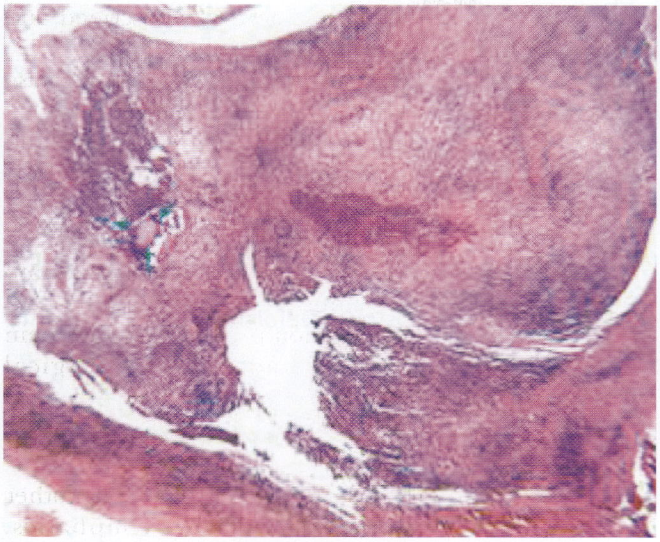

Fig. 10.30: Microscopic features of mycetoma—the tissue above the lower one-fourth of the field is granulation tissue. The two darker zones in the granulation tissue are areas of suppuration. In the zone of suppuration to the left, green arrows identify a colony of organisms. The colony is a "Grain" (mycetoma)

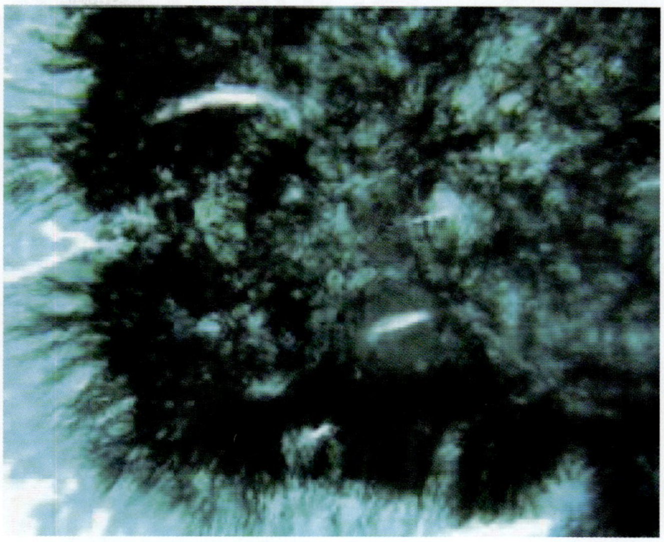

Fig. 10.31: Microscopic features of mycetoma—with a silver methenamine stain, the organisms are filamentous

- Voriconazole is the drug of choice for invasive infections, caused by agents of eumycetoma in immunocompromised patients
- Surgery is recommended for localized mycetoma lesions that can be excised completely without residual disability. Surgical reduction of large lesions can improve the patient's response to medical treatment; however, partial surgical resection without subsequent use of appropriate antimicrobial or antifungal agents is prone to failure
- Amputation is also done for mycetoma in limb extremities
- External beam radiotherapy in doses ranging from 3.5 to 14 Gy has been considered successful treatment in a few selected cases.

Prognosis

- Recovery from mycetoma may take months or years and the infection recurs after surgery in at least 20 percent of cases
- Drug therapy can reduce the chances of a re-established infection
- The extent of deformity or disability depends on the severity of infection; the more deeply entrenched the infection, the greater the damage
- By itself, mycetoma is rarely fatal, but secondary infections can be fatal.

Prevention

Mycetoma is a rare condition that is not contagious, regular aseptic precautions are recommended.

11 Bone Tumors

- Benign Tumors of the Bone
- Malignant Tumors of the Bones
- Dyschondroplasia (Enchondromatosis or Ollier's Disease)
- Paget's Disease (Osteitis Deformans)
- Fibrous Dysplasia

INTRODUCTION

General Principle of Bone Tumors

- Like any other systems in the body, musculoskeletal system may also develop tumors, either as primary or as a secondary, from a distant primary location
- Primary bone tumors may be benign or malignant
- Incidence of bone tumors is very low 1 to 1.5 percent of total malignancies in the body
- Since the cells of skeletal system are derived from mesoderm, primary bone tumors are called "sarcomas"
- Tumors spreading secondarily to the bone are generally primary carcinomas of the breast, kidney, thyroid and lungs. These tumors are called metastatic carcinomas, as the tissue of origin is ectoderm.

Difference between Primary Bone Tumors and Secondary Bone Tumors

Difference between primary and secondary bone tumor is described in Table 11.1

Table 11.1: Difference between primary and secondary bone tumor

Benign	*Malignant*
Slowly growing	Rapidly growing
Well circumscribed	Not well circumscribed
Non-invading	Invading
No or few symptoms	Associated with pain and disability
Does not metastasize	Metastasizes
X-ray shows lesion confined to the bone	X-ray shows ill defined bone lesion, mottled appearance, cortex may be broken

Classification of Bone Tumors (WHO Classification)

Bone Forming Tumors

Benign

- Osteoid osteoma
- Osteoblastoma.

Intermediate

Aggressive (malignant) osteoblastoma.

Malignant

- Central (medullary)
- *Surface (peripheral):* These can further be divided into following types:
  - Parosteal
  - Periosteal
  - High grade surface.

Cartilage Forming Tumors

Benign

- *Chondroma:* These can further be divided into:
  - Enchondroma
  - Periosteal (juxtacortical)
- Osteochondroma
  - Solitary
  - Multiple hereditary
- Chondroblastoma (epiphyseal chondroblastoma)
- Chondromyxoid fibroma.

Malignant

- Chondrosarcoma (primary or secondary)
- Differentiated chondrosarcoma
- Juxtacortical chondrosarcoma
- Mesenchymal chondrosarcoma
- Clear cell chondrosarcoma.

Giant Cell Tumor

Osteoclastoma

Marrow Tumors

- Ewing's sarcoma of the bone
- Neuroectodermal tumor of the bone
- Malignant lymphoma of bone (primary/secondary)
- Myeloma.

Vascular Tumors

Benign

- Hemangioma
- Lymphangioma
- Glomus tumor (glomangioma).

Intermediate

- Hemangioendothelioma
- Hemangiopericytoma.

Malignant

- Angiosarcoma
- Malignant hemangiopericytoma.

Other Connective Tissue Tumors

Benign

- Benign fibrous histocytoma
- Lipoma.

Intermediate

Desmoplastic fibroma.

Malignant

- Fibrosarcoma
- Malignant fibrous histocytoma
- Liposarcoma
- Malignant mesenchymoma
- Leiomyosarcoma
- Undifferentiated sarcoma.

Other Tumors

Benign

- Neurilemmoma
- Neurofibroma.

Malignant

- Chodroma
- Adamantinoma.

Secondary Malignant Tumors

- Thyroid
- Breast
- Lungs
- Kidney
- Prostrate.

■ Lichtenstein Classification of Primary Bone Tumors (Table 11.2)

Table 11.2: Lichtenstein classification of primary bone tumors

Histologic types	***Benign***	***Malignant***
Hemopoietic		*Myeloma*
Chondrogenic	Osteochondroma Chondroma Chondroblastoma Chondromyxoid fibroma	Primary chondrosarcoma Secondary chondrosarcoma Clear cell chondrosarcoma
Osteogenic	Osteoid osteoma Benign osteoblastoma	Osteosarcoma Parosteal osteosarcoma Periosteal osteosarcoma
Unknown origin	Giant cell tumor Fibrous histocytoma	Ewing's tumor Malignant giant cell tumor Adamantinoma
Fibrogenic	Fibroma Desmoplastic fibroma	Fibrosarcoma Malignant fibrous histocytoma
Notochordal		Chodroma
Vascular	Hemangioma	Hemangioendothelioma Hemangiopericytoma
Lipogenic	Lipoma	
Neurogenic	Neurilemmoma	

Briston University Classification (Table 11.3)

Table 11.3: Classification of bone tumors according to Briston University

Origin	*Benign*	*Malignant*
Cartilage	Osteochondroma Chondroma Chondroblastoma Chondromyxoid fibroma	Chondrosarcoma
Bone	Osteoid osteoma osteoblastoma	Osteosarcoma
Bone marrow		Multiple myeloma Malignant lymphoma
Fibrous tissue	Desmoplastic fibroma	Fibrosarcoma
Unknown origin	Giant cell tumor	Malignant giant cell tumor
	Fibrous histocytoma	Ewing's tumor Adamantinoma
Vascular tissue	Aneurysmal bone cyst Hemangioma	
Synovium	Synovioma	Synovial sarcoma

ABC Classification by Charles Price (Table 11. 4)

Table 11.4: ABC Classification of bone tumors by Charles Price

Section	*Benign*	*Malignant*
Section A Angioid tumor	Angioma aneurysmal bone cyst glomus tumor	Angiosarcoma
Section B Bone forming tumor	Osteoma osteoblastoma osteoid osteoma	Osteosarcoma periosteal osteosarcoma
Section C Cartilage forming tumor	Chondroma osteochondroma chondroblastoma	Chondrosarcoma
Section D Dental and allied	Odontogenic cyst ameloblastoma	Malignant odontoma
Section E Embryogenic vestigial tissue		Chondroma
Section F Fibroblastic	Fibroma	Fibrosarcoma
Section H Heterotrophic tissue	Dermoid	Adamantinoma
Section N Nonosseous connective tissue	Lipoma neurofibroma neurolemmoma	Liposarcoma Ewing's sarcoma myeloma
Section S Synovial tissue	Synovioma	Synovial sarcoma
Section U Undifferentiated connective tissue	Osteoclastoma	Malignant osteoclastoma

Parameters of General Principles of Tumors

History

- Pain and mass disability are the usual presenting symptoms
- Anorexia, weight loss and fever are more pronounced in malignant tumors
- Onset is acute in malignant tumors and insidious in benign tumors
- *Age:* Certain tumors have predilection for certain age groups, e.g. Ewing's tumor has predilection for children.

Clinical Examination

- General examination for evidence of anemia, cachexia, lymphadenopathy, etc.
- Local examination, done to know the extent of the plane of the tumor or presence of any pathological fracture
- Joint examination, done to know the involvement of joint and mechanical effect
- Neurological examination, for assessing the damage of peripheral nerves, due to spread of tumors
- Assessment of the status of arterial and venous circulation.

Investigations

Routine Laboratory Investigations

- Hemoglobin is decreased
- Total WBC count and differential count are increased or decreased
- ESR is increased
- Serum calcium and phosphorous are increased
- Serum alkaline phosphatase is increased in tumors, like osteogenic sarcoma
- Serum acid phosphatase is increased in tumors, like metastatic tumors
- Urine analysis.

Special Investigations

- Radiological investigations
- Chest X-ray for evidence of secondaries
- CT scan
- Arteriography
- Ultrasonography
- MRI
- Bone scan
- Biopsy

Biopsy

Types of Biopsy

- Closed
- Open

Tumor Biopsy Rules

- In malignant tumors remove tumor, 'en bloc'
- No transverse incision
- No important neurovascular structures should be exposed
- It should traverse with only one compartment
- Collect the sample from periphery of the tumor
- If bone sample has to be taken, make a small, oval or circular hole in the bone, to prevent pathological fracture.

Staging of Tumors

Ennekings System of Staging (Table 11.5)

- It is based on degree of anaplasia
- It is divided into two types: G1 of low grade and G2 of high grade
- *Tumor location:* Intracompartmental (T1) and extracompartmental (T2)
- *Metastasis:* Absent (M0) and present (M1).

American Joint Committee on Cancer (AJCC) System for Staging Soft Tissue Sarcomas (Table 11.6)

AJCC System for Staging Bone Sarcomas (Table 11.7)

Treatment

Adjuvant Therapy

- Radiation therapy
- Chemotherapy

Table 11.5: Enneking's system of staging

IA	G1	Low grade
	T1	Intracompartmental
	M0	No metastasis
IB	G1	Low grade
	T2	Extracompartmental
	M0	No metastasis
IIA	G2	High grade
	T1	Intracompartmental
	M0	No metastasis
IIB	G2	High grade
	T2	Extracompartmental
	M0	No metastasis
IIIA	G1 or G2	Any grade
	T2	Intracompartmental
	M1	Metastasis
IIIB	G1 or G2	Any grade
	T2	Extracompartmental
	M1	Metastasis

Table 11.6: AJCC system for staging soft tissue sarcomas

Stage	*Grade*	*Size*	*Depth*	*Metastases*
IA	Low	≤ 5 cm	Any	None
IB	Low	> 5 cm	Superficial	None
IIA	Low	> 5 cm	Deep	None
IIB	High	≤ 5 cm	Any	None
IIC	High	> 5 cm	Superficial	None
III	High	> 5 cm	Deep	None
IV	Any	Any	Any	Present

Table 11.7: AJCC system for staging bone sarcomas

Stage	*Grade*	*Site*	*Metastases*
IA	Low	Within cortex	None
IB	Low	Beyond cortex	None
IIA	High	Within cortex	None
IIB	High	Beyond cortex	None
IIIA		Not defined	
IIIB		Not defined	
IVA	Any	Any	Regional lymph nodes
IVB	Any	Any	Distant metastases

Surgical Therapy

- Choice of surgical procedure can be acertained by Enneking's staging of tumors, as suggested below:
  Grade IA : Requires local procedure like curettage
  Grade IB : Wide excision
  Grade IIA : Radical excision
  Grade IIB : Radical amputation
  Grade III : Multiprolonged approach, like surgery, chemotherapy and radiotherapy
- Other surgical procedures include:
  – Curettage
  – Limb-salvage surgeries
  – Resection and reconstruction
  – Amputation

BENIGN TUMORS OF THE BONE

The benign tumors of the bone are:

- Osteoma
- Osteoblastoma
- Osteoid osteoma
- Chondroma
- Chondroblastoma
- Osteochondroma
- Chondromyxoid fibroma
- Aneurysmal bone cyst

■ Osteoma

Definition

An osteoma is a benign slowly growing tumor, occurring in the membranous bones of the skull and face. Usually it is solitary, found in cranial vault, nasal sinuses or bones of jaw.

- *Age:* Onset is in childhood
- *Predominant location:* Frontal and facial bones, usually external, but they may be intracranial, intranasal, intraorbital and within a sinus.

Clinical Features

- It is hard, immovable, mound like or sessile, non-tender swelling, over which the soft tissue is freely movable
- External tumors are asymptomatic. Others produce symptoms referable to the part (e.g. intracranial osteomas cause epileptic seizures and headache).

Pathology

- The most common type of slowly growing osteoma is composed of dense compact bone, covered by a fibrous tissue capsule continuous with the periosteum. The bony structure is continuous with the inner or the outer tables of the skull
- The rapidly growing tumor is composed of a proliferating vascular fibrous stroma, containing newly formed osteoid or osseous spicules.

Treatment

- Once the osteoma has reached a certain size, it remains stationary. It does not undergo malignant change. Excision is indicated, only for symptomatic reasons, rarely for cosmetic reasons
- The defect in the skull is covered with tantalum plate.

■ Osteoid Osteoma

Definition

It is a benign osteoblastic tumor with a well demarcated nidus of less than 1 cm, surrounded by a distinct reactive bone

- *Age:* It is common in young adults between 10 and 25 years of age
- *Sex:* Male preponderance (male to female ratio is 2:1)
- *Sites:* Long bones usually tibia and femur are more commonly affected.

Clinical Features

- The patient complains of vague and intermittent pain, which is more at night
- The pain dramatically decreases after giving aspirin, so much so that this is called as the therapeutic test
- Patient complains of limp due to pain
- There is mild swelling, the local area may be tender, temperature is not raised, the skin is not stretched, shiny or warm
- When the lesion occurs in spine, the patient complains of pain.

Radiology

- The classic radiological presentation of an osteoid osteoma is a radiolucent nidus, surrounded by a dramatic reactive sclerosis in the cortex of the bone
- The center can range from partially mineralized to osteolytic to entirely calcified
- The lesion can occur only in the cortex, in both the cortex and medulla or only in the medulla. The reactive sclerosis may be present or absent.

Differential Diagnosis

- Sclerosing nonsuppurative osteomyelitis of Garre
- Brodie's abscess
- Chronic osteomyelitis with annular sequestrum
- Syphilitic ossifying periostitis
- Eosinophilic granulomas

Treatment

- Complete excision of the nidus immediately and effectively relieves the pain
- Latest treatments are arthroscopically assisted excision for intra-articular situated lesions, CT- guided endoscopic removal, percutaneous excision, MRI guided cryotreatment, CT guided biopsy and thermo-coagulation.

Osteoblastoma

- A benign osteoblastoma also known as osteogenic fibroma of bone or giant osteoid osteoma. It is an uncommon vascular osteoid and bone forming tumor
- It is slow growing and causes symptoms by encroachment on neighboring structures
- *Age:* Young adults, usually less than 20 years of age
- *Sex:* Male to feamale ratio is 2:1
- *Location:* The majority occurs in the spine, affecting the posterior element, the metaphyseal or diaphyseal areas of the long bones of the lower extremities and the small bones of hand and feet.

Clinical Features

Symptoms

- Dull aching pain, not nocturnal or relieved by aspirin

- When the tumor involves cervical or thoracic vertebra, the tumor encroaches the spinal cord, so weakness and paresthesia develops
- Symptoms occur usually from few months to 2 years, before the tumor is discovered.

Signs

Single tender mass is palpable, when the tumor is superficial. Scoliosis and neurological complaints may be present.

Pathology

- Mass is deep red, friable and gritty. It is richly vascular
- Microscopically features, show a loosely fibrillar and vascular tissue, containing numerous dilated thin walled vascular channels
- Within the vascular tissue, a profusion of osteoblast lies between sheets of osteoid and primitive bone trabeculae
- Degree of mineralization of osteoid varies
- In more advanced stages, the primitive osseous tissue undergo osteoclastic resorption and replacement by mature lamellar bone
- Giant cells are prominent, represents osteoclast and macrophages and are unlike those in giant cell tumors
- The stromal cells are compact, round, ovoid or spindly, but are distinct, relatively uniform and mitotic figures are rare.

Radiological Findings

Lesion is essentially radiolucent or mottled, well circumscribed and as it enlarges, the cortex is gradually attenuated, but the tumor is delimited by delicate shell of periosteal bone. Within the tumor, faint stippled densities are noted. Long standing tumors become extremely dense, especially after radiation treatment.

Differential Diagnosis

- Osteoid osteoma
- Osteogenic sarcoma
- Giant cell tumor.

Treatment

- Complete excision, results in cure
- Large defect may be filled with bone grafting
- Radiotherapy to inaccessible tumors.

■ Chondroma

It is also known as enchondroma

- *Age:* 20 to 30 years of age
- *Site:* Phalanges of hand and feet, spine, pelvis, ribs
- *Location:* About two-third of the lesion arise in metaphysic and one-third arise in diaphysis.

Clinical Features

- Slight soreness and severe pain occurs, actual from a pathologic or slowly from malignant transformation
- The phalanges are enlarged as a result of distension of a thinned cortex. In a long bone, no deformity is observed and the tumor remains intramedullary.

Radiological Findings

- X-ray, shows a small translucent loculated or non-loculated area, well demarcated from surrounding bone in a phalanx, the cortex is thinned and expanded. In large long bone cortex is not involved
- The center may exhibit stippling of calcification and striation of fibrous space. No reactive bone formation is present
- In small bones of hand and feet the cortex may be perforated and the shadow of the tumor extends into the soft tissues, although the tumor is benign
- On the other hand, erosion of the cortex in a large tubular bone and spreading externally, strongly suggest malignant change
- This is particularly true, when the borders of the lesion become mottled and hazy.

Pathology

Macroscopically

- The tumor is surrounded by a fibrous capsule, which on cut section displays extensions into the interior, dividing the growth into lobules
- The neoplastic tissue is composed of bluish white translucent cartilage, which contains white areas of calcification and cysts containing gelatinous or myxomatous substance.

Microscopically

- The tumor shows stages of formation of cartilage from embryonic tissue
- The mesenchymal type of tissue is seen only at the periphery of the tumor
- The most mature cartilage is found in the center of the tumor, where it may undergo the usual degenerative changes of cartilage, namely calcification cystic disintegration and myxomatous change
- These chondrocytes are normal in appearance.

Treatment

- Tumor is excised or curetted and the wall cauterized
- The capsule is removed, to reduce the possibility of recurrence
- Large defect is filled with bone graft
- Tumors of long bone should be considered as malignant and radical resection should be done.

Chondromyxoid Fibroma

- Chondromyxoid fibroma or fibromyxoid chondroma is a rare tumor of bone, occurring mainly in adolescent and in young adult
- *Age:* Usually second or third decade and less often in childhood
- *Sex:* No predominance
- *Location:* Most commonly, metaphyseal region of large tubular bone of lower limb. May also involve thin tubular bone, like fibula, phalanx and calcaneum.

Clinical Features

- In adolescent or young adult, the tumor causes mild or no pain
- Slowly increasing local swelling
- Palpable tender mass fixed to underlying bone
- It never metastasizes and sarcomatous degeneration is extremely rare.

Radiological Findings

- The lesion is translucent mass of variable size, usually located eccentrically in the metaphysic
- On the medullary aspect of the lesion, the margin is scalloped and sclerosed
- Over the outer aspect, the cortex is expanded and thinned and may appear interrupted
- In children, at the edge of the tumor, triangular periosteal bone formation, not unlike Codman's triangle often forms
- Within the tumor, a faint trabecular pattern is apparent
- When the tumor involves the narrow tubular bone or small tubular bone, it generally occupies the entire width of the bone, producing fusiform expansion and thinning of cortex.

Treatment

- Local excision and filling of cavity with autogenous bone graft
- Curettage is not sufficient because the tumor may recur
- Wide en bloc excision result in high rate of tumor.

Chondroblastoma

Definition

A chondroblastoma is a cellular, vascular and cartilaginous tumor of young adult, occurring about the epiphyseal line. Destroying cancellous bone and characteristically containing multiple calcium deposits

- *Age:* Onset occurs before obliteration of epiphyseal line from 10 to 20 years
- *Sex:* Male predominance
- *Location:* Ends of long bones, about the knee and humerus
- *Position:* About one side of epiphyseal line, chiefly in the metaphysic, it may extent to epiphysis.

Clinical Features

- Pain, tenderness and swelling in most cases
- Occasionally, limp and joint effusion is present.

Radiological Findings

- Lesion begins or is centered within the epiphysis
- It is oval to round with well defined borders. The epiphysis are opened at the time of initial presentation
- They fill less than one half of the epiphyseal end of the bone. The opposite is true for the GCT.
- It is eccentrically positioned
- Thin ring sclerosis is present around the tumor, with puntated densities in tumor mass.

Treatment

Curettage and obliteration of tumor with bone graft.

Osteochondroma (Exostosis)

Definition

It is benign cartilage capped, protuberance of the metaphysis or diaphysis

- *Age:* With solitary form 75 percent of the patient are 30 years of age or younger. More than 95 percent of patients with multiple lesion are younger than 20 years of age
- *Incidence:* Osteochondroma represents 20 percent of all benign tumors. Solitary osteochondroma represents 7.9 percent and multiple variant represents 0.6 percent
- *Sex:* Male: female ratio is 1.6:1.

Location

- About 80 percent of the lesion occur in long bone, particularly around the knee and in upper humerus
- Pelvis, scapula and ribs are involved in 20 percent of cases
- Usually, osteochondromas are metaphyseal for metadiaphyseal located.

Clinical Features

- Some patients develop pain due to mechanical irritation. Pedunculated osteochondromas can result in irritation of muscle, ligaments or tendons, during motion, nerve compression or fracture through the stalk
- Lumps can be palpated, which can be painful or painless
- It can be associated with aneurysm and bursitis

■ Hereditary Multiple Exostoses

- Hereditary multiple exostoses (HME) is an autosomal dominant condition, associated with short stature, multiple osteochondromas and asymmetrical growth at the knees and ankles. It may lead to deformities
- The leg length inequality is usually about 4 cm and the risk of malignant degeneration is between 1 and 20 percent
- The osteochondromas are located close to the metaphyses and they may be sessile or pedunculated
- The cortex of the lesion is continuous with the cortex of the bone, with a homogeneous continuation of the medulla.

■ Dysplasia Epiphysealis Hemimelica

- Dysplasia epiphysealis hemimelica (DEH) or Trevor disease is characterized by osteochondromas, arising in the epiphyses and thus involving the joint
- The lesions are usually restricted to one side of the body, either left or right. Hence, the name hemimelica is used to reflect involvement of one side of the body
- There may be multiple lesions in a single limb
- DEH usually occurs in infants or young children
- DEH primarily involves one side of an epiphysis, the medial side is affected twice as often as the lateral side
- On macroscopic inspection, the bony lesion is found to be a pedunculated mass closely connected to the epiphysis with a cartilaginous cap
- The histologic appearances are similar to those of an osteochondroma.

■ Multiple Epiphyseal Dysplasia

- Multiple epiphyseal dysplasia is another autosomal dominant condition characterized by the presence of irregular epiphyseal ossification, with intracapsular or periarticular chondromas of the knees and ankles
- This condition is usually present in late childhood
- The spine is usually normal.

■ Dominant Carpotarsal Osteochondromatosis

Introduction

- Dominant carpotarsal osteochondromatosis is another autosomal dominant entity, which Maroteaux and colleagues described in a mother and son
- The osteochondromas are confined to carpotarsal bones
- Maroteaux suggested that dominant carpotarsal osteochondromatosis is a condition distinct from DEH
- Dominant carpotarsal osteochondromatosis is usually sporadic.

Pathogenesis

- Osteochondromas develop due to a beaked failure of constriction, with cortical overgrowth adjacent to the growth plate and subsequent eccentric bony growth from this beak, usually away from the joint
- The excrescence that forms, then continues to grow until the growth plate closes. Growth ceases at puberty
- Malignant degeneration occurs in 1 to 25 percent of cases and should be suspected, if an exostosis rapidly increases in size, especially in an adult
- Spontaneous resolution of osteochondromas has been described
- Osteochondromas that continue to grow after puberty, should raise the possibility of chondrosarcomatous transformation
- The pathogenesis of HME is poorly understood, but many theories have been put forward to explain its development
- The isolation of islets of cartilaginous tissues from the diaphyseal surface of growing cartilage had been hypothesized to cause abnormal osteogenesis
- Further theories postulate that osteochondroma formation is related to a defect in the anchoring of germinal cartilage cells to the physes or to the failure of a thin, cortical sleeve of bone, acting as a structural constraint, with this failure, allowing a spillover of physeal cells onto the metaphysis
- The physical stress theory postulates, that focal accumulations of embryonic connective tissue at sites of tendon attachments are converted to hyaline cartilage.

Theories

- Müller supports a clonal etiology and theorizes that osteochondromas result from a primary defect in periosteal differentiation, in which ectopic collections of cartilage cells arise from the proliferative layer of the metaphyseal periosteum. Multipotent mesenchymal cells in the region of the perichondral groove of Ranvier, have also been implicated in the development of osteochondromas.
- Langenskiöld believes that proliferative interstitial physeal chondrocytes persist in chondrogenesis, as they are transformed into the proliferative layer of the metaphyseal periosteum.
- Clonal karyotypic abnormalities have been documented in osteochondromas. Studies indicate that the cartilaginous portion of the osteochondroma has a clonal or neoplastic origin.
- Porter and Simpson believe that the osteal portion of the osteochondroma, provides only a supportive stroma, an idea that is supported by the fact that

ablation of the cartilage cap alone is followed by cessation of growth of the osteochondroma. Currently, however, no molecular or immunohistochemical data supports this observation.

- *The physical-stress theory:* Postulated by Geschikter and Copeland, states that focal accumulations of embryonic connective tissue at sites of tendon attachments are converted to hyaline cartilage.
- *Theory of histogenesis:* Throughout the life, the deep layer of the periosteum retains the potential for forming cartilage or bone, the cambium layer produces an embryonic tissue that is the common forerunner for bone and cartilage, the tumor may represent a perverted activity of the periosteum, which reverts to its role as perichondrium.
- *Neoplastic theory:* Research has shown loss of heterozygosity at the EXT loci in the cartilaginous cap of osteochondromas and in tissue from chondrosarcomas. Further, clonal karyotypic anomalies have been documented in osteochondromas. These studies indicate that the cartilaginous portion of the osteochondroma has a clonal or neoplastic origin.

Radiological Features

- All osteochondromas solitary or multiple are bony protruberance, showing as a pedunculated stalk or sessile. They typically point away from joint
- The cortical and medullary portion of the tumor is continuous with cortex and medulla of the bone
- The cartilage covering is invisible, unless it is calcified.

Pathology

- An osteochondroma is composed of two basic parts, a cartilage-capped protruberance and its bony stalk
- Bony stalk may be pedunculated or sessile
- The shape of the cap is usually mushroom like and rounded to irregularly bosselated
- On cut section large osteochondroma may demonstrate irregular conglomeration of hard, gritty whitish to yellowish areas, that contain variably sized fragments of translucent to whitish calcified cartilage.

Treatment

Total excision of the tumor.

■ Aneurysmal Bone Cyst

- It is a benign, solitary, expansile and erosive lesion of bone
- One percent of benign bone lesion
- *Age:* Most frequent in children (85% cases are less than 20 years old)
- *Sex:* Female to male ratio is 2:1
- *Location:* Aneurysmal bone cyst (ABC) can be found in any bone of the body. The most common location is metaphysic of the lower extremity long bones, more so than the upper extremity. Approximately one-half of the lesion in flat bones occur in pelvis.

Etiology

- Unknown, but ABC are thought to be a reactive process secondary to trauma or vascular disturbances
- One theory of primary ABC is that these lesions are secondary to increased venous pressure that leads to hemorrhage, which causes osteolysis. These osteolysis can in turn promote more hemorrhage, causing amplification of cyst
- Aneurysmal bone cyst (ABC) can be secondary to underlying disease
- The most common precursor lesion was giant cell tumor (19–39%) of cases, followed by osteoblastoma, angioma and chondroblastoma.

Pathology

- Macroscopically, an ABC is like a blood filled sponge, with a thin periosteal membrane. Soft fibrous walls separate spaces filled with friable blood clot
- Microscopically, the ABC has cystic spaces filled with blood. The fibrous septa have immature woven bone trabeculae as well as macrophages, filled with hemosiderin, fibroblast, capillaries and giant cells.

Clinical Features

- Swelling, tenderness and pain
- Occasionally, there is a limited range of motion due to joint obstruction
- Spinal lesion can cause neurological symptoms secondary to cord compression
- Pathological fractures are rare due to the eccentric location of the lesion.

Differential Diagnosis

- Unicameral bone cyst
- Chondromyxoid fibroma
- Giant cell tumor
- Osteoblastoma
- Telangiectatic osteosarcoma.

Radiographic Features

- ABC is placed eccentrically in the metaphysic and appear osteolytic
- The periosteum is elevated and the cortex is eroded to a thin margin
- The expansile nature of the lesion is often reflected by a "blow-out" or soap bubble appearance
- Pencil-in-cup appearance.

Radiological Classification of Aneurysmal Bone Cyst (Companacci's Classification)

- *Type I:* Cyst in middle with little or no expansion
- *Type II:* Lesion substitutes the whole bone segment
- *Type III:* Eccentric interosseous lesion with little or no expansion
- *Type IV:* Subperosteal cyst and superficial erosion of cortex
- *Type V:* Periosteum eroded and expansion into soft tissue.

Treatment

- Curettage with bone grafting
- Curettage with cementing
- Cryosurgery
- En bloc excision with or without reconstruction of skeletal defect.

MALIGNANT TUMORS OF THE BONES

■ Giant Cell Tumor

Definition

Benign giant cell tumor is an osteolytic tumor, arising from the epiphysis and is common in young adults. Though it is benign, but it is locally malignant

- *Sex:* The male to female ratio is 1.5:1
- *Age:* It is common between 15 and 35 years of age (80% occur, in more than 20 years of age and the average age group is 35 years)
- *Sites:* About 75 percent of GCT occurs in lower end of femur and upper end of tibia
- *Gross structure:* The tumor consists of ragged fibula and distal end of radius.

Pathology

- Friable, bleeding tissue filled with old or fresh blood clot, with various sized cysts and cavities
- Color varies from red and brown
- Epiphyseal end of the bone is distorted
- Tumor extension in the joint cavity is usually not seen and there is no evidence of periosteal reaction
- Microscopically, the tumor is encompassed by a fibrous capsule at the periphery
- Presence of abundant tumor giant cells are quiet characteristic
- These cells are characterized by their larger size, multiple nuclei, which are more than 150 in number, distributed throughout the cell
- Appearance of spindle cell indicate malignant potential.

Histological Grading

Jaffe's Criterion

Grade I

- Presence of characteristic stromal cells <30 percent
- Little intercellular collagen
- Spindle cells are adjacent to the necrotic tissue.

Grade II: Random distribution of giant cells are seen among the stromal cells greater than 30 percent and less than 50 percent.

Grade III: Nuclei of giant cells are identical to those of the stromal cells > 50 percent.

Ennekings Staging of Benign GCT

Stage 1 (Latent)

- Incidence is 10 to 15 percent
- It was discovered accidentally, no symptoms
- Pathological fractures may be present.

Stage 2 (Active)

- Incidence is 70 percent
- Symptomatic, pathological fracture may be present
- Benign.

Stage 3 (Aggressive)

- Incidence is 10 to 15 percent
- Symptomatic rapidly growing
- Benign, cortex is perforated.

Clinical Features

- The course of the tumor is chronic
- Unlike osteogenic sarcoma, pain is not the presenting feature, but history of trauma is there, as the patient complains of swelling, which is situated on one side of the bone
- Skin over the tumor is stretched, but there are no dilated veins
- Tenderness is moderate or absent, egg shell crackling sensation may be present or absent
- Invasion in the joint is rare and joint effusion is rare
- Pathological fracture is a late feature.

Radiological Features (Figs 11.1A and B)

- An osteolytic area is seen near the epiphysis
- The cortex is thin and expanded
- There is no periosteal new bone formation
- Thin septa of bone traverse the interior of bone and gives it "soap bubble" appearance
- The cortex may be disrupted in late stages
- Joint extension is rare.

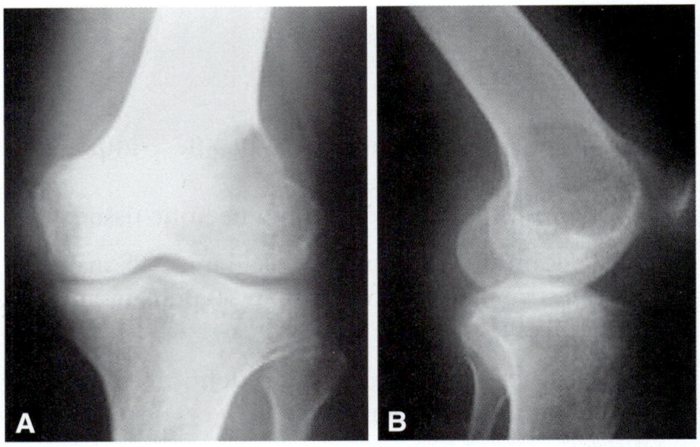

Figs 11.1A and B: Radiological features of GCT

Companacci's Radiographic Grading

Grade I: Cystic lesion
Grade II: Cortex is thin but not perforated
Grade III: Cortex is perforated, with extension in the soft tissue.

Treatment

- Curettage and bone grafting
- En bloc resection
- Curettage and acrylic bone cementation
- Curettage and cryosurgery
- Turnoplasty
- Arthrodesis
- Arthroplasty
- Radiotherapy.

Giant Cell Variance

- Osteoclastoma
- Chondroblastoma
- Aneurysmal bone cyst
- Brown's tumor
- Fibrous dysplasia
- Non-ossifying bone tumor
- Adamantinoma.

■ Osteosarcoma

Definition

It is the most common malignant primary bone tumor, arising from multipotent mesenchymal tissue of bone. It is characterized by direct formation of bone or osteiod, by proliferating tumor cells.

Incidence

- 1/75000 of the population
- Common primary malignant bone tumor next to multiple myeloma
- Occurs in young, between 10 and 20 years, mostly second decade. Rare before 10 years of age. Male predominance, when seen in females, starts at early age.

Sites

- Metaphysis of long bones (90%)
- Distal end of femur
- Proximal end of tibia
- Proximal end of humerus
- May affect the jaws in the aged.

Location

About 52 percent in femur, 9 percent in greater trochanter, 20 percent in tibia and 9 percent in humerus. It is common in the upper aspect, but rare below deltoid tuberosity.

Predisposing Factors

The predisposing factors of the tumors are:

- Virus
  - *DNA virus:* Polyoma and SV-40 virus
  - *RNA virus:* Harvey and Moloney mouse sarcoma virus, known to produce tumors in animals and not in humans
- *Radiation:* A dose of 2000 rads are given, to osteoprogenitor cells situated in the area of active growth, at the metaphysis and malignancy set in
- *Chemicals:* Beryllium compounds, methylcholanthrene, etc.

Clinical Features

- Pain is the initial and dominating symptom
- Bony swelling appears after some week
- Swelling progressively increases in size.

General Examination

- General health deteriorates with anemia, loss of weight and cachexia
- Patient develops pulmonary symptoms, due to secondaries.

On Examination

- Swelling is fusiform
- Skin is stretched, shiny and vascular, with prominent veins
- Swelling is warm to touch and show pulsation, if tumor is highly vascular
- It is firm to hard in consistency
- In late stages, tumor fungates.

Classification of Osteosarcoma

Primary Osteosarcomas

- *Conventional:* They show following characteristics:
  - Osteoblastic poor, 5 years survival rate

– Chondroblastic, 5 years survival rate, 3 times more than osteoblastic variety
– Fibroblastic, 5 years survival rate, 2 times more than osteoblastic variety
– Small cell
– Telangiectatic

- Surface (juxtacortical) osteosarcoma
  – Parosteal osteosarcoma
  – Periosteal osteosarcoma
- High grade surface osteosarcoma.

Secondary Osteosarcoma

- Postirradiation
- Paget's sarcoma
- Solitary/multiple osteochondromatosis
- Bone infarction
- Chronic osteomyelitis
- *Miscellaneous:* GCT, fibrous dysplasia, chondroblastoma, osteoblastoma, etc.

Rare Osteosarcoma

- Li-Fraumeni syndrome (p-53 mutation in association with retinoblastoma)
- Osteosarcoma of the jaw
- Multicentric osteosarcoma.

Other Classifications

Dahlins (Prognostic) Classification

- *Osteoblastic:* Poor 5 years survival rate
- *Chondroblastic:* Five years survival rate, three times more than osteoblastic variety
- *Fibroblastic:* Five years survival rate, two times more than osteoblastic variety.

Geschickter and Copeland Classification

- Sclerosing type
- Osteolytic type
- Mixed type with both osteoblastic and osteolytic variety
- Telangiectatic type.

Lichtensten Criteria

This criteria for identifying osteogenic sarcoma, includes the following:

- Sarcomatous stroma
- Spindle cells
- Direct formation of neoplastic osteoid and bone.

Pathology

- Grossly it is a large tumor, with areas of destruction gives an appearance of "leg of mutton"
- Consistency range from hard to soft
- Color of tumor could be white, if fibroblastic, yellowish-white, if osteoblastic and bluish, if cartilaginous
- At the areas of rapid growth, there are areas of cavitation, necrotic foci and hemorrhages
- Sun ray appearance seen is due to the bone deposition along the vessels
- Codmans triangle is the reactive new bone formation, parallel to the bone.

Histology

- Small spindle cells, with hyperchromatic nuclei
- Shape may be round, cuboidal or columnar
- Cells are pleomorphic in nature
- Giant cells are often present
- Matrix may be myxomatous, cartilaginous or osseous
- Areas of hemorrhages may be present.

Radiological Features (Figs 11.2A and B)

- Tumor arises from metaphyseal region of the bone, either centrally or from cortex
- Mottled area of rarefaction with areas of osteosclerosis
- When it extends beyond the cortex, the periosteum is raised and there is new bone formation in lines at right angle to the cortex. This causes "sun ray appearance" on X-ray.
- Codman's triangle is seen at the junction of normal bone and tumor area, it is a reactive new bone formation subperiosteally.
- Chest X-ray (CXR) may show secondaries in chest.

Treatment

- The aim of treatment is to confirm the diagnosis, to evaluate the spread and to execute adequate treatment
- Confirmation of diagnosis is done clinically, histologically, radiologically and through laboratory findings

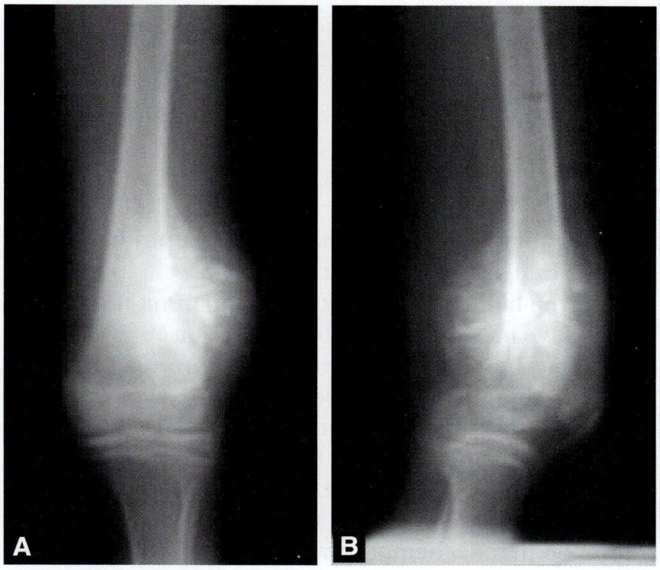

Figs 11.2A and B: Radiological features

- Evaluation of the spread of the tumors is done. Lung is common area of metastasis, CXR should be done. CT and MRI will detect the extent of tumor and soft tissue involvement
- Bone scan will detect skip lesions
- *Surgery:* Early and radical ablation is the surgery of choice. Amputation remains the mainstay
- *Level of amputation*
  - *Upper end of humerus:* Fore quarter amputation
  - *Upper end tibia:* Mid thigh amputation
  - *Upper end femur:* Hind quarter amputation and hip disarticulation
  - *Lower end femur:* Mid-thigh amputation and hip disarticulation.

Newer Techniques

- Limb salvage with tumor endoprosthesis
- In juxta-articular, intraepiphyseal resection and biological reconstruction
- Megavoltage radiotherapy
- Radiation is given preoperatively, to decrease the viable cells that get disseminated into bloodstream
- Useful adjuvant in the treatment of resectable tumors
- Radiation destroys tumor cells, with minimal effect on uninvolved parts
- Total dose is 6,000 to 8,000 rads or 230 rads/day or 1,000 rads/week.

Preliminaries before Irradiation Therapy

- Bone scan are done to detect the skip lesion
- Biopsy scar is limited to less than 2 cm size, to avoid skin necrosis
- Chemotherapy is given to increase the susceptibility of tissue to irradiation.

Chemotherapy

- It is given pre-and postoperatively to control the micrometastasis
- Drugs are methotrexate, citrovorum factor, endoxan and cisplatinum.

Role of Chemotherapy

- After ablation of the primary tumor, it produces a disease-free state for many months
- If given before the metastasis is apparent, it improves the 5 years survival rate by 60 percent
- Chemotherapy started early after the diagnosis destroys the microscopic foci at a stage, when they are most susceptible to the action of drugs
- It prevents metastasis in 60 percent of the cases and the remaining 40 percent become disease-free due to aggressive attack on the metastasis. After metastasis has occurred, chemotherapy decreases the tumor size and enables easy removal.

Immunotherapy

- New concept, the sensitized lymphocytes from the survivors are infused in the patient
- The immunological status is increased, by giving specific antibiotics, BCG vaccine, allogenic sarcoma tumor cell vaccine for 2 years, interferon, etc.
- *Follow up:* Every 6 to 8 weeks for recurrence and metastasis.
- *Prognosis:* Without therapy, death occurs in 6 months to 2 years. With surgery and chemotherapy 5 years disease-free life seen in 70 percent of patients.

■ Ewing's Sarcoma

- Ewing's sarcoma was first described by Ewing in 1928
- It arises from primitive mesenchymal cells of the medullary cavity.
- This is a rare primary malignant bone tumor (10–14%) of all malignant bone tumors, affecting children
- It is a lethal tumor with poor survival rate of 5 years.

Incidence: Common between 4 and 25 years of age group (80%).

Sex: More common in males.

Site: Diaphysis of long bones, i.e. femur, tibia, fibula, humerus, etc. About 20 percent of bone tumors are seen in flat bones.

Clinical Features

On General Examination

Patient has moderate fever, anemia, pain and swelling are the common symptoms.

Local Examination

- Visible or palpable tender swelling
- Rapidly increasing in size
- Raise of local temperature with dilated veins
- Location in rib, may be associated with pleural effusion
- Constitutional symptoms, like fever, sweating, chills, anemia and leukocytosis creates confusion, as it mimics acute osteomyelitis.

Pathology

Macroscopically

- Tumor is pale soft mass, with minimal bone tissue
- Areas of cystic degeneration and hemorrhages
- There is simulation of osteomyelitis by the presence of milky pus, like fluid due to degeneration
- From the medulla, it reaches to the surface through the haversian canals.

Microscopically

- Tumor is very cellular with minimal stromal tissue

- Characteristic cells are small polyhedral, with pale cytoplasm and large nucleus
- Appearance is monotonously uniform
- In some areas, there was pseudorosette formation, simulating rosette formation by neuroblastoma
- Tumor can be differentiated from reticulum cell sarcoma, as it stains for glycogen positively by periodic acid-schiff stain (PAS) and in reticulum cell sarcoma, silver stain is positive.

Investigations

Radiographic Features

- Lesion can be lytic, sclerotic or mixed
- Diaphyseal lesion, with irregular destruction (motheaten appearance or cracked ice appearance) (Fig. 11.3)
- Periosteal new bone formation is in layers giving an "onion peel" appearance
- Permeative margin
- Biopsy is necessary for diagnosis.

Laboratory Tests

- Increased ESR
- Leukocytosis
- Anemia
- Urine for vanillylmandelic acid
- Immunohistochemical markers
- Electron microscopy study
- Tissue for glycogen stain
- Special staining with HBA-71, which recognizes a product of MIC-2 gene has been suggested to be specific for Ewing's sarcoma and neuroectodermal tumors
- Ewing's sarcoma is associated with chromosomal transformation (11 and 22). The tumor markers include, neuron specific enolase, myeloperoxidase.

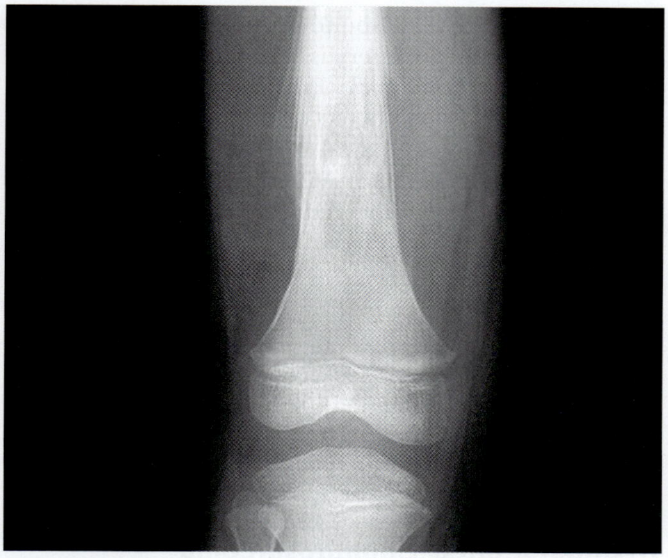

Fig. 11.3: Ewing's sarcoma diaphyseal lesion with onion peel appearance

Differential Diagnosis

- Osteomyelitis
- Osteosarcoma
- Malignant lymphoma.

Treatment

- Tumor is highly sensitive to radiation, it melts like snow
- Combination of radiotherapy and chemotherapy is used
- Even after chemotherapy, recurrence rate is 20 to 30 percent, because of radiation induced sarcomas
- Therefore, surgical resection for the control of primary lesion is used
- *Effective chemotherapy:* Drugs, like ifosfamide, cisplatinum, epipodophyllotoxin for short period of time
- *Radiation:* Highly sensitive, it is mainstay of treatment and dose is 4,000 rads, for entire limb and 1000 rads, as boost to tumor (melts like a snow)
- *Surgery:* Amputation, conservative surgery, like debulking or limb salving surgery
- Unfavorable prognostic factors:
  - Male patient
  - Humerus, if involved
  - Pelvic bone, if involved
  - Distant metastasis
- Primary irradiation with amputation, has two years survival rate of 15 percent
- A combination of chemotherapy, radiotherapy with surgery improves the survival rate of 50 to 75 percent for 3 to 5 years.

■ Chondrosarcoma

- It is malignant slow growing tumor
- It arises from cartilage cell
- It ranges from being locally aggressive, to high grade malignancy.

Incidence: Second in frequency to osteosarcoma.

Site: Common are proximal femur, humerus, ribs, scapula, innominate bones, rare in hand and feet except in calcaneum.

Sex: Males commonly affected than females (about 2%)

Location: Long bone from diaphyseal-metaphyseal region

Age: 20 to 60 years of age, peak in sixth decade.

Types

Primary

- Central (medullary) type
- Juxtacortical (peri/parosteal)
- Clear cell chondrosarcoma
- Mesenchymal chondrosarcoma
- Dedifferentiated chondrosarcoma.

Secondary

Arising from pre-existing benign condition, like exostosis or multiple enchondromas.

Classification of Chondrosarcoma

- *Conventional chondrosarcoma*
  - Borderline: Can be low grade or high grade.
- *Secondary chondrosarcoma*
  - Solitary/multiple exostosis
  - Solitary/multiple enchondromatosis
- *Peripheral chondrosarcoma*
- *Dedifferentiated chondrosarcoma*
- *Miscellaneous*
  - Mesenchymal chondrosarcoma
  - Chondrosarcoma of small bone
  - Synovial chondrosarcoma

Pathology

Macroscopically

- Tumor is lobulated, appears as white or bluish mass
- Firm in consistency
- Areas of myxomatous degeneration and softening
- Irregular patchy areas of calcification seen.

Microscopically

Masses of cartilage cells with more than one nucleus and are hyperchromatic

Histologically

Tumor is based on cellularity, pleomorphism and mitosis

- Grade 1: Low grade
- Grade 2: Intermediate grade
- Grade 3: High grade.

Clinical Features

- Patients complaints of swelling with history of dull aching pain
- Swelling is hard, in consistency with lobulated surface
- Grows very slowly and may causes mechanical restriction of joint movements

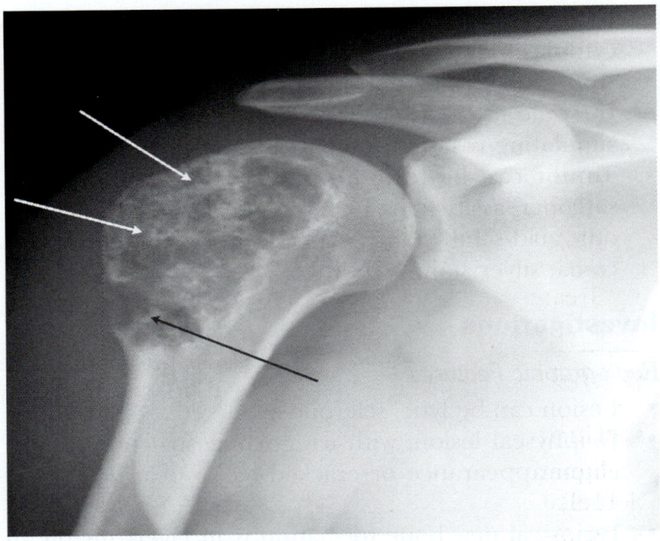

Fig. 11.4: Chondrosarcoma of proximal humerus showing lytic lesion with calcification (cotton wool appearance) lytic lesion (black arrow) speckled calcification (white arrows)

Radiological Features (Fig. 11.4)

Central Tumors

- Central lytic lesion with calcification gives fluffy, cotton wool, popcorn or bread-crumb appearance
- It invades the soft tissue little or no periosteal reaction.

Peripheral Tumors

Very large tumors and central part is calcified.

Treatment

- If tumor does not respond to radiotherapy and chemotherapy, then surgery is the treatment of choice
- *Low and medium grade:* En bloc excision and reconstruction of skeletal defects, endoprosthesis, etc.
- *High grade lesion:* Radical excision and chemotherapy or amputation at appropriate level
- *Palliative radiotherapy:* If tumor is present in inaccessible area.

Prognosis

Prognosis is poor in following cases:

- Axial skeleton and proximal bone tumors
- Childhood and young adults
- Cytologically suggesting high grade malignancy
- Secondary chondrosarcoma
- Survival time after treatment is 10 years.

Dedifferentiated Chondrosarcoma

- Most malignant variety of chondrosarcoma
- Accounts for 10 percent of all chondrosarcoma

- It is second mutation with the pre-existing chondrosarcoma, with the second sarcoma taking on microscopic features of high grade fibrosarcoma or osteosarcoma
- The tumor, thus have a bimorphic histological feature
- Radiographic feature is also dimorphic. Most radiographs show a chondrosarcoma with superimposed destructive area
- Treatment is wide excision and prognosis is poor.

■ Multiple Myeloma

Definition

Malignant tumor arising from plasma cells of reticuloendothelial cells of bone marrow. It can occur as:

- *Solitary plasmocytoma:* Constitutes less than 10 percent of the myelomas. It is a low grade lesion, which involves the younger age group. In about 30 percent of the patients, systemic evidence of multiple myeloma develops
- Multiple myeloma
- *Osteosclerotic myelomas:* It is a rare variant, characterized by sclerotic or mixed sclerotic/lytic lesion, involving spine, pelvis and ribs. Amylodosis leading to chronic inflammatory demyelinating polyneuropathy. Patient may have a polyneuropathy; organomegaly; endocrinopathy; 'M' protein; skin changes (POEMS syndrome)
- *Incidence:* Accounts for 45 percent of total malignant tumors
- *Age:* 50 to 80 years of age. Males are commonly affected (M:F-2:1)
- *Site:* Flat bones, like vertebra, skull, ribs and pelvis where red marrow is present.

Pathology

Grossly

- Tumor is dark red in color
- Soft in consistency and lies within medulla
- The cortex is thin and broken.

Microscopically

- Consist of round cells, with eccentrically placed nucleus with nucleolus
- Chromatin is sparse and is arranged in spokes of wheel fashion
- Perinuclear halo, typical of plasma cell not seen in multiple myeloma.

Associated Pathology

- Interstitial fibrosis in the kidney
- Nodules in the lungs
- Amylodosis may occur.

Clinical Features

General Examination

- Patient becomes severely anemic, loses weight and becomes cachexic
- In the late stages, patient develops hyperazotemia, uremic syndrome, hypercalcemia, hyperuricemic syndrome and hemorrhagic diasthesis.

Signs and Symptoms

- Generalized bone pain and pain in back
- Pain may be intermittent, but later becomes intense
- In the early stages, there are hardly any clinical symptoms
- Late stages, patient's complaint of soft tissue swelling and sign of pathological fracture
- The sternum and ribs may be tender and sign of vertebral collapse present
- Tumor is chronic and tubular block due to protein cast may be seen, causing renal failure (myeloma kidney).

Radiological Features (Fig. 11.5)

- Affected bone shows diffuse osteoporosis or lytic lesion
- Biconcave vertebra and collapse of vertebra.
- Punched out lesion in the skull and pelvis
- In vertebras the rarefaction is extensive, leading to disappearing vertebrae
- Vertebral pedicle involvement is more common and when involved, it is called as pedicle sign (common in secondaries).

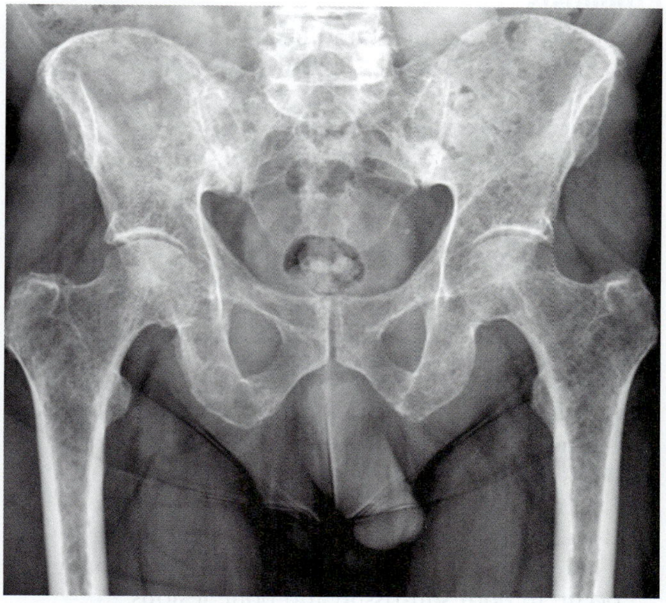

Fig. 11.5: Multiple myeloma: showing diffuse osteoporosis and lytic lesions

Laboratory Findings

- Low hemoglobin
- High ESR
- Increased total protein, A/G ratio is reversed
- Increased serum calcium
- Low to normal alkaline phosphatase, but is raised in pathological fracture
- Urine Bence-Jones proteins are found in 30 percent of patients
- *Serum electrophoresis:* M spike of gamma globulin in 90 percent of cases, e.g. G-60 percent, A-25 percent and others 15 percent
- *Sternal puncture:* Myeloma cell may be seen
- Bone marrow shows, 5 to 100 percent plasma cells
- Bone scan
- Open biopsy
- Serum alpha-2 micro-globulin is increased (tumor marker).

Treatment

- Chemotherapy is the mainstay of the treatment
- Drugs used are melphalan, cyclophosphamide, vincristine, steroids, urethane (SCUM)
- High dose of vincristine, doxorubicin, dexamethasone (VDD) is new and better alternative
- Tumor is radiosensitive and localized lesions are treated with radiation for pain relief.

Surgery

- In case of pathological fractures, intramedullary (IM) nailing and limb salvage surgery
- Decompression of cords in neurological involvement.

Prognosis

- Disease is widespread and fatal
- Death in 3 to 5 years.

Complications

- Pathological fractures of rib
- Spinal cord or nerve root compression
- Renal failure
- Severe infection
- Amyloidosis.

Maffucci's Syndrome

This rare disorder is characterized by the development of multiple enchondromas and soft-tissue hemangiomas of the skin and viscera

- Lesions appear during childhood
- Boys and girls are affected with equal frequency
- There is a strong tendency for malignant change to occur, in both soft-tissue and bone lesions
- The incidence of sarcomatous transformation in one of the enchondromas is probably greater than 50 percent, but fortunately these tumors are not highly malignant
- Patients with Maffucci's syndrome should be monitored regularly throughout life for any changes in either the bone or the visceral lesions.

DYSCHONDROPLASIA (ENCHONDROMATOSIS OR OLLIER'S DISEASE)

This is a rare, but easily recognized disorder, in which there is defective transformation of physeal cartilage columns into bone.

Clinical Features

Typically, the disorder is unilateral, indeed only one limb or even one bone may be involved. An affected limb is short and if the growth plate is asymmetrically involved, the bone grows in a bent fashion. Bowing of the distal end of the femur or tibia is not uncommon and the patient may present with valgus or varus deformity at the knee and ankle. Shortening of the ulna may lead to bowing of the radius and sometimes dislocation of the radial head. The fingers or toes frequently contain multiple enchondromata, which are characteristic of the disease and may be so numerous that the hand is crippled. A rare variety of dyschondroplasia is associated with multiple hemangiomata (Maffucci's syndrome), this is described below. The condition is not inherited. Indeed, it is probably an embryonal rather than a genetic disorder.

Radiological Features

The characteristic change in the long bones is radiolucent streaking, extending from the physis into the metaphysic, the appearance of persistent, incompletely ossified cartilage columns trapped in bone. If only half of the physis is affected, growth is asymmetrically retarded and the bone becomes curved. With maturation the radiolucent columns eventually ossify, but the deformities remain. In the hands and feet, the cartilage islands characteristically produce multiple enchondromata. Beware of any change in the appearance of the lesions after the end of normal growth, as this may be a sign of malignant change, which occurs in 5 to 10 percent of cases.

Treatment

Bone deformity may need correction, but this should be deferred until growth is complete, otherwise it is likely to recur.

■ Dyschondrosteosis

In this disorder, there is also disproportionate shortening of the limbs, but it is mainly the middle segments (forearms and legs), which are affected. It is the commonest of the mesomelic dysplasias and is transmitted as an autosomal dominant defect. Stature is reduced, but not as markedly as in achondroplasia. The most characteristic X-rays changes are shortening of the forearms and leg bones, bowing of the radius and Madelung's deformity of the wrist, which may require operative treatment.

PAGET'S DISEASE (OSTEITIS DEFORMANS)

Paget's disease is characterized by enlargement and thickening of the bone, but the internal architecture is abnormal and the bone is unusually brittle. The condition has a curious ethnic and geographic distribution, being relatively common in North America, Britain, Germany and Australia (more than 3% of people aged over 40 years), but rare in Asia, Africa and the Middle East. There is a tendency to familial aggregation. The cause is unknown, although the discovery of inclusion bodies in the osteoclasts has suggested a viral infection (Rebel et al. 1980).

Pathology

The disease may appear in one or several sites. In the tubular bones, it starts at one end and progresses slowly towards the diaphysis, leaving a trail of altered architecture behind. The characteristic cellular change is a marked increase in osteoclastic and osteoblastic activity. Bone turnover is accelerated, plasma alkaline phosphatase is raised (a sign of osteoblastic activity) and there is increased excretion of hydroxyproline in the urine (due to osteoclastic activity).

In the osteolytic (or vascular) stage, there is avid resorption of existing bone by large osteoclasts, the excavations being filled with vascular fibrous tissue. In adjacent areas, osteoblastic activity produces new woven and lamellar bone, which in turn is attacked by osteoclasts. This alternating activity extends on both endosteal and periosteal surfaces, so the bone increases in thickness, but is structurally weak and easily deformed. Gradually, osteoclastic activity abates and the eroded areas fill with new lamellar bone, leaving an irregular pattern of cement lines that mark the limits of the old resorption cavities. These 'tidemarks' produce a marbled or mosaic appearance on microscopy. In the late, osteoblastic stage the thickened bone becomes increasingly sclerotic and brittle.

Clinical Features

Paget's disease affects men and women equally. Only occasionally does it present in patients under 50 years, but from that age onwards, it becomes increasingly common. The disease may be present for many years remain localized to part or the whole of one bone, e.g. the pelvis and tibia being the commonest sites and the femur, skull, spine and clavicle the next common ones.

Most people with Paget's disease are asymptomatic, the disorder being diagnosed when an X-ray is taken for some unrelated condition or after the incidental discovery of a raised serum alkaline phosphatase level. When patients do present, it is usually because of pain or deformity or some complication of the disease.

The pain is a dull constant ache, worse in bed, when the patient warms up, but rarely severe, unless a fracture occurs or sarcoma supervenes. Deformities are seen mainly in the lower limbs. Long bones bend across the trajectories of mechanical stress, thus the tibia bows anteriorly and the femur anterolaterally. The limb looks bent and feels thick and the skin is unduly warm, hence the term "osteitis deformans". If the skull is affected, it enlarges. The patient may complain that old hats no longer fit. The skull base may become flattened (platybasia), giving the appearance of a short neck. In generalized Paget's disease, there may also be considerable kyphosis, so the patient becomes shorter and ape-like, with bent legs and arms hanging in front of him.

Cranial nerve compression may lead to impaired vision, facial palsy, trigeminal neuralgia or deafness. Another cause of deafness is otosclerosis. Vertebral thickening may cause spinal cord or nerve root compression.

Steal syndromes, in which blood is diverted from internal organs to the surrounding skeletal circulation, may cause cerebral impairment and spinal cord ischemia. If there is also spinal stenosis, the patient develops typical symptoms of spinal claudication and lower limb weakness.

X-ray Findings

The appearances are so characteristic that the diagnosis is seldom in doubt. During the resorptive phase, there may be localized areas of osteolysis, most typical is the flame shaped lesion, extending along the shaft of the bone or a circumscribed patch of osteoporosis in the skull (osteoporosis circumscripta). Later, the bone becomes thick and sclerotic, with coarse trabeculation. The femur or tibia sometimes develops fine cracks on the convex surface stress fractures that heal with increasing deformity of the bone. Occasionally, the diagnosis is made only when the patient presents with a pathological fracture. Silent lesions are revealed by increased activity in the radio nuclide scan.

Biochemistry

Serum calcium and phosphate levels are usually normal. The most useful test is measurement of the serum alkaline phosphatase level, which correlates with the activity and extent of disease. Twenty-four hours urinary excretion of pyridinoline cross-links is a good indicator of disease activity and bone resorption. However, the test is expensive and is, therefore, not used routinely. Patients who are immobilized may develop hypercalcemia.

Complications

- *Fractures:* They are common, especially in the weight-bearing long bones. In the femoral neck, they are often vertical. Elsewhere, the fracture line is usually partly transverse and partly oblique, like the line of section of a felled tree. In the femur, there is a high rate of nonunion, for femoral neck fractures prosthetic replacement and for shaft fractures early internal fixation is recommended. Small stress fractures may be a very painful and they resemble "looser's zones" on X-ray, except that they occur on convex surfaces.
- *Osteoarthritis:* Osteoarthritis of the hip or knee is not merely a consequence of abnormal loading due to bone deformity, in the hip it seldom occurs, unless the innominate bone is involved. The X-ray appearances suggest an atrophic arthritis, with sparse remodelling and at operated joint, vascularity is increased.
- *Nerve compression and spinal stenosis:* Occasionally, this is the first abnormality to be detected and may call for definitive surgical treatment.
- *Bone sarcoma:* Osteosarcoma arising in an elderly patient is almost always due to malignant transformation in Paget's disease. The frequency of malignant change is probably around 1 percent. It should always be suspected, if a previously diseased bone becomes more painful, swollen and tender. Occasionally, it presents as the first evidence of Paget's disease. The prognosis is extremely grave.
- *High output cardiac failure:* Though rare, this is an important general complication. It is due to prolonged increased bone blood flow.
- *Hypercalcemia:* Hypercalcemia may occur, if the patient is immobilized for long. In spite of all these complications, patients with Paget's disease usually come to terms with the condition and live to a ripe old age.

Treatment

Most patients with Paget's disease never have any symptom and require no treatment. Sometimes pain is due to an associated arthritis, rather than bone disease and this may respond to nonsteroidal anti-inflammatory therapy.

Patients should be examined and the alkaline phosphatase level should be measured, at least once a year. Any change in symptoms or a rise in alkaline phosphatase, calls for further investigation and if necessary, more active treatment.

The indications for specific treatment are:

- Persistent bone pain
- Repeated fractures
- Neurological complications
- High-output cardiac failure
- Hypercalcemia, due to immobilization
- For some months before and after, major bone surgery, where there is a risk of excessive hemorrhage.

Drugs that suppress bone turnover, notably calcitonin and bisphosphonates, are most effective, when the disease is active and bone turnover is high.

Calcitonin is most widely used. It reduces bone resorption, by decreasing both the activity and the number of osteoclasts, serum alkaline phosphatase and urinary pyridinoline cross-link levels are lowered. Salmon calcitonin is more effective than the porcine variety, subcutaneous injections of 50 to 100 MRC units are given daily, until pain is relieved and the alkaline phosphatase levels are reduced and stabilized. Maintenance injections once or twice weekly may have to be continued indefinitely, but some authorities advocate stopping the drug and resuming treatment, if symptoms recur. Drug resistance, due to antibody formation may occur, but this will be avoided, when human calcitonin is more generally available.

Bisphosphonates, bind to hydroxyapatite crystals, inhibiting their rate of growth and dissolution. It is claimed that the reduction in bone turnover following their use, is associated with the formation of lamellar rather than woven bone and that, even after treatment is stopped, there may be prolonged remission of disease (Bickerstaff et al. 1990). Etidronate can be given orally (always on an, empty stomach), but dosage should be kept low (e.g. 5 mg/kg per day for up to 6 months), lest impaired bone mineralization results in osteomalacia.

The newer bisphosphonates, such as pamidronate and alendronate are more effective and produce remissions, even with short courses of 1 or 2 weeks. They do not impair bone mineralization and can be repeated if necessary.

Surgery

The main indication for operation is a pathological fracture, which (in a long bone) usually requires internal fixation. When the fracture is treated, the opportunity should be taken to straighten the bone. Other indications for surgery are painful osteoarthritis (total joint replacement), nerve entrapment (decompression) and severe spinal stenosis (decompression). Beware, blood loss is likely to be excessive in these cases. An osteosarcoma, if detected early, may be resectable, but generally the prognosis is grave.

FIBROUS DYSPLASIA

Definition

Fibrous dysplasia or (fibro-osseous dysplasia) is a skeletal developmental anomaly of the bone-forming mesenchyme that manifests as a defect in osteoblastic differentiation and maturation. Thus, leading to replacement of normal marrow and cancellous bone, by immature bone and fibrous stroma

- It is a benign condition, in which normal bone is replaced by fibrous connective tissue, due to a defect in osteoblast differentiation and maturation
- Relatively common disorder of bone, involving the proliferation and maturation of fibroblasts
- Etiology is unknown
- Recognized most frequent during second and third decade of life
- Females affected more than males
- Possible developmental dysplasia
- "Great imitator of bone disease"
- May affect one or more bones
- Less than 1 percent transformation to malignancy.

Three Basic Forms

- Monostotic (70%)
- Polyostotic (27%)
- Polyostotic, with endocrine dysfunction (3%)

Pathological Features

- Normal bone undergoes physiologic resorption and is replaced by irregular shaped woven bone, which is dispersed haphazardly into a predominately fibrous collagenous matrix
- The variable amount of bone, accounts for the range of roentgen density. Radiolucent to ground glass.

Clinical Manifestations

- Signs and symptoms depend on the size, location and number of lesions
- Asymptomatic to intermittent pain
- Local swelling
- Deformity and fracture
- Spontaneous scalp hemorrhage
- Café-au-lait Spots
  - Tanned to dark brown skin lesions and is not raised
  - Fibrous dysplasia "Coast of Maine"
  - Neurofibromatosis "Coast of California"
  - Most common extraskeletal manifestation.
- McCune-Albright syndrome
  - Predominantly in females
  - Consists of:
    i. Polyostotic fibrous dysplasia
    ii. Café-au-lait spots
    iii. Endocrine dysfunction (hyperthyroidism, premature puberty, acromegaly, hyperparathyroidism, Cushing's syndrome and vitamin D resistant rickets).

Laboratory Features

- Normal calcium and phosphorus levels
- Occasional elevations of alkaline phosphatase.

Plain Radiography (Figs 11.6A to C)

First-line of imaging modality.

Advanced Imaging

- Bone scintigraphy, helps to determine activity and areas of skeletal involvement (Fig. 11.7)
- CT scan (Fig. 11.8)
  - Cystic area

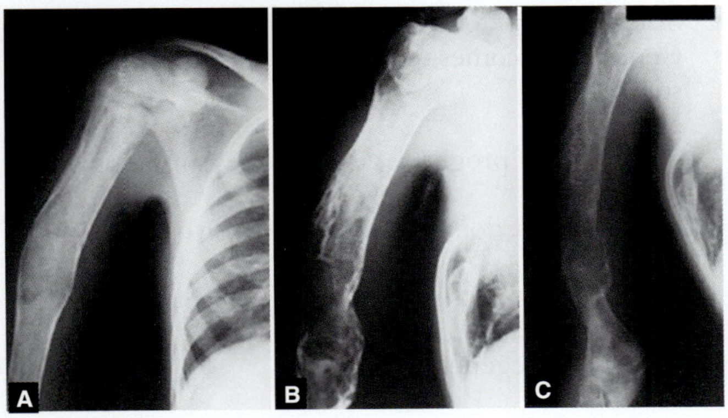

Figs 11.6A to C: Fibrous dysplasia of humerus: the medullary cavity is replaced by fibrous tissue showing ground glass appearance

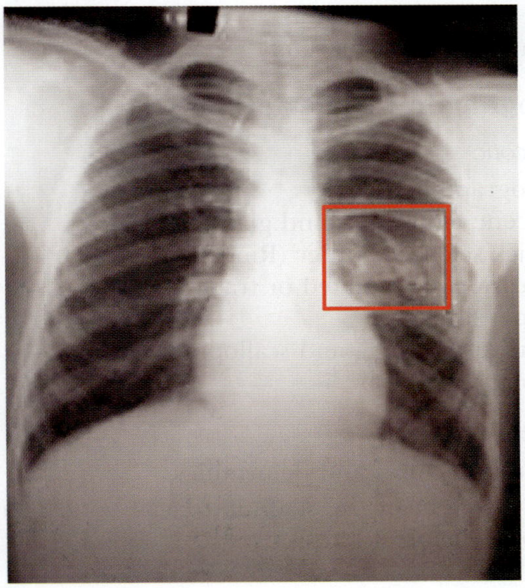

Fig. 11.7: Bone scintigraphy, helps to determine activity and areas of skeletal involvement

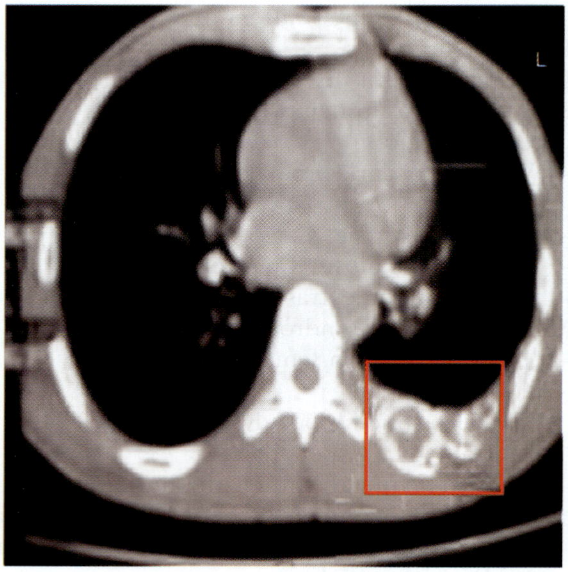

Fig. 11.8: CT scan, showing fibrous dysplasia

- Well defined thick sharp border
- Useful to define extent of craniofacial disease
- *MRI:* Typically moderately low signal T1 and bright or mixed signal on T2.

Skeletal Locations

- *Monostotic:* Proximal femur and ribs
- *Polyostotic:* Femur, skull, tibia, humerus, ribs, etc.
- Most common benign rib lesion
- May demonstrate the "extrapleural sign"
- Diaphyseal-metaphyseal location, typically sparring the subarticular region
- Usually centrally located.

Radiographic Manifestations

Monostotic

- Geographic
- Lucent, smoky (ground glass) (Fig. 11.8)
- Thick sclerotic border (Rind sign)
- Occasionally septated or trabeculated
- Expansile lesion
- Cortical thinning and scalloping
- Elongated lesion.

Polyostotic

- Pseudofractures and deformities
- Involvement of the skull and facial bones, tends to produce more sclerosis
- Pseudoarthrosis
  - Usually lower extremity
  - Fibrous dysplasia and neurofibromatosis most common causes.

Craniofacial Type

- 10 to 25 percent in monostotic
- 50 percent in polyostotic form
- Occurs in an isolated craniofacial form
- *Sites of involvement:* Frontal region, these include following sites:
  - Sphenoid (vestibular dysfunction, tinnitus, hearing loss)
    - Maxillary hypertelorism, cranial asymmetry, facial deformity (i.e. leontiasis ossea)
    - Orbital and periorbital bones, visual impairment, exophthalmos and blindness
    - Ethmoidal bones
    - Cribriform plate, hyposmia or anosmia may result.

Treatment

- Splints and casts
- Curettage and bone grafting
- Bone grafting and stabilization
- En bloc resection
- Osteotomy.

Complications

- Pathological fractures are most common
- Bowing deformities, e.g.
  - Shepherd's crook
  - Leontiasis ossea
- Sarcomatous transformation in 0.5 to 1 percent
  - Fibrosarcoma most common
  - Femur and skull, most common sites.

Prognosis

- Depends on extent and degree of initial skeletal involvement and extraskeletal features
- Size and shape of lesions may change
- Generally becomes quiescent at puberty and remains so
- Monostotic
  - Excellent prognosis, if the bone can be strengthened
  - Usually, it does not change to polyostotic
- Polyostotic
  - Several operative procedures, to achieve bone strength and correct deformity
- Malignant degeneration is rare.

Associated Disorders

Cherubism

- Familial fibrous dysplasia of the jaws (autosomal dominant)
- Begins during 18 months to 2 years and regresses during puberty
- Swelling of the lower face
- "Eyes-raised-to-heaven" sign
- Multilocular cystic lesions, with asymmetric distribution.

Differential Diagnosis

- Eosinophilic granuloma
- Nonossifying fibroma
- Bone hemangioma
- Hyperparathyroidism
- Paget's disease
- Brown's tumor
- Aneurysmal bone cyst.

Mazabraud Syndrome

It is a fibrous dysplasia and soft-tissue myxomas.

12 Gait Analysis

• Gait

■ Gait

Continuous rhythmic alternative movements of lower limbs, in order to propulse the body forward, by moving center of gravity in forward direction with minimal expenditure of energy.

Gait Cycle

It is the duration that occurs from the time, when the heel of one foot strikes the ground to the time at which the same foot contacts the ground again. Normally, the gait cycle is of 1 to 2 seconds.

Two phases of gait cycle are shown in Figure 12.1.

Phases of Gait Cycle

- Stance phase (60% of a gait cycle)
- Swing phase (40% of a gait cycle).

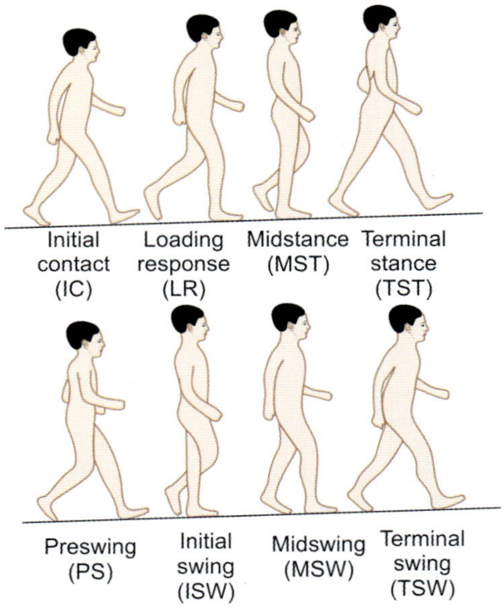

Fig. 12.1: The descriptive phases of a normal gait cycle

Stance Phase

Definition

It is the time during which the limb is in contact with the ground and supporting the weight of the body from heel strike to toe off.

It comprises 60 percent of the gait cycle and is divided into following five phases:

Initial Contact or Heel Strike

- Knee is extended and ankle is in neutral position
- Normally, heel contacts the ground first.

Loading Response or Flat Foot

- Corresponds to the gait cycle's first period of double limb support and ends with a contralateral toe off, when the opposite extremities leaves the ground
- During loading, knee flexes 15°, while ankle plantar flexes 15°, which is an energy conserving mechanism
- Throughout the first phase of stance, hamstrings and ankle dorsiflexors remain active
- Quadriceps and gluteal muscles act during loading and through the early midstance to maintain hip and knee stability.

Midstance

- Begin with contralateral toe off. The center of gravity is directly over the reference foot (stance foot)
- By midstance, the knee is extended and ankle is neutral again
- The triceps surae acts to control tibial advancement (preventing tendency of ankle to dorsiflex, due to body weight and inertia).

Terminal Stance or Heel Off

- Begins when center of gravity is over the supporting foot and ends when contralateral foot contacts the ground
- Terminal stance and midstance are only phases when center of gravity truly lies over the base of support.

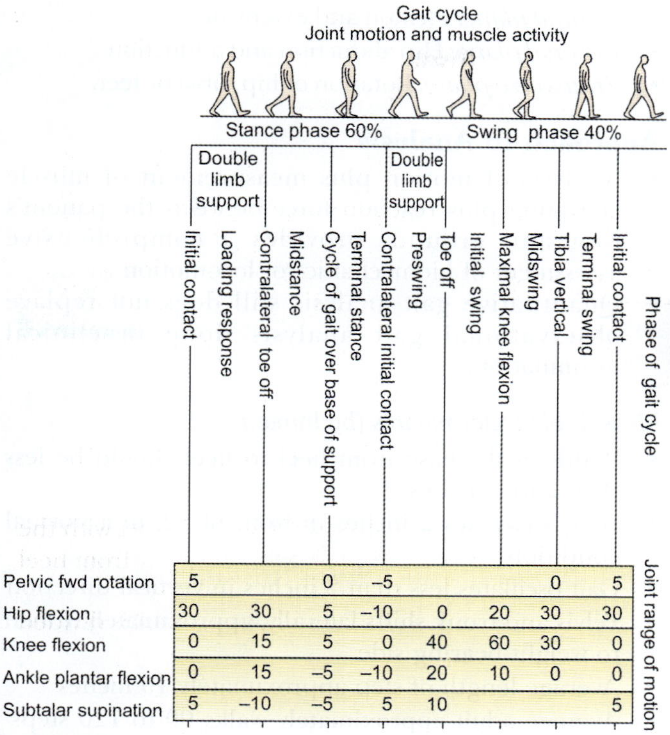

Fig. 12.2: Gait cycle, with different phases and range of motion at various joints

Preswing (Toe Off)

- Begins at contralateral initial contact and ends at toe off
- Preswing corresponds to the gait cycle seconds period of double limb support
- At preswing, knee flexes 35° and ankle plantar flexes at 20°
- In these last phases of stance, the toes, which have been neutral, dorsiflex at the metatarsophalangeal joints.

Swing Phase

Definition

It is the time period during which the limb is off the ground and advancing forward, the body weight is supported by contralateral limb, i.e. acceleration to deceleration. It comprises of 40 percent of gait cycle (Fig. 12.2) and is divided into three phases:

Initial swing or acceleration

- Begins at toe off and continues until maximum knee flexion (60°) occurs
- Contraction of quadriceps initiated before toe off and serves two purposes
  - It prevents heel from rising too high in a posterior direction
  - It helps to initiate forward swing of leg.

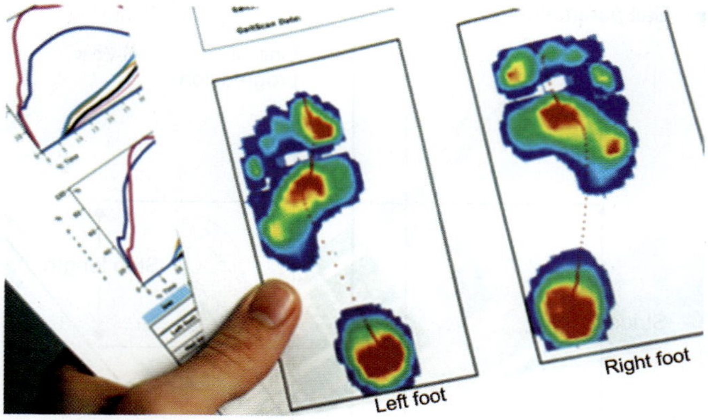

Fig. 12.3: Pressures in the soles of left and right feet

Mid swing

From maximum knee flexion, until the tibia is vertical or perpendicular to the ground.

Terminal swing or deceleration

- Begins, where tibia is vertical and ends at initial contact
- Hamstrings muscles become active, to decelerate forward swing of the leg.

Gait Measurement Technique

- Force
- Motion
- Electromyography
- Energy consumption.

Force/Pressure Measurements

- Glass plate views
- Pressure distribution
- Pressure plates
- Pressure distribution inside a shoe
- Pressure in the soles are seen in Figure 12.3

Motion Measurements

- Goniometers, is used for measuring range of motion
- Electrogoniometers, for joint angle at successive instants
- Conductive walkway, stride length, cadence, velocity, etc.
- Dynamic base, etc.
- Video cameras, for measuring stride length, cadence, velocity, dynamic base, etc.
- *High speed video:* Stop motion measurements
- *Accelerometers:* It is used for measuring accelerations and is comparatively cheaper than other instruments
- Gyroscopes is used for measuring change in orientation
- 3D marker systems, for all possible kinematic measures

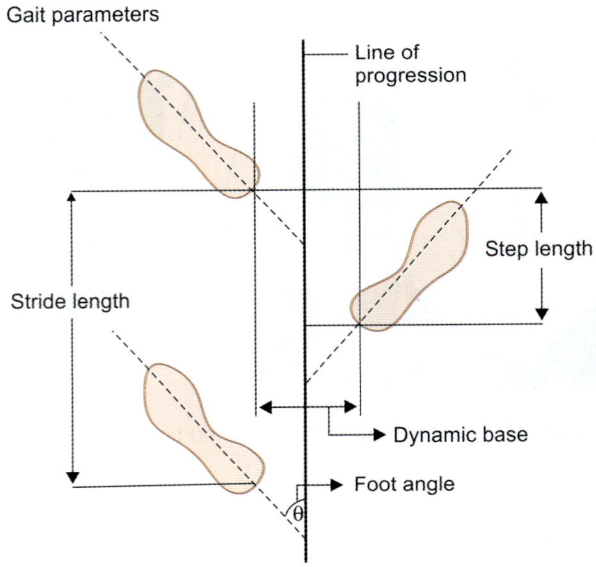

Fig. 12.4: Parameters for gait measurement

Electromyography (EMG) Measurement

- Noisy and qualitative
- Indicator of when the muscle is active
- Surface EMG (most common)
  - Cheap, easy
  - Difficult to interpret because of cross talk and noise
- Fine wire and needle EMG:
  - Penetrate skin
  - Isolate single muscle
  - Mildly painful
  - May change behavior
- Parameters of gait measurement are shown in Figure 12.4.

Energy Consumption Measurement

- *Heart rate:* Cheap and easy
- *Oxygen consumption:* Better indication of relative metabolic state
- Indicator of overall effort
- Often difficult to detect change because of variability.

Gait Energy

- Bipedal gait is inherently unstable and inefficient
- To conserve energy, the movement of joint minimizes the rise and fall of center of gravity, located just anterior to S2 vertebra
- Muscular activities are coordinated
- Inertia is used to its fullest advantage, to lessen the work of walking.

Kinematics

It is defined as the study of the angular rotation of each joint during movement. Kinematics can be observed in three planes:

- *Sagittal plane:* Flexion and extension
- *Coronal plane:* Hip abduction and adduction
- *Transverse plane:* Rotation of hip, tibia or feet.

Approach to Analysis

- Analysis of motion plus measurement of muscle activating plus reaction force between the patient's foot and ground, provides a comprehensive assessment of biomechanics of locomotion.
- Quantitative gait analysis still does not replace observational gait analysis done in clinical examination.

Measurable Determinants (by Inman)

- Width of the base from heel to heel should be less than 2 to 4 inches
- Body's cog lies 2 inches in front of S2, in a normal condition
- Gait oscillates less than 2 inches in vertical direction
- Pelvis and trunk shifts laterally, approximately 1 inch to weight-bearing side
- Average length of step approximately 15 inches
- Average adult approximately walks 90 to 120 steps/min, with average energy cost of only 100 cal/mile
- During swing phase, pelvis rotates 40° forward, while hip joint on the opposite side acts as the fulcrum for rotation.

Gait Abnormalities

Antalgic Gait or Painful Gait

- Due to pain anywhere from foot to hip to spine
- The patient avoids to bear weight on the affected limb (avoid stance phase). Quick, short steps on affected limb, thereby reducing the stance phase and increasing stance phase of unaffected limb
- *Hip abnormality:* The patient leans towards the affected side during stance phase
- *Spine abnormality:* Patient may not walk or walks slowly to avoid pain.

Trendelenburg Gait

- It may be unilateral or bilateral
- When unilateral, the patient leans on the affected side with swaying of the pelvis and shoulder of the uneffected side, as the pelvis drops on the opposite side of the hip and to keep cog over the stance leg. Any condition, in which there is a deficit in the abduction mechanism of the hip joint, medial deviation of the mechanical axis of lower limb and costopelvic impingement, causes this abnormal gait pattern
- Abduction mechanism can be deficit in fulcrum (hip joint), lever arm (neck of femur), power (gluteus

medius), e.g. congenital dislocation of hip, fracture of the neck of femur and polio paralysis.

Stiff Hip Gait

- Patient walks without flexing the hip (about 20° of flexing of hip is essential for normal gait)
- To compensate patient raises pelvis and semi-circumducts the limb to propel forward
- Increase motion of pelvis on lumbar spine during swing.

Stiff Knee Gait

Pelvis raised during swing phase, so that heel clear the floor.

Gluteus Maximus Weakness Gait

- In normal gait gluteus maximus, provides for stability in sagittal plane and for restrain of forward progression. This muscle helps to counteract flexion moment at the hip in early part of stance and restrains the forward movement of femur in late swing in normal gait
- In gluteus maximus, weak trunk must be thrown posteriorly at heel strike, to prevent trunk from falling forward, when there is flexion moment at hip
- Hip in hyperextension, so the center of gravity is behind the joint
- The backward lean is typical of a gluteus maximus weakness gait.

Quadriceps Weakness Gait

- In very weak or paralyzed quadriceps, patient stabilizes his knees for weight-bearing by little leaning on effected side and pressing over the lower thigh by his ipsilateral hand
- Walking on level surface may appear to be normal
- At speed, limb behaves as pendulum, due to full extension of knee joint. This is a preparatory step to heel strike
- At full extension, action of quads is not necessary for stability of knee joint
- If line of gravity is maintained anteriorly to the axis of motion of knee joint, full extension persists through stance phase
- Such a patient however, will be unable to run and may have difficulty in walking on rough or inclined surface and stairs because in those full extension is not attained and knee tends to buckle into flexion.

Spastic Gait

- Spastic muscles does not allow hip and knee to be flexed enough for foot to clear the ground
- Therefore, patient partially drags his weight on the spastic leg. In this attempt, there is some circumduction effect on the lower limb, e.g. hemiplegia, diplegia, cerebral palsy, etc.

High Stepping Gait

Patient flexes the hip and knee excessively, to clear the ground, e.g. foot drop.

Short Limb Gait

- Less than 3.5 to 5.5 percent compensation, by walking on toes on the short limb, flexes the hip and knee of opposite side during stance phase
- Greater than 3.5 to 5.5 percent gait manifests and there is no compensation.

Ataxic Gait

Gait in which foot is raised higher than normal and brought down suddenly in a flapping manner.

Knock Knee Gait

While walking, patient flexes hip slightly, knees points and appose each other, ankles and feet are kept apart with tendency of toeing.

Stamping Gait

Patient raises his feet abnormally high and jerks them forward to strike ground, with a “Stamp”, e.g. sensory ataxia (tabes dorsalis).

Short Shuffling Gait

The patient with stooping body, is propelled forward quickly in successions, as if trying to catch-up with center of gravity, e.g. Parkinsonism.

Gluteus Medius Gait

More or less like Trendelenburg’s gait, occurs in paralysis of gluteus medius.

Cerebeller Gait

Staggering gait, often with tendency to fall to one or other side, forward or backward.

Hysterical Gait

- Diagnosed by exclusion, bizarre and inconsistency. Does not fits with available clinical signs
- History of emotional upset is present.

Wobbling Gait or Chorus Girl Swing

- In bilateral weakness of gluteus medius muscle, gait shows accentuated side-to-side movement
- This gait is also be seen in CDH and coxa vara.

Calcaneal Gait

Patient walks on his broadened heel with a tendency of rotating the foot outwards, tendency of genu recurvatum, with no calcaneal pick up, no push off and is due to weakness of triceps surae.

Scissors Gait

- One leg crosses directly over other with each stapes, like crossing of the blade of scissors due to adductor tightness
- Knee may also be flexed resulting in couching, which lead to couch gait
- During the swing phase, one lower extremity crosses the other leg which is in stance phase
- Seen in cerebral diplegia.

Lathyriatic Gait

Combination of spasticity, hyperabduction and dragging of lower limb elements in the gait.

Helicopod Gait

Legs and feet are thrown in half circles as in hemiplegia.

Drunkers or Reeling Gait

Patient walks irregularly on wide base, swinging side way with out stability and balance, with tendency of falling with each step.

Genu Recurvatum Gait

- In paralysis of hamstring muscle the knee goes for hyperextension, while transmitting weight in mid stance phase
- Seen in poliomyelitis.

Section 2

General Surgery Related to Orthopedics

13 Tetanus

- Types
- Treatment
- Prevention

Introduction

Tetanus is a neurological disorder, characterized by increased muscle tone and spasms. It is caused by tetanospasmin, a powerful protein toxin elaborated by *Clostridium tetani*.

It occurs in several clinical forms, including generalized, neonatal and localized disease. Mortality in developing countries like India is approximately 90 percent and 50 percent in developed countries like USA.

Features of *Clostridium tetani*

- Anerobic, motile, gram-positive and rod like
- Forms an oval and colorless, terminal spores
- Assumes a shape resembling a tennis racket or drumstick (Fig. 13.1)
- Found worldwide in soil, in the inanimate environment, in animal feces and occasionally in human feces
- Spores may survive for years in some environments and are resistant to various disinfectants and to boiling for 20 minutes

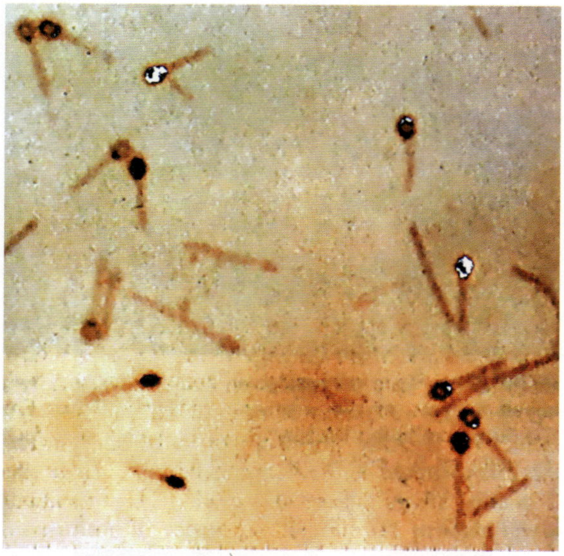

Fig. 13.1: *Clostridium tetani*—shape resembling a tennis racket or drumstick

- Vegetative cells are easily inactivated and several antibiotics, including metronidazole and penicillin are effective against it.

Note: Round terminal spores give cells a "drumstick" or "tennis racket" appearance.

- Tetanus occurs sporadically and almost always affects unimmunized persons, partially immunized persons and fully immunized individuals, who fail to maintain adequate immunity with booster doses of vaccine may be affected as well
- Not contagious from person-to-person
- It is an only vaccine-preventable disease that is infectious but not contagious
- *Temporal pattern:* Peak in winter and summer season
- *Incubation period:* 8 days (3–21 days).

Host Factors

- *Age:* It is a disease of active age (5–40 years), newborn baby, female during delivery or abortion
- *Sex:* Higher incidence in males than females
- *Occupation:* Agricultural workers are at higher risk
- *Rural and urban difference:* Incidence of tetanus in urban areas is much lower than in rural areas
- *Immunity:* Herd immunity does not protect the individual
- *Environmental and social factors:* Unhygienic custom habits and unhygienic delivery practices
- Most cases follow an acute injury (puncture wound, laceration, abrasion or other trauma)
- Abdominal surgeries, anterior/anterolateral approach of spine, foot surgeries, rarely contaminated hand surgeries
- Complicated chronic conditions such as skin ulcers, abscesses and gangrene
- Tetanus has also been associated with burns, frostbite, middle-ear infection, abortion, childbirth, body piercing and drug abuse (notably "skin popping")
- Tetanus is a notifiable disease in many countries.

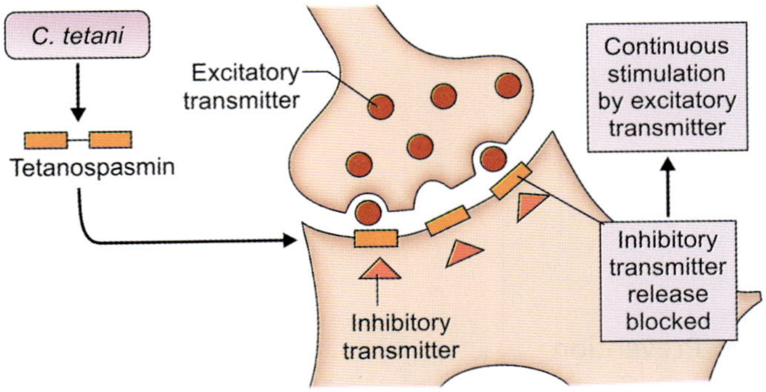

Fig. 13.2: Pathogenesis of *C. tetani*

Pathogenesis

- Entry of *C. tetani* into the body usually involves implantation of spores into a wound (Fig. 13.2). It multiplies and produces a powerful toxin in any deep, contused wound in the presence of dead tissue, foreign bodies and other bacteria. When the oxygen levels of the surrounding tissue is sufficiently low, the implanted *C. tetani* spore then germinates into a new, active vegetative cell that grows and multiplies and most importantly produces toxins
- Cardiotoxin (endotoxin), acts on hemopoetic cells and cardiac tissue
- *Tetanospasmin (exotoxin) acts on CNS:* The effects of this toxin are so severe that the effects of the cardiotoxin is completely masked by it. As growing cells produce tetanospasmin at the wound site, the toxin starts to migrate along nerves and acts mainly on four areas of nervous system, these areas are:
  - Motor end plate
  - Spinal cord
  - Brain
  - Sympathetic system
- The exotoxin produced in the inoculation site inhibits cholinesterase at the motor end plates, resulting in an excess of acetylcholine locally and therefore, a sustained state of tonic muscle spasm
- The exotoxin also travels along the nerves to the central nervous system and causes extreme hyperexcitability of motor neurons in the anterior horn cells, thereby evoking explosive and widespread reflex spasms of muscle in response to sensory stimuli
- Once fixed in the nerve tissue, the toxin can no longer be neutralized by antitoxin
- The shorter the interval between the first symptom and the first reflex spasm, the poorer is the prognosis
- If the interval is less than 48 hours, death is likely
- Wounds containing tetanus organizms may have healed and been forgotten for months or years before some (unknown) change produces the right conditions for the organism to multiply and produce toxin (latent tetanus).

Types

Generalized Tetanus

- Also called descending tetanus
- The most common form of the disease
- Toxin released in the wound enters the lymphatics and bloodstream and is spread widely to distant nerve terminals
- The blood-brain barrier blocks direct entry into the central nervous system
- Characterized by increased muscle tone and generalized spasms
- Median time of onset after injury is 7 days (15% of cases occur within 3 days and 10% after 14 days)
- Short nerves are affected before long nerves, this fact explains the sequential involvement of nerves of the head, trunk and extremities in generalized tetanus.

Signs and Symptoms

- Increased tone in the masseter muscles (trismus or lockjaw) (Fig. 13.3)
- Dysphagia, stiffness or pain in the neck, shoulder and back
- Involvement of other muscles produces a rigid abdomen and stiff proximal limb muscles (the hands and feet are relatively spared)
- *Opisthotonus:* Contraction of the back muscles produces an arched back (Figs 13.4 and 13.5)
- *Risus sardonicus*: Sustained contraction of the facial muscles results in a grimace or sneer (Fig. 13.6)
- Some patients develop paroxysmal, violent, painful, generalized muscle spasms that may cause cyanosis and threaten ventilation.

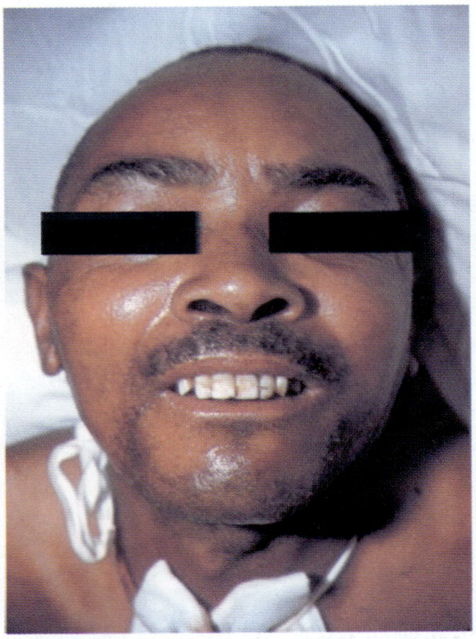

Fig. 13.3: Increased tone in masseter muscle

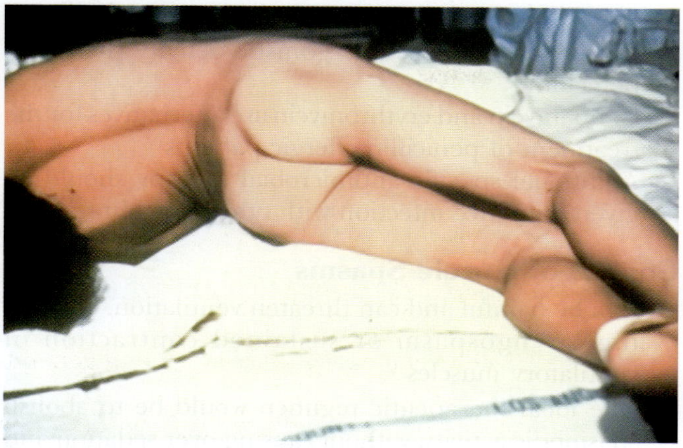

Fig. 13.4: Opisthotonic position after contraction of back muscles (seen from back)

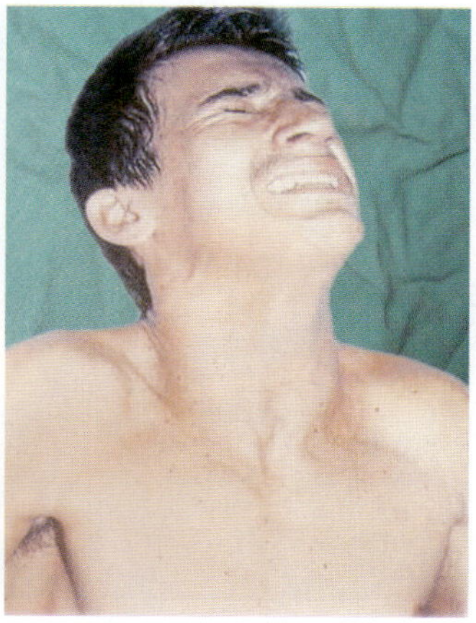

Fig. 13.6: Risus sardonicus, due to sustained facial muscles contraction

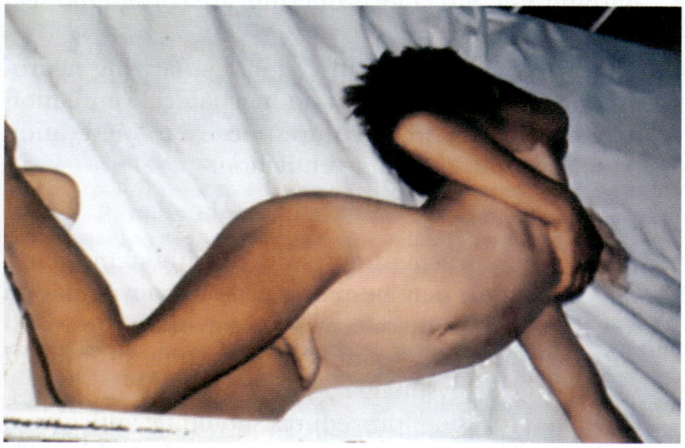

Fig. 13.5: Opisthotonic position (seen from front)

- Spasms occur repetitively and may be spontaneous or provoked by even the slightest stimulation
- A constant threat is reduced ventilation or laryngospasm causing apnea
- The patient may be febrile, although many patients have no fever
- Mentation is unimpaired
- Deep tendon reflexes may be increased
- Dysphagia or ileus may preclude oral feeding
- The severity of illness may be:
  - Mild (muscle rigidity and few or no spasms)
  - Moderate (trismus, dysphagia, rigidity and spasms)
  - Severe (frequent explosive paroxysms)
- *Autonomic dysfunction:* This can occur due to following factors:
  - Labile or sustained hypertension
  - Tachycardia
  - Dysrhythmia
  - Hyperpyrexia, profuse sweating and peripheral vasoconstriction
  - Increased plasma and urinary catecholamine levels
  - Periods of bradycardia and hypotension may also be documented.

Local Tetanus

- Also called ascending tetanus
- Uncommon form
- Toxins travel along the peripheral nerves
- Disease confined to the extremities
- Seen most often in inadequately immunized persons
- May last for months, but usually resolves spontaneously.

Cephalic Tetanus

- Rare form of local tetanus
- Results from head wounds and affects the face
- Most commonly the muscles are innervated by lower cranial nerves
- Can occur in fully immunized persons
- The incubation period is a few days and mortality is high
- The outcome is typically poor
- Mild cases (often associated with otitis media) have more favorable outcomes.

Neonatal Tetanus

- Seen in newborns, when the mother lacks immunity and the umbilical stump becomes contaminated with *C. tetani* spores
- Detected at an early stage, by the refusal of feeds and absence of suckling reflex (Fig. 13.7).

Diagnosis

- Suspected upon exposure to a bite or puncture wound
- Based entirely on clinical findings
- Unlikely, if a reliable history indicates the completion of a primary vaccination series and the receipt of appropriate booster doses

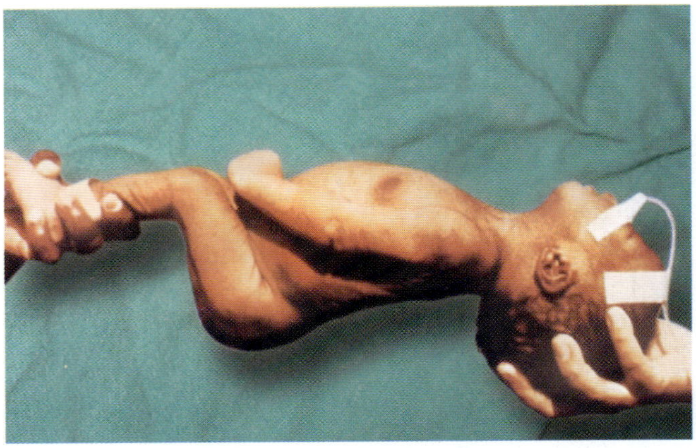

Fig. 13.7: Neonatal tetanus

- Wounds should be cultured in suspected cases
- *C. tetani* can be isolated from wounds of patients, without tetanus and frequently cannot be recovered from wounds of those with tetanus
- The leukocyte count may be elevated
- Cerebrospinal fluid examination yields normal results
- Electromyograms may show continuous discharge of motor units and shortening or absence of the silent interval normally seen after an action potential
- Muscle enzymes levels may be raised
- Serum antitoxin levels of 0.1 IU/ml (as measured by enzyme-linked immunosorbent assay) are considered protective and make tetanus unlikely, although cases in patients with protective antitoxin levels have been reported.

Treatment

The goals of therapy are:

- Eliminate the source of toxin
- Neutralize unbound toxin
- Prevent muscle spasms, while monitoring the patient's condition and providing support, especially respiratory support, until recovery
- Patients should be admitted to a quiet room in an intensive care unit, where observation and cardiopulmonary monitoring can be maintained continuously, but stimulation can be minimized
- Protection of the airway is vital
- Wounds should be explored, carefully cleansed and thoroughly debrided
- Antibiotic therapy is administered to eradicate vegetative cells, i.e. the source of toxin
- The use of penicillin G (10–12 million units IV, given daily for 10 days) has been recommended, but metronidazole (500 mg every 6 hours or 1 gm every 12 hours) is preferred by some experts. On the basis of this drug's excellent antimicrobial activity and the absence of the GABA-antagonistic activity seen with penicillin
- Clindamycin and erythromycin are alternatives for the treatment of penicillin-allergic patients
- Additional specific antimicrobial therapy should be given for active infection with other organims.

Control of Muscle Spasms

- Can be painful and can threaten ventilation, by causing laryngospasm or sustained contraction of ventilatory muscles
- The ideal therapeutic regimen would be to abolish spasmodic activity, without causing over sedation and hypoventilation
- Diazepam, a benzodiazepine and GABA agonist is in wide use
- Barbiturates and chlorpromazine are considered second-line agents
- Therapeutic paralysis with a nondepolarizing neuromuscular blocking agent and mechanical ventilation may be used for spasms unresponsive to medication or spasms that threaten ventilation.

Respiratory Care

- Intubation or tracheostomy, with or without mechanical ventilation, may be required for hypoventilation due to over sedation or laryngospasm or for the avoidance of aspiration by patients with trismus, disordered swallowing or dysphagia
- The need for these procedures should be anticipated and they should be undertaken electively and as early as possible.

Wound Management

- Proper wound management requires consideration of the need for:
  - Active immunization with tetanus toxoid vaccine
  - Passive immunization with TIG
- The dose of TIG for passive immunization of wounds with average severity produces a protective serum antibody level for at least 4 to 6 weeks
- Vaccine and antibody should be administered at separate sites with separate syringes
- In established cases, intrathecal injection of TIG has shown better results than intramuscular injections
- All wounds receive surgical toilet
- Wounds less then 6 hours old, clean, nonpenetrating and with negligible tissue damage
- Dose of tetanus toxoid and anti-tetanus serum (ATS), which must be administered depending upon the immune status of the patient has been described in Tables 13.1 and 13.2 respectively

Table 13.1: Dose of tetanus toxoid, depending upon the immunity category

Immunity category	*Treatment*
A	Nothing more required
B	Toxoid 1 dose
C	Toxoid 1 dose
D	Toxoid complete dose

Table 13.2: Dose of tetanus toxoid and ATS, depending upon the immunity category

Immunity category	*Treatment*
A	Nothing more required
B	Toxoid 1 dose
C	Toxoid 1 dose + human ATS
D	Toxoid complete dose + human ATS

Classification of the Patients, Depending Upon their Immune Status

Class A: Has had complete dose of toxoid or booster dose within past 5 years

Class B: Has had complete dose of toxoid or booster dose within past 5 years, but less than 10 years

Class C: Has had complete dose of toxoid or booster dose more than 10 years ago

Class D: Has not had a complete dose or immunity status unknown.

Course (Manifestation of Disease)

- The course of tetanus extends over 4 to 6 weeks and patients may require prolonged ventilator support
- Increased tone and minor spasms can last for months, but recovery is usually complete
- Death may occur from tetanus, often from cardiac and respiratory effects or secondary complications from the infection.

Prevention

- Spores are extremely stable, although immersion in boiling water for 15 minutes kills most spores
- Exposure to saturated steam under 15 lbs of pressure for 15 to 20 minutes at 121°C is highly effective against spores
- Sterilization by dry heat is slower than by moist heat (1–3 hours at 160°C), but it is also effective against spores
- Ethylene oxide sterilization is also sporicidal
- Sterilization of operation theatre with 500 ml of formalin, 200 g of potassium permanganate/30 cubic meter of space
- All windows and doors are closed except one
- Fissures between the panels of the doors and windows are closed with adhesive tape
- After 12 hours, the doors and windows are opened and the theatre is aired for 24 hours before commissioning it.

Active Immunization

- All partially immunized and unimmunized adults should receive vaccine
- The primary series for adults of tetanus toxoid consists of three doses
  - The first and second doses are given 4 to 8 weeks apart
  - The third dose is given 6 to 12 months after the second.
- A booster dose is required every 10 years.

Passive Immunization

- ATS (equine) 1500 IU (SC) after sensitivity test
- *ATS (human) 250 to 500 IU:* No anaphylactic shock, very safe but costly.

14 Deep Vein Thrombosis

- Venous Anatomy
- Venous Thromboembolism
- Treatment

■ Venous Anatomy

Venous anatomy is divided into the superficial, deep and perforator components. In the lower extremity, the major superficial veins are (Fig. 14.1):

- The greater saphenous vein (located anterior to the medial malleolus and travelling medially to the fossa ovalis in the groin)
- The lesser saphenous vein (posterior to the lateral malleolus, coursing posterolaterally to the popliteal-fossa)
- The posterior arch vein, also called Leonardo's vein (beginning in the medial ankle and joining the greater saphenous vein below the knee)
- The deep veins of the calf typically are duplicated as venae comitantes with numerous communicating branches
- The posterior tibial and peroneal veins also communicate with the soleal sinusoids
- In the thigh, the deep venous system includes the superficial and deep femoral veins that join about 4 cm below the inguinal ligament
- The superficial and deep systems are connected by perforating veins (direct and indirect)
- Most blood flows from the superficial to the deep system via the direct perforators, but indirect perforators (small superficial veins draining into muscles that connect to the deep system via intramuscular veins)
- Blood is propelled toward the heart by compression of the deep veins by calf muscle contractions during walking and flow is unidirectional due to a series of one-way valves (also called as peripheral heart).

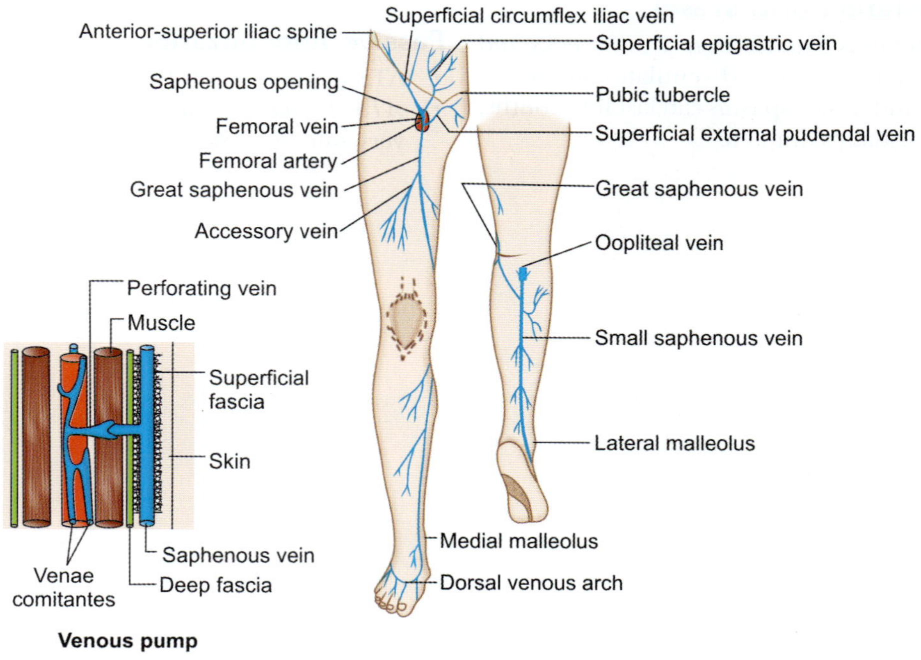

Fig. 14.1: Venous distribution of lower limb

Etiology

- Congenital (although it may present later in life)
- Primary (cause undetermined)
- Secondary (post-thrombotic, post-traumatic or other)
  - Deep venous thrombosis (DVT) accounts for most of the secondary cases and may be responsible for a significant number of other cases because many deep vein thrombi are asymptomatic
  - Diagnosis is made by history, physical examination and non-invasive studies.

History

- A history of any DVT or trauma should be sought, as well as any family history of varicose veins
- Patients may complain of lower-extremity edema, aching, skin irritation or varicose veins. Leg pain is described as a dull ache, worsening at the end of the day and often relieved with exercise or elevation
- In severe cases, individuals can experience acute, bursting pain with ambulation (venous claudication). Prolonged rest and leg elevation (20 minutes) are needed to obtain relief.

Physical Examination

Physical examination reveals, following findings:

- Ankle edema (Fig. 14.2)
- Subcutaneous fibrosis, hyperpigmentation (brownish discoloration secondary to hemosiderin deposition)
- Lipodermatosclerosis
- Venous eczema and dilatation of subcutaneous veins, including telangiectases (0.1–1.0 mm), reticular veins (1–4 mm) and varicose veins (greater than 4 mm)
- Ultimately ulcers develop, typically proximal to the medial malleolus. Any signs of infection should be noted. Arterial pulses should be examined and are usually adequate.

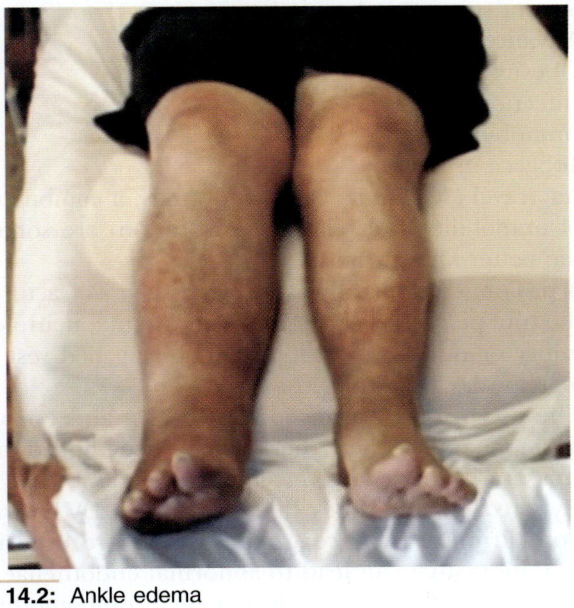

Fig. 14.2: Ankle edema

■ Venous Thromboembolism

Epidemiology

Venous thromboembolism, which includes DVT and pulmonary embolism (PE) is a common cause of death. The true incidence of DVT is difficult to determine because its clinical diagnosis can be inaccurate and it often occurs in the setting of other critical illnesses

- Deep vein thrombosis commonly affects the leg veins (such as the femoral vein or the popliteal vein) or the deep veins of the pelvis
- Occasionally the veins of the arm are affected (if spontaneous, this is known as Paget-Schrötter disease)
- Virchow's triad (Fig. 14.3).

Mechanism

Venous thrombosis occurs via three mechanisms:

1. Decreased flow rate of the blood
2. Damage to the blood vessel wall
3. An increased tendency of the blood to clot (hypercoagulability).

Pathophysiology (Fig. 14.4)

- DVT starts as a platelet nidus, usually in the venous valves of the calf. The thrombogenic nature of the nidus activates the clotting cascade, leading to a thrombus that grows by accumulating more platelets and fibrin (Fig. 14.5)
- The fibrinolytic system is also activated and thrombogenesis and thrombolysis compete for dominance

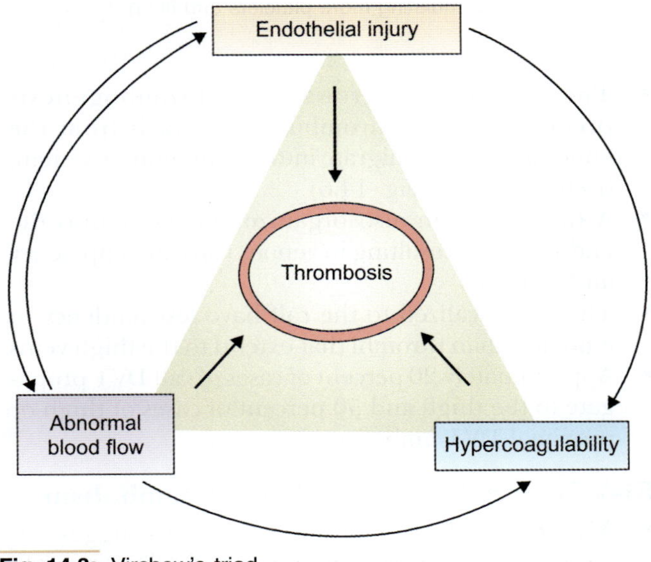

Fig. 14.3: Virchow's triad

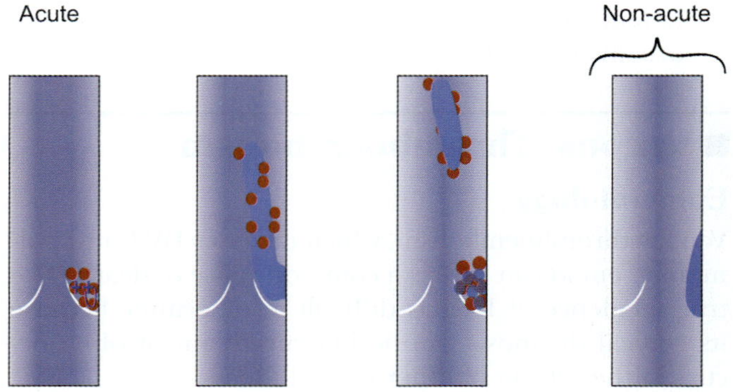

Fig. 14.4: Pathophysiology of DVT

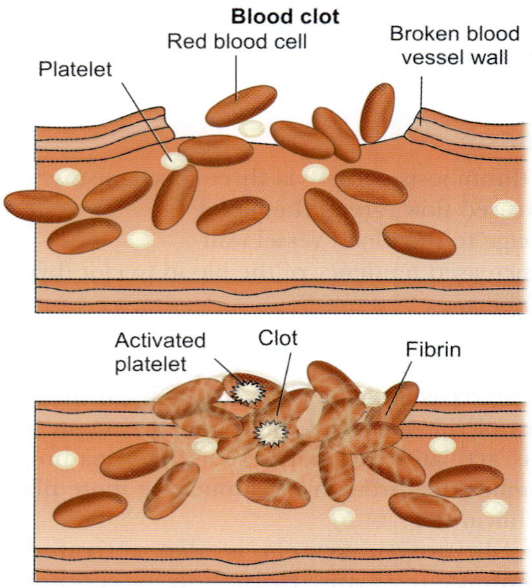

Fig. 14.5: DVT starts as a platelet nidus in the venous valves of the calf. The thrombogenic nature of the nidus activates the clotting cascade, leading to a thrombus that grows by accumulating more platelets and fibrin

- The thrombus grows, if thrombogenesis predominates. A thrombus can detach from the endothelium and migrate into the pulmonary system, becoming a PE (Fig. 14.6)
- A thrombus can also organize and grow into the endothelium, resulting in venous valve incompetency and phlebitis
- Thrombi localized to the calf have less tendency to embolize than thrombi that extend to the thigh veins
- Approximately 20 percent of cases of calf DVT propagate to the thigh and 50 percent of cases of thigh or proximal DVT embolize.

Risk Factors for Venous Thromboembolism

- *Malignancy:* Trousseau was the first to suggest an association between malignancy and a hypercoagulable state when he observed episodic migratory thrombophlebitis in his cancer patients

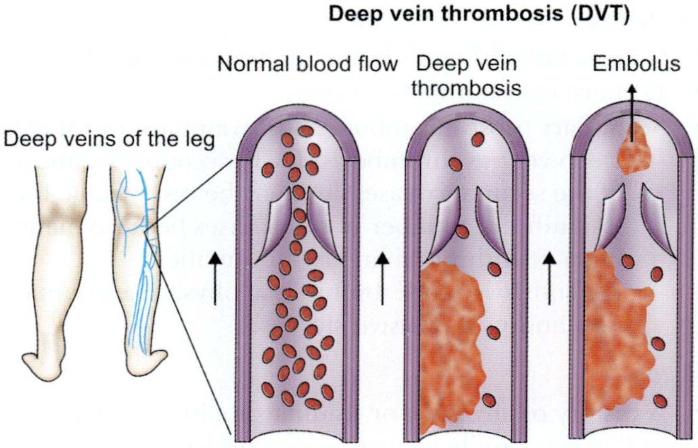

Fig. 14.6: A thrombus detaching from endothelium and migrating to become a pulmonary embolism

- Tumor cell activation, of the clotting cascade can occur directly through interactions with factors VIIa and X and tissue factor (TF). Indirect clotting activation can occur through stimulation of mononuclear cells to produce TF or factor X activators and stimulation of macrophages to produce TF activators.
- *Endothelial injury:* Another mechanism for the association of malignancy and thrombus formation is endothelial injury. Adhesion of tumor cells to endothelium can lead to disruption of endothelial intracellular junctions and expose the highly thrombogenic subendothelial surface.
- *Chemotherapeutic drugs:* These include drugs, such as bleomycin, carmustine, vincristine and adriamycin can also cause vascular endothelial cell damage.
- Recent surgery or hospitalization
- Advanced age
- Obesity
- Infection
- Immobilization
- Tobacco usage
- Air travel ("economy class syndrome", a combination of immobility and relative dehydration) are some of the better known causes
- A prolonged nonambulatory state, such as fracture of the hip, pelvis or leg; multisystem trauma, neurologic injury or other critical injury, requiring bed rest can increase DVT risk (Fig. 14.7)
- The use of oral contraceptives (OCPs) and estrogen hormone replacement therapy have been linked to increased risk of venous thrombus formation
- Hypercoagulable states can also lead to DVT formation. Primary hypercoagulable states are inherited conditions that can lead to abnormal endothelial cell thromboregulation (e.g. decreased thrombomodulin-

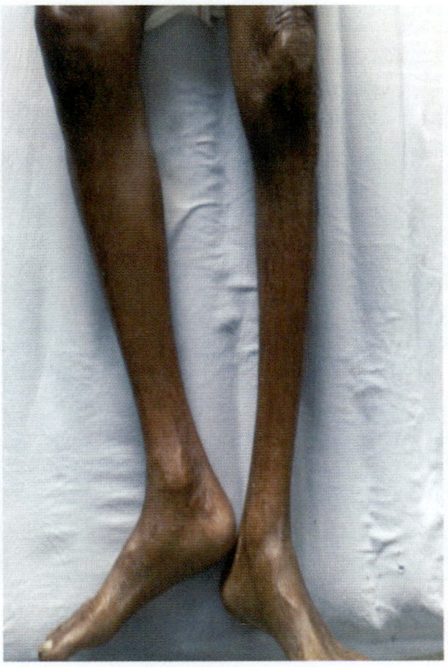

Fig. 14.7: DVT due to prolonged nonambulatory state

dependent activation of protein C, impaired heparin binding of antithrombin III, down-regulation of membrane-associated plasmin production) or decreased thrombogenic inhibitors (e.g. antithrombin III, protein C, protein S).

Hypercoagulable States

- Factor V: Leiden mutation
- Prothrombin gene mutation
- Protein C deficiency
- Protein S deficiency
- Antithrombin III deficiency
- Homocysteine
- Antiphospholipid syndrome

Clinical Presentation

- Pain/swelling of the extremity
- Increased circumference of affected extremity, with respect to the contralateral extremity
- Dilation of superficial veins of the suspected extremity only
- Calf pain on dorsiflexion of the ankle. Positive "Homans' sign" (Pain on dorsiflexion of foot in the calf muscles)
- *Mosses sign:* Squeezing of posterior calf elicits pain
- Palpable "cord", indicates superficial thrombophlebitis
- A more severe presentation of DVT is "phlegmasia cerulea dolens", in which, pain and swelling are accompanied by cyanosis, a sign of arterial ischemia.

Procedure for Predicting the Pretest Probability of Deep Venous Thrombosis (Well's Scoring System)

This has been illustrated in the Table 14.1

Diagnostic Methods for DVT (Flow chart 14.1)

- Clinical findings
- D-dimer
- Blood tests
- Conventional X-ray contrast venogram
- Duplex Doppler ultrasound
- MRI
- Radionuclide methods

Table 14.1: Procedure for predicting the pretest probability of deep venous thrombosis

Clinical characteristic	*Score*
• Active cancer (patient receiving treatment for cancer within the previous 6 months or currently receiving palliative treatment)	1
• Paralysis, paresis or recent plaster immobilization of the lower extremities	1
• Recently bedridden for 3 days or more, or major surgery within the previous 12 weeks requiring general or regional anesthesia	1
• Localized tenderness along the distribution of the deep venous system	1
• Entire leg swollen	1
• Calf swelling at least 3 cm larger than that on the asymptomatic side (measured 10 cm below tibial tuberosity)	1
• Pitting edema confined to symptomatic leg	1
• Collateral superficial veins (non-varicose)	1
• Previously documented DVT	1
• Alternative diagnosis at least as likely as DVT	2
• Clinical probability	Total Score
• DVT unlikely	< 2
• DVT likely	≥ 2

Flow chart 14.1: Diagnostic methods for DVT

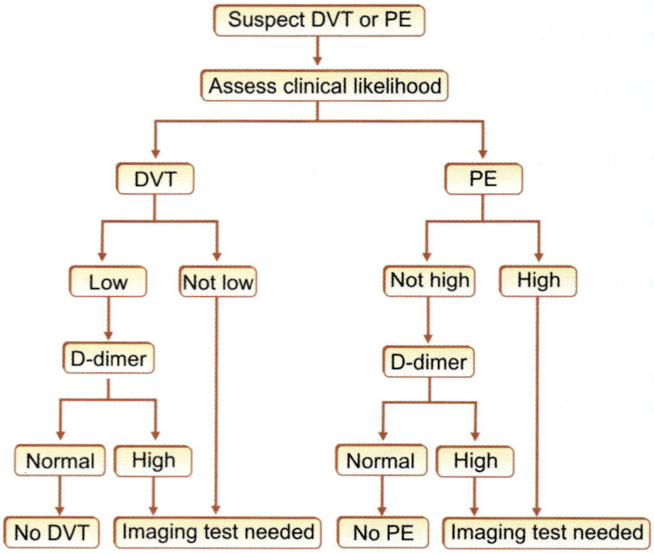

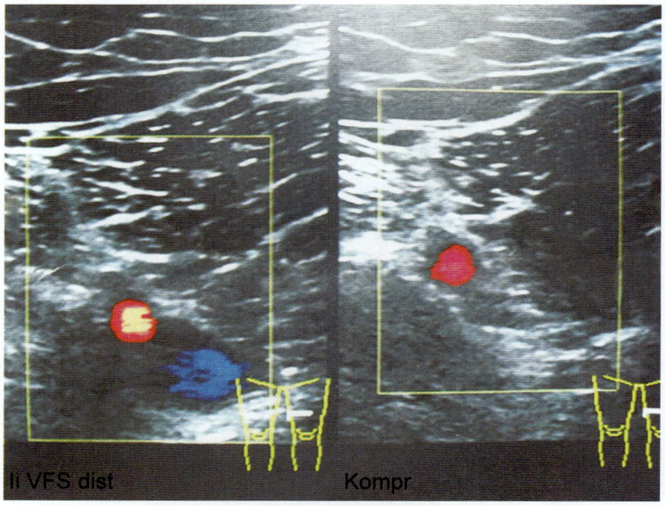

Fig. 14.8: Color Doppler for detecting thrombus

Blood Tests

- The quantitative plasma D-dimer enzyme-linked immunosorbent assay (ELISA) rises in the presence of DVT or PE because of plasmin's breakdown of fibrin
- The D-dimer assay is not specific. Levels increase in patients, with myocardial infarction, pneumonia, sepsis, cancer, during postoperative state and second or third trimester of pregnancy
- *D-dimer:* Blood testing for acute thrombosis
- Degradation product of circulating cross-linked fibrin
- Elevated levels in acute thrombosis
- This cross-linked fibrin degradation product is an indication that thrombosis is occurring and that the blood clot is being dissolved by plasmin
- Various assays not standardized (ELISA, latex and immunofilteration)
- Studies have not looked for presence or absence of both DVT and PE.
- Complete blood count
- Primary coagulation studies
- PT (Prothrombin time)
- Activated plasma thromboplastin time (APTT)
- Fibrinogen
- Liver enzymes
- Renal function
- Electrolytes.

Ultrasonography of the Deep Leg Veins

Criteria for establishing the diagnosis of acute DVT are:

- Lack of vein compressibility (the principal criterion). Vein does not "wink", when gently compressed in cross-section
- Failure to appose the walls of the vein, due to passive distension. Direct visualization of thrombus homogenous low echogenicity and abnormal Doppler flow
- *Dynamics normal response:* Calf compression augments, Doppler flow signal and confirms vein patency proximal
- *Distal to Doppler abnormal response:* Flow blunted rather than augmented with calf compression.

Ultrasound examination (Fig. 14.8)

- The vein is not compressible and thrombus (far left arrow, as seen in Figure 14.8) is visualized directly in the deep venous system
- Superficial femoral vein (SFV)
- Deep femoral vein (DFV).

Venous Doppler

Advantages

- High sensitivity (82–100%) for proximal DVT (thighs and knees) in patients with localizing signs and symptoms
- Fast
- Low cost per procedure.

Drawbacks

- Heavily operator dependent
- Some segments may be "blind" to sampling
- Calf veins usually not studied, but with new generation equipment calf veins can be reliably seen in 60 to 90 percent, if seen Doppler 90 percent sensitive and specific for clot in them.

Magnetic Resonance (Contrast Enhanced)

- When ultrasound is equivocal, magnetic resonance (MR) venography is an excellent imaging modality,

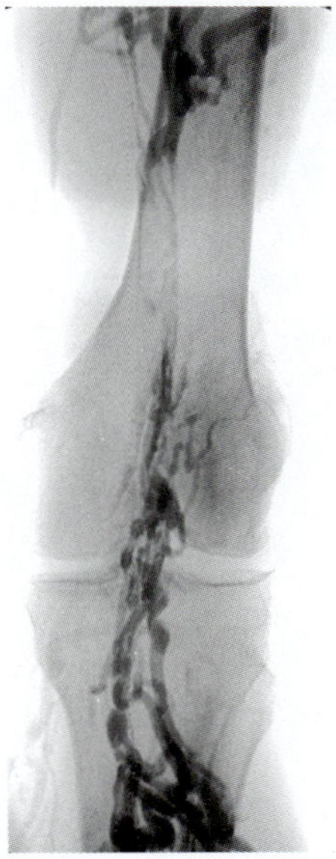

Fig. 14.9: Contrast venography detecting the block in the flow

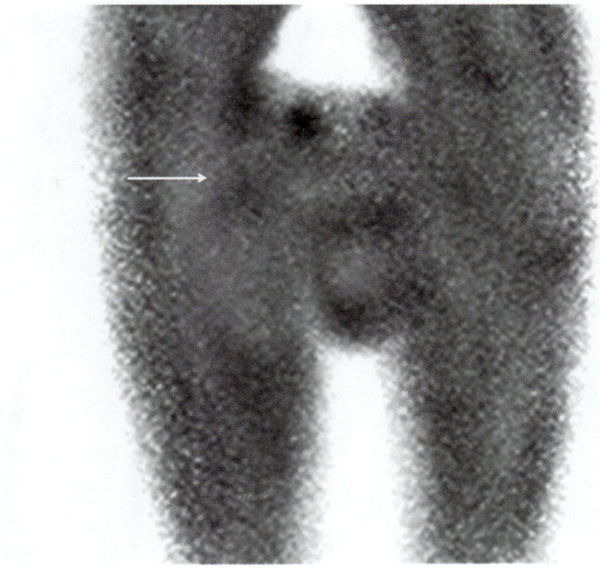

Fig. 14.10: Nuclear venographic image

to diagnose DVT. MR utilizes gadolinium contrast agent, which, unlike iodinated contrast agents used in venography or CT angiography is not nephrotoxic

- MR imaging should be considered for suspected DVT or PE patients, with renal insufficiency or contrast dye allergy. MR pulmonary angiography detects large proximal PE, but is not reliable for smaller segmental and subsegmental PE.

Invasive Diagnostic Modalities

Contrast Phlebography

Venous ultrasonography has virtually replaced contrast phlebography, as the diagnostic test for suspected DVT.

Contrast Venography (Figs 14.9)

- "Gold standard" for imaging DVT, when technically adequate
- Can image entire lower extremities
- Sensitive in asymptomatic patients
- *Limitations*
  - Painful
  - Technically inadequate/difficult to interpret in 10 to 30 percent of cases

Nuclear Venography (Figs 14.10 and 14.11)

- Technitium 99m (Tc-MAA)
- Sensitivity (94%)
- Specificity (92%)
- PRO'S
  - Lung perfusion
  - Iliacs/IVC

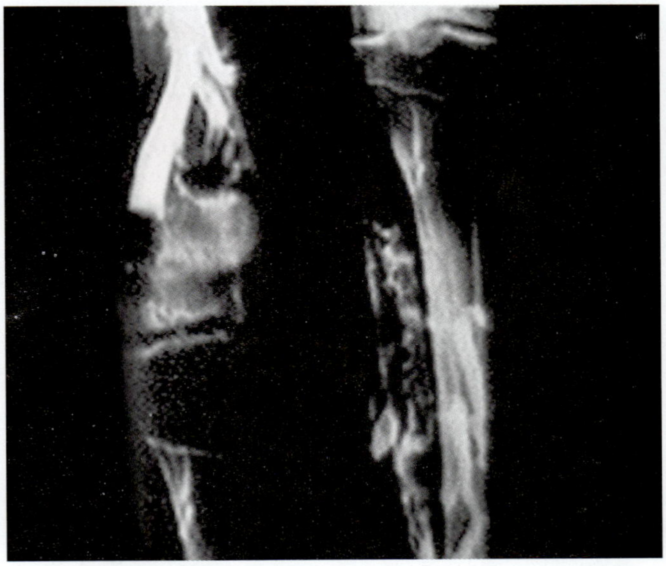

Fig. 14.11: Nuclear scan diagnosing DVT

- CON'S
  - Calf veins
  - Nonobstructing clot without collaterals
- Tc-99m apcitide scintigraphy specific for acute DVT (Figs 14.12A and B)
- Binding to platelet (Fig. 14.13) GPIIb/IIIa
- *Tc-99m apcitide:* Normal biodistribution
- *Tc-99m apcitide:* Positive cases
- For suspected DVT, compression ultrasonography of the femoral, popliteal and calf trifurcation veins is

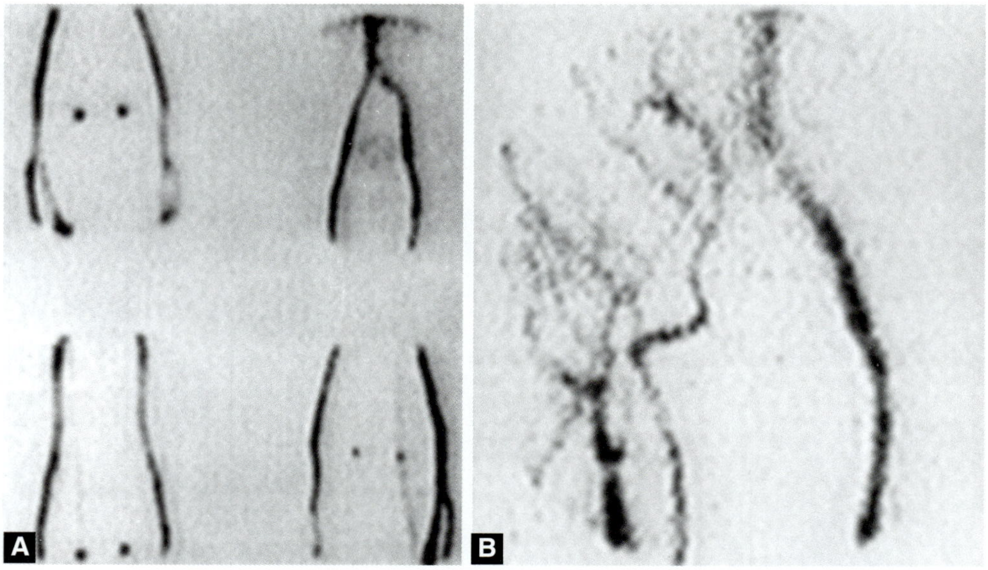

Figs 14.12A and B: Tc-99m apcitide scintigraphy specific for acute DVT

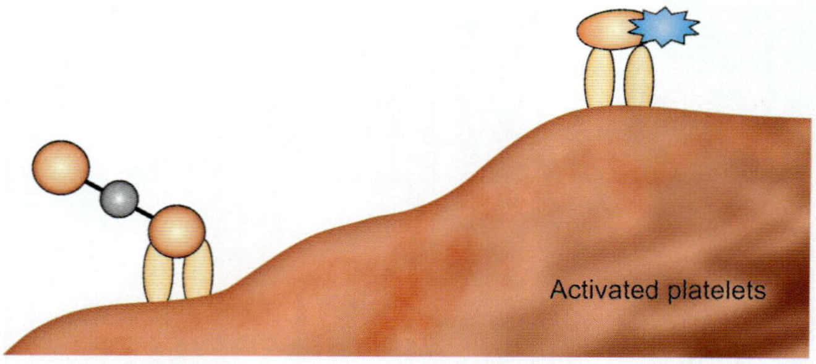

Fig. 14.13: Receptors binding to activated platelets

highly sensitive (greater than 90%) in detecting thrombosis of the proximal veins (femoral and popliteal), but less sensitive (50%) in detecting calf vein thrombosis
- Chest CT can be combined with CT angiography of pelvic and deep thigh veins, to detect DVT as well as PE.

Prophylaxis

- Prophylaxis is achieved by either altering the blood coagulation state, preventing venous stasis or preventing embolization
- Low-dose unfractionated heparin is given subcutaneously at 5,000 units, 2 hours before surgery and every 8 or 12 hours postoperatively. Low-dose heparin reduces the risk of venous thromboembolism by 50 to 70 percent.

Prevention of Venous Thromboembolism (Table 14.2)

Treatment

Hospitalization should be considered in patients with more than two of the following risk factors, as these patients may have more risk of complications during treatment:
- Bilateral DVT
- Renal insufficiency
- Body weight greater than 70 kg/154 lbs
- Recent immobility
- Chronic heart failure
- Cancer
- Anticoagulation is the usual treatment for DVT
- In general, patients are initiated on a brief course (i.e. less than a week) of heparin treatment, while they start on a 3 to 6 months course of warfarin (or related vitamin K inhibitors). Low molecular weight heparin (LMWH) is preferred, though unfractionated heparin is given in patients, who have a contraindication to LMWH (renal failure or imminent need for invasive procedure)
- LMWH displayed the following:
  - Reduced antifactor IIa activity, relative to antifactor Xa activity
  - More favorable benefit-risk ratio in experimental animals
  - Superior pharmacokinetic properties

Table 14.2: Preventive measures of venous thromboembolism in different conditions

Condition	*Prophylaxis strategy*
High-risk general surgery	Mini-UFH + GCS or LMWH + GCS
Thoracic surgery	Mini-UFH + IPC
Cancer surgery, including gynecologic cancer surgery	LMWH, consider 1 month of prophylaxis
Total hip replacement, total knee replacement, hip fracture surgery	LMWH, fondaparinux (a pentasaccharide) 2.5 mg sc, once daily or warfarin (target INR 2.5) (except for total knee replacement)
Neurosurgery	GCS + IPC
Neurosurgery for brain tumor	Mini-UFH or LMWH + IPC + predischarge venous ultrasonography
Anticoagulation contraindicated	GCS + IPC
Mini-UFH: Minidose unfractionated heparin	IPC: Intermittent pneumatic compression devices
GCS: Graduated compression stockings	LMWH: Low-molecular-weight heparin

- LMWHs are derived from heparin, by chemical or enzymatic depolymerization, yielding fragments approximately one-third the size of heparin
- LMWHs have a mean molecular weight of 4,500 to 5,000, with a distribution of 1,000 to 10,000
- Low binding properties of LMWH, to circulating and cellular protein
- Cleared by renal route
- LMWH therapy was started postoperatively, the first dose administered 12 to 24 hours after surgery, which increased the acceptability of prophylaxis
- This approach is particularly appealing in view of concerns about the risk of spinal cord hematoma, when anticoagulant prophylaxis is used in conjunction with spinal anesthesia
- The first dose of LMWH should be delayed, until after the epidural catheter has been removed. When this is not possible, the catheter should be removed at least 8 hours after the last dose of LMWH
- Under these circumstances, other drugs that impair hemostasis (such as nonsteroidal anti-inflammatory agents) should be avoided.

Multiple Trauma

- LMWH (Enoxaparin sodium 30 mg s/c 12 hourly) is the treatment started within 36 hours of multiple trauma
- LMWH (tinzaparin, 175 U/kg s/c 6 hourly) or heparin (50 U/kg IV bolus followed by an infusion of 500 U/kg/day) adjusted to an APTT ratio of 2.0 to 3.0, for prevention of recurrent thromboembolism, major bleeding and death
- Thrombolysis is generally reserved for extensive clot, e.g. an iliofemoral thrombosis
- In the case of known bilateral lower-extremity DVT, the compression device can be placed on the upper extremity
- Pedal compression devices are also effective in patients, whose body habits does not allow conventionally sized devices to fit around their thighs or calves
- Graduated compression stockings are effective in preventing DVT formation, by reducing venous stasis. However, this efficacy has been shown just for calf DVT (Fig. 14.14)
- "Beginning within one month of diagnosis of proximal DVT and continuing for a minimum of one year after diagnosis"
- Intermittent pneumatic compression of the extremities enhances blood flow in the deep veins and increases blood fibrinolytic activity (Fig. 14.15)
- For patients with significant bleeding risk with anticoagulation, pneumatic compression is an effective alternative.

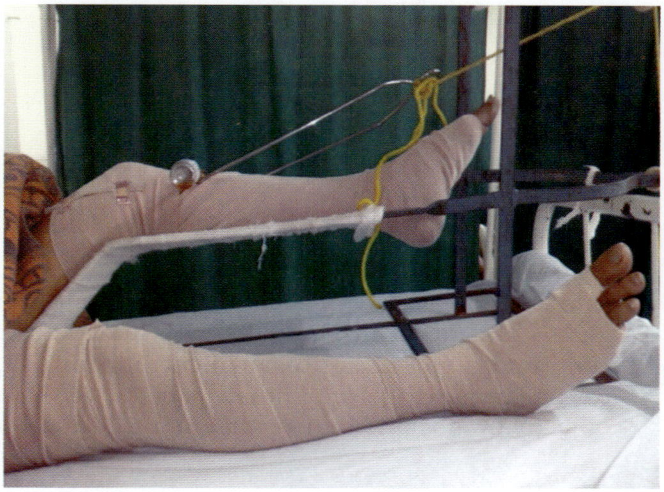

Fig. 14.14: Graduated compression stockings effective in preventing DVT formation

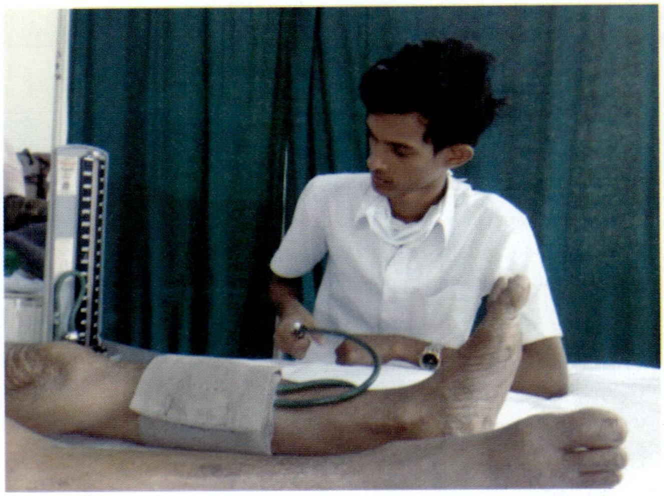

Fig. 14.15: Intermittent pneumatic compression given on extremities

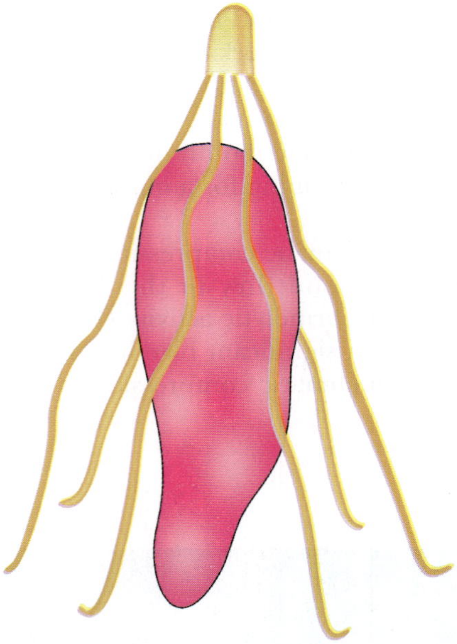

Fig. 14.16: Green field filter

Interventional Techniques

- Caval interruption with intra caval filters
- Inferior vena cava filter reduces pulmonary embolism and is an option for patients with an absolute contraindication to anticoagulant treatment (e.g. cerebral hemorrhage) or those rare patients, who have objectively documented recurrent PE, while on anticoagulation, an inferior vena cava filter (also referred to as a green field filter) may prevent pulmonary embolization of the leg clot (Fig. 14.16)

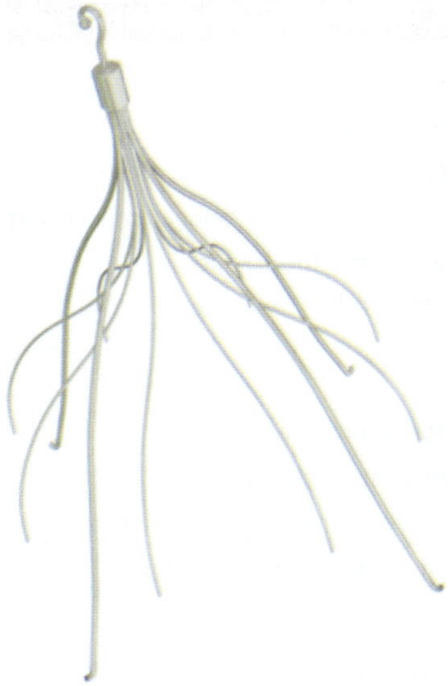

Fig 14.17: Tulip filters

- These filters are themselves potential foci of thrombosis, IVC filters are viewed as a temporizing measure, for preventing life-threatening pulmonary embolism
- The procedure for insertion of intracaval filters is known as sieve procedure.

Types of Filter

- Tulip filter (Fig. 14.17)
- Catheter-directed thrombolysis of acute DVT with or without mechanical thrombectomy devices has been advocated in order to avoid sequele of DVT
  The goals are to restore venous flow, preserve venous valve function, and eliminate the possibility of thromboembolism.
- Thromboembolectomy.

Differential Diagnosis

- Ruptured baker's cyst
- Cellulitis
- Postphlebitic syndrome/venous insufficiency. It presents with leg edema, pain, nocturnal cramping, venous claudication, skin pigmentation, dermatitis and ulceration (usually on the medial aspect of the lower leg)
- Hematoma.

15 Fat Embolism Syndrome

- Treatment

Introduction

History

- First diagnosed in 1873 by Dr Von Bergmann
- In1879, Fenger and Salisbury published description of fat embolism syndrome (FES).

Fat Embolism vs Fat Embolism Syndrome

Fat Embolism (FE)

It is fat in the vascular circulation, which can cause embolic phenomenon. It is more common, i.e. 90% of patients with traumatic injury suffer from it (reports have shown high incidence of fat embolism after fractures and orthopedic surgery).

Fat Embolism Syndrome (FES)

Fat embolism occurs with pattern of symptoms

Incidence: 1 to 3 percent femur fractures and 5 to 10 percent, if bilateral or multiple fractures.

- *Mortality:* 5 to 15 percent
- *Clinical diagnosis*: No specific laboratory test is diagnostic. Mostly associated with long bone and pelvic fractures and more frequent in closed fractures. Single long bone fracture have 1 to 3 percent chance of developing FES and increases with number of fractures.
- *Onset:* 24 to 72 hours from initial insult
- *Causes:* Nontrauma related factors. These include:
  - Pancreatitis
  - Diabetes mellitus
  - Osteomyelitis and panniculitis
  - Bone tumor lysis
  - Steroid therapy
  - Sickle cell hemoglobinopathy
  - Alcoholic liver disease
  - Lipid infusion
  - Cyclosporin asolvent.

Diagnostic Criteria

Gurd criteria (Table 15.1)

- Gurd criteria is most commonly used
- One major and four minor

Schonfeld's criteria: Schonfeld's criteria for diagnosis of fat embolism (Table 15.2)

Table 15.1: Gurd's criteria for diagnosing features of fat embolism

Major criteria	Petechial rash
	Respiratory symptoms—tachypnea, dyspnea, bilateral inspiratory crepitations, hemoptysis, bilateral diffuse patchy shadowing on chest X-ray
	Neurologial signs—confusion, drowsiness, coma
Minor criteria	Tachycardia >120 beat min^{-1}
	Pyrexia >34.9°C
	Retinal changes—fat or petechiae
	Jaundice
	Renal changes-anuria or oliguria
Laboratory features	Thrombocytopenia > 50% decrease on admission value
	Sudden decrease in hemoglobin level >20% of admission value
	High erythrocyte sedimentation rate >71 mm h^{-1}
	Fat macroglobulinemia

Table 15.2: Schonfeld's criteria for diagnosis of fat embolism

	Score
Petechiae	5
X-ray chest diffuse infiltrates	4
Hypoxemia	3
Fever	1
Tachycardia	1
Tachypnea	1
Confusion	1

Pathogenesis (Fat Embolism)

Direct entry of fat globules (fat enters torn venules) predisposed by:

- Torn vessels
- Free fat present
- Temporary rise in marrow pressure above venous pressure
- In orthopedic surgery, echogenic material can be seen in right heart circulation
- *Paradoxical embolism:* Fat embolism in arterial system, e.g. patent foramen ovale.

Pathogenesis (Fat Embolism Syndrome)

- Production of toxic byproducts from triglyceride (TG)/chylomicrons (lipase)
- FES result from degradation of fat from FE to free fatty acids (these have been shown in animal models to cause vasculitis/ARDS). Probably phospholipase A2 (PLA2) and C-reactive protein (CRP) mediated (inflammatory mediated)
- CRP also shown to be elevated in FE and causes fat agglutination (Fig. 15.1).

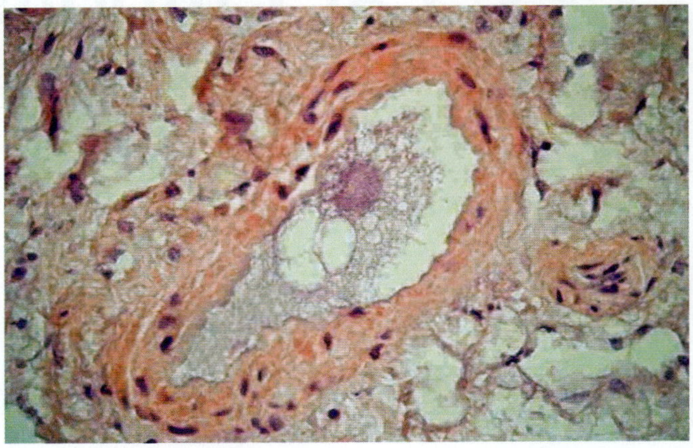

Fig. 15.1: Hematoxylin and eosin stain of a section of the lungs showing a blood vessel with fibrinoid material and an optical empty space indicative of the presence of lipid dissolved during the staining process. This 55-year-old woman died of massive fat embolism after developing pancreatitis due to endoscopic retrograde cholangiopancreaticography
(*Image source:* Pancreatitis with an unusual fatal complication following endoscopic retrograde cholangiopancreaticography)

Pathogenesis of ARDS in Fat Embolism

- Fat emboli obstructs lung vessel (20 μ). Platelets and fibrin adhere there (Fig. 15.2)
- Lipase creases free fatty acid
- Inflammatory changes, leads to endothelial damage, which are contributing factors for acute respiratory distress syndrome (ARDS).

Triad of Fat Embolic Syndrome

- Hypoxemia (Pulmonary)
- Neurological abnormalities (Cerebral)
- Petechial rash (Cutaneous)

Early Signs

- Dyspnea
- Tachypnea
- Hypoxemia
- Pulmonary
- Hypoxia, rales, pleural friction rub, etc.
- ARDS may develop
- Half of patients with fat embolic syndrome requires mechanical ventilation
- Chest X-ray usually normal early on, later may show 'snow storm' pattern, with diffuse bilateral infiltrates (Fig. 15.3)
- *CT chest:* Ground glass opacification, with interlobular septal thickening.

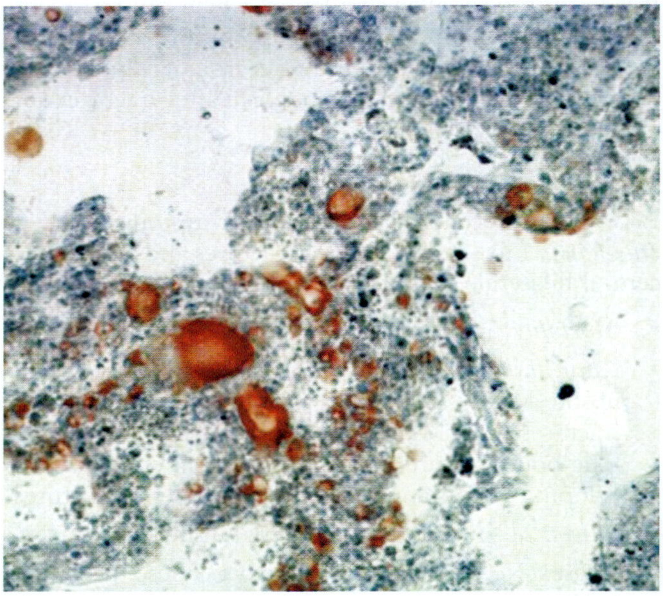

Fig. 15.2: Fat emboli obstruct lung vessel

Neurological Findings

- Usually occur after respiratory symptoms
- *Incidence:* Eighty percent patients with FES
- Minor global dysfunction most common, but ranges from mild delirium to coma
- Seizures/focal deficits not common, but can occur
- Transient and reversible in most cases
- *CT head:* General edema, usually nonspecific
- *MRI brain:* Low density on T1 and high intensity T2 signal, correlates to degree of impairment

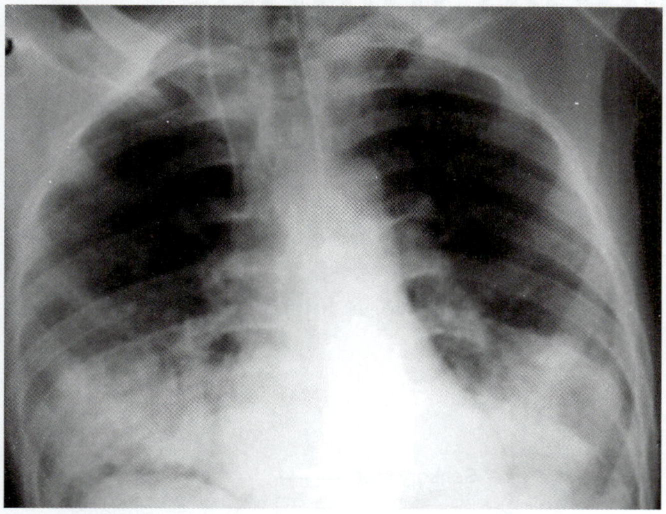

Fig. 15.3: Snow storm pattern, with diffuse bilateral infilterates

Cutaneous Findings

- Rash
- Petechial
- Usually on conjunctiva, mucous membrane, neck and axillae
- Results from occlusion of dermal capillaries, by fat globules and then extravasations of RBC
- Resolves in 5 to 7 days
- Pathognomonic, but only present in 20 to 50 percent of patients.

Other Findings

- Retinopathy (exudates, cotton wool spots, hemorrhage, etc.)
- Lipiduria
- Fever
- Disseminated intravascular coagulation (DIC)
- Myocardial depression (Right heart strain)
- Thrombocytopenia/anemia
- Hypocalcemia.

Laboratory Findings

- Laboratory tests are mostly nonspecific
- Serum lipase level increases in bone trauma, which is often misleading
- Cytologic examination of urine, blood and sputum with Sudan or oil red O staining, may detect fat globules that are either free or in macrophages
- Blood lipid level is not helpful for diagnosis
- Decreased hematocrit occurs within 24 to 48 hours and is attributed to intra-alveolar hemorrhage
- Alteration in coagulation and thrombocytopenia
- In summary, the diagnosis of FES may be difficult, as except petechiae, there are no pathognomic signs.

■ Treatment

- Supportive care
- Early immobilization of fractures reduces incidents of FES
- Open reduction internal fixation (ORIF) over conservative treatment also reduces risk
- Higher incidence rate occurs, when fixation is delayed for more than 24 hours
- External fixation or fixation with plate and screw, produces lesser lung injury than nailing the medullary cavity.

Supportive Care

- Maintenance of intravascular volume, as shock can exacerbate the lung injury caused by FES
- Albumin has been recommended for volume resuscitation in addition to balanced electrolyte solution, as it also binds fatty acids and may decrease the extent of lung injury
- Mechanical ventilation and PEEP may be required to maintain arterial oxygenation.

Steroids

- Steroid prophylaxis is controversial to prevent FES
- Theorized to cause blunting of inflammatory response and complement activation
- Prospective studies suggests that prophylactic steroids benefit high risk patients
- Few studies and small study size, hence remains controversial
- Once FES is established, steroids have not shown to improved outcomes
- Heparin and acetyl salicylic acids have also been proposed for treatment, as they activate lipase and block thromboxane respectively, but no evidence exists for either use in FES.

16 Peripheral Nerve Injuries

- Anatomy
- Management of Nerve Injuries

■ Anatomy

- Each segmental spinal nerve is formed at or near its intervertebral foramen by the union of its dorsal or sensory root, with its ventral or motor root. In most of the thoracic segments, these mixed spinal nerves retain their autonomy and supply one intercostal dermatomal and myotomal segment.
- Other segments of the spinal axis, the spinal nerves join with others to form a plexus that innervates a limb or a special body segment that no longer retains the primitive myomeric pattern.
- A total of 31 mixed spinal nerves leave their respective foramina on each side of the spine, to innervate the homolateral trunk and extremities. They are, 8-cervical; 12-thoracic; 5-lumbar; 5-sacral; 1-coccygeal.

Components of Mixed Spinal Nerve (Fig. 16.1)

Motor

- Several rootlets leave the anterolateral sulcus of the spinal cord and unite to form each motor root
- The fibers traversing these roots arise from the anterior horn cells and innervate the skeletal muscles.

Sensory

- The sensory fibers arise from pain, thermal, tactile and stretch receptors
- Cell bodies for these fibers are located within the dorsal root ganglia, with axons entering the posterolateral sulcus of the cord via several rootlets
- The fibers conveying joint or position sensibility and some tactile fibers turn cephalad in the dorsal columns and do not synapse before reaching the gracile and cuneate nuclei at the cervicomedullary junction
- Pain and temperature fibers synapse in the substantia gelatinosa and cross to ascend in the dorsal spinothalamic tract
- Tactile fibers enter, synapse and cross to ascend in the ventral spinothalamic tract.

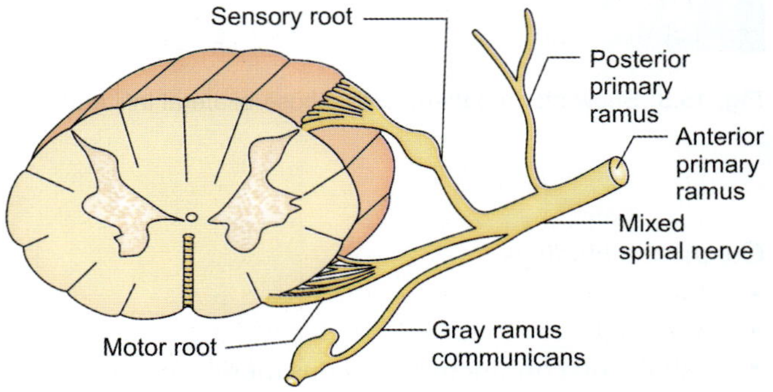

Fig. 16.1: Components of mixed spinal nerve

Sympathetic

- The sympathetic component of all 31 mixed spinal nerves leaves the spinal cord along only 14 motor roots
- The fibers exit from the cord with the 12 thoracic and first 2 lumbar motor roots enter the respective mixed spinal nerve and promptly emerge from it as white rami. The white rami pass anteriorly to the corresponding sympathetic ganglion
- Synapse may occur within the ganglion, with which the ramus is associated and postganglionic fibers pass back to the mixed spinal nerve as a gray ramus
- More often, however, the fibers entering the ganglion via the white rami pass for variable distances up or down the paravertebral chain, to synapse at higher or lower levels
- The postganglionic fibers pass along gray rami to cervical, lower lumbar or sacrococcygeal mixed spinal nerves having no white rami
- Sweat glands, blood vessels and erector pili are innervated also in a segmental pattern
- Mixed spinal nerves, having left the intervertebral foramina, receive their sympathetic component and promptly branch into anterior and posterior primary rami.

Posterior Primary Rami

- Directed posteriorly and supply the paraspinal musculature and the skin along the posterior aspect of the trunk, neck and head
- The upper three cervical posterior rami are larger than their corresponding anterior rami, supplying relatively large areas of the scalp posteriorly and the musculature around the craniocervical junction
- With these exceptions, posterior primary rami are small and the major part of each spinal nerve continues laterally in an anterior primary ramus, to enter a plexus or to become an intercostal nerve.

Anterior Primary Rami

- The cervical, the first thoracic and all the lumbosacral nerves join in the formation of plexuses
- The upper four cervical anterior rami form the cervical plexus
- The lower four cervical and first thoracic anterior rami form the brachial plexus
- The first three and a part of the fourth lumbar anterior rami form the lumbar plexus
- The sacral anterior rami along with the fifth lumbar and a part of the fourth join to form the lumbosacral plexus
- The area of skin supplied by the fibers of a single spinal root is called a dermatome
- Segmental dermatomal patterns are well preserved in the thoracic region, but not in the limbs (Fig. 16.2)
- Migration of the limb buds accounts for the displacement of midcervical dermatomes along the lateral aspect of the arm and radial aspect of the forearm and of the lower cervical and upper thoracic dermatomes along the medial aspect of the arm and the ulnar aspect of the forearm
- Lumbar and sacral dermatomal alignment along the various aspects of the lower extremity is similarly explained
- The line separating the more rostral segmental dermatomes from the more caudal ones is called the axial line and may be followed into the spinal axis.

Microscopic Anatomy (Fig. 16.3)

- Each nerve fiber or axon is a direct extension of a dorsal root ganglion cell (sensory), an anterior horn cell (motor) or a postganglionic sympathetic nerve cell and it is either myelinated or unmyelinated. Sensory and motor nerves contain unmyelinated and myelinated fibers in a ratio of 4:1
- In the unmyelinated or sparsely myelinated fibers, several axons are wrapped by a single Schwann cell. In the more heavily myelinated fibers, the Schwann cell, by rotation forms a multilaminated structure that encloses a myelin sheath around a single axon
- The segment of myelinated nerve fiber enclosed by a single Schwann cell is referred to as an internode with the more heavily myelinated fibers, having the longer internodes (Fig. 16.4). The point at which one Schwann cell ends and the next begins is relatively sparse in myelin and is called the nodal gap or node of Ranvier
- The axon with its Schwann cell and myelin sheath is surrounded by a veil of delicate fibrous tissue called the endoneurium. Seen longitudinally, the endoneurium forms a tube encircling individually the Schwann cell sheaths that cluster together to form a fascicle (or *funicle* as termed by Sunderland)

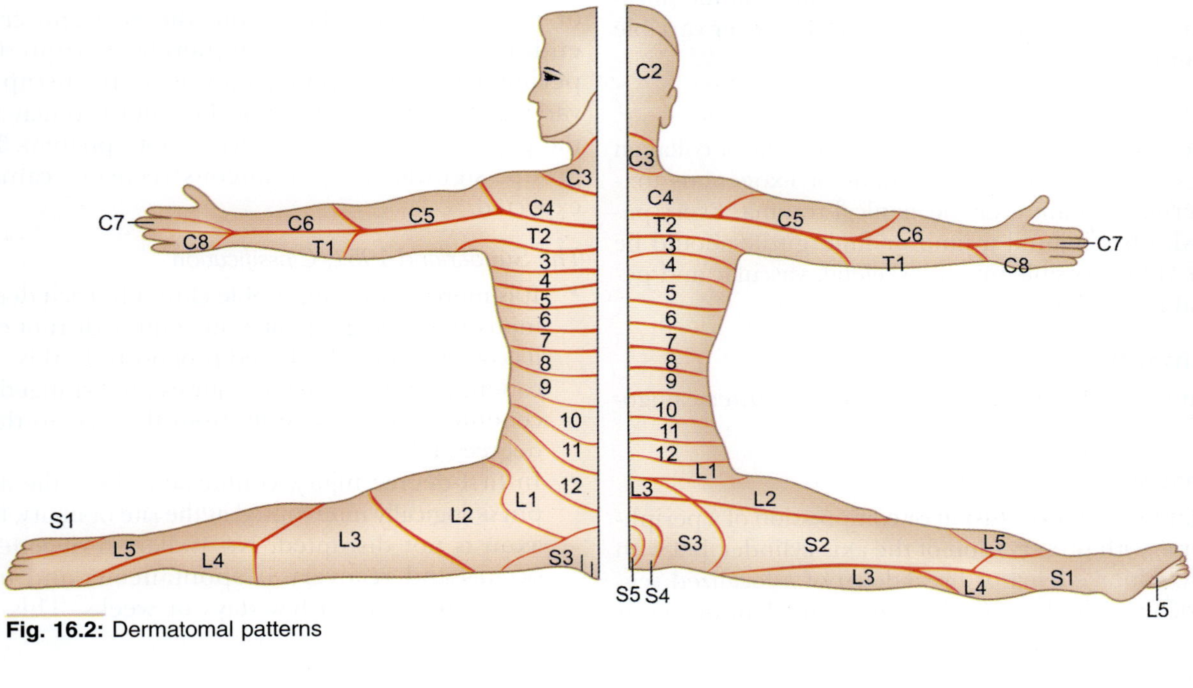

Fig. 16.2: Dermatomal patterns

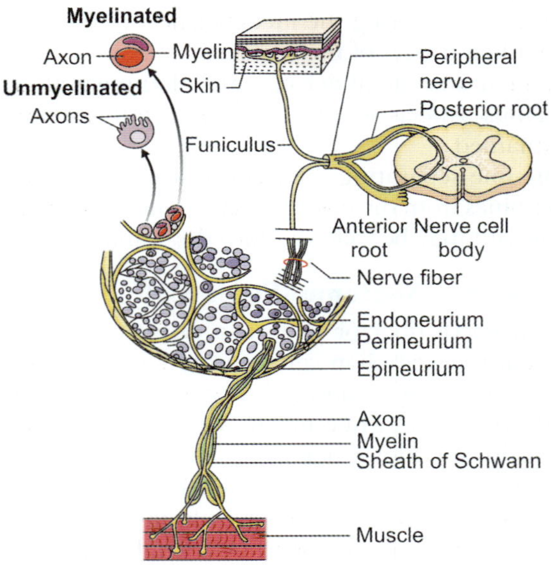

Fig. 16.3: Microscopic anatomy

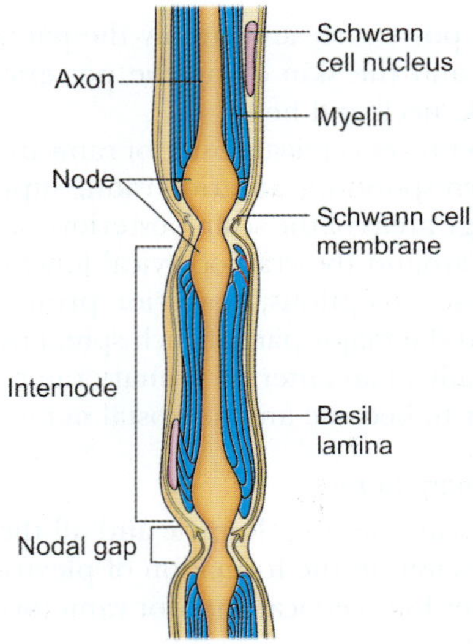

Fig. 16.4: Myelinated nerve fiber

- Each fascicle or separate group of sheathed axons is surrounded by a denser layer of perineurium. The entire group of fascicles with their surrounding perineurium is encased as a mixed spinal or peripheral nerve in a denser epineurium. The blood supply to the peripheral nerve enters through the mesoneurium, which is loose connective tissue extending from the epineurium to the surrounding tissues
- There is an extrinsic (segmental) and an intrinsic (longitudinal) blood supply to each nerve
- The intrinsic blood supply that runs longitudinally within the epineurium, perineurium and endoneurium is fairly extensive and allows surgical mobilization without complete devascularization over variable lengths of nerves.

Etiology

Peripheral nerves can be injured by metabolic or collagen diseases, malignancies, endogenous or exogenous toxins, thermal, chemical or mechanical trauma. Every patient, who has injured a limb or limb girdle should be evaluated for possible musculoskeletal, vascular and peripheral nerve damage.

Classification

Seddon in 1943 divided nerve injuries into three categories:

Neurapraxia

Designating minor contusion or compression of a peripheral nerve with preservation of the axis-cylinder, but with possibly minor edema or breakdown of a localized segment of myelin sheath. Transmission of impulses is physiologically interrupted for a time, but recovery is complete in a few days or weeks.

Axonotmesis

Designating more significant injury with breakdown of the axon and distal wallerian degeneration, but with preservation of the Schwann cell and endoneurial tubes. Spontaneous regeneration with good functional recovery can be expected.

Neurotmesis

Designating a more severe injury, with complete anatomical severance of the nerve or extensive avulsing or crushing injury. The axon, the Schwann cell and endoneurial tubes are completely disrupted. The perineurium and epineurium also are disrupted to varying degrees. Segments of the latter two may bridge the gap, if complete severance is not apparent. In this group, significant spontaneous recovery cannot be expected.

The Sunderland 1951, Classification

- It is more readily applicable clinically, each degree of injury suggesting a greater anatomical disruption with its correspondingly altered prognosis. In this classification, peripheral nerve injuries are arranged in ascending order of severity from the first to the fifth degree (Table 16.1)
- In first-degree injury, conduction along the axon is physiologically interrupted at the site of injury, but the axon is not disrupted. No Wallerian degeneration occurs and recovery is spontaneous and usually complete within a few days or weeks. This injury

Table 16.1: The Sunderland 1951, Classification

Degree of injury		Histopathological changes					Tinel sign	
Sunderland	*Seddon*	*Myelin*	*Axon*	*Endoneurium*	*Perineurium*	*Epineurium*	*Present*	*Progresses distally*
I	Neurapraxia	±					-	-
II	Axonotmesis	+	+				+	+
III	Neurotmesis	+	+	+			+	+
IV	Neurotmesis	+	+	+	+		+	-
V	Neurotmesis	+	+	+	+	+	+	-

coincides with the neurapraxia of Seddon. The loss of function varies. Usually, motor function is more profoundly affected than sensory function. Sensory modalities are affected in order of decreasing frequency as follows: proprioception, touch, temperature and pain. A characteristic of this injury is the simultaneous return of motor function in the proximal and distal musculature

- In *second-degree injury,* disruption of the axon is evident, with Wallerian degeneration distal to the point of injury and degeneration proximal for one or more nodal segments. The integrity of the endoneurial tube (Schwann cell basal lamina) is maintained, providing a perfect anatomical course for regeneration. Any permanent deficit is related to the number of neural somas that die, such death being more common in injuries at the more proximal levels. Clinically, the neurological deficit is complete with loss of motor, sensory and sympathetic function. Motor reinnervation is accomplished in a progressive manner from proximal to distal
- In *third-degree injury,* the axons and endoneurial tubes are disrupted, but the perineurium is preserved. The result is disorganization resulting from disruption of the endoneurial tubes. Scar tissue within the endoneurium can obstruct certain tubes and divert sprouts to paths other than their own. Clinically, the neurological loss is complete in most instances and because of the additional time required for the regenerating axon tips to penetrate the fibrous barrier, the duration of loss is more prolonged than in second-degree injury. Returning motor function is evident from proximal to distal, but with varying degrees of permanent motor or sensory deficit
- In *fourth-degree injury,* the axon and endoneurium are disrupted, but some of the epineurium and possibly some of the perineurium are preserved, so complete severance of the entire trunk does not occur. Retrograde degeneration is more severe after this degree of injury and the mortality among neuronal soma is higher, sometimes resulting in a significant reduction in the number of surviving axons. Essentially, nerve continuity is maintained only by scar tissue, preventing proximal axons from entering the distal endoneurial tubes
- In *fifth-degree injury,* the nerve is completely transected, resulting in a variable distance between the neural stumps. These injuries occur only in open wounds and usually are identified at the time of early surgical exploration. The likelihood of any significant bridging by axonal sprouts is remote and the possibility of any significant return of function without appropriate surgery is equally remote
- *Sixth-degree (Mackinnon)* or *mixed injuries* occur, in which a nerve trunk is partially severed and the remaining part of the trunk sustains fourth-degree, third-degree, second-degree or rarely even first-degree injury. A neuroma in continuity is present and the recovery pattern is mixed depending on the degree of injury to each portion of the nerve. Surgical intervention to correct the fourth-degree and fifth-degree components may sacrifice the function of lesser injured fascicles.

Effect of Peripheral Nerve Injuries Motor

- When a peripheral nerve is severed at a given level, all motor functions of the nerve distal to that level is abolished. All muscles supplied by branches of the nerve distal to that level are paralyzed and become atonic
- Significant electromyography (EMG) changes are not apparent for 8 to 14 days, at which time transient fibrillation potentials on needle insertion may become apparent. Spontaneous fibrillations may become evident after 2 to 4 weeks, coinciding with the onset of atrophic change within the muscle fibers. Atrophy of muscle bulk progresses rapidly to 50 to 70 percent at the end of about 2 months (Sunderland, 1952)
- Atrophy continues at a much slower rate and the connective tissue component of the muscles increases. Striations and motor end plate configurations are retained for longer than 12 months, whereas the empty endoneurial tubes shrink to about one third of their normal diameter (Sunderland and Bradley, 1950). Complete disruption and replacement of muscle fibers may not become complete, until after 3 years.

Table 16.2: Muscle function assessment

M0	*No contraction*
M1	Return of perceptible contraction in proximal muscles
M2	Return of perceptible contraction in proximal and distal muscles
M3	Return of function in proximal and distal muscles of such a degree that all important muscles are sufficiently powerful to act against resistance
M4	Return of function as in stage 3; in addition, all synergistic and independent movements are possible
M5	Complete recovery

Muscle Function Assessment after Peripheral Nerve Injuries (Table 16.2)

Sensory

- Sensory loss usually follows a definite anatomical pattern, although the factor of overlap from adjacent nerves may confuse inexperienced surgeons. After severance of a peripheral nerve, only a small area of complete sensory loss is found. This area is supplied exclusively by the severed nerve and is called the autonomous zone or isolated zone of supply for that nerve
- A larger area of tactile and thermal anesthesia is readily delineated and corresponds more closely to the gross anatomical distribution of the nerve. This larger area is known as the intermediate zone
- When a nerve is intact and the adjacent nerves are blocked or sectioned, an area of sensibility exceeds the gross anatomical distribution of the nerve, then this area is known as the maximal zone.

Sensibility Recovery Sequence

- Myelinated and unmyelinated fibers (restore perception of pain and temperature) and pseudomotor function
- Touch perception
  - Perception of 30 cps of vibratory stimulus
  - Perception of moving touch
  - Perception of constant touch
  - Perception of 256 cps vibratory stimulus.

Sensation Assessment after Peripheral Nerve Injury

S_0: Absence of sensibility in autonomous area
S_1: Recovery of deep cutaneous pain sensibility within autonomous area of the nerve
S_2: Return of some degree of superficial cutaneous pain and tactile sensibility within autonomous area of the nerve
S_3: Return of superficial cutaneous pain and tactile sensibility throughout autonomous area, with disappearance of any previous over response
S_{3+}: Return of sensibility as in stage 3, in addition, there is some recovery of two-point discrimination within autonomous area
S_4: Complete recovery.

Reflex

Complete severance of a peripheral nerve abolishes all reflex activity transmitted by that nerve. This is true in severance of the afferent or the efferent arc. Commonly, however reflex activity is abolished in partial nerve injuries, when neither arc is completely interrupted and is not a reliable guide to the severity of injury.

Autonomic

- Interruption of a peripheral nerve is followed by loss of sweating and of pilomotor response and by vasomotor paralysis in the autonomous zone. The area of anhidrosis usually corresponds to, but may be slightly larger than the sensory deficit
- If the injury is incomplete and especially, if it is associated with causalgia, sweating may be excessive and may involve areas beyond the intermediate zone of the nerve. Vasodilation occurs in complete lesions and the area affected is at first warmer and pinker than the rest of the limb. After 2 to 3 weeks, however, the affected area becomes colder than the adjacent normal areas and the skin may be pale, cyanotic or mottled in an area often extending beyond the maximal zone of the injured nerve. Trophic changes occur commonly and are most evident in the hands and feet. The skin becomes thin and glistening and when subjected to trauma then ordinarily does little harm, it breaks down to form ulcers that heal slowly. The fingernails become distorted, often ridged or brittle and may be lost entirely.

Diagnostic Tests

Diagnostic tests majorly include electrodiagnostic tests. These are explained below:

Nerve Conduction Velocity (Fig. 16.5)

Stimulation of a peripheral nerve by an electrode placed on the skin overlying the nerve readily evokes a response from the muscle innervated by that nerve. This response can be seen, palpated and measured. The nerve is stimulated proximal to distal and across the level of injury, with subsequent distal evoked potential recording, achieved using a needle or surface pick-up electrode (Table 16.3).

Electromyography

- Muscle activity observed with a needle pick-up electrode (e.g. monopolar, concentric, single fiber) placed in myotomes, innervated by an injured nerve provides crucial information

Table 16.3: Nerve conduction velocity

Injury pattern	*Proximal stimulation (Segment A)*	*Immediately after injury distal stimulation (Segment B)*	*Ten days after injury distal stimulation (Segment B)*
Neuropraxia	No response	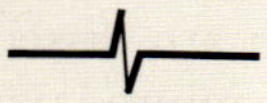	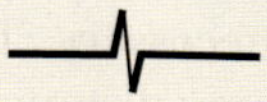
Axonotmesis or Neurotmesis	No response	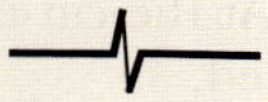	No response

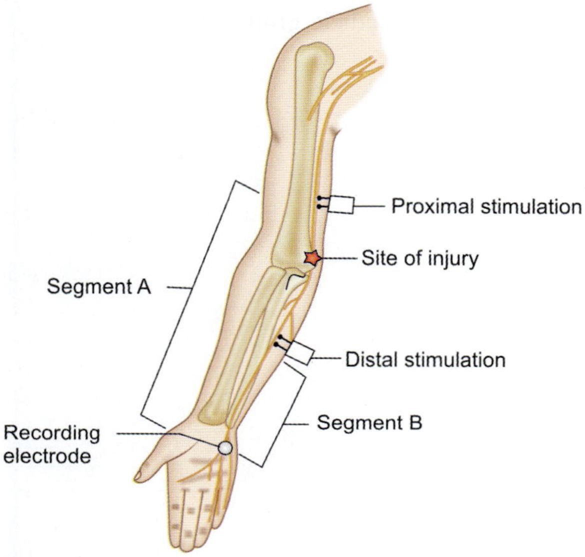

Fig. 16.5: Nerve conduction velocity

- At approximately 10 to 14 days after neural injury, abnormal spontaneous rest potentials (positive sharp waves) appear in innervated myotomes, where axonal injury has occurred. At 14 to 18 days, fibrillations appear. At approximately 3 months after injury, some peripheral neural sprouting has occurred and the motor unit potential amplitude has progressively increased. This is preceded at times by polyphasic configuration potentials. After 2 to 6 months of injury, larger potentials are established and remain so, until the reinnervation is completed, at which time the motor unit potential configuration returns to a more normal appearing pattern.

Tinel Sign

The Tinel sign is elicited by gentle percussion, by a finger or percussion hammer along the course of an injured nerve. A transient tingling sensation should be felt by the patient in the distribution of the injured nerve, rather than in the area percussed and the sensation should persist for several seconds after stimulation. It should be tested for in a distal to proximal direction. A positive Tinel sign is presumptive evidence that regenerating axonal sprouts that have not obtained complete myelinization and progressing along the endoneurial tube.

Sweat Test

The time-honored sweat test (iodine starch test) consists of dusting the extremity with quinizarin powder. Sweating is induced by various means. The powder remains dry and light gray throughout the denervated area and assumes a deep purple color throughout the area of normal sweating.

Skin Resistance Test

The skin resistance test is another method of evaluating autonomic interruption. In it a Richter dermometer is used. The autonomous zone with absence of sweating shows an increased resistance to the passage of electrical current. The adjacent innervated areas have a normal resistance and further decreased resistance in these areas can be elicited by high external temperatures that do not affect the denervated area.

Management of Nerve Injuries

Factors that influence regeneration after neurorrhaphy, are illustrated below:
- Age of the patient
- Gap between the nerve ends
- Delay between the time of injury and repair
- Level of injury
- Condition of the nerve ends
- Experience and techniques of the surgeon.

Technique of Nerve Repair

Endoneurolysis

The epineurium is incised longitudinally proximal to the lesion, beginning not more than 0.5 cm from the level of gross changes in the nerve, as determined by palpation. The flaps of epineurium on each side may be retracted laterally by nylon sutures and are undermined widely. The funiculi are separated, if possible with a pointed or diamond-bladed knife, using sharp or blunt dissection as necessary. Spring-loaded microscissors also are helpful in this dissection. The surgeon constantly should be aware of the possibility of plexus formation between fascicles and protect these.

Partial Neurorrhaphy

When the decision has been made to perform partial neurorrhaphy, the incision is extended longitudinally in the epineurium proximally and distally several centimeters, as necessary. The intact funiculi are dissected out for the same distance. The ends of the injured part of the nerve are resected to normal tissue. At the cut ends, an end-to-end neurorrhaphy is performed.

Complete Neurorrhaphy and Nerve Grafting

Technique of Neurorrhaphy

- Epineurial
- Perineurial
- Interfascicular nerve grafting.

Methods of Closing Gaps between the Nerve Ends

- Mobilization
- Positioning of extremity
- Transposition
- Bone resection
- Nerve grafting
- Nerve stretching and bulb suture
- Nerve crossing (pedicle grafting).

17 Peripheral Vascular Disease

- Peripheral Arterial Disease
- Arterial Disorders
- Arterial Stenosis
- Acute Arterial Occlusion
- Gangrene
- Arteritis
- Vasospastic Conditions
- Frostbite
- Peripheral Venous Disease

Introduction

Peripheral vascular disease refers to any disease or disorder of the circulatory system outside of the brain and heart.

It is divided into two disorders:

1. Arterial disorders
2. Venous disorders

Arterial Disorders

- *Pain:* Aching to sharp brought on by exercise and is relieved by rest.
- *Pulses:* Diminished or absent
- *Edema:* None
- *Skin changes:* Skin become cold, dry, shiny and hairless. Pallor, when elevated and red, when dangling.

Venous Disorders

- *Pain:* Aching, to cramp like, relieved by activity or elevating the extremity
- *Pulses:* Usually present
- *Edema:* Present, increases at the end of the day
- *Skin changes:* Warm, thick, tough, darkened, stasis ulcers.

Peripheral Arterial Disease

Definition

Decreased patency of the arterial supply to the lower extremities, leading to claudication, ischemia and potentially limb loss as well as narrowing of the arteries of the extremities due to atherosclerosis.

Risk Factors

- Positive family history of premature heart attacks or strokes
- Older than 50 years
- Obesity
- Inactive (sedentary) lifestyle
- Smoking
- Diabetes
- High blood pressure
- High cholesterol or LDL (bad cholesterol), plus high triglycerides and low HDL (the good cholesterol)
- Men are slightly more likely affected than women.

Arterial Disorders

Arterial disorders include:

- Arterial stenosis
- Acute arterial occlusion
- Gangrene
- Arteritis

Arterial Stenosis

- The most common cause of peripheral artery disease is due to atherosclerosis
- This is a gradual process, in which a fatty material builds up inside the arteries
- The fatty material mixes with calcium, scar tissues and other substances and then hardens slightly, forming plaques of arteriosclerosis
- These plaques block, narrow or weaken the vessel walls. Blood flow through the arteries can be restricted or blocked totally.

Symptoms and Signs of Arterial Occlusion

Claudication Pain

- It is an intermittent cramp-like pain felt in the muscles that is brought on, by walking, not present on taking the first step and relieved by standing still
- Claudication is the muscle pain due to accumulation of excessive P substance, owing to inadequate blood flow.

- The pain develops only when the muscles are working and disappears when exercise stops. Claudication pain is most commonly felt in calf, but can affect thigh or buttock
- Pain in the buttock, occurring on exercise (walking) and associated sexual impotence, which result from arterial ischemia are given the eponymous title "Leriche's syndrome". Distance walked is called claudication distance
- *Boyd's classification of claudication pain*
  - *Grade 1:* Claudication pain appears, but as the patient continues the exercise claudication pain disappears
  - *Grade 2:* Pain continues and the patient can still walk with effort
  - *Grade 3:* Pain compels the patient to take rest
  - *Grade 4:* Rest pain
- Spinal claudication/neurogenic claudication, is not due to lack of blood supply, but rather it is caused by nerve root compression and/or stenosis of the spinal canal, usually from a degenerative spine
- This may result from many factors, such as bulging disk, herniated disk or fragments from previously herniated disks (postoperative), scar tissue from previous surgeries, osteophytes or other causes
- *Vascular claudication*
  - Arterial pulses are diminished
  - Relieved by rest
  - Typically occurs after activities/ambulation for a distance with resultant vascular insufficiency
  - Not associated with weakness
- *Neuro claudication*
  - Arterial pulses are normal
  - Symptoms may be relieved by sitting down (flexing the spine)
  - Typically, occurs after standing erect or standing and walking
  - Generally associated with weakness.

Rest Pain

It is severe pain felt in the foot at rest, made worse by lying down or elevation of the foot. The pain is worse at night and relieved by hanging the foot out of bed or by sleeping in a chair. It is described "cry of dying nerves".

Coldness, Numbness and Paresthesia

These are common in moderate and severe ischemia, but in the absence of color changes, it is essential to exclude neurological cause (Fig. 17.1).

Color Changes

- Severely ischemic limbs develop purple discoloration on dependency. Bright red color is due to extravasation of RBC through capillary walls

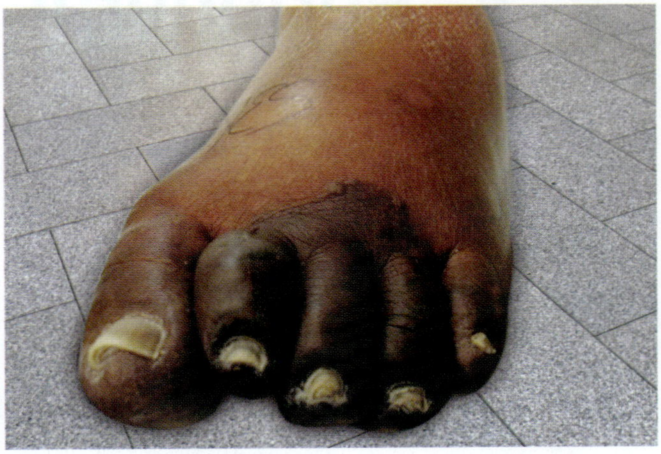

Fig. 17.1: Severe ischemia of the foot

- *Buerger's postural test*: The limb is raised for a minute or two. With a normal peripheral circulation, the toes should remain pink at 90°. In an ischemic limb because arterial pressure is unable to overcome gravity, the elevated leg becomes waxy, cadaveric, white color, best seen on the sole of the foot. The angle to which the leg must be raised before it becomes white, is the vascular angle or Buerger's angle, usually less than 30° in an ischemic limb. When the limb is hung down, it gradually becomes a bluish-red color due to reactive hyperemia
- *Capillary filling*: The time will be longer in case of ischemic limb
- *Cross legged test*: This is to detect popliteal pulsations. The patient is asked to sit with legs crossed one above the other so that popliteal fossa of one leg will lie against the knee of the other leg. Patient's attention is diverted. Crossed leg will show oscillatory movements of the foot, which occur synchronously with the pulse of the popliteal artery
- *Allen's test*: Instruct the patient to clench his/her fist. Using your fingers, apply occlusive pressure to both the ulnar and radial arteries. This maneuver obstructs blood flow to the hand. While applying occlusive pressure to both the arteries, patient should relax his/her hand. Blanching of the palm and fingers should occur. If it does not, you have not completely occluded the arteries with your fingers. Release the occlusive pressure on the ulnar artery. You should notice a flushing of the hand within 5 to 15 seconds. This denotes that the ulnar artery is patent and has good blood flow.

Ulceration and Gangrene

- Ulceration occurs with severe arterial insufficiency and is often present as a painful superficial erosion between toes (Figs 17.2 and 17.3)

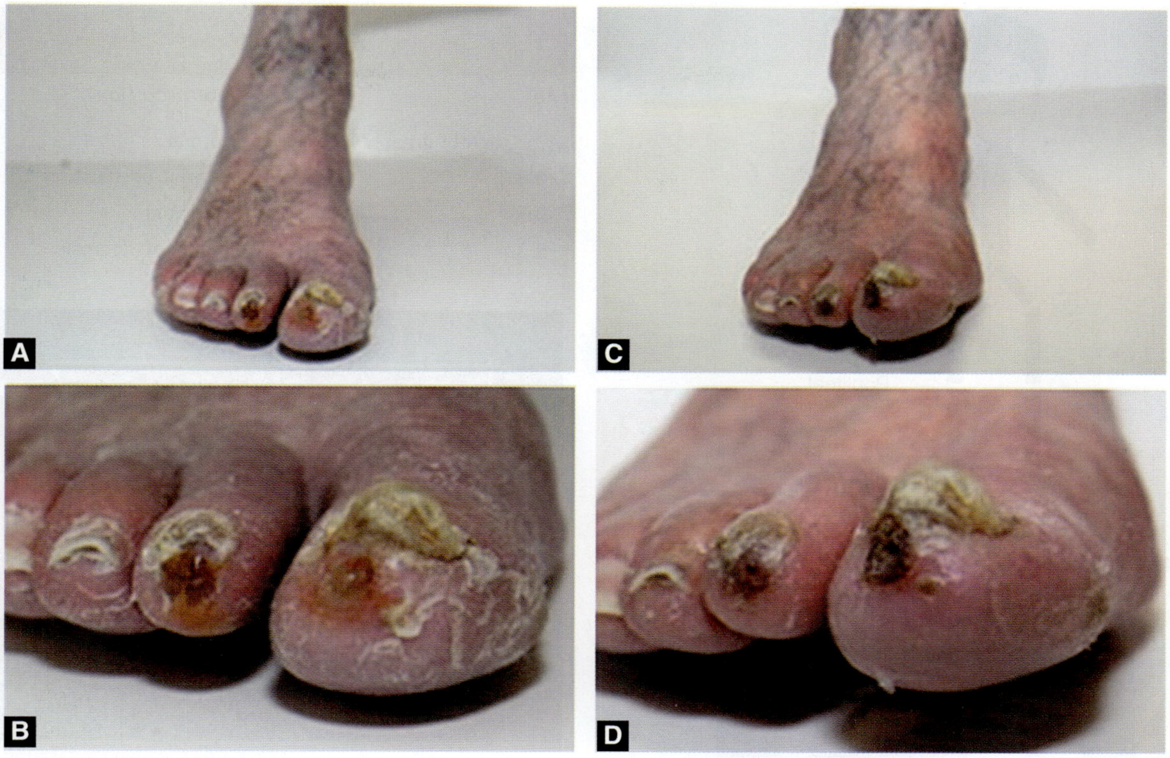

Figs 17.2A to D: Ulceration of the toes

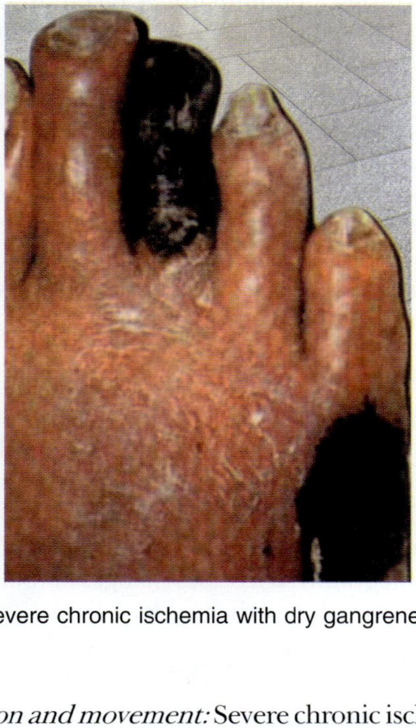

Fig. 17.3: Severe chronic ischemia with dry gangrene

- *Sensation and movement:* Severe chronic ischemia produce hyperesthesia, especially on the borderline skin of gangrene
- *Arterial pulsations:* Arterial pulsation below occlusion are usually absent or diminished in the presence of good collaterals. Expansile arterial pulsation with a mass may indicate an aneurysm
- Other physical findings include, loss of hair, nail changes (brittle nails), pallor on elevation and dependent rubor of the affected extremities.

Symptoms

Symptoms are related to the organ supplied by the artery:

- *Lower limb:* Claudication, rest pain and gangrene
- *Brain:* Transient ischemic attacks and hemiplegia
- *Myocardium:* Angina and myocardial infarction
- *Kidney:* Hypertension or infarction
- *Intestine:* Abdominal pain and infarction.

Physical Signs

- In case of arterial occlusion with normal distal pulses and highly developed collateral circulation (Fig. 17.4)
- *Disappearing pulse:* On exercising till claudication, palpable pulse disappear. Then after 1 to 2 minutes of rest the disappearing pulse reappears
- *Arterial bruits:* Auscultation of subclavian arteries and systolic bruits
- Bruit in neck at the level of mandibular angle, without supraclavicular bruit means carotid artery stenosis.

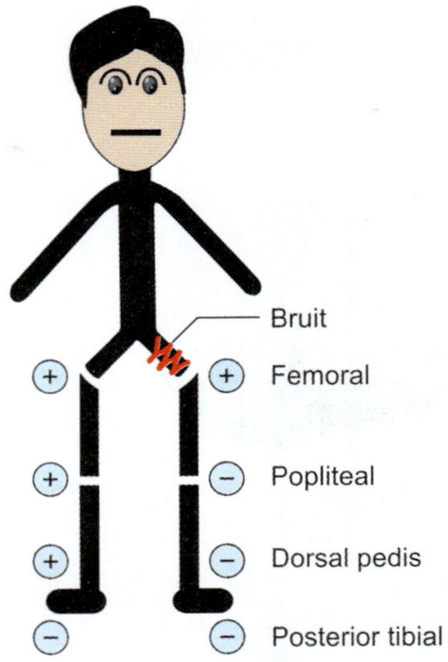

Fig. 17.4: Physical signs, in case of arterial occlusion

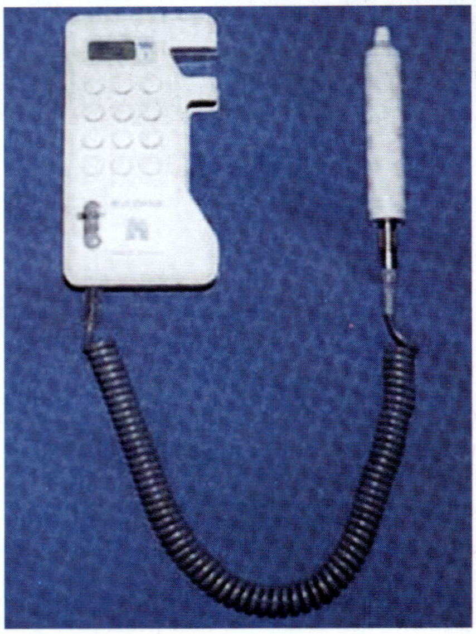

Fig. 17.5: Doppler ultrasound

Diagnosis and Investigations

Routine investigation

- Hemoglobin, full blood count, ESR, plasma fibrinogen, protein electrophoresis, blood and urine glucose, blood lipid profile and exercise ECG

Noninvasive tests

- *Doppler ultrasound:* Use a stethoscope with sphygmomanometer, to assess the systolic blood pressure in relatively small vessels (Fig. 17.5)
- *Ankle brachial index (ABI):* It is the ratio of systolic pressure at ankle artery to that in brachial artery. Numerator is systolic pressure in dorsalis pedis and posterior tibial arteries, denominator is taken as systolic pressure of brachial arteries. ABI values for different conditions are illustrated in the Table 17.1.
- *Duplex imaging:* It provides an image of vessels, which can give detailed knowledge of vessel blood flow and turbulence (Figs 17.6 and 17.7)
- *Color-duplex:* Visualization of blood flow indicates change in direction and velocity of blood flow, increased flow depicts stenosis
- *Treadmill:* It is useful in the assessment of walking distance in claudicants

Table 17.1: ABI values and associated conditions

ABI	*Interpretation*
1 or slightly greater	Normal
<0.8	Arterial obstruction
<0.5	Rest pain
<0.3	Imminent necrosis

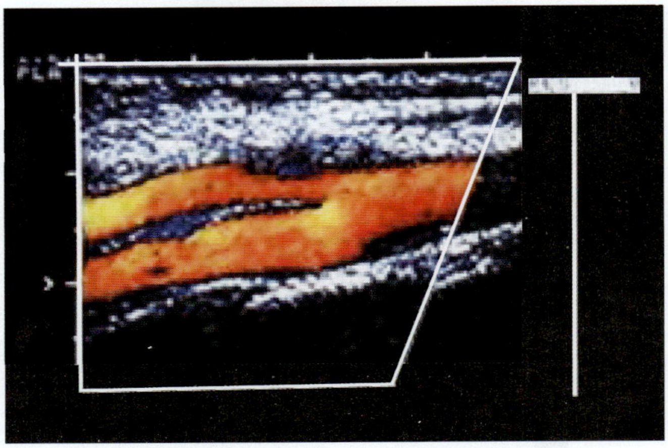

Fig. 17.6: Duplex imaging

Invasive Tests

- *Arterial digital subtraction angiography (DSA):* This technique, which is in widespread use, employs a computer system to digitise the angiographic information (Fig. 17.8)
- Conventional arteriography (Fig. 17.9)
- *Plethysmography:* It assesses changes in volume of a limb or digit over the cardiac cycle.

Management (Arterial Stenosis)

Conservative Treatment

- Stop smoking
- Taking regular exercise within the limits of the pain
- Suitable diet to reduce weight in obese and hyperlipidemics

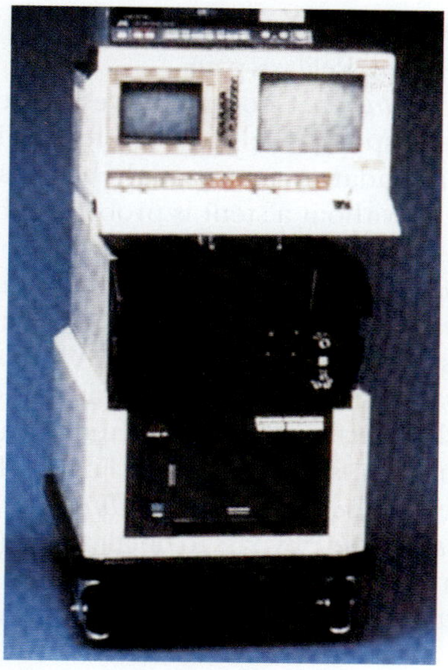

Fig. 17.7: Duplex imaging machine

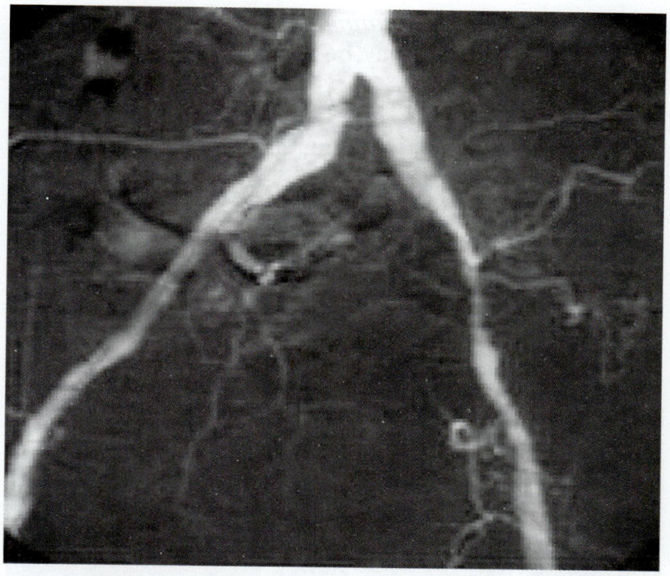

Fig. 17.9: Conventional arteriography

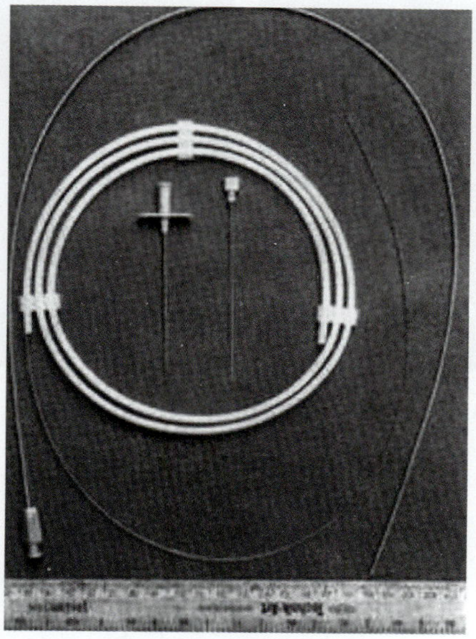

Fig. 17.8: Arterial digital subtraction angiography

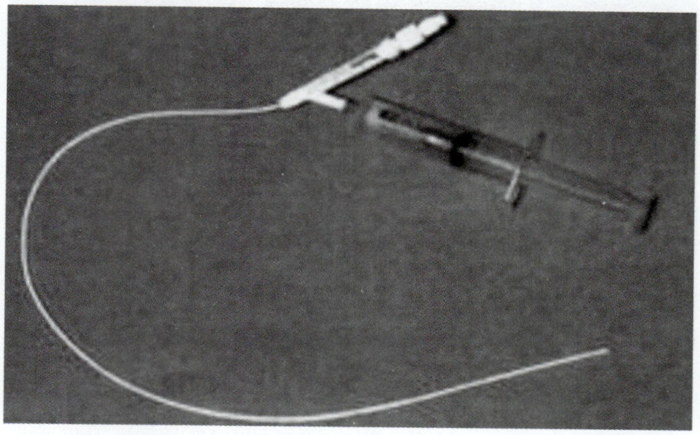

Fig. 17.10: Balloon catheter, used for transluminal angioplasty

- *Heel raise:* Claudication distance may be increased by raising the heels of shoes by 1 cm. The work of the calf muscles is reduced.

Drugs

- Rest pain can be relieved by analgesics and elevation of the head of bed (Buerger's position), pentoxifylline for treatment of intermittent claudication, aspirin in small dose of 150 mg/day to prevent thrombosis
- Two medications have been approved by the United States Food and Drug Administration (FDA) for direct treatment of the symptoms of intermittent claudication
- *Pentoxifylline (Trental):* How this drug helps in intermittent claudication is not completely understood. It is believed to improve blood flow, by decreasing the viscosity of blood and making red blood cells more flexible. With these alterations, the blood can move more easily past obstructions in the blood vessel
- *Cilostazol (Pletal):* This drug keeps platelets from clumping together. This clumping promotes formation of clots and slows down blood flow. The drug also helps to dilate or expand the blood vessels, encouraging the flow of blood.

Nonoperative Procedures to Improve Arterial Flow

- *Transluminal angioplasty:* Inserting a balloon catheter into an artery and inflating it within a narrowed area (Figs 17.10 and 17.11)

- *Percutaneous transluminal angioplasty (PTA):* In this inflatable balloon may be used for stenosis or short occlusions
- *Intraluminal stents:* After balloon dilatation, the vessel may fail to stay dilated then it is possible to keep open lumen by a metal stent (Figs 17.12A and B)
- *Lasers and atherectomy catheters:* Lasers can be used to open occluded arteries, so that a balloon angioplasty catheter can be inserted. Atherectomy catheters actually remove atherosclerotic plaque from arterial wall, either by cutting or extracting.

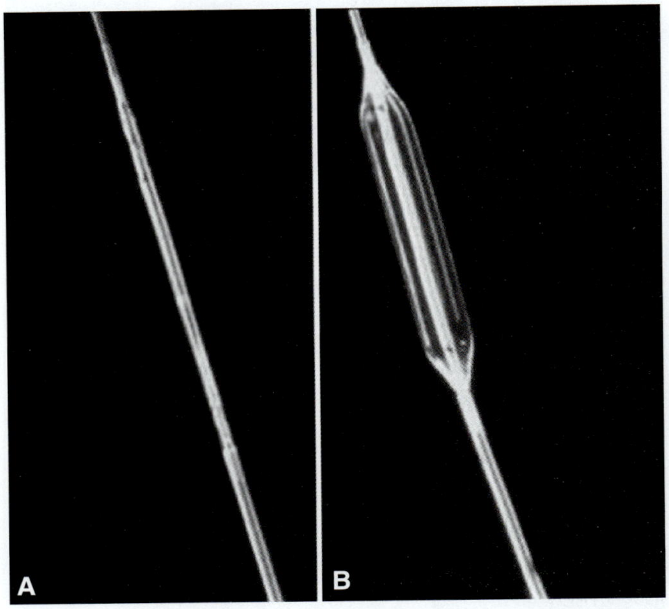

Figs 17.11A and B: Different types of catheter used in transluminal angioplasty

Operations for Arterial Occlusion

- *Sympathectomy:* Relieves pain
- *Aortoiliac occlusion:* Good calibre vessels below the site of disease responds well to aortofemoral bypass. If not, an iliac endarterectomy might be considered, but PTA with or without a stent is probably a better alternative.
- *Superficial femoral and profunda femoris artery occlusion (with unilateral symptoms):* For severe disease angioplasty or bypass may be used. A femoropopliteal bypass graft is the most usual operation (to overcome a blocked superficial femoral artery). Patient's own saphenous vein is the best graft (Figs 17.13A and B).
- *Occlusive disease below the popliteal artery (usually unreconstructable):* Bypass to tibial vessels (down ankle level) can be successful. Long saphenous vein used in the *in situ* fashion, after disrupting the valves with a

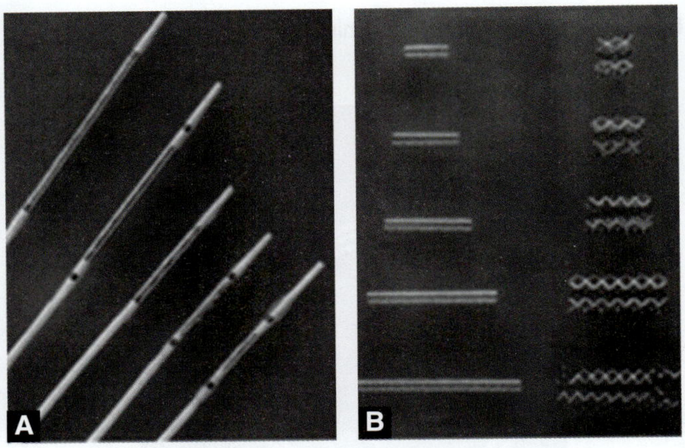

Figs 17.12A and B: Different intraluminal stents

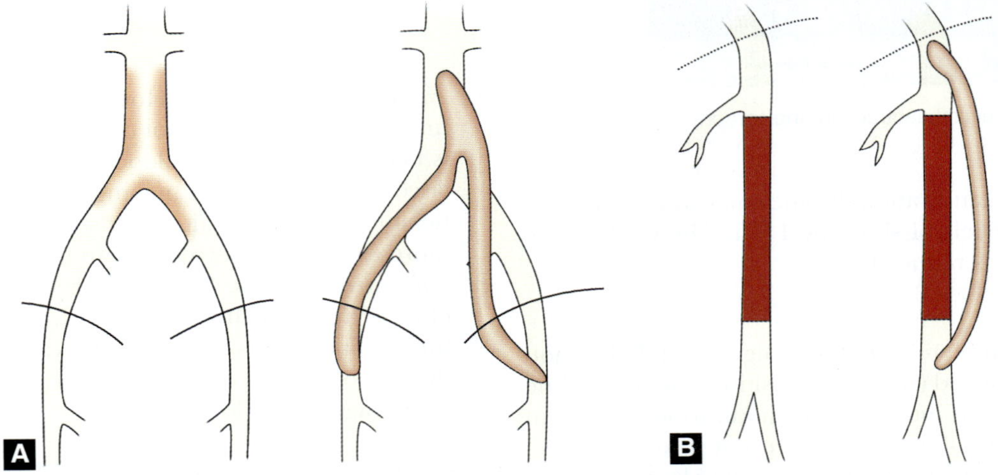

Figs 17.13A and B: (A) Atherosclerotic narrowing of the aortic bifurcation, aorto-bifemoral graft to bypass stenosis; (B) Superficial femoral and profunda femoris stenosis providing poor collateral circulation, femoropopliteal graft used to bypass the occluded area into good "runoff" below

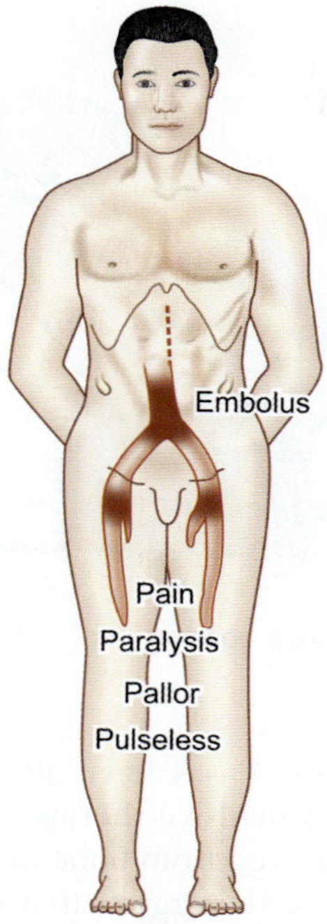

Fig. 17.14: Clinical picture of an acute arterial occlusion

valvulotome. If the saphenous vein is not available a polytetrafluoroethylene (PTFE) graft is used.

Acute Arterial Occlusion

Definition

Sudden occlusion of an artery is commonly due to either emboli or trauma.

Clinical Picture

Six P's (Fig. 17.14)
1. Pain
2. Pallor
3. Pulselessness
4. Paresthesia
5. Paralysis
6. Progressive coldness

Embolic Occlusion

Definition

An embolus is a body, which is foreign to the bloodstream and which may become lodged in a vessel and cause obstruction.

Simple Emboli

- Simple emboli are due to blood thrombus. The sources are most commonly mural thrombus, following a myocardial infarct (a third of cases), mitral stenosis, cardiac arrhythmias (particularly atrial fibrillation) and aneurysms

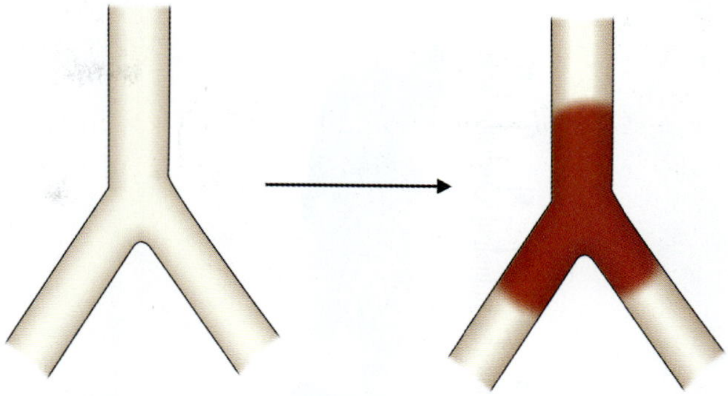

Fig. 17.15: Aortic bifurcation embolus

- Emboli may lodge in any organ including brain, mesentric vessels, spleen, kidneys, lungs, lower limbs, etc. with resultant ischemia (Fig. 17.15)
- The diagnosis can be made clinically in the majority of cases. The patient, who has no previous symptoms of claudication or limb pain and has a source of emboli, suddenly develops severe pain or numbness of the limb, which becomes cold with mottled blue and white discoloration. Movement of the toes becomes progressively more difficult and sensation to touch is lost. Pulses are absent distally.

Treatment

- The immediate administration of heparin 5000 units intravenously, can reduce this extension and maintain patency of the surrounding (particularly the distal) vessels, till the embolus can be treated
- Embolectomy or thrombolysis are the treatments available for patients with limb emboli (Figs 17.16 and 17.17)
- The common thrombolytic agents are streptokinase, urokinase and tissue plasminogen activator (TPA)
- Whichever drug is used, regular angiograms are carried out to check the extent of lysis. Using streptokinase, lysis was usually complete within 48 hours. TPA may achieve lysis within 24 hours and pulse spray TPA may take less than 6 hours.

Air Embolism

Air may be accidentally injected into the venous circulation, e.g. artificial pneumothorax or sucked into an open vein. Thus, venous air embolism occasionally complicates operations on the neck or axilla, if a large vein is inadvertently opened or it may be an accessory cause of death following a cut throat.

Treatment

- *Trendelenburg's position (Fig. 17.18):* It encourages air to pass into the veins of the lower half of the body

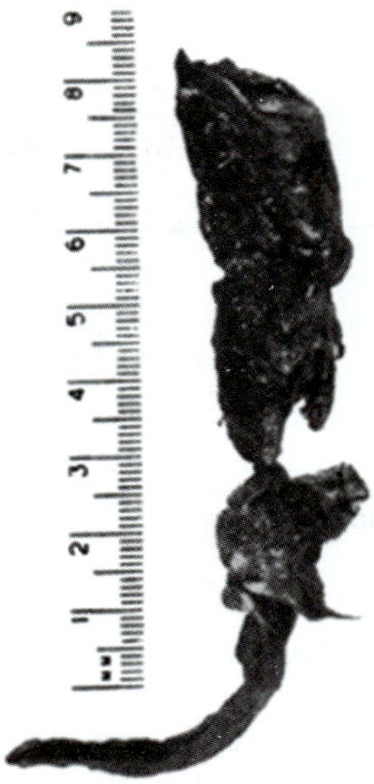

Fig. 17.16: Limb embolus

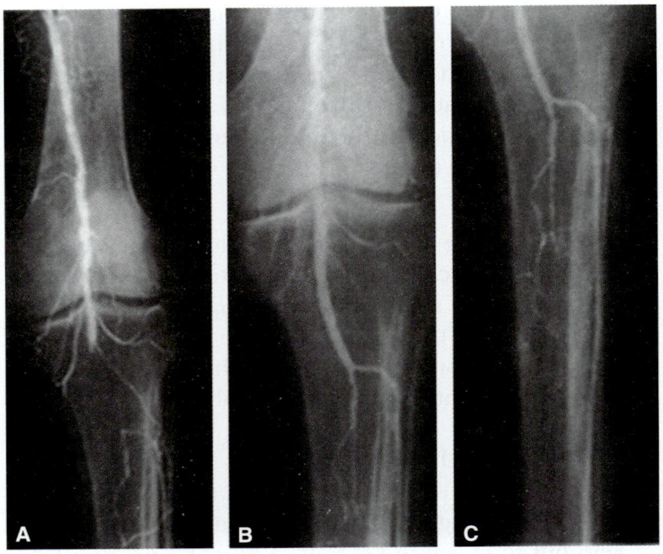

Figs 17.17A to C: (A) Angiography showing blockade; (B and C) Reflow after embolectomy

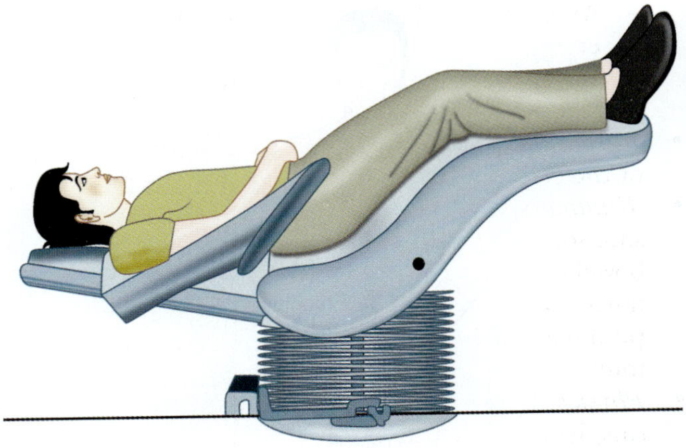

Fig. 17.18: Trendelenburg's position

and the patient is placed on the left side, so that air will float into the apex of the ventricle, away from the pulmonary artery
- Oxygen is administered to counteract hypoxemia and to assist in the excretion of nitrogen. In serious cases, the right ventricle should be aspirated by a needle passed upwards and backwards from below the left costal margin.

Fat Embolism

- This condition, which is more common than generally supposed, usually follows severe injuries with multiple or major fractures. Cases have also been recorded following electroconvulsive therapy
- The fat may be derived from bone marrow or adipose tissue, but recent work suggests that it is metabolic in origin, perhaps by aggregation of chylomicrons
- Symptoms are evident a day or so after injury and two more or less distinct types, cerebral and pulmonary are recognized
- In the cerebral type, the patient becomes drowsy, restless and disorientated (delirium tremens may be suspected). Subsequently, the patient is comatose, the pupils become small and pyrexia ensues
- The pulmonary type is ushered in with cyanosis, which increases in intensity and signs of right heart failure. White froth may occur at the mouth and nostrils
- The sputum should be examined for fat droplets and fat may be excreted in the urine. A fall in the hemoglobin value of the blood is a constant sign. Petechial hemorrhages often occur
- Treatment consists of oxygen, early heparinization and intravenous low molecular weight dextran.

Gangrene

Gangrene implies death with putrefaction of macroscopic portions of tissue. It is commonly seen affecting the distal part of a limb, the appendix or a loop of small intestine and sometimes organs such as the gallbladder, the pancreas or the testis.

Types of Gangrene (Based upon the Cause)

- *Secondary to arterial obstruction*: It can be from disease, for example:
  - Thrombosis of an atherosclerotic artery
  - Embolus from the heart in atrial fibrillation or after coronary thrombosis
  - Arteritis with neuropathy in diabetes
  - Buerger's disease

  - Arterial shutdown in Raynaud's disease or ergotism
  - Effect of intra-arterial injections, i.e. thiopentone and cytotoxic substances
- *Infective:* Boils and carbuncles, gas gangrene, gangrene of the scrotum (Fournier's gangrene), etc.
- *Traumatic:* Due to direct trauma, such as crushes, pressure sores and the constriction groove of strangulated bowel or indirect, due to injury of vessels at some distance from the site of gangrene, e.g. pressure on the popliteal artery, by the lower end of a fractured femur
- *Physical:* For example burns, scalds, frostbite, chemicals, irradiation and electricity
- *Venous gangrene*

Clinical Features of Gangrene

- A gangrenous part lacks arterial pulsation, venous return, capillary response to pressure (color returns), sensation, warmth and function
- The color of the part changes through a variety of shades, according to circumstances (pallor, dusky gray, mottled, purple), until finally taking on the characteristic dark brown, greenish black or black appearance, which is due to the disintegration of hemoglobin and the formation of iron sulfide (See Figs 17.3).

Clinical types: These include following types of gangrene, with their different clinical presentation.

- *Dry gangrene:* Dry gangrene occurs when the tissues are desiccated by gradual slowing of the bloodstream. It is typically the result of atherosclerosis. The affected part becomes dry and wrinkled, discolored from disintegration of hemoglobin and greasy to the touch (Fig. 17.19).
- *Moist gangrene:* This occurs when venous as well as arterial obstruction is present, when the artery is suddenly occluded, as by a ligature or embolus and in diabetes. Infection and putrefaction are always present, the affected part becomes swollen and discolored and the epidermis may be raised in blebs. Crepitus may be palpated, owing to infection by gas forming organisms (Fig. 17.20).

Separation of Gangrene

Separation by Demarcation

- A zone of demarcation between the truly viable and the dead or dying tissue appears first. It is indicated on the surface, by a band of hyperemia and hyperesthesia. Separation is achieved by the development of a layer of granulation tissue, which forms between the dead and the living parts
- In dry gangrene, if the blood supply of the proximal tissues is adequate, the final line of demarcation appears in a matter of days and separation begins to take place neatly and with the minimum of infection (so-called separation by aseptic ulceration)
- In moist gangrene, there is more infection and suppuration extends into the neighboring living tissue, thereby causing the final line of demarcation to be more proximal than in dry gangrene.

Separation by Septic Ulceration

Treatment of gangrene

General principles of treatment includes:

- A limb-saving attitude is needed in most cases of symptomatic gangrene affecting hands and feet
- With arterial disease all depends upon a good blood supply to the limb above the gangrene or whether a poor blood supply can be improved by such measures, as percutaneous transluminal angioplasty or direct arterial surgery
- A life-saving amputation is required for a badly crushed limb, rapidly spreading symptomatic gangrene and gas gangrene

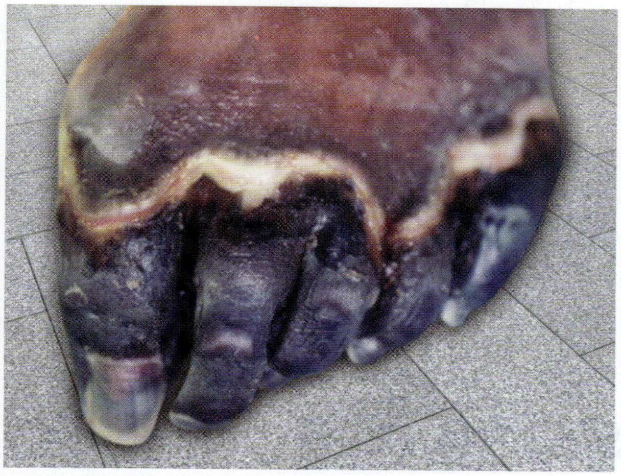

Fig. 17.19: Dry gangrene of the toes

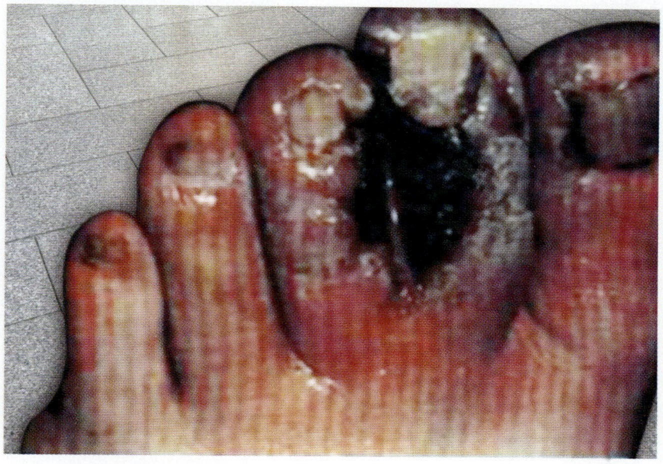

Fig. 17.20: Moist gangrene

General treatment includes
- Treatment of cardiac failure, atrial fibrillation and anemia, to improve the tissue oxygenation
- A nutritious diet is essential in all forms of gangrene and the control of diabetes, when present, are additional items of care

Local treatment includes
- Care of the affected part includes, keeping it absolutely dry. Exposure and the use of a fan may assist in the desiccation and may relieve pain. The limb must not be heated
- A bed-cradle, padded rings, foam blocks and air beds are useful preventive aids
- The release of pus, assists in relief of pain

Arteritis

Thromboangiitis Obliterans (Buerger's Disease) (Fig. 17.21)

- This is a condition characterized by occlusive disease of the small and medium-sized arteries (plantars, tibials, radial, etc.), thrombophlebitis of superficial or deep veins and Raynaud's syndrome, occurring in male patients in a young age group (usually under the age of 30 years) (Fig. 17.22)
- The condition does not occur in women or nonsmokers. It is not as used to be stated more common in Russian and Jews, but cases are seen in different races all over the world.

Histology

Localized inflammatory changes occur in the walls of arteries and veins, leading to thrombosis. The usual symptoms and signs of arterial occlusive disease are present. Gangrene of the toes and fingers is common and progressive (Figs 17.23A to C).

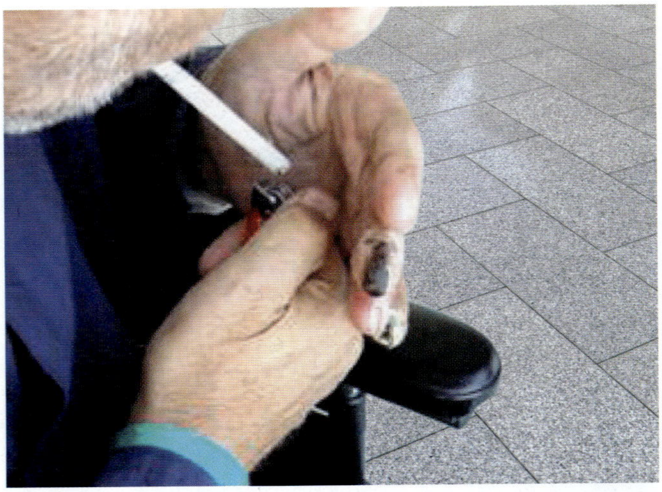

Fig. 17.21: Discolored nails depicting Buerger's disease

Investigations
- A formal vascular assessment should be undertaken, e.g. ESR, autoantibodies, coagulation screening and lipid profile
- Arteriography sometimes shows a characteristic 'corrugation' of the femoral arteries as well as the distal arterial occlusions and helps to distinguish the condition from presenile atherosclerosis.

Treatment
- The treatment is total abstinence from smoking. While this will arrest the disease, it will not reverse established arterial occlusions
- Use of vascular growth factor and stem cell injections have been showing promise in clinical studies

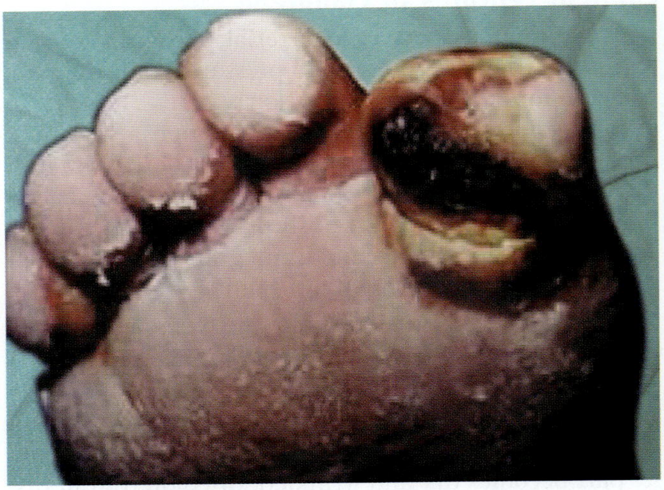

Fig. 17.22: Raynaud's syndrome

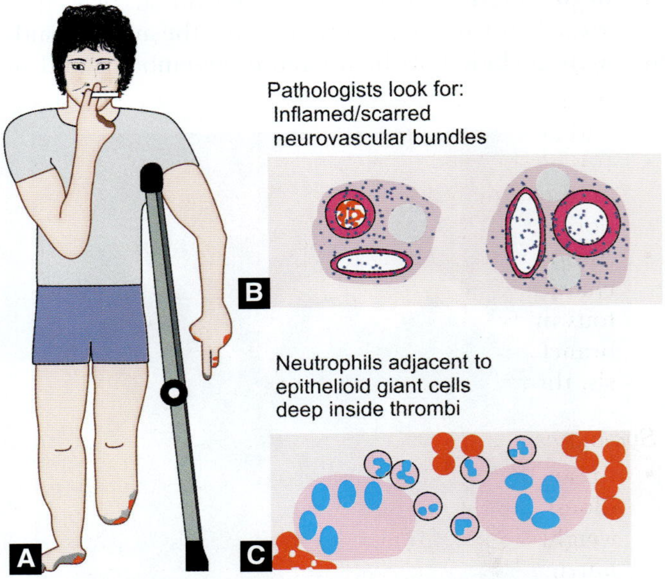

Figs 17.23A to C: Histological changes, seen in Buerger's thromboangiitis obliterans

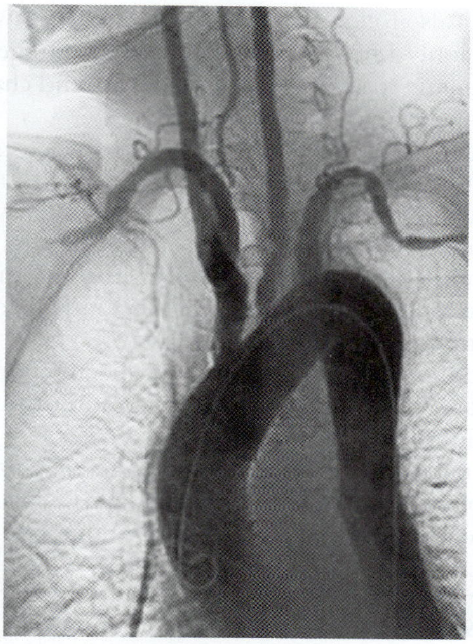

Fig. 17.24: Takayasu's arteritis

- Streptokinase has been proposed as adjuvant therapy in some cases
- Established arterial occlusions may be treated along the usual lines and sympathectomy may be a useful adjunctive procedure. Nevertheless, amputations, conservative, if possible, may eventually be required.

Takayasu's Arteritis (Fig. 17.24)

- Takayasu's arteritis (also known as "aortic arch syndrome" and "pulseless disease") is an inflammatory disease with an unknown cause
- It affects the aorta, the main blood vessel from the heart, as well as the blood vessels that attach to it
- Females are about 8 to 9 times more likely to get it than males. People usually get the disease between 15 and 30 years of age
- It is also known as "pulseless disease" because pulses on the upper extremities, such as the wrist pulse may not be felt
- Although, its etiology is unknown, the condition is characterized by segmental and patchy granulomatous inflammation of the aorta and major derivative branches. This inflammation leads to arterial stenosis, thrombosis and aneurysms.

Symptoms

- About half of all patients develop an initial systemic illness, with symptoms of malaise, fever, night sweats, weight loss, arthralgia and fatigue. There is often an anemia and marked elevation of the ESR
- This is followed by a more chronic stage characterized by inflammatory and obliterative changes in the aorta and its branches
- In the late stage, weakness of the arterial walls may give rise to localized aneurysms
- Raynaud's phenomenon is commonly found in this disease.

Treatment

- The great majority of patients with Takayasu's arteritis, respond to prednisilone. The usual starting dose is approximately 1 milligram per kilogram of body weight per day
- Surgical options may need to be explored for patients, who do not respond to steroids. Reperfusion of tissues can be achieved by large vessel reconstructive surgery, such as bypass grafting

Other Types of Arteritis

Other types of arteritis are encountered in rheumatoid arthritis, diffuse lupus erythematosus and polyarteritis. Treatment is similar.

■ Vasospastic Conditions

Raynaud's Syndrome

Raynaud's syndrome may be:

- Primary
- Secondary

Primary Raynaud's Syndrome

- The primary idiopathic form, usually occurs in young women and affects the upper extremities more than the lower. The peripheral pulses are normal
- The condition is attributable to abnormal sensitivity in the direct response of the arterioles to cold
- When cooled, these vessels constrict and as a result, the part (usually the fingers) becomes blanched and incapable of finer movements
- The capillaries then dilate and fill with slowly flowing deoxygenated blood, the digits therefore becoming swollen and dusky. As the attack passes off, the arterioles relax, oxygenated blood returns into the dilated capillaries and the digits become red (Figs 17.25A to C)
- Thus, the condition is recognized by the characteristic sequence of blanching, dusky cyanosis and red engorgement, often accompanied by pain
- Raynaud's disease or "Primary Raynaud's" is diagnosed, if the symptoms are idiopathic, that is, they occur by themselves and not in association with other diseases. Some refer to primary Raynaud's disease as being allergic to coldness.

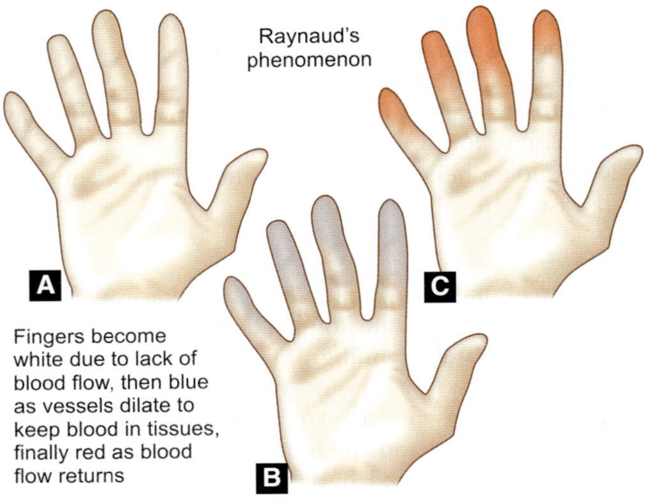

Figs 17.25A to C: Raynaud's syndrome

Conservative Treatment

- Avoid environmental triggers, e.g. cold, vibration, etc. Emotional stress is another recognized trigger
- Quit smoking
- Avoid caffeine, other stimulants and vasoconstrictors.

Treatment

- Treatment for Raynaud's phenomenon may include prescription medicines that dilate blood vessels, such as calcium channel blockers nifedipine or diltiazem
- There is some evidence that angiotensin II receptor, antagonists (Losartan) reduce frequency and severity of attacks
- Fluoxetine, a selective serotonin reuptake inhibitor and other antidepressant medications may reduce the frequency and severity of episodes
- Infusions of prostaglandins, e.g. prostacyclin, may be tried
- In severe cases, a sympathectomy procedure can be performed. Here, the nerves that signal the blood vessels of the fingertips to constrict are surgically cut.

Secondary Raynaud's Syndrome

- Raynaud's syndrome, or "Secondary Raynaud's" occurs secondary to a wide variety of other conditions. This was previously called Raynaud's disease (a term to be avoided).
- Although peripheral vasospasm may be noted in atherosclerosis, thoracic outlet syndrome, carpal tunnel, etc. The term secondary Raynaud's syndrome is most often used for a peripheral arterial manifestation of the collagen diseases, especially progressive systemic sclerosis (scleroderma) and systemic lupus erythromatosis
- It may also follow the use of vibrating tools (when it is commonly known as "vibration white finger"), e.g. pneumatic road drills, mining borers and chain saws, which vibrate at certain frequencies.

Treatment

- Treatment is directed primarily at the underlying condition. The syndrome when secondary to the collagenoses leads frequently to necrosis of digits and multiple amputations. Sympathectomy yields disappointing results and is rarely used.
- Nifedipine, steroids and vasospastic antagonists may all have a place. Patients with vibration white finger should avoid vibrating tools.
- Sildenafil (Viagra) improves both microcirculation and symptoms in patients with secondary Raynaud's phenomenon, resistant to vasodilatory therapy.

■ Frostbite

- Frostbite occurs with exposure of tissues to subfreezing temperatures for a period of several hours
- Short-term exposure to sub-zero temperatures, results in a different form of frostbite, commonly occurring in airplanes at high altitudes and characterized by the term "high-altitude" frostbite
- It has been demonstrated experimentally that cold-induced injury to mammalian tissues begins when the tissue temperature reaches 10°C. At 5°C, cells lose the ability to recover from the freezing process
- The pathophysiologic features of frostbite depend on the degree of cold-induced injury. Initially, vasoconstriction occurs on exposure to the cold. The histologic findings in mild frostbite consist of a low-grade vasculitis
- The process progresses to an intense inflammatory reaction of the intima with severe frostbite
- The capillary endothelium becomes permeable and the resultant extravascular fluid accumulation produces soft-tissue edema
- Thrombi form in the terminal arterioles and capillaries and irreversible tissue necrosis develops
- It is not known, whether the fundamental cold injury occurs as a result of direct freezing with disruption of cell membranes or from ischemic necrosis, secondary to widespread thrombosis of the arterioles and capillaries.

Classification of Frostbite

- First degree injury, consists of edema and redness without necrosis
- In second degree injury, blistering becomes evident
- Third degree injury, constitutes of necrosis of skin

- Fourth degree injury, gangrene develops in fourth degree injury, necessitating amputation of the affected extremity
- A simpler categorization of frostbite divides injuries into superficial and deep classifications. Superficial frostbite involves the skin and superficial subcutaneous tissue, deep frostbite involves the deeper subcutaneous tissue, muscle and even bone.

Treatment

- The treatment of frostbite begins with rapid warming of the injured tissue. The involved body part should be immersed in warm water with a temperature in the range of 40° to 44°C
- Complete rewarming generally requires about 20 minutes. Once warm, the injured extremity should be elevated to minimize the formation of edema and antibiotics with antitetanus therapy are instituted
- The extent of gangrene is difficult to assess early in the course of frostbite. The degree of irreversible injury is often much less than initially feared because the skin may be involved to a much greater extent than the subcutaneous tissue
- For this reason, amputation should be delayed for several weeks, until the precise extent of gangrene can be accurately determined
- If the injury is severe enough to produce tissue necrosis, operative sympathectomy should be performed within the first few days
- Sympathectomy is also useful in alleviating the late sequelae of cold injury, including hyperhidrosis, cold sensitivity and pain.

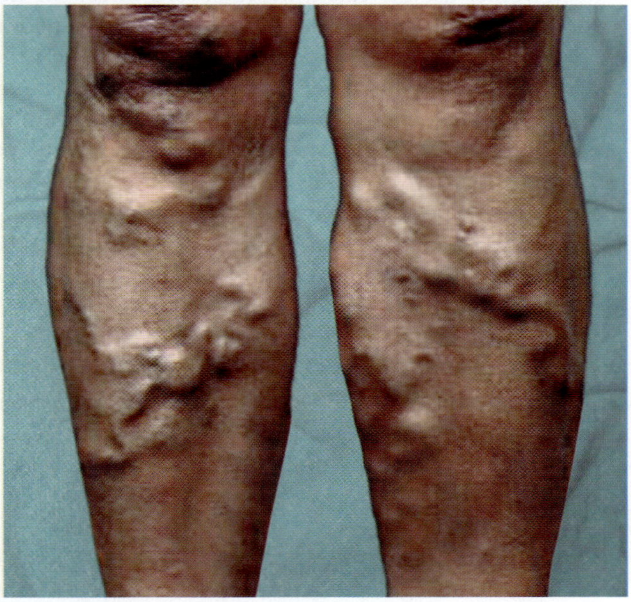

Fig. 17.26: Varicose veins

Peripheral Venous Disease

Venous Incompetence (Varicose Veins)

One of the most common problems with the veins of the leg is failure of their valves. This occurs frequently in the superficial venous system, resulting in varicose veins (Fig. 17.26).

Incidence

In developing countries, where a primitive way of life is maintained, there is a very low incidence of varicose veins. The reasons for this difference are unclear, but are probably related to differences in diet.

Causative Factors

- It is common in people, who have long standing jobs
- *A further major factor is inheritance:* Women in whom neither parent has varicose veins, have a 10 percent risk of developing varices, but when both parents are affected, there is an 80 percent chance. Men are affected less frequently than women.

Mechanism (Figs 17.27A and B)

- The mechanisms that cause the superficial vein valves to fail have not been fully established. What appears to happen, is that first a small gap appears between the valve cusps at the commisure
- This gap widens and more reverse flow (venous reflux) is allowed. The valve cusps degenerate and holes develop in them. Eventually, they disappear completely. The vein below the valve responds by dilating

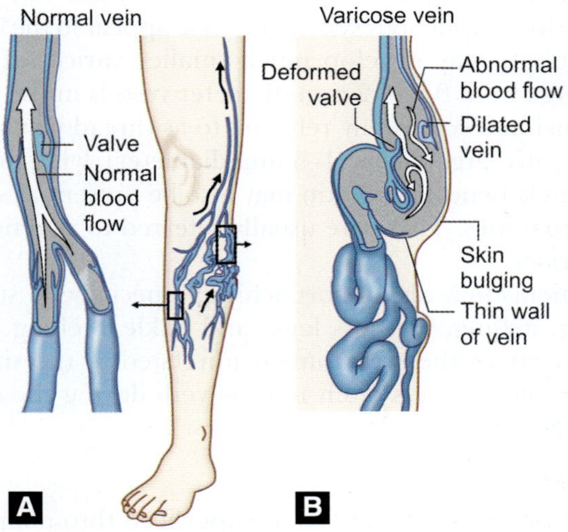

Figs 17.27A and B: Mechanism causing varicose veins

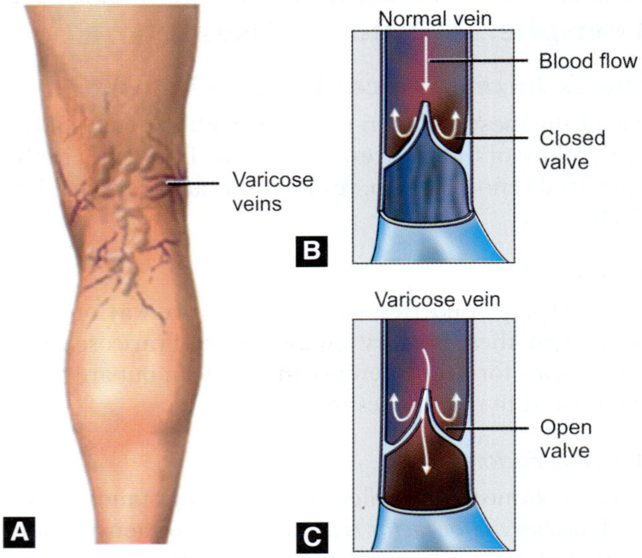

Figs 17.28A to C: Diagrammatic comparison of normal vein and varicose vein

- Varicose veins are thought to develop more often in people, who stand during their work. People who sit or walk are at less risk of developing varices
- They often develop during pregnancy, under the influence of estrogen and progesterone, which cause the smooth muscles in the vein wall to relax.

Clinical Features

- Varices are recognized as tortuous dilated veins in the leg, but physiologically speaking a varicose vein is one, which permits reverse flow through its faulty valves (Figs 17.28A to C)
- Varices of the major tributaries of the saphenous veins or the saphenous veins themselves are large (5–15 mm diameter) and usually start in the calf. Later varices of the long saphenous system may also appear in the thigh
- Patients may develop much smaller varices. These range from 0.5 to 2 mm diameter vessels in the skin, which are commonly referred to as thread veins
- Slightly larger veins (1–3 mm diameter), lying immediately beneath the skin may also be present as small varicosities. These are usually referred to as reticular varices
- Patients may also report aching, especially on standing, itching, "restless legs" and ankle swelling. The severity of the symptoms is unrelated to the size of the veins, and is often more severe during the early stages of development of varices.

Complications

- Thrombosis, referred to as superficial thrombophlebitis
- Spectacular hemorrhage can occur, when large superficial varices are damaged
- The most serious problem is venous ulceration, which complicates varicose veins in less than 5 percent of patients

Venous Incompetence (Deep Vein Incompetence)

Valvular incompetence of the deep veins may develop in the same way as in the superficial venous system, with the degeneration of the valve cusps, resulting in reverse flow in these veins. In other patients, it may develop following a deep vein thrombosis

Clinical Features

- In patients with venous valvular incompetence, the calf muscle increases in size, apparently in response to the greater work in returning blood from the leg
- Ankle edema
- Skin complications, like eczema to severe ulceration
- An early sign of skin injury is brown pigmentation, due to hemosiderin deposition in the skin
- A later and more serious stage is lipodermatosclerosis, in which palpable induration develops in the skin and subcutaneous tissues. This particularly affects the greater area of the leg, just above the malleoli and may be the precursor of leg ulceration
- Contraction of the skin and subcutaneous tissues is seen and the ankle becomes narrower. The combination of a narrow ankle and prominent calf is often referred to as a (Fig. 17.29) "champagne bottle leg"
- *Ambulatory venous hypertension:* Incompetence of the deep veins, usually has a more severe effect on the venous physiology than the superficial venous incompetence, as the deep veins are much larger than the superficial veins. The effect of reverse flow in the deep or superficial veins is to prevent the superficial venous pressure from falling during exercise. This is referred to as ambulatory venous hypertension and is the main cause of venous leg ulceration
- Persistently raised venous pressure tracks back to the microcirculation of the skin and causes skin damage that eventually may result in venous ulceration

Investigation of Venous Disease

A full history should always be taken, enquiring about any injury to the leg or swelling, which may suggest a previous episode of deep vein thrombosis

Clinical Symptoms

- These include, tiredness, aching, tingling and ankle swelling, which get progressively worse towards the end of the day and are relieved by elevating the leg

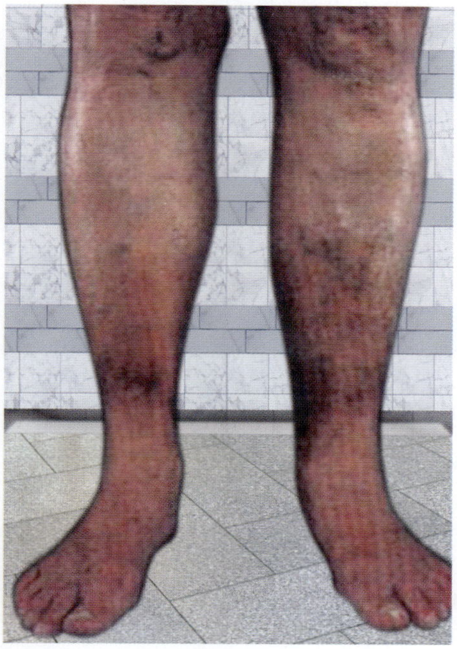

Fig. 17.29: Champagne bottle legs, seen in venous incompetency

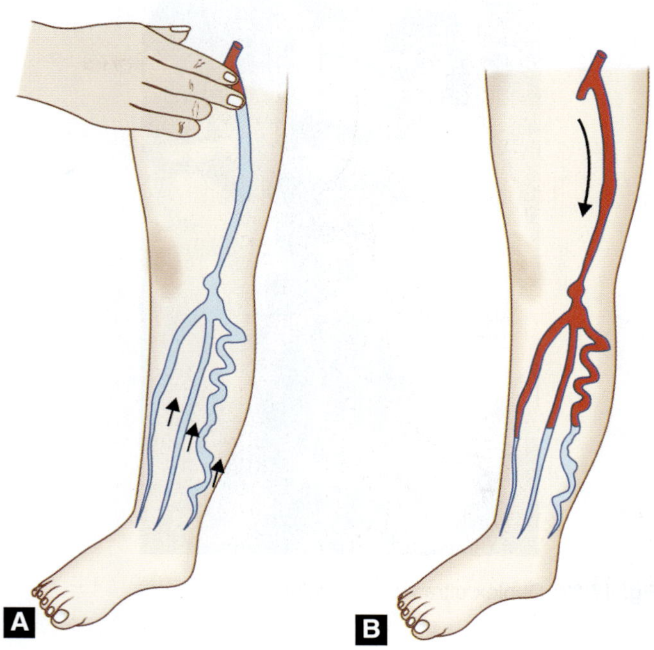

Figs 17.30A and B: Tourniquet test, done for checking venous sufficiencies

- Sometimes patients report cramps in the legs, which are usually worse at night
- Patients with severe deep vein obstruction may also develop bursting pain in the calf on walking, due to the very high venous pressures that may occur under these conditions
- *Venous refilling:* The limb should be elevated for 30 seconds and then laid flat on the bed. Normal refilling occurs within seconds. Reduced venous filling is often present in the severer forms of arterial insufficiency
- *Harvey's sign:* If the two index fingers are placed firmly, side by side on a vein and the finger nearer the heart is moved, so as to empty a short length of vein, the release of the distal finger will allow the speed of venous refilling to be observed. Increased venous return and varicosities of veins are associated with arteriovenous fistulas
- *Tourniquet test (Figs 17.30A and B):* The patient lies and the leg is elevated to empty the veins. The tourniquet is applied high on the thigh and the patient stands again. The speed at which the varices fill is observed. In the case of varices from the long saphenous vein, these fill within a few seconds without a tourniquet, but with the trunk of the long saphenous vein compressed in the thigh, much slower filling takes place over 15 to 20 seconds. The tourniquet is often replaced by the hand of the examiner, used to compress the long or short saphenous vein.

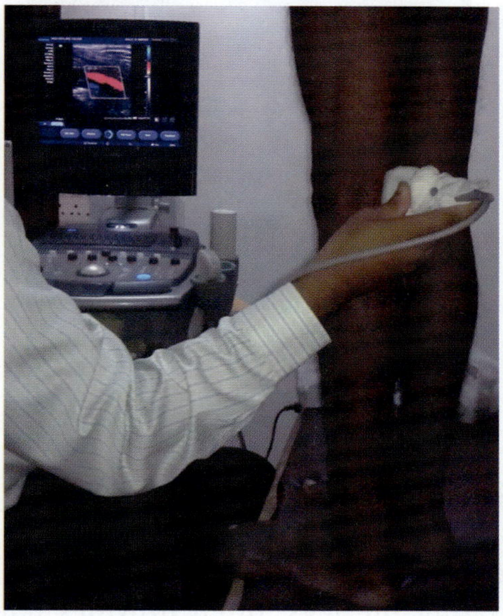

Fig. 17.31: Doppler ultrasound taken, for checking venous sufficiency

Other Investigations

- Doppler ultrasound (Fig. 17.31)
- Duplex ultrasound imaging (Fig. 17.32)
- Venography (Fig.17.33).

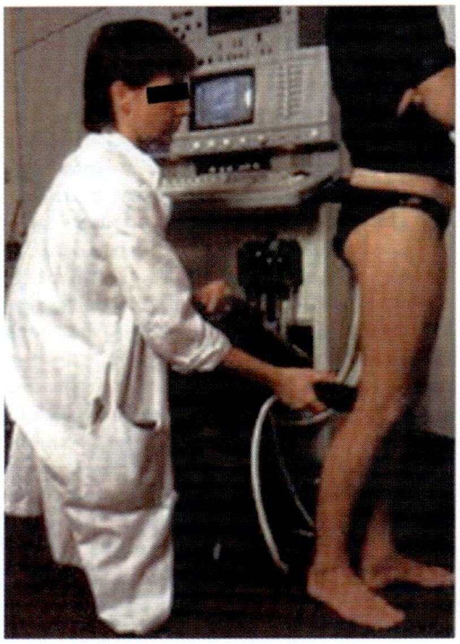

Fig. 17.32: Duplex ultrasound imaging

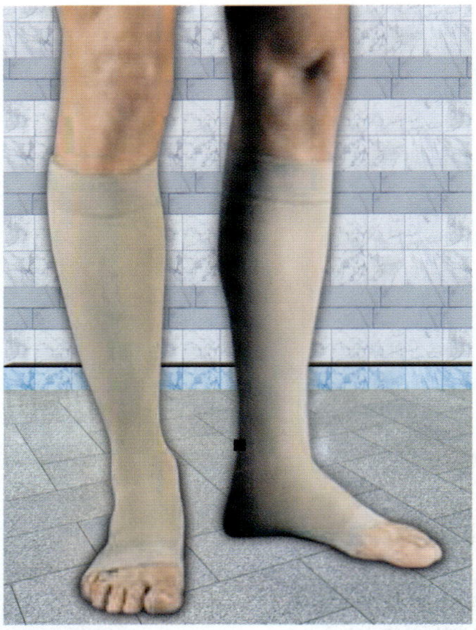

Fig. 17.34: Compression stockings

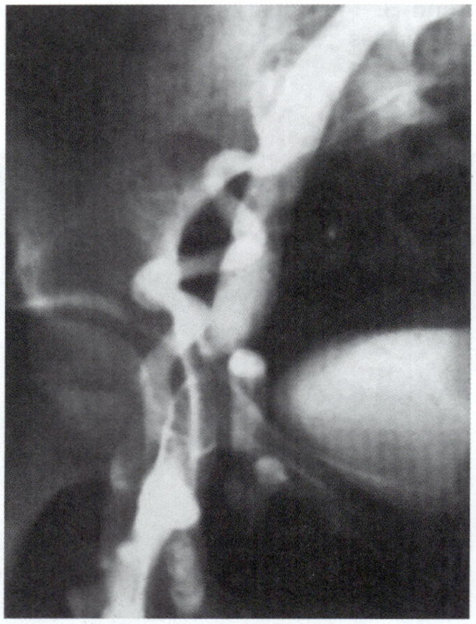

Fig. 17.33: Venograph, showing diseased veins

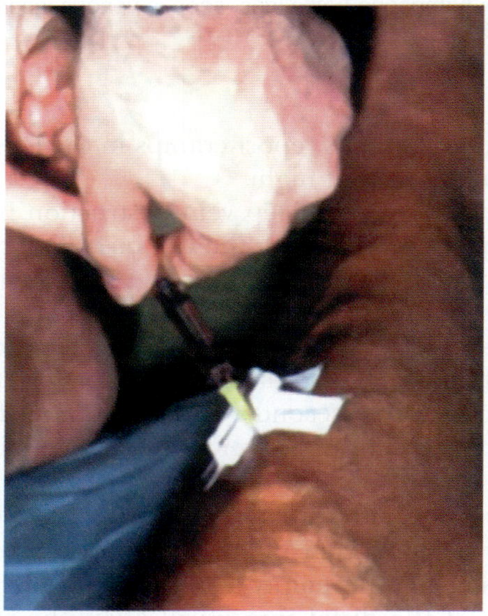

Fig. 17.35: Injection sclerotherapy

Management

- Elevating the legs, often provides temporary symptomatic relief
- *Compression stockings:* The wearing of graduated compression stockings, with a pressure of 30 to 40 mm Hg has been shown to correct the swelling, nutritional exchange and improve the microcirculation in legs, affected by varicose veins (Fig. 17.34).
- Avoid prolonged standing
- *Injection sclerotherapy (Fig. 17.35):* Injection sclerotherapy is best used in the management of small varices and those where the main long and short saphenous veins and their major tributaries are competent. This type of treatment is also effective, where the larger varices have been removed surgically and only small varices remain.
- The basis of sclerotherapy is that a solution, which destroys the endothelial lining of the veins is injected.
- In UK, the most widely employed drug is sodium tetradecyl (STD), which is chemically a soap.
- To be effective, the sclerosant has to be given into an empty vein that is compressed immediately after the injection has been given, to avoid the development of thrombosis within the vein. The complications of

this treatment, include skin pigmentation and ulceration, if the sclerosant is not injected within a vein.

Surgical Treatment of Varicose Veins

- The main principles of surgical treatment are to ligate the source of the venous reflux, usually the saphenous femoral junction (SFJ) or the saphenous popliteal junction (SPJ) and to remove the incompetent saphenous trunks and the associated varices
- Saphenofemoral ligation alone, sometimes referred to as a Trendelenburg procedure is associated with a high rate of recurrence of varices
- Recent research has shown that it is necessary to remove the long saphenous vein, to ensure that as much venous reflux as possible is eliminated
- Similarly, communications between the many deep veins in the popliteal fossa and the short saphenous vein means that some patients develop recurrences in the short saphenous vein, due to the re-establishment of reflux from these veins. This problem may be eliminated by removing the short saphenous vein
- Complications of varicose vein surgery, include:
  - Sensory nerve injury
  - Motor nerve injury
  - Deep vein thrombosis
- *Recurrence:* In recurrence, venous reconstructive surgery can be considered.

Leg Ulcers

The most common cause of leg ulceration in western countries, is venous disease of the lower limb. However, many patients have other causes for their leg ulcer. Some common causes of leg ulcers are shown in Table 17.2

Examination and Investigation

- Venous ulcers, usually lie just proximal to the medial or lateral malleolus, although they may extend to the ankle and dorsum of the foot (Fig. 17.36).

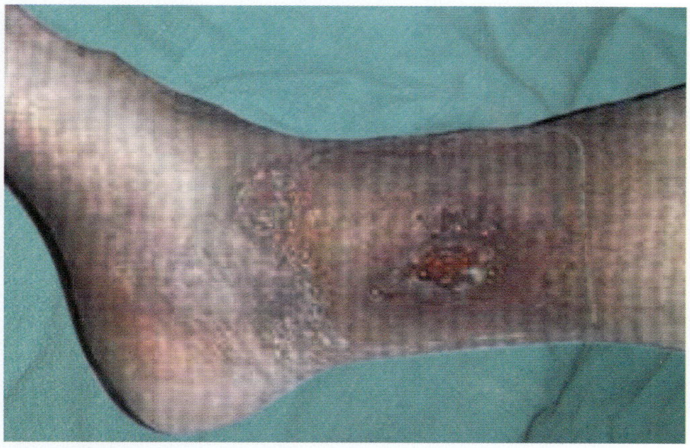

Fig. 17.36: Venous ulcers

Table 17.2: Common causes of leg ulcers

• Venous disease of the lower limb
• Peripheral arterial disease
• Diabetes
• Neuropathy
• Rheumatoid disease
• Autoimmune disease (systemic sclerosis, systemic lupus erythematosus)
• Trauma
• Malignant ulcers (basal cell carcinoma, squamous cell carcinoma, malignant melanoma)
• Infective

- Venous ulcers are accompanied by lipodermatosclerosis and hemosiderosis. The presence of obvious varicose veins should be recorded, although these are often not present or not visible in patients with venous ulcers
- The peripheral pulses should be palpated to assess the peripheral arteries
- The presence of loss of sensation in the foot or area of ulceration should be assessed, especially in a diabetic patient. Diabetic leg ulceration, usually affects the foot and is almost always associated with peripheral neuropathy.

Management of Venous Leg Ulcers

- In patients who have venous ulceration due to superficial venous incompetence alone, varicose vein surgery is effective in producing ulcer healing
- The ulcer is covered by a dressing during surgery and prophylactic antibiotics are given, to prevent infection of the surgical wounds with any bacteria present in the ulcer
- Ulcers managed in this way usually heal rapidly (within 4 weeks) following surgery
- In patients with deep venous insufficiency or who are unfit or unwilling to undergo surgery, standard ulcer management should be used. The mainstay of this is local ulcer management combined with the application of compression. The ulcer is cleaned by soaking in tap water (the use of sterile water is unnecessary) and debriding the ulcer to remove any slough
- The skin of the leg often becomes very scaly beneath compression dressings and should be treated with emulsifying ointment. Topical antibiotics are ineffective in healing leg ulcers and are particularly, likely to produce skin sensitization. They should never be used in the management of venous ulceration
- The most important factor in achieving healing is the use of high levels of compression. The use of dressings alone leads to a very slow rate of ulcer healing. It

has been found that pressures of 30 to 45 mm Hg applied to the ulcer are much more effective than lower levels of compression

- The best known of these techniques is the "four-layer bandage" developed at Charing Cross Hospital in London. This method achieves pressures of 45 mm Hg at the ankle and has been shown to produce healing of 70 percent of venous ulcers within 12 weeks.

Prevention of Recurrence

- Even when healing has been achieved, there is a risk that further ulcers may develop
- Patients with healed ulcers should be encouraged to wear support stockings and rest with their feet elevated, whenever possible
- Drug treatment for leg ulcers
- No drugs have been found, which are more effective than compression bandaging in the management of venous leg ulceration
- Antibiotics have no effect on ulcer healing, but are required if infection develops around an ulcer
- A few drugs have been investigated, to assess their efficacy in venous ulcer healing. These have included aspirin, to pentoxyphylline (Trental, Hoechst), prostaglandin El analogue and diosmin.

18 An Overview of Diabetes Mellitus

- Diabetic Foot
- Diabetic Ulcer

Introduction

- Diabetes mellitus comprises a group of common metabolic disorders that share the phenotype of hyperglycemia
- Several distinct types of diabetes exist and are caused by complex interaction of genetics, environmental factors and lifestyle choices
- Depending on the etiology of diabetes mellitus, factors contributing to hyperglycemia may include reduced insulin secretion, decreased glucose usage and increased glucose production
- Diabetes mellitus is the leading cause of nontraumatic lower extremity amputation in United States
- Foot ulcers and infections are also a major source of morbidity in individuals with diabetes mellitus
- The reasons for the increased incidence of these disorders in diabetes mellitus are complex and involve the interaction of several pathogenic factors, like neuropathy, abnormal foot biomechanics, peripheral vascular disease and poor wound healing. The peripheral sensory neuropathy interferes with normal protective mechanisms and allows the patient to sustain major or repeated minor trauma to the foot, often without knowledge of the injury
- Disordered proprioception causes abnormal weight bearing, while walking and subsequent callus formation or ulceration
- Motor or sensory neuropathy leads to abnormal foot mechanics and structural changes in the foot (hammer toe, claw toe deformity, prominent metatarsal heads, etc.)
- Autonomic neuropathy results in anhidrosis and altered superficial blood flow in the foot, which promotes drying of the skin and fissure formation
- Peripheral vascular disease and poor wound healing impede resolution of minor breaks in the skin, allowing them to enlarge and to become infected
- Approximately 15 percent of individuals with diabetes mellitus, develop foot ulcer and a significant number of these individuals will at sometime undergo foot amputation
- Risk factors for foot ulcers or amputation include:
  - Male sex
  - Diabetes more than 10 years duration
  - Peripheral neuropathy
  - Abnormal structure of foot (bony abnormalities, callus, thickened nails)
  - Peripheral vascular disease
  - Smoking
  - History of previous ulcer or amputation
  - Glycemic control is also a risk factor, each 2 percent increase in the HbA1c increases the risk of a lower extremity ulcer by 1.6 times and the risk of lower extremity amputation by 1.5 times.

Types of Diabetes Mellitus

Two broad categories of diabetes mellitus are type I and type II.

Type I

- Type I A, results from autoimmune beta cell destruction, which usually leads to insulin deficiency
- Type I B diabetes mellitus is also characterized by insulin deficiency as well as tendency to develop ketosis, however immunologic markers indicative of an autoimmune destructive process of beta cells are absent.

Type II

It is a heterogenous group of disorders, usually characterized by variable degrees of insulin resistance, impaired insulin secretion and increased glucose production.

Diagnosis

Revised criteria for diagnosing diabetes mellitus have been issued by panel of experts from National Diabetes Data Group and World Health Organization, these are:

- Either symptoms of diabetes plus random blood glucose concenteration greater than 200 mg% or
- Fasting plasma glucose greater than 126 mg% (fasting is defined as no caloric intake for 8 hours) or
- Two hours plasma glucose greater than 200 mg%, during an oral glucose tolerance test
- Insulin resistance associated with obesity, augments the genetically determined insulin resistance of type 2 diabetes mellitus. Adipocytes secrete a number of biologic products (leptin, tumor necrosis factor, free fatty acids, etc.) that contribute to insulin resistance.

Diabetic Foot

Introduction

- In the diabetic foot, ischemia and infection are serious and sometimes life-threatening conditions, however neuropathy is the most difficult condition to treat
- Neuropathy, angiopathy, retinopathy and nephropathy alone or in combination and in varying degrees of severity may influence the treatment of the diabetic foot
- Neuropathy may be mild with minimal somatic sensory changes and no autonomic nervous system changes
- In its severest form, total anesthesia from the midtibia distally (somatic loss) and complete absence of sweating (autonomic loss), result in a dry, scaly, swollen, clumsy limb that the patient dissociates from the rest of the body because of the loss of the sensory feedback
- Vibratory and position senses are lost early and the patient does not know, where in space the foot is located at a given time. This is especially catastrophic, if the patient also cannot see the foot
- Feet show most severe complications of diabetes, i.e. dry-scaly skin, swelling and venous shunting from autosympathectomy
- Deformity from neuropathic arthopathy in midfoot, with collapse of arch on left foot with prominent bony protrusions medially and plantarward and further deformity from amputation of left fourth toe.

Diabetic Ulcer

- Diabetic ulcers are most common in the forefoot, beneath one of the metatarsal heads or in the interphalangeal joint of the hallux (Figs 18.1 and 18.2)
- If the ulcer is associated with fixed clawing of the toes as a result of intrinsic muscle paralysis of diabetic, somatic or peripheral neuropathy, successful treatment is difficult
- This is especially true if the ulcer is beneath the first metatarsal head (Fig. 18.3), where the sesamoid bones are beneath the skin
- Patient with diabetes mellitus and neuropathy had severe claw toes and shear forces across plantar surface of first metatarsal head, causing recurrent ulceration (Fig. 18.3)
- In approximately 30 percent of the patients with diabetic fore foot, plantar ulcerations, artherosclerosis

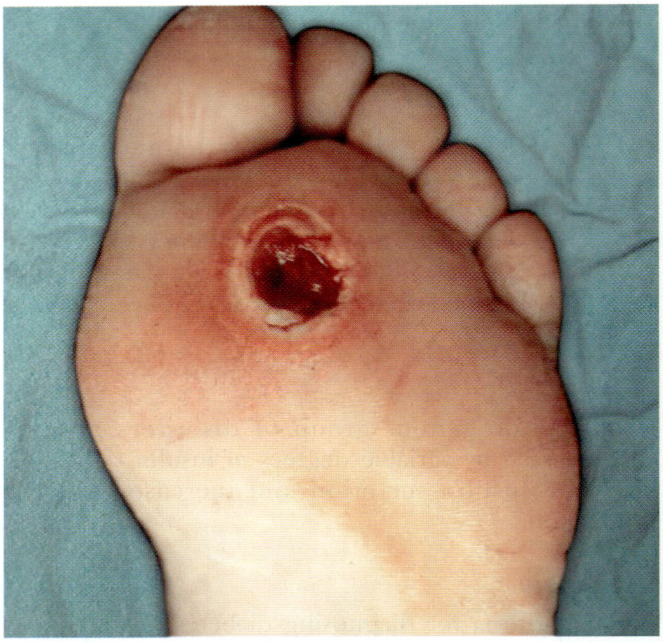

Fig. 18.1: Diabetic ulcer beneath metatarsal heads

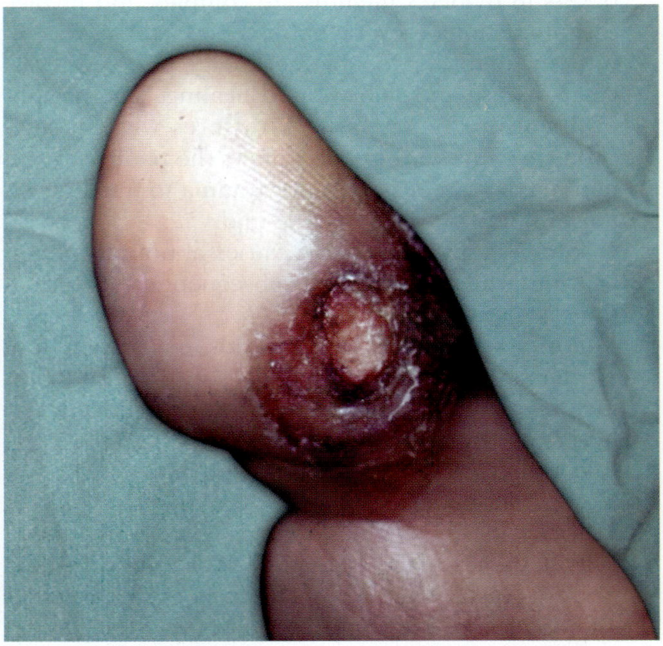

Fig. 18.2: Diabetic ulcer in the interphalangeal joint of the hallux

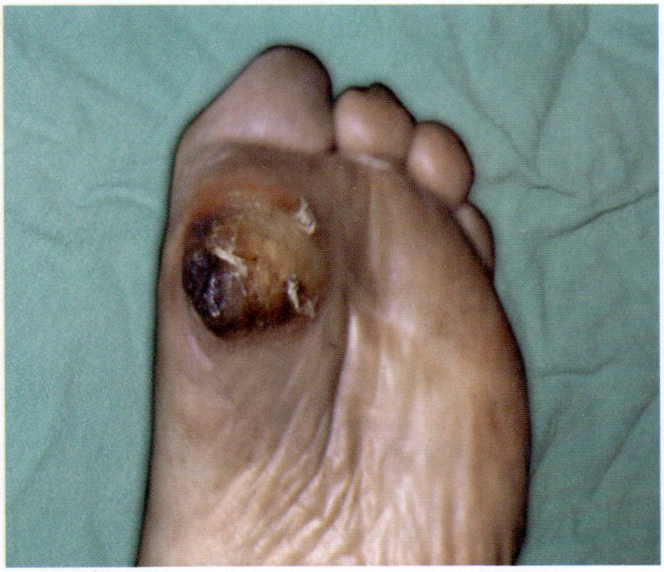

Fig. 18.3: Diabetic ulcer beneath first metatarsal heads and claw toes

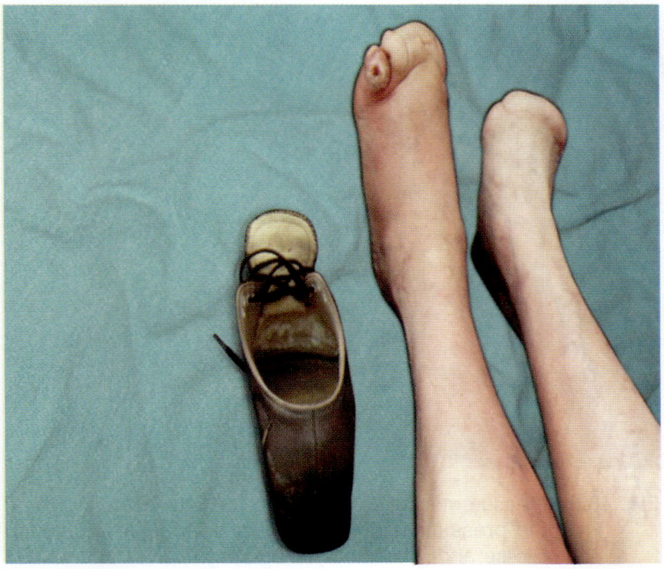

Fig. 18.4: Shoe box filler in right shoe and ulcerated claw toes that duplicate forerunners of previously amputated toes

of the tibial and peroneal arteries contributes to the prolonged healing time

- Patient with diabetes had arteriosclerotic and neuropathic involvement of foot
- Because of recurrent infections and deformities in multiple toes, patient had multiple toes on left amputated and transmetatarsal amputation on right with primary healing
- You can also see the shoe box filler in right shoe and ulcerated claw toes that duplicate forerunners of previously amputated toes (Fig. 18.4).

Classification of Diabetic Ulcers and Diagnostic Aids

- Wagner developed a classification system for diabetic plantar ulcers and a treatment algorithm for each grade of ulcer
- He asserted that the ischemic index derived from Doppler flow pressures is an essential baseline test, to predict ulcer healing and to predict healing of a limited foot amputation, if it becomes necessary
- The ischemic index is the ratio of ankle to brachial pressure (Fig. 18.5). Normal condition on right side of the body with ankle systolic pressure, equal to brachial systolic pressure
- Ankle pressure divided by arm pressure, determines ankle/arm index, in this case 1 (Fig. 18.5)
- On left side ankle/arm index is 0.6, indicating only 60 percent of expected normal flow at rest
- In addition, any gradient greater than 30 mm Hg between two successive cuffs, indicates high grade stenosis or occlusion

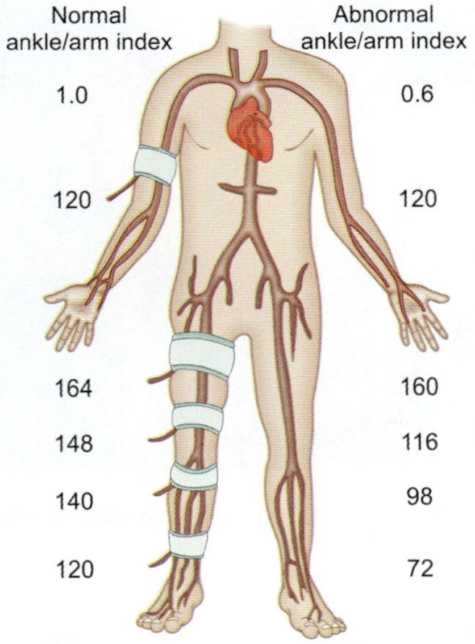

Fig. 18.5: Ischemic indices (both normal and abnormal for different areas), derived from Doppler flow pressures

- In this case, 44 mm Hg high gradient localizes diseased segment to superficial femoral artery
- An ankle to brachial pressure ratio of 0.6, an absolute ankle pressure of 70 mm Hg or more, an absolute toe pressure of 40 mm Hg or more and a transcutaneous oxygen measurement of 30 mm Hg or more are strong indicators that a limited foot amputation should heal
- Measurement of posterior tibial ankle pressure and great toe pressure is shown using Doppler ultrasound device and photoplethysmography (Fig. 18.6).

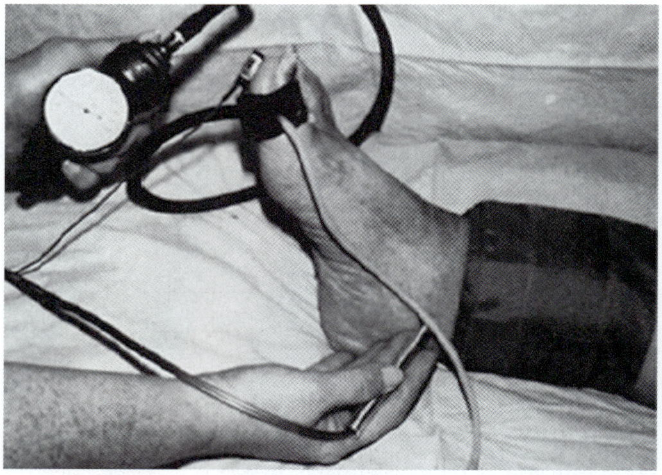

Fig. 18.6: Measurement of posterior tibial ankle pressure and great toe pressure is shown, by using Doppler ultrasound device and photoplethysmography

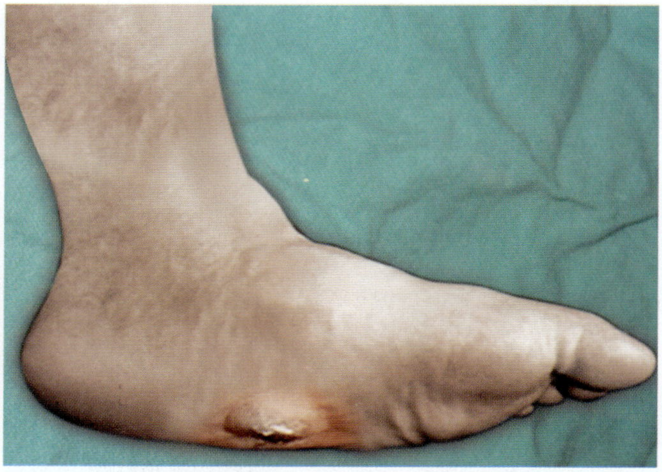

Fig. 18.7: Collapsed midfoot, shown in the figure due to diabetic neuroarthropathy and preulcerative lesion

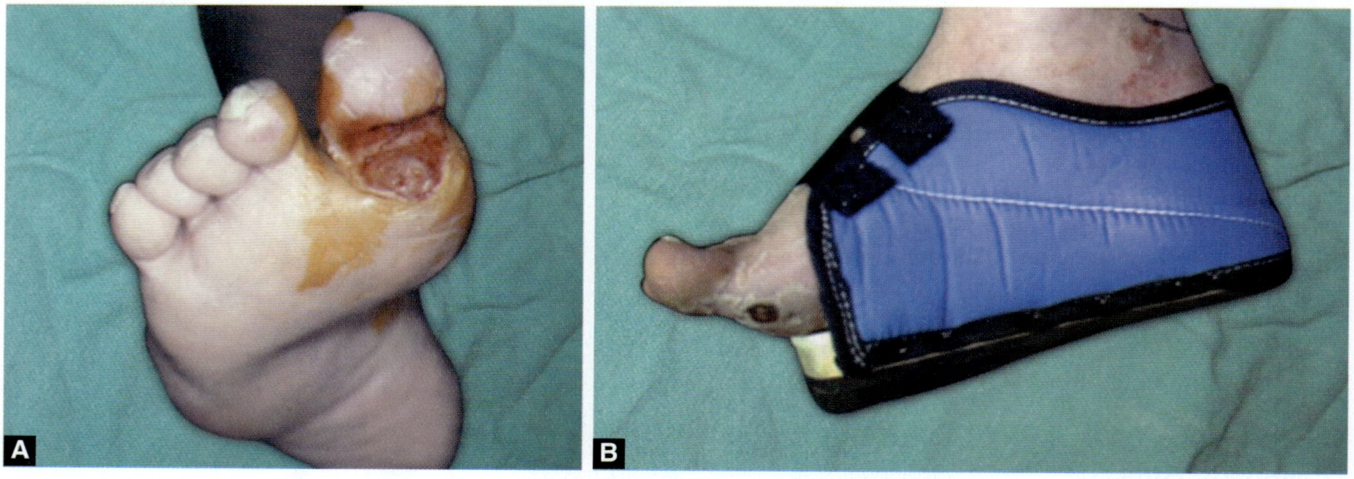

Figs 18.8A and B: (A) Localized superficial ulcer treated in cut-off postoperative shoe; (B) Six weeks in shoe

Wagner Classification of Diabetic Ulcer

- *Grade zero:* Skin intact, but bony deformities produce a "foot at risk" (Fig. 18.7)
- *Grade 1:* Localized superficial ulcer (Figs 18.8A and B)
- *Grade 2:* Deep ulcer to tendon, bone, ligament or joint
- Metatarsophalangeal joint can be dislocated, plantar plate disrupted and bone with tendon is exposed (Figs 18.9A to C)
- *Grade 3:* Deep abscess, osteomyelitis. Diabetic abscess is shown in Figures 18.10A and B
- *Grade 4:* Gangrene of toes or forefoot (Fig. 18.11)
- *Grade 5:* Gangrene of entire foot
- The purpose of this classification is to clarify the prognosis and treatment plan
- In caring for an ulcerated diabetic foot, it is necessary to determine, if the ulcer is primarily neurotrophic or ischemic. If the ulcer is localized or has a deep abscess with multiple tissue plane involvement and if osteomyelitis or pyarthrosis is present, it would allow a reasonable treatment plan.

Brodsky's Classification of Diabetic Ulcer

This does not include gangrene:

- *Grade zero:* Intact skin, but represents a preulcerative lesion with erythema, callus formation and intradermal hemorrhage over a bony prominence
- *Grade 1:* It is a superficial, but full thickness skin ulcer down but not through the subcutaneous tissue

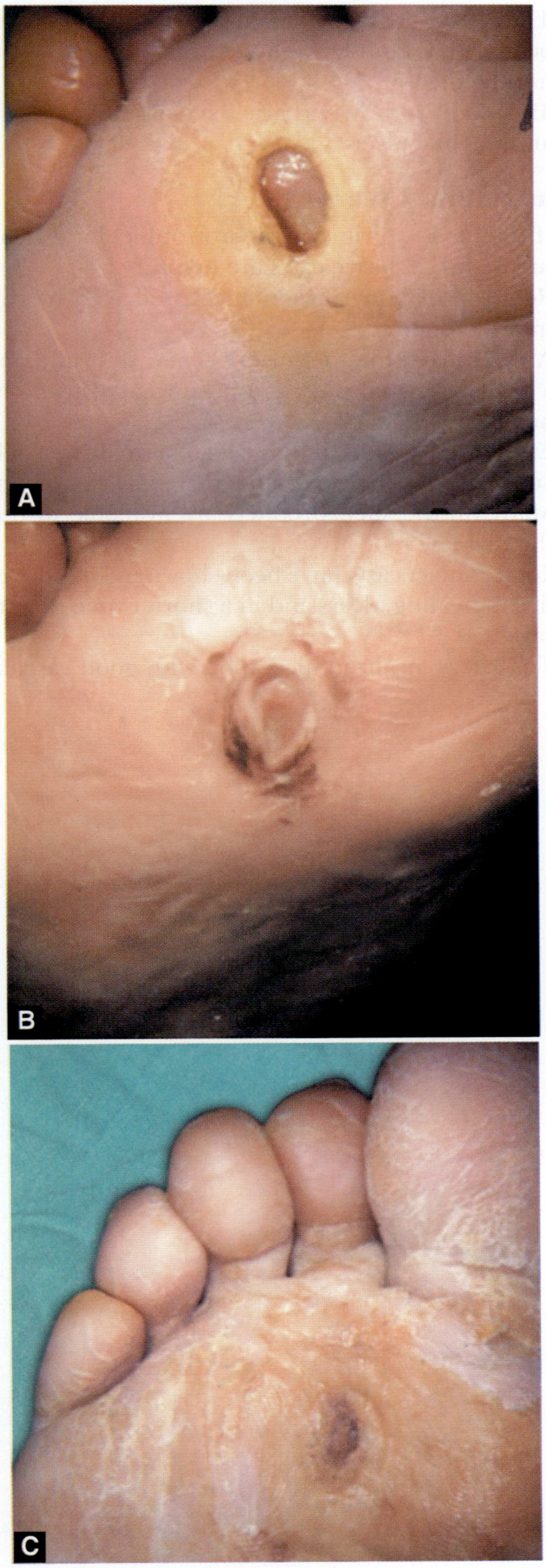

Figs 18.9A to C: (A) Fibrinous bed to deep ulcer over metatarsal head; (B) Shows ulcer has started healing; (C) More rapid healing ensues in occlusive cast

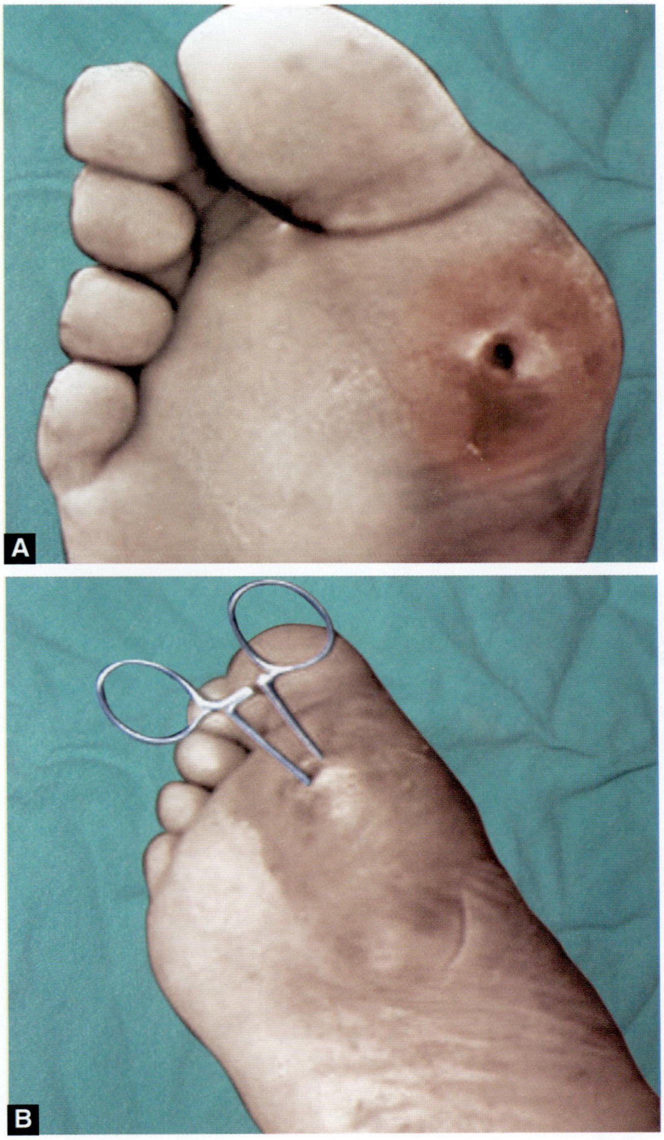

Figs 18.10A and B: Diabetic abscess—(A) Note discoloration proximal to abscess beneath first metatarsal head; (B) Picture showing depth of abscess

- *Grade 2:* Ulceration is down to the tendon and joint capsule, but neither the joint nor the bone is visible
- *Grade 3:* Ulceration implies exposed bone or joint and osteomyelitis or pyarthrosis
- The ulcerated foot, with no palpable pedal pulses needs at least Doppler pressures
- The ischemic index is helpful
- In general, an occlusive cast is not used, if no pedal pulses are present
- Occasionally in limbs, unsuitable for vascular reconstruction with reliable ischemic index of 0.6 or

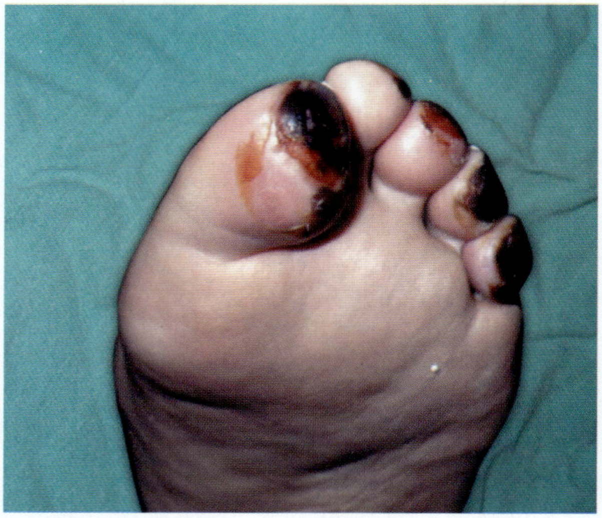

Fig. 18.11: Gangrene of toes, due to diabetes

greater and wound margins that bleed when debrided, an occlusive cast can be used

- The risk of loss of a vascularity, deficient foot in an occlusive cast must be weighed against the risk of leaving the ulcer
- Treatment with hyperbaric oxygen may help to heal an ischemic ulcer

Neuropathic Ulcer

- If the ulcer is primarily neurotrophic, local debridement and occlusive casts are helpful
- Removal of bony prominences, followed by casting may be required
- Any localized forefoot ulcer, 3 cm or less in diameter with good pedal pulses, can be treated in occlusive healing cast
- Even osteomyelitis, if localized to a small area of bone adjacent to the ulcer, can be treated by cast technique
- Many off-the shelf products are available to unload the diabetic foot
- Total contact casts have been shown to be more effective in healing ulcers and in a shorter time than these products
- The key is localized ulceration with good vascularity.

19 Shock

- Types
- Hypovolemic Shock
- Cardiogenic Shock
- Distributive Shock
- Obstructive Shock
- Transient Shock
- Treatment

Introduction

Definition

Shock is a serious, life-threatening medical condition, characterized by a decrease in tissue perfusion to a point, at which it is inadequate to meet cellular metabolic needs.

Types

Hinshaw and Cox Classification

In 1972, Hinshaw and Cox suggested the following classification, which is still used today.

It names four types of shock, these are enumerated below:

- Hypovolemic shock
- Cardiogenic shock
- Distributive shock
- Obstructive shock.

In many patients, shock is a combination of two or more of these four types of shock.

Hypovolemic Shock

- This is the most common type of shock and based on insufficient circulating volume
- Primary cause is loss of fluid from the circulation (most often "hemorrhagic shock").

Causes

- Blood loss following trauma (intra-abdominal, intra-thoracic)
- Blood loss during surgery
- Burns
- Dehydration (vomiting and diarrhea).

Cardiogenic Shock

- This type of shock is caused by the failure of the heart to pump effectively
- This can be due to damage to the heart muscle, most often from a large myocardial infarction
- Other causes of cardiogenic shock include:
  - Arrhythmias
  - Cardiomyopathy
  - Congestive heart failure
  - Commotio cordis
  - Cardiac valve defects.

Distributive Shock

- There is an insufficient intravascular volume of blood
- This form of "relative" hypovolemia is the result of dilation of blood vessels, which diminishes systemic vascular resistance
- Examples of this form of shock are:
  - Septic shock
  - Anaphylactic shock
  - Neurogenic shock.

Septic Shock

- It is caused by an overwhelming systemic infection, resulting in vasodilation leading to hypotension
- Two stages are recognized:
  - Hyperdynamic (warm) septic shock
  - Hypovolemic hypodynamic (cold) septic shock.

Hyperdynamic Septic Shock

- This occurs in patients with serious gram-negative infections
- In this stage, patient has increased cardiac output, with tachycardia and warm dry skin

- The tissue cells get damaged, by anaerobic metabolism (lactic acidosis)
- The capillary membranes, start to leak and endotoxins enter the bloodstream leading to generalized inflammatory state.

Hypovolemic Hypodynamic Septic Shock

- This stage follows, if severe endotoxemia or sepsis is allowed to persist
- Generalized capillary leakage and fluid loss lead to severe hypovolemia, with reduced cardiac output, tachycardia and vasoconstriction
- The systemic infection, induces cardiac depression, pulmonary hypertension, pulmonary edema and hypoxia, which in turn reduces cardiac output further.

Anaphylactic Shock

It is caused by a severe anaphylactic reaction to an allergen, antigen, drug or foreign protein, causing the release of histamine, which causes widespread vasodilation, leading to hypotension and increased capillary permeability.

Neurogenic Shock

- Neurogenic shock is the rarest form of shock. It is caused by trauma to the spinal cord, resulting in the sudden loss of autonomic and motor reflexes below the injury level
- Without stimulation by sympathetic nervous system, the vessel walls relax uncontrollably, resulting in a sudden decrease in peripheral vascular resistance, leading to vasodilation and hypotension
- This term can be confused with spinal shock, which is a recoverable loss of function of the spinal cord after injury and does not refer to the hemodynamic instability.

Obstructive Shock

- In this situation the flow of blood is obstructed, which impedes circulation and can result in circulatory arrest. Several conditions result in this form of shock, e.g. cardiac tamponade, tension pneumothorax, pulmonary embolism, aortic stenosis, etc.
- *Cardiac tamponade:* In this, fluid in the pericardium prevents inflow of blood into the heart (venous return). Constrictive pericarditis, in which the pericardium shrinks and hardens, is similar in presentation
- *Tension pneumothorax:* Due to increased intrathoracic pressure, bloodflow to the heart is prevented (venous return)
- *Massive pulmonary embolism:* It is the result of a thromboembolic incident in the blood vessels of the lungs and hinders the return of blood to the heart
- *Aortic stenosis:* Hinders circulation, by obstructing the ventricular outflow tract.

Transient Shock

- Transitory, i.e. lasts for few seconds to minutes
- Characterized by loss of consciousness, weakness and sinking sensation
- On examination, rapid pulse, low blood pressure and clammy extremities are observed
- Occurs as a result of sudden reduction of venous return, with peripheral pooling of blood, leading to decreased cardiac output
- Rapidly followed by compensation with regulation of blood pressure
- Causes include, trauma, severe pain and emotional over exertion.

Pathophysiology

Flow chart 19.1 shows pathophysiology.

Different Stages of Shock

There are four stages of shock. As it is a complex and continuous condition, there is no sudden transition from one stage to the next

- Stage 1: Initial
- Stage 2: Compensatory (Compensating)
- Stage 3: Progressive (Decompensating)
- Stage 4: Refractory (Irreversible).

Flow chart 19.1: Pathophysiology of shock

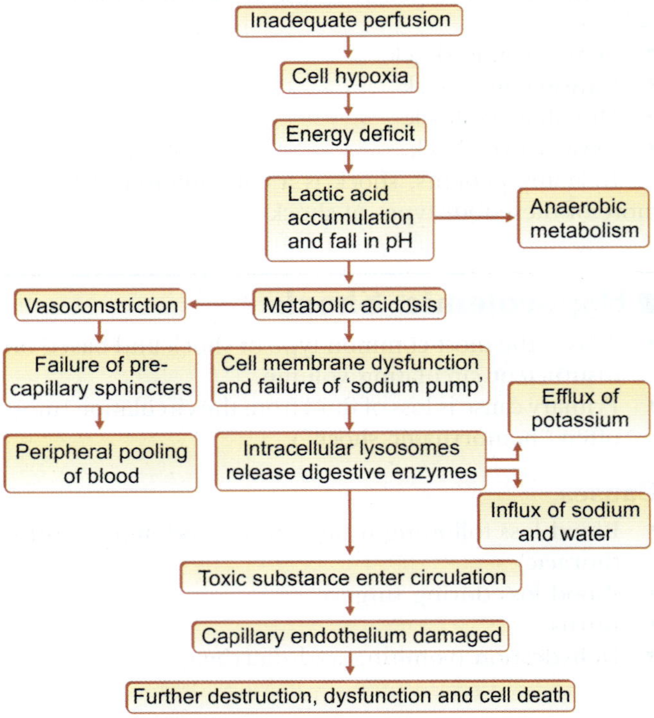

Stage 1 (Initial Stage)

- During this stage, the hypoperfusional state causes hypoxia, leading to the mitochondria being unable to produce adenosine triphosphate (ATP)
- Due to this lack of oxygen, the cell membranes become damaged, they become leaky to extracellular fluid and the cells perform, anaerobic respiration
- This causes a build-up of lactic and pyruvic acid, which results in systemic metabolic acidosis
- The process of removing these compounds from the cells, by the liver requires oxygen, which is absent.

Stage 2 (Compensatory Stage)

- This stage is characterized by the body employing physiological mechanisms, including neural, hormonal and biochemical mechanisms in an attempt to reverse the condition
- As a result of the acidosis, the person will begin to hyperventilate, in order to rid the body of carbon dioxide (CO_2). CO_2 indirectly acts to acidify the blood and by removing it, the body is attempting to raise the pH of the blood
- The baroreceptors in the arteries, detect the resulting hypotension and cause the release of adrenaline and noradrenaline
- Noradrenaline causes predominately vasoconstriction with a mild increase in heart rate, whereas adrenaline predominately causes an increase in heart rate with a small effect on the vascular tone. The combined effect results in an increase in blood pressure. This is known as Cushing's reflex and its triad is the subjective identifying characteristic of this stage
- Renin-angiotensin axis is activated and arginine vasopressin (antidiuretic hormone, ADH) is released to conserve fluid via the kidneys. Also, these hormones cause the vasoconstriction of the kidneys, gastrointestinal tract and other organs, to divert blood to the heart, lungs and brain. The lack of blood to the renal system causes the characteristic low urine production.

Stage 3 (Progressive Decompensating)

- Should the cause of the crisis not be successfully treated, the shock will proceed to the progressive stage and the compensatory mechanisms begin to fail
- Due to the decreased perfusion of the cells, sodium ions build up within, while potassium ions leak out
- As anaerobic metabolism continues, increasing the body's metabolic acidosis, the arteriolar smooth muscle and precapillary sphincters relax, such that blood remains in the capillaries
- Due to this, the hydrostatic pressure will increase and combined with histamine release, this will lead to leakage of fluid and protein into the surrounding tissues. As this fluid is lost, the blood concentration and viscosity increase, causing sludging of the microcirculation
- The prolonged vasoconstriction will also cause the vital organs to be compromised due to reduced perfusion. If the bowel becomes sufficiently ischemic, bacteria may enter the blood stream, resulting in the increased complication of endotoxic shock.

Stage 4 (Refractory or Irreversible)

At this stage, the vital organs have failed and the shock can no longer be reversed. Brain damage and cell death have occurred. Death will occur immediately.

Signs and Symptoms

- The essential signs of shock are seen as tachycardia/tachypnea (compensatory mechanisms), hypotension and signs of poor end-organ perfusion (such as low urine output, confusion or loss of consciousness or failure to compensate)
- Other signs should be looked for, to establish the underlying cause for the shock to guide effective treatment.

Signs of Severity

The severity of shock can be graded 1 to 4, based on the physical signs. This approximates to the effective loss of blood volume. The blood volume does not have to actually be lost from the circulation, as an expansion in the volume of the circulatory system (e.g. in septic shock) will render the patient proportionally hypovolemic.

Grade I

- Up to about 15 percent loss of effective blood volume (~750 ml in an average adult, who is assumed to have a blood volume of 5 liters)
- This leads to a mild resting tachycardia and can be well tolerated in otherwise healthy individuals. In the elderly or those with underlying conditions, such as ischemic heart disease the additional myocardial oxygen demands may not be tolerated so well.

Grade II

- Between 15 and 30 percent loss of blood volume (750–1500 ml) will provoke a moderate tachycardia and begin to narrow the pulse pressure. The time taken for the capillaries to refill after 5 seconds of pressure (capillary refill time) will be extended.

Grade III

- At 30 to 40 percent loss of effective blood volume (1500–2000 ml) the compensatory mechanisms begin to fail and hypotension, tachycardia and low urine output (less than 0.5 ml/kg/hr in adults) are seen.

Grade IV

At 40 to 50 pecent loss of blood volume (2000–2500 ml) profound hypotension will develop and if prolonged will cause end-organ damage and death.

Signs Relating to Different Causes

Hypovolemic Shock

- Anxiety, restlessness, altered mental state, due to decreased cerebral perfusion and subsequent hypoxia
- Hypotension due to decrease in circulatory volume
- A rapid, thready pulse due to decreased blood flow combined with tachycardia
- Rapid and shallow respirations due to sympathetic nervous system stimulation and acidosis
- Hypothermia, due to decreased perfusion and evaporation of sweat
- Thirst and dry mouth, due to fluid depletion
- Fatigue due to inadequate oxygenation
- Cold and mottled skin (cutis marmorata), especially extremities, due to insufficient perfusion of the skin
- Distracted look in the eyes or staring into space, often with pupils dilated.

Cardiogenic Shock

- Similar to hypovolemic shock, but in addition, distended jugular veins due to increased jugular venous pressure
- Weak or absent pulse
- Arrhythmia, often tachycardic.

Obstructive Shock

- Similar to hypovolemic shock but in addition shows other clinical features, like distended jugular veins, due to increased jugular venous pressure
- Pulsus paradoxus, in case of tamponade.

Septic Shock

- Similar to hypovolemic shock except, pyrexia due to increased level of cytokines
- Hypotension, due to systemic vasodilatation
- Warm and sweaty skin, due to vasodilatation.

Neurogenic Shock

- As with hypovolemic shock, but in high spinal injuries may also be accompanied by other signs and symptoms, like profound bradycardia, due to loss of the cardiac accelerating nerve fibers from the sympathetic nervous system at T1-T4
- The skin is warm and dry or a clear sweat line exists, above which the skin is diaphoretic
- Priapism, due to peripheral nervous system stimulation.

Anaphylactic Shock

- Skin eruptions and large welts
- Localized edema, especially around the face
- Weak and rapid pulse
- Breathlessness and cough, due to narrowing of airways and swelling of the throat.

■ Treatment

- Shock requires immediate interventions to preserve life. Therefore, the early recognition and treatment is essential, even before a specific diagnosis is made
- As a general rule, you should treat for a sustained wound and shock
- Most forms of shock seen in trauma or sepsis respond initially to aggressive intravenous fluids (e.g. 1 liter normal saline bolus, over 10 minutes or 20 ml/kg in a child). Therefore, this treatment is usually instituted as the person is being further evaluated
- Re-establishing perfusion to the organs is the primary goal, through restoring and maintaining the blood circulating volume ensuring oxygenation and blood pressure are adequate, achieving and maintaining effective cardiac function and preventing complications
- Patients attending with the symptoms of shock should have, regardless of the type of shock, their airway managed and oxygen therapy initiated. In case of respiratory insufficiency (i.e. diminished levels of consciousness, hyperventilation due to acid-base disturbances or pneumonia) intubation and mechanical ventilation may be necessary.

Treatment (Hypovolemic Shock)

- Limbs should be freed from any tight clothing
- Head in low position, with foot end elevation
- Maintenance of airway. This can be done by:
  - Removing any debris from mouth
  - Suction
  - Endotracheal intubation, if patient is unconscious
- Maintaining breathing
- After monitoring respiratory rate, administration of 100 percent O_2, if there is any sign of respiratory failure (cyanosis, pallor, etc.)
- Endotracheal intubation with assisted ventilation, if necessary
- Tracheostomy
- Maintaining circulation
- Monitoring blood pressure and starting on intravenous fluids immediately
- IV canula (16–18G) to be passed
- If veins are not visible, venesection in anticubital fossa to be done

- In children, intraosseous transfusion can be done (less than 6 years in tibia).

Fluid Selection in Shock

Crystalloids

- NS (0.9%) and Ringer lactate solution
- They expand the interstitial space and not intravascular space
- Dextrose can potentiate ischemia to organs particularly brain, by increasing lactic acid production through anaerobic glycolysis
- Hence, IV fluids containing dextrose are contraindicated in shock (DNS, 5D, 10D, 25D, etc.).

Colloids

- *Albumin* (5–25% solution in isotonic saline)
  – Responsible for 80 percent of osmotic pressure of plasma and is an effective colloid
  – Increases intravenous volume, by an excess of what is transfused (e.g. transfusion of 100 ml of 25 percent albumin increases the intravenous volume of 500 ml)
  – Effect lasts for about 36 hours
  – Adverse effects include, allergic reaction and dilutional coagulopathies.
- *Dextran* (10% solution)
  – Polysaccharide obtained from sugar beets
  – Expands intravenous volume, by twice the volume transfused
  – Effect lasts for about 6 hours
  – Adverse effects include, anaphylaxis, bleeding risks, acute renal failure, interferance with cross matching of blood, as it coats RBC.
- *Heta starch*
  – Synthetic starch available as 6 percent solution
  – Will expand the intravascular volume, by twice the amount transfused
  – Duration of action is around 24 hours
  – Starch is degraded by amylase to small particles and is excreted in urine
  – Adverse effects include, allergic reactions and hyperamylasemia.

Whole Blood Transfusion

- Contains, 350 ml blood and 50 ml anticoagulants (citrate/phosphate/dextrose)
- Stored at 1° to 6°C temperature
- Shelf-life is 21 days
- Should be used after warming to normal body temperature
- Rate is 8 to 15 drops per minute
- Adverse effects include, anaphylactic reactions, thrombocytopenia, hypocalcemia, hypothermia, metabolic acidosis, etc.

Drugs Used in Shock

- Dopamine, 5 to 15 micrograms per kg per minute
- Dobutamine, 2 to 3 micrograms per kg per minute
- Norepinephrine, 15 to 20 micrograms per kg per minute
- Corticosteroids, 100–500 mg
- Antibiotics.

Treatment (Cardiogenic Shock)

- Depending on the type of myocardial infarction, one can infuse fluids
- *Inotropic agents:* Inotropic agents, which enhance the heart's pumping capabilities, are used to improve the contractility and correct the hypotension. Should that not suffice, an intra-aortic balloon pump can be considered (which reduces the workload for the heart and improves perfusion of the coronary arteries) or a left ventricular assist device (which augments the pump function of the heart)
- Use of vasopressing drugs (to induce vasoconstriction)
- Use of pneumatic anti-shock garment (PASG), that compress the legs and concentrate the blood in the vital organs (lungs, heart, brain, etc.)
- Use of blankets to keep the patient warm, e.g. metallic PET film emergency blankets are used to reflect the patient's body heat back to the patient.

Treatment (Distributive Shock)

- In distributive shock caused by sepsis the infection is treated with antibiotics and supportive care is given (i.e. inotropic, mechanical ventilation, renal function replacement)
- Anaphylaxis is treated with epinephrine "adrenaline", to stimulate cardiac performance and corticosteroids, to reduce the inflammatory response
- More suitable would be the use of vasopressors, such as norepinephrine, to decrease vasodilatation.

Treatment (Obstructive Shock)

- In obstructive shock, the only therapy consists of removing the obstruction
- Pneumothorax or hemothorax is treated by inserting a chest tube
- Pulmonary embolism requires thrombolysis or embolectomy
- Cardiac tamponade is treated by draining fluid from the pericardial space through pericardiocentesis.

Treatment (Endocrine Shock)

- The major and generally accepted modalities for treatment of hyperthyroidism, involve initial temporary use of suppressive thyrostatics medication and possibly later use of permanent surgical or radioisotope therapy
- All approaches may cause under active thyroid function (hypothyroidism), which is easily managed with levothyroxine supplementation
- Adrenal deficiencies are often treated with use of corticosteroids.

Complications

- Disseminated intravascular coagulation
- Acute renal failure
- Adult respiratory distress syndrome
- Damage to brain, heart, adrenals and GIT.

Prognosis

- The prognosis of shock, depends on the underlying cause and the nature and extent of concurrent problems
- Hypovolemic, anaphylactic and neurogenic shocks are readily treatable and respond well to medical therapy
- Septic shock, however is a grave condition and with a mortality rate between 30 and 50 percent.
- Prolonged hypovolemia and hypotension carry a risk of respiratory and then cardiac arrest. Perfusion of the brain may be the greatest danger during shock. Therefore, urgent treatment (cessation of bleeding, rapid restoration of circulating blood volume and ready respiratory support) is essential for a good prognosis in hypovolemic shock.

20 Gas Gangrene

- Etiology
- Pathophysiology
- Clinical Features
- Differential Diagnosis
- Prognosis
- Complications

Introduction

- Gas gangrene (Fig. 20.1) is a type of clostridial infection, characterized by rapid and extensive necrosis of muscle, accompanied by gas formation and systemic toxicity and occurs when bacteria invade healthy muscle
- Gas gangrene and clostridial myonecrosis are interchangeable terms used to describe an infection of muscle tissue, by toxin-producing clostridia.

Background

- Louis Pasteur identified the first clostridial species, *Clostridium butyricum* in 1861
- In 1892 and later, Welch, Nuttall and other scientists isolated a gram-positive anaerobic bacillus from gangrenous wounds

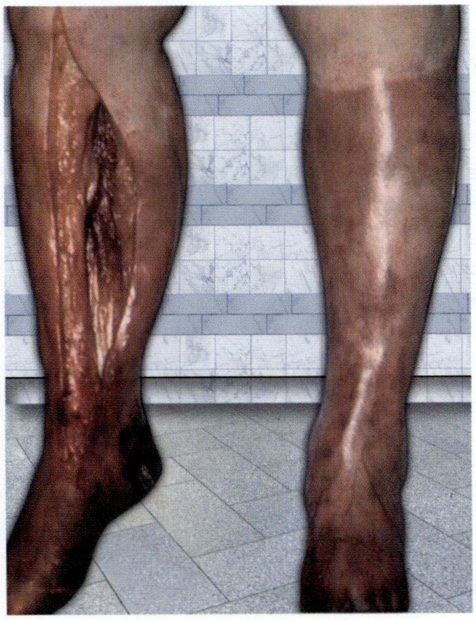

Fig. 20.1: Gas gangrene of lower extremities, due to toxin producing clostridia

- The organism was later renamed *Bacillus perfringens* and then *Clostridium welchii*. The organism is now named *Clostridium perfringens*.

Etiology

- Organisms in the formation of gas gangrene, include spore-forming clostridial species, including *Clostridium perfringens*, *Clostridium septicum* and *Clostridium novyi*, which constitute most of the cases
- Less pathogenic species include *C. histolyticum*
- *C. fallax*, *C. bifermentans* and *C. sporogenes*
- A nonclostridial form also occurs, which is caused by a mixed infection of aerobic and anaerobic organisms
- These organisms are true saprophytes and are ubiquitous in soil and dust
- Clostridia have been isolated from the mucous membranes of humans, including the GI tract and the female genital tract
- Clostridia are obligate anaerobes, but some species are relatively aerotolerant
- A recent clinical series on gas gangrene demonstrated a predominance (83.3%) of aerobic gram-negative bacilli in wound cultures compared with anaerobic gram-positive bacilli
- The most frequently identified aerobic gram-negative bacteria were *Escherichia coli*, *Proteus*, *Pseudomonas aeruginosa* and *Klebsiella pneumoniae*
- Genus *Clostridium* are gram-positive, spore-forming, obligate anaerobes, that are arranged in pairs and short chains with rounded or pointed ends that are ubiquitous and pleomorphic in nature (Fig. 20.2)
- Some species of clostridia, such as *C. novyi* type A are strict anaerobes
- *C. perfringens*, is the most commonly isolated *Clostridium* species and causes around 80 percent of the cases of gas gangrene, usually may be divided into 5 types (A–E), depending on the toxins they produce

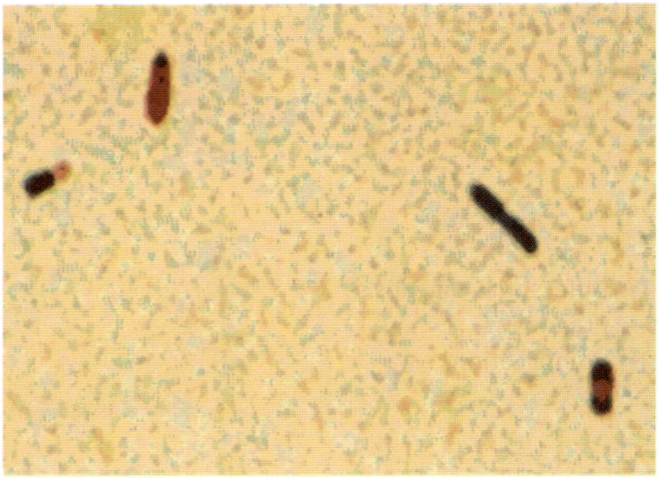

Fig. 20.2: Genus *Clostridium*

- The other 20 percent cases are constituted by *C. novyi* and *C. septicum.*

■ Pathophysiology (Figs 20.3A and B)

- Contamination with clostridial spores, in post-traumatic or postoperative lesions establishes the initial stage of infection
- Local wound conditions are more important than the degree of clostridial contamination in the development of gas gangrene
- Disrupted or necrotic tissue provides the necessary enzymes and a low oxidation/reduction potential, allowing for spore germination
- Foreign bodies, premature wound closure and devitalized muscle, reduce the spore inoculum necessary to cause infection in laboratory animals
- The typical incubation period for gas gangrene is frequently short (i.e. less than 24 hours)
- Self perpetuating destruction of tissue occurs via a rapidly multiplying microbial population and the production of locally and systemically acting exotoxins
- Local effects include necrosis of muscle and subcutaneous fat as well as thrombosis of blood vessels
- Marked edema may further compromise blood supply to the region. Fermentation of glucose is probably the main mechanism of gas production in gas gangrene. In spontaneous gas gangrene, nitrogen is the predominant gas component followed by oxygen, hydrogen and carbon dioxide
- Production of gas begins late and dissects along muscle bellies and fascial planes. These local effects create an environment, which facilitates rapid spread of the infection

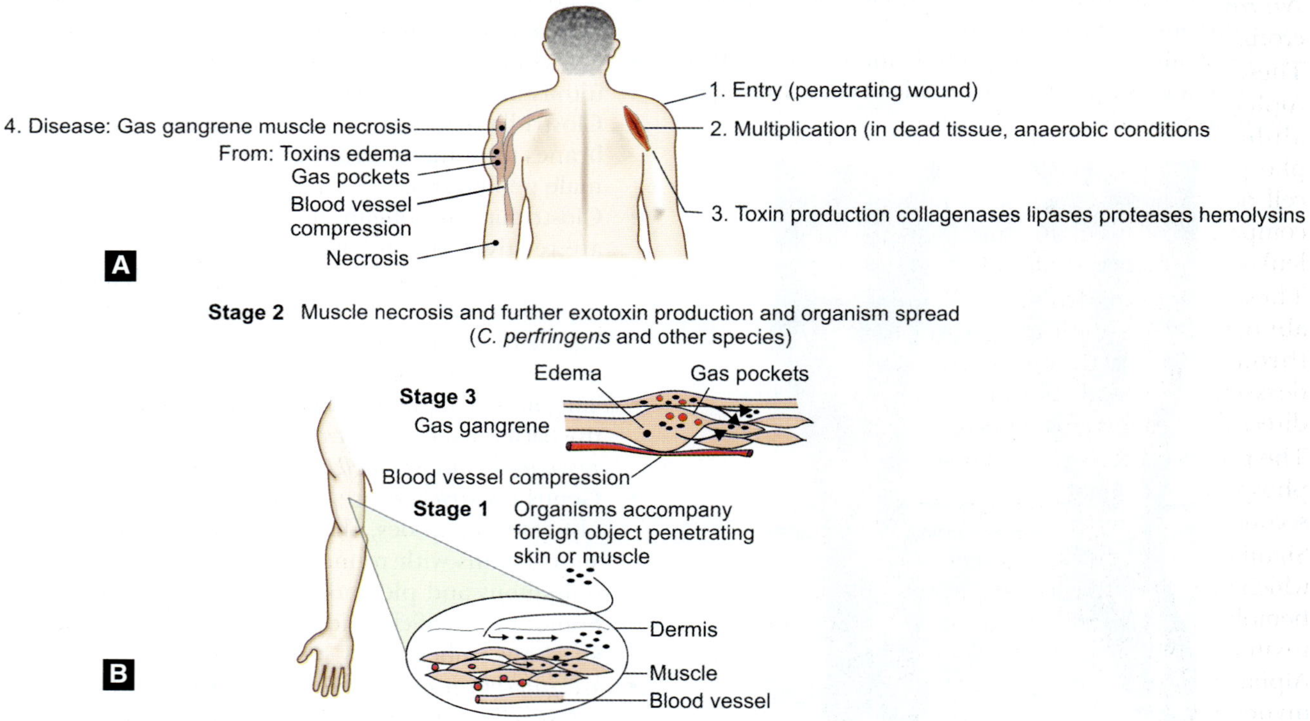

Figs 20.3A and B: Diagrammatic representation of manifestations and stages of gas gangrene

- Systemically, exotoxins may cause severe hemolysis. Hemoglobin levels may drop to very low levels and when occurring with hypotension, may cause acute tubular necrosis and renal failure
- A rapidly progressive infection can quickly result in shock. The mechanism of shock is poorly understood
- Spontaneous gas gangrene is most often caused by hematogenous spread of *C. septicum* from the gastrointestinal tract in patients with colon cancer or other portals of entry
- With *C. perfringens,* the local and systemic manifestations of infection are due to the production of potent extracellular protein toxins by the bacteria.

Exotoxins

Different exotoxins and the biological effects of *C. perfringens* are illustrated below:

- *Alpha toxin:* Lethal, lecithinase, necrotizing, hemolytic and cardiotoxic
- *Beta toxin:* Lethal and necrotizing
- *Epsilon toxin:* Lethal, permease
- *Iota toxin*: Lethal and necrotizing
- *Delta toxin:* Lethal, hemolysin
- *Phi toxin:* Hemolysin, cytolysin
- *Kappa toxin*: Lethal, collagenase, gelatinase, necrotizing
- *Lambda toxin*: Protease
- *Mu toxin*: Hyaluronidase
- *Nu toxin*: Lethal, deoxyribonuclease, hemolytic, necrotizing
- These toxins are lethal, as tested by injection in mice
- Alpha toxin is apparently of utmost importance. The alpha toxin is a zinc metalloenzyme that has phospholipase-C activity (i.e. lecithinase) and causes cell destruction by hydrolysis of key cell membrane components. This toxin can cause lysis of erythrocytes, leukocytes, platelets, fibroblasts and muscle cells
- These toxins hydrolyze cell membranes, cause abnormal coagulation, leading to microvascular thrombosis (further extending the borders of devascularized and thus anaerobic tissue) and have direct cardiodepressive effects
- The products of tissue breakdown, including creatine phosphokinase, myoglobin and potassium, may cause secondary toxicity and renal impairment
- Significant and refractory anemia may also be present, which may be a direct consequence of toxin-mediated hemolysis of RBC, when significant amounts of alpha toxin are released into the bloodstream
- Alpha toxin has negative inotropic effects on cardiac myocytes, contributing to the severe, refractory hypotension seen in some cases of gas gangrene
- Theta toxin causes a cytokine cascade, which results in peripheral vasodilation, similar to that seen in septic shock.

Causes

- Gas gangrene can be classified as post-traumatic, post-operative or spontaneous
- Post-traumatic gas gangrene accounts for 60 percent of all gas gangrene cases. Most of these cases involve automobile collisions
- Other complications of trauma arise from crush injuries, compound fractures, gunshot wounds, thermal or electrical burns and frostbite
- Farm or industrial injuries contaminated with soil are especially prone to developing gas gangrene
- Intramuscular or subcutaneous injections with insulin, epinephrine, quinine or cocaine are rare antecedent events leading to gas gangrene (Fig. 20.4)
- Postoperative clostridial infections follow cases of colon resection, ruptured appendix, bowel perforation and biliary or other GI surgery, including laparoscopic cholecystectomy and colonoscopy
- Septic backstreet abortions are the main cause of uterine gas gangrene
- Spontaneous gas gangrene without external wound or injury occurs frequently in patients, who have serious underlying conditions
- Colorectal adenocarcinoma is the most prevalent risk factor in this group. Hematologic malignancy is also a major premorbid condition
- In children, neutropenia, either induced by chemotherapy or cyclic in nature, represents the single most important risk factor for spontaneous *C. septicum* infections
- The remaining cases are associated with diabetes or neutropenic colitis

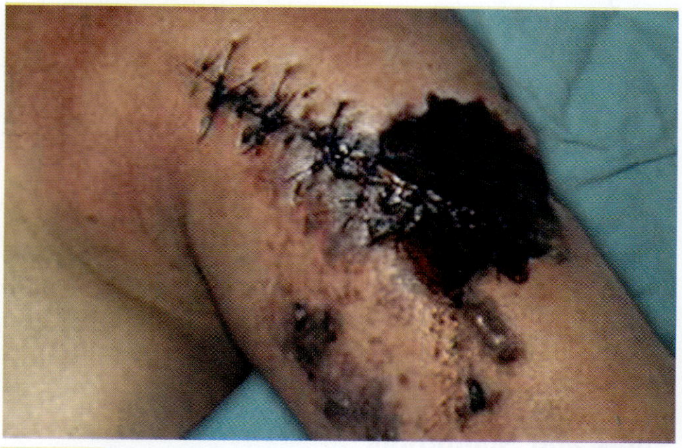

Fig. 20.4: Patient developed gas gangrene after injecting cocaine. *C. septicum* was isolated in both blood and wound cultures

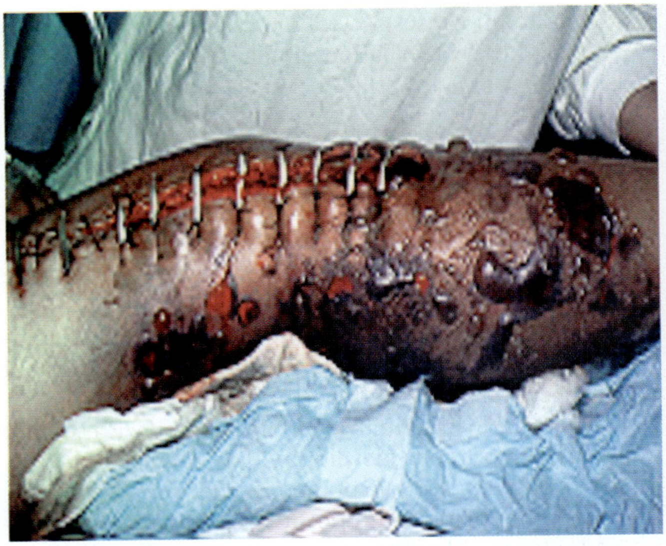

Fig. 20.5: Gas gangrene formed with chronic alcoholism

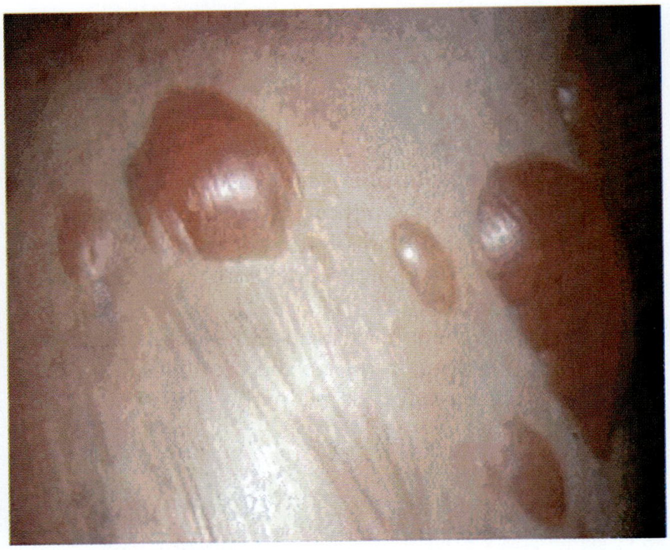

Fig. 20.6: Cutaneous gangrene

- Patients with *C. septicum* infections have overt or occult malignancies approximately 5 times more often, than patients with other clostridial infections.

Risk Factors

- Atherosclerosis
- Burns
- Corticosteroid use
- Diabetes
- Gastrointestinal malignancy
- HIV/AIDS
- Hypoalbuminemia
- Intravenous drug abuse
- Chronic alcoholism (Fig. 20.5)
- Obesity
- Open fractures
- Peripheral vascular disease
- Surgery
- Trauma.

Clinical Features

History

Most patients with post-traumatic gas gangrene have sustained serious injury on the skin or soft tissues or have experienced open fractures. Patients with postoperative gas gangrene have frequently undergone recent surgery of the GI or biliary tract.

Signs and Symptoms

- Typically, gas gangrene begins with the sudden onset of pain in the region of the wound, which helps to differentiate it from spreading cellulitis
- Following pain, local swelling and edema accompanied by a thin often hemorrhagic exudate appear
- Patients frequently develop marked tachycardia
- Elevation in temperature may be only minimal
- Gas usually is not obvious at early stages and may be completely absent
- Frothiness of the wound exudate may be noted
- The skin is tense, white, often marbled with blue and may be cooler than normal
- The symptoms progress rapidly. Swelling, edema, and toxemia increase and a profuse serous discharge appears, having a peculiar sweetish smell
- Gram's staining of the wound exudate shows many gram-positive rods with relatively few inflammatory cells
- Despite hypotension, renal failure and (often) body crepitation, patients with myonecrosis frequently have a heightened awareness of their surroundings until just before death, when they lapse into toxic delirium and coma
- In untreated cases, as the local wounds progress, the skin becomes bronzed, bullae appear, become filled with dark red fluid and are accompanied by dark patches of cutaneous gangrene (Fig. 20.6)
- Gas appears in later phases, but may not be as obvious as in anaerobic cellulitis. Jaundice is rare in wound gas gangrene (in contrast to uterine infections)
- Cases of clostridial myonecrosis without a history of trauma have bullous lesions and crepitation of the skin, they present with a rapidly worsening course that includes myonecrosis, especially of the extremities (Fig. 20.7)

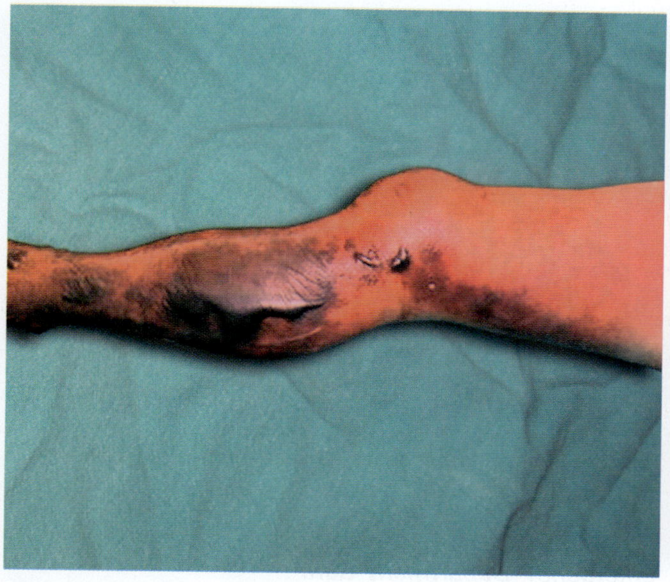

Fig. 20.7: Myonecrosis of extremities

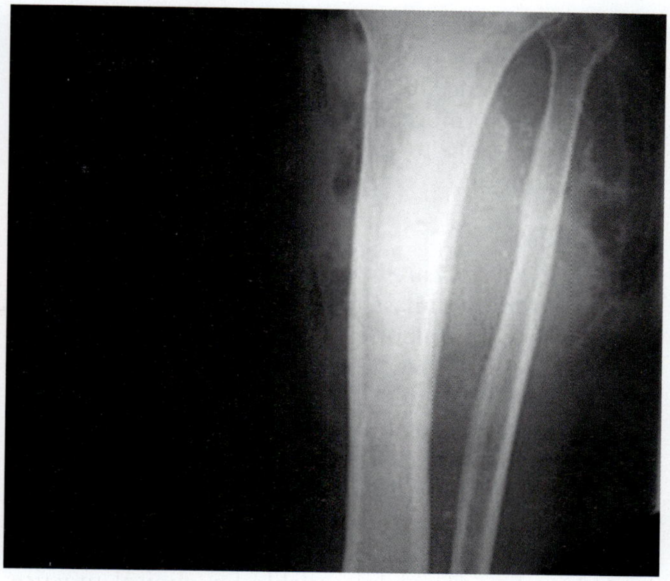

Fig. 20.8: X-ray of extremity taken, with gas gangrene

Differential Diagnosis

- Abdominable abscess
- Anthrax infection
- Pyomyositis (muscle abscess)
- Cellulitis
- Rhabdomyolysis
- Deep venous thrombosis and thrombophlebitis
- Streptococcal (pyogenes) myositis
- Necrotizing cellulitis
- *Vibrio vulnificus* infection
- Necrotizing fasciitis
- Toxic shock syndrome
- Clostridial cholecystitis (emphysematous cholecystitis)
- Other problems to be considered
- Other causes of necrotizing myositis (Group A streptococci, polymicrobial aerobic-anaerobic flora and nonclostridial anaerobes)
- Cutaneous anthrax
- Acute gout
- Familial mediterranean fever
- Septic arthritis
- Pyoderma gangrenosa
- Carcinoma erysipeloids
- Pyomyositis
- Water-borne skin infections (*Vibrio vulnificus, Aeromonas hydrophila, Mycobacterium marinum, etc.*)
- Other causes of soft tissue gas (e.g. pneumomediastinum, pneumothorax, fractured larynx, fractured trachea, etc.).

Laboratory Studies

- Gram stain and culture of bullae fluid, *Clostridia* species are known to be large, gram-positive rods (boxcar appearance)
- The presence of gram-positive or gram variable rods with few white blood cells is indicative of clostridial etiology
- Complete blood count may reveal anemia, thrombocytopenia and evidence of intravascular hemolysis on smear
- *Electrolyte level:* Hyperkalemia can result from cell breakdown. Hypocalcemia may result from subcutaneous fat necrosis
- *Renal panel:* Kidney dysfunction may occur secondary to hypotension, hemoglobinuria and myoglobinuria or direct toxin effect
- *Coagulation panel:* Coagulopathy and thrombocytopenia can also result
- *Liver function tests:* Hyperbilirubinemia and liver dysfunction may result from release of toxins
- *Arterial blood gas determination:* Gas gangrene can cause metabolic acidosis, with significant lactic acidosis secondary to tissue death and ischemia
- *Myoglobin level:* Myoglobinemia and myoglobinuria can result from cellular breakdown
- *Blood cultures:* This may help narrow antibiotic coverage.

Imaging Studies (Fig. 20.8)

- Gas in the soft tissues is neither sensitive nor specific for gas gangrene. Many different bacteria, trauma and visceral perforation can cause soft tissue gas. Plain radiographs or ultrasonography can be used to look for the presence of gas

- Computed tomography or magnetic resonance imaging can help to evaluate the depth of soft tissue inflammation.

Other Tests

- Once *Clostridia* are isolated from culture, identification of the lecithinase function of alpha toxin may be elicited by inoculating blood agar with the isolated bacteria. A double area of hemolysis will develop around the colonies, demonstrating the presence of lecithinase. Inoculation of the colonies with antitoxin will halt the hemolysis
- Rapid detection of alpha-toxin or sialidases (i.e. neuraminidases) in infected tissues through enzyme linked immunosorbent assay (ELISA)
- Although, not widely available for clinical practice, *in vitro* amplification of the alpha-toxin or DNA by polymerase chain reaction (PCR) has been used to isolate clostridial species.

Procedures

- Tissue biopsy with culture and Gram stain is the criterion standard in helping to make the diagnosis of gas gangrene
- Surgical exploration confirms the diagnosis of myonecrosis. Affected muscle appears pale and shows no contractile function, when incised or electrically stimulated
- Under local anesthesia, bedside biopsy with immediate frozen section can be performed, to provide early and accurate diagnosis of gas gangrene
- Patients with gas gangrene frequently develop massive hemolysis, shock, acute respiratory distress syndrome (ARDS) and renal failure, which often requires invasive procedures (e.g. right-sided heart catheterization, mechanical ventilation, hemodialysis, etc.).

Histologic Findings (Fig. 20.9)

Histopathologic findings in gas gangrene consist of widespread myonecrosis, destruction of other connective tissues and a paucity of neutrophils in the infected area. Leukocyte aggregates are found in the border regions.

Treatment

The combination of aggressive surgical debridement and effective antibiotic therapy is the determining factor for successful treatment of gas gangrene.

Prehospital Care

- Oxygenation
- Intravenous (IV) fluids.

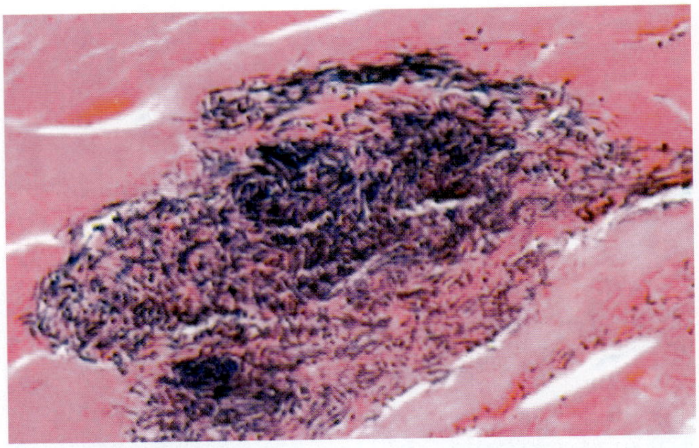

Fig. 20.9: Destructive changes as seen in histological findings in gas gangrene

Emergency Department Care

- Gas gangrene is a true emergency and concurrent evaluation, treatment and coordination of care should be carried out
- *Airway and breathing:* Oxygen and airway management as necessitated
- *Circulation:* Good vascular access and liberal use of intravenous fluids is indicated
- Administer tetanus toxoid, if indicated
- Administer antibiotics
- Correct electrolyte abnormalities
- Check compartment pressures, if severe pain and evidence of compartment syndrome are present with minimal cutaneous evidence of infection.

Antibiotics

- Historically, penicillin G in dosages of 10 to 24 million U/D was the drug of choice. Currently, a combination of penicillin and clindamycin is widely used
- Recent studies show that protein synthesis inhibitors (e.g. clindamycin, chloramphenicol, rifampin, tetracycline, etc.) may be more effective because they inhibit the synthesis of clostridial exotoxins and lessen the local and systemic toxic effects of these proteins
- A combination of clindamycin and metronidazole is a good choice for patients allergic to penicillin
- Although, approved for treating complicated skin and soft-tissue infections, latest antibiotics such as daptomycin, linezolid and tigecycline have not been studied in patients with gas gangrene, therefore they should not be used as primary antibiotics for treating this condition
- *Adjuvant therapy:* Recombinant human activated protein C has been used as an adjuvant therapy for patients with severe sepsis, but aside from the serious

bleeding that may be associated, repeated surgical debridement in patients with gas gangrene requires frequent interruption of the continuous infusion of this product. Therefore, is not widely used.

Surgical Care

- Fasciotomy, for compartment syndrome may be necessary and should not be delayed in patients with involvement of extremities
- Perform debridement, as needed to remove all necrotic tissue
- Exposure of all the affected muscle groups, by long incisions or in the subcutaneous infections, multiple subcutaneous drainage and slough extraction by incisions into the subcutaneous tissue may be done
- Amputation of the extremity may be necessary and life-saving
- Abdominal involvement requires excision of the body wall musculature
- Uterine gas gangrene following septic abortion, usually necessitates hysterectomy.

Hyperbaric Oxygen (HBO)

- Use is controversial
- Can be used to supplement surgical debridement and antibiotics
- Particularly helpful in areas, where complete surgical resection of necrotic tissue is difficult, such as the paraspinal muscles or abdominal wall (Fig. 20.10)
- Potential benefits include improved neutrophil-mediated killing of bacteria, direct bactericidal effect on anaerobes, improved activity of some antibiotics and enhanced wound healing.

Deterrence/Prevention

Avoid suturing wounds, due to a crush injury or open fractures with devitalized muscle and soil contamination.

Prognosis

- Failure to provide an early diagnosis and inadequate surgical intervention are the two most common mistakes in the management of gas gangrene. These are the factors which eventually dictate the outcome

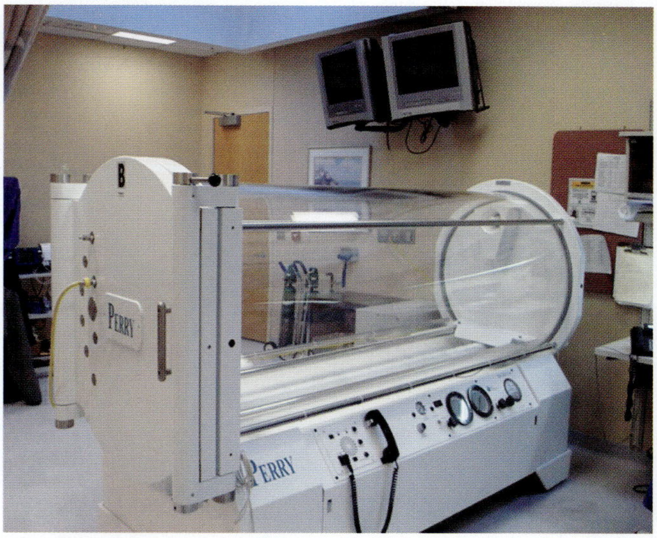

Fig. 20.10: Hyperbaric oxygen, set up

- The prognosis of gas gangrene is better, if the incubation period is shorter than 30 hours, if the patient has limb involvement and if he or she does not have concomitant serious medical conditions or complications (e.g. shock, disseminated intravascular coagulation (DIC), ARDS, renal failure, etc.)
- Spontaneous gas gangrene frequently carries a worse prognosis than other forms of gas gangrene.

Complications

- Massive hemolysis, which may require repeated blood transfusion
- Disseminated intravascular coagulation, which may cause severe bleeding and may complicate aggressive surgical debridement
- Acute renal failure
- Acute respiratory distress syndrome
- Shock
- The most important factors in the successful treatment of gas gangrene are early diagnosis and prompt treatment.

Section 3

Regional Orthopedics

21 Hand and Wrist

ANATOMY OF WRIST

Anatomy

Wrist joint comprises of the distal end of radius and articular disk overlying the distal end of ulna and the scaphoid, lunate and the triquetrum.

It is an ellipsoid variety of synovial joint, where the joint line is obtained by joining the styloid process of the radius and ulna. X-ray of wrist joint is shown in Figure 21.1.

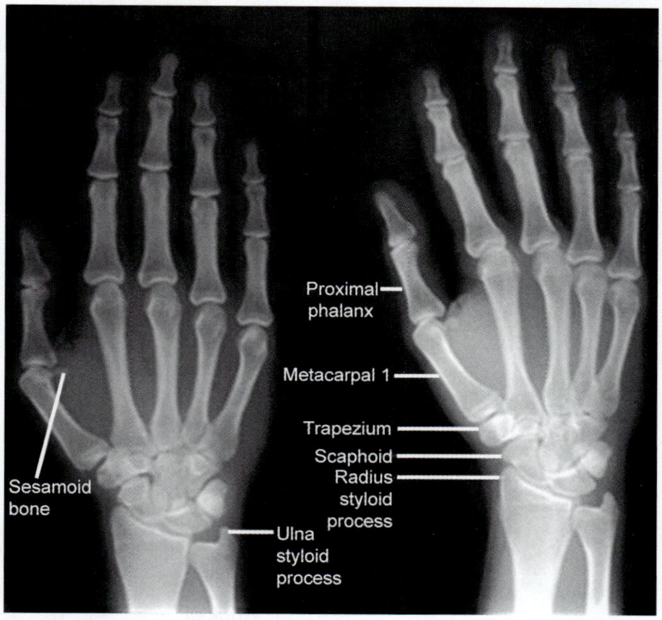

Fig. 21.1: X-ray showing wrist joint

Surface Landmarks

Important surface landmarks of this joint includes:
- Radial styloid process
- Lister's tubercle
- Head of ulna
- Anatomical snuffbox
- Lunate fossa
- Thenar and hypothenar eminences
- Distal wrist flexion crease

Lister's tubercle: It is dorsal prominence over the distal aspect of the radius, which redirects the extensor pollicis longus.

Lunate fossa: It is a palpable depression found in the line with the third metacarpal. The lunate bone lies directly below this depression.

Anatomical snuffbox: It is formed ulnarly, by the third dorsal compartment (extensor pollicis longus), radially by the first dorsal compartment (abductor pollicis longus, extensor pollicis brevis) and proximaly by the extensor retinaculum.

Osteology and Joint Anatomy

The skeletal components (Fig. 21.2) of wrist joint include:

- Distal radius and ulna
- Carpal bones
- Proximal ends of the five metacarpal bones
- The carpal bones are arranged into proximal and distal rows. The midcarpal joint is the articulation between these rows.

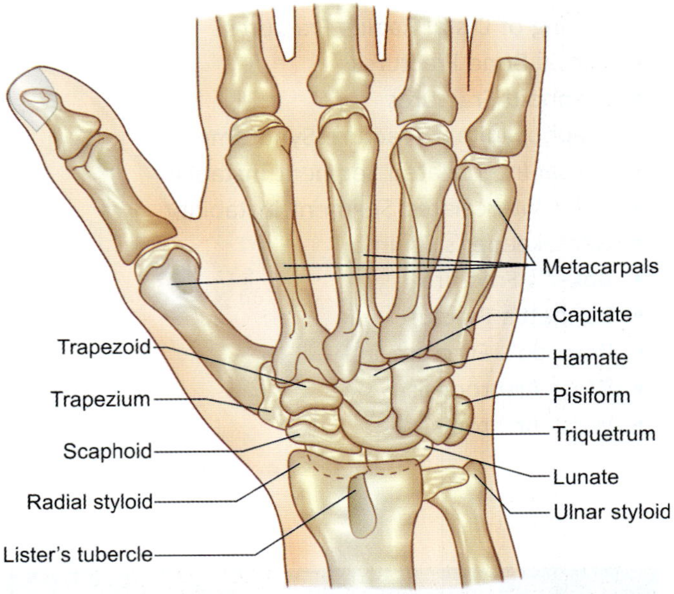

Fig. 21.2: Skeletal components of the wrist joint

- The proximal row is formed by scaphoid, lunate, triquetrum and pisiform and has no muscular attachments.
- The distal row is formed by trapezium, trapezoid, capitate and hamate.
- The articulation of distal radius is composed of two fossae:
  - Ovoid shaped lunate fossa
  - Triangular shaped scaphoid fossa, which articulates with the lunate and scaphoid bones respectively (Fig. 21.3).

Distal Radioulnar Joint

- On the ulnar aspect of the distal radius, sigmoid notch articulates with the distal ulna to form distal radioulnar joint (DRUJ).
- It is a pivot joint, which permits pronation and supination of the wrist joint.
- Other movements at wrist joint are flexion and extension, radial deviation and ulnar deviation.

Triangular Fibrocartilage Complex

- Triangular fibrocartilage complex (TFCC) (Fig. 21.4) consists of following structures:
  - Ulnolunate ligament
  - Ulnotriquetral ligament
  - Ulnarcollateral ligament
  - Sheath of the extensor carpi ulnaris

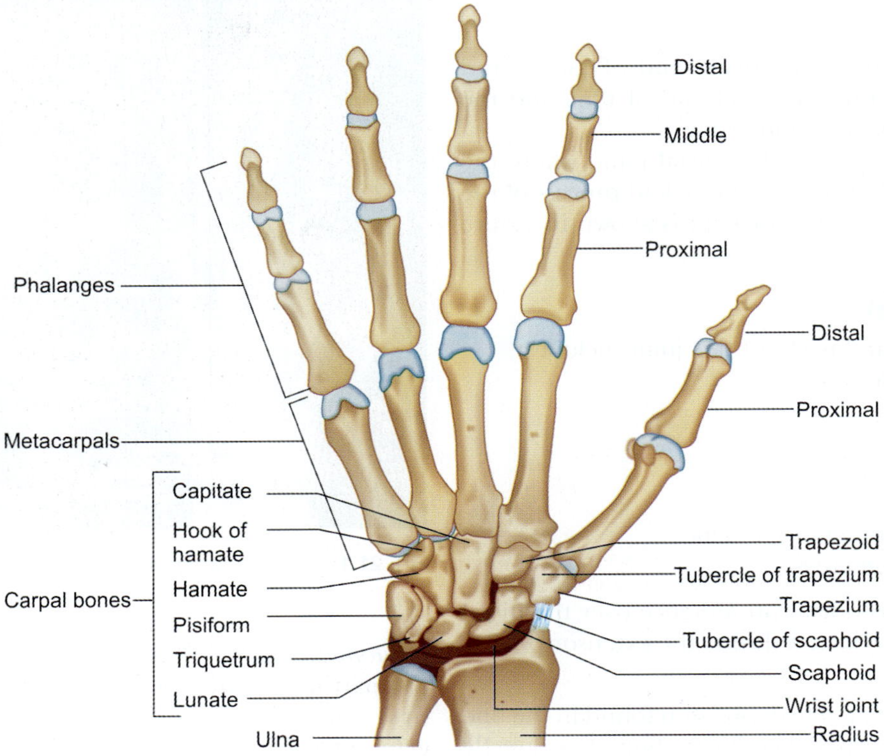

Fig. 21.3: Lunate fossa and scaphoid fossa

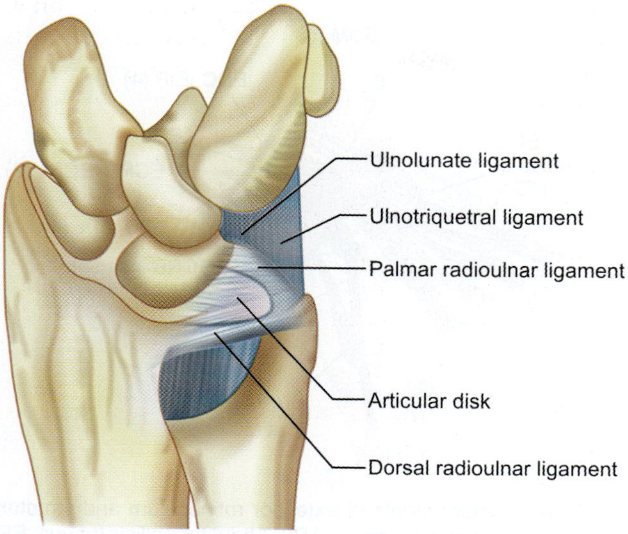

Fig. 21.4: Triangular fibrocartilage complex

- Dorsal radioulnar ligament
- Palmar radioulnar ligament

- DRUJ is primarly stabilized by TFCC. Additional stability is imparted by joint capsule, interosseous membrane, pronator quadratus and extensor carpi ulnaris.
- Between the head of the ulna and the carpus, there is a fibrocartilageous plate, which is a fan shaped structure spreading from ulnar styloid process to the rim of the radial sigmoid notch.
- The peripheral attachment of the TFCC has a good vascular supply and can heal after surgery.
- The central area of the triangular plate is avascular and tears do not heal.
- The articular surface of the distal radius is typically tilted with:
  - 22° of radial inclination (RI)
  - 12 mm of radial length (RL)
  - 11° of radial tilt (RT)
- These are the various angles to assess in distal radial fractures (Figs 21.5A to D).

Ligament Anatomy

- Wrist joint ligaments are divided into following sub-components:
  - Extrinsic and intrinsic
  - Palmar and dorsal
  - Extrinsic ligaments span the radiocarpal and midcarpal joints, whereas the intrinsic ligaments connects the carpal bones.
  - The extrinsic palmar radiocarpal ligaments originating from the distal radius and travel towards the scaphoid, lunate and capitate (Fig. 21.6).

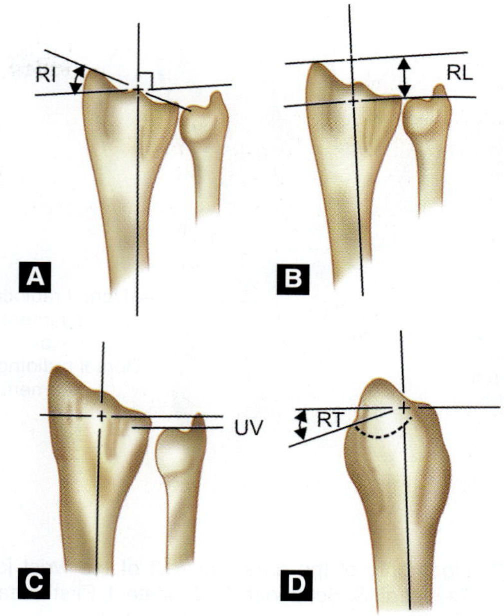

Figs 21.5A to D: Various angles for assessing distal radius fractures

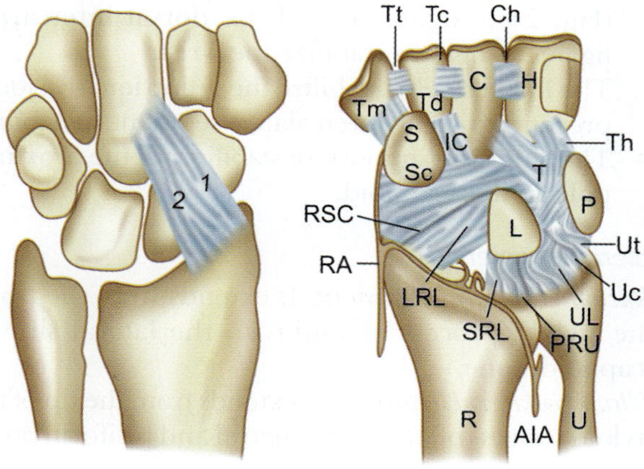

Fig. 21.6: Wrist from palmar perspective—*Bones:* C. Capitate; H. Hamate; L. Lunate; P. Pisiform; R. Radius; S. Scaphoid; Td. Trapezoid; Tm. Trapezium; U. Ulna; *Arteries:* AIA. Anterior interosseous artery; RA. Radial artery. *Ligaments:* Ch. Capitohamate; LRL. Long radiolunate; PRU. Palmar radioulnar; RSC. Radioscaphocapitate; Sc. Scaphocapitate; SRL. Short radiolunate; Tc. Triquetrocapitate; Th. Triquetrohamate; Tt. Trapezio-trapezoid; Uc. Ulnocapitate; Ul. Ulnolunate; Ut. Ulnotriquetral; T. Triquetrum; IC. Intercarpal

- The radial most extrinsic ligament, the radio-scaphocapitate (RSC) ligament originates from the radial styloid, travels across the wrist and distal pole of the scaphoid, crosses the capitate and coalesces with the ulnocapitate ligament.

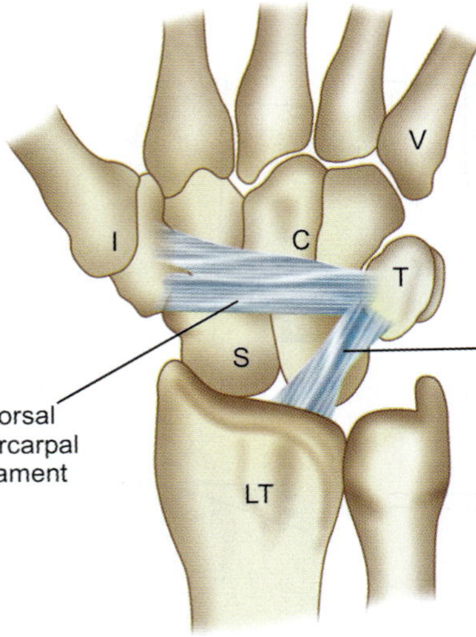

Fig. 21.7: Ligaments of the dorsal aspect of the wrist joint—T. Triquetral; S. Scaphoid; C. Capitate; I. First metacarpal; V. Fifth metacarpal; LT. Lunotriquetral

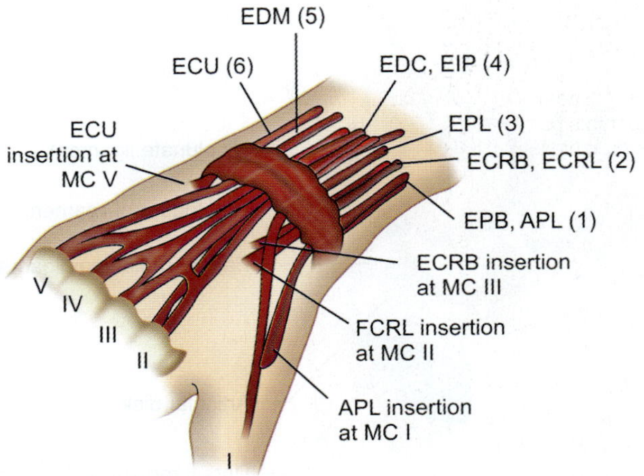

Fig. 21.8: Compartments of extensor retinaculum and structures passing through it—APL. Abductor pollicis longus; EPB. Extensor pollicis brevis; FCRL. Flexor carpi radialis longus; ECRB. Extensor carpi radialis brevis; EPL. Extensor pollicis longus; ED. Extensor digitorum; EI. Extensor indicis; EDM. Extensor digitorum minimi; ECU. Extensor carpi ulnaris

- Dorsally, the dorsal radiotriquetral (radiocarpal) (Fig. 21.7) ligament and the dorsal intercarpal ligament help to stabilize the wrist.
- The former helps stabilize the lunotriquetral joint, preventing volar intercalated segment instability.
- The latter is an important stabilizer of the proximal pole of the scaphoid.

Collateral Ligaments

- *Radial collateral ligament*: It extends from the tip of the styloid process of radius to the lateral side of scaphoid bone.
- *Ulnar collateral ligament:* It extends from the tip of the styloid process of ulna to triquetral and pisiform bone.

Retinaculum Anatomy

Two retinaculum are present in the wrist joint:
1. Extensor retinaculum
2. Flexor retinaculum

Extensor Retinaculum

- Deep fascia on the back of the wrist is thickened to form it, which holds the extensor tendons in place.
- It is an oblique band, which is 2 cm broad directed downwards and medially.
- *Attachments of extensor retinaculum:*
  - *Laterally:* To the lower part of the anterior border of radius
  - *Medially:* To the styloid process of ulna, triquetrum and pisiform bone
- *Compartments of extensor retinaculum (Fig. 21.8):* There are six osteofascial compartments formed over the back of the wrist. Structures passing through each compartment from lateral to medial side are given in Table 21.1.

Table 21.1: Structures passing through six osteofacial compartments in lateral to medial fashion

Compartment	Structures passing through it
I	Abductor pollicis longus and extensor pollicis brevis
II	Flexor carpi radialis longus and extensor carpi radialis brevis
III	Extensor pollicis longus
IV	Extensor digitorum, extensor indicis, posterior interosseous nerve and anterior interosseous artery
V	Extensor digitorum minimi
VI	Extensor carpi ulnaris

Flexor Retinaculum

- This is a strong fibrous band, which bridges the anterior concavity of the carpus and converts it into a tunnel, i.e. the carpal flexor tunnel
- *Attachments of flexor retinaculum:*
  - Laterally, it is attached to the tubercle of scaphoid and crest of the trapezium
  - Medially, it is attached to pisiform bone and the hook of the hamate.
- *Structures passing through flexor retinaculum:* These can be superficial or deep sitted structures:
  - Structures passing superficial to flexor retinaculum: Tendon of palmaris longus, palmar

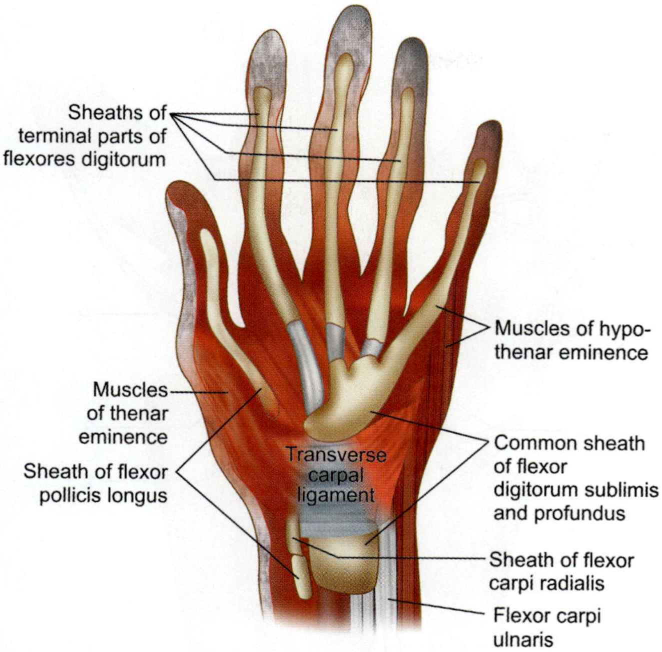

Fig. 21.9: Boundaries of flexor retinaculum

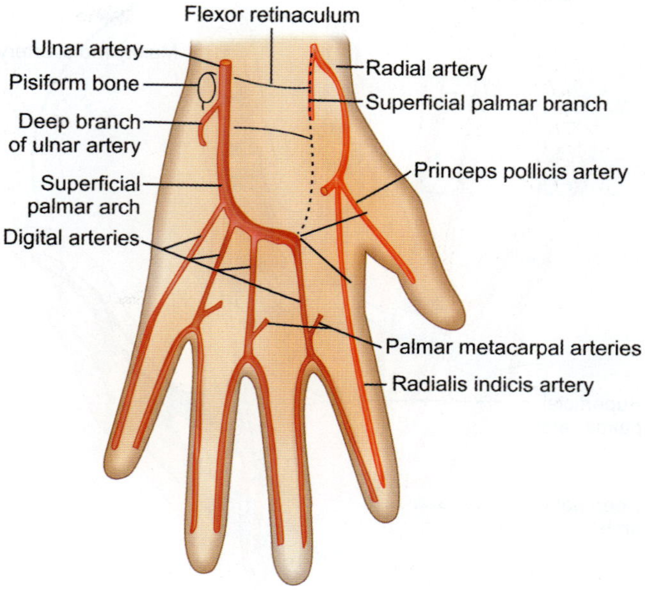

Fig. 21.10: Superficial palmar arch—formation and branches

cutaneous branch of median nerve, palmar cutaneous branch of ulnar nerve and ulnar vessels
  - Structures passing deep to flexor retinaculum: Median nerve, tendons of flexor digitorum superficialis, tendon of flexor digitorum profundus, tendon of flexor pollicis longus, ulnar bursa and radial bursa
- *Guyon's canal:* Lies ulnar to the carpal cannal and contains ulnar nerve and ulnar artery
- *Boundaries of flexor retinaculum (Fig. 21.9)*
  - *Floor:* Transverse carpal ligament (between pisiform and hook of the hamate)
  - *Roof:* Volar carpal ligament and palmaris brevis
  - *Radially:* Hook of hamate and the digital flexor tendons
  - *Ulnarly:* Pisiform, flexor crapi ulnaris and abductor digiti minimi.

Vascular Anatomy

Blood supply to the hand is by radial and the ulnar arteries, which form two interconnected vascular arches. These are:

- Superficial palmar arch
- Deep palmar arch

Superficial Palmar Arch

- *Formation:* It is formed as the direct continuation of ulnar artery beyond the flexor retinaculum (Fig. 21.10). On the lateral side, the arch is completed by one of the following branches of the radial artery:
  - Superficial palmar branches
  - Radialis indices
  - Princeps pollicis
- *Relations of the superficial palmar arch:* It lies deep to palmaris brevis and palmar aponeurosis (Fig. 21.10).
- Medial three and half fingers are supplied by ulnar artery and lateral one and a half fingers are supplied by radial artery.

Deep Palmar Arch

- This arterial arch provides second channel connecting the radial and ulnar arteries in the palm. It is situated deep to the long flexor tendon.
- *Formation*: Formation is done by the terminal part of radial artery and is completed medially by the deep palmar branch of the ulnar artery (Fig. 21.11).
- *Branches of deep palmar arch:* It gives off three palmar metacarpal arteries, which run distally in the second, third and fourth spaces. Dorsally, the arch gives off three perforating arteries. Recurrent branches arise from concavity of the arch and supply carpal bones (Fig. 21.11).

Vascular Supply of Wrist Joint

Vascular supply of wrist joint is shown in Figure 21.12.

Surgical Approaches to Wrist

- Dorsal approach to the wrist
- Volar approach to the wrist
- Volar approach to scaphoid
- Dorsolateral approach to scaphoid

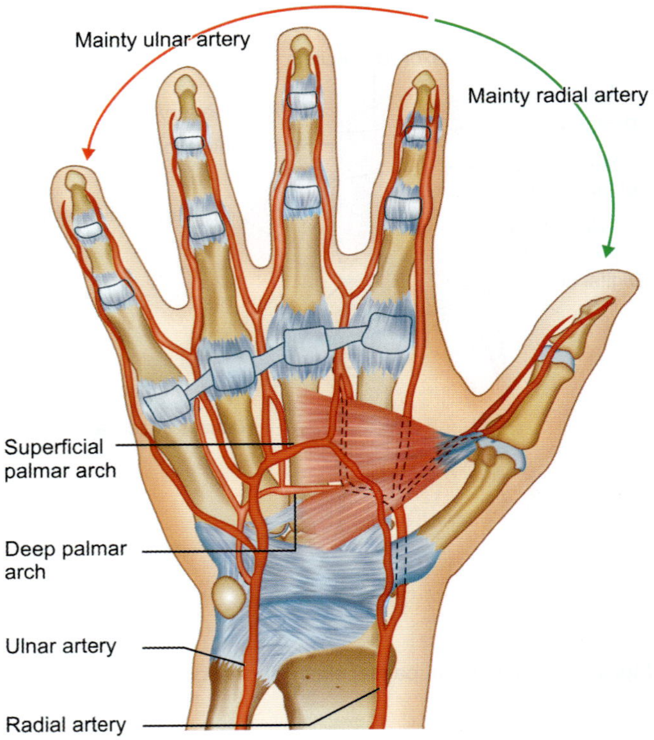

Fig. 21.11: Deep palmar arch: Formation and its branches

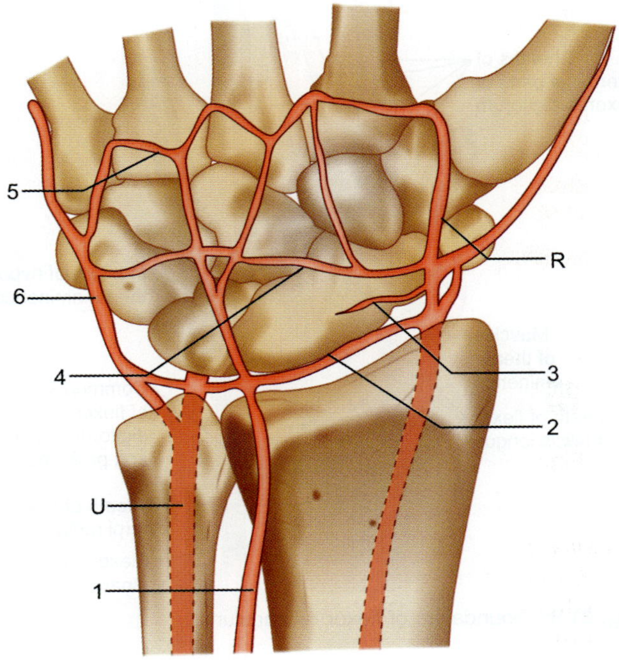

Fig. 21.12: Vascular supply of wrist joint—R. Radial artery; U. Ulnar artery; 1. Dorsal branch of anterior interosseous artery; 2. Dorsal radiocarpal arch; 3. Branch to dorsal ridge of scaphoid; 4. Dorsal intercarpal arch; 5. Basal metacarpal arch; 6. Medial brach of ulnar artery

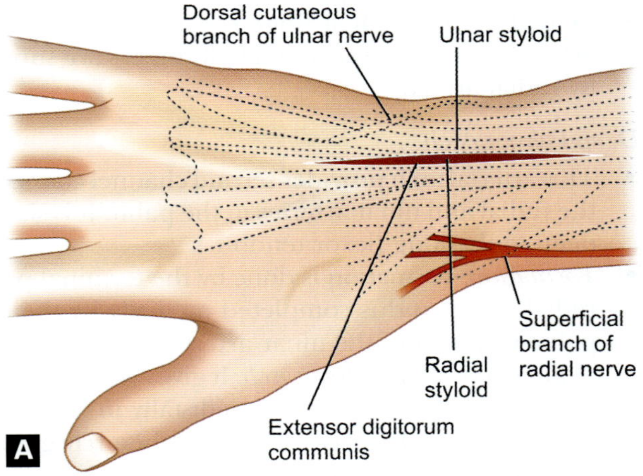

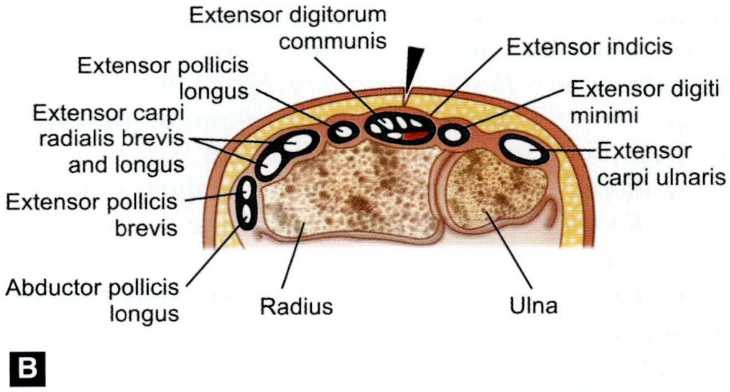

Figs 21.13A and B: Surgical approach to wrist in dorsal fashion

Dorsal Approach to the Wrist

Dorsal approach to wrist is shown in Figures 21.13A and B.

Indications

- Synovectomy
- Repair of extensor tendons in case of rheumatoid arthritis.
- Dorsal stabilization of wrist
- Wrist fusion
- Excision of lower end of radius for benign and malignant tumor.
- Open reduction and internal fixation for certain distal radial and carpal fractures and dislocation.
- Proximal row carpalectomy

Position

- Patient supine
- Arm on arm table
- Forearm in supination

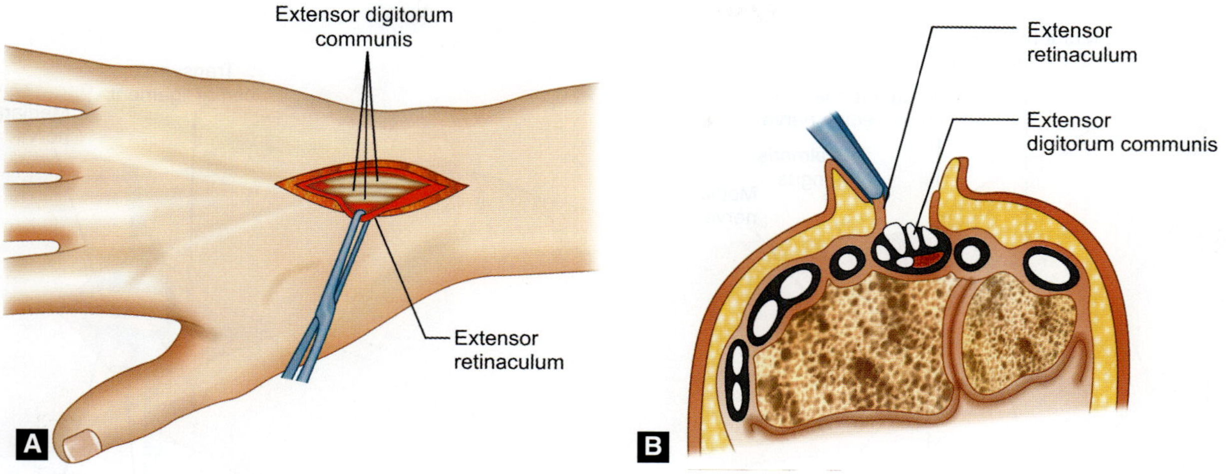

Figs 21.14A and B: Incision of extensor retinaculum

Landmarks
- Radial styloid process
- Ulnar styloid process
- Lister's tubercle

Incision
- Take a 8 cm longitudinal incision on dorsal aspect of wrist, crossing midway between radial styloid and ulnar styloid.
- Incision begins 3 cm proximal to wrist joint and ends 5 cm distal to it.

Internervous plane: There is no true internervous plane.

Superficial and deep surgical dissection: It involves following steps:
- Incise the skin, subcutaneous tissue and fat to expose the extensor retinaculum.
- Extensor retinaculum is visualized and incised between third and fourth dorsal compartment (Figs 21.14A and B).
- Extensor pollicis longus is retracted radially and fourth compartment is retracted laterally.
- Subperiosteal dissection is continued to expose distal radius and carpal capsule.
- A longitudnal incision is taken over the the joint capsule on dorsal aspect of radius and carpus.
- Dissect below the capsule towards radial side of the radius to expose entire distal end of radius and carpal bones (Fig. 21.15).

Dangers
- The superficial radial nerve emerges just above the wrist joint before travelling to the dorsum of the hand. Cutting a cutaneous nerve may result in a painful neuroma.
- Radial artery, crosses the wrist joint on its lateral aspect and is at high-risk of injury.

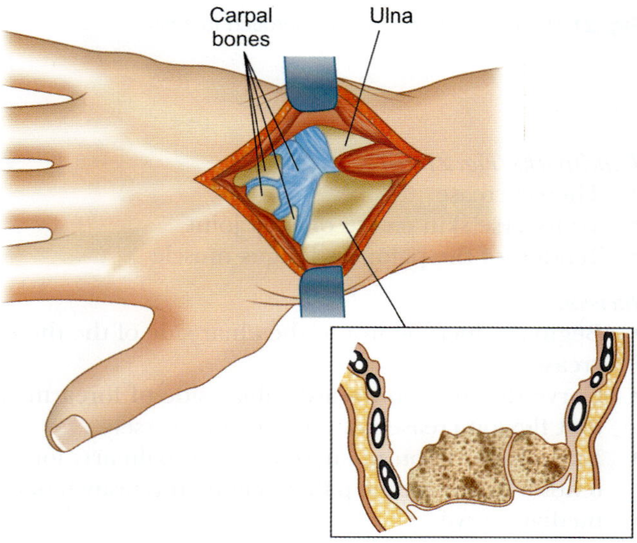

Fig. 21.15: Exposure of distal end of radius and carpal bones after dissection is made below the capsule

Volar Approach to the Wrist

Indications
- Decompression of median nerve
- Synovectomy
- Excision of tumors within the carpal tunnel
- Repair of lacerated tendon and nerves with in carpal tunnel
- Open reduction and internal fixation of some fractures of distal radius and carpal bones.

Position of the patient
- Place the patient in supine position
- Rest the hand in supinated position on arm board

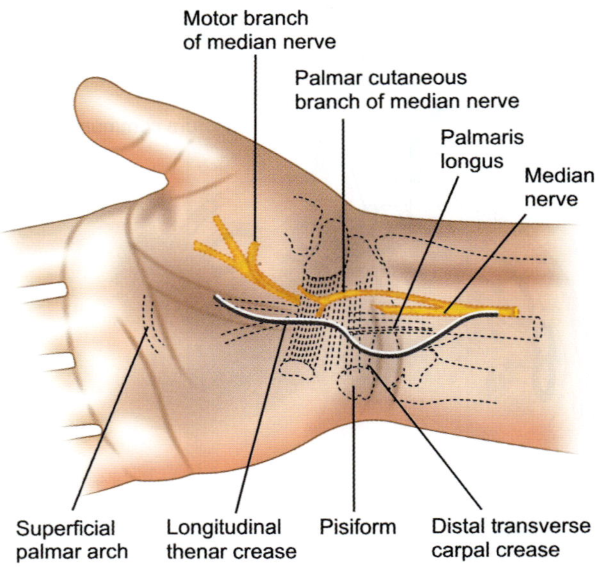

Fig. 21.16: Landmarks of volar approach to wrist

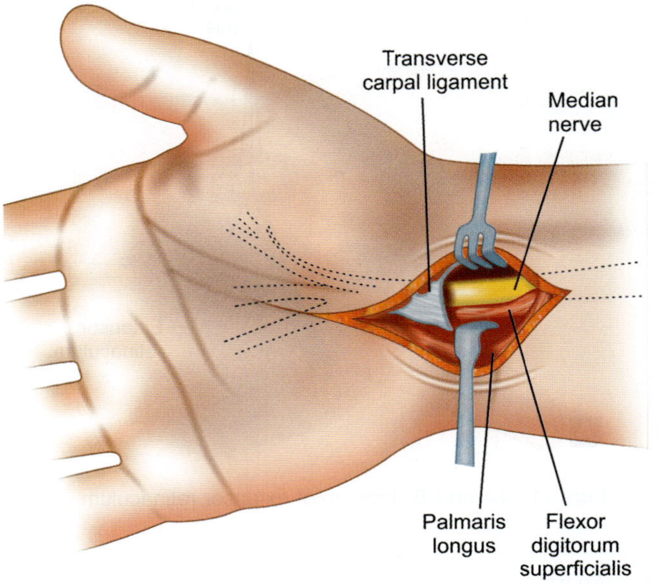

Fig. 21.17: Median nerve between tendon of palmaris longus muscle and flexor carpi radialis muscle

Landmarks (Fig. 21.16)
- Thenar crease
- Transverse skin crease of wrist joint
- Tendon of the palmaris longus muscle

Incision
- Begin the incision just to the ulnar side of the thenar crease
- Curve the incision towards ulnar side of forearm, so that flexion crease not crossed transversely
- Incision made on ulnar side of the palmaris longus tendon to protect the palmar cutaneous branch of the median nerve.

Internervous plane: There is no intervenous plane

Superficial and deep surgical dissection
- Incise the skin and subcutaneous tissue.
- Identify superficial palmar fascia and tendon of palmaris longus.
- Superficial palmar fascia incised.
- Retract the palmaris tendon to the ulnar side.
- Identify median nerve between tendon of palmaris longus muscle and flexor carpi radialis muscle (Fig. 21.17).
- Flexor retinaculum identified and cut along the length of the retinaculum.
- Median nerve retracted radially.
- Later base of the carpal tunnel is incised longitudinally to expose the volar aspect of the carpus and distal radioulnar joint (Fig. 21.18).

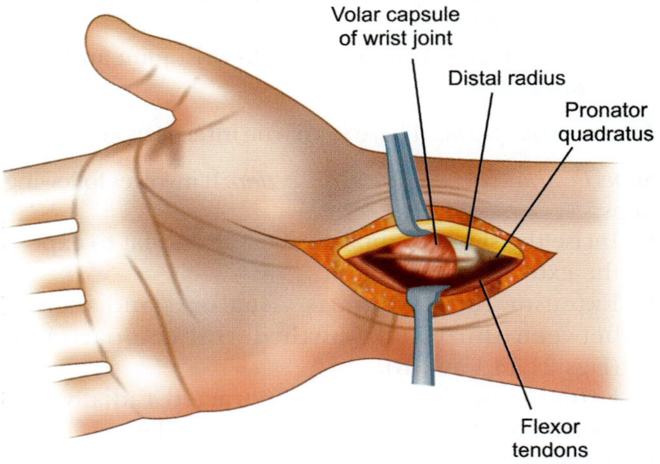

Fig. 21.18: Exposure of volar aspect of carpus and distal radioulnar joint is done after longitudinal incision

Volar Approach to the Scaphoid

It is also known as "Russe" approach (Fig. 21.19).

Indications:
- Bone grafting for nonunion of scaphoid
- Excision of proximal 1/3rd of scaphoid
- Excision of radial styloid

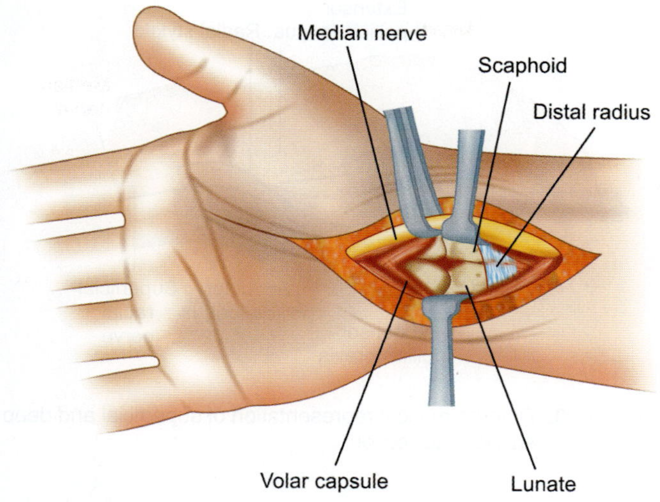

Fig. 21.19: Volar approach to scaphoid. It is also known as "Russe" approach

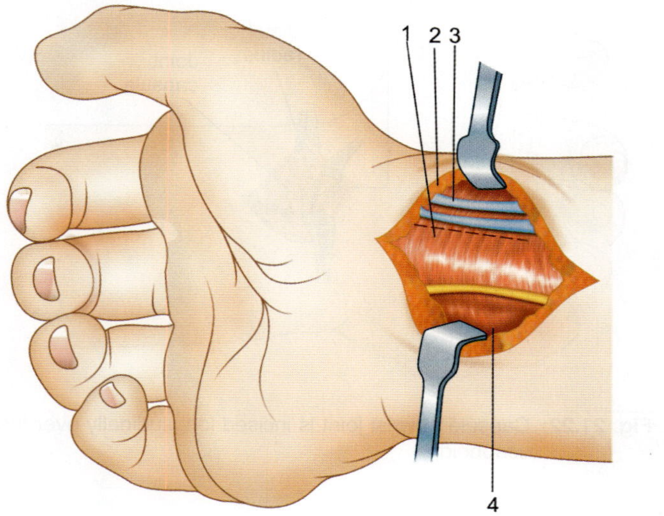

Fig. 21.21: Superficial and deep surgical dissection of the volar approach—1. Palmar cutaneous branch of median N; 2. Fascia over flexor carpi radialis; 3. Radial artery and venae comitantes; 4. Palmaris longus

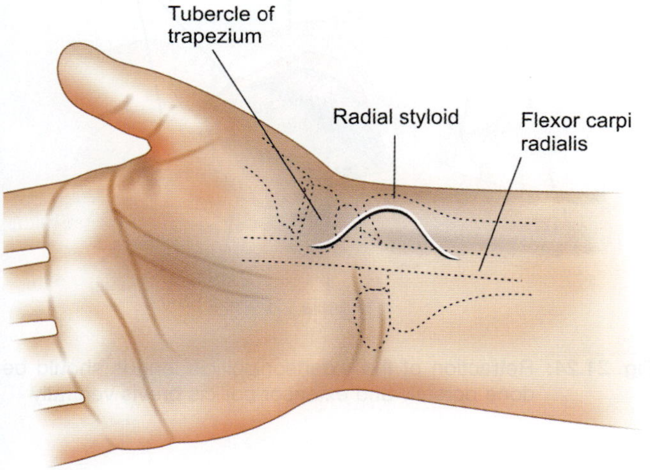

Fig. 21.20: Landmarks of volar approach to scaphoid

Procedure

Open reduction and internal fixation (screw fixation) for fracture of scaphoid.

Position

Supinate the forearm.

Landmarks (Fig. 21.20)

Tuberosity of the scaphoid (palpate it just distal to the skin crease of wrist joint) at level of tubercle of trapezium. Flexor carpi radialis tendon (flexor carpi radialis muscle crosses the scaphoid before inserting into the base of second and third metacarpal).

Incision

Vertical or curvilinear incision 2 to 3 cm long. Base the incision on the scaphoid tuberosity and extend it proximally between tendon of flexi carpi radialis muscle and radial artery. Incision should cross the wrist crease at 45° angle.

Internervous plane: No internervous plane because the only muscle mobilized is flexor carpi radialis, which is supplied by median nerve.

Superficial and deep surgical dissection (Fig. 21.21)

- Incise skin, subcutaneous tissue and deep fascia
- Identify the radial artery on the radial aspect
- Retract the radial artery and subcutaneous tissue radially
- Identify the tendon of flexor carpi radialis muscle, trace it distally and free it from flexor retinaculum after incising it
- Retract it medially, to expose the wrist joint
- Incise the capsule of the wrist joint longitudinally over the scaphoid (Fig. 21.22)
- Place the wrist in marked dorsiflexion to get a better view of the joint.

Dangers

- Radial artery lies laterally and is prone to be incised.
- Care should be taken to prevent palmar cutaneous branch of median nerve (in superficial dissection).

Advantages

- It avoids damaging the dorsal blood supply to the bone's proximal half.
- Avoids damage to superficial branch of radial nerve.

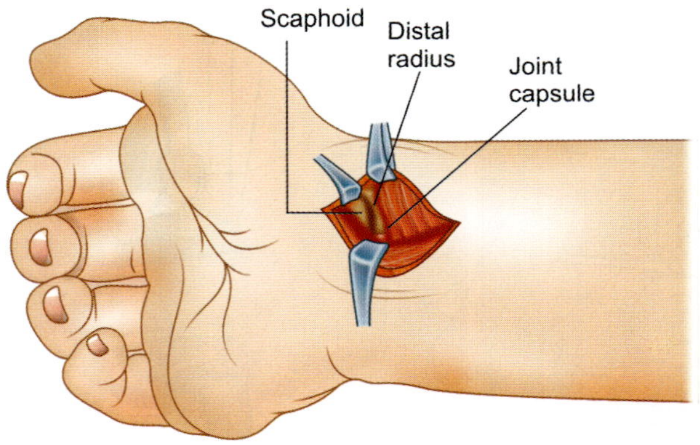

Fig. 21.22: Capsule of wrist joint is incised longitudinally over the scaphoid

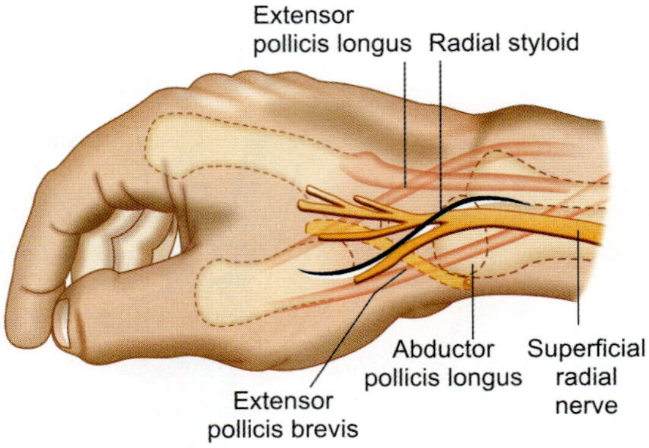

Fig. 21.23: Diagrammatical representation of superficial and deep surgical dissection

Dorsolateral Approach to the Scaphoid

Indications
- Bone grafting for nonunion scaphoid
- Excision of proximal fragment of scaphoid
- Excision of radial styloid
- Open reduction and internal fixation of fracture of scaphoid.

Position: Pronate the forearm.

Landmarks
- Radial styloid process
- Anatomical snuffbox.

Incision
- "S" shaped incision centered over snuffbox.
- Cut should extend from base of 1st metacarpal to 3 cm above the snuff box.

Internervous plane: No true internervous plane.

Superficial and deep surgical dissection (Fig. 21.23)
- Cut skin and subcutaneous tissue
- Identify tendon of extensor pollicis longus (dorsally) and extensor pollicis brevis (ventrally)
- Open fascia between the two tendons
- Retract the extensor pollicis longus dorsally and extensor pollicis brevis ventrally (Fig. 21.24)
- Identify radial artery lying on the bone and retract it radially
- Incise capsule of the wrist joint longitudinally
- Expose the articulation between distal end radius and proximal end of scaphoid
- Place the wrist in ulnar deviation to expose the joint completely (Figs 21.25A to C).

Dangers
- Superficial radial nerve is at risk during exposure (because it lies directly over the tendon of extensor pollicis longus muscle and can get cut during mobilization of extensor pollicis tendon)
- Incising the nerve may produce:
  - Neuroma
  - Hypoesthesia (area on dorsal aspect of hand).

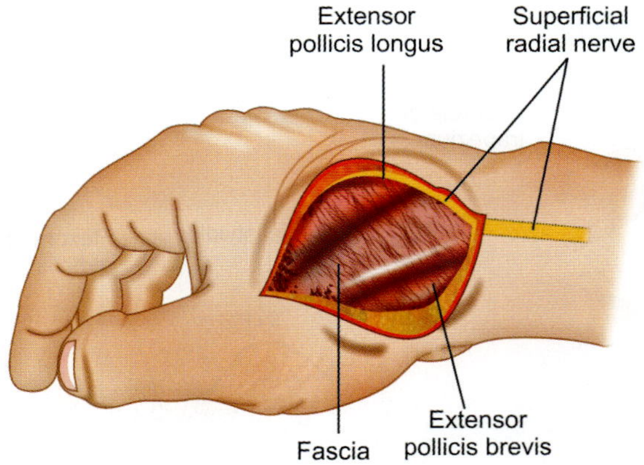

Fig. 21.24: Retraction of the extensor pollicis longus should be done dorsally and extensor pollicis brevis ventrally

EXAMINATION OF WRIST JOINT

■ Introduction

Wrist joint as shown in Figure 21.26 is a synovial joint of ellipsoid variety. It is formed by inferior surface of lower end of radius, articular disk of inferior radioulnar joint, scaphoid, lunate and triquetral bone.

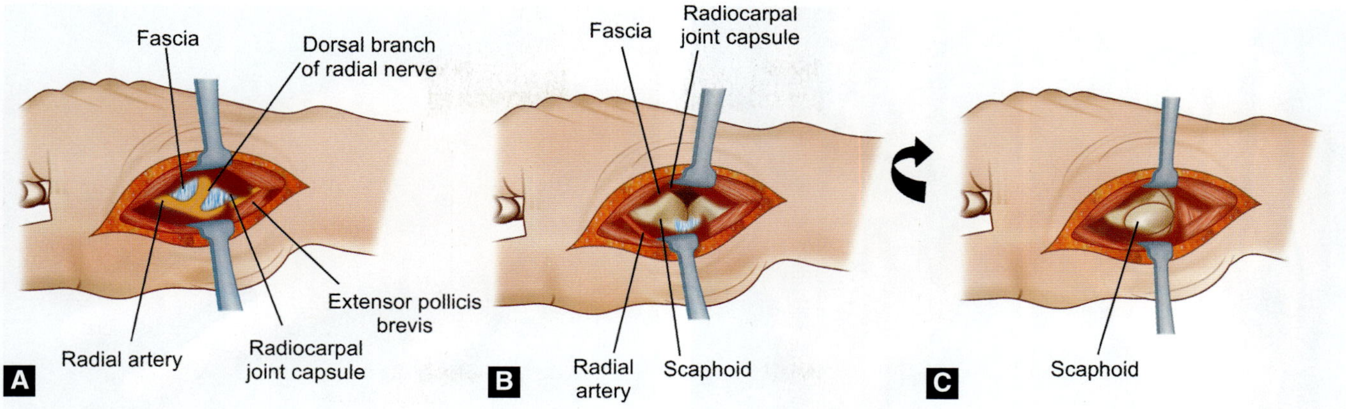

Figs 21.25A to C: Radial artery should be identified and retracted radially. After longitudinal incision of wrist joint capsule, articulation between distal end radius and proximal end of scaphoid should be exposed

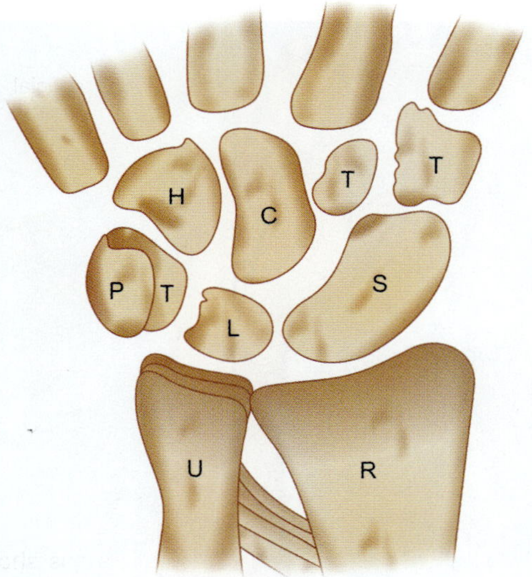

Fig. 21.26: Wrist joint—S. Scaphoid; L. Lunate; T. Triquetrum; P. Pisiform; T. Trapezium; T. Trapezoid; C. Capitate; H. Hamate; R. Radius; U. Ulna

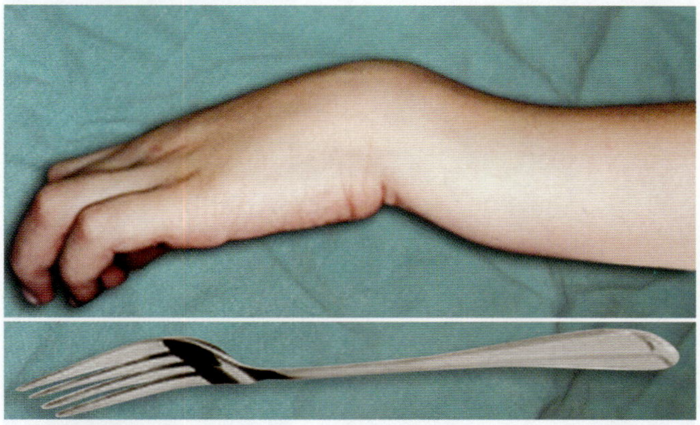

Fig. 21.27: Dinner fork deformity in Colle's fracture

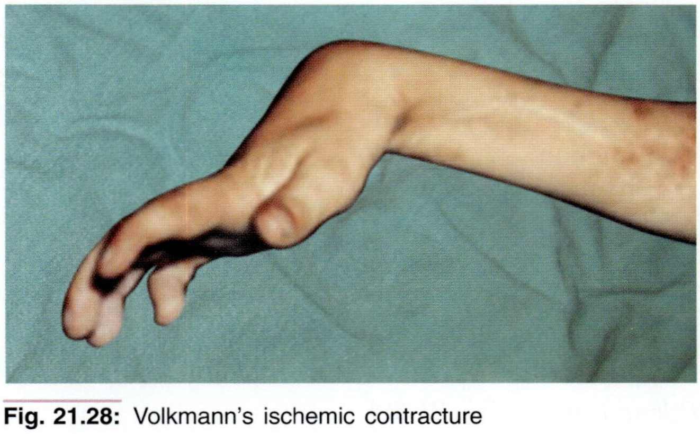

Fig. 21.28: Volkmann's ischemic contracture

History

Patient with any wrist pathology usually presents with a history of:

- Swelling, trauma
- Deformity
- Restricted movements, etc.

Attitude

- Dinner fork deformity, e.g. Colle's fracture (Fig. 21.27)
- Flexion contracture of wrist and finger, e.g. Volkmann's ischemic contracture (VIC) (Fig. 21.28).

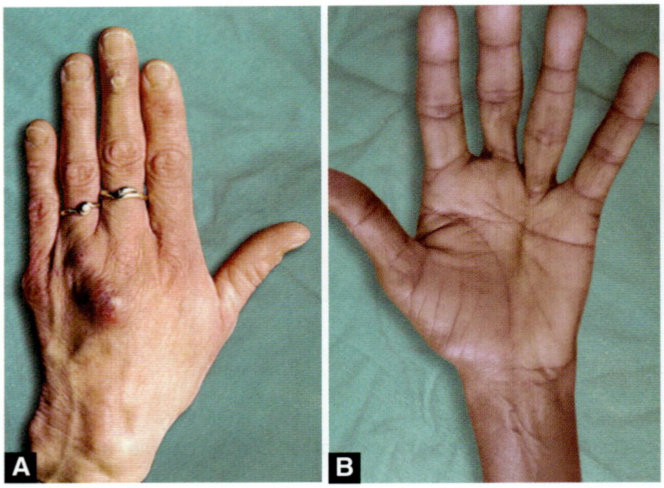

Figs 21.29A and B: Generalized inspection of the dorsal surface of the wrist

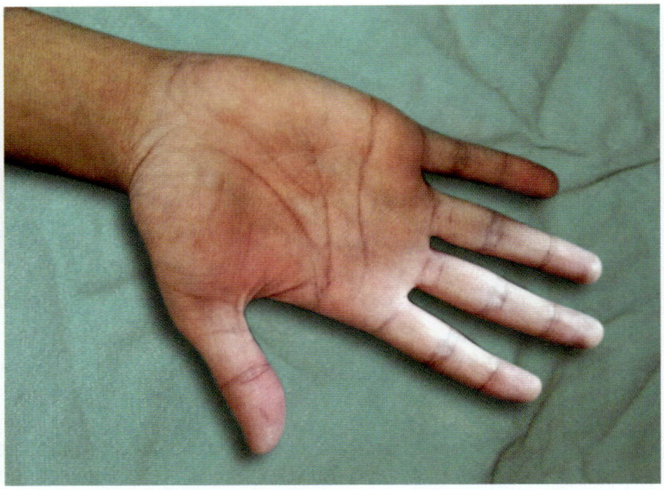

Fig. 21.31: Hypothenar eminence

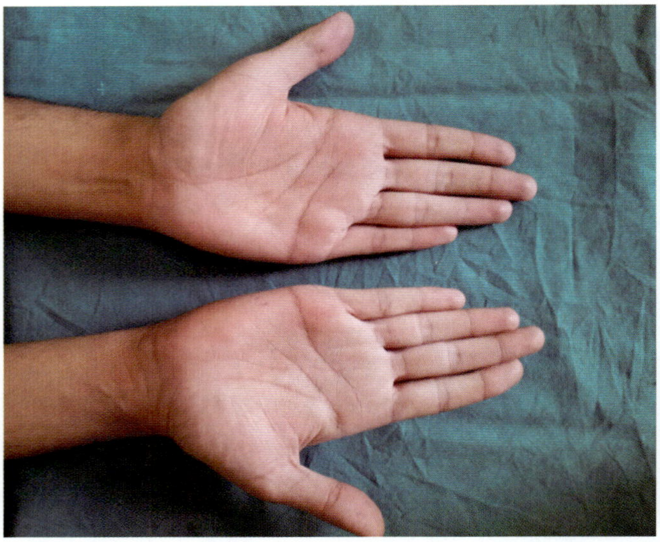

Fig. 21.30: Inspecting palmar surface of the wrist and hands for any pathological signs

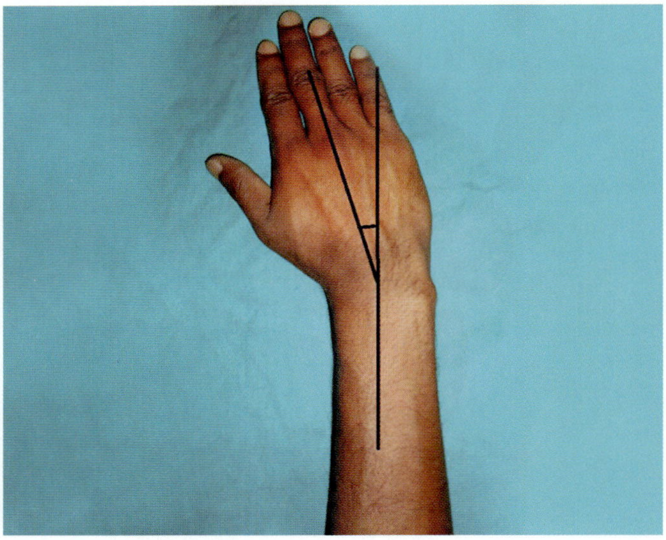

Fig. 21.32: Measuring radial deviation

Inspection

Dorsal Surface

Localized

- Ganglion
- Rheumatoid nodule
- Tumor

Generalized (Figs 21.29A and B)

- Traumatic
- *Skin Condition:* Any scar, sinuses, venous prominence, contracture, etc.

Palmar Surface (Fig. 21.30)

- Swelling
- Muscle wasting, e.g. RA, TB
- Anterior tilting, e.g. Smith fracture
- Posterior tilting, e.g. Colle's fracture.

Radial Surface

Swelling in anatomical snuffbox.

Ulnar Surface

Hypothenar eminence (Fig. 21.31).

Deformity

- Radial deviation (Fig. 21.32), e.g. in Colle's fracture
- Ulnar deviation (Fig. 21.33), e.g. rheumatoid arthritis.

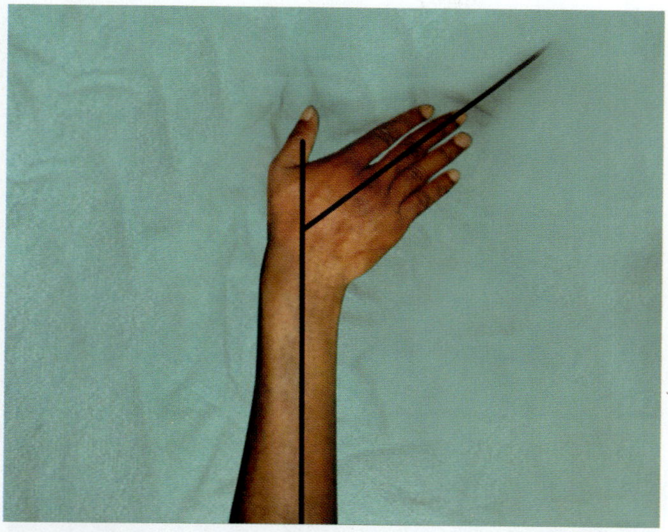

Fig. 21.33: Measuring ulnar deviation

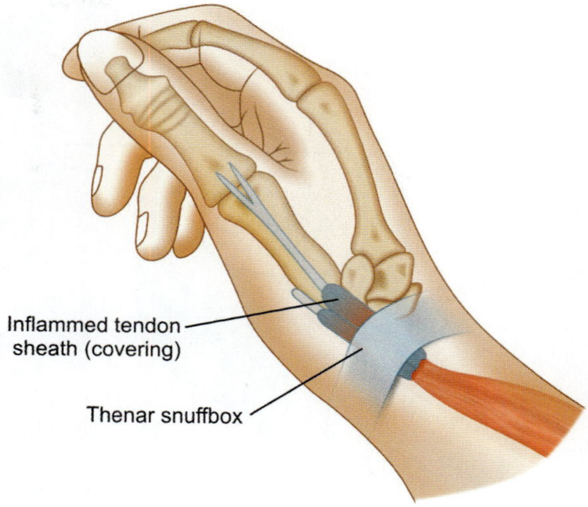

Fig. 21.35: De Quervain's disease

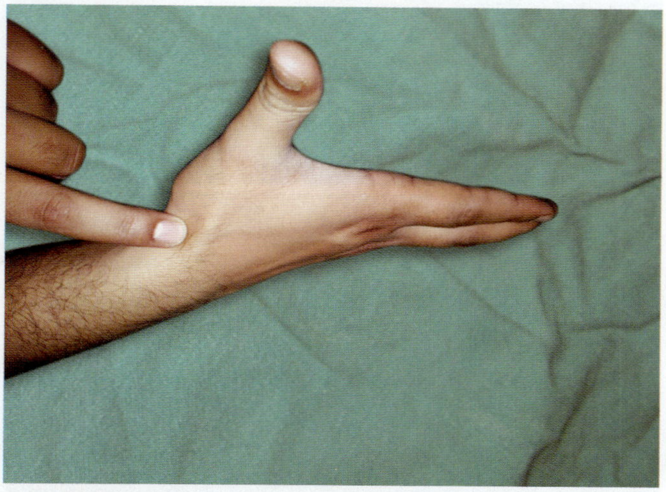

Fig. 21.34: Tenderness present over anatomical snuffbox: scaphoid fracture

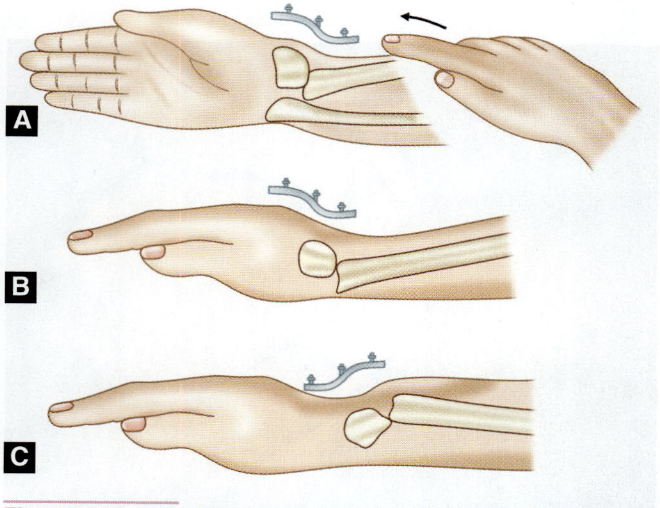

Figs 21.36A to C: Step sign—(A) Lateral step-up; (B) Posterior step-up; (C) Posterior step-down

Palpation

Superficial

- *Temperature:* Hypo/hyperthermia
- Anesthesia
- Bony projection
- Radial pulse

Deep

- *Palpate ulnar and radial styloid process:* Normally, radial styloid process is 1 cm distal to the ulnar styloid process (Fig. 21.34). Tenderness present over anatomical snuff box, indicates scaphoid fracture.
- *De Quervain's disease (Fig. 21.35):* Tenderness present oversheath of abductor pollis longus and extensor pollicis brevicis:
- *Step sign:* In case of any injury to the wrist joint, note for step sign (Figs 21.36A to C), pass down your index finger on outer aspect of forearm over radial shaft. In case of outer shift of lower fragment (Fig. 21.36A), finger will step over the hard underlying structure and can be seen on dorsal aspect also (lateral step-up). In Colle's fracture (posterior stepping up) (Fig. 21.36B) and reverse in Smith's (posterior stepping down) (Fig. 21.36C).
- *Styloid process of radius and ulna (Fig. 21.37):* Patient forearm is pronated. Wrist is in neutral position. Support the palm in one hand.
- Put thumb and index fingertip of opposite hand on two sides of wrist from dorsal aspect. Gently squeeze

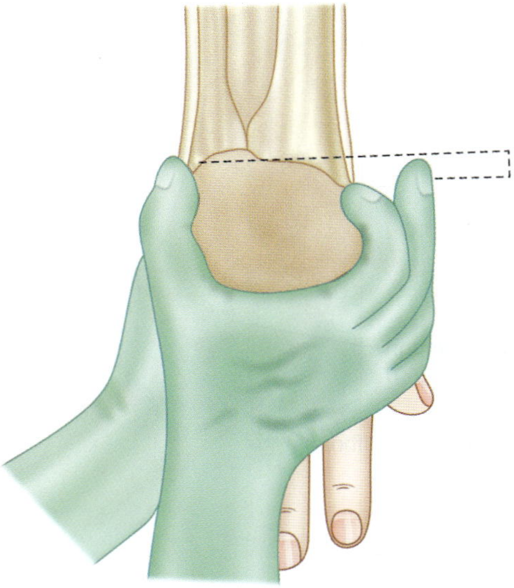

Fig. 21.37: Styloid process of radius and ulna

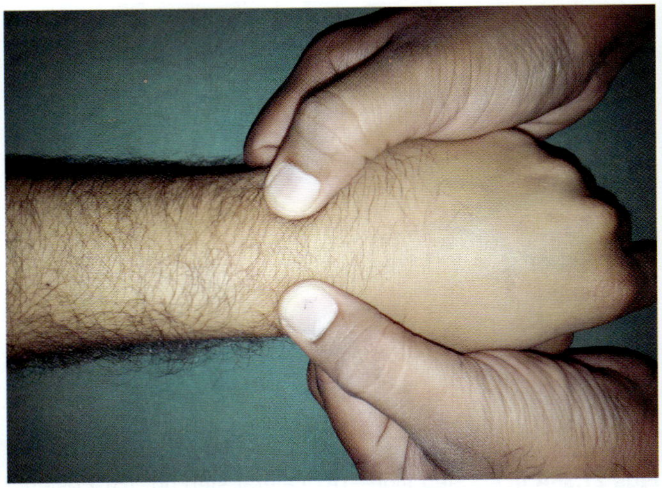

Fig. 21.38: Palpation of joint line (wrist)

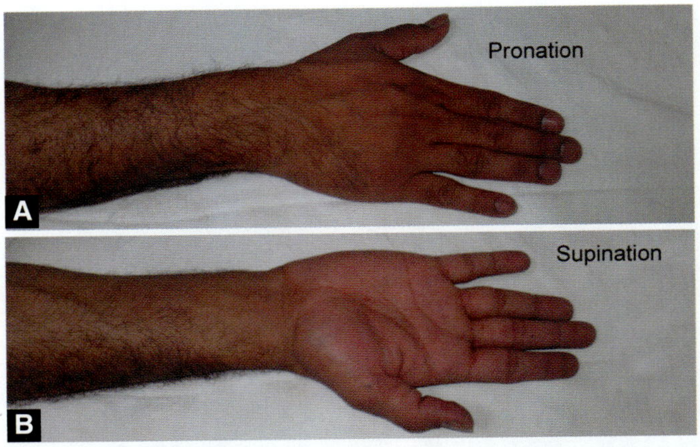

Figs 21.39A and B: Pronation and supination movement of wrist

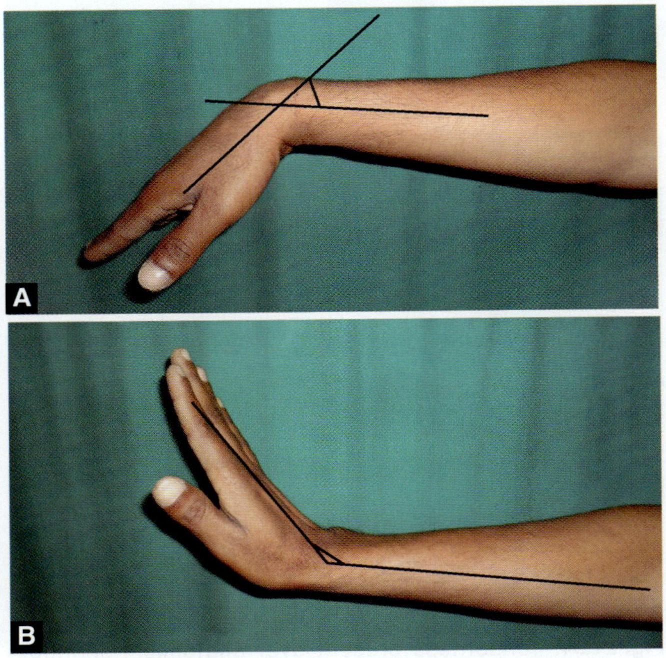

Figs 21.40A and B: Dorsiflexion, palmar flexion of wrist

within and at the same time shift your fingertip proximally styloid process will be felt.

- *Palpation of joint line (Fig. 21.38)*
- *Crepitus radioulnar joint (Figs 21.39A and B):* Place index finger and thumb overjoint, then, supinate and pronate the wrist. Crepitus comes when joint is disorganized.
- *Crepitus radiocarpal joint:* Encircle the wrist with the hand and ask the patient to dorsiflex, palmarflex, radial deviate, ulnar deviate the wrist (Figs 21.40A and B). Osteoarthritis of wrist is uncommon but occurs after scaphoid and distal radius fracture and Kienbock's disease.

Range of Motion

Palmar Flexion

- *Normal range:* 75°
- *Screening test:* Ask the patient to put the backs of the hands in contact and then to bring forearm into horizontal position (Figs 21.41A and B).

Dorsiflexion

- Measured with goniometer (Fig. 21.42)
- Normal range: 75°
- Restricted in:
  - Ankylosis of joint secondary to infection
  - Reduced Colle's fracture

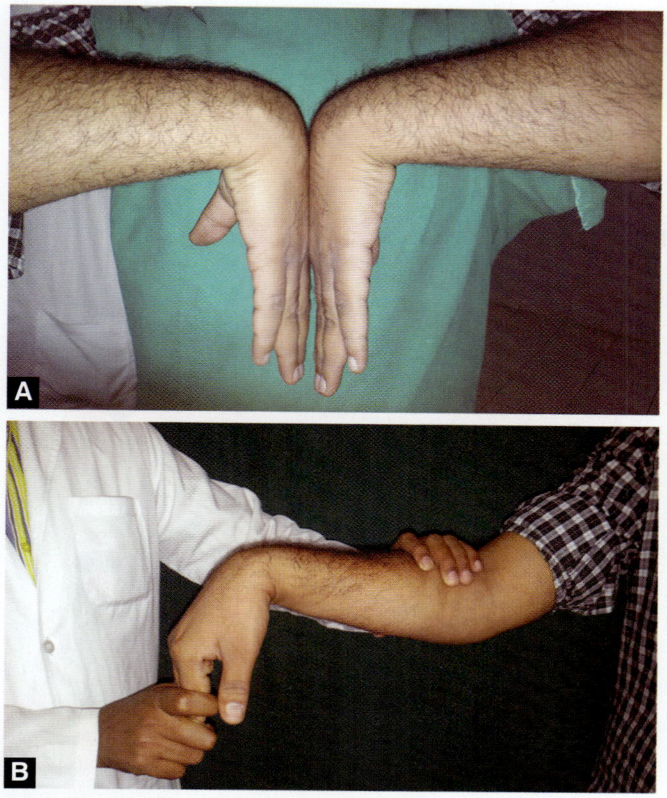

Figs 21.41A and B: Screening test for palmar flexion

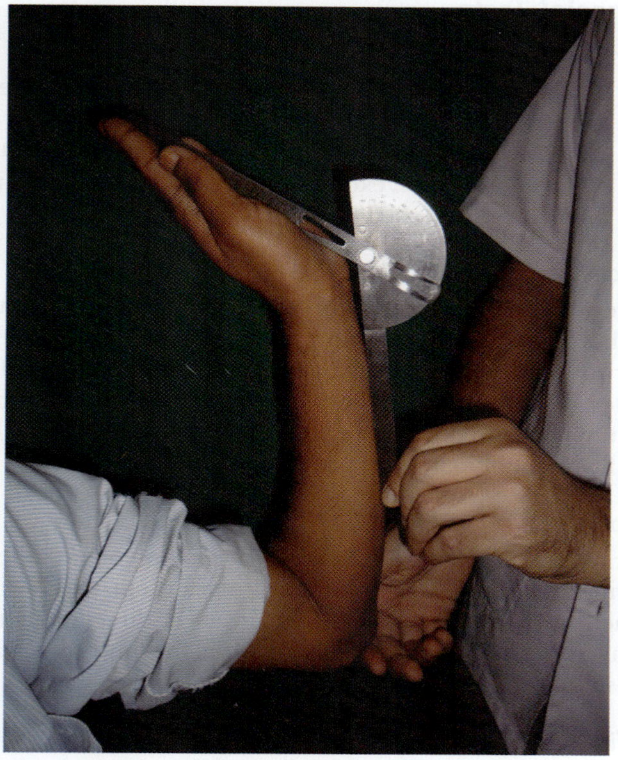

Fig. 21.42: Measurement of dorsiflexion with goniometer

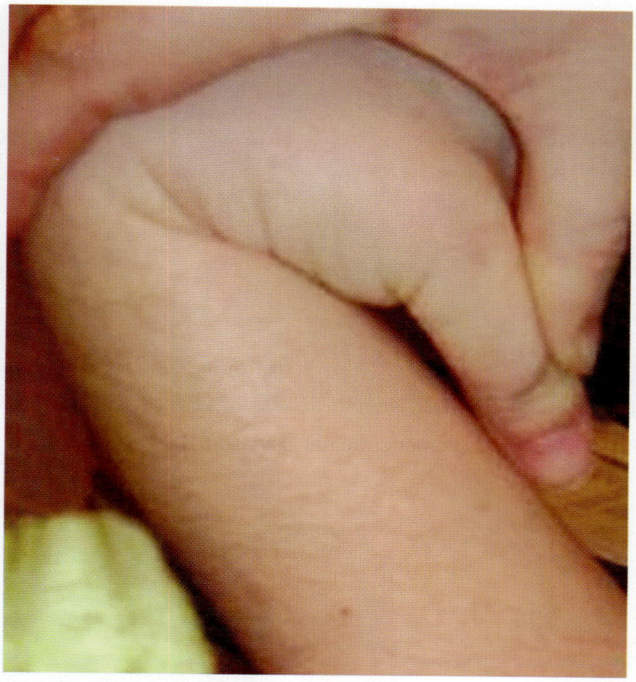

Fig. 21.43: Depiction of joint hypermobility

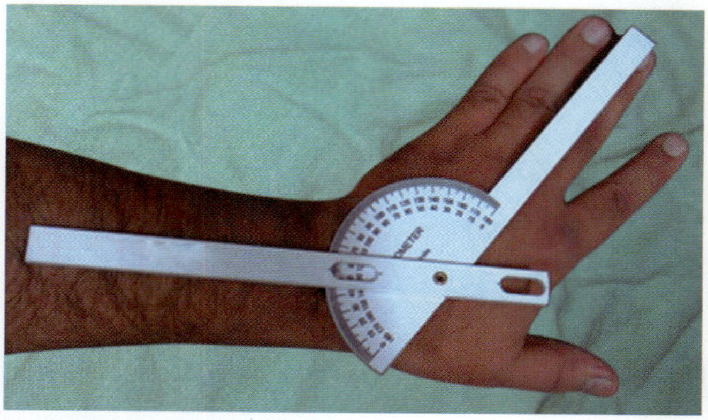

Fig. 21.44: Radial deviation

Joint Hypermobility (Fig. 21.43)

Try to bring the thumb into contact with forearm and measure gap. Average separation is 4.5 cm at 17.5 years. It increases with age due to loss of elasticity of ligament.

Radial Deviation (Fig. 21.44)

It is an angle formed between forearm and middle metacarpal. Normal range is 20°.

Ulnar Deviation (Fig. 21.45)

- *Normal range:* 35°
- It is measured with goniometer

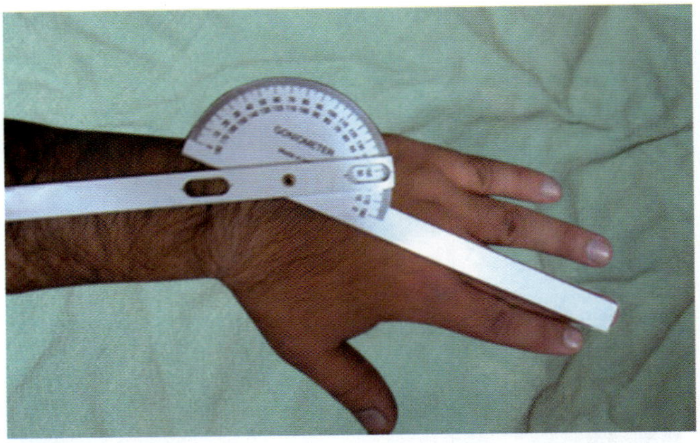

Fig. 21.45: Measurement of ulnar deviation

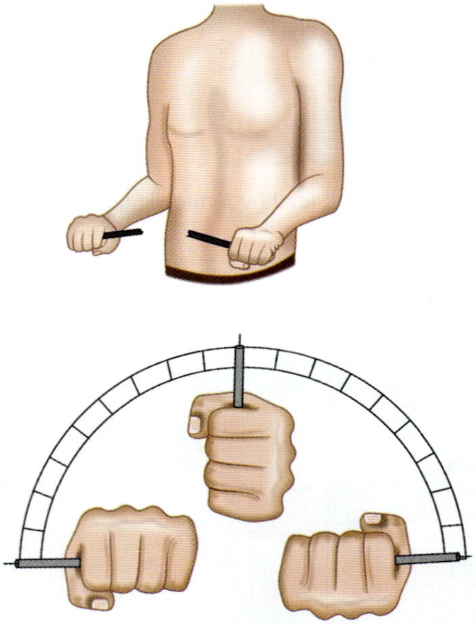

Fig. 21.46: The elbow range of motion in supination and pronation

Supination

- *Normal range:* 90°
- It is defined by the degree to which radius can rotate over ulna
- *Tests*: Tell the patient to hold the pencil in each hand, then move both forearm simultaneously into supination (Fig. 21.46). Normally, pencils are parallel to floor.

Pronation

Ask the patient to flex elbow to 90° at his waist fist holding the pencil. Ask the patient to rotate his fist from fully supinated position until his palm faces downward. Normally, palm faces downwards and pencil parallel to floor (Fig. 21.46). Any dissimilarty implies restricted ROM.

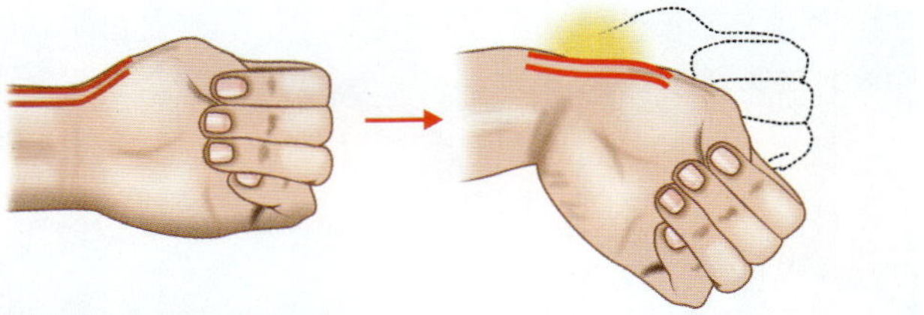

Fig. 21.47: Finkelstein's test

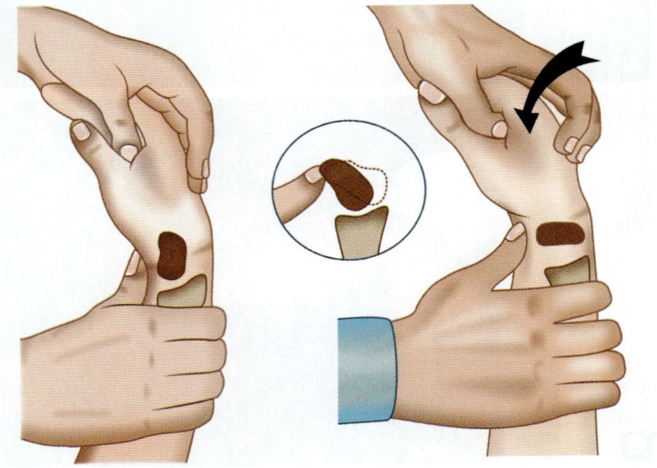

Fig. 21.48: Watson's test

Special Tests

Finkelstein's Test (Fig. 21.47)

- Ask the patient to flex the thumb and close the finger over it
- Now, move the hand in ulnar deviation in De Quervains disease, excruciating pain accompanies this maneuver. It is used for carpal instabilities.

Watson's Test (Fig. 21.48)

Press the thumb against tubercle of scaphoid. With the other hand palamarflex and radially deviate the patient wrist. A click sound should be felt. The scaphoid subluxate over distal radius and reduction occurs if pressure of thumb is slacked. Accompanying pain is confirmatory. It is for scapholunate instability.

Ballottement Test (Fig. 21.49)

Triquetral and lunate are grapsed with thumb and index finger. An attempt is made to displace them relative to each other, first in dorsal then in volar direction note any associated pain and crepitus. It is for lunotriquetral instability.

Midcarpal Instability (Fig. 21.50)

With one hand steady the forearm and with other hand grasp the patient's hand. Push the carpus against radius

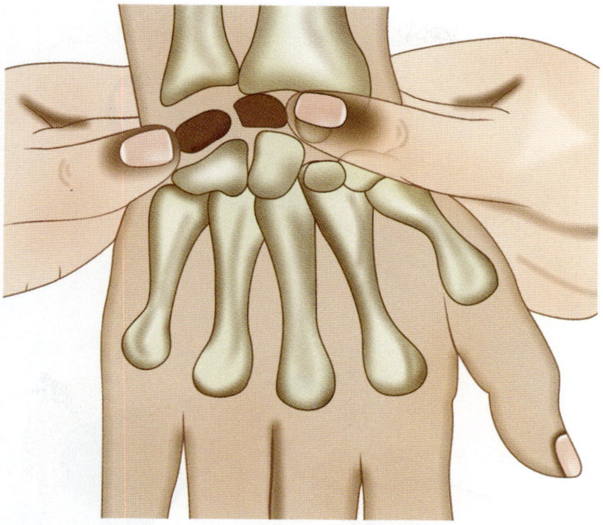

Fig. 21.49: Ballottement test

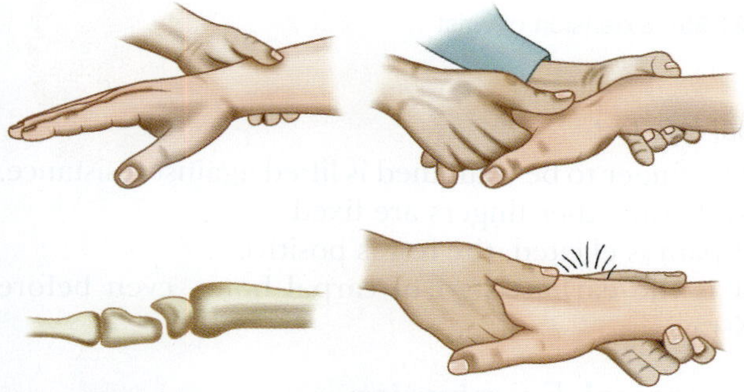

Fig. 21.50: Test for midcarpal instability

and gently swing the wrist from position of full ulnar deviation to full radial deviation. The test is positive, if this normal smooth movement is irregular.

Test for DRUJ Laxity (Fig. 21.51)

- It is to test weakness of wrist. Clicking sensation is present, if ulnar nerve involvement is present.
- *Procedure*: Steady the carpus with one hand, the other hand use to hold distal ulna and attempt to move in dorsal and then volar direction. Note, if any click sensation and complain of pain, then compare other side.

Allen Test (Figs 21.52A to D)

- It determines patency of radial and ulnar arteries
- *Procedure*: To perform this test, open and close the fist several times. Squeeze the fist tightly so that venous blood comes out of palm. Place your thumb over radial artery, index and middle finger over ulnar arterty. Press them against underlying bone to occlude them.

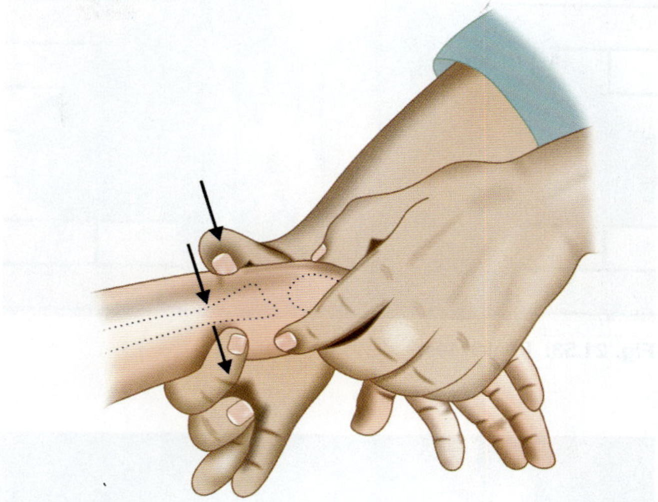

Fig. 21.51: Test for DRUJ laxity

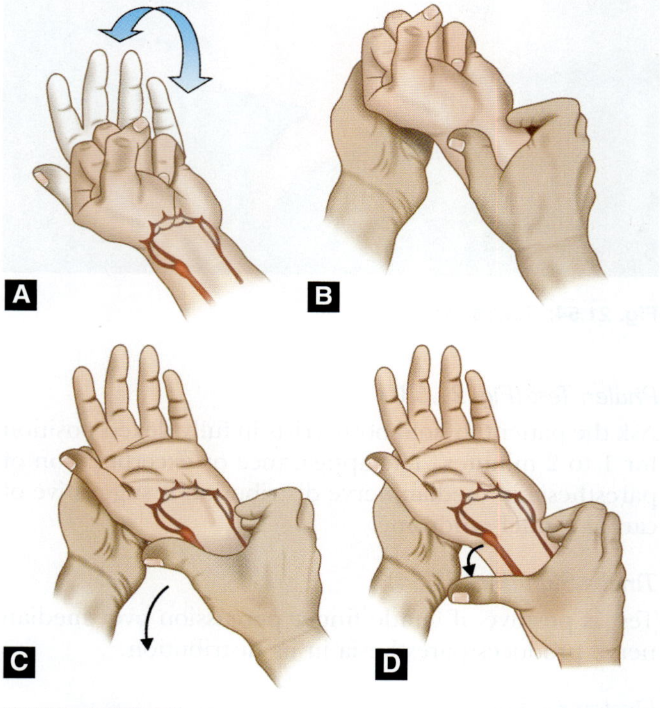

Figs 21.52A to D: Procedure to perform Allen's test

Instruct the patient to open his palm. It should be pale. Release one of the artery at wrist, while maintaining pressure over other. Normally, hand flushes immediately. If flushed slowly, then released artery is partially or completely occluded, so other artery should be tested. Similarly, other hand should be checked for comparison.

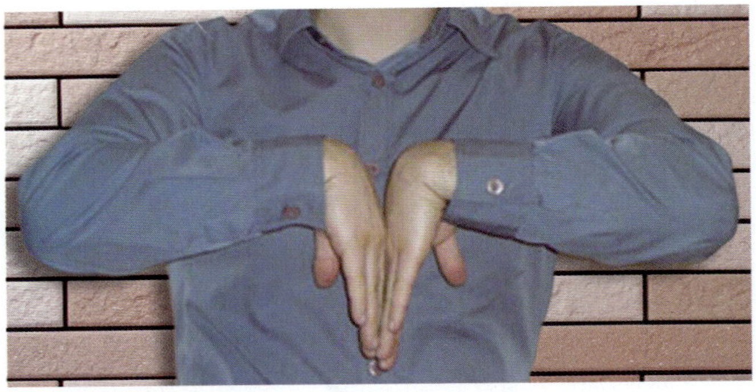

Fig. 21.53: Phalen test

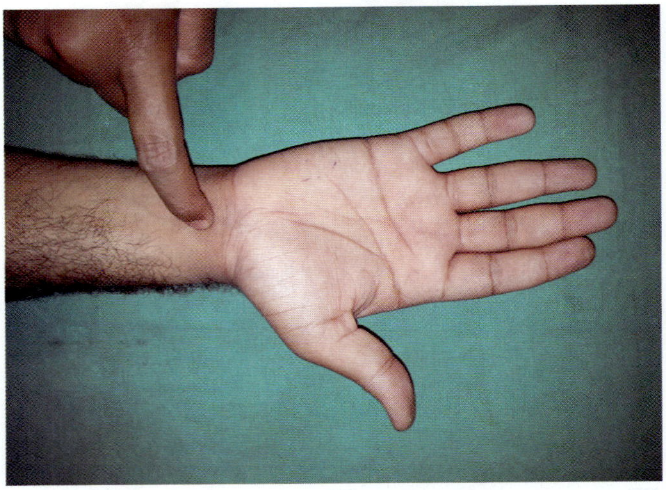

Fig. 21.54: Tinel's sign

Phalen Test (Fig. 21.53)

Ask the patient to hold both wrists in fully flexed position for 1 to 2 minutes. The appearance or excerberation of paresthesia in median nerve distribution is suggestive of carpal tunnel syndrome.

Tinel's Sign (Fig. 21.54)

Test is positive, if gentle finger percussion over median nerve produces paresthesia in its distribution.

Finsterer's Sign

- Percuss at the head of third metacarpal bone with the arm pronated
- If produces pain, then it suggests Keinbock's disease of lunate

Maisonneuve's Sign

- Arm is pronated with elbow flexed
- The hand and wrist are actively dorsiflexed
- If marked hyperextension of wrist is seen, then the test is positive
- It is seen in old malunited Colles.

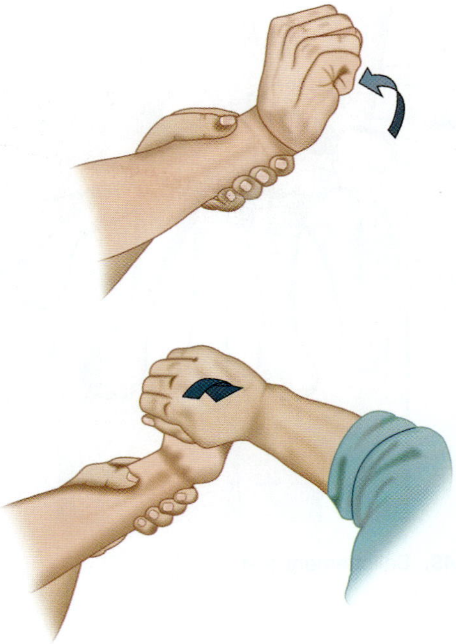

Fig. 21.55: Extension of wrist

Carpal Lift Test

- The finger to be examined is lifted against resistance, while the other fingers are fixed
- If pain is elicited, the test is positive
- It is the earliest sign of carpal bone, even before X-ray.

Neurological Examination

Muscle Power

- Wrist extensor (C6)
- Wrist flexor (C7)
- Supination (C5, C6)
- Pronation (C6, C8, T1)

Sensory Examination

Reflex

- *Wrist extensors (C6) (Fig. 21.55):* Primary extensor and their nerve supply:
  - *Extensor carpi radialis longus:* Radial nerve (C6, C7)
  - Extensor carpi radialis brevis: Radial nerve (C6, C7)
  - *Extensor carpi ulnaris:* Radial nerve (C7)
- *Wrist flexion (Fig. 21.56) (C7):* Primary flexors are:
  - *Flexor carpi radialis:* Median nerve (C7)
  - *Flexor carpi ulnaris:* Ulnar nerve (C8)

Pronation

1. Primary pronator are:
   - *Pronator teres:* Median nerve (C6)
   - *Pronator quadratus:* Anterior interosseous branch of the median nerve (C8, T1)
2. Secondary pronator, is flexor carpi radialis

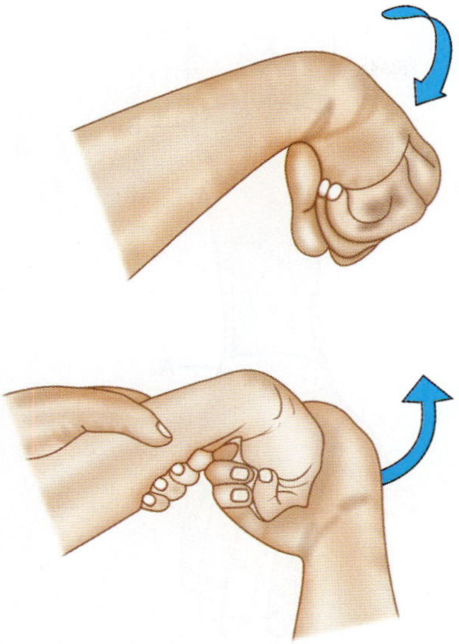

Fig. 21.56: Muscle test for wrist flexion

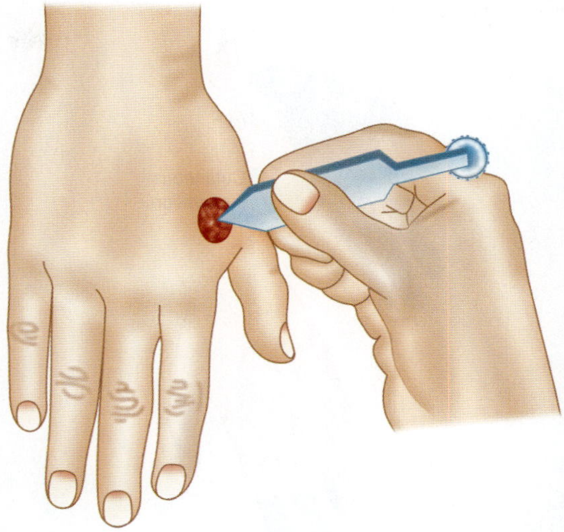

Fig. 21.58: Web space between thumb and index finger is supplied by the radial nerve

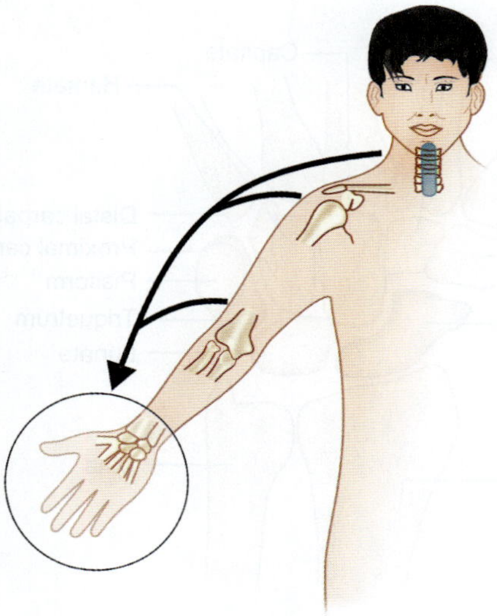

Fig. 21.57: Other joints, e.g. cervical spine, shoulder and elbow that need to be examined along with the wrist joint

Supination

1. Primary supinator are:
   Biceps, e.g. musculocutaneous nerve (C5, C6)
   Supinator, e.g. radial nerve (C6)
2. Secondary supinator is brachioradialis

Other Joints Examinations (Fig. 21.57)

- While examining wrist joint, attention must also be paid to:
  - Cervical spine
  - Shoulder
  - Elbow
- Evaluate causes of wrist pain:
  - Herniated cervical disk
  - Osteoarthritis.

Sensation

Radial Nerve

It supplies the dorsum of hand on the (Fig. 21.58):

- Radial side of third metacarpal
- Dorsal surface of thumb
- Index finger
- Middle finger
- Web space between thumb and index finger (Fig. 21.58).

Median Nerve

It supplies hand on the (Fig. 21.59):

- Radial portion of palm
- Palmar surface of thumb
- Index and middle finger
- It also supplies phalanges of these finger.

Ulnar Nerve

It supplies hand on the (Fig. 21.60):

- The ulnar surface of hand (both dorsal and palmar surface)
- Ring and little finger
- Its purest area is on the volar surface of tip of little finger.

Circumferential Measurement (Fig. 21.61)

- Done at joint level, i.e. the tape passing around both styloid tips
- Second measurement is at the level of the mid forearm
- Look for any wasting and compare with the other side.

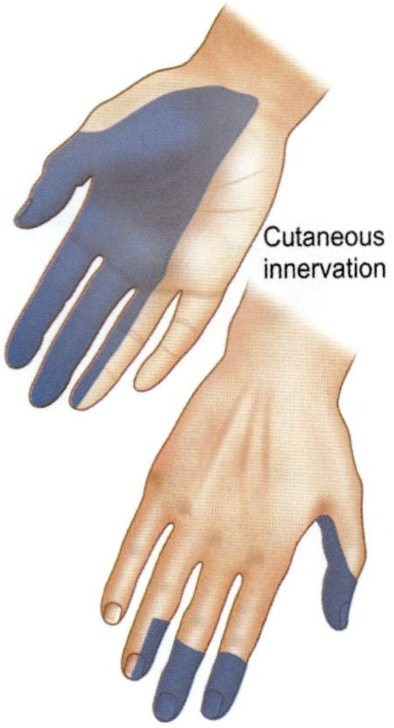

Fig. 21.59: Area supplied by median nerve

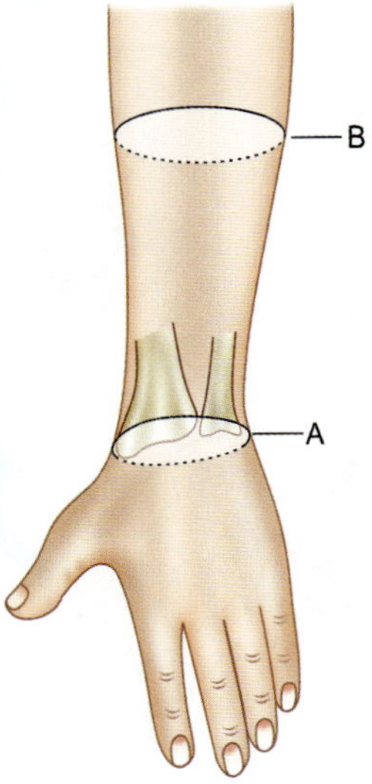

Fig. 21.61: Circumferential measurement—A. Joint level, B. Level of mid forearm

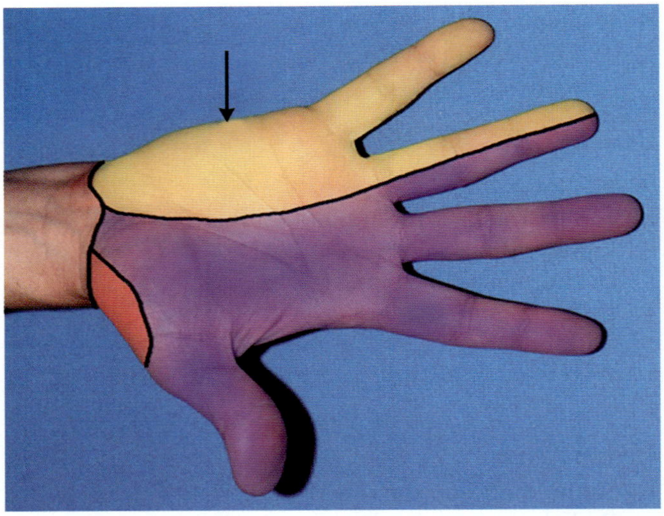

Fig. 21.60: Area supplied by ulnar nerve

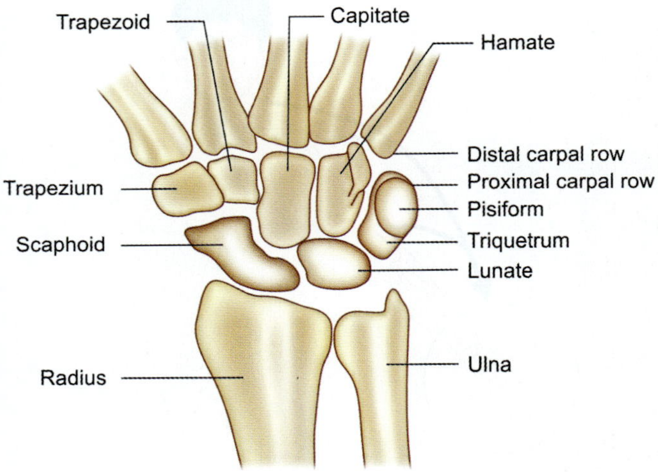

Fig. 21.62: Anteroposterior view of wrist, note the gap between the carpals

Radiology of Wrist

Anteroposterior View

- In anteroposterior view, identify carpal bones and note their shape, density and position
- There are eight carpal bones (Fig. 21.62) in two rows. They are as follows:
  - Pisiform
  - Triquetrum
  - Lunate
  - Scaphoid
  - Trapezium
  - Trapezoid
  - Capitate
  - Hamate
- Note smooth curve between proximal and distal rows of carpus. The distal end of ulna stops short of the radius, to make room for triangular fibrocartilage (Fig. 21.63)
- If there is widening of gap between scapholunate and lunotriquetral, obtain additional view in full radial and ulnar deviation and compare with other side.

Radial Inclination (Fig. 21.64)

- It is an angle between distal articular surface of radius and radial shaft

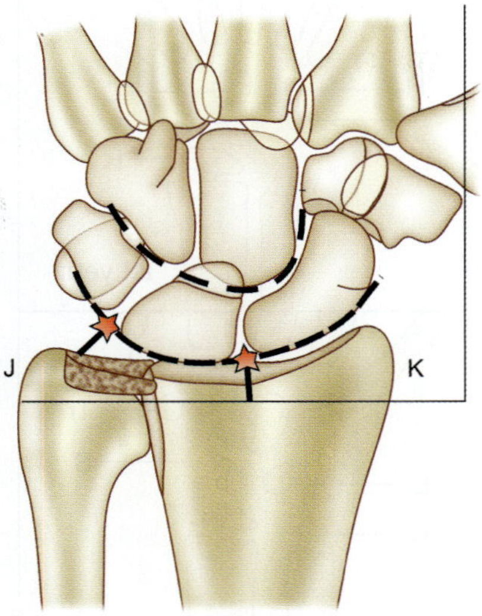

Fig. 21.63: Distal end of ulna stops short of the radius to make room for triangular fibrocartilage—J. Ulna styloid, K. Radial styloid

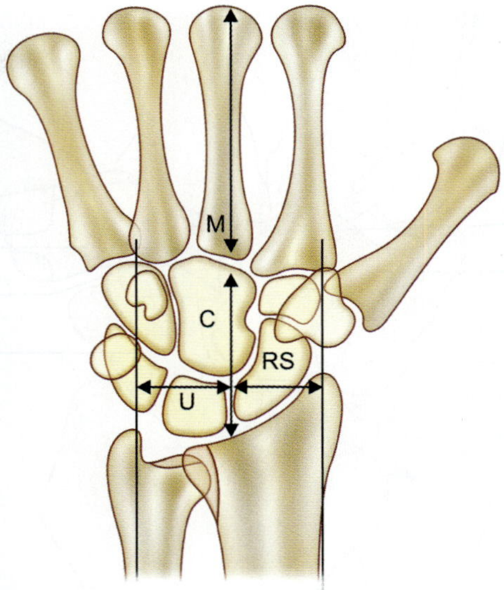

Fig. 21.65: Assessment of carpal height and drift—M. Middle metacarpal; C. Capitate; RS. Radial styloid; U. Ulnar axis; C. Triquetral

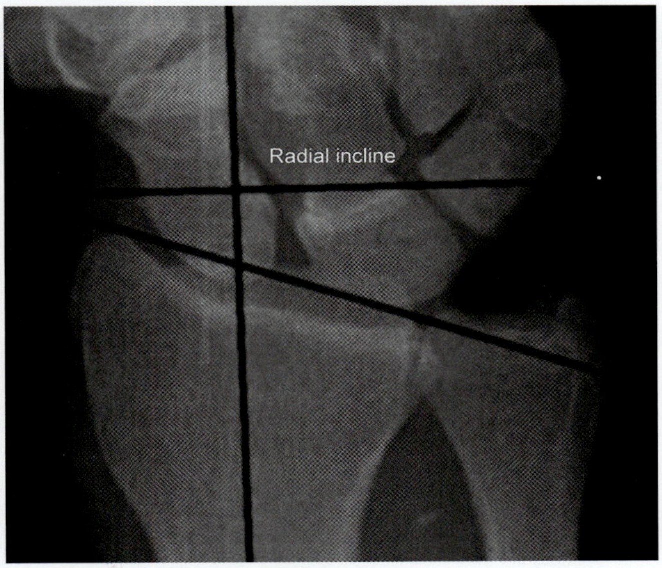

Fig. 21.64: Radial inclination

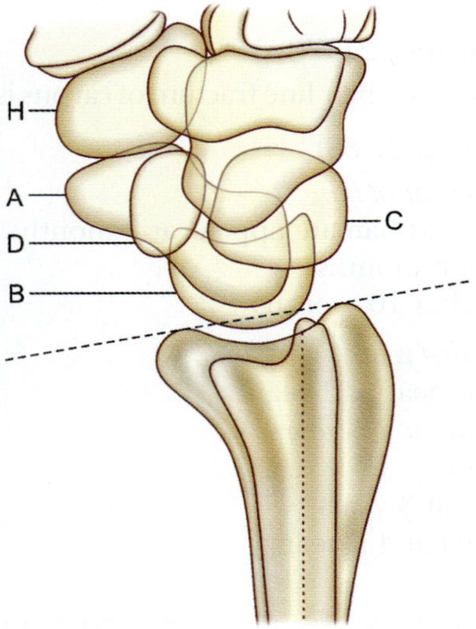

Fig. 21.66: Structures seen on lateral radiograph—H. Trapezium; A. Tubercle and body of scaphoid; D. Pisiform one; B. Crest of lunate; C. Triquetral

- It is decreased after Colle's fracture
- Normal range is 19 to 25°.

Assessment of Carpal Height and Drift (Fig. 21.65)

A line drawn through middle metacarpal (M), carpus (C) and its distance from radial styloid (RS), ulnar axis (U) expresses these ratio as:

- Carpal height ratio: C/M (Normal: 0.51–0.57)
- Chamy measurement: U/M (Normal: 0.25–0.31)
- McMurty's index: U/M (Normal: 0.27–0.33)

Lateral Radiograph

- Structures seen on lateral radiograph (Fig. 21.66) are as follows:
  - Trapezium
  - Tubercle and body of scaphoid
  - Pisiform bone
  - Crest of lunate
  - Triquetral
- The plane of wrist joint normally tilted at 5° anteriorly

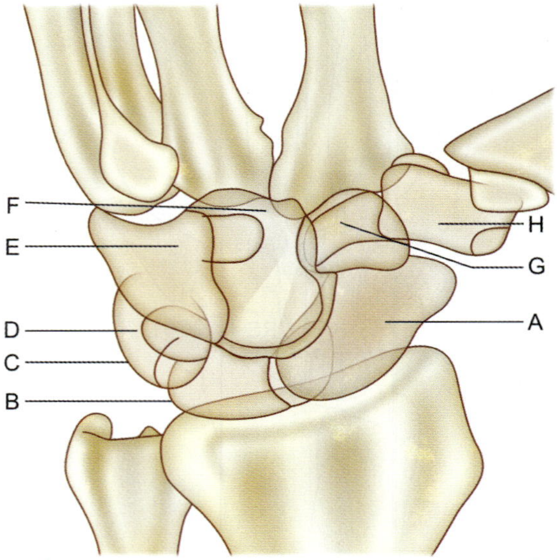

Fig. 21.67: Wrist shown in oblique view—A. Tubercle of scaphoid; B. Creast of lunate; C. Triquetral; D. Pisiform; E. Hamate; F. Capitate; G. Trapezoid; H. Trapezium

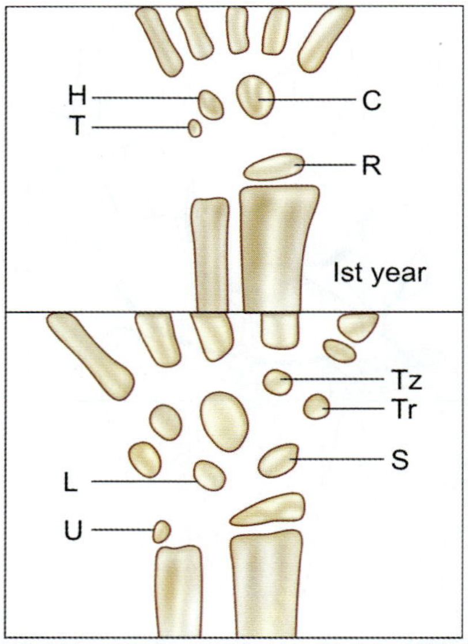

Fig. 21.68: Ossification in first year and after first year of life—H. Hamate; C. Capitate; R. Radial styloid; Tz. Trapezium; T. Triquetrum; L. Lunate; U. Ulnar styloid; S. Scaphoid; Tr. Trapezoid

Oblique View (Fig. 21.67)

This is taken, when hair line fracture of carpus is suspected.

Ossification (Fig. 21.68)

I. *In the first year of life*
- Capitate and hamate appear at 2 months
- Radius at 6 months
- Triquetral at 10 months

II. *After the first year*
- Lunate appear at 2 years
- Trapezium at 2.5 years
- Trapezoid
- Scaphoid at 3 years
- Distal ulna at 4.5 years

CONGENITAL DEFORMITIES OF HAND

Introduction

A congenital disorder involves defects or damage to a developing fetus. It may be the result of:
- Genetic abnormalities
- The intrauterine environment
- Errors of morphogenesis
- Chromosomal abnormality.

Congenital Deformities of Hand

Swanson, Barsky and Entin classification
- Failure of formation (Arrest of development)
- Failure of differentiation (or separation)
- Duplication
- Overgrowth
- Undergrowth
- Congenital constriction band syndrome
- Generalized skeletal abnormalities.

Incidence and prevalence: 11 per 10,000 population

Most common anomalies
- Syndactyly
- Polydactyly
- Camptodactyly
- Clinodactyly
- Congenital amputations
- Radial clubhand.

Embryology

- The arm arises as a small bud of tissue on the lateral body wall beginning on 26th day of gestation, preceding leg bud formation by only 24 hours
- "Proximal-to-Distal" growth and development fashion
- Growth occurs under apical ectodermal ridge, which produces fibroblast growth factor
- By day 31 of gestation, hand paddle is present
- Programmed cellular death and fissuring of hand paddle is completed by day 36, with central rays forming first, followed by preaxial and postaxial digits
- This is followed by development of:
  - Chondral elements
  - Endochondral ossification
  - Joint, muscle and vascular development
  - The entire process is completed by 8 weeks of gestation.

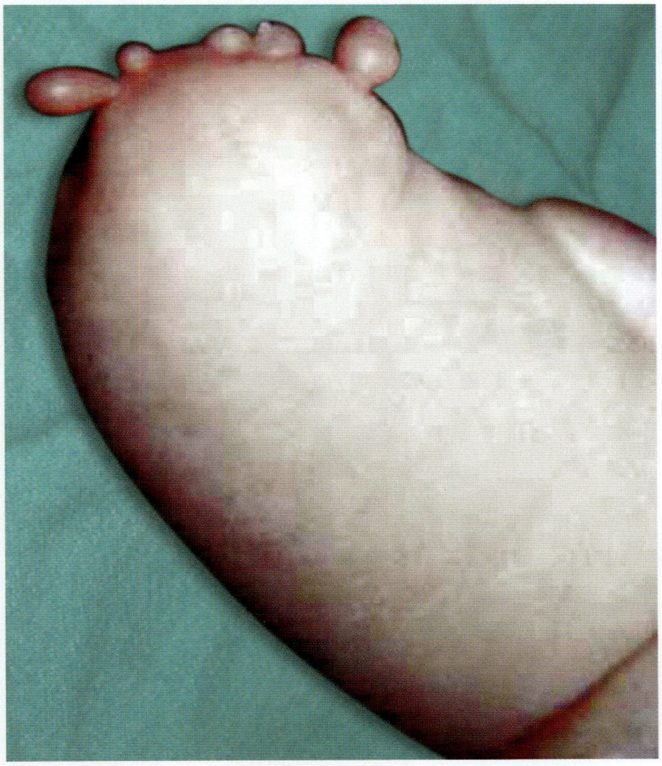

Fig. 21.69: Failure of formation

Failure of Formation or Arrest of Development (Fig. 21.69)

The upper limb can fail to develop either:
- Transversely
- Longitudinally.

Transverse Deficiencies

- These include deformities in which there is complete absence of parts distal to some point on the upper extremity, producing amputation-like stumps
- Further classification is by naming the level at which the remaining stump terminates
- Ninty-eight percent are unilateral and the most common level is upper 1/3rd of forearm.

Causes

- Failure of apical ectodermal ridge, possibly secondary to infarct
- Use of misoprostol, to induce abortion
- Usually, slightly bulbous, well-padded stump is present, while in more distal deficiencies, rudimentary vestigial digital 'Nubbins' are present
- Hypoplasia of more proximal muscles helps differentiate these deficiencies from deficiencies associated with congenital bands
- Usually, forearm is 7 cm at birth and no more than 10 cm in adults.

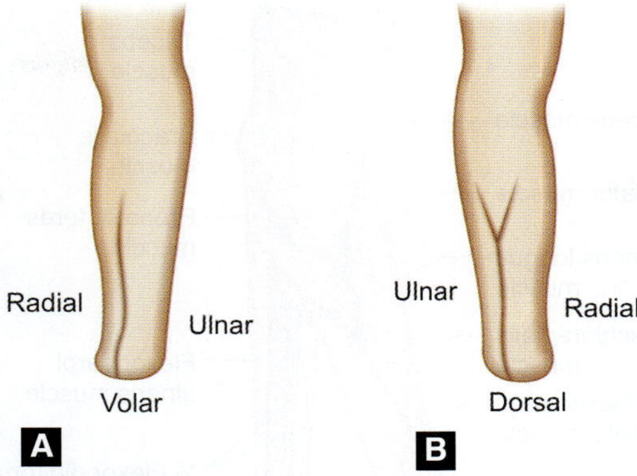

Figs 21.70A and B: Incisions on flexor/volar and dorsal surfaces of forearm

Management

I. *Prosthetic management:* It is useful for patients who do not require surgery:
- *Timing:* At the time of crawling and certainly at the time of independent ambulation. The fitting of upper limb prosthesis should complement and enhance the normal developmental milestones.
- Choice of prosthesis depends on following:
  - Level of amputation
  - Age
  - Mental capacity of child
  - Socioeconomic conditions.

II. *Surgical management:* Krukenberg reconstruction and Nathan and Trung modification (Figs 21.70 to 21.72)
- It consists of separation of radius and ulna to allow a sensate, "Chop-Stick" like forearm
- Best in bilateral below-elbow amputation
- Prosthesis can still be used for cosmesis
- Surgical prerequisites are:
  - Stump length of 8 cm from insertion of biceps
  - Normal forearm musculature
  - Patient and family should be willing to undergo this disfiguring operation, to improve function.

Procedure of Krukenberg reconstruction (Figs 21.70 to 21.72)
Skin closure on flexor surface of forearm elliptical area, indicates location of any needed split-skin grafts

Metacarpal lengthening
- It is usually reserved for transverse deficiencies at level of metacarpophalengeal joints in a child with at least one remaining digit
- *Ideal age:* 5 to 11 years
- Matev (1967) described osteotomy of digital ray, with gradual distraction and subsequent bone grafting for a deficient thumb
- An ideal of 4 to 5 cm of length can be gained, but improved function and cosmesis may not be achieved.

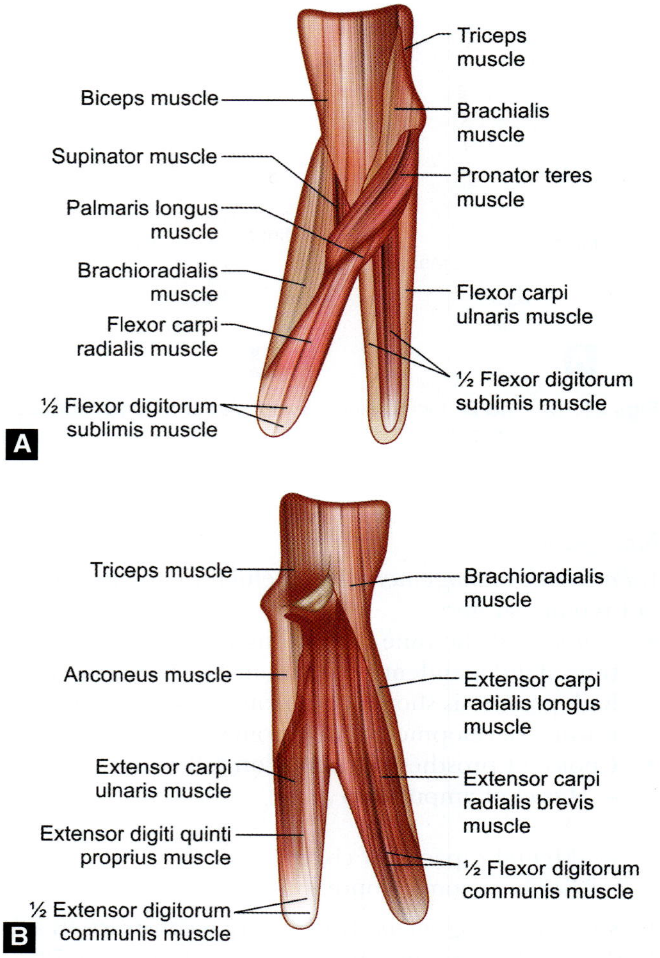

Figs 21.71A and B: Forearm muscles have been separated into two groups

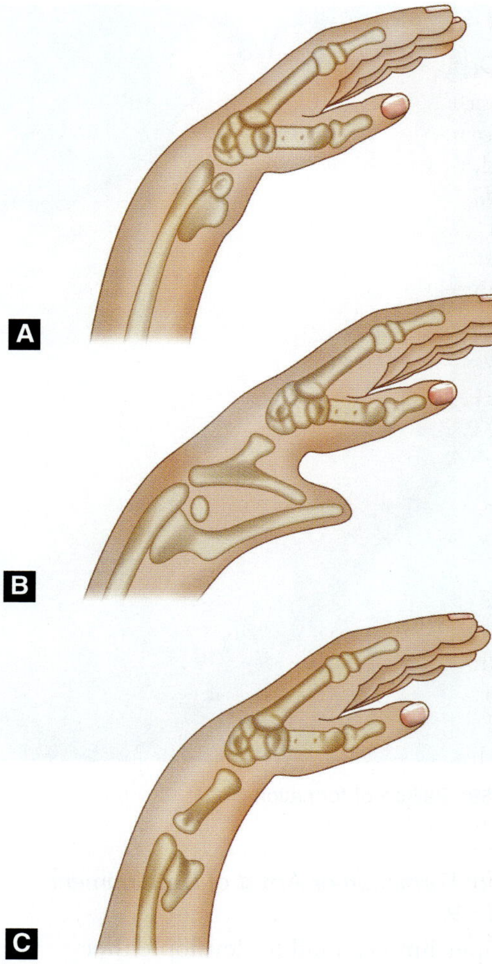

Figs 21.73A to C: Different types of longitudinal deficiencies

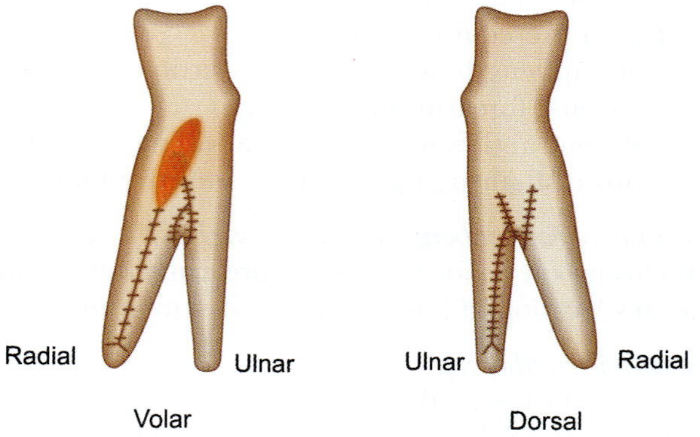

Fig. 21.72: Skin closure on flexor surface of forearm elliptical area

Longitudinal Deficiencies (Figs 21.73A to C)

It includes all failure-of-formation anomalies that are not transverse deficiencies. These include:

- Phocomelia
- Radial ray dysplasia
- Ulnar ray dysplasia
- Central dysplasia

Phocomelia

Phocomelia is a greek word, meaning "Seal Limb" or "Flipper".

There are three anatomical patterns:

Type 1: Complete phocomelia with absence of all limb bones proximal to hand

Type 2: Absence or extreme hypoplasia of proximal limb bones with forearm and hand attached to trunk

Type 3: Hand attached directly to humerus

Treatment

- Usually conservative
- Surgery indicated only for shoulder instability, limb shortening or inadequate thumb opposition
- Prosthesis may help to certain extent.

Radial Club Hand

Radial Deficiencies

- Include all malformations with longitudinal failure of formation of parts along the pre-axial or radial border of upper extremity
- *Radial club hand:* Deficient or absent thenar muscles, shortened, unstable and absent thumb, shortened and absent radius
- Thalidomide may play a role in its occurrence.

Heikel's classification of radial dysplasia (Figs 21.74A to D)
Type 1: Short distal radius
Type 2: Hypoplastic radius
Type 3: Partial absence of radius
Type 4: Total absence of radius

Manske's modified classification of radial longitudnal deficiency (Table 21.2)

Management

- *Nonsurgical management:* Immediately after birth, early casting and splinting is done. A light, molded plastic short-arm splint is applied along radial side of forearm and removed only for bathing, until infant begins to use his hands and then it is worn only at night. There is no satisfactory conservative treatment for associated significant thumb deformities.
- *Surgical management*: Ideal age: 3 to 6 months. Pollicization, if indicated, follows at 9 to 12 months.

Specific Contraindications

- Severe associated anomalies, not compatible with life
- Inadequate elbow flexion
- Mild deformity with adequate radial support
- Older patients, who are well-adjusted.

Procedures to be Considered

- Centralization of the hand
- Centralization of the hand and tendon transfers
- Pollicization for reconstruction of thumb with radial clubhand
- Opponensplasty
- Triceps transfer to restore elbow flexion

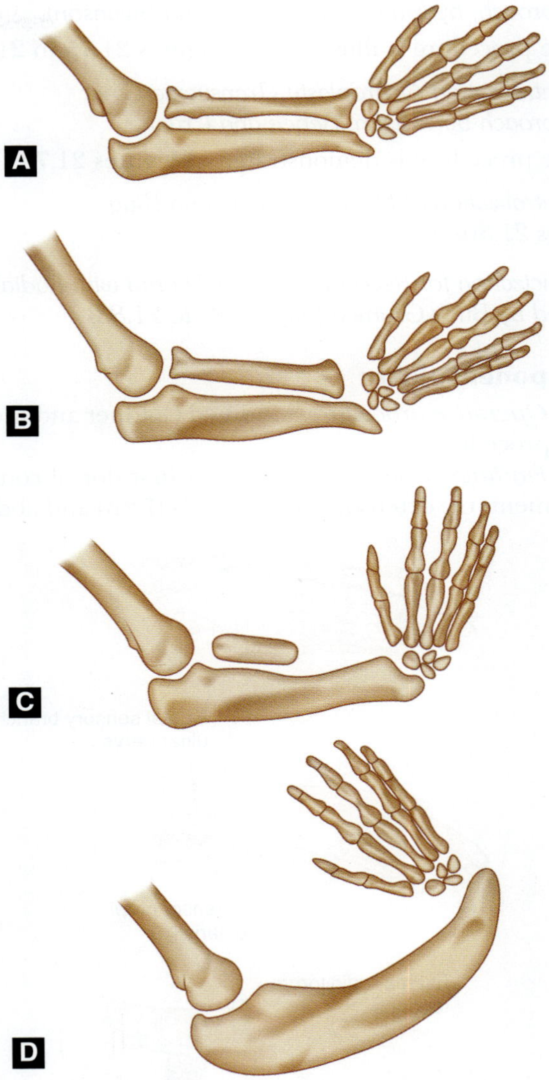

Figs 21.74A to D: Different types of radial dysplasia—(A) Type 1. Short distal radius; (B) Type 2. Hypoplastic radius; (C) Type 3. Partial absence of radius; (D) Type 4. Total absence of radius

Table 21.2: Manske's modified classification of radial longitudinal deficiency

Type	*Thumb*	*Carpus*	*Distal radius*	*Proximal radius*
N	Hypoplastic or absent	Normal	Normal	Normal
0	Hypoplastic or absent	Absence, hypoplasia or coalition	Normal	Normal, radioulnar synostosis, or congenital dislocation of radial head
1	Hypoplastic or absent	Absence, hypoplasia or coalition	> 2 mm shorter than ulna	Normal, radioulnar synostosis, or congenital dislocation of radial head
2	Hypoplastic or absent	Absence, hypoplasia or coalition	Hypoplasia	Hypoplasia
3	Hypoplastic or absent	Absence, hypoplasia or coalition	Physis absent	Variable hypoplasia
4	Hypoplastic or absent	Absence, hypoplasia or coalition	Absent	Absent

Centralization Arthroplasty (Transverse Ulnar Approach, by Manske, McCarroll and Swanson)

The procedure is illustrated in Figures 21.75 to 21.78

Centralization Arthroplasty (Transverse Ulnar Approach by Watson, Bebee and Cruz)

The procedure is demonstrated in Figures 21.79A to G

Centralization of Hand by Bayne and Klug (Figs 21.80A to C)

Pollicization for Reconstruction of Thumb with Radial Club hand by Buck-Grumco (Figs 21.81 to 21.83)

Opponensplasty

- *Operative procedure:* Modified Goldner and Riordan procedure
- *Findings:* Complete absence of first dorsal compartment, i.e. extensor pollicis brevis (EPB) and abductor

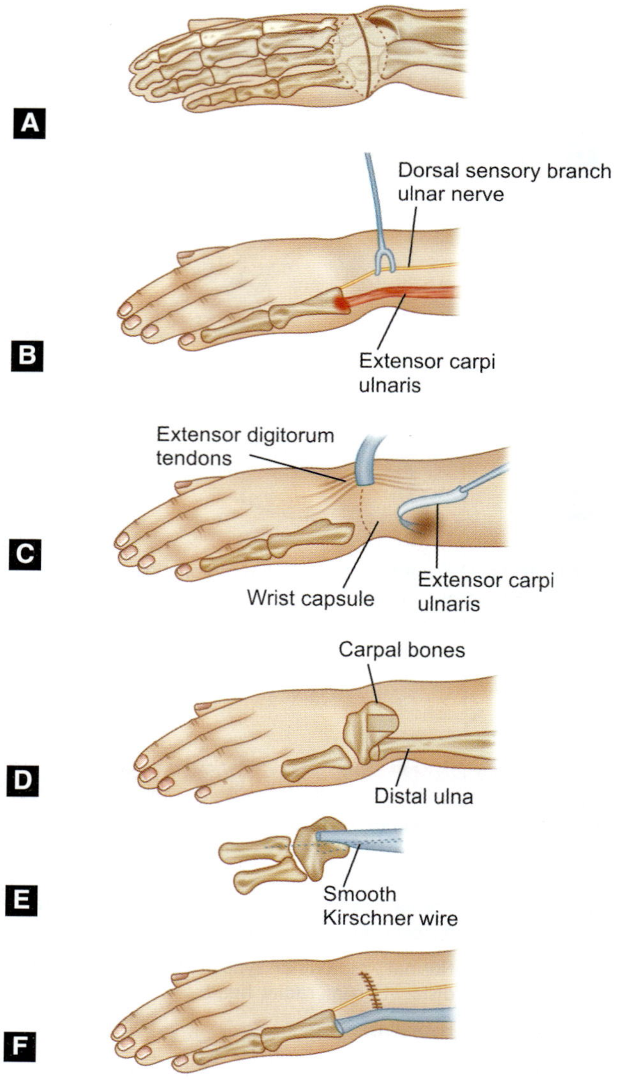

Figs 21.75A to F: Different steps of centralization arthroplasty

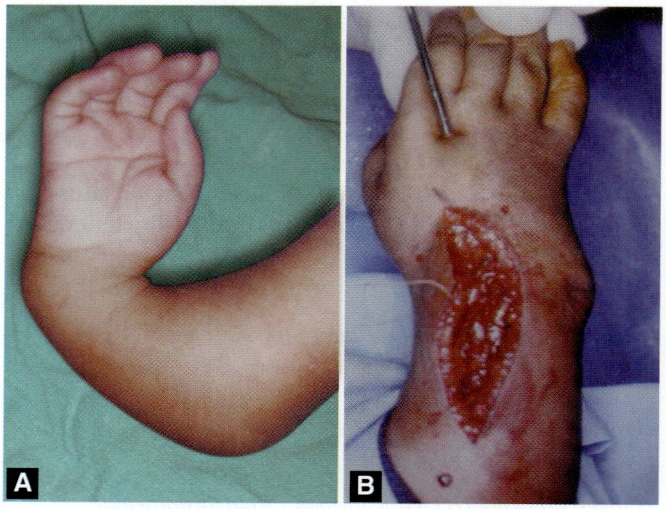

Figs 21.76A and B: Centralization arthroplasty, transverse ulnar approach by Manske, McCarroll and Swanson

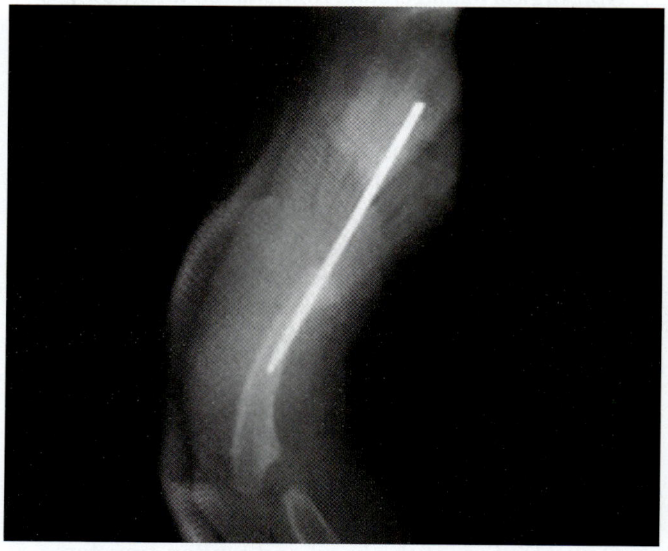

Fig. 21.77: X-ray taken after performing centralization arthroplasty

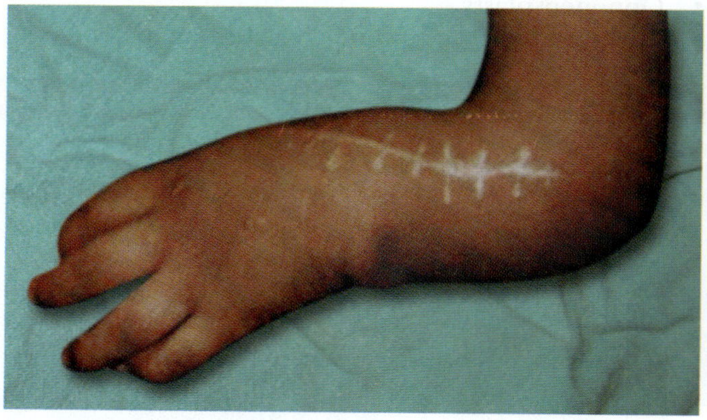

Fig. 21.78: Centralization arthroplasty performed, by transverse ulnar approach

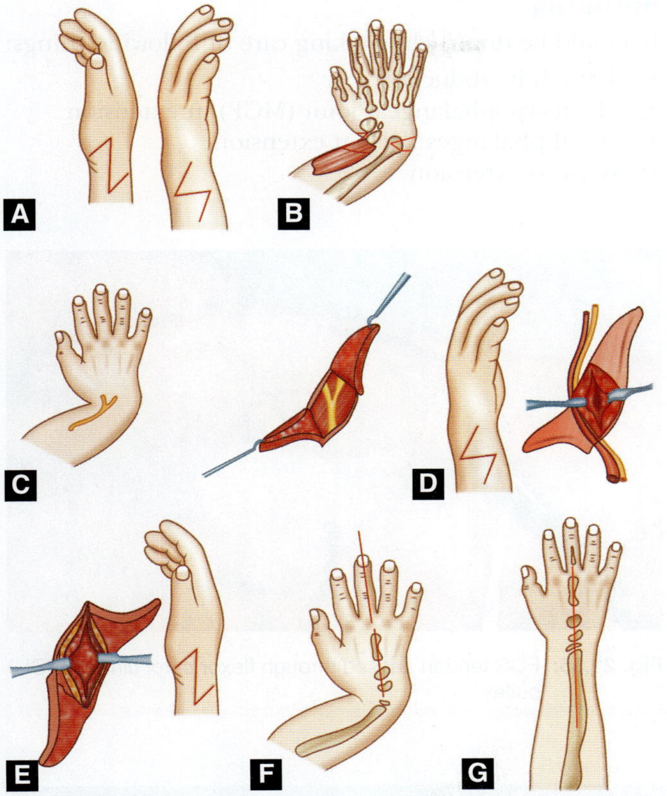

Figs 21.79A to G: Different steps of centralization arthroplasty (transverse ulnar approach by Watson, Bebee and Cruz)

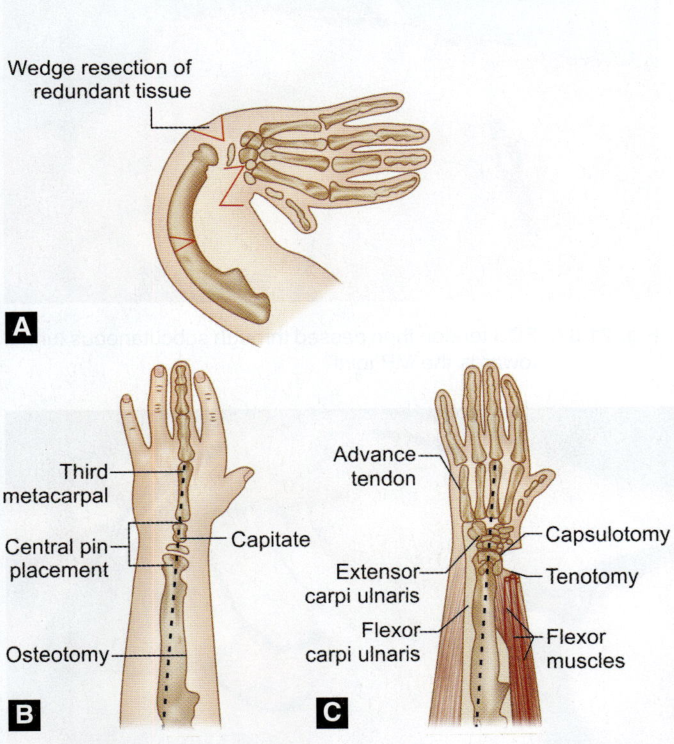

Figs 21.80A to C: Different steps of carrying out centralization of hand procedure as given by Bayne and Klug

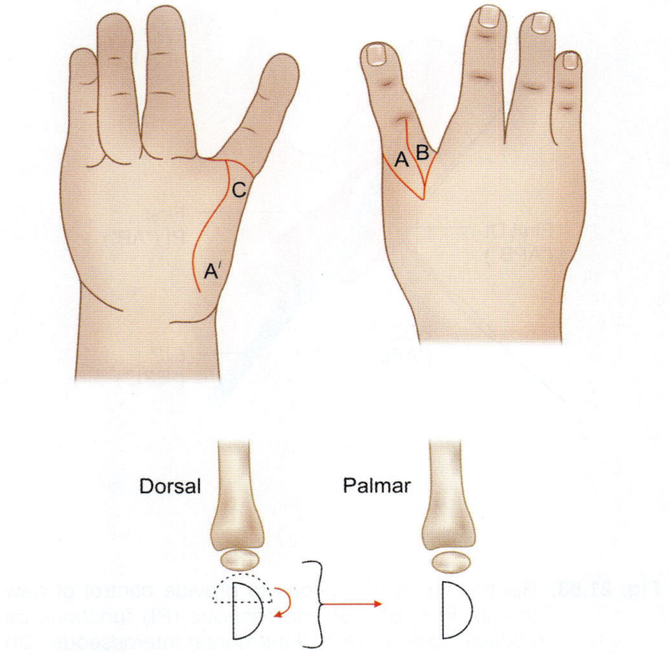

Fig. 21.81: Pollicization of index finger—A. Palmar skin incision; B. Dorsal skin incision; C. Rotation of metacarpal head into flexon to prevent postoperative hyperextension

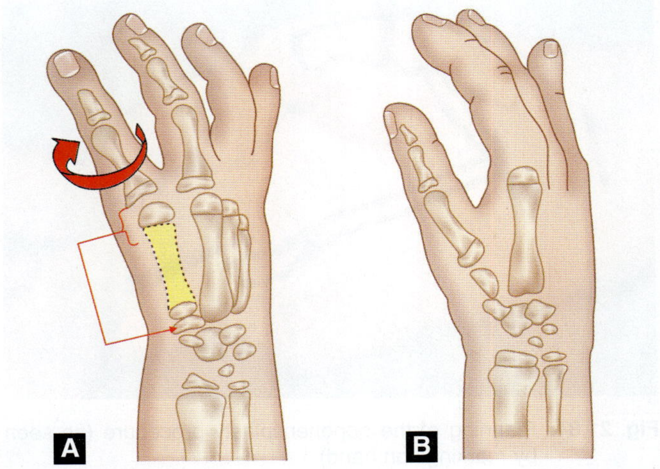

Figs 21.82A and B: (A) Index finger rotated about 160° along long axis; (B) Final positioning in about 40° of palmar abduction with metacarpal head secured to metacarpal base or carpus

pollicis longus (APL) and hypoplastic extensor pollicis longus (EPL).

- *Plan*: Rerouting of ring finger flexor digitorum superficialis (FDS) tendon and then attaching it to extensor pollicis longus (EPL) and base of proximal phalanx of thumb through transosseous tunnel (Fig. 21.84).
- The procedure is demonstrated in Figures 21.85 to 21.89.

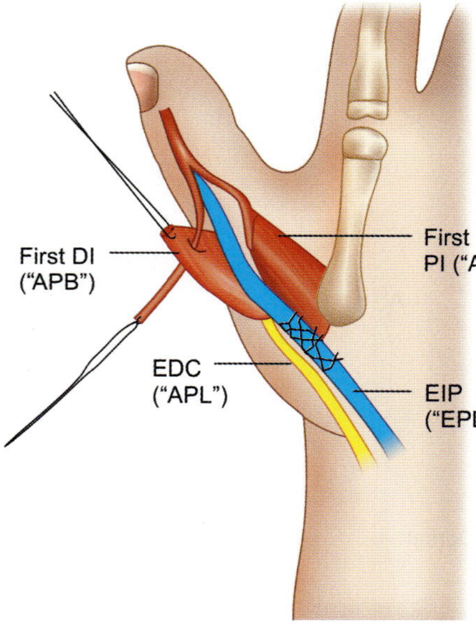

Fig. 21.83: Reattachment of tendons to provide control of new thumb. First palmar interosseous (PI) functions as adductor pollicis (AP); First dorsal interosseous (DI) as abductor pollicis brevis (APB); Extensor digitorum communis (EDC) as abductor pollicis longues (APL); and extensor indicis proprius (EIP) as extensor pollicis longus (EPL)

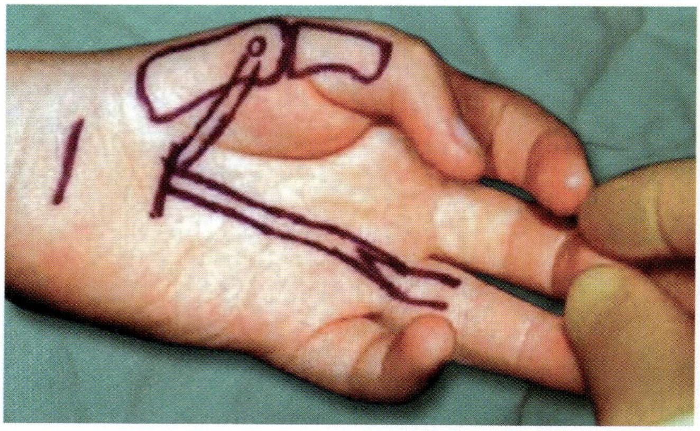

Fig. 21.84: Planning of the opponensplasty procedure (as seen by markings on hand)

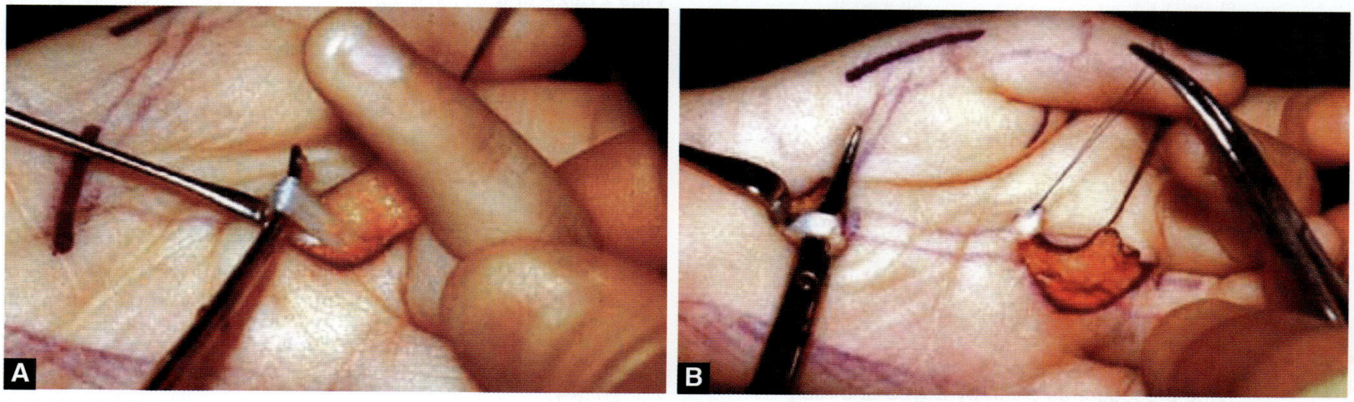

Figs 21.85A and B: The two slips of FDS detached from ring finger

Splinting

It should be done, while taking care of following things:

- Thumb in abduction
- Metacarpophalangeal joint (MCP) in extension
- Distal phalanges (DP) in extension
- Wrist in extension

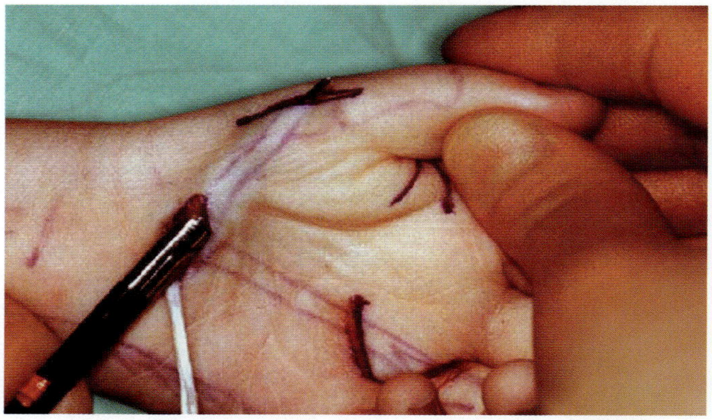

Fig. 21.86: FDS tendon passed through flexor carpi ulnaris (FCU) pulley

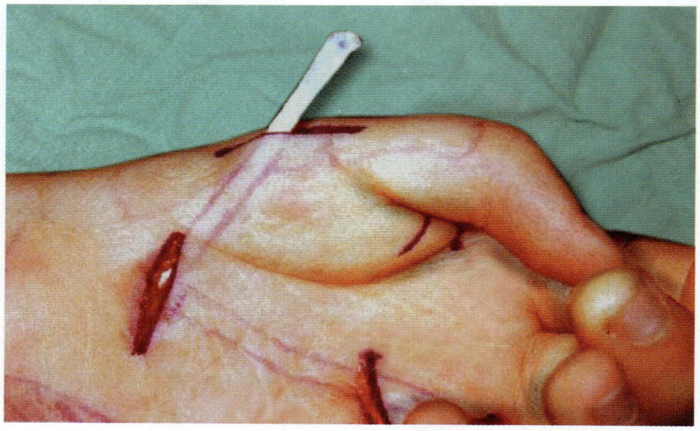

Fig. 21.87: FDS tendon then passed through subcutaneous tunnel towards the MP joint

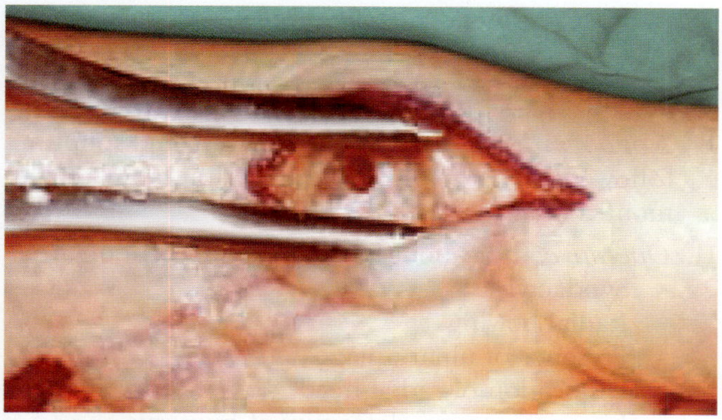

Fig. 21.88: A transverse hole drilled into the proximal phalanx and one slip of FDS attached to it

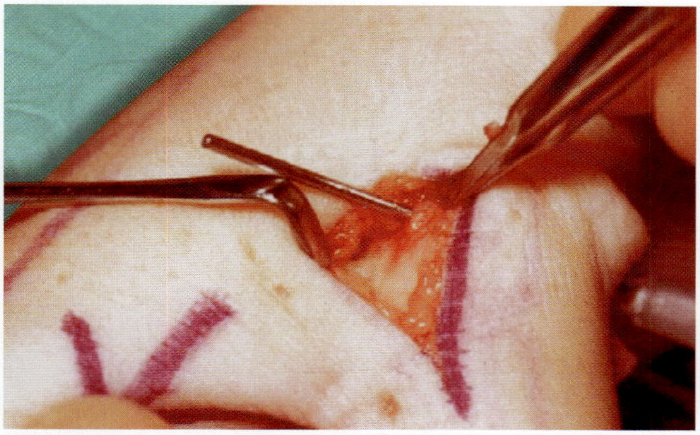

Fig. 21.89: The second slip attached to the EPL tendon

Cleft Hand

Central Deficiencies

- Also known as “ectrodactyly”, “crab claw” or “lobster claw” (Fig. 21.90)
- Cleft deficiencies of the hand include malformations, in which there is a longitudinal failure of formation of the second, third or fourth ray
- It also includes a one-digit (fifth-ray) hand
- Two main patterns of occurrences are:
  - Typical pattern of central deficiency, with central V-shaped cleft (Fig. 21.91).
  - Atypical pattern of central deficiency with U-shaped defect, involving index, long and ring fingers (Fig. 21.92).

Flatt’s classification of central deficiencies (Figs 21.93A to C)

Treatment

- No definitive treatment
- Operative treatment must be Tailor-made
- Surgical reconstruction includes:
  - Closure of cleft
  - Release of syndactyly
  - Correction of thumb adduction contracture
  - Removal of deforming bony elements
  - Correction of delta phalynx

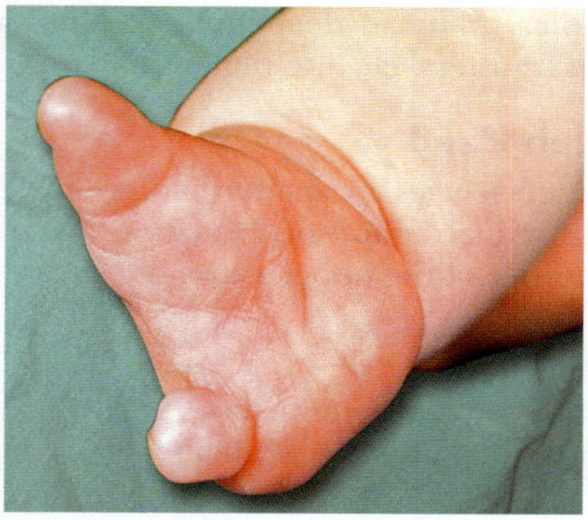

Fig. 21.90: Cleft hand

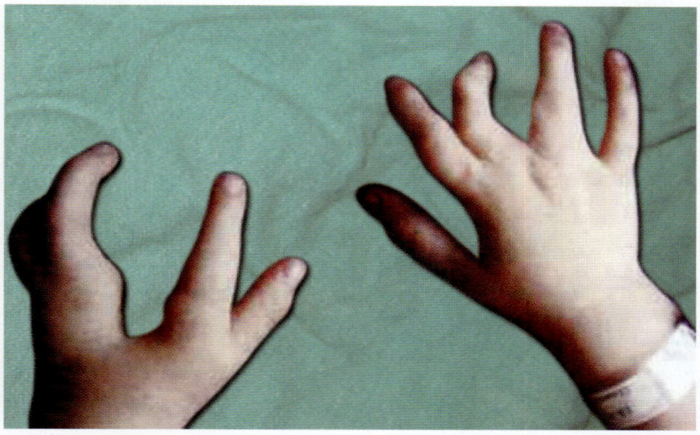

Fig. 21.91: Typical pattern of central deficiency with central V-shaped cleft

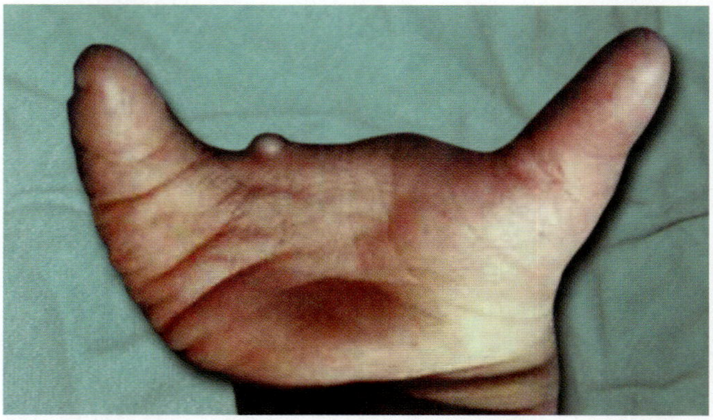

Fig. 21.92: Atypical pattern of central deficiency with U-shaped defect, involving index, long and ring fingers

- In atypical pattern, deepening of palm for grasp, tendon transfers, etc. are required.

Ulnar Club Hand

- Ulnar deficiencies are malformations, in which there is longitudinal failure of formation along the post-axial border of the upper extremity
- Other terms used are:
  - Dysmelia
  - Paraxial ulnar hemimelia
  - Congenital absence of ulna.

Swanson's Classification of Ulnar Deficiency (Figs 21.94A to D)

Treatment

I. *Nonoperative:* Serial corrective casting and splinting, followed by surgery if indicated, for more than 6 months of age

II. *Operative:* Indications for surgical intervention are:
  - Syndactyly
  - Radial bowing
  - Presence of ulnar anlage
  - Dislocation of radial head
  - Internal rotation deformity of humerus.

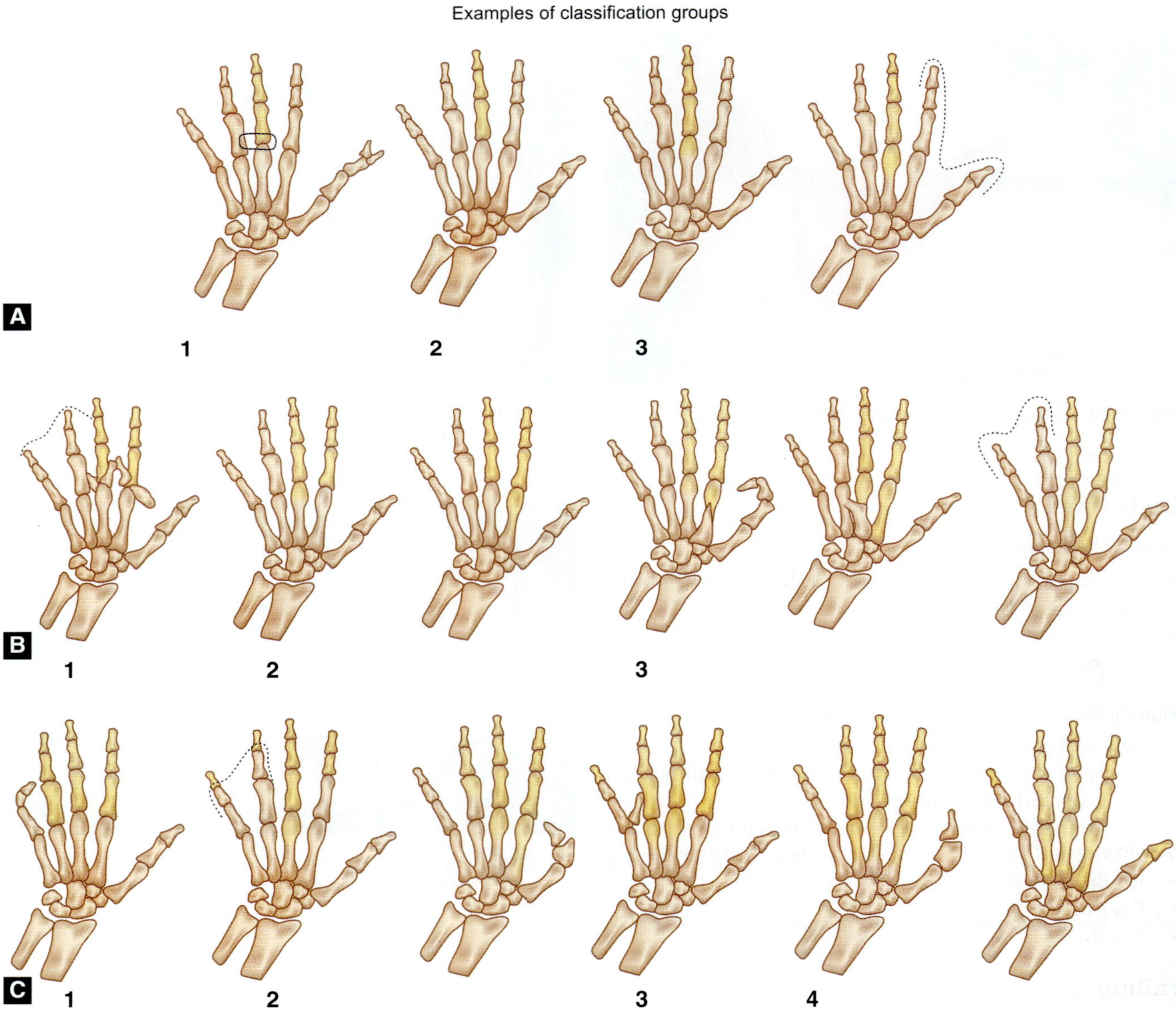

Figs 21.93A to C: Flatt's classification of central deficiencies

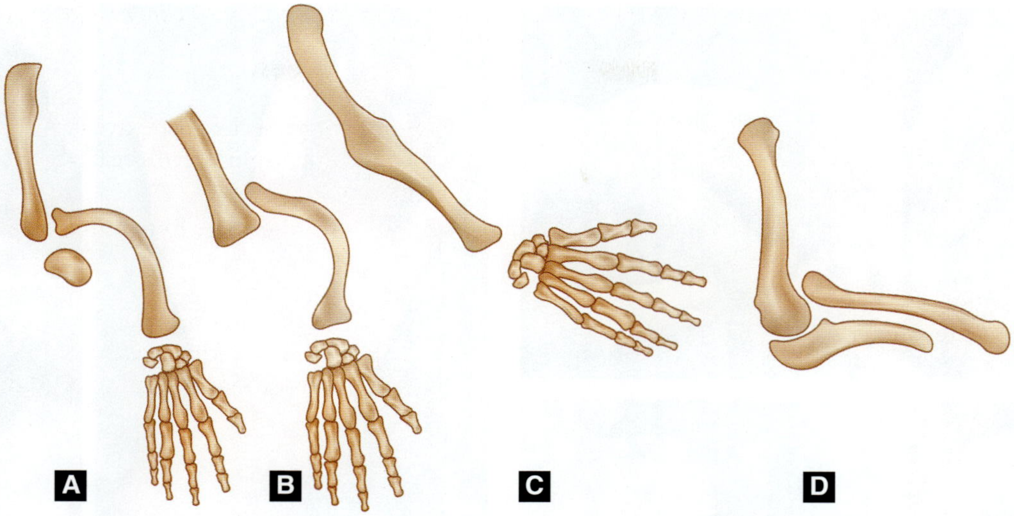

Figs 21.94A to D: Swanson's classification of ulnar deficiency—(A) Hypoplasia or partial defect of ulna; (B) Total defect of ulna; (C) Partial or total defect of ulna, with humeroradial synostosis; (D) Total or partial defect of ulna, with congenital amputation at wrist

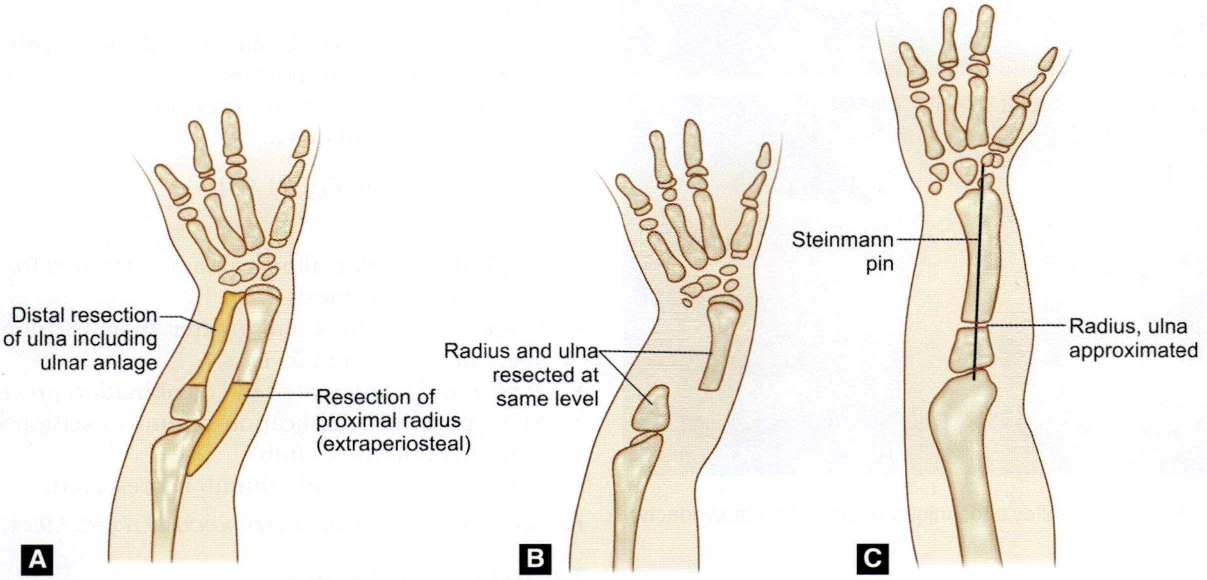

Figs 21.95A to C: Different steps of surgical correction of ulnar club hand: Creation of one-bone forearm—(A) Resection of distal ulnar anlage and proximal radius (shaded areas); (B) Alignment of distal radius and proximal ulna; (C) Kirchner wire extending into carpals used to stabilize radial and ulnar segments

Surgical Procedures

- Rotational osteotomy of first metacarpal
- Excision of ulnar anlage
- Creation of one-bone forearm (Figs 21.95A to C).

Failure of Differentiation

- Syndactyly
- Alpert syndrome

Syndactyly

Syndactyly word derived from Greek "συν" meaning together or plus "δακτυλος" meaning finger, is a condition where two or more digits are fused together.

Treatment

Intraoperative or Whitey's technique: The procedure is illustrated in Figures 21.96A to C.

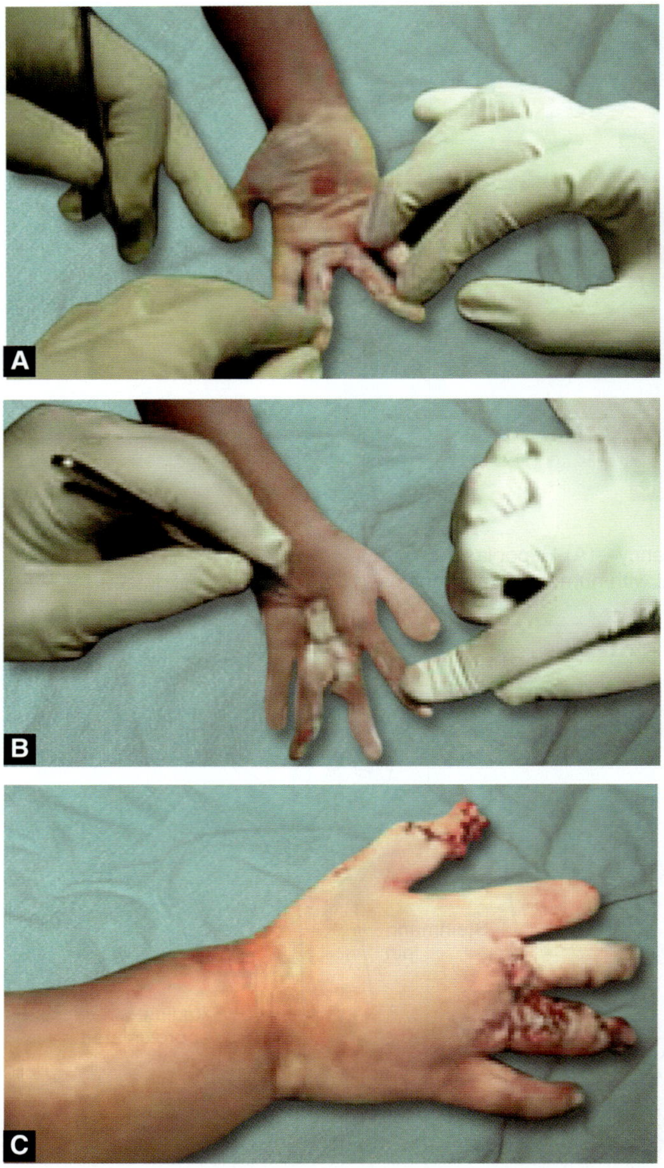

Figs 21.96A to C: Whitey's technique of correction of syndactyly

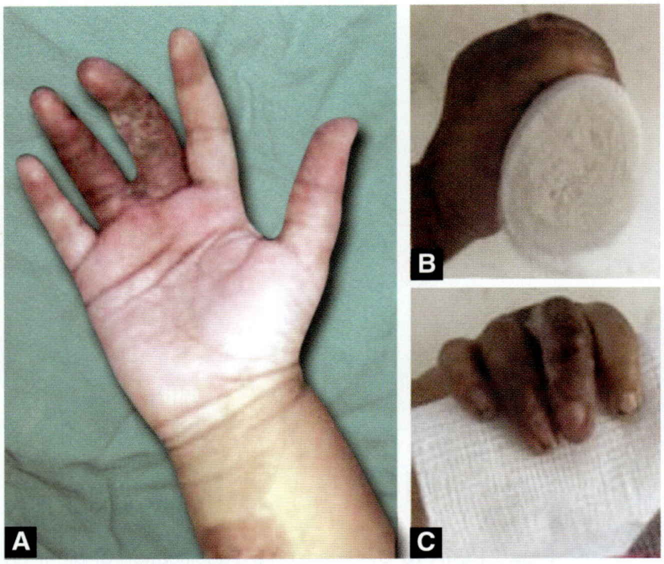

Figs 21.97A to C: Postoperative follow-up after correcting syndactyly

Postoperative follow-up: This has been shown in Figures 21.97A to C.

Duplication

- Polydactyly
- Bifid thumb

Polydactyly

- Preaxial polydactyly, e.g. bifid thumb
- Central polydactyly, e.g. duplication of index, middle or ring finger
- Postaxial polydactyly, e.g. duplication of little finger
- Ulnar dimelia, e.g. mirror hand.

Bifid Thumb

- Complete or partial duplication of the thumb
- *Incidence:* 1/3000 live births
- Seventy percent cases are unilateral
- Exact cause is unknown.

Wessel Classification (Fig. 21.98)

Treatment

- Surgical correction almost always warranted for better function and cosmesis
- Surgery generally, done greater than 18 months of age, but not beyond 5 years
- Type 1 and 2 are treated by "combination procedure"
- More proximal duplication requires excision of the more hypoplastic thumb
- Usually, the ulnar side thumb is preserved.

Bilhaut-Cloquet "combination procedure" (Figs 21.99A and B).

Triphalangeal Thumb

- It has three phalanges instead of normal two (Fig. 21.100)
- These are of two types:
  - Wedge-shaped extraossicle: Angular deformity
  - Normal-sized extraossicle: "Five-finger hand"
- Also classified as "opposable and nonopposable".

Treatment

Nonoperative treatment: It is not very useful

Operative treatment (Figs 21.101A to D): Goals of an operative treatment are:

- Correction of angular deformity
- Restoration of normal length

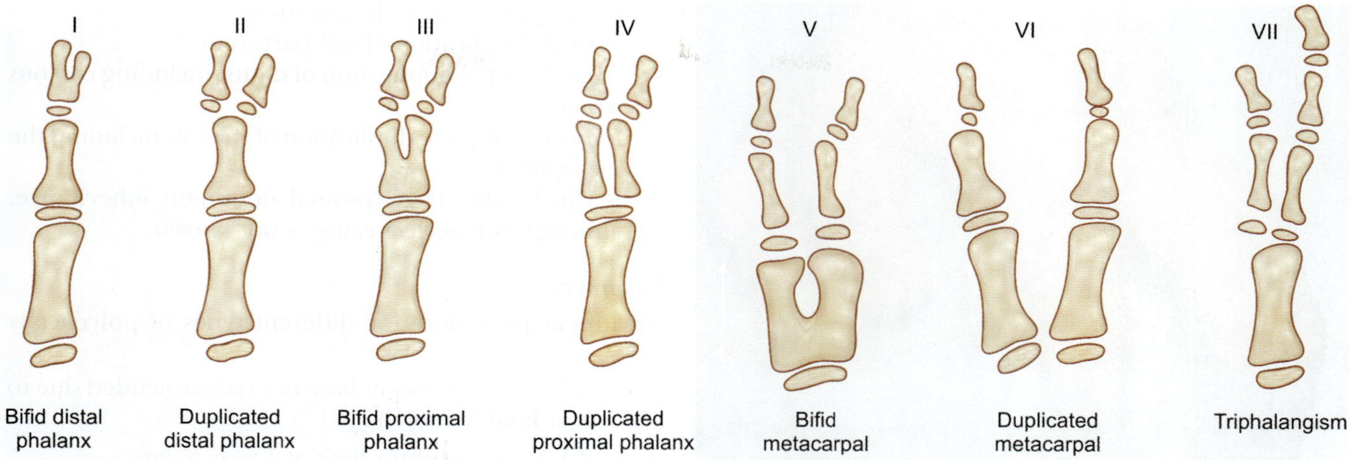

Fig. 21.98: Wessel's classification of bifid thumb

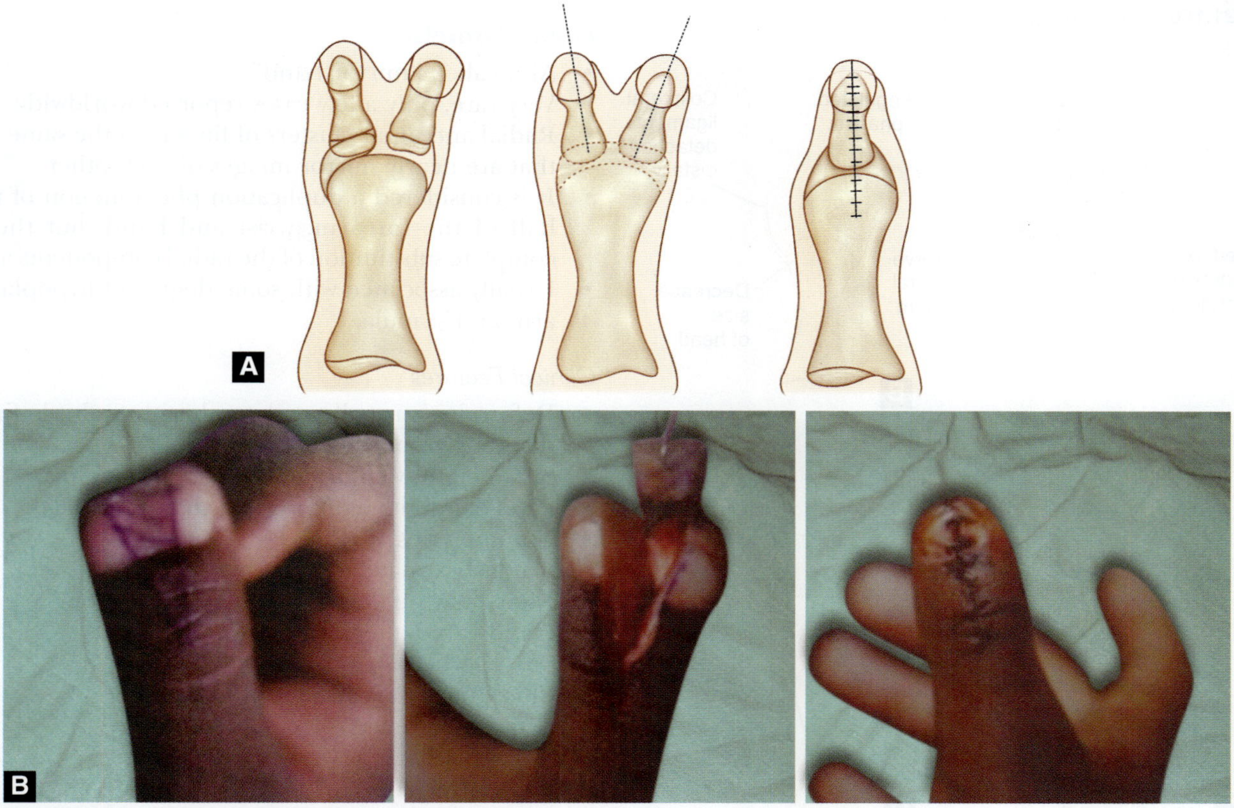

Figs 21.99A and B: Bilhaut-Cloquet "combination procedure"

- Correction of web contracture
- Improvement of opposition
- Adequate stability of the thumb.

Central Polydactyly

- Duplication of index, middle or ring finger
- Usually associated with complex syndactyly
- *Most common:* Type 2, concealed within syndactyly between long and ring fingers.

Treatment

- *Isolated central polydactyly:* Excision of most hypoplastic digit
- *Central polysyndactyly:*
  - Reconstruction with excision of extradigit or
  - Creation of three-fingered hand
  - To be done at 6 months of age, to prevent further angular deformity

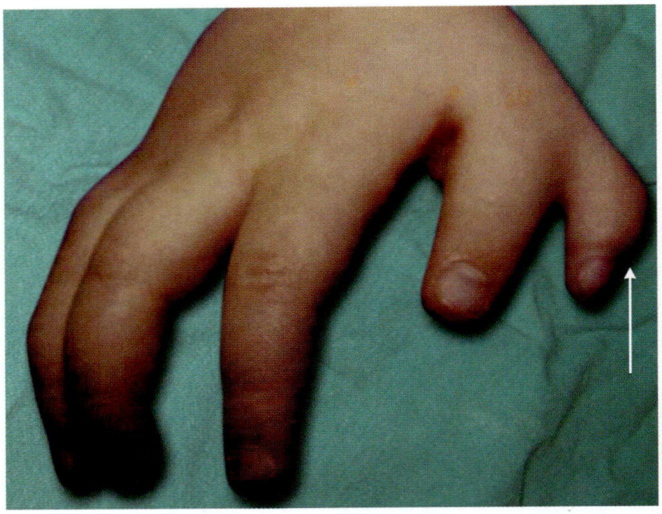

Fig. 21.100: A triphalangeal thumb

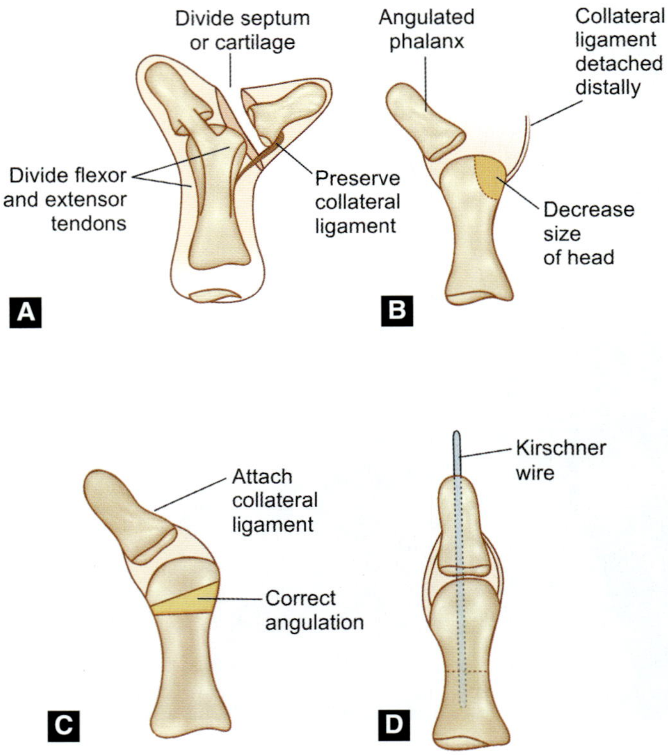

Figs 21.101A to D: Operative procedure for correcting triphalangeal thumb

- Amputation of functionless digits may be performed later.

Postaxial Polydactyly

Duplication of Little Finger

- Most common in black population (1 per 300 live births)
- Stelling and Turek classification:
  Type 1: Duplication of soft parts only
  Type 2: Partial duplication of digits, including osseous structures
  Type 3: Complete duplication of the ray, including the metacarpal
- It can be due to autosomal dominant inheritance, although the perfect cause is not known.

Treatment

Treatment procedure for different types of polydactyly are:

Type 1: Use of ligatures at base not recommended due to reports of fatal hemorrhage

Type 2: Excision of extra digit at 1 year of age

Type 3: No definitive treatment.

Ulnar Dimelia

- Also called "mirror hand"
- Very rare, only a few cases reported worldwide
- Radial and ulnar clusters of fingers in the same hand that are nearly mirror images of each other
- It is considered a duplication phenomenon of ulnar half of the forearm, wrist and hand, but there is complete substitution of the radial components as well
- Usually associated with some degree of hypoplasia of arm and scapula.

Clinical Features

- Deformity is usually unilateral, with multiple fingers dangling from the palm
- Six to eight, wellformed fingers in same plane
- Postaxial digits more normal than preaxial
- Thumb is absent
- Syndactyly may be present
- Digits may be flexed, absence of extensors
- Hand is radially deviated
- Wrist and elbow are thick
- Elbow motion is decreased
- Arm is shortened
- Ulna and ulnar carpal bones are completely duplicated
- Distal ulnar epiphysis is broadened
- At the elbow, each of the duplicated ulna articulate with humerus separately
- No capitellum on distal humerus.

Treatment

- Parents encouraged to maintain passive range of motion in fingers, wrist, elbow and shoulders by gentle stretching exercises, until child reaches 2 years of age
- Child should be carefully observed during play, to see which radial digit may function best as the opposable thumb

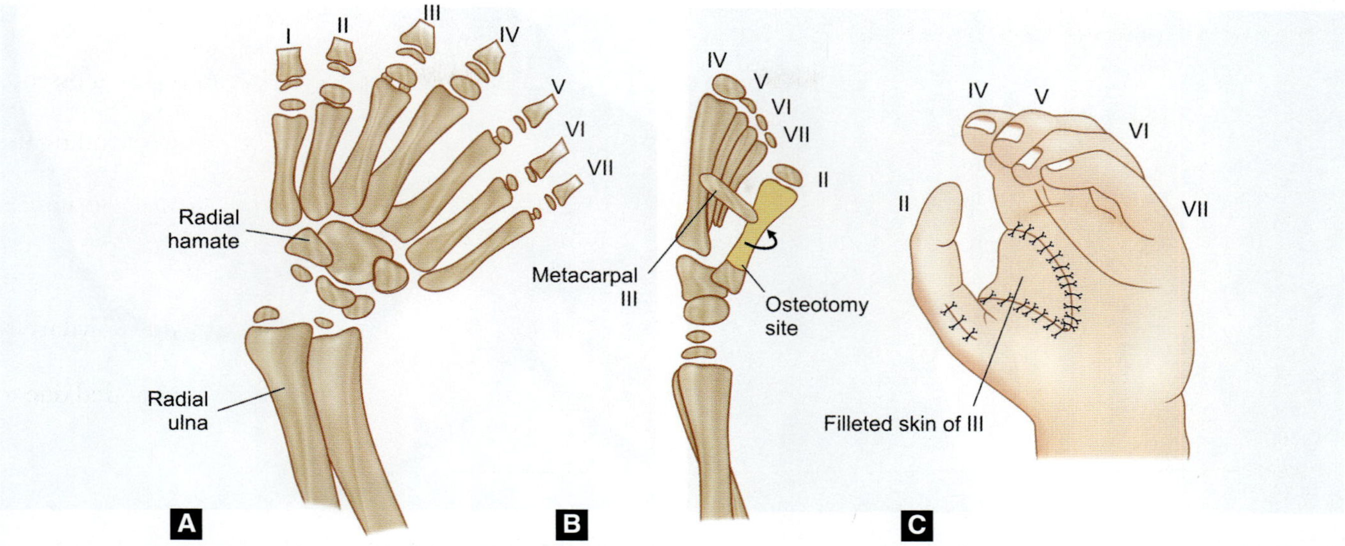

Figs 21.102A to C: Hand reconstruction (by Entin et al.)

- Surgery should be done early, to prevent psychological trauma to parents and child
- The reconstruction of hand as described by *Entin*, et al. is shown in Figures 21.102A to C.

Overgrowth: Macrodactyly

- A rare congenital anomaly, in which there is enlargement of the finger
- Incidence (0.9%)
- Index finger most commonly involved (Fig. 21.103)
- *Barsky classification:* They are of two types:
  - *Static enlargement:* Enlargement of the digit, without further growth with growth of the child
  - *Progressive enlargement:* Continuous growth of the digit with the growth of the child
- Usually unilateral, involves greater than two fingers
- With advancing age, the enlarged digits begin to lose function
- The phalanges are always involved and metacarpals may be involved
- If thumb is involved, usually an abduction and hyperextension deformity results.

Treatment

Nonsurgical methods are unsatisfactory

Operative procedure:

- Indications for surgery are:
  - Excessive enlargement
  - Angulation
  - Carpal tunnel syndrome
  - Causalgia
- Procedure is called "debulking"
- Most common complication is recurrence.

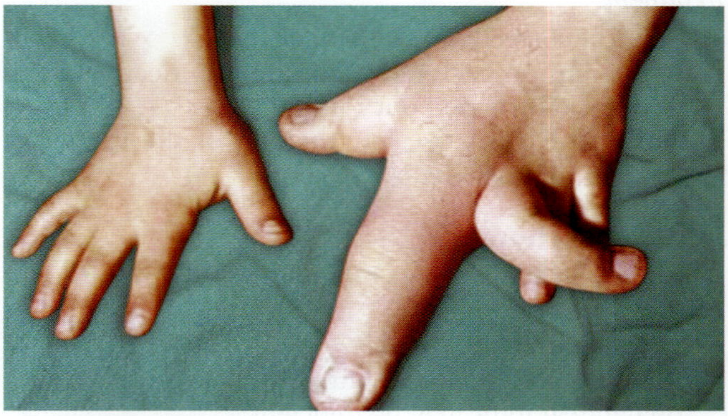

Fig. 21.103: Macrodactyly—Overgrown index finger

Undergrowth: Hypoplastic Thumb (Fig. 21.104)

- Short thumb
- Adducted thumb
- Abducted thumb
- Floating thumb (pouce flottant)
- Absent thumb
- Clasped thumb
- Hypoplastic hands and digits
- Hypoplastic thumb
- Some degree of deficiency in its anatomical parts, e.g. osseous, musculotendinous or ectodermal.

Short Thumb

If normal thumb extends to the level of proximal interphalangeal joint of the index finger, if it is shorter than this, it is considered a "short thumb".

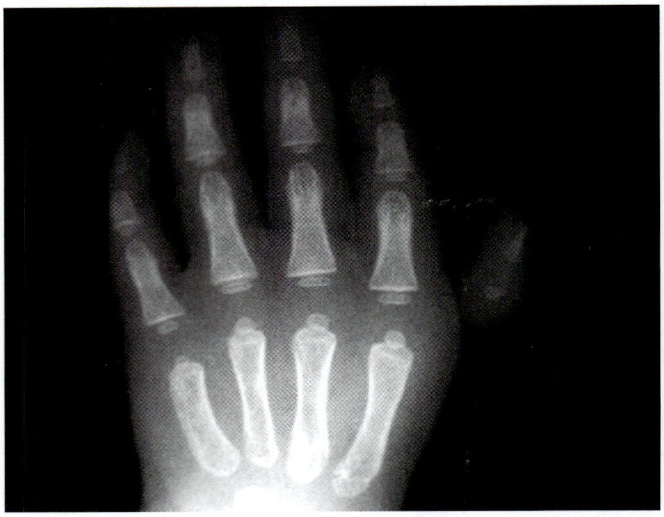

Fig. 21.104: X-ray showing hypoplastic thumb

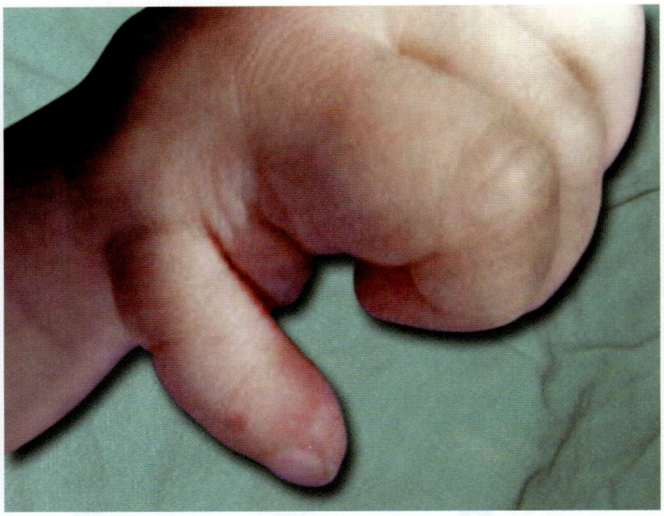

Fig. 21.105: A floating thumb

Treatment

- Surgical correction rarely indicated
- If prehension is significantly limited, deepening of web space is carried out
- This created relative lengthening of the thumb in relation to other digits.

Adducted Thumb

- Absence or deficiency of thenar muscles, resulting in deficient opposition
- FPL often absent
- Radial collateral ligament of thumb's metacarpophalangeal joint may be deficient
- Deformity is transmitted as autosomal dominant trait
- It is usually unilateral.

Treatment

Goals of the treatment are:

- Reconstruction of adducted thumb
- Correction of adduction contractures.

Procedure

Huber, Littler and Cooley procedure: Ring finger's flexor superficialis tendon opponensplasty and abductor digiti quinti opponensplasty.

Abducted Thumb

- Described by Tupper in 1969
- Also called "pollex abductus"
- Results from abnormal insertion of FPL into an otherwise normal EPL muscle
- This results in marked abduction of proximal phalynx of thumb
- Extremely rare, only few cases are reported.

Treatment

- Many treatments have been proposed
- Release of bifurcated tendon insertion and reattachment to metacarpal neck
- Release of tendon, distally withdrawal at wrist reattachment to distal phalynx
- Also required release of radial collateral ligament and reefing of ulnar collateral ligament of metacarpophalangeal joint.

Floating Thumb: Pouce Flottant (Fig. 21.105)

- Small and slender thumb that seems to dangle from radial border of hand
- There are two phalanges, a finger nail and no metacarpophalangeal joint and first metacarpal.

Treatment

- Amputation, followed by pollicization of index finger
- In bilateral cases, pollicization of one side should be performed early.

Absent Thumb

- It is most severe manifestation of hypoplastic thumb
- Associated with radial ray deficiencies, ring D chromosomal abnormalities, trisomy 18 syndrome, etc.

Treatment

Choice between two procedures:

- Pollicization of index finger
- Recession of index finger (Figs 21.106A to C)
- Done at 6 to 12 months of age, to allow some growth of hand before surgery.

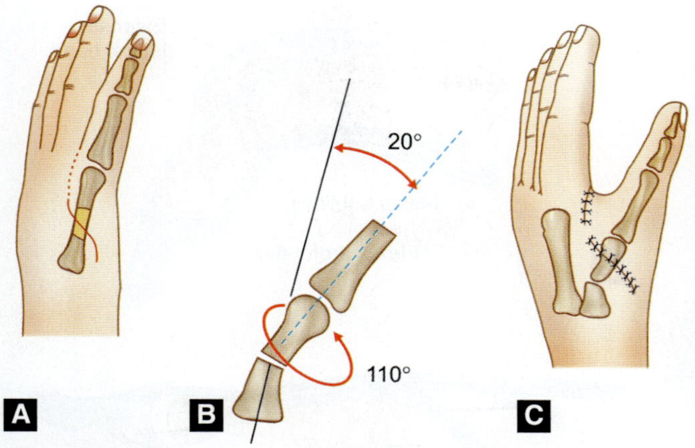

Figs 21.106A to C: Recession of index finger

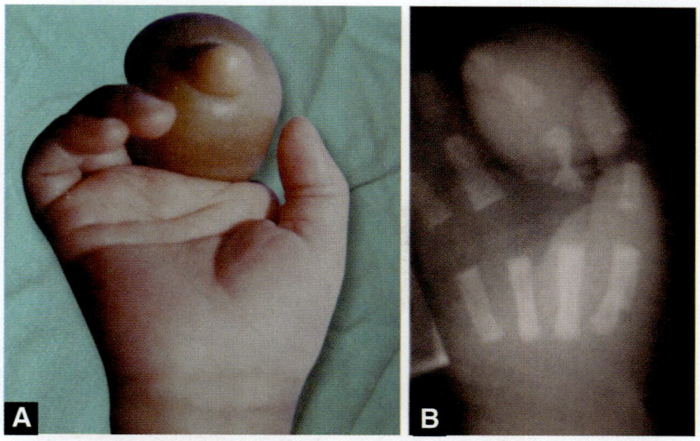

Figs 21.107A and B: (A) Congenital ring syndrome; (B) X-ray image of the ring syndrome

Congenital Clasped Thumb

- Thumb is positioned in adduction and extreme flexion at metacarpophalangeal joint
- Weckesser, Reed and Heiple classification:
  Group 1: Deficient extension only
  Group 2: Flexion contracture with deficient extension
  Group 3: Hypoplasia of thumb, including tendon and muscle deficiencies
  Group 4: Other deformities.

Treatment

Nonoperative: Early splinting in extension and abduction

Operative: Useful donor tendons for inadequate EPL muscle are:

- Palmaris longus
- Brachioradialis
- Extensor carpi radialis longus
- Extensor indicis proprius
- Flexor superficialis
- Significant web space reconstruction may also be required.

Congenital Ring Syndrome (Figs 21.107A and B)

- Occurs when deep cutaneous creases encircle a limb, as if a string was tightly tied around it
- Other common terms are streeter bands, annular grooves and intrauterine amputations.

Patterson Classification

Type 1: Simple ring, usually transverse or oblique around a digit

Type 2: Deeper ring with abnormality of part distally, usually lymphedema

Type 3: Fenestrated syndactyly or lateral fusion of adjacent digits at their distal ends, with proximal fenestrations between intervening skin and soft tissue

Type 4: Intrauterine amputation (Guillotine amputation).

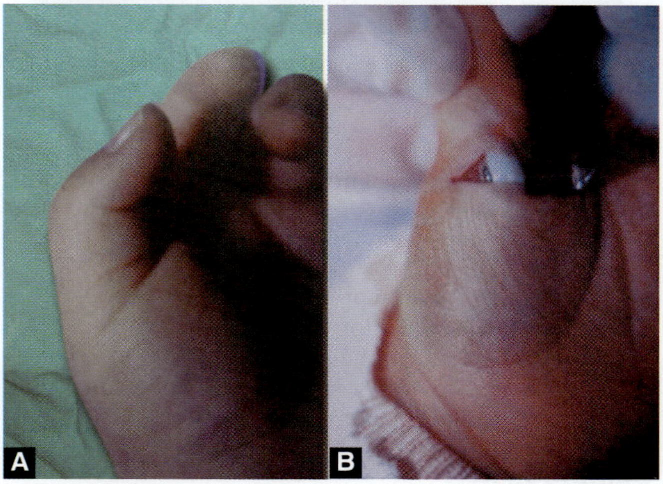

Figs 21.108A and B: (A) Trigger thumb and (B) A1 pulley

Treatment

- Superficial bands do not require any treatment
- Deeper bands require staged excision of one half of groove, with Z-plasty closure, followed by another surgery 2 to 3 months later.

Generalized Skeletal Abnormalities

- Congenital trigger digits
- Camptodactyly
- Kirner deformity
- Delta phalynx
- Madelung deformity.

Congenital Trigger Digits (Figs 21.108A and B)

- When normal gliding movement of flexor tendon is impeded within digital flexor sheath
- In contrast to adult condition (stenosing tenovaginitis), it shows persistent flexion deformity rather than "triggering"

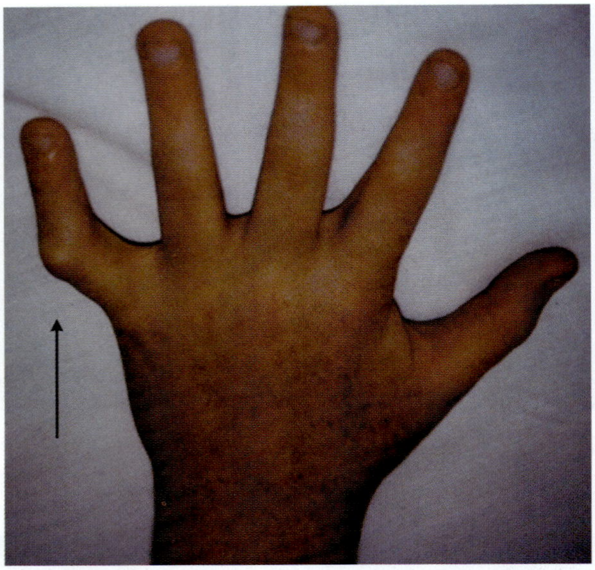

Fig. 21.109: Camptodactyly, with flexed proximal interphalangeal joint of little finger

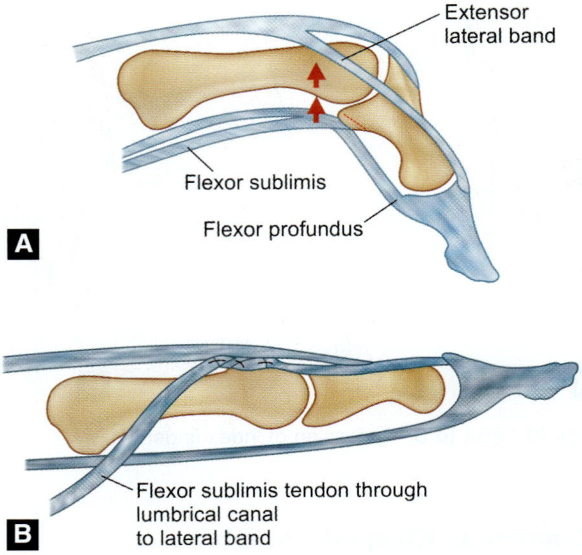

Figs 21.110A and B: Millesi and Lankford procedure for correcting camptodactyly

- Sheath is narrowed and thickened, with occasional ganglion cyst.

Treatment

- Conservative treatment is tried first
- Surgery not delayed for greater than 3 years
- Surgery at first year of age, if multiple digits involved
- Surgical release of first annular pulley is done
- May also be done percutaneously.

Camptodactyly

- Flexion deformity of proximal interphalangeal joint, that usually involves only little finger (Fig. 21.109)
- Should be distinguished from clinodactyly, in which finger is bent radially or ulnarly.

Classification

- *Type 1:* Occurs in infancy and affects both sexes equally. More common (80%)
- *Type 2:* Occurs during adolescence and affects girls. Less common (20%).

Cause

Exact cause although not known, it may be due to:

- Relative imbalance between flexors and extensors
- Relative shortening in flexor superficialis muscle tendon group
- Contractures of collateral ligaments or volar plate
- Insufficient palmar skin
- Congenital fibrous substrata in subcutaneous tissues.

Treatment

- For mild deformity, no treatment is advised
- In age less than 4 years
  - In patients, where deformity disappears with wrist flexion, release of sublimis tendon may correct the deformity
- In age greater than 4 years
  - Release of flexor digitorum sublimis muscle and transfer to extensor apparatus is done as given by Millesi and Lankford (Figs 21.110A and B).

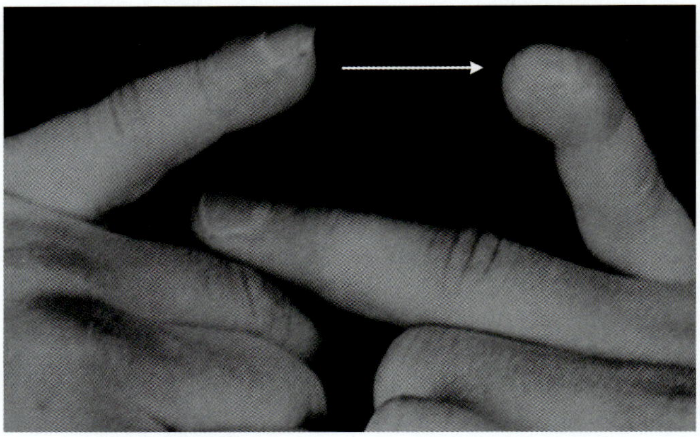

Fig. 21.111: Kirner deformity

Kirner Deformity (Kirner, 1927)

- Palmar and radial curving of distal phalanx of little finger (Fig. 21.111)
- Appears when child 8 to 10 years old and appears as a beaked little fingertip, with increased convexity of finger nail
- Fingertip curves radially and towards the palm
- Usually bilateral and symmetrical

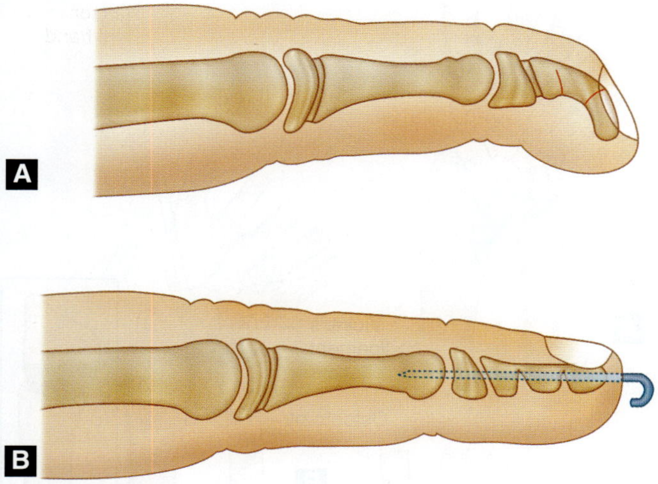

Figs 21.112A and B: Correction of Kirner deformity by osteotomy

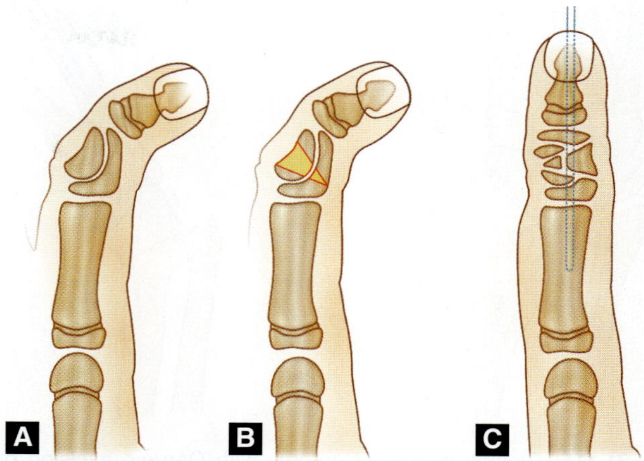

Figs 21.113A to C: Reverse wedge osteotomy, for correcting delta phalanx

- Usually not painful, though progressive
- *X-ray:* Broadened epiphysis, irregularities of metaphysis and typical curvature of distal phalanx.

Treatment

- Mild deformities warrant a conservative treatment
- Severe deformities in skeletally mature patients, require one or more osteotomies of terminal phalanx (Carstam and Eiken) (Figs 21.112A and B)
- No effective treatment for correction of nail deformity.

Delta Phalanx

- Abnormal, trapezoidal phalanx that appears triangular on radiographs
- It derives its name from a Greek letter "delta"
- Abnormal epiphysis is "J" or "C"shaped and brackets on one side of phalanx
- Delta phalanx causes an angular deformity of digit in frontal plane
- Most common site is proximal phalanx of ring finger.

Treatment

- *Reverse wedge osteotomy (Carstam and Theander):* This is shown in the Figs 21.113A to C.

MADELUNG DEFORMITY

Introduction

Abnormality of palmar ulnar part of distal radial physis, in which progressive ulnar and volar tilt develops at distal radial articular surface with dorsal subluxation of distal ulna. It was described by Malgaigne in 1855 and by Madelung in 1878 (Figs 21.114A and B).

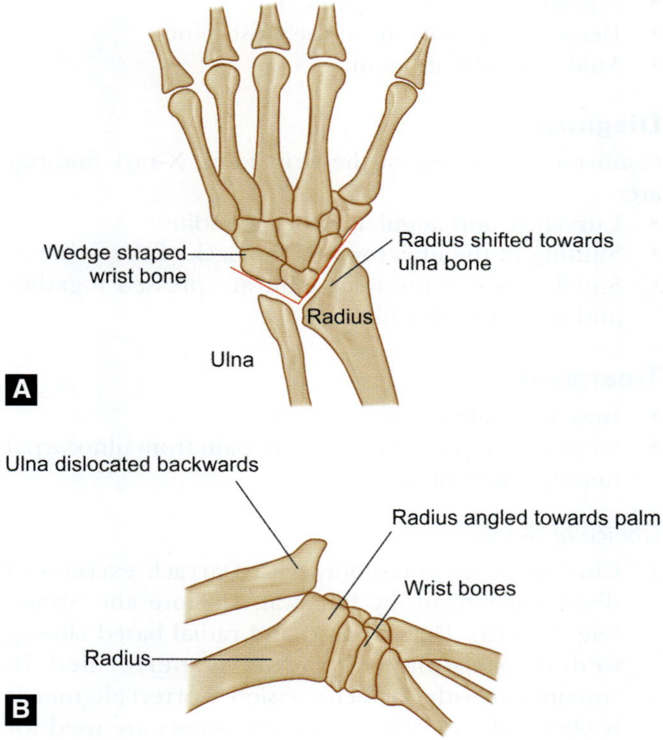

Figs 21.114A and B: Madelung deformity

Vender and Watson Classification

- Post-traumatic
- Dysplastic
- Genetic
- Idiopathic.

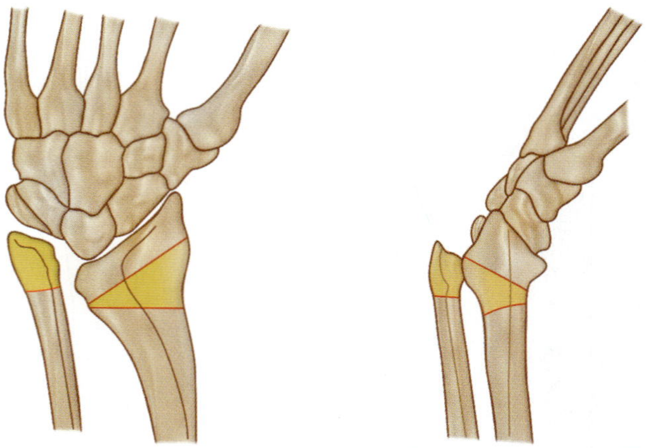

Fig. 21.115: Closing wedge osteotomy with Darrach excision of distal ulnar head, by Ranawat, DeFiore and Straub

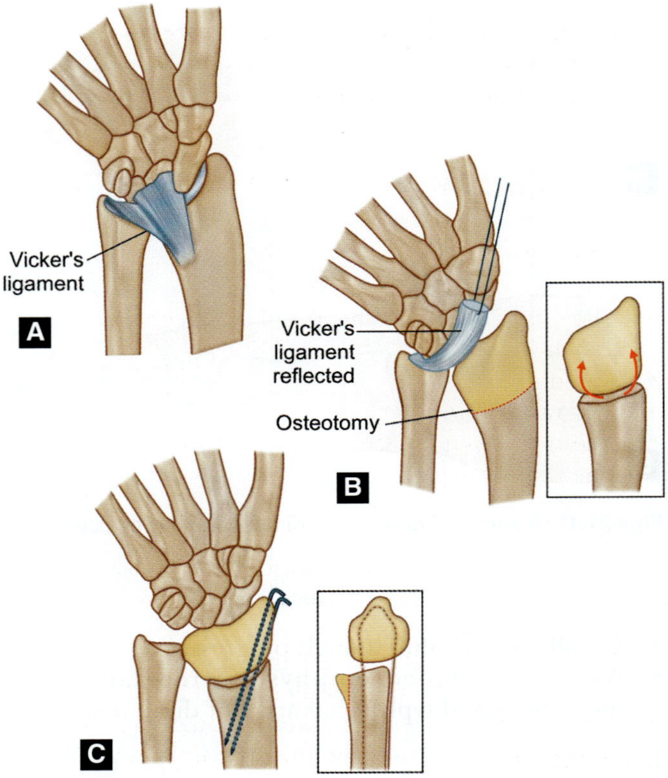

Figs 21.116A to C: Dome osteotomy and excision of Vickers ligament, by Carter and Ezaki

Symptoms

- A gradually worsening deformity
- Decreased movement in the wrist joint
- Mild-to-moderate pain.

Diagnosis

Confirmed by X-rays of the wrist joint. X-rays findings are:

- Curvature and angulation of the radius
- Shifting of the ulna towards the back of the wrist
- Small bones of the wrist joint are pressed together and appear wedge like.

Treatment

- Initially treated conservatively
- Surgery indicated due to severe pain from ulnocarpal impingement of carpus.

Choice of Surgery

1. Closing wedge osteotomy with Darrach excision of distal ulnar head, by Ranawat, DeFiore and Straub (Fig. 21.115): Dorsal based and radial based closing wedge osteotomy of radius is performed in conjunction with Darrach excision. Correct alignment is obtained and plate along with screws are used for fixation.
2. Dome osteotomy and excision of Vicker's ligament, by Carter and Ezaki (Figs 21.116A to C): Ligament of Vicker's is excised, biplanar dome osteotomy is made in metaphysic, distal fragment is rotated at osteotomy site and secured with Steinmann pins.

HAND INFECTIONS

■ Introduction

Hand infections occur commonly due to following reasons:

- It is frequently injured
- It is infrequently infected
- Has abundant blood supply.

Potential Problems

- *Confined spaces*
  - Joints
  - Tendon sheaths
  - Compartments and bursae.
- *Local factors*
  - Soft tissue damage
  - Amount or virulence of organism
  - Type or amount of foreign material.
- *Systemic factors*
  - Malnutrition
  - Alcoholism

- Diabetes mellitus
- Steroids
- Immunosuppression.

Anatomy

The spaces of hand are of practical significance because they may become infected and in consequence become distended with pus. The important spaces are:

- The superficial pulp spaces of the finger
- The synovial tendon sheaths of the second, third and fourth finger
- The ulnar bursa
- The radial bursa
- The midpalmar space
- The thenar space.

Superficial Pulp Space

- The pulp space of the fingers is a closed fascial compartment situated in front of the terminal phalanx of each finger.
- Each space is subdivided into numerous smaller compartments by fibrous septa (Fig. 21.117).
- Accumulation of inflammatory exudate within these compartments causes the pressure in the pulp space to rise quickly
- In children, pressure on the blood vessels could result in necrosis of diaphysis
- The close relationship of the proximal end of the pulp space to the digital synovial sheath accounts for the involvement of the sheath in the infectious process, when the pulp-space infection has been neglected.

Synovial Tendon Sheath

- The common synovial sheath for the flexor tendons is a synovial sheath in the carpal tunnel
- It contains tendons of the flexor digitorum superficialis and the flexor digitorum profundus, but not the flexor pollicis longus
- The sheath which surrounds the flexor digitorum extends downward about half-way along the metacarpal bones, where it ends in blind diverticula around the tendons to the index, middle, and ring fingers. It is prolonged on the tendons to the little finger and usually communicates with the mucus sheath of these tendons
- Untreated infection of the synovial sheaths can impair hand function.
- Infection of the synovial sheaths of the thumb or little finger may spread readily into the palm and even into the forearm (space of parona) (Fig. 21.118).

Ulnar and Radial Bursae

- The common and pollicial sheaths are frequently referred to in clinical writing as the ulnar and radial bursae, respectively
- These two sheaths project proximally, a short distance above the flexor retinaculum and they usually communicate with each other in the carpal tunnel
- Hence, infection of the synovial sheaths of the thumb or little finger may spread readily into the palm and even into the forearm.

Ulnar Bursa

- Common flexor synovial sheath (ulnar bursa)
- The long flexor tendons of the fingers (flexor digitorum superficialis and profundus) are enclosed in a common synovial sheath, while passing deep to the flexor retinaculum
- The sheath has a parietal layer, lining the walls of the carpal tunnel and a visceral layer closely applied to the tendons
- From the arrangement of the sheath, it appears that the synovial sac has been invaginated by the tendons from its lateral side
- In hands, the tendons of the flexor digitorum superficialis and profundus muscle invaginate a common synovial sheath from the lateral side

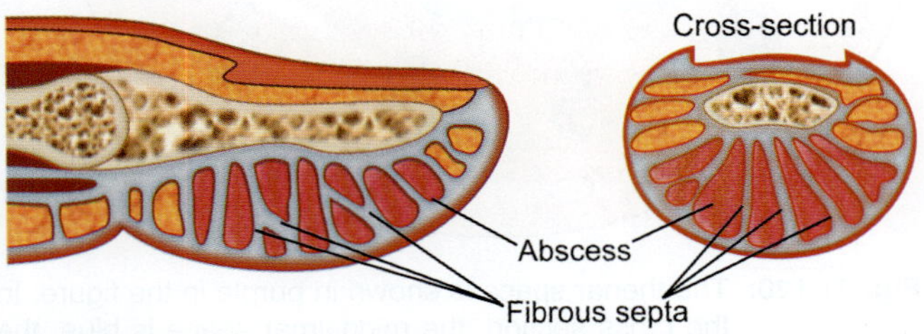

Fig. 21.117: Superficial pulp space and subdivided smaller compartments divided by fibrous septa

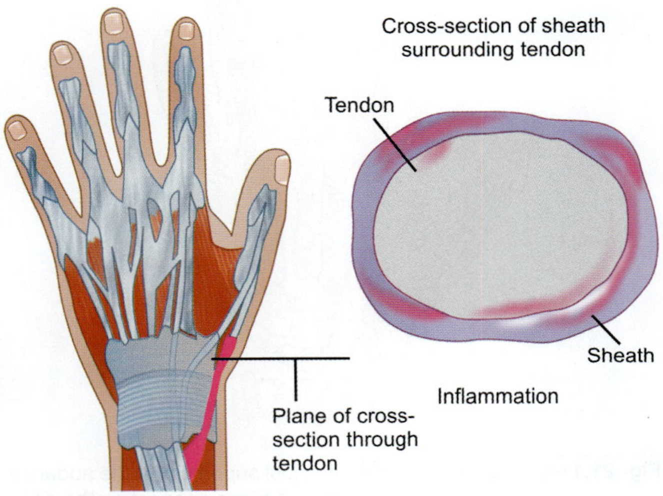

Fig. 21.118: Routes through which infection of synovial sheath of thumb will spread

- Medial part, common sheath extends distally on the tendons of little finger
- Lateral part, it stops on the middle of palm
- Distal ends of index, middle and ring finger acquire digital synovial sheaths.

Radial Bursa

- The synovial sheath of the tendon of flexor pollicis longus forms the radial bursa.
- This sheath is usually separate, but may communicate with the common sheath behind the retinaculum.
- Superiorly, it is coextensive with the common sheath and inferiorly, it extends up to the distal phalanx of the thumb.
- Flexor pollicis longus tendon has its own synovial sheath that passes into the thumb, which allows the long tendons to move smoothly.
- Synovial sheath of the flexor pollicis longus (radial bursa) communicates with the ulnar bursa, at the level of wrist in about 50 percent of subjects.

Mid Palmar Space (Mid Central Palmar Space)

- Contains three to five flexor tendons, two to four lumbricals, superficial palmar arch, three to five digital vessels and nerves.
- Communicates through the subcutaneous tissues at webs and extends dorsally to common flexor sheaths.
- *Location:* The midpalmar space lies posterior to the long flexor tendons to the middle, ring and little fingers. It lies in front of the interossei and the third, fourth and fifth metacarpal bone.
- *Boundaries*
  - *Anterior:* Flexor tendons of medial three fingers is surrounded by synovial sheaths (ulnar bursa)
  - *Posterior:* Third, fourth and fifth, metacarpal bones with its interossei muscles
  - *Medially:* Hypothenar muscles
  - *Laterally:* Septum separating it from thenar space
  - *Distally:* Communicate with web spaces
  - *Proximally:* Communicate with parona space

Thenar Space (Lateral Central Palmar Space)

- It contains, tendons of flexor pollicis longus, flexor digitorum superficialis and profundus to index finger, palmar digital nerves and vessels to thumb and radial side of index finger.
- Communicates through web of thumb and under flexor retinaculum.
- *Location:* The thenar space lies posterior to the long flexor tendons of the index finger and in front of the adductor pollicis muscle.
- *Boundaries*
  - *Radial:* Thenar eminence, radial bursa
  - *Ulnar:* Middle metacarpal, ulnar bursa
  - *Superficial:* Carpal tunnel
  - *Deep:* Adductor pollicis
- The thenar space lies just superficial to the adductor pollicis muscle, forming a plane connecting the deep aspects of the radial bursa and the ulnar bursa. Abscess or space occupying lesions may spread transversely through the thenar space, deep in the palm between the thumb and the carpal tunnel (Figs 21.119 and 21.120).

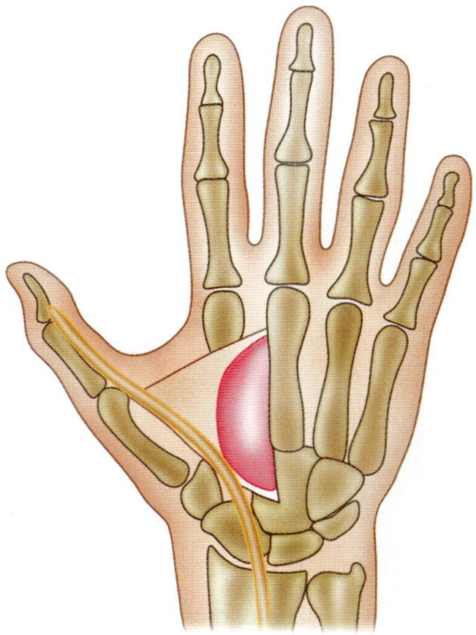

Fig. 21.119: The thenar space lying just superficial to the adductor pollicis muscle, forming a plane connecting the deep aspects of the radial bursa and the ulnar bursa

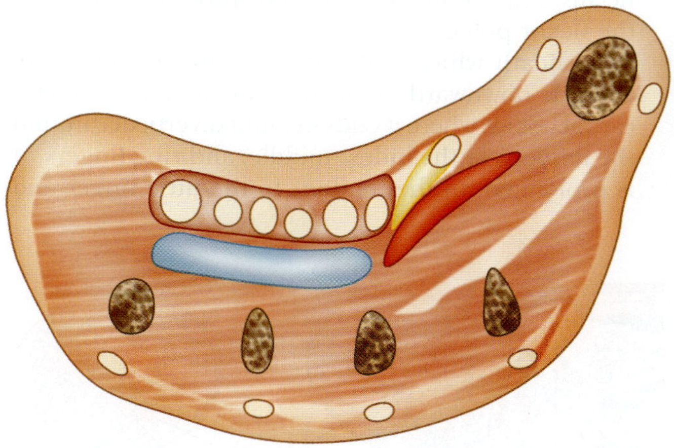

Fig. 21.120: The thenar space is shown in purple in the figure. In the cross section, the midpalmar space is blue, the radial bursa is light blue and the ulnar bursa is red

Overview

- Cellulitis
- Paronychia or eponychia
- Felon
- Herpetic whitlow
- Flexor tenosynovitis
- Deep fascial space infections
- Septic arthritis
- Osteomyelitis
- Fight bites.

Principles of Management of Hand Infections

- Rest, elevation and immobilization
- Antibiotics after culture and sensitivity
- Incision and drainage
- Tetanus prophylaxis.

Cellulitis of the Hand

- Involves only the skin, erythema, edema and pain of localized area (Fig. 21.121).
- One must rule out that deeper structures are not involved. Beware of the dorsal hand cellulitis
  - Full painless ROM of digits, hand and wrist
  - No tenderness on palpation of deeper structures.

Causative Organisms

- *Streptococcus pyogenes*
- Occasionally, *Streptococcus aureus.*

Treatment

- Splint and elevate
- *Warm soaks:* Open wounds
- *Irrigating catheters (Wicks):* Closed wounds
- Gentle ROM
- Culture specific antibiotics.

Paronychia

- Localized superficial infection or abscess of the lateral nail fold
- Most common infection in the hand
- Caused by frequent trauma to area
- Swelling and tenderness of the soft tissue next to the nail fold (Fig. 21.122)
- May have associated cellulitis
- If extends to overlying proximal nail, it is called eponychia.

Causative Organisms

- *S. aureus*: Thumb sucking, nail biting and is an anaerobes
- Chronic infection by *Candida.*

Treatment

- *Early cellulitis:* Warm soaks, elevation, antibiotics
- *Late or fluctuant cellulites:* Treatment include:
  - Marsupialization
  - Partial nail removal (Figs 21.123A and B)
- Mostly resolve in 5 to 10 days.

Complications

Osteomyelitis of distal phalanx.

Felon

Infection of the pulp of the distal finger or thumb (Fig. 21.124)

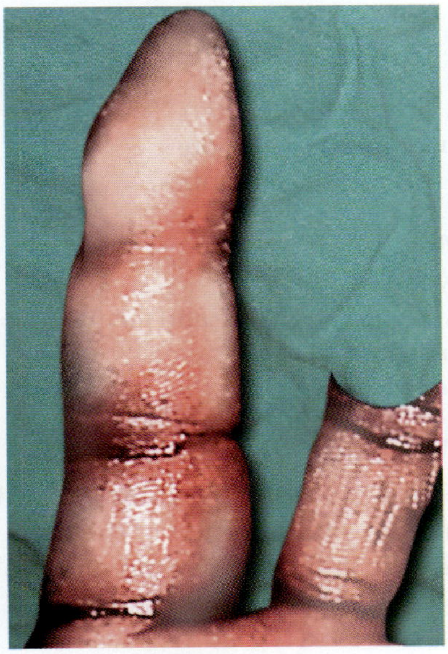

Fig. 21.121: Cellulitis of hand

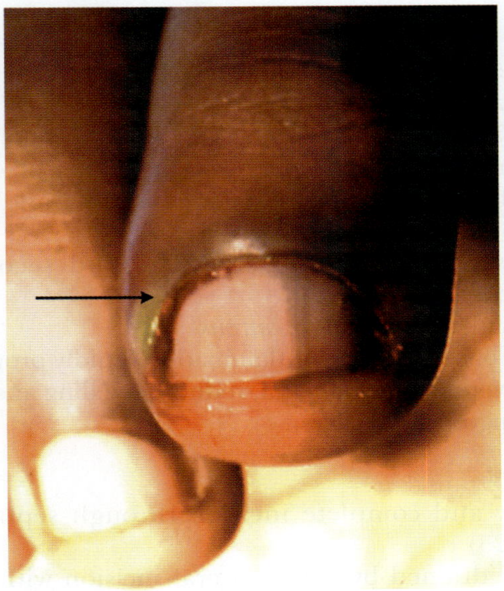

Fig. 21.122: Swelling and tenderness of the soft tissue next to the nail fold in paronychia

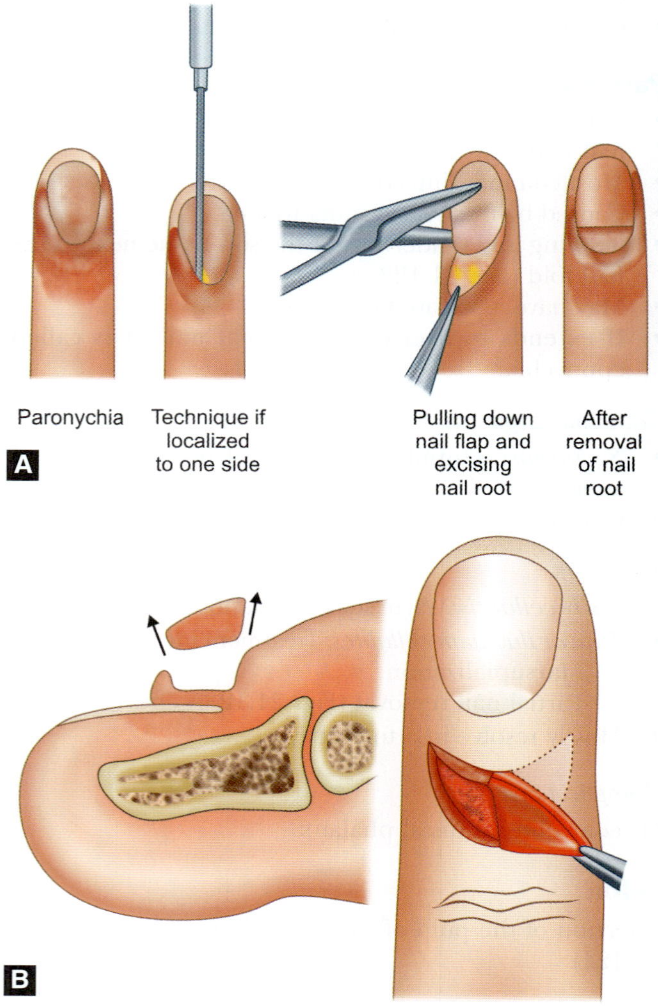

Figs 21.123A and B: Partial nail removal procedure

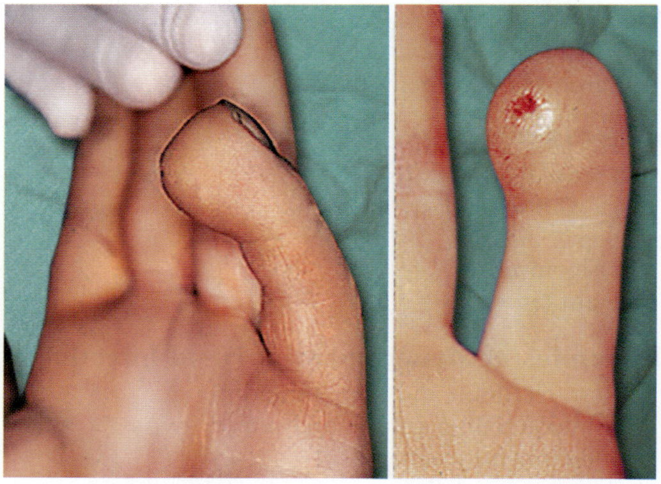

Fig. 21.124: Felon, with infection of the pulp of the distal finger or thumb

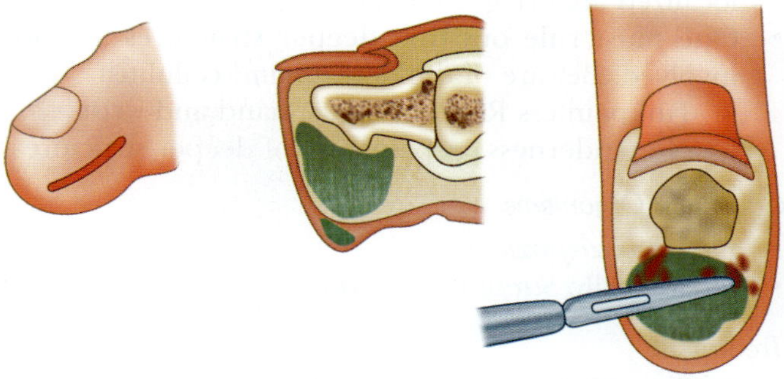

Fig. 21.125: Felon: Pus drained by incision made on the septa

- Septa
  - Facilitate infection
  - Inhibit drainage, but acts as a barrier protecting the joint space and tendon sheath and limits proximal spread
- Caused by penetrating trauma and secondary infection
- Causative organism: *S. aureus*
- Area of cellulitis and inflammation rapidly progresses to severe throbbing, pain, redness, swelling and tense feeling of distal finger.

Treatment

- Early and complete incision through septa (Fig. 21.125)
- Most drained by single lateral incision with blunt dissection, also volar approach (Fig. 21.126)
- Send cultures
- Irrigate, dress, elevate, etc.
- Re-evaluate in 24 to 48 hours
- Culture specific IV antibiotics.

Complications

- Osteomyelitis
- Necrosis of palmar surface and formation of sinus tract
- Septic arthritis
- Flexor tenosynovitis

Herpetic Whitlow

- Herpes simplex virus (HSV) infection of distal finger
- Most common viral infection of the hand
- Caused by direct inoculation through broken skin:
  - Kids with herpetic gingivostomatitis
  - Adults more likely HSV 2
  - Health care workers
- Single finger involved

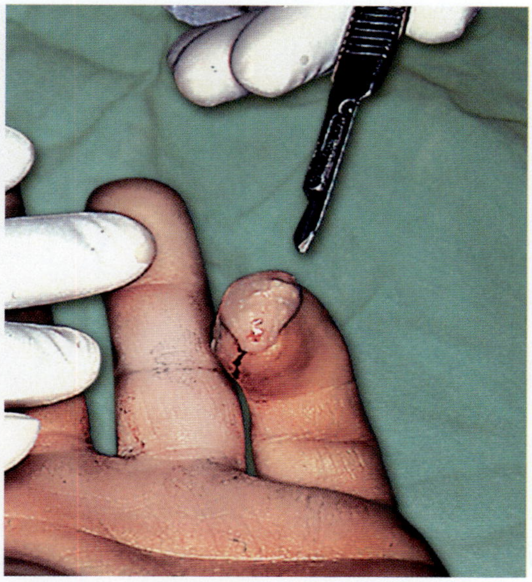

Fig. 21.126: Pus drainage by single lateral incision with blunt dissection (volar approach)

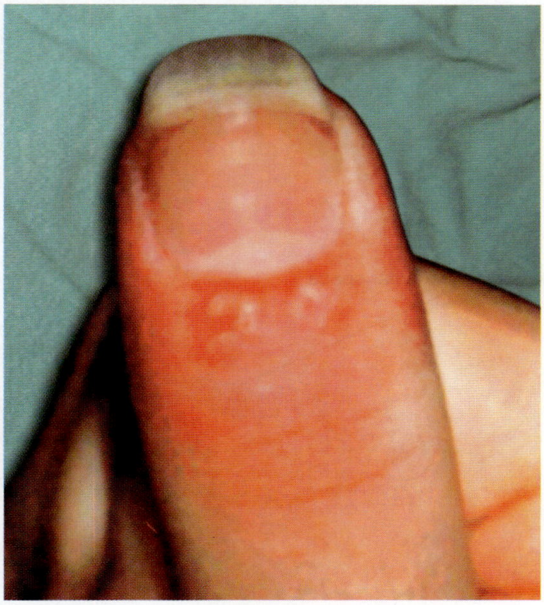

Fig. 21.127: Vesicles in herpetic whitlow

- Pain, pruritis and swelling
- Vesicles (Fig. 21.127)
- Coalescence over 2 weeks
- Ulcer formation
- Hemorrhagic base
- May look like a felon, but drainage is contraindicated
- Careful history should be taken
- Tender distal finger, but soft pulp space
- Resolves spontaneously in 3 to 4 weeks

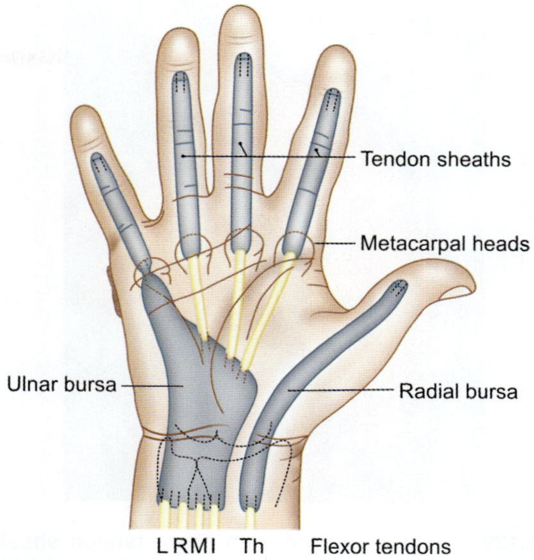

Fig. 21.128: Flexor tendon sheaths and radial or ulnar bursae, involved most commonly in tenosynovitis: L. Little finger; R. Ring finger; M. Middle finger; I. Index finger; Th. Thumb

- Prevent oral inoculation, by covering with a dry dressing. Acyclovir is given, only if immunocompromised or frequent infections.

Flexor Tenosynovitis

- This is a surgical emergency and should act quickly, to preserve function of digit and hand
- Usually involves flexor tendon sheaths and radial and ulnar bursae (Fig. 21.128)
- Infection spreads along course of flexor tendon sheaths, which may spread to midpalmar, thenar and lumbrical compartments (Fig. 21.129)
- *Kanavel's signs* (Fig. 21.130)
  - Finger in slight flexion
  - Fusiform swelling
  - Pain with extension
  - Tenderness along tendon sheath
- Caused by penetrating trauma to sheath
- Consider disseminated *Gonococcal* infection, if no trauma is there and person is sexually active.
- *Causative organisms: S. aureus* (anerobes, gram-negatives).

Clinical Features

- Tenderness along course of tendon
- Symmetric swelling of the finger
- Pain on passive extension
- Flexed posture of finger.

Treatment

- Splint and elevate
- Incision and drainage (Fig. 21.131)

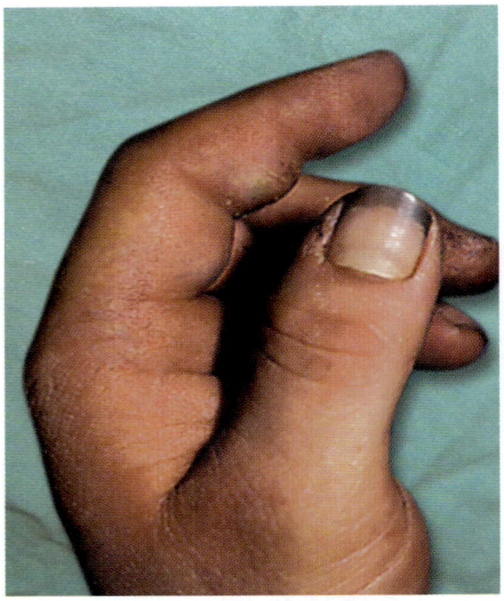

Fig. 21.129: Infection spread from flexor tendon sheaths to midpalmar, thenar and lumbrical compartments

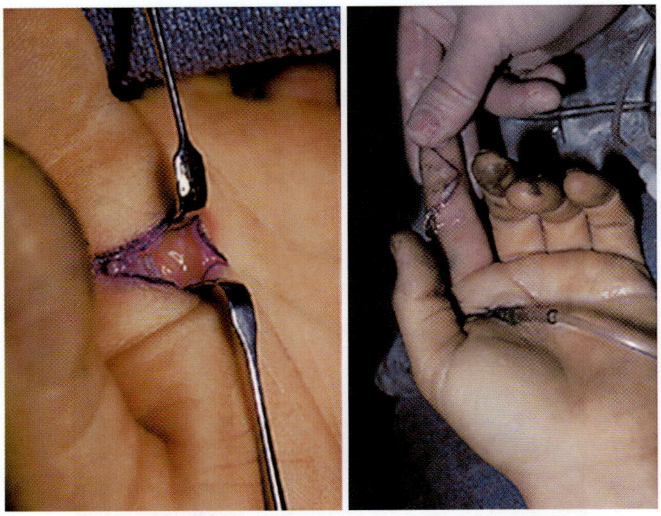

Fig. 21.131: Incision and drainage of pus in infected tenosynovitis

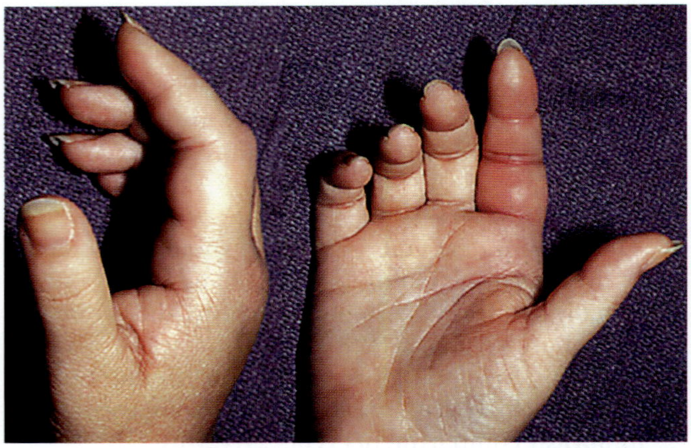

Fig. 21.130: Kanavel's signs

- Irrigation
- IV antibiotics

Deep Fascial Space Infection

- Palm is relatively fixed, the infection is seen on the dorsal side of the hand
- Four potential spaces, shown in Figures 21.132A to C
  - Dorsal subaponeurotic space
  - Subfacial web space
  - Thenar space
  - Midpalmar space.

Route of Infection

- Direct penetrating trauma
- Contiguous spread
- Hematogenous spread.

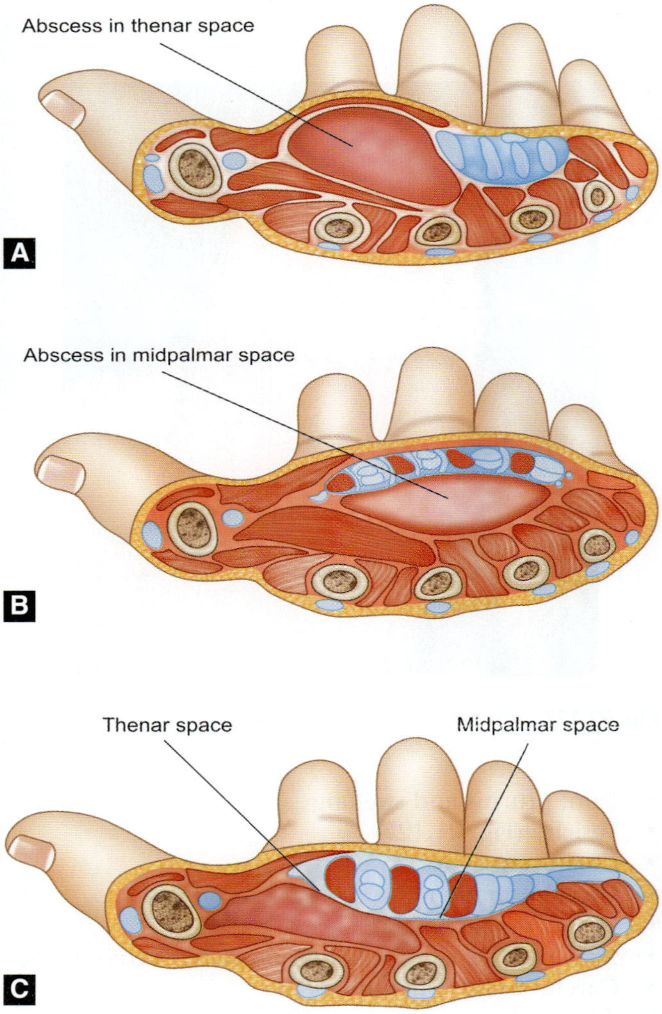

Figs 21.132A to C: Four potential deep fascial spaces

Causative Organisms

- *S. aureus, Streptococcus*
- Occasionally coliforms and anerobes.

Dorsal Subaponeurotic Abscess

- Swelling and erythema on dorsum of hand
- Pain with passive movement of extensor tendons
- Looks like cellulitis.

Subfacial Web Space Infection

- Secondary to infection of palmar blisters
- Spreads dorsally "collar button abscess" (Figs 21.133A and B).

Thenar Space Infection

- Pain and swelling of thenar eminence and first web space (Figs 21.134A and B)
- Can be from tenosynovitis of second digit with rupture proximally
- Thumb is held, abducted and flexed.

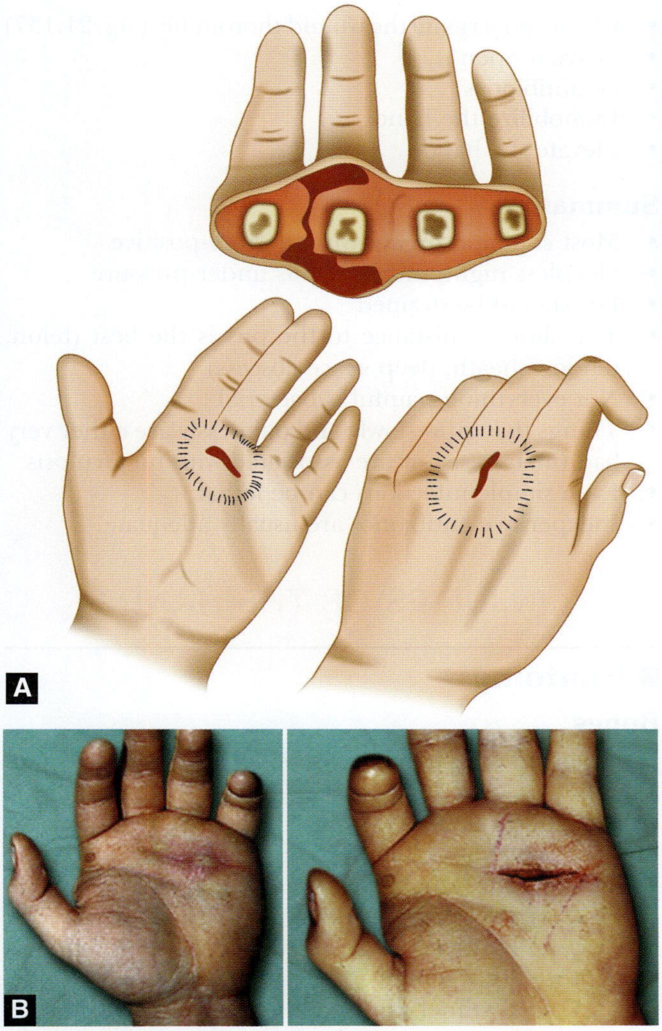

Figs 21.133A and B: Collar button abscess

Midpalmar Infection

- Loss of normal hand concavity
- Tenderness of central palm
- Pain with movement of third and fourth digits
- Can be from tenosynovitis of third, fourth and fifth digits.

Treatment

- Incision and drainage (Fig. 21.135)
- Culture sensitivity
- IV antibiotics
- Resting splint.

Septic Arthritis

- Any joint may be involved
- Can spread from direct inoculation, from penetrating trauma or contiguous spread
- Causative organism: *S. aureus* (rarely others).

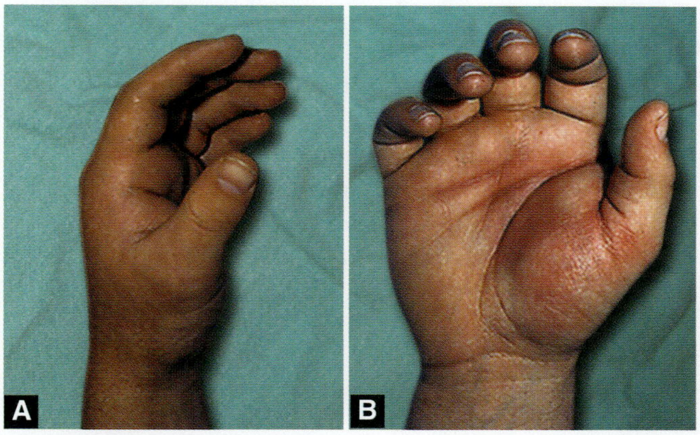

Figs 21.134A and B: Pain and swelling of thenar eminence and first web space

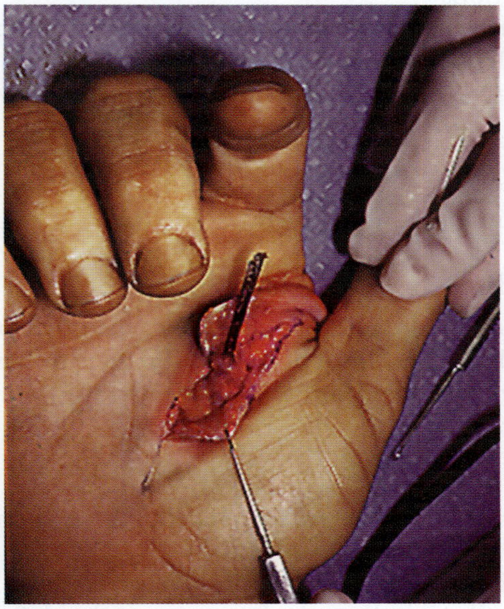

Fig. 21.135: Incision and drainage

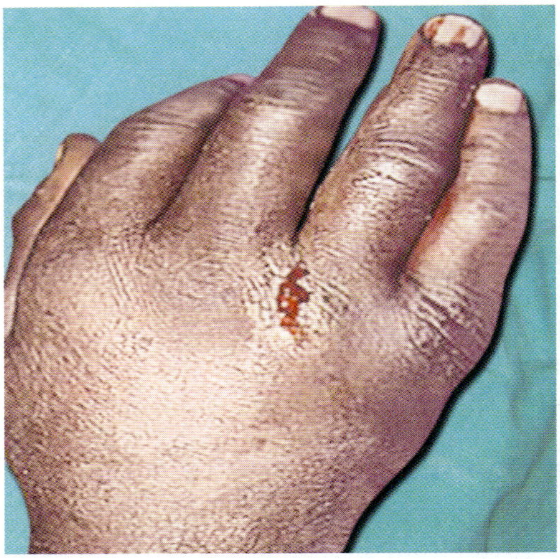

Fig. 21.136: Puncture wound, with surrounding area of cellulitis

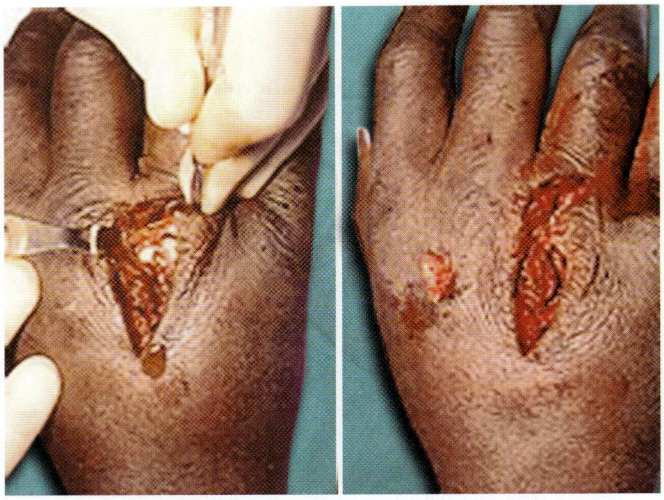

Fig. 21.137: Clean and irrigate the wound thoroughly

Clinical Features

- Joint is red, swollen, tender and localized (unlike flexor tenosynovitis)
- May have overlying puncture wound
- Held in position to maximize joint volume
- Very painful passive flexion and axial load
- Diagnozed by arthrocentesis.

Treatment

- IV antibiotics
- Open drainage.

Osteomyelitis

- Most common with open fractures or soft tissue infections
- Fever, redness, swelling, warmth, tenderness, pseudo-paralysis (in kids)
- *Plain film:* Bony destruction or periosteal elevation.

Treatment

- Debridement
- IV Antibiotics (long-term).

Fight Bites

- During fights, when a person bites the other person's hand, the oral flora of the incisors gets deposited in the deep layers, thus facilitating rapid spread of infection.

Physical Examination

- Puncture wound with area of cellulitis surrounding it (Fig. 21.136)
- Tendon may be visible inside the wound
- Plain film is indicated, often associated with fractures.

Treatment

- Clean and irrigate the wound thoroughly (Fig. 21.137)
- Leave it open
- IV antibiotics
- Immobilize the hand
- Elevate the hand.

Summary

- Most common organisms are gram-positive
- Sleepless night, indicates pus under-pressure
- Pus should be drained
- The shortest distance to the pus is the best (felon, tendon sheath, deep space abscess)
- Not everything painful is bacterial
- Things that grow slowly and painlessly are either very bad (metastasis) or are associated with tuberculosis
- Even simple infections can be lethal
- Inexpensive antibiotics are usually adequate.

INJURIES OF THE HAND

Anatomy

Bones

Hand consist of 27 bones. Wrist bones are shown in Figure 21.138.

- Phalangeal bones (14)
- Metacarpal bones (5)
- Carpal bones (8)
  - Carpal bones are made up of two rows of four bones bridged by flexor retinaculum which forms the carpal tunnel
  - Carpal tunnel consist of the median nerve and the nine long flexor of the fingers.

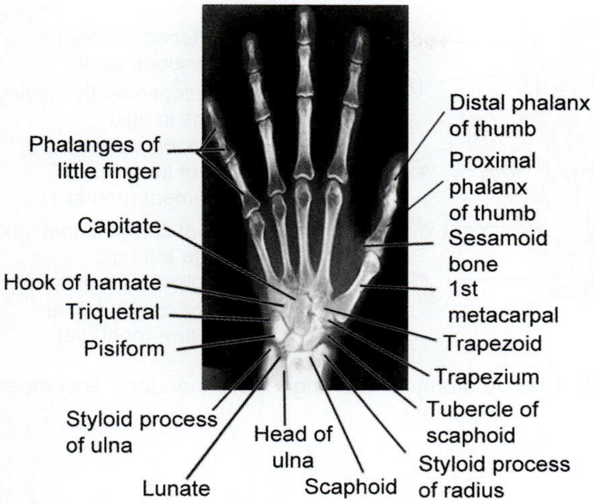

Fig. 21.138: Anatomy of the hand

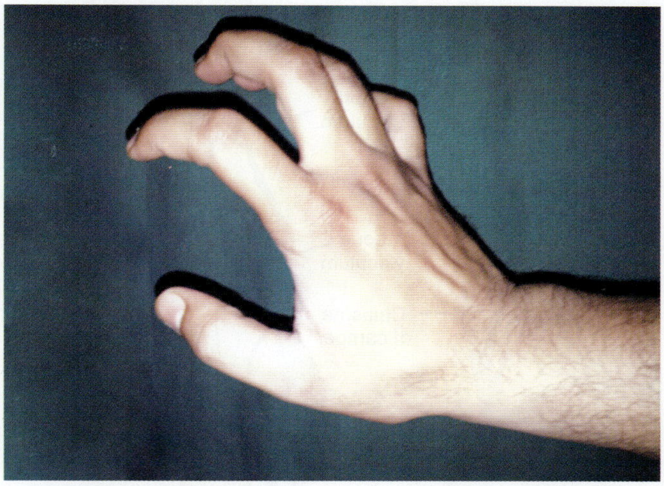

Fig. 21.139: Extensor tendons, passes under the extensor retinaculum, separates it into six compartments

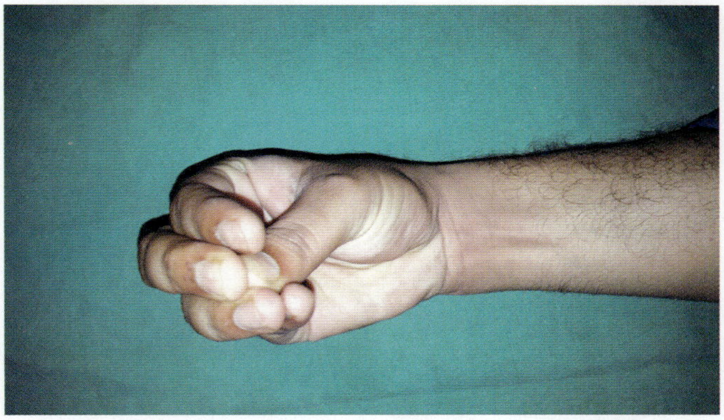

Fig. 21.140: Flexor carpi radialis, flexor carpi ulnaris and palmaris longus tendons are visible and are prime flexors of the wrist

Intrinsic Muscles

- Intrinsic muscles have their origins and insertions within the hand. Consist of the following muscles:
  - Thenar
  - Hypothenar
  - Adductor pollicis
  - Interossei
  - Lumbricals.

Extensor Tendons

- Courses over the dorsal side of the forearm, wrist and hand.
- Nine extensor tendons pass under the extensor retinaculum and separate it into six compartments (Fig. 21.139).
- The tendons that are palpated, with thumb abducted and extended, form an anatomical snuffbox
- Extensors digitorum communis are connected by junctura and because of this, a complete tendon laceration proximal to the junction may still result in normal extensor function.

Flexor Tendons

- Courses over the volar side of the forearm, wrist and hand
- Unlike the extensor tendons, the flexor tendons are enclosed in synovial sheaths, making them prone to deep space infections.
- Flexor carpi radialis, flexor carpi ulnaris and palmaris longus, primarily flex the wrist (Fig. 21.140).
- Nine flexor tendons pass through the carpel tunnel:
  - One tendon (FPS) goes to the base of the distal phalanx of the thumb
  - The other four digits has two tendons each (FDS and FDP)

Flexor Digitorum Superficialis (FDS)

- *Origin (two muscle bellies):* Medial epicondyle and radial shaft
- Insert into the middle phalanx of the four fingers (Fig. 21.141).

Flexor Digitorum Profundus (FDP)

- *Origin:* Ulna and interosseous membrane
- Inserts at the base of the distal phalanx (Fig. 21.141)

Tendon Sheets

Anatomy of the synovial sheaths of the fingers and the radial and ulnar bursae is depicted in (Fig. 21.142).

Zones (by Milford)

- The anatomy of the finger flexor tendons encompasses five zones, each of which is separated from the others by anatomic landmarks (Figs 21.143 to 21.145)

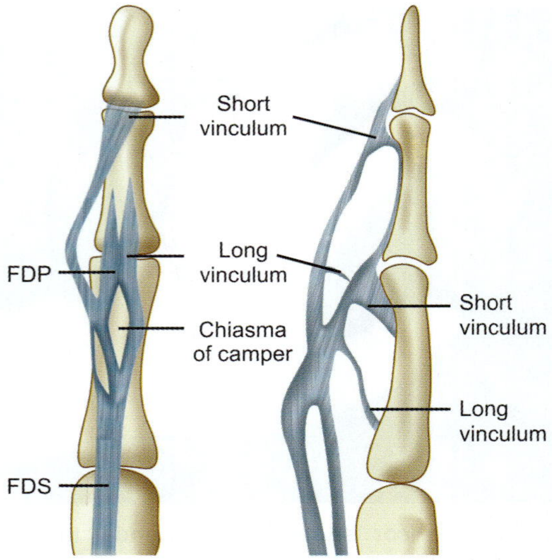

Fig. 21.141: Insertion of FDS into the middle phalanx of the four fingers and insertion of FDP at the base of the distal phalanx

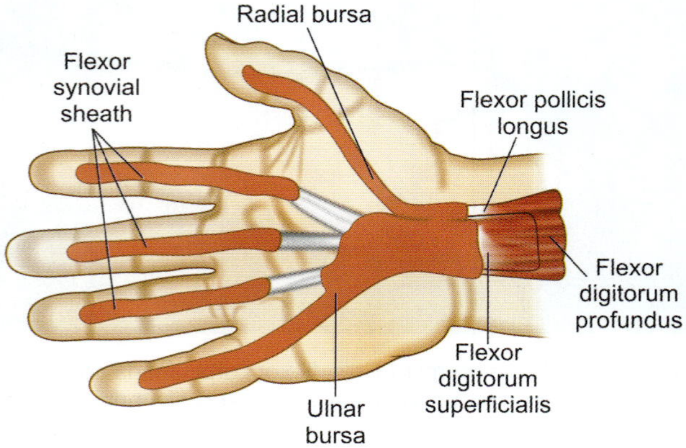

Fig. 21.142: Anatomy of the synovial sheaths of the fingers and the radial and ulnar bursae

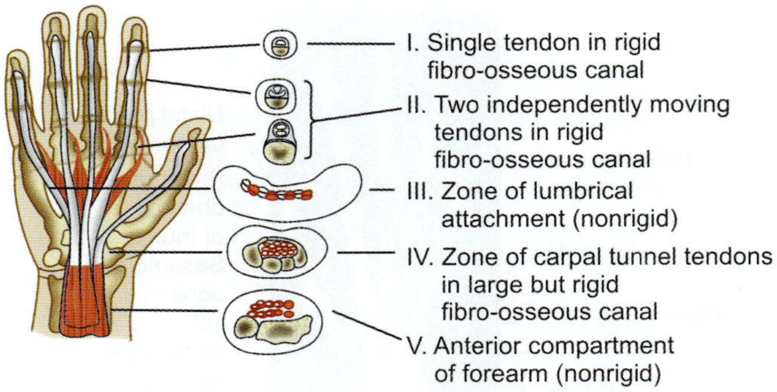

Fig. 21.143: Anatomy of the finger flexor tendons encompasses five zones

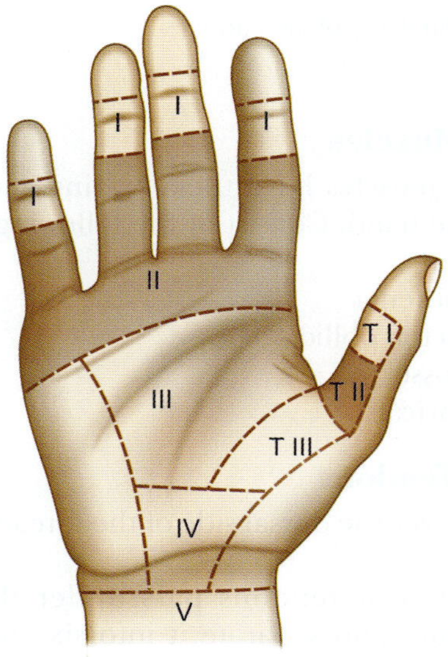

Fig. 21.144: Five zones of finger flexor tendons

- All the zones must be treated differently, in cases of tendon laceration.

Zone I

- It is the area distal to the insertion of the superficialis tendon
- Although the profundus tendon is still enclosed tightly within a fibro-osseous sheath here, it runs alone
- Therefore, the prognosis for the repair of lacerations in this zone is better than that for zone 2, although not as good as that for zones III, IV and V.

Zone II

- Stretches from the distal palmar crease to the middle of the middle phalanx
- In this area, the two tendons for each finger run together in a common fibro-osseous sheath
- The sheaths run from the level of the metacarpal heads (the distal palmar crease) to the distal phalanges. They are attached to the underlying bone and prevent the tendons from bowstringing
- Thickenings in the fibrous flexor sheath act as pulleys, directing the sliding movement of the tendons
- There are of two types, viz. annular and cruciate
- *Annular pulleys*: These are composed of a single fibrous band (ring). Cruciate pulleys have two crossing fibrous strands (cross)
- Annular pulleys include the following (Fig. 21.146)
  - The A1 pulley, which overlies the metacarpophalangeal joint. It is incised during trigger finger release
  - The A2 pulley, which overlies the proximal end of the proximal phalanx. It must be preserved (if at all possible) to prevent bowstringing

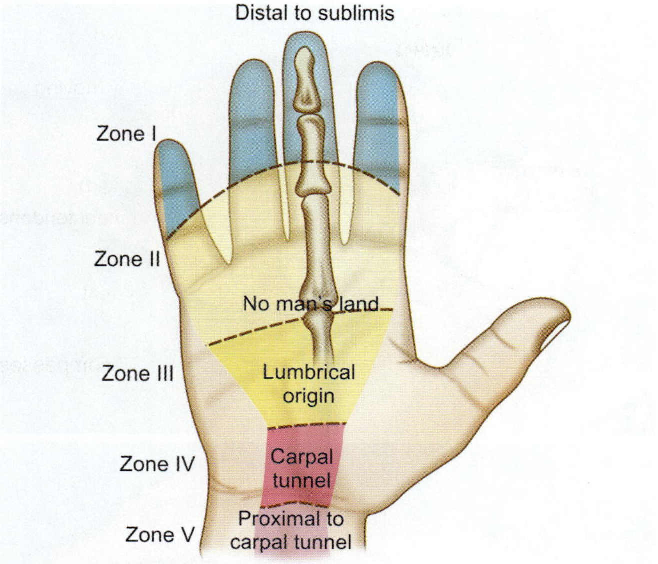

Fig. 21.145: Zones of the finger flexor tendons—Zone I. Distal to superficialis tendon; Zone II. Distal palmar crease to PIP crease; Zone III. Palm; Zone IV. Within the carpal tunnel; Zone V. Forearm proximal to the carpal tunnel

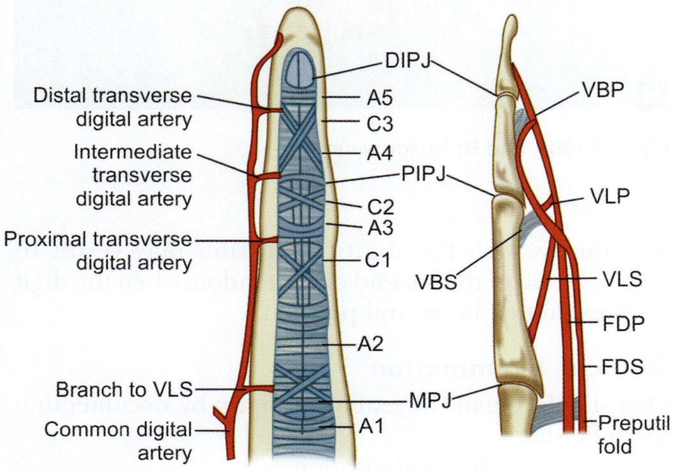

Fig. 21.146: Annular pulleys and cruciate pulleys

- The A3 pulley, which lies over the proximal interphalangeal joint
- The A4 pulley, which is located about the middle of the middle phalanx. It must be preserved to prevent bowstringing.

- *Cruciate pulleys:* None of which are critical for flexor function, include the following (Fig. 21.146):
  - The C1 pulley, which is located over the middle of the proximal phalanx
  - The C2 pulley, which is located over the proximal end of the middle phalanx

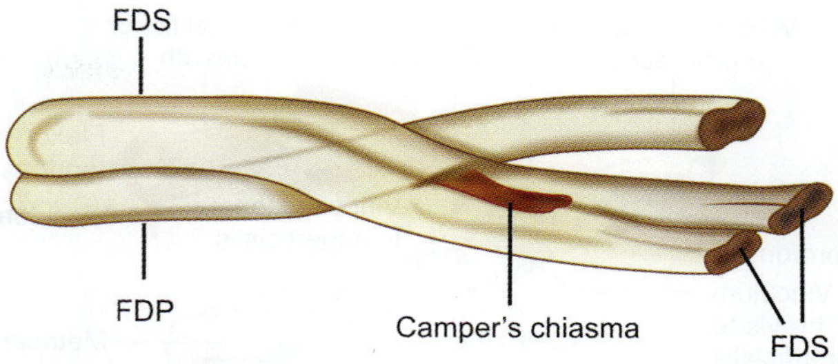

Fig. 21.147: Diagram showing FDS divides and passes around the FDP tendon to reunite at "Camper's chiasma"

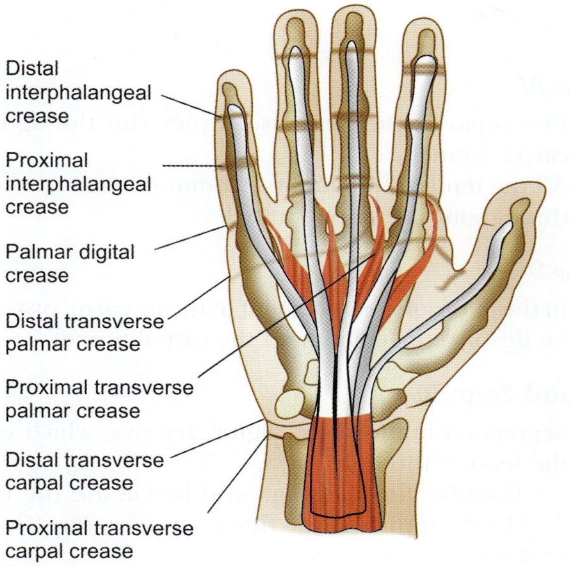

Fig. 21.148: Lumbricals originate from radial side of FDP

  - The C3 pulley, which is located over the distal end of the middle phalanx
- Over the proximal phalanx, FDS divides and passes around the FDP tendon, the two portions of the FDS reunite at "Camper's chiasma" (Figs 21.147)
- Repairs in this zone have the worst prognosis of all the zones. It has been nicknamed "no man's land" by Bunnell.

Zone III

- It is the zone of the lumbrical origin
- Lumbricals originate from radial side of FDP (Fig. 21.148)
- The tendons of the lumbricals pass along the radial sides of the metacarpophalangeal joints, before they insert into the dorsal expansion.
- They pass volar to the axes of the metacarpophalangeal joints. Thus, they act as flexors of those joints, even as they extend the interphalangeal joints.

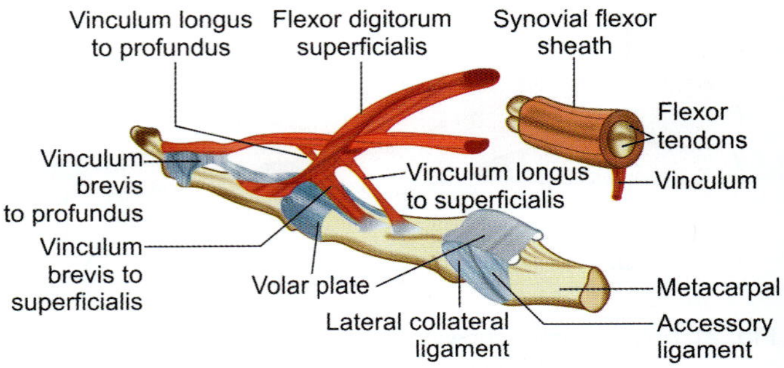

Fig. 21.149: Vincula longa and brevia are the main blood supplies to the flexor tendons

Zone IV

- Encompasses the tendons, as they run through the carpal tunnel.
- All the tendons remain in a common synovial sheath throughout the carpal tunnel.

Zone V

It's in the anterior compartment of the forearm, proximal to the flexor retinaculum and the carpal tunnel.

Blood Supply

- Segmental branches of digital arteries, which enter the tendon through:
  - *Vincula:* Vincula longa and brevia are the main blood supplies to the flexor tendons (Fig. 21.149)
  - Osseous insertions
- Synovial fluid diffusion.

Hand Injuries

Etiology

- Needle puncture
- Blade, knife cut, broken glass or edge of metal
- Burn, road traffic accidents and explosion
- Boxing and allied sports
- Machine parts, e.g. fan belt, grinding mechanism, guillotine, hot press machine, like those used in sealing wrappers and those used in plastic manufacturing industries.

Classification

- Tidy wound
- Untidy wound (Figs 21.150A and B)
- Injury may involve, nerves, tendons, intrinsic hand muscles as well as bones and joints.

Principles of Evaluation

- The position of the hand at the time of injury should be determined.

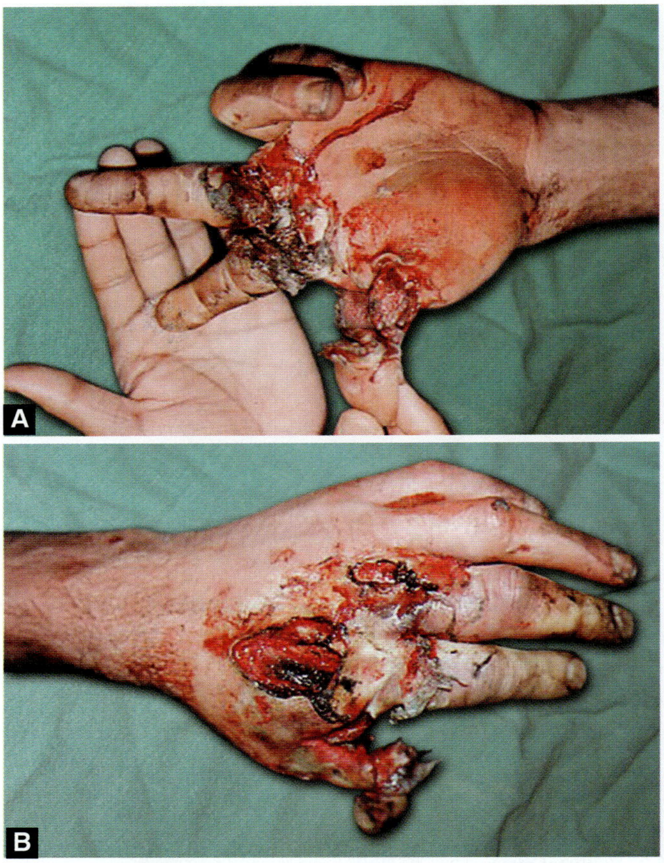

Figs 21.150A and B: Untidy wound

- Injuries with the digits in flexion may result in retraction of the cut end of the tendon, when the digit is examined in neutral position.

Clinical Examination

One should detail the extent of injury by documenting the following:

- Amount of devascularization
- Status of the skin
- Posture of the fingers
- Presence of deformity
- Active bleeding
- Bilateral grip strength
- ROM and strength should be tested against resistance.

Radiography

- X-rays should include PA, lateral and oblique views
- Rule out dislocations and fractures.

Nerve Testing—Motor

Test for Median Nerve

- Have the patient flex the distal phalanx of the thumb against resistance. Test opposition by touching the tip of the thumb to the tip of the little finger. The patient will be unable to oppose against resistance, if median nerve function is lost

- Test thumb abduction by placing the hand palm up and raising the thumb to the perpendicular while palpating the belly of the abductor pollicis muscle to insure it is contracting.

Test for Ulnar Nerve

- Spread the fingers apart against resistance and then push them together against resistance
- Test the hypothenar muscle, extend the fingers and then move the fifth finger away from the others
- Test thumb adduction (ulnar nerve innervates the adductor pollicis muscles), bring the thumb tightly against the side of the index finger. Adductor strength can be further tested by interposing a piece of paper between the thumb and the side of the index finger and then trying to pull the paper away.

Test for Radial Nerve

- Extend the fingers and wrist
- With the thumb in the hitchhiking position, test its resistance to further extension.

Nerve Testing—Sensory

- Determined by two-point discrimination
- Normal two-point discrimination is less than 6 mm at the fingertips and is often less than 2 mm. Both injured and non-injured fingers must be compared
- Repeat two-point discrimination testing two to four times on each side of the digit (80% accuracy is considered acceptable)
- A sensory deficit implies a potential digital artery laceration because of the close proximity of the two.

Nerve Injury Management (Table 21.3)

Tendon Testing

- Full ROM of each tendon against resistance should be assessed and compared with the uninjured side.

Table 21.3: Seddon's classification of nerve injuries, their treatment and prognosis

Seddon's classification of nerve injury	Disruption	Treatment	Prognosis
I Neuropraxia	Minimal axonal	Conservative	Complete in days or months
II Axonotmesis	Total axonal	Conservative	Complete in months
III Neurotmesis	Axon, endoneurium perineurium	Repair	Moderate reduction of function

- Important to test resistance because up to 90% of a tendon can be lacerated with preservation of ROM without resistance.
- Pain along the course of the tendon, during resistance testing suggests a partial laceration even if the strength appears adequate.

Flexor Digitorum Superficialis

Flexor digitorum superficialis (FDS) is tested by flexing the proximal interphalangeal (PIP) against resistance, while the remaining fingers are held (Fig. 21.151).

Flexor Digitorum Profundus

Flexor digitorum profundus (FDP) is tested by flexing the DIP against resistance, while the MP and PIP are held in extension (Fig. 21.152).

Tenodesis Effect

Passive extension of the wrist does not produce the normal "tenodesis" flexion of the fingers, if flexors are injured (Fig. 21.153).

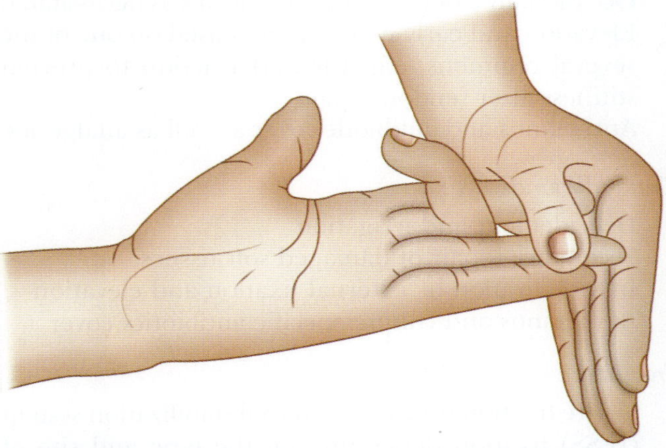

Fig. 21.151: Testing FDS, by flexing the PIP against resistance

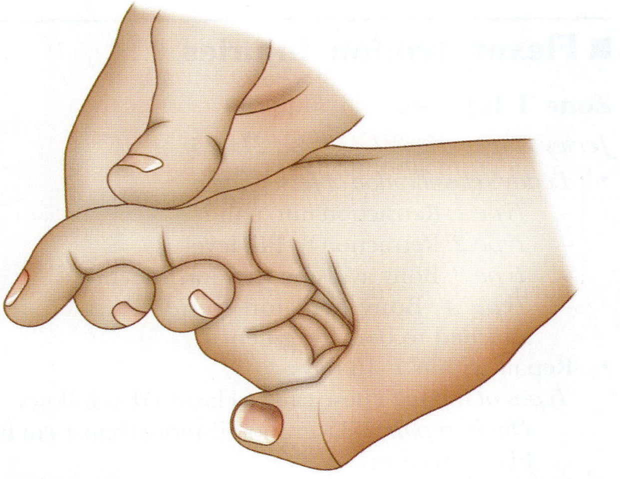

Fig. 21.152: FDP is tested by flexing the DIP against resistance

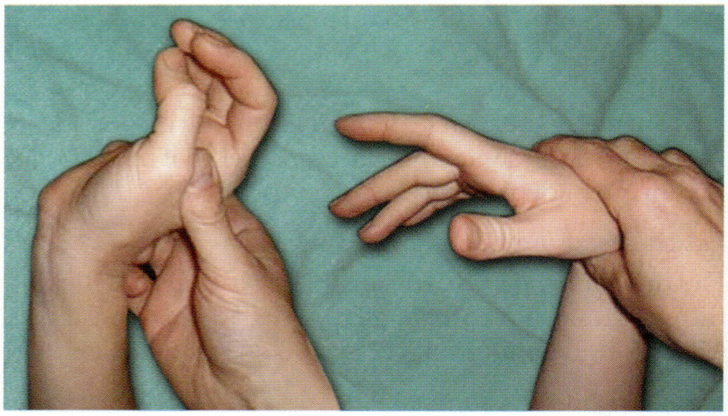

Fig. 21.153: Tenodesis effect

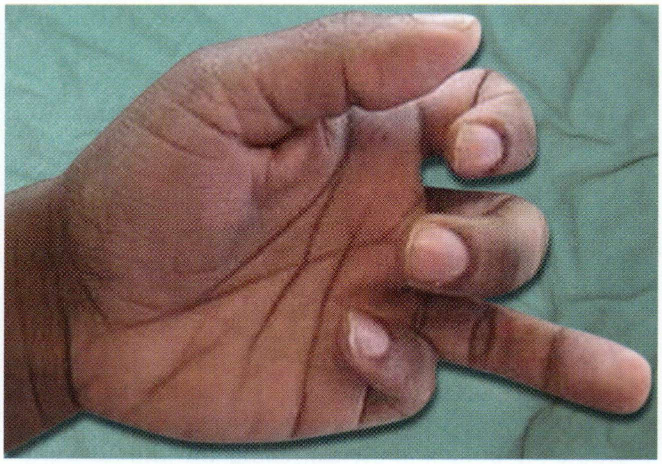

Fig. 21.154: Jersey finger

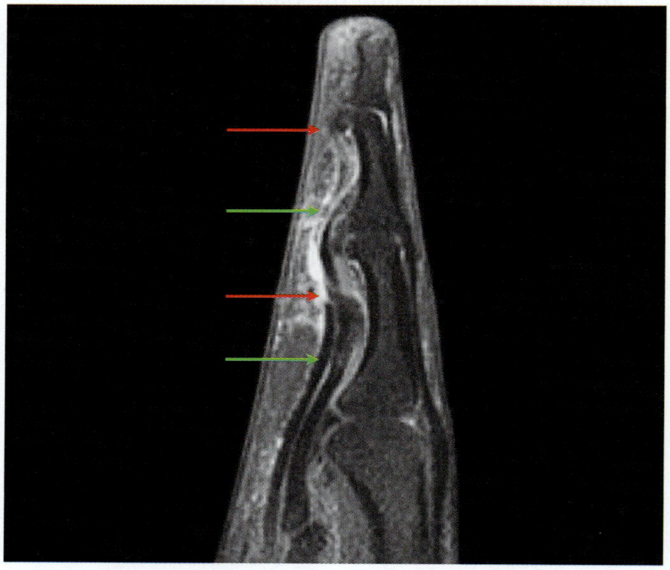

Fig. 21.155: The sagittal image of the ring finger reveals the gap (red arrows) between the torn ends of the FDP and also depicts the intact flexor digitorum superficialis tendon (green arrows)

Principles of Treatment of Hand Injury

Tidy Wounds

- Early debridement, irrigation and primary repair of damaged structures including soft tissue cover. Occasionally a delayed primary closure is necessitated
- Elevation and early mobilization based on one of the several regimens, e.g. Kleinert traction to prevent stiffness after tendon repair
- Antitetanus and antibiotic cover as well as analgesics.

Untidy Wounds

- Debridement and irrigation
- Secondary repair of damaged soft tissues
- Immobilization by external fixation and elevation
- Antitetanus and culture specific antibiotics cover.

Fractures

- K-wire fixation or Joshi's external stabilization system (JESS) fixation depending on the type and site of injury
- Immobilization by plaster of Paris (POP) slab or cast.

■ Flexor Tendon Injuries

Zone 1 Injuries

Jersey Finger (Figs 21.154 and 21.155)

- *Leddy's classification of Jersey finger*
  - *Type 1:* Retraction into palm
  - *Type 2:* Retraction to PIP level
  - *Type 3:* Bony avulsion (tendon attached)
  - *Type 4:* Bony avulsion (tendon attached not attached to bony fragment).
- Repair within 7–10 days
  Types of repair: These can be classified as follows:
  - *Direct repair:* If laceration is more than 1 cm from FDP insertion
  - *Tendon advancement:* If the laceration is less then 1 cm from insertion (Figs 21.156A to D)
  - Previously advocated for zone 1 repairs, as moving the repair site out of the sheath was felt, to decrease adhesion formation.

Disadvantages

- Shortening of flexor system
- Contracture
- Quadriga effect

Quadriga Effect

- If FDP tendon advanced too distally
- Entire muscle bells gets pulled distally

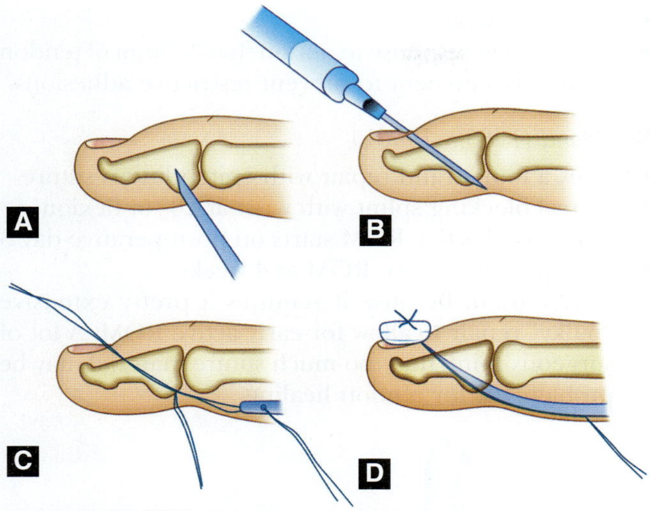

Figs 21.156A to D: Tendon advancement

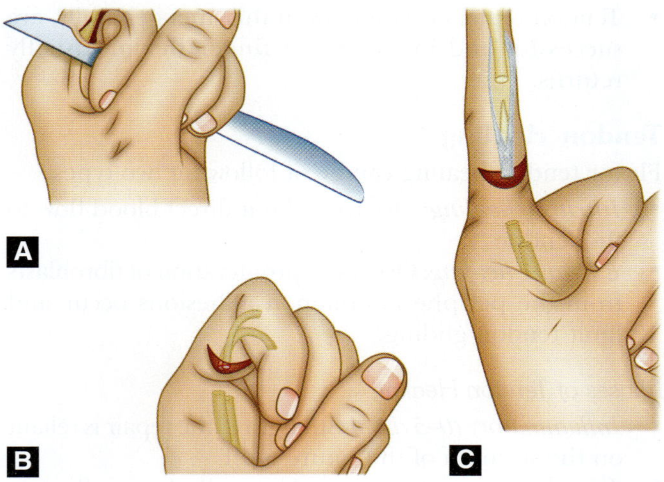

Figs 21.157A to C: Injury (lacerated) in this zone causes tendons to retract

- Tendon excursion of FDP of other digits is limited
- Loss of grip strength.

Zone 2 Injuries

- Deep and superficial flexor gliding inside tendon sheets
- Traditionally "no man's land", stiffness after repair
- Injury (lacerated) in this zone causes tendons to retract (Figs 21.157A to C).

Partial Lacerations

- No repair if 40% of the tendon intact
- Potential complications:
  - Triggering
  - Tendon entrapment
- Evaluate for the risk of triggering debride, if necessary
- Dorsal block splinting with wrist in 10° of flexion for 6 to 8 weeks
- It is better not to fix a partial laceration because the dissection necessary to fix it, might cause too much scarring, which might outweigh the benefit.

Complete Lacerations

- Repair of the flexor tendons by multiple strand sutures
- Ultimate strength and repair is proportional to number of strands
- Six and eight strand repairs are strongest, but have got a disadvantage of increased adhesion formation, due to increased tendon handling.
- Usually, four strand repair provides adequate strength.

Injuries to Both FDP and FDS

- Fix FDP and FDS
- As the blood supply to the FDP tendon is jeopardized, if the FDS is not also fixed (due to the vinculae anatomy).

Complications

- Stiffness
- Rerupture
- Tenolysis may be required in an estimated 18 to 25 percent of patients
  - No earlier than 3 months after repair
  - If no ROM, improvement for 1 to 2 months.

Zone 3 Injuries

- Lumbrical muscle bellies usually not sutured because this can increase the tension of these muscles and result in a "lumbrical plus" finger (paradoxical proximal interphalangeal extension on attempted active finger flexion).

Zone 4 Injuries

- Tendon repairs carried out in zone 4 have a good prognosis, but not as good as the prognosis of those carried out in zone 5, because the tendons are enclosed in a fibro-osseous tunnel
- The tunnel must be opened for repairs and adhesions may form after surgery.

Zone 5 Injuries

- In this zone 5, distinct tendons run into the hand toward the digits
- Each finger has two tendons, one each from the flexor digitorum superficialis muscle and the flexor digitorum profundus muscle
- The thumb has one long flexor, the flexor pollicis longus
- The tendons in zone 5 are not enclosed in a tight canal, but are surrounded by a synovial sheath in the distal part of the forearm

- Tendon repairs carried out in this area generally, are successful and independent finger flexion usually returns.

Tendon Healing

Flexor tendon healing can be of following two types:

- *Intrinsic healing*: Occurs without direct blood flow to the tendon
- *Extrinsic healing*: Occurs by proliferation of fibroblasts from the peripheral epitenon adhesions occur and limit tendon gliding.

Phases of Tendon Healing

- *Inflammatory (0–5 days):* Strength of the repair is reliant on the strength of the suture itself.
- *Fibroblastic (5–28 days):* Also called as collagen-producing phase.
- Remodelling (28 days–4 months)

Postoperative Rehabilitation

- Evaluate the range of motion of the repaired fingers
- Too much motion, indicates rupture of the tendon
- To little motion, indicates stiffness.

Postoperative Protocols

- *Kleinert:* Active extension, passive flexion by rubber bands (Figs 21.158 and 21.159).
- *Duran:* Controlled passive motion methods
- *Strickland:* Early active ROM

Kleinert: Goal is to achieve full active ROM, by 10–12 weeks.

Duran Protocol (Figs 21.160 and 21.161)

- Dorsal splint in 20° wrist flexion
- No rubber bands
- Passive flexion
- Designed in response to notion that 3–5mm of tendon gliding is sufficient to prevent restrictive adhesions.

Strickland (1980's–1990's)

- Uses a four strand repair with epitendinous suture
- Dorsal blocking splint with wrist at 20° of flexion
- Supervised active ROM starts on postoperative day 3
- Unsupervised active ROM at 4 weeks
- Rarely used, because it requires a pretty extensive "bulky" repair to allow for early active ROM. A lot of surgeons think that too much suture material may be problematic for tendon healing.

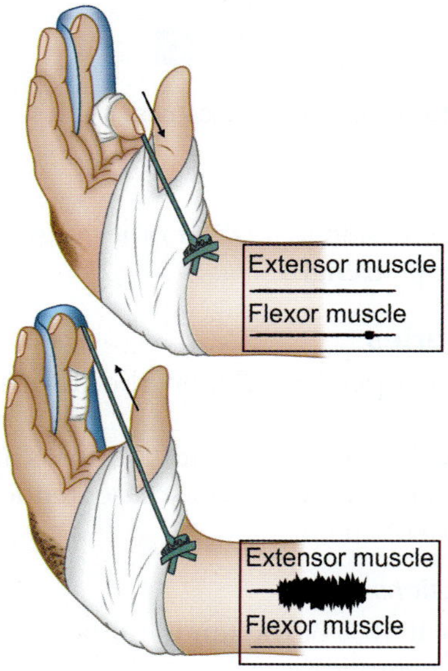

Fig. 21.159: Mechanism of Kleinert protocol of active extension and passive flexion by rubber bands

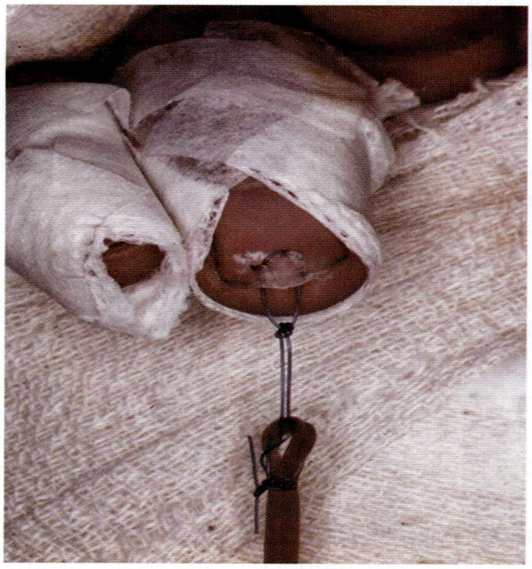

Fig. 21.158: Active extension, passive flexion by rubber bands

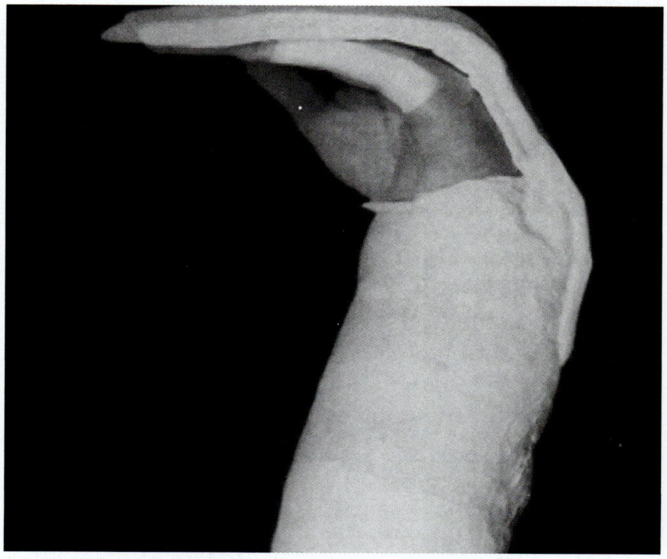

Fig. 21.160: Dorsal splint in 20° of wrist flexion

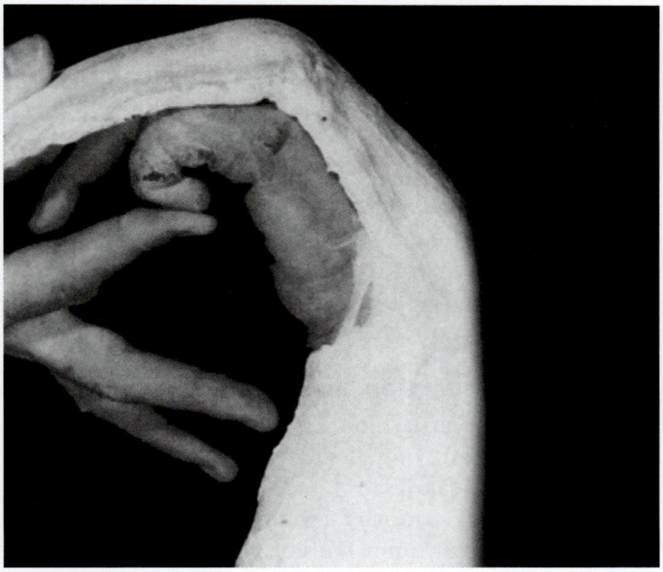

Fig. 21.161: Passive flexion exercises are performed, to promote tendon gliding and to prevent restrictive adhesions

In children

- They are usually not able to reliably participate in rehabilitation programs
- No benefit to early mobilization in patients under 16 years
- Immobilization greater than 4 weeks may lead to poorer outcomes.

Delayed Reconstruction

Single Stage Tendon Grafting

Indications for single stage tendon gliding are:

- Segmental tendon loss
- Delay in definitive repair (greater than 3–6 weeks)
- Patient should be having:
  - Full passive range of motion (PROM)
  - Competent pulleys
- Graft donors are:
  - Palmaris longus
  - Plantaris
  - Long toe extensors
  - Flexor digitorum superficialis
  - Extensor indicis proprius
  - Extensor digiti minimi.

Two Stage Reconstruction

Indications for two stage reconstructions are:

- Extensive soft tissue scarring
  - Crush injuries
  - Associated fractures, nerve injuries, etc.
- Loss of significant portion of pulley system.

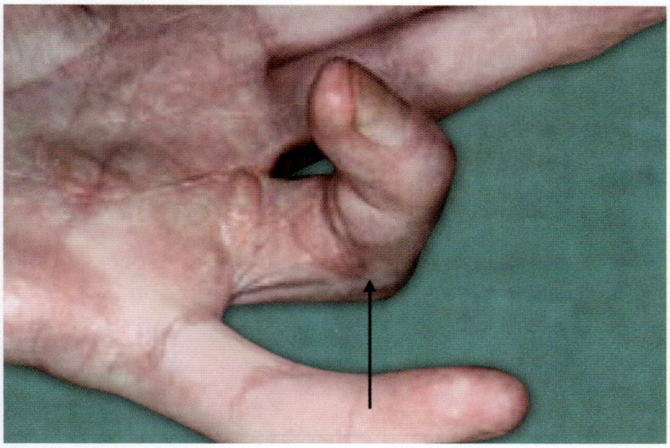

Fig. 21.162: Joint contracture, after reconstruction

Stages of Reconstructions

Stage 1

- Excision of tendon remnants
- Hunter rod then placed through pulley system and fixed distally
- Reconstruct pulleys as needed, if implant bowstrings.

Stage 2

- Implant removal and tendon graft insertion
- FDS transfer from adjacent digit described
- *Postoperative:* Early controlled motion for 3 weeks, then slow progression to active motion.

Complications

- Joint contracture (Fig. 21.162)
- Adhesions
- Rupture
- Bowstringing
- Infection.

Amputation and Replantation

- Care of amputated part needs to be done. The part should be:
  - Washed gently with saline
  - Wrapped in moist saline gauze
  - Tucked into polythene bag (or bread wrapper)
  - Put in a container of a mixture of ice block and water.
- Absolute contraindications to replantation:
  - Concomitant life threatening injury
  - Inhibiting systemic illness
  - Severe crushing
  - Extreme contamination
  - Prolonged ischemia time
  - Multiple levels injures
  - Previous surgery to the amputated part.

Replantation

Steps followed are illustrated below as:
- Bone shortening and fixation
- Arterial repair
- Venous anastomosis
- Nerve and tendon repair
- Skin closure

Note: The reader is requested to refer other special books on hand surgery for details of reimplantation.

GANGLIONIC CYSTS OF THE WRIST

■ Introduction

- It is a type of mucinous filled cyst which is found adjacent to joint capsule or tendon sheath.
- It consists of an outer fibrous coat and an inner synovial lining along with a clear, colorless, gelatinous fluid
- Ganglions usually occurs singly, but may be multilocular
- More common in women.

Age

- Seventy percent occur between the second and fourth decades
- Ganglions occurring at DIP joint (mucus cyst) are associated with osteoarthritis and occur at older ages
- Rarely seen in children.

Location

- Frequent in hand and wrist (Fig. 21.163), less often in ankle, foot and knee
- Most common soft tissue mass of hand is ganglion
- *Dorsal ganglion*: 60–70 percent of all ganglia occur over scapholunate ligament
- V*olar ganglion*: 20 percent of all ganglia occur at volar wrist (Fig. 21.164). Most common site is at volar wrist crease between the flexor carpi radialis (FCR) and abductor pollicis longus (APL) at the scaphotrapezoid joint.

Differential Diagnosis

- Synovial sarcoma
- Extraskeletal chondrosarcoma
- Avascular necrosis (AVN)
- Venous aneurysm.

Clinical Presentation and Examination

- Dorsal wrist pain, which is made worse with repeated use; a slow growing, localized swelling, with mild aching and weakness
- Cyst is firm, smooth, rubbery, rounded, slightly fluctuant and at times tender
- Cysts will transilluminate
- It is usually fixed but may be slightly movable, if it involves tendon sheath
- Mass may become obvious with wrist flexion
- Palpation of cyst with compression may not only increase the extent of the cyst, but also the direction of pedicle.

Occult Ganglia

- Source of similar symptoms occur especially in young gymnasts. Discomfort is usually maximal in extension
- Point tenderness is directly overs capholunate interval
- Attempt to palpate mass overs capholunate ligament, with wrist in volar flexion.

Radiographs

- Usually negative
- Arthrography is usually not helpful
- Dorsal ganglions may be found with scapholunate diastasis.

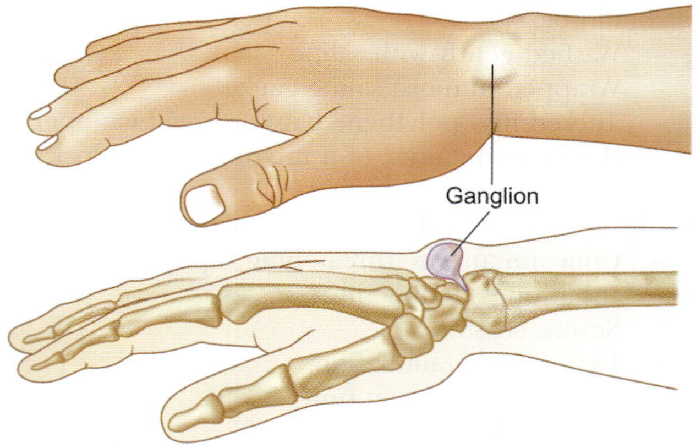

Fig. 21.163: Ganglion on wrist

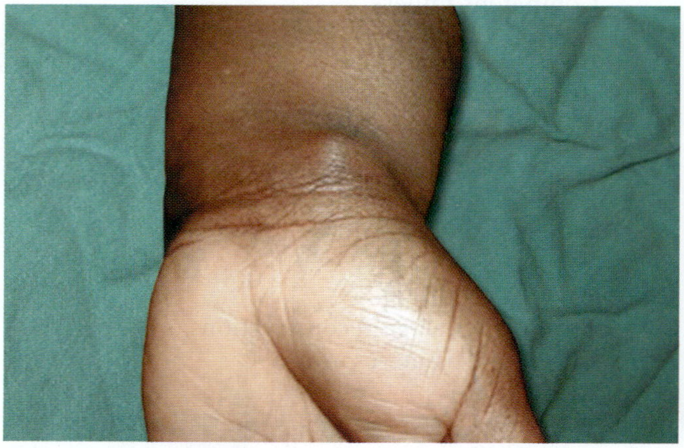

Fig. 21.164: Volar ganglion

Surgical Treatment

- Aspiration
- Complete excision
- In a few cases, cysts return following needle aspiration or surgical treatment.

DISTAL RADIOULNAR JOINT

■ Carpal Bones

There are eight carpal bones, arranged in two rows, as shown in Figure 21.165.

Proximal Row (Lateral to Medial)

- Articulates with inferior surface of lower end of radius and articular disk of inferior radioulnar joint.
  - Scaphoid (S)
  - Lunate (L)
  - Triquetral (Tq)
  - Pisiform (P)

Distal Row (Lateral to Medial)

- Articulates with the base of metacarpals
  - Trapezium (Tm)
  - Trapezoid (Td)
  - Capitate (C)
  - Hamate (H)

■ Ligaments

There are 33 ligaments around the wrist. These can further be classified as follows:

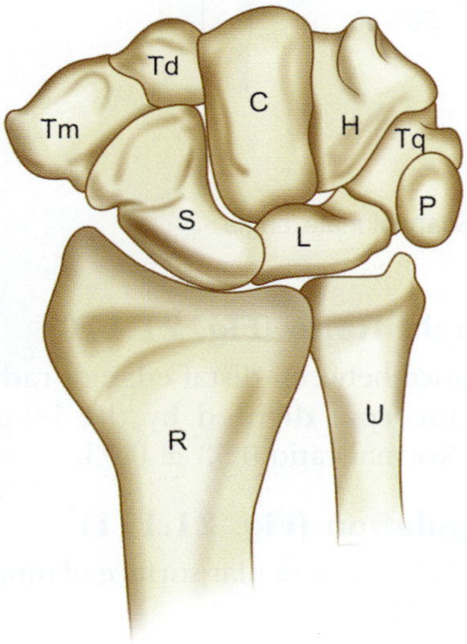

Fig. 21.165: Radiocarpal joint—C. Capitate; H. Hamate; L. Lunate; P. Pisiform; S. Scaphoid; Td. Trapezoid; Tm. Trapezium; Tq. Triquetrum; R. Radius; U. Ulnar

Taleisnik and Kelly's Classification

I. Extrinsic ligaments
II. Intrinsic ligaments.

Extrinsic Ligaments

These are radiocarpal and carpometacarpal ligaments (Fig. 21.166). These can further be divided into ligaments on volar and dorsal aspects.

i. Volar ligaments
ii. Dorsal ligaments.

i. *Volar ligaments*: Extrinsic ligaments on volar aspects are enumerated below:
   - Radioscaphocapitate
   - Long radiolunate
   - Radioscapholunate (ligamnent of Testut)
   - Short radiolunate
   - Ulnolunate
   - Ulnotriquetral
   - Ulnocapitate.

ii. *Dorsal ligaments: These include following ligaments*
   - Dorsal intercarpal
   - Dorsal radiotriquetral

Intrinsic Ligaments (Fig. 21.167)

These are intercarpal ligaments and include following ligaments:

- Scapholunate
- Lunotriquetral

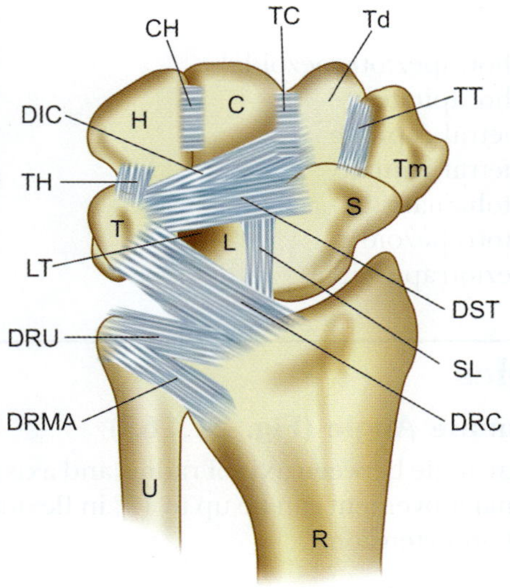

Fig. 21.166: Wrist from dorsal perspective—*Bones:* C. Capitate; H. Hamate; L. Lunate; R. Radius; S. Scaphoid; T. Triquetrum; Td. Trapezoid; U. Ulna; *Ligaments:* CH. Capitohamate; DIC. Dorsal intercarpal; DRC. Dorsal radiocarpal; DRMA. Dorsal radial metaphyseal; DRU. Dorsal radioulnar; LT. Lunotriquetral; SL. Scapholunate; TC. Trapezocapitate; TH. Triquetrohamate; TT. Trapeziotrapezoid; Tm. Trapezium; DST. Dorsal scaphotriquetral

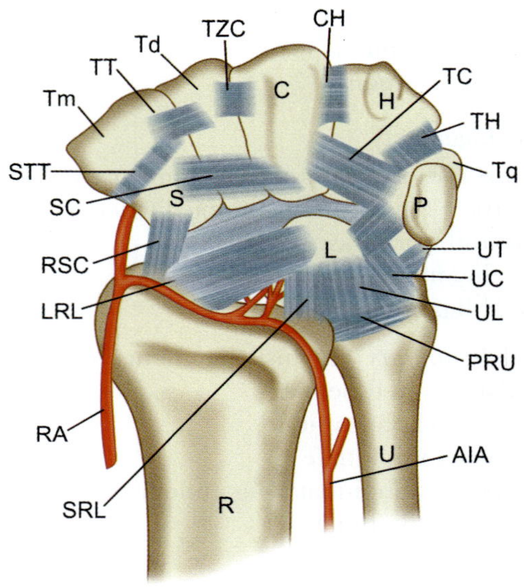

Fig. 21.167: Wrist from palmar perspective—*Bones:* C. Capitate; H. Hamate; L. Lunate; P. Pisiform; R. Radius; S. Scaphoid; Td. Trapezoid; Tm. Trapezium; Tq. Triquetrum; U. Ulna, *Ligaments:* CH. Capitohamate; LRL. Long radiolunate; PRU Palmar radioulnar ligament; RSC. Radioscaphocapitate; SC. Scaphocapitate; SRL. Short radiolunate; STT. Scaphotrapeziotrapezoid; TZC. Trapezocapitate; TC. Triquetrocapitate; TH. Triquetrohamate; TT. Trapeziotrapezoid; UC. Ulnocapitate, UL. Ulnolunate; UT. Ulnotriquetral; RA. Radial artery; AIA. Anterior interosseous artery

- Scaphotrapeziotrapezoidal
- Scaphocapitate
- Triquetral capitate
- Triquetral hamate
- Capitohamate
- Capitotrapezoidal
- Trapeziotrapezoidal

■ Angles

Radiolunate Angle (Fig. 21.168)

- It is an angle between axis of radius and axis of lunate
- Normal movement can be up to 15° in flexion and up to 20° in extension.

Capitolunate Angle

- It is an angle between axis of capitate and axis of lunate
- There is some abnormality, if movement is more than 15°.

Scapholunate Angle (Fig. 21.169)

It is an angle between axis of lunate and axis of scaphoid. Normal range 30–70°.

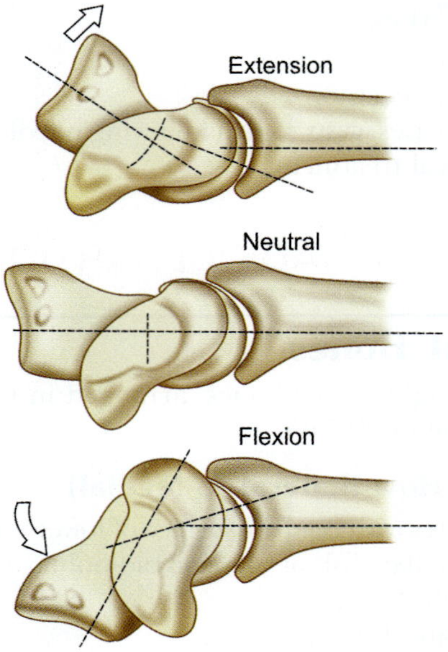

Fig. 21.168: Radiolunate angle

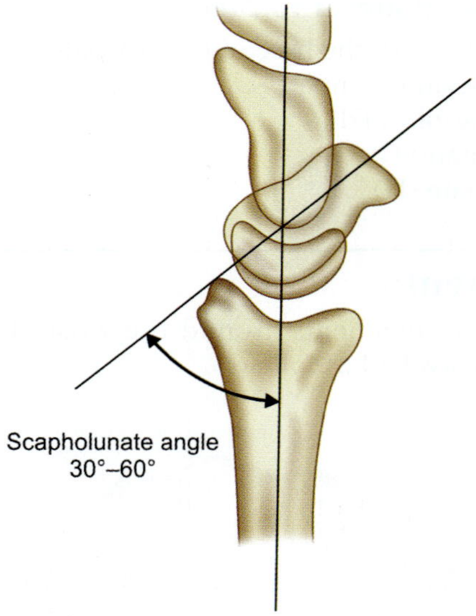

Fig. 21.169: Scapholunate angle

Carpal Height Ratio (Fig. 21.170)

It is the distance between distal edge of radius and base of third metacarpal divided by the length of third metacarpal. Normal ratio 0.53 ± 0.03.

Radial Angulation (Fig. 21.171)

It is an angle between articular surface of ulna and radius. Normal range 23°.

Palmar Angulation (Fig. 21.172)

It is an angle between axis of radius and axis of lunate in lateral view. Normal range 11°.

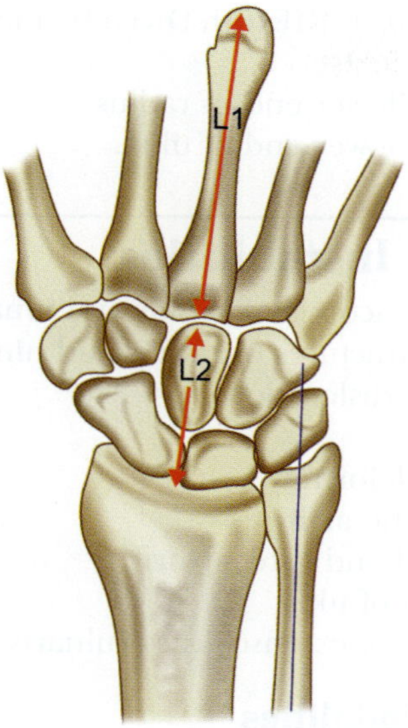

Fig. 21.170: Carpal height ratio—L1. Length of the third metacarpal; L2. Distance between distal edge of radius and base of third metacarpal

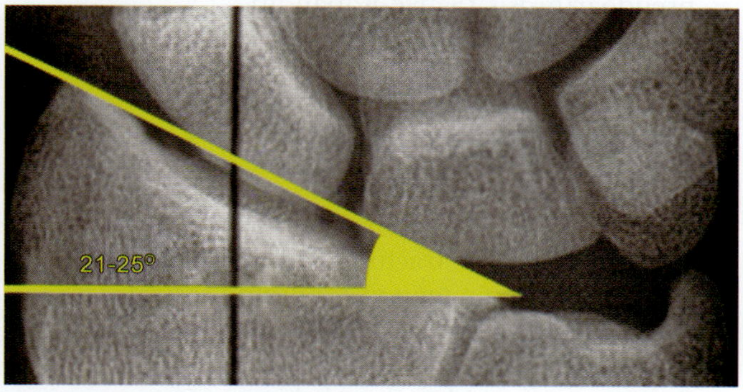

Fig. 21.171: Radial angulation

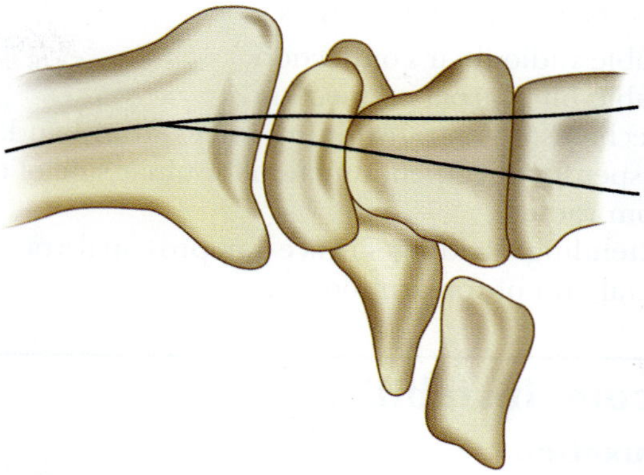

Fig. 21.172: Palmar angulation

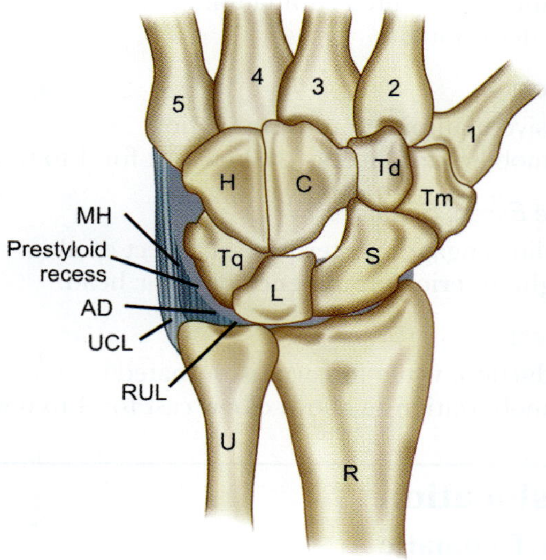

Fig. 21.173: Components of triangular fibrocartilage complex. AD. Articular disk; MH. Meniscus homologue; RUL. Dorsal and volar radioulnar ligaments; UCL. Ulnar collateral ligament. Other structures shown are metacarpal bones (1,2,3,4, and 5), Carpal bones; C. Capitate; H. Hamate; S. Scaphoid; Td. Trapezoid; Tq. Triquetrum; R. Radius; U. Ulna; L. Lunate; Tm. Trapezium

Radial Length

It is the distance between radial styloid and ulnar styloid. Normal length is 12 mm.

Anatomy of Distal Radioulnar Joint

Distal radioulnar joint (DRUJ) is a pivot type synovial joint, where head of ulna articulates with ulnar notch of radius. It consists of the following features:

- *Articular disk:* Fibrocartilage apex attached to the base of styloid of ulna and base to lower margin of ulnar notch of radius.
- *Capsule:* Upper part is weak and evaginated by synovial membrane, forming recessus sacciformis.
- Triangular fibrocartilage complex of Werner and Palmar.

Triangular Fibrocartilage Complex

Triangular fibrocartilage complex (TFCC). It begins on ulnar side of lunate fossa of radius and attaches to ulnar head and base of ulnar styloid (Fig. 21.173).

It has following components:

- Volar and dorsal radioulnar ligament
- Ulnar collateral ligament
- Meniscal homologue
- Articular disk
- Extensor carpi ulnaris sheath
- Ulnolunate ligament
- Ulnotriquetral ligament.

It consists of following features:

- Stable radioulnar connection
- Stable ulnocarpal connection
- Mechanism for transmitting forces from hand.
- Suspensory ligament function for ulnar side of carpus from radius.
- Extending dividing surface for proximal row across distal end of forearm bones.

Acute Instability

Subluxation

There can be two reasons for subluxation:

Forcible Excess Pronation

- Radius engages ulnar prominence
- Painful and limited supination
- No deformity.

Treatment

- Passive manipulation to supination
- Immobilization in above elbow cast for 4 to 6 weeks.

Forcible Excess Supination

- Radius engages posterolateral aspect of ulna
- Slight anterior prominence of ulnar head.

Treatment

- Reduction, while forearm is pronated
- Immobilization in above elbow cast for 4 to 6 weeks.

Dislocation

Acute Traumatic

- Complete volar or dorsal displacement of ulna, associated with disruption of volar or dorsal radioulnar capsular ligament.
- Radiocarpal unit displaces, abducted fixed inferior end of ulna
- Excessive prominence of ulnar head and narrow wrist.

Treatment

- Reduction by pressure on ulna and above elbow cast for 4 to 6 weeks.

Associated Instability

- Galleazzi fracture:
  - Fracture of lower third radius with dislocation of DRUJ
  - *Treatment:* ORIF with plating
  - If DRUJ not reduced, fixation with K-wire for 6 weeks in supination.
- Essex Lopresti fracture dislocation
  - Fracture radial head or neck with disruption of DRUJ with interosseous membrane tear.
  - *Treatment:* ORIF with DRUJ fixation by K-wire for 6 weeks
- Fractures of lower end of radius
- Fractures of lower end of ulna.

Chronic Instabilities

- Malunited fractures of radius and ulna
- Nonunited fractures of radius and ulna
- Undetected dislocations
- TFCC tear
- Madelung deformity
- Post-traumatic arthritis
- Rheumatoid and osteoarthritis
- Subluxation of ulna
- Subluxation of extensor carpi ulnaris tendon.

Treatment Modalities

- Ulnar hemiresection-interposition arthroplasty (Bowers)
- Ulnar shortening procedures
- Distal radioulnar arthrodesis with distal ulnar pseudoarthrosis (Sauve-Kapandji).
- Procedures to stabilize DRUJ.

Ulnar Hemiresection Interposition Arthroplasty (Bowers) (Figs 21.174 and 21.175)

Indications

- Unreconstructable fractures of ulnar head
- Ulnocarpal impingement syndrome
- Rheumatoid arthritis
- Chronic painful TFCC tear
- Post-traumatic and osteoarthritis

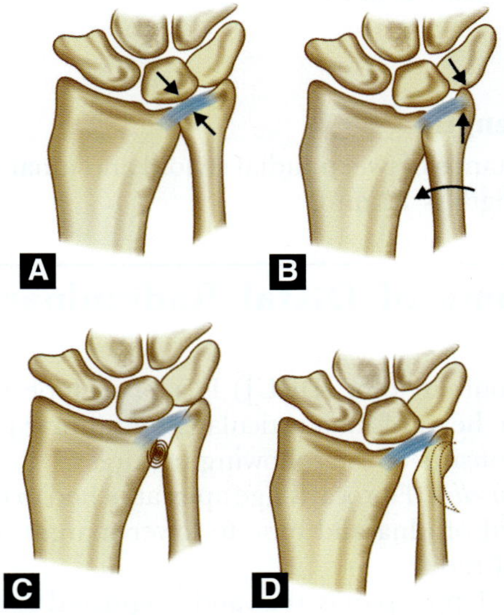

Figs 21.174A to D: Steps followed, while performing ulnar hemiresection interposition arthroplasty (Bowers arthroplasty)

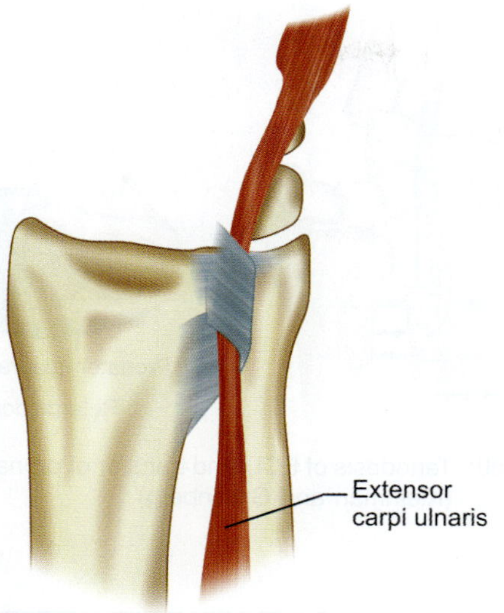

Fig. 21.175: Ulnar hemiresection interposition arthroplasty (Bowers)

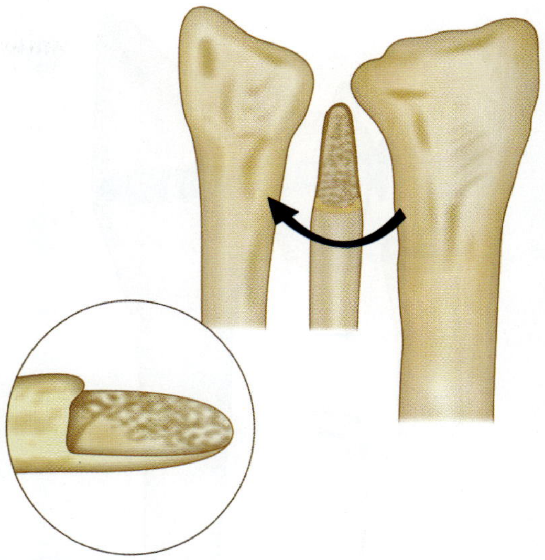

Fig. 21.177: Matched resection (Watson)

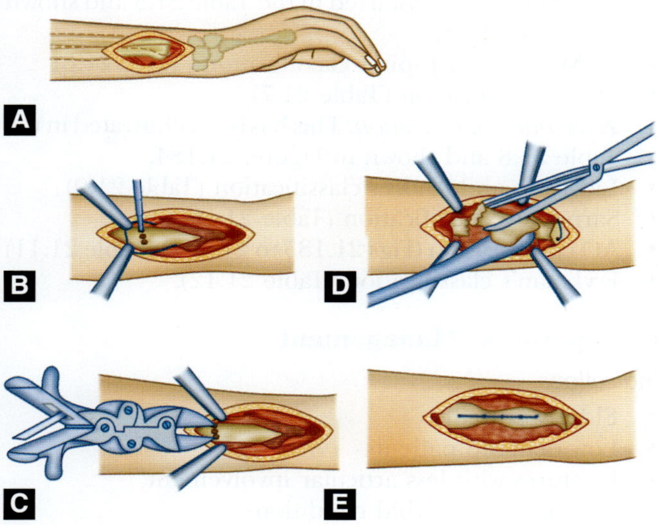

Figs 21.176A to E: Darrach resection

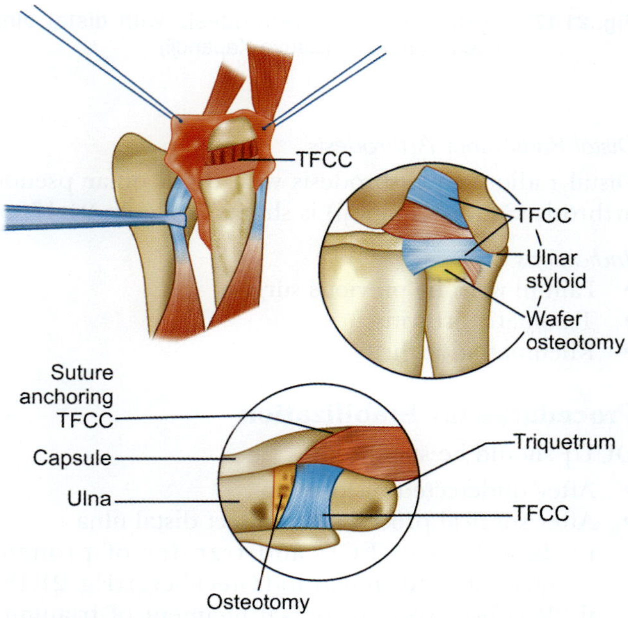

Fig. 21.178: Wafer resection (Feldon)

Ulnar Shortening Procedure

Darrach Resection (Figs 21.176A and E)

Indications

- Malunited Colle's fracture
- Malunion or nonunion of radius
- Abnormality of growth of distal radius.

Matched Resection (Watson) (Fig. 21.177)

Indications

- Rheumatoid arthritis
- Trauma.

Wafer Resection (Feldon) (Fig. 21.178)

Indications

- TFCC tear
- Ulnar impaction syndrome.

Milch Cuff Resection (See Figs 21.208A to C)

Indications

- Malunited Colle's fracture
- Malunion or nonunion of radius
- Cessation or abnormality of growth of distal radius.

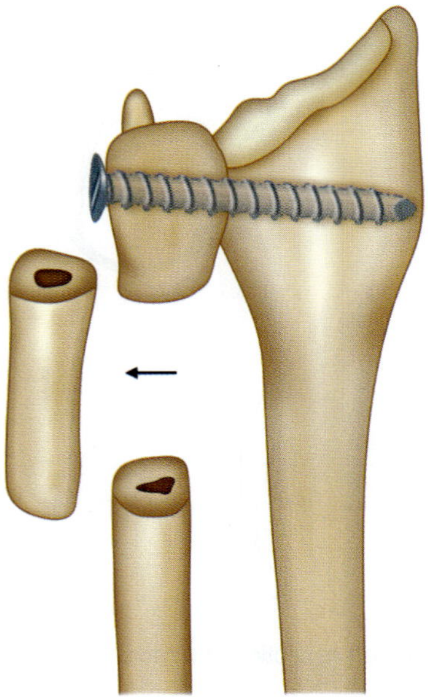

Fig. 21.179: Distal radioulnar arthrodesis with distal ulnar pseudoarthrosis (Sauve-Kapandji)

Distal Radioulnar Arthrodesis

Distal radioulnar arthrodesis with distal ulnar pseudoarthrosis (Sauve-Kapandji) is shown in Figure 21.179.

Indications

- Painful wrist by previous surgery
- Traumatic arthritis
- Rheumatoid arthritis.

Procedures for Stabilization

DUUJ should be stabilized:

- After undetected dislocation
- After surgical procedure to resect distal ulna
  i. Tenodesis of ECU and transfer of pronator quadratus (Kleinman and Greenberg) (Fig. 21.180)
  ii. Reconstruction of dorsal ligament of triangular fibrocartilage complex (Scheker) (Figs 21.181A to G).

DISTAL RADIUS FRACTURES

To be effective, a classification system must accurately categorize the fracture type and injury severity to serve as a guideline for treatment and prognosis.

Although many classification systems have attempted to provide a more accurate representation of various distal radius fracture patterns, some have proven more useful than others in guiding treatment and predicting outcome.

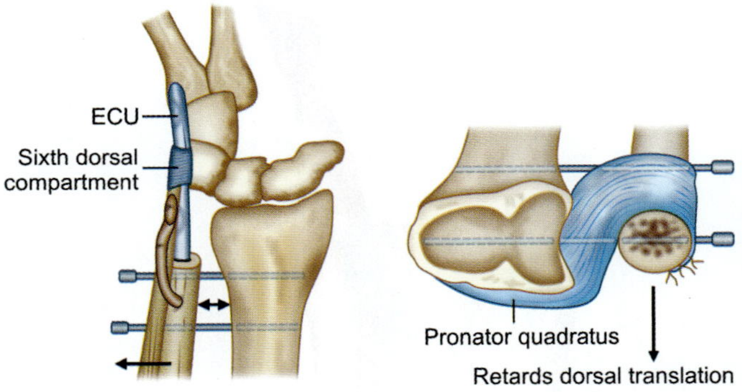

Fig. 21.180: Tenodesis of ECU and transfer of pronator quadratus (Kleinman and Greenberg)

Classification

- *Gartland and Werley classification:* This has been illustrated in the Table 21.4 and shown in Fig. 21.182.
- *Melone's classification:* Intra-articular fractures are classified, as demostarted in the Table 21.5 and shown in Figure 21.183.
- McMurtry and Jupiter classification (Table 21.6)
- Mayo classification (Table 21.7)
- *Fernandez classification:* This has been illustrated in the Table 21.8 and shown in Figure. 21.184.
- Lidstrom and Andres classification (Table 21.9)
- Sarmiento classification (Table 21.10)
- AO classification (Figs 21.185 to 21.187) (Table 21.11)
- Frykman's classification (Table 21.12).

Nonoperative Management

Indications

- Elderly patients
- Low demand patients
- Fractures with less articular involvement
- Associated comorbid conditions
- Fractures which can be maintained in acceptable position.

Guidelines for Reduction

- Radial shortening less than 5 mm at distal radioulnar joint
- Radial inclination on posteroanterior radiographs greater than 15°
- Sagittal tilt on lateral projection between 15° dorsal tilt and 20° volar tilt
- Intra-articular stepoff or gap less than 2 mm of radiocarpal joint
- Articular incongruity less than 2 mm of sigmoid notch of distal radius.

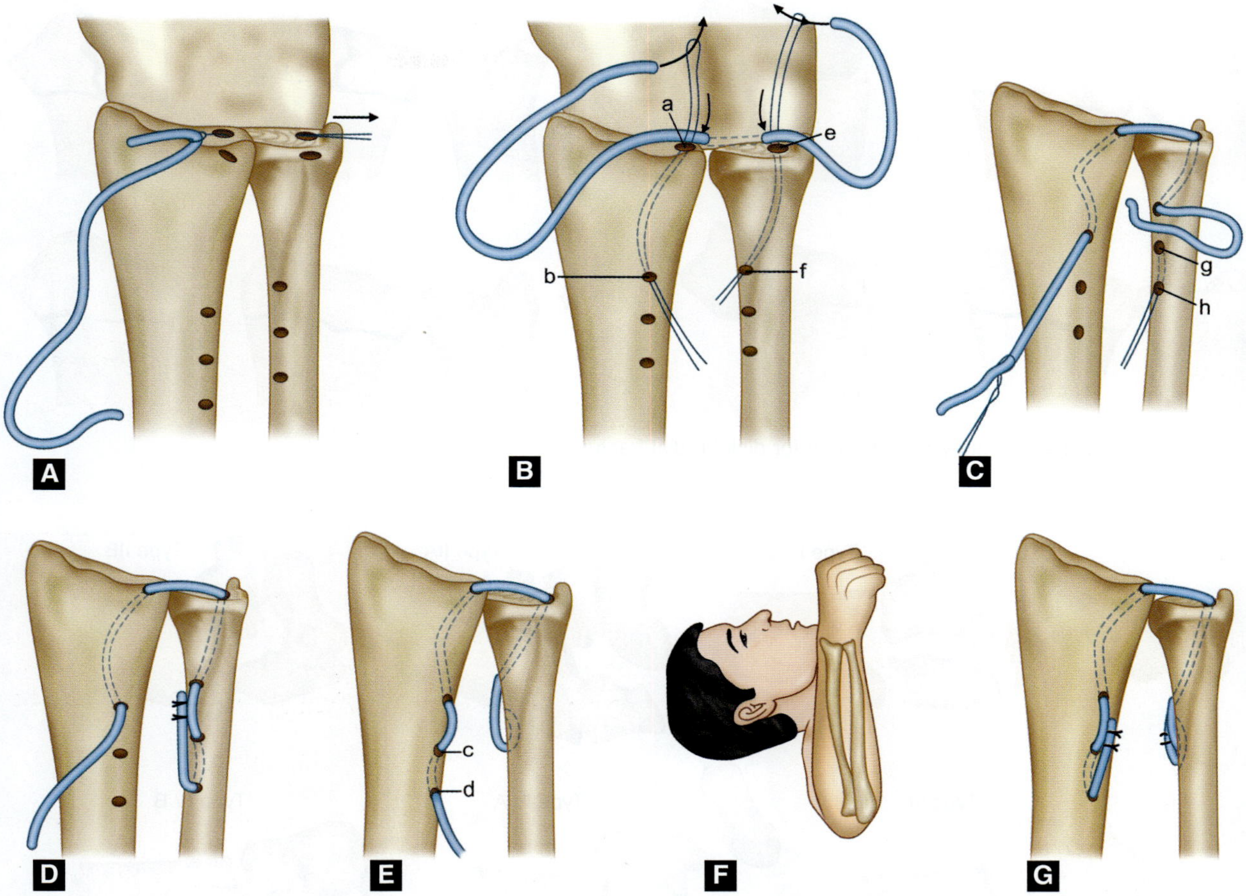

Fig. 21.181A to G: Schekar technique—(A) Tendon graft is drawn through casulotomies; (B) Ends of tendon graft inserted into loops of wire emerging from tunnels in ulnar fovea and dorsal lip of sigmoid notch of radius; (C) Tendon graft is drawn through two distal tunnels; (D) Ulnar end of tendon graft is threaded through second tunnel and sutures to itself; (E) Tendon graft is pulled between middle and distal hole in metaphysic of radius to ensure that full tension has been applied between fovea and sigmoid notch; (F) With tension applied to radial end of tendon graft while forearm is supinated, joint stability is tested through full range of motion; (G) On radial side, graft is sutures to itself with forearm is supinated, completing reconstruction of dorsal ligament

Table 21.4: Gartland and Werley classification of distal radius fractures

Group 1	Simple Colle's fracture
Group 2	Comminuted Colle's fracture with undisplaced intra-articular fragments
Group 3	Comminuted Colle's fracture with displaced intra-articular fragments

Table 21.5: Melone's intra-articular fractures classification

Type I	Minimal comminution-stable
Type II	Comminuted-stable Displacement of medial complex: Posterior: Die-punch, barton Anterior: Smith
Type III	Displacement of medial complex as a unit + anterior spike
Type IV	Wide separation or rotation of the dorsal fragment and palmar fragment rotation

Reduction Techniques

Typical dorsally angulated fractures with minimal displacement of volar cortex:

- Adequate analgesia
- Longitudinal traction
- Increase the dorsal angulation (to unlock volar cortex if overlapped)
- Direct pressure on the distal fragment to correct the angulation
- Palpate the volar and dorsal rim (estimation of correction).

Cast Application (Fig. 21.188)

- Mechanical analogy in reducing Colle's fracture (Disimpaction reduction, locking the fracture by pronation)
- The squeezing grip is for reduction and for molding the cast into an oval cross-section

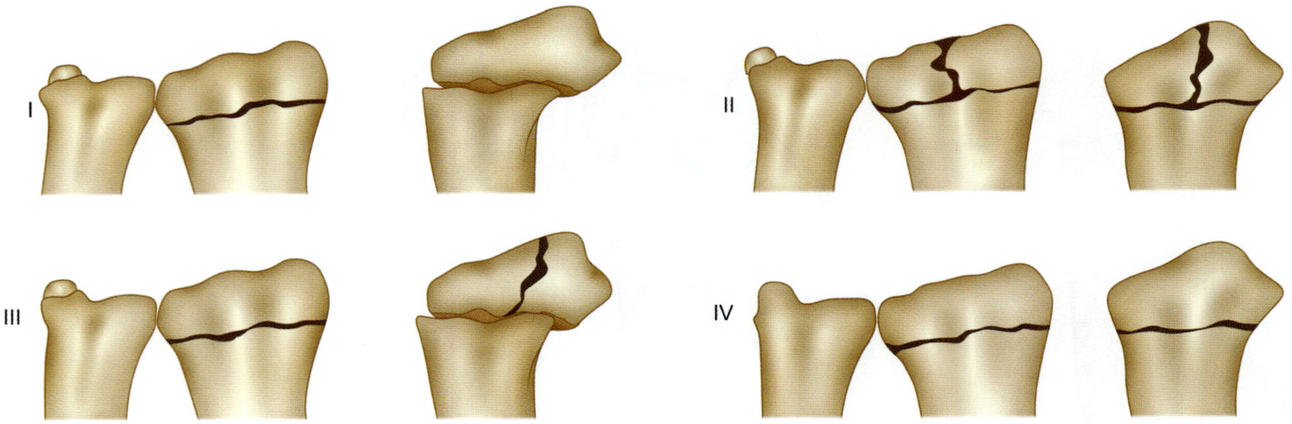

Fig. 21.182: Gartland and Werley classification for distal radial fractures

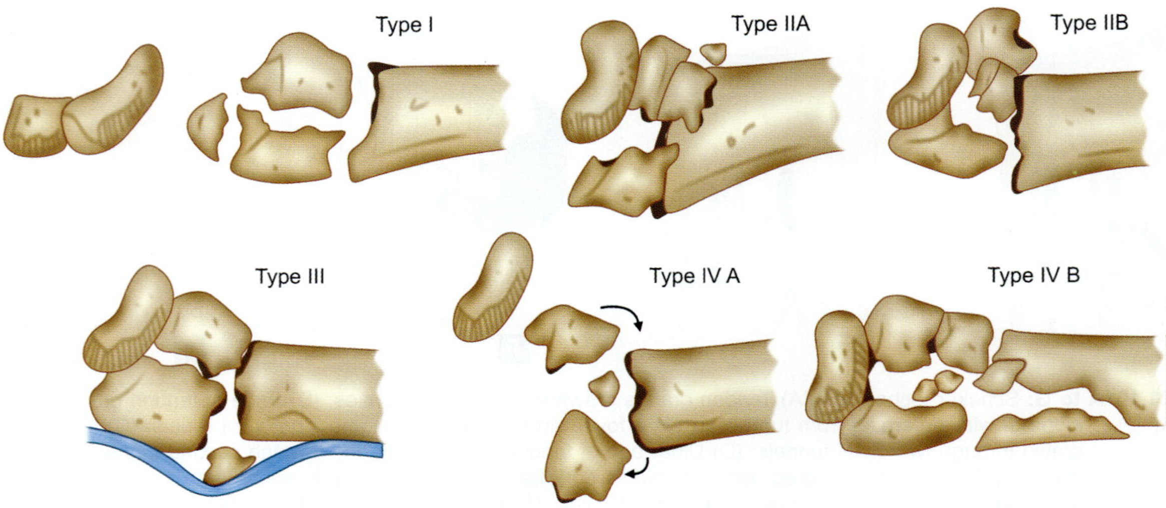

Fig. 21.183: Melone's classification

Table 21.6: McMurtry and Jupiter classification

Group 1	2 parts: (The opposite portion of the radiocarpal joint remains intact) • Dorsal barton • Volar barton • Chauffeur • Die-punch
Group 2	3 parts: The lunate and scaphoid facets separate from each other and the proximal portion of the radius
Group 3	4 parts: Groups 2 + lunate facet fractured in dorsal and volar fragment
Group 4	5 parts or more

Table 21.7: Mayo classification

Type I	Extra-articular radiocarpal
Type II	Intra-articular radioulnar
Type III	Intra-articular scaphoid fossa of distal radius
Type IV	Intra-articular, scaphoid fossa, lunate fossa and sigmoid fossa of the distal radius

- If the thenar eminence is liberated from the plaster with the object of encouraging movement in the thumb, a pressure sore often results at the proximal part of the aperture. This is inevitable, if the radius collapses towards the ulna.
- By incorporating the whole thumb, as in the scaphoid cast, a pressure sore at the base of the thumb is avoided.
- Showing the ideal shape of the cast for function of the hand. Full opposition of the thumb is imperative.
- X-ray appearance of a Colle's plaster in strong ulnar deviation, as shown in Figure 21.189.

Follow-up and Aftercare

- Follow-up radiographs to assess for redisplacement and healing
- Loss of reduction most commonly occurs during the second week of cast treatment or later, especially in the elderly osteopenic patient

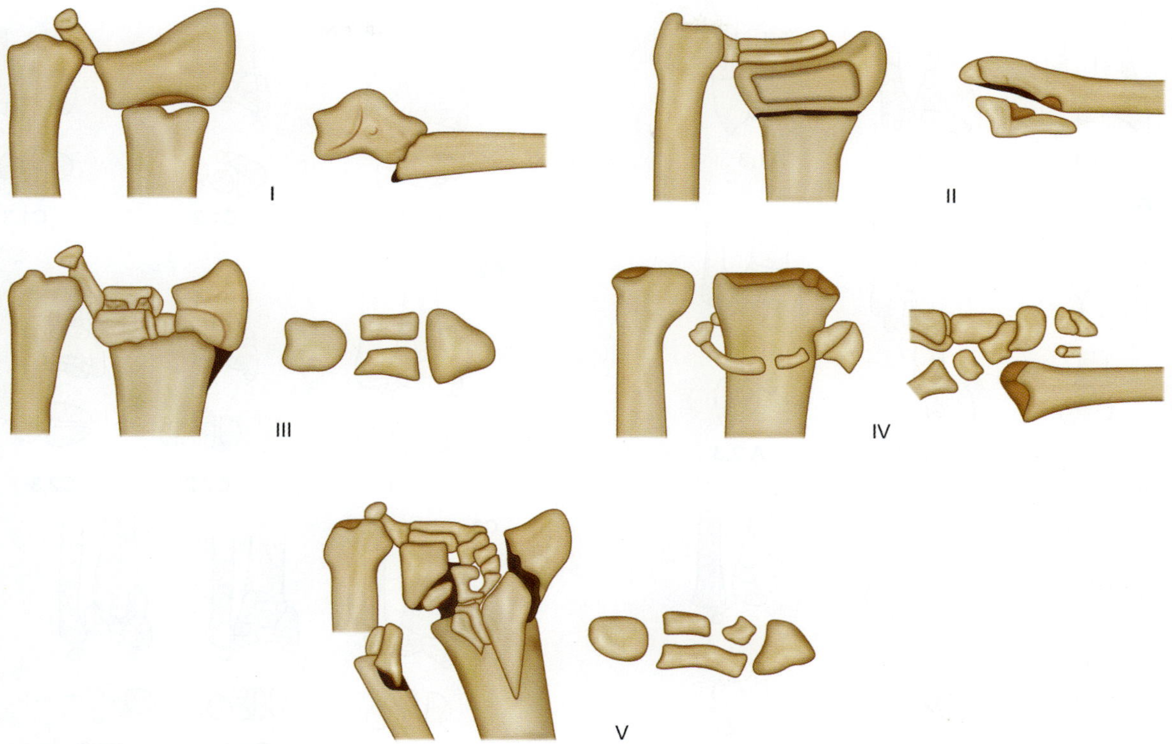

Fig. 21.184: Fernandez classification

- This suggests that the timing and number of follow-up visits needs to be individualized to both the patient and fracture
- For those fractures that are less stable, immobilization for at least six weeks is indicated.

Table 21.8: Fernandez classification

Type I	Metaphyseal bending fractures
Type II	Shearing fractures
Type III	Compression of the articular surface without the characteristic fragmentation
Type IV	Avulsion fractures or radiocarpal fracture dislocations
Type V	Combined injuries with significant soft tissue involvement due to high energy nature of these fractures

Table 21.9: Lidstrom and Andres Classification

Group 1	Undisplaced
Group 2a	Dorsal angulation, extra-articular
Group 2b	Dorsal angulation, intra-articular but without gross separation of fragments
Group 2c	Dorsal angulation plus dorsal displacement, extra-articular
Group 2d	Dorsal angulation plus dorsal displacement, intra-articular but without gross separation of fragments
Group 2e	Dorsal angulation plus dorsal displacement, intra articular with separation of fragments

Table 21.10: Sarmiento classification

Group 1	Nondisplaced fractures without radiocarpal joint involvement
Group 2	Displaced fractures without radiocarpal joint involvement
Group 3	Nondisplaced fractures with radiocarpal joint involvement
Group 4	Displaced fractures with radiocarpal joint involvement

Table 21.11: AO classification

Group 1	Extra-articular
Group 2	Partial articular
Group 3	Complete articular
C1	Simple articular and metaphyseal
C2	Simple articular and complex metaphyseal
C3	Complex articular and complex metaphyseal

Table 21.12: Frykman's classification

Type I	Extra-articular
Type II	Extra-articular fracture with ulnar styloid fracture
Type III	Radiocarpal articular involvement
Type IV	Radiocarpal involvement with ulnar styloid fracture
Type V	Radioulnar involvement
Type VI	Radioulnar involvement with ulnar styloid fracture
Type VII	Radiocarpal and radioulnar involvement
Type VIII	Radiocarpal and radioulnar involvement with ulnar styloid fracture

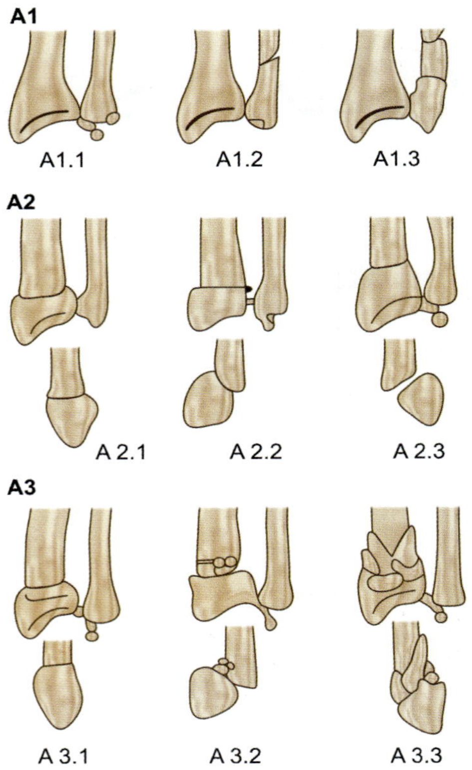

Fig. 21.185: AO classification, A. Extra-articular

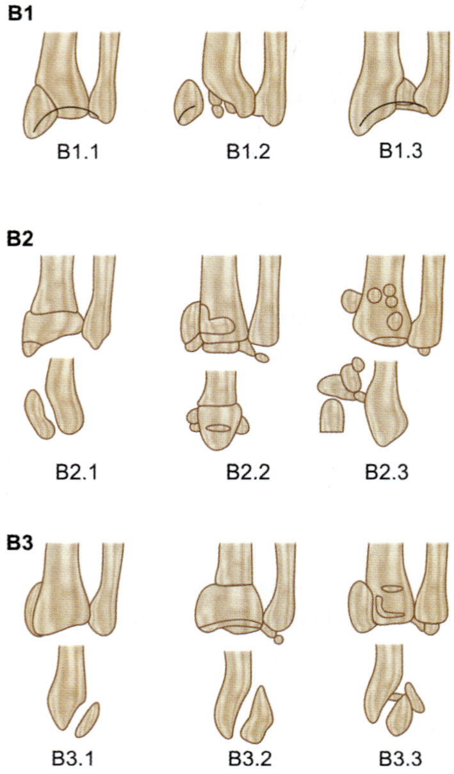

Fig. 21.186: AO classification, B: Simple articular

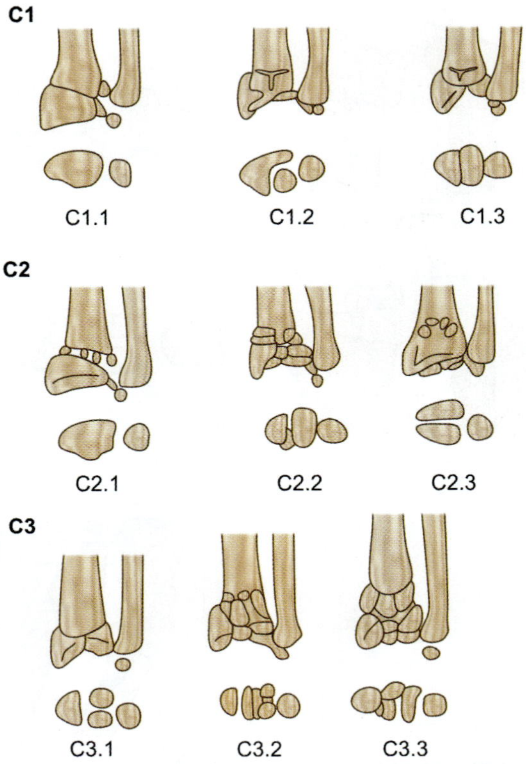

Fig. 21.187: AO classification, C: Complex articular

Predicting Successful Nonoperative Treatment

- Careful patient selection
- Initial satisfactory reduction
- Maintenance of reduction throughout the follow-up period to final fracture healing
- At present, we can conclude that radial shortening followed by dorsal comminution is most predictive of instability
- Increasing age significantly increases the risk of both early and late loss of reduction, even with minimal initial displacement
- In recent times, adjunctive modalities such as ultrasound and electrical stimulation have been postulated to quicken healing and subsequently prevent redisplacement.

Complications

- May be associated with the injury itself, its management or failure to restore the anatomy
- Some of the common complications are:
  - Compression neuropathies, which can be acute or delayed
  - Malunion
  - Midcarpal instability
  - Post-traumatic arthritis
  - Residual wrist and hand stiffness
  - Attrition ruptures of the EPL

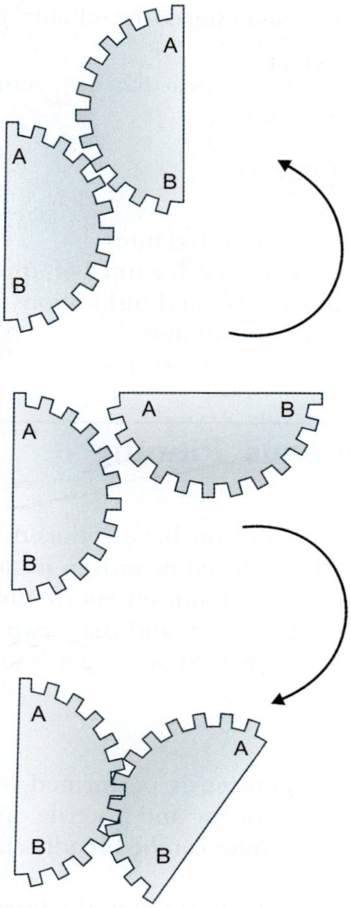

Fig. 21.188: Cast application

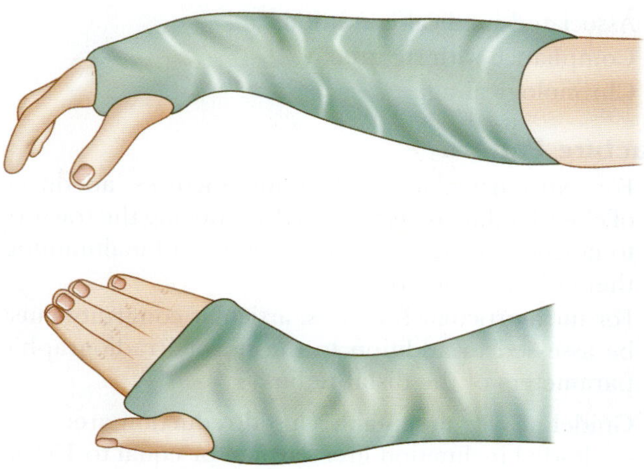

Fig. 21.189: Colle's plaster in strong ulnar deviation

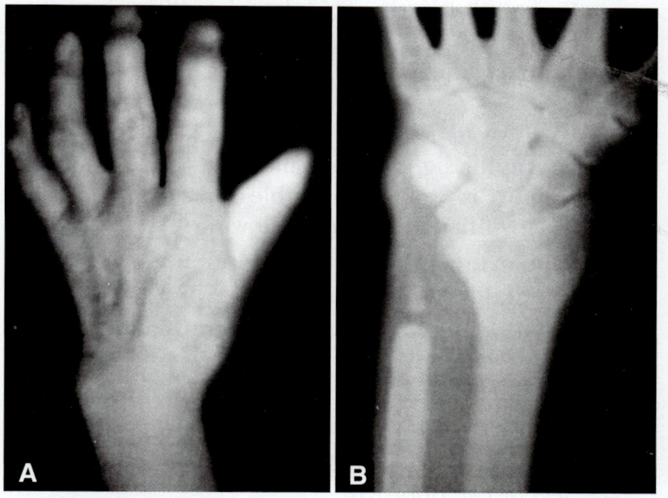

Figs 21.190A and B: Ugly deformity of radial deviation corrected by cosmetological resection of lower end of ulna

- Complex regional pain syndrome (CRPS) Type 1 and 2
- Ugly deformity of radial deviation is cosmeticologically corrected by resection of lower end of ulna (Figs 21.190A and B). This also restores full rotation and abolishes residual pain round the prominent head of the ulna.

Outcomes

- Preservation of radial length is most important for the preservation of function, followed by palmar angulation
- Loss of radial length can lead to ulnar impaction or dysfunction of the DRUJ, with limited range of motion in pronation and supination, depending on the volar or dorsal subluxation of the ulnar head within the sigmoid notch
- Residual dorsal angulation can precipitate ulnar impaction, midcarpal instability and altered stress concentrations, which may lead to early arthritis
- Poor outcomes are more common in malunions and include at least one of the following:
  - DRUJ pain
  - Nerve compression
  - Radial deviation of the wrist
  - Osteoarthritis
  - Dorsal angulation
  - Reduced grip strength
  - Prominent ulnar styloid.

Indications for Surgery

- Patient factors
- Fracture pattern
- Fracture stability
- Associated injuries.

Patient Factors

- Lifestyle
- Mental attitude

- Associated medical conditions
- Compliance with treatment
- Chronological age.

Fracture Pattern

- For extra-articular distal radius fractures, adequacy of closed reduction is assessed by reducing the fracture to normal radiographic parameters and maintaining them till the fracture heals.
- For intra-articular fractures, articular congruity must be assessed in addition to the normal radiographic parameters of the distal radius.
- Guidelines for acceptable closed reduction are:
  - Radial inclination greater than or equal to 15° on PA view
  - Radial length less than or equal to 5 mm shortening on PA view
  - Radial tilt less than 15° dorsal or 20° volar tilt on lateral view
  - Articular incongruity less than 2 mm of stepoff.

Fracture Stability

- Radiographic signs that should alert the surgeon that the fracture is probably unstable and closed reduction will be insufficient include following:
  - Palmar metaphyseal comminution
  - Initial dorsal tilt greater than 20°
  - Initial displacement (fragment translation) greater than 1 cm
  - Initial radial shortening greater than 5 mm
  - Intra articular disruption
  - Associated ulna fracture
  - Severe osteoporosis
- Other factors that influence the stability of distal radius fractures are:
  - Radiocarpal intra-articular involvement
  - Age of the patient.

Associated Injuries

- Open fractures
- Bilateral distal radius fractures
- Ipsilateral concomitant fractures of upper extremity
- Carpal bone fractures and dislocations
- Acute median nerve dysfunction
- Raised compartment pressures.

■ Percutaneous Pinning

Indications

- Younger patients who have reduced or reducible fractures with predicted or proven instability
- Fractures without significant shortening, comminution of the volar cortex and that have failed closed reduction or redisplaced with regards to dorsal angulation.

Technique

- Percutaneous pinning is performed with adequate anesthesia, fluoroscopy and a sterile operating environment. Techniques can be broadly classified into:
  - Extrafocal
  - Intrafocal (passing through the fracture site)
- Irrespective of the preferred method of fixation, the selected technique should achieve fracture stability, minimize injury to nerves, vessels and tendons as well as avoid injury to the articular surface. This technique is illustrated in Figures 21.191 to 21.194.

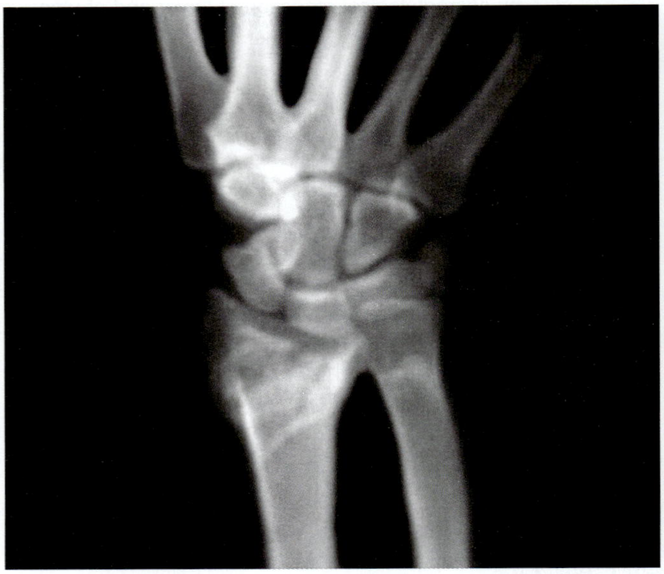

Fig. 21.191: Distal radial fracture before percutaneous pinning

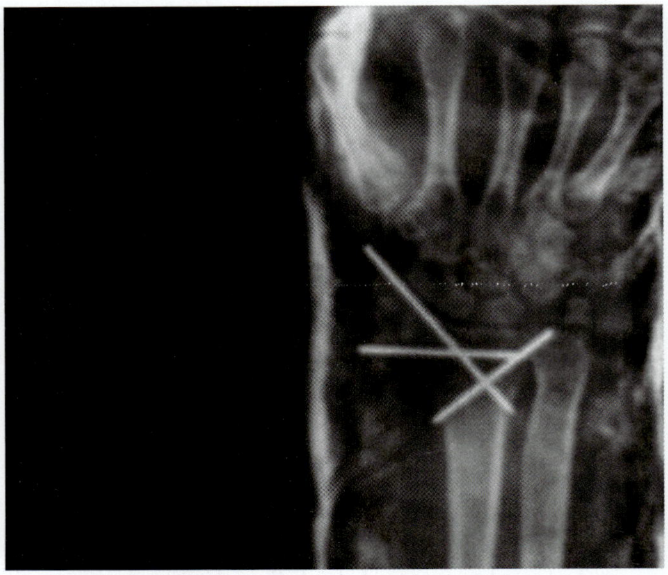

Fig. 21.192: Distal radial fracture after percutaneous pinning

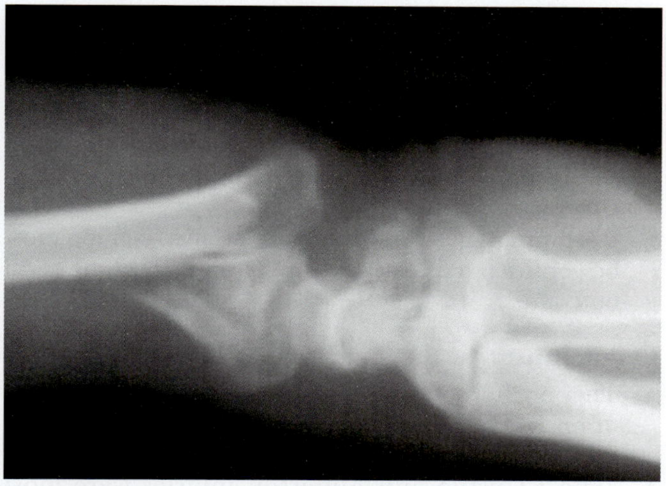

Fig. 21.193: Distal radial fracture before percutaneous pinning (lateral view)

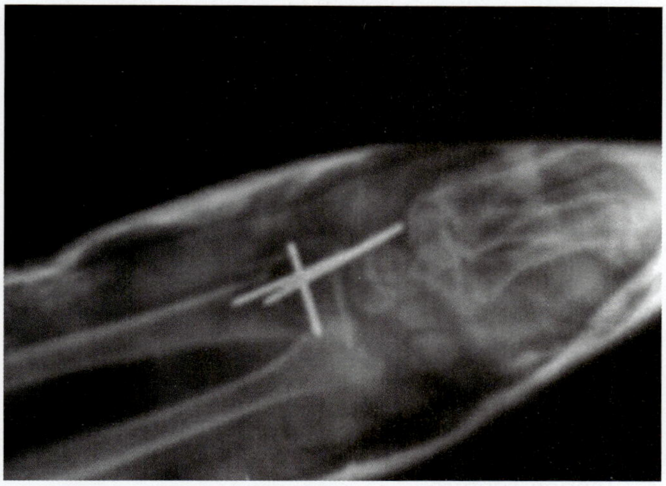

Fig. 21.194: Distal radial fracture after percutaneous pinning lateral view

Complications

Includes those previously described in nonoperative treatment as well as those directly attributed to the use of percutaneous pins such as:

- Tendon tethering, injury or rupture
- Pin migration
- Nerve injury
- Pin site infection
- Superficial radial nerve irritation and injury.

Summary

- Percutaneous pinning demonstrates good reproducible outcomes with minimal risk in appropriately selected fracture patterns. It is well suited for younger patients who have unstable, but reducible extra or intra-articular distal radial fractures.
- This technique can provide adequate fracture stability and soft tissue and vascular preservation in addition to minimal patient morbidity, which may facilitate a more rapid return to function compared with more invasive methods of treatment.

COMPLICATIONS AND MANAGEMENT OF DISTAL RADIUS FRACTURES

Introduction

- Fractures occur at the distal end of the radius more commonly than at any other location. They comprise about 10 to 12 percent of all fractures. The reported complication rate vary from 6 to 60 percent.
- McKay and colleagues reviewed the overall incidence of complications after distal radius fracture in their literature and subsequently in their series of 250 consecutive patients treated for distal radius fractures. The results are shown in Table 21.13.

Immediate Complications

- Nerve injury
- Open injury
- Compartment syndrome
- Skin injury during manipulation
- Missed associated injury.

Nerve Injury

- Incidence of nerve injuries varies from 0 to17 percent
- The median nerve is the most commonly involved, followed by the radial and the ulnar nerves (Fig. 21.195)
- The radial nerve's sensory branch is particularly vulnerable to injury during the K-wire fixation, as the nerve exists beneath the dense fascia between the tendons of brachioradialis and extensor carpi radialis longus

Table 21.13: Complications and incidences of distal radius fractures

Complication	*Incidence*
Ligament damage	98%
Arthritis/arthrosis	7-65%
Loss of motion (marked deformity, decreased ROM)	2-31%
Osteomyelitis	4-9%
Malunion	5%
Others like delayed union, nerve compression, neuritis hardware complications tendon rupture, radioulnar disturbance	0.5-1.2%

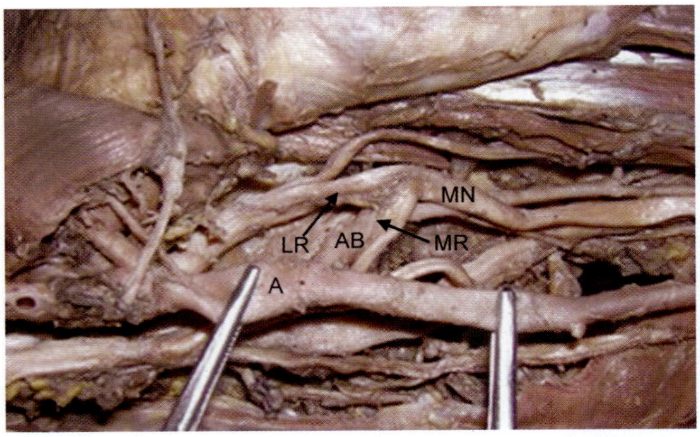

Fig. 21.195: Dissection showing median nerve and adjoining structures— A. Third part of axillary artery; AB. Anomalous branch; MR. Medial root of median nerve; LR. Lateral root of median nerve; MN. Median nerve

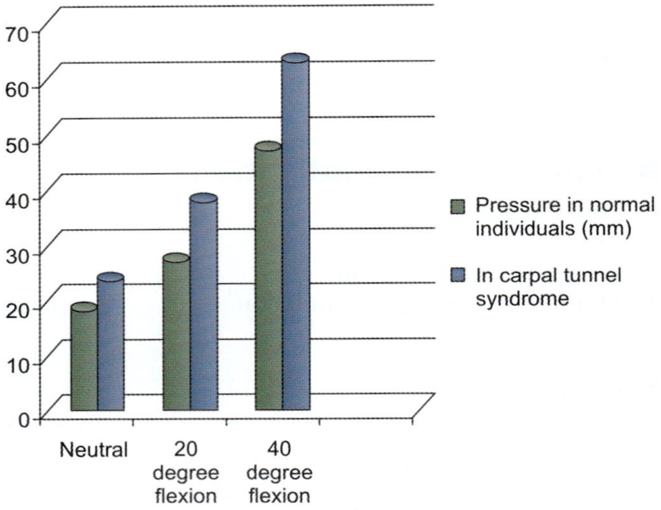

Fig. 21.196: Carpal tunnel pressure variations, as studied by Gelberman and colleagues

- Neuromas in this area are particularly troublesome because they can be irritated by rubbing against shirt cuffs, watches and bracelets.

Carpal Tunnel Syndrome

- Acute carpal tunnel syndrome is more common in patients, who have more severe and comminuted fractures. It may also occur in those people, who undergo multiple closed reduction attempts
- Gelberman and colleagues studied the mean carpal tunnel pressures and made the following graph (Fig. 21.196).

How to Avoid?

- Careful examination of the patients to rule out neurological injury
- Splinting and casting to be avoided in extreme wrist flexion
- Encourage patients to keep the hand elevated and actively flex and extend their fingers
- In patients with significant hand and wrist swellings splints or bivalved casts should be used rather than circumferential casts
- If symptoms get worse then surgical intervention must be considered as early release has a better long-term outcome.

Open Injury

- They are infrequent and the largest reported series of open fractures included 18 consecutive patients collected over 8 years
- Type I Gustilo and Anderson injuries were most common with an incidence of 50 percent followed by Type III with 34 percent and lastly Type II with 16 percent. Four patients in this series had nerve and tendon injuries and two had vascular injuries
- They were promptly irrigated, debrided, intravenous antibiotics were given and tetanus status was assessed in emergency. Fracture was stabilized and patients were subjected to multiple operative procedures
- Eight out of 18 patients developed postoperative infections (5 soft tissues and 3 osteomyelitis) and 5 developed a nonunion.

■ Early Complications (Less than 6 Weeks)

- Cast issues
- Loss of reduction
- Infection
- Tendon rupture.

Cast Issues

- Depending upon the degree of swelling the full cast and noncircumferential splint should be applied
- Cast should support the fracture and permit free movement of the fingers and thumb
- Patient should be encouraged to exercise the fingers, to prevent stiffness and reduce the risk of dystrophy.

Loss of Reduction

- Charnley's three-point fixation technique is recommended to support the fracture within the cast
- MacKenney reported following findings in case of early instability:
  - Ten times more common in patients, greater than 80 years age
  - Six times more common in fractures with dorsal comminution
  - Five times more common in fractures maintaining 5–10° of dorsal angulation

– Greater risk of displacement with percutaneous K-wire in older individuals and fractures with dorsal comminution.

Infection

- Compound fractures and fractures treated operative are at risk for infection
- Largest reported series of compound fractures reported 44 percent infection rate with 62 percent of infections involving the soft tissues and 38 percent as osteomyelitis
- A randomized trial reported that buring K-wire percutaneously reduces the risk of infection by half.
- Percutaneous K-wires should not be used to supplement internal fixation because this can act as a pathway for superficial infection to spread to the deeper tissues and bone
- Soft tissue infections should be treated with oral antibiotics and those involving the bone, causing osteomyelitis requires surgical intervention.

Tendon Rupture

- It may occur as an early or as a late complication.
- Extensor pollicis longus tendon is the most commonly ruptured tendon (Fig. 21.197)
- The ruptured tendon usually cannot be repaired and function can be well-restored by performing an extensor indicis proprius transfer.

Late Complications (Greater than 6 Weeks)

- Nerve complications and CRPS
- Arthrosis
- Nonunion/delayed union
- Malunion.

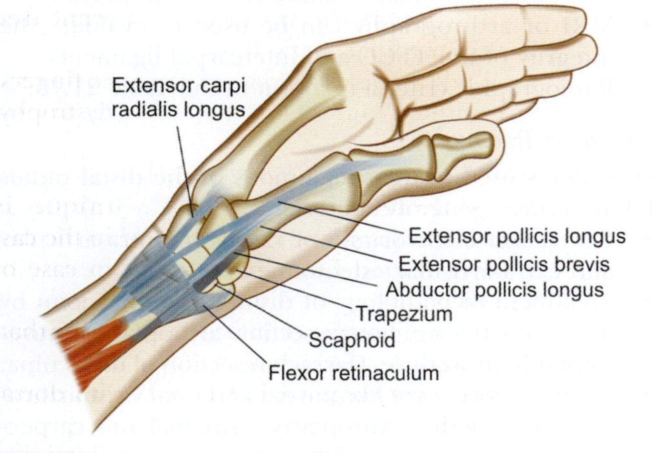

Fig. 21.197: Different tendons of hand

Complex Regional Pain Syndrome (CRPS)

- It refers to a pattern of symptoms and signs that are disproportionate to those from the degree of trauma, leading to functional impairment. It was formerly referred to as reflex sympathetic dystrophy (RSD) and symptoms include:
  – Increased pain
  – Swelling, stiffness, discoloration and hyperhidrosis
  – Osteoporosis
- The condition was first observed by Mitchell, Morehouse and Keen in 1867. Mitchell coined the term "Causalgia", a Greek word meaning "burning pain".
- Other eponyms in the literature are Sudeck's atrophy, shoulder-hand syndrome and Leriche post-traumatic pain syndrome.
- CRPS type I now replaces RSD and CRPS type II replaces causalgia.
- Various theories have been proposed including short-circuiting effects at the area of injury, permitting irritation of the sensory afferent fibers by the efferent sympathetic impulses, periarteritis involving the vessels around the injured neural segments and abnormal feedback into the internuncial centers of the spinal cord.
- Lankford stated that the following triad must be present to develop RSD:
  – Persistent painful stimulus
  – Diathesis (inherent sympathetic overactivity or insecure fearful personality)
  – Abnormal sympathetic reflex.

Classification

Lankford further classified RSD in order of increasing severity as shown in Table 21.14.

Clinical Features

- Excruciating burning pain often described as having superimposed throbbing, aching, bursting pressure

Table 21.14: Lankford classification of RSD

Type	*Cause*
Minor causalgia	Injury to purely sensory nerve, cutaneous branch of median, radial nerve
Minor traumatic dystrophy	Minor crush injuries, sprains and fractures
Shoulder-hand syndrome	Proximal injury to neck, chest, shoulder or visceral lesion like cervical disk, heart attack, stroke, pancoast tumor
Major traumatic dystrophy	Severe crush injuries or Colle's fracture
Major causalgia	After injury to major mixed nerve (median nerve)

with a knifelike stabbing, twisting or crushing component. It usually begins around the first week.
- Clinical picture in early stage is that of pain and vasomotor instability with sympathetic overactivity, edema, redness, increased warmth, hyperhidrosis and stiffness.
- Intermediate stage starts by around third month and is characterized by pale and dry extremity with increasing stiffness and trophic changes. Patient may be comfortable at rest but pain persists on motion.
- Late stage is seen around the end of first year and is characterized by stiff, cool, atrophic and osteoporotic extremity.

Investigations

- Three phase radionucleotide bone scan can aid in early diagnosis. A diffusely increased uptake in the delayed images was found to be diagnostic of RSD with a sensitivity of 96 percent and specificity of 98 percent.
- In severe causalgia local anesthetic block of the second and third sympathetic ganglia also confirms the diagnosis.

Treatment of CRPS

- No specific treatment.
- Early sympathetic (Stellate ganglion) block with physical therapy is widely recommended
- Surgical preganglionic sympathectomy in resistant cases.

Arthrosis

- A review of patients at a mean of 6.7 years after an intra-articular fracture of the distal radius fractures found that 65 percent had radiographic evidence of post-traumatic arthrosis.
- Fractures with residual radiocarpal incongruity had a higher rate of radiographic arthrosis.
- It is a challenge in young patients and treatment options include activity modification, oral analgesics, splinting or surgery.
- Surgical options include partial or complete wrist fusions with arthroplasty.

Nonunion or Delayed Union

- Fractures with no radiographic signs of bridging trabeculae across the fracture site at 4 months are categorized as delayed unions and as nonunions after 6 months, although later is uncommon.
- Factors affecting it are open fractures, severe comminution, infection, devascularization of the bone ends, overdistraction of fracture, with inadequate stabilization, diabetes, prolapsed vertebral disk (PVD), peripheral neuropathy, smoking and alcoholism.
- Diagnosis may be confirmed through mobility of the fracture noted on lateral radiographs of wrists in dorsiflexion and volar flexion. CT scan helps to confirm diagnosis and surgical planning.
- Surgical treatment includes wrist arthrodesis/bone grafting stabilization with internal fixation as a single stage procedure or primary distraction lengthening with tenotomy of brachioradialis with secondary stabilization and bone grafting.

Malunion and Its Management

Despite improved treatment since early 1980's, malunion remains to be a common cause of residual disability after distal radius fractures. It can be caused due to failure to achieve or maintain an accurate reduction or by inadequate duration or type of immobilization. It is associated with extra-articular deformities, intra-articular malalignment, distal radioulnar incongruity or instability or a combination of these features.

Clinical Evaluation

- Pain, stiffness, weakness and cosmetic deformity are common complaints in patients with distal radial malunion
- Decreased wrist flexion is typical in dorsally tilted malunions and extension is limited with volarly tilted malunions. Loss of radial inclination may cause impaired ulnar deviation. Incongruity at distal radioulnar joint leads to decreased pronation and supination with supination more affected
- Grip strength is impaired because of a combination of pain and altered wrist mechanics.

Radiographic Evaluation

- Plain anteroposterior and lateral radiographs of both wrists in are in neutral rotation. Uninjured wrist is used as a template for surgical reconstruction if osteotomy is chosen.
- CT scan to evaluate potential for conguity of the distal radioulnar joint and malunions of ulnar styloid.
- MRI or arthrography can be used to evaluate the integrity of the TFCC and intercarpal ligaments.
- Radiographic criteria is shown in the Table 21.15.

Operative Treatment

Procedures used to treat malunions of the distal radius fall into three general categories:

- Correction of deformity of radius by intra-articular and extra-articular osteotomies.
- Treatment of pathology of distal radioulnar joint by ulnar shortening, hemiresection arthoplasty, Sauve-Kapandji procedure, Darrach resection of distal ulna.
- Salvage procedures like partial and total wrist arthrodesis, total wrist arthroplasty, proximal row carpectomy.

Table 21.15: Radiographic criteria

Radiographic criterion	*Acceptable measurement*
Radioulnar length	Radial shortening of < 5 mm at distal radioulnar joint compared with contralateral wrist
Radial inclination	Inclination of > 15 degrees on posteroanterior film
Radial tilt	Sagittal tilt on lateral projection between 15-degree dorsal tilt and 20-degree volar tilt
Articular incongruity	Incongruity of intra-articular fracture < 2 mm at radiocarpal joint

I. *Extra-articular malunion with dorsal angulation (Figs 21.198 and 21.199)*

- Osteotomy and grafting is the most commonly performed procedure and is indicated in patients younger than 45 years. It can be performed in older patients with good bone quality and high functional demands.
- Contraindications are active RSD, acceptable function despite deformity, poor soft tissue envelope, severe osteopenia, advanced radiocarpal/intercarpal arthritis.
- Wrist is immobilized for 2 weeks in a volar plaster splint and 2 weeks ROM exercises are begun. No lifting work is allowed until osteotomy has healed radiographically.

II. *Extra-articular malunion with volar angulation (Figs 21.200A to E)*

- Indications and contraindications are similar to that of dorsal osteotomy and plating
- Volar open wedge osteotomy with bone grafting and plating is advocated
- Postoperational volar splint for 2 weeks should be advised. If lengthening of 10 mm or more is necessary, then 6 weeks or below elbow cast is worn. Activities against resistance and manual labor are not permitted until union has been confirmed radiographically.

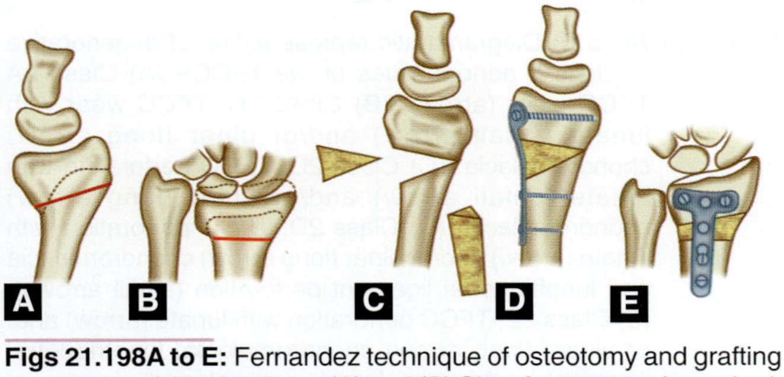

Figs 21.198A to E: Fernandez technique of osteotomy and grafting of distal radius—(A) and (B) Site of osteotomy is marked; (C) Osteotomy is opened dorsally and graft is prepared; (D) and (E) Graft is inserted and plate applied

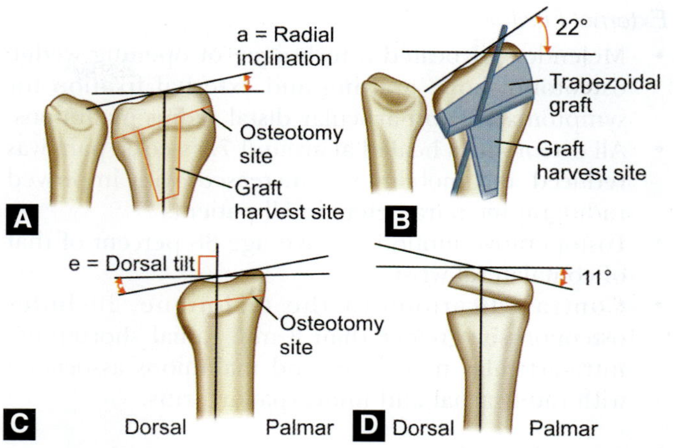

Figs 21.199A to D: Trapezoidal osteotomy of distal radius—(A) Preoperative posteroanterior view with decreased radial inclination, osteotomy and trapezoidal graft site are outlined; (B) Postoperative posteroanterior view shows normal radial tilt and single "caging" pin; (C) Abnormal dorsal tilt of radial articular surface reverses all loads across carpals and does not tolerate loading in active patients; (D) Postoperative lateral view shows restorations of 11° of palmar tilt before insertion of graft

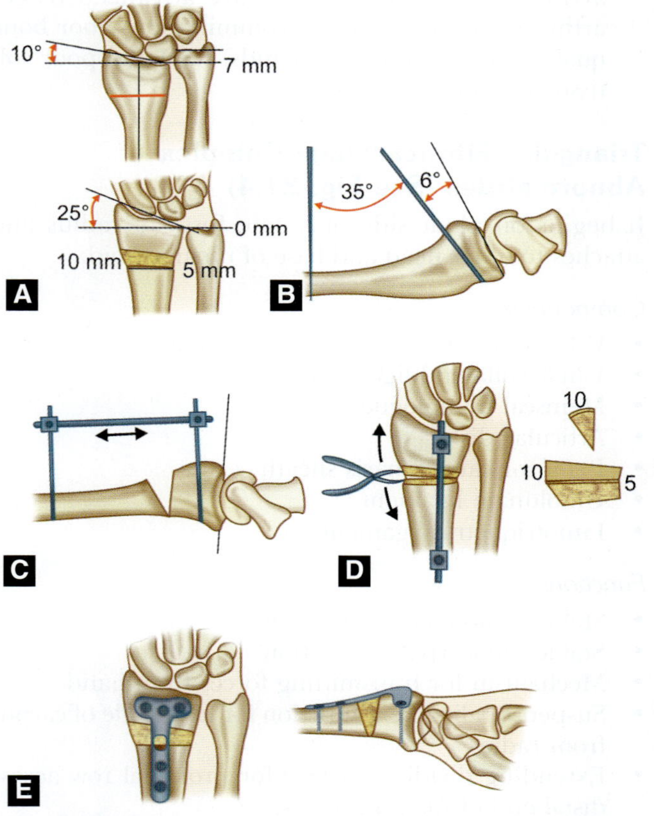

Figs 21.200A to E: Volar osteotomy for malunited distal radial fracture—(A) Preoperative planning; (B) K-wire drilled into radial shaft proximal to osteotomy site; (C) Fixator used to maintain corrected alignment; (D) Osteotomy wedged open with lamina; (E) Iliac graft inserted and osteotomy stabilized with T-plate

External Fixator

- Melendez advocated a technique of opening wedge osteotomy, bone grafting and external fixation for symptomatic extra-articular distal radius malunions
- All osteotomies healed at around 7.5 weeks, pain was reduced and mobility was increased, with improved radiographic parameters in all patients
- Postoperative motion was average 88 percent of that of contalateral wrist
- Contraindications to the technique, includes osteoporosis, greater than 8 mm radial shortening, intra-articular malunions and malunions associated with radiocarpal and midcarpal arthritis.

Intra-articular Malunions

- They lead to functional disability and the procedures in this group are divided into:
  - Prevent post-traumatic arthritis (osteotomies).
  - Salvage procedures (carpal arthrodesis, proximal row carpectomy, wrist arthroplasty).
- Intra-articular osteotomies are indicated in young, active patients with high functional demands, greater than 2 mm stepoff, no evidence of post-traumatic arthritis. Contraindications are advanced osteoarthritis, massive articular comminution, poor bone quality, low functional demands, RSD and poor soft tissue coverage.

Triangular Fibrocartilage Complex Abnormalities (See Fig. 21.4)

It begins on ulnar side of lunate fossa of radius and attaches to ulnar head and base of ulnar styloid.

Components

- Volar and dorsal radioulnar ligament
- Ulnar collateral ligament
- Meniscal homologue
- Articular disk
- Extensor carpi ulnaris sheath
- Ulnolunate ligament
- Lunotriquetral ligament

Functions

- Stable radioulnar connection
- Stable ulnocarpal connection
- Mechanism for transmitting forces from hand
- Suspensory ligament function for ulnar side of carpus from radius
- Extending dividing surface for proximal row across distal end of forearm bones.

Classification

Triangular fibrocartilage complex (TFCC) abnormalities are illustrated in the Table 21.16 and Figures 21.201 to 21.203:

Table 21.16: Classification of TFCC abnormalities

Class 1	**Traumatic**
A.	Central perforation
B.	Ulnar avulsion With distal ulnar fracture Without distal ulnar fracture
C.	Distal avulsion
D.	Radial avulsion With sigmoid notch fracture Without sigmoid notch fracture
Class 2	**Degenerative (Ulnocarpal abutment syndrome)**
A.	TFCC wear
B.	TFCC wear Plus lunate and/or ulnar chondromalacia
C.	TFCC perforation Plus lunate and/or ulnar chondromalacia
D.	TFCC perforation Plus lunate and/or ulnar chondromalacia Plus lunotriquetral ligament perforation
E.	TFCC perforation Plus lunate and/or ulnar chondromalacia Plus lunotriquetral ligament perforation Plus ulnocarpal arthritis

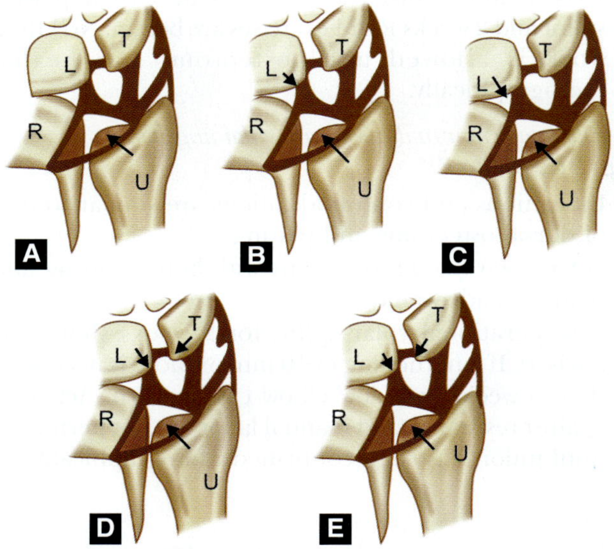

Figs 21.201A to E: Diagrammatic representation of degenerative or class 2 abnormalities of the TFCC—(A) Class 2A TFCC wear (arrow); (B) Class 2B, TFCC wear with lunate (small arrow) and/or ulnar (long arrow) chondromalacia; (C) Class 2C, TFCC perforation with lunate (small arrow) and/or ulnar (long arrow) chondromalacia; (D) Class 2D, TFCC perforation with lunate (arrow) and/or ulnar (long arrow) chondromalacia and lunotriquetral ligament perforation (small arrows); (E) Class 2E, TFCC perforation with lunate (arrow) and/or ulnar (long arrow) chondromalacia, lunotriquetral ligament perforation (small arrows) and ulnocarpal arthritis

Key: L. Lunate; R. Radius; T. Triquetrum; U. Ulna

I. *Ulnar hemiresection interposition arthroplasty (Bowers) indications*
- Unreconstructable fractures of ulnar head
- Ulnocarpal impingement syndrome
- Rheumatoid arthritis
- Chronic painful TFCC tear
- Post-traumatic and osteoarthritis.

II. *Matched resection (Watson) (See Fig. 21.177)*

Matched distal ulnar resection. Ulna is resected 5 to 6 cm and shaped to match contour of radius through full supination and pronation. Distal resected ulna should be at level of radial articular surface. Large cancellous surface adheres to ulnar sling mechanism

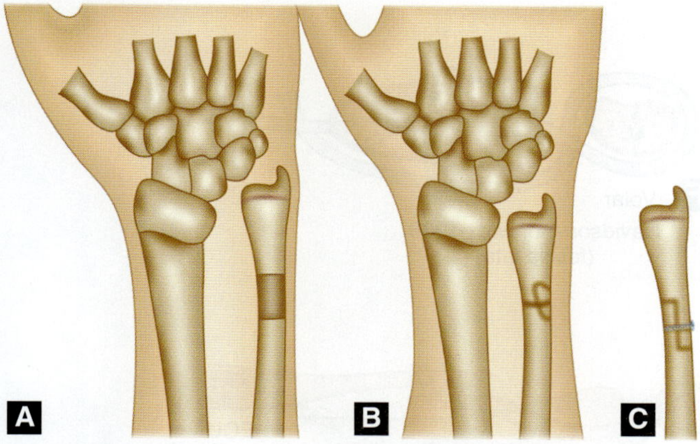

Figs 21.207A to C: Milch cuff resection of ulna—(A) Shaded area indicates bone to be resected; (B) Ends of ulna apposed, correcting disproportion in length of radius and ulna; (C) More stable fixation secured by step-cut procedure and fixation with one screw

Indications
- Rheumatoid arthritis
- Trauma

III. *Milch cuff resection (Figs 21.207A to C)*

Indications
- Malunited Colle's fracture
- Malunion or nonunion of radius
- Cessation or abnormality of growth of distal radius

IV. *Ulnar shortening procedures—Darrach resection*

Indications
- Malunited Colle's fracture.
- Malunion or nonunion of radius
- Abnormality of growth of distal radius

V. *Distal radioulnar arthrodesis with distal ulnar pseudo-arthrosis (Sauve-Kapandji) (Figs 21.208A and B)*

Indications
- Painful wrist by previous surgery
- Traumatic arthritis
- Rheumatoid arthritis

VI. *Procedures to stabilize DRUJ*

Indications
- After undetected dislocation
- After surgical procedure to resect distal ulna.

Methods
- Radioulnar tenodesis (Figs 21.209A to H)
- Reconstruction of dorsal ligament of TFCC (Scheker)
- Radioulnar tenodesis procedures using extensor carpi ulnaris (ECU), extensor digitorum communis (EDC) and extensor digiti minimi (EDM)

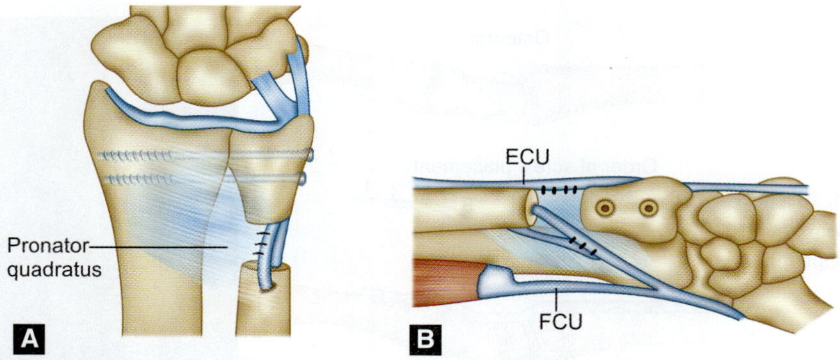

Figs 21.208A and B: Distal radioulnar arthrodesis with distal ulnar pseudoarthrosis (modified Sauvé-Kapandji procedure)—(A) Posterior view of wrist with two screws fixing ulnar head to sigmoid notch; after resection, gap, which measures 10 mm, is filled with pronator quadratus; (B) Lateral view of wrist showing stabilization of proximal ulnar segment with distally based slip of flexor carpi ulnaris tendon (FCU). Nonunion gap is filled with pronator quadratus, which is sutured to tendon sheath of extensor carpi ulnaris muscle (ECU)

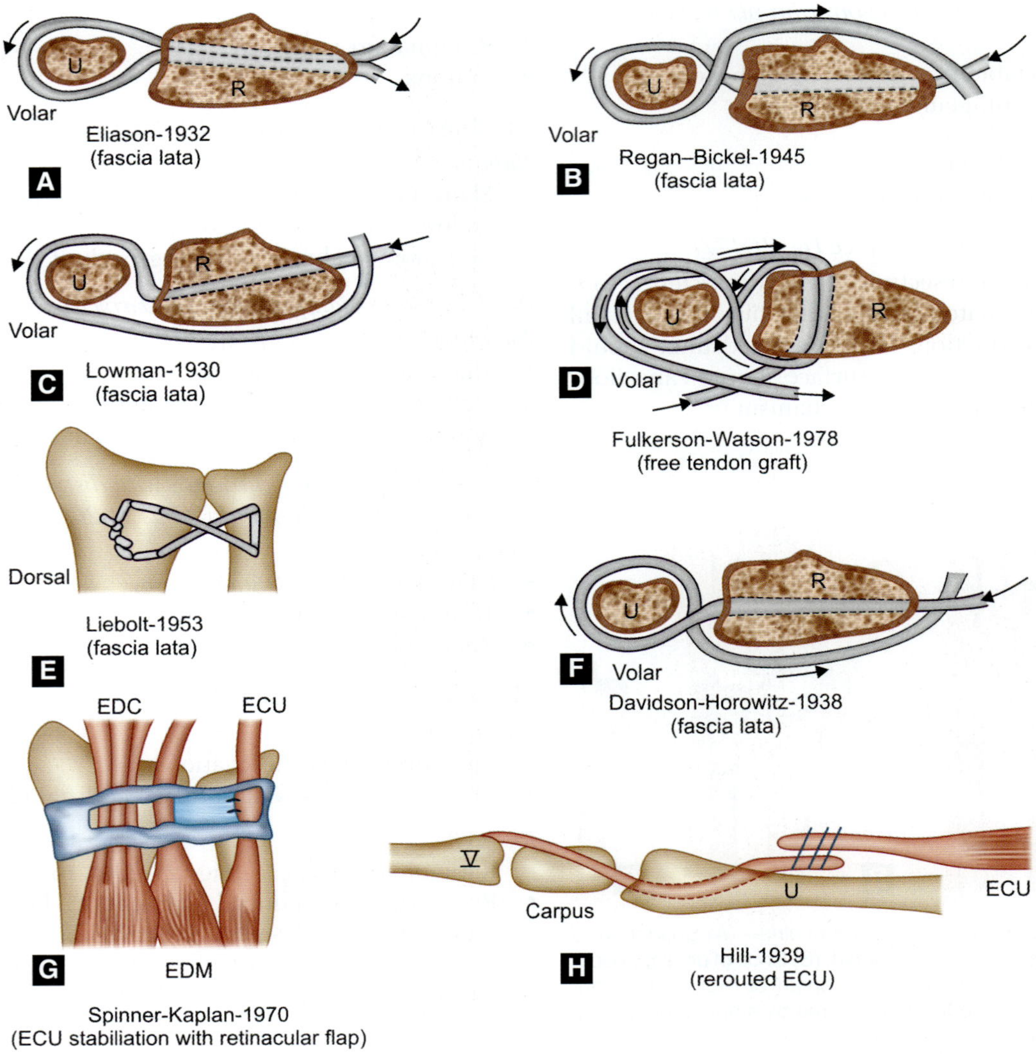

Figs 21.209A to H: Different methods of radioulnar tenodesis

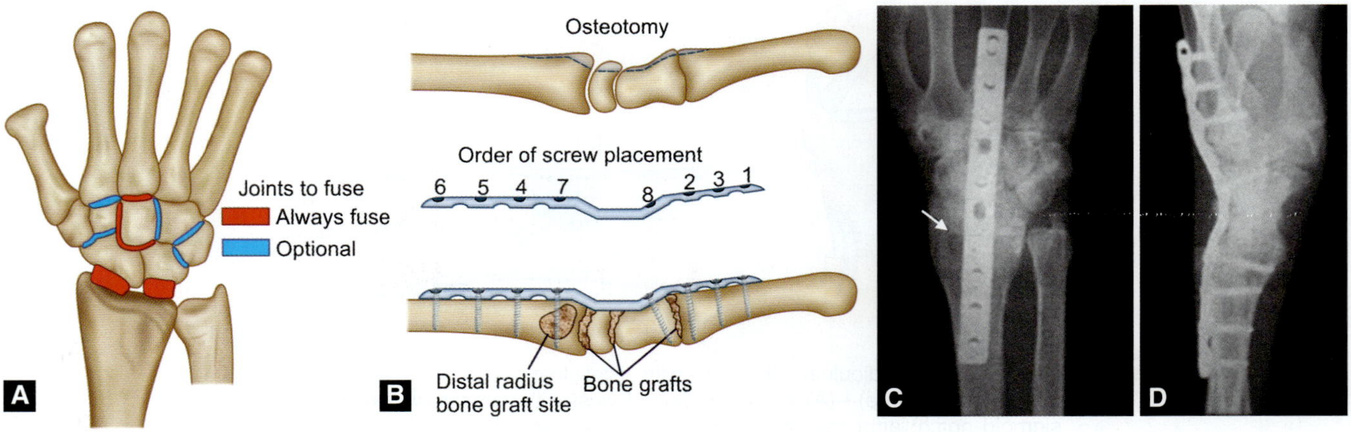

Figs 21.210A to D: Wrist fusion with bone grafting and plate fixation—(A) Rigid fusion column through carpus to metacarpal must coincide with the plate placement. All joints spanned directly by plate should be fused if desired; (B) Dorsal cartilage is denuded and plate is applied from distal to proximal, spanning local radial bone graft augmentation; (C) and (D) Placement of 3.5 mm dynamic compression plate, note local distal radial bone graft portal (arrow) and thickness of plate distally

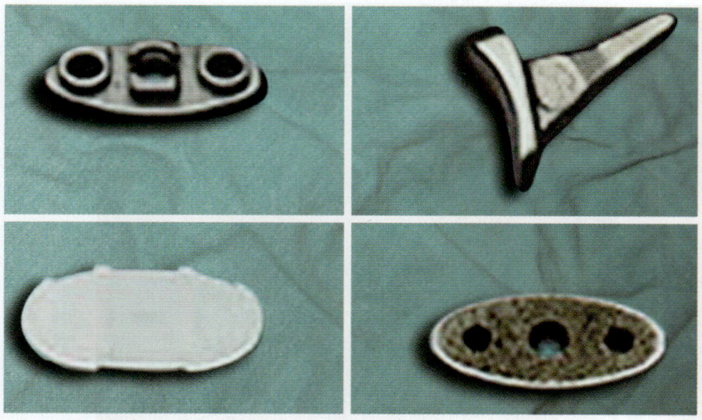

Fig. 21.211: Different types of Menon prosthesis

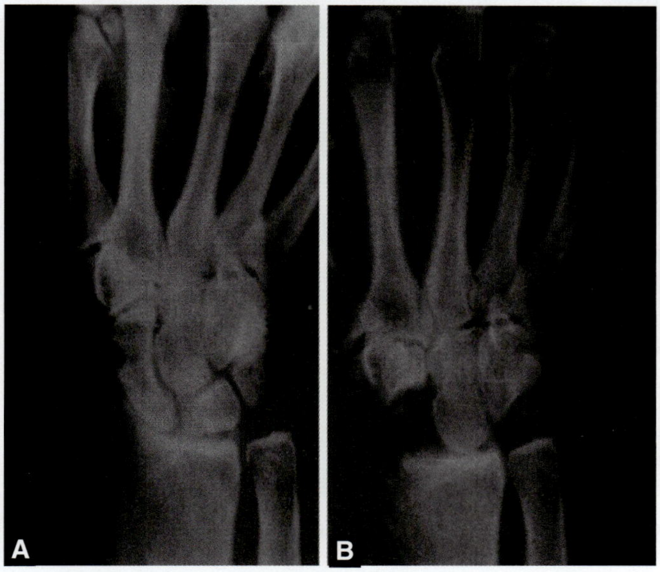

Figs 21.212A and B: (A) Degenerative arthritis limited to the radioscaphoid and radiolunate joints; (B) Postoperative radiograph depicting proximal row carpectomy with radial styloidectomy

- Salvage procedures (Figs 21.210A to D):
  - Wrist arthrodesis, partial and total
  - Total wrist arthroplasty (Fig. 21.211)
  - Proximal row carpectomy (Figs 21.212A and B)

Future Trends

Future trends are as follows (Figs 21.213 to 21.219):

- Computer assisted surgeries (Figs 21.213A to D)
- Bone graft alternates like carbonated hydroxyapatite and calcium phosphate (Figs 21.214A to D)

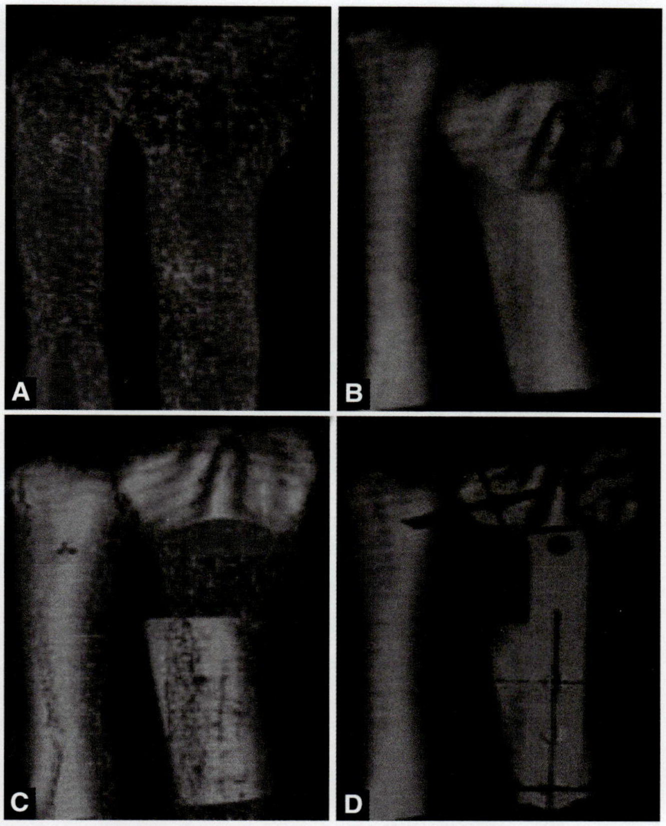

Figs 21.213A to D: Computer-assisted distal radius osteotomy planning—(A) Computer-assisted 3-D surgical planner use contralateral wrist as a template; (B) The malunited wrist; (C) Virtual osteotomy and is aligned; (D) The surgical planner then digitizes a plate onto the realigned radius and saves the coordinates and orientation of the screw holes for intraoperative referencing

- Volar fixed-angle plate osteosynthesis (Figs 21.215 to 21.217)

Computer assisted surgeries (Figs 21.213 to 21.216)

Volar fixed angle plates (Figs 21.217).

Summary

Sumptomatic distal radius malunion algorithms are explained in the following Flow charts 21.1 to 21.3.

The treatment of distal radius malunions is continually evolving. The advent of new computer technologies, plating systems and bone graft substitutes will likely have a significant impact upon the way distal radius malunions are corrected in the near future. But prevention of malunions through optimal fracture management remains the best option.

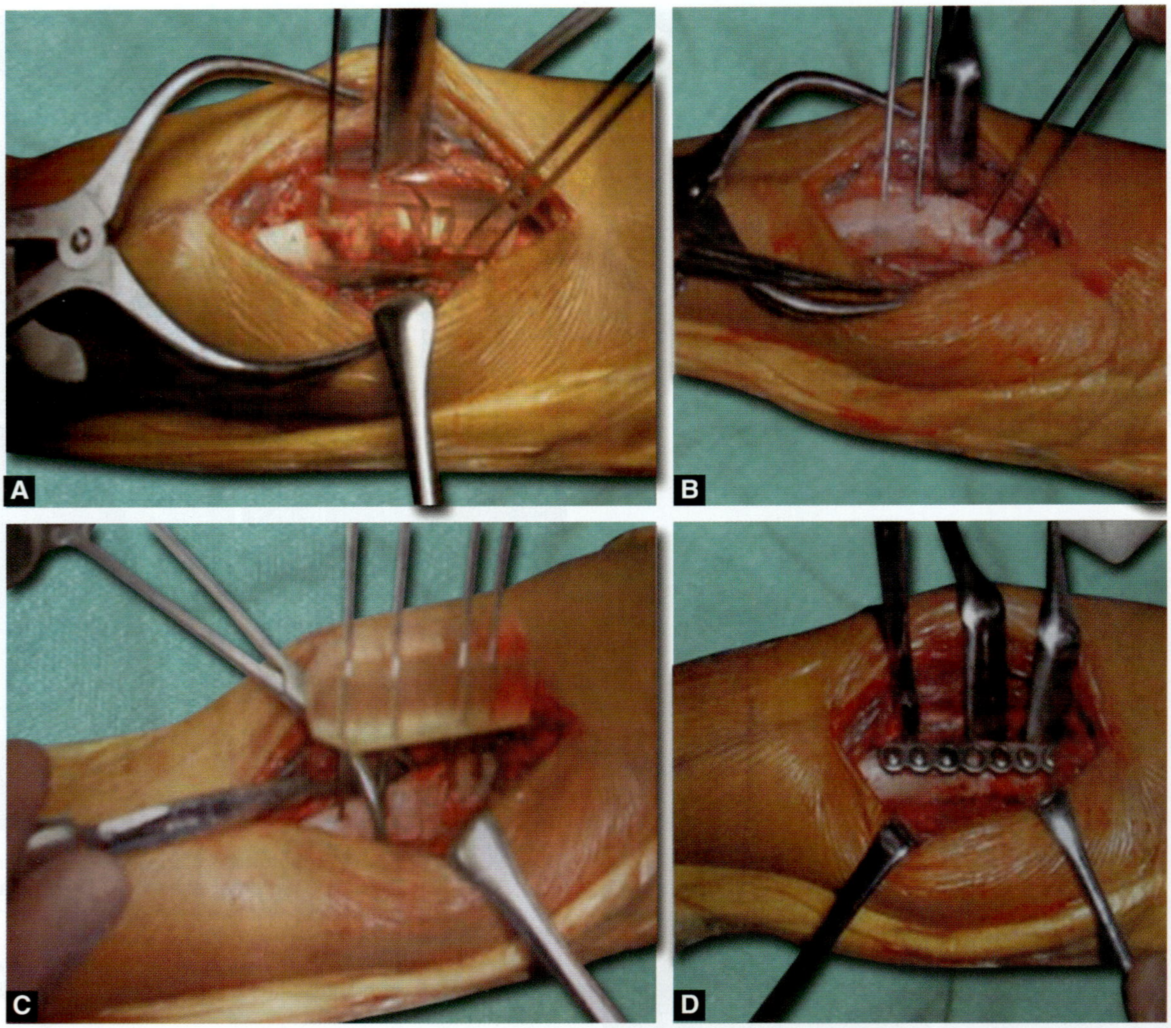

Figs 21.214A to D: Bone graft alternates like carbonated hydroxyapatite and calcium phosphate fracture fixed with recon plate

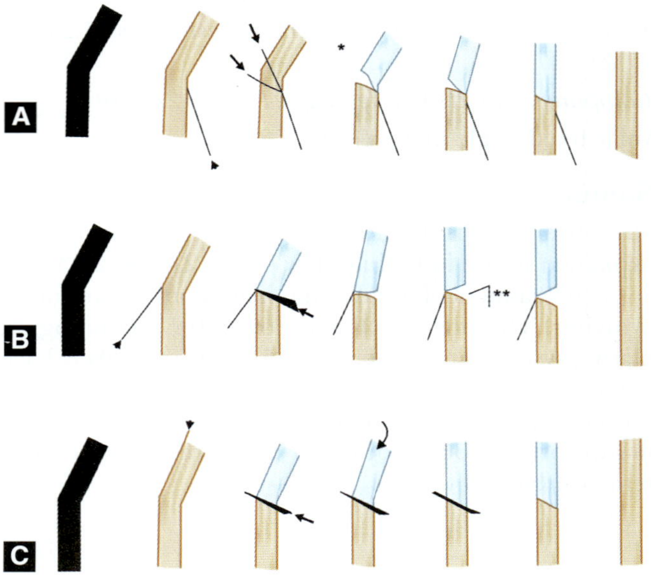

Figs 21.215A to C: The bent cylinders represent the deformed bones. Different deformities can show a similar silhouette (the left figures of A, B, C). The 3-D relationship between the bone and deformity axis (arrowhead of each figure) suggests the most appropriate methods of correction—(A) When the axis runs along the concave side of the deformity, a closing osteotomy after removal of a wedge (asterisk) brings about the roation of the bone segment around the deformity axis, thereby completing the correction; (B) When the deformity axis is along the convex side, opening wedge ostetomy followed by wedge-shaped bone-grafting (double asterisks is considered appropriate; (C) If the deformity axis is displaced from the bone, a closing or opening wedge osteotomy with shortening or lengthening is appropriate. The osteotomy planes are indicated by arrows

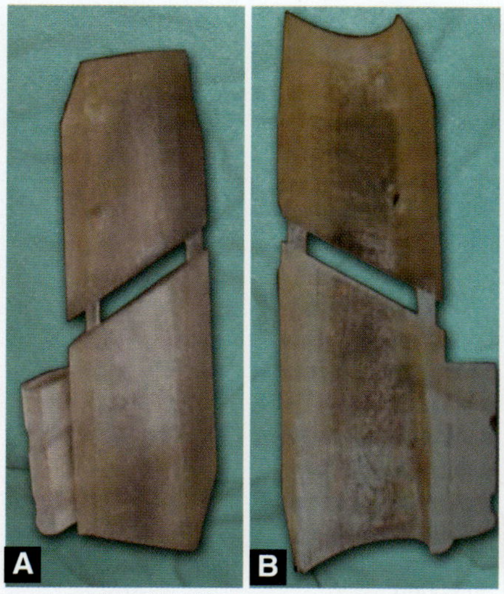

Figs 21.216A and B: The osteotomy template was embodied as a real plastic model—(A) The surgeon's side; (B) The template

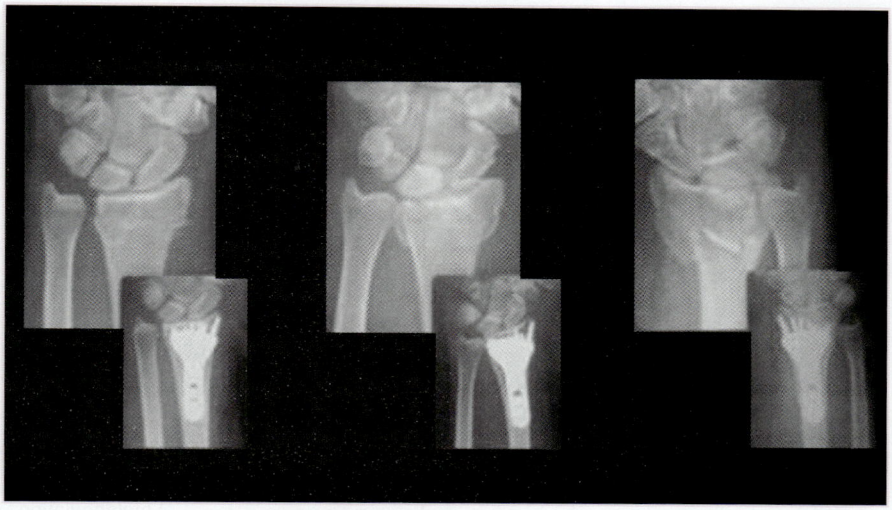

Fig. 21.217: Different types of volar fixed angle plates applied for correcting distal radial fractures abnormalities

Flow chart 21.1: Symptomatic distal radius malunion algorithm no. 1

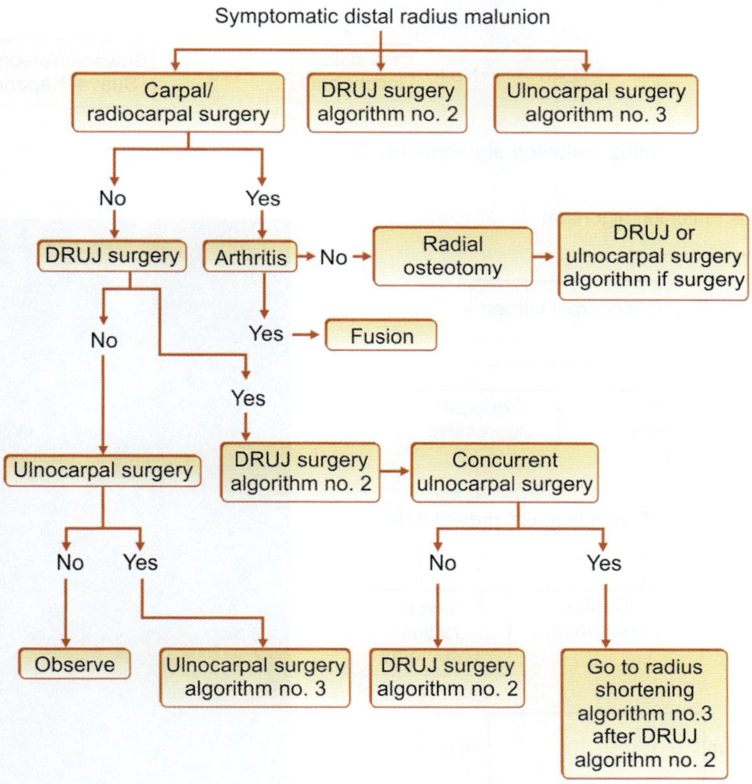

Flow chart 21.2: Symptomatic distal radius malunion algorithm No. 2

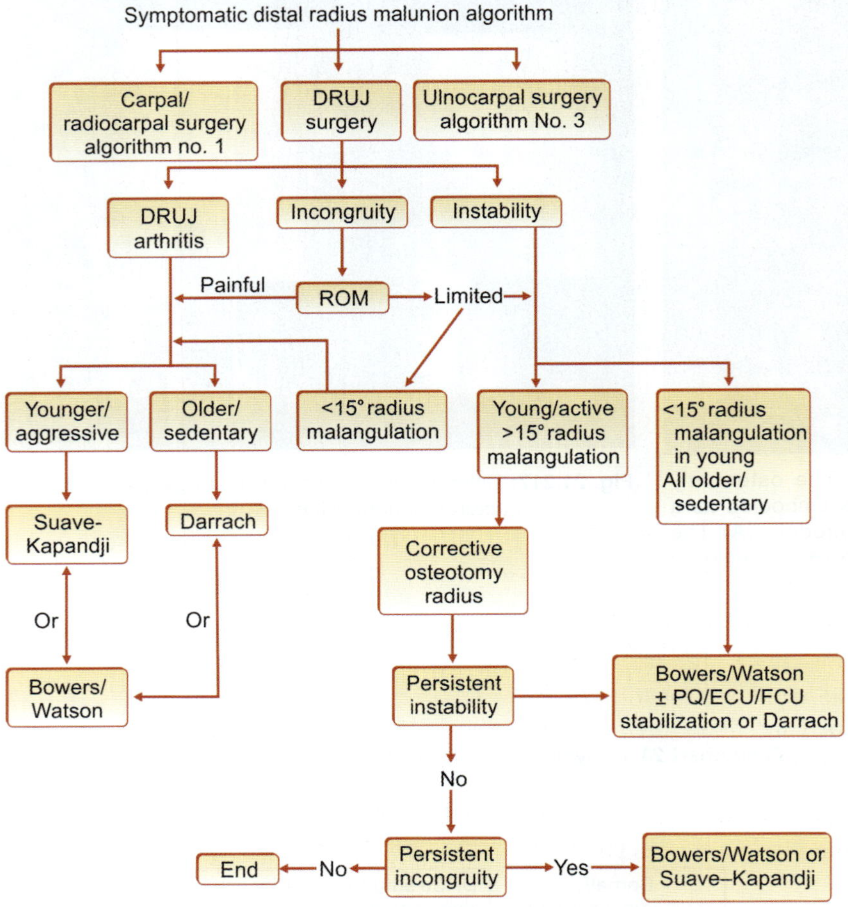

Flow chart 21.3: Symptomatic distal radius malunion algorithm no. 3

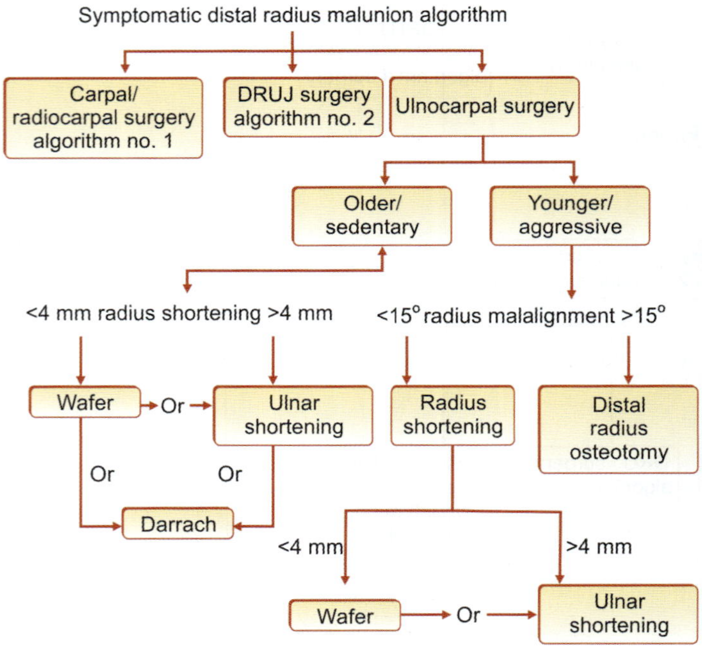

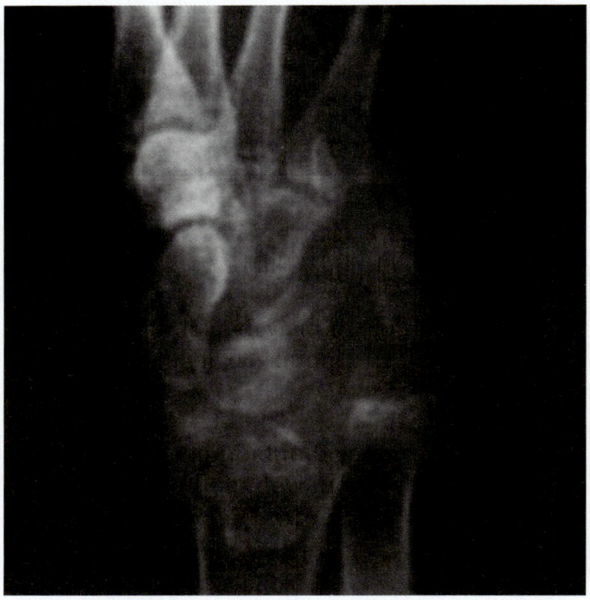

Fig. 21.218: Preoperative X-ray of wrist (AP view)

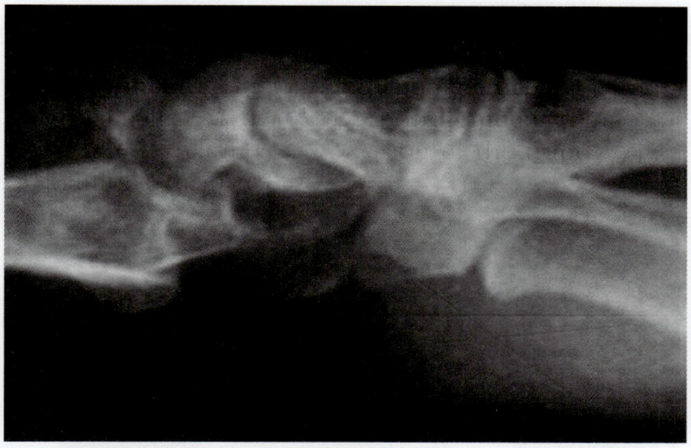

Fig. 21.219: Preoperative X-ray of wrist lateral view

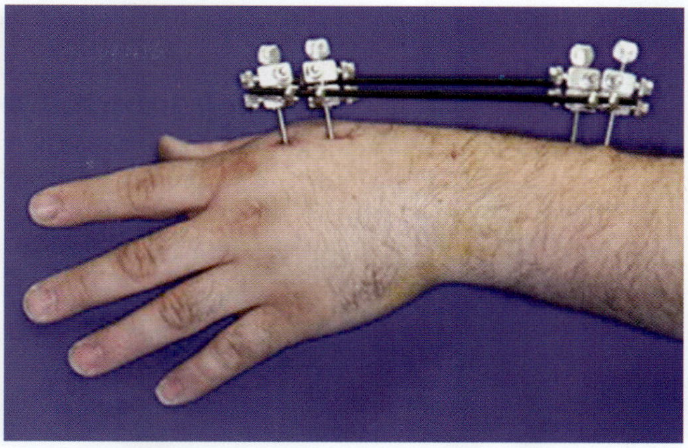

Fig. 21.220: Static external fixation

EXTERNAL FIXATION OF DISTAL RADIUS FRACTURES

Introduction

They are the most common fractures that occur in patients between ages 15 and 75 years. Many methods are there for treating displaced distal radius fractures (Figs 21.219 and 21.220).

All forms of treatment involve obtaining fracture reduction, which may then be maintained by:
- Casting
- Functional bracing
- External fixation
- Percutaneous pinning
- Internal fixation
- Combination of these methods.

We will be discussing the indications and techniques of fracture treatment with external fixation and when they are required, adjuvant with percutaneous pins.

Indications

- Unstable or open fractures
- Fractures occurring in patients with multiple injuries
- Loss of reduction following closed orthopedic treatment
- Bilateral fractures of distal radius
- Acceptable reduction parameters are explained in the Table 21.17.

Types of External Fixation

- Static external fixator
- External fixator with bone grafting
- External fixation with distractor
- Dynamic external fixator
- Roger Anderson external fixator
- Combined external fixation with plating and K-wires.

Table 21.17: Radiographic parameter for finding acceptable reduction of radial fractures

Radiographic parameter	*Normal*	*Acceptable*
Radial length	Plus or minus 2 mm comparing level of lunate facet to ulnar head	No more than 2 mm shortening relative to ulnar head
Radial inclination	20° as measured from lunate facet to radial styloid	No less than 10°
Lateral tilt	11° of volar tilt	Neutral
Intra-articular step or gap	None	Less than 2 mm of either

Static External Fixator (Fig. 21.220)

- Initially, a closed reduction maneuver should be performed to corrrect significant deformity. An assistant provides counter traction at the elbow and the surgeon manipulates the hand and wrist first with inline traction. Most fractures can be reduced with slight volar and ulnar deviation of hand and wrist
- When the provisional reduction is achieved the external fixator can be applied. Two pins are inserted into the radial shaft proximal to the zone of injury in the posterolateral aspect of the middle third of radius.
- The distal pins are inserted in the posterolateral aspect of second metacarpal shaft, which is subcutaneous
- Two pins inserted in each bone, should be in parallel direction, the plane of pins should be varied to construct a quadrangular frame (Fig. 21.221)
- For the second metacarpal, the pins are radially based to avoid injury to extensor mechanism (Fig. 21.222).
- The reduction is verified using the image intensifier and once achieved, a second bar is added to frame construct and tightened (Figs 21.223 and 21.224)
- When applying the external fixator, extreme positions of the wrist should be avoided. The goal is to restore

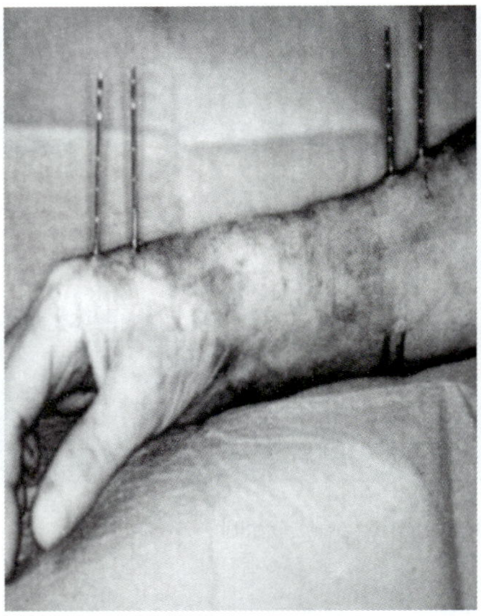

Fig. 21.221: Two pins are inserted in each bone in parallel direction, the plane of pins are varied to construct a quadrangular frame

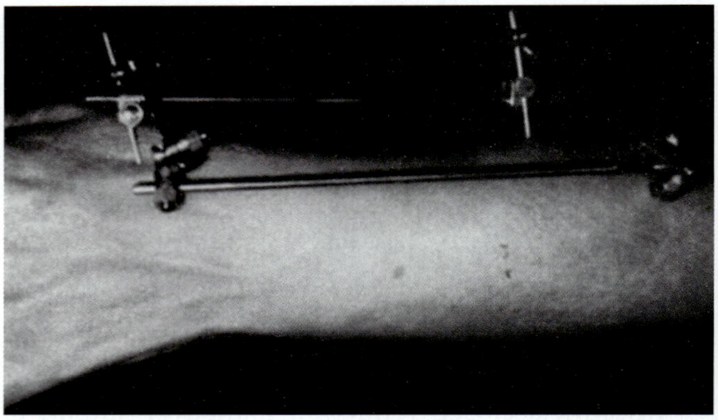

Fig. 21.222: Pins are radially based for second metacarpal, to avoid injury to extensor mechanism

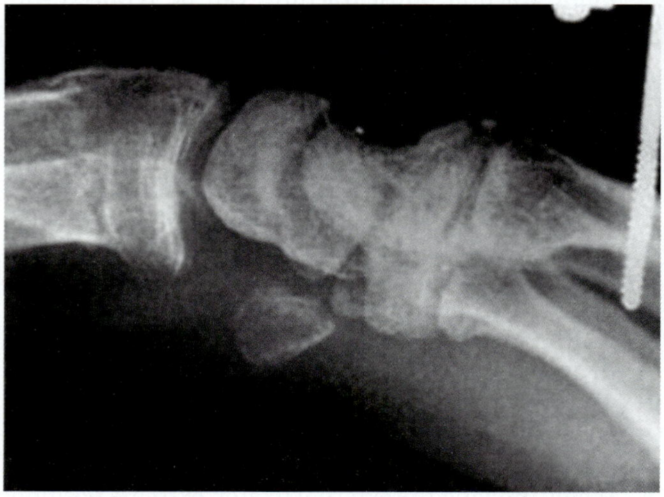

Fig. 21.223: Postoperative radiograph (lateral view)

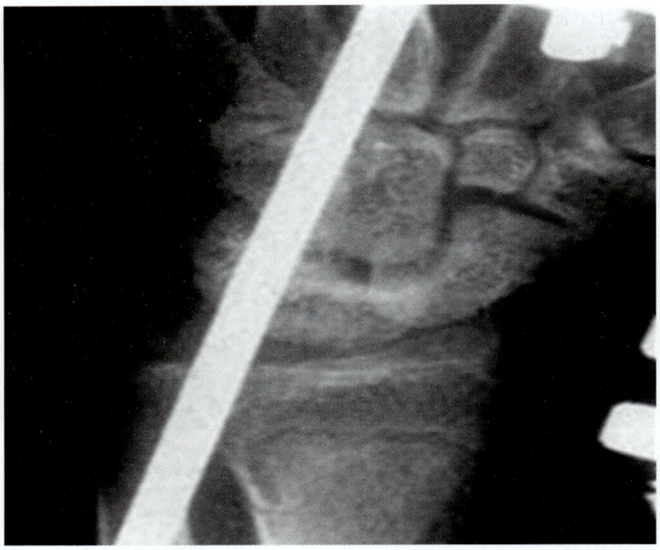

Fig. 21.224: Postoperative radiograph (AP view)

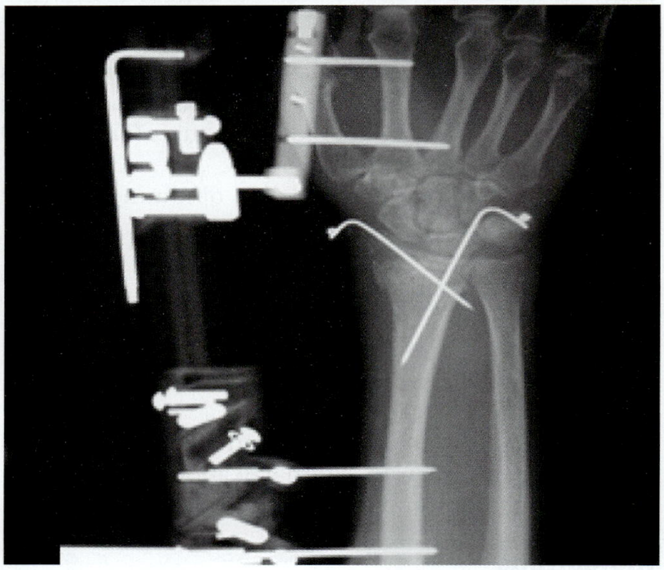

Fig. 21.225: Reduction using percutaneous pins with external fixator

radiographic parameters, most importantly the radial length
- The reduction, especially residual intra-articular deformity, must be finely tuned using percutaneous pins or bone grafting (Fig. 21.225).

Postoperative Care

- Dress the pin sites with the vaseline coated gauze and wrap the forearm and wrist in soft bandage.
- Keep the sites clean and dry daily

- Patients who have isolated injury can be discharged on the same day from hospital, whereas others stay longer depending on the associated injuries
- Patients are asked to return to clinic within 2 weeks and again 6 weeks postoperatively
- At each visit, plain radiographs are taken, the frame and radiographs are usually removed on sixth week, if the radiographs shows fracture union and a supervised physiotherapy program is initiated to regain the wrist motion and strength (Figs 21.226A to D)
- Treating displaced distal radius fractures, including those with an articular component, with external fixation and percutaneous pins yields good results.
- Patients experienced improvement in function and pain scores at all points of follow-up
- Grip strength is also superior in those treated with external methods

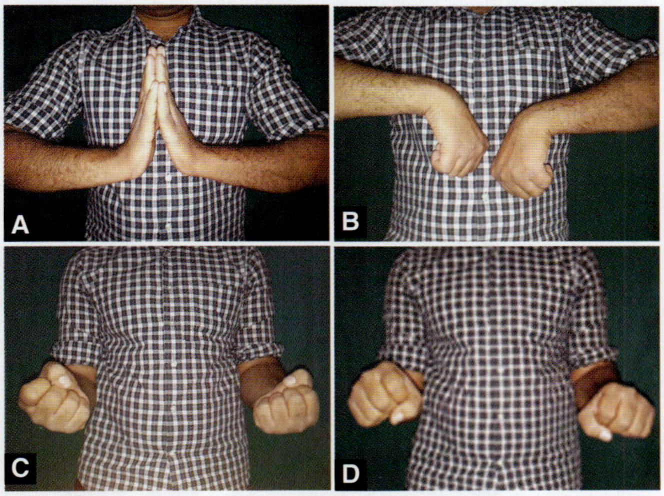

Figs 21.226A to D: Wrist exercises initiated after fracture union to increase strength

- Pin tract infections can be treated with an oral antibiotic prescription and local pin care. Fractures are usually healed by 6 to 8 weeks.

Dynamic External Fixator

- The rationale of this device is a ball joint at proximal part of capitate at the capitolunate joint, since this is the center of rotation of wrist
- Advantage of this design is early motion of wrist and hand without any loss of reduction
- The device is placed in radial or coronal plane to permit the movements. Proximal pins are placed in radial bone in perpendicular direction and distal pins are placed in first and second metacarpal bone or second metacarpal bone (Figs 21.227A and B).

External Fixation with Bone Graft

- Severerly displaced communited Colles fracture, tend to heal with malunion (Figs 21.228A and B)

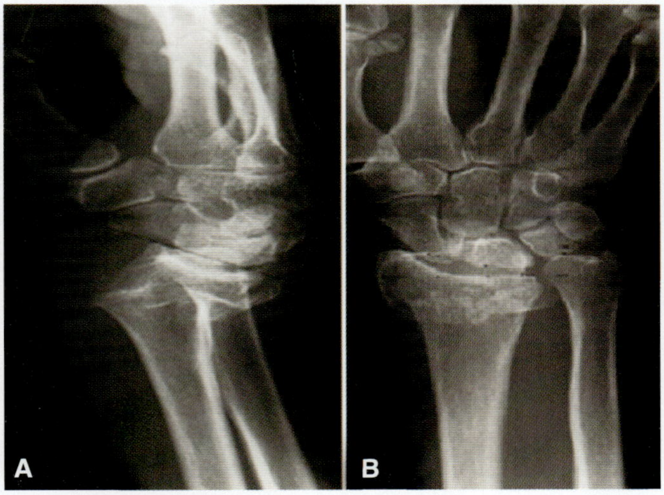

Figs 21.228A and B: Preoperative X-rays

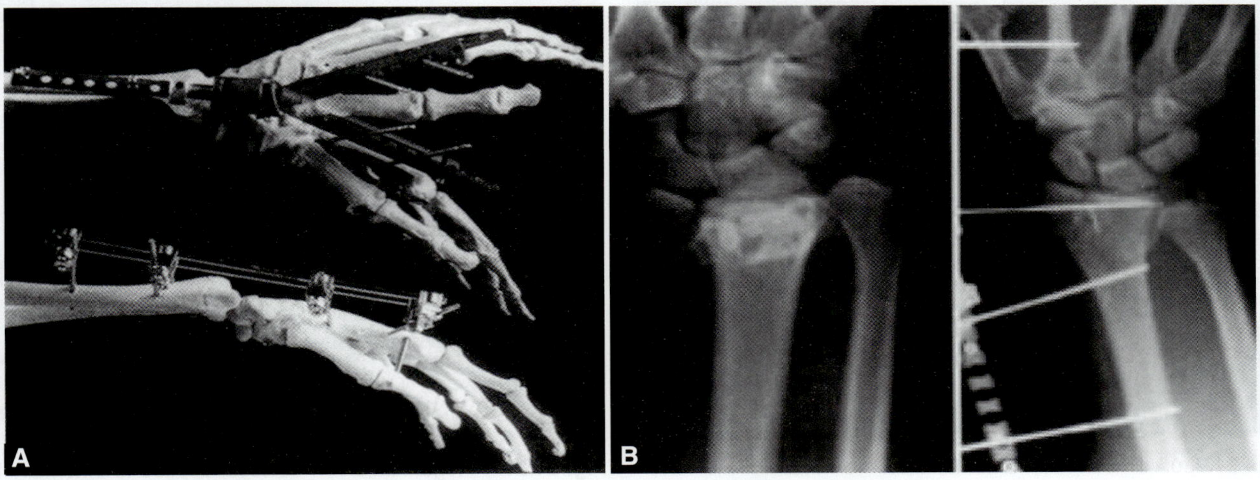

Figs 21.227A and B: Proximal pins are placed perpendicularly and distal pins are placed in first and second metacarpal bone

- Several methods were tried, like plasters, percutaneous K-wires and external fixation. More recently, the option of primary bone grafting has been explored
- Cancellous bone grafting has both mechanical effects and biological effects, giving intrinsic stability to fracture and speeding the healing process (Figs 21.229A and B) and after external fixator removal (Figs 21.230A and B)
- We insert a distractor rod instead of a connecting rod in the fixator frame (Figs 21.231)
- Principle is distraction could be manually adjusted to aid in the healing process of the fracture union.

Roger Anderson Device (Fig. 21.232)

It consists of series of pins and rods interconnected with movable clamps, giving a three dimensional configuration to the fixator. The pins are placed at 45° angulation to the shaft (Figs 21.233 and 21.234).

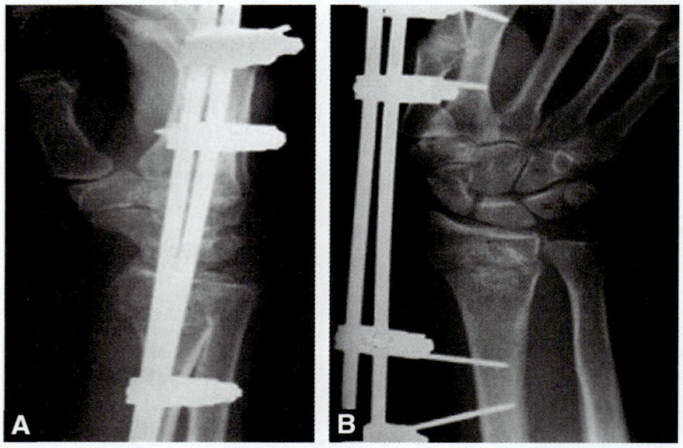

Figs 21.229A and B: Postoperative X-rays

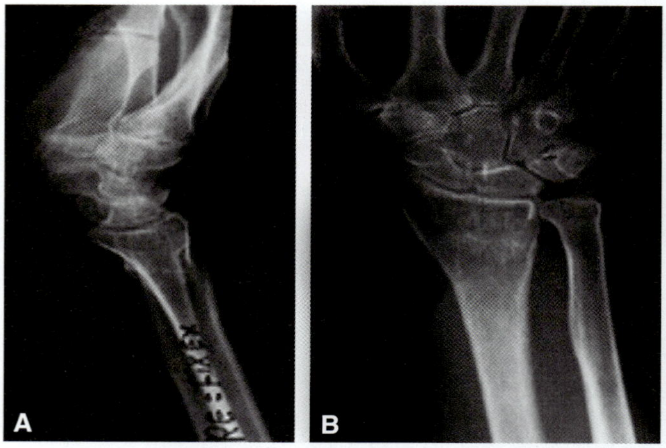

Figs 21.230A and B: After external fixator removal

AO External Fixator (Figs 21.235 and 21.236)

Prerequisites

- Severe communition of fracture
- Extension of fracture to radiocarpal joint
- Dorsal angulation more than 25°
- Articular step off more than 2 mm

Technique

- 2.5 mm partially threaded AO half pins are used.
- Pins are placed 20 to 30° off the perpendicular plane, this is done to give convergence to the frame, so that it prevents the loosening of pins.

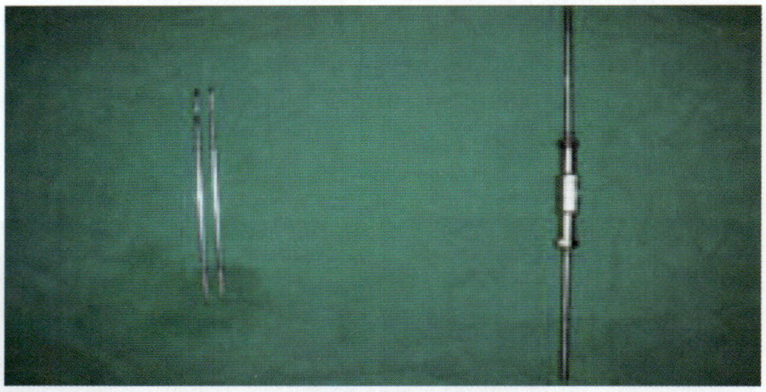

Fig. 21.231: Schanz screws and distraction rod

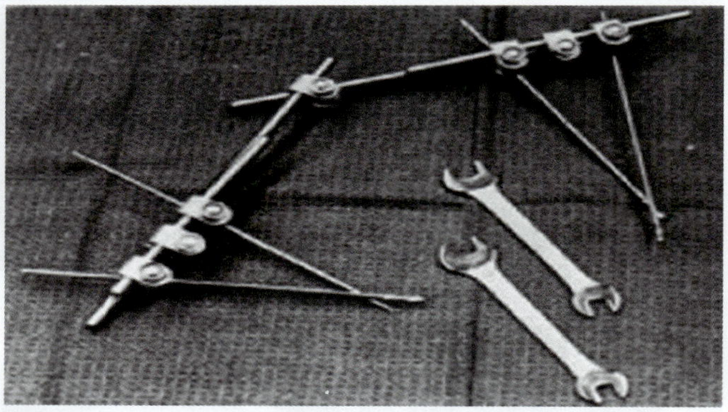

Fig. 21.232: Roger Anderson devices

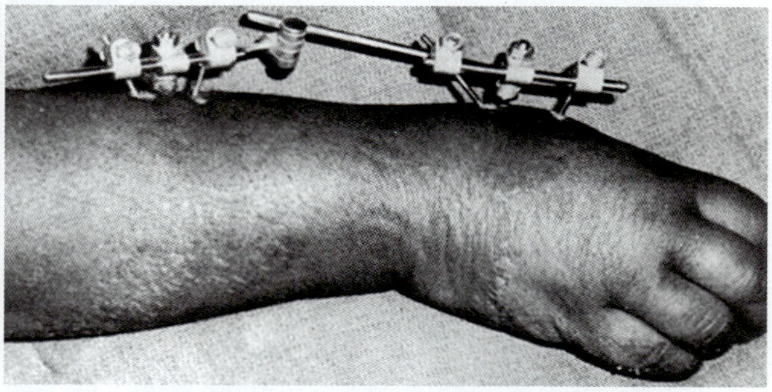

Fig. 21.233: Roger Anderson devices, applied to externally fixing the fractures fragments

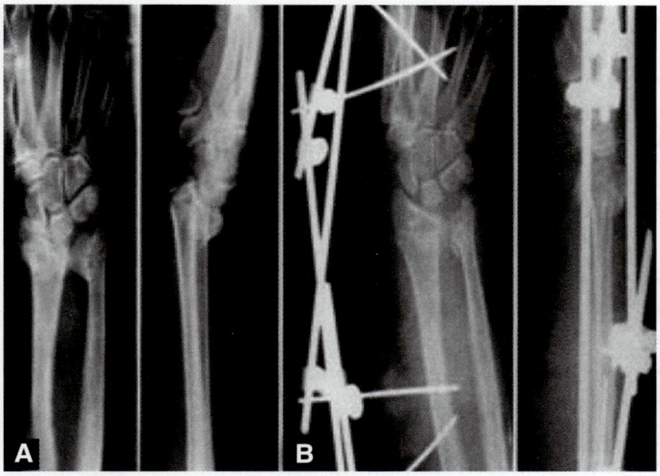

Figs 21.234A and B: (A) Preoperative X-ray (AP and lateral view); (B) X-ray showing Roger Anderson external fixators are applied

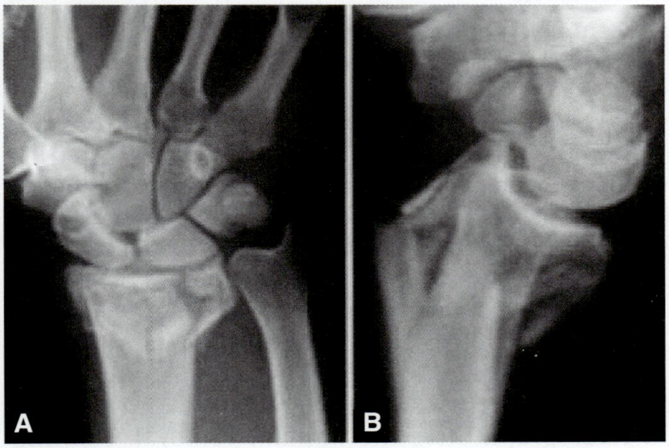

Figs 21.235A and B: Preoperative X-rays—(A) AP view; (B) Lateral view

- Overdrilling of the pins should be avoided, to stripping of threads in far cortex by the smooth shaft of the pins, likewise unicortical placement of pins should also be avoided.

Discussion

- External fixation supplemented with percutaneous pins is an excellent option for treating displaced fractures of the distal radius with reliably good results, showing a low operation rate and a low complication rate.
- The key to success is to restore the anatomic parameters of the distal radius while minimizing insult to the soft tissue envelope.

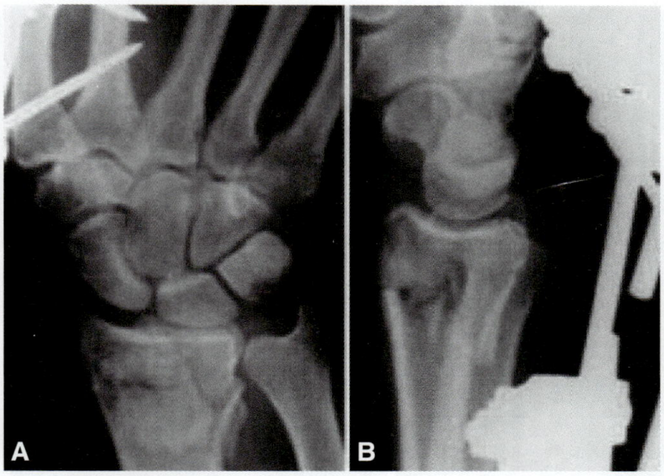

Figs 21.236A and B: Postoperative X-ray, with AO fixator applied—(A) AP view; (B) Lateral view

PLATING OF DISTAL RADIUS FRACTURES

■ Introduction

No area in fracture management has had a recent explosion of treatment modalities as in distal radius plating. A drift from dorsal to volar plating has occurred. Segment specific fixation has been the new mindset. Other novel approaches for proposed problems include locking plates, nail-plate combinations and others. Here, some of these approaches are outlined.

Indications for Open Reduction

- Type 2 distal radius fractures (Fernandez classification)
- Type 3 distal radius fractures
- Unstable distal radius fractures
- Partial volar or dorsal (B-type intra-articular fractures)
- Radial styloid fractures
- Lunate fossa split and displaced
- Intra-articular comminuted C2–C3 fractures.

Plating Techniques (See Fig. 21.263)

- Volar plating
- Dorsal plating
- Combined volar and dorsal plating
- Distraction plate fixation
- Fragment specific fixation.

Volar Plating

Surgical approach

AO type C distal radius fracture (Figs 21.237 and 21.238)

- Plate is placed

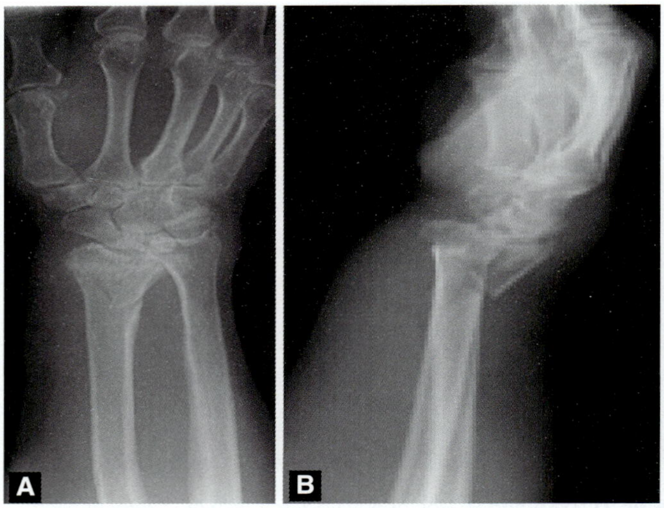

Figs 21.237A and B: Preoperative X-ray of AO type C distal radius fracture—(A) AP view; (B) Lateral view

- A screw is placed in central oval hole (Fig. 21.239)
- In each of the distal slot, smooth peg is placed, followed by lag screw to engage the dorsal fragment (Fig. 21.240)
- Screws are then placed proximal to holes of the plate (Fig. 21.241)
- Brachioradialis and pronator quadratus are sutured
- Postoperative X-rays after volar plating are shown in Figures 21.242 to 21.244

Postoperative care

- Patient with stable radioulnar joint are placed in wrist splint
- After 1 week, a fabricated wrist splint is used, during which hand range of motions are started and continued for 6 weeks
- After 6 weeks splint is removed and strengthening exercise program is begun
- Unrestricted activities are allowed after 12 weeks
- Patients with DRUJ derangement are placed in supination splint, for 6 weeks, later gentle active pronation and supination exercises are done till another 6 weeks
- After 12 weeks unrestricted activities are begun.

Dorsal Plating

Dorsally displaced distal radial fracture are shown in Figures 21.245A and B.

Surgical approach (Fig. 21.246)

- Incision taken midway of radial and ulnar styloid (Fig. 21.247)
- Extensor retinaculum incised, extensor communis and extensor indicis exposed (Fig. 21.248)
- Fourth compartment muscles are retracted (Fig. 21.249)
- Dorsal radiocarpal ligament and extensor tendons are elevated
- Extensor tendons in their compartments have been elevated to expose the distal end of the radius.
- Using a low profile plate, stabilization of fracture is done (Fig. 21.250).

Postoperative care

- Wrist is immobilized in a volar splint
- Active and passive finger movements are encouraged
- Active and active assisted motions are done after 1 week
- Passive and grip strengthening exercises are started after 6 weeks
- Patients were followed up with serial radiographs.

Combined Dorsal and Volar Plates Fixation

Indications

- Complex fragmentation of both articular surface and the metaphysis
- AO type C 3.2 fracture
- Percutaneous pinning was attempted, but did not restore the alignment (Fig. 21.251)
- Note, the inability of K-wires to control the fragments, when there is a metaphyseal comminution (Fig. 21.252)
- A second procedure of dorsal plate fixation resulted in volar translation of fragments because of absence of volar metaphyseal support (Figs 21.253A and B) Application of second volar plate has improved the alignment. The functional result was rated good according to system of Gartland and Werley. Radiograph after the implant removal, showing healing with reasonable alignment (Fig. 21.254).

Distraction Plate Fixation

- Indicated in fractures of distal end radius with extensive metaphyseal and diaphyseal communition (Figs 21.255 and 21.256).

Surgical Technique (Figs 21.257 and 21.258)

- Distal incision is made first over the long finger metacarpal
- Proximal incision is made over dorsal aspect of radial shaft at the anticipated levels of proximal portion of plate
- The level of incision and length of plate are chosen by utilizing flouroscopy, while holding the plate against the skin to appropriate level of metacarpal and ensuring that at least four holes of plate are proximal to fracture site (Fig. 21.257). Intraoperative

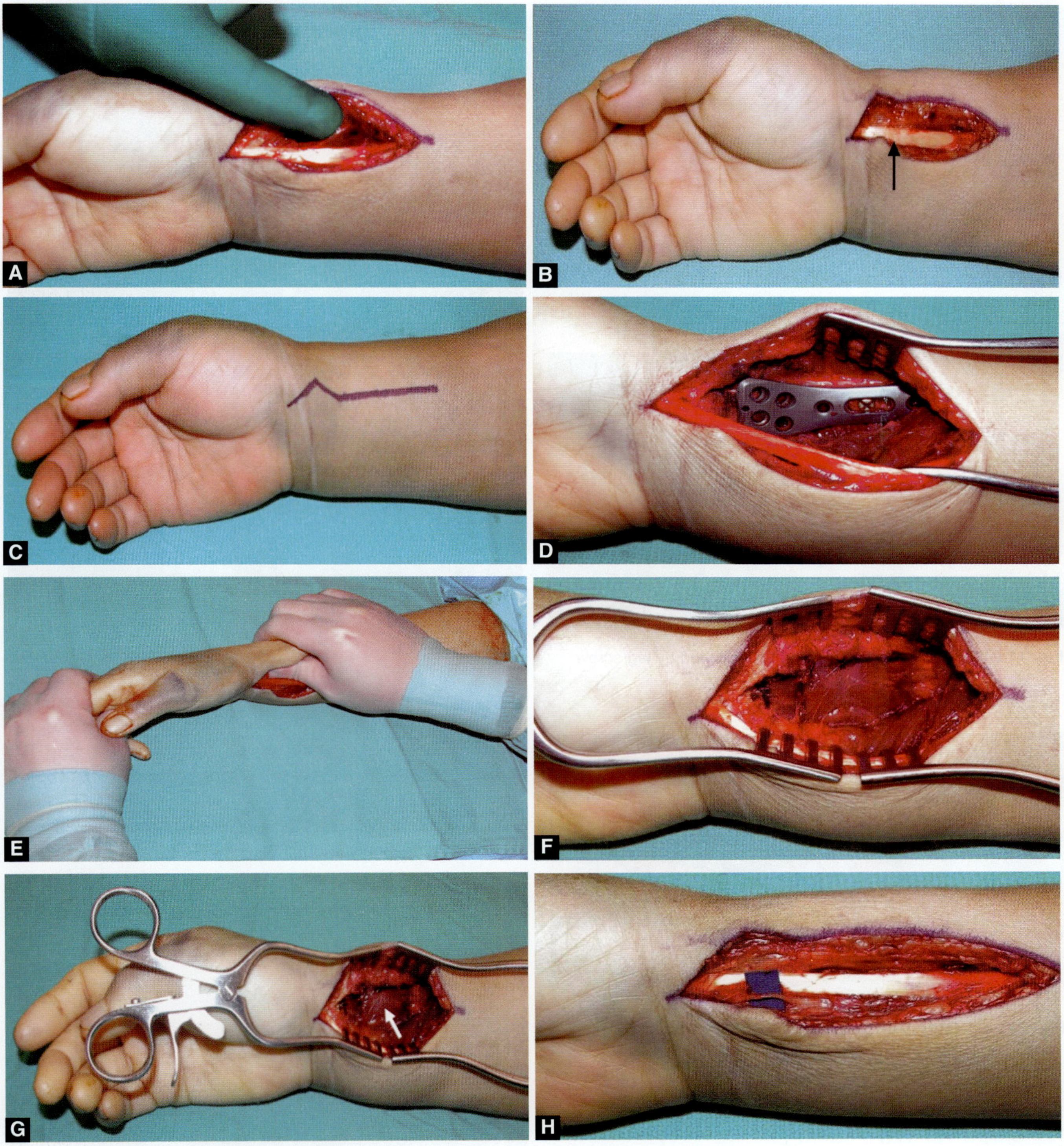

Figs 21.238A to H: Surgical approach (AO type C, distal radius fracture)

radiographs taken to check the collect alignment are shown in Figures 21.259A and B.

- *Postoperative radiographs (Fig. 21.260):* At 4 months, X-rays show maintenance of radial length and palmar tilt with the union of fracture and bridging of bone defect.
- Range of motion of operated wrist compared to the normal wrist is shown in Figures 21.261A to D.

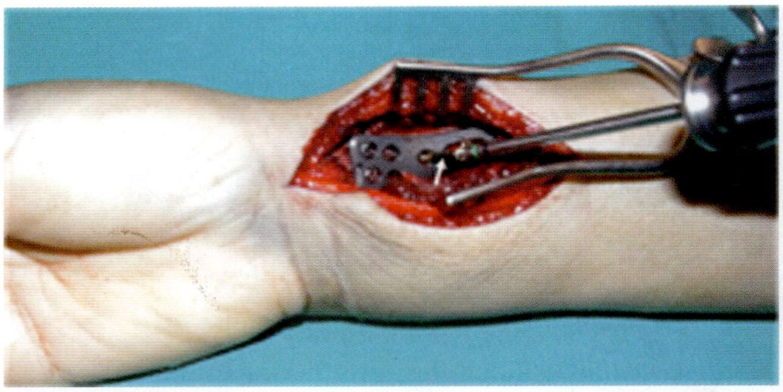

Fig. 21.239: A screw is placed in central oval hole

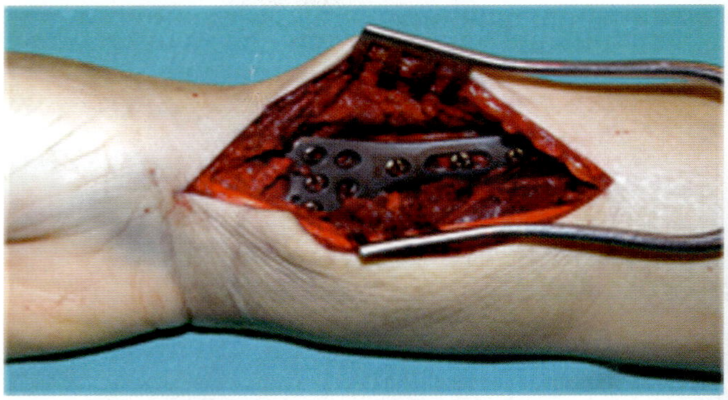

Fig. 21.240: Placement of smooth peg, followed by lag screw

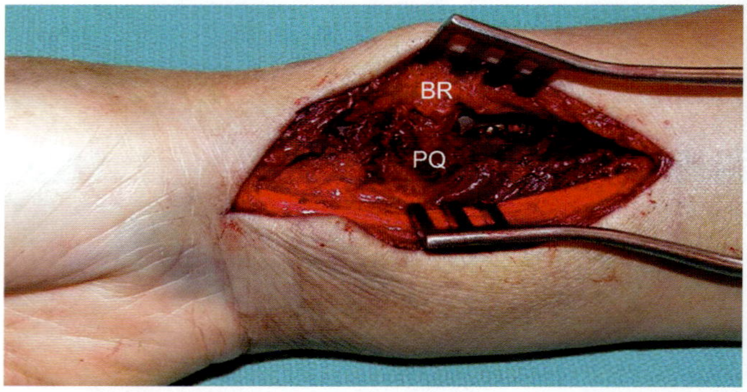

Fig. 21.241: Placement of screws proximal to holes of the plate—BR. Brachioradialis; PQ. Pronator quadratus

- Dorsal plate (Fig. 21.262) placements are associated with high rate of complications, like stiffness of joint, tenosynovitis and tendon rupture (Figs 21.263 and 21.264)
- The effect of attendant scar is difficult to separate from actual location of dorsal plate
- A volar plate (See Fig. 21.262) placement through flexor carpi radialis approach affords a soft tissue layer between the skin and the plate (See Fig. 21.258)

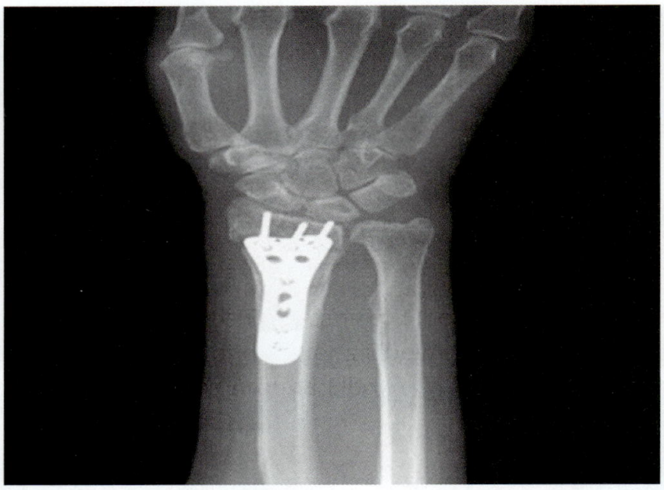

Fig. 21.242: PA view after surgery

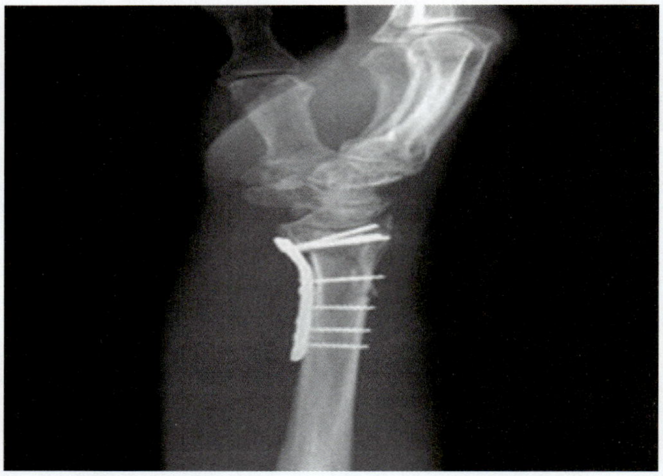

Fig. 21.243: Lateral view after plating

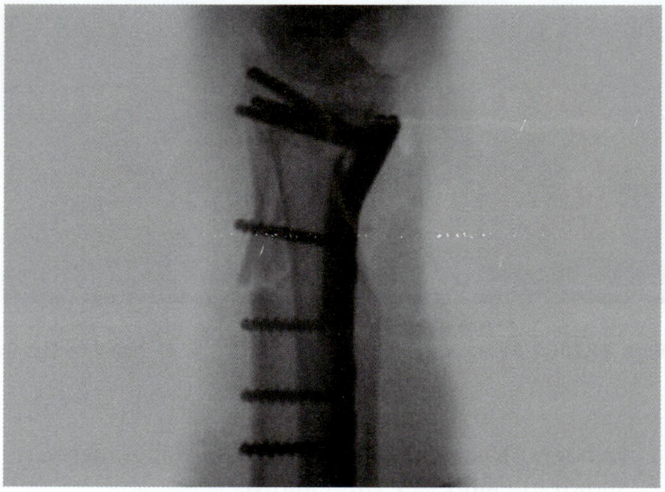

Fig. 21.244: Lateral view, showing anatomic reduction, protrusion of peg in dorsal cortex less than 1 mm

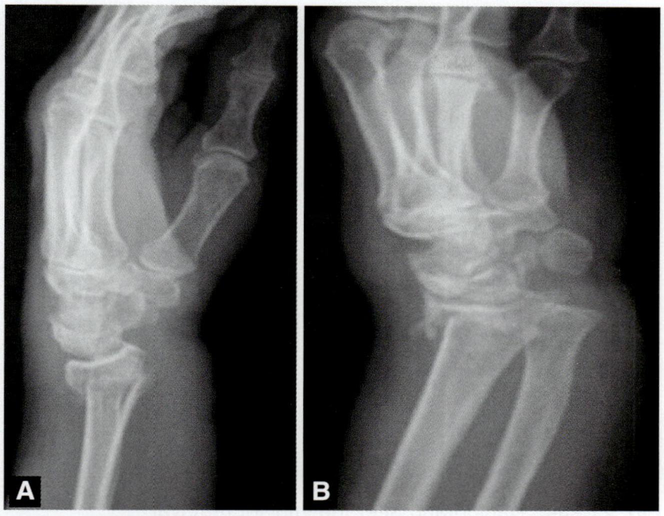

Figs 21.245A and B: Dorsally displaced distal radial fractures

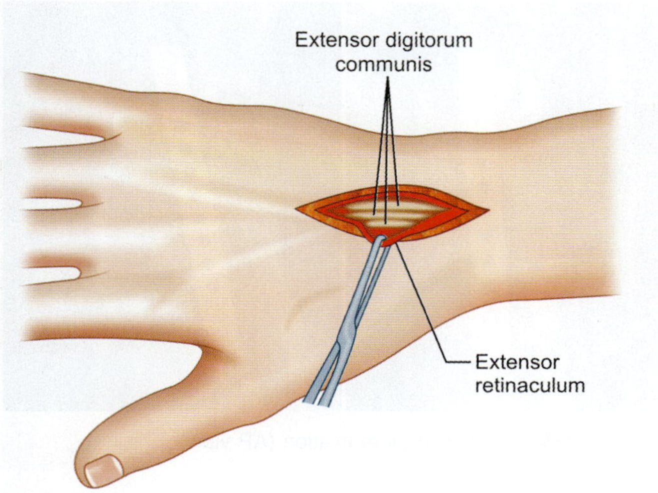

Figs 21.246: Surgical approach for dorsal plating

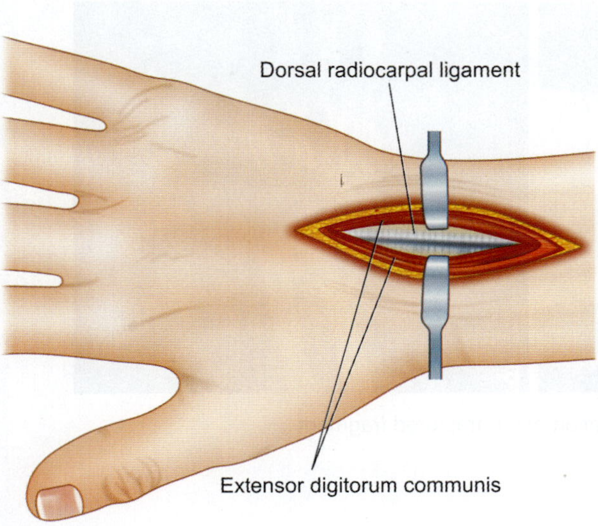

Fig. 21.247: Site of incision (midway to radial and ulnar styloid)

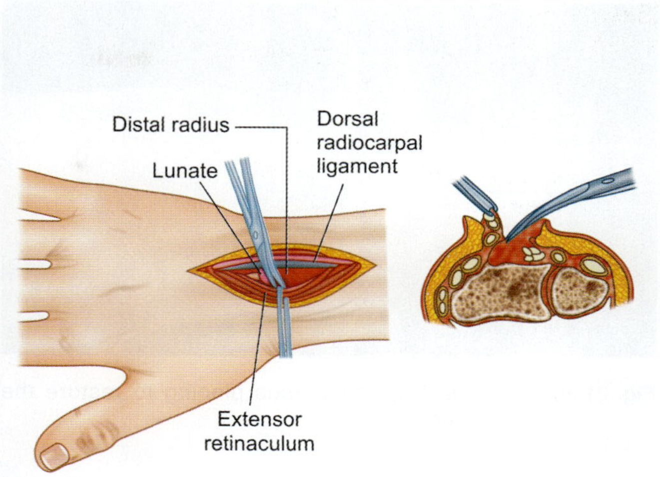

Fig. 21.248: Extensor communis and extensor indicis are exposed, by making incision through extensor retinaculum

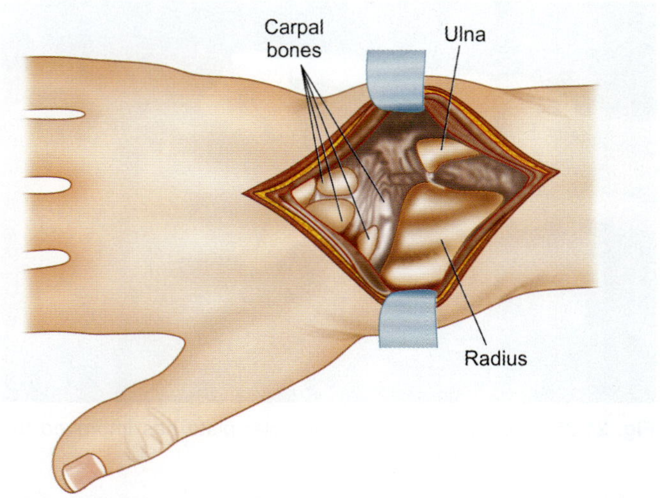

Fig. 21.249: Muscles of fourth compartment are retracted

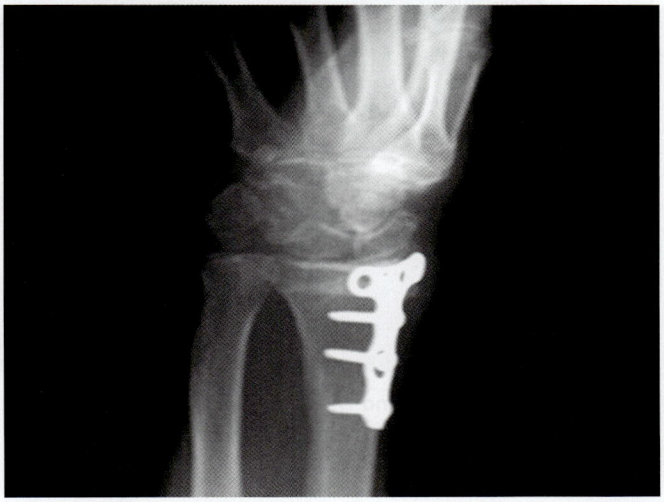

Fig. 21.250: Postoperative X-ray taken after dorsal plating

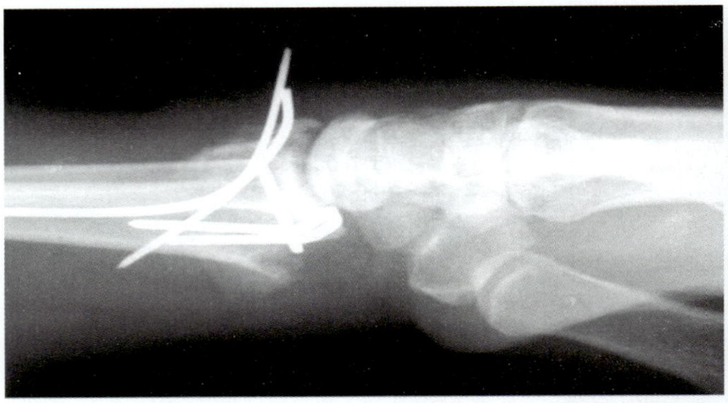

Fig. 21.251: Failure of percutaneous pinning to restore the alignment

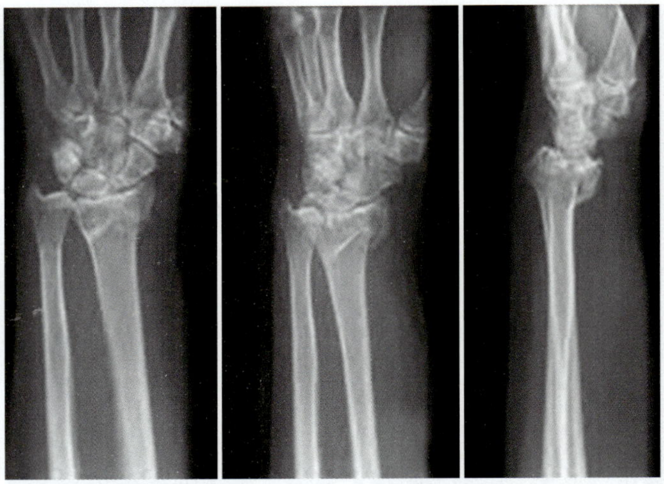

Fig. 21.254: Radiograph after the implant removal

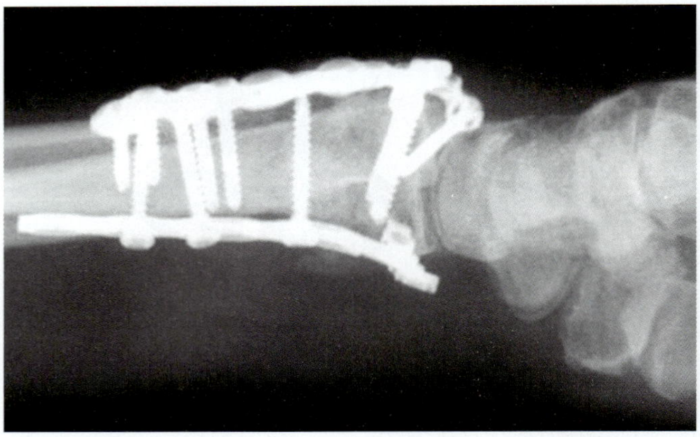

Fig. 21.252: Application of second volar plate has improved the alignment

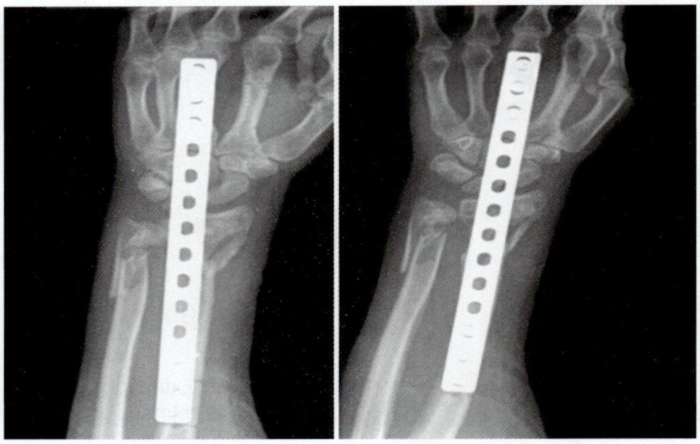

Fig. 21.255: Distraction plate fixation (AP view)

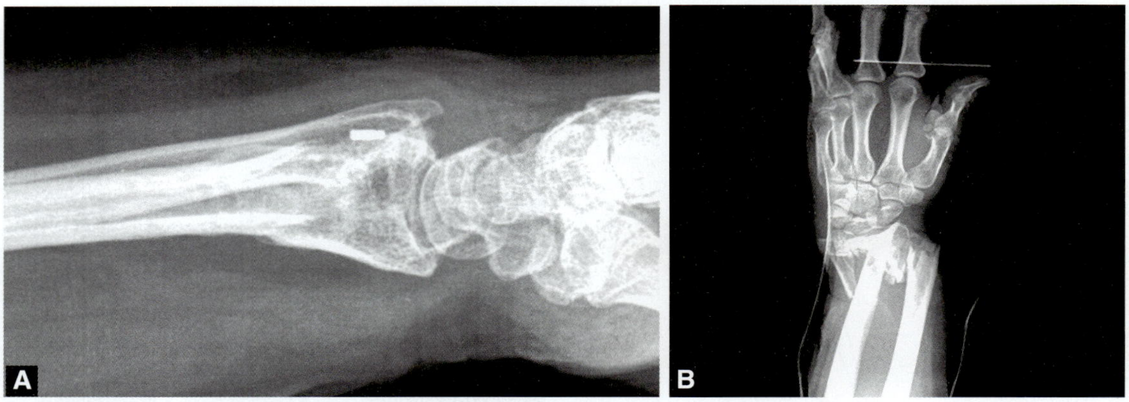

Figs 21.253A and B: Dorsal fixation resulted in volar translation of the fractured fragment

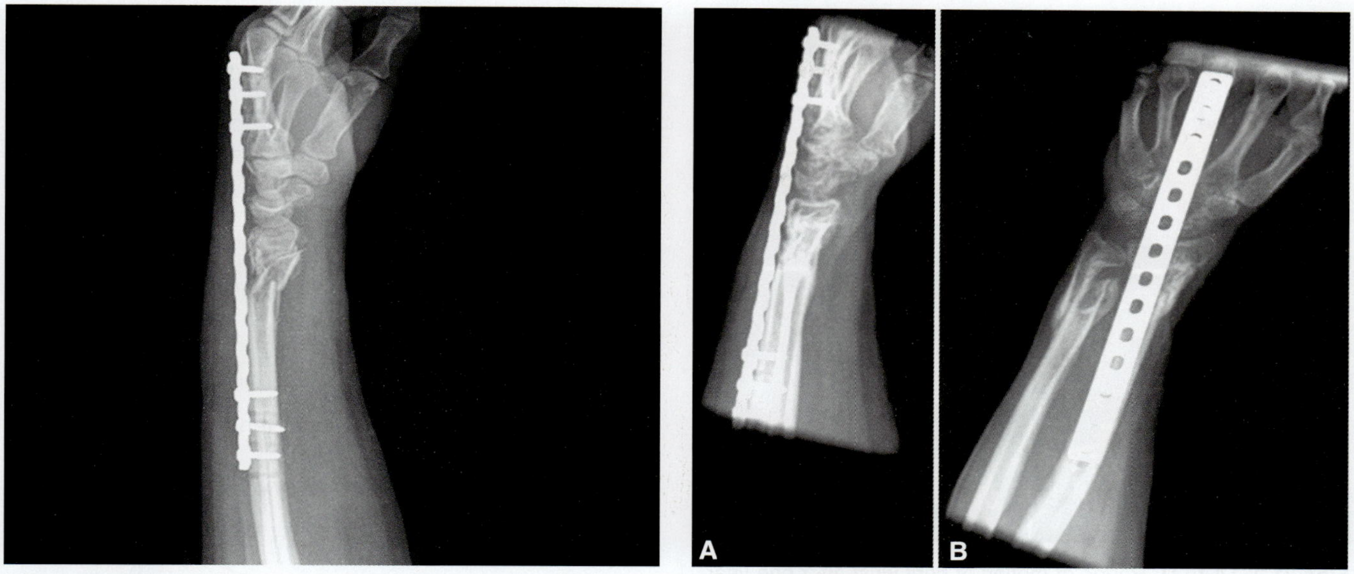

Fig. 21.256: Distraction plate fixation (an oblique view)

Figs 21.259A and B: Intraoperative radiographs

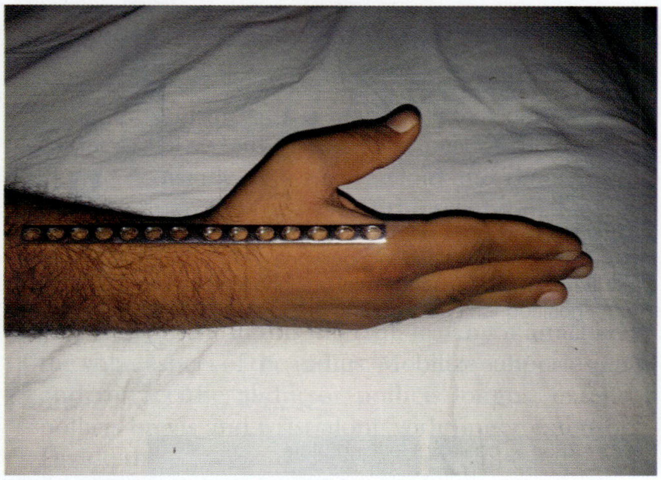

Fig. 21.257: Measurement taken for the length of the plate

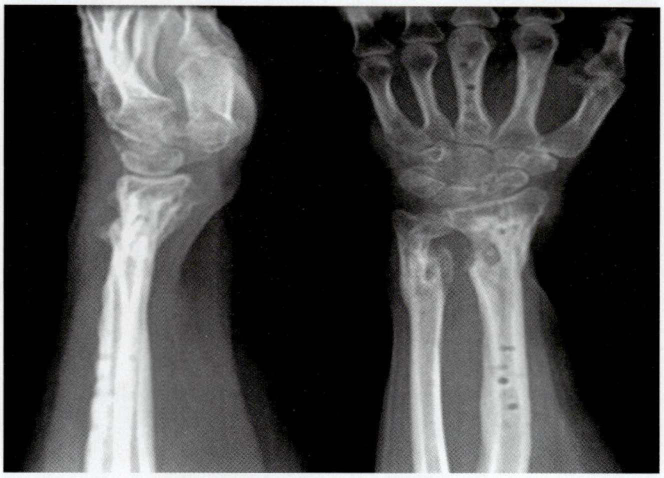

Fig. 21.260: Postoperative radiographs taken after removal of implant

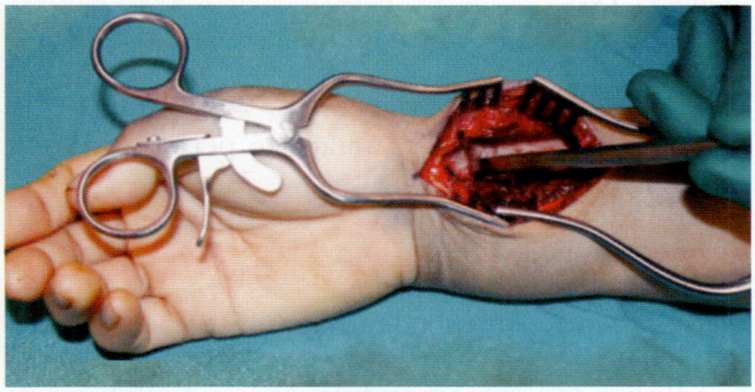

Fig. 21.258: A volar plate placement through flexor carpi radialis approach showing elevating pronator quadratus with an periosteal elevator

- With the advent of new fixed angle plates designs, volar fixation has become the standard approach for distal radius fractures with joint congruity.

Volar Plates

Volar plates generally fall into four functional categories:
- Buttress plates with or without distal screws
- Tine or blade plates
- Fixed angled locking plates
- Polyaxial locking plates (Fig. 21.265).

Different types of volar plates most commonly used are summarized below:
- AOVL: AO 3.5 mm small fragment locking plate
- AOV: AO 3.5 mm small fragment plate

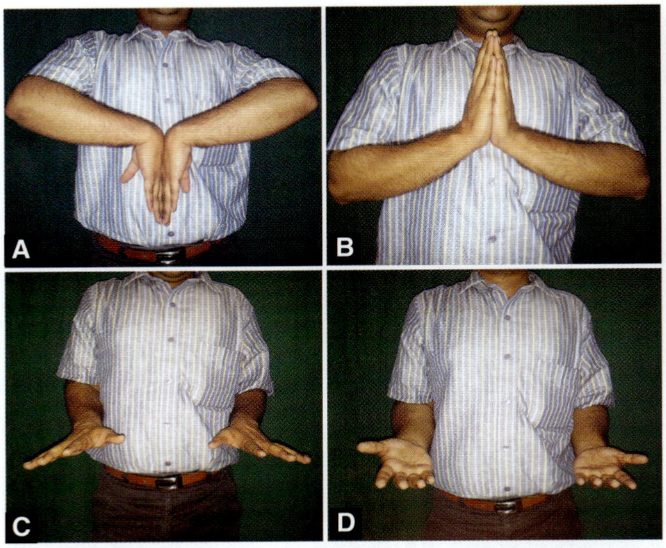

Figs 21.261A to D: Range of motion of right wrist after one year

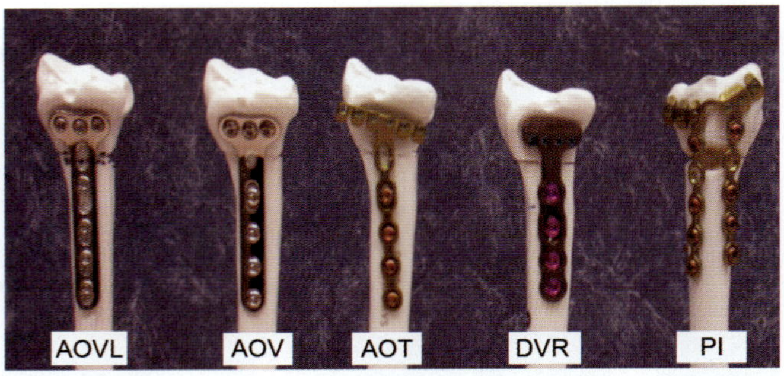

Fig. 21.262: Different types of volar and dorsal plates

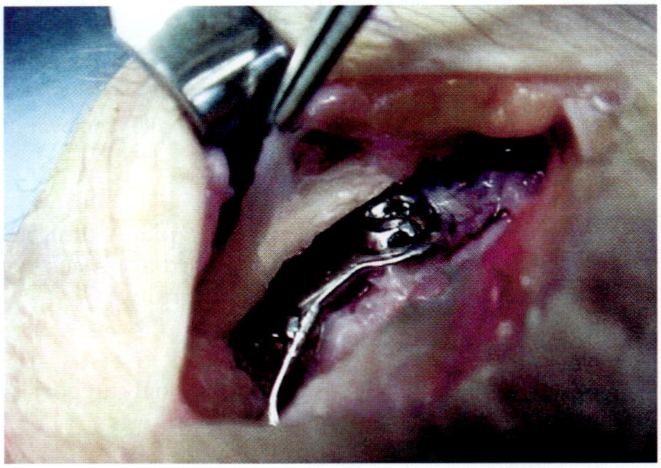

Fig. 21.263: Extensor tenosynovitis and extensor tendons directly gliding over the dorsal plate

- AOT: AO T-Plate
- DVR: Hand innovations distal single row locking plate
- PI: AO PI plate.

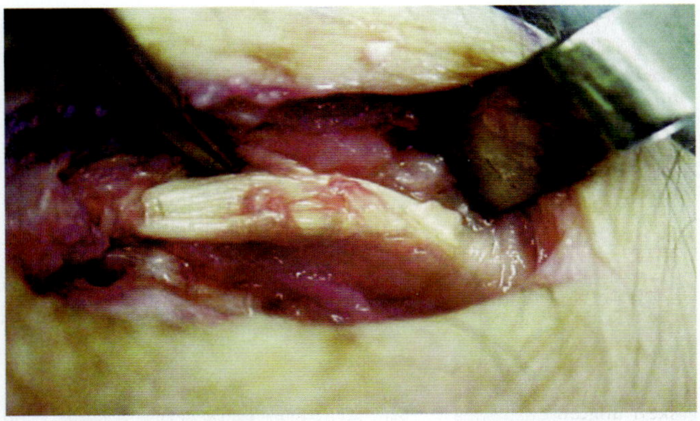

Fig. 21.264: After implant removal tendons showing visible attritional changes

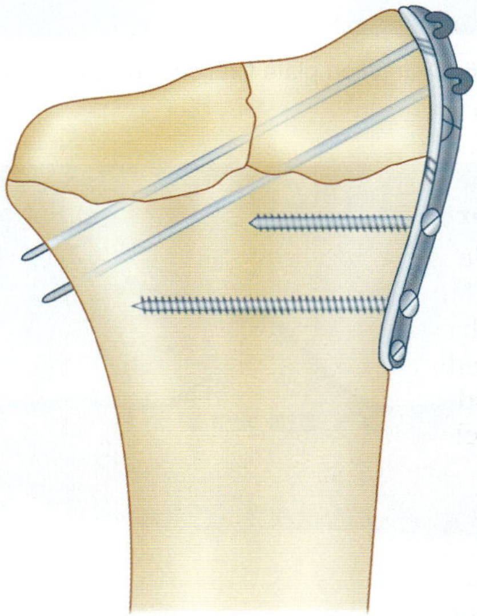

Fig. 21.265: A polyaxial locking plate

Advantages of locking plates over non-locking plates (Table 21.18)

- Produces fixation in bone defects and osteopenic bones
- Early range of motion
- Locked plate as an advantage to perform indirect reduction
- Provide an advantage even for communited osteoporotic fractures
- Fragment specific fixation
- Designed to independently stabilize each fracture element
- Subchondral support and rigidity can be enhanced
- Increased rigidity provided by implants placed orthogonal planes, taking into consideration complex three dimensional geometry of the distal radius.

Table 21.18: Advantages and disadvantages of different locking and non-locking plates

Plates	Advantage	Disadvantage
Buttress plates	Traditional plate design. Can be used with or without distal screw fixation in distal fragment	Since the screws are not locked into plate construct they do not resist angular motion effectively
Blade plates	They offer high strength and stiffness	Having to be placed in a position predetermined to shape and position of times
Fixed angled locking plates	Improved strength and resists angular motion	Fixed trajectory
Polyaxial locking plates	Independent trajectory, matching the distal fixation to variable geometry and surface contour	They tend to be thicker and prominent

Common Fracture Types and Chosen Treatment (Table 21.19)

Summary

With wide array of options and approaches means that almost all distal radius fractures can be fixed and held in place with open reduction and internal fixation. Whether this procedure is required or can reliably be accomplished with good functional outcome, is open to debate until clinical relevant questions are answered.

CARPAL BONE FRACTURES

Anatomy

Carpal bones and adjoining bones, X-rays are shown in Figures 21.266 and 21.267.

Lunate Fractures

Introduction

The lunate is the fourth most fractured carpal bone (following the scaphoid, triquetrum and trapezium) (Fig. 21.268). They often are not diagnosed initially and present delayed as lunate osteonecrosis, which is also known as Kienbock's disease.

Anatomy

- The lunate is shaped like a crescent (Fig. 21.269)
- *Carpal keystone:* Since it resides within a protected concavity of the distal radius (lunate fossa) and is integral in the flexion/extension arc and the radial/ulnar deviation arc, at both the radiocarpal and midcarpal joints.

Table 21.19: Common fracture types and their chosen treatment

Fracture type	Chosen treatment
Extra-articular Intra-articular	A volar fixed angled locking plate
Partial (B-type) volar	A volar buttress plate
Partial (B-type) dorsal	A volar fixed angled or polyaxial plate
Radial styloid	A volar fixed angled locking plate or fragment specific fixation
Lunate fossa	A volar fixed angled locking plates or polyaxial locking plates. Communition necessitates dorsal reduction then a fragment specific fixation
Lunate fossa split and displaced	A volar locking plate or polyaxial locking plate (Complex intra-articular fractures different plate designs and alternate fixation options should be available
Communited (C2-3)	An extended volar locking plate plus or minus dorsal plates in fragment specific manner
Communited (C2) osteoporotic	Extended volar locking plate or distal radius bridge plate
Communited with non-reconstructable dorsal rim	Volar plate with dorsal Pi Plate extending over the first carpal row

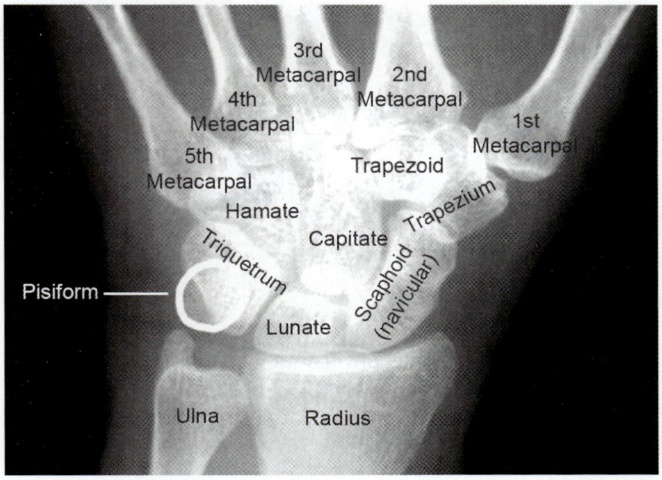

Fig. 21.266: Identification of carpal bones on X-rays AP view

- The lunate is attached to the scaphoid and triquetrum via interosseous ligaments.
- Distally, it is concave and articulates with the convex head of the capitates and proximally, it articulates with the lunate facet of the distal radius.
- It is supplied by a proximal carpal vascular arcade, volarly and dorsally. There are three variable intralunate anastomoses.

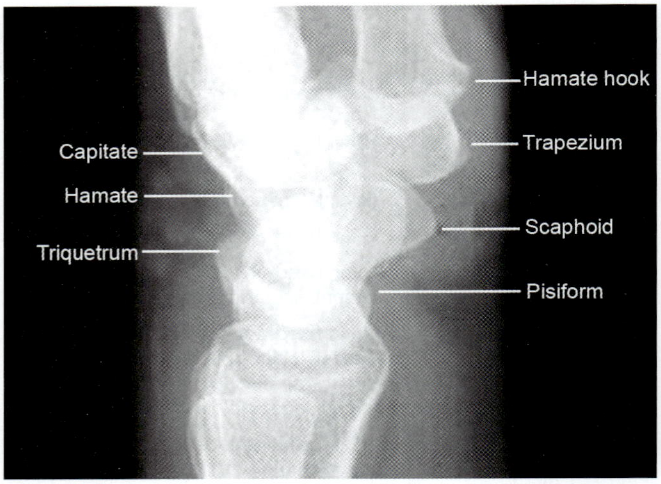

Fig. 21.267: Identification of carpal bones on X-rays lateral view

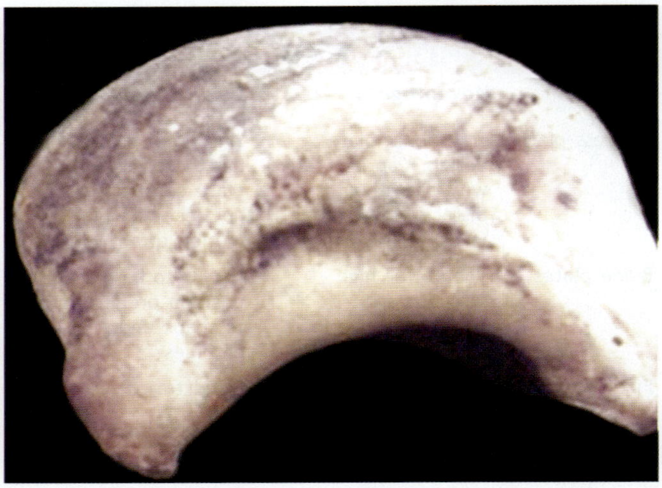

Fig. 21.269: Lunate is shaped like a crescent

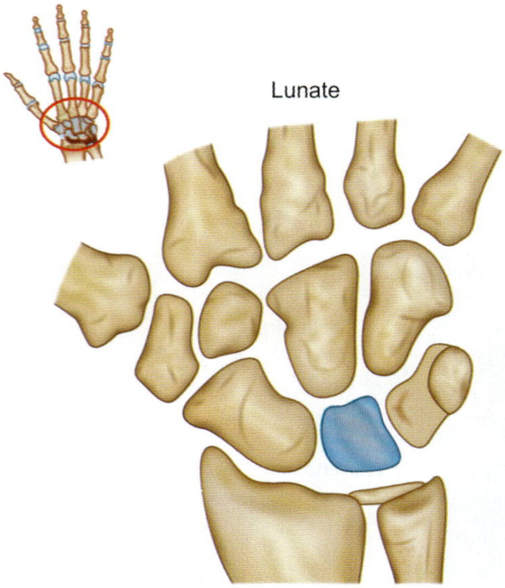

Fig. 21.268: Carpal bones of wrist with lunate (proximal row)

Table 21.20: Classification of different types of lunate fractures

Teisen classification	*Anteroposterior view*	*Lateral view*	*Type*
I			Volar pole
II			Chip fracture
III			Dorsal pole
IV			Sagittal
V			Transverse

Mechanism of Injury

The mechanism of injury is typically a fall onto an outstretched hand, with a hyperextended wrist or during a forceful push with an extended wrist.

Classification

Lunate fractures can be classified into five groups, this is illustrated in Table 21.20:

- Frontal fractures of the palmar pole, with involvement of the palmar nutrient arteries
- Osteochondral fractures of the proximal articular surface, without substantial damage to the nutrient vessels
- Frontal fractures of the dorsal pole
- Transverse fractures of the body
- Transarticular frontal fractures of the body of the lunate.

Presentation

- Patients often present with central dorsal wrist pain, loss of motion at the wrist and diminished grip strength
- Tenderness is demonstrated with direct palpation of the dorsal aspect of the lunate.

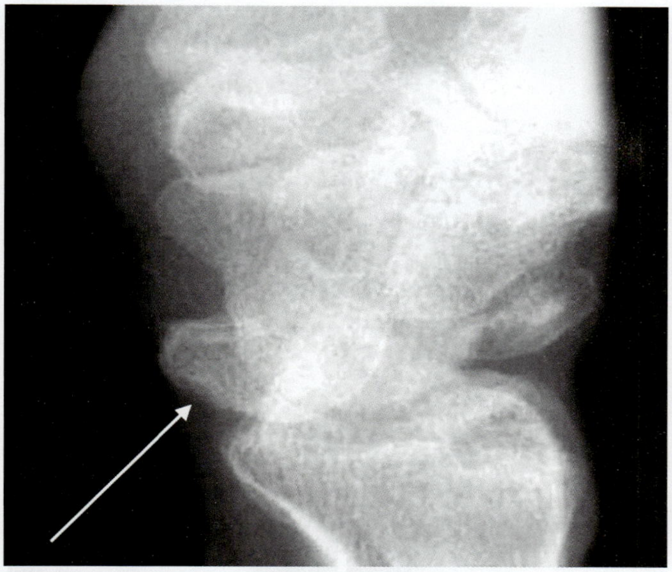

Fig. 21.270: Radiographs of the wrist, often inadequate to detect a lunate fracture (arrow), due to overlapping radiodensities

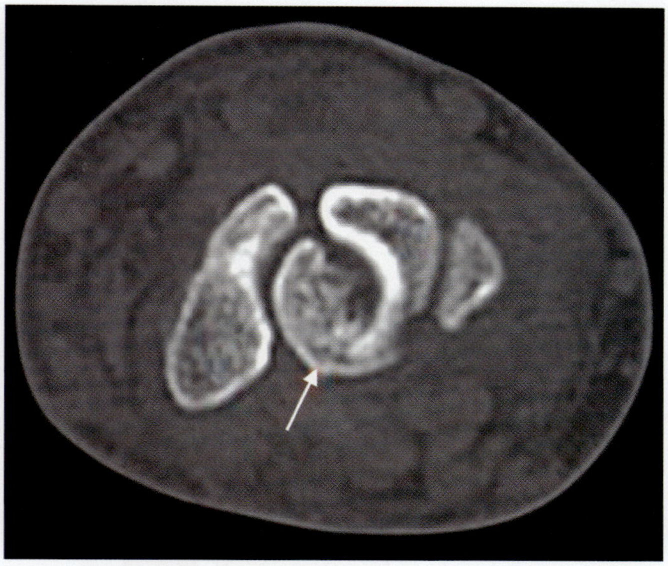

Fig. 21.271: MRI demonstrating healing, vascular injury and signs of osteonecrosis on the fracture site arrow showing a vascular necrosis of lunate

Diagnosis

- Standard PA and lateral radiographs of the wrist are often inadequate to detect a lunate fracture because of overlapping radiodensities (Fig. 21.270)
- Oblique views may be slightly more helpful, however, MRI, CT scans are often needed
- MRI is also helpful for evaluating healing, vascular injury and signs of osteonecrosis (Fig. 21.271).

Treatment

- Nondisplaced fractures can be treated with cast immobilization. Follow-up must proceed at close intervals to monitor healing and possible progression to Kienbock disease
- Displaced or angulated fractures require surgical apposition to allow healing of the vascular supply to the lunate.

Complications

Kienbock's Disease (Figs 21.272A and B)

- It is an osteonecrosis of the lunate and can lead to devastating advanced collapse and radiocarpal arthrosis.
- Surgical intervention may be necessary to relieve the severe pain.
- The options for surgical management of Kienbock' disease includes:
  - Radial wedge osteotomy
  - Radial shortening
  - Ulnar lengthening
  - Salvage procedures, such as arthrodesis or proximal row carpectomy.

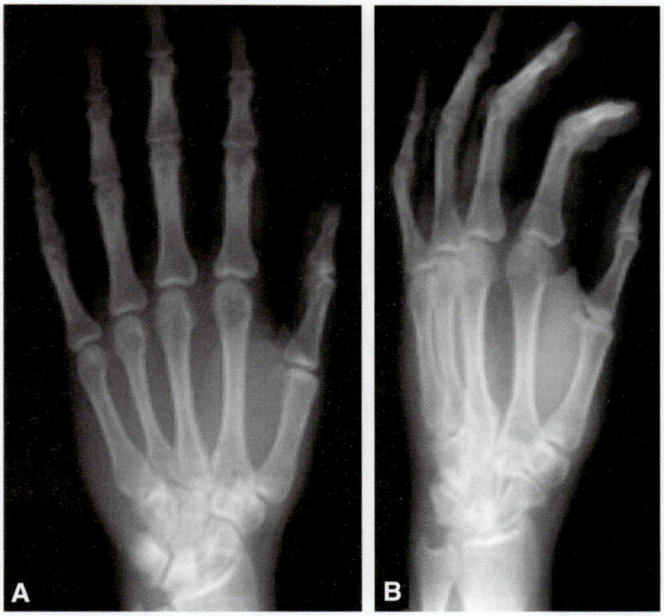

Figs 21.272A and B: Radiographs showing Kienbock's disease

■ Triquetral Fractures

Introduction

The triquetrum is reported as the second or third most common carpal fracture, representing 3 to 4 percent of all carpal bone injuries. It is the second most common carpal fracture in sports (Fig. 21.273).

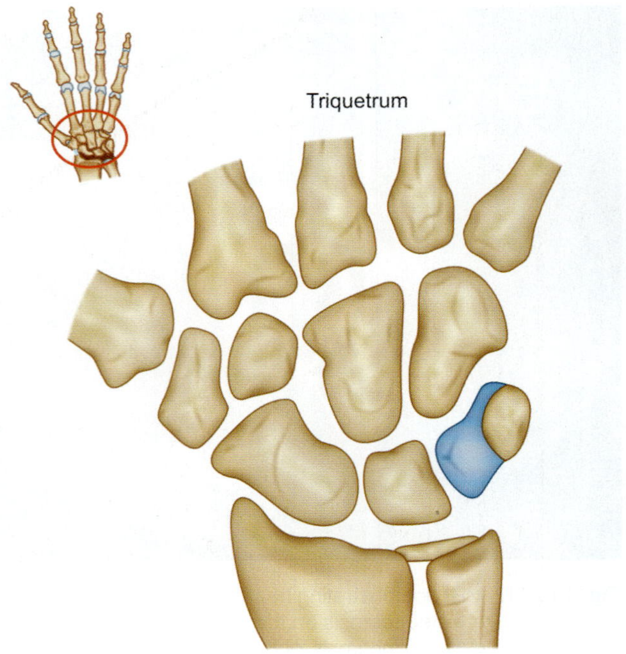

Fig. 21.273: Triquetrum bone

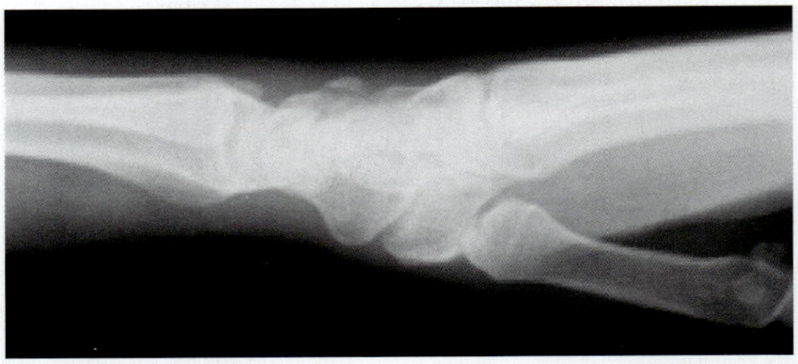

Fig. 21.274: Chip (dorsal cortical) fractures

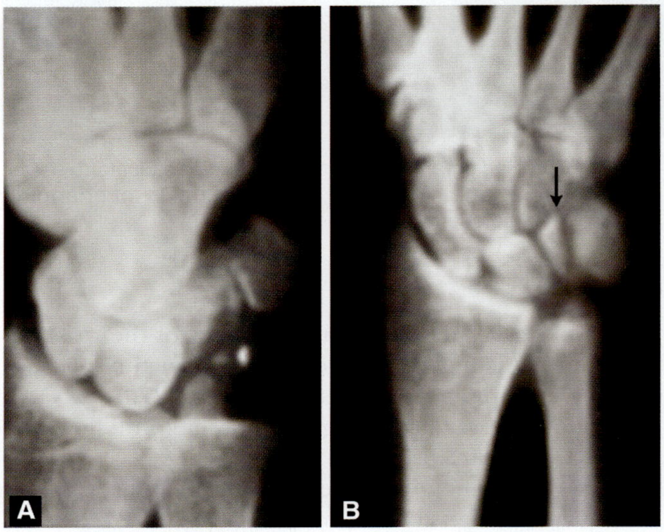

Figs 21.275A and B: Arrow shows midbody fracture

Anatomy

- The triquetrum is located just distal to the ulna and the triangular fibrocartilage complex and proximal to the base of the hamate
- The triquetrum articulates on its radial side with the lunate, to which it is attached by the lunotriquetral ligament. On the volar (palmar) aspect, there is an articulation with the pisiform.

Mechanism of Injury

- Triquetral fractures typically occur from a hyper-extension injury, with the wrist in ulnar deviation. However, injury can also occur with hyperflexion
- The dorsal surface of the triquetrum may be fractured by means of impingement from the ulnar styloid (chisel effect), shear forces or avulsion from strong ligamentous attachments.

Classification

Triquetral fractures can be divided into two types:

- *Chip (dorsal cortical) fractures:* A chip fracture typically occurs with a wrist hyperextension (dorsiflexion) and ulnar deviation injury (Fig. 21.274).
- *Midbody fracture:* This type of fracture is usually the result of a direct blow or may occur in conjunction with a perilunate dislocation (Figs 21.275A and B).

Presentation

- A history of injury and pain on the ulnar aspect of the wrist
- On examination, there will be pain and point tenderness, either dorsally or on the ulnar border of the wrist about 1–2 cm distal to the most distal aspect of the ulna or the ulnar styloid, respectively. The triquetrum is most easily palpated with the wrist in radial deviation.

Diagnosis

- Triquetral body fractures are best visualized on anteroposterior and oblique views (Fig. 21.276)
- Dorsal chip fractures are best detected on a pronated lateral projection that projects the dorsal triquetrum away from the adjacent carpal bones (Fig. 21.276)
- CT scan and or MRI confirms the diagnosis in suspicion cases.

Treatment

- Immobilization in a cast for a period of 4 to 6 weeks, usually leads to good long-term functional outcomes for isolated triquetrum fractures.

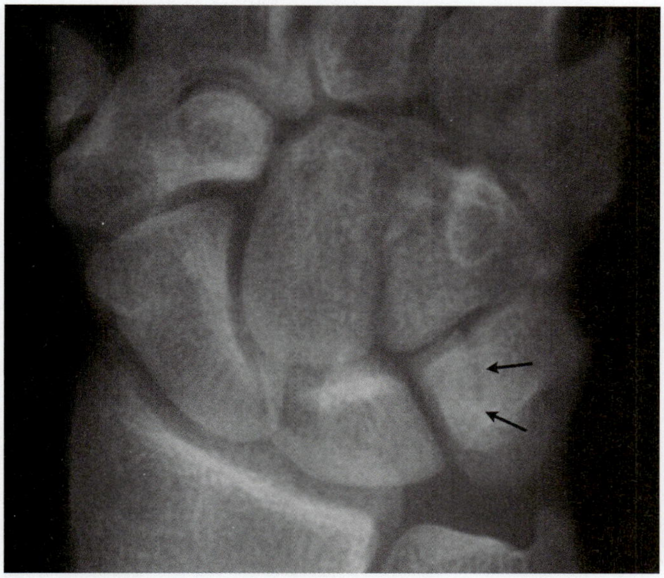

Fig. 21.276: X-ray AP view, arrows showing triquetral body fracture

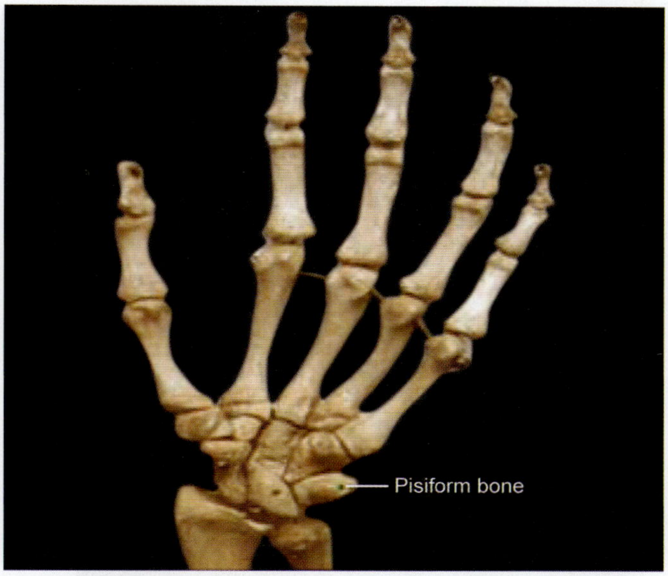

Fig. 21.277: Location of pisiform bone

- Fractures in association with perilunate dislocation or those with more than 1 mm of displacement, probably should be considered for surgical treatment to maximize long-term wrist function.
- A persistently symptomatic chip fracture may require excision.

Complications

- The deep branch of the ulnar nerve lies in close proximity to the triquetrum and may be compromized in triquetral fractures, with resultant motor impairment
- Pisotriquetral arthritis, secondary to a triquetral malunion can occur. Treatment can be by pisiform excision.

Pisiform Fractures

Introduction

The pisiform is a sesamoid bone in the flexor carpi ulnaris tendon (Fig. 21.277). It means "pea-shaped". This carpal bone is rare to fracture. Often pisiform fractures are associated with injuries of distal radius, hamate or triquetrum.

Anatomy

- With the exception of the pisotriquetral ligament and the articular surface with the triquetrum, the pisiform is entirely embedded in the tendon of the flexor carpi ulnaris
- It also serves as the proximal origin of the flexor digiti minimi. The vascular supply to the pisiform is via the ulnar artery with its circumferential foramina on the nonarticular surface.

Mechanism of Injury

The mechanism of injury is usually by a direct blow to the palm, when the wrist is dorsiflexed pulling the pisiform against the triquetrum.

Classification (Figs 21.278A to C)

Class A: Avulsion fracture
Class B: Transverse body fracture
Class C: Comminuted fracture.

Presentation

- Pain and swelling at the palmar and ulnar aspects of the wrist
- Tenderness on palpation of the pisiform and over the hypothenar eminence
- Presentation is often delayed, when in isolation and it can be overlooked, when the pisiform fractures are in association with other injuries.

Diagnosis

- Fractures may be missed on AP view. Special views are required to see the pisiform injuries
- A lateral view of the wrist with the forearm in 20 to 45° supination and carpal tunnel views are useful
- When in question, a CT may be required to make the diagnosis (Figs 21.279 and 21.280)

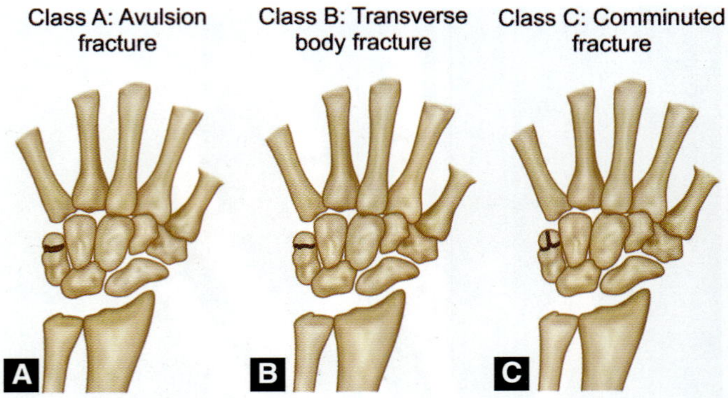

Figs 21.278A to C: Classification of different types of pisiform fractures

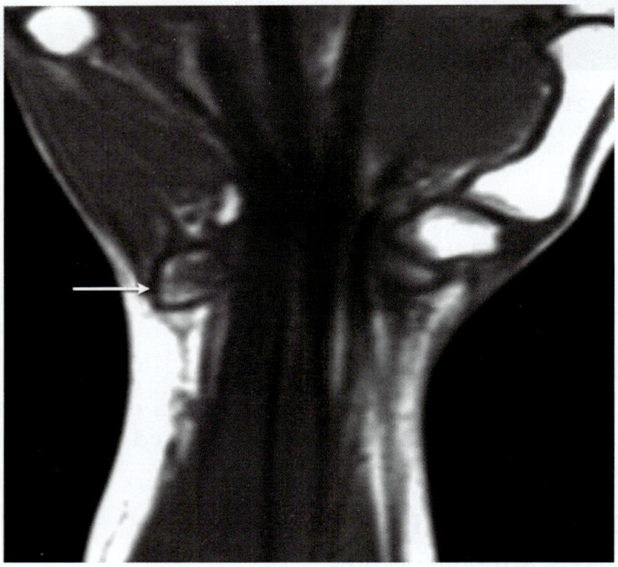

Fig. 21.279: CT scan used for making diagnosis, for detecting with arrow showing pisiform bone fracture

- If subluxation of the pisotriquetral joint is suspected, the diagnosis is made when one or more of the following are present: a joint space less than 4 mm in width, loss of parallelism of the joint surfaces greater than 2° proximal or distal over-riding of the pisiform, amounting to more than 15 percent of the width of the joint surfaces.

Treatment

- Generally, cast immobilization is warranted as a first line treatment. The cast should be in ulnar deviation with 30° of flexion
- If the fracture progresses to a symptomatic nonunion, the pisiform can be excised.

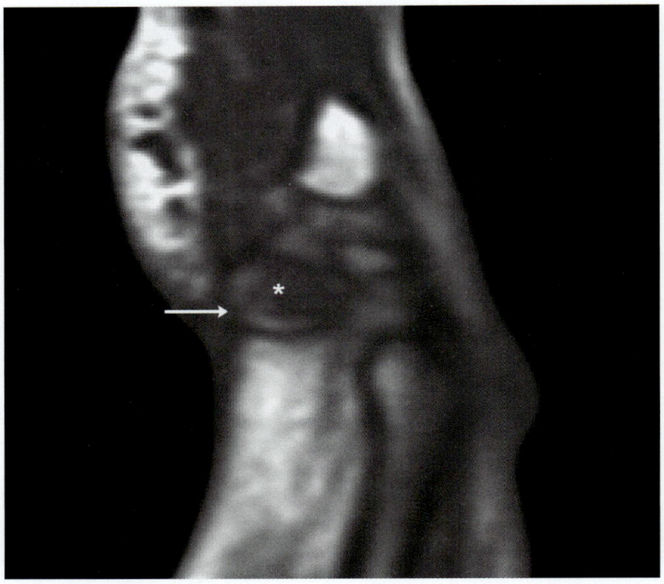

Fig. 21.280: CT Scan with star (*) showing pisiform and arrow indicates pisciform bone fractures

Complications

- *Nonunions:* In nonunions, bone should be excised. Loss of grip strength occurs after excision, but the difference between hands is not significant.
- *Pisotriquetral joint degeneration:* It can also be treated with pisiform excision.

Trapezium Fractures

Introduction

Fractures of the trapezium account for 1 to 5 percent of all carpal fractures.

Anatomy

- The trapezium is on the radial side of the distal carpal row (Fig. 21.281). It articulates distally with the thumb metacarpal and proximally with the scaphoid and the trapezoid
- It forms a double saddle articulation with the base of the thumb metacarpal, allowing motion in two planes, both flexion/extension and abduction/adduction
- The volar beak ligament from the metacarpal to the trapezium, is a key structure in maintaining joint stability and resisting dorsal radial subluxation during key pinch
- A longitudinal ridge is present on the volar surface, which serves as attachment for the transverse carpal ligament.

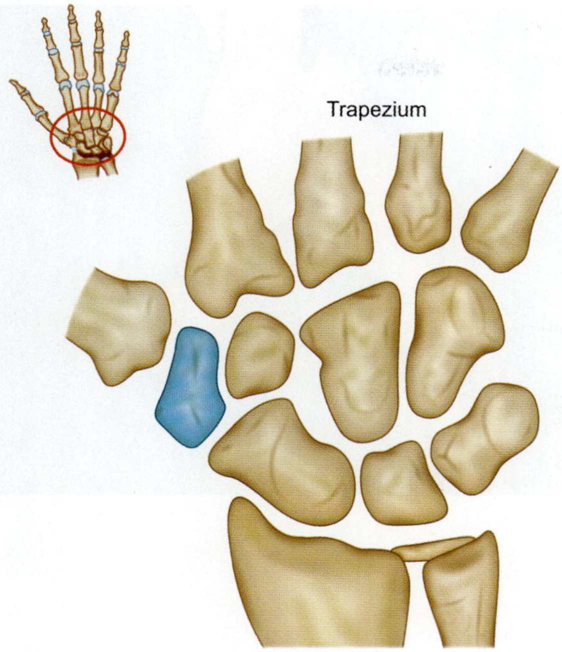

Fig. 21.281: Trapezium bone (on the radial side of the distal carpal row)

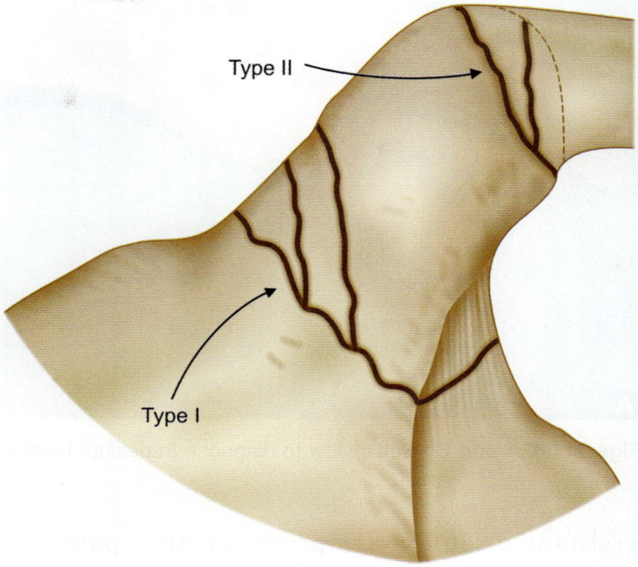

Fig. 21.282: Trapezial ridge fractures

Mechanism of Injury

- Axial loading of the first metacarpal in the adducted position, typically causes vertical fractures through the articular surface of the trapezium
- Avulsion fractures are caused by capsular and ligamentous attachments that are overloaded in forceful deviation, traction or rotation
- A direct injury from a blow to the thenar eminence or an avulsion of the transverse carpal ligament will cause a ridge fracture.

Classification

- *Trapezial ridge fractures* (Fig. 21.282)
  - Type I: Basal
  - Type II: Apical
- *Trapezial body fractures*
  - Vertical
  - Horizontal
- *Marginal trapeziometacarpal fractures*

Presentation

- Pain and weakness with pinching (making an ok sign or touching the thumb to the tip of the fifth digit)
- Pain with resisted wrist flexion from a dorsiflexed start position may indicate a fracture of the trapezial ridge.

Diagnosis

Special views are required to view the trapezium fractures. These are:

- *Bett's view*: It is obtained with the elbow raised from the cassette, the thumb extended and abducted, the hand somewhat pronated and the hypothenar eminence resting on the plate. The center beam is directed to the Scaphotrapeziotrapezoid (STT) joint. (Figs 21.283A and B)
- *A carpal tunnel view* is mandatory when a fracture of the trapezial ridge is suspected. When there is uncertainty, CT scanning can be diagnostic.

Treatment

- Undisplaced body and marginal trapeziometacarpal fractures can usually be treated with plaster immobilization in a thumb spica cast for 4 weeks, followed by intermittent protective splinting and gradual mobilization
- Displaced body fractures must be exposed surgically open reduction and internal fixation with screws or Kirshner wires
- Type I ridge fractures heal with immobilization, while type II fractures are much likely to heal with immobilization, symptomatic management is therefore advised.
- Fractures that remain symptomatic after a period of splinting are treated by surgical excision of the ununited fragment through a palmar approach.

Complications

Progressive degenerative changes of trapeziometacarpal joint is the consequence of intra-articular fractures. With

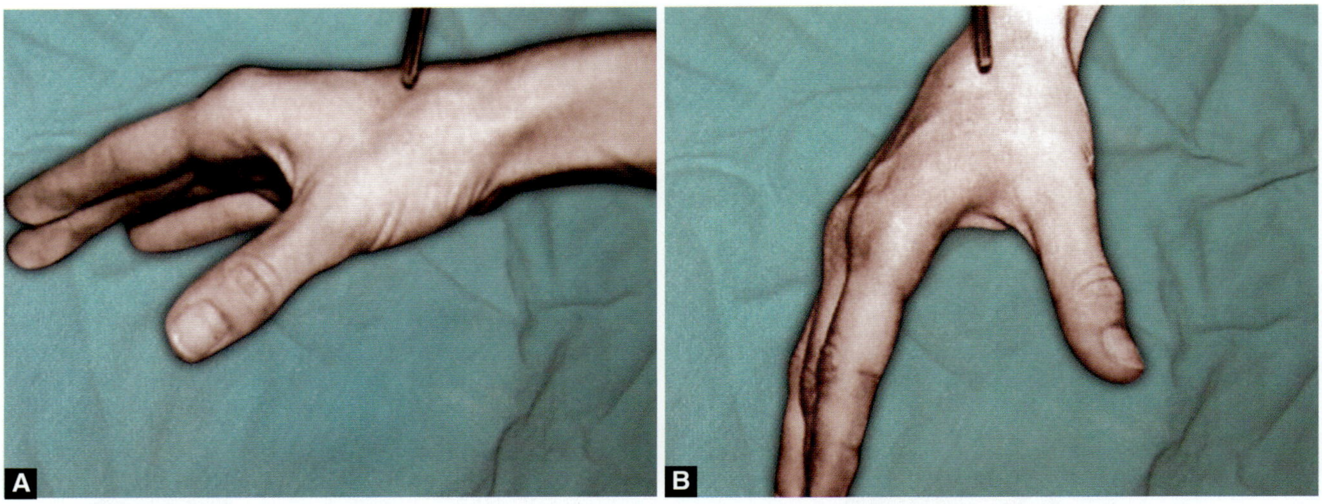

Figs 21.283A and B: Bett's view to diagnose trapezium fracture

persistant disabling symptoms (aching pain and weakness), trapeziometacarpal arthrodesis or excisional arthroplasty of the trapezium is carried out.

Trapezoid Fractures

Introduction

Trapezoid fractures are the least common carpal fractures of the wrist, involving less than 1 percent of all carpal fractures.

Anatomy

The wedge-shaped trapezoid is in the distal carpal row and articulates distally with the index-metacarpal base, radially with the trapezium, ulnarly with the capitate and proximally with the scaphoid (Fig. 21.284).

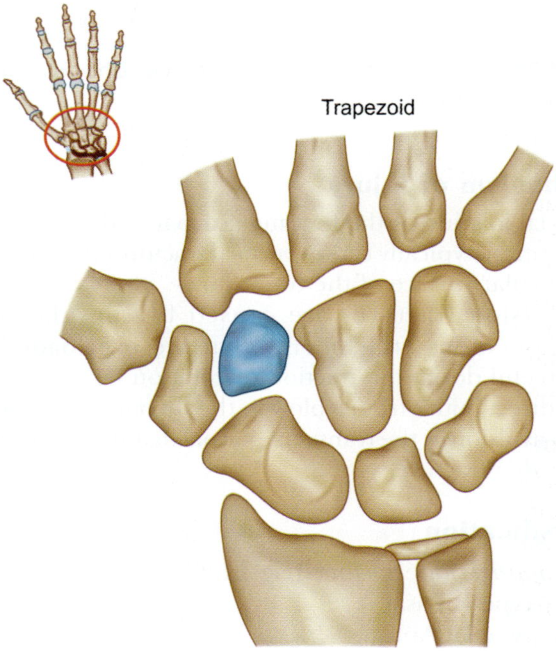

Fig. 21.284: A wedge shaped trapezoid bone (distal carpal row)

Mechanism of Injury

- Fractures of the trapezoid generally occur with axial loading of the second (index) metacarpal or may rarely occur secondary to direct dorsal trauma
- Wrist hyperflexion with dorsal loading of the index metacarpal and index finger hyperextension with wrist hyperextension, have been suggested as mechanisms and likened to the effect of a nutcracker
- More typically, with a dorsally applied force to the distal aspect of the index metacarpal, a dislocation will occur with the proximal aspect of the metacarpal slipping volar (palmar) to the trapezoid.

Classification

- Vertical fracture
- Osteoligamentary avulsion injury.

Presentation

- Patients will usually have some degree of swelling on the dorsum of the hand and point tenderness dorsally just proximal to the second metacarpal base
- Resisted wrist dorsiflexion may cause pain as the extensor carpi radialis inserts on the proximal aspect of the index metacarpal, which is closely fixed to the trapezoid by firm intercarpal ligamentous attachments.

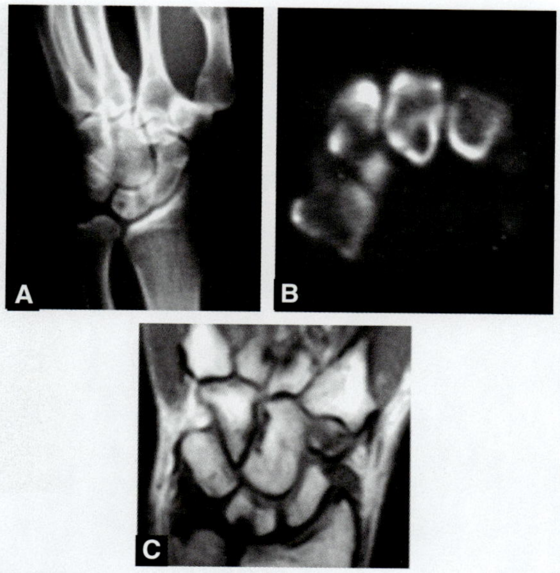

Figs 21.285A to C: (A) and (B) X-rays, showing trapezoid dislocation or fracture; (C) CT scan

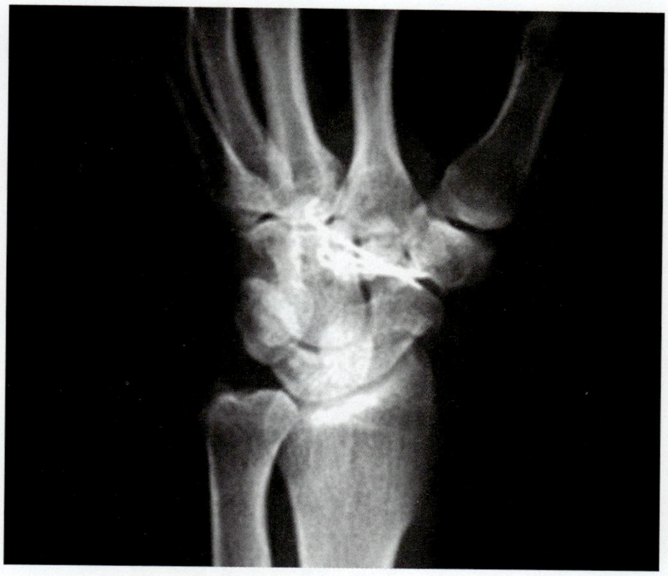

Fig. 21.286: Large fragment of displaced fracture of trapezoid bone

Diagnosis

- A trapezoid dislocation or fracture dislocation is seen on the anteroposterior X-ray, as a loss of the normal relationship between the second metacarpal base and the trapezoid (Figs 21.285A and B).
- The trapezoid may be superimposed over the trapezium or the capitate and the second metacarpal may be proximally displaced.
- Diagnosis and analysis are best achieved with the CT scans (Fig. 21.285C).

Treatment

- *Undisplaced fracture:* Cast immobilization
- *Displaced fracture:*
  - *Small fragment:* Closed reduction and casting
  - *Large fragment:* Open reduction and internal fixation (Fig. 21.286)
- *In chronic injuries:* Open reduction, bone grafting and carpometacarpal arthrodesis.

Complications

- Malunion
- Delayed union
- Nonunion.

■ Capitate Fractures

Introduction

The capitate is the largest carpal bone. Injuries to the capitate are often part of complex injuries. Capitate fractures are sometimes seen along with scaphoid waist fractures or distal radius fractures.

Anatomy

The capitate articulates distally with the bases of the third and fourth metacarpals and proximally with the scaphoid and lunate. The trapezoid and the hamate are lateral (radial) and medial, respectively (Fig. 21.287).

Classification

- Capitate fractures are classified by the anatomic location of the fracture, along with what other concomitant injuries may be present.
- The combination of a capitate fracture and a scaphoid waist fracture is known as scaphocapitate syndrome. The force of injury in this syndrome can propagate leading to perilunate dislocation as well.

Mechanism of Injury

- Direct blow or crushing injuries. These are usually associated with injuries to the metacarpals and other carpal bones.
- A fall with the wrist in dorsiflexion, forcing the capitates onto the dorsal rim of the radius. The dorsal border of the radius will impinge on the capitates and cause a fracture through its waist.
- Scaphocapitate syndrome

Note: Refer to scaphocapitate fracture syndrome on page No. 335.

Presentation

Patients typically present with wrist pain after an acute injury and a careful examination can pinpoint the area to the capitate.

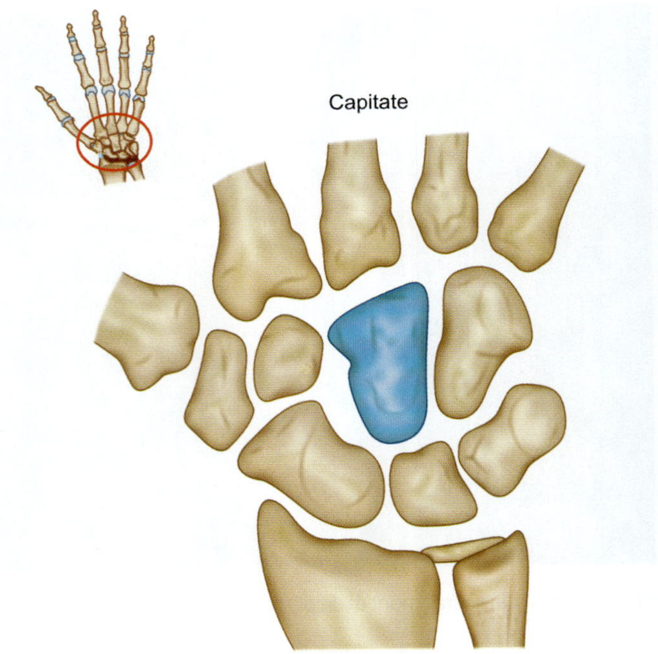

Fig. 21.287: Capitate bone

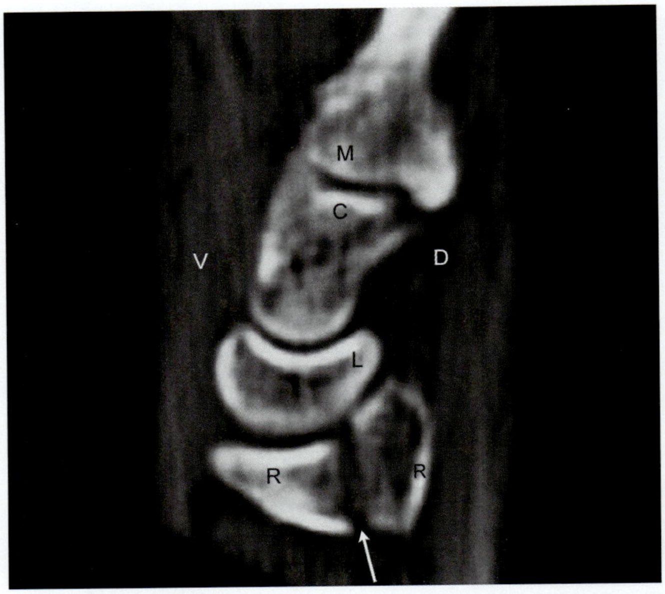

Fig. 21.288: Standard scaphoid views, lateral views to look for rotation or displacement—M. Metacarpal; C. Carpal; L. Lunate; R. Radius; V. Volar; D. Dorsal and arrow shows radius fracture

Diagnosis

- Standard scaphoid views, lateral views to look for rotation or displacement (Fig. 21.288).
- CT scan and MRI aid in accurate diagnosis.

Treatment

- *Nondisplaced capitate fractures:* They need to be immobilized in a short arm thumb spica with the wrist in slight dorsiflexion and the thumb immobilized to the IP joint for 8 weeks.
- *Displaced capitate fractures:* Closed reduction followed by immobilization should be attempted first. If unsuccessful, surgical fixation with a K-wire or a screw, with bone graft, added for significant comminution.

Scaphocapitate Syndrome

- If diagnosed within 3 to 4 weeks of injury, open reduction is carried out through a dorsal approach with internal fixation for one or both fractures, depending on stability. Cast immobilization is continued until both fractures have healed.
- For fractures diagnosed late, treatment becomes a matter of judgement. If the scaphoid has healed or is healing in a satisfactory position, watchful waiting may be appropriate in as much as some patients will remain symptom free or have tolerable symptoms for many years, despite of capitate head displacement. Patients seen late with significant symptoms and malalignment of both the scaphoid and capitate are probably best treated by a salvage procedure, such as midcarpal-arthrodesis.

Complications

- Malunion or avascular necrosis
- Post-traumatic arthritis
- Fibrosis after the injury may result in a median nerve neuropathy or a carpal tunnel syndrome.

Hamate Fractures

Introduction

The hamate is the most ulnar carpal bone on the distal row (Fig. 21.289). Hamate fractures account for 2 to 4 percent of the carpal fractures. Hamate fractures mainly occur in two locations, the hook of the hamate or the body.

Anatomy

- The body of the hamate articulates distally with the bases of the fourth and fifth metacarpals, radially with the capitate and proximally with the triquetrum and lunate
- The hook of the hamate (hamulus) is the distal border of Guyon's canal, which contains the ulnar artery and nerve. With injury of the hamate one should always assure vascular patency and that sensation is intact in the fifth digit and the ulnar border of the fourth
- The hook of the hamate develops from an ossification center separate from the body of the hamate. In some adults, it persists as the os hamulus proprius. This normal variant can present a potential diagnostic pitfall, if misinterpreted as a hamate fracture or nonunion

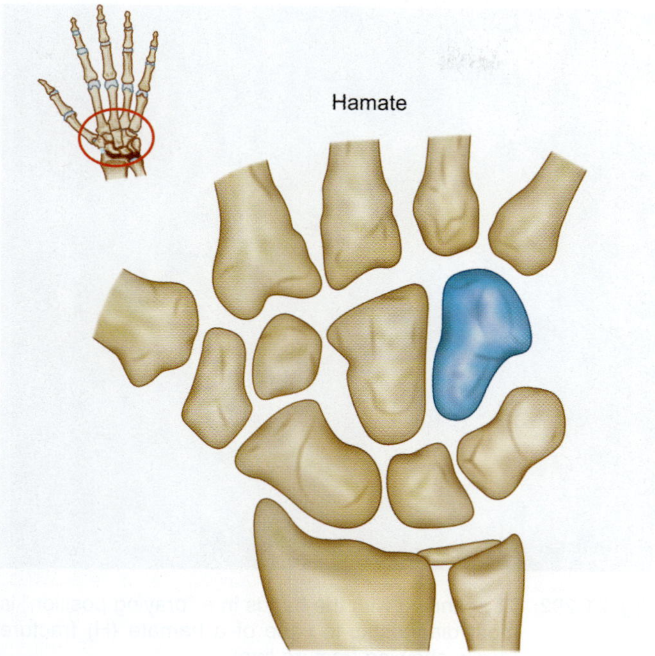

Fig. 21.289: Hamate bone (distal carpal row on ulnar side)

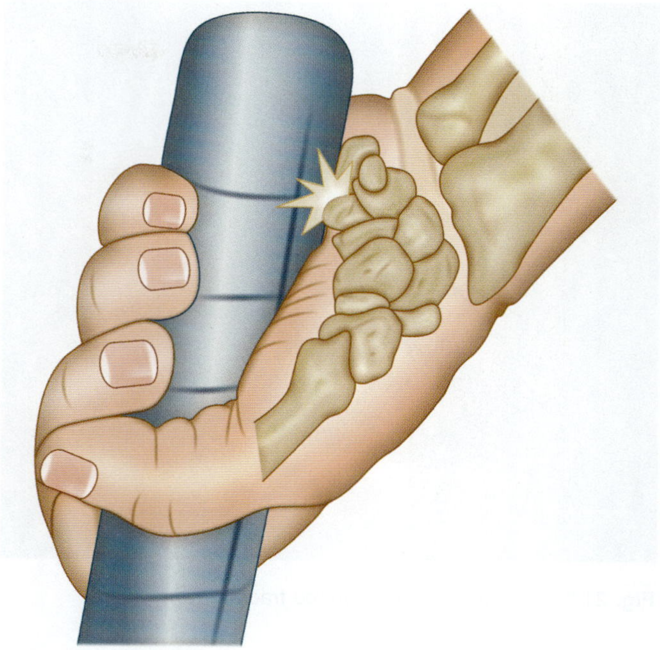

Fig. 21.290: In sports, fracture of the hook of the hamate results, when a club, racquet or bat is forced into the palm, exerting direct pressure on the hypothenar eminence and thus the hamulus

- Attachments to the hamate include the transverse carpal ligament and flexor carpi ulnaris
- The blood supply to the hamate is variable with 70 percent having only vascular supply to the body, predisposing hook fractures to nonunion.

Mechanism of Injury

- Fractures of the hook of the hamate are more common.
- Fall on the outstretched hand that puts the transverse carpal ligament in tension and causes avulsion of the hook from the body
- In sports, fracture of the hook of the hamate results, when a club, racquet or bat is forced into the palm, exerting direct pressure on the hypothenar eminence and thus the hamulus. This typically occurs on the nondominant hand (Fig. 21.290)
- Fractures of the hamate body are less common and can be associated with fifth or sometimes fourth metacarpal fractures.

Classification

Fracture of hamate body

- *Vertical fracture:* These can be on either the ulnar or radial side of the hamulus.
- *Horizontal fracture:* Fracture of the hook (hamulus) of the hamate.

Presentation

- Ulnar sided wrist pain and point tenderness over the hook of the hamate.
- In acute injuries, pain is present with palpation in hypothenar area.
- Pain also may be present with resisted flexion of the fourth and fifth fingers.

Diagnosis

- Standard radiographs of the wrist (AP and lateral) may be insufficient to make the diagnosis and a carpal tunnel or 45° supination oblique view may be required (Fig. 21.291)
- A special view (Papilion et al.), involving a lateral radiograph with the thumb maximally opposed (to move it out of the way) and the wrist in ulnar deviation, hand slightly supinated to bring the hook into greatest profile
- CT scanning with the hands in a praying position is the most sensitive diagnostic study. When in doubt of hook fractures versus os hamulus proprius, an MRI may distinguish the acuity of the injury (Fig. 21.292).

Treatment

- Acute injuries can be treated closed with cast immobilization

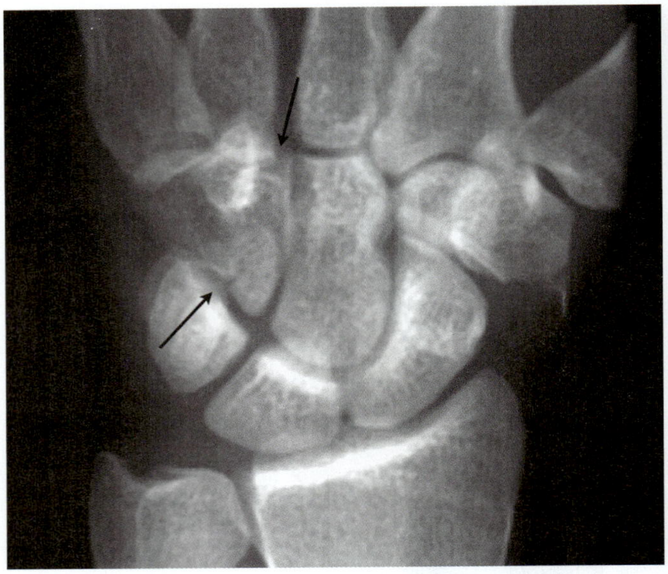

Fig. 21.291: X-ray showing hamate fracture (arrows)

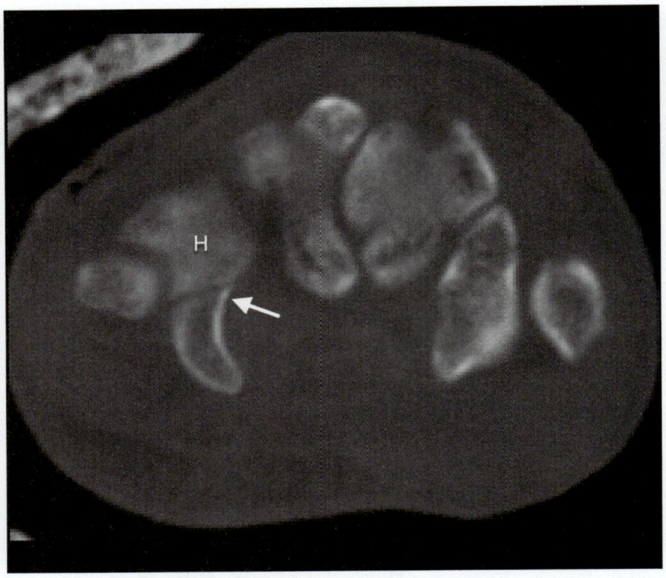

Fig. 21.292: CT scanning with the hands in a "praying position" is most diagnostic, in case of a hamate (H) fracture (arrow showing fracture line)

- Hook of the hamate nonunions can be excised with small fragments or fixed with bone graft and screws, when fragments are large enough
- Displaced hamate body fractures may either be precutaneously pinned or fixed with an open reduction.

Complications

- Nonunion may occur with vascular disruption
- Ulnar neuropathy may have profound affects
- Flexor tendon rupture over the bony prominence is not an uncommon complication.

SCAPHOID FRACTURES

■ Anatomy

It is irregularly shaped tubular bone, twisted and bent into "S" shaped. More than 80 percent of its surface is being covered by articular cartilage, which reduces its capacity for periosteal healing and increases chances of nonunion.

It articulates with the distal radius and four of the carpal bones. Scaphoid moves with nearly all carpal motions. Thus, any change in its articular surface will cause severe secondary changes in the carpus.

Blood Supply of Scaphoid

Blood supply of scaphoid bone is shown in Figures 21.293A and B.

Signs and Symptoms of Scaphoid Fractures

Symptoms

- Pain in wrist due to fall on outstretched hand
- Usually associated with hyperextension injury and slight radial deviation of the wrist.

Signs

- Tenderness of anatomical snuffbox and scaphoid tubercle
- Pain with axial compression of thumb
- ROM is reduced and painful at extremes of motion
- Loss of wrist extension suggests nonunited scaphoid fractures, associated with carpal collapse deformity and palmar capsular contracture.

Diagnosis

X-rays

Various views of scaphoid, in which X-rays can be taken are enumerated below and also shown in Figures 21.294 to 21.297:

- Posteroanterior ulnar deviation
- Radial oblique ulnar deviation
- True lateral
- Posterior oblique
- Motion views of scaphoid in flexion extension, along with radial and ulnar deviation will demonstrates fracture displacement.

Reasons of misdiagnosis of scaphoid fracture on X-ray

- A dark line formed by dorsal lip of radius overlapping the scaphoid

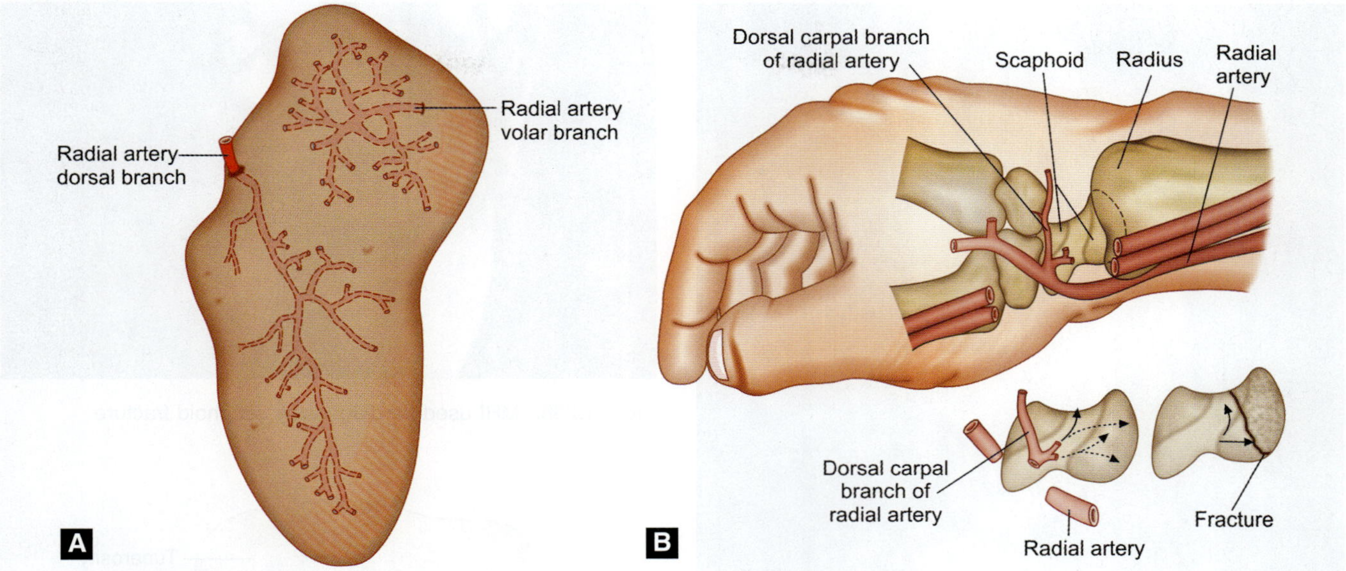

Figs 21.293A and B: Blood supply of scaphoid

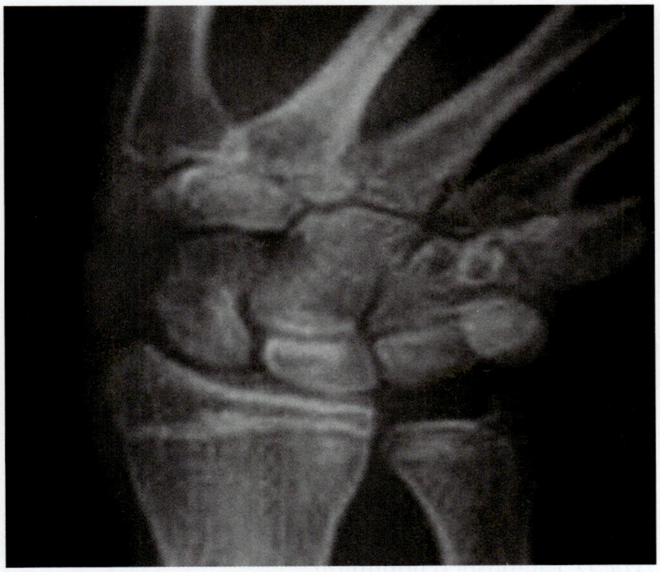

Fig. 21.294: Normal posteroanterior radiograph of scaphoid (right)

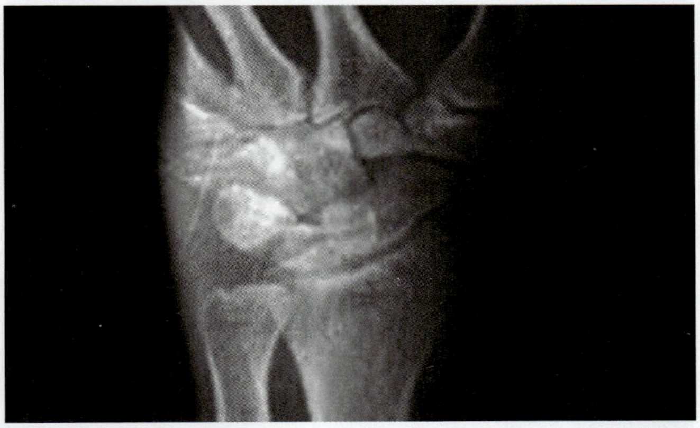

Fig. 21.295: Normal anterior oblique radiograph of scaphoid (left)

- Presence of white line formed by proximal end of scaphoid tuberosity
- Dorsal ridge may appear bent in semisupinated view.

MRI

It is gold standard for diagnosing carpal and wrist injury at an early stage. It is the most effective way of diagnosing scaphoid fractures (Fig. 21.298).

Classification

Classification of Scaphoid Fractures by Anatomic Location (Fig. 21.299)

- Proximal pole fracture
- Waist fracture
- Distal body fracture
- Tuberosity fracture

Cooney, Dobyns and Linscheild Classification of Scaphoid Fracture (Fig. 21.300)

- Undisplaced and stable
- Displaced and unstable

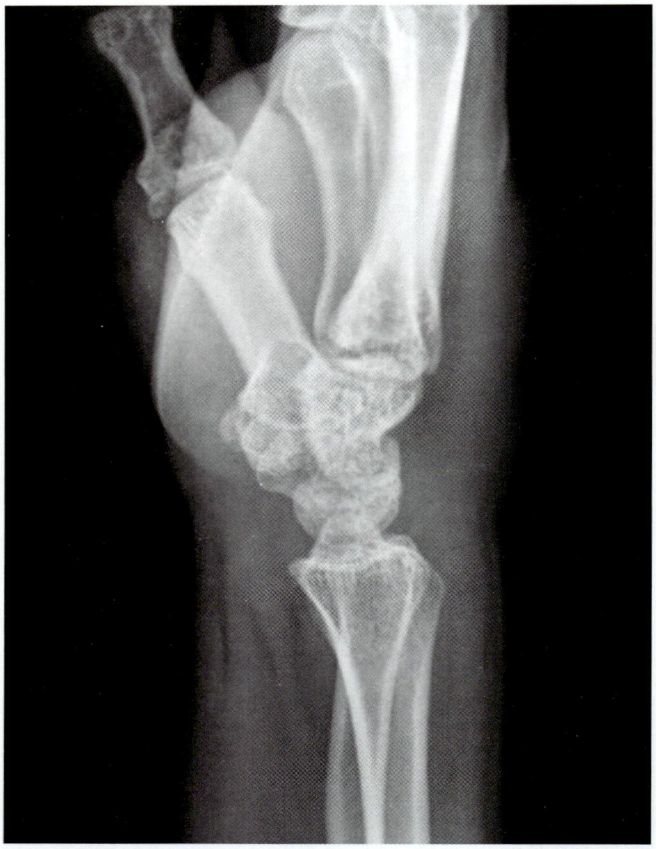

Fig. 21.296: Normal lateral radiograph of wrist

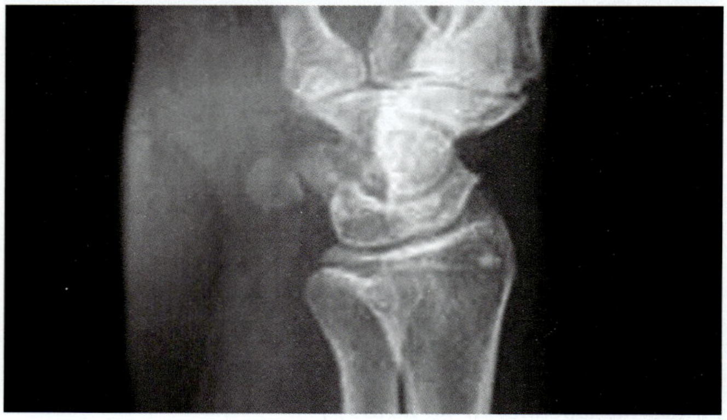

Fig. 21.297: Normal posterior oblique radiograph of wrist

Herbert and Fisher's Classification (Fig. 21.301)

Type A: Stable acute fractures

- A1: Fracture of tuberosity
- A2: Incomplete fracture through waist

Type B: Unstable acute fractures

- B1: Distal oblique fractures
- B2: Complete fracture of waist
- B3: Proximal pole fracture

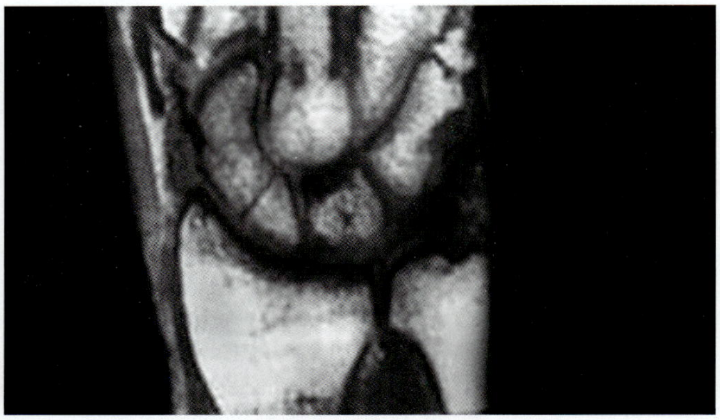

Fig. 21.298: MRI used for diagnosing scaphoid fracture

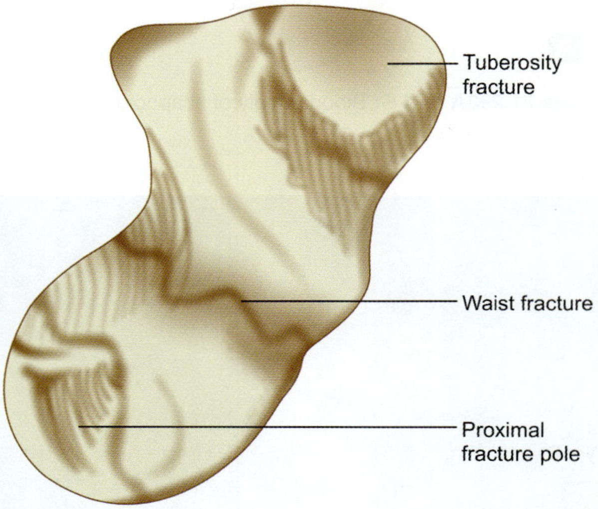

Fig. 21.299: Classification of scaphoid fractures by anatomic location

- B4: Trans-scaphoid perilunate fracture dislocation
- B5: Comminuted fractures

Type C: Delayed union

Type D: Established nonunion

- D1: Fibrous nonunion
- D2: Pseudoarthrosis

Treatment

- Nondisplaced stable fractures
- Displaced stable fractures

Treatment for Nondisplaced Stable Scaphoid Fractures

Nonoperative treatment

It is usually recommended. Prognosis is better, if fracture is diagnosed early.

Early diagnosis

- *Forearm cast or munster type cast (Fig. 21.302):* It is given from just below the elbow proximally to the base of

Scaphoid nonunion associated with the location of fracture and amount of displacement

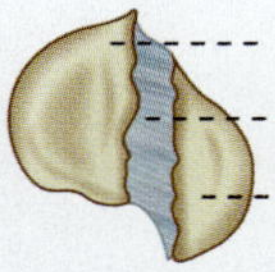

Location	Number of fracture	Percentage of union
Distal third	2	100
Middle third	56	80
Proximal third	32	64

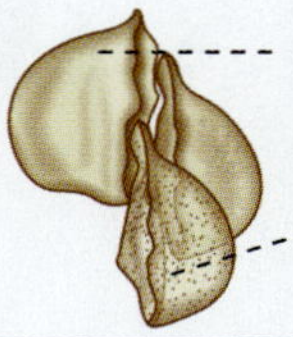

Displacement	Number of fracture	Percentage of union
Stable	48	85
Unstable	42	65

Fig. 21.300: Cooney, Dobyns and Linscheild classification of scaphoid fractures

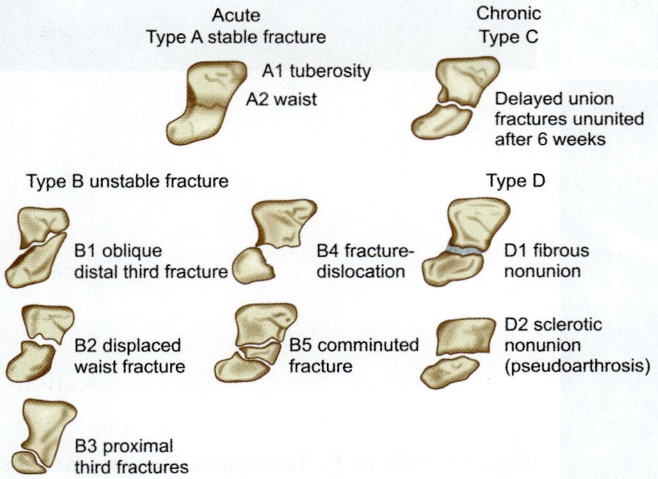

Fig. 21.301: Herbert and Fisher's classification of scaphoid fracture

thumbnail and proximal palmar crease distally. Wrist in slight radial deviation and in neutral flexion. Thumb is maintained in functional position

- *Colle's cast:* It may be given for stable nondisplaced fractures
- *Above elbow cast:* Earlier above elbow cast was also given for fracture of scaphoid. The cast is kept for 10–12 weeks. During this time, fracture is observed radiologically for healing. In case of query fracture, cast is applied and X-ray is taken after 2 weeks.

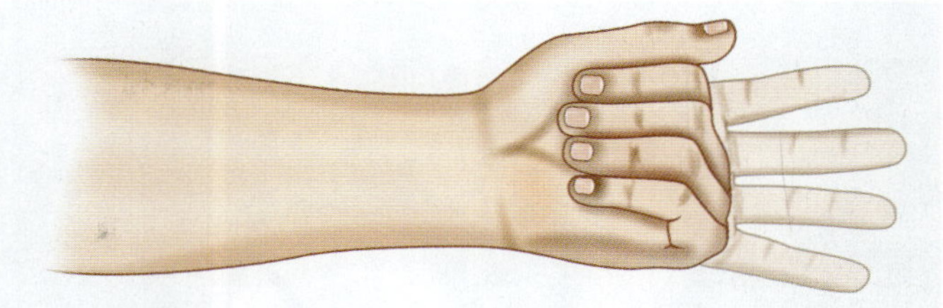

Fig. 21.302: Forearm cast or munster type cast

Delayed diagnosis

- *Middle third stable fracture:* It is diagnosed after 1 to 6 months of injury. It is treated with cast immobilization. It usually takes 19 weeks to unite as compared to average of 10 weeks for acute fractures.
- *Proximal third fracture:* Its prognosis is less favorable, but initial long arm thumb spica cast may be justified for 6 weeks.

Operative (Nondisplaced Stable)

Indications

- Diagnosis is delayed
- Fracture is in proximal third
- Collapse or angulation of the fracture fragment, if found during regular radiological evaluation.
- Due to joint stiffness, muscle atrophy and inability to use the hand during and after prolonged immobilization, operative treatment may be considered in some patients, e.g. young laborers or athletes.

Operative technique: Percutaneous fixation technique for nondisplaced stable scaphoid fracture. This technique is illustrated in Figures 21.303A to F.

Treatment for Displaced Stable Scaphoid Fractures

Criteria for fracture to be displaced unstable (Figs 21.304A to C)

- Displacement greater than 1 mm in AP or oblique view
- Lunocapitate angulation greater than 15°
- Scapholunate angulation greater than 45° in lateral view
- Lateral intrascaphoid angle greater than 45°
- AP intrascaphoid angle less than 35°

It is usually treated operatively or and if done with Herbert differential pitch bone screw/AO screw/Acutrak screw, percutaneous fixation of the fracture can also be done.

Advantages of Surgery

- Reduces the time of external fixation
- Provides relatively strong internal fixation
- Produces compression at fracture site
- These screws can be used with bone graft to correct scaphoid angulation.

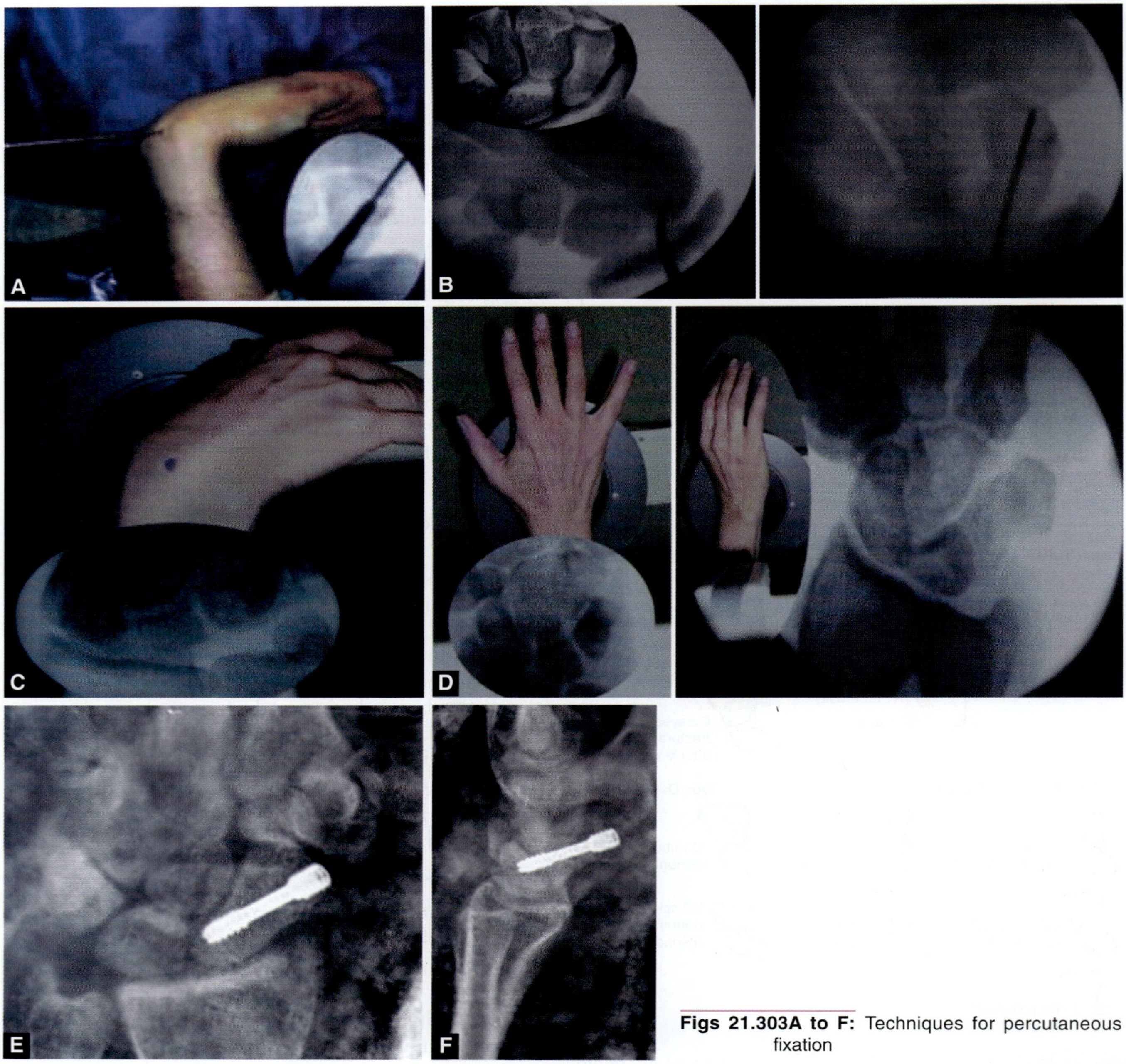

Figs 21.303A to F: Techniques for percutaneous fixation

Exposure of Scaphoid

- *Volar approach (Figs 21.305A to D):* Used for scaphoid fracture at or distal to the waist.
- *Dorsal approach (Fig. 21.306):* Used for proximal pole noncomminuted fractures. Extend skin incision from radial styloid to ulnar styloid. Make parallel incisions on external retinaculum on each side of external digitorum tendon. Open the dorsal capsule by radially creating base flap and expose fracture.
- *Dorsolateral approach (Figs 21.307A to C)*

■ Scaphoid Nonunion

Nonunion is influenced by:

- Delayed diagnosis
- Gross displacement
- Associated injuries of carpus
- Impaired blood supply

Radiographic Findings

- Arthritis
- Radioscaphoid narrowing

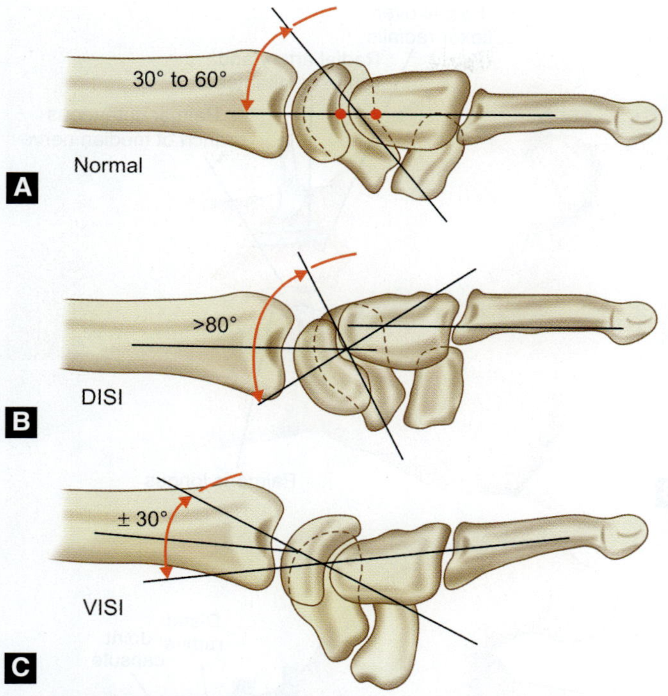

Figs 21.304A to C: Criteria for fracture to be displaced unstable

- Capitolunate narrowing
- Cyst formation
- Pronounced dorsal intercalated segment instability is also called scaphoid nonunion advanced collapse pattern.

Differentiation Between Acute Fracture and Nonunion

- Acute fracture is represented by a single line through bone, occasionally with dorsoradial comminution and dorsal angulation.
- Nonunion will show resorption at the fracture site, subchondral sclerosis and displacement on both PA and lateral X-rays.

Stages of Scaphoid Nonunion

Different stages of scaphoid nonunion are shown in Figure 21.308.

Treatment

Algorithm for treatment of scaphoid nonunion (Flow chart 21.4)

Following operations can be useful for scaphoid nonunion:

- Radial styloidectomy
- Excision of proximal fragment, distal fragment or entire scaphoid
- Proximal row carpectomy
- Bone grafting
- Vascularized bone grafting
- Partial and total wrist arthrodesis.

Radial Styloidectomy

Image of wrist joint following radial styloidectomy is shown in Figure 21.309.

Indications

- Arthritic changes in scaphoid fossa. It is indicated with any grafting of scaphoid or excision of its ulnar fragment.
- Older patients with radioscaphoid arthritis and when the proximal fragment not loosen.

Procedure

- Resect enough of the styloid to remove the entire articulation with the scaphoid.
- Preserve palmar radiocarpal ligaments to avoid ulnar translocation of the carpus.

Excision of Proximal Fragment

Indications

- The fragment is one-fourth or less of the scaphoid.
- Above indication and fragment is sclerotic, comminuted or severly displaced
- The fragment is one-fourth or less of the scaphoid and grafting has failed
- Arthritic changes are present in the region of radial styloid.

Excision of the Distal Scaphoid

Indicated in scaphoid nonunions with radioscaphoid arthritis.

Proximal Row Carpectomy

It is reconstructive procedure for post-traumatic degenerative conditions in the wrist, involving the scaphoid and lunate.

Indications

- In patients who have limited requirements for wrist mobility and accept mild persistent pain
- Useful in treating severe open carpal fracture dislocation with significant comminuted fractures of scaphoid and lunate (Figs 21.310A and B).

Procedure

- Excision of the triquetrum, lunate and entire scaphoid is done
- If the distal scaphoid pole is left, radial styloidectomy should be done to avoid impingement of the distal scaphoid pole and trapezium on the radial styloid.

Contraindications

- Severe arthrosis at capitolunate joint

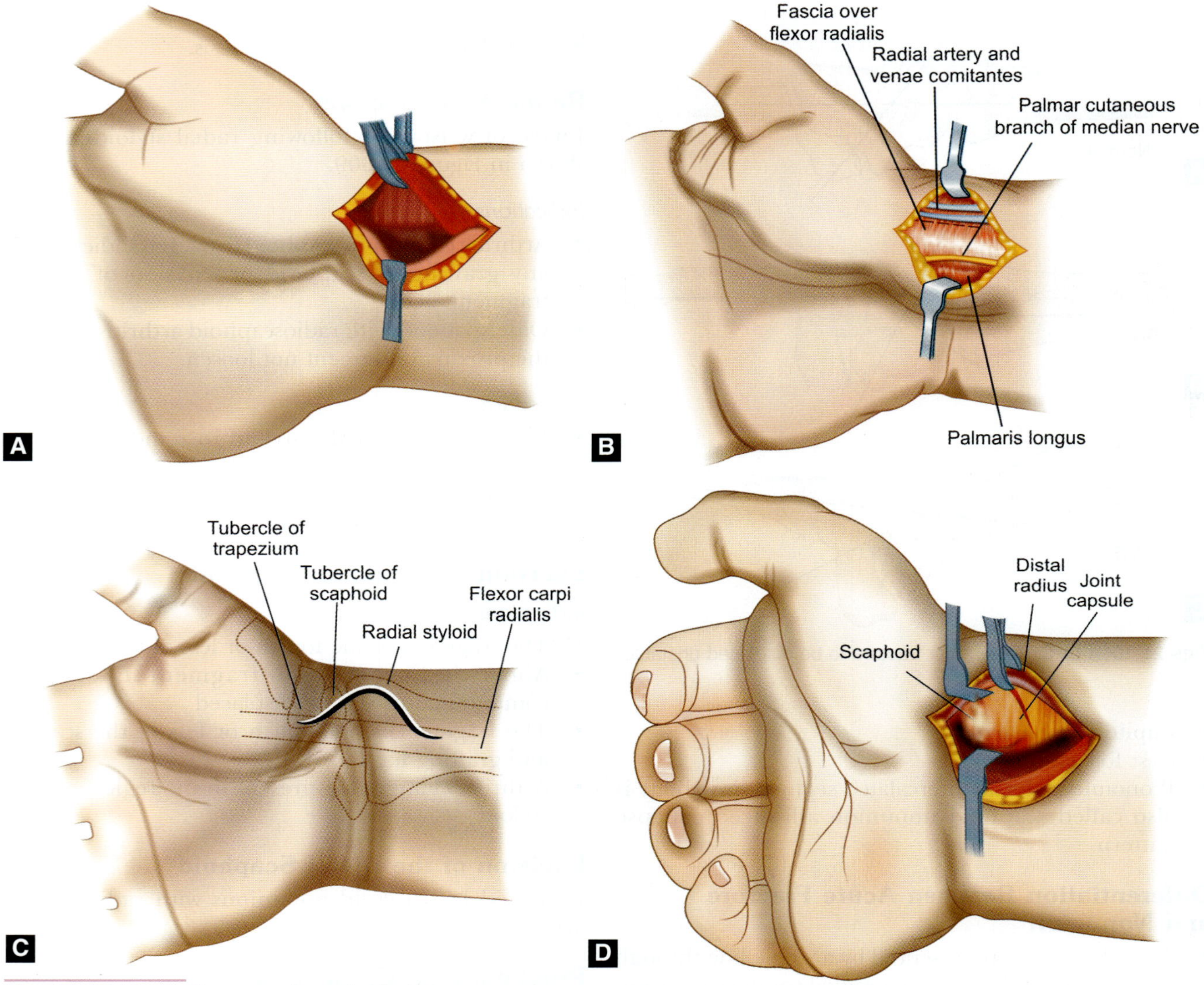

Figs 21.305A to D: Exposure of scaphoid—Volar approach

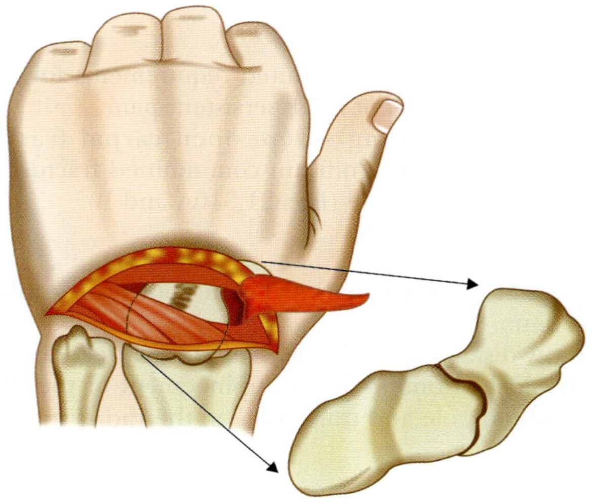

Fig. 21.306: Dorsal approach to expose scaphoid bone

- If mild arthrosis than carpectomy is done with excising proximal pole of capitate and cover that with dorsal capsular flap.

Grafting Operations

- Cancellous bone grafting for scaphoid nonunion that do not have shortening or angulation (Fig. 21.311)
- It was first describe by Matti and modified by Russe.
- It is done with or without fixation of scaphoid with screw.

Malpositioned Nonunion of Scaphoid Fractures

- Nonunions of scaphoid fractures on X-ray have resorption or comminution, with resulting shortening and angulation, with dorsal and radial convexity (humpback deformity)
- CT scan in the sagittal and coronal planes shows this deformity (Figs 21.312A to F).

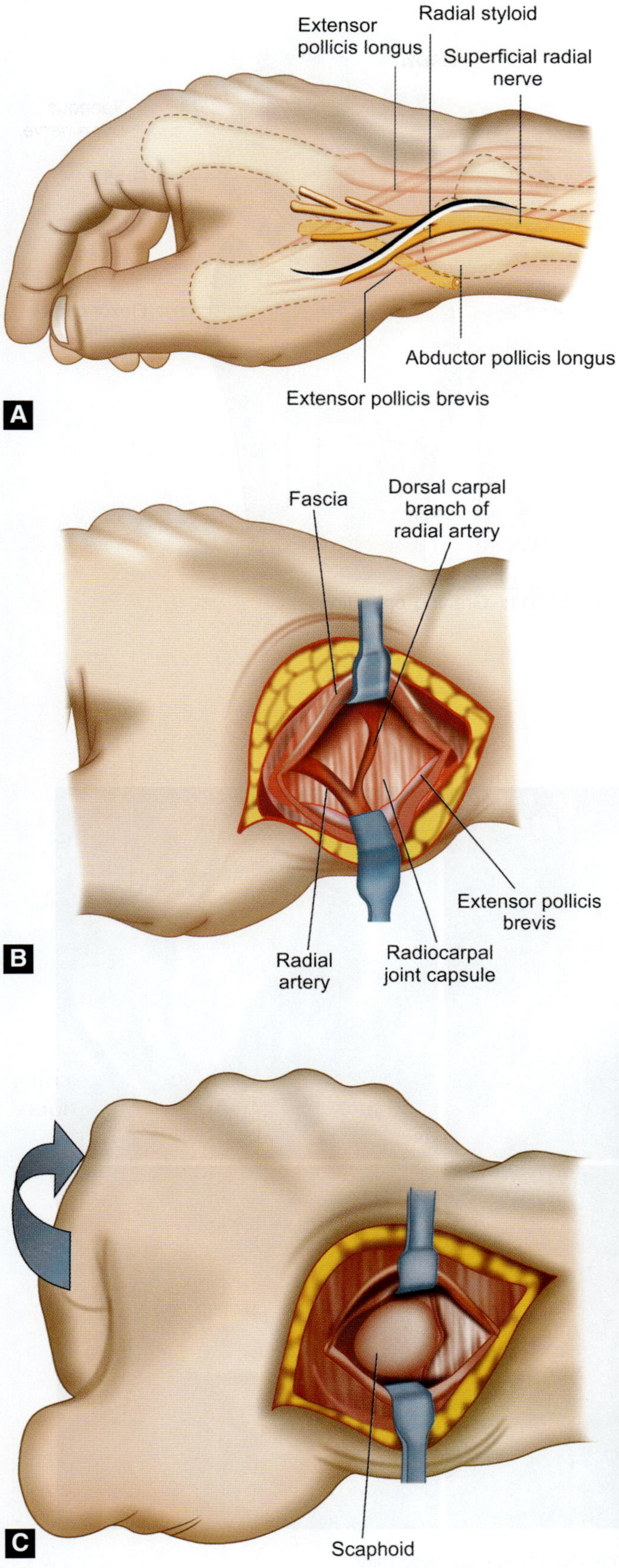

Figs 21.307A to C: Dorsolateral approach to expose scaphoid bone

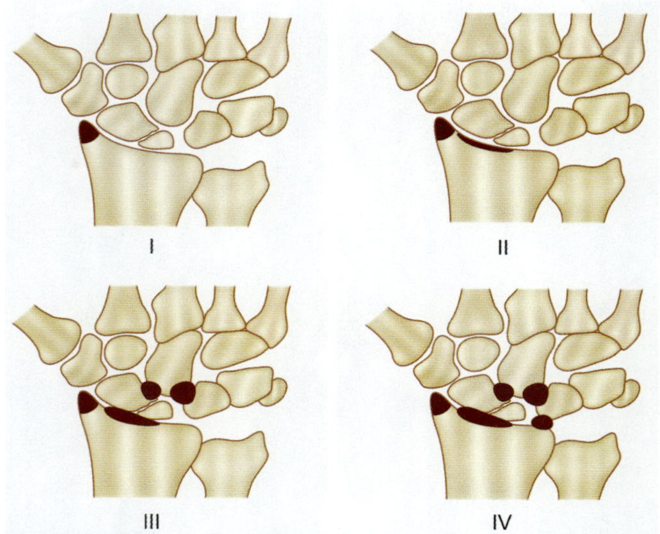

Fig. 21.308: Stages of scaphoid nonunion advanced collapse. Stage I. Arthritis at radial styloid; Stage II. Scaphoid fossa arthritis; Stage III. Capitolunate arthritis. Stage IV. Diffuse arthritis of carpus

Flow chart 21.4: Algorithm for treatment of scaphoid nonunion

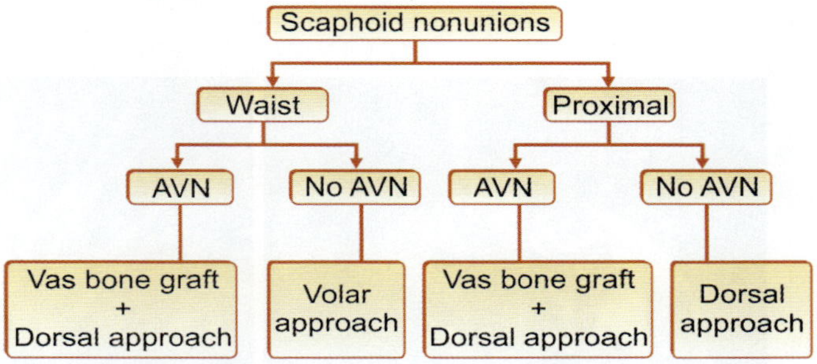

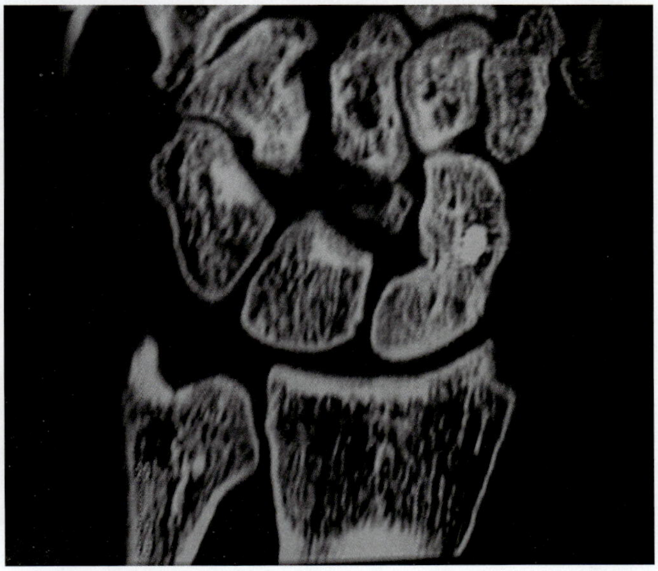

Fig. 21.309: Image of the wrist joint, illustrating radial styloidectomy

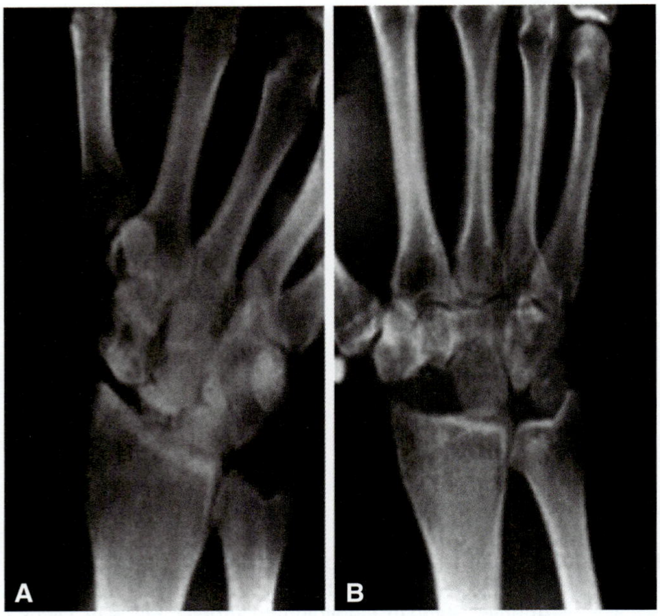

Figs 21.310A and B: X-ray showing open carpal fracture dislocation with significant comminuted fracture of scaphoid and lunate

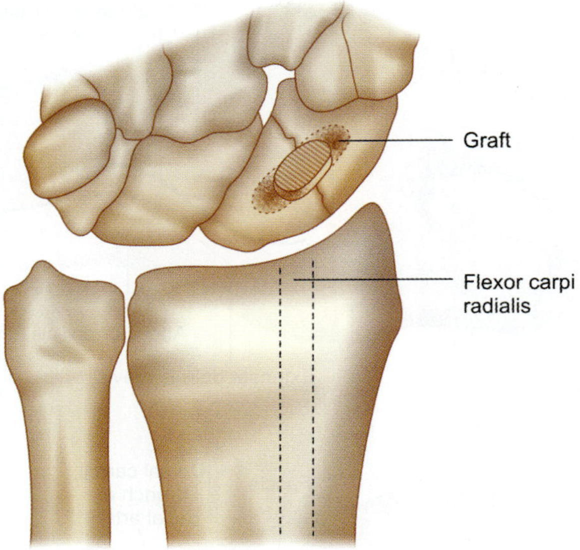

Fig. 21.311: Grafting operations

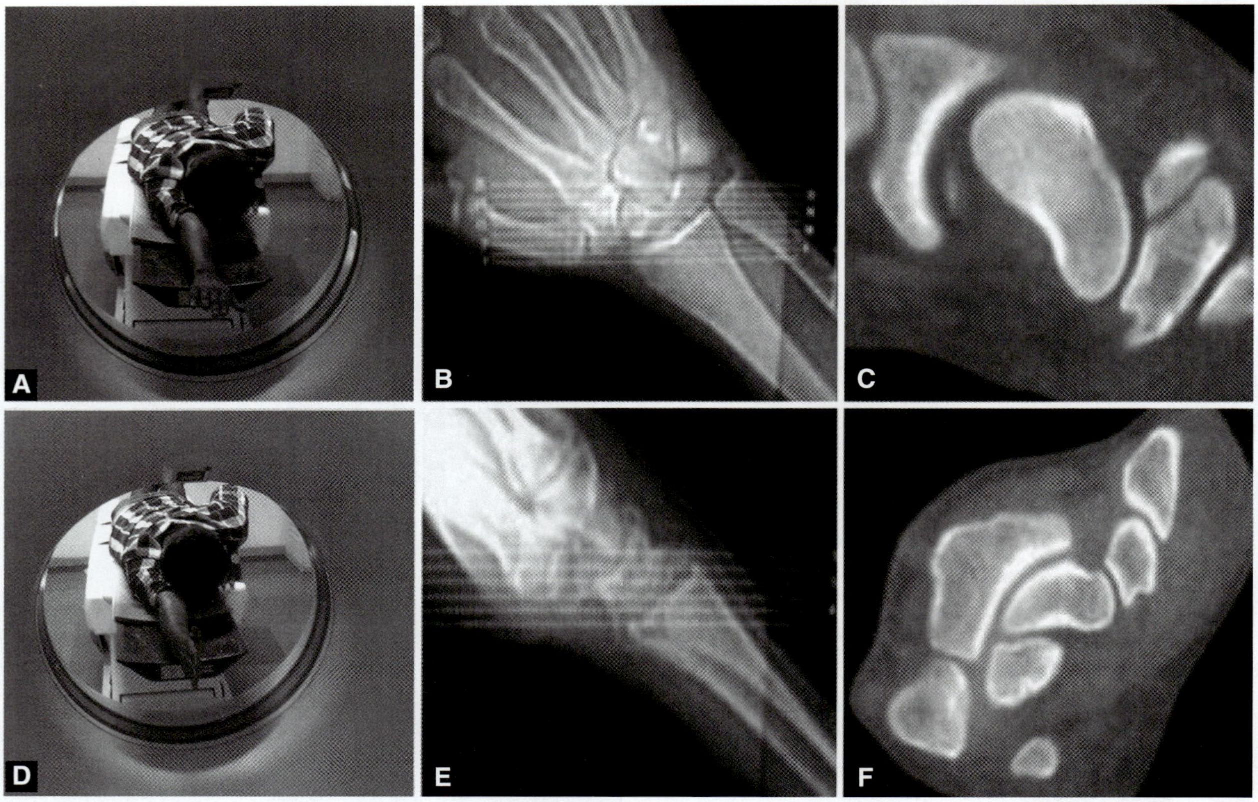

Figs 21.312A to F: CT scan in the sagittal and coronal planes showing, humpback deformity

Fernandez Technique

- Trace the uninjured wrist with measurement of scaphoid length and scapholunate angle
- Calculate the resection area and type of graft to be used

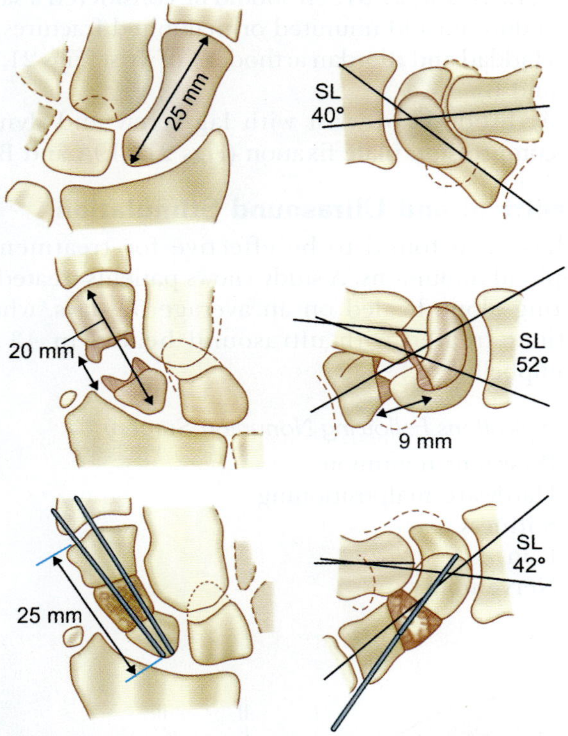

Figs 21.313A to C: (A) Tracing of uninjured wrist with measurement of scaphoid length and scapholunate angle; (B) Calculation of resection area and type of graft to be used; (C) Definitive diagram of operation

- Definitive diagram of operation is shown in Figures 21.313A to C.

Tomaino Technique

Diagrammatic representation of Tomaino technique is shown in Figures 21.314A to D.

Stark Technique (Figs 21.315A to C)

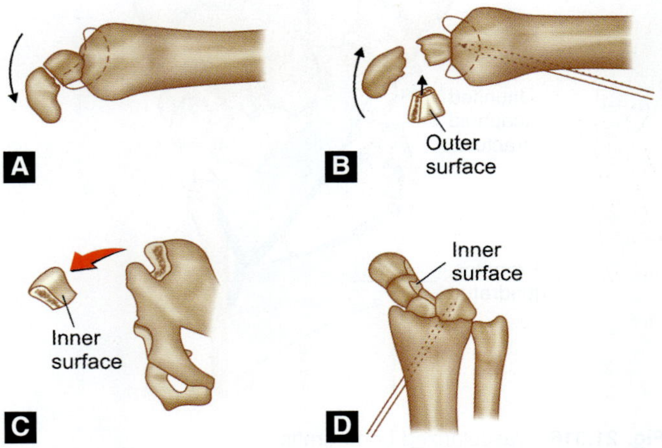

Figs 21.314A to D: Tomaino technique—(A) Lunate extension, dorsal intercalated segment instability with scaphoid nonunion; (B) With wrist extension, radiolunate joint is pinned. Scaphoid opens at nonunion site; (C) Tricortical corticocancellous graft is harvested; (D) Graft is placed after that herbert whipple screw is placed and lunate transfixation pin is removed

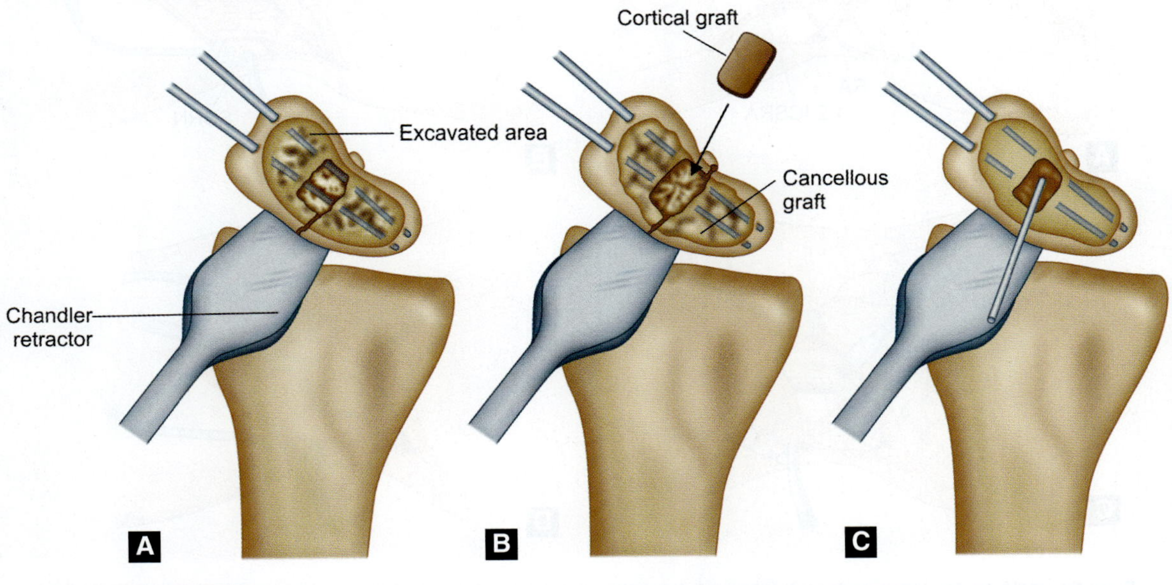

Figs 21.315A to C: Stark technique—(A) Excavation of scaphoid and placement of K wires; (B) Bone graft inserted into cavity; (C) K wire inserted to stabilize the bone graft

Vascularized Bone Grafts (Fig. 21.316)

Kawai and Yamamoto reported the use of a pedicle bone graft using a segment of the pronator quadratus. Their technique can be useful in difficult nonunions.

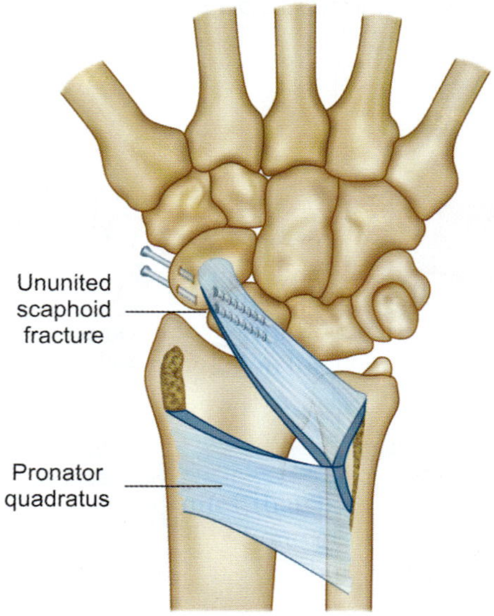

Fig. 21.316: Vascularized bone grafts

Zaidemberg et al. used a vascularized bone graft from the distal dorsolateral radius, as shown in the Figures 21.317A to D.

Arthrodesis of the Wrist

Different representations of wrist arthrodesis is shown in Figs 21.318 and 21.319. It should be considered a salvage procedure for old ununited or malunited fractures.

- Haddad and Riordan arthodesis of wrist (Figs 21.318A and B)
- Arthrodesis of wrist with lag screw and dynamic compression plate fixation (Figs 21.319A and B).

Electrical and Ultrasound Stimulation

It has been found to be effective for treatment for scaphoid nonunions. A study shows patients treated with casting alone healed on an average 62 days, whereas patient treated with ultrasound healed in 43 days (Campbell et al.)

Complications Following Nonunion Surgery

- Persistent nonunion
- Hardware malpositioning
- Stiffness
- Pain
- Nerve injury

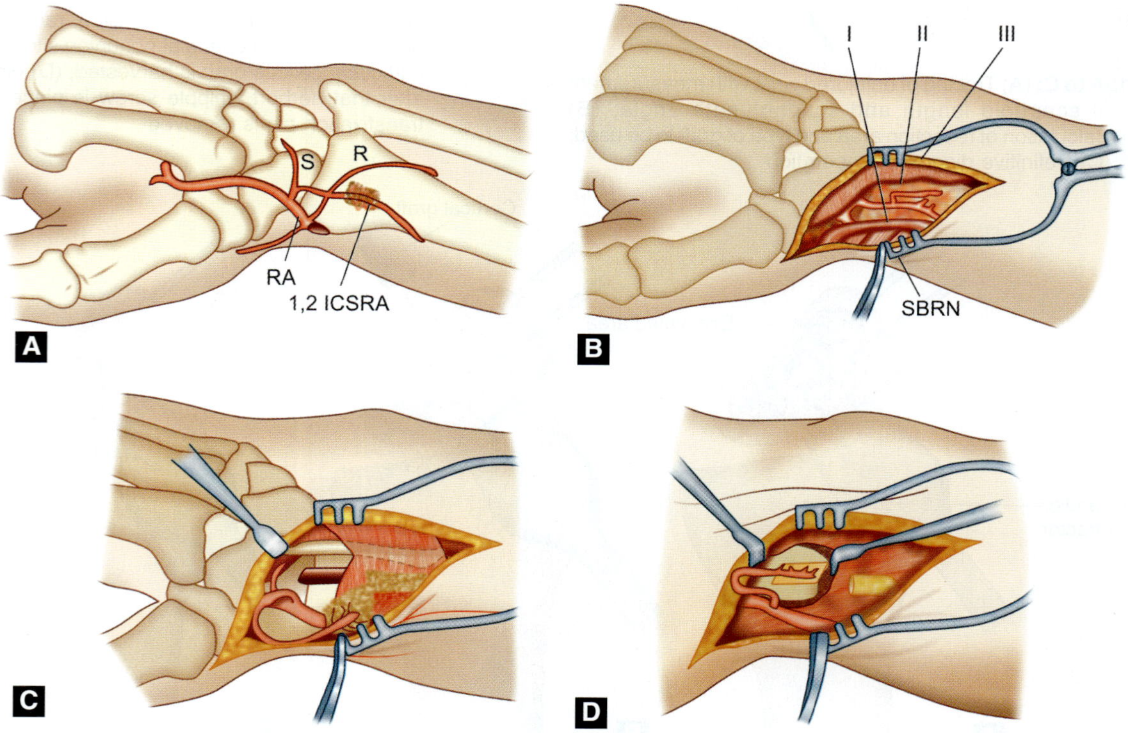

Figs 21.317A to D: Vascularized bone graft from the distal dorsolateral radius

SCAPHOCAPITATE FRACTURE SYNDROME

Introduction

The scaphocapitate fracture syndrome associated with perilunar dislocation of the carpus is uncommon. There has been some discussion concerning the mechanism of the injury.

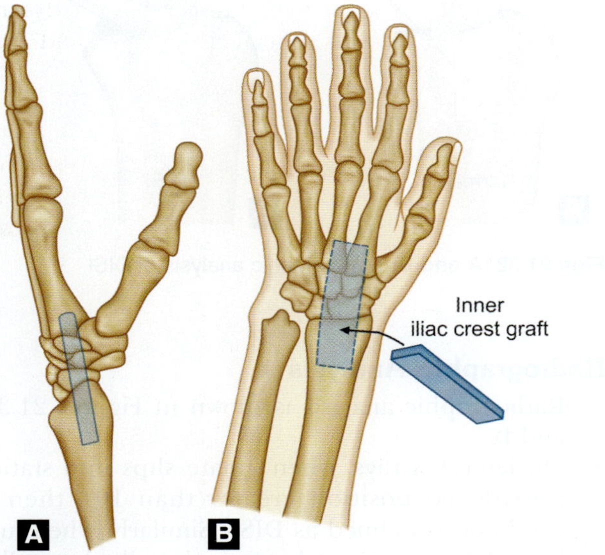

Figs 21.318A and B: Haddad and Riordan arthrodesis of wrist—(A) Radial view, showing slot cut in distal radius, carpal bones and second and third metacarpal; (B) Dorsal view, showing shape of the graft and its final position

Mechanism of Injury

Stein and Siegel (1969) said that during hyperextension of the wrist the scaphoid bone, which connects the proximal and distal rows of the carpus may be fractured (Fig. 21.320A). The lunate bone rotates dorsally on a transverse axis, so that its dorsal lip comes to lie under the dorsal edge of the lower radial articular surface.

The capitate bone rotating dorsally with the lunate bone, comes to lie with its long axis perpendicular to the long axis of the radius. A continuation of this hyperextension force causes the dorsal surface of the neck of the capitates to come into contact with the dorsal edge of the lower radial articular surface leading to fracture (Fig. 21.320B).

If the wrist continues into further hyperextension, the proximal fragment of the capitate is rotated through 90° (Fig. 21.320C). When the wrist returns to the neutral position, the proximal fragment of the capitate assumes a position of 180° rotation in relation to the main fragment of the capitate (Fig. 21.320D).

The axis of this rotation has been discussed by several authors (Fenton 1956, Adler and Shaftan 1962, Stein and Siegel 1969). Stein and Siegel believed that the rotation occurs in the transverse axis. Fenton described two cases of scaphocapitate fracture, not associated with perilunar dislocation, in which the proximal fragment of the capitate had rotated through 180°. He believed that the rotation of the proximal fragment occurred through an axis perpendicular to the palm because the initial displacement of the wrist was one of extension and radial deviation, during which the apex of the radial styloid impinged on the lateral surface of the body of the scaphoid bone, causing it to fracture.

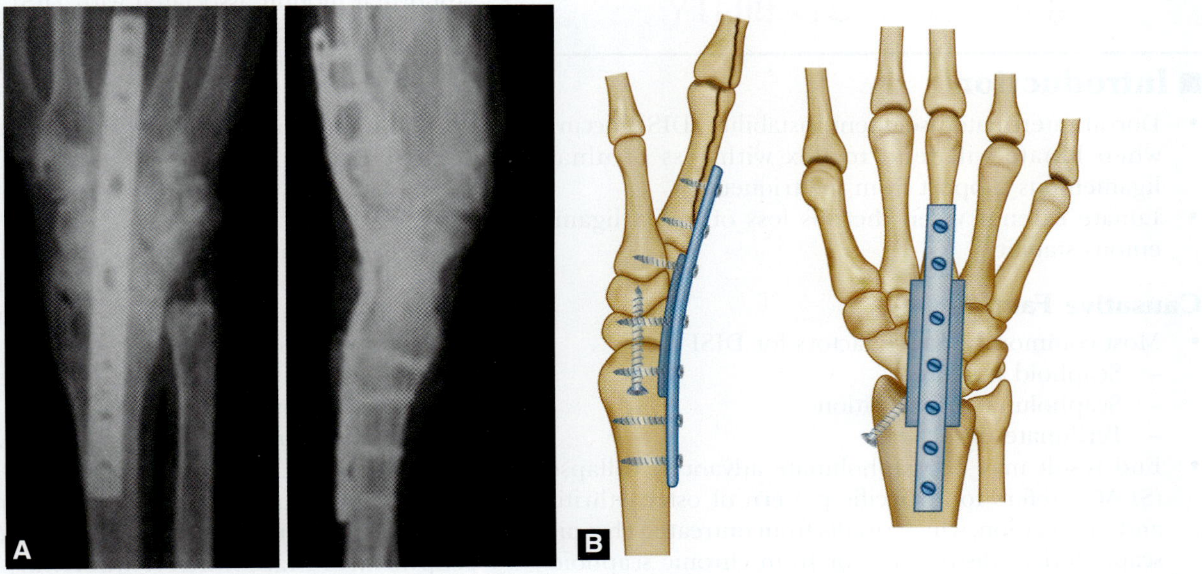

Figs 21.319A and B: Arthrodesis of wrist with lag screw and dynamic compression plate fixation

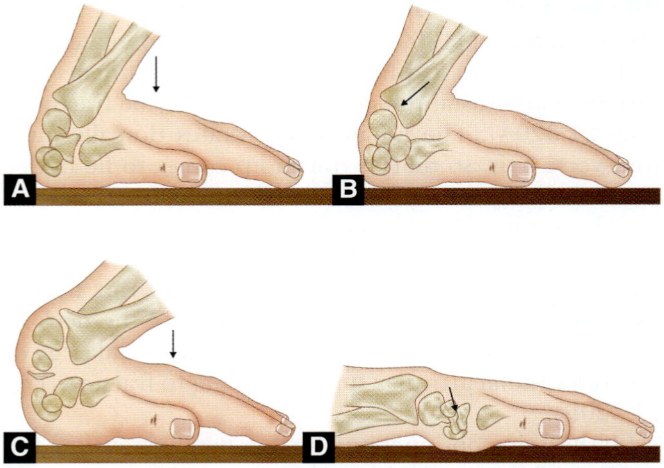

Figs 21.320A to D: (A) During hyperextension of the wrist the scaphoid bone may get fractured; (B) If hyperextension force is continued, then dorsal surface of the neck of the capitates to come into contact with the dorsal edge of the lower radial articular surface leading to fracture; (C) If further hyperextension in continued, then the proximal fragment of the capitate is rotated through 90°; (D) As wrist returns to neutral position, the proximal segment of capitate rotates at 180° in relation to the main fragment of capitate

If the force was great enough, the adjacent capitate bone was fractured at the same level as that of the scaphoid bone and a continuation of the force caused the proximal fragment of the capitate to rotate in a perpendicular plane.

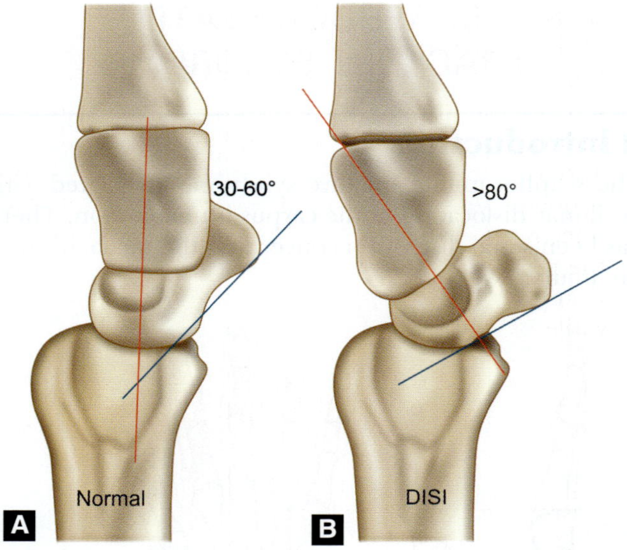

Figs 21.321A and B: Radiographic analysis of DISI

DORSAL INTERCALATED SEGMENT INSTABILITY

Introduction

- Dorsal intercalated segment instability (DISI) occurs when lunate will tend to flex with loss of ulnar ligamentous support from the triquetrum
- Lunate extends when there is loss of radial ligamentous stability.

Causative Factors

- Most common causative factors for DISI are:
  - Scaphoid fracture
  - Scapholunate dissociation
  - Perilunate dislocation
- End result may be scapholunate advanced collapse (SLAC), refers to a specific pattern of osteoarthritis and subluxation, which results from untreated chronic scapholunate dissociation or from chronic scaphoid nonunion.

Radiographic Analysis

- Radiographic analysis is shown in Figures 21.321A and B.
- On lateral X-rays, when lunate slips into statically dorsiflexed position greater than 10°, then this condition is defined as DISI. Similarly, when lunate lies palmar to capitate, but faces dorsally, then collapse pattern is also consistent with dorsiflexion instability
- DISI deformity is also present, when the scapholunate angle is greater than 60° (signifying scapholunate dissociation. Scapholunate dissociation has been called the "Terry Thomas" sign in which the scapholunate interval is greater than 2 mm)
- Abnormal motion associated with DISI and scapholunate dissociation can lead to degeneration and collapse of the medial scaphoid, lateral lunate and radiocarpal joint. This degeneration is termed scapholunate dissociation with advanced collapse (SLAC) of wrist.

Treatment

- Acute ligamentous disruption is usually treated with direct ligamentous reapproximation and repair
- When ligamentous repair is not possible, but degenerative changes have not occurred, ligamentous reconstruction, dorsal capsular ligamentodesis or intercarpal fusions may be considered
- *In case of degenerative changes (as seen on X-ray):* When radioscaphoid change is present, but the articular surface of the capitate retains its normal articular cartilage, proximal row carpectomy (removal of scaphoid, lunate and triquetrum) will allow preservation of wrist motion, as the capitate's head

shifts proximally to articulate within the ulnar fossa of the distal radius
- When degenerative change is present at the capitate's lunate portion of the midcarpal joints, in addition to radioscaphoid change, the scaphoid may be excised and intercarpal fusion of the capitate, lunate, triquetrum and hamate will be accomplished. This selective intercarpal fusion provides motion through the residual radiolunate articulation
- Complete wrist fusion provides reliable pain relief, while permanently sacrificing wrist motion.

VOLAR INTERCALATED SEGMENT INSTABILITY

Introduction

- Volar inercalated segment instability (VISI) consists of volar flexion of the lunate, relative to the longitudinal axis of the radius and capitate, when the wrist rests in a neutral position
- Lunate will tend to flex, when there is loss of ulnar support from the triquetrum. It may result from disruption of radial carpal ligaments on ulnar side of wrist and is characterized by scapholunate angle less than 30° (Figs 21.322A and B)
- Volar flexion instability pattern is usually associated with triquetrolunate dissociation or triquetral-hamate instability
- The dorsal radial triquetral and triquetroscaphoid ligaments have an increased space (increased "V") between them.

Static VISI

- When lunate slips into a statically fixed position greater than 15° of flexion, then it is called static VISI

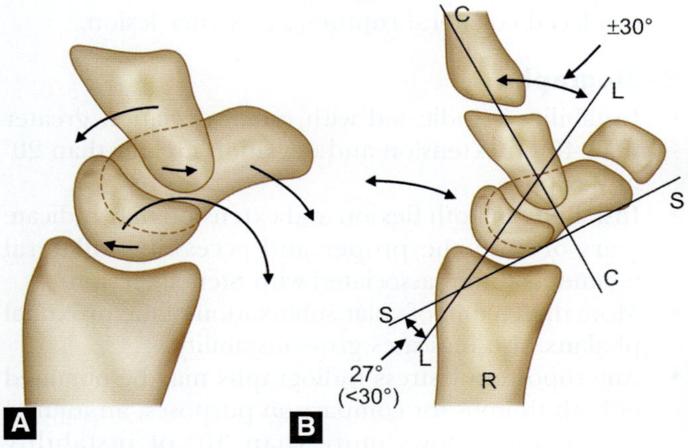

Figs 21.322A and B: VISI characterized by scapholunate angle greater than 30°

- *Early treatment:* Closed reduction and casting (with or without K wires).

Dynamic VISI

- Normal wrist may assume a VISI pattern when relaxed, however this is not considered abnormal unless it is symptomatic
- Etiology may be a laxity in the volar capitotriquetral ligament. These patients may note pain on volar stress testing
- Radiographs may show a widening between the capitate and the triquetrum, when wrist is placed in radial deviation
- *Treatment:* Capitolunate fusion.

Radiographs

- Lateral view of wrist (Fig. 21.323)
- *Capitolunate angle*
  - Wrist must be placed in a neutral position
  - Normally the distal radius, lunate, capitate and third metacarpal are colinear, however in VISI, there is a zig-zag deformity pattern, so that the lunate is volar flexed in relation to the capitates.

Management

Space of Poirier (it lies at the volar aspect of the proximal capitate, lying between the volar radiocapitate and volar radiotriquetral ligament) is reinforced and is closed, which closes down the space between the triquetrohamate and triquetrocapitate ligaments.

GAMEKEEPER'S THUMB

Introduction

Injury to the ulnar ligament of thumb joint or ulnar collateral ligament is commonly referred to as Gamekeeper's thumb or Skier's thumb (Figs 21.324A and B).

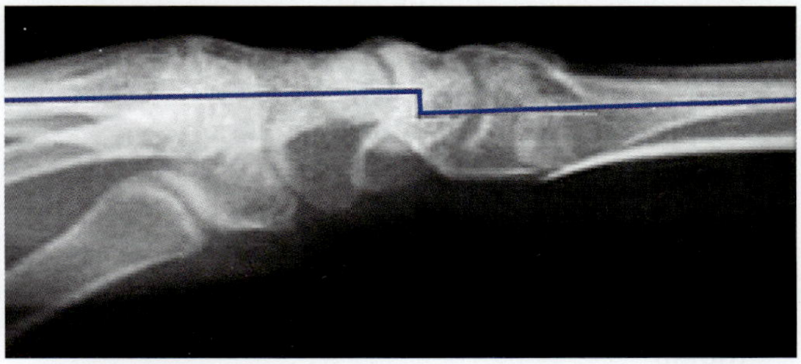

Fig. 21.323: Lateral view of the wrist in VISI

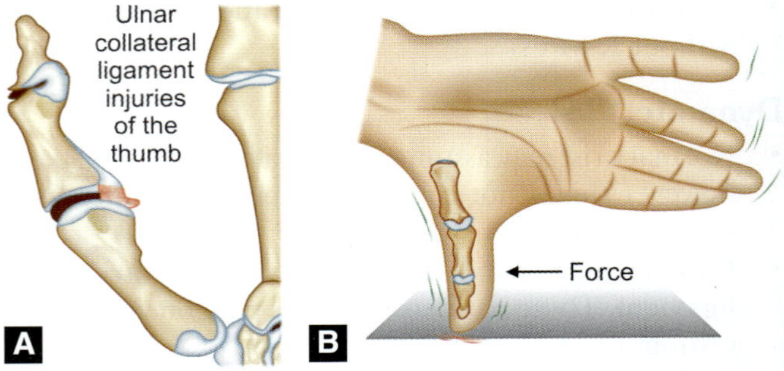

Figs 21.324A and B: (A) Injury to the ulnar collateral ligament in Gamekeeper's thumb; (B) Mechanism of injury

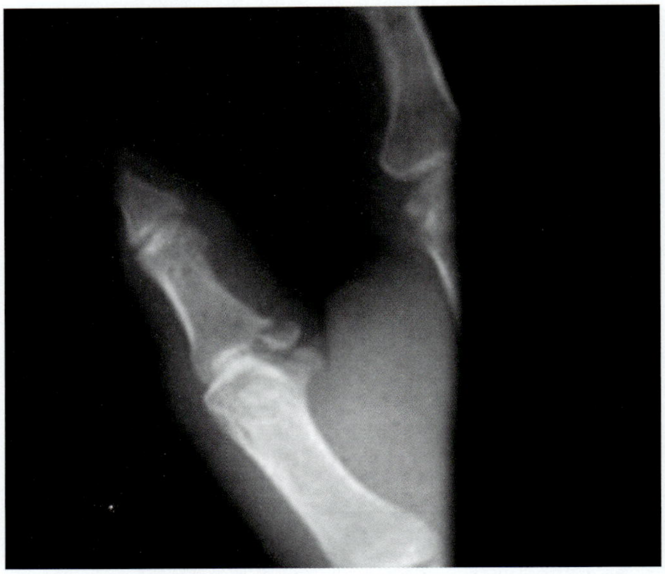

Fig. 21.325: X-ray showing Gamekeeper's fracture

It involves injury to ulnar collateral ligament of thumb's MCP joint, causing instability at that joint. Original it is referred to a chronic injury brought on by chronic stretch of the ulnar collateral ligament, which nearly always separates from the base of first phalanx of the thumb. It frequently becomes lodged between adductor pollicis aponeurosis and its normal position (Stener lesion).

A spectrum of ulnar instability may exist, depending on whether there is an additional injury to the adductor aponeurosis and volar plate.

Stener Lesion

It occurs when torn distal edge of collateral ligament displaces superficially and proximally to the adductor aponeurosis. Proximal margin of aponeurosis slides distal to insertion of ligament.

Creation of Stener lesion requires significant radial deviation of phalanx (up to 60°) along with combined tears of the proper and accessory collateral ligaments, in order for the ligament to be displaced above the adductor aponeurosis. Ruptured end of ligament is no longer in contact with its area of insertion of the phalanx and therefore healing can not occur.

Gamekeeper's Fracture (Fig. 21.325)

- Even slightly displaced Gamekeeper's fractures tend to do well with immobilization
- Conservative indications for surgery include, fractures with more than 30 percent of the joint surface and significant displacement or malrotation
- Avoid stress testing of these fractures, since it can lead to fracture displacement.

Physical Examination

- Examination should begin with normal uninjured thumb
- Note the stability of the uninjured MP joint as well as its ROM
- Look for a supination deformity of the joint (which may be associated with palmar subluxation of the joint) and stability
- This is generally performed in conjunction with X-rays
- Local anesthetic block is required for patient's comfort
- Gamekeeper's fracture is a contraindication to stress testing (but stress testing can proceed with nondisplaced avulsion fractures)
- Stability is documented with stress radiographs.

Palpation

- Determine point of maximum tenderness, noting that generally, the ligament tears distally off the proximal phalanx
- Palpation of torn ligament ends, may identify displaced collateral rupture, i.e. Stener lesion.

Radiographs

- Instability is indicated with radial deviation greater than 40° in extension and deviation greater than 20° in flexion
- Instability in both flexion and extension may indicate tears of both the proper and accessory collateral ligaments (often associated with Stener's lesion)
- More than 3 mm of volar subluxation of the proximal phalanx also indicates gross instability
- Anteroposterior stress radiographs may be obtained of both thumbs for comparison purposes, an injured thumb that shows more than 30° of instability compared with the uninjured side indicates a complete rupture.

Treatment

Nonoperative Treatment

- Treat with a short arm cast with a thumb spica
- Complications of nonoperative treatment are:
  - Main complication is failure of ligament to heal, resulting in instability of joint
  - Gross instability is usually caused by Stener's lesion

Surgical Treatment

Indications for surgery are:

- Gross radiographic instability (which usually represents tears of both the proper and the accessory collateral ligaments)
- Presence of palpable torn ligament ends (Stener's lesion)
- With excessive swelling the Stener's may not be palpable
- Occassionally, significant ligamentous injury may occur without immediate gross instability due to swelling and muscle spasm
- Consider re-examing patients in 5 to 7 days and if motion has not been regained and swelling has not improved consider surgical fixation.

Surgical treatment for injuries of less than 2 to 3 weeks old

- Acute complete rupture of the ulnar collateral ligament should be treated with surgical repair of the ligament. The detached tendinous insertion of the adductor muscle can be advanced and reattached to furnish a dynamic reinforcement
- If the repair is done several months after the injury, a graft can be used to replace the ligament. The graft can be boxlike, with a strip of fascia or palmaris longus tendon passed through the proximal and distal attachments of the ligament or the extensor pollicis brevis tendon, either split or in total, can be threaded through bone and attached by pull-out sutures to reconstruct the ligament.

Chronic Gamekeeper's thumb

- Proximal phalanx tends to volarly subluxate and rotate
- Deformity develops as a result of damage to ulnar collateral ligament and dorsal capsule
- In addition to dorsal joint support provided by capsule, EPB and EPL tendons also contributes to the dorsal stability of MP joint
- When ulnar collateral ligament ruptures, ulnar side of phalanx tends to displace volarly and rotate into supination
- With repeated radial stress, dorsal expansion may attenuate and allow EPL to shift ulnarly, compromising its extension effect on the joint
- *Management:* An MP joint with chronic instability and a small flexion arc should be considered for MP joint arthrodesis.

BOXER'S FRACTURE

Introduction

- Metacarpal neck fracture involving little finger (Fig. 21.326)
- Only collateral ligaments remains attached to the proximal phalanx and therefore metacarpal head is free from any proximal stabilizing influence
- Metacarpal head tilts volarly, causing joint to lie in hyperextension and collateral ligaments become slack.
- If joint is allowed to remain in hyperextension, collateral ligaments will shorten, leading to limited MCP flexion
- Little finger CMC articulation allows flexion extension arc of 20 to 30° in addition to a rotatory motion facilitating little finger opposition to thumb
- Ring metacarpal provides 10 to 15° of mobility.

Differential Diagnosis

- *Transverse metacarpal shaft fracture:* This fracture may be amenable to a four holed plate.
- *Fracture of metacarpal head:* It is an infrequent variant of Boxer's fracture. In this injury, impact is received directly on metacarpal head, producing fracture through joint surface. It requires operative fixation.

Radiographs

- True lateral radiograph is necessary with these fractures, in order to measure the angle of displacement of the distal fragment.

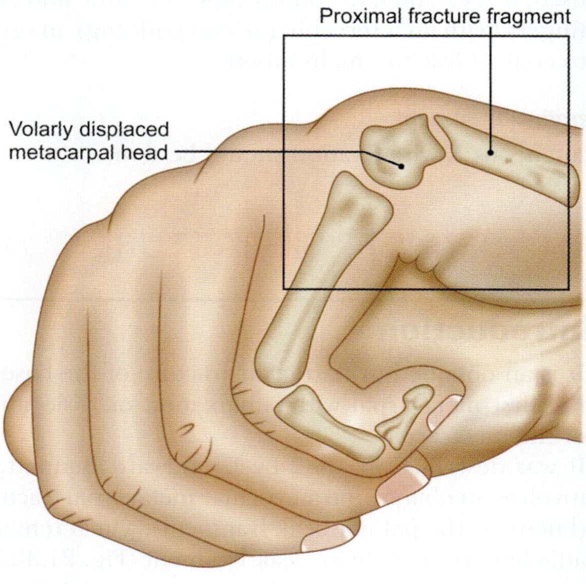

Fig. 21.326: Boxer fracture—Metacarpal neck fracture of little finger

- Normal metacarpal neck angle is about 15° and therefore a measured angle on film of 30° is actually 15°.
- When displaced, angulate with dorsal angulation at fracture line and distal metacarpal head displaces towards palmar side.

Treatment

Nonoperative Treatment

- Clawing results from the palmar displacement of the metacarpal head and resulting imbalance of extrinsic tendons
- May have cosmetic deformity, but leads to good function.

Methods of reduction

- As collateral ligaments are the only remaining attachment to metacarpal head, collaterals must be placed in a tightened position to control distal fragment and achieve reduction
- MP joint is flexed at 90° to produce tightening of MP collateral ligaments
- Flexed metacarpal is directed dorsally, which effects reduction of metacarpal head by correction of volar angulation
- *Acceptable reduction:* Following points need to be considered, while accepting the reduced fragment:
  - On lateral view, if angulation greater than 30–40°, a functional deficit (pseudoclawing) may result. Percutaneous pin fixation may be considered then
  - On AP view, little or no angulation should be accepted, since this indicates malrotation of the digit
- *Casting technique:* No matter what casting technique is used, it is essential to "buddy tape" the little and ring fingers (with an intervening of cast padding), in order to control fracture malrotation.

Operative Treatment

Percutaneous K-wire fixation should be done.

BENNETT'S FRACTURE

Introduction

- It is an oblique intra-articular fracture of the base of the first metacarpal with subluxation or dislocation of the metacarpal.
- It was described in 1882 by Dr Edward Bennett. It involves an oblique intra-articular metacarpal fracture (known as the palmar beak fragment), which remains attached to the palmar beak ligament (Fig. 21.327).

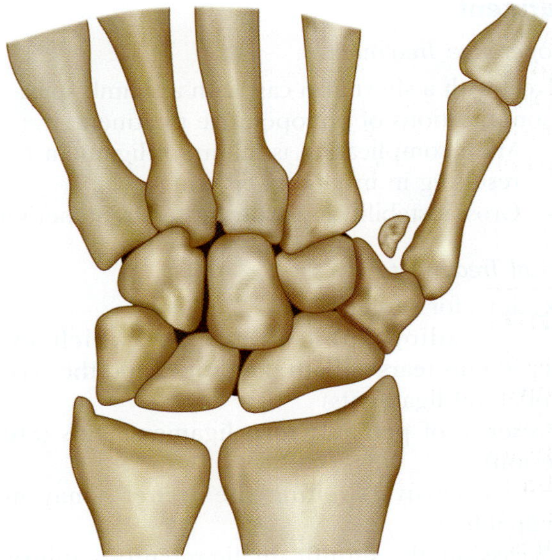

Fig. 21.327: Palmar beak fragment

Mechanism of Injury

- Injury results from axial blow, directed against the partially flexed metacarpal (i.e. from fist fights). Fracture starts at ulnar base of thumb metacarpal, as palmar ulnar aspect of thumb is normally stabilized by strong ligaments
- Disruption of the ulnar fragment destabilizes thumb and volar fracture fragment remains attached to CMC, by volar anterior oblique ligament. Anterior oblique ligament anchors volar lip of metacarpal to tubercle of the trapezium, hence small volar lip fragment remains attached to anterior oblique ligament, which is attached to trapezium
- Distal metacarpal fragment (containing most of articular surface) is displaced proximally, radially and dorsally by pull of APL. It is also rotated in supination by the pull of APL. Metacarpal head is displaced into palm by pull of ADP.

Radiographs

- Oblique fracture line with a triangular fragment at ulnar base of metacarpal
- Triangular fragment remains attached to trapezium with proximal displacement of the metacarpal.

Treatment

- Closed manipulation and casting
- Closed reduction and percutaneous K-wire fixation
- Open reduction and internal fixation with a K-wire or a screw.

Complications

- Malunion with persistent subluxation may progress to painful arthritis of the carpometacarpal joint
- Osteoarthritis, due to improper alignment of the joint surfaces. Treatment by excision of the trapezium in painful arthritis cases.

ROLANDO'S FRACTURE

■ Introduction

It was described in 1910 by Dr Rolando:

- Involves three part fracture, at base of first metacarpal (Fig. 21.328)
- In addition to volar lip fracture (as seen with Bennett's fracture), there is also large dorsal fragment, resulting in "Y" or "T" shaped intra-articular fracture
- It is a comminuted intra-articular fracture at the base of thumb metacarpal, even if "Y" or "T" is not present
- It is uncommon, but has a worse prognosis than Bennett's fracture.

Treatment

Nonoperative Treatment

- May be indicated in highly comminuted fracture
- Mold in thumb spica for 3–4 weeks and then begin ROM.

Surgical Treatment

- Indicated for presence of large volar and dorsal fragments amenable to fixation
- Fracture reduction and K-wire fixation
- If radial fragment is large, consider using 2.0 mm cortical lag screw
- Immobilization is required for 6 weeks.

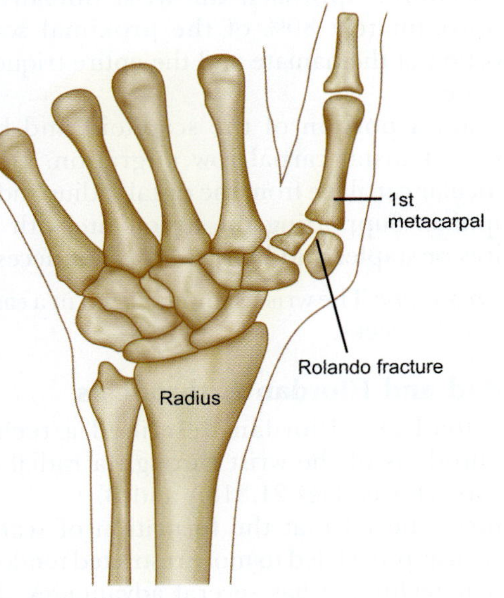

Fig. 21.328: Rolando fracture

WRIST ARTHRODESIS

■ Introduction

- Due to recent trend towards reconstructive surgery, arthrodesis of the wrist is performed less often now, than it was a few decades ago. However, it still remains an important procedure
- Arthrodesis of the radiocarpal joint has evolved over the last 50 years. The trend has been toward increasing stability in the method of fixation. Early procedures used cortical or cancellous bone grafting with limited fixation methods such as pins or screws
- Campbell and Keokarn described an inlay bone grafting technique of wrist fusion in 1964. Haddad and Riordan applied this technique through a lateral (radial) approach. Various fixation methods have been described including screws, multiple staples and multiple Steinmann pins
- In 1970, the AO group described a rigid fixation method, using a dynamic compression plate.

Dynamic Compression Plate

Advantages

- Excellent fusion rates
- Decreased incidence of malposition
- Increased stability allowing early rehabilitation
- Requires less bone grafting than other methods and usually an adequate amount of graft can be harvested from the distal radius.

Indications

- Post-traumatic arthritis
- Neoplastic lesions
- Severely comminuted intra-articular fractures
- Rheumatoid arthritis
- Wrist or hand paralysis
- Spastic hemiplegia
- Failed total joint arthroplasty
- Failed limited arthrodesis.

Contraindications

Includes an open physis of the distal radius. The distal radial physis closes at approximately 17 years of age and care should be taken not to damage it in patients under this age.

Position

- This is usually 10 to 20° of extension (dorsiflexion) with the long axis of the third metacarpal shaft aligned with the long axis of the radial shaft and neutral to 5° of ulnar deviation. Clinically, it is determined by the position that the wrist normally assumes with the fist strongly clenched

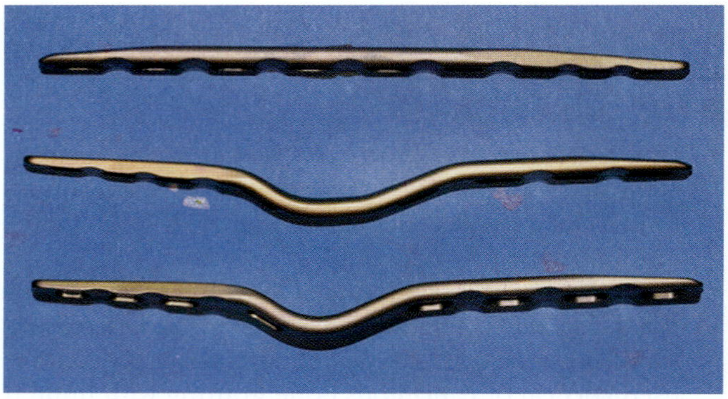

Fig. 21.329: Different types of AO plates

- If bilateral wrist fusions are indicated, the position of the wrists should be determined by the needs of the patient. The neutral position for both wrists is thought to provide maximal function.

Techniques

- Of the many techniques that have been described, most include the use of a bone graft. The iliac crest is the most common donor site, but bone graft may be obtained from the distal radius, ulna, tibia or rib
- The distal radius may be exposed through a dorsal, ulnar or radial (lateral) approach. Dorsal approach is the most commonly used approach.

AO Plates (Fig. 21.329)

- Straight plate use large intercalary graft required
- Long carpal bend in large wrist
- Short carpal bend in short wrist.

Plate Fixation

- Curvilinear skin incision is given, beginning with 2 cm, extending over the distal radioulnar joint and ending over the midshaft of the second and third metacarpals
- Protect the branches of the superficial cutaneous nerve. Make a longitudinal incision between the tendons of the extensor digitorum communis, which are retracted in the ulnar direction and the extensor pollicis longus, which is retracted in the radial direction
- An I-shaped incision is made in the capsule, crossing proximally over the radiocarpal joint and distally over the carpometacarpal joints
- Remove Lister's tubercle and the dorsal cortices of the carpal bones, to allow flat apposition of the precontoured plate
- Denude the radiocarpal and intercarpal joint surfaces of cartilage and fill the gaps with cancellous bone harvested from the excised bone and distal radial metaphysic
- A 3.5 mm cortex lag screw may be placed through the radial styloid in the capitate, to pull the carpus against the radial styloid and help prevent impingement of the distal radioulnar joint
- Secure the appropriate precontoured plate to the dorsal aspect of the third metacarpal. Ensure that the distal end of the plate is centered on the metacarpal.
- Mark the position of the distal hole and remove the plate. Drill a 2.0 mm hole in a dorsal to volar direction, centered in the midline of the metacarpal. Replace the plate, measure, tap and fill the distal hole with a 2.7 mm screw
- Fill the remaining metacarpal holes and compress the radiocarpal and intercarpal joints. This is done using a 3.5 mm screw, placed in compression mode through the second most distal hole in the radius. Fill the remaining holes and close the capsule over a small suction drain.

After Treatment

- A cast is applied from the upper arm to the tips of the fingers and thumb, with the elbow at right angle, the forearm in neutral position and the wrist in 10–15° of extension
- The fingers and thumb should be slightly flexed. To allow for swelling, the dorsum of the cast is windowed.
- At 3 weeks a short cast below the elbow, just proximal to the metacarpophalangeal joints, is applied with the wrist in the correct position
- Support is continued until firm fusion is present, usually at 10 to 12 weeks.

Fusion with Proximal Row (Carpectomy)

- This technique was described by Louis (Figs 21.330A and B)
- *Procedure:* Approach the wrist dorsally. Remove approximately 80% of the proximal scaphoid, a portion of the hamate and the entire triquetrum and lunate
- Retain a portion of the scaphoid and hamate to prevent distal carpal row migration. Denude the articular cartilage from the distal radius and proximal capitate. Supporting the fusion site with Kirschner wires or staples and bone graft is not necessary.

After treatment: The wrist is immobilized in a cast or splint for 12 to 16 weeks.

Haddad and Riordan Arthrodesis

- Haddad and Riordan described a technique of arthrodesis of the wrist through a radial or lateral approach (see Figs 21.318A and B)
- They believed that the formation of scar with the dorsal approach led to more restricted tendon gliding.
- Their technique has several advantages. The distal radioulnar joint is not entered, the extensor tendons

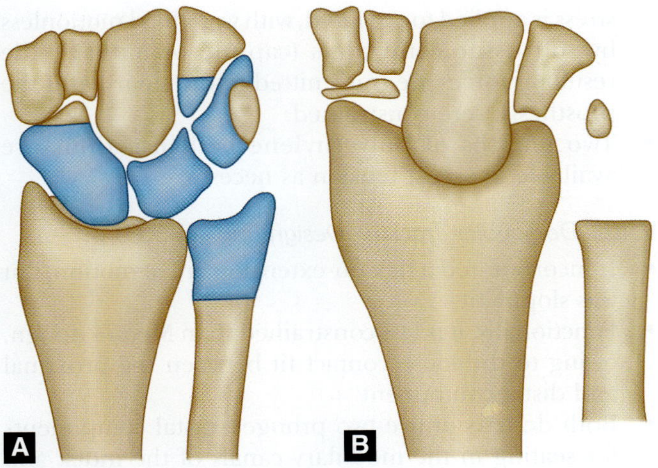

Figs 21.330A and B: Fusion with proximal row after carpectomy—(A) Carpectomy (as shown by the shaded portion) performed; (B) Fusion being performed with proximal row

to the digits are not disturbed as much and because dorsal thickening is avoided, the appearance of the wrist is not altered.

Technique

- J-shaped skin incision is made, 2.5 to 4 cm proximal to the radial styloid midlateral aspect of the forearm, extend it distally across the styloid and then curve it dorsally to end at the base of the second metacarpal
- Mobilize and retract the superficial branch of the radial nerve. Identify the interval between the first and second dorsal compartments and incise the dorsal carpal ligament in this interval, leaving it attached to the volar aspect of the radius. Mobilize subperiosteally and retract the abductor pollicis longus, extensor pollicis brevis and wrist along with finger extensors
- Divide the extensor carpi radialis longus tendon just proximal to its insertion on the base of the second metacarpal, leaving a stump distally, so that it can be sutured later
- Remove the capsule from the radiocarpal, the intercarpal and the second carpometacarpal joints. Locate the dorsal branch of the radial artery, then ligate and divide it
- Denude the radiocarpal joint of articular cartilage and subchondral bone. Harvest iliac bone graft. With the wrist in 15° of dorsiflexion, cut a slot in the distal end of the radius, the carpal bones and the bases of the second and third metacarpals
- Do not cut through the medial cortex of the radius and enter the distal radioulnar joint. Then place the graft in the prepared bed. If the wrist is unstable, insert another added Kirschner wire obliquely or longitudinally, to engage the base of the second metacarpal and the distal radius
- Cut off the wire under the skin at the palm, to be removed 6 to 8 weeks later. Close the dorsal carpal ligament deep to the abductor pollicis longus and extensor pollicis brevis. Suture the extensor carpi radialis longus tendon and close the wound over a drain.

After Treatment

- Above elbow cast should be applied with elbow at a right angle, the forearm in neutral position and the wrist in 10 to 15° of extension. The fingers and thumb are slightly flexed
- At third-week, below elbow cast is applied just proximal to the metacarpophalangeal joints, with the wrist in the correct position
- Support is continued until firm fusion is present, usually at 10 to 12 weeks.

Watson and Wendor Arthrodesis

Watson and Wendor reported a technique using a radial incision and incorporating iliac bone graft into the fusion site and securing it in place with two removable Kirschner wires.

Technique

- Make a longitudinal incision radially extending 6 cm from the distal radius to the distal second metacarpal. Protect the superficial radial nerve and deep branch of the radial artery. Free and retract the extensor pollicis brevis and abductor pollicis longus in the palmar direction. Retract the extensor pollicis longus and extensor carpi longus with brevis.
- Lift the origin of the first dorsal interosseous from the second metacarpal. Fashion a groove extending 2 cm from distal radius to 1 cm of the second and third metacarpals, by drilling multiple holes and connecting them.
- This trough should include the scaphoid, capitate, lunate and trapezoid. The depth of the groove should be just through the metacarpals and even throughout.
- Place an outer cortical piece of iliac bone graft into the trough with the cancellous side down. Lock the graft into place by bringing the wrist from ulnar deviation to the neutral position. Secure the graft into position, by passing Kirschner wires through the distal radius and graft proximally and the metacarpals and graft distally.

After Treatment

Long arm cast is applied incorporating the thumb, index and long fingers. This is replaced at fourth-week by a short arm splint, which is used for an additional 2 to 4 weeks. The Kirschner wires are removed once the fusion site is solid.

Complications

- Painful hardware
- Tendon adhesions or ruptures
- Early wound infection
- Metacarpophalangeal joint stiffness
- Carpal tunnel syndrome
- Reflex sympathetic dystrophy
- Nonunion
- Persistent pain

WRIST ARTHROPLASTY

- The goal is to provide a mobile, stable and painless wrist with reasonable durability.
- If bilateral bony procedures on the wrist joint are necessary, arthroplasty on at least one side should be considered.
- In some cases, arthroplasty may be indicated initially because eventual collapse of the opposite wrist may require reconstruction.

■ Total Wrist Arthroplasty

- Total wrist arthroplasty is surgical resection of all or a portion of carpus, removal of the articulating surface of the radius and usually the ulna as well, so that it could be replaced with an articulated implant (Fig. 21.331).
- The concept of using an articulated non-hinged prosthesis in the wrist was developed by Meuli in Switzerland and by Voltz in Arizona, in early 1970's.

First Designs

Meuli's Ball and Socket Trunnion Design (Fig. 21.332)

- Allows rotation within the articulation in functional mode. Distal cup firmly encompasses the ball and if stress is applied to the hand, with wrist held motionless by soft tissue constraints (capsule or muscle), the resultant forces are transmitted to the stems, as if the prosthesis were constrained
- Two lengths of polyethylene ball insertions are available to adjust tension as necessary.

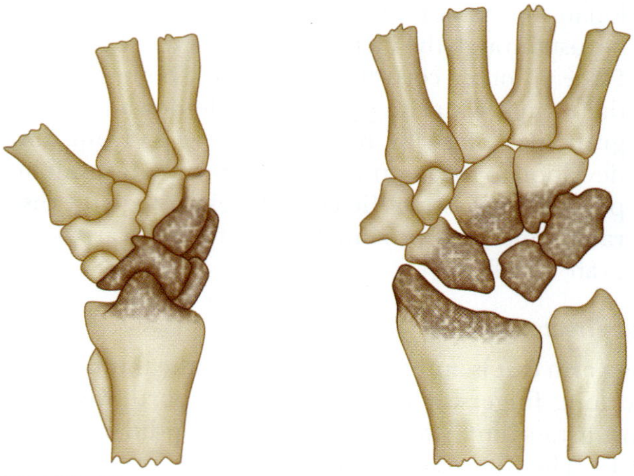

Fig. 21.331: Total wrist arthroplasty: Surgical resection of all or a portion of carpus (as shown by the shaded portions)

Voltz's Dorsovolar Tracking Design (Fig. 21.333)

- It incorporated a flexion-extension arc of motion, but was sloppy fit
- Functionally, it is less constrained than Meuli's design, owing to the loose contact fit between the proximal and distal component
- Both designs utilize two pronged distal components for seating in the modulary canals of the index and long metacarpals.

Problems with Arthroplasty

- *Balancing:* With both the prosthetic designs patients developed ulnar deviation, deformity and contractures (Fig. 21.334)
- *Infection:* Requires prosthetic removal

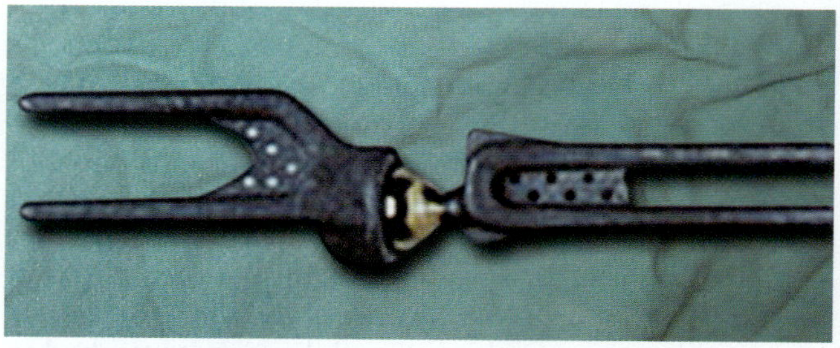

Fig. 21.332: Ball and socket trunnion design

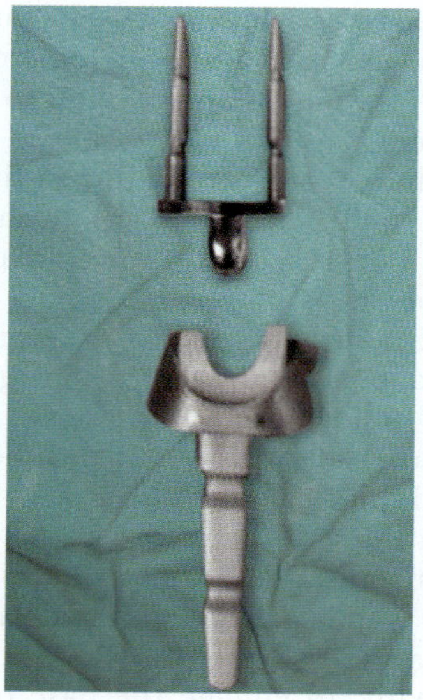

Fig. 21.333: Dorsovolar tracking design

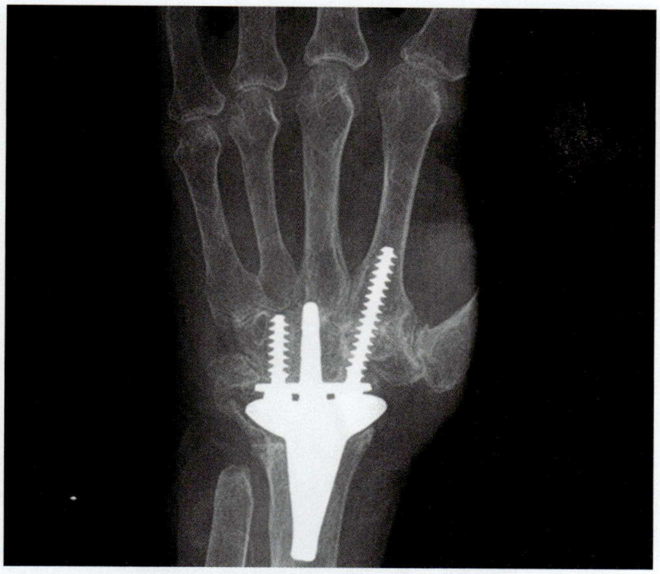

Fig. 21.334: Ulnar deviation after total wrist arthroplasty

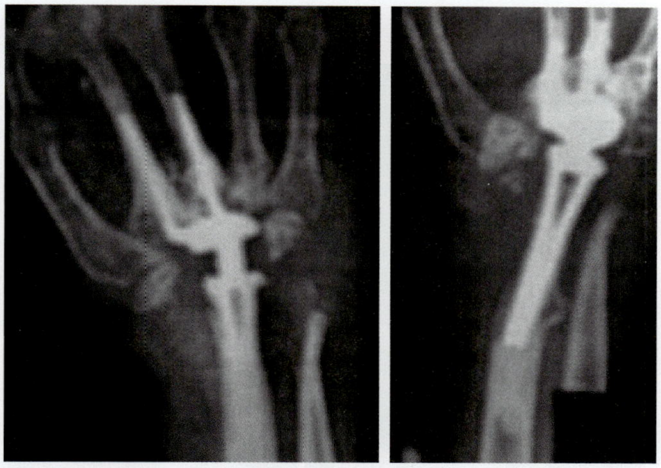

Fig. 21.335: Stem fixation problem after arthroplasty

- *Dislocation with deformity:* Requires revision surgery
- *Stem fixation problem:* Loosening of the distal component and stress shielding of the proximal component (Fig. 21.335)
- With the Meuli's design, distal component loosens as it tends to migrate volarly into the carpal canal. This may cause symptoms of the median neuropathy or ruptures of the flexor tendon at the edge of the prosthesis (Fig. 21.336).

Salvage

Salvage following total wrist arthroplasty done by arthrodesis with bone grafting (Fig. 21.337).

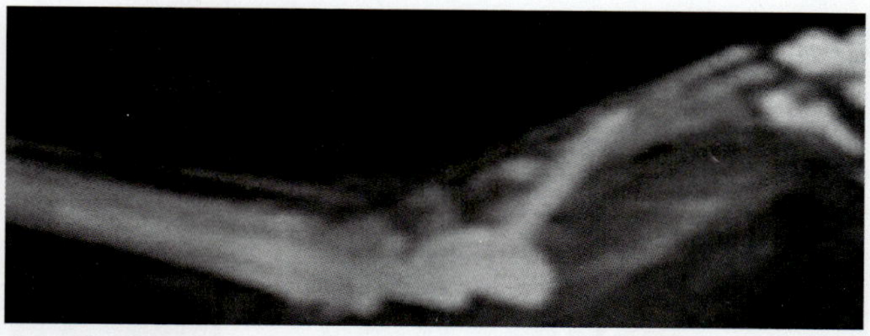

Fig. 21.336: Meuli's design with distal component loosening and volar migration into carpal canal

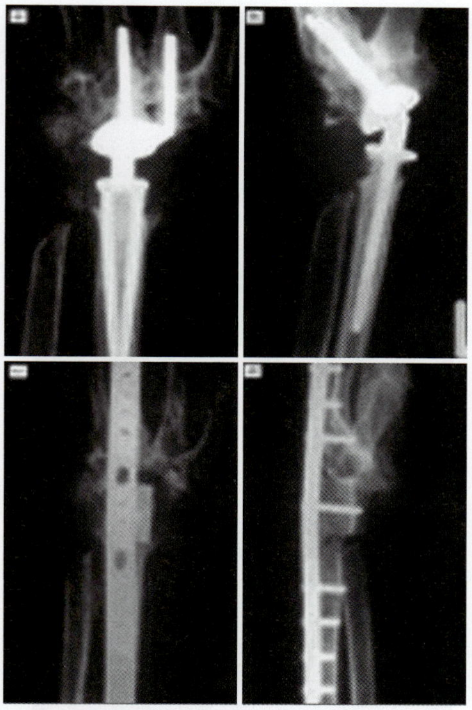

Fig. 21.337: Salvage after arthroplasty done by arthrodesis with bone grafting

Current Considerations

As a result of deterioration with the first generation of implants other designs were being developed in an attempt to improve durability, balance and function.

- *Guepar prosthesis by Alnot:* It is backed with polyethylene component proximally and is fixed with screws distally (Fig. 21.338).
- *Clayton and Ferlic prosthesis:* Clayton and Ferlic developed prosthesis for biologic fixation with proximal ball and distal cup portion.
- *Menon's prosthesis:* It has metal backing at the radial component and screw fixation distally (Fig. 21.339).

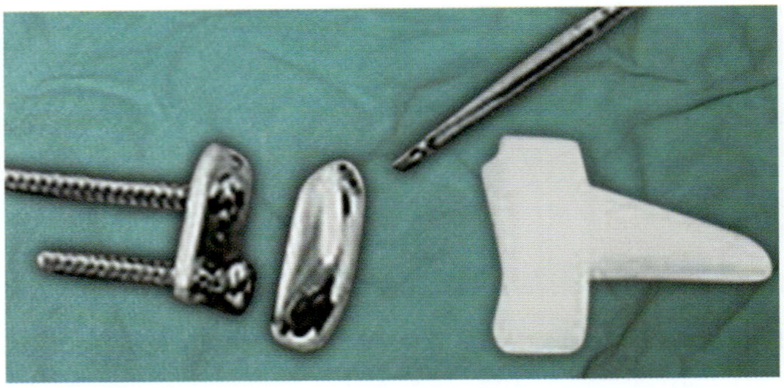

Fig. 21.338: Guepar prosthesis

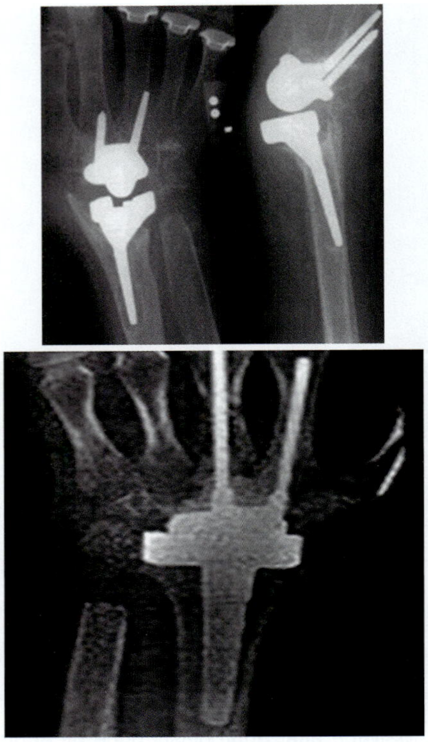

Fig. 21.339: Clayton and Ferlic prosthesis

- *Biaxial wrist prosthesis:* The radial component stem is offset radially and the metacarpal component is curved to match the shape of the long metacarpal (Figs 21.340 and 21.341).

Procedure

- Make curved dorsal longitudinal incision, preserving the veins and sensory nerves. Split the dorsal retinaculum over the extensor digitorum tendons and reflect it to the radial side. Detach the dorsal capsule from the radius and reflect it distally as a widely based flap. Detach the radial collateral ligament from the radius and carefully protect the abductor pollicis longus and extensor pollicis brevis tendons

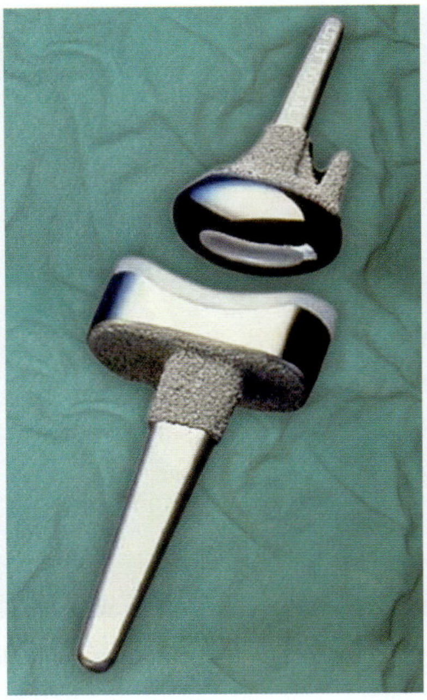

Fig. 21.340: Biaxial wrist prosthesis

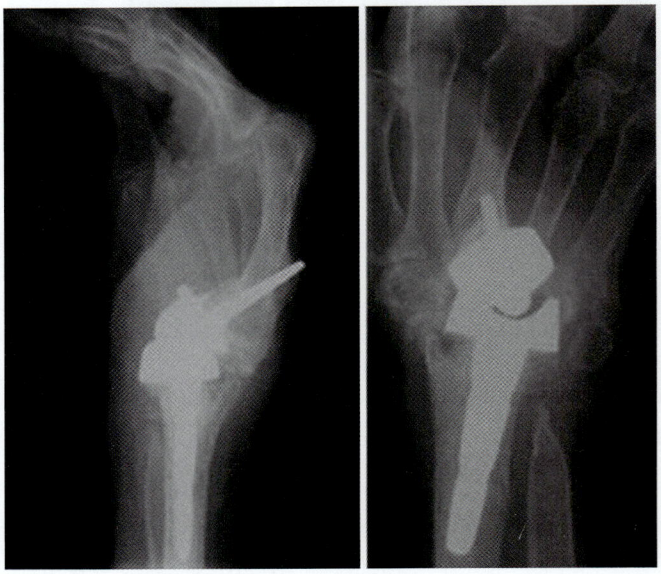

Fig. 21.341: X-ray of biaxial wrist prosthesis

- Now-hyperflex the radiocarpal joint, to expose the distal radius. Remove the lunate, the proximal half of the scaphoid and the radial side of the triquetrum. Resect the radial styloid in line with the distal articular surface of the radius at 90° to the long axis of the radius. Preserve as much cortical bone as possible to provide support. When the joint is dislocated, resect more of the radius as necessary. Align the wrist and prepare the capitate and the base of the third metacarpal to receive the prosthesis

- To ensure proper placement of the reamer in the medullary canal of the third metacarpal, insert a Kirschner wire and check its position by roentgenograms. Then ream with an awl or if necessary, with a power reamer. Do not perforate the metacarpal shaft. The size of the third metacarpal shaft will determine the size of the prosthesis. Use this shaft for size and then ream the radius to fit the opposite stem of the prosthesis. Smooth the base of the capitate and radius, to eliminate any sharp bony edges that could cause a prosthetic fracture. Use metal sleeve "grommets" as needed. Seat the prosthesis against the radius and capitate, so that there is no tendency for buckling
- Align the hand on the wrist, avoiding ulnar deviation or flexion. See that passive flexion and extension of about 30° each are possible without blockage. Strip the volar capsule, if it is too tight. Next resect the distal ulna. Close the capsule with sutures passed through holes drilled in the dorsal cortex of the distal radius. Reattach the collateral ligament of the radius and realign the dorsal retinaculum under the finger and wrist extensors
- Relocate the extensor carpi ulnaris tendon dorsally, to prevent it from functioning as a wrist flexor. If it has shifted palmarward, pass it through a pulley created from a segment of the dorsal retinaculum if necessary. Repair any extensor tendons as indicated and close the wound loosely. Insert a suction drain and apply a bulky dressing and a plaster splint.

After Treatment

- The splint is worn for 5 to 6 weeks
- At third week, limited wrist motion is started and at fourth week active motion is begun.
- A total motion of 60° is considered satisfactory and 95 percent of patients obtain relief from pain.

Contraindications for Arthroplasty

- Chronic subluxation
- Poor bone
- Prior infection
- Impaired motor or neurologic function
- Use of walker or cane
- Impaired wrist extensor tendons.

22 Elbow

- Anatomy, Biomechanics and Examination of the Elbow
- Congenital Anomalies Around the Elbow Joint
- Trauma to Elbow-fractures Around Elbow
- Myositis Ossificans
- Volkmann's Ischemic Contracture
- Osteochondritis Dissecans of Elbow
- Tennis Elbow and Golfer's Elbow
- Inflammations Around Elbow
- Elbow Arthrodesis
- Elbow Arthroplasty
- Tumors Around the Elbow

ANATOMY, BIOMECHANICS AND EXAMINATION OF THE ELBOW

Anatomy

The elbow joint, although a single synovial cavity is made up of three distinct articulations:

- *The humeroulnar:* Between the trochlea of the humerus and the trochlear notch of the ulna (a hinge-joint)
- *The humeroradial:* Between the capitulum and the upper concave surface of the radial head (a ball and socket joint)
- *The superior radioulnar:* Between the head of the radius and the radial notch of the ulna, the head being held in place by the tough annular ligament (a pivot joint)
- The capsule of the elbow joint is closely applied around this complex articular arrangement
- The nonarticular medial and lateral epicondyles are extracapsular
- The capsule is thin and loose anteriorly and posteriorly, to allow flexion and extension, whereas it is strongly thickened on either side to form the medial and lateral collateral ligaments
- *Two set of movements takes place at the elbow:*
  - Flexion and extension at the humeroulnar and humeroradial joints (Figs 22.1A and B)
  - Pronation and supination at the proximal radioulnar (in conjunction with associated movements of the distal radioulnar joint) (Figs 22.2A and B).

Muscles Acting on Elbow

Muscles acting on the elbow are shown in Table 22.1.

Collateral Ligaments of Elbow

Medial Collateral Ligament Complex (Fig. 22.3)

The anterior component is the most easily identifiable. It is the major portion that inserts along the medial aspect of the coronoid process. It is taut with the elbow in flexion and in extension. The posterior component is taut during flexion.

Lateral Ligament Complex (Fig. 22.4)

- The radial collateral ligament arises from the lateral epicondyle and inserts into the annular ligament along with fibers of the capsule
- The lateral ulnar collateral ligament consists of posterior fibers of the radial collateral ligament, which extend superficial to and across the annular ligament, inserting in a tubercle on the crista supinatorius of the ulna
- The accessory lateral collateral ligament arises from the lateral epicondyle and inserts into the inferior margin of the annular ligament. It is taut when the elbow is stressed in varus
- The annular ligament arises and inserts on the anterior and posterior margins of the lesser sigmoid notch of the ulna and stabilizes the radial head adjacent to the ulna
- In extension, the anterior capsule provides approximately 70 percent of soft-tissue restraint to distraction
- Valgus stress in extension is divided equally among the medial collateral ligament, capsule and joint surfaces
- Varus stress in extension is limited equally by the joint articulation, lateral collateral ligament and capsule

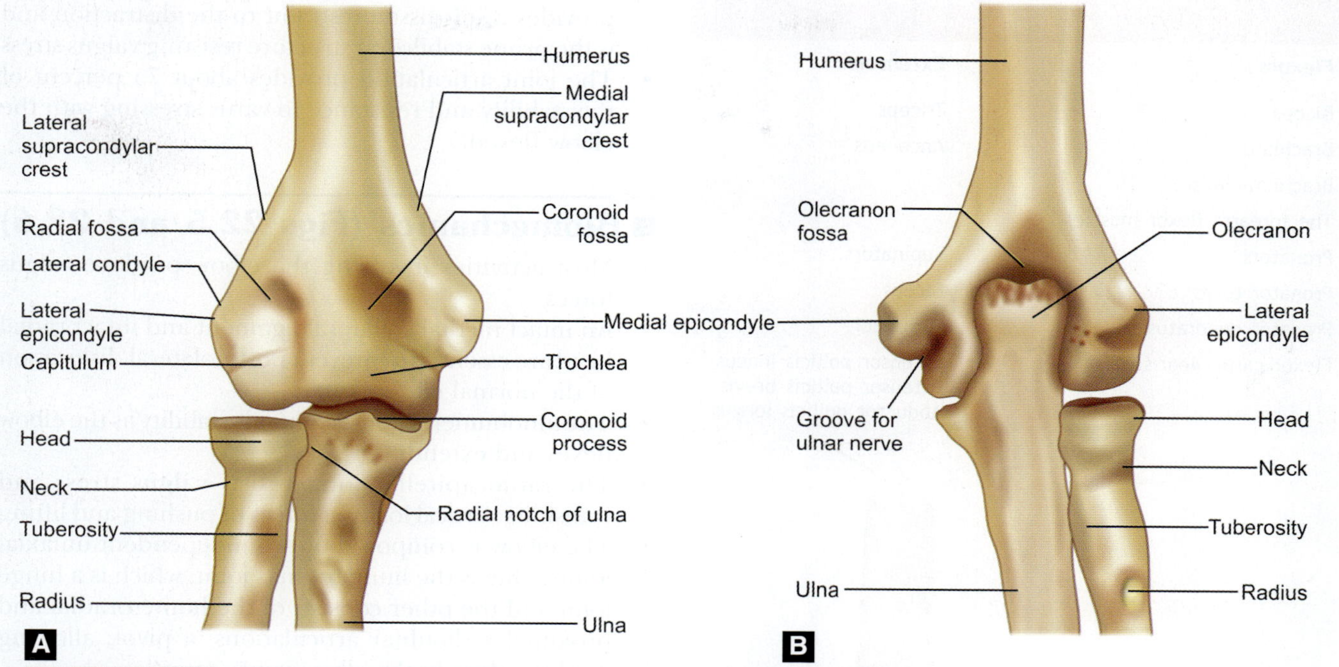

Figs 22.1A and B: View of elbow joint in extension— (A) Anterior view; (B) Posterior view

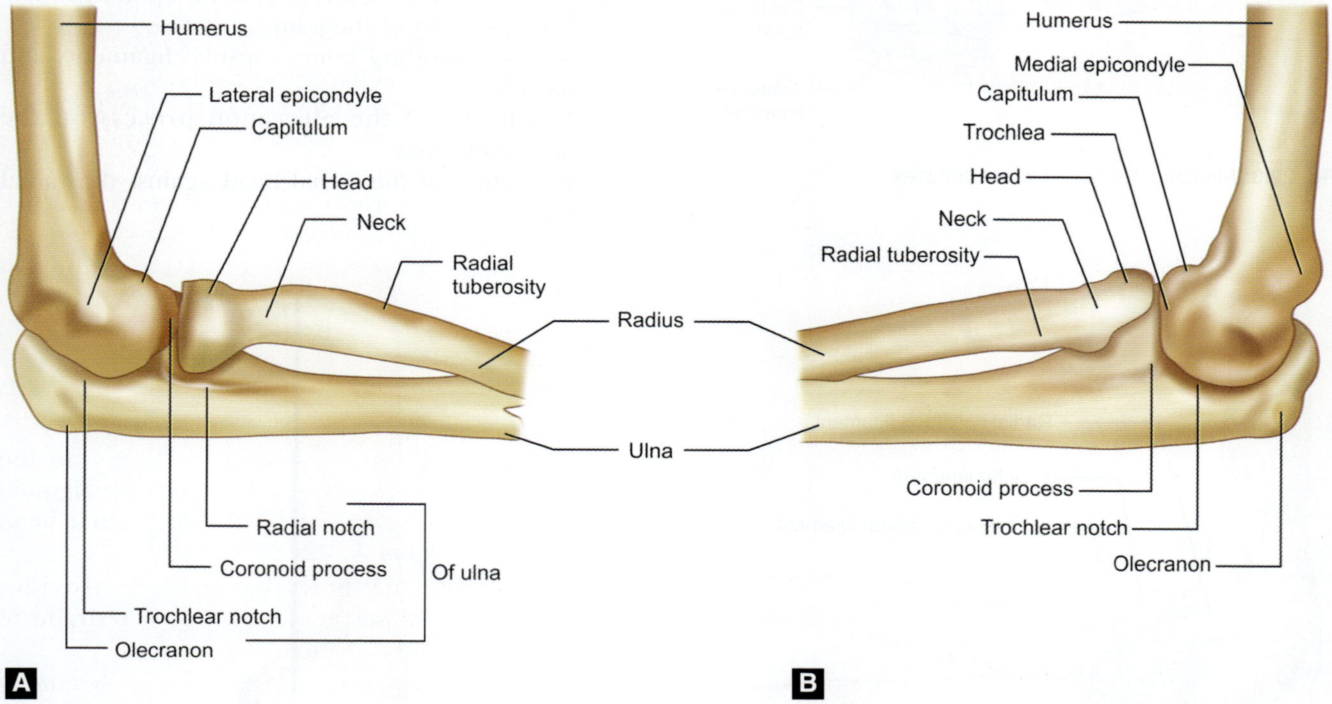

Figs 22.2A and B: View of elbow joint in 90° flexion—(A) Lateral view; (B) Medial view

Table 22.1: Different muscles acting on the elbow	
Flexors	***Extensors***
Biceps	Triceps
Brachialis	Anconeus
Brachioradialis	
The forearm flexor muscles	
Pronators	Supinators
Pronator teres	Biceps
Pronator quadratus	Supinator
Flexor carpi ulnaris	Extensor pollicis longus Extensor pollicis brevis Abductor pollicis longus

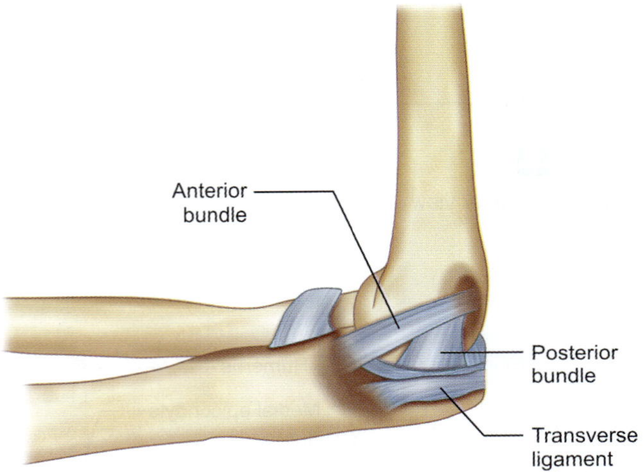

Fig. 22.3: Medial collateral ligament complex

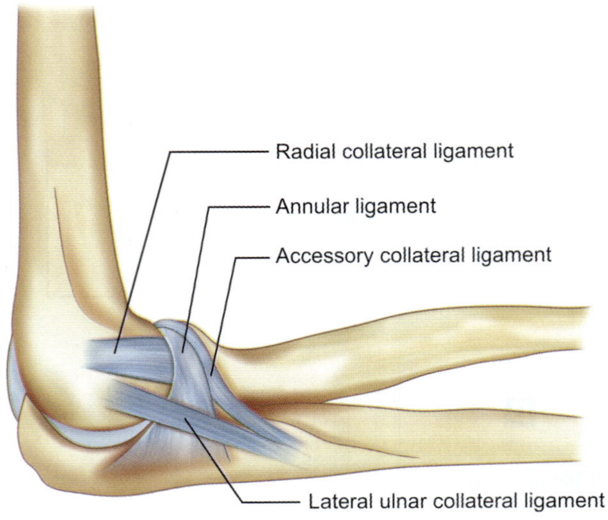

Fig. 22.4: Lateral ligament complex of elbow

- In flexion, the medial collateral ligament complex provides a soft-tissue restraint to the distraction and is the prime stabilizing structure resisting valgus stress
- The joint articulation provides about 75 percent of the stability and resistance to varus stressing with the elbow flexed.

■ Biomechanics (Figs 22.5 and 22.6)

- Most activities involving the elbow produce valgus forces
- An intact medial collateral ligament and intact radial head are essential to prevent posterolateral dislocation of the normal elbow joint
- The ulnohumeral joint maintains stability as the elbow flexes and extends
- The radiocapitellar joint resists valgus stress and transmits vertical loading forces of pushing and lifting
- The elbow is composed of two independent uniaxial joints. One is the humeroulnar joint, which is a hinge joint and the other consists of the humeroradial and proximal radioulnar articulations, a pivot, allowing 2° of freedom in the elbow joint
- Motion in the elbow involves rotation of the ulna around the humerus, during flexion and extension and rotation of the radius around the ulna, during supination and pronation
- The anatomical restraints of elbow motion include:
  - The geometry of the joint
  - The surrounding bone, capsule, ligaments and muscles
  - Impaction of the olecranon process on the olecranon fossa
  - Impaction of the radial head against the radial fossa

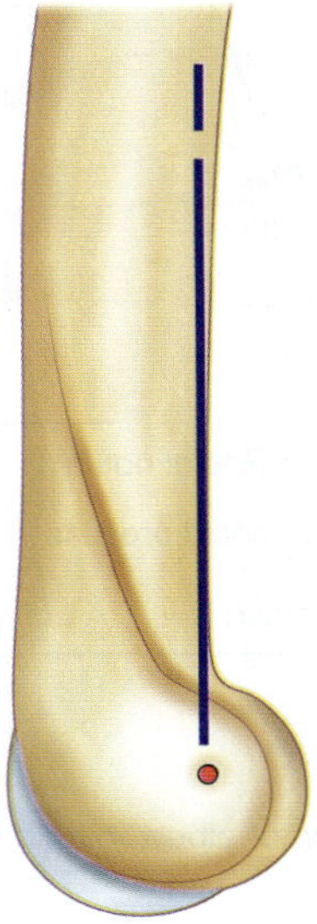

Fig. 22.5: Instant center of extension and flexion of elbow at the center of trochlea (as viewed from lateral aspect)

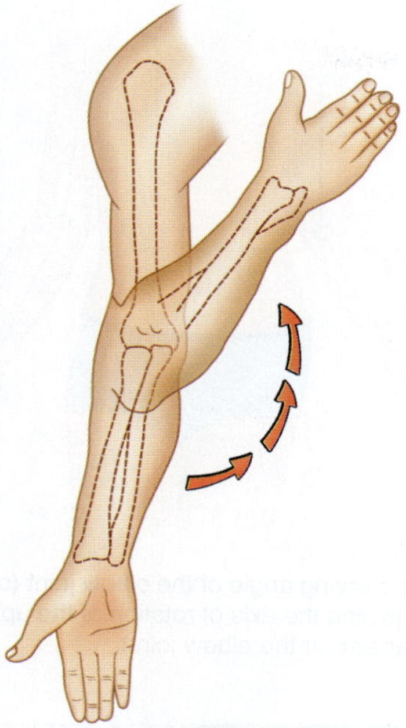

Fig. 22.6: Axis of elbow rotation

- Rotation is limited by passive resistance of the stretched muscles, ligaments and impingement of the flexor pollicis longus against the finger flexors
- The instant center of flexion and extension for the elbow at the center of concentric circles formed by the lateral projection of the capitulum and trochlea of the distal humerus is about 2 to 3 mm in diameter and is located in the center of the trochlea, when viewed from the lateral aspect (Fig. 22.5). The axis of rotation of the elbow lies anterior to the humeral midline and on a line drawn along the anterior cortex of the humerus.
- Morrey and Chao found that the carrying angle varied from 11° of valgus with the elbow in full extension to 6° of varus with the elbow in full flexion (Fig. 22.6)
- The contact surfaces of the elbow change with different elbow positions. In full extension, the contact surfaces are on the inferomedial aspect of the ulna and in other positions, most of the joint contact occurs along the trochlear notch, which passes from posterolateral to anteromedial
- Electromyographic studies of elbow muscle activity show that the brachialis is active in most ranges of elbow motion and is the "workhorse" of flexion
- The joint surfaces slide until the extremes of full flexion and extension are reached and then bony impingement occurs
- The transverse axis of rotation of the radiohumeral joint coincides with the ulnohumeral axis. The longitudinal axes of the forearm passes through the radial head proximally and the ulnar head distally and is oblique to the longitudinal axes of the radius and ulna
- The normal range of motion of the elbow is from 0° (full extension) to approximately 150° (full flexion)
- The forces around the elbow joint forces are greatest in extension. The flexed elbow being able to tolerate higher loads than the extended.
- Elbow joint forces also are found to be greatest in pronation
- Maximal elbow flexion strength occurs at 90°. One third to one half of the maximal lifting force can be generated with the elbow in an extended or a 30° flexed position.
- A force three times the body weight can be developed in the elbow joint during strenuous lifting. Considerable rotatory torque is developed at the distal humerus, when the elbow is flexed to 90° and force is applied to the hand from the side.
- Tensile forces on the medial collateral ligament can approach two times the body weight and compressive forces on the radial head can approach three times the body weight
- If the radial head is excised, humeroradial force is transmitted to the ulna and the medial collateral ligament tension adds to the humeroulnar force, which may concentrate the entire load on the lateral edge of the coronoid process. This may apply a force of nine times the body weight to the medial collateral ligament.

■ Examination

Inspection (Figs 22.7 to 22.10)

- Focus at the attitude of the upper limb and look for:
  - Generalized swelling
  - Muscle wasting
- Earliest clinical sign of effusion is filling of hollows, which is seen in fixed elbow above the olecranon (Fig. 22.7)
- Look for any localized swellings around the elbow (Fig. 22.8), e.g. rheumatoid nodules or olecranon bursitis
- Look for any scars or sinuses (Fig. 22.9)
- *The carrying angle (Fig. 22.10):* The normal carrying angle is 11° in males and 13° in females. Look for varus (decreased carrying angle) or valgus (increased carrying angle) deformities at the elbow, by extending both the upper limbs fully and comparing them. In cases of fixed flexion deformity of the elbow, the carrying angle cannot be determined and one should not comment on the valgus or varus deformity.

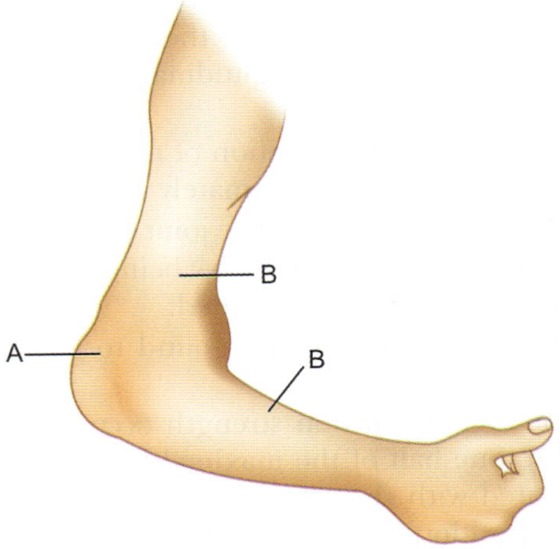

Fig. 22.7: Earliest sign of effusion, hollows of elbow above olecranon gets filled— A. Swelling; B. Hollow

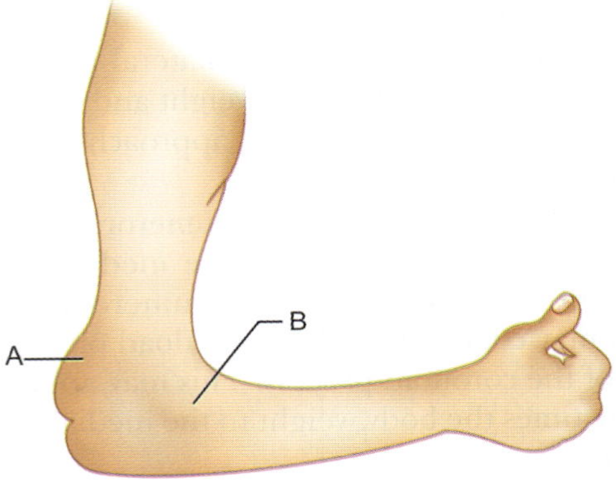

Fig. 22.8: Inspect for any localized swelling around elbow joint, A and B. Swelling

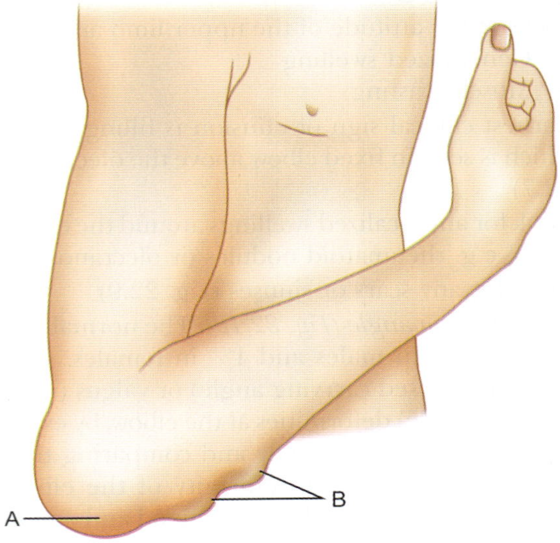

Fig. 22.9: Inspection done for scars and sinuses—A. Scar; B. Sinuses

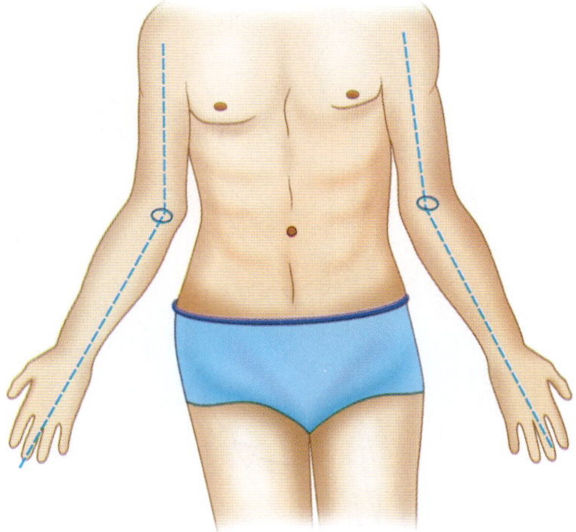

Fig. 22.10: The carrying angle of the elbow joint (seen as a dotted line joining the axis of rotation of the upper arm and the lower arm at the elbow joint)

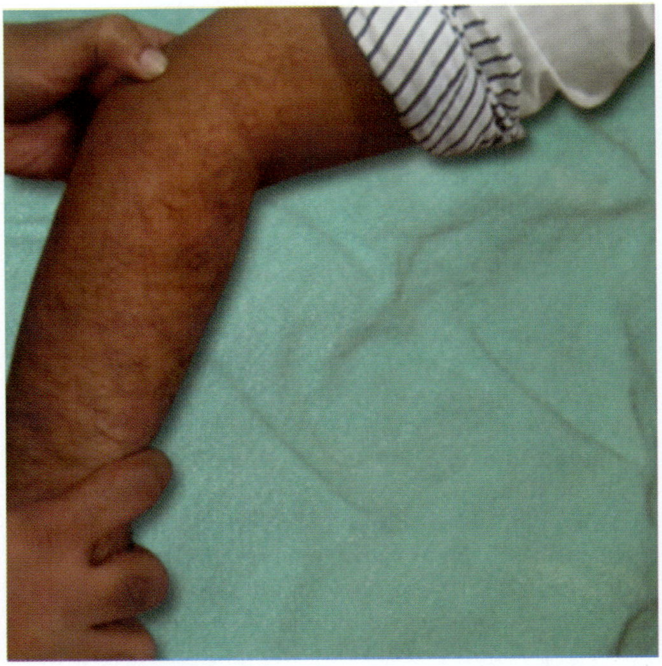

Fig. 22.11: Eliciting tenderness over lateral epicondyle

Palpation

- Look for local rise in temperature
- Look for joint line tenderness
- Palpate the three prominent bony landmarks, i.e. the medial epicondyles, lateral epicondyles and the olecranon
- Sharply localized tenderness at the lateral epicondyle is almost diagnostic of tennis elbow (Fig. 22.11)
- Sharply localized tenderness at the medial epicondyle is almost diagnostic of golfers' elbow

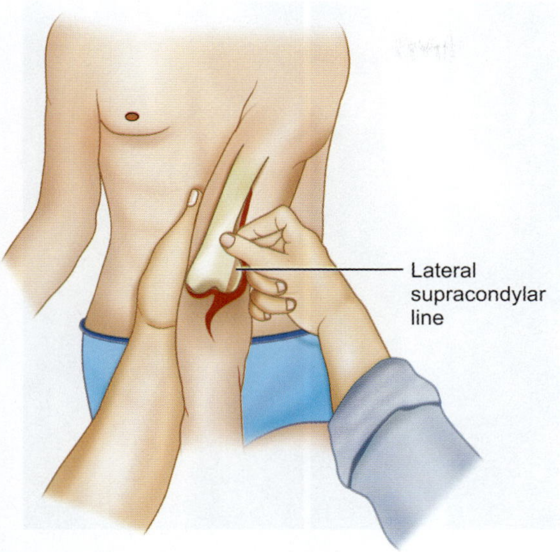

Fig. 22.12: Palpating the supracondylar ridge

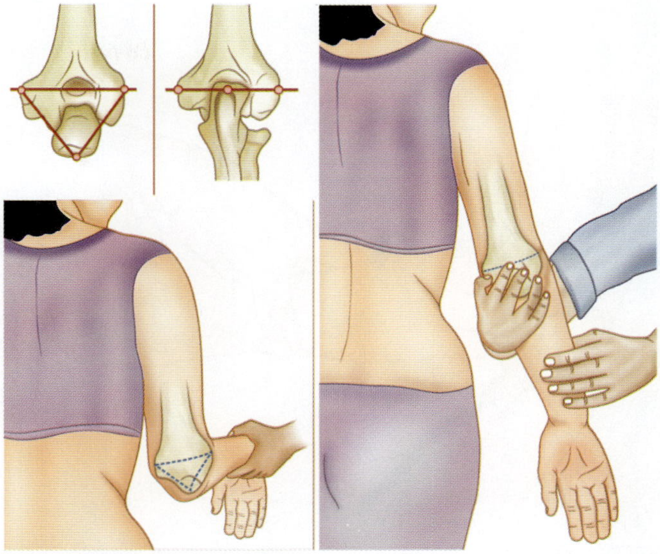

Fig. 22.13: Isosceles triangle of elbow

- Tenderness over the olecranon is uncommon, except after trauma or infected olecranon bursitis
- Palpate the supracondylar ridge of humerus (Fig. 22.12) and look for any thickening, suggestive of old supracondylar fractures.

Isosceles Triangle of the Elbow

- When the elbow is flexed, the olecranon and the medial and lateral epicondyles form an isosceles triangle, as shown in Figure 22.13
- These three points come to lie in a straight line, when the elbow is extended
- Altered distance between the two condyles and olecranon is seen in intercondylar fractures or isolated fracture of medial or lateral condyle
- Palpate the lateral epicondyle of the humerus and distally the elbow joint, 1 cm more distal to it feels a firm rounded structure under the thumb. This is the radial head
- Now pronate and supinate the forearm and feel its movement under the thumb (Fig. 22.14)
- Palpate the thumb firmly into the space on the lateral side of elbow between the radial head and humerus, any tenderness here is common after injuries to the radial head, osteoarthritis and osteochondritis dessicans (Fig. 22.15)
- For abnormal position of radial head, as occurs in dislocated radial head, one must look for ulnar Bow sign, as explained ahead
- The relationship is disturbed in any pathological condition, such as intercondylar fracture of the humerus, elbow dislocation, etc. (Fig. 22.16)
- Reversal of triangle is seen in posterior dislocation of elbow (Fig. 22.17)

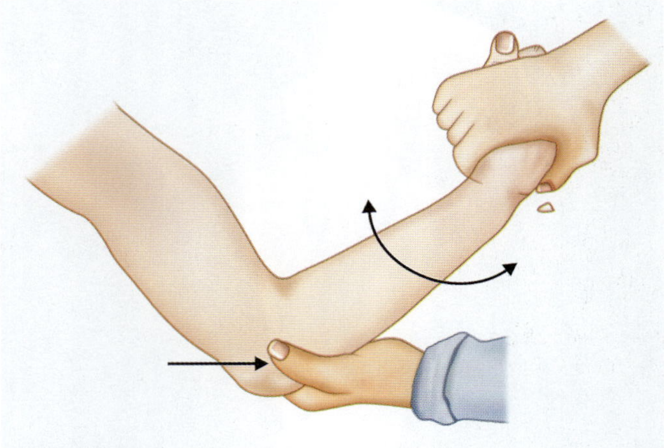

Fig. 22.14: Pronating and supinating the forearm and palpating its movement under the thumb

- There may be an associated Monteggia fracture or dislocation.

Ulnar Bow Sign

It is an undetected, isolated radial head dislocation. The shape of ulna indicated persistent plastic deformation of the ulna (Figs 22.18 and 22.19)

- The ulnar bow line is drawn between the distal ulna and olecranon, defines the ulnar bow
- The ulnar bow sign is deviation of more than 1mm of ulnar border from the reference line
- Palpate the front of the elbow on both sides of the biceps tendon, while flexing and extending the elbow through 20° (Fig. 22.20)

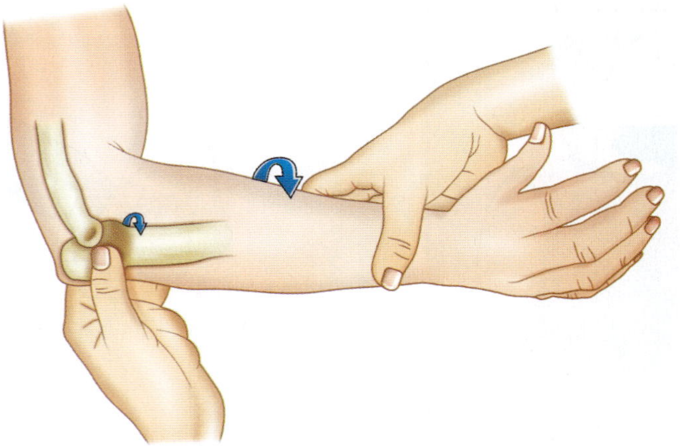

Fig. 22.15: Palpation of the thumb firmly into the space on the lateral side of elbow between the radial head and humerus

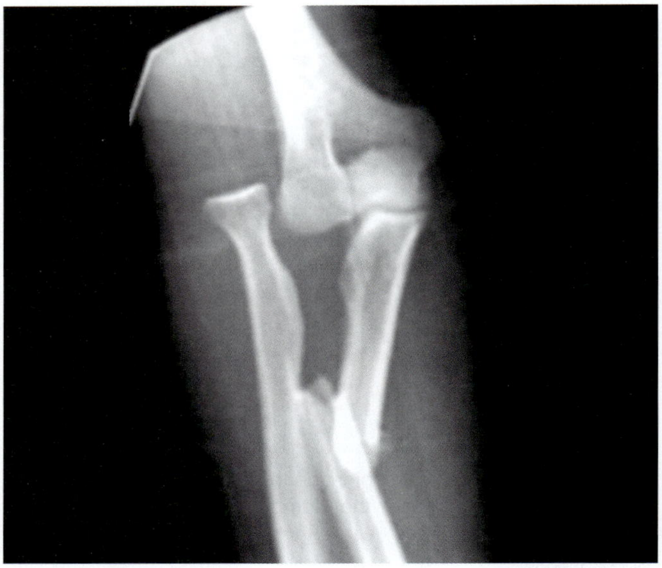

Fig. 22.16: Disturbed anatomy of the isosceles triangle of elbow in case of fracture forearm

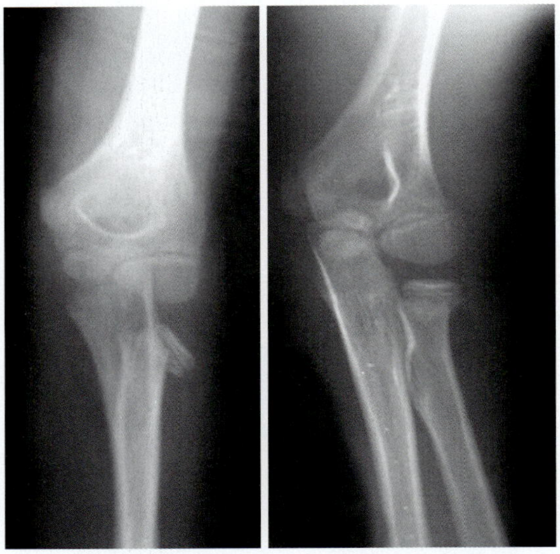

Fig. 22.17: Disturbed anatomy of the isosceles triangle of elbow in case of elbow dislocation

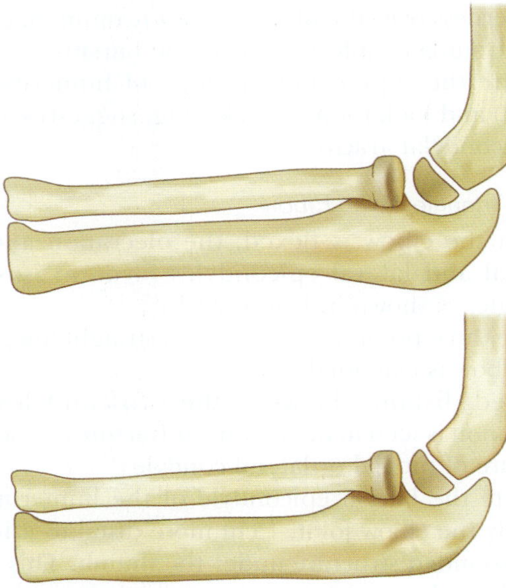

Fig. 22.18: Ulnar bow sign

- Notice any abnormal masses or thickening of bone (myositis ossificans, loose bodies or osteochondritis dessicans)
- Look for synovial thickening, doughy.

Movements

- The normal range of motion of flexion (Fig. 22.21). Movements of elbow flexion 135° and extension 0°-5°.
- The normal range of motion of pronation and supination is 90° (Fig. 22.22)
- The range of motion testing should be done passively as well as actively.

Additional Tests

Mills' Maneuver (Fig. 22.23)

- Flex the elbow and fully pronate the hand
- Now extend the elbow
- Pain over the lateral epicondyle is almost diagnostic of tennis elbow
- As an alternative, pain may be sought by pronating the arm with the elbow fully extended (Fig. 22.24)

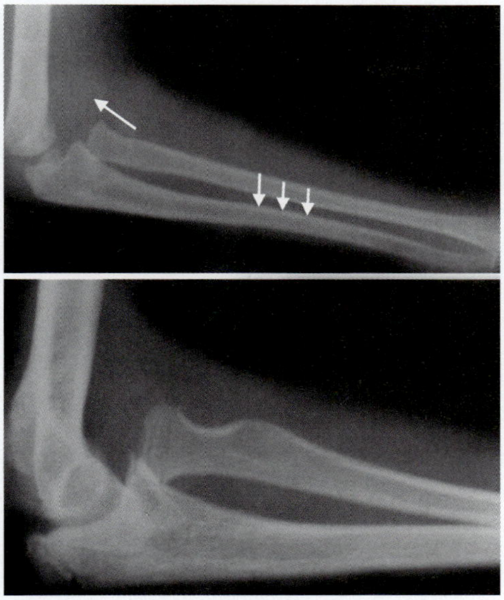

Fig. 22.19: X-ray showing ulnar bow sign

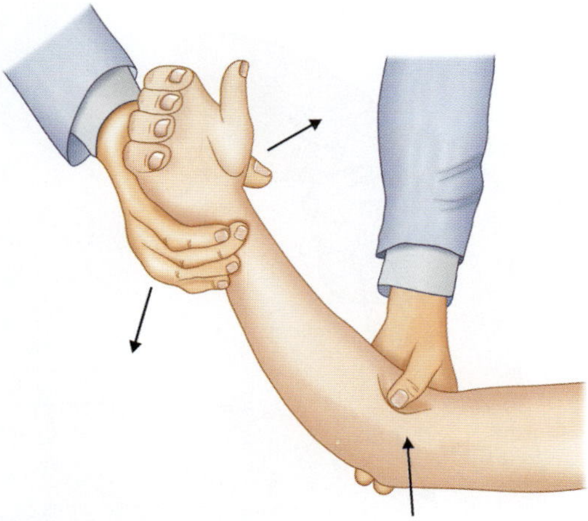

Fig. 22.20: Demonstrating the ulnar bow sign

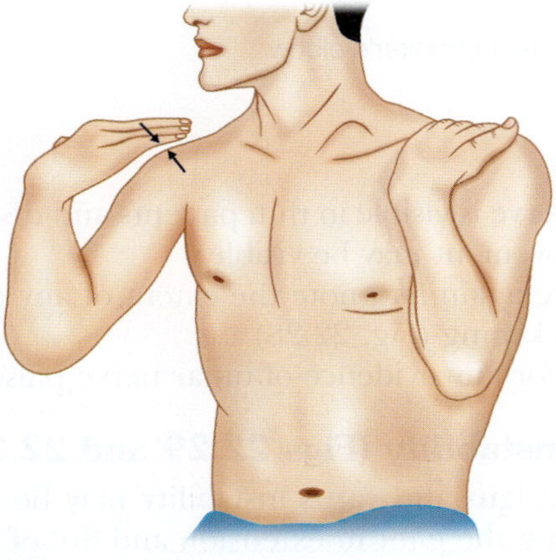

Fig. 22.21: Flexion movement of elbow joint

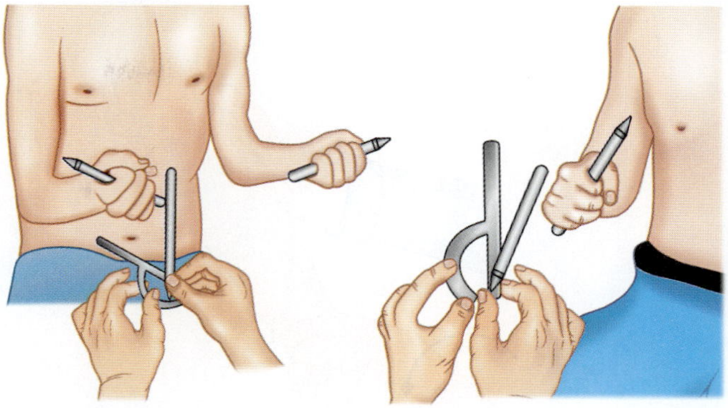

Fig. 22.22: Supination and pronation movements of elbow

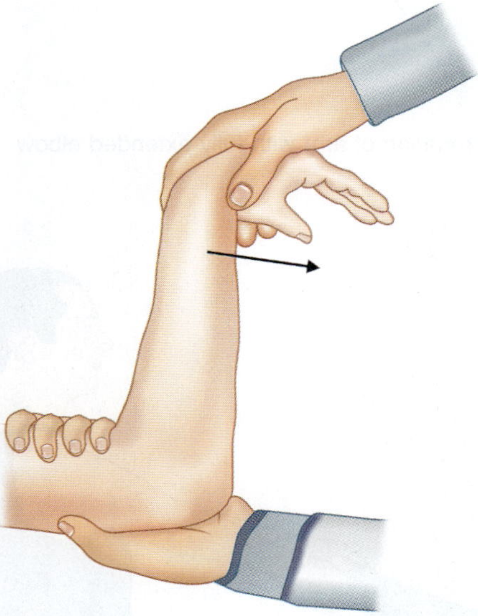

Fig. 22.23: Mills' maneuver

Chair Test (Fig. 22.25)

- Ask the patient to attempt to lift the chair (3.5 kg) with the elbows extended and the shoulders flexed to 60°
- Difficulty in performing this maneuver, with complaint of pain on the lateral aspect of the elbow is suggestive of tennis elbow.

Thomsen's Test or Cozen's Test (Fig. 22.26)

- Ask the patient to clench the fist, dorsiflex the wrist and extend the elbow
- Try to force the hand into palmar flexion, while the patient resists
- Severe pain over the lateral epicondyle is suggestive of tennis elbow
- Also repeat the test, this time attempting to flex the extended middle finger rather than the wrist.

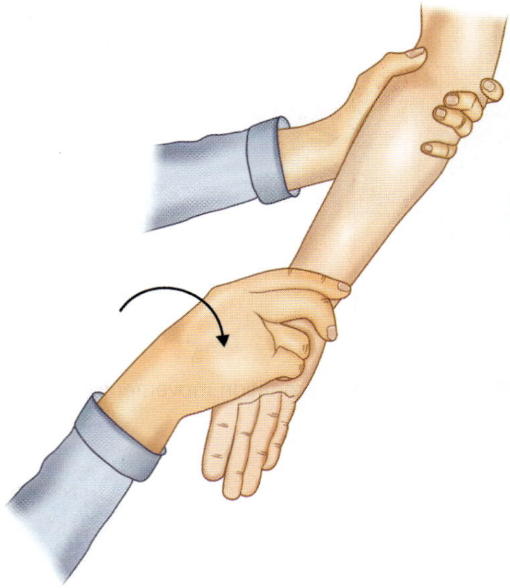

Fig. 22.24: Pronation of arm with fully extended elbow

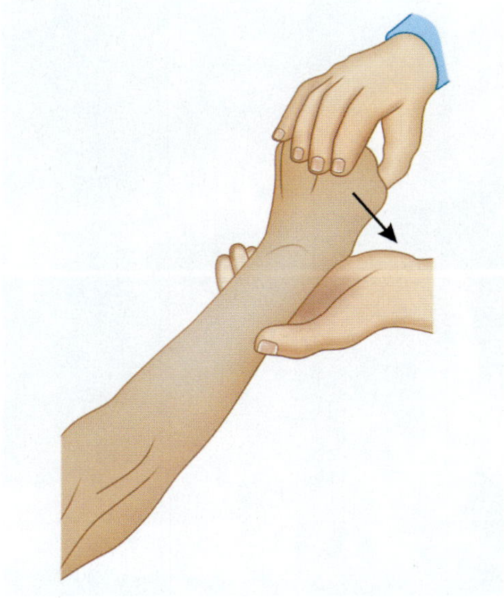

Fig. 22.26: Thomsen's test (Cozen's test)

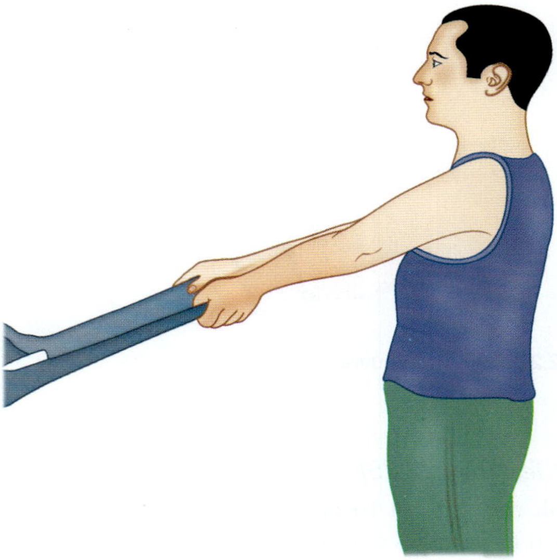

Fig. 22.25: Chair test

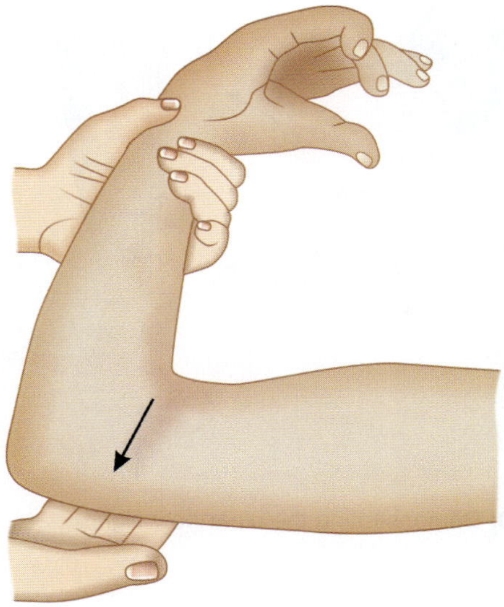

Fig. 22.27: Test of golfer's elbow

Golfer's Elbow (Fig. 22.27)

- Flex the elbow, supinate the hand and then extend the elbow
- Pain over the medial epicondyle is very suggestive of golfer's elbow.

Ulnar Nerve Palsy (Fig. 22.28)

- Inspect the medial side of the joint carefully, while the patient flexes and extends the elbow
- The nerve is visible in thin patients and displacement on movement may be visible
- Palpate again and note the extent of any tenderness or thickening (Fig. 22.28)
- Look for any evidence of ulnar nerve palsy.

Elbow Instability (Figs 22.29 and 22.30)

- Both valgus and varus instability may be elicited by stressing the joint in extension and 30° of flexion

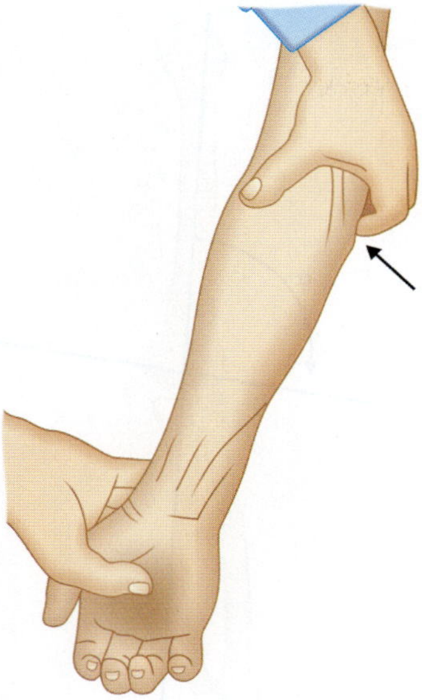

Fig. 22.28: Palpating ulnar nerve on the medial aspect of the joint

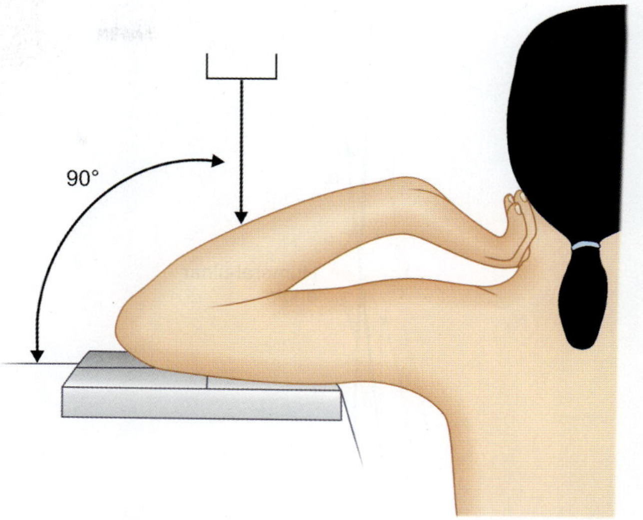

Fig. 22.30: Procedure for testing elbow instability, when extension is not possible

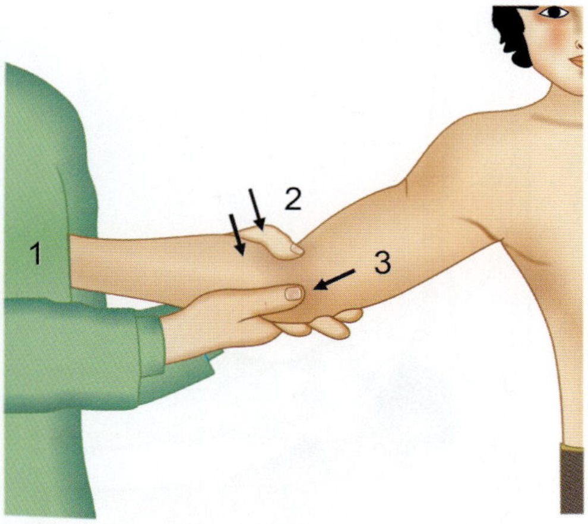

Fig. 22.29: Test for elbow instability—1. The fixed arm; 2. The valgus force; 3. Opening up of the medial joint space

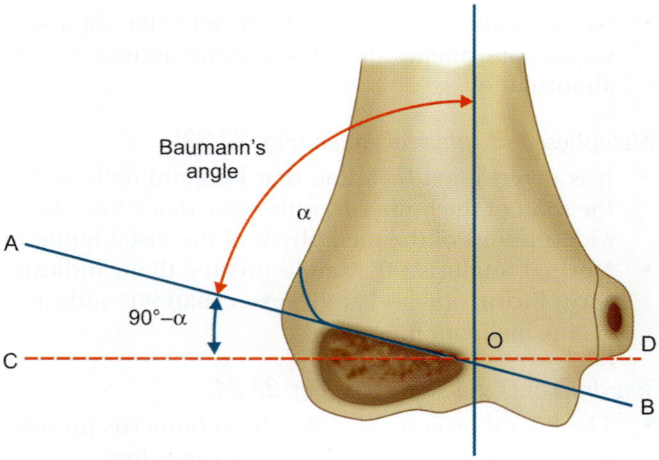

Fig. 22.31: Baumann's angle

- Any gap or opening up of the joint space is noted, as shown in Figure 22.29
- Another method for finding joint instability, mainly carried out in children, where extension is not possible due to pain is shown in Figure 22.30
- The radius or ulna and their relation to each other is seen
- The humerus is overlapped, but the supracondylar fractures can be visualized with the displacements.

Angles Around Elbow

Baumann's Angle (Fig. 22.31)

- It is the angulation of the physeal line between the lateral condyle and the distal humeral metaphysis
- The ossification center of the lateral condyle extends into the radial or lateral crista of trochlea. This line forms an angle with long axis of the humerus called the Baumann's angle.
- Different Baumann's angles and its significance
  - Normal Baumann's angle is 72°
  - Angle greater than 81° is cubitus varus
  - Angle less than 61° is cubitus valgus
  - A change in 5° of Baumann's angle corresponds to 2° change in clinical carrying angle.

Humeral-Ulnar Angle (Fig. 22.32)

- It is determined by lines longitudinally bisecting the shaft of humerus with shaft of ulna.

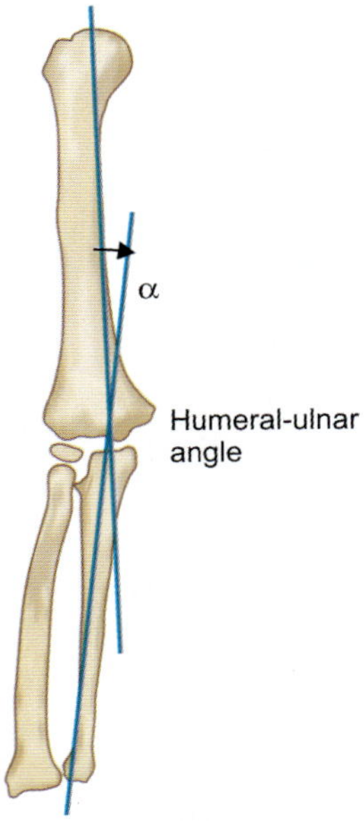

Fig. 22.32: Humeral-ulnar angle

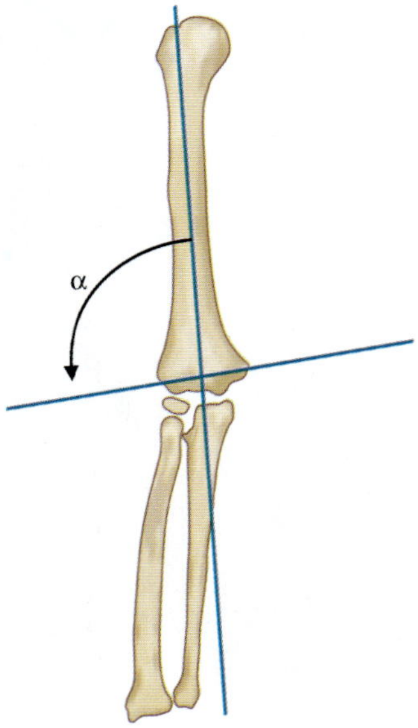

Fig. 22.33: Metaphyseal-diaphyseal angle

- Normal value is 12° to 18°. A greater value signifies a valgus abnormality and a lesser value signifies a varus abnormality.

Metaphyseal-diaphyseal Angle (Fig. 22.33)

- It is determined by a line that longitudinally bisects the shaft of the humerus, with a line that connects the widest points of the metaphysis of the distal humerus
- Normal angle is 90°. Angle greater than, indicates varus inclination and angle lesser than 90° indicated valgus inclination.

Teardrop of Distal Humerus (Fig. 22.34)

- The lateral projection of the distal humerus presents a teardrop like shadow above the capitulum
- On a true lateral film, the teardrop should be well-defined
- *Significance:* Teardrop is disturbed in fractures of distal end of humerus.

Shaft-condylar Angle

- On lateral X-ray, there is angulation of 40° between the long axis of humerus and long axis of lateral condyle
- *Significance:* It defines extension and flexion type of injury
- If angle is less than 40°, extension deformity is present. If angle greater than 40° flexion deformity is present.

Anterior Humeral Line (Fig. 22.35)

- If a line is drawn along the anterior border of the distal humeral shaft, it should pass through the middle third of ossification center of the capitulum

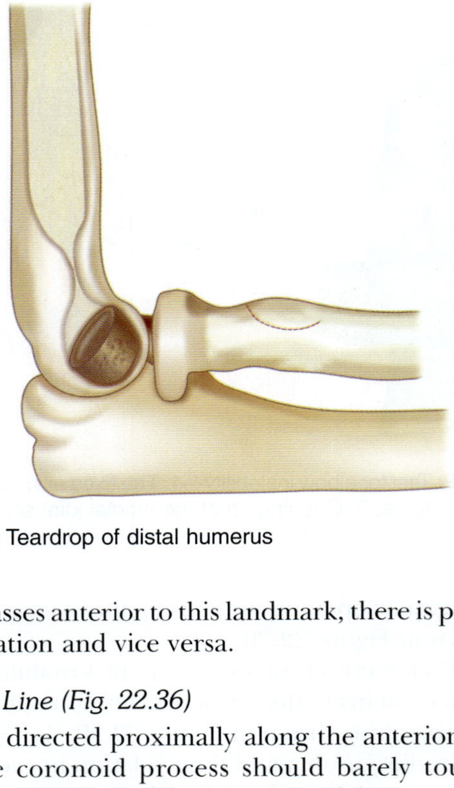

Fig. 22.34: Teardrop of distal humerus

- If it passes anterior to this landmark, there is posterior angulation and vice versa.

Coronoid Line (Fig. 22.36)

- A line directed proximally along the anterior border of the coronoid process should barely touch the anterior portion of the lateral condyle
- Posterior displacement of the lateral condyle projects the ossification center posterior to this coronoid line.

Crescent Sign

In varus deformity, part of ulna overlies distal humeral epiphyses producing crescent sign. This is shown in Figure 22.37.

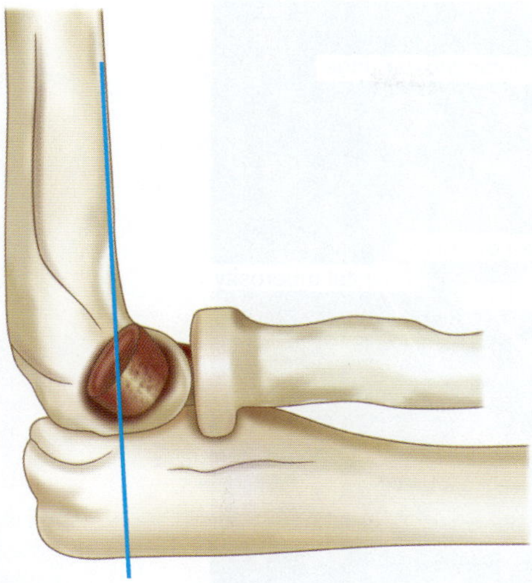

Fig. 22.35: Anterior humeral line

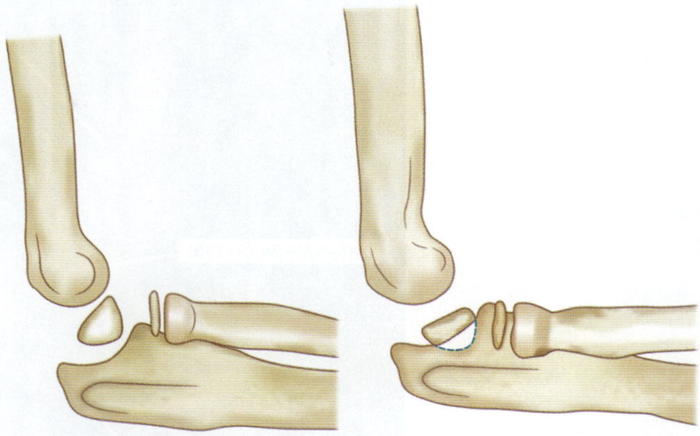

Fig. 22.37: Crescent sign

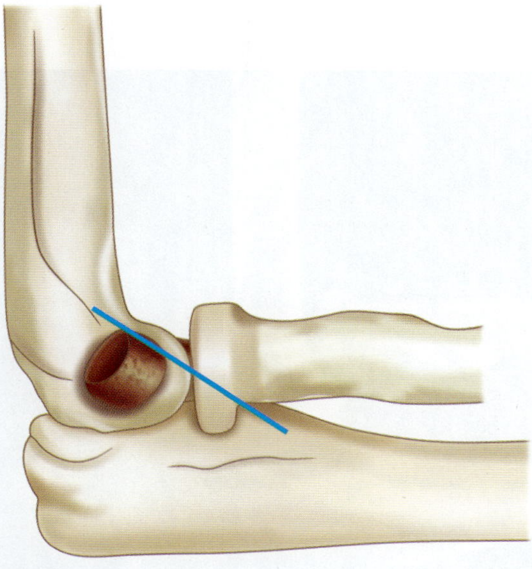

Fig. 22.36: Coronoid line

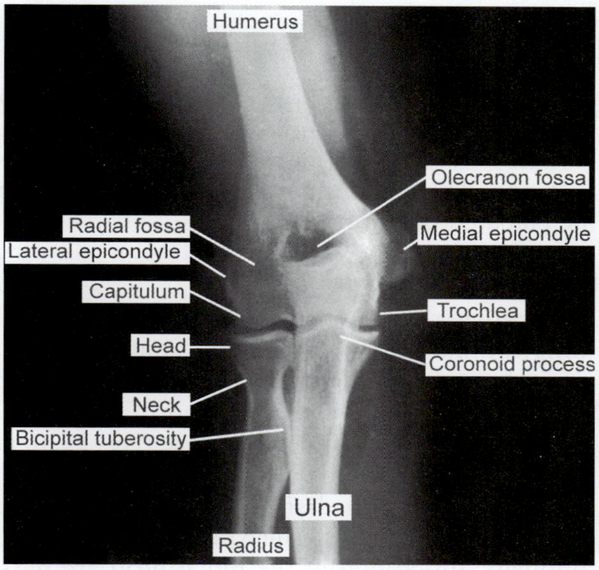

Fig. 22.38: X-ray of the elbow

Radiological Findings

Normal lateral X-ray of the elbow (Figs 22.38 and 22.39).

CONGENITAL ANOMALIES AROUND THE ELBOW JOINT

■ Congenital Radial Head Dislocation

- Congenital dislocation of the radial head was described by McFarland. The direction of the displacement of the radial head may be anterior, posterior or lateral
- Condition is often unilateral
- The abnormality is usually not detected at birth, but is diagnosed later on in childhood when the elbow is examined following some minor injury
- Usually the elbows are asymptomatic. A complaint of stiffness may be reason of visit to physician in some cases.
- The ulna is bowed, in the direction of convexity depending on the type of dislocation:
  - Anterior dislocation—ulnar bow is forward
  - Posterior dislocation—ulnar bow is backward
  - Lateral dislocations—ulnar bow is laterally

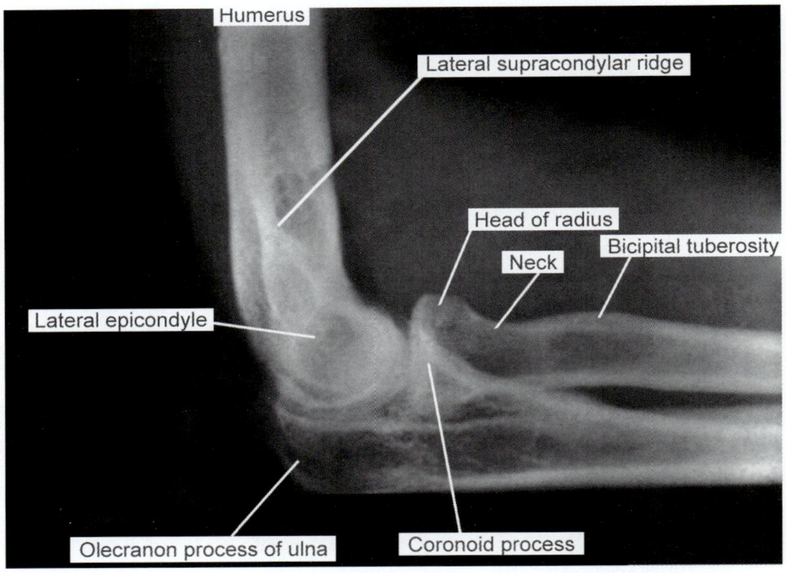

Fig. 22.39: Normal lateral X-ray of the elbow

- In anterior dislocations, the range of elbow flexion is limited and the radial head may be palpated in the cubital fossa. In posterior dislocations, the elbow will not extend fully and the prominent radial head may be palpated posteriorly.

Radiographs

- In a normal elbow, a line drawn through the longitudinal axis of the radial shaft bisects the capitulum of the humerus. This normal finding is absent in this condition. The head of the radius is dome shaped on its superior surface (Figs 22.40 and 22.41)
- It is important to distinguish traumatic from congenital dislocations. The types of injury that cause traumatic dislocation of the radial head are missed Monteggia fracture dislocations, fracture of the radial neck, pulled elbow and occasionally a primary traumatic dislocation of the radial head with other associated injury
- In the newborn and infant, arthrography of the elbow is helpful in the definitive diagnosis of radial head dislocation.

Treatment

- When the diagnosis is made in the newborn or young infant, closed reduction may be attempted
- The posteriorly dislocated radial head is reduced by supination of the forearm and extension of the elbow
- The anteriorly dislocated radial head is reduced by flexion of the elbow

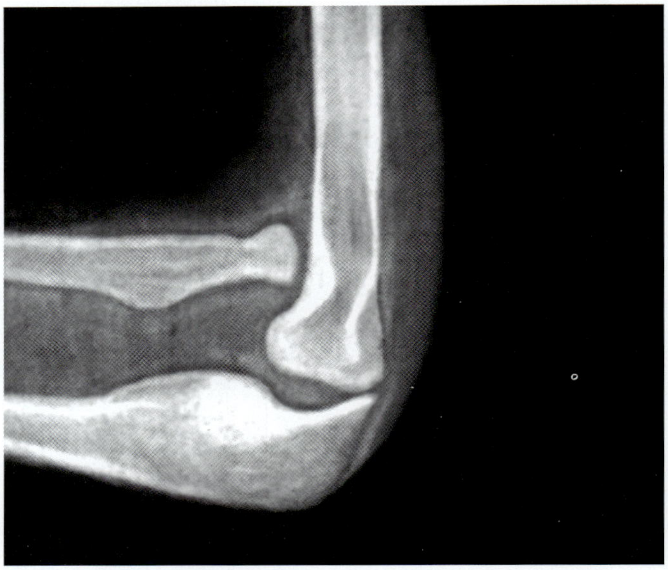

Fig. 22.40: Diagrammatic representation of the superior surface of dome-shaped head of the radius

- Reduction is maintained in an above elbow cast for 4 to 6 weeks
- Closed reduction is often unsuccessful
- In children up to three years of age, open reduction should be carried out
- In the older children, it will be impossible to reduce the radial head
- The dislocation is left alone until late adolescence, when if symptoms warrant, the radial head is excised

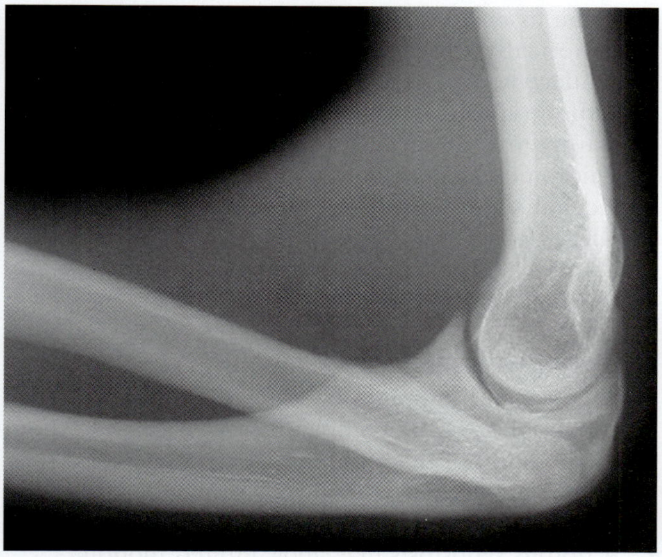

Fig. 22.41: X-ray of the elbow joint showing dome-shaped head of the radius on its superior surface

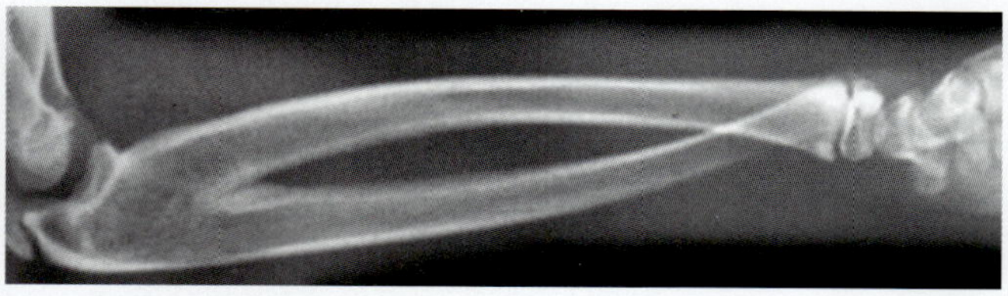

Fig. 22.42: Congenital radioulnar synostosis

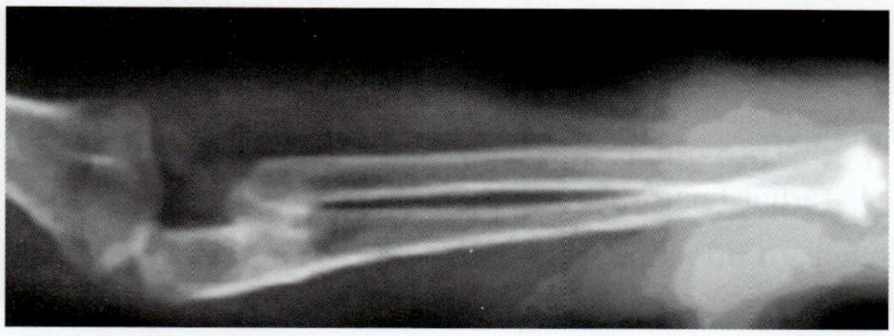

Fig. 22.43: Post-traumatic radioulnar synostosis

■ Congenital Radioulnar Synostosis

- Synostosis or osseous union, of any two adjacent bones can involve any part of the upper extremity. Synostosis between the radius and ulna can take two forms:
  - Congenital (Fig. 22.42)
  - Post-traumatic (Fig. 22.43)
- The degree of fusion in radioulnar synostosis varies and may or may not involve the radial head.

Etiology

Congenital

- In 1793, Sandifort provided the initial description of congenital radial-ulnar (radioulnar) synostosis
- This condition is caused by a failure of segmentation between the radius and ulna
- Embryologically, the upper limb bud arises from the unsegmented body wall between 25 and 28 days
- The elbow becomes visible in 34 days and the humerus, radius and ulna become visible in 37 days
- Initially, the three cartilaginous analogs of the humerus, radius and ulna are connected before segmentation. Therefore, for a short time, the radius and ulna share a common perichondrium.
- Abnormal events at this time can lead to a failure of segmentation
- The duration and severity of the insult can determine the degree of subsequent synostosis
- Endochondral ossification then proceeds and the cartilaginous synostosis ossifies, either partially or completely, in the longitudinal or transverse plane
- In the forearm, congenital radioulnar synostosis usually occurs between the proximal radius and ulna
- Although the condition is present at birth, it usually is not discovered until early adolescence, when the patient presents with a lack of pronation and supination
- Initially, the union may be more of a synchondrosis, but as the skeleton matures, the osseous bridge between the radius and ulna becomes more apparent
- Usually, motion between the two adjacent bones, if existent, is minimal.

Post-traumatic

- It is a separate entity from the congenital form, having a different cause, treatment and prognosis.
- The traumatic form can occur anywhere between the radius and ulna along the length of the interosseous membrane
- The most common cause of post-traumatic radioulnar synostosis is an operatively treated forearm fracture
- Patients with high-energy, comminuted, open fractures appear to be more likely to develop this complication
- Monteggia and proximal forearm fractures also appear to have a higher incidence of synostosis
- The use of bone graft and screws protruding through the opposite cortex also increases the incidence of synostosis
- Additionally, radioulnar synostosis is described as a consequence of soft-tissue injury, reconstructive procedures or any trauma causing hematoma formation between the radius and ulna or injury to the interosseous membrane

- Patients with closed head injuries (skull/cranial trauma) appear to be more prone to this complication, presumably for the same reason that they develop heterotopic ossification.

Classification

Wilkie described two types of congenital synostosis, based on the proximal radioulnar junction

- In type 1, complete synostosis has occurred, with the radius and ulna fused proximally for a variable distance
- In type 2, there is less involvement and may exist as a partial union. Type 2 involves the region just distal to the proximal radial epiphysis and is associated with radial head dislocation.

Cleary and Omer described four types of congenital synostosis, as follows:

- Fibrous synostosis
- Bony synostosis
- Associated posterior dislocation of the radius
- Associated anterior dislocation of the radius

Simmons and colleagues considered congenital synostosis to be a spectrum of anomalies in which the synostosis occurred in varying lengths, with or without involvement of the radial head.

Post-traumatic radioulnar synostosis has been classified into the following three types, based on location:

- *Type 1 :* Least common, occurs in the distal forearm
- *Type 2 :* Occurs in the mid-forearm
- *Type 3 :* Occurs in the proximal forearm

Frequency

- Congenital radioulnar synostosis occurs rarely, with approximately 350 cases reported in the literature. The rarity of this condition often leads to a delayed clinical diagnosis
- Cleary and Omer reported an average patient age at diagnosis of 6 years, with a range of from 6 months to 22 years
- There is no sex predilection in congenital radioulnar synostosis and no particular inheritance pattern is apparent
- 60 percent of cases are bilateral
- Because congenital radioulnar synostosis is caused by an *in utero* insult, its association with other abnormalities is not surprising
- About one-third of cases are associated with general skeletal abnormalities, such as hip dislocation, knee anomalies, clubfoot, polydactyly, syndactyly, Madelung deformity, ligamentous laxity, thumb hypoplasia, carpal coalition and problems of the cardiac, renal, neurologic and GI systems
- Some associated abnormalities and syndromes are genetically determined, including acrocephalo-syndactyly, Apert syndrome, Carpenter syndrome, arthrogryposis, mandibulofacial dysostosis, William syndrome, Klinefelter syndrome, Holt-Oram syndrome, microcephaly, multiple exostoses and fetal alcohol syndrome. In 20 percent of their patients, Cleary and Omer found a genetic basis for an autosomal dominant form (with variable penetrance) of congenital radioulnar synostosis.

Pathophysiology

- The skeletal anomaly includes varying degrees of proximal radial and ulnar fusion, with or without involvement of the radial head
- If the radial head is involved, it may be dislocated anteriorly or posteriorly
- A fibrous synostosis may allow limited motion
- Regional soft-tissue hypoplasia is often present in severe cases, including when atrophy and fibrosis of the brachioradialis, pronator teres, pronator quadratus and supinator muscles occur
- The interosseous membrane also may be abnormal.

Presentation

- Functional deficits associated with congenital radioulnar synostosis depends on the severity of the deformity and on whether or not it is bilateral
- In cases involving severe fixed forearm pronation deformity, the patient cannot compensate for the resulting functional limitations by using scapular and glenohumeral motion
- The forearm usually lies in the pronated or hyperpronated position (See Fig. 22.42)
- Radioulnar synostosis occurs as either a congenital or a post-traumatic condition (See Fig. 22.43)
- Radioulnar synostosis occurs as either a congenital or a post-traumatic condition
- The degree of fusion in radioulnar synostosis varies and may or may not involve the radial head
- Hypermobility at the midcarpal and radiocarpal joints can disguise this lack of forearm rotation, particularly with neutral or mild pronation deformities
- There is usually full or nearly full elbow range of motion, with flexion contractures rarely exceeding 30°
- An abnormal carrying angle of the elbow or a shortening of the forearm may be observed
- Pain is usually not a presenting symptom until the teenage years, when progressive and symptomatic radial head subluxation may be noted
- This accounts for the delayed clinical diagnosis in many cases, but it also indicates that function may be satisfactory

- The disability is most significant in bilateral cases with severe pronation
- Children may initially have a reduced radial head and in adolescence may develop symptomatic radial head subluxation. Therefore, radiographic follow-up is necessary.

Indications for Surgical Treatment

- Indications for surgical treatment of congenital radioulnar synostosis still remain somewhat controversial but are related to bilaterality and to the degree of deformity
- Patients with neutral rotation, mild pronation or rare supination positions can compensate somewhat with ipsilateral shoulder motion. Wrist hypermobility allows further functional compensation.
- Severe pronation deformities (specifically those >60°) cause significant functional difficulty, especially with activities requiring supination
- Therefore, indications for surgery must be determined based more on individual functional limitations than on absolute forearm position
- It is recommended that surgery be performed in childhood before patients are of school going age
- In patients with symptomatic subluxation of the radial head, the radial head may be excised at maturity
- Appropriate workup includes plain radiography performed in orthogonal planes (e.g. posteroanterior and lateral views).

Contraindications for Surgical Treatment

The only contraindication to surgical correction is the presence of milder deformity in an older patient, if the patient has only minimal functional deficit and has already made adjustments in his/her activities to accommodate the synostosis.

■ Congenital Ankylosis of the Elbow Joint

Congenital ankylosis of the cubital joint is extremely rare.

- When reporting one case, *Romanus* (1933) had been able to collect only 23 cases formerly described in the literature
- *Frostad* (1940) reported five cases of bilateral ankylosis in adults.

Anatomical Findings

- In all of the formerly reported cases, except one, the radius had been found to be the chief bone in the formation of the ankylosis, merging broadly with osseous connection directly into the humerus
- In one case, the ulna was ankylotically joined with the humerus, while the radius articulated freely with both
- The brachialis muscle is poorly developed, biceps, the long head of triceps and the muscles of the forearm originating at the humerus, are all present
- This finding is not surprising, as these muscles also exert their effect on the shoulder and the wrist joint, respectively, and thus maintain some activity despite a stiff elbow
- The presence of these muscles is of the greatest importance to a successful operative treatment of a congenital ankylotic elbow.

Treatment

- In schools of surgery and in textbooks it seems to be an established rule that in cases of congenital ankylosis of the elbow, arthroplasty should be postponed until the patient reaches adult age, partly because of the close relationship between the epiphysis and the joint
- But especially because of the difficulties connected with the after-treatment in children, there are a number of important daily tasks which these patients cannot perform
- For example, they cannot wash the face or neck, the upper part of the chest or back. They cannot shave, wash their teeth or comb their hair. They cannot button their coats or upper part of the vest. They all have difficulties in eating. They have to bend the head forward in order to meet the spoon or fork
- So, surgeons feel that operation should be performed in early childhood, before atrophy of the muscles had time to occur.

TRAUMA TO ELBOW-FRACTURES AROUND ELBOW

■ Surgical Anatomy

Medial and lateral columns diverge from humeral shaft at 45° angle. The columns are the important structures for support of the "distal humeral triangle".

■ Mechanism of Injury

The fracture is related to the position of elbow flexion, when the load is applied, as shown in Figures 22.44A to C.

■ Evaluation

Physical Examination

- Soft tissue envelope
- Vascular status, e.g. radial and ulnar pulses
- Neurological status
  - *Radial nerve:* Most commonly injured

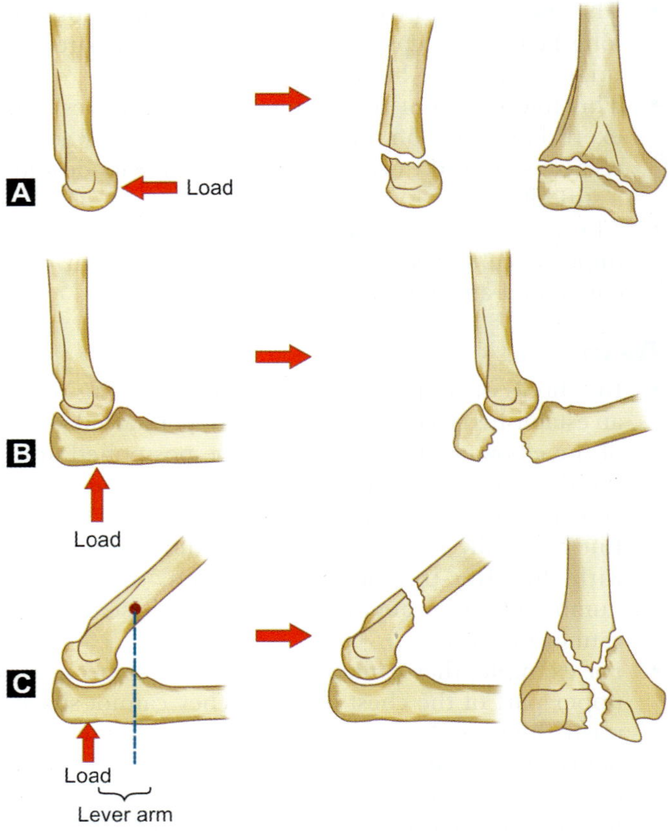

Figs 22.44A to C: Different mechanisms of elbow injury

– *Median nerve:* Rarely injured
– *Ulnar nerve*

Radiographic Examination

- Anteroposterior and lateral radiographs
- Traction views are necessary to evaluate intra-articular extension and for preoperative planning. Traction removes overlap.
- CT scan is also helpful in selected cases, e.g. comminuted capitulum or trochlea.

Fractures at Distal End of Humerus

- Supracondylar fractures
- Transcondylar fractures
- Intercondylar fractures
- Fractures of the condyles (lateral and medial)
- Fractures of the articular surfaces (capitulum and trochlea)
- Fractures of the epicondyles
- Fractures of the radial head
- Fractures of olecranon
- Monteggia fracture dislocation
- Fractures at the distal end of humerus.

■ Classifications

OTA Classification

Humerus, Distal Segment (13)

Types: These are shown in Figures 22.45A to C and are of the following types:

- Extra-articular fracture (A2)
- Partial articular fracture (B1)
- Complete articular fracture (C2)

Anatomical Classification

- Supracondylar fractures
- Transcondylar fractures
- Intercondylar fractures; fractures of the condyles (lateral and medial)
- Fractures of the articular surfaces (capitulum and trochlea)
- Fractures of the epicondyles.

■ Treatment Principles

- Anatomic articular reduction
- Stable internal fixation of the articular surface
- Restoration of articular axial alignment
- Stable internal fixation of the articular segment to the metaphysis and diaphysis.
- Early range of motion of the elbow.

Technical Objectives for Fixation of Distal Humerus Fractures

- Every screw should pass through a plate
- Every screw should engage a fragment on the opposite side that is also fixed to a plate
- As many screws as possible should be placed in the distal fragments
- Each screw should be as long as possible
- Every screw should engage as many articular fragments as possible
- Plates should be applied such that compression is achieved at the supracondylar level for both the columns
- Plates used must be strong enough and stiff enough to resist breaking or bending before union occurs at supracondylar level
- AO implants.

■ Supracondylar Fractures

Careful neurovascular examination of the arm is essential, especially in extension-type (apex anteriorly angulated) supracondylar fractures. The brachial artery may be lacerated by the proximal fracture fragment, either at the time of injury or during reduction and a compartment

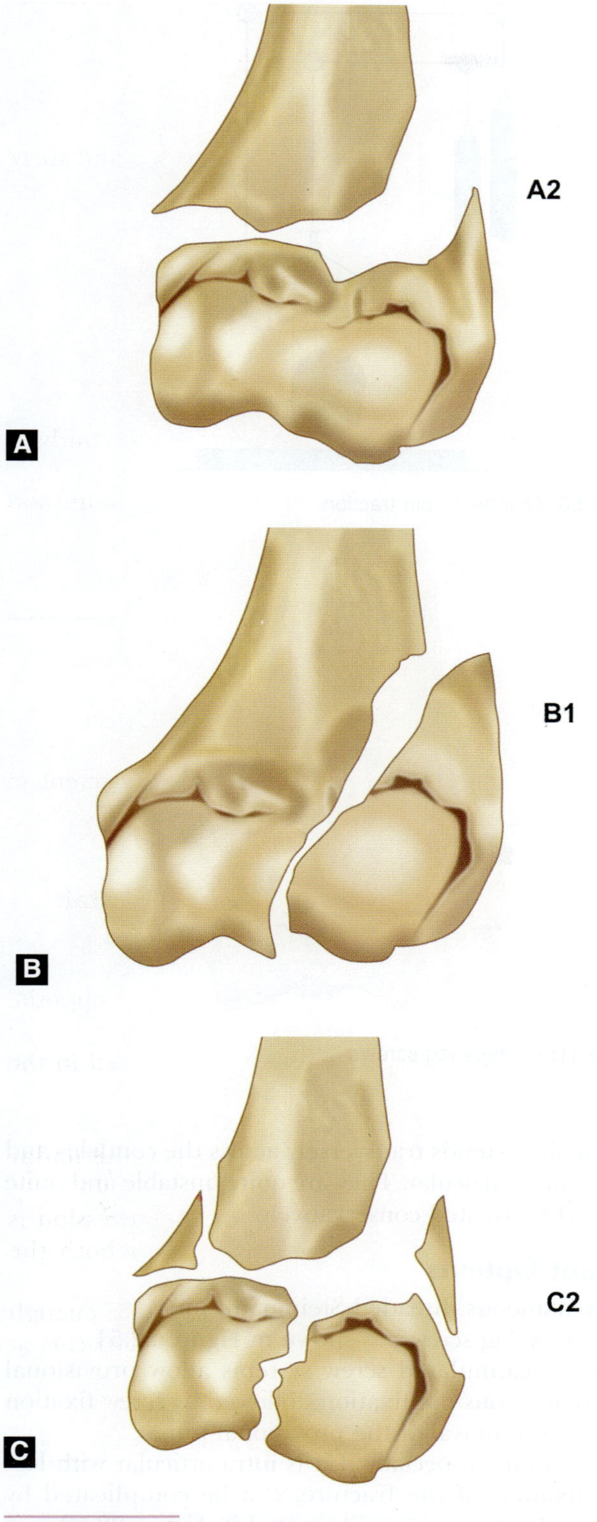

Figs 22.45A to C: Orthopedic Trauma Association classification of distal humerus—(A) Extra-articular fracture; (B) Partial articular fracture; (C) Complete articular fracture of distal humeral segment

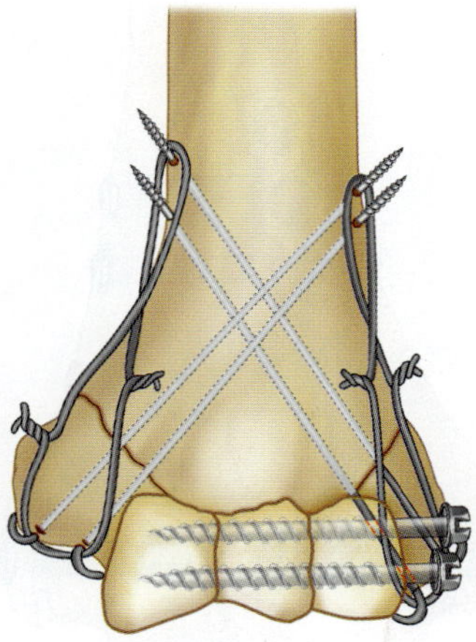

Fig. 22.46: Crossed screws or crossed threaded pins

syndrome may develop. All three major nerves that cross the elbow can be injured, but the radial and median nerves are those most commonly affected.

Treatment

Conservative

- Hanging arm cast
- Overhead olecranon skeletal traction

Open Reduction and Internal Fixation

They are used as a rule only in the presence of neurovascular damage or when a satisfactory position of the fracture is not obtained by closed methods.

- *Crossed screws or crossed threaded pins (Fig. 22.46):* The screws or pins should be placed in the medial and lateral pillars and should engage the posterior cortex of the bone. Over-drilling of the distal fragment may be done, to allow compression, when the screws are tightened.
- *Hand contoured plates (Fig. 22.47):* When one or both columns are comminuted, hand-contoured plates can be used to reconstruct the humeral pillars.
- *Precontoured plate fixation:* It is illustrated in Figures 22.48A and B. Goal should be to stabilize rigid internal fixation, as shown in Figure 22.49.
- *Olecranon pin traction (Fig. 22.50):* If operative treatment is postponed because of severe swelling, trauma, contused skin or the patient's overall condition, displaced supracondylar fractures, side arm or overhead olecranon pin traction should be done until operative treatment can be performed.

■ Transcondylar Fractures

They are often grouped with supracondylar fractures. Rare injury requires special consideration. The fracture

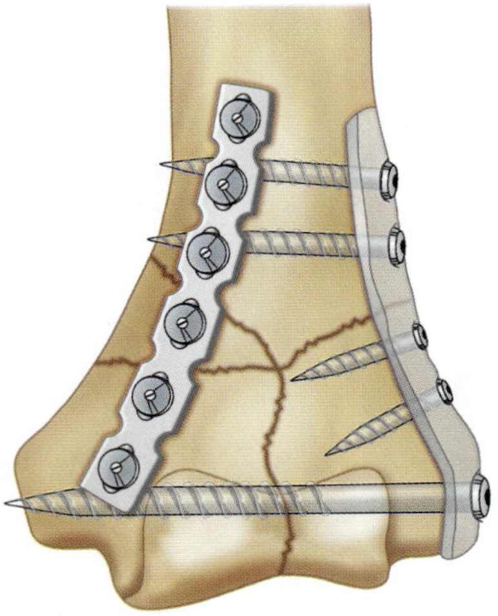

Fig. 22.47: Hand contoured plates

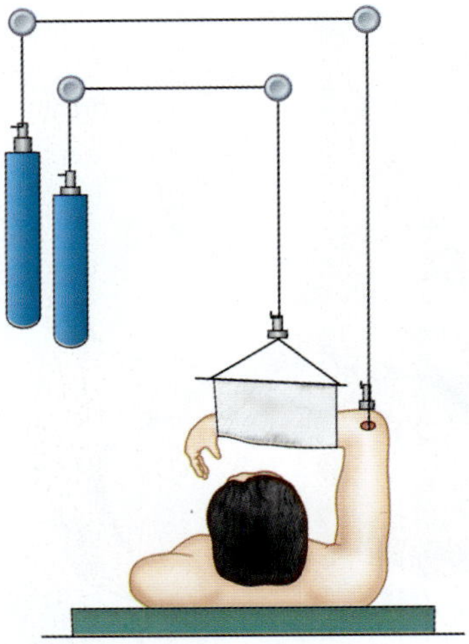

Fig. 22.50: Olecranon pin traction

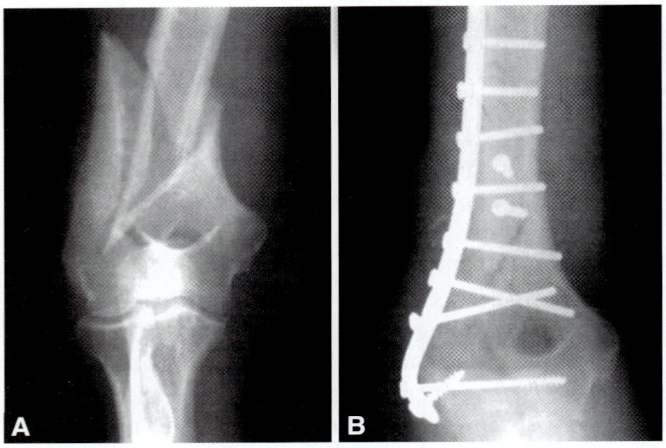

Figs 22.48A and B: X-ray showing precontoured plate fixation

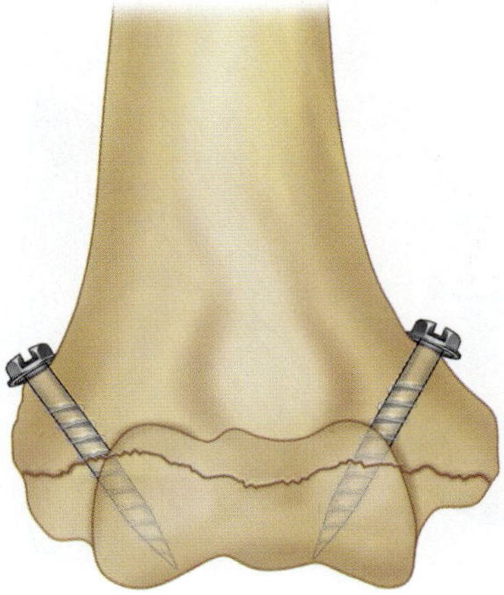

Fig. 22.51: AO type lag screws

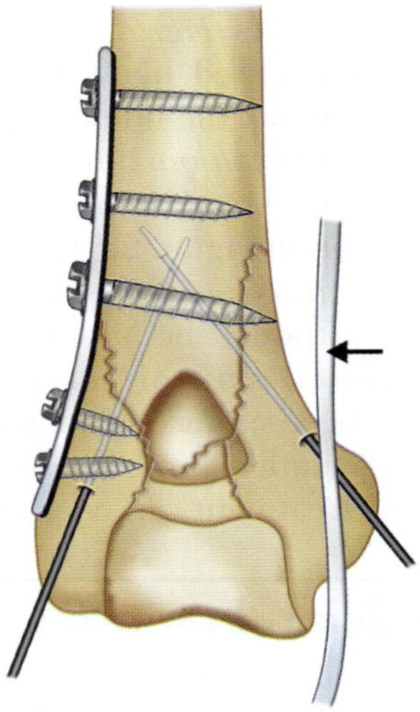

Fig. 22.49: Precontoured plate fixation used to stabilize rigid internal fixation

line usually extends transversely across the condyles and often is intra-articular. They are quite unstable and unite slowly when treated conservatively.

Implant Options

- Percutaneous threaded Steinmann pins.
- AO type lag screws, as shown in Figure 22.51.
- Newer cannulated screw systems allow provisional percutaneous pin fixation, followed by screw fixation without removal of the provisional pins.
- This injury, especially if it is intra-articular with loss of fixation of the fracture, can be complicated by avascular necrosis, as illustrated in Figure 22.52.

■ Intercondylar Fractures

Most difficult challenge of the fractures is of the lower end of the humerus.

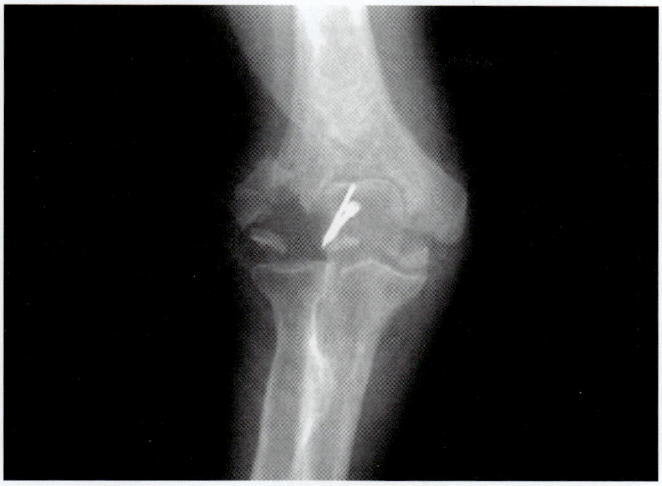

Fig. 22.52: Avascular necrosis in case of intra-articular fracture, with loss of fracture fixation

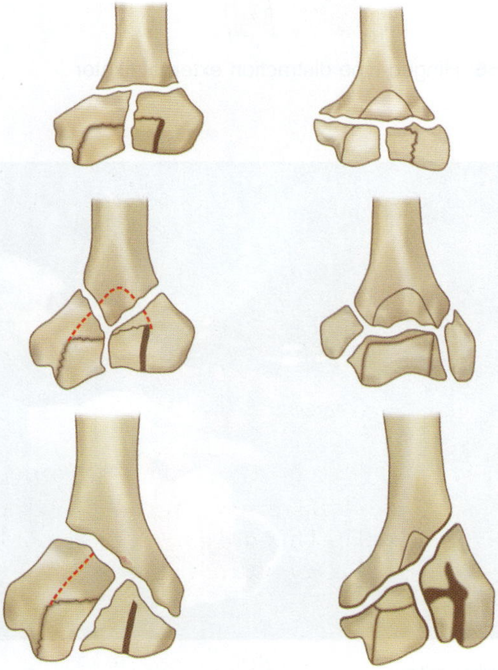

Fig. 22.53: Mehne and Matta classification system

Classification

Mehne and Matta Classification System (Fig. 22.53)

According to pattern of fracture line in the distal humerus.

Classification of Riseborough and Radin (Fig. 22.54)

Type I: Fractures involving minimally displaced articular fragments

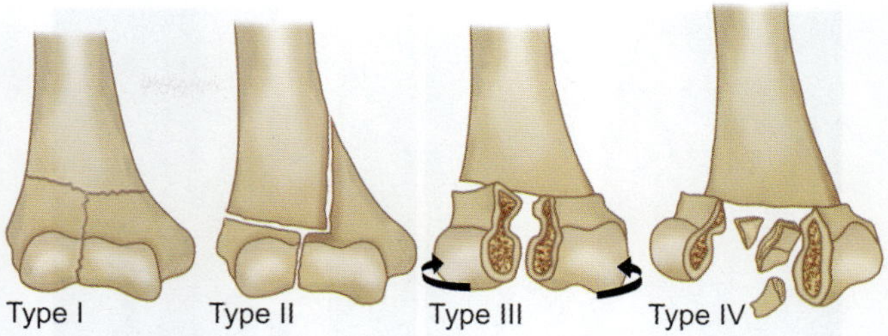

Fig. 22.54: Riseborough and Radin classification

Type II: Fractures involving displaced fragments that are not rotated

Type III: Fractures involving displaced and rotated fragments

Type IV: Fractures involving comminuted fracture fragments.

Treatment

Type I Fractures

Plaster splint immobilization, with gradual motion being permitted, once sufficient healing has occurred.

Types II and III Fractures

- ORIF especially, when patient is young and active
- Open fractures up to Gustilo type II
- Surgery is best performed within the first 24 to 48 hours.

Type IV Fractures "A Bag of Bones" (Figs 22.55A and B)

- Usually treated nonoperatively by:
  - Sling and early motion if the patient is elderly
  - Skeletal traction through an olecranon pin, if the patient is younger.
- When the patient is young, open reduction and internal fixation of two or three of the major articular fragments, as shown in Figure 22.55B is done, followed by skeletal traction and early motion may be preferred. Hinged-type distraction external fixator that allows early motion can be a satisfactory treatment option for intercondylar fractures, for which total reconstruction is not possible, as shown in Figures 22.56 and 22.57, besides it is more cost effective than traction and may yield similar results. Open reduction and fixation of Y fracture is shown in Figure 22.58.

Comminuted Fractures

If there is comminution of pillars hand contoured, one-third tubular plate is applied to the medial edge of the medial humeral pillar and a contoured reconstruction plate may be applied to the posterior aspect of the lateral humeral pillar, as illustrated in Figure 22.59.

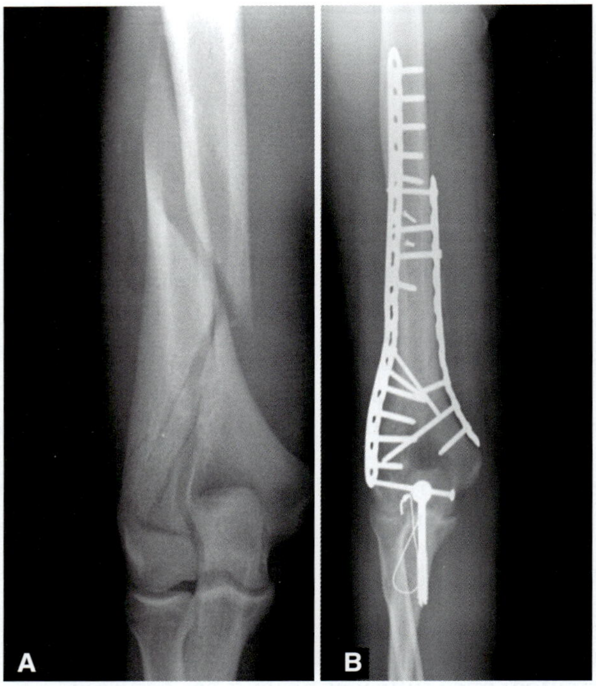

Figs 22.55A and B: (A) Intercondyle fracture; (B) Fixed by ORIF

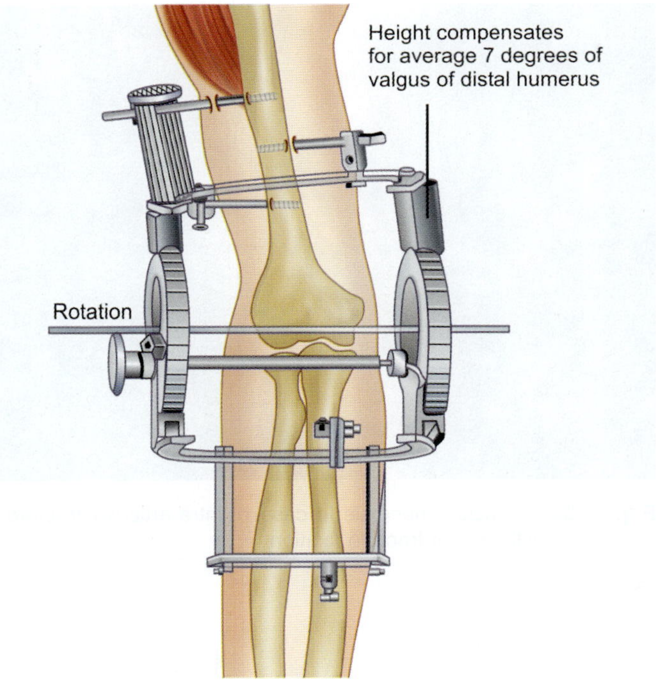

Fig. 22.56: Hinged-type distraction external fixator

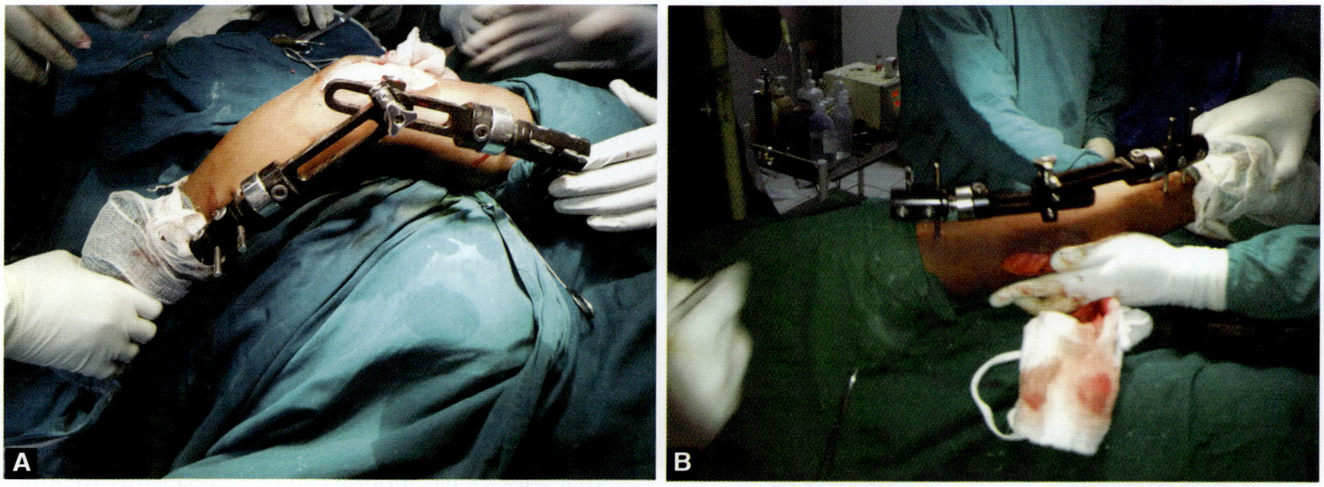

Figs 22.57A and B: AO elbow hinge fixator—(A) Elbow at flexion; (B) Extended elbow

Lateral Comminution (Figs 22.60 to 22.63)

If the medial pillar is not severely comminuted, a rigid, prebent plate can be applied alone to the lateral pillar.

Minifragment

After Treatment

- Light posterior plaster splint is applied from the posterior axillary fold to the palm of the hand
- At 7 days, the posterior plaster splint is removed periodically and gentle active and active-assisted exercises are carried out
- By 3 weeks, the posterior plaster splint can be removed and arm is supported by a sling with active motion in the elbow as pain permits
- Vigorous stretching by a therapist, forced motion, whether active or passive and manipulation under anesthesia are contraindicated, as it may result in increased periarticular hemorrhage and fibrosis, heterotrophic calcification, increased joint irritability and decreased rather than increased motion.

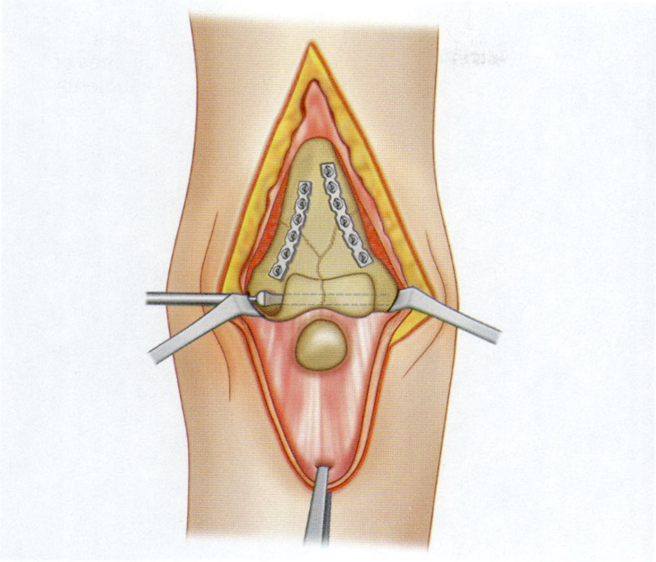

Fig. 22.58: Open reduction internal fixation of Y fracture of distal humerus

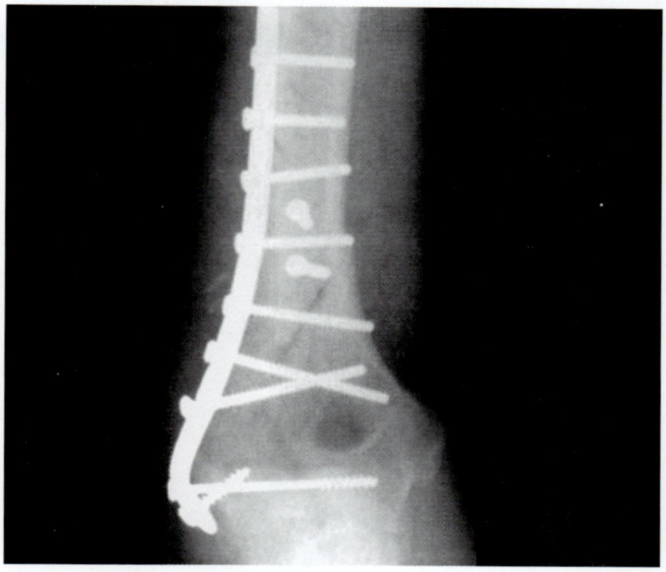

Fig. 22.60: Precontoured DuPont plate fixation

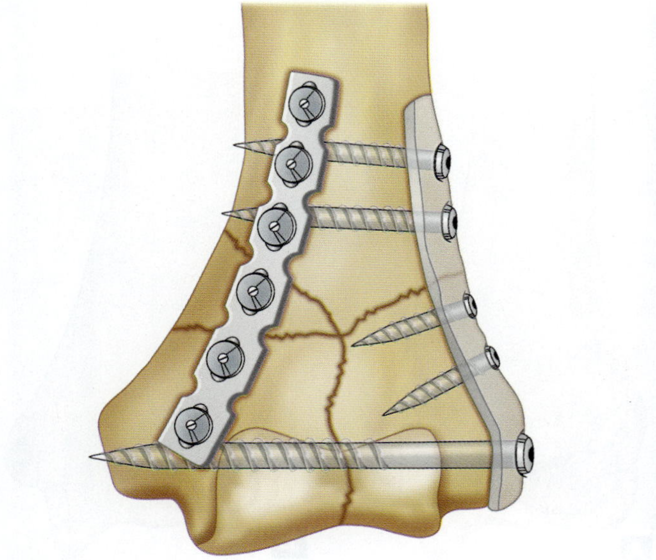

Fig. 22.59: Contoured reconstruction plate is applied to the posterior aspect of lateral humeral pillar

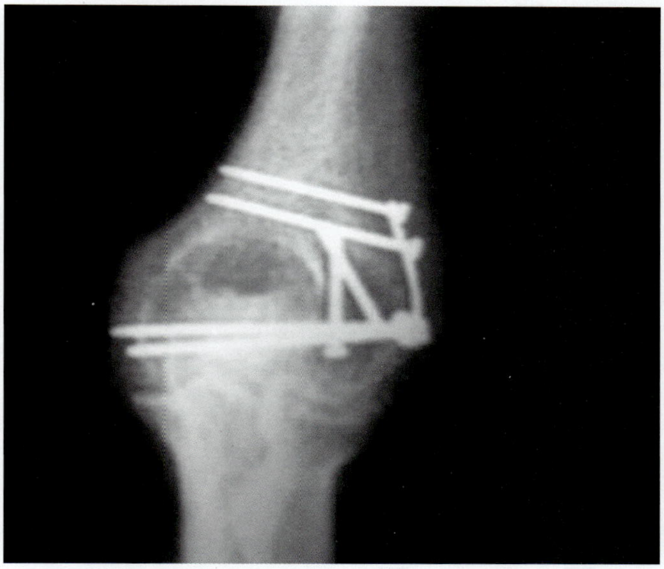

Fig. 22.61: AP view showing precontoured plate applied to lateral pillar

■ Fractures of Condyles of Humerus (Medial or Lateral)

Isolated fractures of the medial or lateral condyle of the humerus in adults are uncommon. When the condyle is displaced, open reduction and internal fixation are the best treatment. Lateral condylar fractures are more common than medial. Mechanism of injury is abduction or adduction of forearm with elbow in extension.

- Medial condyle fractures include trochlea and medial epicondyle fractures, as shown in Figure 22.64.
- Lateral condyle fracture include lateral epicondyle and capitulum fractures.

Classification

Milch Classification

Type I: In the type I fracture, the fracture line courses medially to the trochlea through and into the capitellar-

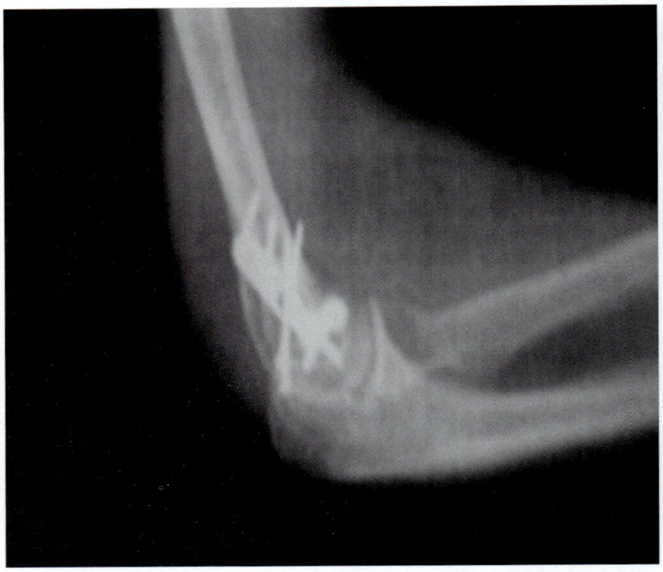

Fig. 22.62: Lateral view showing precontoured plate applied to lateral pillar

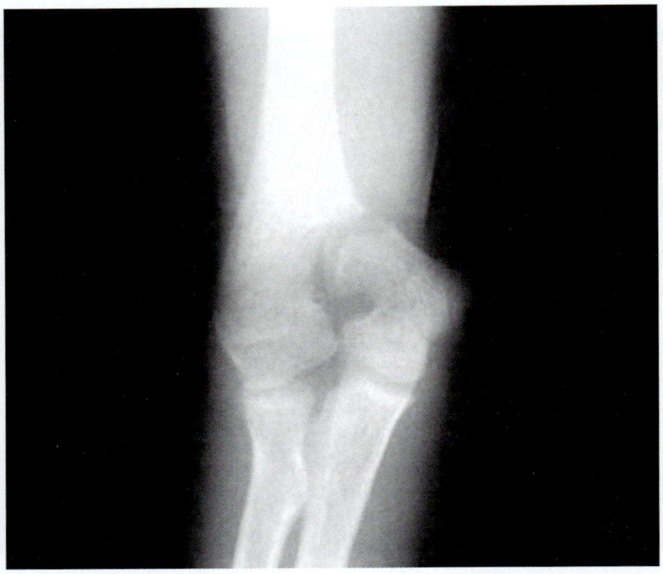

Fig. 22.64: X-ray showing medial condyle fracture including lateral epicondyle and capitulum fractures

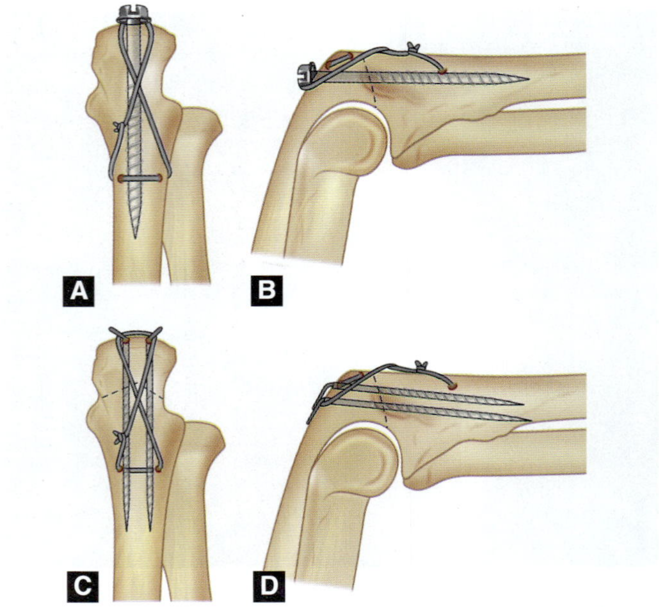

Figs 22.63A to D: Tension band wiring and screw

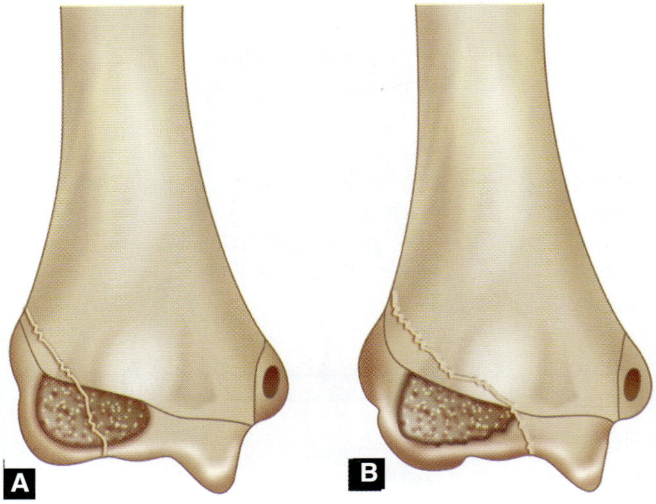

Figs 22.65A and B: (A) Type I fracture of lateral condyle according to Milch classification; (B) Type II fracture

trochlear groove. This type of fracture is rare because of the location of the fracture line. It is a true Salter-Harris type IV fracture but is frequently stable.

Type II (Figs 22.65A and B): In the type II fracture described by Milch, which is more common, the fracture line extends into the area of the trochlea and produces inherent instability of the elbow because of the ability of the distal fragment and the forearm not only to angulate, but also to translate into a lateral position.

Classification of Lateral Condylar Fractures According to the Amount of Displacement

- Undisplaced
- Moderately displaced
- Completely displaced and rotated.

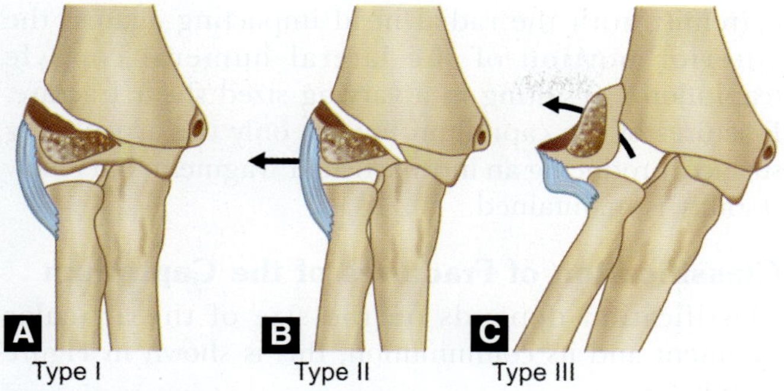

Figs 22.66A to C: Radiographic criteria of determining fracture stability

Radiographic Criteria of Determining Fracture Stability According to Finnbogason et al. (Figs 22.66A to C)

Finnbogason et al. described radiographic criteria for determining fracture stability, which they used in planning the initial treatment.

Type I: Fracture through the lateral humeral condyle with minimal lateral gap—a stable fracture.

Type II: Fracture through the lateral humeral condyle to the epiphyseal cartilage with a lateral gap—a fracture with undefinable risk.

Type III: Fracture through the lateral humeral condyle with the fracture gap as wide laterally as medially—a fracture with high risk of later displacement.

Treatment

Nonoperative treatment is indicated in nondisplaced or minimally displaced fractures. Consists of posterior splinting with elbow in 90° flexion, with forearm in supination in lateral condylar fracture and pronation in medial condylar fractures.

Operative consists of screw fixation with or without collateral ligament repair, with attention to rotational axis restoration.

Prognosis depends on

- Degree of comminution
- Accuracy of reduction
- Stability of internal fixation (Figs 22.67 and 22.68).

Complications

Improper reduction in failure of fixation may result in cubitus valgus and tardy ulnar palsy in lateral condyle fractures.

Medial condyle fractures

- Post-traumatic arthritis, especially in fractures involving the trochlea groove.
- Ulnar nerve symptoms with excess callus formation in malunion.
- Cubitus varus

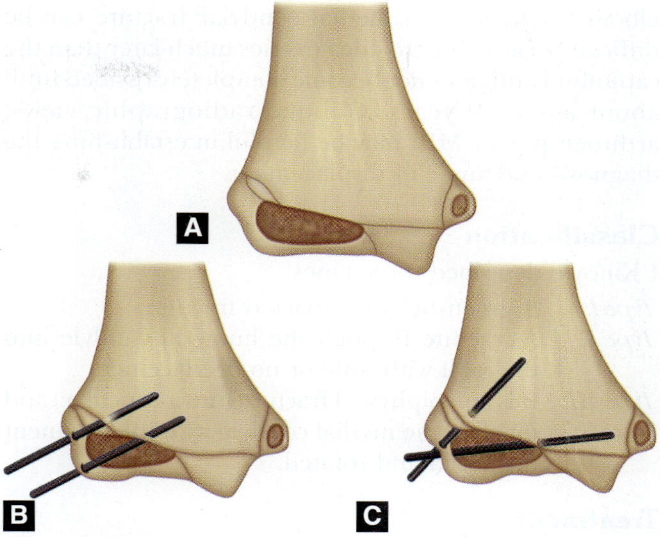

Figs 22.67A to C: Stability of internal fixation

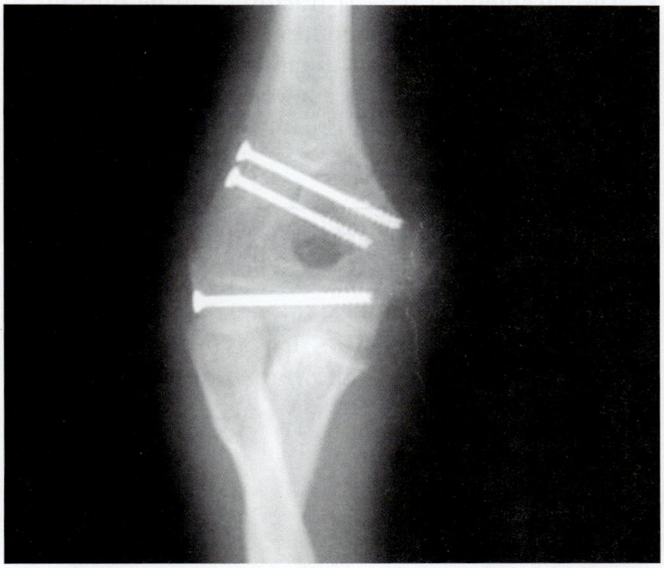

Fig. 22.68: X-ray showing securing of fractured condyle to uninvolved condyle with lag screws

After Treatment

- Usually fixation is sufficiently rigid to permit early active motion.
- After treatment is similar to that described for intercondylar fractures, but usually rehabilitation advances at a more rapid pace.

■ Medial Condyle Fractures

Fractures of the medial humeral condyle in adults and children are among the least common injuries of the elbow. Diagnosis of a medial condylar fracture can be difficult because the trochlea ossifies much later than the capitulum and does not become completely ossified until about age of 9 years. Oblique radiographic views, arthrography or MRI may be helpful in establishing the diagnosis and angle of displacement.

Classification

I Kilfoyle described three types:

Type I: A greenstick or impacted fracture

Type II: A fracture through the humeral condyle into the joint with little or no displacement

Type III: It is an epiphyseal fracture (intra-articular) and involves the medial condyle with the fragment displaced and rotated.

Treatment

- Type I and undisplaced type II fractures can be treated by observation and posterior splinting with elbow in 90° flexion.
- Displacement of type II fractures can be difficult to determine; if displacement is suspected, open reduction and internal fixation are appropriate to avoid growth disturbance and nonunion.
- Type III fractures should be treated by open reduction and internal fixation.

■ Fractures of Articular Surface of Distal Humerus

Fracture of the capitulum is one of the most common purely intra-articular fractures that occur about the elbow. It usually is caused by a fall on the outstretched upper extremity, with the radial head impacting against the anterior portion of the lateral humeral condyle (capitulum), resulting in a varying sized shear fracture. Fractures of the capitulum involve only the articulating surface, producing an intra-articular fragment, but elbow stability is maintained.

Classification of Fractures of the Capitulum

Classification depends on the size of the articular fragment and its comminution, this is shown in Figure 22.69:

Type I fracture (Hahn-Steinthal): A large fragment of bone and articular cartilage

Type II fracture (Kocher-Lorenz): A small shell of bone and articular cartilage

Type III fracture: Comminuted fracture.

Treatment

- Closed reduction, usually not successful
- Open reduction with and without internal fixation, done for type I and II (large fragment)
- *Excision of the fragments:* Type II and most of type III fractures
- *Insertion of prosthesis:* Not proven successful or practical in literature.

Technique

With a small AO lag screw/Herbert screw as shown in Figure 22.70, secure the fragment in place and countersink the screw head by over-drilling the posterior cortex.

New implants (Fig. 22.71): A small osteochondral fracture is being fixed with absorbable screws.

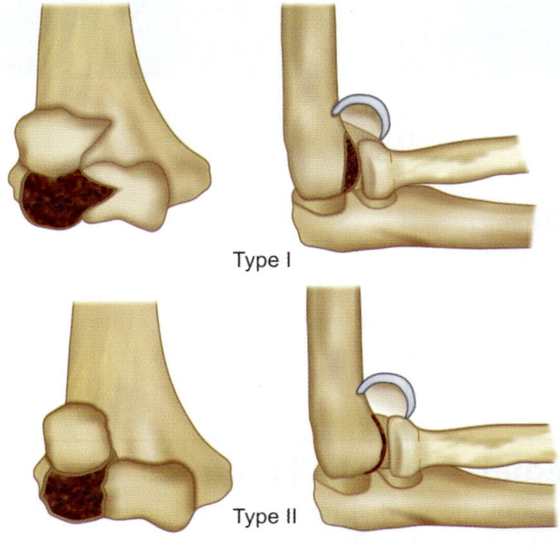

Fig. 22.69: Type I and type II capitulum fractures

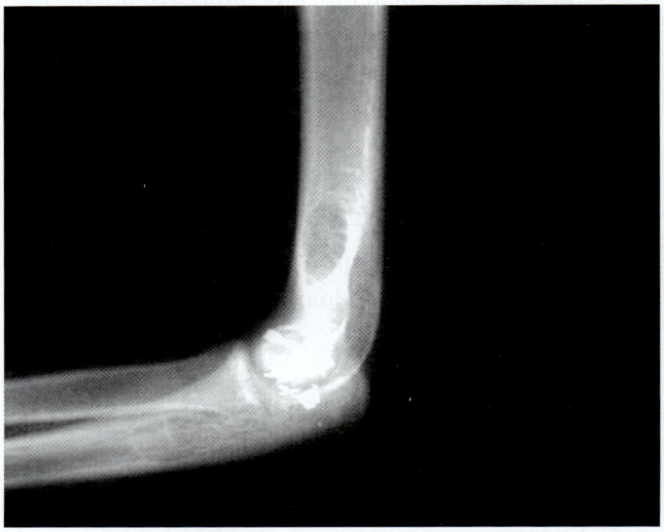

Fig. 22.70: Osteochondral fracture, fixed by absorbable screws

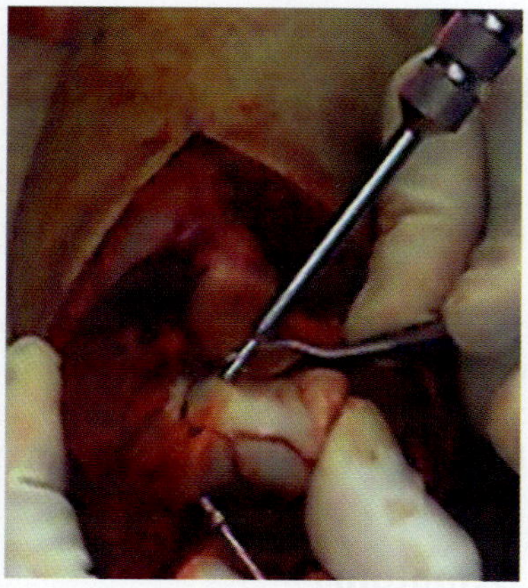

Fig. 22.71: Osteochondral fracture fixation with screws

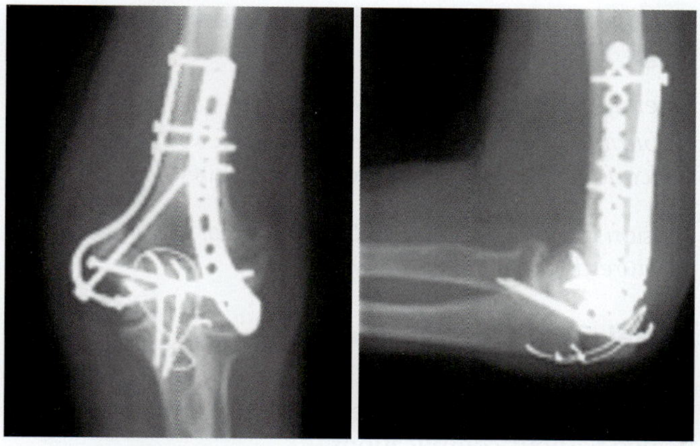

Fig. 22.72: Bone graft with revision plating

Outcomes: Outcomes are based on pain and function. Flexion is the first to return usually, within the first-two months. Extension usually takes 4 to 6 months to return. Supination/pronation is usually unaffected.

Complications

Painful retained implant is the most common complaint. Common locations are olecranon and medial implant. Implant removal is done after fracture union. One plate at a time in bicolumnar fractures. Removal of both plates with a single surgery is a fracture risk.

Ulnar Nerve Palsy

It can be due to:
- Operative manipulation
- Hardware prominence
- Inadequate release

Prevention is the best treatment.

Heterotopic Ossification

- It occurs in up to 50 percent of cases after treatment of distal humerus fractures.
- Hastings and Graham functional classification system

Class I: These fractures are associated with no functional limitations.

Class II: These can further be classified into following types:

IIA: Functional limitation of flexion and extension;

IIB: Functional limitation of supination and pronation

Class III: These fractures are associated with ankylosis that eliminates elbow ROM.

Preventive measures

- Early operative treatment (24 to 48 hours)
- Nonsteroidal anti-inflammatory drugs (NSAIDs)
- Low-dose radiation therapy
- Continuous passive ROM exercises.

Treatment

- *Indomethacin:* Recommended dose is 75 mg orally BD for 3 weeks.
- Low-dose radiation therapy, single doses of 600 to 700cGy. The timing of the irradiation (preoperative vs postoperative) does not seem to affect operative outcomes.
- Operative excision of heterotopic ossification is recommended 12 months after the injury.

Failure of Fixation

- Associated with stability of operative fixation
- K-wires fixation alone is inadequate
- If diagnosed early, revision fixation indicated
- Late fixation failure must be tailored to radiographic healing and patient symptoms.

Nonunion of Distal Humerus

Nonunion of distal humerus is uncommon and is usually a failure of fixation. Symptomatic treatment is required. A bone graft with revision plating, is generally used to correct it as shown in the Figure 22.72.

Nonunion of Olecranon Osteotomy

- Rates as high as 5 percent or more
- Treated with bone graft and revision tension band technique
- Excision of proximal fragment is salvage
- Fifty percent of olecranon must remain for joint stability.

Infection

Highest for open fractures, no style of fixation has a higher rate than any other.

Lateral Epicondyle and Capitulum Fracture (Figs 22.73 to 22.75)

Lateral Approach (Figs 22.74A and B)

Capitulum: Posterior to anterior lag screws
Epicondyle: Screw and buttress plate healed.

Tension Band Screw and ORIF for Medial Column Fracture (Figs 22.75A and B)

Distal, Two Column Fracture (Figs 22.76 to 22.79)

Prognosis: Healed lacks 20° flexion and extion. Osteotomy healed without complications.

Radial Head Fractures (Figs 22.80A and B)

Mode and Mechanism of Injury (Fig. 22.81)

The radial head fractures, when it collides with the capitulum. This can occur with a pure axial load (Essex-Lopresti injury), a valgus load with a posterolateral rotatory (elbow dislocation) type of load or as the radial head dislocates posteriorly as part of a posterior Monteggia fracture or posterior olecranon fracture-dislocation.

Signs and Symptoms

- It is painful because the elbow joint is usually distended with blood

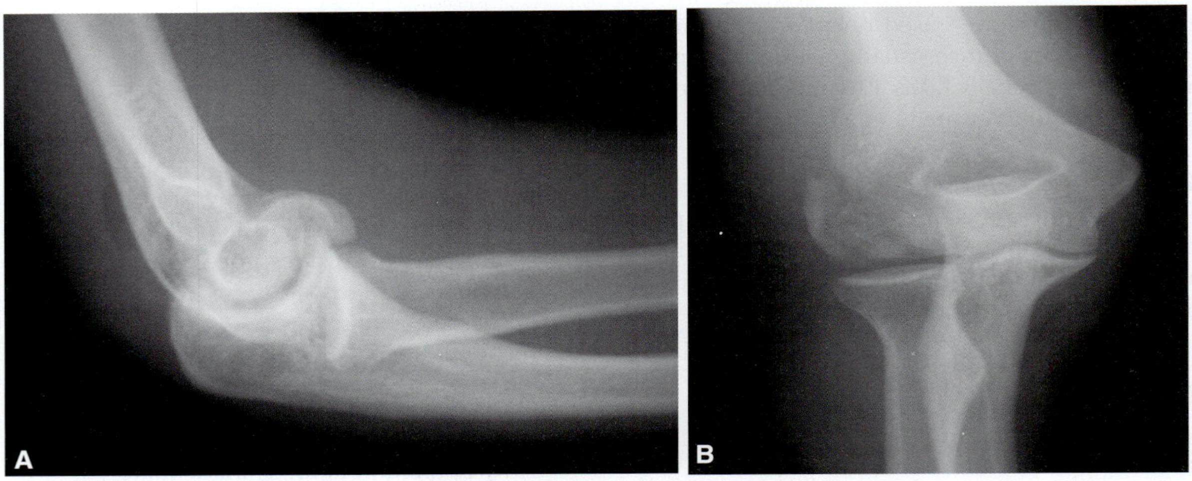

Figs 22.73A and B: Lateral epicondyle and capitulum fracture—(A) Lateral view; (B) AP view

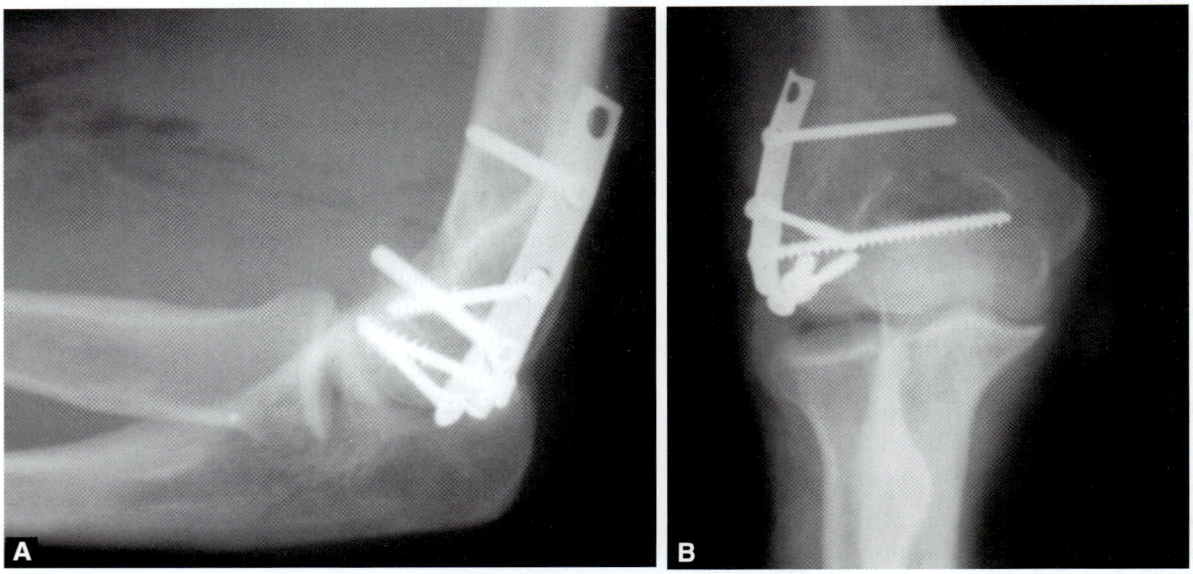

Figs 22.74A and B: Lateral approach for treating lateral epicondyle and capitulum fracture—(A) Lateral view; (B) AP view

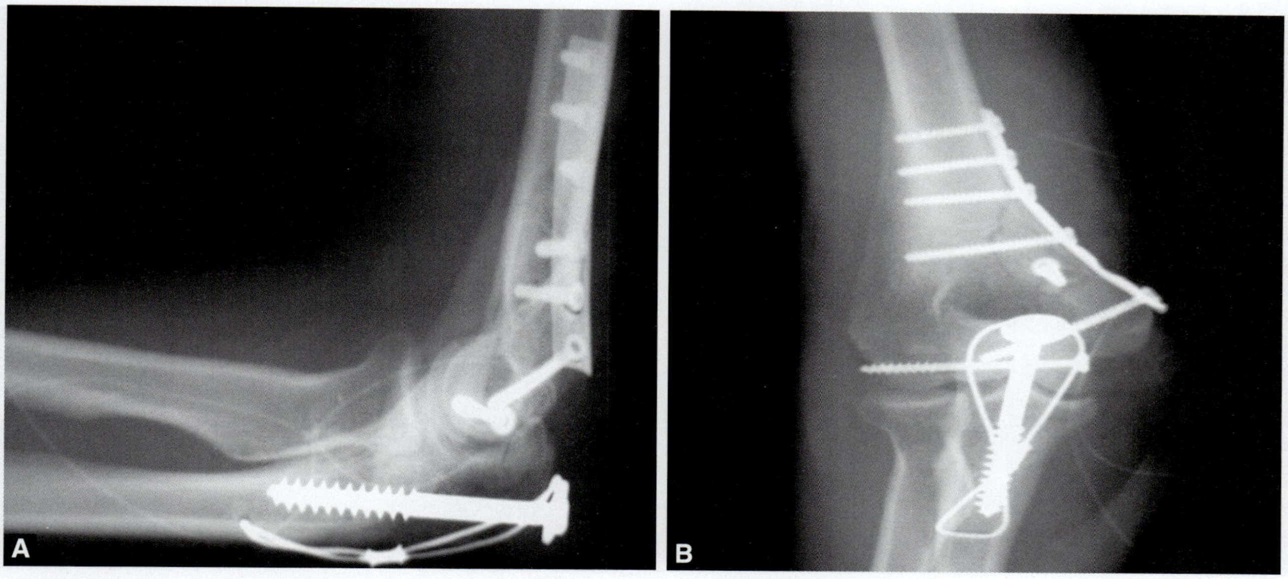

Figs 22.75A and B: Tension band screw and ORIF medial column fracture—(A) Lateral view; (B) AP view

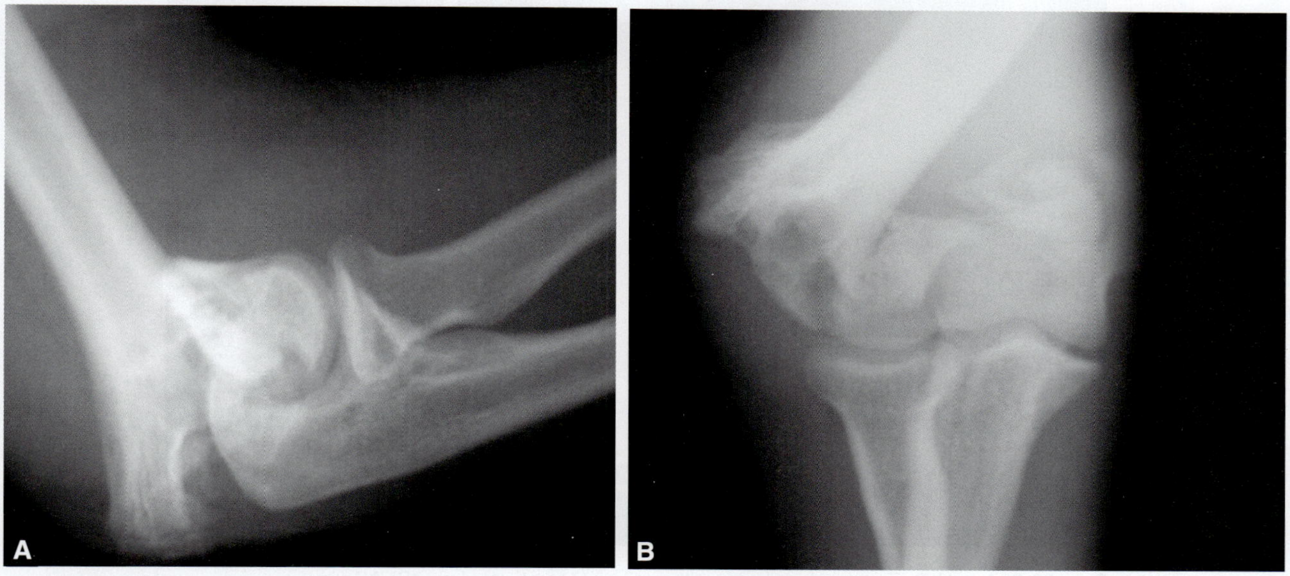

Figs 22.76A and B: Distal, two column fracture

- Variable amount of swelling and ecchymosis, which may correspond with the degree of associated ligament injury
- There is often crepitation of the radial head with forearm rotation and occasionally a fracture fragment will block forearm rotation.

Associated Injuries

- Fracture of the radial head associated with rupture of the MCL
- Concomitant fracture of the radial head and capitulum
- Posterior dislocation of the elbow with fracture of the radial head
- Posterior dislocation of the elbow with fracture of the radial head and the coronoid process (the so-called terrible triad of the elbow)
- Posterior Monteggia fractures, including posterior olecranon fracture-dislocations
- Essex-Lopresti lesions and variants

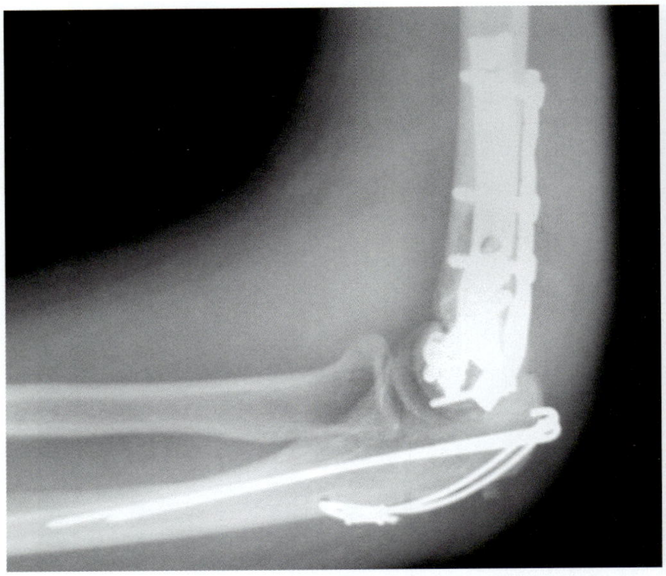

Fig. 22.77: Transverse intra-articular approach

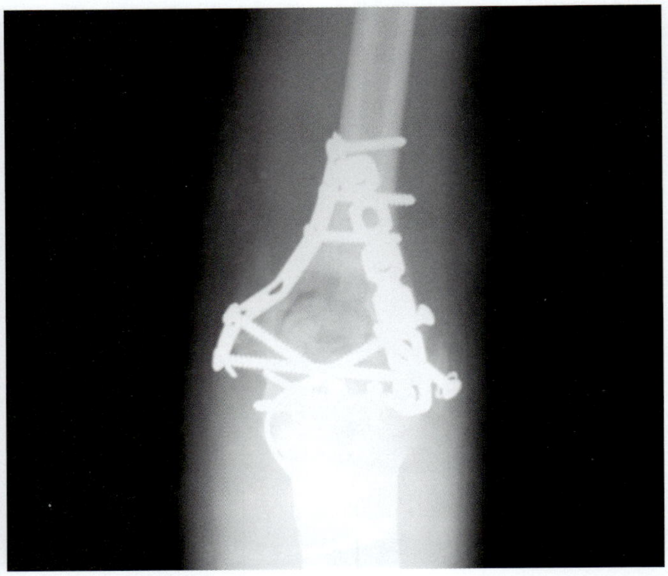

Fig. 22.78: Lag screw and bicolumn plating

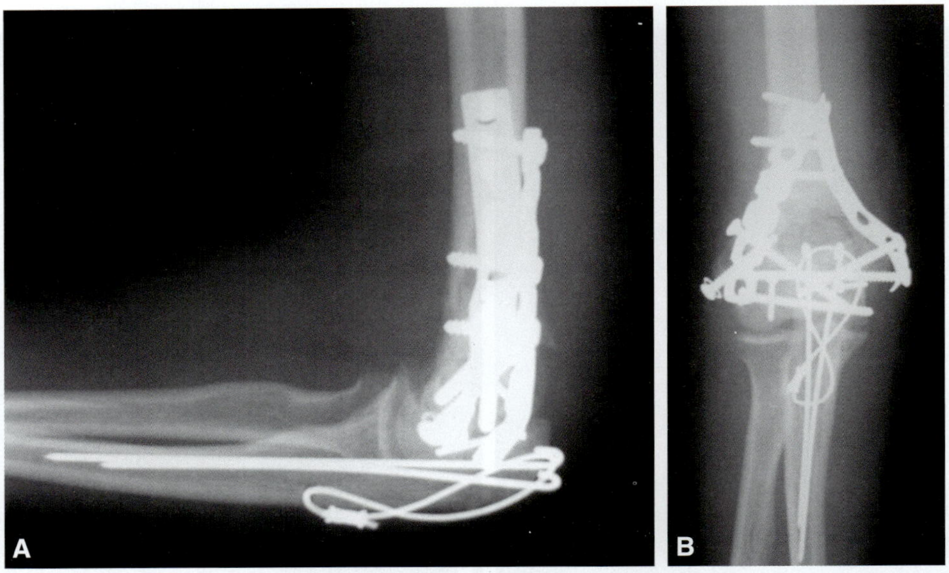

Figs 22.79A and B: Tension band wire with cable—(A) Lateral view; (B) AP view

Classification

In 1924, speed proposed a classification based on the amount of radial head involvement, marginal or complete and the degree of displacement.

In 1954, Mason further subdivided the classification into three groups:

Type I: Small or marginal fractures with minimal displacement

Type II: Marginal fractures with displacement

Type III: Comminuted fractures.

Modified Mason's Classification

Type I (Fig. 22.82)

- Nondisplaced or minimally displaced fracture of head or neck
- Forearm rotation (pronation/supination) is limited only by acute pain and swelling
- Intra-articular displacement of the fracture is less than 2 mm.

Type II (Fig. 22.83)

- Displaced fracture of the head or neck

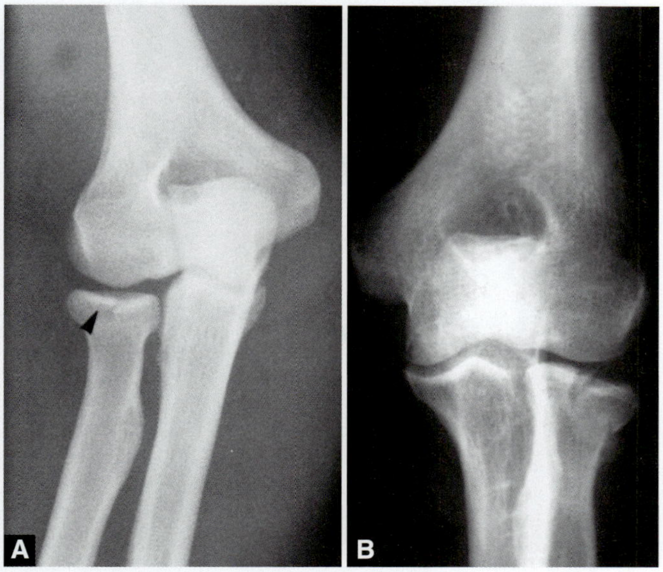

Figs 22.80A and B: Radial head fracture

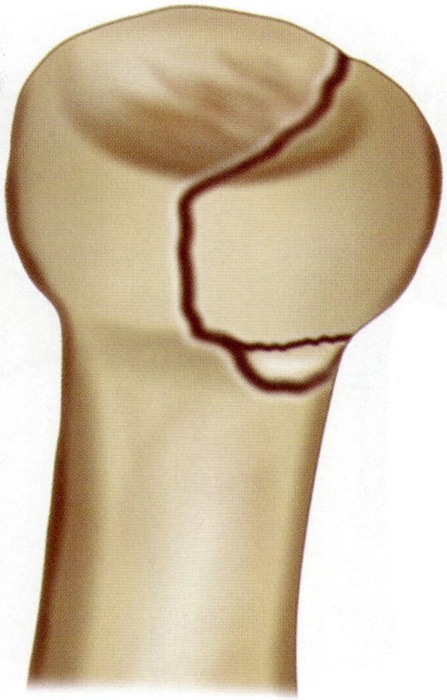

Fig. 22.82: Modified Mason's type I fracture of radial head

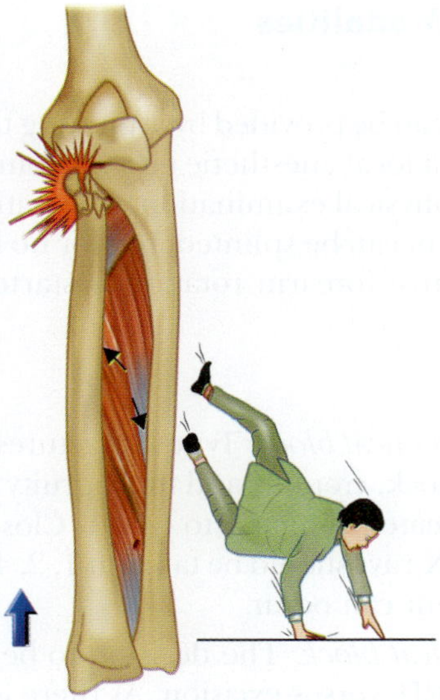

Fig. 22.81: Mechanism of radial head injury due to collision of radial head with capitulum

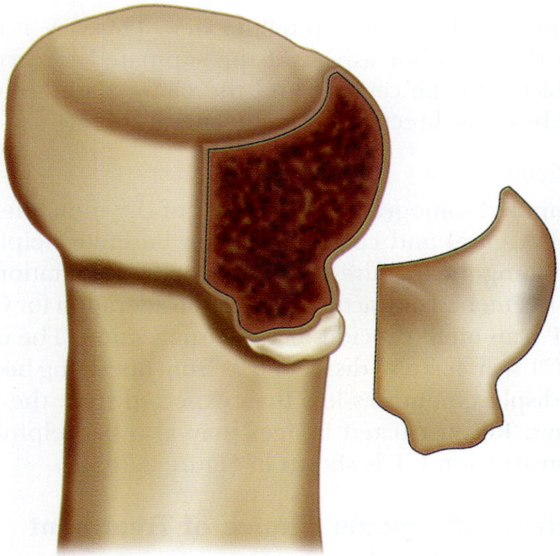

Fig. 22.83: Modified Mason's type II fracture of radial head

- Motion may be mechanically limited with or without significant joint incongruity
- Can be repaired by open reduction with internal fixation.

Type III (Fig. 22.84)

Severely comminuted fracture of the radial head and neck.

Type IV

Comminuted fracture with elbow dislocation.

Radiographic Examination

Plain Films

X-rays in the anteroposterior, lateral and oblique planes of the elbow are usually sufficient to diagnose the fracture. However, if a fat pad sign is present without a noticeable fracture, a radiocapitellar view may be helpful. The radiocapitellar view is taken with the forearm in neutral rotation and the X-ray tube angles cephalad. An alternative technique to demonstrate difficult minimally or nondisplaced fractures of the radial head is the

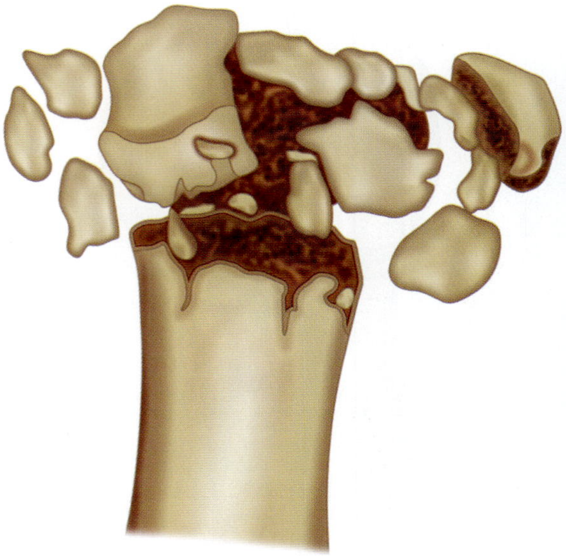

Fig. 22.84: Modified Mason's type III fracture of radial head

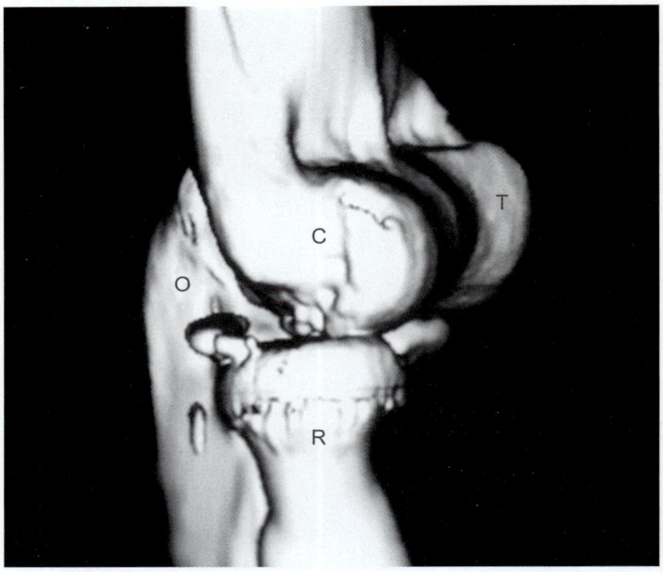

Fig. 22.85: Radial head comminuted fracture—R. Radius; C. Capitulum; T. Trochlea; O. Olecranon

modified radial-head capitellum view. This view is taken with the posterior aspect of the supinated forearm, in contact with the cassette and the elbow slightly flexed. The beam is directed 45° mediolateral (MLat).

CT Scan

Computed tomography (CT) scans of the radial head in axial, sagittal and coronal cuts can be quite helpful in estimating the fracture size, degree of fragmentation and displacement. For fractures under consideration for ORIF, a CT scan often provides better visualization. The use of the CT scan has also dissuaded us from operating because the displacement was less than expected from the plain X-rays. Reconstructed images may also be helpful. 3D reconstruction CT is shown in Figure 22.85.

Factors Influencing Choice of Treatment

Depends on High or Low-demand Elbow

An ideal high-demand patient is typically considered young and athletically active, as compared to a low-demand patient, who would be elderly and less likely to stress the elbow physically. For low-demand patients excision without prosthetic replacement is often well tolerated. If replacement is needed in the low-demand elbow, to obtain acute instability, there is less likely to be a problem of long-term wear.

In the younger, high-demand patient, metallic radial head replacement poses more potential for long-term failure. In considering radial head arthroplasty, the patient must be counseled carefully about the risks of loosening the radiocapitellar wear and ultimate removal.

Treatment Modalities

Type I

Relief of pain can be provided by aspirating the hematoma and injecting a local anesthetic into the joint, thus aiding in the initial physical examination. The patient is given a sling or the arm can be splinted, but for no longer than 3 to 4 days. Active forearm rotation is started as soon as tolerated.

Type II

Without mechanical block: Type II fractures that have no mechanical block, crepitus and incongruity of less than 2 mm can be treated similarly to type I. Close follow-up is required and X-rays should be taken at 1, 2, 4 and 6 weeks, as displacement can occur.

With mechanical block: The decision to be made in this situation is ORIF versus excision. As there is no evidence of associated interosseous injury, radial head arthroplasty is not a consideration. Patient selection is crucial.

With associated injury: Associated injury can be interosseous ligament tear. In that case preservation of the radial head (or radial head function with a prosthesis) is crucial in this setting. Excision of the radial head may lead to symptomatic proximal migration of the radius.

Elbow dislocation (with or without coronoid fracture): In most instances the combination of elbow dislocation and radial head fracture does not result in gross instability or recurrent dislocation. If radial head fracture displacement requires open treatment, it is preferable to preserve the radial head, if technically possible.

Type III (Unrepairable)

Fractures of the radial head and neck with extensive comminution and displacement, but without concomitant elbow dislocation or longitudinal dissociations, should undergo early excision as the treatment of choice. These patients do not require radial head replacement. They should begin early active motion.

With associated injury: With interosseous ligament tear, the fractured native radial head must be excised, to permit early motion and a metallic radial head implanted, to stabilize the forearm.

■ Open Reduction and Internal Fixation

There are three major technical challenges:

1. Reassembling the fractured radial head
2. Securing the fractured radial head to the radial neck
3. Ensuring that the implants do not interfere with pronation and supination.

The radial head should be approached laterally, just anterior to the anconeus. The structure at risk is the posterior interosseous nerve. Once the fracture is thoroughly exposed, the pieces should be repositioned to reconstruct the radial head, small Kirschner wires can be used to temporarily hold the fracture.

Safe Zones for ORIF (Figs 22.86A to C)

Based on anatomic dissections, there is a safe zone of hardware placement, comprising approximately 90°, centered about the equator in the neutral position. If this zone is used, normal headed screws and plates can be placed without fear of impinging in the proximal radioulnar joint. If the fracture is limited to the radial head, without extension to the radial neck, the Herbert screw can be used and placed below the chondral surface. Absorbable pins have also been used.

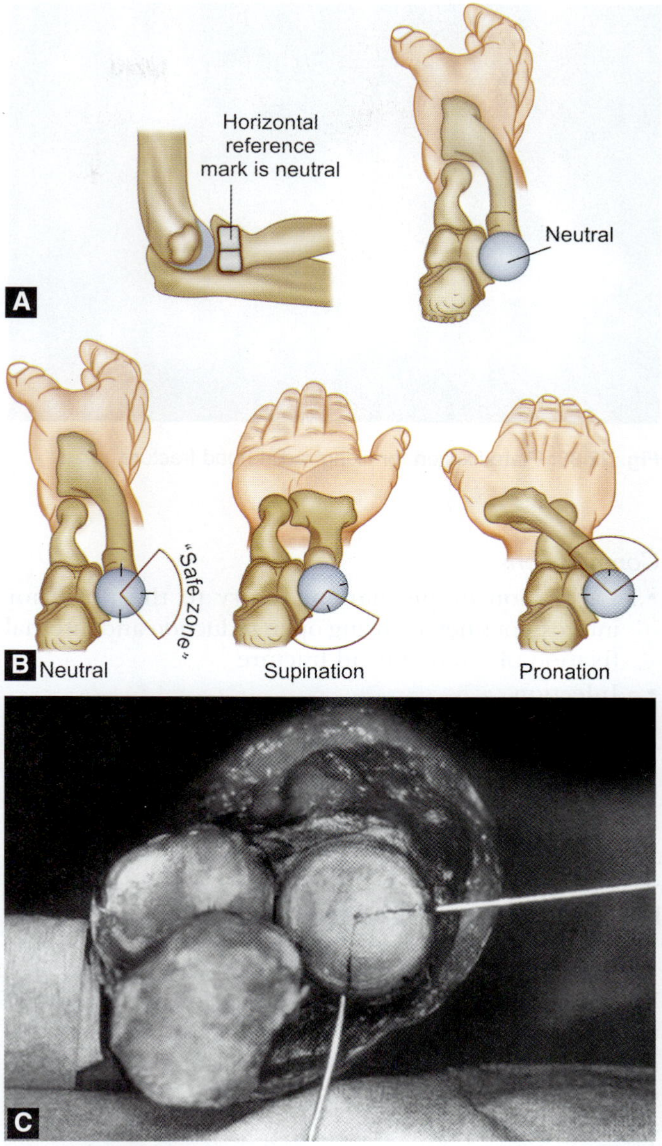

Figs 22.86A to C: Safe zones for ORIF, approximately 90° centered about the equator in the neutral position

Screw Fixation

Figure 22.87 shows screw fixation.

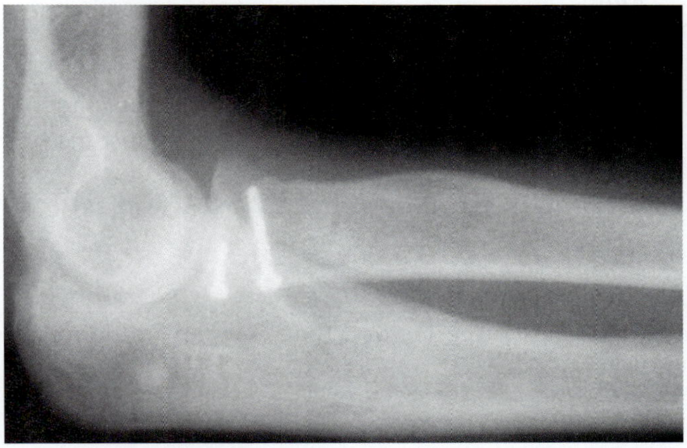
Fig. 22.87: Correcting radial head fracture by screw fixation

Plate Fixation

Figure 22.88 represents plate fixation.

Prosthetic Replacement

A metal prosthesis is inserted, when there is elbow or forearm instability and in most young and active patients.

Excision

The fragments are excised and the neck smoothed off. In the setting of an olecranon fracture-dislocation or posterior Monteggia injury, it may be useful to seal the end of the radius with bone wax. The LCL complex should be repaired if injured. There are various designs of prosthesis avilable—vitallium, silastic, metallic, bipolar.

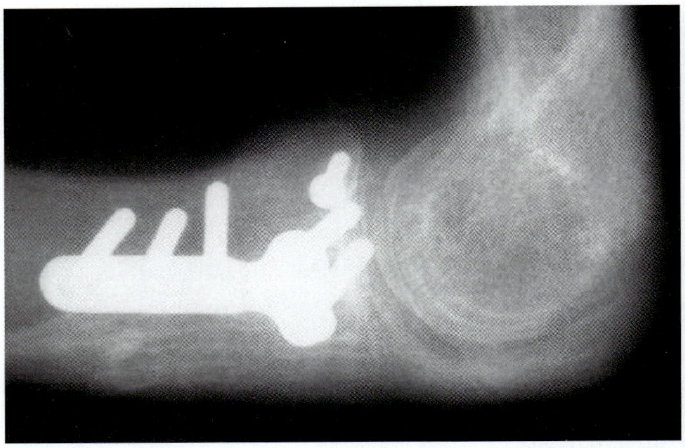

Fig. 22.88: Plate fixation for fixing radial head fracture

Complications

- Laceration or permanent injury to the posterior interosseous nerve during open reduction and internal fixation of a radial head fracture
- Infection
- Malunion
- Nonunion (rare)
- Pain
- Pronation—supination restriction.

Olecranon Fractures (Figs 22.89A and B)

Fractures of the olecranon can be caused either by direct trauma, such as falling on the tip of the elbow or by indirect trauma, such as falling on a partially flexed elbow, with indirect forces generated by the triceps muscle avulsing the olecranon.

Clinical Features

- Swelling due to hemorrhagic effusion of the elbow joint
- Pain on movement
- Tenderness
- Palpable defect may be noted at the fracture site
- Inability to extend the elbow actively against gravity.

Radiological Studies (Figs 22.90A and B)

Classification

Mayo classification (Fig. 22.91)

Distinguishes three factors, that have an influence on treatment.
These are:

- Fracture displacement

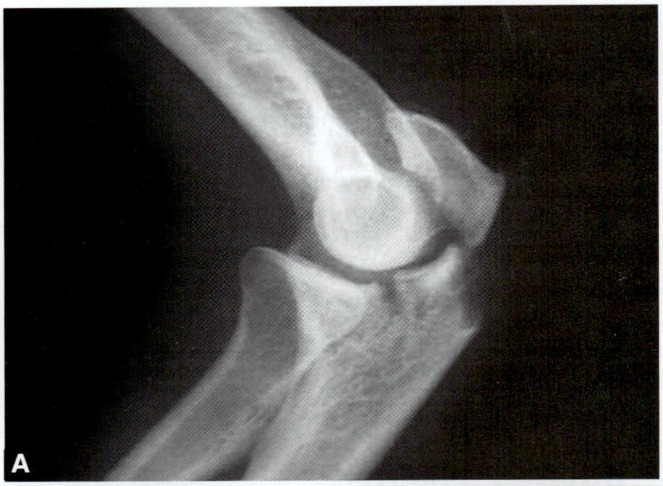

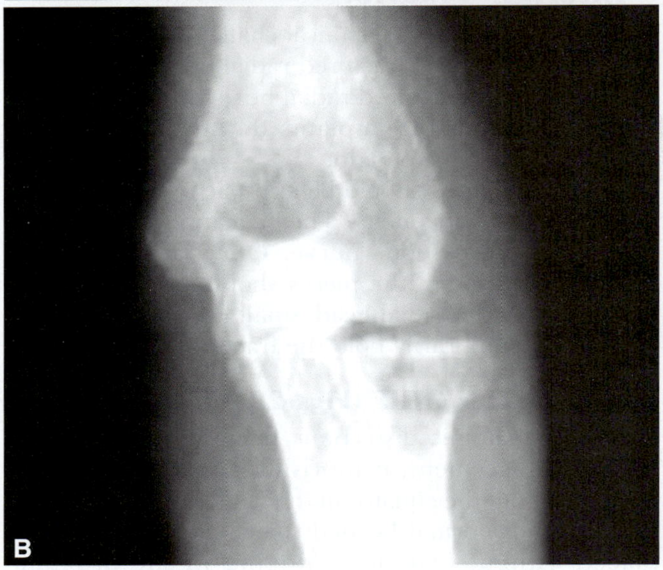

Figs 22.89A and B: X-ray showing olecranon fracture

- Comminution
- Ulnohumoral stability

Type I: Nondisplaced or minimally displaced

- Noncomminuted (Type IA)
- Comminuted (Type IB)

Type II: Fractures have displacement of proximal fragment, without elbow instability.

- Noncomminuted (Type IIA)
- Comminuted (Type IIB)

Type III: Fractures feature instability of ulnohumoral joint and require surgical treatment.

Colton classification

Type I (Nondisplaced)

- Less than 2 mm of displacement
- No increase in displacement with flexion of 90 degrees
- Patient able to extend their arm against gravity

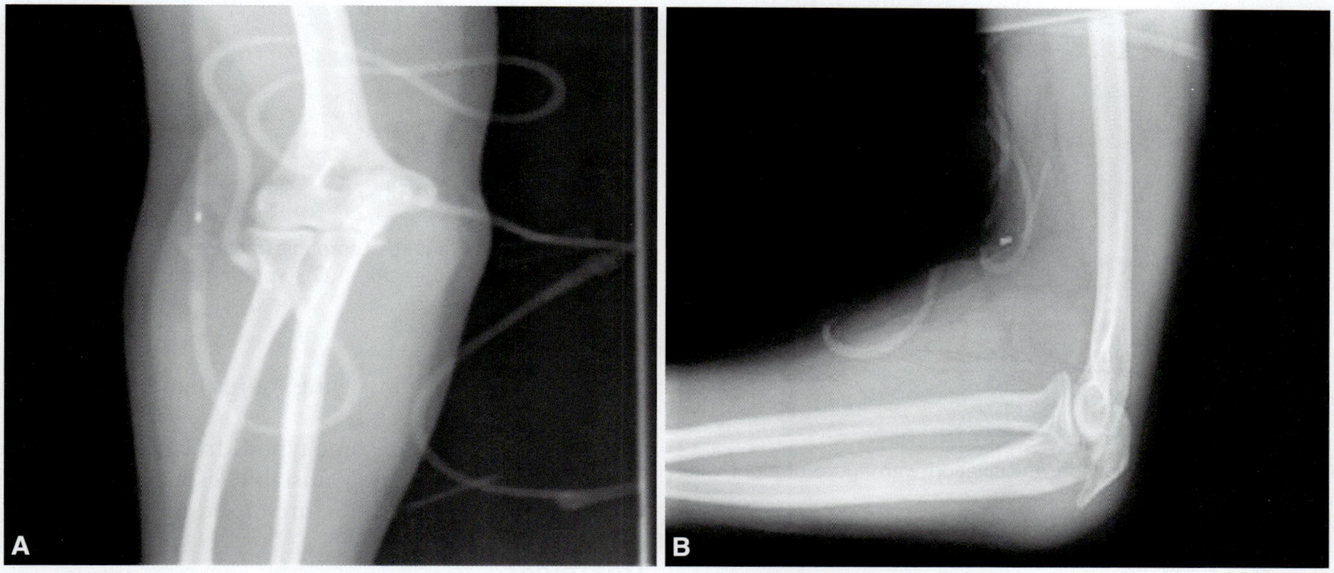

Figs 22.90A and B: X-rays showing olecranon fractures—(A) AP view; (B) Lateral view

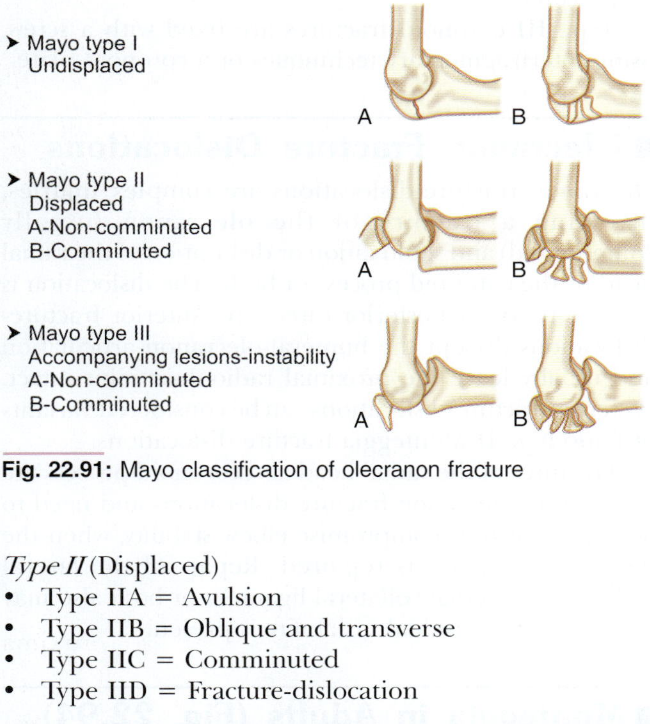

Fig. 22.91: Mayo classification of olecranon fracture

Type II (Displaced)
- Type IIA = Avulsion
- Type IIB = Oblique and transverse
- Type IIC = Comminuted
- Type IID = Fracture-dislocation

Fractures were classified by Schatzker; based on fracture pattern and mechanical considerations, as to the type of internal fixation required for repair:
- Transverse
- Transverse impacted
- Oblique
- Comminuted
- Oblique distal
- Fracture dislocation.

Operative Treatment

The methods of operative treatment commonly used are:
- Open reduction and fixation with a figure-of-eight wire loop
- Medullary fixation
- A combination of intramedullary pin or screw and tension bands
- Contoured plate and screws
- Excision of the proximal fragment

Open reduction and internal fixation and excision of the olecranon fragments have their advocates. Advocates of open reduction and internal fixation claim that this method provides an anatomical reduction of the bony fragment and a congruous articular surface, rigid fixation allows for an early range of motion, elbow stability is preserved and the extensor power of the triceps muscle is maintained.

Open Reduction and Fixation with Figure-of-eight Wire Loop (Fig. 22.92)

Open reduction and fixation with figure-of-eight wire loop is applicable to fractures of the olecranon that are not comminuted and that are well proximal to the coronoid process. This fixation is used most commonly for avulsion and transverse fractures, but may be combined with intramedullary fixation in comminuted fractures and fracture-dislocations.

Intramedullary Fixation

Displaced olecranon fractures fixed with intramedullary Kirschner wires and tension band wiring or long intramedullary cancellous screw fixation combined with a figure-of-eight wire.

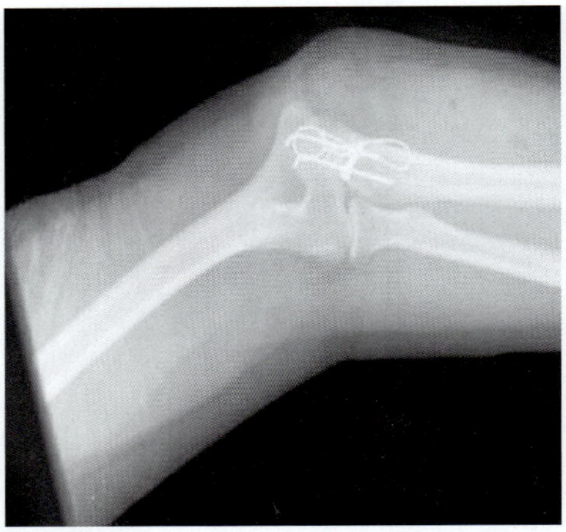

Fig. 22.92: Open reduction and fixation with figure-of-eight wire loop

Plate Fixation

If comminution with bone loss prevents use of a tension band compression technique because of the possibility of shortening of the olecranon, hand-contoured plates and screws provide rigid fixation, applied most easily on the posterior surface and unicortical screws are used near the articular surface.

Excision of Proximal Fragment

Excision of a proximal fragment has several advantages. First, the possibility of nonunion is eliminated and only the triceps tendon must become anchored to the distal fragment. The possibility of traumatic arthritis resulting from irregularity of the articular surface is minimized. This method can be used, only if enough of the olecranon is left to form a stable base for the trochlear excision of olecranon fragments, we consider it the method of choice in the following circumstances:

- In severely comminuted fractures, in which open reduction and internal fixation are not technically possible.
- In nonarticular fractures
- After failed open reduction and internal fixation
- In nonunions
- In type III open fractures, or if local soft-tissue conditions are precarious and the subcutaneous location of the internal fixation devices might present a problem.

Fractures of the Coronoid Process (Figs 22.93A to C)

Classification by Regan and Morrey

Type I: A small chip fracture

Type II: A fracture involving less than 50 percent of the process

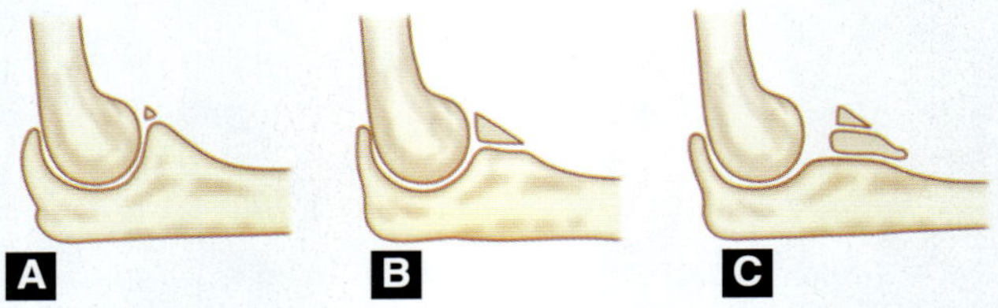

Figs 22.93A to C: Fracture of coronoid fracture—(A) Type I fracture; (B) Type II fracture; (C) Type III fracture

Type III: A fracture involving more than 50 percent of the process.

Type III and some type II fractures render the elbow extremely unstable, especially if there is an associated fracture of the radial head.

Treatment

Type I and type II coronoid fractures are fixed with heavy suture woven into the brachialis and coronoid insertions, passed through two drill holes in the proximal ulna, and tied securely.

Type III coronoid fractures are fixed with a screw, using interfragmentary techniques or a coronoid plate.

Olecranon Fracture Dislocations

Olecranon fracture-dislocations are complex injuries, involving a fracture of the olecranon (usually comminuted) and subluxation or dislocation of the radial head or the coronoid process or both. The dislocation is in an anterior or posterior direction (Anterior fracture-dislocations disrupt the humeral-olecranon articulation and usually leave the proximal radioulnar joint intact. Posterior fracture-dislocations can be considered variants of Bado type II Monteggia fracture-dislocations.

Fractures of the radial head and coronoid process are common in olecranon fracture dislocations and need to be treated, if they compromise elbow stability, when the olecranon fracture is repaired. Repair of the lateral collateral or medial collateral ligament or both also may be necessary if residual instability is present.

Monteggia in Adults (Fig. 22.94)

Fractures of the proximal third of the ulna with dislocation of the radial head. The combination of injuries known as a Monteggia fracture-dislocation is an often treacherous condition to treat. This combination of fracture of the ulna with dislocation of the proximal end of the radius with or without fracture of the radius usually can be treated conservatively in children, but routinely requires open reduction in adults.

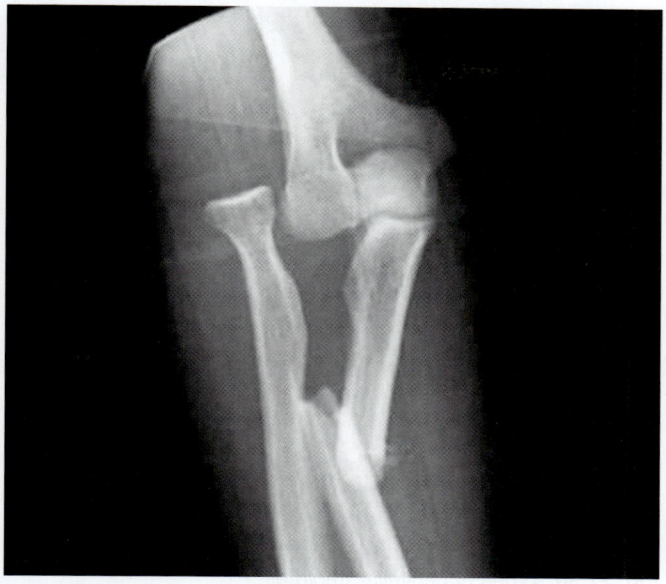

Fig. 22.94: Monteggia fracture dislocation

Classification

Bado suggested classification into four types:

Type 1: Fracture of the middle or proximal third of the ulna with anterior dislocation of the radial head and characteristic apex anterior angulation of the ulna.

Type 2: Fracture of the middle or proximal third of the ulna (the apex usually is posteriorly angulated) with posterior dislocation of the radial head and often a fracture of the radial head.

Type 3: Fracture of the ulna, just distal to the coronoid process with lateral dislocation of the radial head.

Type 4: Fracture of the proximal or middle third of the ulna, anterior dislocation of the radial head and fracture of the proximal third of the radius below the bicipital tuberosity.

Type 1 far exceeds all others in frequency. Several mechanisms of injury probably exist, including direct blows to the ulnar aspect of the forearm and a fall with hyperpronation or hyperextension, with the strong supinating force of the biceps pulling the radial head anteriorly as the fracture of the ulna is produced by the compression forces of the fall.

Most of type 1 injuries can be treated by rigid fixation of the fracture of the ulna, closed reduction of the radial head and immobilization of the elbow for 6 weeks in a position of flexion above 90° with the forearm supinated. Nonunions of the ulna, synostosis and limitation of elbow motion are the factors primarily responsible for poor results, head can be reduced by closed methods, open reduction of the dislocation is not indicated, but the fracture of the ulna is rigidly fixed. In the proximal third of the ulna, where the medullary canal is large, a compression plate is used. In the middle third, where the medullary canal is small, either a compression plate or a triangular intramedullary nail is used.

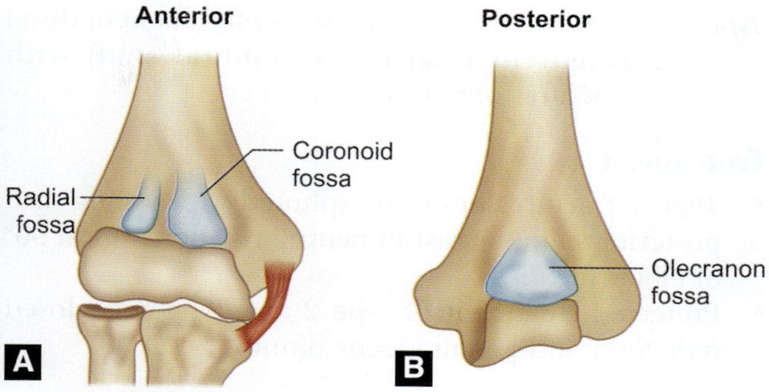

Figs 22.95A and B: (A) Anterior view of elbow joint, showing radial and coronoid fossa; (B) Posterior view of elbow joint, showing olecranon fossa

Fractures in Children

- Extremely common 15 percent of all fractures in pediatric patients
- Most common fractures in children are supracondylar fractures, lateral condyle fractures, medial epicondyle fractures and transphyseal fractures
- Evaluation of pediatric patient
- A gentle approach with parent and child is always best.
- Cubital fossa must be checked for any tenting of skin that would indicate that fracture has punctured the brachialis, which would be difficult for reduction (Figs 22.95A and B)
- Signs and symptoms of compartment syndrome must be ruled out
- Finger flexion must be assesed for anterior interosseous nerve palsy
- If a child has a warm hand with a good capillary refill a vascular injury is unlikely.

Supracondylar Fractures

It is most common elbow fracture in children. Mechanism of injury is an extension on distal humerus, causing an extension-type fracture. A flexion type fracture may occur with a direct blow to the elbow with elbow flexed.

Gartland classification for extension type supracondylar humerus fractures:

Type 1: Fracture is a nondisplaced fracture and difficult to detect on X-rays.

Type 2: Fracture has the posterior periosteum intact, connecting the distal fragment and humeral shaft.

Type 3: Fracture has a complete displacement of distal fragment relative to humeral shaft with fractures of both cortices.

Treatment

- Type 1 fracture should be splinted with a long arm posterior splint or cast in neutral rotation and in 90° of elbow flexion.
- Preferred treatment of type 2 and type 3 is closed reduction and percutaneous pinning.

Complications

- Early complications are attributable to neurovascular compromise.
- Compartment syndrome
- Volkmans ischemic contracture
- Malunion, usually cubitus varus due to rotational malrotation
- Stiffness is rare.

Radial Head and Neck Fractures

Children with radial neck fractures usually are 4 to 14 years old, primarily because ossification of the radial head usually does not begin before 5 years of age. The normal anatomical angulation of the radial neck in children has been erroneously diagnosed as a buckle fracture in this area. Most fractures in children are of the radial neck and not the radial head. Fractures of the epiphysis of the radial head are usually Salter-Harris type IV fractures. Most radial neck fractures occur through the metaphysis, but they can occur through the physis, with a metaphyseal spike of bone producing a characteristic Salter-Harris type II epiphyseal injury.

Type A: Salter-Harris type I and II injuries of the proximal radial epiphyses.

Type B: Salter-Harris type IV injuries of the proximal radial epiphysis.

Type C: Fractures involving only the proximal radial metaphysis.

Type D: Fractures occurring when a dislocated elbow is being reduced.

Type E: Fractures occurring in conjunction with the elbow dislocation.

Capitellar Fractures

This fracture was first described in 1853 by Hahn. This fracture has only one portion of lateral column and not epicondyle or metaphysic. It's an uncommon fracture, not many reports are presented. A small series was presented by Johnsson.

Morphology

Basically it is a terminal intra-articular fracture. It can be due to a fall on hand, either extension or flexion.

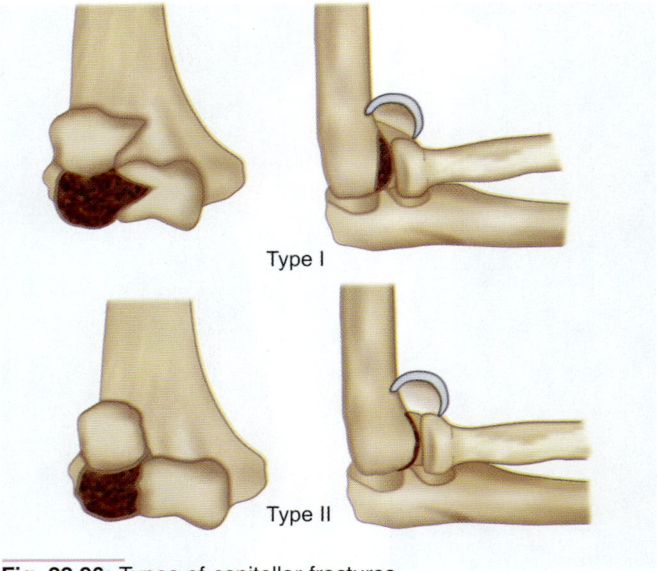

Fig. 22.96: Types of capitellar fractures

Two types (Fig. 22.96):
- Hahn-Steinthal (type I)
- Kocher-Lorentz (type II)

Hahn-Steinthal

Injury in extension are more common. A large portion of capitellum with a small piece of trochlea attached.

Kocher-Lorentz

Articular chip fracture, with small subchondral bone. It may be associated with ulnar collateral injury.

Clinical Features

- X-rays AP and lateral views are important
- Restricted elbow movements
- Tenderness
- Loss of rotatory movements
- Fractured chip generally migrates anteriorly and superiorly
- Double arch sign (Fig. 22.97).

■ Fractures of Lateral Condyle of Humerus

Most common distal humeral epiphyseal fracture (16-18%). Approximate average age is 6 years

The pertinent anatomical considerations in lateral condylar fracture include:
- Capitulum, lateral epicondyle and soft tissue attached to it namely extensors and supinators.
- Difficult to diagnose and have propensity for late displacement.

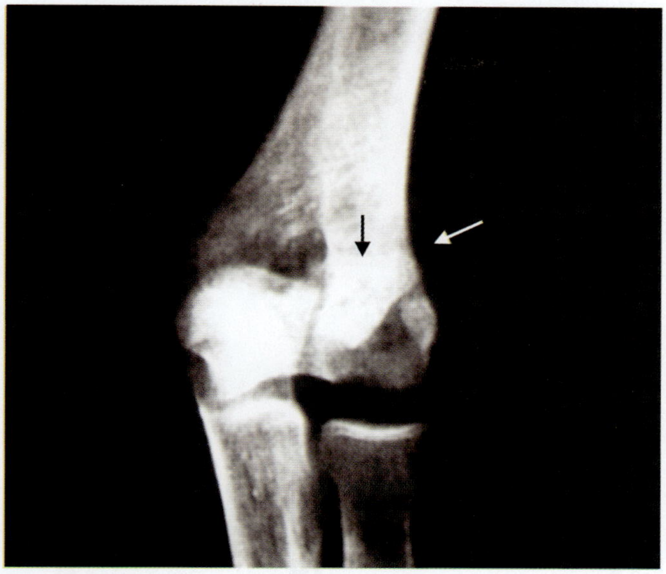

Fig. 22.97: Double arch sign

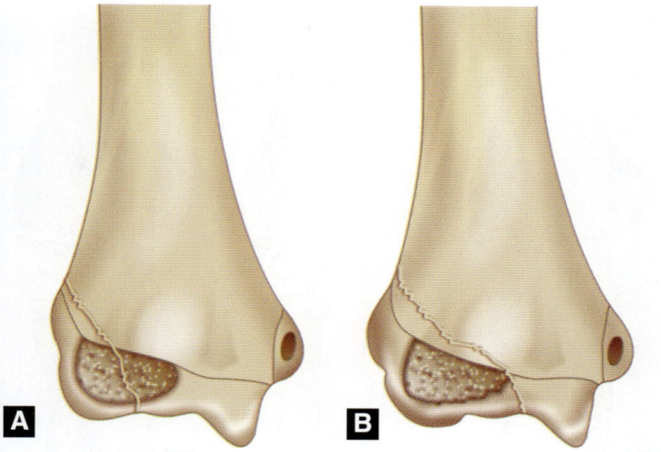

Figs 22.98A and B: (A) Milch type I lateral condylar fracture; (B) Type II fracture

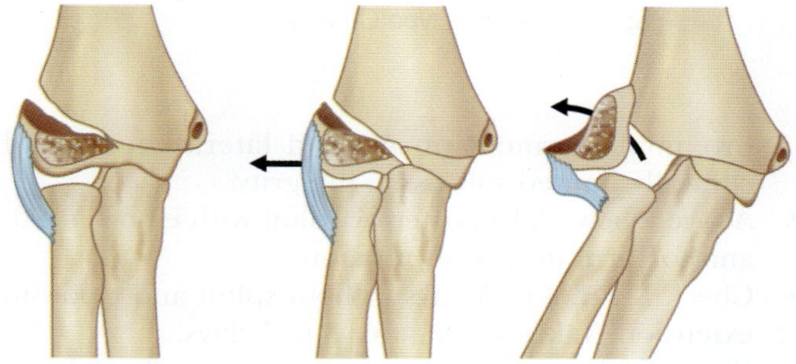

Fig. 22.99: Different types of lateral condylar fractures

Mechanism of Injury

- Pulloff or Avulsion theory (most common)
- Elbow forced in varus along with extensor
- Muscles and lateral collateral ligaments applies an avulsion force to the lateral condyle (Milch type II)
- Pushoff theory (less common)
- Fall on palm with elbow flexed, the radial head is forced against the capitulum and may cause Milch type I fracture.

Classification

Milch Classification (Figs 22.98 and 22.99)

- Milch type I lateral trochlear ridge is left intact
- Milch type II (more common).

Anatomical Location

- Salter-Harris type II (milch type II)
- Salter-Harris type IV (milch type I)

Signs and Symptoms

- Distortion of elbow is less due hematoma
- Location of soft tissue swelling concentrated over lateral aspect of distal humerus
- Undisplaced fractures, produce local tenderness
- *Displaced and rotated fracture:* Some amount of crepitus with the movement of fragment.

Radiography

Finnbogason et al. described roentgenographic criteria for determining fracture stability, which they used in planning and initial treatment.

Type A (Fig. 22.100A): Fracture through the lateral humeral condyle with minimal lateral gap—a stable fracture.

Type B (Fig. 22.100B): Fracture through the lateral humeral condyle to the epiphyseal cartilage with a lateral gap—a fracture with undefinable risk.

Type C (Fig. 22.100C): Fracture through the lateral humeral condyle, as shown in Figures 22.100A to C with the fracture gap as wide laterally as medially—a fracture with high risk of later displacement.

MRI

- Diagnosis of minimally displaced fracture
- To distinguish between this fracture and fracture of entire distal humeral physis.

Arthrogram

Determines the stability of nonossified articular cartilage of trochlea.

Treatment

Immobilization

- If fracture is minimally displaced on X-ray (i.e. metaphyseal fragment is less than 2 mm from the

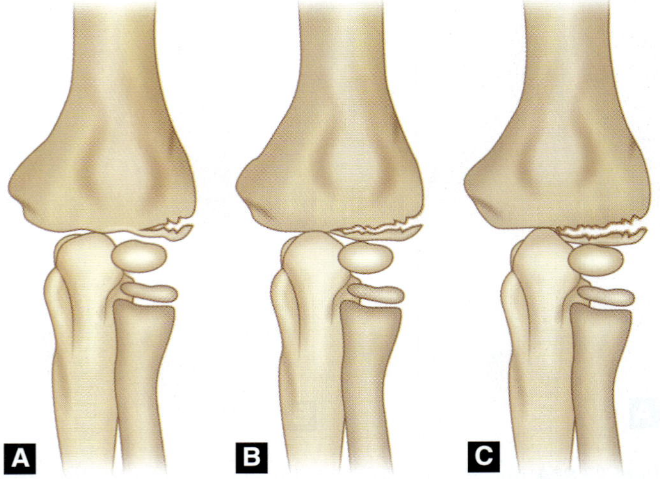

Figs 22.100A to C: Roentgenographic criteria for determining fracture stability—(A) Type A stable fracture with minimal lateral gap; (B) Type B fracture through the lateral humeral condyle to the epiphyseal cartilage with a lateral gap; (C) Unstable type C fracture

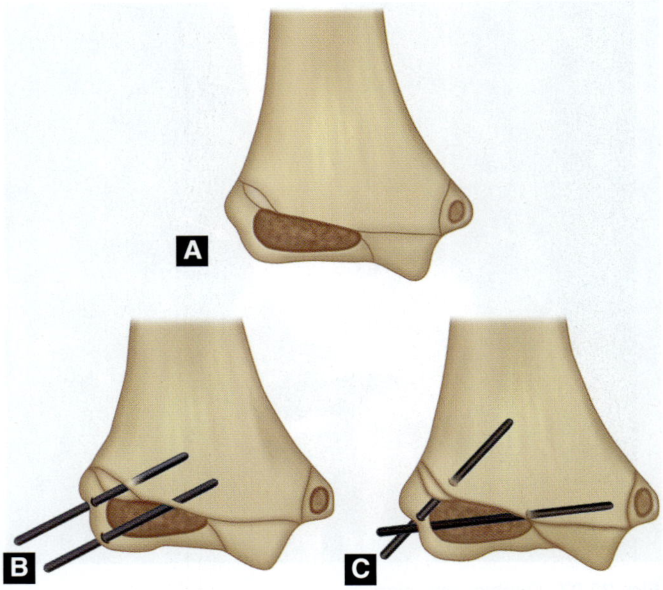

Figs 22.101A to C: Percutaneous pinning of stage II displacement

proximal fragment on AP and lateral views) and clinically limited soft tissue integrity.
- Above elbow (A/E) posterior splint with elbow in 90° and forearm in neutral rotation.
- Check X-ray, 3 to 5 days without splint and elbow in extension. Taken again after 3 to 5 days.
- If no displacement A/E cast for at least 3 weeks or until fracture union is apparent.

Percutaneous Pinning
- Stage II displacement (2-4 mm), with varus stress views under anesthesia by arthrography, as shown in Figures 22.101A to C.
- If fracture is stable then percutaneous pinning is indicated.

Open Reduction Internal Fixation
- All fracture with stage III displacement
- *Approach:* Kochers lateral J
- *Fixation:* Suture fixation, which is inadequate
- Smooth pin fixation, preferably with two pins, either through the epiphysis or through the metaphyseal spike, as shown in Figures 22.102A and B.
- Screw fixation, preferably through the metaphyseal area.

Complications

Biological Problems
- Lateral spur formation
- Cubitus varus
- Cubitus valgus (Fig. 22.103)

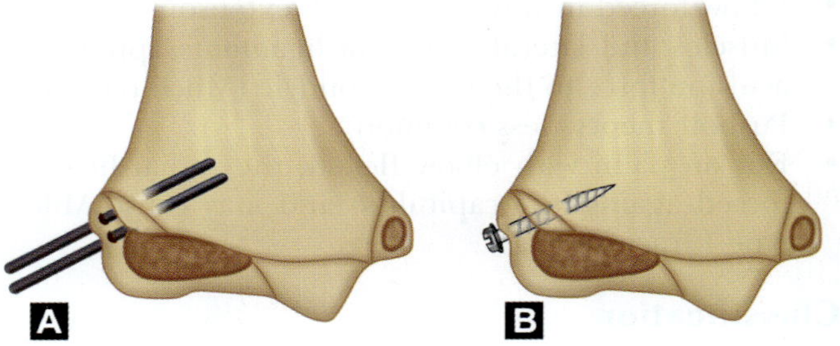

Figs 22.102A and B: Open reduction internal fixation—(A) Pin fixation; (B) Screw fixation

Technical Problems (Fig. 22.104)
- Nonunions/delayed union
- Fishtail deformity
- Tardy ulnar nerve palsy
- Myositis ossificans
- Osteonecrosis of condylar fragment

Nonunion: Flynn et al. criteria, if fracture has not united by 12 weeks it is classified as nonunion. Criteria outlined by Flynn et al. for surgical treatment include:
- A large metapyseal fragment
- Displacement of less than 1 cm from joint surface
- An open viable lateral condyle physis

Open reduction and internal fixation with bone grafting for nonunion or delayed union of minimally displaced fractures is the main line of treatment for these fracture.

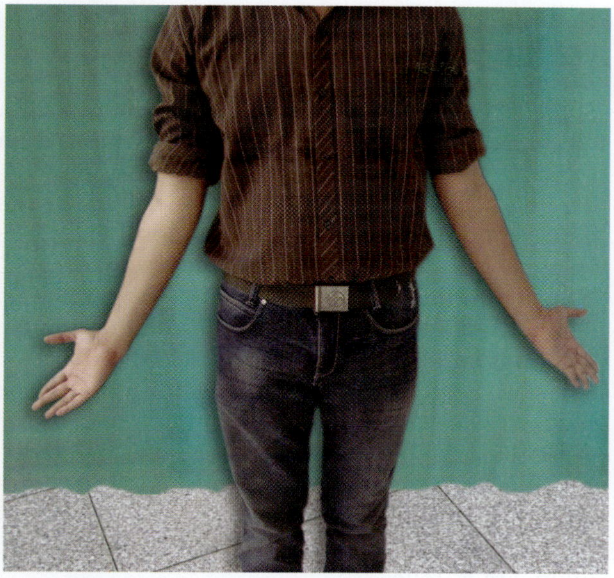

Fig. 22.103: Cubitus valgus

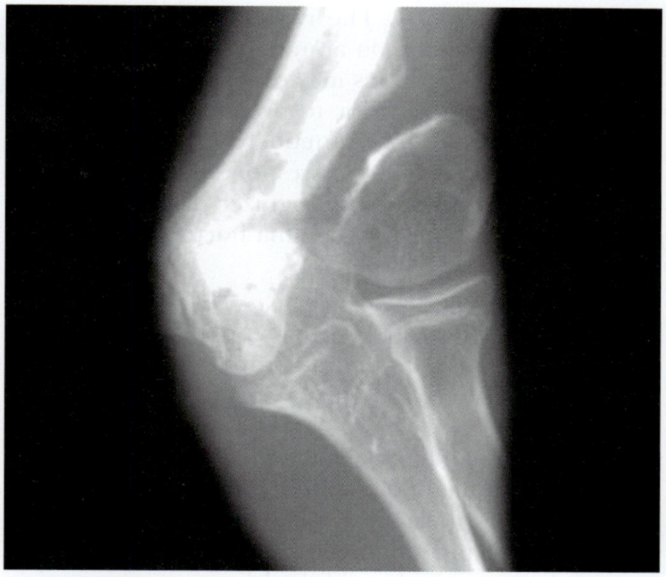

Fig. 22.104: Nonunion of lateral condylar fracture

Monteggia in Children

Introduction

The eponym Monteggia fracture is most precisely used to refer to a dislocation of the proximal radioulnar joint in association with a forearm fracture. These injuries are relatively uncommon, accounting for less than 5 percent of all forearm fractures. The ulna fracture is usually clinically and radiographically apparent. Findings associated with the concomitant radial head dislocation are often subtle and can be overlooked.

The keys to successful diagnosis of a Monteggia fracture are clinical suspicion and radiographs of the entire forearm and elbow. Properly assessing the nature of this injury in a timely fashion is imperative, in order to prevent permanent disability or limb dysfunction.

History

In 1814, Giovanni Battista Monteggia of Milan first described this fracture, as a fracture to the proximal third of the ulna with associated anterior dislocation of the radial head. Interestingly, he described this injury pattern in the preroentgen era, based solely on the history of injury and on physical examination findings. However, this particular fracture pattern only accounts for about 60 percent of these types of injuries. More than 150 years later in 1967, Bado coined the term Monteggia lesion and classified the injury into four types.

Classification by Bado

Type I: Fracture of the proximal or middle third of the ulna with anterior dislocation of the radial head.

Type II: Fracture of the proximal or middle third of the ulna with posterior dislocation of the radial head.

Type III: Fracture of the ulnar metaphysis with lateral dislocation of the radial head.

Type IV: Fracture of the proximal or middle third of the ulna and radius with anterior dislocation of the radial head.

The basis of the Bado classification is in the recognition that the apex of the fracture is in the same direction as the radial head dislocation. The first challenge is correctly assessing the extent and nature of the injury. The ulna fracture is usually noted, commonly in the proximal third of the ulna. The olecranon, mid and distal shafts may be involved. Some injuries associated with radiocapitellar dislocation (such as the transolecranon fracture-dislocation of the elbow) are mislabeled as Monteggia lesions, when in fact the proximal radioulnar joint remains intact. The Monteggia lesion is most precisely characterized as a forearm fracture in association with dislocation of the proximal radioulnar joint.

The radial head dislocation may not be apparent and may be missed, if the elbow is not included in the radiograph. Whenever a fracture of a long bone is noted, the joints above and below should be evaluated using radiographs in orthogonal planes (planes at 90° angles to each other). If one of the forearm bones is injured, look for injury in the other bone and associated joints of the forearm, elbow and wrist. This principle also applies to Galeazzi fractures, the eponym used to refer to a fracture of the distal radius and concomitant dislocation of the distal radioulnar joint. Separate radiographs should be taken of the elbow. The radial head should point towards the capitellum on all radiographs of the elbow. Unrecognized dislocations may result from reduction of the dislocated radius prior to presentation. This may occur in the field spontaneously or as a result of manipulation by emergency responders. The treating physician may reduce an unrecognized dislocation, while reducing or immobilizing the ulna fracture.

Frequency

Fixation to stabilize the ulna and prevent further displacement forces on the radiocapitellar joint. Closed Monteggia fractures in pediatric patients are generally treated in a closed fashion. A posterior long-arm splint with the elbow in 90° of flexion and full supination is the immobilization method of choice for types I, III and IV. Type II injuries (posterior lesions) are best splinted in Monteggia fractures comprise less than 5 percent of forearm fractures, with published literature supporting 1-2 percent. Of the Monteggia fractures, Bado type I is the most common (59%), followed by type III (26%), type II (5%), and type IV (1%). Monteggia fractures are one third as common as the more familiar Galeazzi fractures.

Etiology

Monteggia fractures are primarily associated with falls on an outstretched hand with forced pronation. If the elbow is flexed, the chance of a type II or III lesion is greater. In some cases, a direct blow to the forearm can also produce similar injuries.Penrose considered type II lesions a variation of posterior elbow dislocation. Bado believed that the type III lesion, the result of a direct lateral force on the elbow was primarily observed in children. In essence, high-energy trauma (e.g. motor vehicle collisions) and low-energy trauma (e.g. a fall from standing) can result in the described injuries. A high index of suspicion therefore, should be maintained with any ulna fracture.

Pathophysiology

The forearm structures are intricately related and any disruption to one of the bones affects the other. The ulna and radius are in direct contact with each other only at the proximal and distal radioulnar joints. However, they are unified along their entire length by the interosseous membrane. This allows the radius to rotate around the ulna. When the ulna is fractured, energy is transmitted along the interosseous membrane, displacing the proximal radius. The end result is a disrupted interosseous membrane proximal to the fracture, dislocated proximal radioulnar joint and dislocated radiocapitellar joint.

Clinical Features

- Elbow pain
- Elbow swelling
- Deformity
- Crepitus
- Paresthesia or numbness
- Some patients may not have severe pain at rest, but elbow flexion and forearm rotation is limited and painful.
- The dislocated radial head may be palpable in the anterior posterior, or anterolateral position.
- In type I and IV lesions, the radial head can be palpated in the antecubital fossa.
- The radial head can be palpated posteriorly in type II lesions and laterally in type III lesions.
- The skin should be closely inspected to ensure an open fracture is not present.
- Pulses and capillary refill should be documented.
- A negligible hematoma may be present at the site if no direct trauma is associated.
- Monteggia fractures in children based on type of ulnar injury are as follows:
  - Plastic deformation
  - Incomplete (greenstick or buckle) fracture
  - Complete transverse or short oblique fracture
  - Long-oblique or comminuted fracture

Treatment

Indications for treatment of Monteggia fractures are based on the specific fracture pattern and the age of the patient (i.e. pediatric or adult). Most pediatric fracture patterns can be managed conservatively with closed reduction and long arm casting. However, most adult fractures require open reduction and internal fixation techniques. The radial head dislocation should be reduced emergently. Closed reduction under sedation should be performed within 6 to 8 hours of the injury. This is usually achieved with supination of the forearm, but it may require traction and direct pressure on the radial head.

If closed reduction is unsuccessful, the patient should be taken to the operating room within this same time frame for open reduction. Delay in reduction of the radius may lead to permanent articular damage, further nerve injury or both. An open fracture requires emergent operative intervention. In closed injuries, once the radial head is reduced, the forearm is splinted and operative fixation of the ulna fracture may be carried out in an elective fashion for closed injuries. Adults usually require operative internal 70° elbow flexion with supination.

Imaging Studies

Plain Radiography (Figs 22.105 to 22.107)

Views of the forearm in AP and lateral are needed with the wrist and elbow joints included. The evaluating physician should also obtain separate radiographs of the elbow, to assess the proximal radioulnar joint, ulnohumeral articulation and the radiocapitellar joint.

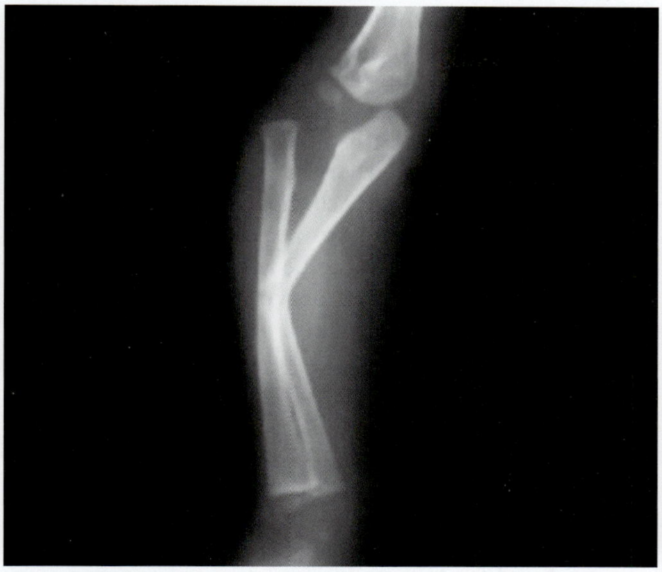

Fig. 22.105: X-ray showing Monteggia fracture dislocation

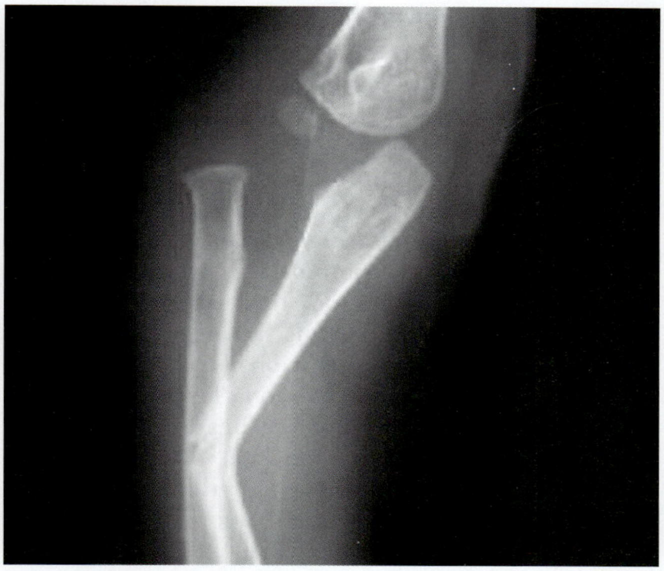

Fig. 22.106: Magnified view of Figure 22.105

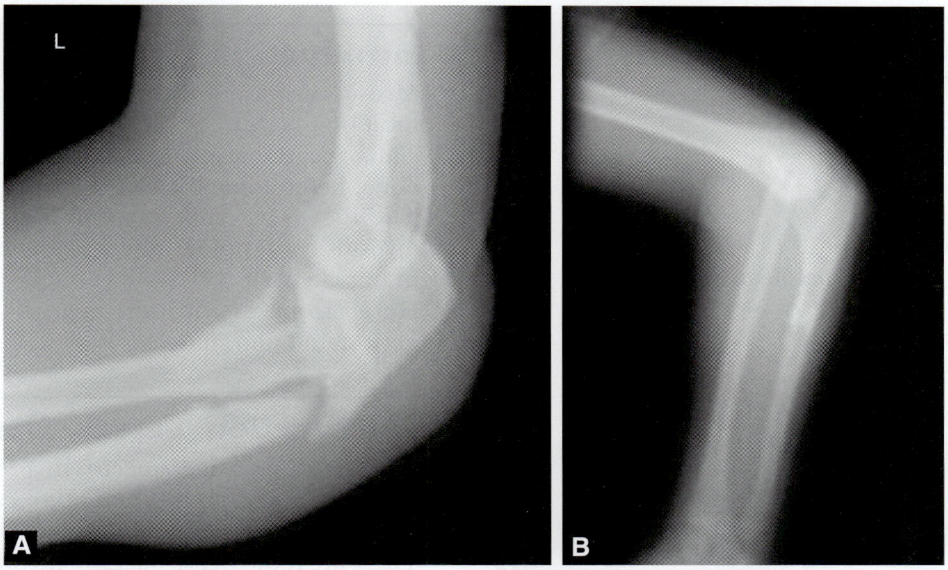

Figs 22.107A and B: Lateral X-ray taken, showing Monteggia fracture dislocation

The ulna fracture is usually obvious, but the findings associated with the radial head dislocation may be subtle and overlooked. To assess the radiocapitellar joint, draw a line parallel to the long axis of the radius. This line should point directly at the capitulum on any projection of the elbow.

The radial head dislocation almost always points in the same direction as the apex of the ulna fracture. In children, recognizing a plastic deformation of the ulna, which may also lead to radial head dislocation is important.

Nonoperative Management

Nonoperative treatment is successful for most Monteggia injuries in children because the majority of the fractures are inherently stable, they require a shorter time for both the osseous and the ligamentous injuries to heal, they can be immobilized for the duration of the initial healing period (3-6 weeks) with little trouble regaining motion lost through stiffness and they may have the potential for remodeling of mild residual angular deformities (less than 10°).

Surgical Management

Open fractures require emergent surgical consultation. The initial treating physician may reduce the radial head dislocation and splint this fracture. Unless the fracture is open, surgical treatment is performed on an elective basis. While, most adults require operative treatment, most pediatric fractures are treated closed. Operative fixation of complete fractures of the ulna with proximal radioulnar joint dislocation is recommended in children. The complete disruption of bone continuity is likely to be associated with substantial soft tissue trauma in these injuries. Shortening and angulation of complete fractures after cast immobilization is common. Anatomic reduction of the ulnar fracture and radial head often requires operative treatment.

Transverse and short oblique fractures are adequately treated with intramedullary wire fixation. Intramedullary wires, however cannot be relied on to maintain reduction of complete fractures that are either long oblique in pattern or comminuted. These fractures are likely to displace or even shorten and therefore, should be fixed with a plate and screws, as shown in Figures 22.108A and B.

Complications

- Infection
- Bleeding
- Malunion
- Nonunion
- Nerve injury
- Redislocation of the radial head
- Radioulnar synostosis
- Chronic pain

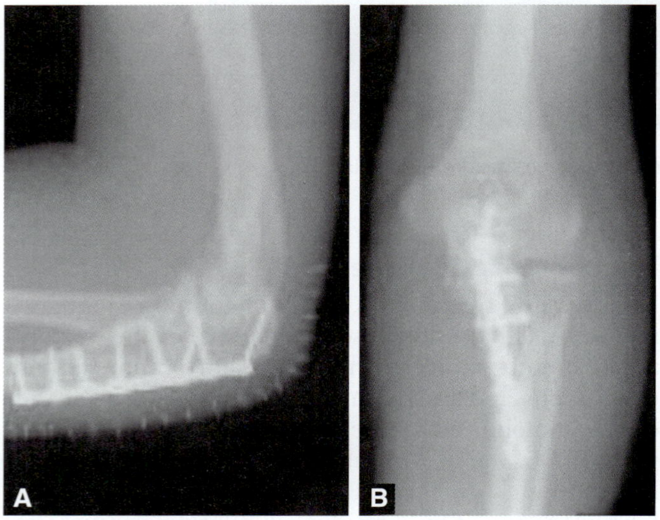

Figs 22.108A and B: Plate and screw fixation of Monteggia fractures

Many of the complications listed are significantly reduced with timely diagnosis, adequate reduction, stable surgical fixation and appropriate postoperative care. Most nerve injuries are neurapraxias, and function usually returns within 1-6 months. Baseline electrodiagnostic studies are obtained early. If nerve function does not return within 2-3 months, surgical exploration may be indicated. If the nerve injury results from reduction or operative treatment, it should be addressed immediately.

Prolonged or complete nerve dysfunction requires early splinting and therapy and may result in the need for tendon transfers. If the radial head dislocates after surgery, improper ulnar reduction must be considered. If this is the case, the hardware should be removed and a proper reduction of the ulna should take place. If dislocation of the radial head is recognized more than 6 weeks after the surgery, a radial head excision should be performed. A nonunion or malunion complication can be considered for bone grafting.

MYOSITIS OSSIFICANS

Introduction

- Myositis ossificans refers to bone formation in atypical location
- Three terms that are used interchangeably are ectopic bone, heterotopic bone and Myositis ossificans
- The first two terms have similar connotation, but myositis ossification usually refers to bone formation in muscle itself
- Heterotopic ossification involves tendons, fascia periosteum and muscle.

Calcification Versus Ossification

- Calcific deposits do occur in tendons, articular cartilages, synovium, articular capsule typically consists of calcium pyrophosphates
- These are radio dense but have no trabecular structure and no true bone matrix is formed
- Ectopic calcification as opposed to ossification affects tissues including skin, brain, kidneys and conjunctiva
- Ectopic calcification occur when there is an increase in serum calcium level such as: Hyperparathyroidism, renal failure, dermatomyositis, scleroderma and following tuberculosis infection.

Types of Myositis Ossificans

There are two types of myositis ossificans:

- Myositis ossificans traumatica
- Myositis ossificans progressiva

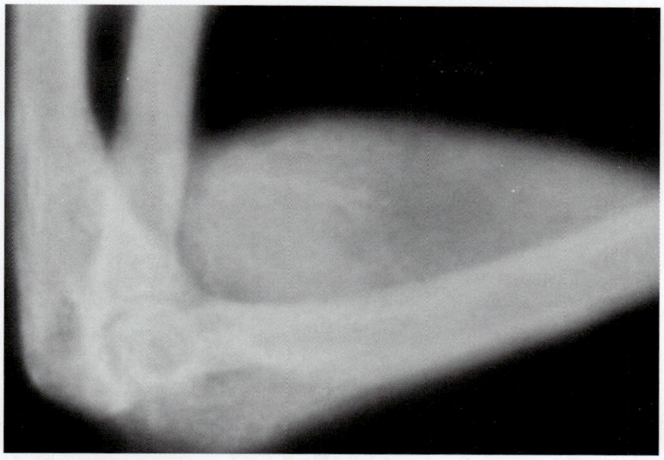

Fig. 22.109: Myositis ossificans traumatica

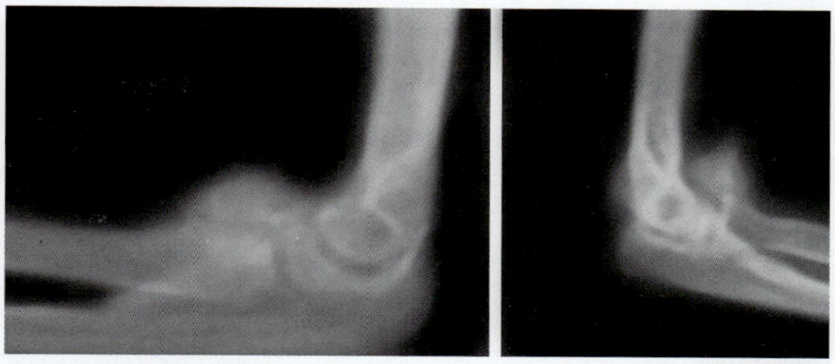

Fig. 22.110: Radial head fracture with dislocation develops a typical pattern of myositis ossificans

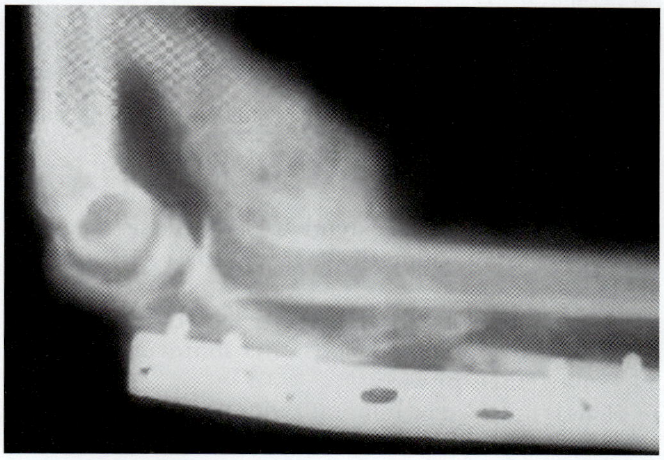

Fig. 22.111: Myositis ossification in a patient with elbow dislocation proximal ulna fracture

Myositis Ossificans Traumatica

It is a reactive lesion occurring in the soft tissues and at times in bone periosteum. It is characterized by fibrous, osseous and cartilaginous proliferation of the subperiosteal hematoma and followed by metaplasia (Fig. 22.109).

Patients who are at risk of developing myositis ossificans are suffering from:

- Elbow trauma
  - Open elbow dislocations which require multiple debridements
  - Elbow dislocations associated with fractures requiring ORIF
  - Radial head fractures treated with surgery more than 24 hours after injury
  - Failed internal fixation about the elbow requiring revision fixation within 3 months
- Distal biceps tendon repair
- Traumatic brain and spinal cord injury
- Burn patients
  - Third degree burns over 20 percent of total body area
  - Third degree burns over the elbow
  - Long periods of bed confinement
  - A hematoma seems to be a necessary prerequisite for myositis ossificans
  - The muscles most often involved are: Brachialis, anticus, quadriceps femoris and adductor muscles of thigh. It is significant that these muscles gain attachment to the bone over a wide area suggesting that the periosteum participates to some extent in the process.
- The region of elbow is a favorite site, ill advised forcible manipulation to increase elbow movement will cause a wide spread involvement (Fig. 22.110).
  Radial head fracture with dislocation develops a typical pattern of myositis ossificans (Fig. 22.110).
  Myositis ossification in a patient with elbow dislocation proximal ulna fracture (Fig. 22.111).
  Entire brachialis muscle has been replaced after head injury without elbow trauma
- Myositis ossification in a patient's third degree burn (Fig. 22.112).

Pathogenesis

- The process is alteration within the ground substance of connective tissue with a striking proliferation of mesenchymal cells
- Degeneration and necrosis of the tissue, disrupted muscle fibers retract followed by histocytic invasion for removal of necrotic debris
- Fibroblasts from endomysium invade the damaged area and rapidly form broad sheets of immature fibroblasts at the same time mesenchymal cells proliferate within the injured connective tissue this histological picture may erroneously diagnosed as fibrosarcoma
- Sarcolemmic nuclei at the ends of the damaged muscle fibers begin to proliferate and chains and columns of plump polyhedral cells appear followed by production

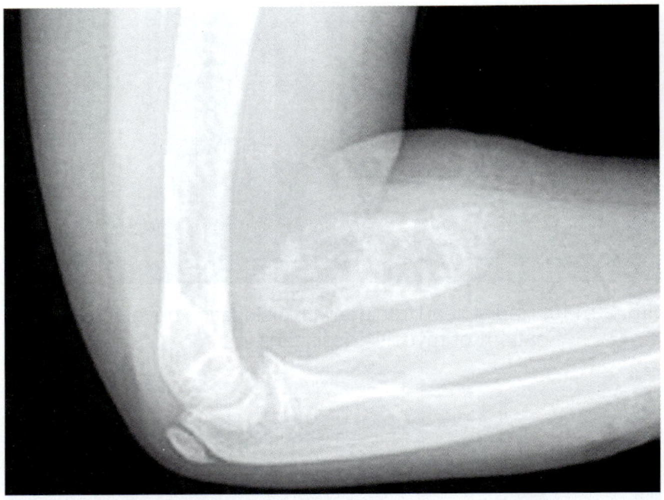

Fig. 22.112: Myositis ossification in a third degree burn patient

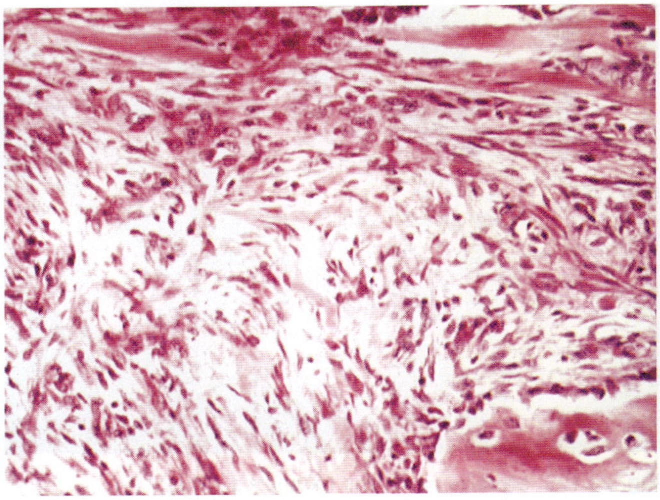

Fig. 22.113: Histological appearance of myositis ossificans

of sarcoplasm which extends as buds, the sarcolemmic nuclei cluster within the center of these sarcoplasmic masses

- The ground substance increase in amount and enclose more mesenchymal cells this material becomes homogenous or waxy
- This is followed by mineralization and bone is formed mineralization occurs periphery to center.

Microscopic Appearance

- Zone phenomenon is of great diagnostic importance
- The central highly cellular region is surrounded by a second zone of fibroblastic tissue and this in turn enveloped by a third zone of mature well oriented bone
- This zonal phenomenon which is not present in soft tissue sarcomas classifies the lesion as benign and obviates the need for radical measures
- When ossification has developed the "tumor" is at least 3 to 4 weeks old
- The cellular inner zone illustrates numerous cells with occasional atypical mitotic figures and variations in size and shape of the cells. The histological appearance is sarcomatous (Fig. 22.113)
- The middle zone shows osteoid formation with a fibrovascular back ground (Fig. 22.114)
- The outer zone illustrates mature fairly well oriented peripheral bone. The fibrous stoma appears more mature than at the center of the lesion (Fig. 22.115).

Clinical Picture

- Pain and loss of range of motion are the common presenting complaints during the evolution of ectopic bone formation

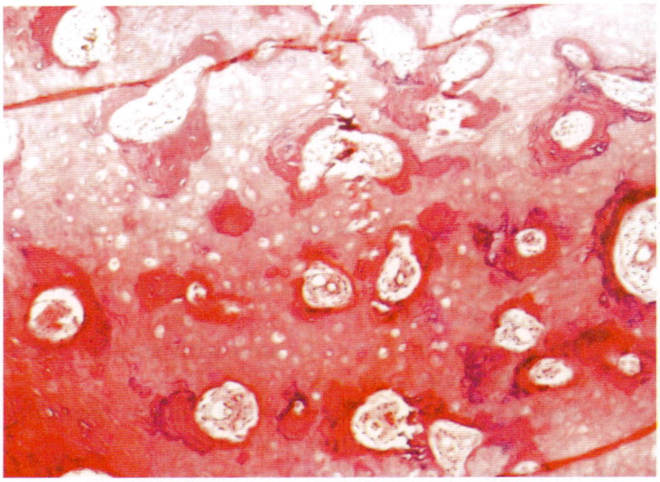

Fig. 22.114: Osteoid formation with fibrovascular background

- On physical examination, there may be swelling, erythema and local warmth of the affected joint
- During formation of extraosseous mass the elbow area is quite swollen and tender, so active and passive movements are reduced
- As pain and swelling are reduced, a circumscribed indurated later hard tumor mass is palpable over the elbow
- Active extension of the joint is limited by virtue of in elasticity of the muscle and flexion is prevented by obstruction offered by the mass
- Aggressive physical therapy with passive stretching beyond the pain free arc of motion, only exacerbates the formation of ectopic bone

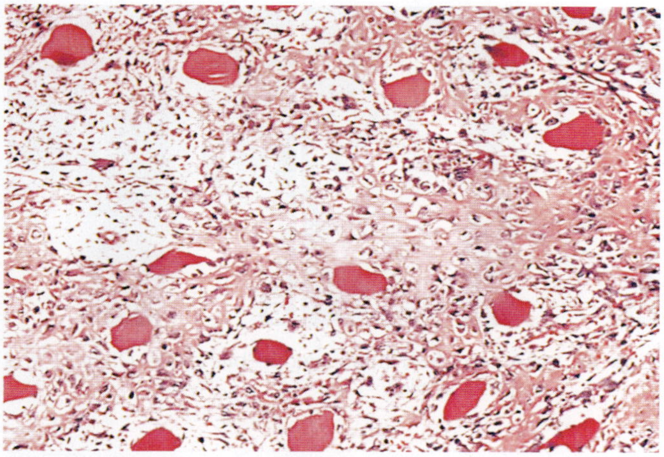

Fig. 22.115: Fibrous stroma appearing more mature at the center of lesion

- Presentation can be confused with cellulitis, deep infection, thrombophlebitis and reflex sympathetic dystrophy.

Physical Examination

- *X-ray:* Shows findings between 4 to 5 weeks
- Biopsy
- Serum alkaline phosphatase
- Technicium bone scan is markedly positive during the formation of ectopic bone and usually remains positive for a prolonged period of time
- An increased incidence of the human leukocyte antigen HLA-B18 in a group of CNS injury has been reported.

Treatment

Acute Stages

Conservative treatment is the method of choice and consists of following:

- Immobilization of elbow by splints
- *Drugs:* Diphosphonate therapy, calcitonin, NSAID's
- *Physiotherapy:* Active physiotherapy is encouraged and passive stretching is avoided
- Manipulation is done under general anesthesia: Adhesions should be snapped abruptly and should not be broken gradually.

Chronic Stages

Surgery is the treatment of choice:

- Not all ectopic bone formation about the elbow requires surgical treatment. The goal of surgery is to restore functional motion
- Careful clinical evaluation should be performed to ensure if ectopic bone itself is blocking motion
- In traumatic conditions, tomograms are necessary to know the congruency of joint surfaces. If joint surfaces are not congruent, total elbow arthroplasty or distraction arthroplasty may be required
- In general, it is better to wait for 9 to 12 months after injury to allow maturation of the ectopic bone. Maturation is judged by plain radiographs.

Principles of Surgery

- Remove ectopic bone at its narrowest portion and with least risk of articulation
- Atraumatic handling of all tissues should be done
- Careful homeostasis
- Suction drainage of the wound
- Postoperative compressive dressing
- Avoiding the creation and deposition of bone dust in the joint by use of osteotomes rather than saws and meticulous lavage
- Avoid injury to cartilage by excision of enough bone to initiate some motion and define joint line, once some motion is initiated additional bone is resected as necessary.

Postoperative Management

- In case of myositis ossificans, surgical field is treated with 700 cgy radiation
- Otherwise 75 mg of indomethacin is prescribed 3 weeks before and 8 weeks after surgery
- Elbow is managed with continuous motion and splints
- When motion goals are not met examination under anesthesia is performed 6 weeks after surgery.

Myositis Ossificans Progressiva

Myositis ossificans progressive; Munchmeyer disease (Fig. 22.116): Progressive, diffuse myositis ossifications was the term applied to this disease by Munchmeyer in 1869. This is a rare congenital condition is autosomal dominant. It is characterized by progressive ossification within the muscles and certain specific skeletal abnormalities.

Skeletal abnormalities include: (Figs 22.116 to 22.118)

- Monophalangeic great toe
- Short first metacarpal bone
- Microdactyly
- Malformation of little finger
- Reduction defects of all limbs
- Abnormalities of cervical vertebrae

Clinical Features

- Progressive ossification occurs in discrete episodes often precipitated by minor trauma such as knock or IM injection
- The region becomes swollen, tender and inflamed. Patient may be pyrexial. As the swelling subsides, muscle mass is replaced by bone
- As the disease progresses, there is interface with the function of the affected muscle leading to progressive immobility

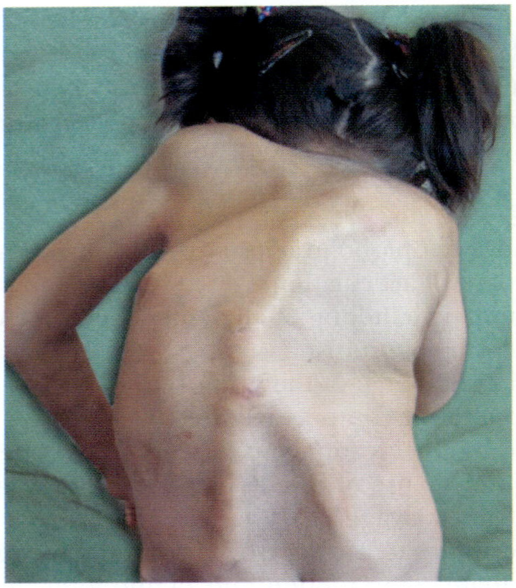

Fig. 22.116: Myositis ossificans progressiva

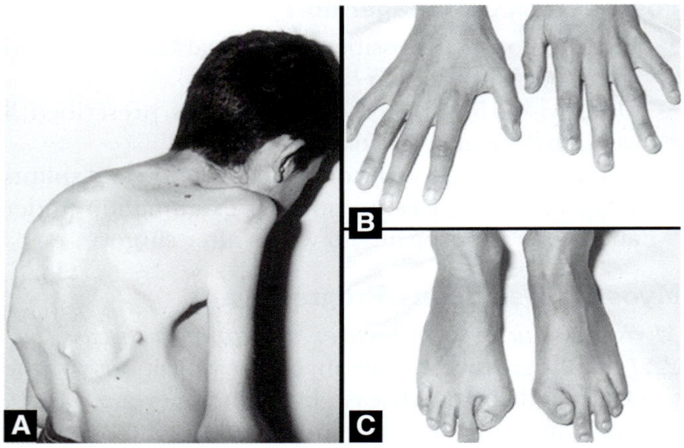

Figs 22.117A to C: (A) Dorsal view of patient of 13 years; (B) Hands to show bilateral clinodactyly of the fifth finger; (C) Typical deformity of the feet (bilateral short hallux valgus)

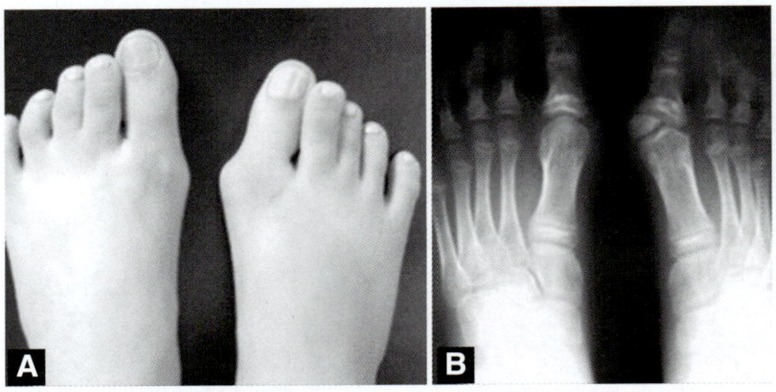

Figs 22.118A and B: Hallux valgus bilateral—Clinical and radiological view

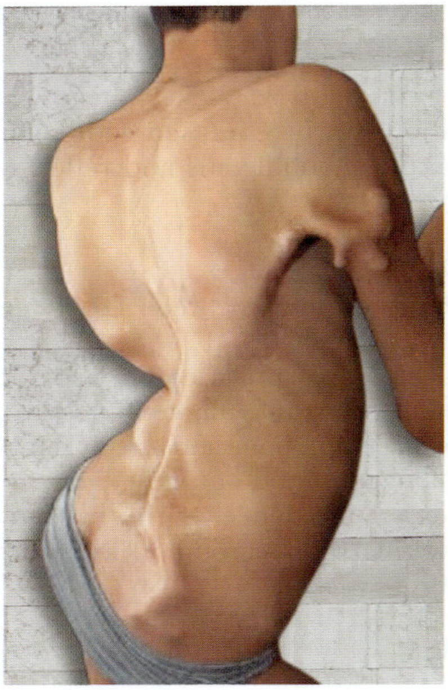

Fig. 22.119: Ossification involving muscles of head and back in early childhood

- Ossification characteristically involves the muscles of head and back in early childhood followed by shoulder and arms and hips (Fig. 22.119)
- There is characteristic sparing of muscles of facial expression, diaphragm, laryngeal muscles, tongue and the small muscles of hand and feet.

Pathology

- The striking feature of the disease is the replacement of muscle, tendon and aponeurosis by masses of bone
- Study of early lesions show that actual bone deposits are not laid down within the actual muscle fiber but in the connective tissue between fibers this lead to alternative name fibrous dysplasia ossificans progressiva
- The only laboratory finding is raised eosinophilic count.

Treatment

- There is no effective treatment which will prevent episodes of ossification
- Diphosphanates have been used but had proved disappointing
- Corticotroponin seems to have an effect of decreased eosinophilic count and joint motion may increase.

Ulnar Neuropathy

- Ulnar neuropathy may occur as a result of compression in the cubital tunnel from ectopic bone

- Ulnar neuropathy is more common in myositis ossificans followed by brain injury. It also occurs after burns and trauma as well.
- Treatment consisted of ulnar nerve transportation anteriorly. Simple subcutaneous translocation is necessary.

VOLKMANN'S ISCHEMIC CONTRACTURE

Introduction

- In 1875, Volkmann described a contracture of muscles of the wrist and fingers, which followed tight bandaging of the arm in the treatment of fractures about the elbow
- Volkmann's contracture (Fig. 22.120) results from acute ischemia of the muscles of the forearm

Etiology

- Fractures (Supracondylar fracture)
- Crush injuries
- Sympathetic cause (Intimal tear→ Sympathetic stimuli Vessel constriction → Mechanical block → Ischemia)
- Other causes which result in compartment syndrome and lead to Volkmann's ischemic contracture:
  - External compression (e.g. tight bandaging)
  - Internal bleeding (e.g. hemophilia)
  - Burns
  - Excessive exercise
  - Snake bites
  - Intra-arterial injections of drugs or sclerosing agents
  - Infections

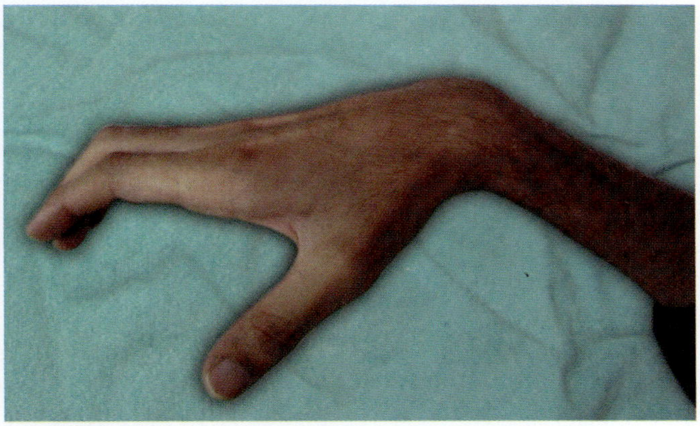

Fig. 22.120: Volkmann's contracture

Pathology

Ischemia necrosis/ infarct fibrosis contracture

Eaton and Green's traumatic ischemia-edema cycle in Volkmann contracture:

- Any situation that causes a decrease in compartment size or increase in compartment pressure can initiate compartment syndrome
- As the intracompartmental pressure increases, capillary blood perfusion is reduced to a level that cannot maintain tissue viability
- The increase in interstitial pressure overcomes the intravascular pressure of the small vessels and capillaries, causing the walls to collapse and impeding local blood flow
- The local tissue ischemia leads to local edema, which increases intracompartmental pressure
- Traumatic ischemia-edema cycle in Volkmann contracture is shown in Figure 22.121.
- Volkmann's contracture is the result of infarction produced by a segmental arterial spasm of the main artery to an extremity with reflex spasm of the collateral circulation (Fig. 22.122)
- Ischemia is produced and the muscle bellies demand the greatest amount of blood and therefore the most vulnerable tissue to its loss are first affected
- The infarct takes the form of an ellipsoid with its axis in the line of the anterior interosseous artery and with its central point a little above the middle of the forearm
- The greatest damage is at the center and usually falls most heavily on flexor digitorum profundus and flexor pollicis longus, which are often necrotic
- The median nerve runs near the center of the ellipsoid and may exhibit profound ischemia

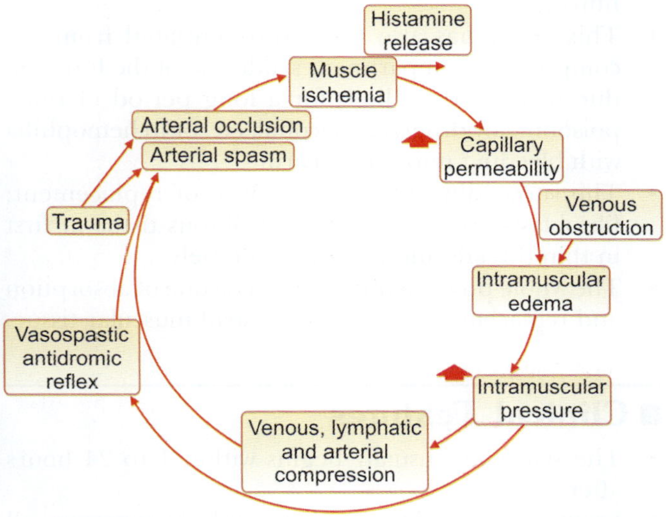

Fig. 22.121: Traumatic ischemia-edema cycle

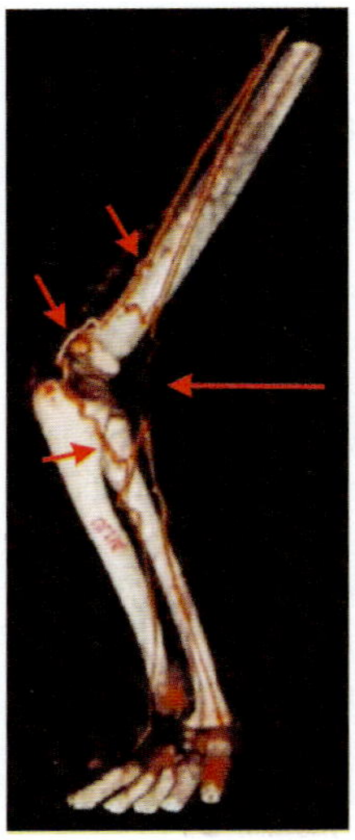

Fig. 22.122: A 6-year-old girl with Volkmann's ischemic contracture. Upper extremity volume-rendered MDCT angiogram shows occlusion of distal brachial artery and reconstitution of ulnar and radial arteries, mainly by recurrent branch of deep brachial artery (*short arrows*) and small antecubital collaterals (*long arrow*).

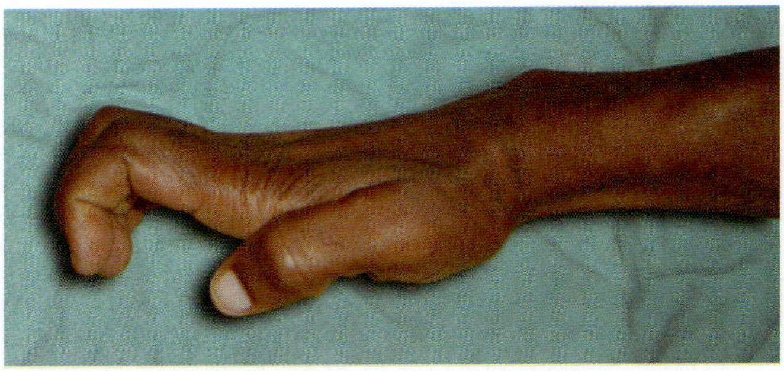

Fig. 22.123: Claw hand deformity (fingers extended at MCP joint and flexed at IP joints)

- The ulnar nerve tends to be less severely affected. It gets involved when extensive fibrosis of the surrounding muscles occurs.
- The most extensive degeneration occurs in the center of the muscle sequestrum and cellular activity and fibrosis takes place only at the periphery, which is surrounded by a sheath of dense fibrous tissue
- In the center of the mass, the muscle fibers lose their nuclei along with cross striations and fuse into a homogenous mass. As the periphery is approached some signs of function are preserved and there is an area of intense cellular activity, both fibroblastic and phagocytic
- This picture is in contrast to muscle degeneration from all other causes, such as denervation and sepsis, in which the appearance is one of diffuse interfibrillar fibrosis
- This entity has also to be differentiated from the compression compartment syndrome of the forearm, due to lying on a limb for a long period of time, poisoning by drugs, e.g. alcohol, etc. or in hemophilia with bleeding into the forearm
- The succeeding phases are those of replacement: fibroblasts appear and deposit fibrous tissue at first in thin threads and later more densely
- The whole process thus seems to be one of absorption and replacement by fibrosis of dead muscular tissue.

Clinical Features

- The symptoms usually begins within 1 to 24 hours after injury
- Severe pain, pallor, paralysis, pulselessness are all present in a greater or lesser degree
- Pallor is usually the first change and it is often striking; pressure on a nail will readily show whether the circulation is impaired
- The pulse distal to the obstruction is invariably absent
- Often there is intense pain, especially on attempted movement and numbness in the fingers; ultimately voluntary movement is totally abolished
- Within 2 days the swelling reduces and the muscles become hard, fibrosed and resistant
- As the fibrosis increases, the deformity becomes obvious, especially the flexion of fingers
- Characteristic deformity: *Intrinsic minus position* (also known as "claw hand") (Fig. 22.123).

Various Degrees of Deformity

- *Mild degrees:* Are often brought to the consultant several years after the injury to the elbow. The patient may be unable to extend the fingers completely but yet may possess a considerable range of movement when the wrist is flexed. It is usually possible to straighten the fingers completely with the wrist fully flexed
- *Severe type:* Fully developed deformity with characteristic attitude
- Severe type complicated by nerve involvement, either a median or ulnar nerve, which are coincidentally involved:
  - In the absence of direct damage, however, either nerve may be implicated in the actual ischemic contracture
  - The median nerve is frequently compressed, where it passes between the two heads of pronator teres and the ulnar nerve may suffer from the contraction of the fibrous tissue which surrounds it; in each case the signs are those of an incomplete nerve lesion—usually partial anesthesia and paralysis of the small muscles of the hand
  - In addition, the nutrition of the limb is impaired, the hand is cold and blue, and trophic ulceration occurs.

There are three levels of severity in Volkmann's contracture:

1. *Mild:* Flexion contracture of two or three fingers only with no or limited loss of sensation
2. *Moderate:* All fingers are flexed and the thumb is stuck in the palm; the wrist may be stuck in flexion and there is usually loss of some sensation in the hand
3. *Severe:* All muscles in the forearm that both flex and extend the wrist and fingers are involved; this is a severely disabling condition:
   - When the damage is reversible, a limited number of muscle fibers die and they are gradually replaced by new ones growing longitudinally, along the surviving sarcolemmal tubes
   - When the damage is irreversible, all grades of fibrosis are present up to almost complete fibrous replacement.

Prognosis

- Early intervention produces good results
- Outlook is grave in severe types and in cases with accompanying nerve involvement.

Prophylaxis

- In all cases of elbow injury look out for pain, stiffness, swelling, cyanosis or lividity of the fingers or obliteration of the radial pulse
- First step, if the event has followed a fracture, is to see if the fragments are displaced. If they are, a further reduction should be carried out at once. Even if they have not moved, it is wise to extend the limb slightly because this is followed occasionally by relief of the spasm. Failure of the pulse to return within a few minutes is an indication for immediate operation.

Treatment

Acute Stage

- The goal of treatment is to restore adequate circulation before irreparable damage is done and thus to avert contracture deformities
- Time is a major factor. The condition is a progressive one in which more and more damage is done
- All measures favoring circulation generally are of great value, e.g. elevation of the part, removal of any splint or circular bandage and application of mild external warmth. The contralateral limb or other limbs may be warmed
- Emergency fasciotomy is required to prevent progression to Volkmann's ischemic contracture. Decompression is performed via volar or dorsal approach. Medial nerve decompression throughout its course is essential, especially in high-risk areas, including deep to the lacertus fibrosus; between the humeral and ulnar heads of the pronator teres, the proximal arch and deep fascial surface of the flexor digitorum superficialis; and in the carpal tunnel.
- The next logical step is the interruption of the sympathetic reflex supply by ganglion injection or arteriectomy. The appearance of Horner's syndrome is the evidence of a successful cervical sympathetic block
- If the circulation does not improve immediately, the artery should be exposed (preferred method nowadays)
- Two percent Papaverine test
- Segmental resection of the spasmotic artery at the fracture site results in interruption of the sympathetic reflex, which in turn leads to vasodilation of the collaterals
- If fracture fragments are not reduced perfectly (as shown on X-ray), attempt should be made to complete the reduction by open operation with wire external fixation.

Fully Developed Stage

Physiotherapy

The first step in treatment is to prevent contractures and maintain a supple joint with a full range of movements and so a splint is applied which makes use of elastic traction to prevent the muscles contraction, while at the same time permitting the joints of the fingers and wrist to be moved if necessary passively, to prevent them from becoming stiff.

Operative Treatment

- A great variety of operations have been recommended for this condition, from tenoplasty, bone section and excision of elbow joint to muscle sliding operation described by Max page
- In every case, operation should be preceded by a course of thorough stretching (physiotherapy)
- Max page described a muscle slide operation in which a straight incision is made from just above the medial epicondyle downward for about 10 cm on the medial aspect of the forearm and the flexor muscles, arising from the medial epicondyle of the humerus and upper ends of the radius and ulna, are erased from their origins by a periosteal elevator. The hand and fingers are then hyper extended and in this way the muscle origin is dragged downwards. The muscles obtain, in time, a new origin lower down the forearm. Watch out for ulnar nerve during operation. The after treatment consists of careful splinting of hand and fingers and physiotherapy.
- Littlewood recommended lengthening of all the shortened tendons. But lengthening of the tendons weakens the power of the muscles. It should be

attempted only if the contraction is limited to one or two of the forearm muscles.

- Shortening of bones of the forearm by resection of 2 to 2.5 cm from each bone is liable to be followed by non union due to trophic changes in the arm
- Seddon achieve good results by completely excising the belly (or the scar representing it) of every muscle that has been completely destroyed, except for flexor carpi ulnaris because of the danger to the ulnar artery. Reconstructive procedures carried out by transplanting living muscles to replace the dead ones.
- Tendon transfers or tenotomies appear to be most rational but they have the risk of recurrence because of contractures
- In very severe deformity cases arthrodesis of the wrist can be done, particularly where it has been necessary to use extensors for giving flexion to various digits.

Treatment of Nerve Complications

Neurolysis and Grafting

- When there is clinical evidence of nerve involvement, which does not show any sign of improvement, after a reasonable period of 2 or 3 months of physiotherapy, the nerves should be exposed at the sites where they are more likely to be compressed
- The median nerve should be free from the callus of the fracture and also released from compression as it passes under the superficial head of pronator teres
- The ulnar nerve is freed through out the length the flexor muscle bellies
- If the nerves have suffered irreversible damage, they should be dealt with grafts
- General physiotherapy should afterwards be carefully carried out, the muscles at the same time being protected from overstretching by adequate splints.

OSTEOCHONDRITIS DISSECANS OF ELBOW

Osteochondritis

Definition

It is a derangement of the normal process of bone growth which occurs at various ossification centers during the period of greatest activity.

Etiology

Vascular Changes

Interruption of the blood flow occurs by infarction, occlusion or malformation of vessels leading to osteochondrosis. For example, Perthe's disease, Freidberg infarction of metatarsal head, OCD of capitulum.

Trauma

In small proportion of cases history of significant trauma be elicited. For example, Osgood schlatterds, OCD of capitulum

Hormonal Features

Hormone changes during periods of altered growth give rise to increased osteogenic proliferation these rapidly dividing cells are more susceptible to trauma or ischemia, e.g. severely affected dyschondrotic epiphysis such as capital femoral epiphysis in gaucher's disease when exposed to normal weight bearing.

- Traction epiphysitis of 5th metatarsal base (Iselin disease)
- Osteochondritis of metatarsal head (Freiberg infarction)
- Osteochondritis of navicular bone (Kohler's disease)
- Osgood-Schlatter disease
- OCD knee
- OCD patella
- Legg-Calvé-Perthes syndrome

Osteochondritis of Elbow

- It is also known as little leaguer's elbow
- Overuse and resultant chronic lateral impaction will lead to OCD capitulum, radial head or medial epicondyle
- Age group: Adolescent 12 to 16 years. Commonly in baseball pitchers and gymnasts.
- It is bilateral in 20 percent
- It accounts for 6 percent of all cases of OCD.

Pathology

- Repeated valgus stress and tenuous blood supply within the capitulum is the reason for frequent occurrence of OCD in this location
- Increased rotatory, compressive or axial loads generated during the acceleration and deceleration phases
- Will cause radiocapitullar compressive and shearing forces.

Clinical Presentation

- Pain
- Impaired range of motion elbow
- Radiographic signs (Figs 22.124 and 22.125).

X-ray Elbow AP and Lateral AP in 45° Flexion

- Degenerative changes in elbow
- Diameter of radial head increased
- Loose body.

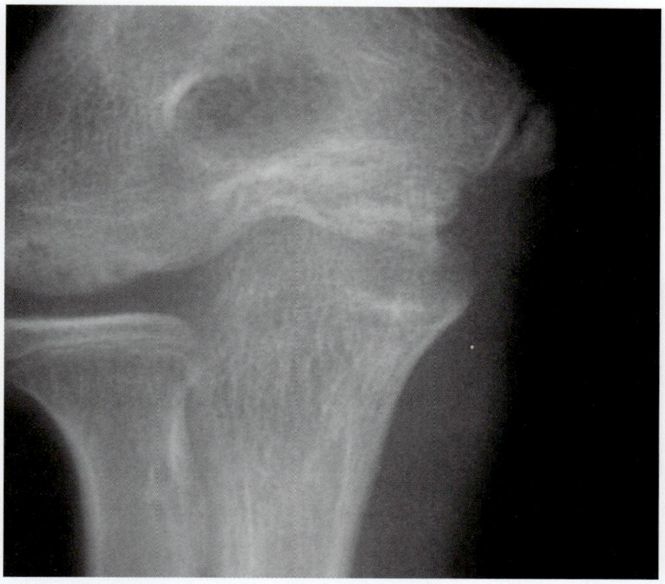

Fig. 22.124: Radiological sign in AP (see text)

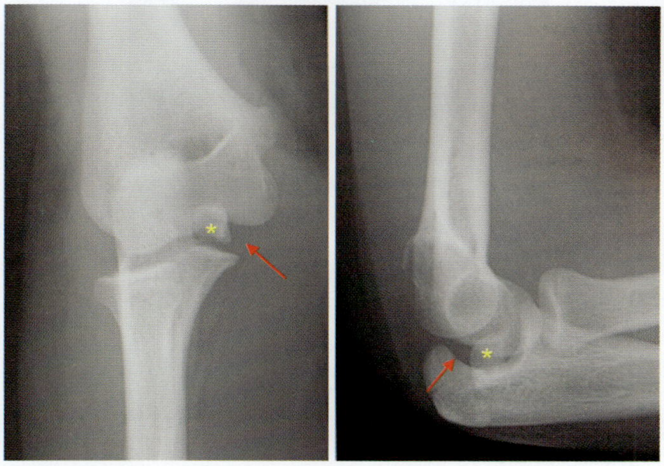

Figs 22.125: OCD of elbow arrows showing osteochondral fragament

ICRS Classification

- *ICRS OCD I:* Indicates a stable lesion with a continuous but softened area covered by intact cartilage
- *ICRS OCD II:* A lesion with partial discontinuity that is stable when probed
- *ICRS OCD III:* A lesion with a complete discontinuity that is not yet dislocated
- *ICRS OCD IV:* An empty defect as well as a defect with a dislocated fragment or a loose fragment lying within the bed.

Although routine anteroposterior radiographs (Figs 22.126 and 22.127) show only slight radiolucency (arrowheads) in the capitulum, anteroposterior

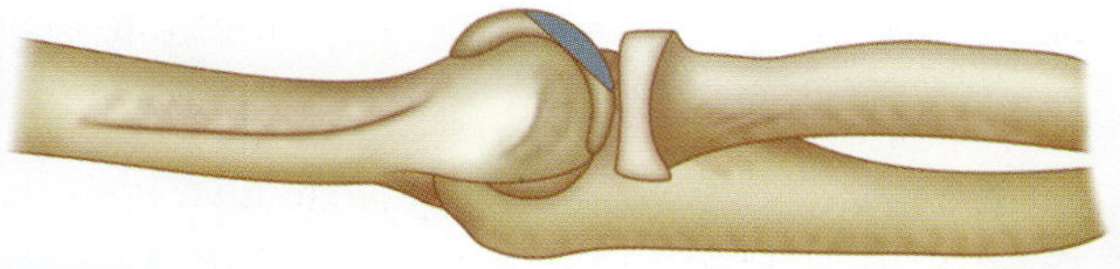

Fig. 22.126: Blue color showing osteochondral defect in extension

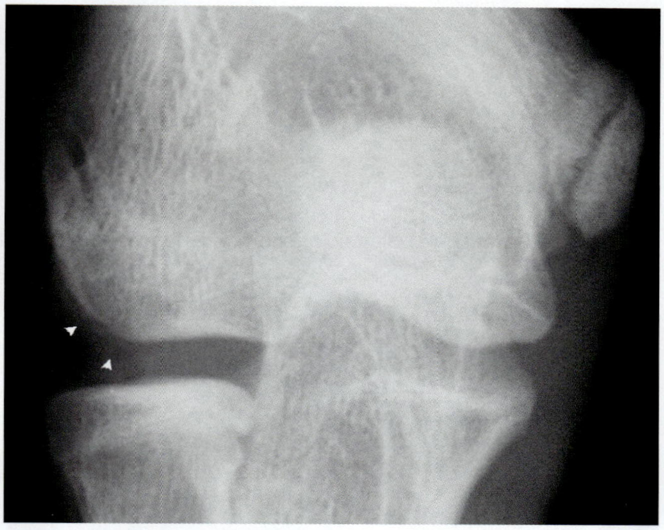

Fig. 22.127: X-ray showing osteochondral defect in full extension

radiographs of the elbow in 45° of flexion (Figs 22.128A and B) clearly show nondisplaced fragments (arrowheads) of the capitulum and avulsion (arrow) of the medial epicondyle.

MRI is Gold Standard for Diagnosing OCD (Fig. 22.129)

Grading system (Figs 22.130 to 22.133)

G 1: Hyaline cartilage covering lesion remains intact
G 2: Enhancing zone of separation but they are stable
G 3: Fluid in zone of separation, unstable
G 4: Loose body.

Treatment

- Conservative
- Operative

Conservative

Indications

- Stable lesion
- No loose body

Mode of treatment

- Rest
- Splinting
- Symptomatic treatment

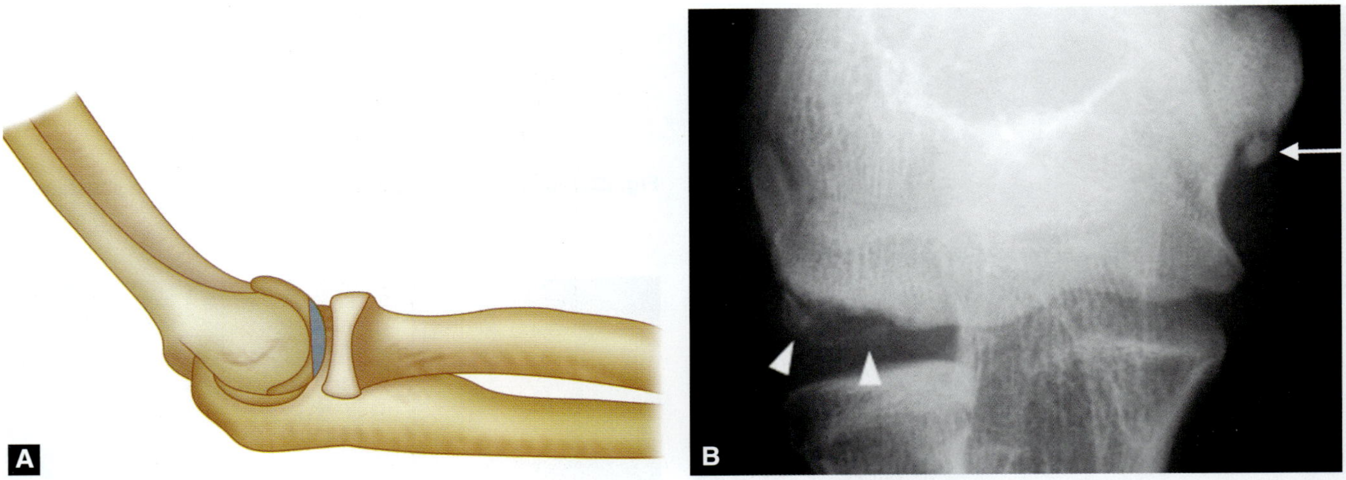

Figs 22.128A and B: (A) Blue color showing osteochondral defect in 45° flexion; (B) X-ray showing osteochondral defect in 45° flexion

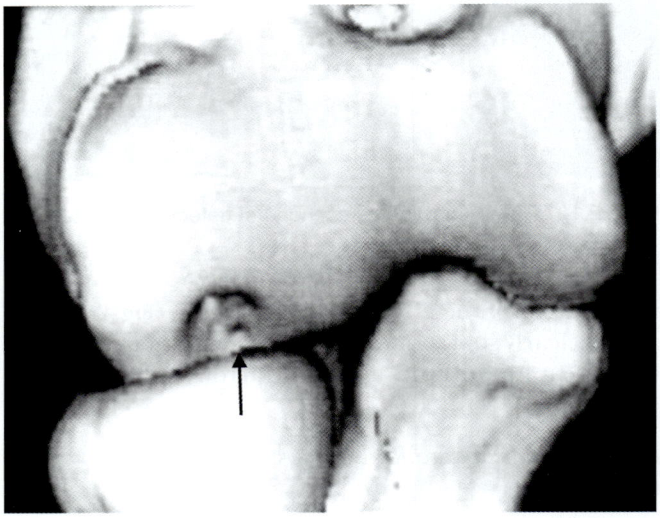

Fig. 22.129: MRI showing OCD

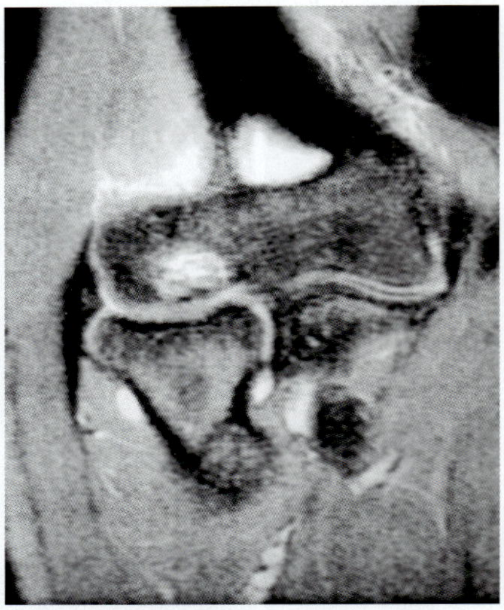

Fig. 22.130: Grade 1

Operative

Indications
- Unstable lesions
- Loose body

Mode of treatment
- Treated with internal fixation of unstable fragment with Herbert screw or using pull out wires
- Bone grafting
- Arthroscopy

Arthroscopic procedures are the following:
- Partial synovectomy
- Excision of loose body
- Drilling the crater
- Fixing unstable viable fragment
- Osteotomy of capitulum

Proposed treatment (Table 22.2).

Case with Pictorial Description (Figs 22.134A to E)

TENNIS ELBOW AND GOLFER'S ELBOW

Introduction

Lateral epicondylitis (Fig. 22.135) *(tennis elbow),* a familiar term used to describe myriad symptoms around the lateral aspect of the elbow, occurs more frequently in nonathletes than athletes, with a peak incidence in the early fifth decade and a nearly equal gender incidence:
- Lateral epicondylitis can occur during activities that require repetitive supination and pronation of the

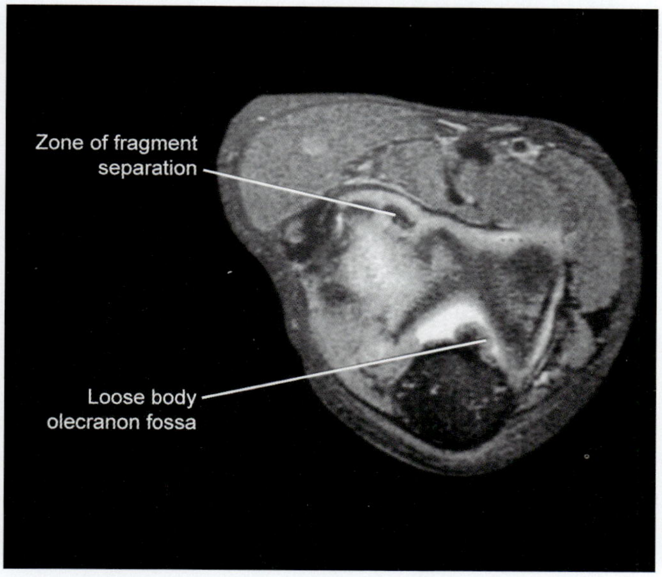

Fig. 22.131: Grade 2

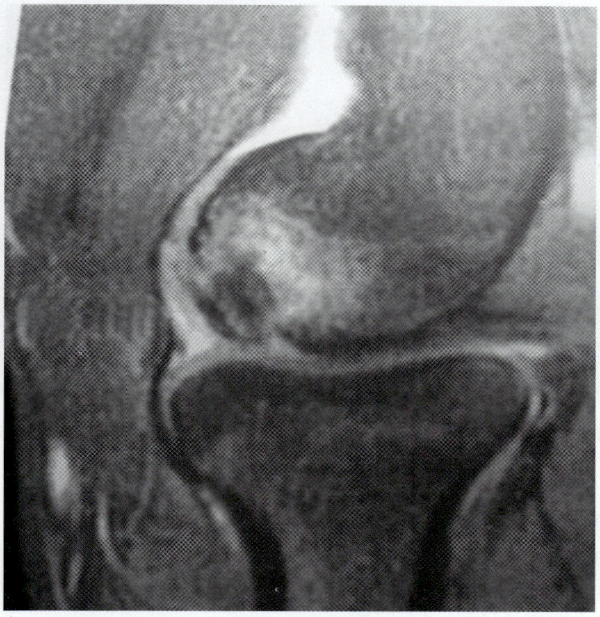

Fig. 22.132: Grade 3

forearm with the elbow in near full extension (Fig. 22.136)

- Although originally described as an inflammatory process, the current consensus is that lateral epicondylitis is initiated as a microtear, most often within the origin of the extensor carpi radialis brevis. Microscopic findings show immature reparative tissue that resembles angiofibroblastic hyperplasia (Fig. 22.137).

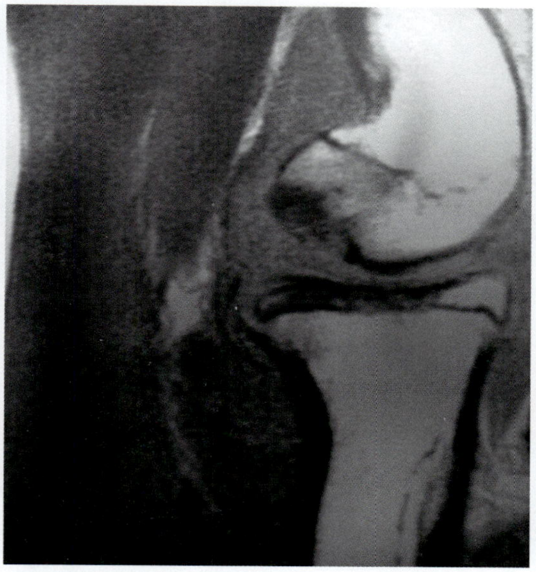

Fig. 22.133: Grade 4

Table 22.2: Proposed treatment of osteochondritis

ICRS classification	*Capitullar growth plate*	*ROM*	*Preferred treatment*
1 (Stable)	Open	Normal	Elbow rest
2 (Stable)	Closed	Restricted	Fixation and bone peg graft
3 (Unstable)			Fixation/bone peg/iliac bone graft
4 (Unstable)			Fragment removal and reconstruction for large defect

Pathology

The pathological process mainly involves the origin of the extensor carpi radialis brevis, but can involve the tendons of the extensor carpi radialis longus and the extensor digitorum communis.

Diagnosis

The diagnosis of tennis elbow is made by localizing discomfort to the origin of the extensor carpi radialis brevis. Tenderness is present over the lateral epicondyle approximately 5 mm distal and anterior to the midpoint of the condyle. Pain usually is exacerbated by resisted wrist dorsiflexion and forearm supination.

Thomson's Test or Cozen's Test

Refer text page No. 355 and See Fig. 22.26

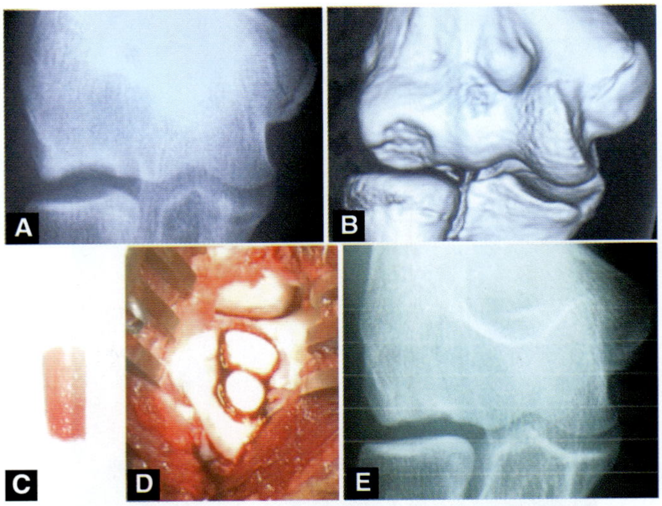

Figs 22.134A to E: A 12-year-old male baseball player with a grade III osteochondritis dissecans lesion of the right elbow with a closed capitellar growth plate. Anteroposterior radiograph with the elbow in 45° of flexion (A) and three-dimensional computed tomographic image (B) made at the time of initial presentation show the defect of the capitulum. Removal of free bodies and reconstruction of the articular surface (D) with use of osteochondral plug grafts (C) was performed. Anteroposterior radiograph with the elbow in 45° of flexion, made 5 months after the surgery, shows union of the osteochondral plug grafts and flattening of the capitular subchondral bone (E)

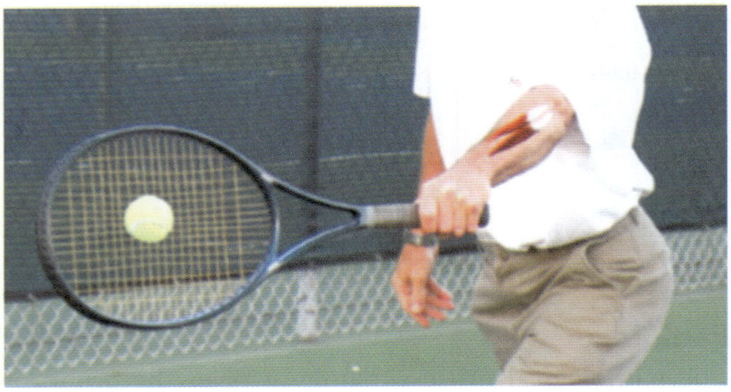

Fig. 22.135: Tennis elbow

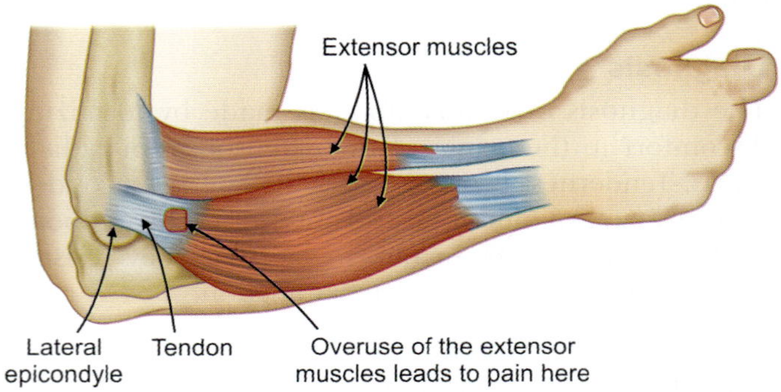

Fig. 22.136: Mechanism causing tennis elbow

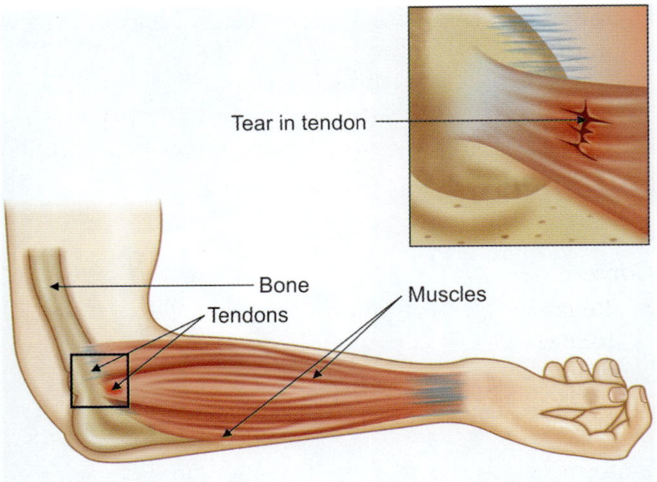

Fig. 22.137: Microscopic findings show immature reparative tissue that resembles angiofibroblastic hyperplasia

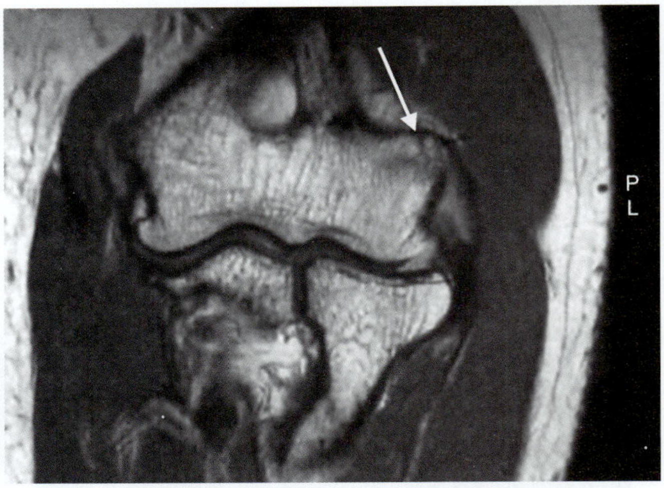

Fig. 22.138: Arrow showing tendon thickening and bone edema

Investigations

Plain radiographs usually are negative; occasionally calcific tendinitis may be present. MRI shows tendon thickening (Fig. 22.138)

Differential Diagnosis

Other entities that can produce pain in this general vicinity are:

- Osteochondritis dissecans of the capitulum
- Lateral compartment arthrosis
- Varus instability
- *Radial tunnel syndrome:* It is a compressive neuropathy of the posterior interosseous nerve caused by any of four different anatomical structures in the radial tunnel, including a fibrous band near the anterior aspect of the radial head, a vascular leash of the recurrent radial artery, the distal extensor carpi

radialis brevis tendon margin or the supinator margin at the arcade of Frohse.

- The pain of radial tunnel syndrome is located 3 to 4 cm distal to the lateral epicondyle and may be reproduced with long finger extension against resistance.

Treatment

Conservative

- Regardless of the underlying cause, nonoperative treatment is successful in 95 percent of patients with tennis elbow.

Initial nonoperative treatment includes rest, ice, injections and physical therapy with ultrasound, iontophoresis, electrical stimulation, manipulation, soft-tissue mobilization, friction massage, stretching and strengthening exercises along with counterforce bracing. One or two local injections of a steroid preparation with local anesthetic like lignocain to the area of maximal tenderness are helpful (Fig. 22.139).

- If prolonged (6 to 12 months) nonoperative treatment is ineffective, operative treatment may be considered; it is effective in 90 percent of properly selected patients.

Surgical Treatment

Numerous surgical procedures have been described for the treatment of tennis elbow

- Mills and later Wadsworth advocated manipulation under anesthesia, especially in patients with concomitant flexion contractures. The technique involves sudden, forcible, full extension of the elbow with the wrist and fingers flexed and the forearm pronated to place the extensor carpi radialis brevis and extensors under tension. An audible, palpable snap frequently can be elicited.
- Almquist, et al. described epicondylar resection with anconeus muscle transfer for chronic lateral epicondylitis
- Nirschl and colleagues described lateral tennis elbow as angiofibroblastic hyperplasia (A-F hyperplasia) of the extensor carpi radialis brevis (ECRB) and on occasion, a small area of the anteromedial border of extensor digitorum communis (EDC) (Figs 22.140A and B)

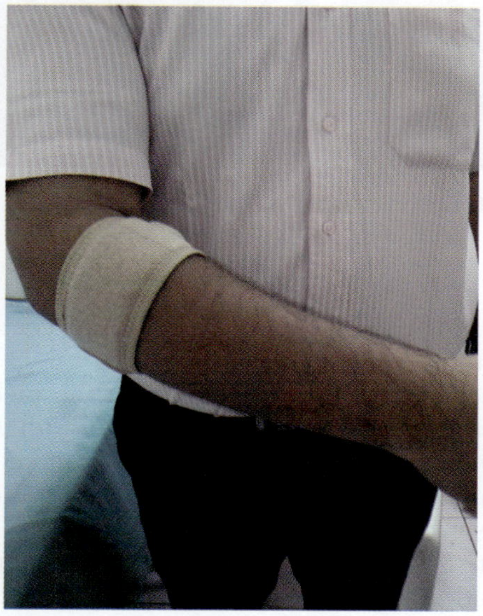

Fig. 22.139: One or two local injections of a steroid preparation with local anesthetic like lignocain to the area of maximal tenderness are helpful

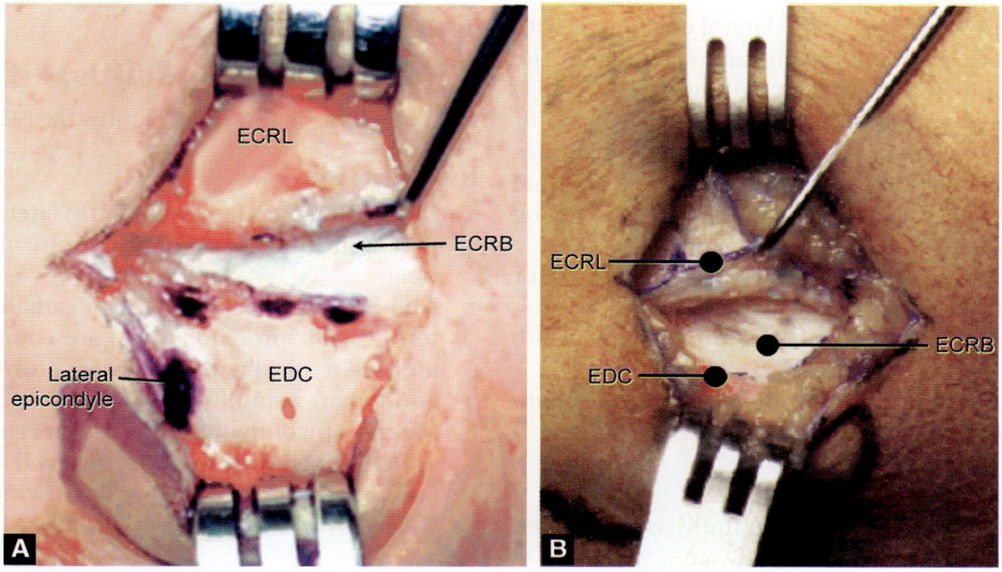

Figs 22.140A and B: Tennis elbow according to Nirschl and colleagues

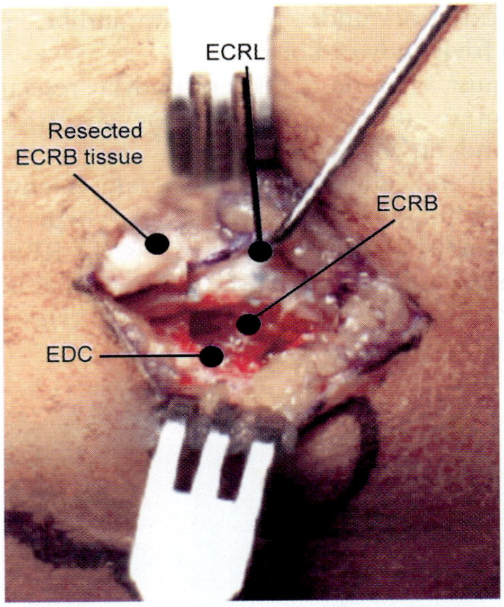

Fig. 22.141: Decortication of a small area of the lateral epicondyle with a rongeur or osteotome

- Make a gently curved incision 5 cm long centered over the lateral epicondyle
- Incise the deep fascia in line with the incision and retract it. Identify the extensor carpi radialis longus and the origin of the extensor digitorum communis, which partially obscures the origin of the deeper extensor carpi radialis brevis
- Elevate the brevis portion of the conjoined tendon at the mid-portion of the lateral epicondyle toward the elbow joint
- As normal-appearing Sharpey fibers are elevated, excise abnormal-appearing tendon. The diseased tissue may appear fibrillated and discolored and may contain calcium deposits.
- Decorticate a small area of the lateral epicondyle with a rongeur or osteotome, taking care not to enter the joint and damage the articular cartilage (Fig. 22.141)
- Suture the remaining normal tendon to the fascia or periosteum, or attach it with nonabsorbable sutures through drill holes in the epicondyle. The use of suture anchors has been reported to be successful in attaching the tendon.
- Close the extensor carpi radialis longus and extensor digitorum communis interval with absorbable sutures. Close the skin incision with subcuticular nylon 4-0 sutures and adhesive strips.
- Apply a dressing and a posterior splint with the elbow in 90° of flexion and palmar flexion

Rehabilitation

- A long-arm splint that includes the wrist is applied and worn for 7 days
- The elbow is flexed at 90°. After 7 days, passive range of motion is started and done three times daily by the patient.
- Between the passive exercise periods, the arm is held at rest in a long-arm elbow splint
- The splint is removed at 4 weeks and the patient begins mild nonresistive range-of-motion exercises, progressing to resistive range of motion at 6 weeks
- The patient may resume full activities as soon as tolerated, although heavy or strenuous activities should be delayed for 10 to 12 weeks
- The rehabilitation protocol is not time dependent, but rather goal dependent, with patients passing from one phase to the next after certain goals have to be met

Rehabilitation Protocol for Epicondylitis

Phase 1: Acute

Goals

- Reduce inflammation and pain
- Promote tissue healing
- Retard muscular atrophy

Phase 2: Subacute

Goals

- Improve flexibility
- Increase muscular strength and endurance
- Increase functional activities and return to function

Phase 3: Chronic

Goals

- Improve muscular strength and endurance
- Maintain and enhance flexibility
- Gradually return patient to sport or high-level activities.

■ Golfer's Elbow (Medial Epicondylitis)

Golfer's elbow is shown in Figures 22.142A and B.

Introduction

- Medial epicondylitis is similar to lateral epicondylitis, although much less common and more difficult to treat
- The origin of the flexor carpi radialis and pronator teres (flexor pronator mass) are commonly involved and less typically, the flexor digitorum superficialis and flexor carpi ulnaris (Figs 22.142 and 22.143)
- Medial epicondylitis frequently occurs in overhead athletes, including athletes involved in racket sports and others who participate in activities that create a valgus force at the elbow (Figs 22.144 and 22.145).

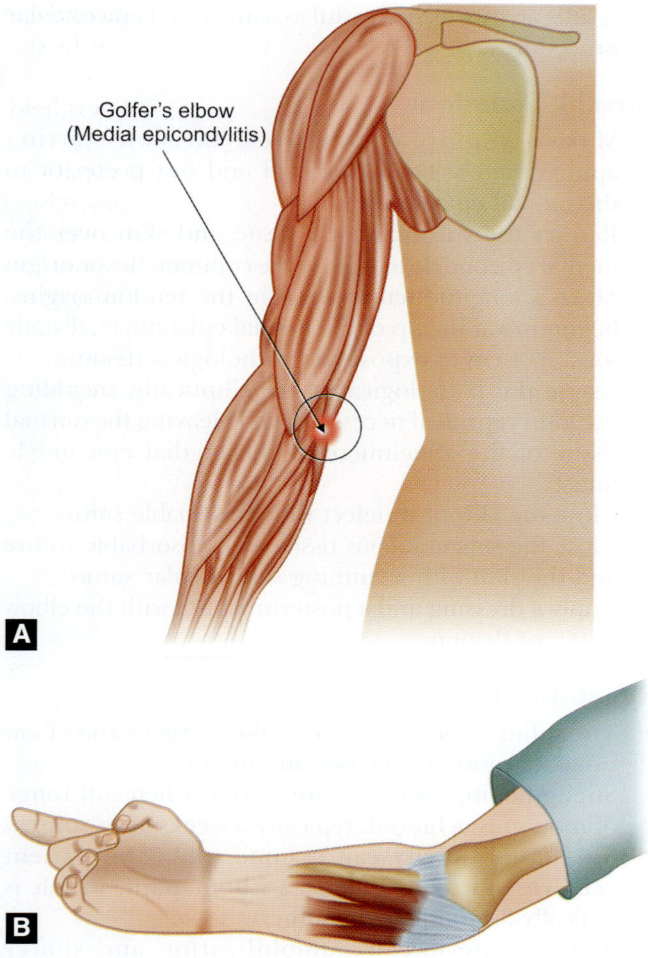

Figs 22.142A and B: Golfer's elbow

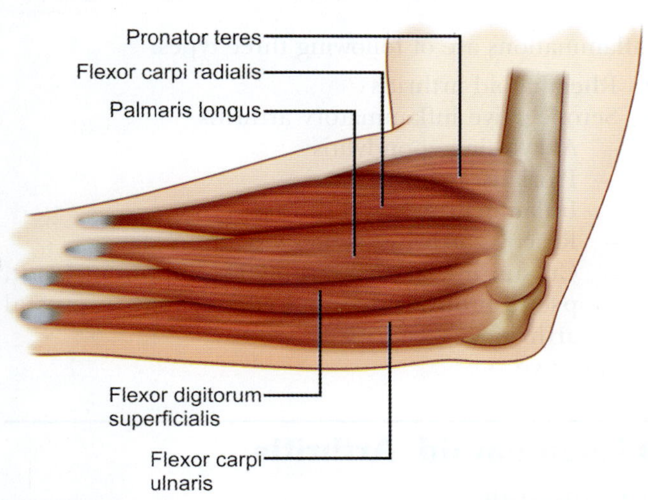

Fig. 22.143: Common muscles involved in golfer's elbow

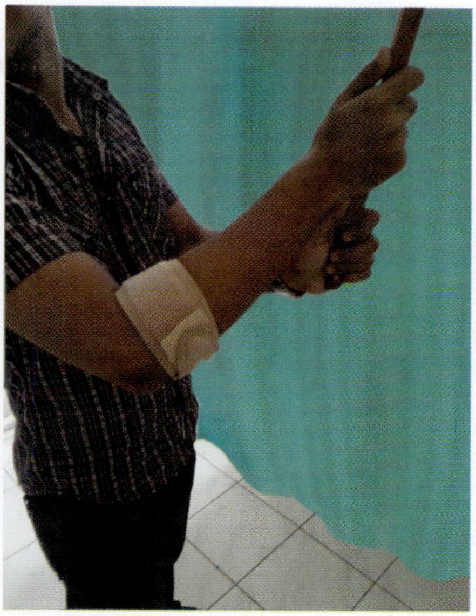

Fig. 22.144: Medial epicondylitis frequently occurs in activities that create a valgus force at the elbow

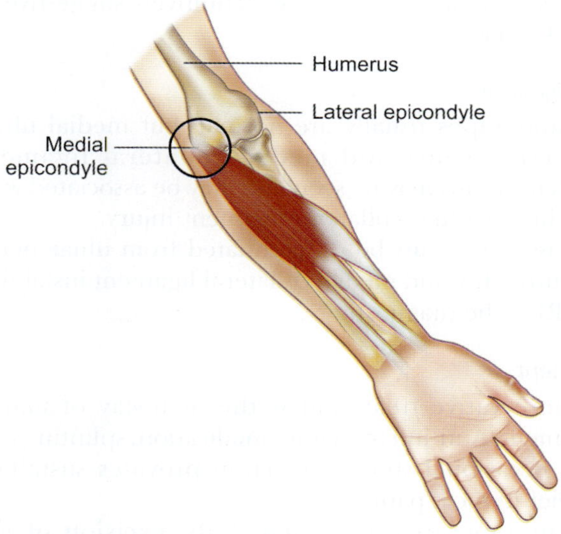

Fig. 22.145: Medial epicondylitis occurring after a valgus force at the elbow

Clinical Features

- Physical examination usually reveals pain along the medial elbow that becomes worse on resisted forearm pronation or wrist flexion
- The area of maximal tenderness is approximately 5 mm distal and anterior to the midpoint of the medial epicondyle
- Loss of range of motion and a flexion contracture may be present.

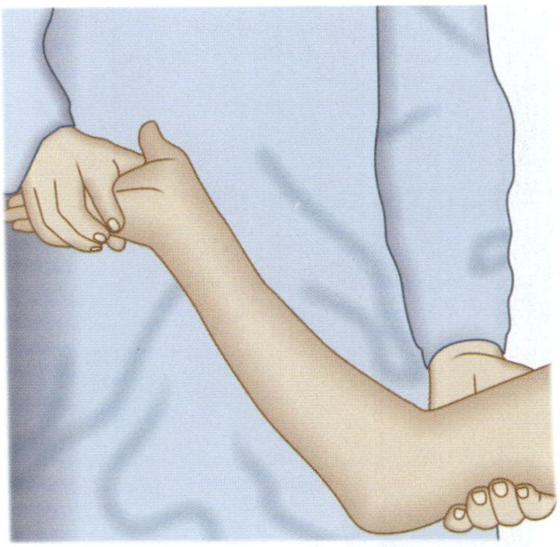

Fig. 22.146: Test for diagnosing golfer's elbow

Diagnosis

Test for Diagnosing Golfer's Elbow (Fig. 22.146)

Flex the elbow, supinate the hand and extend the elbow. Pain over medial epicondyle is definitively suggestive of golfer's elbow.

Investigations

- Radiographs usually are normal, but medial ulnar traction spurs and medial collateral ligament calcifications may be seen and may be associated with a chronic ulnar collateral ligament injury
- This entity must be differentiated from ulnar nerve neuropathy and medial collateral ligament instability MRI is the diagnostic

Treatment

- Conservative treatment is the mainstay of management. Anti-inflammatory medication, splinting and an occasional steroid injection provides sustained relief in most patients
- If nonoperative treatment fails, excision of the diseased tendon origin and reattachment usually are successful. Techniques range from a percutaneous release to open debridement with or without release of the flexor pronator origin.
- Vangsness and Jobe described release of the flexor pronator origin, excision of the pathological tissue and reattachment of the flexor pronator origin to bleeding bone. Nirschl preferred excising the pathological tissue of the flexor-pronator origin in a manner that leaves normal tissue intact and repairing the subsequent defect. The ulnar nerve should be decompressed and transposed in patients who have ulnar nerve symptoms preoperatively. Epicondylectomy also can be done, but no more than 20 percent of the epicondyle should be removed. Overall, the results are not as successful as with lateral epicondylar procedures.

Nirschl Technique

- Make a slightly curved 5 cm incision starting approximately 1 cm proximal and just posterior to the medial epicondyle
- Retract the subcutaneous tissue and skin over the medial epicondyle to expose the common flexor origin
- Make a longitudinal incision in the tendon origins, beginning at the tip of the medial epicondyle, distally for 3 to 4 cm to expose the pathological tissue
- Excise the pathological tissue elliptically, including the joint capsule if necessary, while leaving the normal tissue of the attachment to the medial epicondyle intact
- Close the elliptical defect with absorbable suture
- Close the subcutaneous tissue with absorbable suture and the skin with a running subcuticular suture
- Apply a dressing and a posterior splint with the elbow in 90° of flexion.

Rehabilitation

- The splint is removed 1 week after surgery and elbow range-of-motion exercises are initiated
- Strengthening exercises are started when full range of motion is achieved, typically 3 weeks after surgery
- Strenuous activity can resume when the patient achieves normal strength without pain, which is typically 3 months after surgery
- A longer period of immobilization and slower progression of rehabilitation are indicated in patients who had ulnar nerve transposition.

INFLAMMATIONS AROUND ELBOW

Inflammations are of following three types:

- Rheumatoid arthritis
- Seronegative inflammatory arthritis
  - Ankylosing spondylitis
  - Psoriatic arthritis
  - Inflammatory bowel disease
  - Reactive arthritis (Reiter's syndrome)
  - Crystalline arthropathies (Metabolic)—Gout, pseudogout, calcium hydroxyapatite crystal arthritis
- Infective.

■ Rheumatoid Arthritis

Introduction

Rheumatoid arthritis is a disease of chronic poly-articular inflammation that leads to joint swelling, joint deformity, loss of joint function and extra-articular manifestations.

This disease occurs worldwide and has a prevalence of about 0.5 to 2 percent.

Etiopathogenesis

- The etiology is unknown
- The genetic predisposition, the involvement of activated immune cells, the clonal expansion of the cells in the pathologic lesions and the response to immunosuppressive therapy suggest that this disease is immune mediated. (*MHC class II DR-4 gene*, people who are HLA DRB4 positive are more likely to develop erosive, disabling disease but only one-third of RA patients are DRB4 positive)
- Nongenetic factors include infections (streptococci, parvovirus, Epstein-Barr virus, *Proteus mirabilis*) pregnancy, smoking and others
- Endocrinal (Adrenocortical steroids)
- Cross reaction to self-antigens (in synovial tissues) triggers autoimmune response
- In the early stages, edema, microvascular proliferation and T-lymphocyte infiltration occur in the subsynovial tissues
- Followed by synovial lining cell proliferation
- Synovial infiltration by B-cells, macrophages and fibroblasts
- B-cells develop into plasma cells and reside in the synovium chronically, producing *rheumatoid factor*, leading to complement activation
- The lymphocytes produces hydrolases, DNAase, proteinases which accumulate in the synovial fluid and articular cartilage, leading to destruction of tissues
- In chronic RA, this proliferative granulation tissue called pannus, advances across the joint surface, destroying marginal articular cartilage and invading subchondral bone
- Pannus attached to the joint capsule, ligament and tendons results in joint deformity
- Active inflammation is accompanied by attempted repair and collagen production may become dominant, leading to fibrosis and joint contractures.

Clinical Features

Clinical features of RA are shown in Figures 22.147A and B.

- The presentation of RA can be variable
- Patients present with a symmetric polyarthritis, can present with a single joint swelling (21%), few swollen joints (44%) or a more typical polyarthritis (35%)
- The onset may be acute (days or weeks) in about half of the patients, insidious in the other half
- The joint reacts to an insult in a limited number of ways. (Stiffness, pain, tender, swelling, loss of function)
- Stiffness and pain in the morning, lasting 1 or more hours, improving with low-grade activity

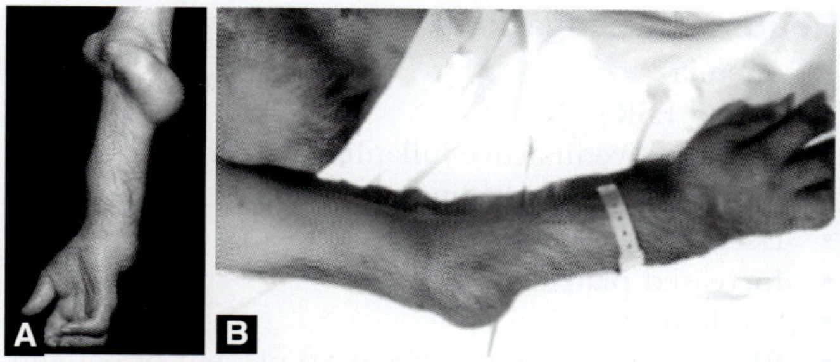

Figs 22.147A and B: Clinical features of rheumatoid arthritis

- The hands and wrist are the most common joints involved. Elbow involvement has been reported in 20 to 65 percent of patients with RA
- The earliest change noted in the elbow is loss of extension
- There is loss of the groove on either side of the olecranon
- Large cystic swellings can occur
- The inflammation in RA goes through intermittent exacerbations and remissions
- In chronic cases fatigue, malaise, fever, weight loss and lymphadenopathy, may be present
- In long standing cases nodules may occur, typically along the olecranon border, spine, occiput, achilles tendon or extensor surfaces of the hands and feet and other areas exposed to mechanical pressure
- Nodules can be observed in tendon sheaths, heart (arrhythmias and heart blocks), lungs (pleural effusion and fibrosis), liver, eyes and the meninges.

American College of Rheumatology Classification Criteria for Rheumatoid Arthritis

- Morning stiffness in and around joints lasting at least one hour.
- Arthritis of three or more joint areas PIP, MCP, wrist, elbow, knee, ankle and MTP joints of either or same side
- Arthritis of joints of the hands at least one joint area involved
- Symmetric arthritis symmetric involvement of the two sides (PIP, MCP and MTP joint involvement does not require absolute symmetry)
- Rheumatoid nodules observed by a physician
- Serum rheumatoid factor in levels above the normal population
- X-ray changes should include typical erosions and/or juxta-articular osteoporosis.

Criteria for Diagnosis

- *Classic:* Any seven criteria for at least 6 weeks
- *Definite:* Any five criteria for at least 6 weeks
- *Probable:* Any three criteria for at least 4 weeks.

Routine Investigations

- Anemia
- Raised ESR
- CRP positive in active inflammatory stages
- Increased serum alkaline phosphatase
- Decreased serum albumin
- Increased platelets
- Serological
- RF tests are positive in about 80 percent of patients with RA
- Positive ANA occurs in 40 percent
- Anticitrullinated cyclic peptide (anti-CCP) antibody can be positive early in RA when the rheumatoid factor is negative
- Synovial fluid analysis:
  - Sugar normal
  - Proteins slightly decreased
  - Increased counts
  - Positive rheumatoid factor
- Histology (Fig. 22.148)
- Lymphoid proliferation
- Inflammatory granulation tissue (pannus)
- Pannus invades into articular cartilage, subchondral region
- X-ray (Fig. 22.149)
- Juxta-articular osteoporosis
- Erosion of joint margin
- Joint space is decreased
- Deformities of joints
- Subchondral erosion and cyst formation
- Fibrous and bony ankylosis develop in late stages.

Criteria for Diagnosis

- Morning stiffness
- Pain on motion or tenderness in at least one joint
- Swelling (soft tissue thickening or fluid; not bony outgrowth alone) in at least one joint continuously for not less than 6 weeks
- Swelling of at least one other joint
- Symmetrical joint swelling
- Subcutaneous nodules
- X-ray changes typical of rheumatoid arthritis
- Positive latex fixation test
- Poor mucin clot
- Characteristic histological changes in synovial membrane
- Characteristic histological changes in nodules

Management

Aims of Treatment

- To keep inflammatory treatment to minimum
- To keep constitutional symptoms to minimum
- Appropriate splinting to prevent deformities
- Surgical measures to correct deformity.

Circumstances in which a more aggressive clinical course of rheumatoid arthritis should be suspected:

- Positive rheumatoid factor and anti-CCP antibodies in high titer
- Elevated inflammatory markers (ESR and CRP)
- Presence of shared epitope alleles (HLA-DRB1 0401 and HLA-DRB1 0404)
- Presence of bony erosions (Plain X-rays or MRI)
- Degree of functional disability.

Drug Therapy

- Analgesics and anti-inflammatory: NSAIDs—aspirin/ibuprofen/diclofenac sodium

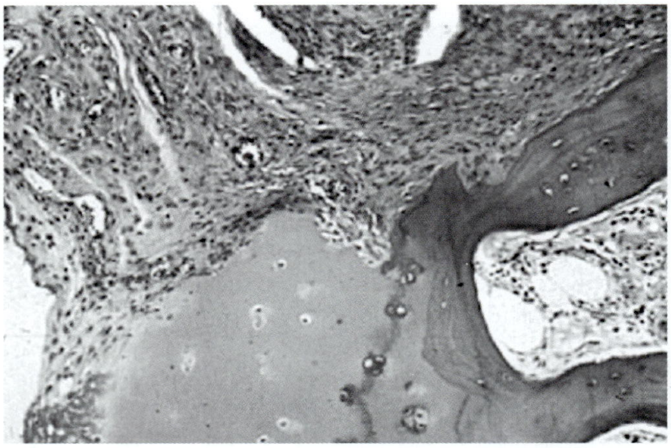

Fig. 22.148: Histology

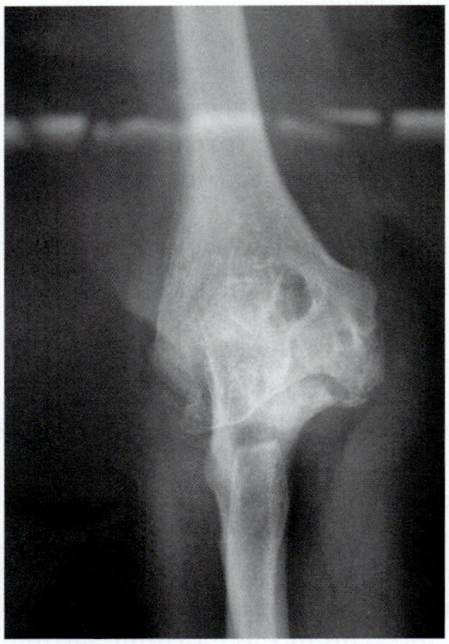

Fig. 22.149: X-ray showing rheumatoid arthritis

- DMARD's
  - Injectable gold and oral gold (sodium aurothiomalate)
  - D-penicillamine (T cell suppressor)
  - Sulphasalazine antimalarials (interference with antigen processing)
  - Dapsone and levamisole
  - Methotrexate (inhibit dihydrofolate reductase)
  - Corticosteroids
  - Leflunomide inhibits the enzyme dihydro-orotate dehydrogenase, thus leading to inhibition of pyrimidine synthesis. This inhibition, in turn, inhibits both T- and B-cell function.
- Immunomodulators
  - Etanercept, anakinra
- Physiotherapy and occupational therapy
- Surgery
  - Synovectomy
  - Osteotomy
  - Arthrodesis
  - Arthroplasty
- Seronegative inflammatory arthritis
- Refers to a group of conditions in which clinical evidence of noninfectious, active inflammation is noted in the joints, but serum autoantibodies, such as rheumatoid factor (RF) or anticyclic citrullinated peptide antibodies (anti-CCP), are absent
- They present with pain, limited motion and swelling of the affected joint, in the absence of trauma.

They are classified for descriptive propose as:

- Spondyloarthropathies
  - Ankylosing spondylitis
  - Inflammatory bowel disease
  - Psoriatic arthritis
  - Reactive arthritis (Reiter's syndrome).
- Crystalline arthropathies
  - Gout
  - Pseudogout
  - Calcium hydroxyapatite crystal arthritis.

Spondyloarthropathies

- They share an increased prevalence of the HLA class IB-27
- Classically, the spondyloarthropathies manifest as an inflammatory arthritis of the spine and sacroiliac joints, but an asymmetric peripheral arthritis can occur
- A key clinical feature distinguishing SpA from RA is the presence of *enthesitis* (inflammation that is located at the sites of ligamentous insertion into bone, such as the Achilles tendon or plantar fascia).

Clinical differences between spondyloarthropathies and rheumatoid arthritis.

Table 22.3: Elbow involvement in spondyloarthropathies

Spondyloarthropathy	*Frequency of elbow involvement*
Ankylosing spondylitis	12%
Psoriatic arthritis	25%
Inflammatory bowel disease	35%
Reactive arthritis	Uncommon

Elbow Involvement in Spondyloarthropathies (Table 22.3)

Management

- NSAIDs reduces pain and inflammation
- Synovial fluid aspiration and local corticosteroid injection
- Systemic corticosteroid therapy in severe cases and extra-articular involvement
- Sulfasalazine, methotrexate
- Anti-TNF therapy (Etanercept, infliximab and adalimumab) in severe cases
- Cutaneous psoriasis frequently responds to topical preparations and especially well to weekly pulse methotrexate.

Crystalline Arthropathies

- Crystalline arthropathies are a group of inflammatory arthritides associated with crystal deposition in the synovial space
- Patients frequently present with an acute painful monoarthritis, which often is indistinguishable from septic arthritis.

Gout

Introduction

- It is metabolic disorder manifesting in the primary and secondary forms characteristic by hyperuricemia and joint lesions
- Gout is a common condition associated with the deposition of monosodium urate (MSU) crystals in the synovial fluid, synovial tissue and surrounding soft tissues. MSU crystals are by-products of an aberrant uric acid metabolism.

Etiopathogenesis

- The actual cause is unknown
- Hereditary
- Risk factors for gout include hypertension, renal insufficiency, obesity, type 2 diabetes mellitus, ethanol intake, lead exposure and use of diuretics, particularly thiazide diuretics
- *Age:* 2nd and 4th decade

- *Sex:* Males are more affected
- Adrenocortical insufficiency (ACTH precipitates attacks)
  Secondary gout—It occurs due to renal insufficiency, hematological disturbances, etc.
- MSU crystals deposited in articular cartilage
- The crystals enter the joint space and synovial fluid
- They erode the cartilage and subchondral bone leading to punched out lesions
- Urate crystals stimulate inflammatory reactions resulting in further damage
- Crystals are deposited in synovium and other soft tissues like bursa and subcutaneous tissue forming tophi
- Elbow is involved in 17 to 33 percent cases of gout.

Clinical Features

- It occurs mostly in men, in third or fourth decade
- The condition may present clinically as an acute attack or chronic gout
- The most commonly affected joint in gout is the metacarpophalangeal joint of big toe
- The attack is characteristic by sudden onset of excruciating pain at night with marked swelling and redness of joint of big toe
- The attack may subside in a week
- The arthritis shows remission and exacerbation and gradually becomes chronic
- In chronic stage, there is deposition of urate salts in the juxta-articular tissue of the involved joint or the subcutaneous tissue of the ear or in olecranon bursa
- These lumps are called gouty tophi
- After certain attacks the joint develops features of secondary osteoarthritis.

Laboratory Investigations

- Raised ESR
  - Leukocytosis
  - Raised serum uric acid (>7 mg/dl) sometimes the levels may be normal
  - Synovial fluid analysis
- Needle shaped negatively birefringent MSU crystals (Fig. 22.150)
- Synovial membrane shows deposition of crystals, leukocyte infiltration with crystals, occasional pannus formation
- X-ray (Fig. 22.151)
- In chronic stage, the characteristic punched out appearance of the periphery of the articular cartilage in the metatarsophalangeal joints
- Tophi may be seen as radiopaque shadow in the juxta-articular tissue
- In late stages, degenerative changes with narrowing of joint space and sclerosis.

Treatment

- Anti-inflammatory drugs like indomethacin in high doses is given
- Colchicine is the specific drug for acute gout. It is both analgesic and diuretic. It's dose is 1 mg/2 hourly.
- Uricosuric drugs like probenecid is given in conjunction with colchicine dose is 0.5 to 1 gm daily
- Allopurinol is given to inhibit the synthesis of uric acid. Dose is 300 mg daily
- Surgical procedures for excision of tophaceuos deposits can be done.

Pseudogout

Introduction

It is a form of arthritis due to deposition of crystals of calcium pyrophosphate dehydrate (CPPD) in the synovium or the articular cartilage or menisci.

Clinically, the acute attack resembles gout but the serum uric acid is normal.

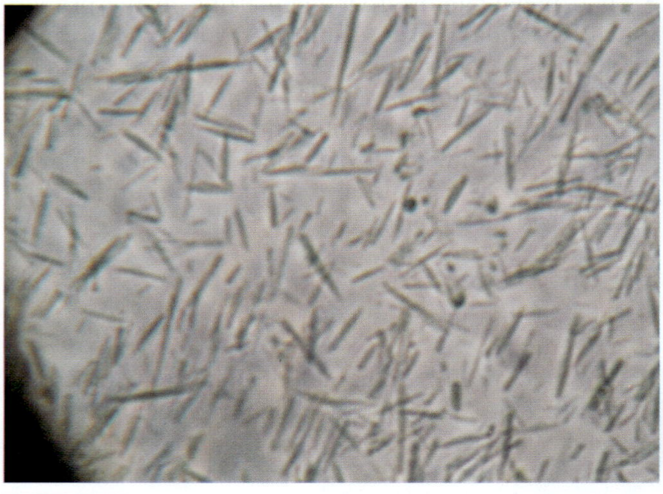

Fig. 22.150: Needle-shaped negatively birefringent MSU crystals

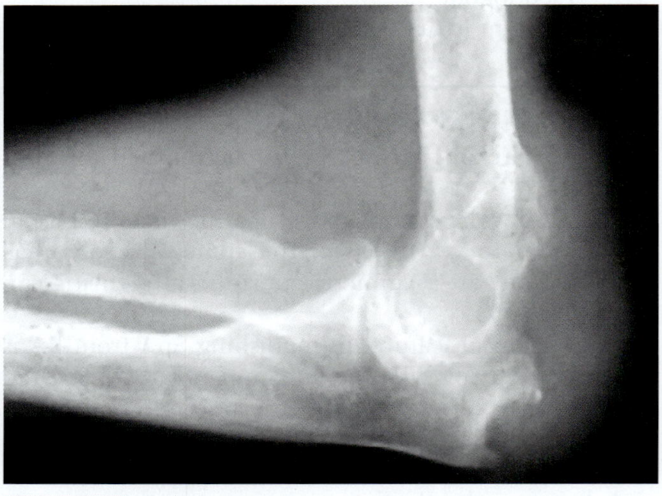

Fig. 22.151: X-ray showing gout of elbow joint

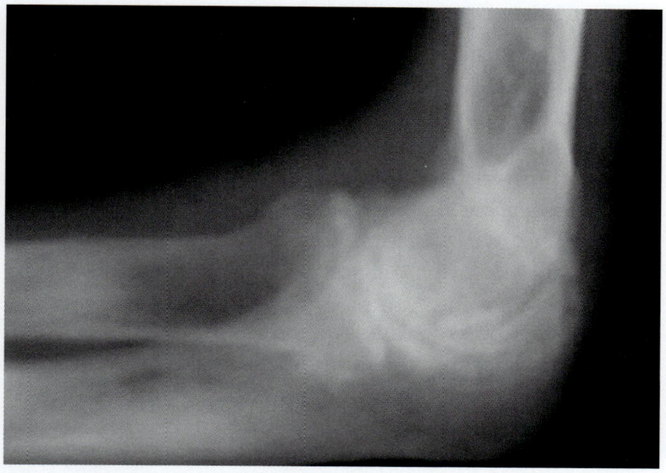

Fig. 22.152: X-ray spots showing calcified spots in articular surfaces

Synovial fluid analysis shows positively birefringent CPPD crystals, that are rhomboid shaped and exhibit positive birefringence undercompensated polarized light, appearing blue. The condition responds to indomethacin.

Radiograph shows calcified spots in articular cartilage (Fig. 22.152).

Treatment
- NSAIDs
- Responds well to indomethacin.

Hydroxyapatite Crystals Deposition Disease

- It may present as primary crystal induced arthropathy or secondary to trauma or degenerative joint disease
- Hydroxyapatite crystal are deposited in soft tissue of joint space, rotator cuff tendons or bursa
- Shoulder and knee are commonly involved
- Hydroxyapatite crystals are nonbirefringent
- Radiologically, the disease appears as radiopaque calcification in a local tumor mass like fashion
- Treatment is with NSAIDs, colchicine and oral as well as intra-articular corticosteroids with physiotherapy
- Large tumor mass like deposits may sometime need excision

Infections

- Osteomyelitis
- Septic arthritis
- Septic olecranon bursitis
- Bone infection occurs
  - Hematogenously
  - By direct inoculation after open fracture or surgery
  - By contiguous spread from a local process

Hematogenous Infections

- Hematogenous infection is the most common type of osteomyelitis
- In the growing child, the end-arterial loop of the metaphyseal bone causes sluggish bone blood flow. The lack of phagocytic activity in these loops allows maturation of a septic thrombus at the arterial site. The abscess spreads through the haversion system into the subperiosteal space.
- As the metaphysis is not intra-articular in the elbow, the abscess does not spread to the joint
- Acute hematogenous osteomyelitis is most common in children younger than 3 and older than 7 years of age
- The first group is vulnerable owing to the lack of acquired host immunity; the second age group corresponds to the time of rapid growth
- Elbow is involved in 8 percent of the cases
- The most common pathogen causing acute hematogenous osteomyelitis is *Staphylococcus aureus*
- Opportunistic organisms are isolated in the debilitated patient and *Pseudomonas aeruginosa* is most commonly associated with drug addiction or chronic draining wounds.

Direct Inoculation

- Direct inoculation is a relatively common cause of infection of the elbow joint
- The thin soft tissue coverage predisposes to compound fractures that may become secondarily infected
- Elective nonprosthetic surgery of the elbow region has been associated with an infection rate of about 2 to 4 percent, significantly greater than the commonly quoted 1 percent for elective orthopedic procedures.

Spread from a Contagious Focus

- Infection by spread from a contiguous focus occurs at the elbow from a septic joint or from an infected olecranon bursa
- These circumstances are most commonly noted in a patient with rheumatoid arthritis.

Clinical Features and Diagnosis

- Local pain, warmth and swelling
- Irritability, restlessness, headache, vomiting, convulsion, chills, fever
- In children, a predisposing, traumatic event is common, remote septic foci identification is difficult
- Afebrile in few cases
- Overlying skin becomes shiny, red and edematous
- Discharging sinus may be present
- The elbow is held in flexion and pseudoparalysis or reflex inhibition may be present.

Physical Examination

- The specific point of maximal tenderness should be determined by gentle palpation. The focus of the septic process can often be accurately localized in this way, even before radiographic changes are apparent.
- Gentle passive motion of the joint should be done. With joint infections, all motion is resisted; with metaphysealoste omyelitis, gentle, supported passive motion is possible.

Laboratory Studies

- Complete blood count, including differential and erythrocyte sedimentation rate is a more sensitive tool raised in about 80 percent cases (markedly raised in joint infections than bone)
- C-reactive protein
- Blood culture
- Pus culture sensitivity
- Synovial fluid analysis (if joint infection is suspected)
- Plain X-rays. Not helpful in early detection. After 7 to 14 days, osteoporosis may be present, followed by periosteal elevation or erosions (Fig. 22.153)
- CT scan helps document sequestra
- MRI for detection of the septic process, is most helpful to determine the extent of damage
- Bone scan (99mTc)
- Leukocyte scanning technique
- Ultrasonography is an effective, noninvasive method to assess soft tissue involvement
- PCR.

Treatment

- Prolonged immobilization is to be strictly avoided. In the acute phase of treatment, the joint should be splinted, elevated and put to rest. As the process resolves, gentle active motion is encouraged as soon as possible. Continuous passive motion may prove to be beneficial in some patients to avoid ankylosis or adhesions.
- In cases that are diagnosed early, antibiotics alone may be adequate
- Surgery is indicated when there is no response to parental antibiotic therapy after 36 to 48 hours

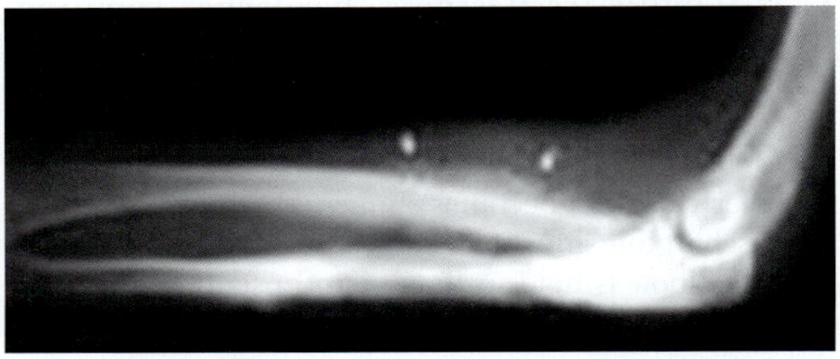

Fig. 22.153: Plain X-ray

- Intravenous antibiotics should be continued for about 3 weeks. Oral agents can be used for an additional 4 weeks.
- Infection involving bone may become subacute or chronic and in this instance, incision and drainage with limited bone debridement and secondary soft tissue healing may be necessary
- An extensive debridement of bone severely impairs function because the joint becomes dysfunctionally unstable
- If soft tissue coverage is a problem, the flexor carpi ulnaris muscle pedicle flap may be used for coverage of the proximal ulna and elbow. Flap brings improved blood supply as well as soft tissue coverage.

Septic Arthritis of the Elbow

- Elbow septic arthritis occurs in 12 to 18 percent diagnosed cases of septic joints
- Peak incidence is at extremes of life
- The frequent association of elbow septic arthritis with rheumatoid arthritis is well recognized
- Thirty-three percent of septic joints in patients with rheumatoid arthritis involved the elbow
- *Staphylococcus aureus* more common (60 to 80%), *Streptococcus* (20%), *Pneumococcus* (10%), *Gonococcus, E. coli, H. influenzae* is common in children less than 2 years of age
- *Predisposing factors:* Trauma, diabetes, steroid therapy, malignancy, HIV (drug addicts and hemophilics), etc.

Routes of Entry

- Primary focus is in respiratory system, GIT, urinary system, etc.
- Pyogenic osteomyelitis
- Punctured wound
- Pneumonia, typhoid, etc.
- Primary focus in joint

Pathogenesis

- The presence of bacteria in the joint initiates local reaction
- The synovial membrane becomes hyperemic, edematous and proliferates
- Infiltration by the leukocytes, producing mediators of inflammation and proteolytic enzymes
- The articular cartilage and bones are destroyed leading to fibrosis and ankylosis.

Clinical Features

- Constitutional symptoms are chills, fever, sweats, malaise, anorexia and in infants refusal to feeds, vomiting, etc.
- Pain gradually increases in intensity over several hours and becomes excruciating

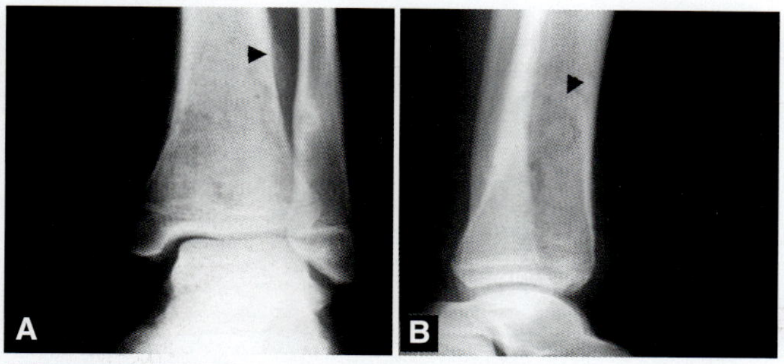

Figs 22.154A and B: X-ray showing periosteal reaction

- Pain accentuates on movement of joints and thus limits the movement
- Swelling and redness around elbow
- Local raise in temperature and tenderness present
- The patient holds the limb in position of maximum capacity to reduce the intra-articular pressure and thus minimizes pain. (50 to 80° of flexion).
- WBC'S (polymorphs 80%) are raised to 50,000 to 100,000
- ESR is raised
- HB is decreased
- Blood culture is positive in 35 to 50 percent of cases
- CRP is positive
- *Synovial fluid aspiration* is critical for diagnosing and treatment of septic arthritis (Figs 22.154A and B)
- X-ray shows increased joint space (ballooning), anterior or posterior fat pad sign, juxta-articular osteopenia, articular cartilage destruction, fibrous and bony ankylosis in later stages
- Gallium or labeled white cell scans may be more specific than technetium scans
- MRI lacks the specificity of distinguishing septic from nonseptic fluid but can assist in the diagnosis of a contiguous osteomyelitis.

Treatment

- Initial specific antibiotic treatment is first based on the gram stain
- Immobilization in initial period with splint/slab. Early mobilization is recommended.
- If infection is suspected and no organism is isolated, initial antibiotic treatment should be based on age and presentation
- In initial stages joint fluid aspiration, lavage, followed by local antibiotic (cefazolin) injection
- Arthroscopic/Arthotomy debridement is done in those who are not responding immediately to the initial aspiration, lavage and antibiotic injection
- Infections that are subacute, postoperative or due to direct inoculation, adequate clearance by aspiration is not reliable and drainage by arthroscopy is preferred (Fig. 22.155)
- If extra-articular involvement is present, arthrotomy may be necessary, so that early motion is begun.

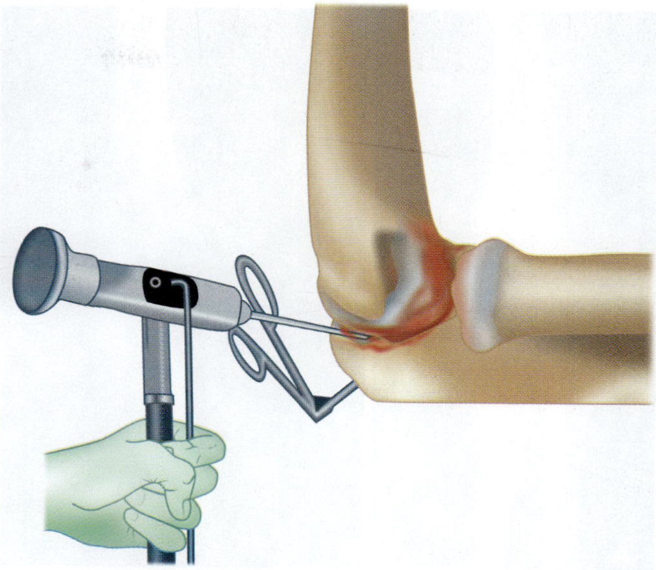

Fig. 22.155: Arthroscopic debridement

Early motion helps in

- Prevents adhesions and pannus
- Improves nutrition of cartilage
- Enhances clearance of exudates including lysozomal enzymes
- Stimulates the living chondrocytes.

Tuberculosis of Elbow

Introduction

Tuberculosis of the elbow is rare and constitutes nearly 2 to 5 percent of all skeletal tuberculosis.

The sites are:

- Olecranon
- Humerus
- Synovium of radius
- Pulmonary tuberculosis is present in only about half of the cases
- Atypical *Mycobacterium* infection, for example, *M. kansasii*, may also occur, both from direct inoculation and from lung involvement and may become slowly progressive over many years.

Clinical Features

- Pain
- Swelling
- Limitation of movements

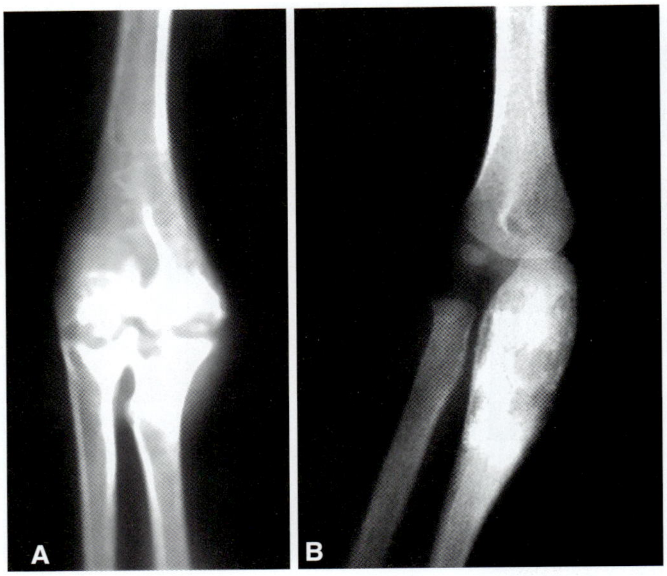
Figs 22.156A and B: Radiology

- Wasting of arm and forearm muscles
- Lymphadenopathy
- Sinus.

Radiology (Figs 22.156A and B)

- Destruction commonly in olecranon/humerus
- Generalized demineralization and fuzziness of joint margins
- Articular cartilage is usually spared
- Subperiosteal new bone formation on the ulna resembling (spinaventosa) or humerus
- Pathological posterior dislocation.

Treatment

- Chemotherapy is the mainstay of treatment
- Plaster in 90° of flexion and mid-prone position of the forearm is advisable
- As pain reliefs, splint is advisable for 6 to 9 months
- For residual dysfunction synovectomy with or without radial head excision
- Excision arthroplasty in advanced arthritis/ankylosis
- Rarely arthrodesis of elbow is justified for heavy manual work.

■ Nonbacterial Infections

- Coccidioidomycosis caused by *Coccidioides immitis* has been reported in the elbow infections
- The treatment recommended is synovectomy with intravenous amphotericin B for the disseminated disease.

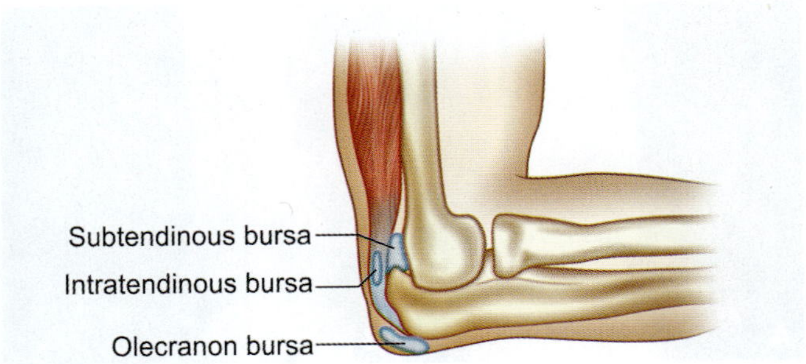

Fig. 22.157: Olecranon bursitis

Bursitis

- Olecranon bursitis (Fig. 22.157) is the most commonly involved site followed by the bicipital radial bursa. Inflamed medial epicondylar bursa is associated with chronic subluxation of the ulnar nerve
- Olecranon bursa is not present at birth and has been shown to develop after the 7th year
- Olecranon bursitis is caused by a number of pathologic conditions that are traumatic (overuse or direct impact), inflammatory (RA, gout, pseudogout), infectious or noninfectious
- It has been associated with dialysis in the ipsilateral extremity
- Inflammation of the superficial olecranon bursa can also result from direct trauma or repetitive stress—*miner's elbow* or *student's elbow*
- Use of anticoagulants increases the possibility of hemobursitis.

Clinical Presentation

- A distended olecranon bursa is usually painless unless it is associated with a septic or crystalline inflammatory process (Fig. 22.158)
- The bursa may rupture and dissect proximally, presenting as triceps swelling
- In patients with rheumatoid arthritis, the bursa may also communicate with the joint, dissect anteriorly and distally into the forearm or even rupture and present as a subcutaneous fullness over the subcutaneous border of the ulna.
- When the bursitis is symptomatic, flexing elbow to more than 90° causes most symptoms (Fig. 22.159)
- In acute septic olecranon bursitis, diffuse swelling is noted about the distal arm and the proximal forearm.

Lab Investigations

- Raised ESR in septic and inflammatory conditions
- Synovial fluid aspiration
- Crystals

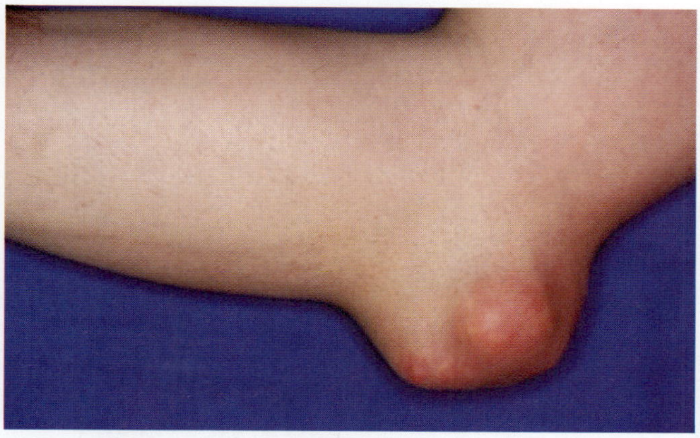

Fig. 22.158: Distended olecranon bursa

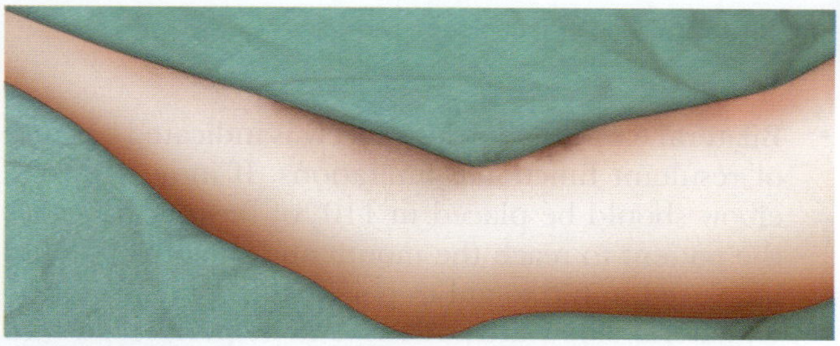

Fig. 22.159: In symptomatic bursitis, elbow cannot be flexed to more than 90°

- In subacute and chronic nonspecific cases TLC is 800 to 900 cells (monocyte predominance)
- X-ray olecranon spur in chronic cases, punched out bony erosions in gout (Fig. 22.160).

Treatment

Acute Bursitis

- Control of any underlying systemic or inflammatory process is the obvious first step in treatment
- If the bursa is not painful, local measures to prevent injury are all that is required (splinting and compression)
- Acute traumatic or idiopathic bursitis is also treated symptomatically with elbow pads
- If pain in the bursa prevents daily or occupational activity, aspiration and corticosteroid injection are indicated.

Chronic Bursitis

- Chronic recurrent or painful olecranon bursitis may require more definitive measures
- A 16-gauge indwelling needle/suction irrigation system, that maintains drainage with a compressive dressing for about 3 days, has been cited as being effective in reducing recurrence of bursal swelling

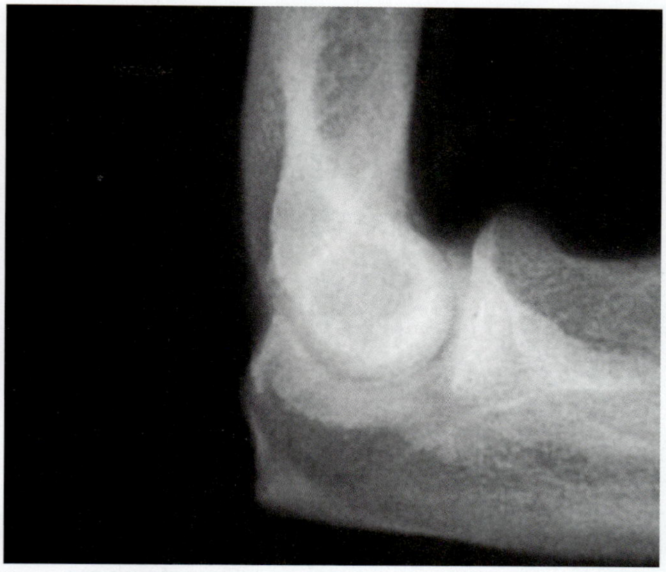

Fig. 22.160: X-ray showing olecranon spur in chronic cases

- When the process is refractory to nonoperative measures and is interfering with occupational or daily activities, operative intervention should be considered
- Operative
  - Endoscopic procedures
  - *Open:* A longitudinal incision medial to the midline or a transverse incision has been recommended. All bursal tissue is removed and the joint is immobilized in flexion or extreme flexion for approximately 2 weeks. Freeing the bursa from the skin can devitalize the skin over the olecranon process or can cause problems with healing.

Quayle and Robinson method (Figs 22.161A and B).

ELBOW ARTHRODESIS

Introduction

- Designed to produce bony ankylosis of a diseased joint. It often is a satisfactory solution for infection, tumors, trauma, paralytic conditions and for certain patients with osteoarthritis and rheumatoid arthritis
- Arthrodesis often results in stiffness in adjacent joints and in the lower extremity energy requirements for ambulation usually are increased
- Arthrodesis can be intra-articular, extra-articular or combined
- Extra-articular techniques are especially useful in treating children, since much of children's joint surfaces are cartilage and in treating patients who have large amounts of necrotic bone or active infection, as in tuberculosis

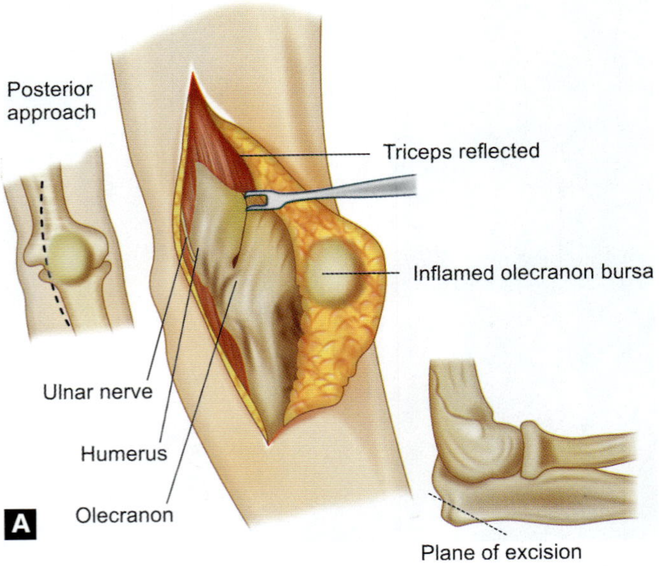

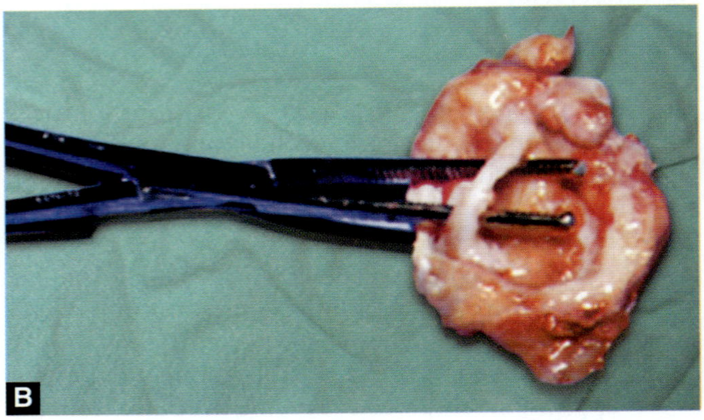

Figs 22.161A and B: Quayle and Robinson method

- Intra-articular techniques permit greater correction of deformity and are satisfactory, if adequate areas of healthy bone surfaces can be apposed
- If adequate bone is not available locally, bone grafts, preferably autogenous, cancellous bone, should be added.

Indications

- Reserved for patients with *painful arthritis* who are not candidates for total elbow arthroplasty, especially those who place high demands on the upper extremities, such as manual laborers
- Persistent infection, including tuberculosis, which historically was the main indication for this procedure
- Severely comminuted, intra-articular fractures of the distal humerus not amenable to repair and may be indicated *after failed total elbow arthroplasty*

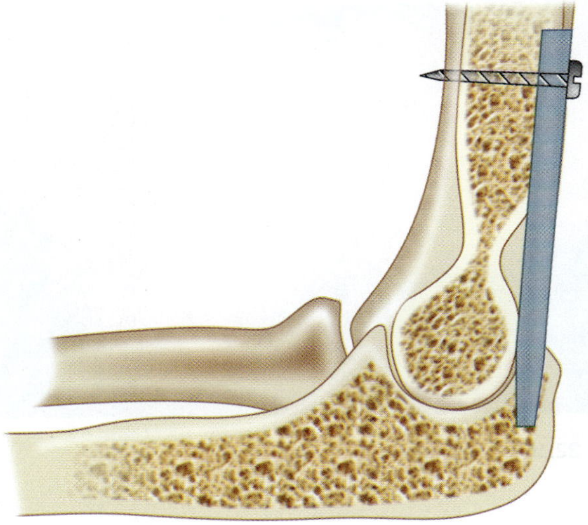

Fig. 22.162: Steindler technique

- Bilateral elbow arthrodesis rarely is indicated because of resultant functional limitations. If indicated, one elbow should be placed in 110° of flexion to permit the patient to reach the mouth and the other should be placed in 65° to aid in personal hygiene.
- Unilateral elbow arthrodesis is to be performed *with 90° of flexion at the elbow*, although many surgeons simulate the position of arthrodesis by splints before actual surgery.

Technique

Shown by Steindler (Fig. 22.162)

- Posterolateral incision from a point 10 cm above the elbow to a point 2.5 cm below the olecranon
- Dissect the triceps tendon from its insertion on the olecranon process
- Then excise the articular cartilage of the semilunar notch of the olecranon and the trochlear surface of the humerus and "fish scale" the subchondral bone
- Before entering the elbow obtain a graft from the upper half of the tibia, approximately 1.5 cm wide and 9 cm long
- With the elbow in flexion, fit the graft into the olecranon cleft and then, after extending the elbow to the position of fusion, place it in its humeral bed
- Insert one or two screws through the graft into the humerus to make it secure and pack the ulnohumeral joint with cancellous bone from the proximal end of the tibia
- (Steindler) after treatment
- Above elbow cast with forearm in neutral rotation for 8 weeks
- Corset till osseous union.

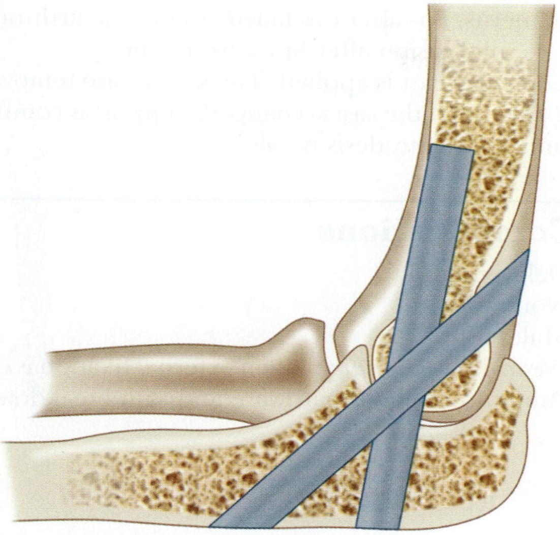

Fig. 22.163: Technique shown by Britton

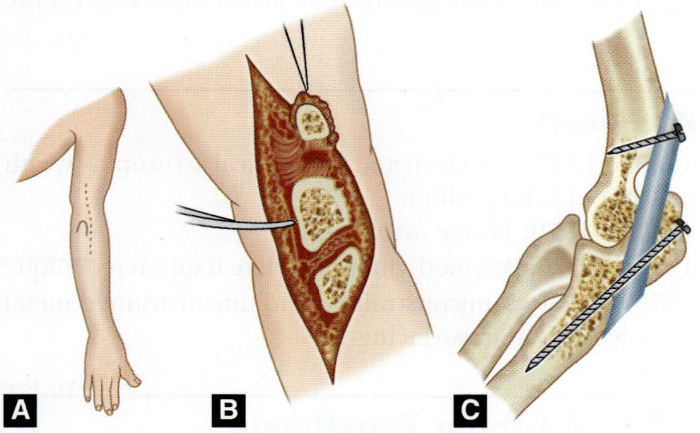

Figs 22.164A to C: Technique shown by Staples

Shown by Britton's (Fig. 22.163)

- Two tibial grafts crossed in shape of letter 'X'
- No important anatomical structure encountered
- Considerable latitude possible as elbow in flexion, the vessels and nerves in cubital fossa displaced forward.

Shown by Staples (Figs 22.164A to C)

- Posterior longitudinal incision and isolate and retract the ulnar nerve. Osteotomize the olecranon
- Denude the elbow joint of cartilage and cut the distal posterior surface of the humerus. Pack iliac bone chips in the joint
- Anchor the graft above with one screw. Then replace the olecranon process and fasten it with a second screw that passes through the olecranon and the lower end of the graft and into the upper end of the ulna.

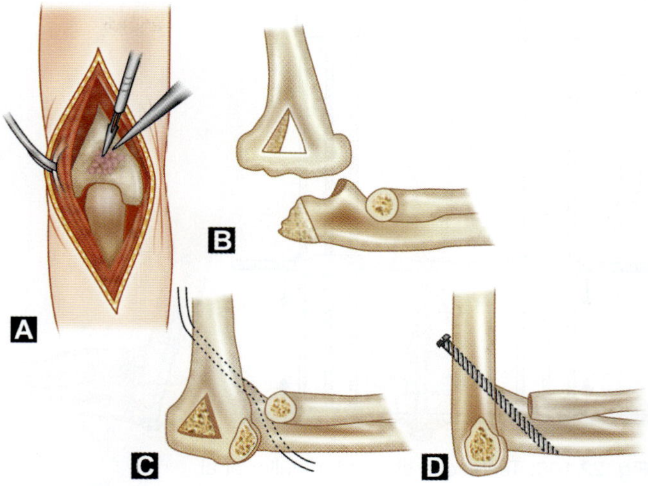

Figs 22.165A to D: Technique shown by Arafiles

Shown by Arafiles (Figs 22.165A to D)

- Technique for fusion in tuberculous arthritis of elbow
- Isolation of ulnar nerve, splitting and release of triceps tendon from olecranon and posterior synovectomy
- Excision of radial head and anterior synovectomy; shaping of olecranon and creation of triangular hole through distal end of humerus
- Insertion of olecranon through hole in distal end of humerus, screw fixation, medial and lateral epicondylectomy and anterior transposition of ulnar nerve. Resulting bone chips are used to fill any ground stump of olecranon
- Completed fusion with screw fixation
- After treatment (Arafiles)
- The elbow is immobilized in a long arm cast for 3 months and in a removable splint for another month
- Hand and shoulder exercises are begun soon after surgery.

Shown by Müller et al. (Fig. 22.166)

- Expose the elbow posteriorly as described in previous techniques
- Fashion a squared-off shelf in the proximal ulna and resect the distal end of the humerus to fit it
- Resect the radial head at the level of the biceps tuberosity. Insert a Steinmann pin from the olecranon into the medullary canal of the humerus to temporarily stabilize the arthrodesis in the desired position.
- Then, insert a Steinmann pin transversely through the olecranon in line with the anterior cortex of the humerus
- Remove the transfixing medullary pin and replace it with a cancellous screw and washer

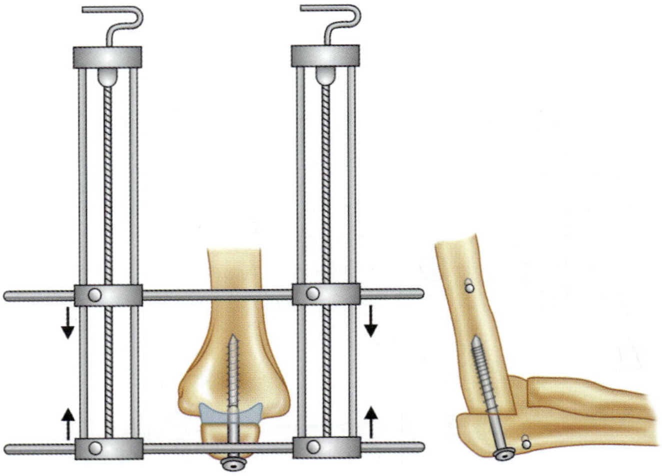

Fig. 22.166: Technique shown by Müller et al.

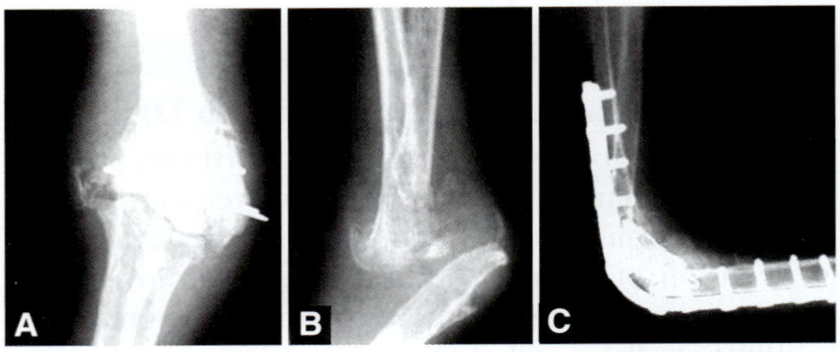

Figs 22.167A to C: (A) Traumatic arthritis after severely comminuted fracture of distal humerus; (B) After two failed attempts at arthrodesis; (C) Solid fusion after Spier technique

- Insert another transverse Steinmann pin through the humerus and use an external fixator to apply compression across the arthrodesis. Close the wound in layers overdrains
- The fixator and pins are removed at 6 to 8 weeks and a long arm cast is worn until the arthrodesis is solid.

Shown by Spier (Figs 22.167A to C)

- Expose the elbow posteriorly. Osteotomize the olecranon and humerus to fit as in the AO technique.
- Contour an 8 to 12 hole AO plate to achieve the desired degree of flexion at the elbow and secure it to the humerus posteriorly by the standard AO technique
- Secure a tensioning device to the ulna and the distal end of the plate and apply compression to the arthrodesis site
- Accessory cancellous screws may be used for additional stability if needed
- Apply bone graft about the fusion
- As shown in Figures 22.167A to C, A is traumatic arthritis after severely comminuted fracture of distal humerus. B is after two failed attempts at arthrodesis. C is solid fusion after Spier technique
- Long arm cast is applied. The sutures are removed at 2 weeks and the cast is changed. Support is continued until the arthrodesis is solid.

Complications

- Delayed union
- Nonunion
- Malunion
- *Neurovascular injury:* When external fixation is done
- Painful prominent hardware and skin breakdown.

ELBOW ARTHROPLASTY

Introduction

Arthroplasty is an operation to restore stability and pain-free motion to a joint and function to the muscles, ligaments and other soft tissue structures that control the joint.

History

1885 to 1947: Resection and anatomical arthroplasty with or without interposition
1947 to 1970: Hinge arthroplasty
1970 to 1975: Polymethylmethacrylate fixation technique
1975 till now: Semiconstrained and unconstrained metal to polyethylene resurfacing.

Ideal Elbow Prosthesis

- Should sacrifice as little bone as possible
- Stable
- Durable and inert
- Leave minimal dead space
- Easy to implant
- Carrying angle with built in laxity
- No pain
- Mobile

Types of Arthroplasty

- Interpositional (fascial) arthroplasty
- Resection arthroplasty
- Debridement arthroplasty
- Implant arthroplasty
- Constrainedmetal on metal
- Semi constrainedmetal to high density polyethyene with a locking pin or a snapfit device

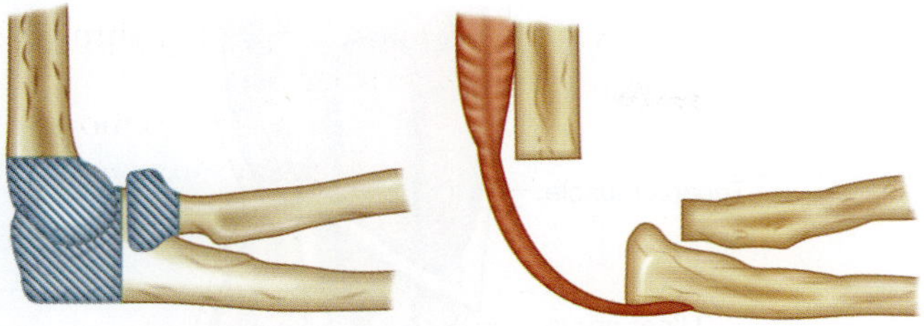

Fig. 22.168: Resection arthroplasty

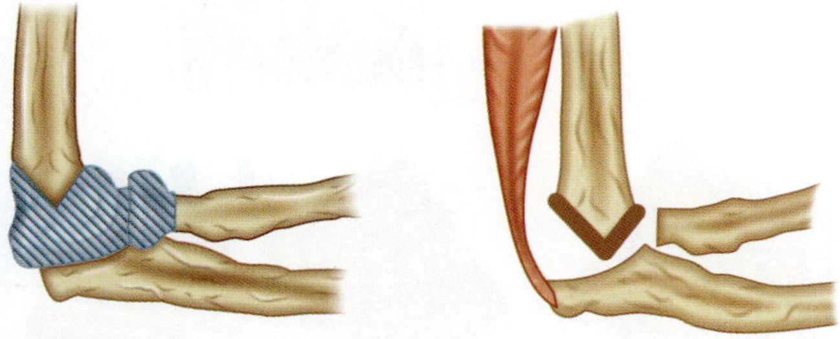

Fig. 22.169: Functional arthroplasty

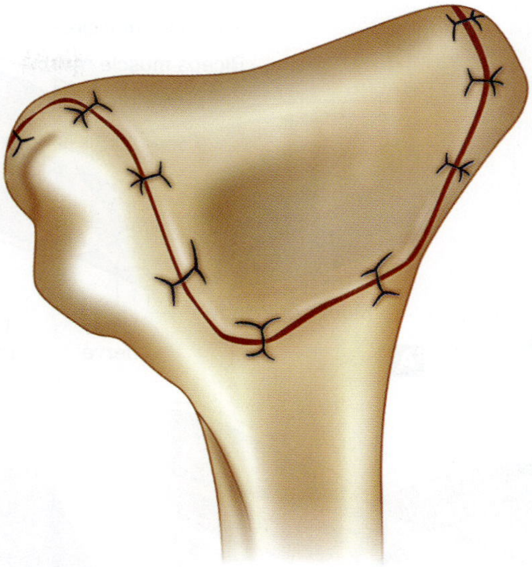

Fig. 22.170: Interposition arthroplasty

- Unconstrained/resurfacing arthroplasty—metal on high density polyethylene without a locking pin or a snapfit device.

Resection Arthroplasty

It is shown in Figure 22.168.

- Verneuil first used this technique in 1860
- Resection of distal humerus, ulna and radius
- Used for ankylosis of elbow after refractory sepsis, rheumatoid arthritis
- Used to treat instability of elbow joint
- Salvage procedure.

Functional Arthroplasty

It is shown in Figure 22.169.

- It was advocated by Hass
- It is a variation of resection arthroplasty
- Wedge shaped section of humerus is taken
- Used in painful ankylosis of elbow without sepsis and as a salvage procedure after infection or failed arthroplasty.

Interposition Arthroplasty (Figs 22.170 and 22.171)

- Murphy 1902 described interposition arthroplasty using fascia lata and fat
- Lexer, in 1909, described fascia lata and vastus externus as interposition material
- Campbell described use of other material like tin, zinc, silicone, celluloid, linoleum rubber, skin
- Used in painful ankylosis of elbow without sepsis
- After myositis ossificans
- Septic arthritis after a period of 6 months to 1 year.

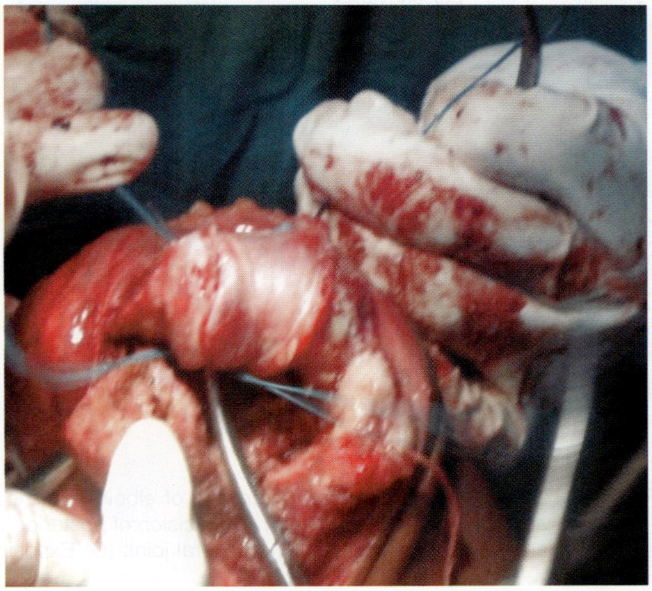

Fig. 22.171: Interposition arthroplasty of elbow

Debridement Arthroplasty

Debridement arthroplasty of elbow is shown in Figures 22.172A to G.

Implant Arthroplasty

Indications

- Pain, instability and bilateral elbow ankylosis
- Bony/fibrous ankylosis with elbow in poor functioning position
- Failed elbow arthroplasty of any type

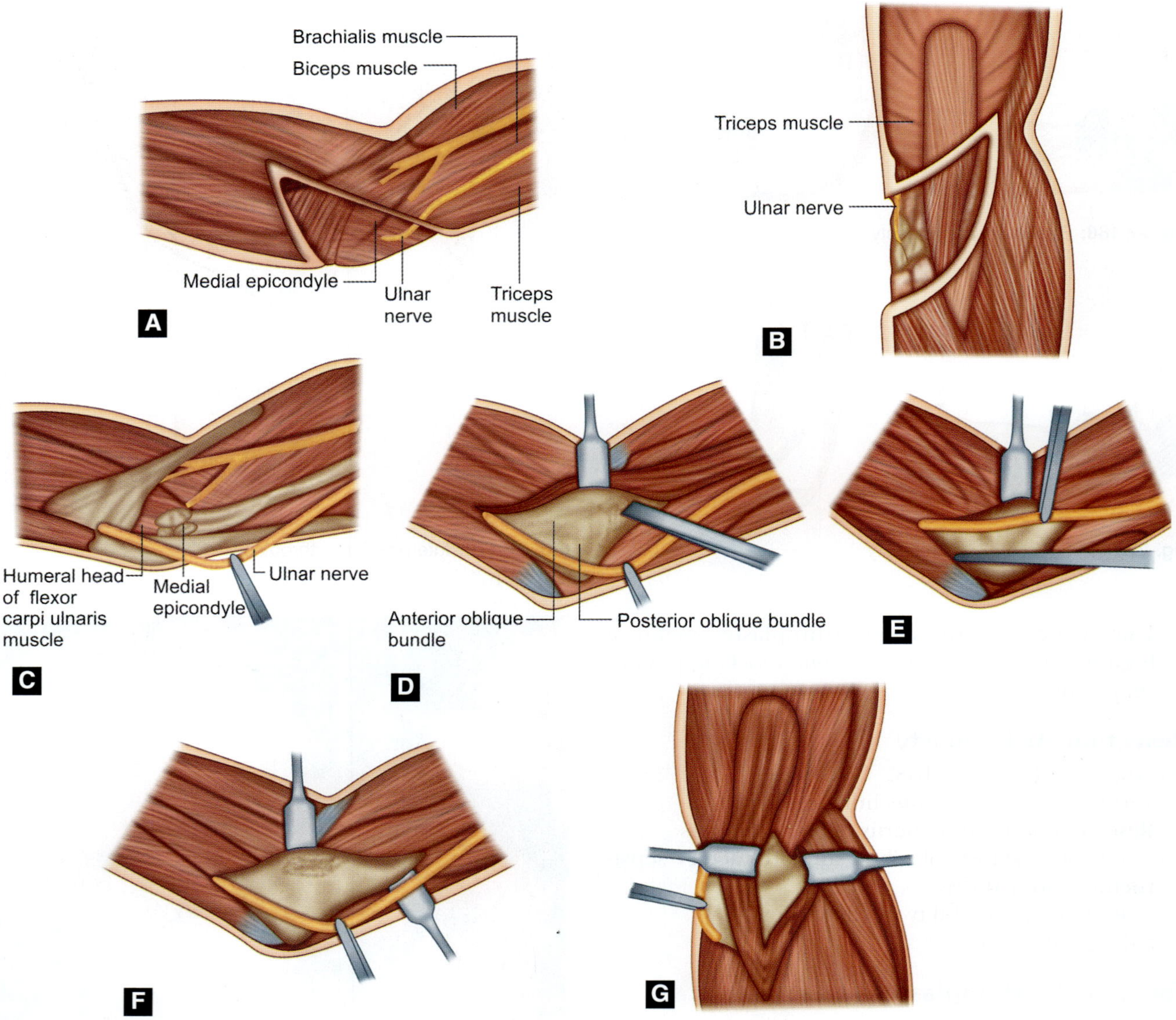

Figs 22.172A to G: Debridement arthroplasty of elbow—(A and B) Incision; (C) Elevation of flexor pronator origin; (D) Exposure of anterior elbow compartment; (E) Excision of posterior oblique bundle and posterior capsule; (F) Exposure of anterior, medial and posterior aspects of ulnohumeral joint; (G) Exposure and excision of osteophytes on lateral aspect of olecranon fossa

- Loss of bone stock due to trauma, tumor or infection
- Painful and disabling rheumatoid arthritis.

Hinged Prosthesis: Constrained (Fig. 22.173)

- Skin breakdown
- Triceps tendon rupture
- Failure due to implant loosening
- Used as salvage procedure.

New Designs (Fig. 22.174)

- Semiconstrained
- Totally unconstrained or snap fit.

Unconstrained Prosthesis (Fig. 22.175)

- Two part device
- Without pin, link
- Anatomical design
- Require intact ligaments, capsules.

Contraindications

- History of previous sepsis
- Ankylosis of the ipsilateral shoulder
- Presence of a neuropathic joint
- Excessive loss on either side of the joint
- Poor functioning flexor and extensor mechanism.

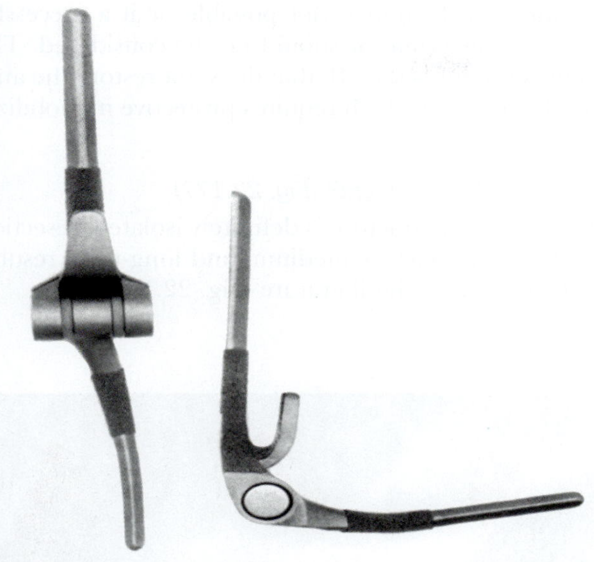

Fig. 22.173: Hinged prosthesis: constrained

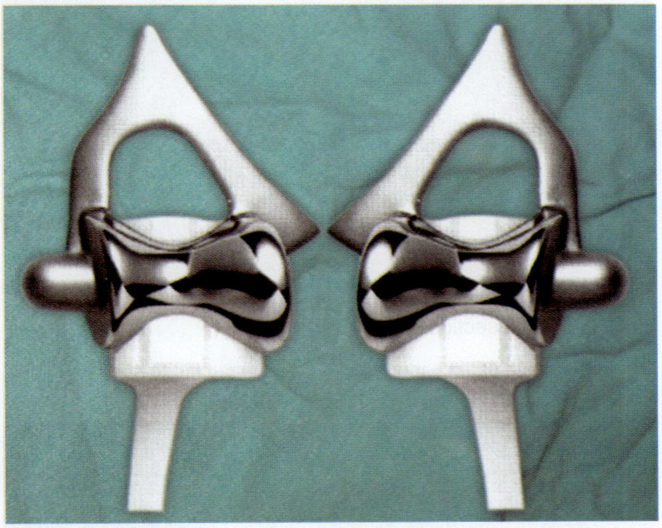

Fig. 22.174: Newer designs

Implant Arthroplasty—Complications

- Rarely requiring surgery
- Nerve paresthesias
- Wound problems
- Fracture humerus
- Fracture ulna
- Usually requiring surgery
- Nerve entrapment
- Triceps problems
- Ankylosis
- Usually requiring revision
- Loosening (semiconstrained)
- Instability (unconstrained)

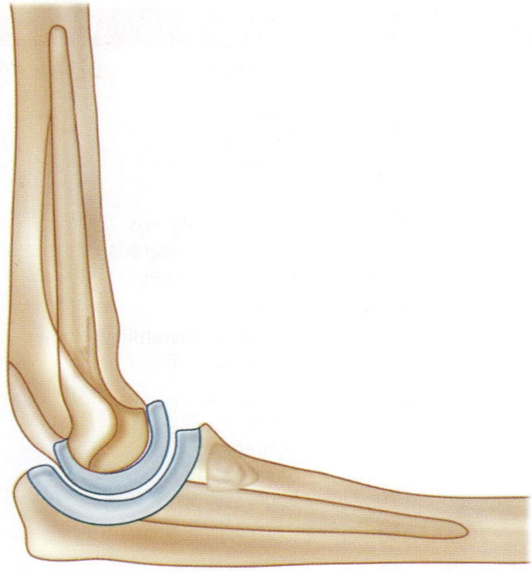

Fig. 22.175: Unconstrained prosthesis

- Infection
- Fracture and loosening.

Rating System for Arthroplasty

Morrey Classification System

Good Results

- No radiological change at the bone cement- prosthesis interface
- No pain
- More than 90° flexion
- 60° of pronation and supination

Fair Result

- 1 mm widening of bone cement prosthesis interface
- Mild pain
- 50 to 90° flexion
- <40° pronation and supination

Poor Result

- > 2 mm widening of bone cement prosthesis interface. Pain limiting activity
- < 50° of flexion and extension
- < 40° pronation and supination

Mayo Elbow Performance Index (Table 22.4)

Radial head implant arthroplasty (Figs 22.176A and B)

Regardless of whether the fracture is an isolated injury or associated with other lesions, internal fixation is the preferred option, providing that stable anatomical reduction can be achieved, so as to enable an exercise regime to be instituted immediately.

Table 22.4: Mayo elbow performance index			
Function	*Points*	*Definition*	*Points*
Pain	45	None Mild Moderate Severe	45 30 15 0
Motion	20	Arc >100 degrees Arc 50-100 degrees Arc <50 degrees	20 15 5
Stability	10	Stable Moderate instability Gross instability	10 5 0
Function	25	Comb hair Feed Hygiene Shirt Shoe	5 5 5 5 5
Total	100		
Excellent result	>90		
Goods result	75-89		
Fair result	60-74		
Poor result	<60		

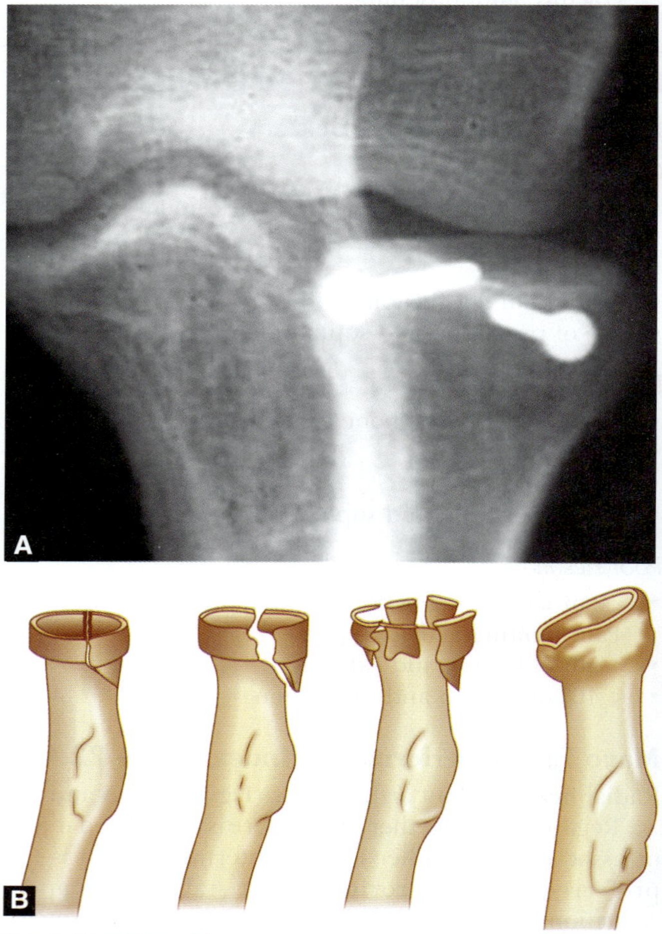

Figs 22.176A and B: Radial head implant arthroplasty

If internal fixation is not possible or if a successful outcome is uncertain, it should not be considered. The patient is not helped by IF that does not restore the anatomical pattern or which requires protective immobilization.

Resection or Replacement? (Fig. 22.177)

If the radial-head fracture is definitely isolated, resection should give satisfactory medium- and long-term results, as documented in the literature (Fig. 22.178).

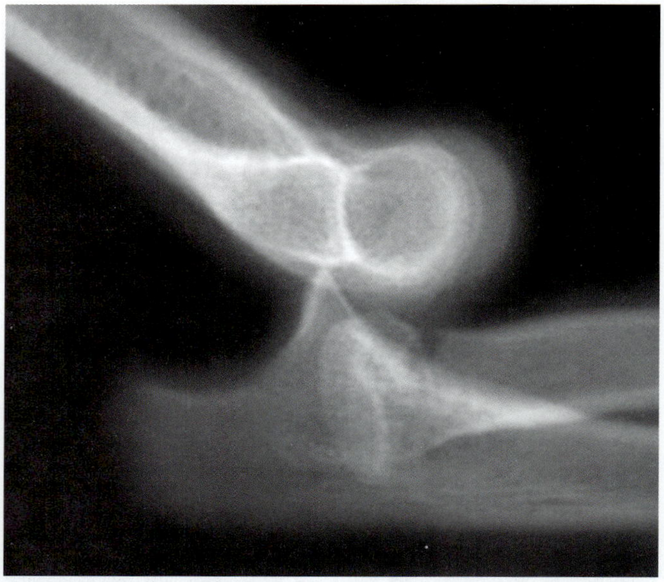

Fig. 22.177: Resection or replacement

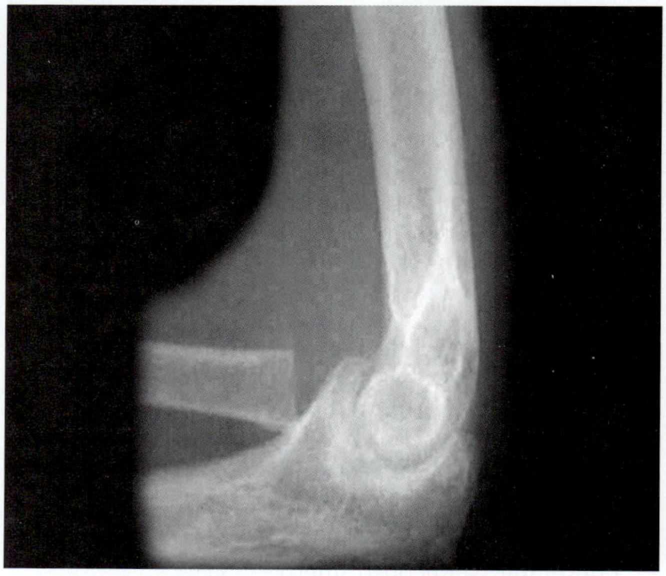

Fig. 22.178: X-ray showing elbow after radial head resection

If, however, the radial-head fracture is associated with other destabilizing injuries, resection may be expected to lead to complications.

Among the early complications are the recurrence of a dislocation, as well as early instability or the failure of an overstressed fixation construct.

Signs of mediolateral instability, recurrent valgus instability and posteromedial OA, anteroposterior instability with recurrence of subluxation or even dislocation and proximal-distal instability, with disturbance of the inferior radioulnar joint (Fig. 22.179).

Procedure of Elbow Arthroplasty (Figs 22.180 to 22.190)

Complications

- Stiffness
- Valgus instability
- Recurrent dislocation
- Cartilage damage
- "Floating radial head prosthesis" is seen when the implant is sitting too high

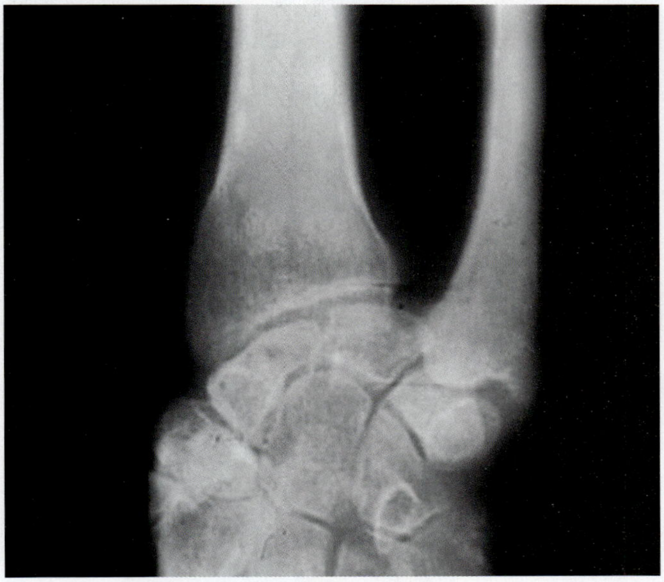

Fig. 22.179: Disturbed inferior radioulnar joint

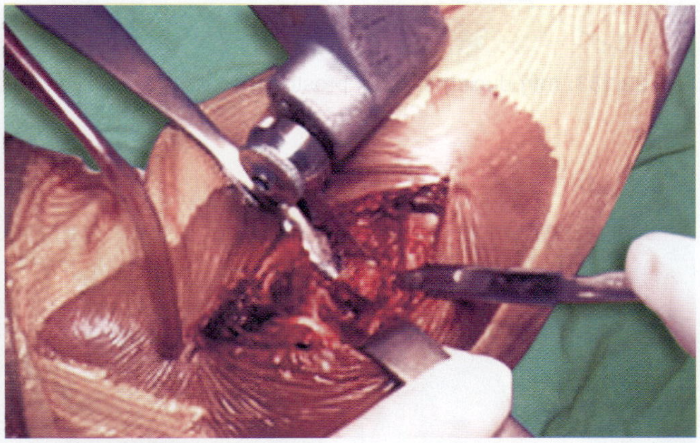

Fig. 22.181: Cutting the remaining part of radial neck

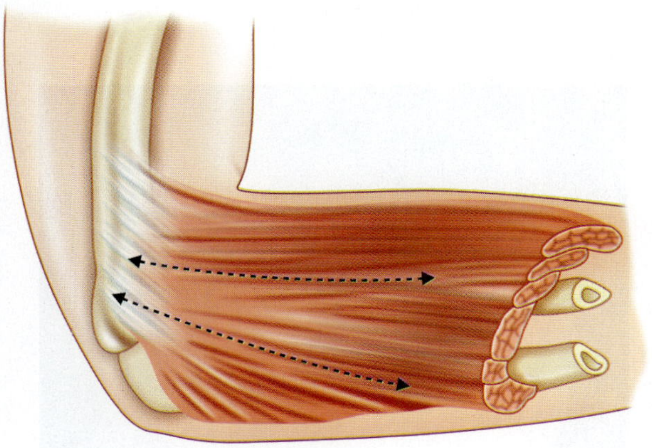

Fig. 22.180: Internervous plane for exposure of radius plane between extensor carpi radialis brevis and extensor digitorius communis

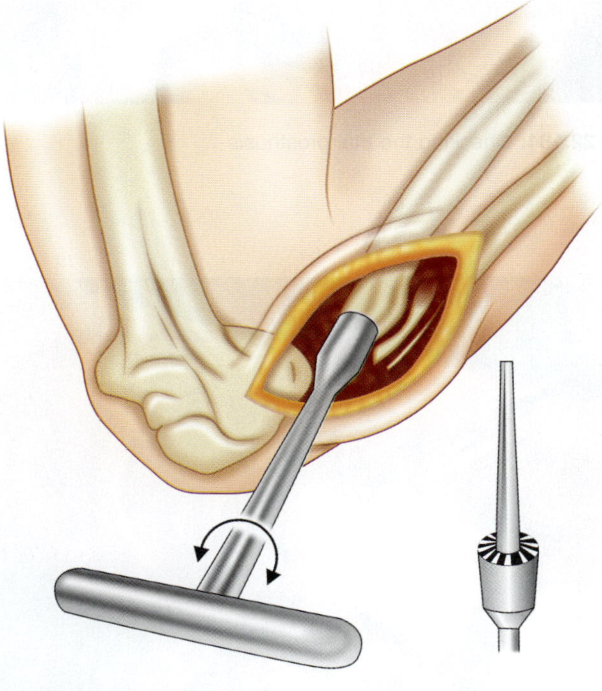

Fig. 22.182: Reaming of proximal radius

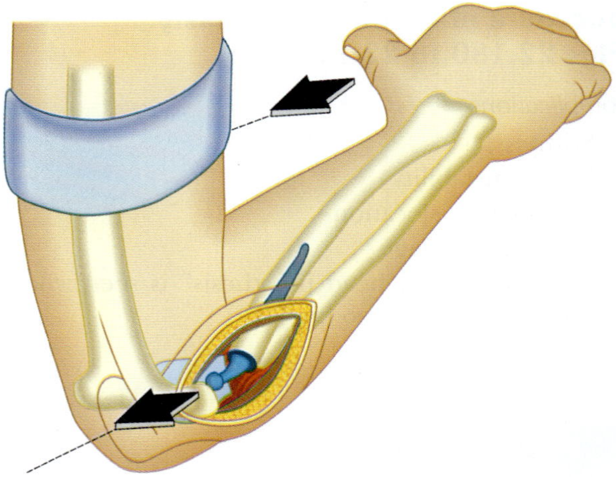

Fig. 22.183: Introducing the trial prosthesis

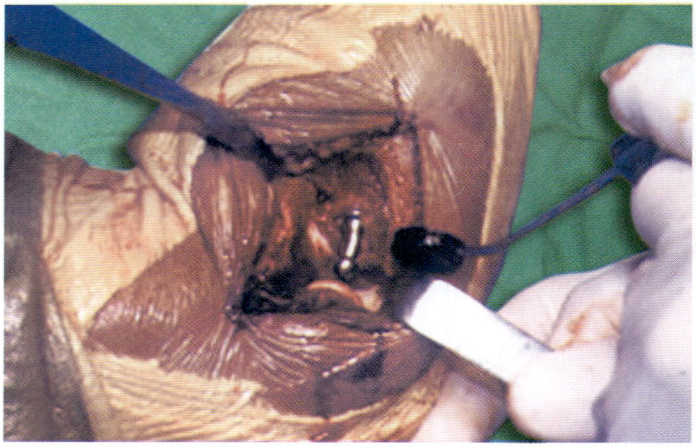

Fig. 22.184: Checking the trial prosthesis

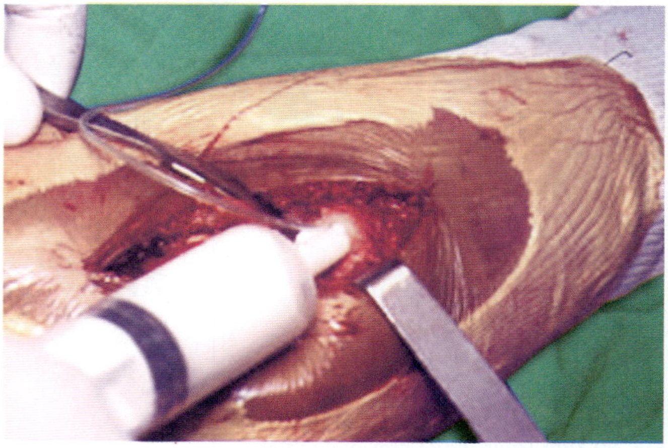

Fig. 22.185: Cementing of proximal end of radius

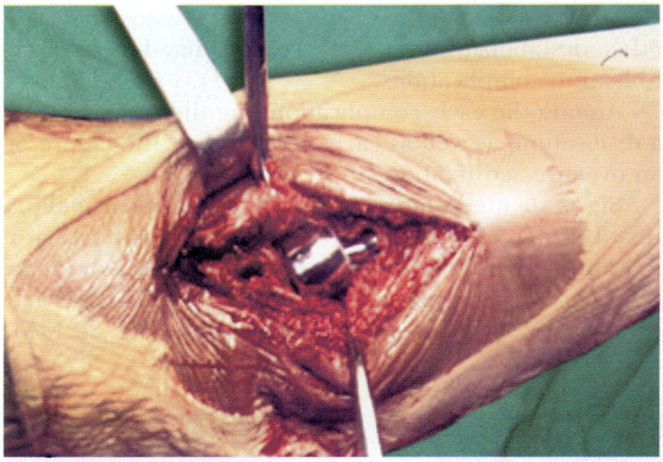

Fig. 22.186: Implanting the prosthesis

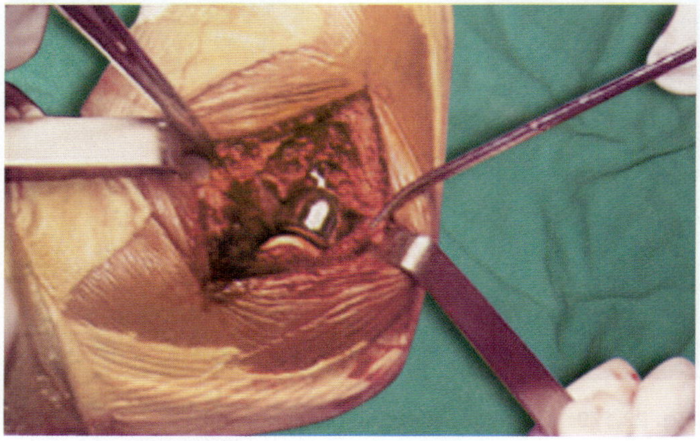

Fig. 22.187: Prosthesis after reduction

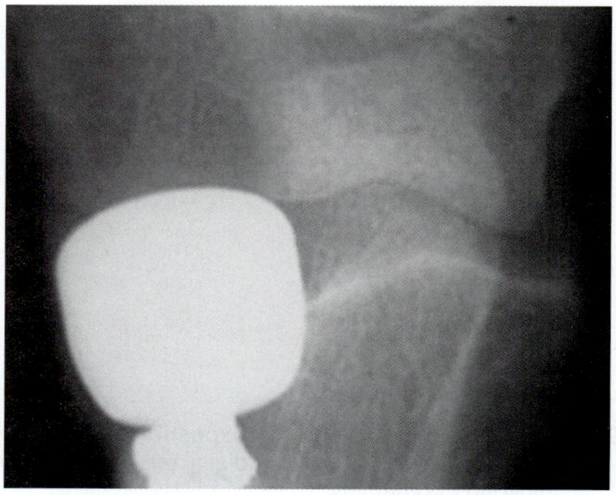

Fig. 22.188: Conforming the position of the prosthesis with X-ray

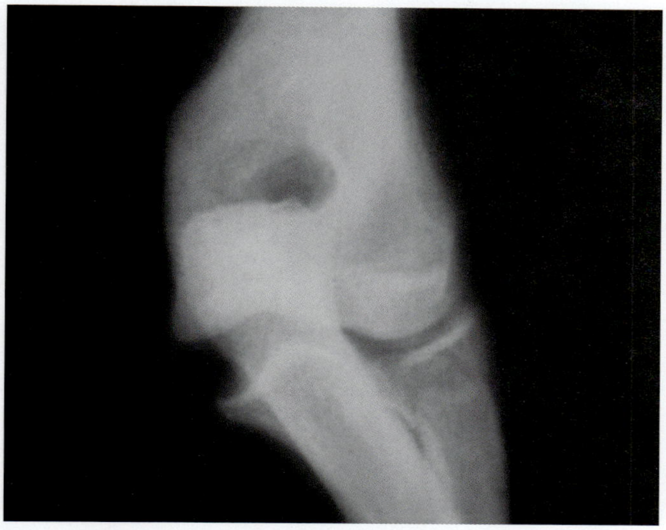

Fig. 22.189: Preoperative X-ray of radial head fracture

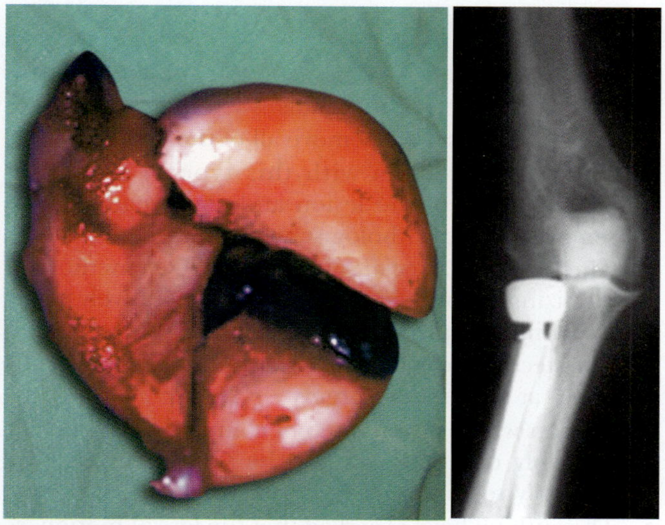

Fig. 22.190: Excised radial head and postoperative X-ray

TUMORS AROUND THE ELBOW

Tumors around the elbow are broadly divided into three categories:

1. Bone tumors
2. Soft tissue tumors
3. Metastatic tumors.

Bone Tumors

They are classified into two categories:
- Benign
- Malignant.

Benign Bone Tumors

Osteoid Osteoma

- This small benign bone tumor occurs in patients of any age, most commonly children and young adults
- Shows predilection for male sex

Clinical features

- Unremitting pain is a usual symptom for which the patient seeks medical attention
- Progressive loss of motion may also be a characteristic feature
- Pain during the night is particularly prominent
- Aspirin may afford very dramatic relief of pain, a fact that may even suggest the diagnosis of osteoid osteoma
- Occasionally, the pain may be experienced at a site remote from the lesion
- Another peculiar feature of this tumor is its occasional association with atrophy of the adjacent soft tissues.

Common sites of lesion in elbow are shown in Figure 22.191.

Pathoanatomy

- The osteoid osteoma, by definition, is small, usually no more than 1.5 cm in diameter
- When osteoid osteoma occurs at or near the elbow joint, there is characteristic loss of some flexion or extension, but pronation and supination are preserved
- In addition, there may be a synovial reaction that may further confuse the diagnosis
- The most striking feature of these tumors is the prolonged average time required for making the diagnosis
- Osteoid osteoma is small when first encountered and remains small.

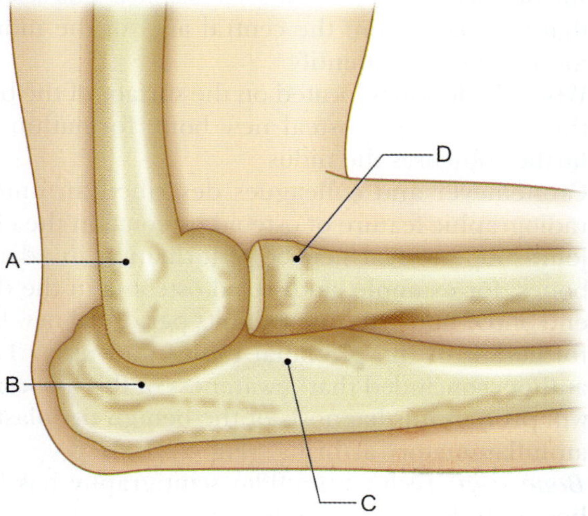

Fig. 22.191: Common sites of lesions in elbow—A. Lower end of humerus; B. Olecranon process; C. Coronoid process; D. Radial head

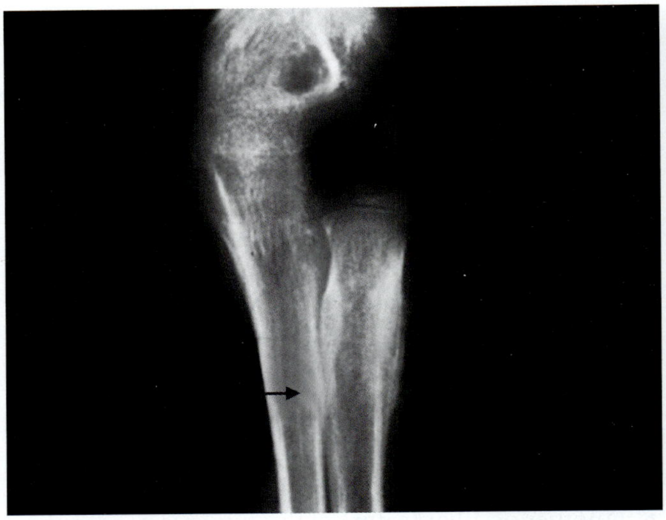

Fig. 22.192: Tumor lesion seen as a small nidus in X-ray film

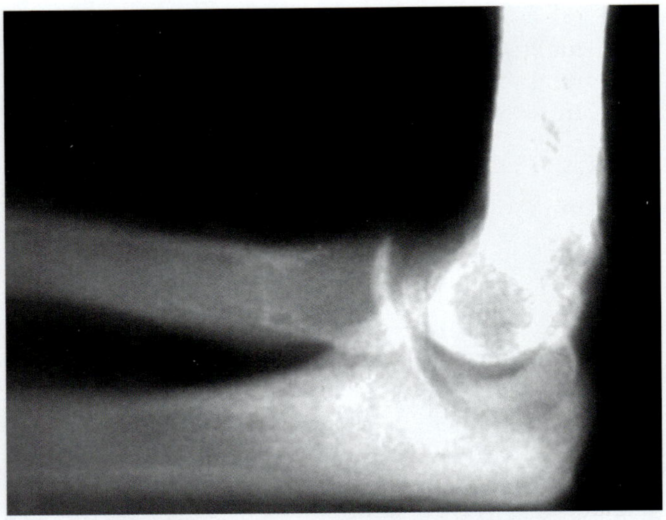

Fig. 22.193: An osteoid sarcoma in the distal end of humerus exhibiting periosteal new bone formation

Histopathology

- There is usually some sclerotic bone surrounding a central nidus
- This nidus may be somewhat redder than the surrounding cortical bone and has been described as having the appearance of a small cherry
- Microscopic examination of the surrounding bone shows no unusual features; the nidus itself consists of a network of osteoid trabeculae.

Imaging

- *Plain radiographs:* It may or may not reveal the presence of the tumor
- The lesion typically appears as a central small nidus (Fig. 22.192) which is a radiolucent area usually surrounded by an area of sclerosis, it is this sclerosis that is usually seen; the central area of the nidus is more difficult to identify
- When the lesion is located on the surface of the bone, there may be periosteal new bone formation that further obscures the nidus
- Cronemeyer and colleagues described an unusual radiographic feature of osteoid osteoma in the elbow joint-subperiosteal new bone formation in adjacent bones; for example, an osteoid osteoma in the distal end of the humerus that exhibits periosteal new bone formation in the proximal radius and ulna. These authors concluded that "awareness of this association will prevent misdiagnosis of the benign neoplasm as an inflammatory arthritis" (Fig. 22.193)
- *Bone scan:* Technetium-99m scintigraphy has been helpful in locating these lesions.
- CT scan is today's diagnostic standard.

Treatment

- In the past, the treatment of osteoid osteoma was surgical excision of the nidus
- It is not necessary to remove all of the sclerotic bone.
- The main problem with this type of surgery is identification of the lesion and confirmation of its removal by the pathologist, which may be difficult
- Ghelman and associates have described a method for localizing an osteoid osteoma intraoperatively, using a scintillation probe
- This technique may simplify the localization of the lesion at the time of surgery
- Patients whose lesions are not completely excised will probably continue to have the same pain and will probably require a second operation
- The authors have observed that the loss of motion, so characteristic of this lesion at the elbow, resolves with removal of the nidus. Hence, capsular release is not necessary as an adjunctive procedure
- At present, the treatment of choice for most lesions is radiofrequency obliteration performed under CT direction.

Osteoblastoma

- Osteoblastoma is an uncommon osteoid tissue forming primary neoplasm of the bone, categorized as a benign bone tumor
- It resembles osteoid osteoma in some respects but is larger (>2 cm)
- Unlike osteoid osteoma:
  - Osteoblastoma occurs in older adolescents and young adults.

- Osteoblastoma usually does not cause localized night pain, and when pain occurs, it is usually not relieved by salicylates (aspirin).
- Intense bony reaction that is seen with osteoid osteoma, does not occur with osteoblastoma.
- Osteoblastoma is more often located in the posterior elements of vertebra.
- Osteoblastoma will not resolve spontaneously.

- If the lesion is superficial, the patient may have localized swelling and tenderness
- In rare cases, malignant transformation is possible.

Histopathology

- Reveals scattered mitotic figures
- Proliferation of immature plump osteoblasts
- Prominent vascular and stromal tissue component; giant cells and broad osteoid seams.

Imaging

- X-rays show radiolucent lesion which is surrounded by a thin margin of reactive bone that may have expanded—aneurysmal appearance (Fig. 22.194)
- Bone scan shows intense radioisotope uptake that helps to localize the lesion
- CT scan confirms preoperative diagnosis and helps to determine surgical approach
- Angiography is used for staging aggressive tumors.

Treatment

- En bloc marginal excision is treatment of choice.
- Active tumors are likely to recur if intracapsular resection is performed
- Risk of recurrence after marginal excision of aggressive stage 3 is 30 to 50 percent
- Radiation therapy or chemotherapy is not effective.

Osteochondroma

- Osteochondroma is probably the most common benign bone tumor, but it is not very commonly encountered in the elbow
- The tumor may be found in a patient of any age, but it usually stops growing when skeletal maturity is reached
- An osteochondroma may arise from the surface of any bone but most commonly does so in the metaphyseal region of long bones
- The tumor tends to project away from the joint along the direction of attached muscles.

Clinical features

- The osteochondroma is not inherently painful but causes symptoms by pressure on adjacent structures
- Osteochondromas (Fig. 22.195) in the region of the elbow may cause mechanical difficulties; specifically, interference with the motion of the elbow joint
- In addition, the cartilage cap may impinge on important neurovascular structures.

Histopathology

- The tumor may be pedunculated on a stalk or may be sessile and have a broad base
- The tumor is covered by a cartilage cap, which, if becomes markedly thickened, suggests the possibility of sarcomatous transformation
- If it is more than 1 cm thick, the risk of secondary chondrosarcoma is relatively high
- In children, the cartilage cap is normally thicker than in adults
- Probably less than 1 percent of osteochondromas ever become malignant

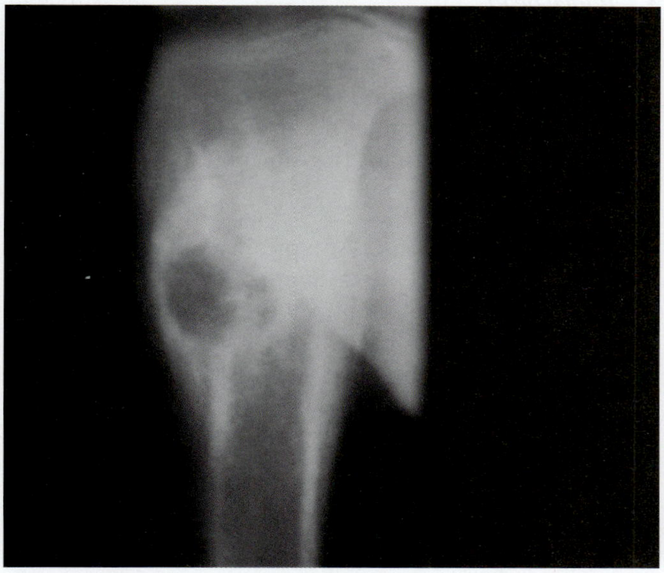

Fig. 22.194: X-ray showing radiolucent lesion, surrounded by a thin margin of reactive bone

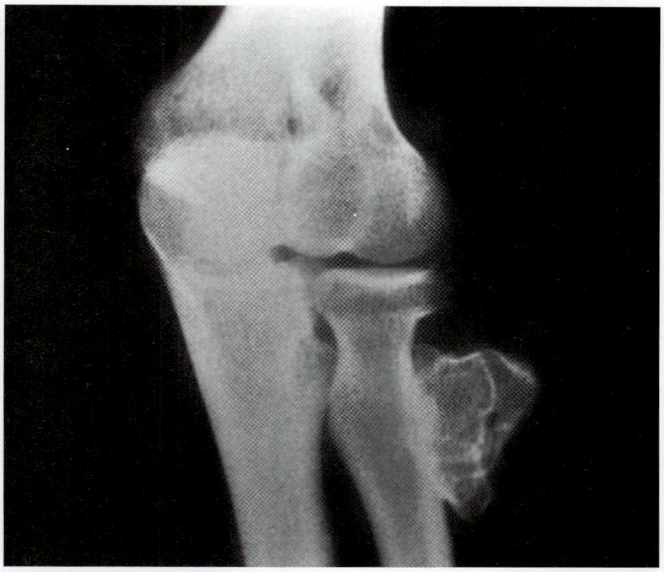

Fig. 22.195: Osteochondroma in a 23-year-old woman showing radial shaft with cortical and medullary bone extending into tumor

- Multiple osteochondromas sometimes occur, a condition that tends to be familial
- When multiple bones are involved, there may be some element of dysplasia with the deformity and the elbow can be severely involved.

Treatment

- If there are symptoms or mechanical or cosmetic difficulties, complete excision of the osteochondroma, together with the overlying cartilage cap, is performed
- Excision commonly involves the use of an osteotome to shave the lesion level with the underlying cortical bone. Such simple excision generally results in cure, although local recurrence may occasionally be noted, indicating that part of the cartilaginous cap was left behind
- If the cap is thicker than 1 cm in an adult, the lesion must be carefully studied histologically to exclude the possibility of a sarcoma.

Giant Cell Tumor (Fig. 22.196)

- Benign giant cell tumors are occasionally encountered in the region of the elbow
- Shows predilection for female sex
- Occur commonly in persons older than 20 years (differentiate from aneurysmal bone cyst)
- Giant cell tumors nearly always occur in the epiphyseal region and may extend to the articular surface of the bone

Classification by Campanacci, et al.

- Grade I: Tumors are radiologically indolent
- Grade II: Radiologically aggressive but the tumor has not yet broken through cortical bone
- Grade III: Radiologically aggressive with breach in the cortex

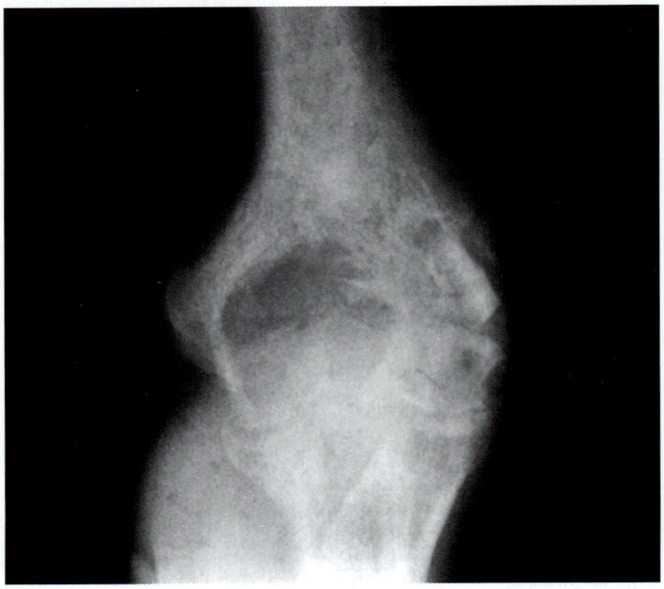

Fig. 22.196: Giant cell tumor

Histopathology

- Grossly, the tumor consists of a red, soft tissue that typically extends up the subchondral bone at the articular surface
- Microscopically, a giant cell tumor shows a combination of giant cells and mononuclear cells, with a more or less uniform distribution of the giant cells.

Treatment

- The extent of surgery required to eradicate giant cell tumors is somewhat controversial.
- *Distal end of humerus*
  - Excision by curettage will suffice in grade I lesion
  - In other grades; total excision of the distal end of humerus with allograft replacement is considered (creates a very serious problem for the reconstructive surgeon)
  - Excision by curettage in other locations results in a local recurrence rate of approximately 25 percent. It is probably reasonable to accept this risk and to try curettage for the first treatment because the alternative of resection of the distal end of the humerus is so drastic.
  - However, if the tumor has already broken through the cortex into the surrounding soft structures, curettage is unlikely to be effective.
- *Proximal end of ulna*
  - Curettage might be more reasonable because there is more bone to work with; hence, a larger margin of normal bone can be included in the resected specimen, whether resection is done by curettage or actual excision
  - Whenever possible, packing the tumor cavity with methylmethacrylate has proven to be effective.
- *Radial head*
  - Simple excision (especially in cases of small tumors).
- Radiation therapy for benign giant cell tumors should be avoided, if possible, because of significant risk of subsequent malignant transformation.

Aneurysmal Bone Cyst

- An aneurysmal bone cyst typically contains abundant benign giant cells in scattered zones
- It is different from giant cell tumor because it nearly always contains blood-filled spaces, is somewhat fibrogenic and usually has zones with osteoid formation and trabeculae of bone
- Occurs usually in persons younger than 20 years of age
- The lesion is usually metaphyseal in location.

Clinical Features

- Pain
- Swelling.

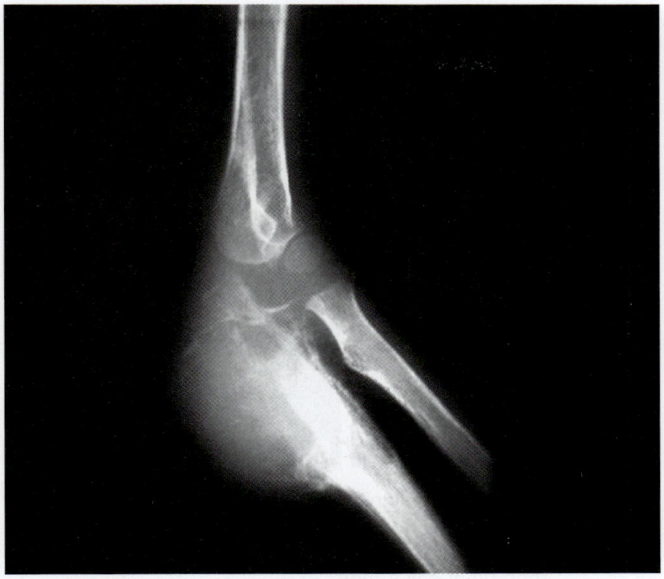

Fig. 22.197: Radiograph image of aneurysmal bone cyst

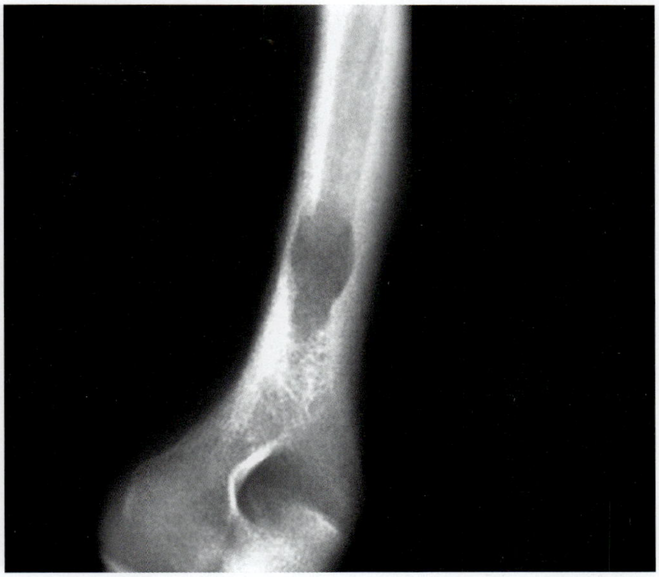

Fig. 22.198: Histiocytosis X-ray producing a well-defined rarefaction of the humeral shaft. This completely benign lesion is associated with a good prognosis, especially if it is solitary

Histopathology

- An aneurysmal bone cyst contains anastomosing cavernous spaces that usually constitute the bulk of the lesion.
- The spaces are usually filled with unclotted blood, which may well up into, but does not spurt from the tumor, when it is unroofed.
- The most important factor to recognize histologically is the benign quality of the constituent cells.

Imaging: (Fig. 22.197)

- *Plain radiographs:* The disease area consists of a zone of rarefaction, which is usually well circumscribed, eccentric and associated with an obvious soft tissue extension of the process
- Classically, the soft tissue extension is produced by bulging of the periosteum and a resultant layer of radiographically visible new bone that delimits the periphery of the tumor
- Fusiform expansion may be produced, especially when small bones are affected.

Treatment

- Curettage and bone grafting are usually required
- Twenty-five percent of these cases will recur and require additional surgery.

Other Benign Bone Tumors and Tumor Simulators (Figs 22.198 to 22.202)

- A number of lesions may occur in any bone and may simulate or mimic a primary bone tumor
- Benign cartilage tumors are very rare at the elbow.

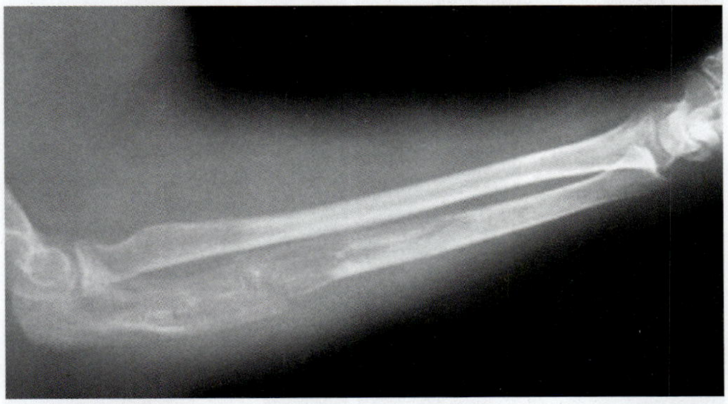

Fig. 22.199: Paget's disease of the proximal two-thirds of the ulna. This classic lesion is associated with pathologic fracture and extends to the end of the bone. Paget's disease of bone is very rare in patients younger than 40 years of age

■ Malignant Bone Tumors

Lymphoma

- Lymphoma tends to occur in middle-aged or elderly adults (Fig. 22.203)
- The tumor may arise primarily in any bone, including bones in the region of the elbow

Clinical Features

- Patients with lymphoma generally present with pain and swelling in the region of the lesion.

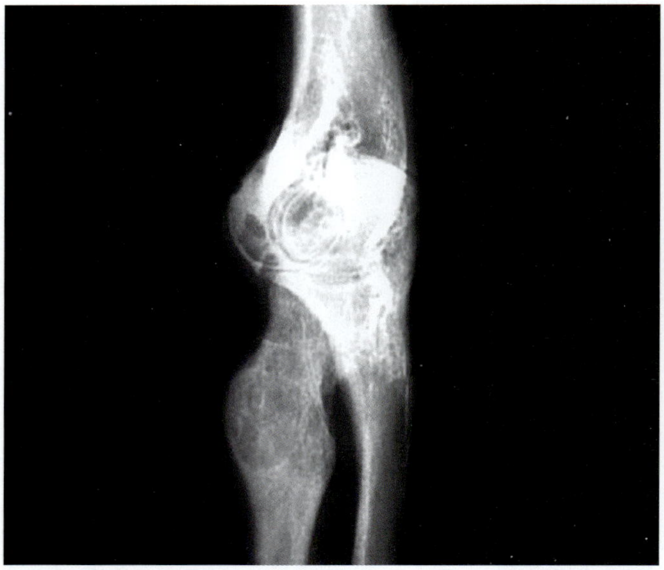

Fig. 22.200: Fibrous dysplasia producing extensive changes on both sides of the joint

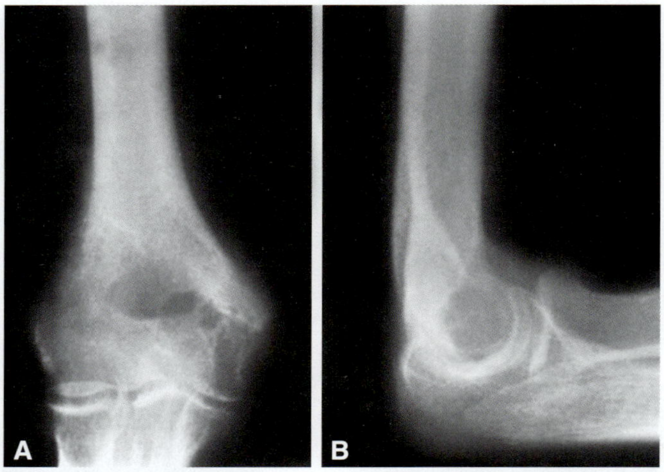

Figs 22.202A and B: Benign chondroblastoma of the distal end of the humerus in a 25-year-old man. Note the discrete zone of rarefaction. Such lesions are more innocuous than giant cell tumors

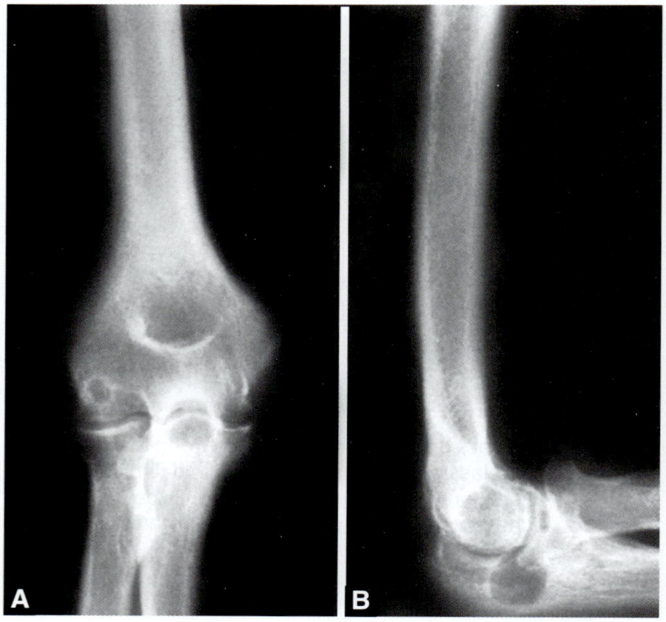

Figs 22.201A and B: Cyst of upper part of the ulna secondary to degenerative joint disease at the elbow

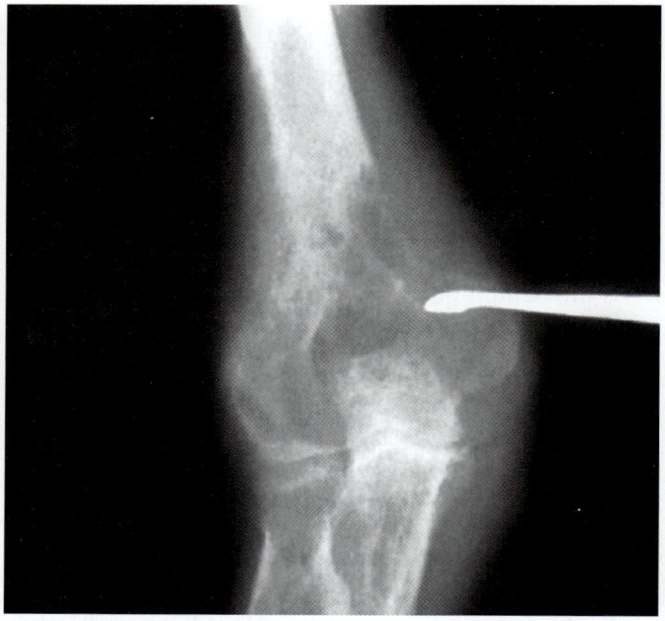

Fig. 22.203: Malignant lymphoma producing malignant-appearing destruction of the distal part of the humerus in a 60-year-old woman

Radiographic Features

- Diffuse, destructive, mottled appearance with indistinct margins
- Variable degrees of sclerosis may be present in the lesion; the cortical bone is usually eroded and the tumor may extend into the adjacent soft tissues
- Periosteal new bone formation, usually is not a prominent feature.

Histopathology

- Grossly-lymphoma tissue is usually gray or white and very soft.
- *Microscopically*
  - malignant lymphomas fit into the group of small round cell tumors
  - Under low power, the tumor shows a permeative pattern

– The infiltrate tends to fill up the marrow cavity without destroying medullary bone.

Treatment

- Lymphoma is generally treated with radiation therapy, if there is only a solitary lesion of bone
- Radiation therapists generally try to avoid circumferential treatment of an extremity to allow some normal lymphatic channels to remain open. Failure to do so may result in significant swelling distal to the treatment area.
- It may be difficult or impossible to avoid treating the entire circumference of the extremity in the region of the elbow
- In addition, when radiation exceeds approximately 4000 rad, radiation therapists generally try to direct treatment away from the articular surface
- There is no clear-cut or obvious advantage to the use of adjunctive chemotherapy at the time of initial treatment if only a solitary lesion is present

Prognosis

- If the disease is localized to one site, the prognosis is excellent
- About a fourth of patients will have multiple bones involved
- If there are other sites, such as liver, spleen or lymph nodes, the survival rate decreases dramatically

Ewing's Sarcoma

- Ewing's sarcoma may arise in any bone, including those in the region of the elbow
- Children are more frequently affected than adults (Fig. 22.204).

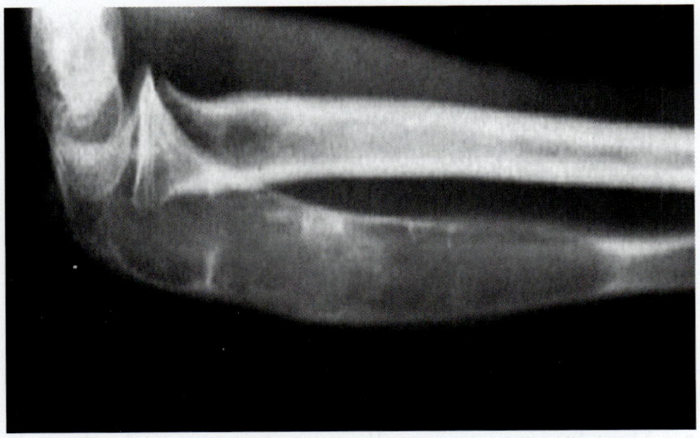

Fig. 22.204: Recurrent Ewing's sarcoma with a cyst-like lesion of the upper half of the ulna in a 21-year-old woman. The original tumor had been treated 10 years previously

Clinical Features

- Pain
- Swelling
- Fever
- Raised ESR

Radiographic Features

- Mottled or moth-eaten destructive lesion that may contain both lytic and blastic areas
- There is frequently periosteal reactive new bone, which may form layers, forming the "onion skin" appearance that is reported to be typical of this disease
- The radiographic appearance combined with the presence of fever and an elevated erythrocyte sedimentation rate may lead to the erroneous diagnosis of osteomyelitis.

Histopathology

- Grossly, Ewing's sarcoma may be very soft or even semiliquid; indeed, the appearance may simulate the purulence of infection
- Microscopically, Ewing's sarcoma is very cellular, composed of small round cells that are remarkably similar to one another.

Treatment

- The local lesion is generally treated with radiation therapy and systemic combination chemotherapy is generally used in an attempt to prevent micro-metastases
- Resecting malignant tumors in the region of the elbow is generally avoided because it is difficult to achieve adequate margins in this region without damaging important normal structures
- Even if an adequate resection could be achieved, satisfactory reconstruction would be difficult or impossible
- Therefore, the treatment for Ewing's sarcoma is radiation therapy
- A major side effect is soft tissue fibrosis causing a stiff joint.

Osteosarcoma

- Osteosarcoma (Fig. 22.205) is the most common bone malignancy except for myeloma
- About one-half of these tumors are predominantly fibrous or cartilaginous and others are predominantly bone forming. *Hence, they are subclassified into:*
  - Fibroblastic
  - Chondroblastic
  - Osteoblastic

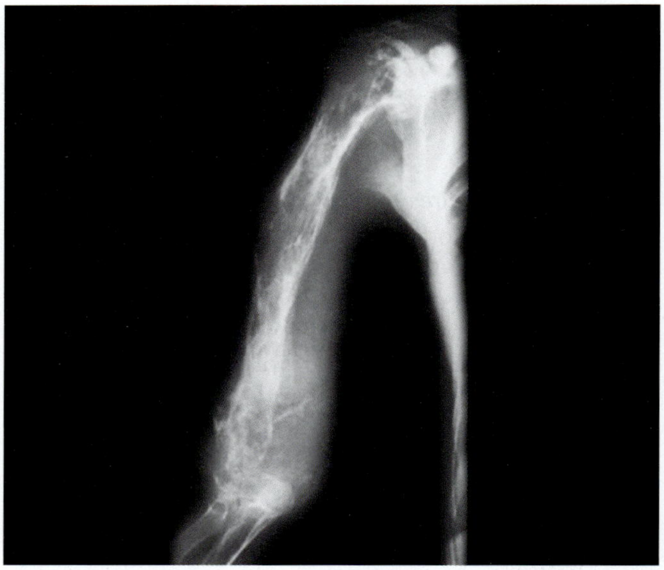

Fig. 22.205: Grade IV osteosarcoma of the distal end of the humerus in a patient with Paget's disease of the entire bone

- This subclassification may be important because the osteoblastic subtype appears to have a worse prognosis than the other two subtypes.

Diagnosis

- Radiographically
  - Appears to be aggressive, with evidence of cortical destruction and reactive periosteal new bone formation
  - In the distal humerus, the classic "sunburst" appearance may be evident
  - The precise extent of the lesion may not be apparent on plain radiographs
  - The tumor can usually be more accurately assessed with a technetium or gallium bone scan
  - *CT scan:* Determine the extent of soft tissue involvement
  - *MRI:* Determine both the extent of soft tissue involvement and the extent of intramedullary involvement.
- Biopsy
  - The reactive new bone formation at the periphery of the lesion should not be sampled for biopsy because this will simply lead to confusion in the interpretation of the histological findings
  - If there is a soft tissue extension of the tumor, this is the area which is best for biopsy because it is usually the most malignant and the easiest to process in the pathology laboratory

Treatment

- It is a radioresistant malignant bone tumor
- Hence, the usual treatment of osteosarcoma is surgical ablation
- In the past for many years amputation was carried out
- Today the majority of patients with osteosarcoma can be managed with various limb salvage procedures
- Neoadjuvant chemotherapy is generally employed before one proceeds with surgery and additional chemotherapy is usually offered after surgery.

Prognosis

The prognosis for patients with osteosarcoma today is much improved; 70 to 90 percent of such patients may be long-term survivors.

Metastatic Tumors

- There is no particular predilection for metastatic disease to involve the elbow
- Yet extensive destruction is observed on occasion from several tumor types
- Treatment is most commonly joint replacement
- Patients do well in general with this palliative treatment
- Complications relate to nerve dysfunction and stiffness.

Soft Tissue Tumors

They are classified into:
- Benign
- Malignant

Benign Soft Tissue Tumors

Lipoma

- Lipoma is probably the most frequently encountered benign soft tissue neoplasm and is the most common tumor in the elbow region
- It is usually solitary but multiple lipomas have occurred
- The tumor is simply a localized collection of adipose tissue that is histologically and chemically similar to ordinary fat.

Clinical Features

- Most lipomas are small, asymptomatic and relatively dormant in that they seem to remain approximately the same size
- Occasionally, however, the tumor may grow and become symptomatic

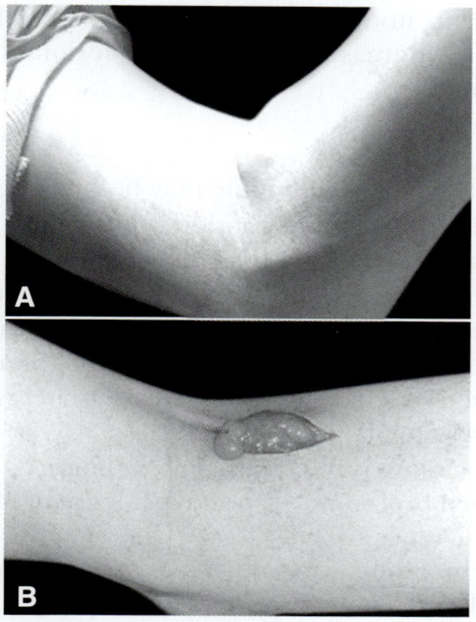

Figs 22.206A and B: (A) Expanding, prominent soft tissue mass in the cubital space; (B) It was found to be a benign lipoma

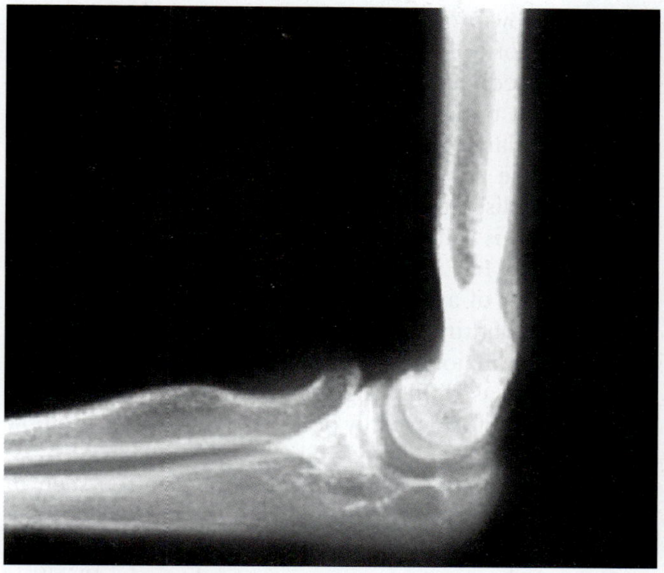

Fig. 22.207: Pigmented villonodular synovitis in a 17-year-old girl, with a 3-year history of pain and swelling. Note cystic erosions

- If there is trauma to the area, necrosis may develop within the lipoma and this is usually symptomatic
- Most lipomas consist almost entirely of adipose tissue; however, there may be increased vascularity, in which case the lesion is referred to as angiolipoma.

Diagnosis

- Mainly on clinical examination
- In some lipomas (Figs 22.206A and B), which do not have the clinical characteristics of the usual subcutaneous lipoma, may require further diagnostic modalities.

Treatment

Surgical excision should be considered for lipomas that:

- Increase in size
- Symptomatic or cosmetically undesirable
- Interfere with function
- In situations when the diagnosis is not certain
- Simple marginal excision should be carried out
- The vulnerability of the neurovascular structures is of particular concern for lipoma of the antecubital space
- When a lipoma is located within the belly of a muscle, it may be necessary to sacrifice some normal muscle tissue on all aspects to minimize the risk of local recurrence
- At the elbow, this can cause permanent stiffness.

Ganglion

- A ganglion is a cystic lesion generally found in the hands, wrists and feet, but it may be found less commonly in the region of the elbow
- The lesion may occur within a tendon, in a muscle or even on occasion in bone.

Treatment

- Symptomatic treatment (not all ganglia require excision)
- Simple excision.

Myxoma

- A myxoma occasionally occurs in the soft tissues at the elbow
- It is soft, well-circumscribed and myxoidal
- A myxoma is relatively small and is usually encountered in the superficial soft tissues.

Histologically

The lesion is hypocellular and contains stellate cells in a myxoid stream.

Treatment

Wide excision (because marginal resection tends to recur).

Pigmented Villonodular Synovitis

- Pigmented villonodular synovitis (PVNS) (Fig. 22.207) is a locally destructive fibrohistiocytic proliferation, characterized by many villous and nodular synovial protrusions, which affects joints, bursae and tendon sheaths
- PVNS was first described by Jaffe, Lichtenstein and Sutro in 1941, who used this name to identify the lesion because of its yellow-brown, villous, and nodular appearance

- The yellow-brown pigmentation is due to excessive deposits of lipid and hemosiderin
- Shows predilection for female sex with 2:1 ratio
- Clinically, there are two forms of the disease:
  - Nodular (or) localized
  - Diffuse
- When a discrete intra-articular mass is present, the condition is called 'localized pigmented villonodular synovitis'. (In European literature—'pigmented giant cell tumor of articulations')
- When the entire synovium of the joint is affected and there is a major villous component, the condition is referred to as 'diffuse pigmented villonodular synovitis'
- The diffuse form usually occurs in the knee, hip, elbow or wrist
- The nodular or localized form is most often seen in the fingers and is the second most common soft tissue tumor of the hand, exceeded only by the ganglion
- One of the most characteristic findings in PVNS is the ability of the hyperplastic synovium to invade the subchondral bone, producing cysts and erosions.

Clinical Features at the Elbow

- Mild pain
- Joint swelling
- Increased thickening of the synovium
- Restriction of joint motion
- Knee joint is most commonly affected and patients present with bloody joint effusion. In fact, the presence of a serosanguinous synovial fluid in the absence of a history of recent trauma should strongly suggest the diagnosis of PVNS. The synovial fluid contains elevated levels of cholesterol and fluid reaccumulates rapidly after aspiration.

Imaging

- *X-ray:* Cystic erosions on either side of the joint
- When erosions are found and there is no loss of joint space and no demineralization of the surrounding bone, the diagnosis should be suspected
- In most cases of pigmented villonodular synovitis, however, there is no bony erosion but there is evidence of lobular swelling of the soft tissues
- *Arthrography:* Reveals multiple lobulated masses with villous projections, which appear as filling defects in the contrastfilled suprapatellar bursa
- *CT scan:* Demonstrates the extent of the disease
- *MRI:* Useful in making the diagnosis (also in defining the extent of the disease).

Histopathology

- Microscopic study shows a stromal background of reticulin and collagen fibers, in which various different cells may be found
- The firm, nodular lesions have more collagenous stroma, whereas the soft villous lesions have less stroma.

Treatment

- Nodular form—the nodule may be simply excised
- Diffuse form—simple excision is likely to be followed by local recurrence
- Radiation therapy has been attempted (but there is no convincing evidence that such treatment will actually eliminate the disease and prevent local recurrences. High doses of radiation are avoided at the elbow joint)
- Synovectomy is the treatment of choice:
  - Open procedure reported incidence of 33 percent recurrence
  - Arthroscopic procedure—less recurrence (hence, today's treatment of choice)
- If synovectomy leads to symptomatic local recurrence, arthrodesis is considered in most joints
- At the elbow, however, because this joint does poorly with an arthrodesis, replacement arthroplasty would appear to be the treatment of choice.

Synovial Chondromatosis

- Synovial chondromatosis (also known as synovial osteochondromatosis or synovial chondrometaplasia) is a benign, tumorous, multifocal, chondromatous or chondro-osseous metaplastic proliferation involving the subsynovial connective tissue of joints, tendon sheaths or bursae
- Knee is the most commonly affected joint, but the process can involve any joint
- It is almost invariably monoarticular; rarely, multiple joints may be affected
- The average age of the patients is about 40 years
- Men are affected more often than women.

Clinical Features

- Pain
- Swelling
- Joint effusion
- Tenderness
- Limited range of motion in the joint
- Soft tissue mass.

Imaging

- *On X-ray (Fig. 22.208):* Radiopaque joint bodies, which are calcified cartilaginous bodies (may/may not reveal on X-ray—depends upon the degree of calcification)
- CT and MRI scans useful in visualizing even non-calcified bodies and also help in location and extent of the disease process (bony erosion)

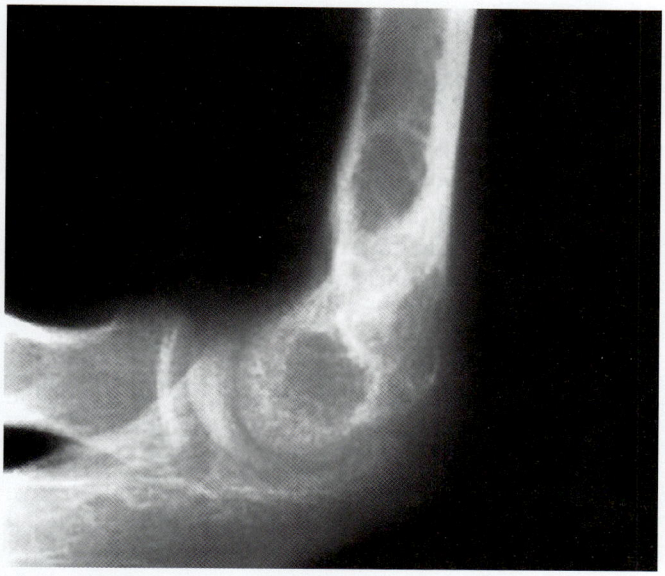

Fig. 22.208: Synovial chondromatosis of the elbow. Note that a small mineralized focus is evident in the antecubital fossa

- Diagnostic arthrotomy or arthroscopy is indicated when the radiographic diagnosis is indefinite and symptoms persist without any other obvious cause.

Joint Loose Bodies

Fibrous, bony, cartilaginous and osteocartilaginous fragments in a synovial joint. Major causes are osteochondritis dissecans, synovial chondromatosis, osteophytes (degenerative arthritis), fractured articular surfaces and damaged menisci.

Histopathology

- Microscopically, many cartilaginous nodules are observed as they form beneath the thin layer of cells that line the surface of the synovial membrane
- These nodules are highly cellular and the cells themselves may exhibit a moderate pleomorphism, with occasional plump and double nuclei
- Although such cytologic atypia mainly indicates an actively growing cartilaginous focus, an erroneous diagnosis of malignancy may sometimes be considered. (However, evidence of aggressive growth (invasion) and lack of attachment of a lesion to the synovial lining support the diagnosis of malignancy)
- The cartilaginous nodules, which often are undergoing calcification and enchondral ossification, may detach and become loose bodies
- The loose bodies continue to be viable and may increase in size as they receive nourishment from the synovial fluid
- Synovial chondromatosis may undergo malignant change to chondrosarcoma

Treatment

- Consists of removing any loose osteochondromatous bodies and the involved synovium, from which they arise
- Arthroscopic complete synovectomy is today's choice of treatment
- If the condition recurs, due to left out nests of synovium, revision arthroscopic synovectomy or maybe even arthrotomy can be done
- Long-standing synovial osteochondromatosis creates secondary osteoarthritis.

Other Non-neoplastic Benign Conditions Mimicking Tumors

- *Myositis ossifications (heterotopic or ectopic ossification):* May occur near the elbow, either in muscle or in other soft tissue. In its early or "florid" stage, there may be such pronounced cellular activity that it may be mistaken for sarcoma
- *Proliferative fasciitis:* Poorly defined small mass showing prominent mitotic activity; has been mistaken for entities such as liposarcoma or fibrosarcoma. The rapidly proliferating cells again do not show true anaplasia
- *Proliferative myositis:* There is a tumefactive, intramuscular proliferation of benign fibroblastic cells, but no discernible osseous metaplasia. Mitotic activity may be pronounced, making it possible to mistake this lesion for a malignant tumor.

■ Malignant Soft Tissue Tumors

Synovial Sarcoma

- Synovial sarcoma or synovioma, is a malignant soft tissue tumor that usually arises near but not in a joint; about 70 percent of lesions involve the lower extremity, most commonly the thigh, but this tumor does occur in the region of the elbow
- Despite its name, it does not arise from synovium, although it may originate from any other structure, including joint capsules, bursae and tendon sheaths
- Because of the similarity between cells of this tumor and primitive synoviocytes, the term synovial cell sarcoma has been used
- Young or middle-aged adults seem to be most commonly affected.

Clinical Features

- Diffuse or discrete soft tissue swelling or mass
- Progressive pain
- Tenderness.

Imaging

- On plain radiographs, synovial sarcoma show evidence of calcification.

- When calcification is found in a soft tissue tumor, synovial sarcoma should be included in the differential diagnosis
- A periosteal reaction may also be observed
- This tumor can invade the bone occasionally
- CT and MRI scans effectively demonstrates the extent of the soft-tissue mass, calcifications and bone invasion.

Histopathology

- The tumor is lobular, circumscribed and gray; may contain areas of calcification, hemorrhage, necrosis or cyst formation
- Several subtypes of synovial sarcoma have been recognized. Among them are biphasic or bimorphic (fibrous and epithelial), monophasic and poorly differentiated types
- Classically, synovial sarcoma has a bimorphic histologic pattern; that is, a combination of slender spindle cells and larger epithelial-appearing cells that may form glands or even show squamous change
- The monophasic synovial sarcoma is composed of interdigitating fascicles and "ball-like" structures formed by the spindle cells.

Treatment

- In the past, local excision of the tumor was done resulting in local recurrence
- Today, the treatment of choice is combination of radiation therapy and surgery. (With this approach local recurrence occurs in only about 5 percent of cases).

Liposarcoma

- Liposarcomas may arise in any part of the body and are occasionally found at the elbow
- Older adults are more commonly affected than younger persons
- A lipoma that shows evidence of growth should be suspected of being malignant.

Imaging

- X-rays are not as diagnostic for liposarcoma as they are for lipoma, but the combination of more dense and less dense tissues may be characteristic of liposarcoma
- CT scan is very helpful not only in defining the extent of the lesion but also in showing relative densities.

Histopathology

- The pathologic diagnosis of liposarcoma may be difficult, especially when the lesion is histologically of low-grade
- Microscopically, liposarcomas are recognized because of their component of malignant lipoblasts
- The diagnostic procedure of choice for liposarcoma is open biopsy. (With superficial, small, fatty tumors, excisional biopsy is recommended for diagnosis. In large; >3 cm and deep tumors, diagnosis and treatment may involve open incisional biopsy followed by definitive resection)
- Fine-needle aspiration or biopsy should be followed by histologic and immunohistochemical examination. (Immunohistochemical examination aids in excluding other sarcomas).

Treatment

- For liposarcomas, radiation therapy may be a valuable adjunct to surgery, especially in those of the myxoid variant
- Although surgical resection is the mainstay of curative treatment, patients with large high-grade liposarcomas may benefit from multimodality treatment with chemotherapy and radiation
- This is difficult to do with tumors in the region of the elbow and amputation may be necessary.

Malignant Fibrous Histiocytoma

- Malignant fibrous histiocytoma (MFH), described by O'Brien and Stout in 1964, is the most common soft-tissue sarcoma of late adult life
- It is now the most commonly encountered malignant soft tissue tumor of the extremities
- This tumor can arise in any age group.

Clinical Features

Painless enlarging soft tissue mass.

Imaging

- Radiographs may reveal a nonspecific soft-tissue mass, often greater than 5 cm in diameter
- It can be detected by MRI, but a biopsy is required for definitive diagnosis
- Central necrosis is often evident, especially on larger masses.

Histopathology

- Grossly, this tumor is usually soft and pink or yellow
- Microscopically, the tumor contains both fibroblast like and histiocyte like cells in varying proportions, with spindled and rounded cells exhibiting a storiform arrangement.
- Several histological subtypes have been described:
  - Storiform/pleomorphic MFH (current WHO classification: undifferentiated high-grade pleomorphic sarcoma)
  - Myxoid MFH (current WHO classification: myxofibrosarcoma)

- Giant cell MFH (current WHO classification: undifferentiated pleomorphic sarcoma with giant cells)
- Inflammatory MFH (current WHO classification: undifferertiated pleomorphic sarcoma with prominent inflammation)
- Angiomatoid fibrous histiocytoma (formerly known as angiomatoid MFH) is now classified by the WHO as a tumor of uncertain differentiation.

Treatment

- Relatively small tumors may be excised with a margin of normal tissues on all aspects
- Larger lesions or those that are histologically higher grade require a more aggressive approach—a course of preoperative radiation therapy using approximately 5000 rad, followed after several weeks by excision of the lesion with a margin of normal tissue on all aspects
- Chemotherapy remains controversial in MFH
- The usual site of metastatic disease is the lungs, and metastases should be resected if possible.

Epithelioid Sarcoma

- Epithelioid sarcoma is a rare, slowly growing malignant tumor that usually begins in the superficial tissues of the hand or forearm and may occur at the elbow (Figs 22.209A and B)
- This rare malignant tumor occurs in adolescents and young adults
- The tumor spreads along fascial and neurovascular structures with formation of satellite nodules
- Multiple recurrences are known to occur in this tumor
- Lymphatic or hematogenous metastasis to the scalp, lymph nodes and lungs occur frequently.

Histopathology

- The tumor is made up of small, poorly defined tumor nodules composed of epithelioid cells or histiocytic aggregates
- Sometimes, central necrosis in these aggregates of cells suggests that the disease is a granulomatous infection
- Rarely, the tumor erodes into underlying bones.

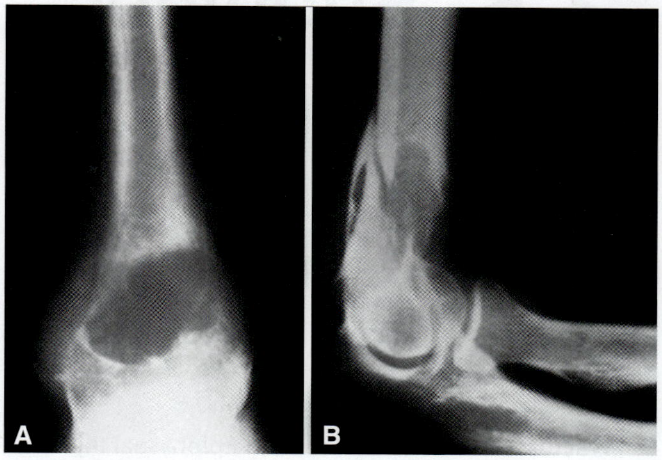

Figs 22.209A and B: Epithelioid sarcoma that has eroded into and destroyed much of the distal part of the humerus in a 27-year-old woman

Treatment

- Marginal or intralesional excision almost always results in tumor recurrence and subsequent disease progression
- Treatment for cure requires wide excision
- Regional lymph node dissection should be included as lymph node metastasis is common in epithelioid sarcoma
- Surgical excision is combined with radiotherapy.

■ Hematopoietic Involvement

- Although certainly not characteristic, the elbow may be involved from hematopoietic neoplastic processes
- The key feature is having a level of suspicion
- A history of pain, often at night, without an easily identified or explained cause is almost always present for infection or neoplasm
- Diagnosis may be made by open biopsy or arthroscopy
- Treatment is as for the underlying pathology.

23 Shoulder

- Normal Anatomy and Biomechanics of Shoulder Joint
- Examination of Shoulder
- Congenital Anomalies of Shoulder
- Fractures Around Shoulder and Epiphyseal Injuries
- Shoulder Dislocation
- Rotator Cuff Tears
- Shoulder Arthrodesis
- Shoulder Arthroplasty
- Inflammations Around Shoulder
- Tumors Around the Shoulder
- Brachial Plexus Injury and its Management
- Thoracic Outlet Syndrome

NORMAL ANATOMY AND BIOMECHANICS OF SHOULDER JOINT

Introduction

Knowledge of normal anatomy and biomechanics of the shoulder joint provides a foundation for evaluation and treatment of shoulder disorders.

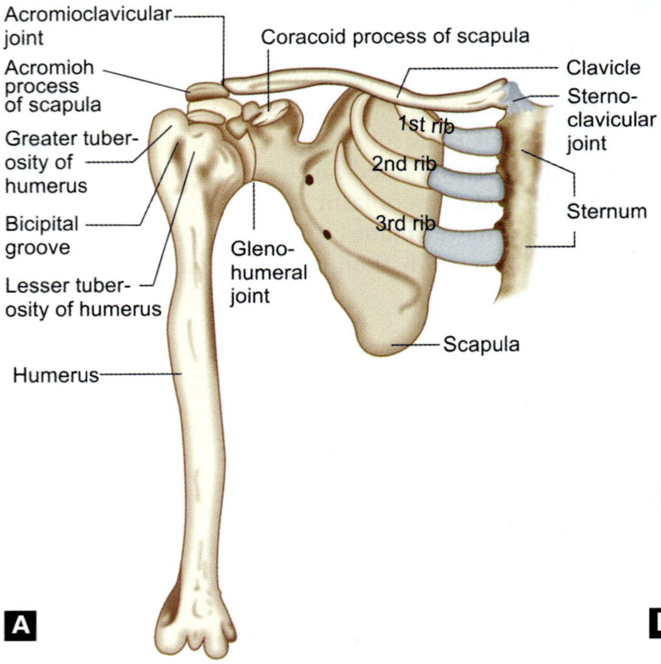

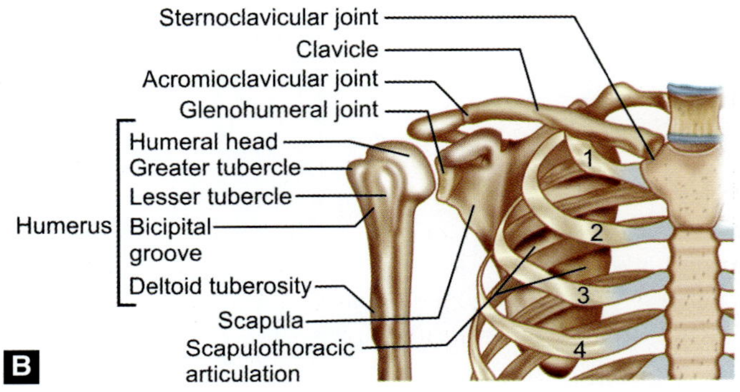

Figs 23.1A and B: Anatomy of shoulder girdle

Shoulder Girdle

Shoulder girdle is described in Figures 23.1A and B.

- Glenohumeral joint
- Acromioclavicular joint
- Sternoclavicular joint
- Scapulothoracic joint
- Subacromial space

Scapulohumeral Muscles

Muscles of anterior and posterior shoulder girdle are shown in Figures 23.2A and B, respectively.

Intrinsic Muscles

- Rotator cuff muscles
- Deltoid
- Pectoralis major
- Teres major

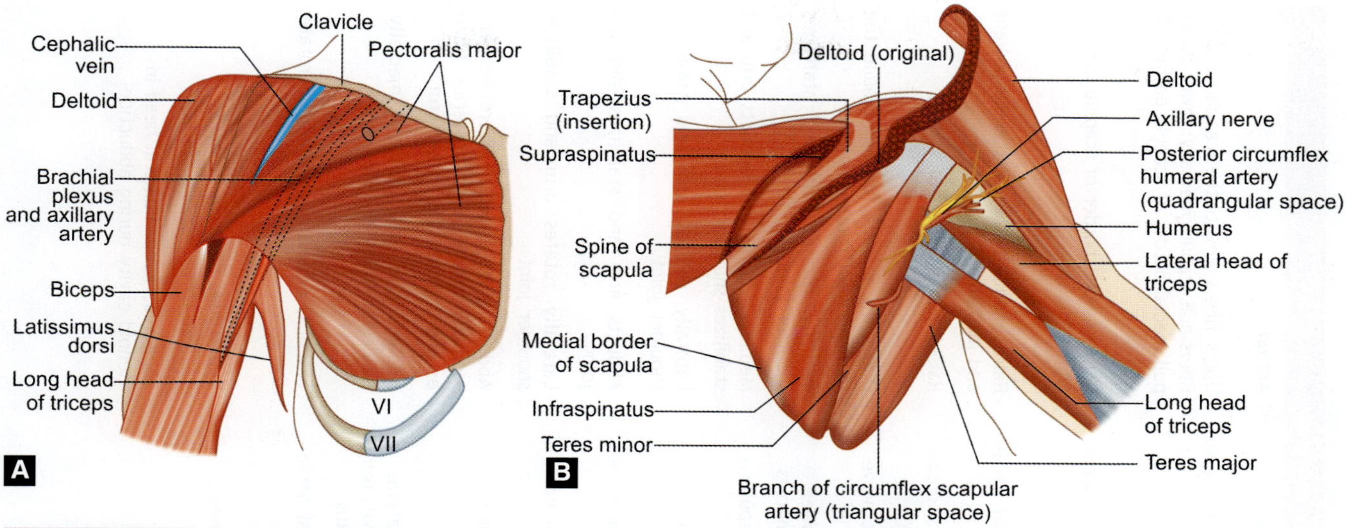

Figs 23.2A and B: (A) Anterior musculature of shoulder girdle; (B) Musculature of posterior shoulder girdle

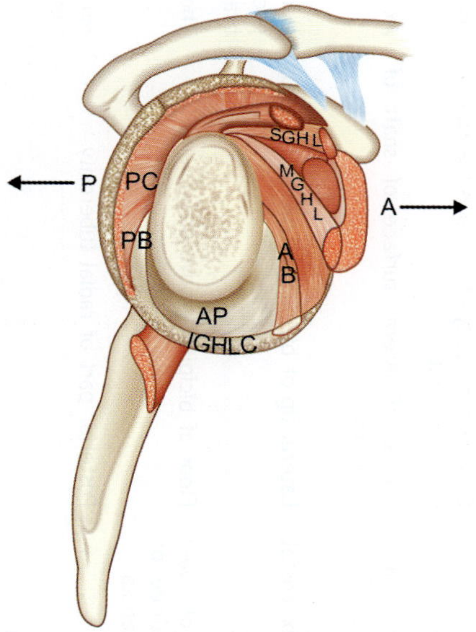

Fig. 23.3: Capsuloligamentous structures—MGHL. Middle glenohumeral ligaments; IGHLC. Inferior glenohumeral ligament complex; AB. Anterior band; PB. Posterior band; AP. Axillary pouch; SGHL. Superior glenohumeral ligament; PC. Posterior capsule

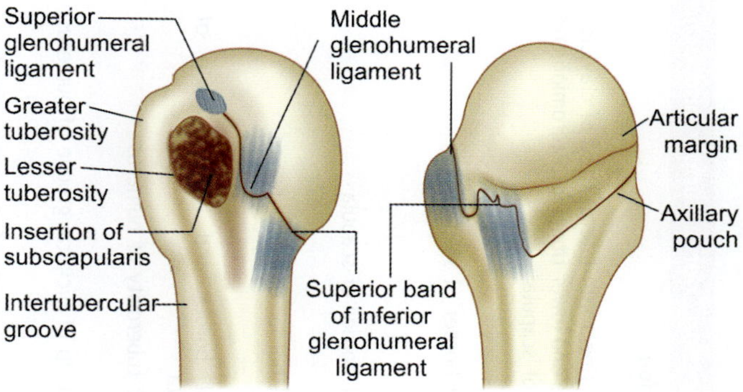

Fig. 23.4: Ligaments of shoulder joint—showing various attachments of glenohumeral ligaments

- Latissimus dorsi
- Biceps brachii

Extrinsic Muscles

Origin, insertion, nerve supply and action of extrinsic muscles are illustrated in Table 23.1. Important extrinsic muscles of the shoulder girdle are:

- Rhomboids major and minor
- Levator scapulae
- Trapezius
- Serratus anterior

Capsuloligamentous Structures (Figs 23.3 to 23.6)

Glenohumeral Ligaments

- Superior glenohumeral ligament (SGHL)
- Middle glenohumeral ligament (MGHL)
- Inferior glenohumeral ligament complex (IGHLC)
  - Anterior band
  - Posterior band
  - Axillary pouch

Coracohumeral Ligaments

Coracohumeral ligaments are shown in Figures 23.5 and 23.6.

- Anterior band
- Posterior band

Table 23.1: Origin, insertion, nerve supply and action of extrinsic muscles

Muscle	*Origin*	*Insertion*	*Nerve supply*	*Action*
Trapezius	Medial 1/3rd of superior nuchal line of occipital bone Spinous process and supraspinous ligaments of T1-T12	Upper fibers into lateral third of clavicle; middle and lower fibers into acromion and spine of scapula	Spinal accessory nerve	Upper fibers elevate the scapula; middle fibers pull scapula medially; lower fibers pull medial border of scapula downward
Rhomboid minor	Ligamentum nuchae and spines of seventh cervical and first thoracic vertebrae	Medial border of scapula	Dorsal scapular nerve	Raises medial border of scapula upward and medially
Rhomboid major	Second to fifth thoracic spines	Medial border of scapula	Dorsal scapular nerve	Raises medial border of scapula upward and medially
Levator scapulae	Transverse processes of first four cervical vertebrae	Medial border of scapula	C3 and C4 and dorsal scapular nerve	Raises medial border of scapula
Serratus anterior	Upper eight ribs	Medial border and inferior angle of scapula	Long thoracic nerve	Draws the scapula forward around the thoracic wall; rotates scapula
Subscapularis	Subscapular fossa	Lesser tuberosity of humerus	Upper and lower subscapular nerves	Medially rotates arm and stabilizes shoulder joint
Teres major	Lower third of lateral border of scapula	Medial lip of bicipital groove of humerus	Lower subscapular nerve	Medially rotates and adducts arm and stabilizes shoulder joint
Teres minor	Upper two-thirds of lateral border of scapula	Greater tuberosity of humerus; capsule of shoulder joint	Axillary nerve	Laterally rotates arm and stabilizes shoulder joint
Supraspinatus	Supraspinous fossa of scapula	Greater tuberosity of humerus; capsule of shoulder joint	Suprascapular nerve	Abducts arm and stabilizes shoulder joint
Infraspinatus	Infraspinous fossa of scapula	Greater tuberosity of humerus; capsule of shoulder joint	Suprascapular nerve	Laterally rotates arm and stabilizes shoulder joint
Deltoid	Lateral third of clavicle, acromion, spine of scapula	Middle of lateral surface of shaft of humerus	Axillary nerve	Abducts arm; anterior fibers flex and medially rotate arm; posterior fibers extend and laterally rotate arm
Pectoralis major	Clavicle, sternum and upper six costal cartilages	Lateral lip of bicipital groove of humerus	Medial and lateral pectoral nerves from brachial plexus	Adducts arm and rotates it medially; clavicular fibers also flex arm
Latissimus dorsi	Iliac crest, lumbar fascia, spines of lower six thoracic vertebrae, lower three or four ribs and inferior angle of scapula	Floor of bicipital groove of humerus	Thoracodorsal nerve	Extends, adducts and medially rotates the arm
Biceps brachii short head	Tip of coracoid process	Posterior part of radial tuberosity	Musculocutaneous nerve	Supination, flexor of elbow
Long head	Supraglenoid tubercle of scapula			Long head keeps humeral head in glenoid cavity during abduction

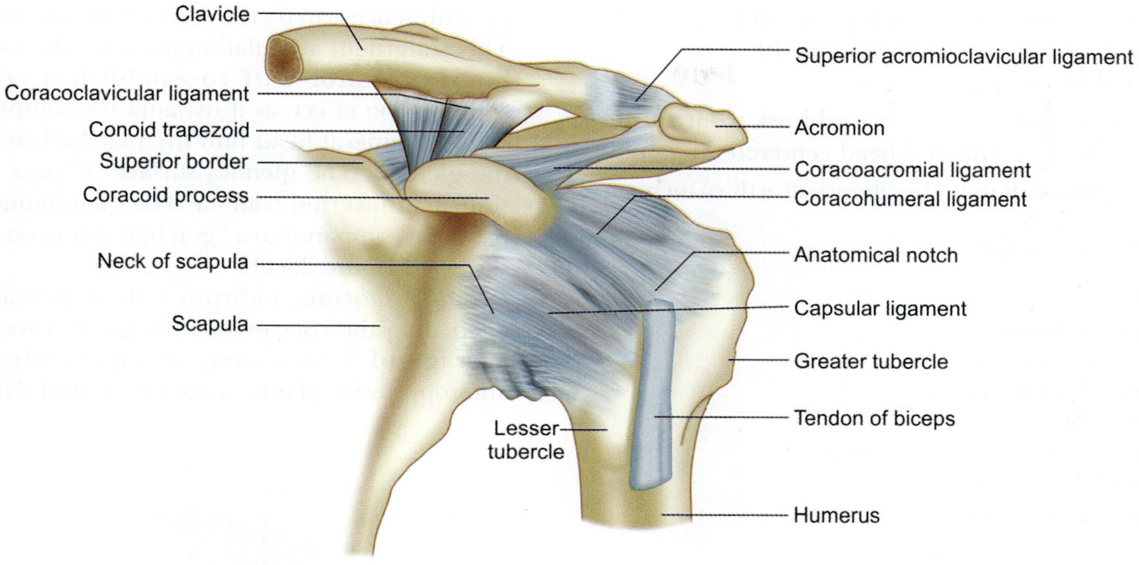

Fig. 23.5: Ligaments of shoulder joint showing attachments of coracohumeral ligaments

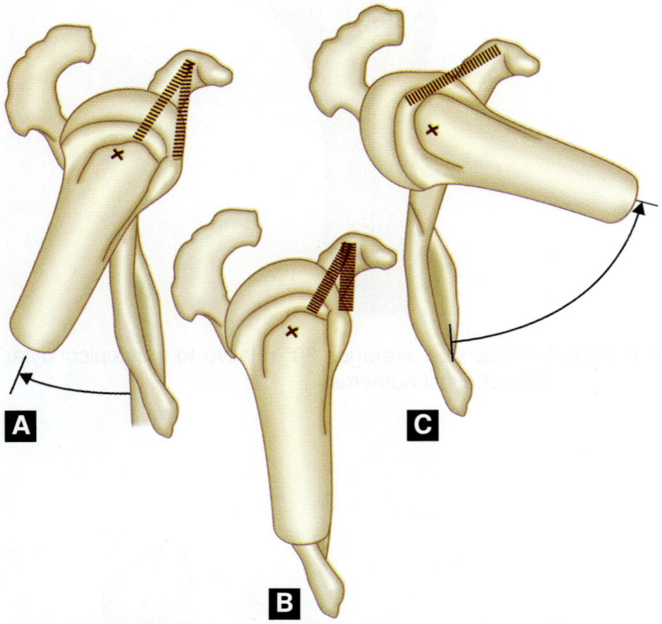

Figs 23.6A to C: Actions of various bands of coracohumeral ligaments

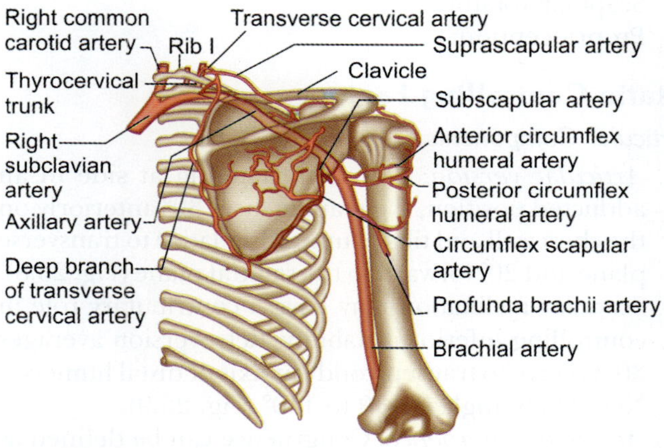

Fig. 23.7: Blood supply of the shoulder joint

■ Blood Supply (Fig. 23.7)

Biomechanics of Shoulder Joint

Glenohumeral Motion

Saha, described movements at shoulder joint in three phases:

Phase I

First 60° of flexion or 30° of elevation of humerus involves 15° of movement of clavicle at sternoclavicular joint.

Phase II

Consists of subsequent movement of 90° flexion or abduction. Scapula and clavicle elevate 5° for every 10° of glenohumeral movement.

Phase III

Completes movement of humerus to elevated position, elevation of scapula is now twice that of glenohumeral joint, without further elevation of clavicle. Clavicle rotates along its long axis to permit elevation of scapula.

Normal Movements at Shoulder Joint

- Abduction: 0 to 170°
- Adduction: 0 to 50°
- Flexion: 0 to 165°
- Extension: 0 to 60°

- External rotation at 90° abduction: 100°
- Internal rotation at 90° abduction: 70°
- Circumduction.

Normal arthrokinematics: Combines rotation and translation, to keep humeral head centered on glenoid.

Capsular tightness: Resulted in abnormal arthrokinematics.

Controlling Factors

Static Factors

- Articular component
  - Articular version
  - Articular congruence
  - Glenoid labrum
- Negative intra-articular pressure
- Adhesion-cohesion
- Capsules and ligaments
- Rotator cuff

Dynamic Factors

- Rotator cuff
- *Biceps brachii*
- Scapular rotators
- Proprioception

Static Controlling Factors

Articular Components

- *Articular version:* With arm hanging at side in an adducted position, the scapula faces 30° anteriorly on the chest wall and tilts 3° upwards relative to transverse plane and 20° forward to the sagittal plane (Fig. 23.8). Scapular inclination may have a contributary role in controlling inferior instability. Retroversion averages 30° relative to transepicondylar axis of distal humerus. Neck shaft angle is 130 to 140° (Fig. 23.9).
- *Articular congruence*: Congruence can be defined as the difference in the radii of humeral head and glenoid articulating surfaces, glenohumeral articulating surfaces are shown in Figure 23.10. Closer the difference is to 0°, the more congruent is the joint. This congruent articulation provides the foundation for the rotator cuff to establish a concavity-compression effect, as it dynamically compresses the convex humeral head into the matched concavity of the glenoid. The glenoid surface is "pear shaped", similar to inverted comma. The glenohumeral joint has been compared to a "golf ball sitting on a tee", as shown in Figure 23.11.
- *Glenoid labrum:* Labrum enhances stability by deepening the concavity of the glenoid socket to an average of 9 to 5 mm, in superoinferior and anteroposterior planes, as demonstrated (Fig. 23.12).

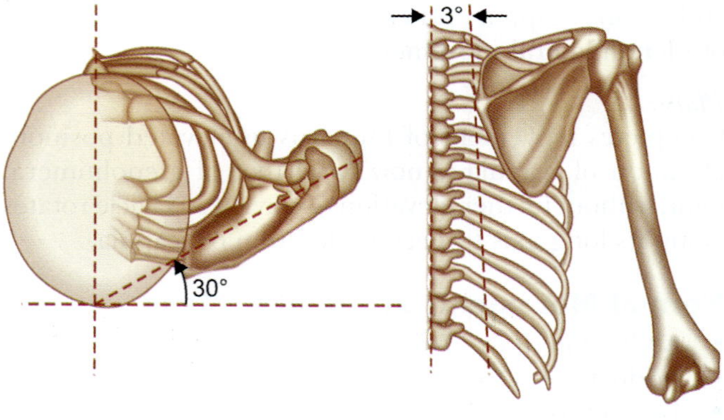

Fig. 23.8: Humeral articular version

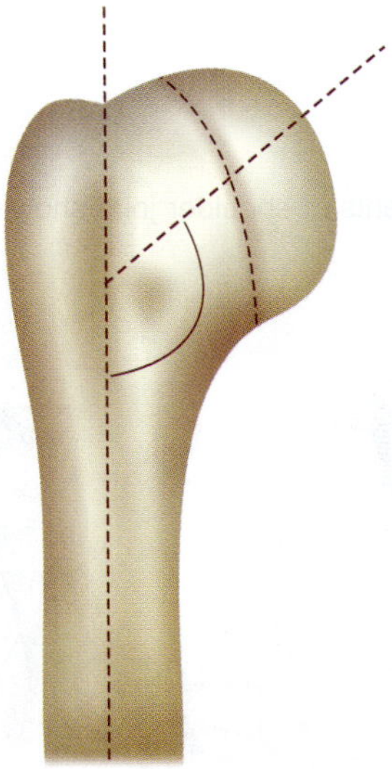

Fig. 23.9: Retroversion averages 30° relative to transepicondylar axis of distal humerus

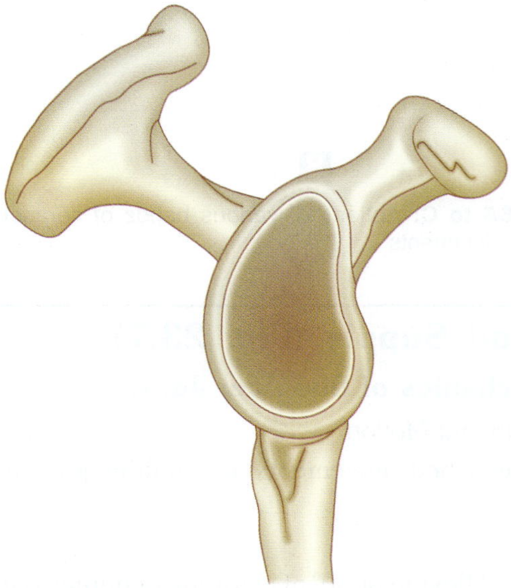

Fig. 23.10: Articular surface of glenohumeral joint

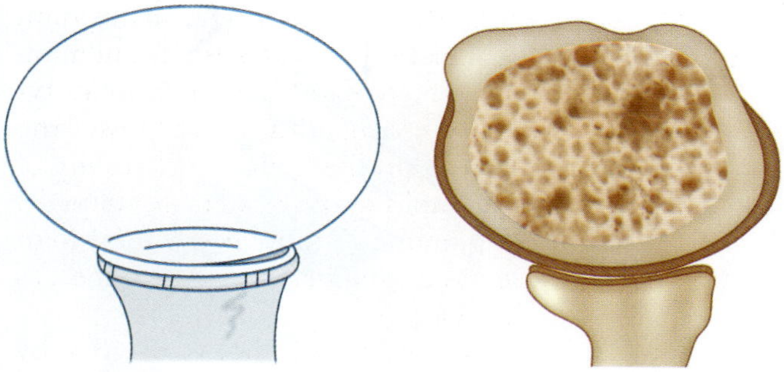

Fig. 23.11: Glenohumeral joint, compared to a golf ball sitting on a tee

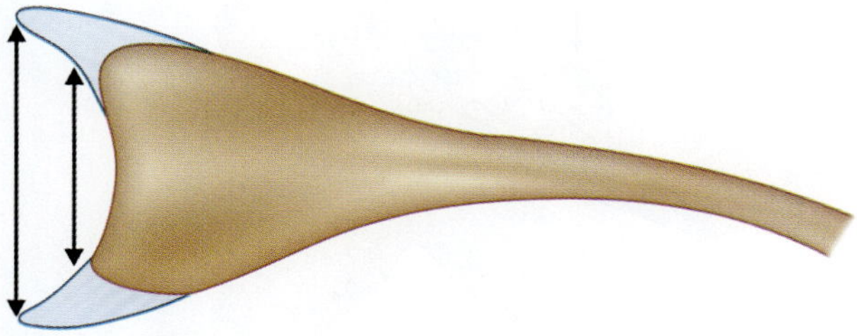

Fig. 23.12: Deepening of concavity of glenoid socket by glenoid labrum

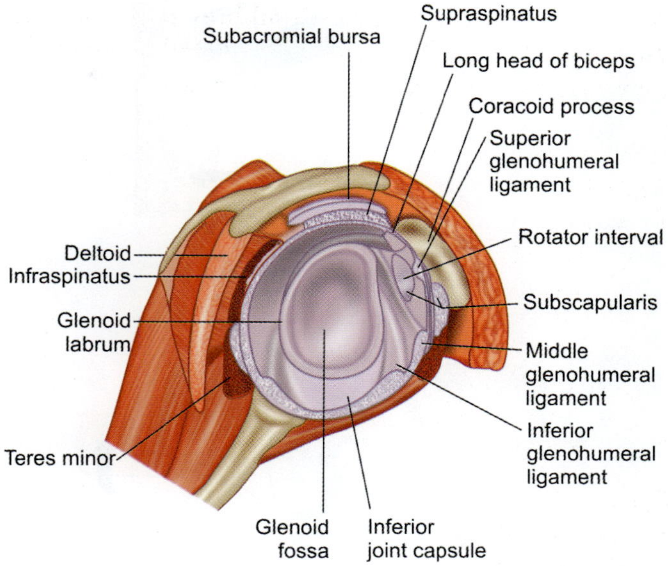

Fig. 23.13: Capsuloligamentous structure of glenohumeral joint

Loss of labrum decreases the depth of socket by 50 percent in either direction. Functionally it acts as "chok-block", preventing the head from slipping over the edge of the glenoid. Labrum acts to increase the surface area of contact, acting as a load-bearing structure.

- *Negative intra-articular pressure:* In normal shoulder, relative vacuum exists as a result of high osmotic pressure in the interstitial tissue, causing water to be drawn out of the glenohumeral joint. As articular surfaces are pulled apart, a suction effect develops to resist further displacement. It becomes important when the rotator cuff is not contracting or when tension has not developed in the superior and coracohumeral ligaments.
- *Adhesion-cohesion:* Glenohumeral joint contains 1 ml of synovial fluid that provides articular nourishment through diffusion and lubrication through several mechanisms. Viscous and intramolecular forces help to create this adhesion-cohesion effect. Negative intra-articular pressure and adhesive forces resulting from presence of synovial fluid between the articular surfaces, contribute static restraints when capsule is lax and muscles are inactive.
- *Capsuloligamentous structure:* Various capsuloligamentous structures are shown in Figure 23.13. Restraints to various movements, by these capsuloligamentous structures are described below:
  – Restraints to external rotation (Fig. 23.14): Dependent on arm position, this is illustrated in Table 23.2:
  – Restraints to internal rotation (Fig. 23.15): Dependent on arm position
  This is illustrated in Table 23.3:
  – Restraints to inferior translation (Fig. 23.16): Dependent on arm position, this is illustrated in Table 23.4.
- *Rotator cuff function:*
  – Approximates humerus, to function
  – Supraspinatus assists deltoid in abduction
  – Subscapularis, infraspinatus and teres minor depresses humeral head
  – Subscapularis:
    a. Effective restraint to external rotation, with arm at side (Fig. 23.17A).

Table 23.2: Structures causing restrainting to external rotation at different arm position

Arm position/angle	*Restrained structures*
At 0°	SGHL, CH and subscapularis
45°	SGHL and MGHL
90°	Anterior band IGHLC

Key: CH. Coracohumeral; IGHLC. Inferior glenohumeral ligament complex; MGHL. Middle glenohumeral ligament; SGHL. Superior glenohumeral ligament

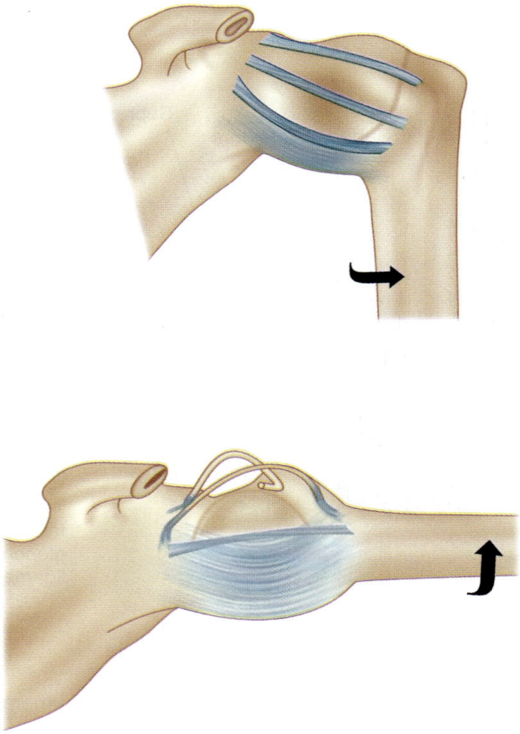

Fig. 23.14: Restraints to external rotation

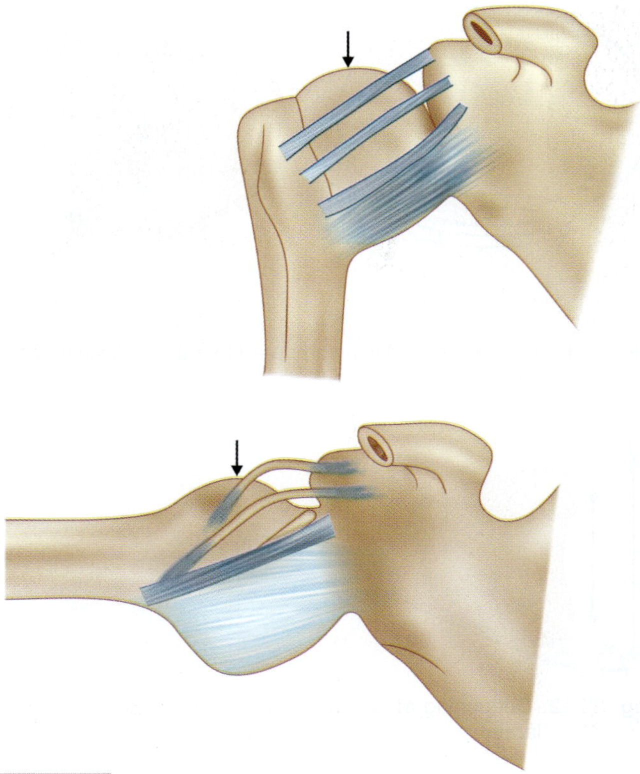

Fig. 23.16: Restraints to inferior translation

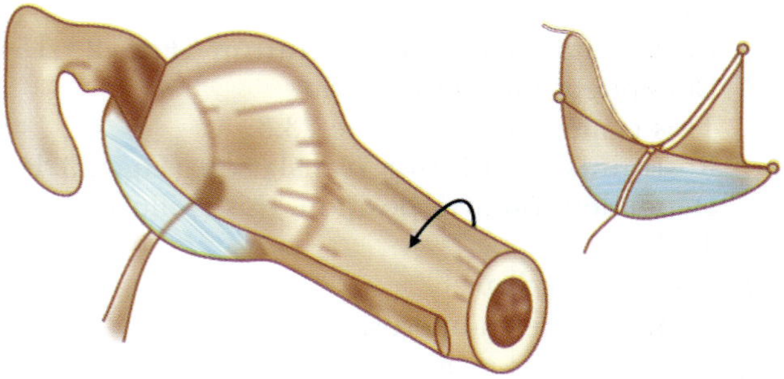

Fig. 23.15: Restraints to internal rotation

b. Ineffective restraint to external rotation, with arm abducted to 90° (Fig. 23.17B).
   - Infraspinatus/Teres minor: Reduces strain on anterior band of IGHLC. Hamstrings of glenohumeral joint.

Dynamic Stability Factors

Long Head of Biceps Brachii (Fig. 23.18)

- Biceps tendon force increases torsional rigidity to external rotation
- No effect on strain of IGHLC
- Effect lost with SLAP (Superior labral tear from anterior to posterior) lesion

Table 23.3: Structures causing restrainting to internal rotation at different arm position

Arm position/angle	*Restrained structures*
At 0°	Posterior band IGHLC
45°	Anterior and posterior band IGHLC
90°	Anterior and posterior band IGHLC

Table 23.4: Structures causing restrainting to inferior translation at different arm position

Arm position/angle	*Restrained structures*
At 0°	SGHL and CH
90°	IGHLC

- Biceps becomes more important anterior stabilizer as capsuloligamentous stability decreases
- Biceps tended to stabilize the shoulder (Fig. 23.19) joint anteriorly, when the arm was internally rotated and served as a posterior stabilizer when humerus is externally rotated.

Force Couples

Force couples acting on glenohumeral joint are:

- *Transverse plane:* Subscapularis versus infraspinatous (Fig. 23.20A)

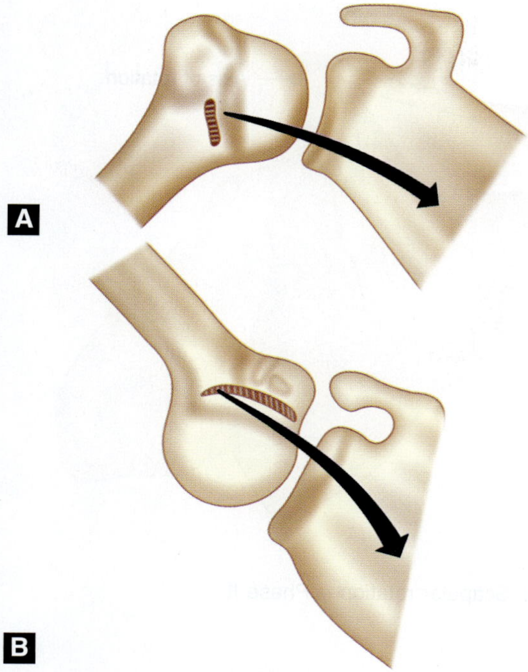

Figs 23.17A and B: Subscapularis action—(A) Effective restraint to external rotation, with arm at side; (B) Ineffective restraint to external rotation, with arm abducted to 90°

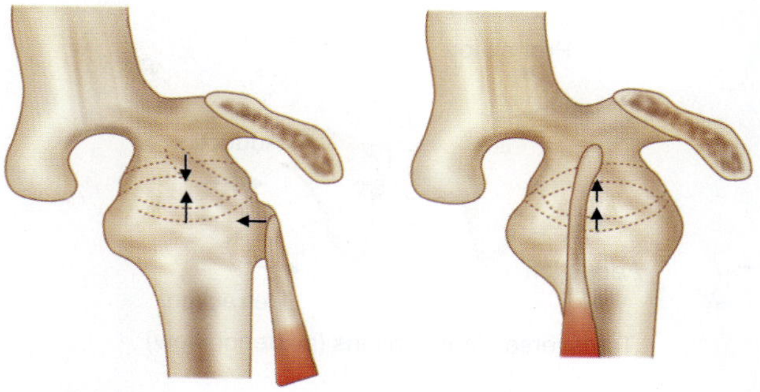

Fig. 23.19: Action of biceps as dynamic stabilizer of shoulder joint

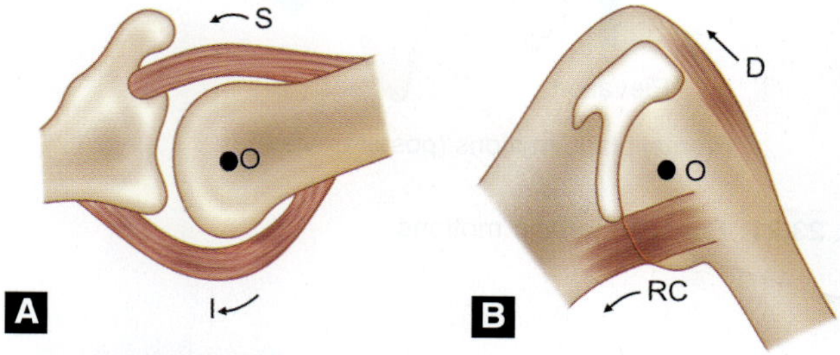

Figs 23.20A and B: Force couples acting on glenohumeral joint—(A) Subscapularis versus infraspinatous; (B) Deltoid versus inferior RC muscles

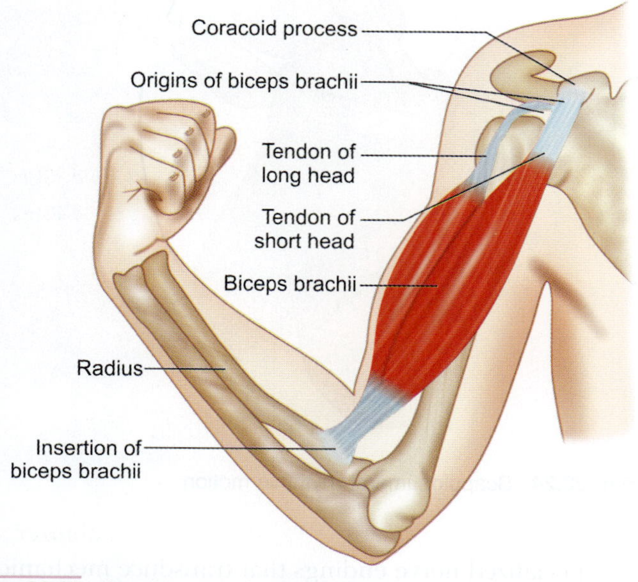

Fig. 23.18: Attachments of the long head of biceps brachii

- *Coronal plane:* Deltoid versus inferior rotator cuff (RC) muscles (Fig. 23.20B).

Scapulothoracic Muscles

- Trapezius
- Serratus anterior
- Rhomboids
- Levator scapulae
- Pectoralis minor
- Subclavius
- Scapulothoracic motion (Fig. 23.21) are:
  - Elevation/depression
  - Protraction/retraction
  - Upward/downward rotation

Biomechanics of Scapular Rotation

- Scapulothoracic motion occurs as part of closed kinetic chain involving:
  - Acromioclavicular (AC) joint
  - Scapuloclavicular (SC) joint
- *Scapular rotation:* Different phases of scapular rotation are:

  Phase I: Upper and lower portions of trapezius and serratus anterior produce upward rotatory force on scapula. Motion at AC joint is prevented by coracoclavicular ligament. Rotation of scapula occurs as elevation of clavicle at SC joint (Fig. 23.22).

  Phase II: Further motion at SC joint prevented by costoclavicular ligament. Continued upward rotation of scapula pulls on costoclavicular ligament, causing posterior rotation of clavicle. Posterior rotation of clavicle allows further upward rotation of scapula (Fig. 23.23).

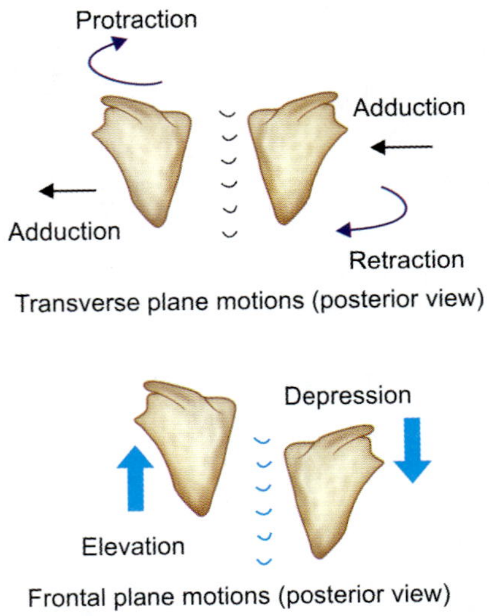

Fig. 23.21: Scapulothoracic motions

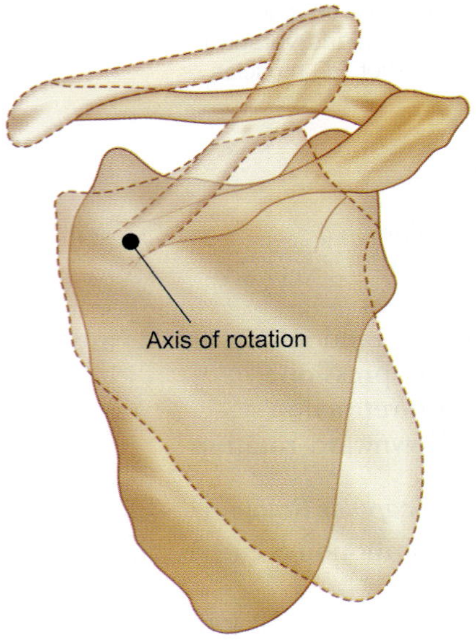

Fig. 23.22: Scapular rotation—Phase I

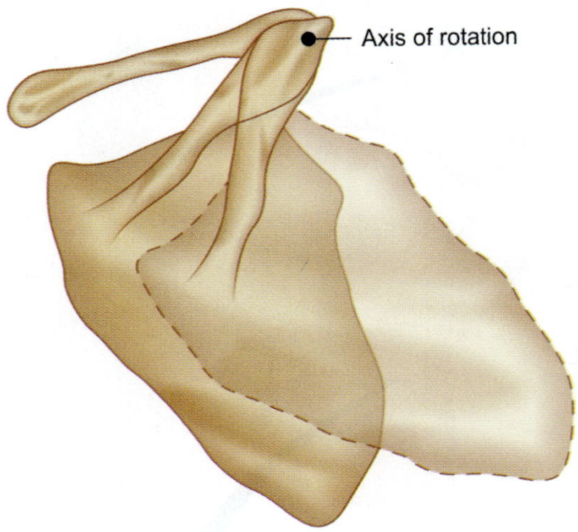

Fig. 23.23: Scapular rotation— Phase II

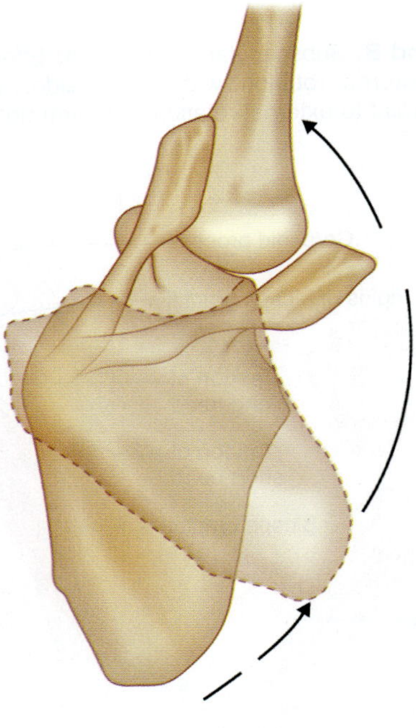

Fig. 23.24: Scapulohumeral rhythmic motion

- Scapular rotation is necessary to:
  - Enhance glenohumeral stability
  - Elevate acromion to avoid impingement
  - Maintain effective length tension relationship of scapulohumeral muscles.
- *Proprioception:* The perception of the joint position and joint motion is termed as proprioception. Proprioceptive interaction between ligaments and muscles mediate a protective mechanism against capsular failure and instability. Mechanoreceptors are specialized nerve endings that transduce mechanical deformation into electric signals that transmit information about joint position and motion.
- *Force couple at scapulothoracic joint*
  - Serratus anterior produces anterolateral movement of inferior angle.
  - Upper trapezius pulls scapula medially
- *Scapulohumeral rhythm:* Total elevation is 120° at GH joint and 60° at scapulothoracic (ST) joint (Fig. 23.24).

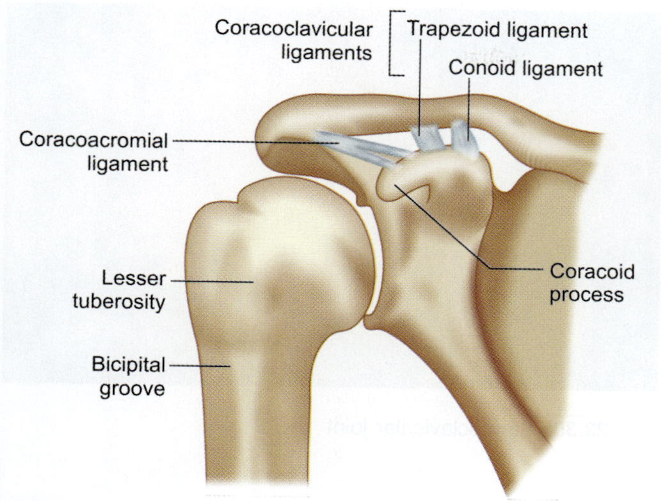

Fig. 23.25: Acromioclavicular joint and adjoining structures

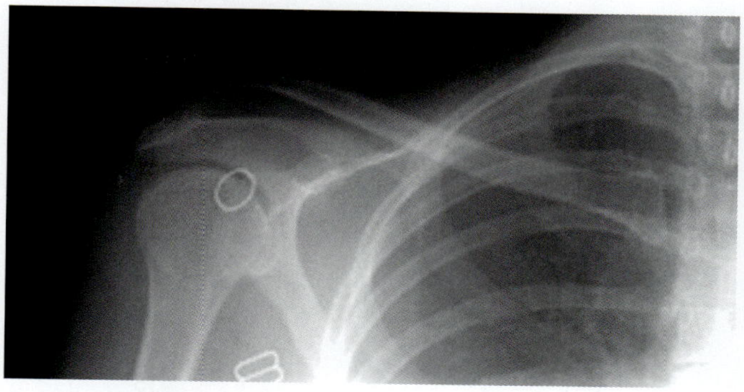

Fig. 23.26: X-ray showing acromioclavicular joint

Acromioclavicular Joint

It is shown in Figures 23.25 and 23.26 and consists of:

- Joint capsule
- AC ligaments
- Intra-articular disk
- Coracoclavicular ligaments:
  - Conoid (medial)
  - Trapezoid (lateral)
- Diarthrodial joint between medial facet of acromion and the lateral (distal) clavicle
- Contains intra-articular disk of variable size
- Thin capsule stabilized by ligaments on all sides:
  - AC ligaments control horizontal (anteroposterior) displacement
  - Superior AC ligament is most important
- Normal anatomy of AC joint, shown in Figure 23.27
- Normal inclination of AC-sternoclavicular joint, is shown in Figure 23.28.
- Stability provided by ligaments (Fig. 23.29):
  - Horizontal stability controlled by AC ligament
  - Vertical stability controlled by coracoclavicular ligament
- Movements
  - Axial rotation of clavicle (spin)
  - Angulation between scapula and clavicle.

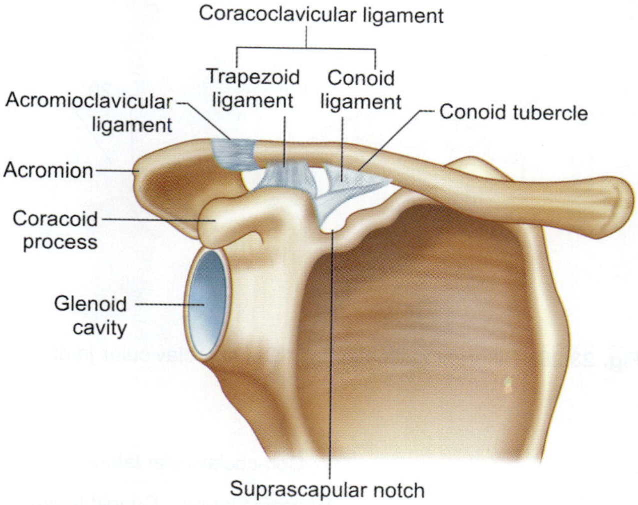

Fig. 23.27: Normal anatomy of AC joint

Sternoclavicular Joint

Sternoclavicular (SC) joint is shown in Figure 23.30. SC joint consist of following structures:

- Joint capsule
- Anterior and posterior SC ligaments
- Intra-articular disk
- Interclavicular ligament
- Costoclavicular ligament

Anatomy of Sternoclavicular Joint

- The anatomy of the sternoclavicular (SC) joint is shown in Figure 23.31.
- It is a diarthrodial joint
- It is a saddle shaped joint
- Poor congruence
- *Intra-articular disk ligament:* It divides SC joint into two separate joint spaces.
- *Costoclavicular ligament (rhomboid ligament):* Short and strong and consist of an anterior and posterior fasciculus.
- *Interclavicular ligament:* Connects the superomedial aspects of each clavicle with the capsular ligaments and the upper sternum.
- *Capsular ligament:* Covers the anterior and posterior aspects of the joint and represents thickenings of the

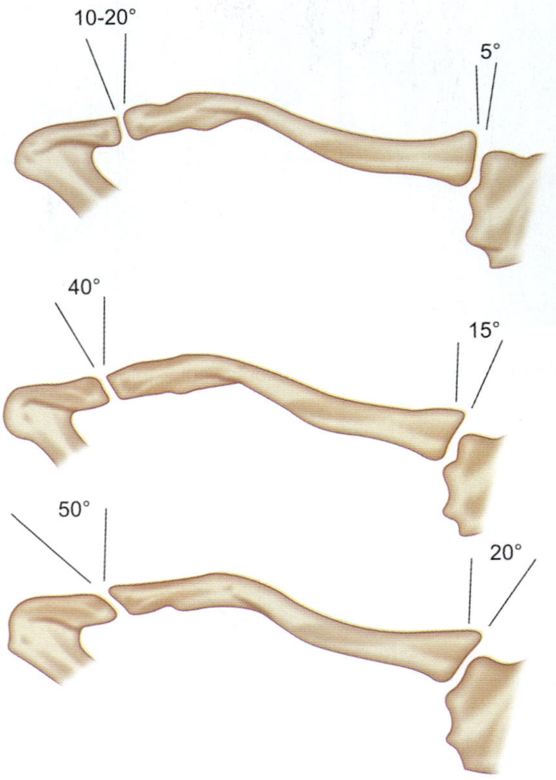

Fig. 23.28: Different inclination of AC-sternoclavicular joint

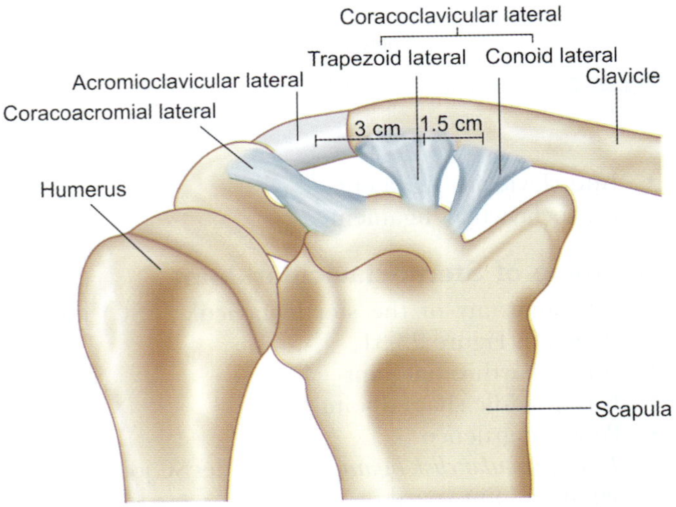

Fig. 23.29: Stability provided by ligaments

joint capsule. The anterior portion of the ligament is heavier and stronger than the posterior portion.

- *Movements (Figs 23.32A and B):* Different SC joint movements are:
  - Protraction/retraction

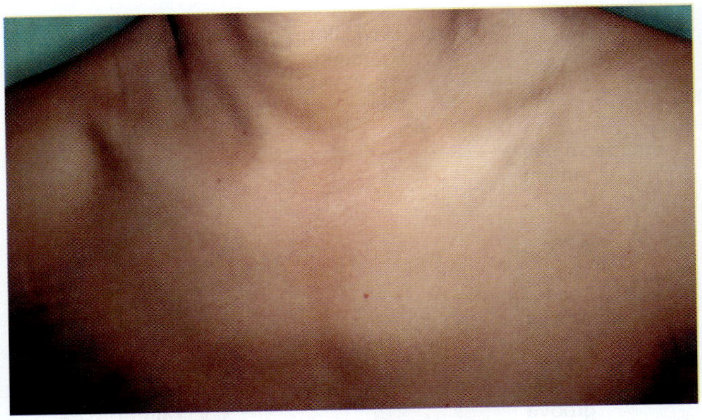

Fig. 23.30: Sternoclavicular joint

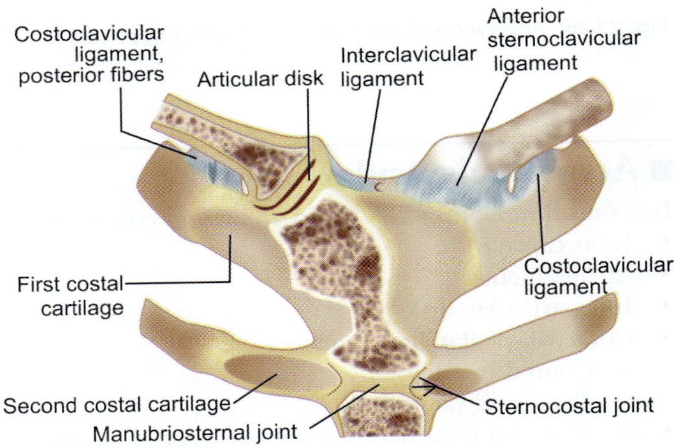

Fig. 23.31: Anatomy of sternoclavicular joint

  - Elevation/depression
  - Axial rotation (spin)

EXAMINATION OF SHOULDER

Inspection

From Front

A. Prominent sternoclavicular joint, e.g. subluxation.
B. Deformity of clavicle, e.g. old fracture.
C. Prominent acromioclavicular joint, e.g. subluxation or osteoarthritis.
D. Deltoid wasting, e.g. disuse/axillary nerve palsy. Methods of inspection of the shoulder joint from front is shown in Figure 23.33.

From Side (Fig. 23.34)

Any swelling of the joint suggesting infection or inflammatory reaction.

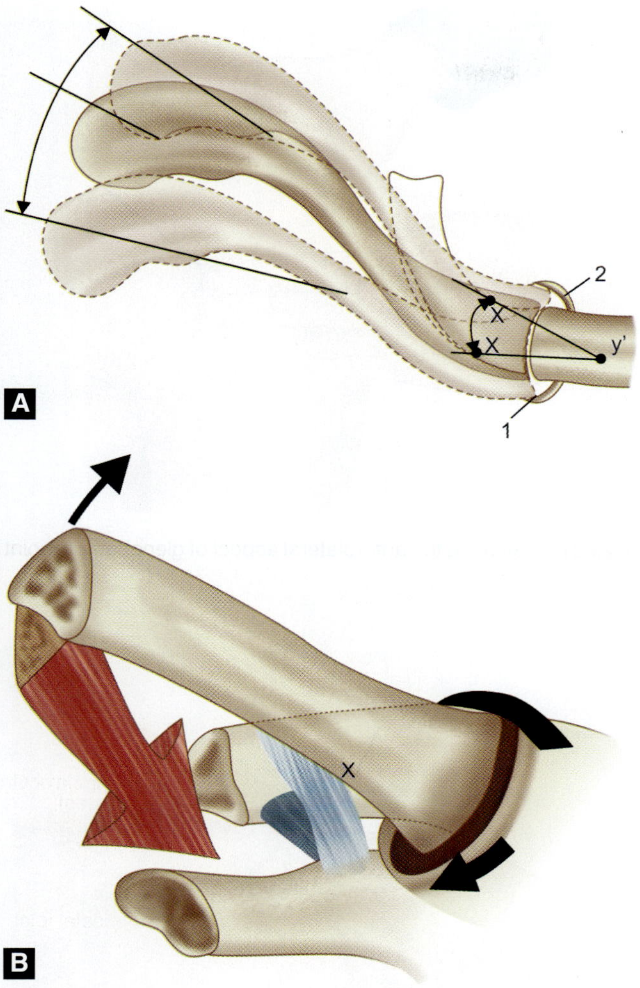

Figs 23.32A and B: Movements of sternoclavicular joint

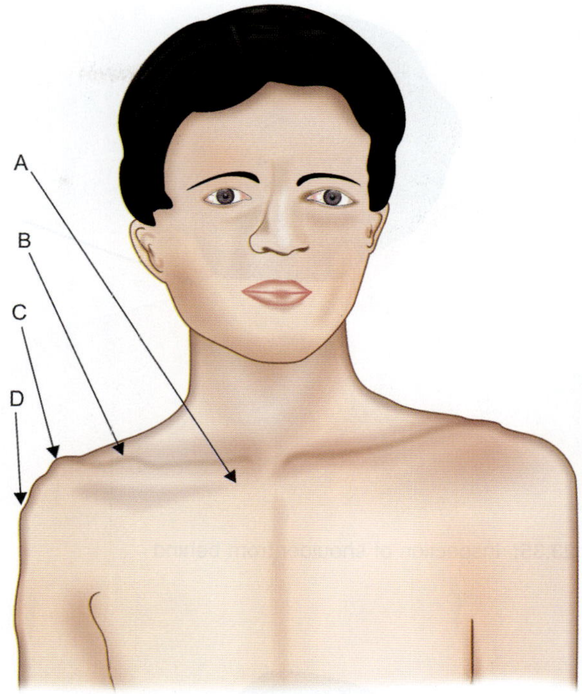

Fig. 23.33: Inspection of shoulder joint from front—A. Prominent sternoclavicular joint; B. Clavicular deformity; C. Prominent acromioclavicular joint; D. Deltoid wasting

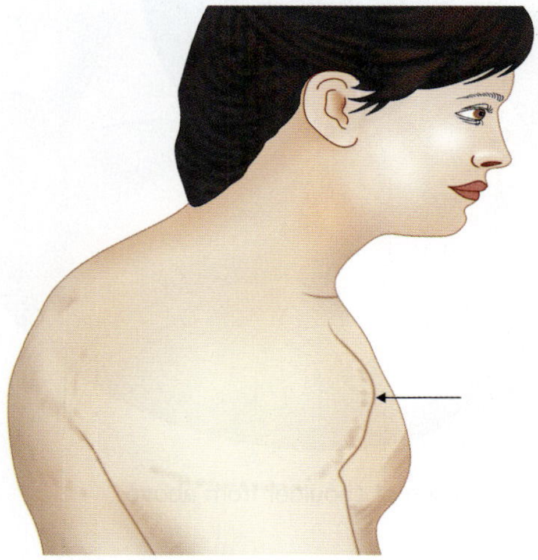

Fig. 23.34: Inspection of shoulder from side

From Behind (Fig. 23.35)

While inspection of the shoulder from behind, one needs to answer the following questions:

- Is the scapula normally shaped and situated?
- Is it small and positioned high?

From Above (Fig. 23.36)

While inspecting the shoulder from above one has to take note of the following:

- Swelling of the shoulder
- Deformity of the clavicle
- Asymmetry of supraclavicular fossa.

Palpation

- Palpate the anterior and lateral aspects of glenohumeral joint (Fig. 23.37). Diffuse tenderness suggestive of infection or calcifying supraspinatus tendinitis.
- Tenderness over the acromioclavicular joint is found after recent dislocation and osteoarthritis (OA) of the joint, as shown in Figure 23.38. Lipping is palpable and crepitus may be detected when arm is abducted.
- Press acromion and abduct the arm, as illustrated in Figure 23.39. Tenderness is present in cases of tear and inflammatory lesions involving rotator cuff.

Movements

- Abduct both the arms, observe the smoothness of movement and range achieved (Fig. 23.40).

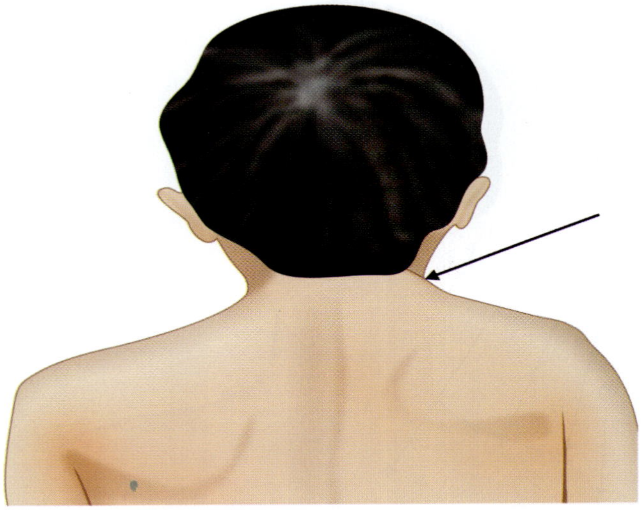
Fig. 23.35: Inspection of shoulder from behind

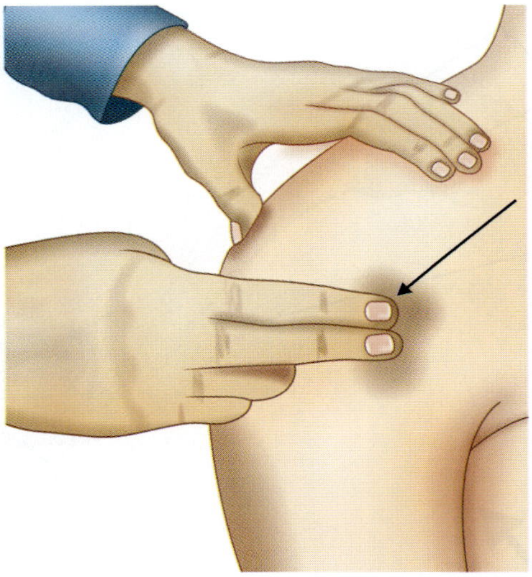
Fig. 23.37: Palpating the anterolateral aspect of glenohumeral joint

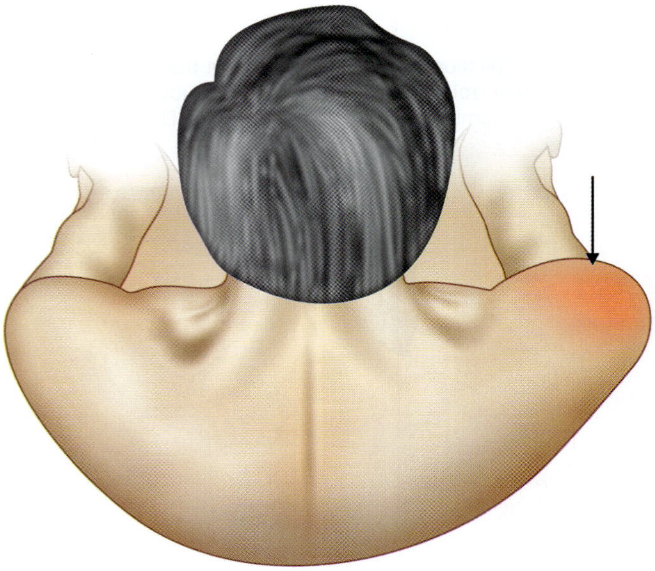
Fig. 23.36: Inspection of shoulder from above

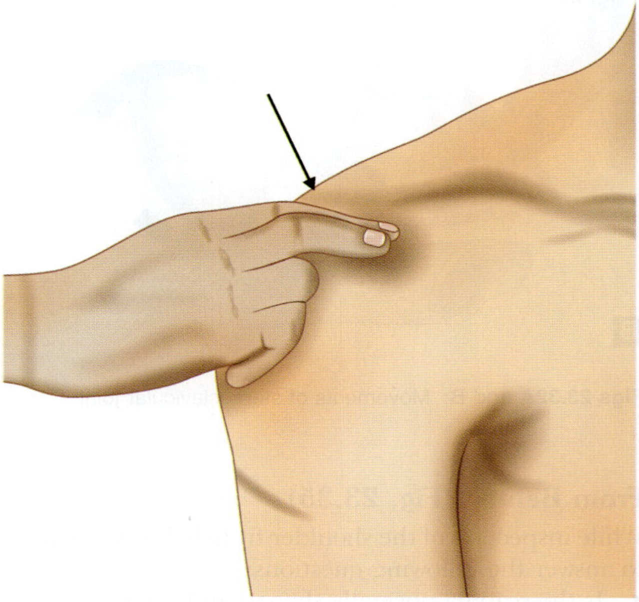
Fig. 23.38: Acromioclavicular joint palpation

- Difficulty in abducting the arm is suggestive of shoulder cuff tear (Fig. 23.41).

Pain During Abduction (Fig. 23.42)

A. Pain during arc of 70 to 120° suggests, shoulder cuff impingement in region of acromion.
B. Pain during later phase of abduction (above 120°) suggests shoulder cuff impingement in region of acromioclavicular joint or coracoacromial ligament.

Shoulder Evaluation

Active Range of Motion (ROM)

- Flexion of 180°
- Extension of 50°
- Abduction of 180°
- Adduction of 40°
- Internal rotation of 90°
- External rotation of 90°

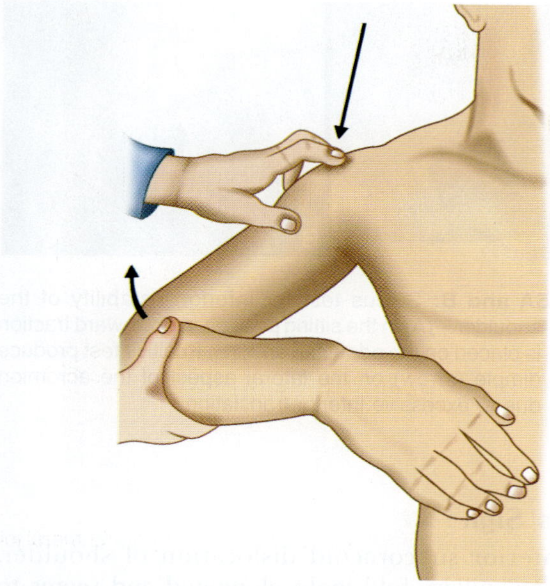

Fig. 23.39: Pressing acromion while simultaneously abducting the arm

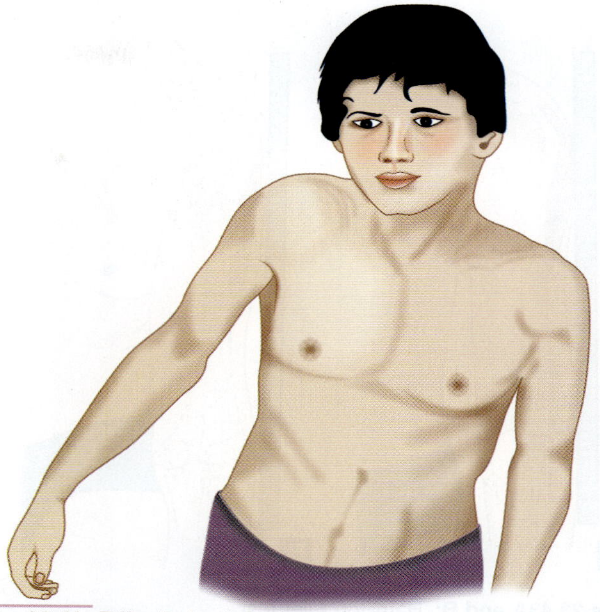

Fig. 23.41: Difficulty in abducting arm due to shoulder cuff tear

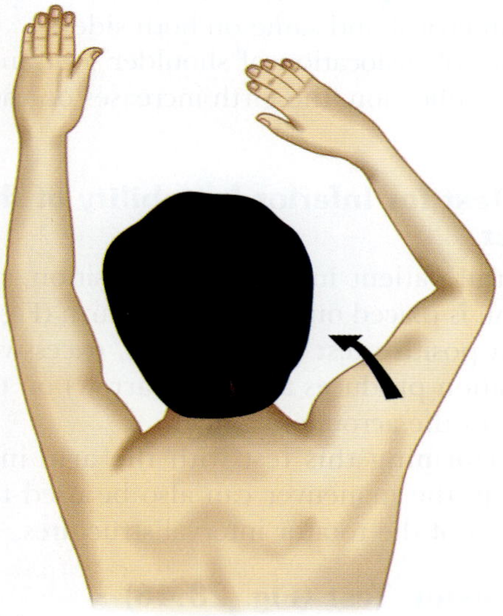

Fig. 23.40: Both arms abducted

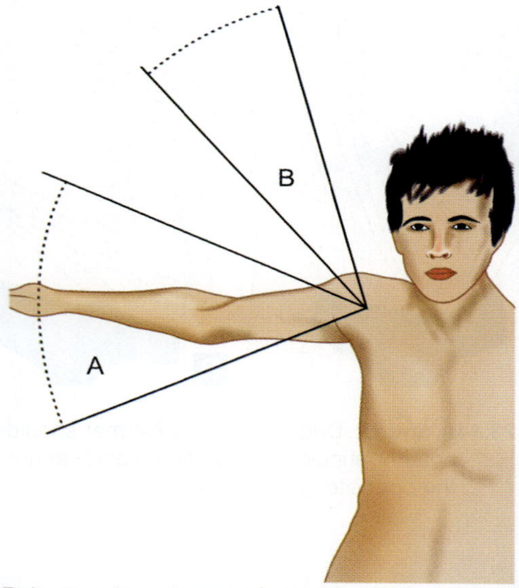

Fig. 23.42: Pain at various ranges of shoulder abduction suggests different joint involvement

Manual Muscle Testing

Five Points Grading System

- Grade 5 = Complete ROM against gravity, with full resistance
- Grade 4 = Complete ROM against gravity, with some resistance
- Grade 3 = Complete ROM against gravity, with no resistance
- Grade 2 = Complete ROM, with gravity omitted
- Grade 1 = Some muscle contractility with no joint motion
- Grade 0 = No muscle contractility.

■ Special Tests

Hamilton Ruler Test (Figs 23.43A and B)

- In normal shoulder ruler cannot touch acromial process and lateral epicondyle of humerus because of

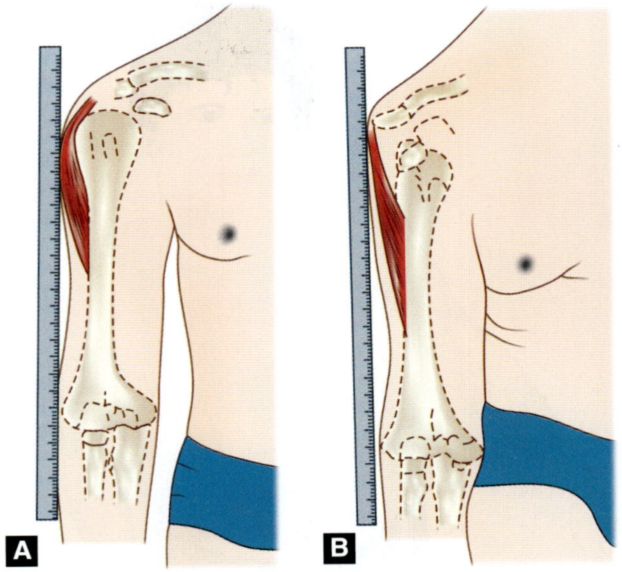

Figs 23.43A and B: Hamilton ruler test

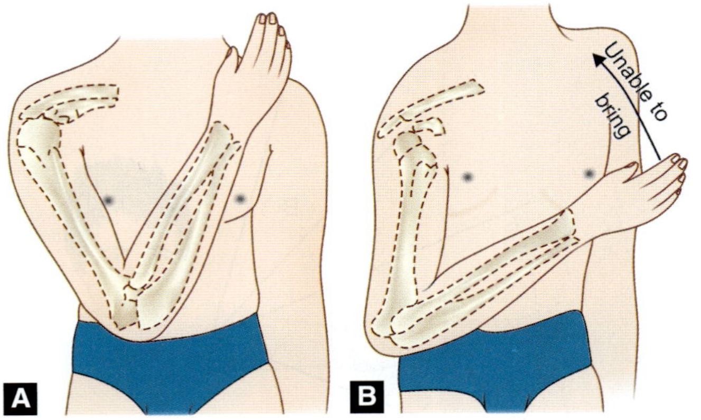

Figs 23.44A and B: Duga's test: (A) Normal shoulder; (B) With anterior shoulder dislocation, hand cannot be taken to the opposite shoulder

prominence of bulge of deltoid supported by head of humerus.

- Ruler touches both the points in dislocation of shoulder absence of head, polio paralysis and dissolution of humeral head in septic arthritis.

Duga's Test (Figs 23.44A and B)

- Normally after full flexion at shoulder, the elbow can be brought to near about midplane and hand to top of the opposite shoulder top.
- In dislocation of shoulder joint, full flexion of shoulder joint cannot be achieved, elbow cannot be brought to midbody plane and hand cannot be taken to opposite shoulder.

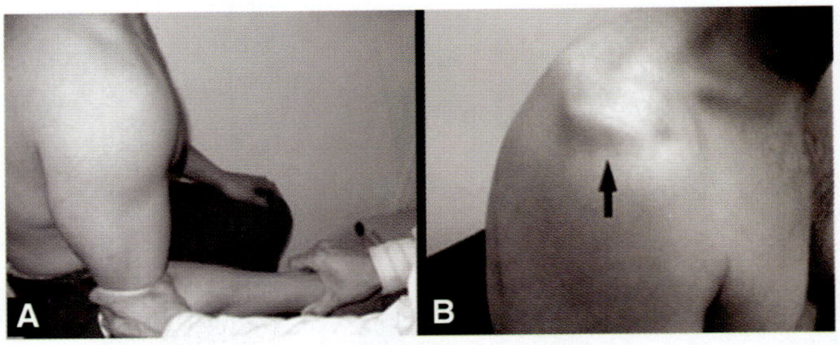

Figs 23.45A and B: Sulcus test for inferior instability of the shoulder—(A) In the sitting position, a downward traction is placed on the adducted arm; (B) Positive test produce dimple (arrow) on the lateral aspect of the acromion due to excessive inferior translation

Bryant's Sign

- In anterior subcoracoid dislocation of shoulder, anterior axillary fold looks elongated and seems to be at lower level.

Callaway's Test

- Normally the girth from axillary base to shoulder top is symmetrical and same on both sides.
- In cases of dislocation of shoulder jont and axillary abscess collection, the girth increases on the affected side.

Sulcus Test for Inferior Instability of the Shoulder

- With the patient in the sitting position, downward traction is placed on the adducted arm (Fig. 23.45A).
- With a positive test (Fig. 23.45B), excessive inferior translation produces a dimple (arrow) on the lateral aspect of the acromion.
- By performing this test with the arm in external rotation, the maneuver can also be used to test the integrity of the rotator interval structures.

Apprehension Test (Fig. 23.46)

- Stand behind the patient; abduct the shoulder to 90°.
- Externally rotate shoulder and push head of the humerus forward
- Apprehension, fear, refusal is evident of chronic anterior instability of shoulder
- Pain felt in minor subluxation.

Relocation Test (Fig. 23.47)

Apprehension test done in recumbent position:

- Abduct and externally rotate the shoulder.
- Press down on upper arm if pain is present, this stabilizes head of humerus in glenoid. When subluxation is imminent, this relieves the pain.
- Release of downward pressure with return of pain is confirmatory to anterior instability.

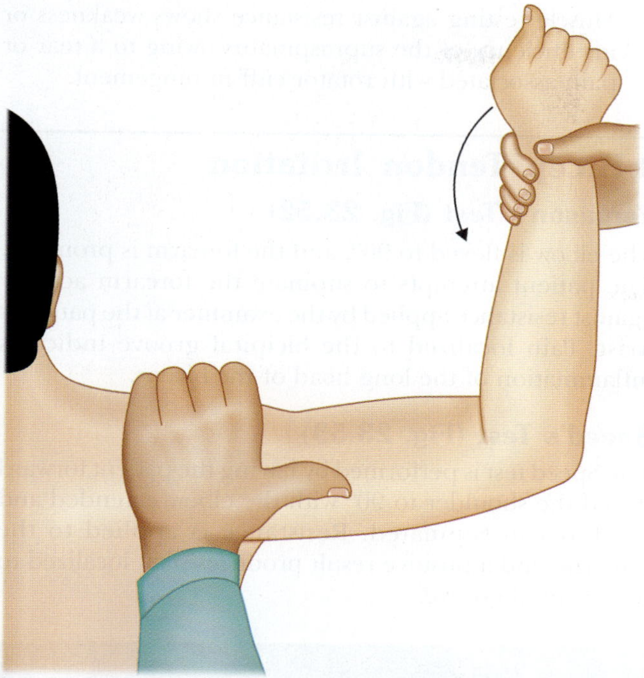

Fig. 23.46: Apprehension text

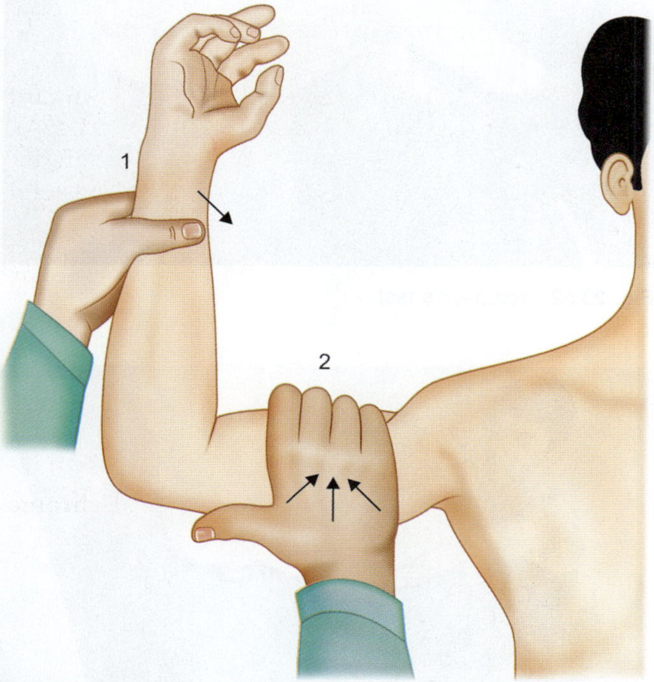

Fig. 23.47: Relocation test performed to detect shoulder instability—(1) Abduct and externally rotate the arm with one hand; (2) Apply downward pressure on arm and look for relief of pain

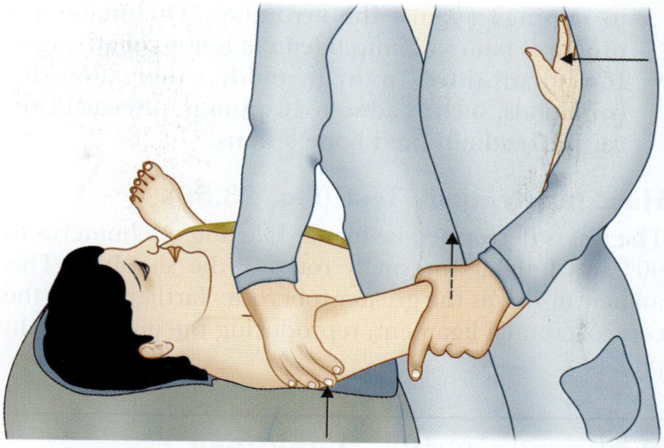

Fig. 23.48: Drawer's test of Gerber and Ganz

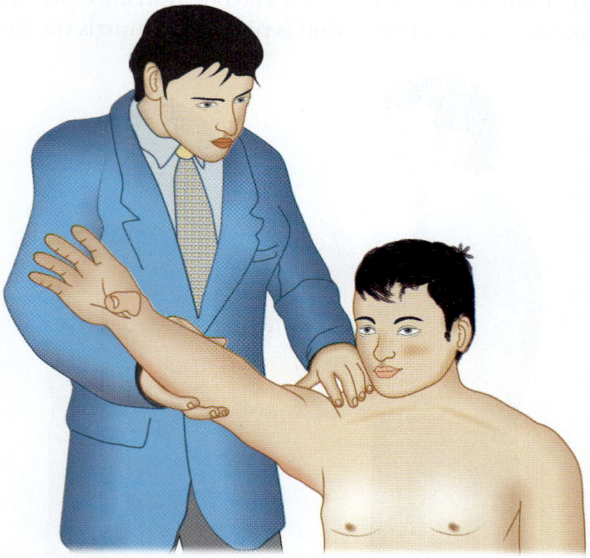

Fig. 23.49: Neer's test

Drawer's Test of Gerber and Ganz (Anterior Glenohumeral Instability) (Fig. 23.48)

- Patient rests in supine position and arm relaxed with shoulder in 90° of abduction, slight flexion and external rotation
- Scapula is steadied on coracoid then move the humeral head
- Any movement or click confirms instability. Axial X-ray should be taken.

Neer's Test (Fig. 23.49)

- With the patient seated, the examiner raises the affected arm in forced forward elevation while stabilizing the scapula, causing the greater tuberosity

to impinge against the acromion. This maneuver produces pain with impingement lesions of all stages.
- It also produces pain in many other shoulder conditions, such as adhesive capsulitis, osteoarthritis, calcific tendinitis and bone lesions.

Hawkins-Kennedy Test (Fig. 23.50)

The test is performed by forward flexing the humerus to 90° and forcibly internally rotating the shoulder. This maneuver drives the greater tuberosity farther under the coracoacromial ligament, reproducing the impingement pain.

Supraspinatus Weakness

Jobe's Test (Fig. 23.51)

- The test is performed by placing the shoulder in 90° of abduction and 30° of forward flexion and internally rotated so that the thumb is pointing towards the floor.
- Muscle testing against resistance shows weakness or insufficiency of the supraspinatus owing to a tear or pain associated with rotator cuff impingement.

Bicep Tendon Irritation

Yergason's Test (Fig. 23.52)

The elbow is flexed to 90°, and the forearm is pronated. The patient attempts to supinate the forearm actively against resistance applied by the examiner at the patient's wrist. Pain localized to the bicipital groove indicates inflammation of the long head of the biceps.

Speed's Test (Fig. 23.53)

The Speed test is performed by having the patient forward flexed the shoulder to 90° with the elbow extended and the forearm supinated. Resistance is applied to the forearm, and a positive result produces pain localized to the bicipital groove.

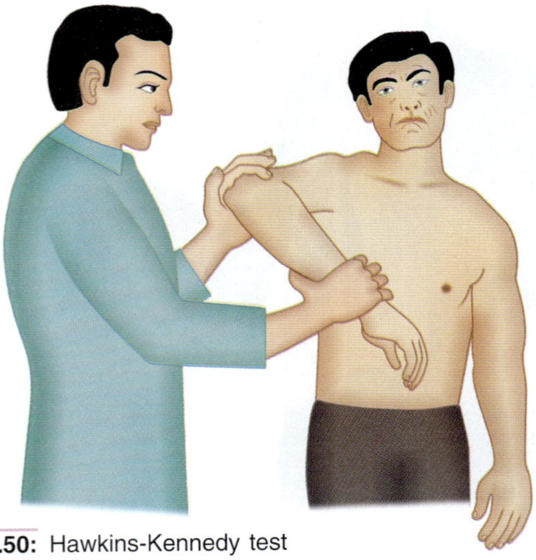

Fig. 23.50: Hawkins-Kennedy test

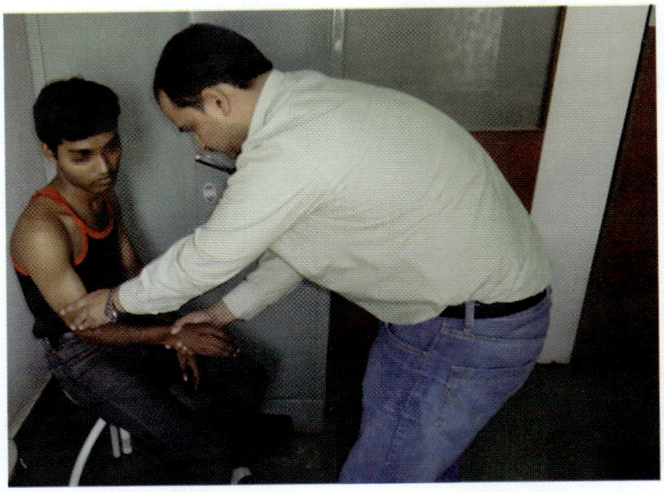

Fig. 23.52: Yergason's test

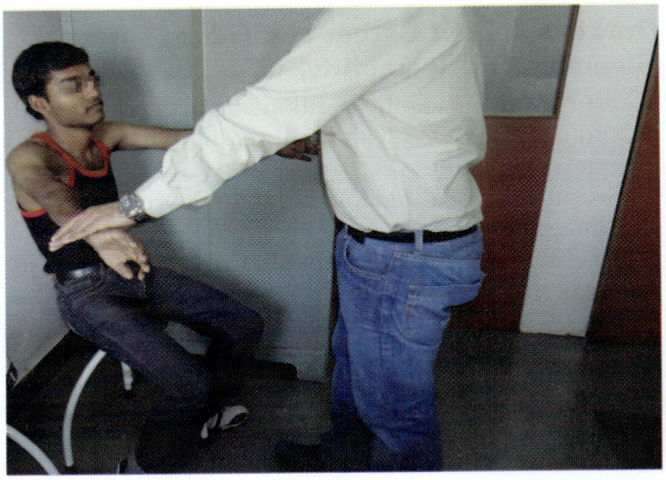

Fig. 23.51: Jobe's test

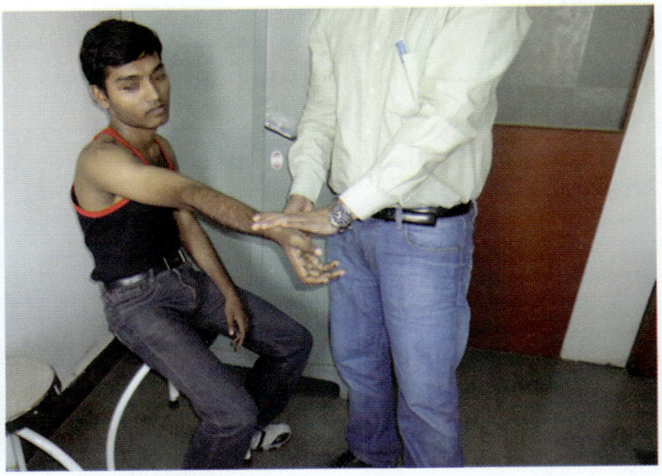

Fig. 23.53: Speed's test

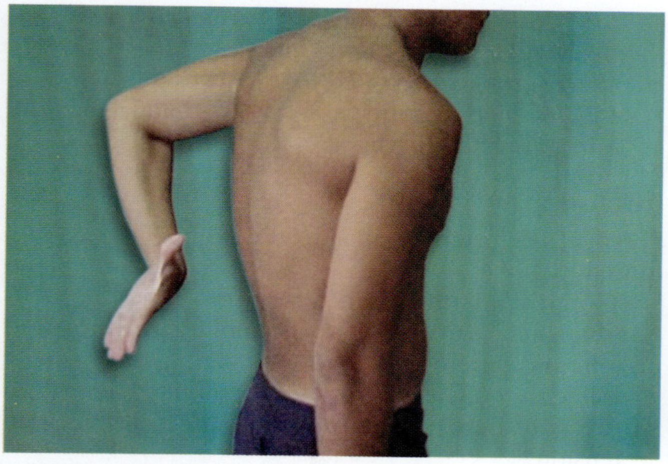

Fig. 23.54: Lift-off test

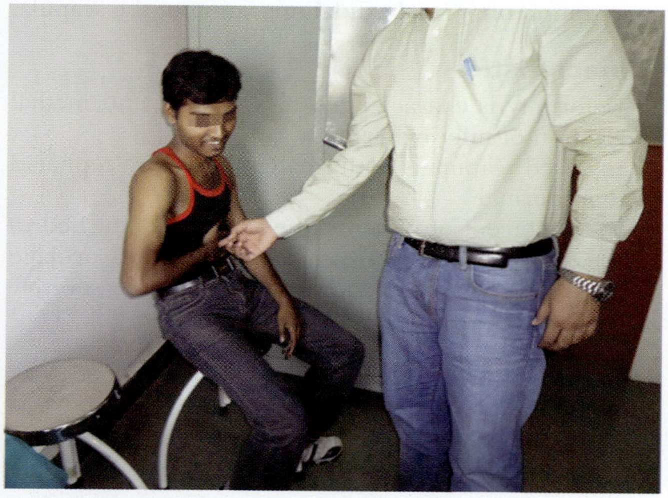

Fig. 23.55: Belly-press test

■ Tests for Evaluating Rotator Cuff Integrity

Lift-off Test (Fig. 23.54)

Patient sitting or standing, arm is internally rotated and dorsum of hand is placed against the lower back. If patient is unable to lift the dorsum of hand from the back, the test is positive.

Belly-press Test (Fig. 23.55)

Patient presses the abdomen with the flat of the hand and attempts to keep the arm in maximum internal rotation. If active internal rotation is strong elbow does not drop backwards.

In case of weakened subscapularis, maximal internal rotation can not be maintained and elbow drops behind the trunk.

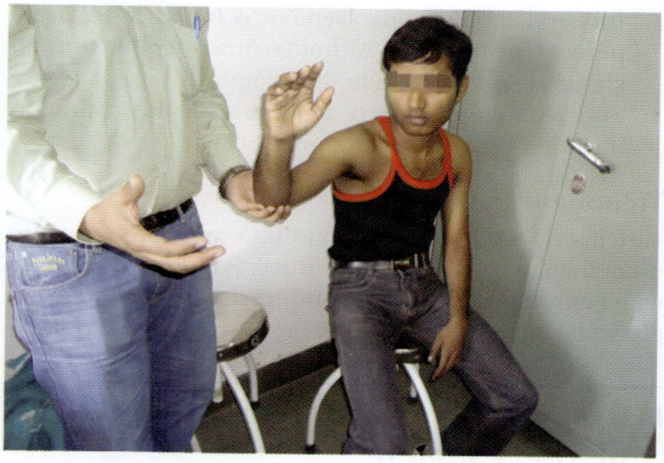

Fig. 23.56: Drop sign

Drop Sign (Fig. 23.56)

Patient is sitting with his/her back to the examiner.

Affected arm is held at 90° of elevation in scapular plane and in almost full external rotation with elbow flexed at 90°. Patient asked to maintain this position actively as the examiner releases the wrist, while supporting the elbow, which is a function of infraspinatus. Sign is positive if *lag* or *drop* occurs.

CONGENITAL ANOMALIES OF SHOULDER

Congenital anomalies of shoulder are classified into two subgroups: (1) Common malformations of the shoulder and (2) Rare anomalies.

■ Cleidocranial Dysostosis

- Cleidocranial dysostosis is a hereditary disorder that affects bones formed by intramembranous ossification.
- The skull, clavicles, ribs, teeth and pubic symphysis are most commonly affected.
- Enlarged head and forward-sloping shoulders are the typical clinical features.
- The range of shoulder function in this condition is vast.
- Patients with this syndrome have been reported to work as heavy laborers without shoulder complaints, whereas others report glenohumeral instability.
- The outer third of the clavicle is the most commonly affected portion, and the medial aspect is usually normal.
- The middle part of the clavicle can also be absent with spared medial and lateral portions.
- In either scenario, the missing portion of clavicle is replaced by fibrous tissue.

- Bilateral shoulder involvement is found in 82 to 90 percent of patients. Although uncommon, normal clavicles do not exclude this diagnosis.
- Two separate reports of families with this condition included members with normal clavicles.

Treatment

Patients do well with this condition and rarely require other than dental treatment. Surgery is indicated for those with neurologic or vascular compression secondary to the clavicular malformation or to prevent skin breakdown.

Congenital Pseudarthrosis of the Clavicle

- Easily mistaken for a fracture of the clavicle anomaly does not show evidence of callus formation
- No or minimal resulting loss of function is thought to occur
- The abnormality occurs unilaterally on the right-side, however, left-sided and bilateral pseudarthrosis have also been reported
- A bump in the midclavicular region is palpable and grossly seen, and smooth ends are apparent on radiographs
- Thoracic outlet syndrome has been reported to be secondary to the pseudarthrosis.

Treatment

Benign neglect has generally been accepted as treatment of this entity. Due to reports of thoracic outlet syndrome, some authors have proposed early excision and bone grafting in younger patients (Figs 23.57A and B).

Sprengel's Shoulder

History

- *1863:* Eulenberg first described three cases of congenital elevated scapulae

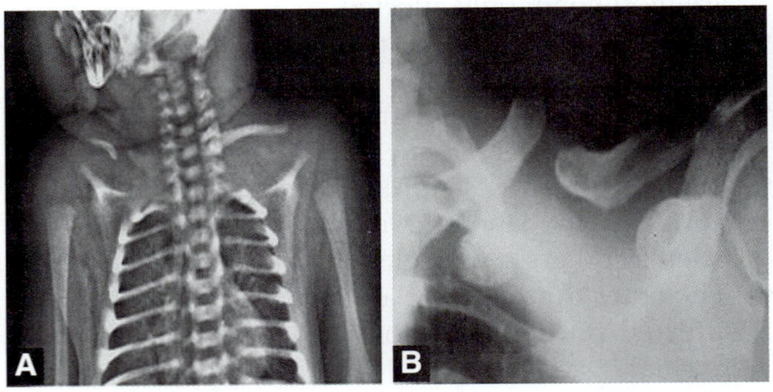

Figs 23.57A and B: (A) The right side is most commonly involved in congenital pseudarthrosis of the clavicle; (B) Note the anterosuperiorly displaced sternal fragment that can manifest as a palpable lump

- *1880:* Willett and Walsham described the first case involving an omovertebral bone
- *1891:* Sprengel described four cases
- *1891:* Kolliker reported several cases and labeled the deformity after Sprengel.

Etiology

Sprengel's deformity is a failure of descent of the scapula caused by:

- Too great an intrauterine pressure
- Abnormal articulations of scapula with the spine (omovertebral bone)
- Defective musculature of the scapulothoracic region
- Arrest of development due to ineffective muscular tension.

Introduction

Uncommon congenital anomaly which arises from interruption of normal caudal migration of the scapula.

Characteristics

- Deformity is characterized by elevation and medial rotation of inferior scapula
- Involved scapula is both smaller and more cephalad than normal
- In 30 percent of patients, the scapula is attached to the cervical spine by an omovertebral bone, cartilage or fibrous tissue, which, when present, can severely limit scapulothoracic motion.

Associated Anomalies

- Absence/Fusion of ribs
- Cervical ribs
- Klippel-Feil syndrome
- Congenital scoliosis with hemivertebrae
- Cervical spina bifida
- Syringomyelia
- Paraplegia
- Platybasia
- Situs inversus
- Mandibulofacial dysostosis
- Clavicular abnormalities
- Cardiac anomalies like atrial septal defect (ASD) ventricular septal defect (VSD), etc.
- Kidney malformations.

Pathology

- The scapula appears at the 5th week of gestation at C5–T1. It then migrates to the adult position by birth to T2–T7
- Some have bony articulations with the spine via omovertebral bones
- *Others have defective musculature:* Trapezius, rhomboids, levator scapula are most commonly affected while others, like pectoralis major/minor, latissimus dorsi,

sternocleidomastoid, serratus anterior, are less commonly affected
- The affected muscles undergo degeneration, necrosis, fibrosis and secondary contracture
- Also the scapula is hypoplastic on the affected side.

Clinical Features

- Most common congenital deformity of the shoulder
- Asymmetry of shoulder (in unilateral cases)
- Female:male ratio is 3:1
- Left scapula is more commonly affected than right scapula
- Neck appears fuller and shorter on the affected side
- Clavicle tilted superiorly about 25° rotated down and away from spine
- Decreased abduction, lateral motion and rotation of scapula are limited with decreased scapulothoracic motion
- Glenohumeral joint is normal with normal range of motion (ROM).

Clinical Presentation (Fig. 23.58)

- Deformity tends to be painless, and many patients are not diagnosed until adolescence
- Due to scapular asymmetry, some patients are mistaken for having scoliosis
- Minor asymmetries commonly seen between right and left scapula should not be designated as having Sprengel's deformity
- Look for loss of shoulder abduction and forward flexion
- If an omovertebral bone is present, abduction of the shoulder is commonly limited to less than 90°.

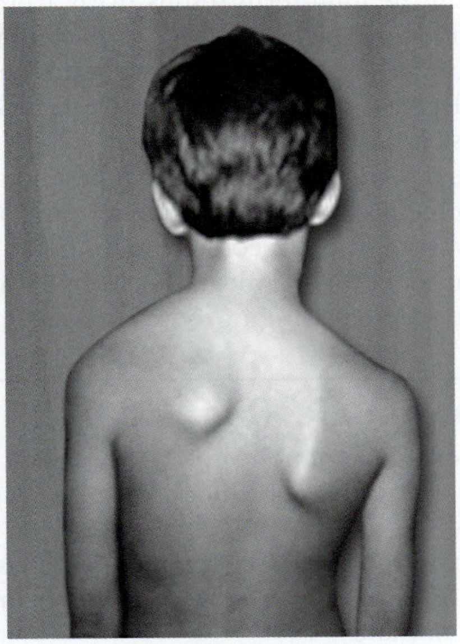

Fig. 23.58: Clinical presentation of Sprengel's deformity

Radiographic Findings

Associated radiographic findings for Sprengel's shoulder are summarized as below:
- Elevated scapula (Fig. 23.59)
- Associated bony deformities
- *Best views:* AP of both shoulders with arms abducted and adducted maximally
- Lateral cervical and thoracic spine to look for other abnormalities
- Oblique and lateral of scapula to show omovertebral bone (one-third of cases) (Fig. 23.60).

Cavendish Classification

- *Grade I:* Very mild
  - Shoulders appear symmetrical when clothed
- *Grade II:* Mild
  - Superomedial angle of scapula is visible as a lump in the web of the neck

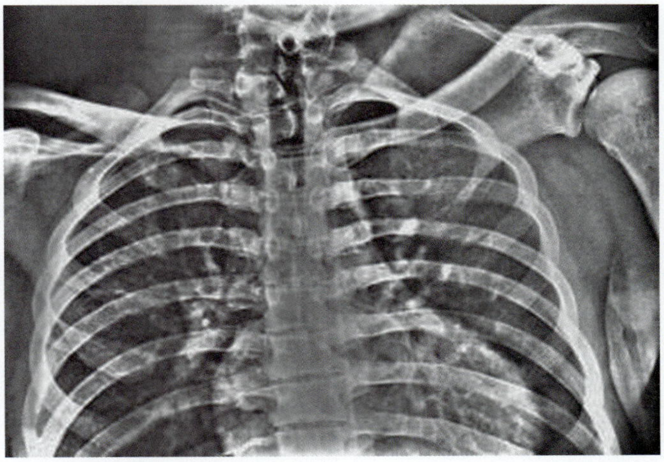

Fig. 23.59: X-ray showing elevated scapula in case of Sprengel's deformity

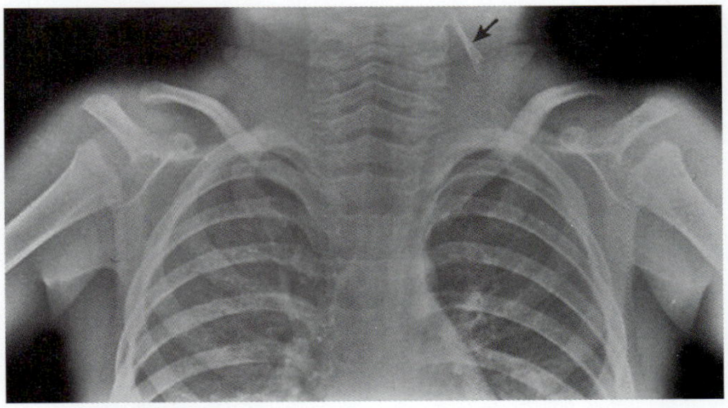

Fig. 23.60: On the left side, an omovertebral bone (arrow) connects the transverse process of the lower cervical spine of C6 with the superomedial angle of the scapula

- *Grade III:* Moderate
  - Shoulder joint is elevated by 2 to 5 cm
  - Deformity is easily visible
- *Grade IV:* Severe
  - Superior angle is near the occiput
  - Severe webbing of the neck.

Treatment

Goals

- Correct deformity
- Improve function
- Improve cosmesis
- Physical-therapy to maintain ROM preoperative and improve strength.

Factors in Considering Surgical Correction

- *Cosmesis*
  - Cavendish Grade III or IV
- *Functional*
  - Omovertebral bone or scapulothoracic fibrous adhesions have better outcomes and improve function with resection
- *Associated anomalies*
  - That is treat scoliosis at the same time
- *Age of patient*
  - Although somewhat controversial most agree 3 to 8 years of age.

Nonsurgical Treatment

As passive stretching exercises advocated in the past are not successful, treatment is primarily surgical.

Surgical Treatment

- *Timing*
  - Surgery is indicated for children between 3 and 8 years of age without significant deformities, both functional and cosmetic.
  - Patients older than 8 years of age are not good candidates for scapular displacement procedures.
- *Options*
  - Detachment of medial and superior scapular muscles, repositioning scapula caudal and subsequently reattaching the muscles to lowered scapula.

Woodward Procedure

- Procedure has 80 percent satisfactory functional and cosmetic results
- Increase shoulder abduction following surgery, ranges from 34 to 60°
- Child's age at operation and differing methods of measurement play largest role in accounting for these differences
- Younger patients obtain better motion and postoperative correction
- Caudal displacement of scapula is reported to be 1.9 times vertebral body heights in one series and 4 cm in another.

Technique (Figs 23.61A to C)

- Involves resection of omovertebral bone and division of vertebral attachments of trapezius, rhomboids and levator scapula
- Scapula is subsequently rotated and translated caudally
- Detached muscle's origins are then sutured to more inferior vertebral spinous processes.

Postoperative Phase (Figs 23.62A and B)

- Three weeks of postoperative immobilization are required
- Osteotomy of clavicle may be required to prevent compression of nerve/vein (N/V) structures against first rib
- Postoperative improvement in shoulder abduction is maintained, although some loss of scapular translation can occur in first four months postoperatively.
- One-third of patients will have widening of their surgical scars, which can be cosmetically disturbing.
- X-ray taken, demonstrates:
  - Elevated left scapula worse than right
  - No evidence of omovertebral bone on either side
- Thoracic kyphosis—no other spinal abnormalities.

Modified Woodward Procedure with Clavicular Osteotomy and Morcellation on Left Side (Fig. 23.63)

Conclusion

- In a recent article from the Alfred I, duPont Institute reviewing the long-term results (with average follow-up period of 8 years) of the modified Woodward procedure in 15 patients, there was improved cosmesis with a decrease of at least one Cavendish Grade in all patients
- Average scapular lowering of 2.7 cm, and an average improvement in shoulder abduction by 35°
- There were only minor complications noted including: one transient brachial plexus palsy; one widened scar and one scapular winging.

■ Os Acromiale (Fig. 23.64)

- Failure of the acromion process to fuse
- It is more common in black patients and in male patients
- The acromion is formed from three ossification centers. Failure of any of these centers to unite causes an os acromiale
- The most common site of persistent cartilage is between the meta-acromion and the mesoacromion.

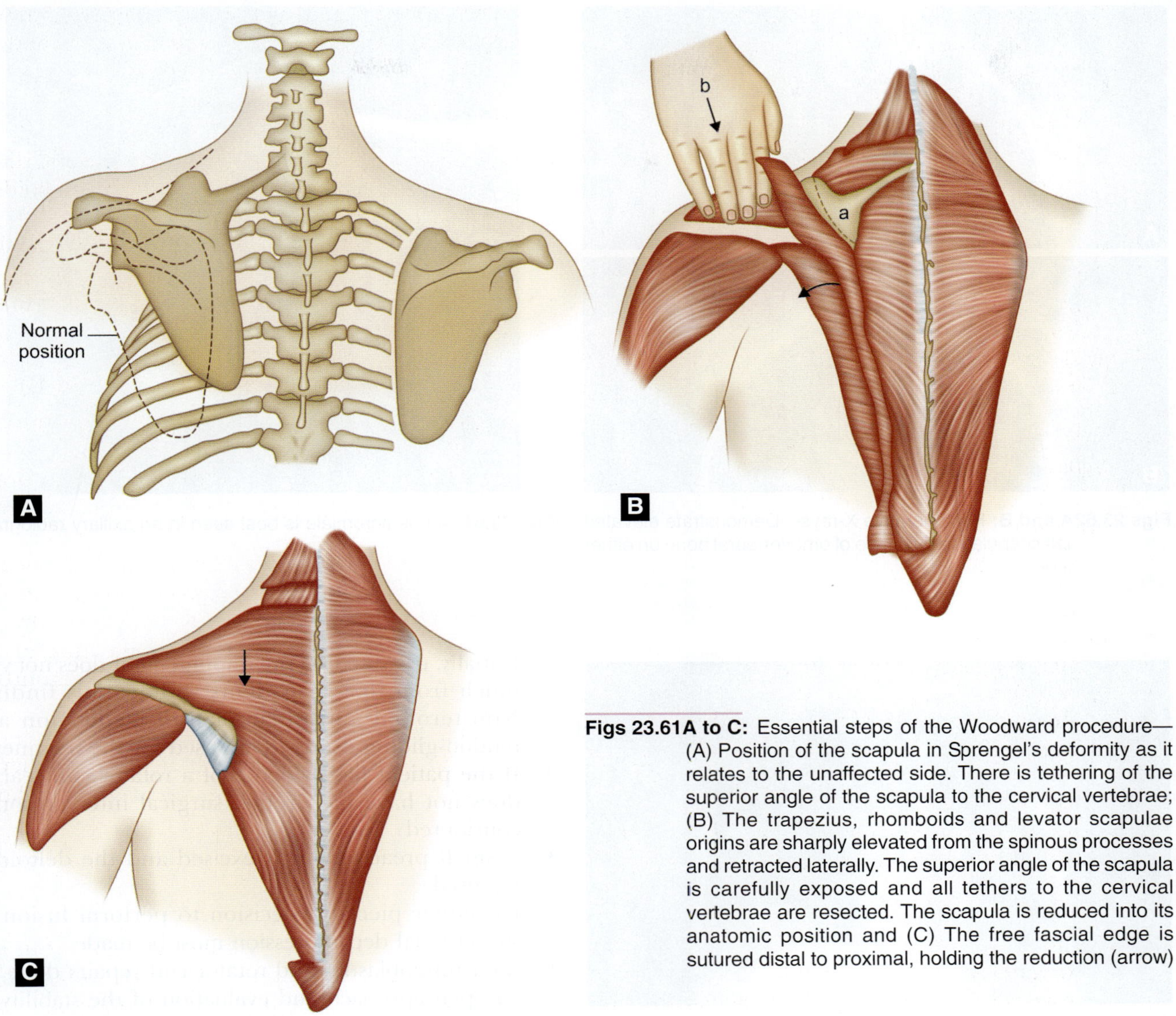

Figs 23.61A to C: Essential steps of the Woodward procedure—(A) Position of the scapula in Sprengel's deformity as it relates to the unaffected side. There is tethering of the superior angle of the scapula to the cervical vertebrae; (B) The trapezius, rhomboids and levator scapulae origins are sharply elevated from the spinous processes and retracted laterally. The superior angle of the scapula is carefully exposed and all tethers to the cervical vertebrae are resected. The scapula is reduced into its anatomic position and (C) The free fascial edge is sutured distal to proximal, holding the reduction (arrow)

- It has been suggested that a more posteriorly situated acromioclavicular joint in relation to the anterior acromial edge is a predisposing factor to the development of an os acromiale
- The acromion process should get fully ossified by 25 years of age
- Os acromiale is bilateral in 33 to 62 percent of cases
- Most often the abnormality is asymptomatic and is an incidental discovery
- The acromion has three separate ossification centers. The most common site of os acromiale is between the mesoacromion and the meta-acromion. Basic-acromion (BA), Mesoacromion (MSA), Meta-acromion (MTA), Preacromion (PA) (Fig. 23.65).

Treatment

- Symptomatic os acromiale falls into two categories:
  - *First group:* Those associated with pain at the unstable segment
  - *Second group:* Those associated with symptoms of impingement
- The first group of patients must be managed conservatively with a sling, if seen acutely after trauma, followed by early mobilization. Persistent pain that lasts longer than three months and limits work or activities of daily living is an indication for surgery
- The second group of patients undergone a more complex treatment protocol

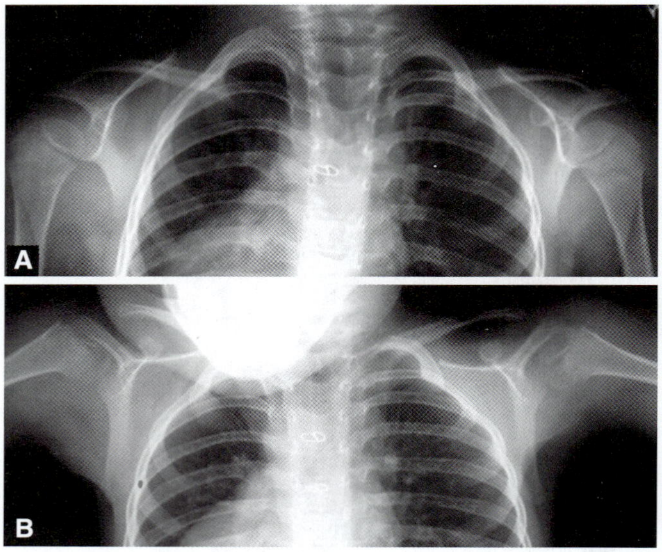

Figs 23.62A and B: Postoperative X-rays—Demonstrate elevated left scapula, no evidence of omovertebral bone on either side

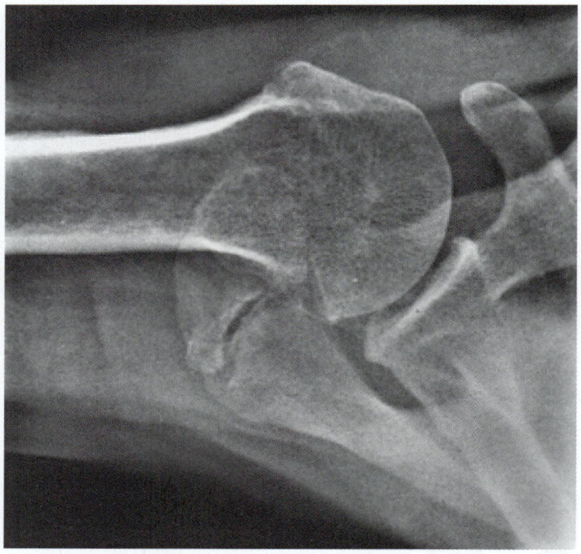

Fig. 23.64: An os acromiale is best seen in an axillary radiograph

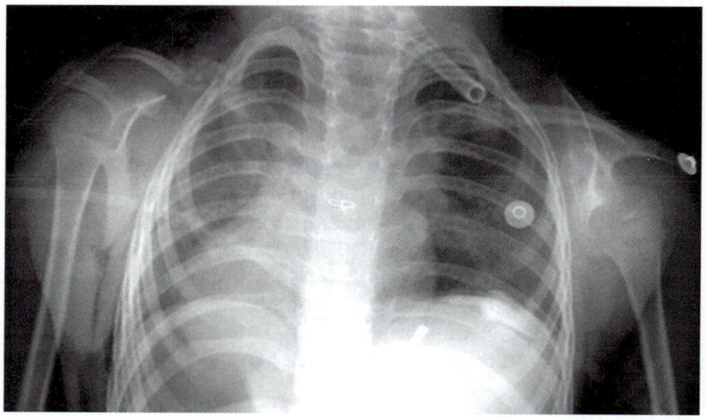

Fig. 23.63: Postoperative X-ray modified Woodward procedure with clavicular osteotomy and morcellation on left side

- Initially, treatment of the impingement does not vary much from that in patients without this finding. Nonsteroidal anti-inflammatory medication and tendon-gliding exercises are used for the treatment
- If the patient has evidence of a rotator cuff tear or does not have pain relief, surgical intervention is considered
- A small preacromion is excised and the deltoid is repaired
- For larger pieces, a decision to perform fusion or subacromial decompression must be made
- All acromioplasties and rotator cuff repairs done via an open approach and evaluation of the stability of the os is performed. If the os acromiale is stable to palpation, a standard acromioplasty is performed. If

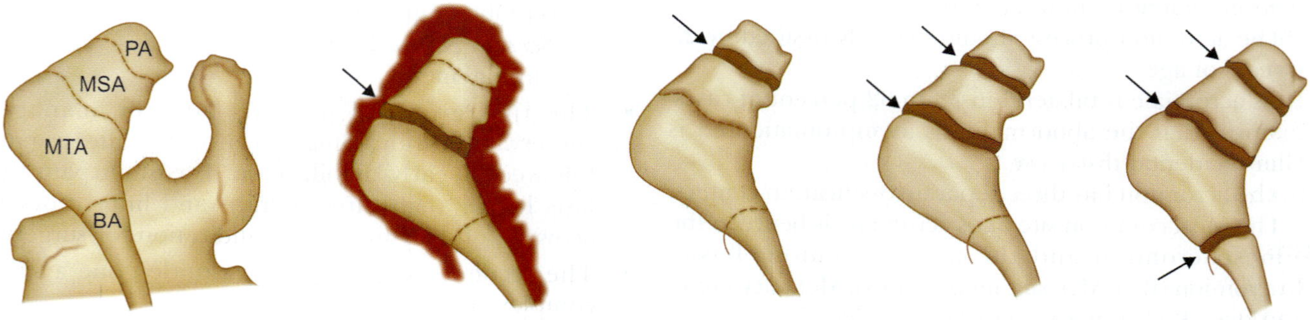

Fig. 23.65: Separate ossification centers of os acromiale (arrows)

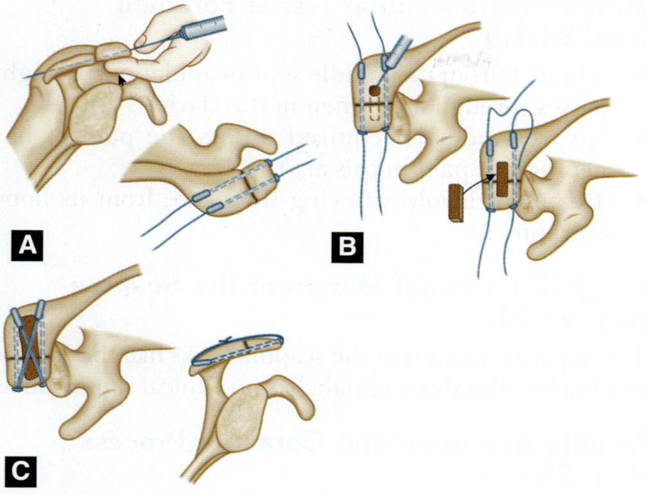

Figs 23.66A to C: Different steps followed in repair of an unstable os acromiale (arrows)

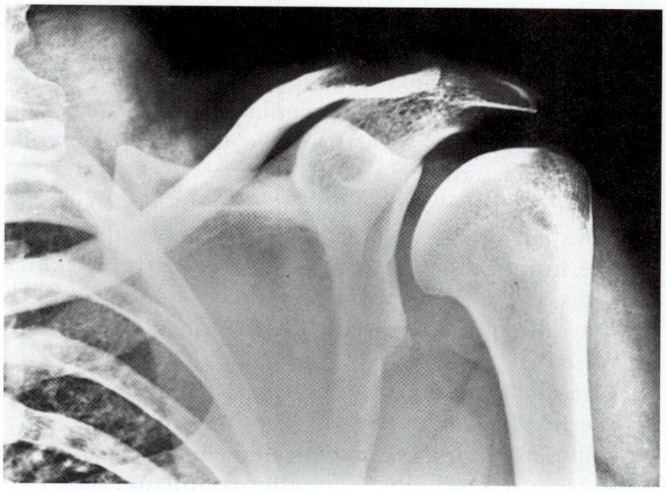

Fig. 23.67: Varying degrees of glenoid flattening are seen in glenoid hypoplasia

the segment has motion with palpation, a *fusion operation* is undertaken

Steps followed in repair of an unstable os acromiale (Figs 23.66A to C):

- Guidewires for two 4.0 mm cannulated screws are placed in the free fragment in an anterior-to-posterior direction (top). The fragment is reduced and the guidewires are advanced across nonunion site (bottom).
- Two distally threaded screws are inserted to compress the reduction.
- Cancellous bone graft obtained from the hip is placed on the superior surface of the acromion. Large nonabsorbable suture is placed through each screw and secured in a figure-of-eight manner.

■ Glenoid Hypoplasia

- Glenoid hypoplasia (Fig. 23.67) results from failure of the inferior glenoid to develop.
- The true incidence is uncertain, and the diagnosis is often made on the basis of routine chest radiographs.
- Patients might complain of pain and limited abduction in the second through fifth decades of life.
- Instability of the glenohumeral joint is reported to be found in a subgroup of patients.
- Glenoid hypoplasia is most commonly bilateral and noted commonly in men.

Treatment

- In these types of patients, avoidance of manual labor and overhead activities are commonly suggested.
- Arthroscopic debridement of the ragged articular cartilage to alter symptoms.

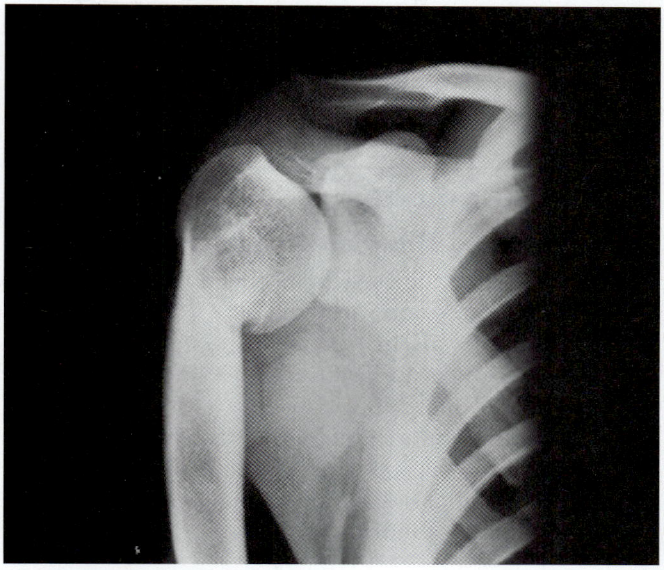

Fig. 23.68: X-ray showing a typical appearance of humerus varus

- Arthroplasty as treatment of the secondary degenerative arthritis but its having a limited result.
- In hemiarthroplasty, it requires revision of total shoulder or bipolar arthroplasty due to pain.
- *Total shoulder replacement:* When nonoperative treatment has failed, total shoulder replacement is the only treatment.

■ Humerus Varus (Fig. 23.68)

- The humeral neck-to-shaft angle is generally considered to be 140° in a normal shoulder.

- When the proximal humeral growth plate is disturbed during growth or development, the neck and shaft angle can be dramatically reduced.
- Premature closure of the medial growth plate results in a differential growth of the lateral and medial humeral lengths.
- Kohler defined a neck-to-shaft angle less than 90°, elevation of the greater tuberosity above the top of the humeral head and reduction of the distance between the articular surface and the lateral cortex as the radiographic criteria for diagnosis of humerus varus.
- Patients have either a decreased ability to perform overhead activities or pain from impingement.
- Compensation by the unaffected shoulder can result in overuse tendinitis as another complaint.
- Trauma during birth or early life may be the underlying cause of idiopathic humerus varus. It occurs unilaterally.
- Several other processes can be responsible for humerus varus, including thalassemia, skeletal dysplasia, neoplasm, osteomyelitis, cerebral palsy, arthrogryposis and brachial plexus injuries.

Therefore, the underlying cause of humerus varus must be investigated before treating the deformity.

Rare Anomalies

Duplicated and Bifurcated Clavicle (Fig. 23.69)

- Duplication of the clavicle has been described in the literature with some variation.
- Complete duplication of the clavicle has been described once and caused no symptoms in that patient.
- In a few cases, bifurcation of the clavicle has also been described in which there is duplication of either the lateral or medial side. Duplication of the clavicle is an extremely rare abnormality.

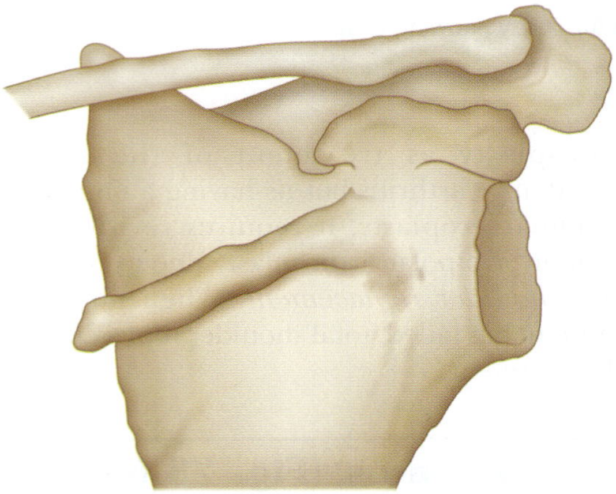

Fig. 23.69: The lateral end of the extraclavicle attaches to the base of the coracoid process

Middle Suprascapular Nerve Foramen (Fig. 23.70)

- A branch from the middle suprascapular nerve might passes through a foramen in the clavicle.
- No treatment is required unless the patient has neurogenic pain in this area.
- Treatment involves freeing the nerve from its bony entrapment.

Clasp-like Cranial Margin of the Scapula (Fig. 23.71)

The superior margin of the scapula looks like the handle of a bucket. But this anomaly has no clinical significance.

Double Acromion and Coracoid Process (Fig. 23.72)

Reported only once, this malformation restricted motion of the shoulder but required no treatment.

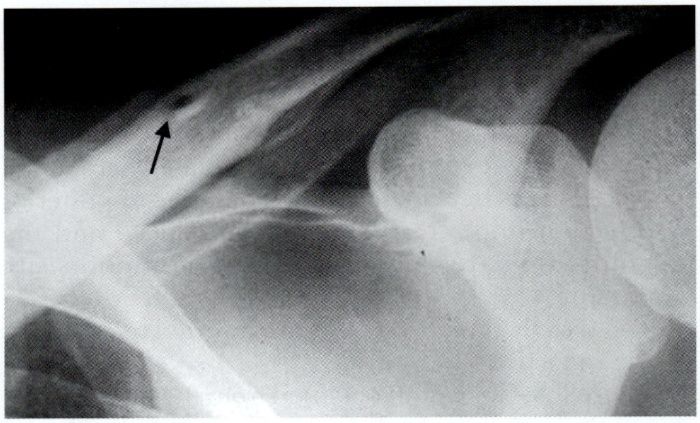

Fig. 23.70: This clavicle has a large foramen (arrow) through which supraclavicular nerve passes

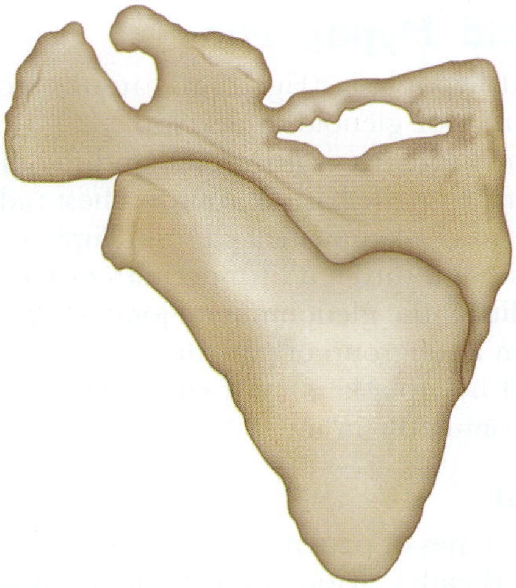

Fig. 23.71: Clasp-like cranial margin of the scapula

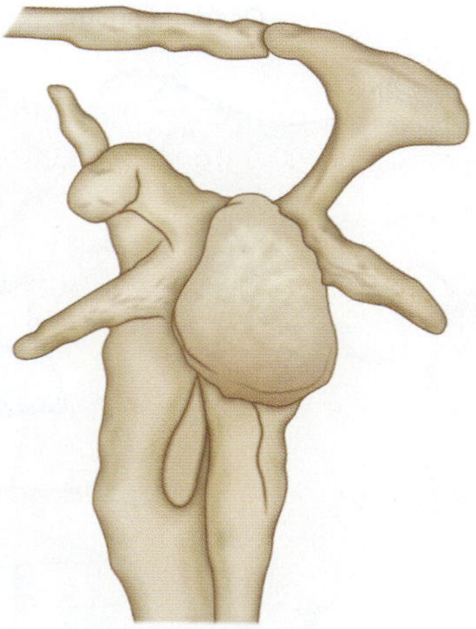

Fig. 23.72: The double acromion and coracoid processes shown here have been identified only once

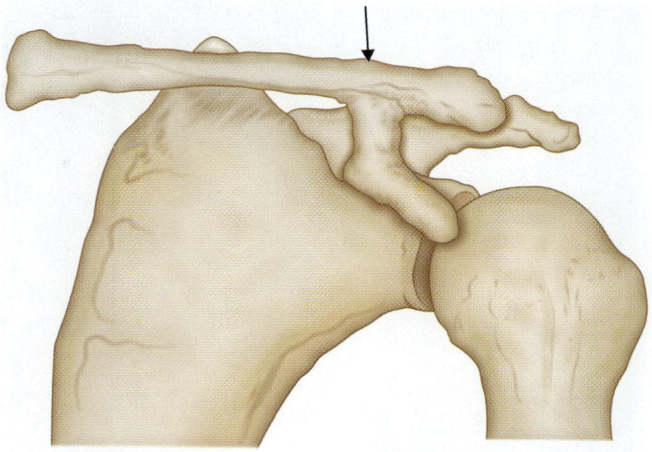

Fig. 23.74: Rarely, a solid bony strut (arrow) connects the coracoid to the clavicle

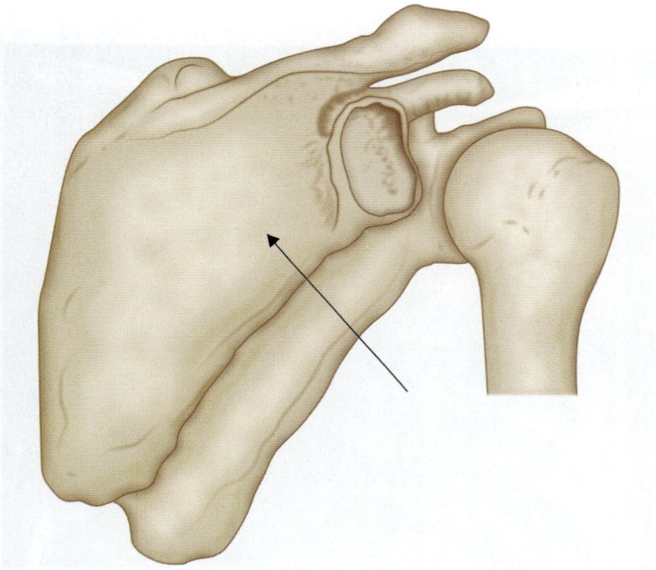

Fig. 23.73: Arrow showing duplicated scapulas (reported only thrice)

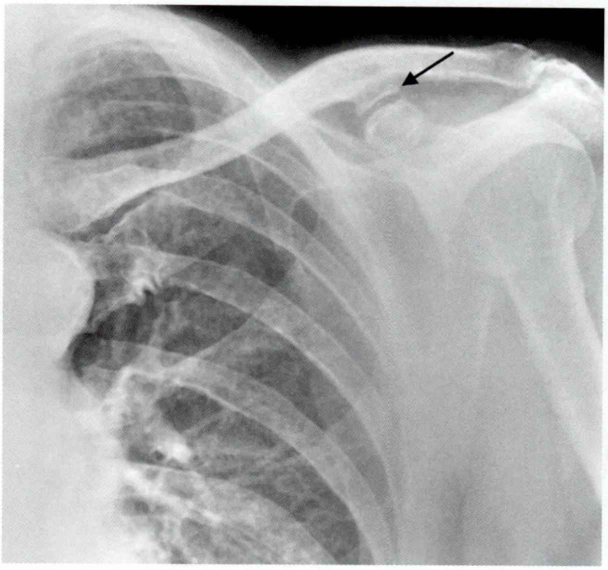

Fig. 23.75: Both the coracoid and the clavicular projections may be covered with cartilage and form a true diarthrodial joint (arrow) with an articular capsule

Duplicated Scapula (Fig. 23.73)

- Multiple humeri and forearm bones are commonly associated.
- Fusion of the two scapulae has been reported to be successful in patients whose motion is restricted.

Coracoclavicular Joint or Bar (Figs 23.74 to 23.76)

- The coracoclavicular ligaments may be replaced by an articulation or a bony bar.
- Symptomatic patients might complain of neurovascular compression, restriction in range of motion or pain from arthritis of the joint.
- When symptomatic, the articulation or bar may be excised.

Coracosternal Bone

- A bony bridge originating from the base of the coracoid and extending cephalad and medially has been reported in one patient with Sprengel's deformity.

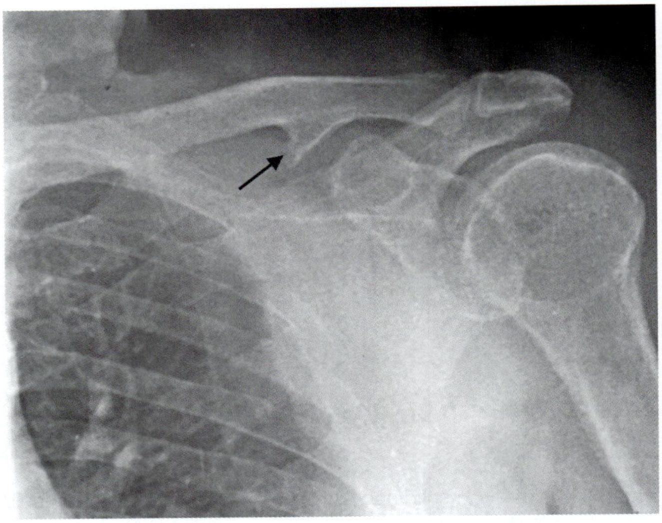

Fig. 23.76: A triangular bony overgrowth under the clavicle (arrow) may be present with its apex directed down toward the coracoid

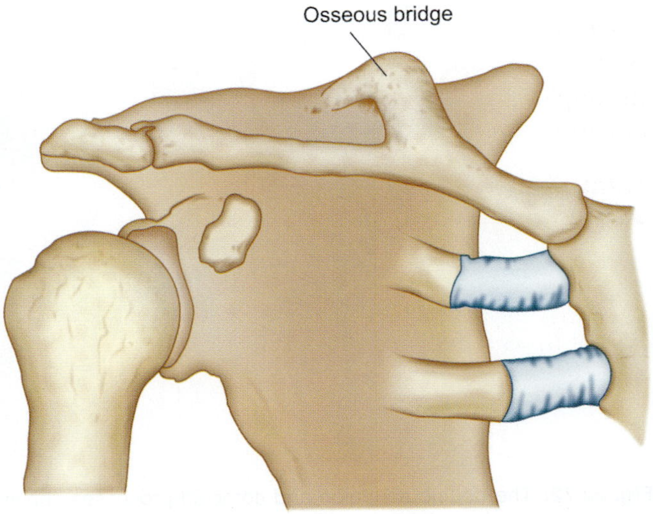

Fig. 23.78: An osseous bridge can extend from the midportion of the clavicle to the spine of the scapula

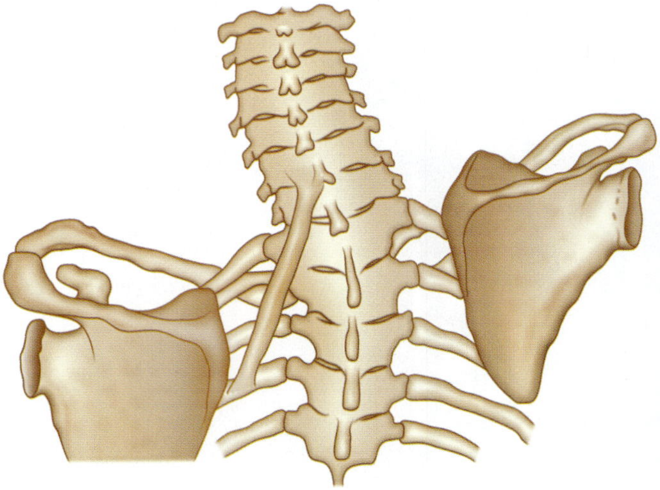

Fig. 23.77: The costovertebral bone ties together the bifid spinous process of the sixth cervical vertebra and the fourth rib

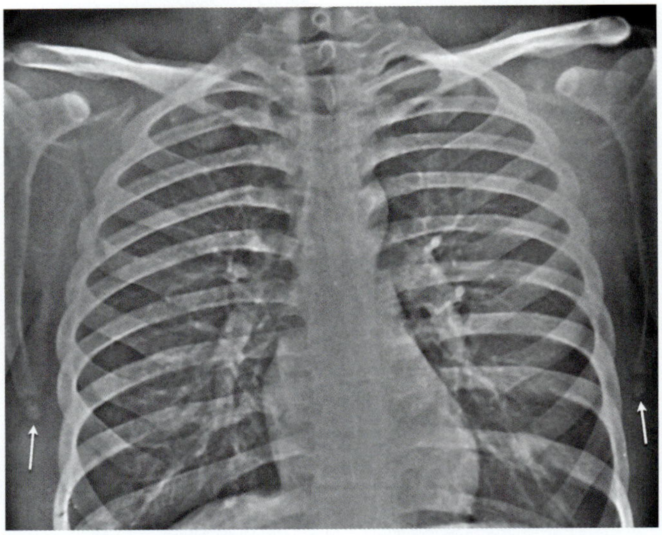

Fig. 23.79: An infrascapular bone (arrows) is present bilaterally in this patient

- It was thought to be the persistence of a mesenchymal coracosternal connection normally seen in an early embryologic stage.

Ligamentous Connecting Bands: Costocoracoid, Costosternal, Costovertebral (Fig. 23.77)

- The three abnormal costocoracoid, costosternal and costovertebral fibrous connections can lead to progressive deformity and dysfunction of the upper extremity
- Excision of the offending structure can provide improved function and prevent further deformity.

Osseous Bridge from Clavicle to Spine of Scapula (Fig. 23.78)

Compression of neurovascular structures and restriction of motion require excision of this structure.

Infrascapular Bone

Infrascapular bone is a normal variant of scapula ossification, represents the attachment of the teres major muscle and may be misinterpreted as a fracture (Fig. 23.79).

Notched Inferior Angle of the Scapula (Fig. 23.80)

Incomplete development of the inferior scapula results in a misshapen scapula.

Dentated Glenoid (Fig. 23.81)

- Incomplete development of the inferior glenoid results in a rippled appearance of the glenoid.
- Fusion of the growth plates usually resolves this appearance, but it can continue to be present in adulthood.

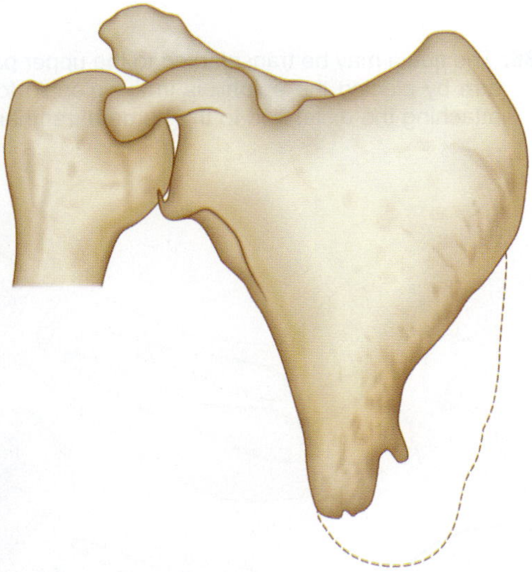

Fig. 23.80: A notched inferior angle of the scapula probably represents an absence of the ossification nucleus of the inferior angle of the scapula

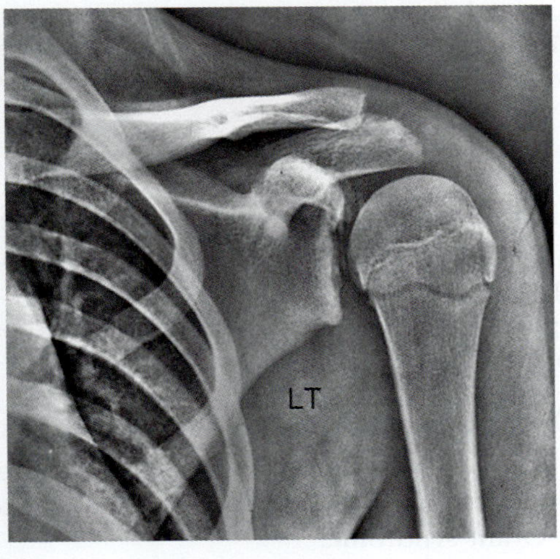

Fig. 23.81: The epiphyseal annular ring of the glenoid it has not fused and appears to be rippled or dentated (the letters LT indicate that the radiograph is of the left shoulder)

Phocomelia (Figs 23.82 to 23.87)

- Absence of the entire upper extremity or severe shortening of the limb with absent portions was a major health catastrophe during the 1950s with the use of thalidomide in pregnant women
- Currently, phocomelia is rare
- The function of the remnant limb dictates intervention
- Preservation of functional fingers can allow improved prosthetic use
- Unsightly and nonfunctioning limbs may be candidates for amputation

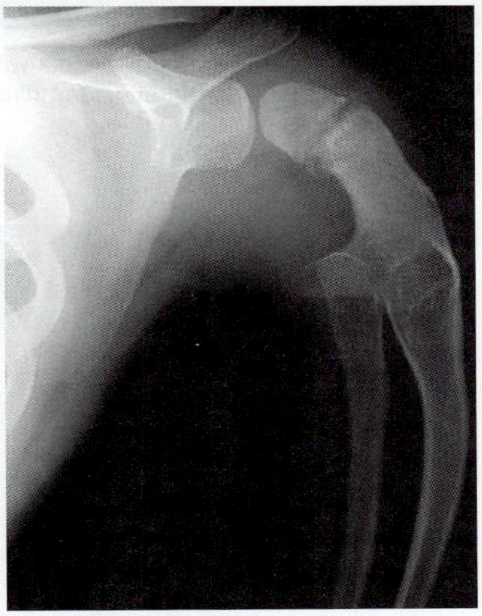

Fig. 23.82: This child with phocomelia has a fairly well-developed shoulder with a small humerus and fused elbow

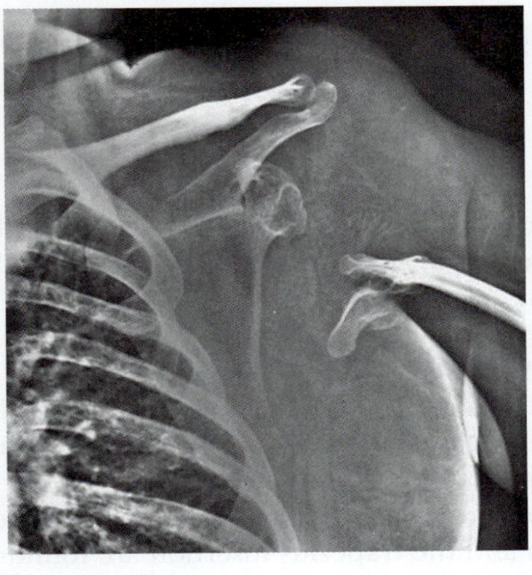

Fig. 23.83: An abnormal glenoid articulates with only a deformed, short distal end of the humerus and a one-bone forearm in this patient with phocomelia

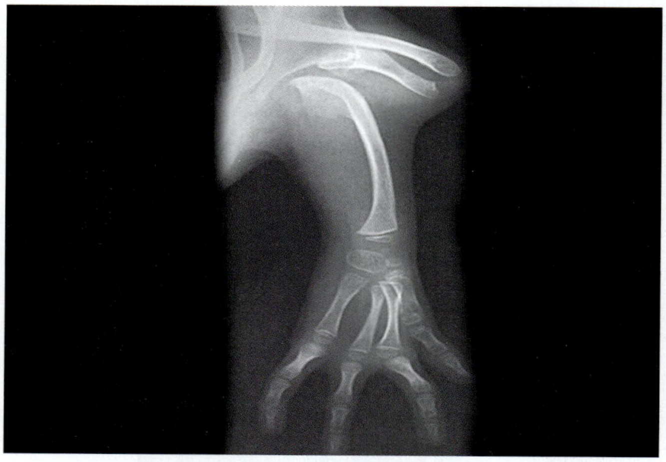

Fig. 23.84: This child has a poorly formed scapula with part of an elbow articulating inside the shoulder joint and only a radius in the forearm

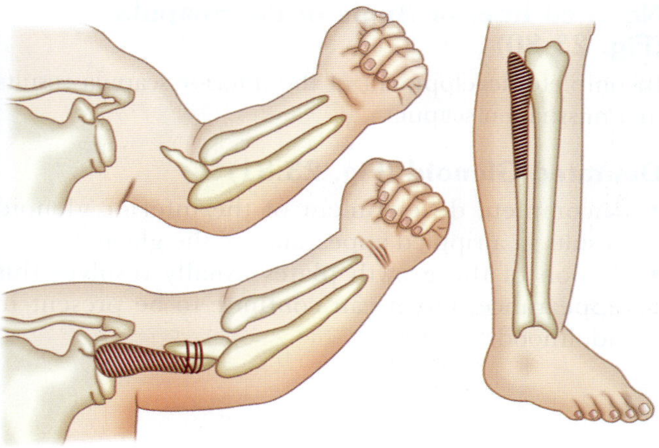

Fig. 23.86: The fibula may be transplanted to the upper part of the arm by placing the epiphysis in the glenoid fossa and attaching the distal end to the humeral remnant

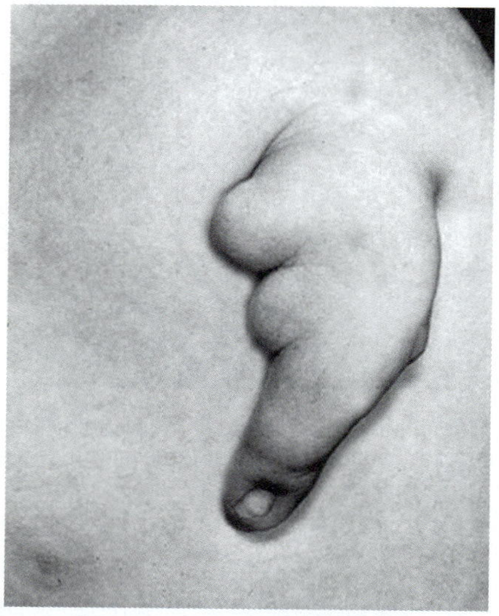

Fig. 23.85: In an extreme case of phocomelia, sometimes only a finger attaches to the trunk

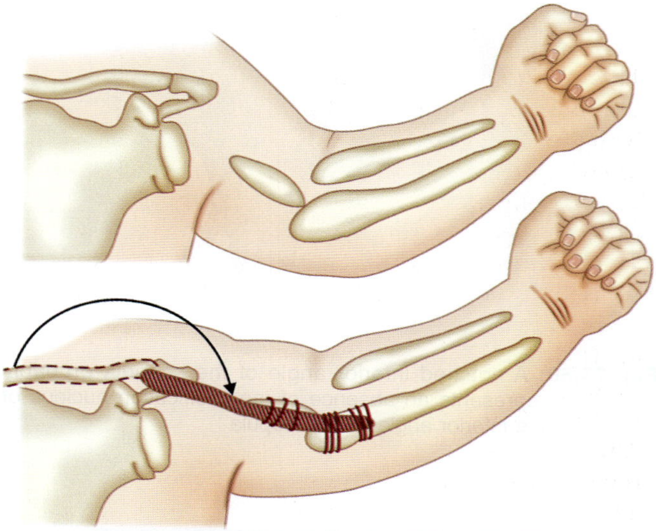

Fig. 23.87: Transposition of the clavicle is accomplished by exposing it subperiosteally and using the sternal end to lengthen the humerus

- Bone transport has been used to lengthen the affected limb, as have vascularized fibula and clavicle grafts.

Absence of the Acromion Head

- Bilateral absence of the acromion has been reported in a few cases and a familial association has been identified
- The coracoacromial ligament is absent and the deltoid origin and the trapezius insertion are found both on the lateral clavicle and on the scapular spine
- The lateral end of the clavicle is blunted, and both the clavicle and coracoid process are hypertrophied.
- Clinical appearance and range of motion of the shoulders were normal, although mild superior translation of the humeral head was noted in one patient.
- Congenital absence of the humeral head has been reported twice.

Holt-Oram Syndrome

- The condition involving multigenerational cardiac and upper extremity congenital anomalies is termed Holt-Oram syndrome.
- These scapular abnormalities are similar to Sprengel's deformity are the most common shoulder manifestation.

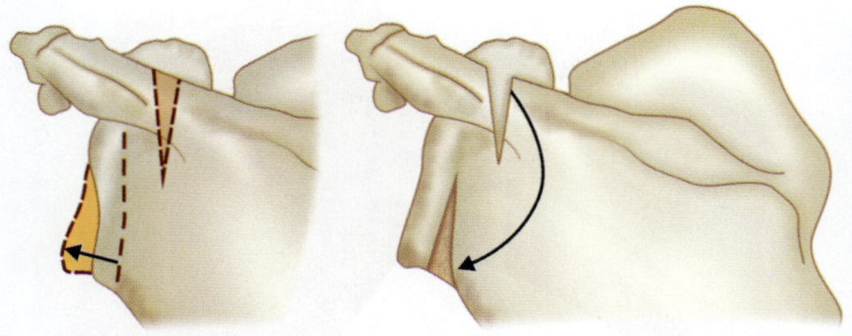

Fig. 23.88: For correction of the shoulder deformity in the Nail-Patella syndrome, an opening wedge osteotomy of the inferior glenoid with bone from the spine of the scapula works well

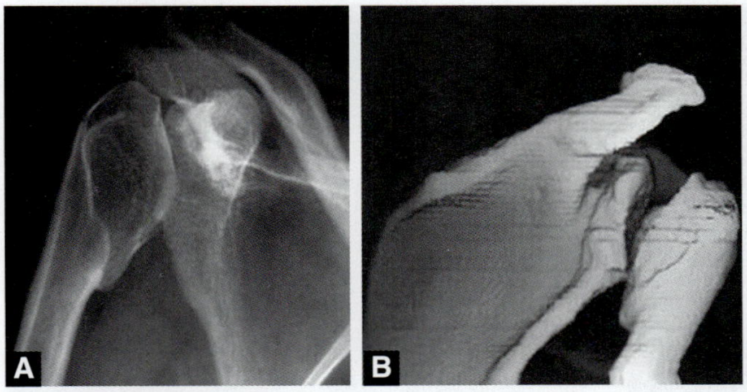

Figs 23.89A and B: (A) This 23-year-old man with Apert's syndrome has flattening of the humeral head with arthropathy; (B) CT scan with three-dimensional reconstruction shows the abnormalities even more dramatically

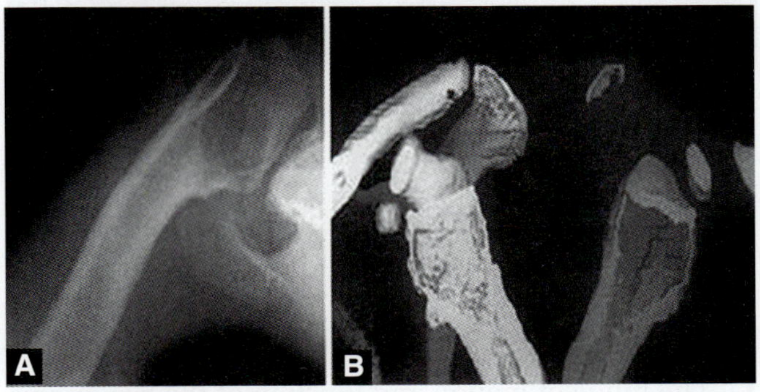

Figs 23.90A and B: (A) The left shoulder of a man with Apert's syndrome; (B) CT scan with three-dimensional reconstruction

- Misshapen clavicles, acromia and humeral heads have also been reported.
- Inheritance is autosomal dominant.

Nail-Patella Syndrome (Fig. 23.88)

- This autosomal dominant syndrome is a relatively common entity in England
- Nail-Patella syndrome is also known as onycho-osteodysplasia
- The main features of Nail-Patella syndrome are:
  - Absent or hypoplastic nails, typically more severe on the radial side of the hand
  - Dysplasia of the patella and lateral femoral condyle of knee
  - Dysplasia of the capitellum and radial head of the elbow
  - Dysplasia of the iliac crests.
- Although not the main abnormality of the disease, the scapula and the humerus are often misshapen.
- The proximal end of the humerus is often small and directed superiorly
- The glenoid is often small and directed laterally or inferiorly
- A small acromion, a prominent lateral clavicle, and a small coracoid complete the bony abnormalities often found
- Some patients complain of impingement-like pain with use of the extremity
- *On examination:* Glenohumeral joint is prominent anteriorly and unstable.
- Double osteotomy of the scapula that successfully relieved the pain of a patient, when nonoperative treatment has failed.

Oto-onychoperoneal Syndrome

- This rare syndrome is characterized by dysmorphic facial features with characteristic ear abnormalities, nail hypoplasia, absent or hypoplastic fibulae and shoulder anomalies. It is thought to be an autonomic recessive disorder
- Shoulder abnormalities include straight clavicles, fibrous fusion of the distal clavicle and the scapular spine, and an abnormal acromioclavicular joint.

Apert's Syndrome (Figs 23.89 and 23.90)

- Apert's syndrome is typically thought of for the hand manifestation, acrocephalosyndactyly
- However, several authors have reported that the shoulder is often affected
- The shoulder is reduced but subluxates anteriorly
- The humeral head and glenoid are dysplastic, and the acromion is sometimes enlarged
- The function and pain typically worsen with age as the joint surfaces degenerate and the joint continues to subluxate.

Multiple Epiphyseal Dysplasia (Fig. 23.91)

- A defect in the ossification center of the epiphysis results in multiple joint involvement with this disease.
- Patients commonly have shoulder manifestations that fall into two categories:

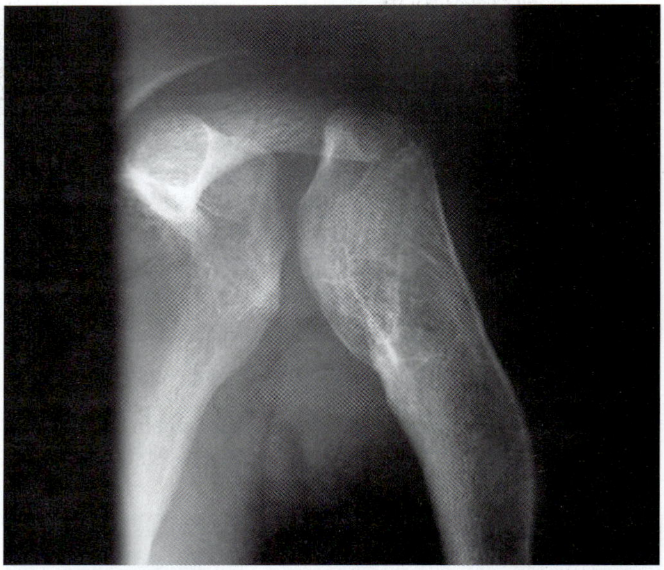

Fig. 23.91: Typical hatchet head shoulder

- Mild abnormalities that lead to glenohumeral arthritis
- Severe failure of epiphyseal development

- Both the groups typically have pain in the fifth and sixth decades of life
- The range of motion and function of the two groups are vastly different
- Mildly affected shoulders have nearly normal motion initially but lose motion and become painful overtime
- Severely deformed shoulders lack motion from an early age but are not painful until later in life.

Pelvis-shoulder Dysplasia

- Pelvis-shoulder dysplasia, also known as scapuloiliac dysostosis or Kosenow's syndrome. It is an autosomal dominant condition characterized by extreme hypoplasia of the scapulae and ilea.
- The scapular body and glenoid display severe hypoplasia, and the acromion and coracoid may be normal.
- The clavicles many times appear elongated but can also be hypoplastic. Cases without shoulder girdle involvement have been reported.
- Anomalies of the eyes, ears, vertebrae, ribs and upper and lower limbs, along with severe lumbar lordosis and hip dislocation, have been reported.

Congenital Dislocation of the Shoulder

- Whether congenital dislocation of the shoulder is a real entity is controversial
- The presence of a dislocated shoulder in a child is often associated with brachial plexus injury or arthrogryposis multiplex congenital

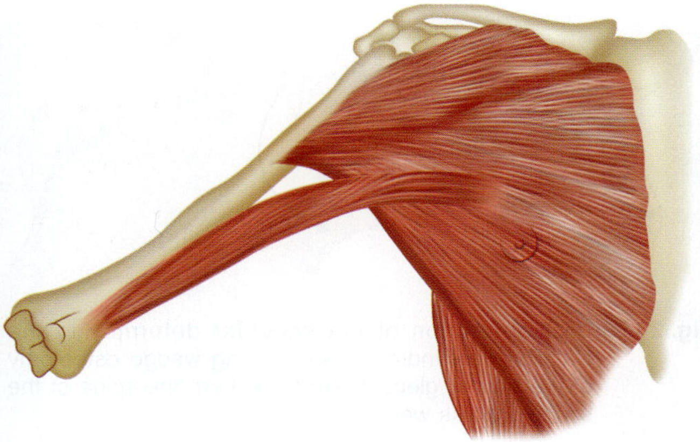

Fig. 23.92: The chondroepitrochlearis muscle originates on the anterior chest wall and inserts along the medial epicondyle

- If a congenital shoulder dislocation is confirmed, closed reduction is the preferred treatment
- Failure of closed reduction can necessitate open reduction.

Chondroepitrochlearis Muscle (Fig. 23.92)

- Reports of this muscle have come mainly from examining the remains of fetuses that died of multiple anomalies
- The muscle arises from the pectoralis major fascia and inserts into the medial brachial fascia
- The chondroepitrochlearis muscle is thought to represent an abnormal insertion of the pectoralis major muscle because of its innervation by the pectoral nerves
- In those rare patients who have this muscle and suffer from restricted range of motion, excision is warranted. As a secondary gain, improved appearance of the axilla should also occur.

Subscapularis-teres-latissimus Muscle (Fig. 23.93)

- This anomalous muscle arises from the lateral border of the scapula, subscapularis or latissimus dorsi and inserts into the lesser tuberosity with the tendon of the subscapularis
- The muscle may be responsible for compression of the brachial plexus in the axilla
- However, no reports of the clinical importance of this muscle have been published.

Coracoclaviculosternal Muscle (Fig. 23.94)

- A single case was reported, describes a muscle originating at the tip of the coracoid and inserting into the anterior clavicular facet
- The patient was asymptomatic.

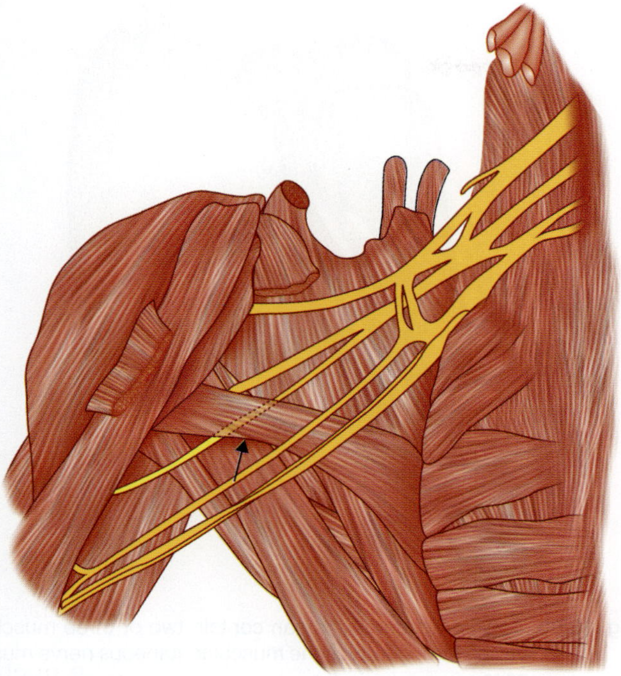

Fig. 23.93: The subscapularis-teres-latissimus muscle (arrow) penetrates the brachial plexus and can lie on top of the axillary, lower subscapular, thoracodorsal or radial nerves

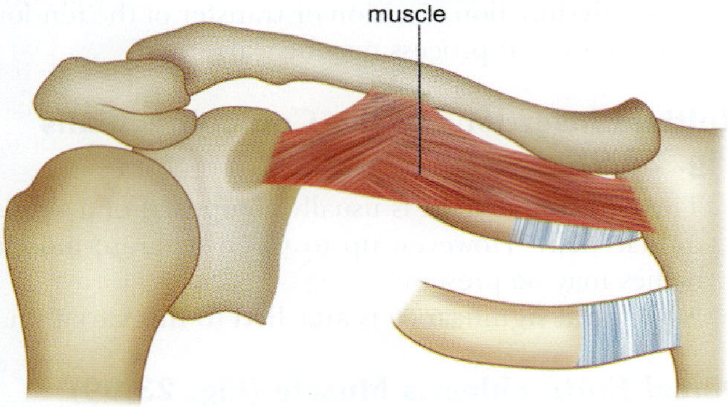

Fig. 23.94: The coracoclaviculosternal muscle originates from the anterior margin of the coracoid process and inserts into the clavicular facet of the sternum

Deltoid Muscle Contracture

- Fibrosis and subsequent contracture of the deltoid most commonly follow intramuscular injection
- Numerous drugs have been implicated
- A rarer condition is a development of a deltoid contraction without an antecedent history of injection
- In either case, range of motion does not improve greatly with physical therapy

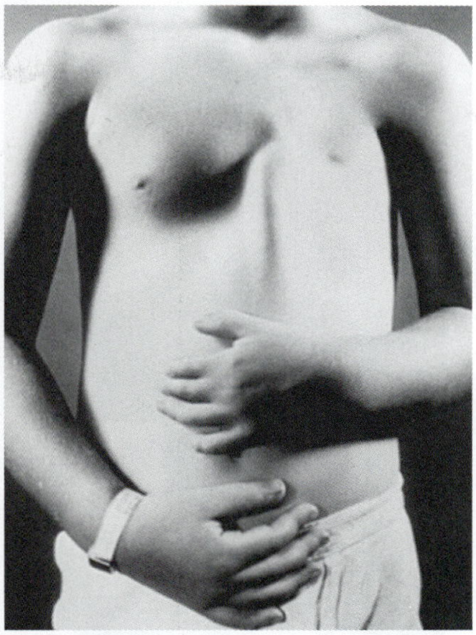

Fig. 23.95: A typical patient with Poland's syndrome

- Surgery is indicated for patients who have an abduction contracture greater than 25° and have experienced progressive deformity
- Release of the fibrotic bands with or without transfer of the posterior deltoid has been recommended.

Poland's Syndrome (Figs 23.95 and 23.96)

- Absence of the pectoralis major muscle causes relatively little disability
- The remnant pectoralis major tendon can form an axillary web that can limit shoulder motion
- Excision of the aberrant tendon and Z-plasty lengthening can greatly benefit a patient in this instance
- The term Poland's syndrome should be reserved for patients with an absent pectoralis major and ipsilateral syndactyly
- The underlying ribs, fascia or breast might also be abnormally formed
- Breast reconstruction may be of cosmetic benefit for female patients
- Shoulder dysfunction is unusual unless it is associated with an axillary web, but associated conditions are common.

Pectoralis Minor Insertion into the Humerus (Fig. 23.97)

- The pectoralis minor usually inserts onto the coracoid process.
- However, it occasionally passes the coracoid process, travels with the coracohumeral ligament and inserts onto the humeral head.

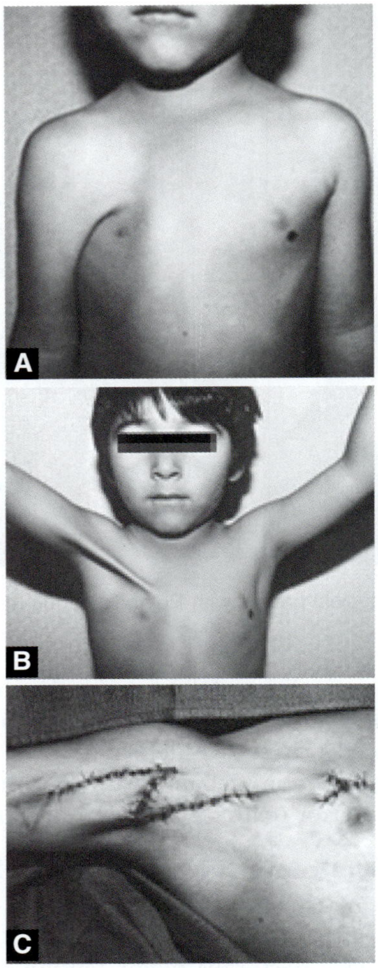

Figs 23.96A to C: (A) This boy has an axillary fold contracture; (B) The axillary fold limited abduction and extension of the shoulder; (C) The contracture was easily corrected by excising the fibrous remnant and closing with a Z-plasty

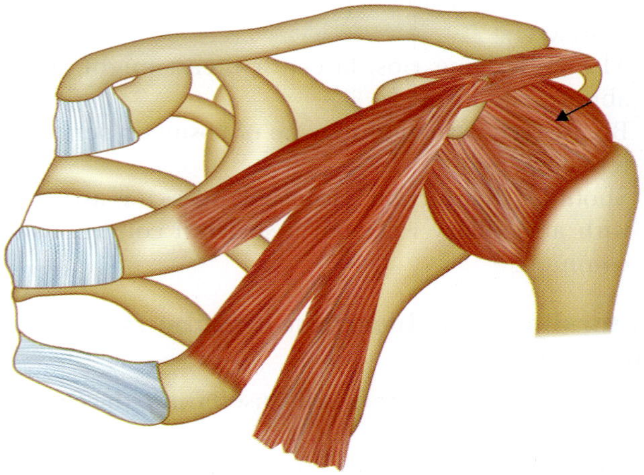

Fig. 23.97: The tendon of the pectoralis minor can pass over the coracoid process and insert into the humeral head (arrow). A bursa can form under the tendon and cause an impingement syndrome

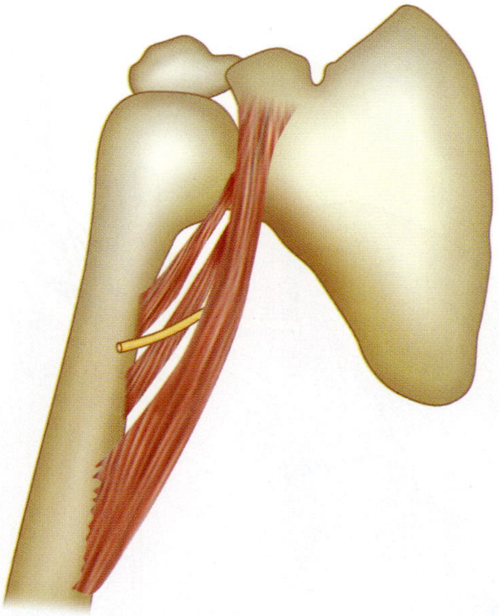

Fig. 23.98: The coracobrachialis can contain two or three muscle bellies through which the musculocutaneous nerve must pass

- The abnormal slip has been identified as a site of compression for neurovascular structures, as well as a possible cause of impingement.
- When the pectoralis minor inserts abnormally and causes dysfunction, excision or transfer of the tendon to the coracoid process may be warranted.

Multiple Insertions of the Coracobrachialis (Fig. 23.98)

- The coracobrachialis is usually composed of a single muscle belly. However, up to three separate muscle bellies may be present.
- No clinical significance is attached to this variation.

Dorsal Epitrochlearis Muscle (Fig. 23.99)

- The latissimus dorsi muscle often has an associated muscle that originates from the tendon of the latissimus dorsi and inserts into the brachial and forearm fascia, the humerus and the lateral epicondyle.
- In contrast to the chondroepitrochlearis muscle, the dorsal epitrochlearis muscle is innervated by the radial nerve and occurs in 18 to 20 percent of people.
- No clinical significance has been identified for this muscle.

Axillopectoral Muscle (Fig. 23.100)

- Langer's armbogen, Langer's arm arch and axillopectoral muscle are names attributed to the anomalous portion of the latissimus dorsi

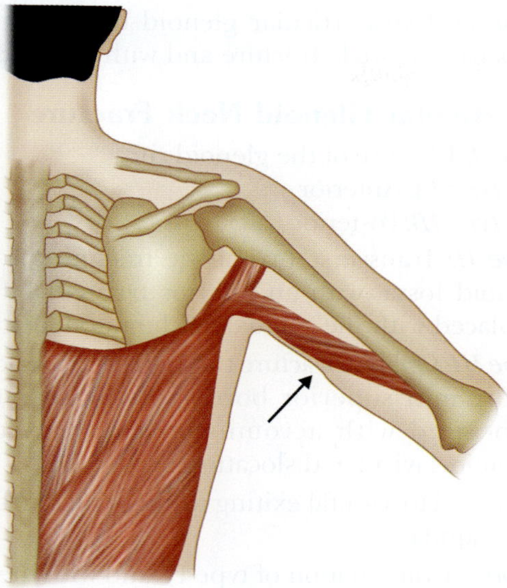

Fig. 23.99: The dorsal epitrochlearis muscle (arrow) originates from the tendon of the latissimus dorsi and inserts onto the brachial and forearm fascia, the humerus, the lateral epicondyle, and the olecranon

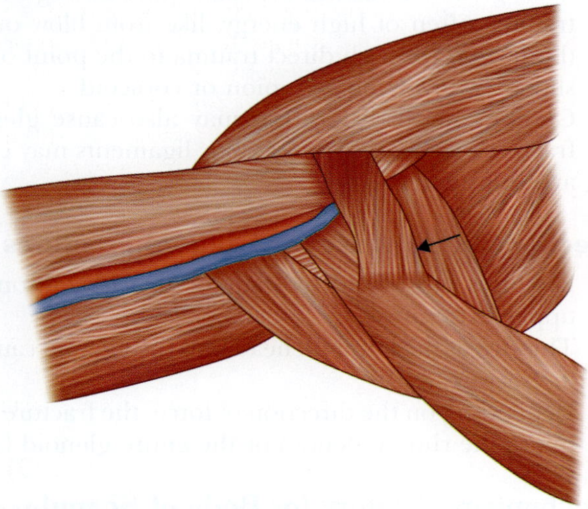

Fig. 23.100: The axillopectoral muscle (arrow) extends from the latissimus dorsi and inserts into the pectoralis major. It overlies the neurovascular bundle in the axilla

- The slip of the latissimus dorsi courses along the inferior border of the axilla and inserts into the pectoralis major muscle
- The muscle, which becomes tight with abduction and external rotation, overlies the neurovascular structures in the axilla
- The muscle is innervated by the pectoral nerve
- The anomaly occurs in 4 to 7.7 percent of the population and is usually asymptomatic.

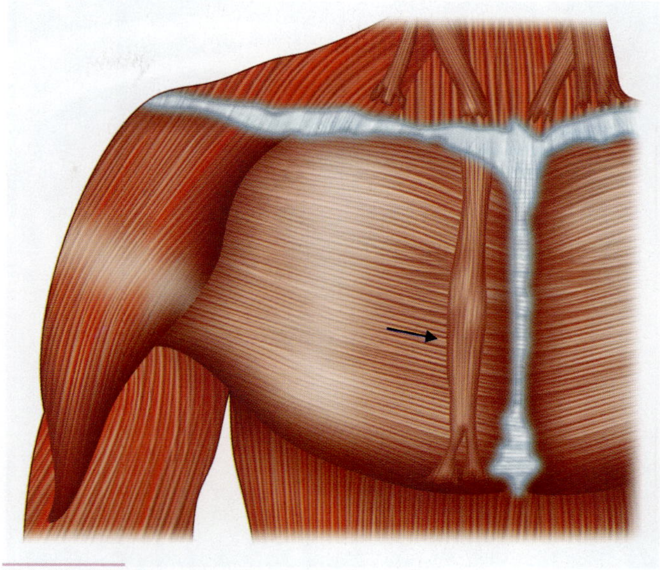

Fig. 23.101: The sternalis muscle (arrow)

Sternalis Muscle (Fig. 23.101)

- The sternalis is a long thin muscle that extends from the sternocleidomastoid to the rectus abdominis along the sternum
- The muscle is superficial and medial to the pectoralis major muscle
- The sternalis is twice as commonly unilateral as bilateral and occurs equally in male and female patients.

FRACTURES AROUND SHOULDER AND EPIPHYSEAL INJURIES

Introduction

Fractures in children involve proximal humeral epiphysis. They are mostly managed by closed reduction and conservative measures and sometimes by open reduction. Fractures around shoulder are common injuries and occur in all age groups.

Classification

- Fractures of scapula
- Fractures of clavicle
- Fractures of the proximal humerus.

Fractures of Scapula (Fig. 23.102)

Injury to the scapula is rare because it is well protected by multiple layers of muscle and other soft-tissues. Only 1 percent of all fractures involve scapula. However, when scapular injuries occur, they are almost certainly a result

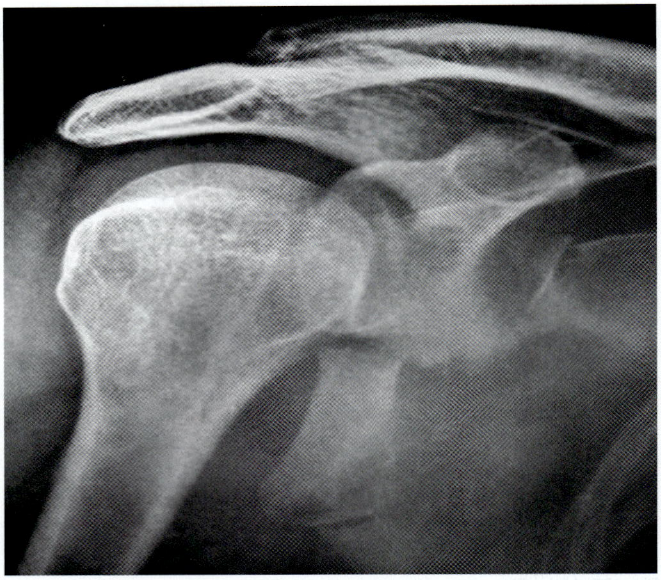

Fig. 23.102: X-ray showing fractured scapula

of high energy trauma and may be associated with significant injuries to other major organ systems. Therefore, all children with apparently isolated scapular fractures should be evaluated for the presence of potentially life-threatening visceral injuries that require further intervention.

■ Classification of Fractures of Scapula

Idenberg's Classification

Fractures of the scapula are described by anatomic area for ease of discussion, i.e. body and spine, glenoid (scapular) neck, intra-articular glenoid, coracoid and acromion. The neck and the body are the most commonly involved areas. Skull fractures may also occur.

Acromial Fracture

- *Type I:* Minimally displaced
- *Type II:* Displaced but does not reduce subacromial space
- *Type III:* Displaced with narrowing of the subacromial space.

Coracoid Fracture

- *Type I:* Fracture proximal to coracoclavicular ligaments
- *Type II:* Fracture distal to coracoclavicular ligaments.

Extra-articular Glenoid Neck Fracture

- *Type I:* Extra-articular glenoid neck fracture without associated clavicle fracture or acromioclavicular (AC) separation
- *Type II:* Extra-articular glenoid neck fracture with associated clavicle fracture and with AC separation.

Intra-articular Glenoid Neck Fracture

- *Type I:* Fracture of the glenoid rim
  - *Type IA:* Anterior
  - *Type IB:* Posterior
- *Type II:* Transverse or oblique fracture through the glenoid fossa, with an inferior triangular fragment displaced with the subluxated humeral head
- *Type III:* Oblique fracture through the glenoid, exiting at the mid superior border of the scapula,often associated with acromioclavicular fracture or acromioclavicular dislocation
- *Type IV:* Horizontal exiting through medial border of the scapula
- *Type V:* Combination of type IV and with the fracture separating the inferior half of glenoid
- *Type VI:* Severe communition of the glenoid surface.

Mechanism of Injury for Scapular Fracture

- The scapula is subject to indirect injury, through axial loading on the outstretched arm, involving scapular neck, glenoid and intra-articular space through direct trauma, often of high energy, like from blow or fall (body) and through direct trauma to the point of the shoulder, involving acromion or coracoid
- Glenohumeral dislocation may also cause glenoid fracture. Traction by muscles or ligaments may cause avulsion injuries.

Mechanism of Injury for Glenoid Fractures

- Fractures of glenoid typically occur with fall on the upper extremity
- This drives the humeral head into the glenoid causing its fracture
- Depending on the direction of force, the fracture may injure the rim of glenoid or the entire glenoid fossa.

Mechanism of Injury for Body of Scapula

- Fractures of the body of scapula occur via direct impact or avulsion mechanisms
- The direct impact mechanism is typically of high energy and rarely an isolated injury
- The avulsion type fractures may occur at any point of the several muscle attachments on the scapula
- Child abuse must be excluded as a cause for scapular injury when no clear traumatic cause is evident.

Signs and Symptoms of Fractured Scapula

- The typical presentation is with the arm held adducted against chest wall and protected from all movements, abduction is specially painful
- Local tenderness is present

- With a displaced scapular neck or acromial fracture, the shoulder may appear flattened
- Ecchymosis is less than what might be expected from the degree of bony injury present, especially compared, with the fracture of the upper humerus
- With deep inspiration, pain may be caused by the pull of attached muscles with a coracoid fracture (pectoralis minor) or due to body fracture (serratus anterior)
- The clinician should always be aware of the possibility of an associated pneumothorax either, immediate or delayed
- With body fractures especially, deep swelling may be quite painful, producing, "pseudorupture of the rotator cuff"
- In this syndrome, there is weak rotator cuff function and loss of active arm elevation, which is probably due only to inhibition of muscle contractions from intramuscular hemorrhage, it usually resolves within few weeks
- This syndrome can be differentiated from a true rotator cuff tear by identifying the fracture radiographically and noting that swelling present with this pseudorupture syndrome exceeds that normally seen with a cuff tear.

Associated Injuries (Fig. 23.103)

- Pneumothorax, ipsilateral rib fractures, etc.
- Pulmonary contusion can be present, which is a life-threatening problem
- Fracture clavicle is frequently present with glenoid or glenoid neck
- Brachial plexus injury, which is usually a supraclavicular type with poor prognosis.

Treatment

- Most scapular fractures are treated by supporting the upper extremity in a sling and by providing an early active motion
- Open reduction with or without internal fixation is rarely required for fractures of the scapula
- Computed tomography (CT scan) is often necessary for accurate assesment of these injuries

Following fractures of scapula require open reduction and internal fixation:

Fractures of the Acromion and Lateral Scapular Spine

Significantly displaced fractures of the acromion and lateral scapular spine, with retraction of the fragment and encroachment on the subacromial space. These fractures are extremely rare.

If the subacromial space is significantly compromised, causing impingement of the tuberosities during abduction, open reduction and internal fixation using K-wires or screws and plates may be indicated.

Fractures of Coracoid with Acromioclavicular Separation

When fracture of coracoid occurs with dislocation of outer end of clavicle, open reduction internal fixation (ORIF) of coracoid with screw or heavy suture and repair of acromioclavicular ligament should be done.

Glenoid Rim Fractures (Figs 23.104 to 23.107)

They are generally associated with traumatic dislocation of the shoulder. If a glenoid rim fracture involves one fourth of the articulating surface, open reduction and

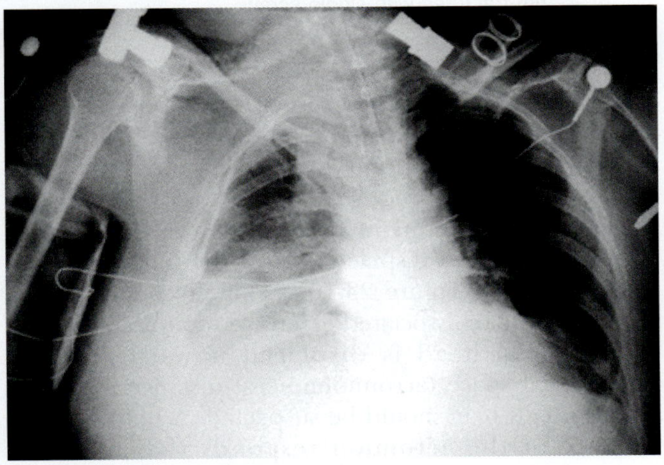

Fig. 23.103: Radiograph of multiple trauma patient with a fractured scapular neck, associated upper extremity fractures and pulmonary contusion

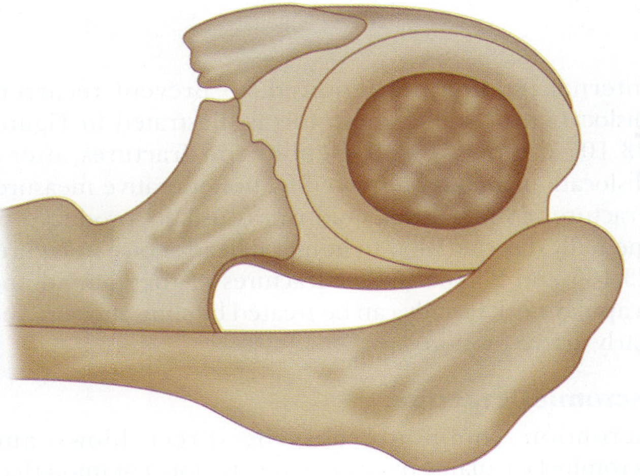

Fig. 23.104: Fracture of anterior glenoid rim

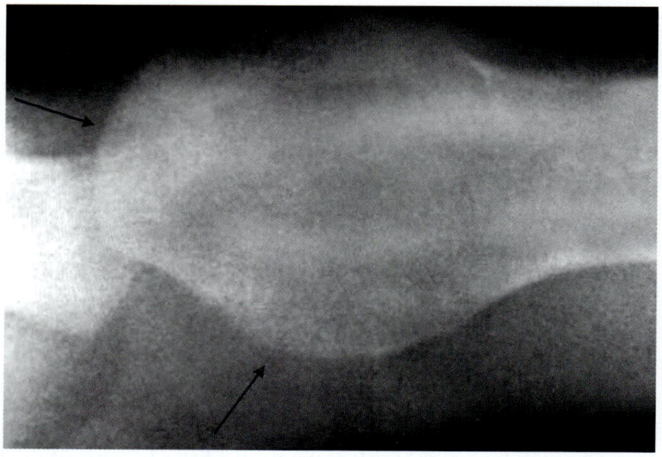

Fig. 23.105: Large anterior glenoid rim fractures with associated posterior Hill-Sachs lesion (arrows)

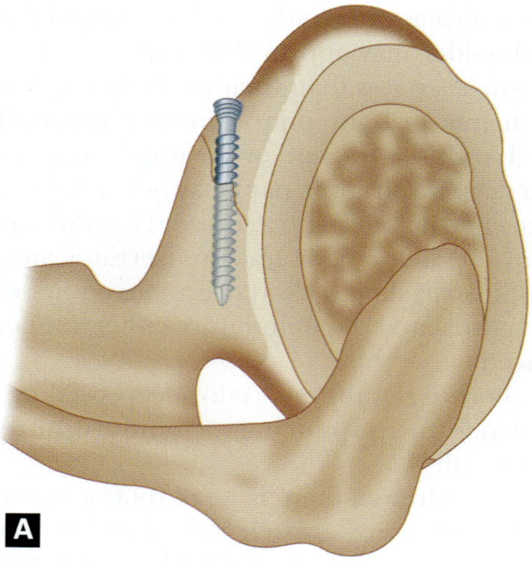

A

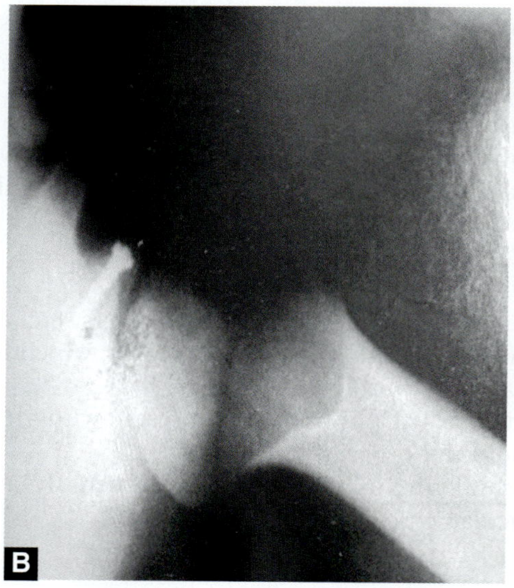

B

Figs 23.107A and B: Open reduction and internal fixation of glenoid rim fractures with single screw

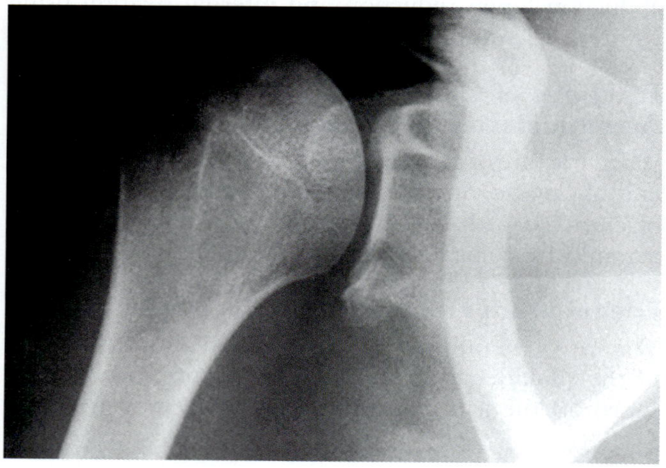

Fig. 23.106: Anteroposterior (AP) view of the glenoid showing an anteroinferior glenoid fracture

internal fixation are required, to prevent recurrent dislocation or subluxation, this is illustrated in Figures 23.107A and B. Small glenoid rim fractures after a dislocation should be treated by nonoperative measures Fracture of anterior glenoid rim is usually produced by medially directed blow to humeral head shown in Figures 23.105 and 23.106. Other fractures of the glenoid and scapular neck usually can be treated by sling support and early active motion.

Acromial Fracture

Acromion commonly absorbs direct blows and acromioclavicular separation is much more common than the fracture of the acromion. Most acromial fractures are minimally displaced. Commonly the fracture line is little lateral to acromioclavicular joint, causing confusion with os acromiale. The fractured base of acromion is well seen on a true (tangential) scapular lateral view. A displaced acromial fracture is a candidate for an open reduction (Fig. 23.108).

Another mechanism of an acromial fracture is traumatic superior displacement of the humeral head, this is shown in Figure 23.109. This mechanism often also results in an associated extensive rotator cuff tear. If the humeral head is displaced upward into the subacromial space (acromiohumeral distance reduced), a rotator cuff tear should be suspected. A nondisplaced fracture of the acromion responds well to initial symptomatic treatment and the use of the sling for three weeks. Displaced fractures require reduction and fixation with tension band wire technique or screws to eliminate impingement or to reduce the acromioclavicular joint.

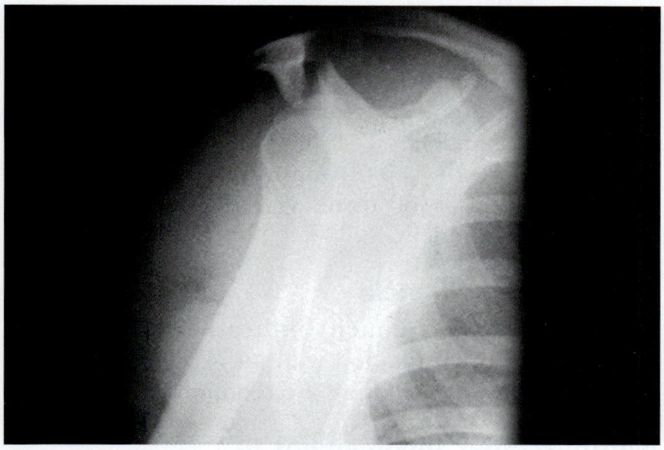

Fig. 23.108: A displaced acromial fracture

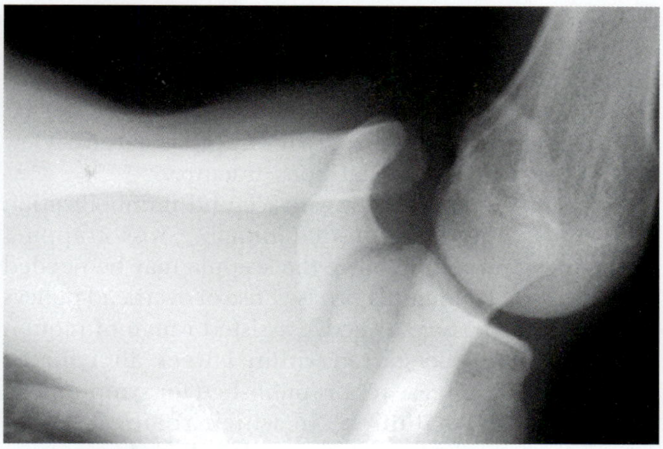

Fig. 23.110: Stryker notch view, showing fracture of the base of coracoid

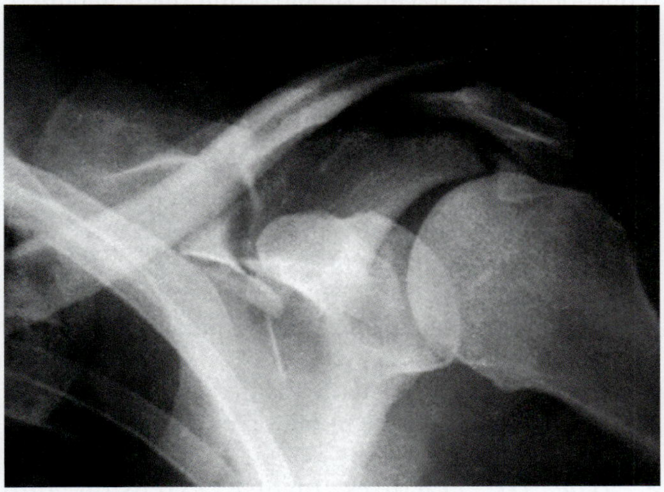

Fig. 23.109: Superior displacement of the humeral head due to some trauma

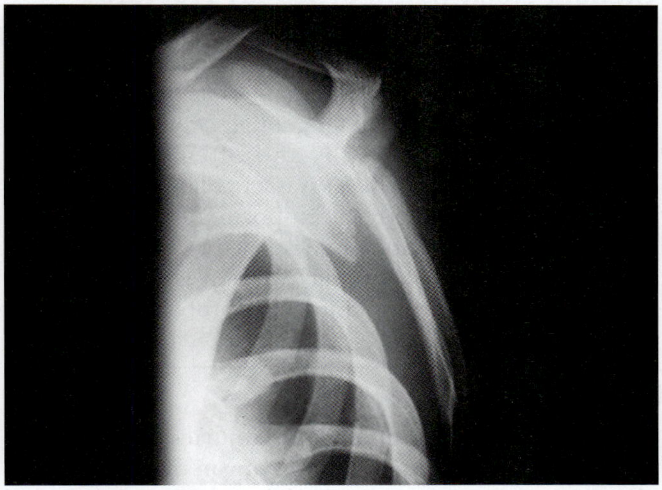

Fig. 23.111: X-ray of scapular lateral view showing displaced scapular body fracture

Coracoid Fracture

Fractures of the coracoid may be isolated, occuring from direct blow to it or to the point of the shoulder. Coracoid fracture may also occur in association with acromioclavicular dislocation. The coracoid tip may be avulsed by muscle pull of the biceps and coracobrachialis or from direct contact from a dislocating humeral head. A fracture of the base of coracoid is best seen on Stryker notch view shown in Figure 23.110.

Coracoid fracture occurs most commonly through the coracoid base and is minimaly displaced unless significant acromioclavicular separation occurs. For an isolated coracoid fracture no specific treatment is needed because anatomic alignment is not essential for either of adequate function or healing.

Indications for Surgery with Coracoid Fracture

- For a displaced coracoid fracture with third degree acromioclavicular separation, acromioclavicular fixation should be done
- If there is obstruction to the reduction of anterior shoulder dislocation
- Displaced fracture of coracoid involving the glenoid fossa
- In third degree acromioclavicular separation asociated with coracoid fracture is an indication for open reduction and threaded steinmann pin fixation of the acromioclavicular joint.

Scapular Body Fracture (Fig. 23.111)

Direct violence and sudden contraction of divergent muscles may cause fractures of the body of the scapula.

Other causes include electrical shock treatments and seizures. In the immediate treatment of these fractures, no reduction is attempted. Restoration of the normal bony anatomy is not necessary for good function in a healed scapular body fracture. A true scapular lateral view showing displaced scapular body fracture.

Symptomatic treatment with ice and immobilization for comfort is all that is needed initially. Cross strapping with adhesive, to immobilize the scapula may be needed in some cases. Pendulum exercises, use of overhead pulleys and a further passive or active assisted range of motion program should be started within 1 week after injury. Earlier there was a case report published for symptomatic scapular body malunion, in which removal of rib prominences and portion of scapula relieved symptoms and improved range of motion. Operative fixation with bone graft has been reported in some cases of nonunion.

Glenoid Neck (Extra-articular) Fracture

A fracture of the neck of scapula is the second most common pattern of scapular fracture, occuring from direct trauma, a fall on the point of shoulder, or a fall on the outstreched hand. True AP, tangential scapular lateral and axillary lateral radiographs and often CT scans are necessary to confirm the extra-articular nature of the fracture and verify the reduced position of the humeral head. Reduction of scapular neck fracture and restoration of the glenoid to its anatomic position is not necessary. Sling immobilization for comfort is probably enough.

■ Fracture Clavicle

One of the most common bony injuries, which rarely requires an open reduction. Mechanism of injury: Direct blow and fall on outstreched hand. Mostly treated conservatively.

May require ORIF in following cases:
- Nonunion
- Neurovascular involvement
- Fracture of lateral end near the acromioclavicular joint in an adult
- Persistent wide separation of the fragments with interposition of soft tissue
- Floating shoulder.

Nonunion of Clavicle

This is the most frequent indication for an open reduction. Internal fixation with an intramedullary pin or a plate and bone grafting are required.

Neurovascular Involvement in Fractured Clavicle

Neurovasular compromise not easily resolved by reduction of the fracture. It requires an immediate open reduction and the fracture should be internally stabilized, if open reduction is done.

Fracture of the Lateral End of Clavicle Near the Acromioclavicular Joint in an Adult

Neer's Classification of Clavicle Fractures

- Neer identified five types of lateral clavicular fractures
- *Type I:* Is minimally displaced and lateral to coracoacromial ligament
- *Type IIA:* Unstable lateral clavicular fractures, coracoacromial ligaments and acromioclavicular joint capsule are intact (Fig. 23.112)
- *Type IIB:* Unstable lateral fracture with disruption of coracoacromial ligament but acromioclavicular joint capsule is intact (Fig. 23.113)
- *Type III:* Fractures involve extension into acromioclavicular joint

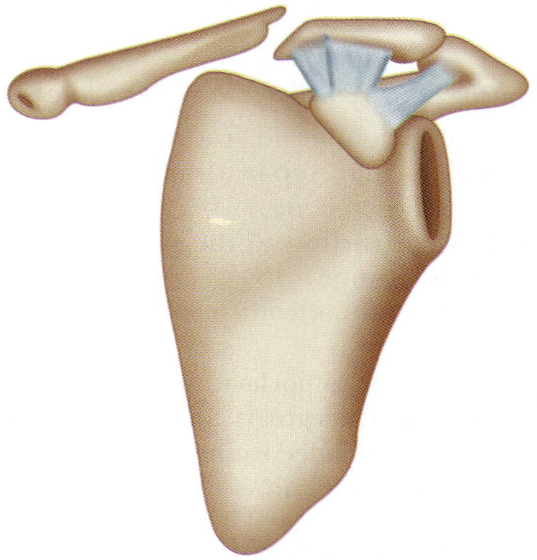

Fig. 23.112: Neer's type IIA, unstable lateral clavicle fracture. Coracoacromial ligaments and joint capsule are intact

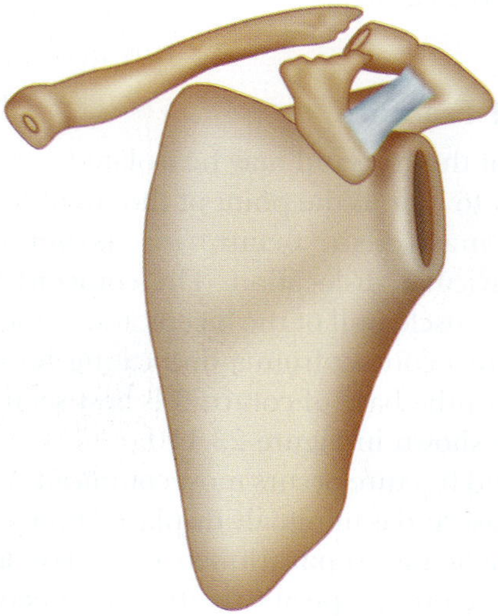

Fig. 23.113: Type IIB unstable lateral fracture with disruption of coracoacromial ligament. Acromioclavicular joint capsule is intact

- *Type IV:* Fractures involve a distal fracture with periosteal sleeve disruption
- *Type V:* Fractures are similar to type II fractures and involve an avulsion, leaving only an inferior cortical fragment attached to the coracoclavicular ligaments.

Surgical Techniques used for Displaced Lateral Clavicular Fractures

- Plate and screw fixation for more medial fractures
- Transacromial K-wires and tension band wires
- Horizontal figure of eight wires or polydioxanone suture (PDS), ethicon.
- Single transacromial Knowles pin.
- Coracoclavicular ligament reconstruction with mersilene tape, dacron arterial graft material, or PDS bands.
- Internal fixation of a fracture is often combined with coracoclavicular ligament reconstruction to improve the chances of good result.

Floating Shoulder

Fracture of the clavicle and surgical neck of scapula make the scapular fractures unstable. The weight of the arm and shoulder girdle muscles that insert into the proximal humerus rotate the glenoid fragment anteromedially. In this case open reduction and internal fixation of clavicular fractures with a 3.5 mm plate and screws to prevent malunion of the scapular fracture and drooping of shoulder is recommended. This can be illustrated in Figures 23.114A to D.

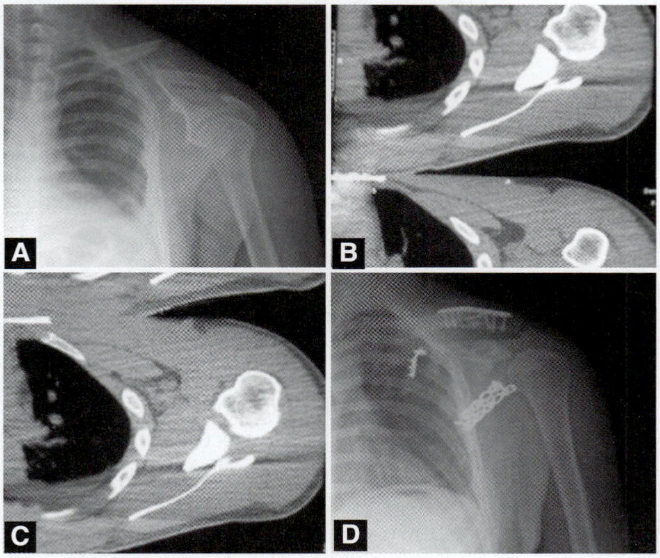

Figs 23.114A to D: X-ray and CT scan images of floating shoulders —(A) Widely displaced floating shoulder injury; (B and C) CT scans showing anteromedial displacement of glenoid fragment; (D) Clavicular and scapular fractures after repair

Intramedullary compression clavicular nail used for widely displaced middle-third of clavicle as shown in Figure 23.115. For intramedullary fixation of the clavicle, the pin must be strong enough to withstand unsupported weight of the upper extremity without bending or breaking. It should be threaded or lateral end should be bent to 90° to prevent medial migration to vital structures.

Rockwood developed an intramedullary clavicular nail with a lateral compression nut. When tightened, the nut allows compression across the fracture site. Precontoured clavicle plate, which is used for widely displaced middle-third clavicle fractures as illustrated in Figure 23.116.

Intramedullary Fixation of Clavicle

- Over the fracture site make a 2.5 cm long incision
- Pass steinman pin of 3.2 mm into the medial fragment
- Remove the pin and pass it laterally into the lateral fragment to emerge in till conoid tubercle

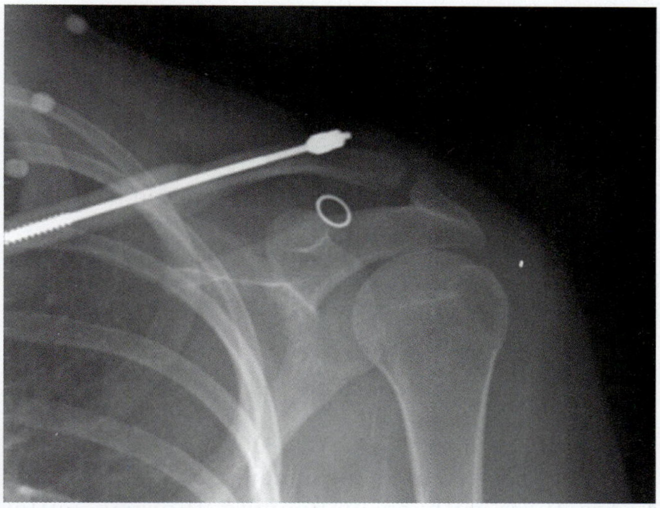

Fig. 23.115: Intramedullary compression clavicular nail used for reducing widely displaced middle-third of clavicle

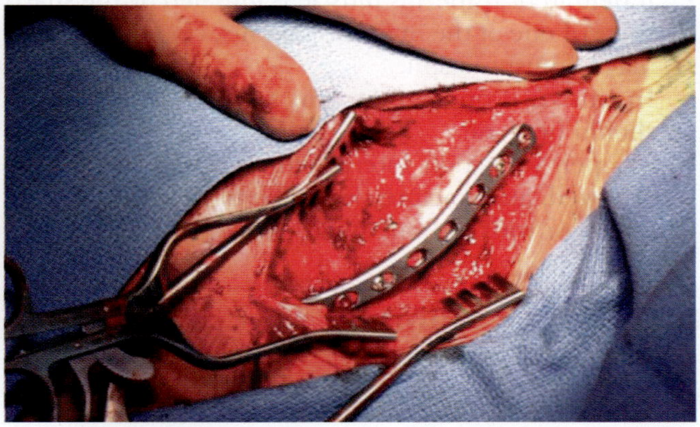

Fig. 23.116: Precontoured clavicle plate, used for widely displaced middle-third clavicle fractures

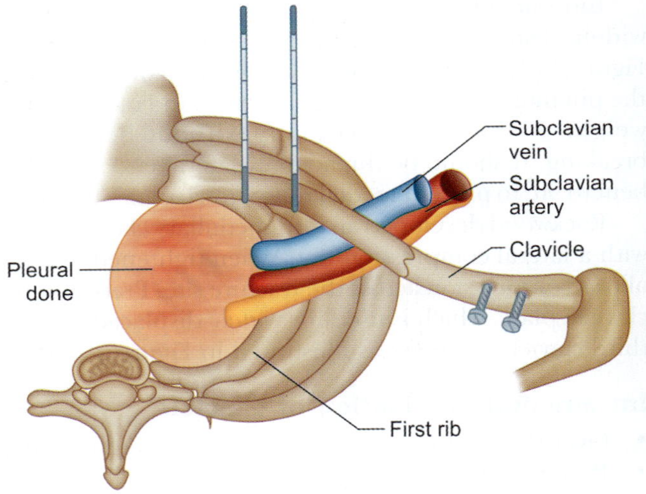

Fig. 23.117: Pin fixation in external fixation of clavicle

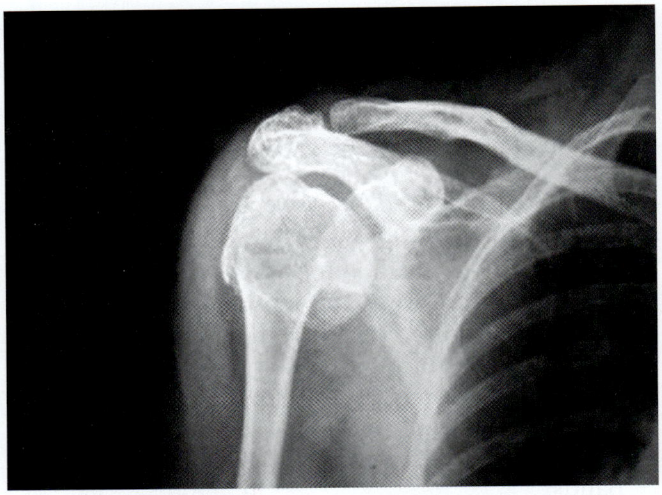

Fig. 23.118: X-ray depicting proximal humeral fracture

- Now take a threaded steinman pin and drill it retrogressively into the lateral fragment.
- Reduce the fracture and drill the pin into the medial fragment.
- Alternatively 2 mm K-wires can be used.
- Method of pin fixation in case of external fixation of clavicle fractures is depicted in Figure 23.117.

Indications for External Fixation in Clavicle Fractures

- Open fractures
- Closed fractures with major displacement and overlying skin damage.
- Multiple trauma
- Painful delayed union or nonunion
- Fractures with accompanying thoracic outlet syndrome.
- A persistent wide separation of the fragments with interposition of soft tissue.
- If deltoid or trapezius muscle is impaled by the sharp spike of one of the major fragments, closed reduction may be unsuccessful.
- In this case open reduction and internal fixation should be done.
- At open reduction interposed soft tissue should be removed, and fracture should be fixed with plates or screws or with intramedullary pins.

■ Proximal Humeral Fractures (Fig. 23.118)

Pathomechanics

Most fractures of the proximal humerus are a result of indirect force, such as a fall on the outstreched hand rather than a direct blow to the shoulder. The origin of a proximal humeral fracture is due to combination of factors, which include relatively osteoporotic bone (in the elderly), direct contact against the adjacent acromion or glenoid rim and forceful pull of the rotator cuff muscles and extrinsic muscles, such as the pectoralis major. The muscular pull of adjacent tendon attachments on humeral fracture fragments, determines the patterns of displacement, as shown in Figure 23.119.

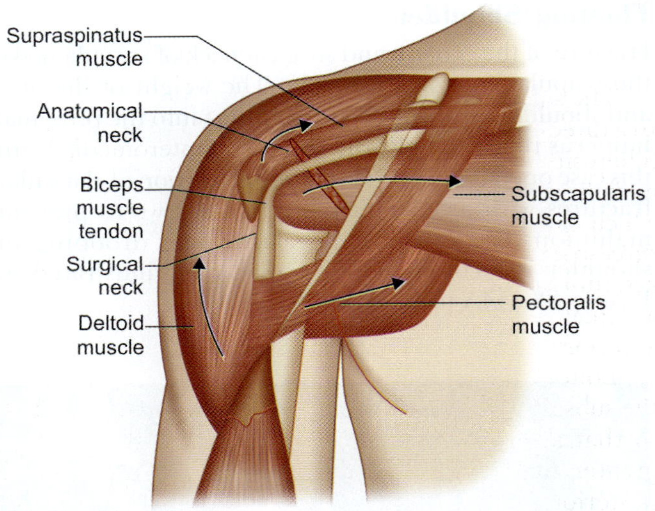

Fig. 23.119: Muscular pull of adjacent tendon attachments on humeral fracture fragments, determines the patterns of displacement as shown by the arrows

The pectoralis major pulls the humeral shaft anteriorly and medially. The supraspinatus and infraspinatus pull the greater tuberosity posterosuperiorly, depending on the integrity of their tendinous insertion. Displacement of the fracture fragments depends on the pull of the muscles of rotator cuff and pectoralis major.

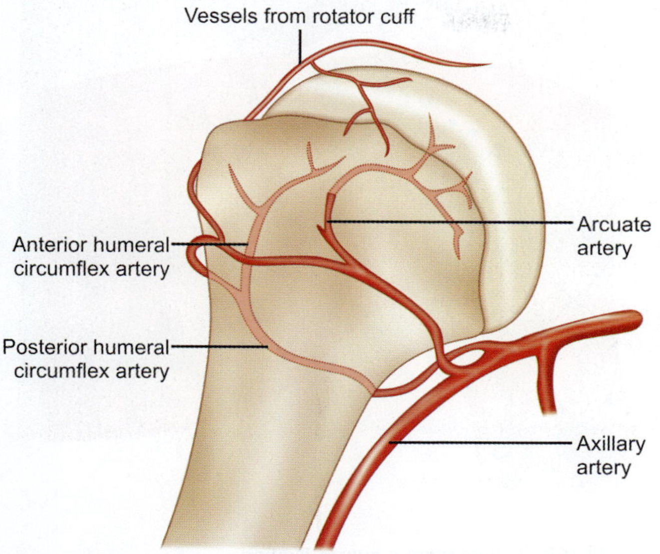

Fig. 23.120: Blood supply of the humeral head

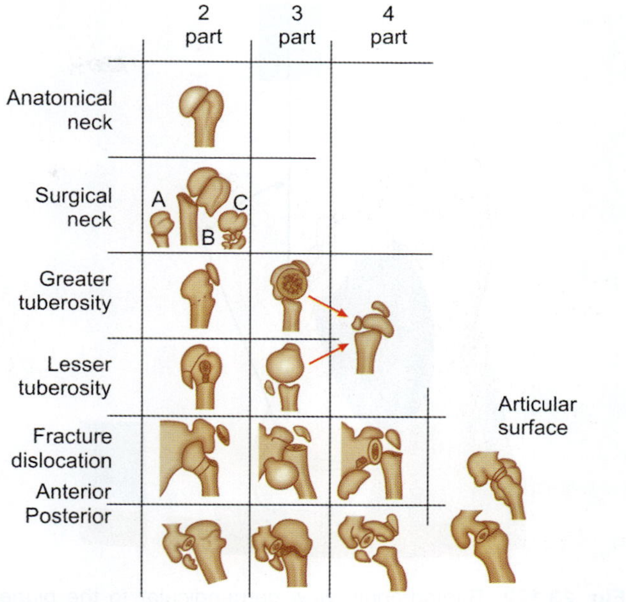

Fig. 23.121: Neer's terminology of four segment classification of displaced fractures

The subscapularis pulls the lesser tuberosity medially. In a three-part fracture with the displacement of the lesser tuberosity, the humeral head will be externally rotated away from the glenoid by the pull of greater tuberosity, which remains attached to the articular segment. Top three-part fracture with greater tuberosity remaining intact, supraspinatus and infraspinatus externally rotate the articular fragment, so that articular segment is oriented anteriorly and lesser tuberosity is displaced medially.

Bottom three-part fracture with lesser tuberosity intact, the subscapularis internally rotates the articular segment so that articular segment is oriented posteriorly. The greater tuberosity fragment is pulled superiorly and posteriorly.

Classification

Classification is based on four-part anatomy of proximal humerus:

1. The humeral head
2. The lesser tuberosity
3. The greater tuberosity
4. The proximal humeral shaft.

Criteria for displacement: Greater than 1 cm of separation of a part or angulation of 45°. Osteonecrosis is most likely after displaced four-part fractures (Fig. 23.120).

Neer's Classification of Proximal Humeral Fractures (Fig. 23.121)

He described the fracture can be two part, three-part or four-part. He also described the key segment displaced in each two pattern, segment named is one which is displaced. Two-part surgical neck fractures can be:

- Impacted
- Unimpacted
- Comminuted

All three-part patterns have displacement of the shaft segment. In four-part pattern, all segments are displaced. Fracture dislocations are identified by the anterior or posterior position of articular segment. Large articular surface defects require separate recognition.

Signs and Symptoms

- In most cases of proximal humeral fractures, there is significant swelling and pain. It may be associated with ecchymosis
- As the swelling subsides over the first 2 to 4 weeks, ecchymosis changes from the classic blue bruising to green and then yellow and may move distally down the arm
- Patients may occasionally note tingling or numbness in the extremity, which may be related to brachial plexus stretch.

Physical Findings

Intially other injuries of the neck or chest wall should be excluded, since this association is common with proximal humeral fractures, especially if high energy trauma, such as motor vehicle accident has occurred. Neurovascular evaluation is the next step.

Radiographic Evaluation

Special radiographic view perpendicular to the plane of scapula, to show glenohumeral joint in profile, as illustrated in Figure 23.122.

Radiographic view parallel to the plane of scapula is taken to show anterior and posterior displacement.

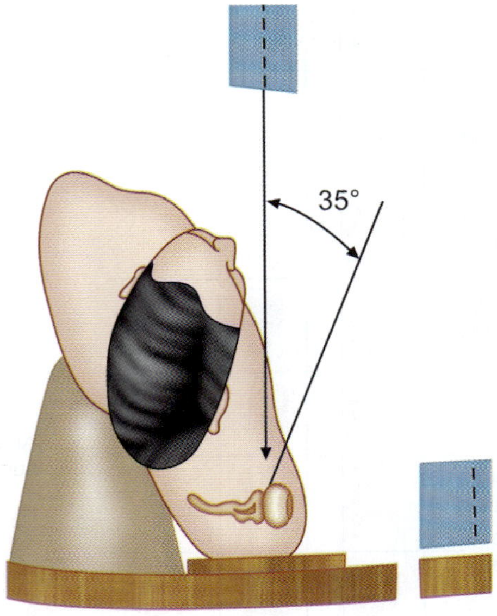

Fig. 23.122: Radiographic view perpendicular to the plane of scapula

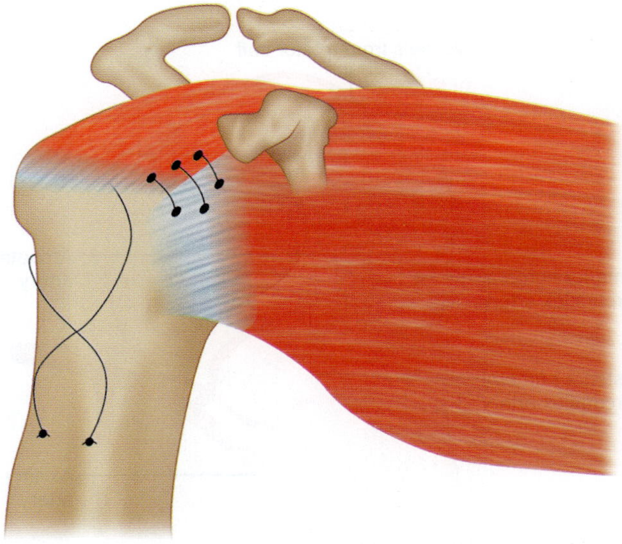

Fig. 23.123: Transosseous suture fixation

Nonoperative Treatment

- Nonoperative treatment can obtain a functional and painless extremity, in most proximal humeral fractures.
- The range of motion of the shoulder joint accommodates moderate angular deformity without significant functional loss.
- Neer described acceptable angulation as less than 45° and less than 1 cm of displacement.
- The first step in treatment decision making is to determine, if displacement and angulation are acceptable for a particular patient.
- The second step is to determine, if humeral head and shaft move as a unit.
- If both of these conditions are present, then fracture is stable and is in an acceptable position.
- A sling is used for comfort, and a physical therapy regimen with pendulum exercises is started.
- If humeral head and shaft do not move as a unit, physical therapy can be delayed for 2 to 4 weeks, in patients who are poor surgical candidates.
- In young active patients, early operative fixation should be considered.

Operative Treatment

Indications

- Displaced two-part surgical neck fractures
- Displaced (>5 mm) greater tuberosity fracture.
- Displaced three-part fractures
- Displaced four-part fractures in young patients.

Types of Fixation

- Transosseous suture fixation
- Percutaneous pinning
- Intramedullary nailing
- Type of fixation depends on patient's age, activity level, bone quality, the fracture type and associated fractures.

Transosseous suture fixation (Figs 23.123 and 23.124)

Exellent results have been obtained in patients with two part and three part proximal humeral fractures treated with suture fixation. Transosseous nonabsorbable sutures incorporate rotator cuff to increase fixation and help control tuberosity fragments. This has been illustrated in Figure 23.124.

The use of strong nonabsorbable suture provides the advantage of incorporating the rotator cuff insertion to increase fixation in patients with poor bone quality. The level of soft-tissue dissection is not extensive, and osteonecrosis is low with these techniques. Since, it is a nonrigid construct, loss of reduction can occur.

Percutaneous pinning (Fig. 23.125)

Percutaneous pinning has the advantage of avoiding further damage to the soft tissue envelope blood supply to the humeral head. The procedure is technically challenging, loss of fixation and pin track infections are common complications. Terminally threaded schanz pins and bicortical pins inserted from greater tuberosity to the medial humeral shaft add stability. Percutaneous pinning is contraindicated in fractures with metaphyseal

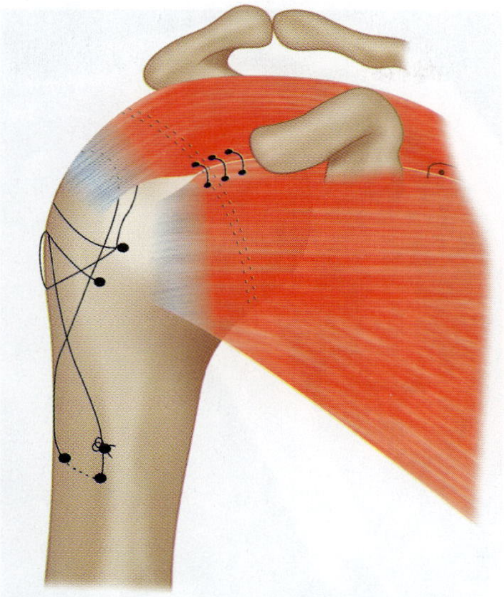

Fig. 23.124: Transosseous nonabsorbable sutures incorporate rotator cuff to increase fixation

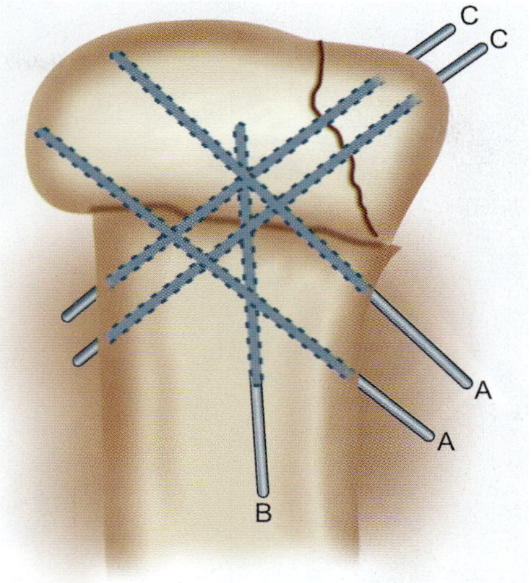

Fig. 23.126: Various methods of placement of percutaneous pins for fracture fixation—A. Two are passed through lateral aspect of the shaft, just above deltoid insertion; B. One is placed through anterior cortex; C. Two pins are inserted retrograde, to reduce and repair this fracture component

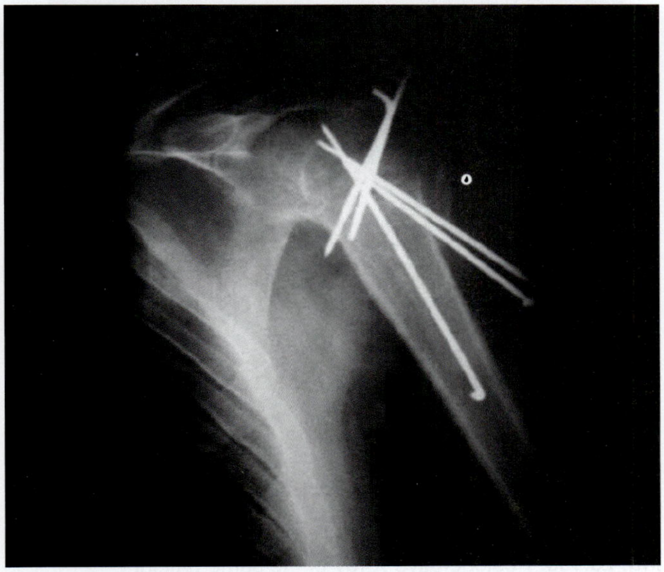

Fig. 23.125: X-ray showing percutaneous pinning: Two part proximal humerus fracture stabilized with pins

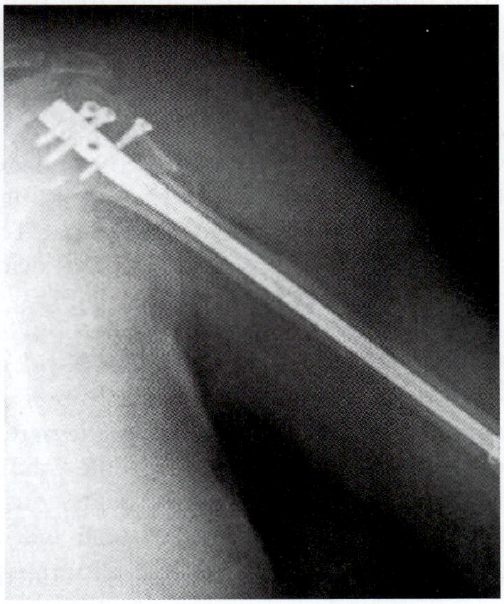

Fig. 23.127: Intramedullary nailing

comminution. Methods of placement of percutaneous pins for fracture fixation shown in Figure 23.126.

Intramedullary nailing (Fig. 23.127)

Intramedullary nailing provides more stable fixation than percutaneous pinning, but less than the locked plate fixation. Insertion of an intramedullary nail into the proximal humerus, violates the rotator cuff. This can lead to postoperative shoulder pain. The advantage of this technique includes preservation of soft tissues.

Plate and Screw Constructs (Fig. 23.128)

This provides the most stable fixation of the three fixation methods. Locked plates add stability, especially in an osteoporotic bone. Open reduction and rigid fixation allows accurate reduction and stabilization of the tuberosities. Historically, plate fixation of the proximal humerus has many complications with malunion and nonunion caused by poor fixation in humeral head.

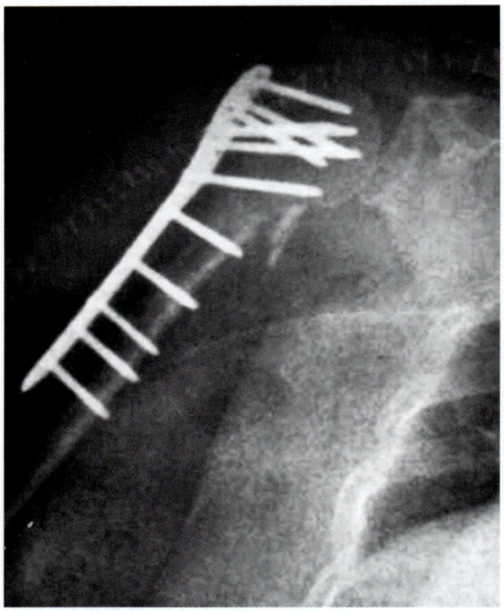

Fig. 23.128: Plate and screw constructs

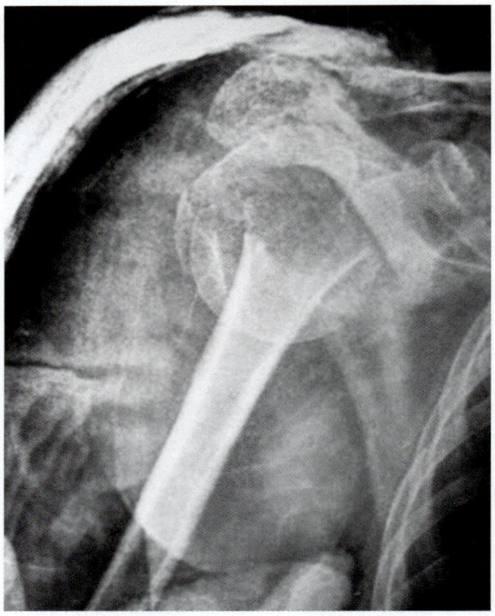

Fig. 23.129: Preoperative X-ray of fractured surgical neck of humerus

Extensive tissue dissection increases the possibility of osteonecrosis of humeral head, leading to a painful and functionally limited shoulder joint. Locked proximal humeral plate is the implant of choice in proximal humeral fractures. Another problem with open reduction and locked plating includes extensive exposure, required for plate application that carries risk of damage to the neurovascular structures, especially the ascending branch of lateral circumflex artery. The most frequent complication of plate fixation is infection and osteonecrosis of humeral head.

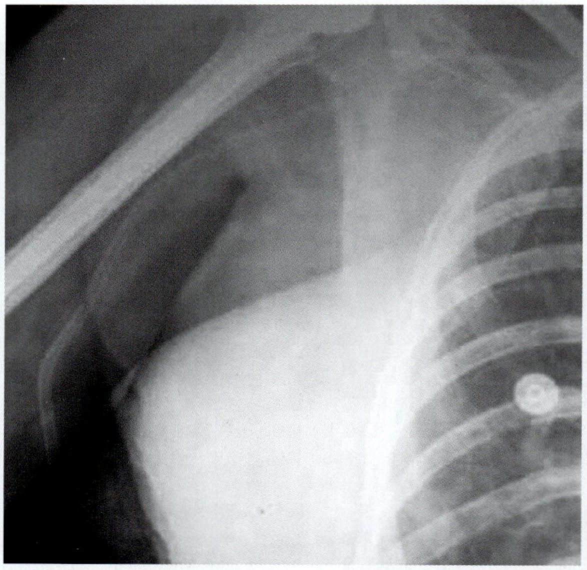

Fig. 23.130: Postoperative X-ray of the same patient

Fixation of Specific Fractures Types (Figs 23.129 and 23.130)

Two parts greater tuberosity fractures: They are treated operatively, when displacement is greater than 1 cm. These fractures are stabilized with transosseous sutures or occasionally with screws in larger fragments.

Two parts surgical neck fractures: Closed reduction and percutaneous pinning have been reported to be successful in fractures that are reducible and are not comminuted. Complicatons such as loss of fixation, pin migration, infection and malunion have made rigid intramedullary nailing the preffered technique. Widely displaced fractures, fractures with comminution and irreducible fractures are stabilized with the locked plate construct. Improved proximal fixation of these systems has increased stability, so that immediate postoperative range of motion is allowed.

Three parts proximal humerus fractures: These fractures in elderly patients with osteopenic bone may require hemiarthroplasty, but for most of these fractures plate fixation is the preffered procedure. The rigid fixation provided with locking plates allows early range of motion which is one of the goals of operative treatment.

Four parts proximal humeral fractures: These fractures treated nonoperatively have poor outcome. Poor bone quality make fixation difficult, vascular insult to the articular surface increases the risk of osteonecrosis of the humeral head. In young active patients, open reduction and plate fixation usually are successful, if soft tissue stripping is kept to minimum to avoid further damage to the humeral blood supply. Rigid fixation with locking plates currently is the procedure of choice for four parts proximal humeral fractures in young active patients. Hemiarthroplasty is a good option in elderly patients with low functional demands. Head of the humerus is removed and replaced with Neer's prosthesis.

Fractures of the Proximal Humerus in Children

Fractures of the proximal humerus are relatively uncommon injuries of childhood. Fractures in this region have enormous potential to heal and remodel, more than anywhere else in the body, mainly due to the thick periosteum at the proximal humerus and proximity to the physis.

Thus, proximal humeral fractures in children can be expected to heal without significant residual functional or cosmetic deficits in most cases.

Mechanism of Injury

Fractures of the proximal humerus can be a common birth related injury. As an infant is passing through the birth canal, the arm may be placed in a variety of abnormal positions that can result in separation through the physis of the proximal humerus.

These fractures are generally believed to be resulted from hyperextension and/or rotation of the arm during passage through the birth canal. Hyperextension or rotation of the ipsilateral arm may result in proximal humeral or physeal injury during birth this has been depicted (Fig. 23.131).

In older children, the predominant cause of fractures in proximal humerus is trauma. In this age group, these fractures can involve the metaphysis, the physis or both. Proximal humerus fractures are typically moderate to high energy injuries and are typically seen in motor vehicle crashes and sporting activities (Fig. 23.132).

Blunt trauma from contact sports may result in fracture of the proximal humerus in children, as shown in Figure 23.133. Less often, pediatric proximal humeral fractures in newborns result from other conditions, such as malignant or benign tumors and pituitary gigantism. This can also be a complication of radiaton therapy to the shoulder region. In addition, shoulder joint neuropathy secondary to Arnold-Chiari malformation, myelomeningocele or syringomyelia is also etiologic factor in case of proximal humeral fractures.

Signs and Symptoms

- Clinical features of proximal humeral fractures in newborns may be subtle and not readily identified.
- Infant may be irritable when there is a movement of upper extremity
- Infant may refuse to move the arm giving appearance of paralysis called pseudoparalysis

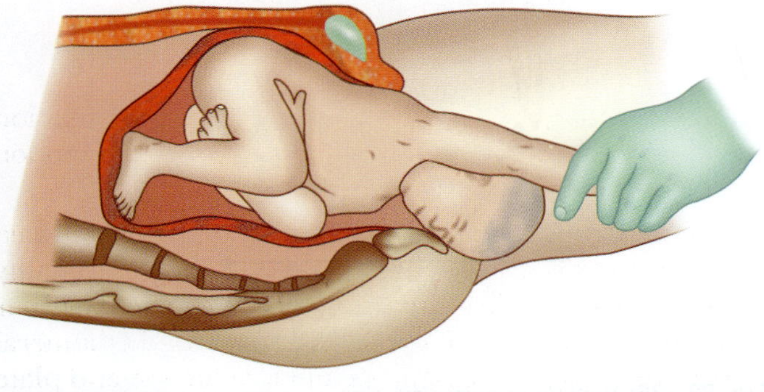

Fig. 23.131: Proximal humeral or physeal injury during birth due to hyperextension or rotation of the ipsilateral arm

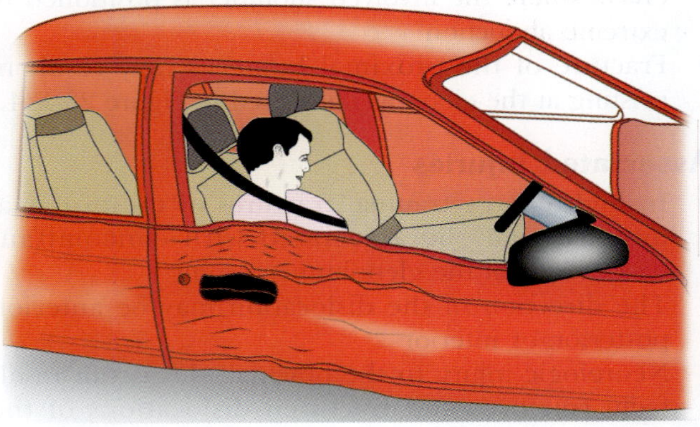

Fig. 23.132: Motor vehicle crashes may result in proximal humeral fractures

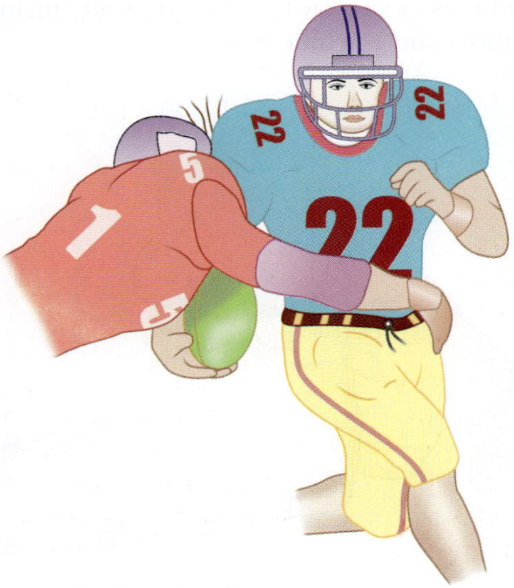

Fig. 23.133: High contact sports may resulted in fracture of the proximal humerus

- Older children typically reports a history consistent with a proximal humeral fracture, immediate development of moderate to severe global shoulder pain exacerbated by motion of the arm
- They also present with obvious deformity or fullness in anterior shoulder region, with the overall contour of the shoulder altered in comparison with the contralateral uninjured shoulder
- The arm is internally rotated against the abdomen and the patient usually refuses to use the involved arm
- Pain, swelling and ecchymosis are present to some degree
- The internally rotated position of the injured extremity is due to pull of the pectoralis major muscle on the distal fragment
- Some children with the fractures of the greater tuberosity have an unusual presentation of luxatio erecta where the involved shoulder is positioned in extreme abduction
- Fracture of the proximal humerus may result in twisting at the elbow as illustrated in Figure 23.134.

Associated Injuries

- In high energy trauma, fractures of the proximal humerus may be associated with concomitant dislocations of the glenohumeral joint
- The direction of the dislocation may be anterior, posterior, or inferior
- Neurologic injury to the brachial plexus can result from fractures and fractured dislocations of the proximal humerus
- Typically these nerve deficits are transient and full function typically returns in less than 6 months
- Fractures of the proximal humerus in children can also be associated with other injuries, including rib fractures and pneumothorax.

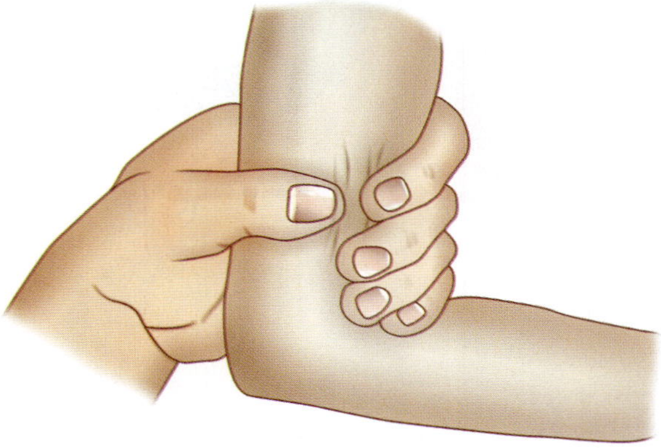

Fig. 23.134: Twisting at the elbow due to fracture of the proximal humerus

Diagnosis and Classification

The proximal humeral epiphysis is not visible on plain X-rays, until about 6 months of age. On an AP X-ray, a change in the positional relationship between the proximal humeral metaphysis and the scapula and acromion is often visible in proximal humeral fractures. A "vanishing epiphysis sign", as shown in Figure 23.135 is seen in posteriorly displaced physeal fractures of the proximal humerus.

On an AP X-ray, epiphysis appears to vanish when it is displaced posteriorly. Because some lesser tuberosity fractures may be visible only on axillary lateral view, X-ray of lateral view should be included whenever possible. When adequate X-rays cannot be obtained, CT is useful in evaluating proximal humeral fractures. CT may be especially useful in characterizing posterior fracture dislocations.

If the child continues to report shoulder pain despite negative radiographic and CT results, an occult fracture must be ruled out. For this purpose, magnetic resonance imaging (MRI) can be diagnostic, due to its ability to identify the intramedullary signal change of edema and the fracture plane. A bone scan may also be useful in equivocal cases. However, due to the normally increased radionuclide uptake at the physis of the proximal humerus, additional uptake due to a fracture may be difficult to interpret.

Classification

Fractures of the proximal humerus in the pediatric population are categorized by their anatomic location. The fractures may involve the physis, the metaphysis, the lesser tuberosity or the greater tuberosity.

Fractures involving the physis are classified according to the Salter-Harris classification (Figs 23.136A to D).

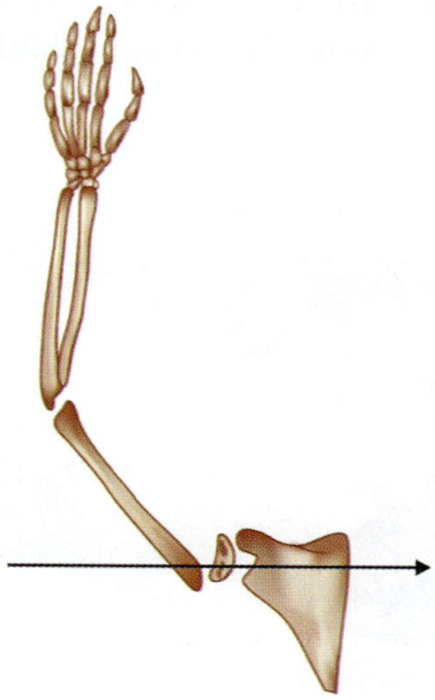

Fig. 23.135: Vanishing epiphysis sign

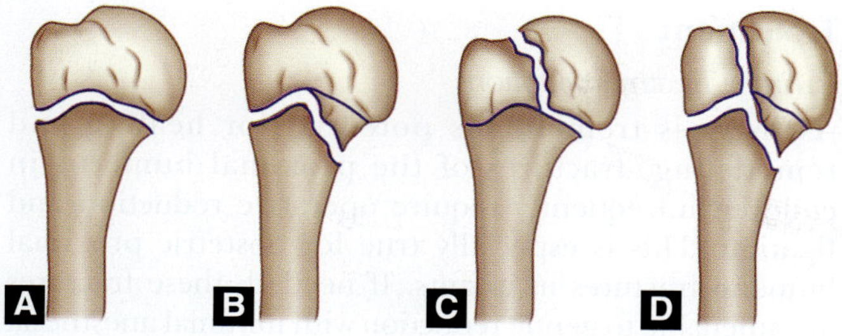

Figs 23.136A to D: Salter-Harris classification—(A) Salter-Harris type I; (B) Salter-Harris type II; (C) Salter-Harris type III; (D) Salter-Harris type IV

Salter-Harris type I injuries: These are associated with fractures through the physis. Occur mostly in patients under 5 years of age.

Salter-Harris type II injuries: Associated with the fracture line, exiting through the metaphysis and are occasionally associated with an additional anterolateral bony fragment.

Salter-Harris type III injuries: Associated with the fracture line exiting through the epiphysis. Rarely occur in the proximal humerus of children and have been reported with and without concomitant glenohumeral dislocation.

Salter-Harris type IV injuries: Involving both the metaphysis and the epiphysis of the proximal humerus, though have not been reported in children.

The articular surface of the proximal humerus covers most of the medial aspect of the epiphysis, as well as the proximal medial corner of the metaphysis. The glenohumeral joint capsule surrounds the articular surface, such that most of the medial epiphysis and the proximal medial corner of the metaphysis are intra-articular.

Anatomy of Proximal Humerus

Anatomy of proximal humerus with prominent demarcation of joint capsule and physis is being shown in Figure 23.137.

Fractures of the metaphysis occur mostly in children of 5 to 12 years of age and are categorized by their anatomic location and the degree of displacement. This rather unexpected finding has been attributed to the rapid metaphyseal growth that occurs during this age, which in turn results in a relative structural weakness of the metaphysis. The anatomic location is described in relation to the major deforming forces in the region, namely the insertions of the pectoralis major and the deltoid muscles.

Presence or absence of other fractures in the ipsilateral upper extremity must also be documented, because segmental fractures may require alternative treatments. Other isolated fractures of the proximal humerus may include the greater and the lesser tuberosities.

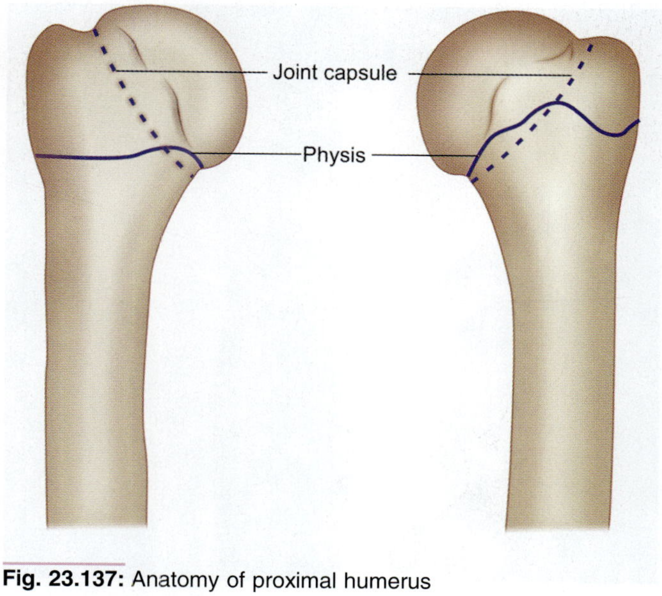

Fig. 23.137: Anatomy of proximal humerus

Physeal Fractures of the Proximal Humerus

Healing undisplaced fracture of proximal humerus in a five years old child is shown in Figure 23.138.

The degree of displacement in proximal humerus fractures is classified with respect to the shaft diameter of the humerus.

Grade I: There is up to 5 mm of displacement.

Grade II: In this fractures are displaced by up to one-third of humeral shaft diameter.

Grade III: Fractures are displaced by up to two-thirds of the humeral shaft diameter.

Grade IV: Displacement of greater than two-thirds of the shaft diameter is classified as a grade IV injury.

In addition to the degree of displacement, fractures in this region typically demonstrate concomitant angular deformities. Proximal humeral fractures are typically moderate to high energy injuries and are frequently seen in motor vehicle crashes and sporting activities. Approximately 50 percent of shoulder girdle fractures in children have been reported to be associated with sporting and playing activities.

Athletic activities associated with proximal humeral fractures, include contact sports (football, hockey), horseback riding (fall from horses), gymnastics (upper extremity impact and weight bearing) and baseball (repetitive throwing).

Surgical and Applied Anatomy

The proximal humeral ossification center cannot be seen on plain X-rays until about 6 months of age. In addition to the proximal humerus, both the greater and lesser tuberosities contain their own separate ossification

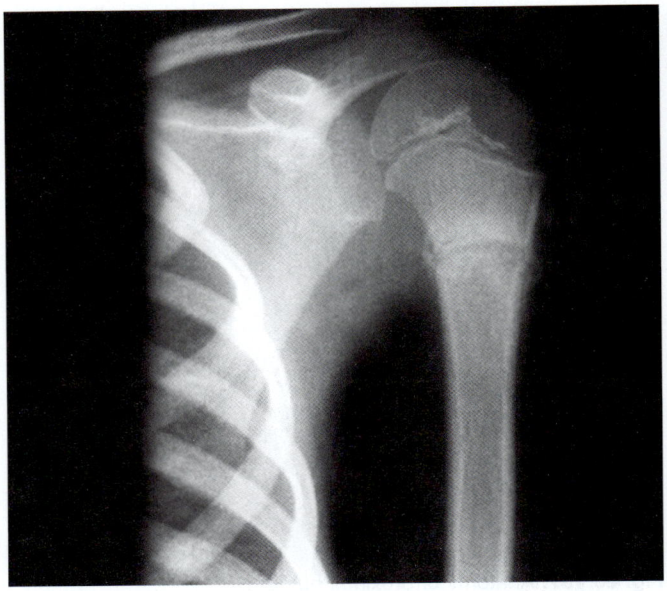

Fig. 23.138: Healing undisplaced fracture of the proximal humerus in a five years old child

centers. The ossification center for the greater tuberosity appears at around 1 to 3 years of age, while the ossification center for the lesser tuberosity takes form at around 4 to 5 years of age.

The two tuberosities typically coalesce between 5 to 7 years of age and subsequently fuse with the humeral head at around 7 to 13 years of age. The proximal physis of the humerus continues to be active well into the teenage years and is ultimately responsible for approximately 80 percent of the overall humeral growth. Interestingly, longitudinal growth at the proximal humeral physis changes during development, such that it is responsible for only 75 percent of humeral growth before the age of two, but up to 90 percent of growth after the age of 11.

For girls, this growth continues until around 14 years of age, with subsequent fusion of the epiphysis with the shaft at 14 to 17 years of age. For boys, growth continues until about age of 16, after which closure of the physis begins. For most boys, the proximal humeral physis is closed by about 18 years of age. The extracapsular location of the proximal humeral physis makes this structure susceptible to injury.

Physeal fractures are thought to occur through the zone of hypertrophy and provisional calcification, while relatively sparing the cells in the resting and proliferative zones. Salter-Harris type I or II fractures in children have high remodeling potential and rarely result in growth arrest. Sling and swathe for immobilization of proximal humerus fractures.

Treatment

Current Treatment Options

As there is tremendous potential for healing and remodeling, fractures of the proximal humerus in children infrequently require operative reduction and fixation. This is especially true for obstetric proximal humeral fractures in infants. If needed, these fractures are amenable to gentle reduction with minimal anesthesia or sedation.

Proximal humeral fractures in this age group heal quite rapidly, typically within 2 to 3 weeks and result in no residual functional or cosmetic deficits. Nondisplaced or minimally displaced proximal humeral fractures (Neer's grades I and II) in older children and adolescents should also be treated nonoperatively. Initial management of these fractures involves sling and swathe immobilization followed by protected motion. Overall, nonoperative treatment provides excellent long-term results.

The remodeling potential of the fracture in young children is significant, but decreases with the increasing age of the child. Hence, the degree of acceptable displacement and angulation also changes with the age of the child. Generally, relative greater displacement and angulation can be accepted in younger children. For fractures in children under the age of 11, good to excellent long-term outcomes have been reported regardless of the fracture displacement. Various types of shoulder immobilization to maintain reduction have been advocated and include sling and swathe, thoracobrachial bandage (Velpeau), hanging arm cast, shoulder spica cast, salute position shoulder spica cast and Statue of Liberty cast.

Grossly displaced or angulated proximal humeral fractures (Neer's grades III and IV) in children over the age of 11 are managed with fracture reduction and sometimes with specialized immobilization. Multiple maneuvers exist for the reduction of pediatric proximal humeral fractures. Most fractures can be reduced by applying longitudinal traction to the arm, while positioning it in abduction, flexion and external rotation.

If this maneuver does not sufficiently reduce the fracture, better reduction can be obtained by moderate abduction, flexion to 90° and external rotation. Alternatively, the fracture can be reduced by direct manual manipulation of the fragments, while the arm is placed in marked abduction of about 135°, slight flexion of about 30° and longitudinal traction. Some fractures cannot be adequately reduced because of a barrier at the fracture site. Anatomic structures that can prevent reduction of proximal humeral fractures, include the periosteum, the shoulder joint capsule and the bicep's tendon. In these situations, open reduction through a small deltopectoral incision is needed to remove the obstacles to reduction.

Proximal humeral fractures that have significant displacement (Neer's grades III and IV) and angulation in patients over 11 years of age are the fractures that typically undergo reduction to improve fracture alignment. General anesthesia is typically necessary for patient comfort and for adequate muscle relaxation due to the difficulties that can be encountered in obtaining and maintaining an acceptable reduction.

Reduction is performed with longitudinal traction on the injured limb, while the arm is placed in abduction, external rotation and flexion, to align the distal fragment with the epiphysis. Increasing the abduction up to 90° and flexion up to 90°of the distal fragment, may be necessary to reduce the fracture. For fractures requiring operative reduction, percutaneous Kirschner wire stabilization is routinely used. The starting point for percutaneously placed implants is at the lateral cortex of the distal fragment, near the insertion of the deltoid muscle and aimed obliquely into the humeral epiphysis. At least two pins of 0.062 or 0.078 inches and preferentially three pins are used and typically allow adequate stabilization. The Kirschner wires may be cut beneath the level of the skin or may be left through the skin and protected with Jergen's balls. The arm is placed into a shoulder immobilizer, with the arm at the patient's side, while the patient is under general anesthesia. The implants can usually be removed as early as 4 weeks after surgery after documenting healing on X-ray.

Complications

In children with multiple traumas, the diagnosis can be delayed due to the need to focus on more life or limb threatening problems and the absence of any dramatic limb malalignment. Even after the diagnosis of proximal humeral fracture is made, full evaluation and characterization of the fracture pattern can remain incomplete because of inadequate radiographic studies. A high index of suspicion, thorough physical examination and insistence on high quality X-rays must be present to ensure prompt diagnosis and treatment of proximal humeral fractures. Neurologic injury to the brachial plexus can result from fractures and fractured dislocations of the proximal humerus.

Most nerve deficits can be diagnosed immediately because the clinical signs are readily apparent. Rarely, however, nerve deficits from proximal humeral fractures can evolve slowly and delay the diagnosis. Typically, these nerve deficits are transient and full function typically returns in less than 6 months. If the neurologic deficit persists longer than 3 months, further evaluation with electromyography is warranted. If no evidence of nerve recovery or regeneration is present, nerve exploration, repair and grafting can be considered. Salvage operations for permanent nerve deficits include proximal humeral osteotomy and muscle or tendon transfers.

Fractures of the proximal humerus in children can also be associated with other injuries, including rib fractures and pneumothorax. In adults, these fractures have been associated with disruptions and thrombosis of the axillary vessels as well. Operative fixation of proximal humeral fractures with pins and wires has been associated with hardware migration, which can be fatal. Therefore, serial radiographic monitoring of the hardware after shoulder operations is essential.

Late Complications

Humerus varus after trauma is a rare complication that typically affects neonates and children under 5 years of age. Children with humerus varus have a significant decrease in the humeral neck shaft angle and shortening of the upper extremity. Although shoulder abduction may be moderately limited, most children with humerus varus have only mild functional deficits and do not require surgical correction of the deformity. If, however, active abduction and flexion are severely limited, corrective osteotomy of the proximal humerus can produce good results.

Osteonecrosis of the humeral head after proximal humeral fractures occurs frequently in adults, but is rare in children. Even after acute disruption of the vascular supply to the proximal humeral epiphysis, subsequent remodeling and revascularization usually occur in children and that lead to excellent clinical results. Similarly, glenohumeral subluxation after proximal humeral fractures is a rare complication in the pediatric population that typically results in good clinical outcomes. These children are best treated with a short period of immobilization followed by early physical therapy and rehabilitation.

SHOULDER DISLOCATION

Dislocation of the shoulder was described in the Edwin Smith Papyrus (3000 BC). Shoulder joint is the most common joint to be dislocated in human body. Males to females ratio is 5:1 and is most common in 20 to 30 years of age group.

Classifications of Shoulder Dislocation

On the Basis of Duration

- Acute
- Chronic

On the Basis of Occurrence

- Single
- Recurrent

On the Basis of Mechanism

- Traumatic
- Atraumatic

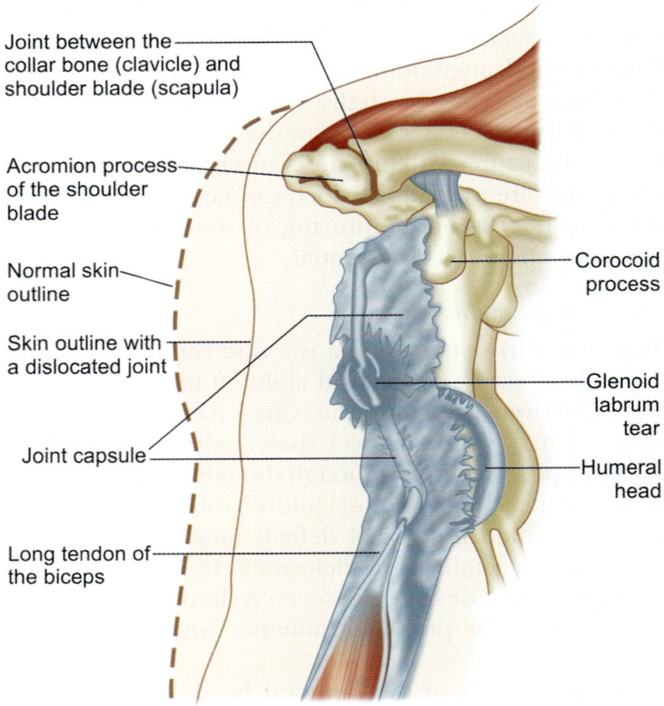

Fig. 23.139: Structures affected and joint position after anterior shoulder dislocation

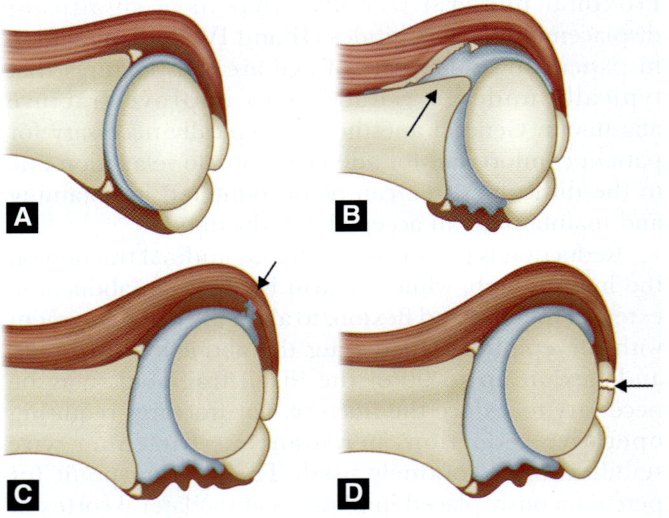

Figs 23.140A to D: Structures affected due to anterior shoulder dislocation—(A) Normal; (B) Glenoid labrum and adjoining periosteum are stripped from the front of the neck of scapula; (C) Anterior capsule is ruptured; (D) Anterior capsule is torn with a fragment of bone from the lesser tuberosity

On the Basis of Direction

- Anterior
- Posterior
- Inferior (subluxatio erecta)
- Transthoracic

■ Anterior Dislocation (Fig. 23.139)

About 95 percent cases of shoulder dislocation are the anterior dislocations. Depending on the location, it can be classified as:

- Preglenoid
- Subcoracoid
- Subclavicular

When the anterior capsule is torn or avulsed from the bone, the joint is dislocated. Head of humerus lies in front of glenoid fossa of scapula below the clavicle and coracoid process of the scapula. Mechanism of injury is abduction and lateral rotation or extended arm. Shoulder injury associated with fall on an out stretched hand. May be direct, when there is a blow from behind to the shoulder. Glenoid labrum and adjoining periosteum are stripped from the front of the neck of scapula. Anterior capsule is ruptured. Anterior capsule is torn with a fragment of bone from the lesser tuberosity, as illustrated in Figures 23.140A to D.

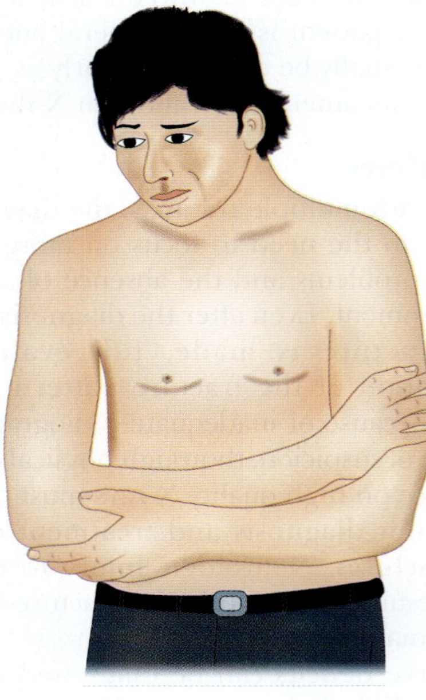

Fig. 23.141: A typical position of arm, held by the patient after anterior shoulder dislocation

Clinical Features

- Joint loses its round outline or normal contour (as the head of humerus does not occupy normal position and is displaced forward and medially)
- *Position of the arm (Fig. 23.141):* Patient holds the injured limb with other hand close to the trunk. The shoulder is abducted and the elbow is kept flexed

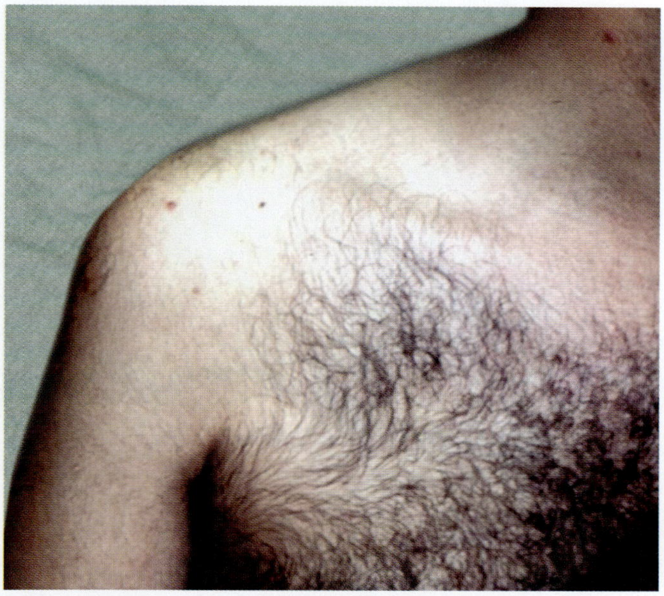

Fig. 23.142: Loss of the contour of the shoulder may appear as a step

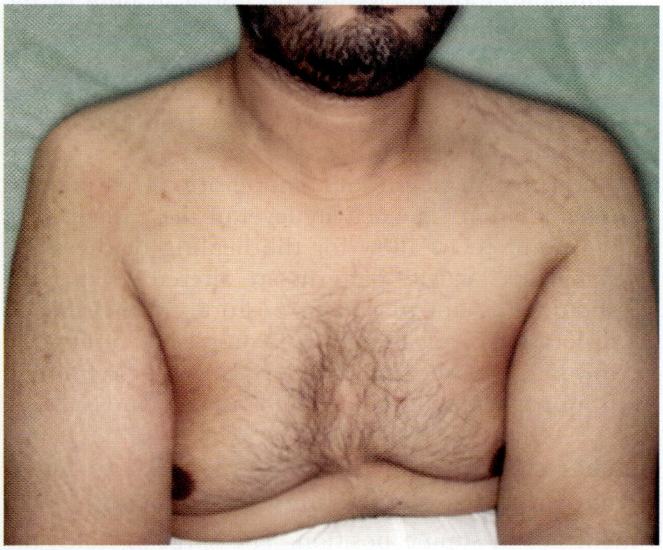

Fig. 23.143: Anterior bulge of the head of humerus is visible

- Loss of the contour of the shoulder may appear as a step this can be seen in Figures 23.142 and 23.143
- Anterior bulge of the head of humerus may be visible or palpable
- A gap can be palpated above the dislocated head of the humerus (Fig. 23.144).

Special Tests

Hamilton Ruler Test

See Figure and text on page No. 451 and 452

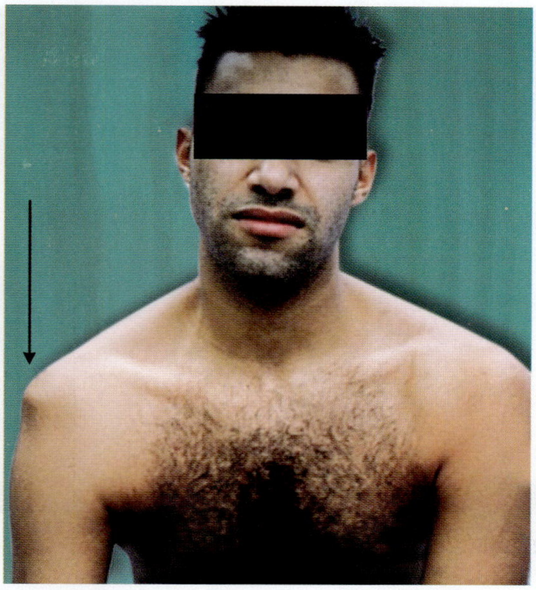

Fig. 23.144: Prominent acromion process and palpable gap above the dislocated head

Duga's Test

See Figure and text on page No. 452

Bryant's Sign

See text on page No. 452

Callaway's Test

See text on page No. 452

Apprehension Test

See Figure and text on page No. 452 and 453

Relocation Test

See Figure and text on page No. 452 and 453

Drawer Test of Gerber and Ganz (Anterior Glenohumeral Instability)

See Figure and text on page No. 453

Crank Test (Fig. 23.145)

The shoulder is abducted and externally rotated, such that it is in a position vulnerable to dislocation. With an anteriorly directed force on the posterior humeral head, the instability is accentuated to cause the sensation of apprehension.

Examination for Nerve and Vascular Injuries (Before and Postreduction)

Lesion of inner cord of plexus: It includes paralysis of small muscles of hand with loss of sensation of the medial side of hand and forearm.

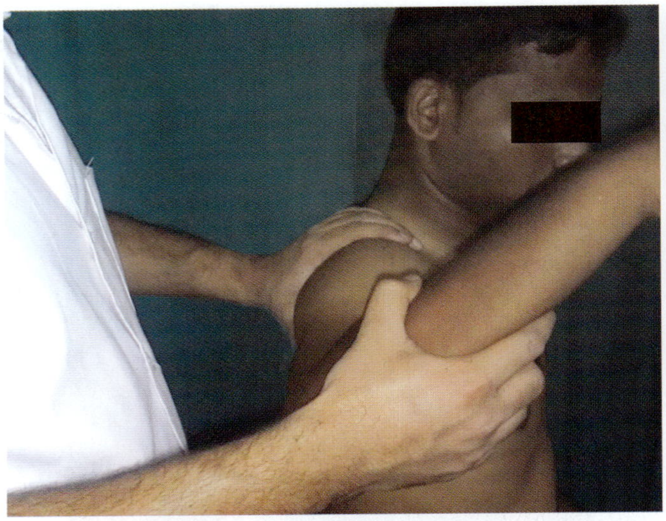

Fig. 23.145: Crank test

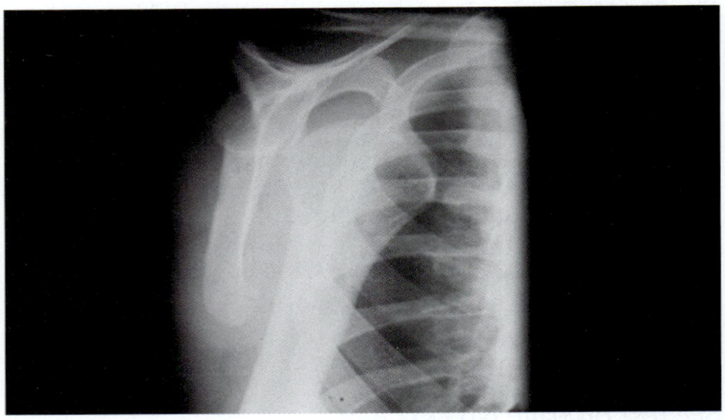

Fig. 23.146: X-ray shows anterior shoulder dislocation (lateral view)

Lesion of posterior cord of plexus: It includes paralysis of extensors of forearm with wrist drop.

Lesion of outer cord of plexus: It is difficult to recognize.

Vascular injury: Examine limb for injury to axillary vessels, which may be compressed or even ruptured.

■ X-rays (Figs 23.146 and 23.147)

Management of Anterior Shoulder Dislocation

- It's an emergency and should be reduced in less than 24 hours or there may be avascular necrosis of the head of humerus.
- Following reduction, the shoulder should be immobilized and strapped to the trunk for 3 to 4 weeks and rested in a collar and cuff.

Treatment

- Nonoperative
- Operative

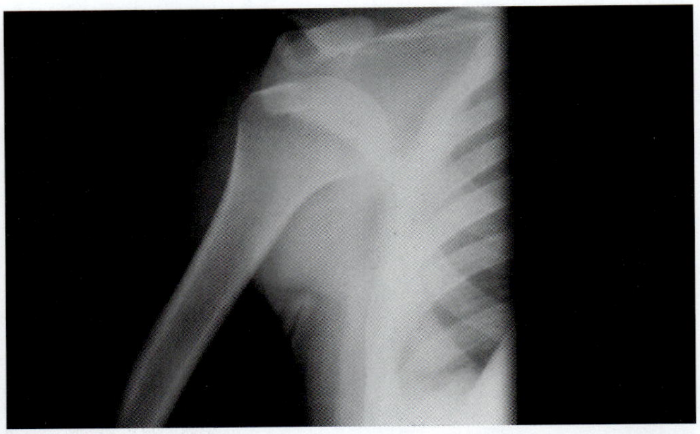

Fig. 23.147: X-ray shows anterior shoulder dislocation (AP view)

Nonoperative Treatment

Nonoperative management of patients with glenohumeral instability relies on the principles of immobilization, protection and rehabilitation.

- Immobilization allows for general recovery of the shoulder from the traumatic incident. In addition, immobilization allows for the initial healing of the static stabilizers.
- The second principle of nonoperative treatment is protection. A brief period of immobilization is designed to protect the shoulder from additional episodes of instability.
- The third principle of nonoperative treatment is rehabilitation. The activity level of the patient must be modified to allow for the healing of the static stabilizers. Activity patterns are altered, so that the shoulder is not placed in positions vulnerable to dislocation. Typically, this is accomplished by limiting the range of shoulder motion as well as refraining from participating in any high-risk activities.

Kocher's Manipulation (Figs 23.148A to D) (Elaborated for Right Sided Dislocation)

Patient lies in supine position. The surgeon holds the patients elbow with his right hand and wrist with his left hand, gentle traction is applied to humerus in the line in which it is lying, while traction is maintained humerus is externally rotated, adducted and medially rotated.

Hippocrate's Method (Figs 23.149A and B)

Uses inferior traction on the arm against the counter traction provided by the foot on the thorax, as shown in Figure 23.149A. Do not place the foot in the axilla, as this could cause damage to the underlying neurovascular structures. A modification of this technique uses a hand held sheet around the thorax to provide countertraction (Fig. 23.149B).

Stimson Technique (Fig. 23.150)

It is used for closed shoulder reduction. With the patient in prone position, weight is hung from the wrist to distract the shoulder joint. Eventually, with sufficient fatigue in the shoulder musculature, the joint can be easily reduced.

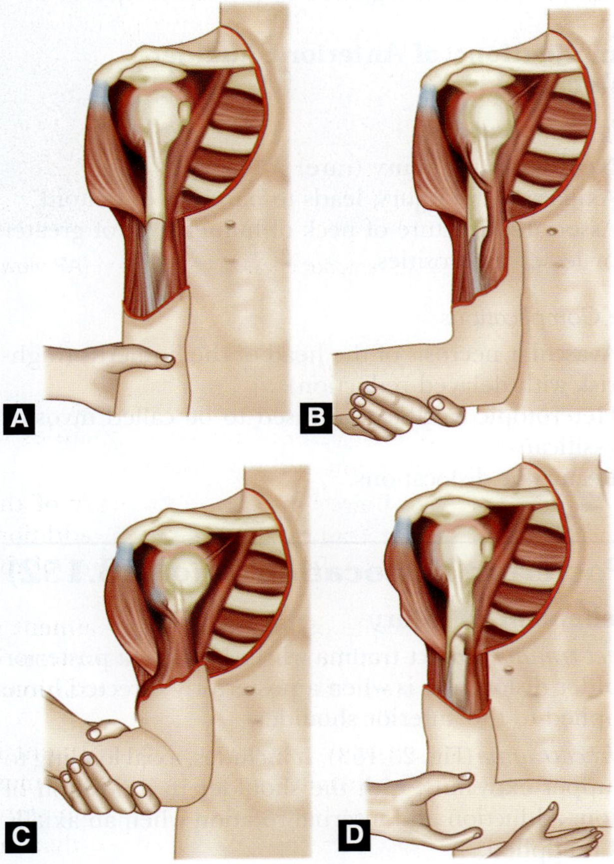

Figs 23.148A to D: Kocher's manipulation, elaborated for right-sided dislocation

Milch Technique

Another commonly used reduction maneuver is the Milch technique. Unlike some of the other maneuvers, this technique relies on shoulder position rather than distraction. The maneuver can be performed with the patient in either supine or prone position.

Upon administration of analgesia and moderate traction, the arm is abducted and externally rotated. The dislocated humeral head is then manually manipulated back into the joint. Various authors have reported that this method is associated with a high rate of success and minimal complications.

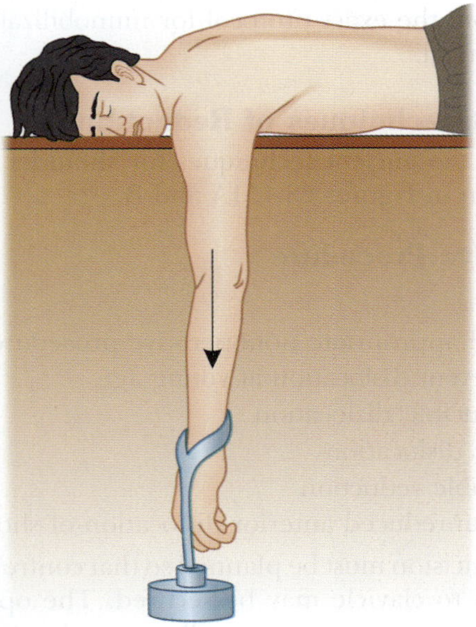

Fig. 23.150: The Stimson technique for closed shoulder reduction using weight hung from wrist to distract shoulder joint

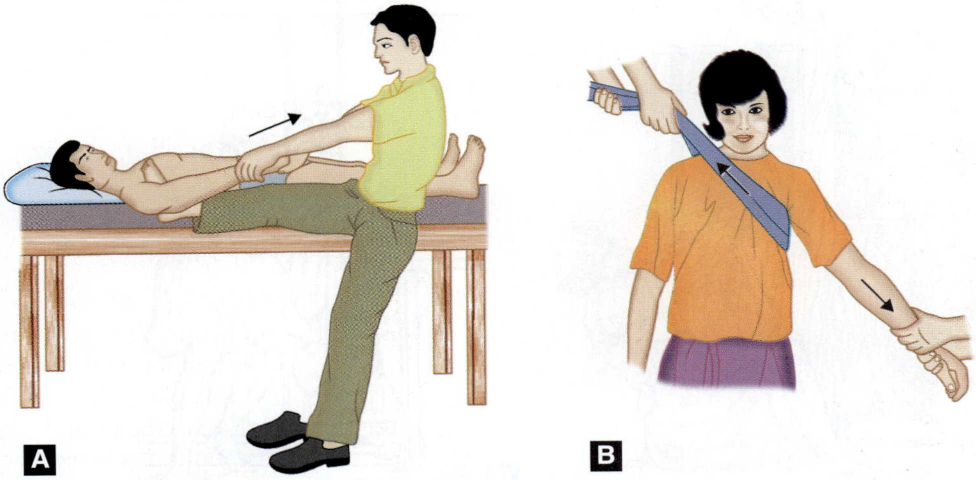

Figs 23.149A and B: (A) Hippocrate's method, inferior traction on the arm against the counter traction provided by the foot on the thorax; (B) Modified, hand held sheet around the thorax to provide countertraction

New Method

The surgeon stands behind the seated patient and inserts his flexed forearm into the axilla of the affected shoulder. His free hand applies traction on the flexed forearm of the patient. The surgeon's forearm pulls in a proximal and lateral direction and levers the head of the humerus into the socket.

The method is relatively atraumatic, provides more direct control of the limb and applies more effective forces than the Kocher, Stimson or Hippocratic maneuvers. After a successful closed reduction that is confirmed by X-rays, the arm should be immobilized for a period of time. Although most surgeons agree that a brief period of immobilization is required for patient's comfort and protection, the exact protocol for immobilization is still controversial.

Ancient Techniques of Reduction

Some of the ancient techniques for shoulder reduction are shown in Figures 23.151A and B.

Operative Procedure

Indications

- Failed appropriate nonoperative procedure
- Recurrent dislocation at young age
- Irreducible dislocation
- Open dislocation
- Unstable reduction
- Late unreduced anterior dislocation of shoulder.

The incision must be planned so that control of vessels proximal to clavicle may be secured. The operation is designed as an exposure of axillary vessels. Once vessels and nerves are exposed and retracted, head of humerus is exposed by dividing the tightened subscapularis and anterior capsule. The head of humerus is then guided outwards and backwards to glenoid fossa. After protection in a sling with the arm bound to the body for 3 weeks, movements are then regained by physiotherapy.

Complications of Anterior Shoulder Dislocation

Early Complications

- Neurovascular injury (rare)
- Axillary nerve injury, leads to paralysis of deltoid.
- Associated fracture of neck of humerus or of greater or lesser tuberosities.

Late Complications

- Avascular necrosis of the head of the humerus (high-risk with delayed reduction).
- Heterotopic calcification (used to be called myositis ossificans)
- Recurrent dislocations.

■ Posterior Dislocation (Fig. 23.152)

Mechanism of Injury

Direct trauma: Direct trauma which leads to a posterior shoulder dislocation is when a posteriorly directed force is applied to the anterior shoulder.

Indirect trauma (Fig. 23.153)*:* It includes, axial loading to the upper extremity, with the shoulder in a position of flexion, adduction and internal rotation when an axially load is applied.

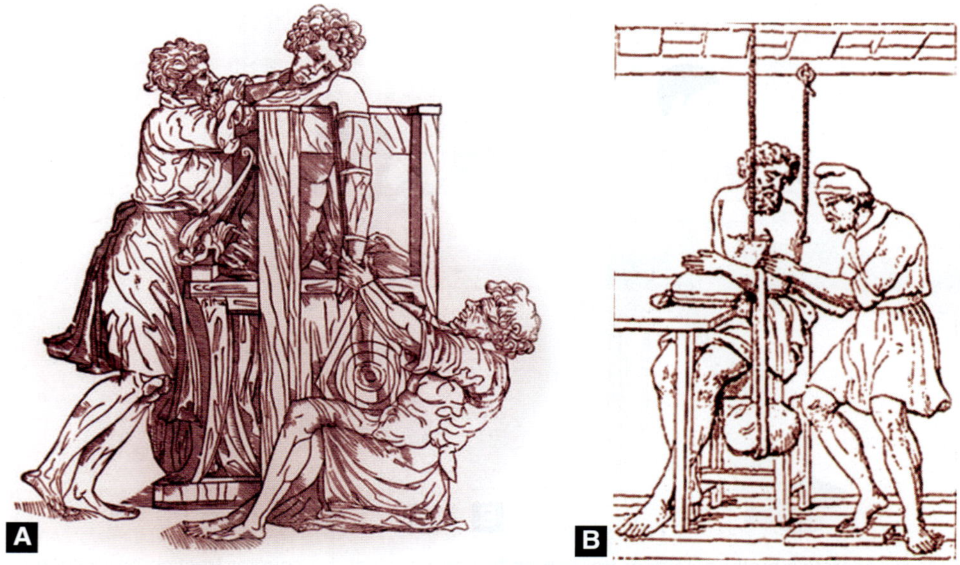

Figs 23.151A and B: Ancient techniques of shoulder reduction for anterior dislocation

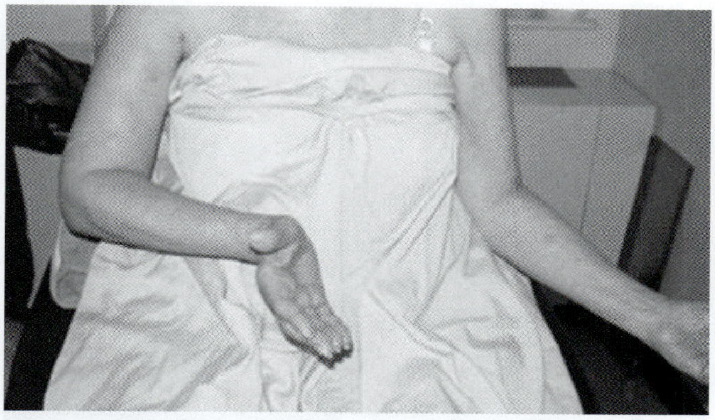

Fig. 23.152: Posterior dislocation of shoulder

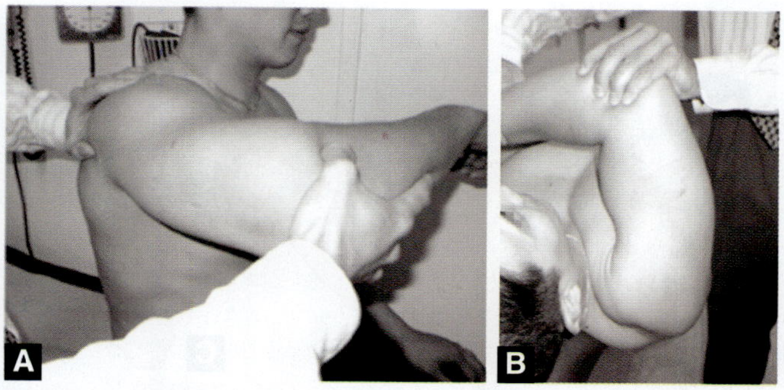

Figs 23.154A and B: Jerk test for posterior dislocation of shoulder—(A) Patient tested in sitting; (B) Supine position

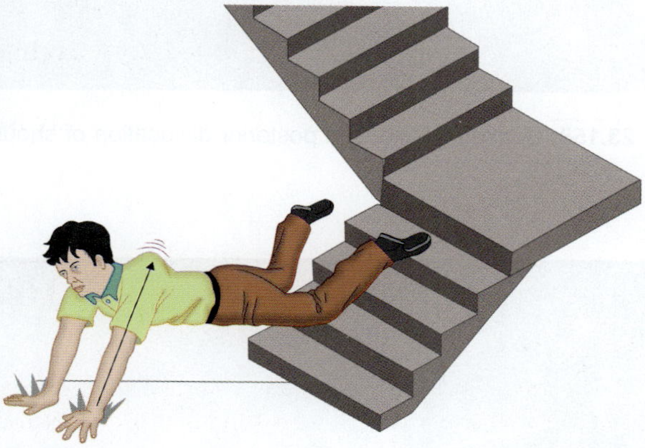

Fig. 23.153: An axial load to the arm, when the shoulder is in flexion, adduction and internal rotation places the humeral head in a position susceptible to posterior dislocation

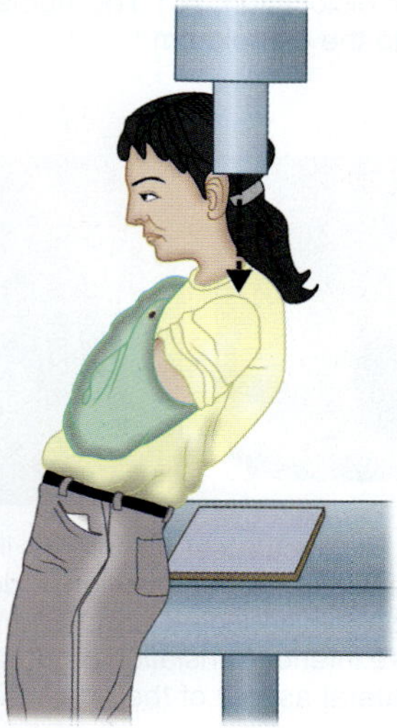

Fig. 23.155: Positioning of the patient for the Velpeau axillary lateral view X-ray

Common Causes of Injury

- *Seizures and electrocution*: These causes produce a violent muscular contraction, during which the internal rotators overwhelm the external rotators.
- Posterior shoulder dislocations can also be associated with:
  - Lesser tuberosity fractures of the humerus
  - Glenoid rim fractures
  - Humeral head and shaft fractures
  - Recurrent instability
  - Rarely, neurovascular injury.

Jerk Test

With the patient in either sitting (Fig. 23.154A) or supine (Fig. 23.154B) position, the arm is abducted and internally rotated. An axial load is then placed on the humerus while the arm is moved horizontally across the body. With a positive test, patients demonstrate a sudden jerk, when the humeral head slides off, of the back of the glenoid and when it is reduced back onto the glenoid. Positioning of the patient for the velpeau axillary lateral view X-ray is shown in Figure 23.155.

■ Inferior Dislocation (Figs 23.156A to C)

Inferior dislocations (also known as luxatio erecta) typically result from a hyperabduction force that levers the humeral head out inferiorly, as the humeral neck impinges on the acromion. Inferior shoulder dislocations can be associated with:

- Rotator cuff tears
- Proximal humerus fractures
- Neurovascular injuries
- Compressive neuropathy
- Thrombosis of the axillary artery.

Sulcus Test

The sulcus test for inferior instability of the shoulder is demonstrated in Figures 23.157A and B. By performing this test with the arm in external rotation, the maneuver can also be used to test the integrity of the rotator interval structures.

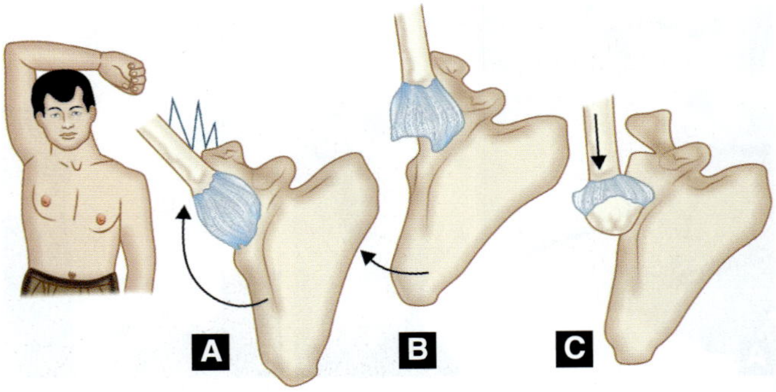

Figs 23.156A to C: Locked inferior dislocation of the glenohumeral joint or luxatio erecta—(A) With hyperabduction of the arm, the lateral acromion acts as a lever against the proximal humerus to dislocate the shoulder inferiorly; (B) After dislocation; (C) The humeral head is locked inferior to the glenoid rim

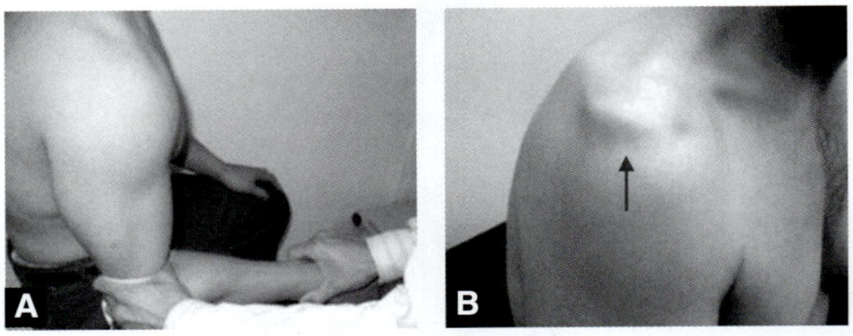

Figs 23.157A and B: Sulcus test for inferior instability—(A) With the patient in the sitting position, a downward traction is placed on the adducted arm; (B) With a positive test, excessive inferior translation produces a dimple (arrow) on the lateral aspect of the acromion

Possible Complications of Shoulder Dislocations

Bankart lesion (Fig. 23.158): It is a permanent anterior defect of labrum.

Hill-Sachs lesion (Fig. 23.159): These are caused by compression of the cancellous bone against anterior glenoid rim, creating a divot in the humeral head.

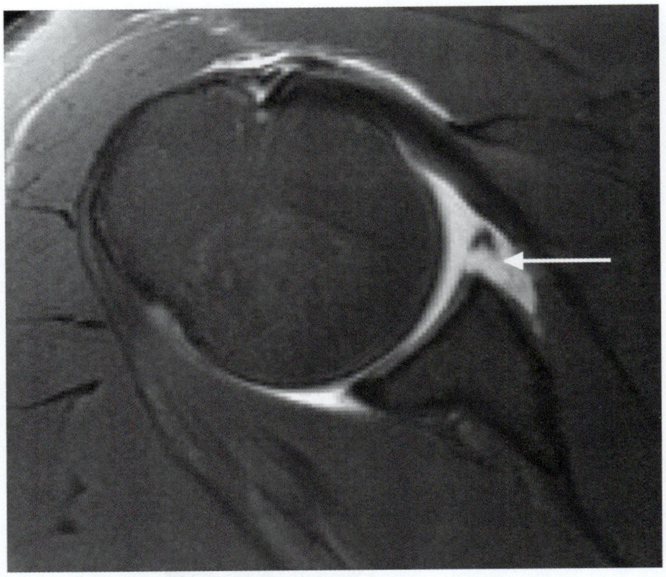

Fig. 23.158: Bankart's lesions in posterior dislocation of shoulder

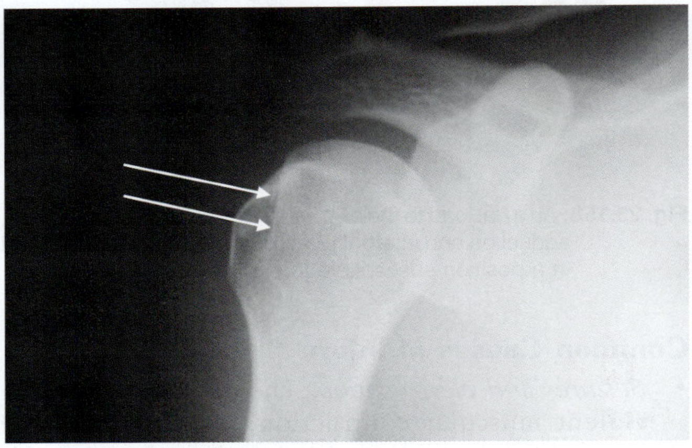

Fig. 23.159: X-ray shows Hill-Sachs lesion after posterior shoulder dislocation

X-rays (Figs 23.160 to 23.162)

Anteroposterior View

Technique for obtaining anteroposterior (AP) (upper panel) and true AP (lower panel), X-rays of the shoulder. In an AP view, the X-ray actually represents an oblique view of the shoulder joint. In a true AP view, the X-ray beam is parallel to the joint so that there is minimal overlap between the humeral head and the glenoid surface.

Apical Oblique View

Radiographic technique for apical oblique view of shoulder, is been demonstrated in Figures 23.163A and B. With patient seated and injured shoulder adjacent to vertical cassette, chest is rotated to 45° in oblique position. Beam is directed 45° caudally, passing longitudinally through scapula, which rests at 45° angle on thorax, while extremity is adducted.

West Point View

Radiographic technique for west point view of shoulder to show glenoid labrum lesions, is shown in Figure 23.164. With patient prone and pillow beneath shoulder, cassette is placed superior to shoulder. Ninty degree abduction at shoulder and cassette at 25° medial and 25° cephaled, to see anterior and posterior glenoid.

Stryker Notch View (Fig. 23.165)

Patient lies in supine position. Overhead abduction, with hand overforehead. Cassette is below the shoulder. This is done to see inferior glenoid.

Other investigations include:
- Arthrogram
- MRI
- Ultrasound

Recurrent Instability

The procedure for recurrent instability should include the following factors:
- It should has a low recurrence rate
- Accompanied with low complication rate
- There should be low reoperation rate
- It does not of harm (arthritis)
- It helps and maintains motion
- It should be applicable in most of the cases
- It allows observation of the joint
- It should corrects the pathological condition
- It should not be too difficult.

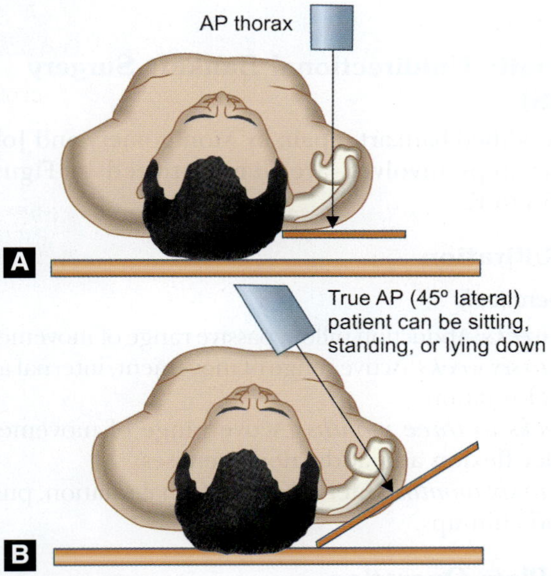

Figs 23.160A and B: Positions for taking X-ray in posterior shoulder dislocation— (A) AP view, upper panel; (B) True AP view, lower panel

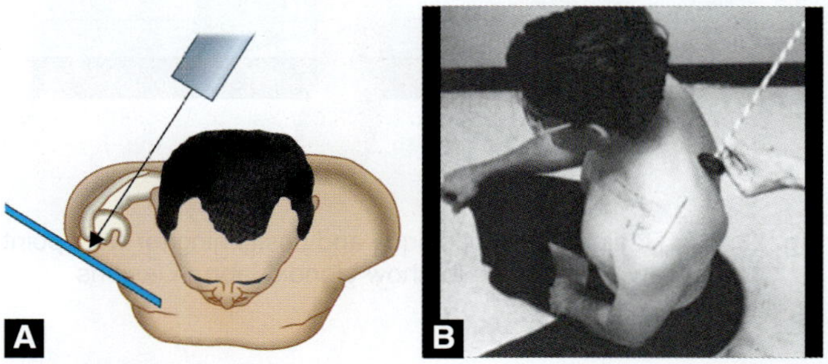

Figs 23.162A and B: Technique for obtaining a scapula lateral, known as the Y-view X-ray—(A) With the cassette placed on the lateral aspect of the shoulder; (B) The X-ray beam is directed parallel to the plane of the scapula

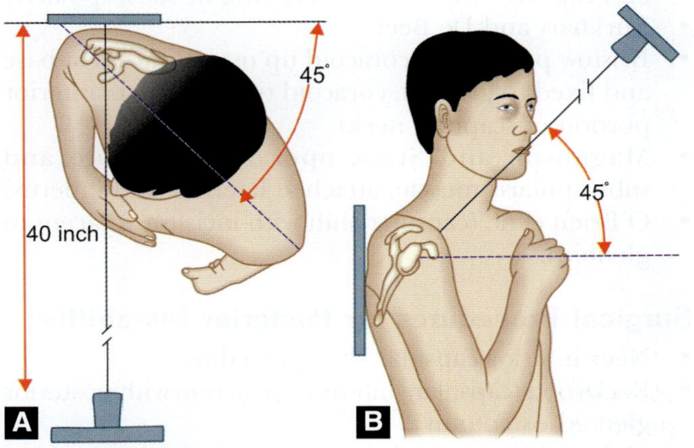

Figs 23.163A and B: Radiographic technique for apical oblique view of shoulder—(A) A view from above; (B) A view from side

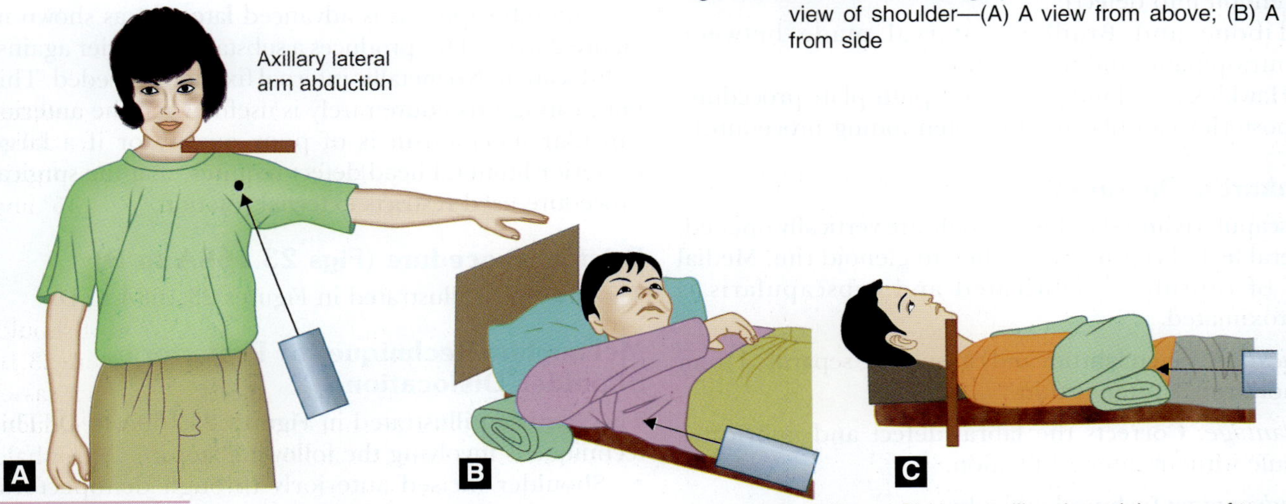

Figs 23.161A to C: Techniques for obtaining axillary view X-rays—(A) Lateral view; (B and C) X-ray axillary lateral, in case of trauma

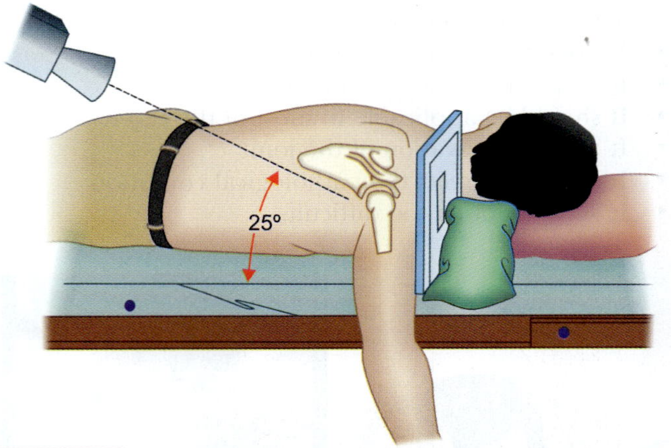

Fig. 23.164: Radiographic technique and positioning for west point view of shoulder, to show glenoid labrum lesions

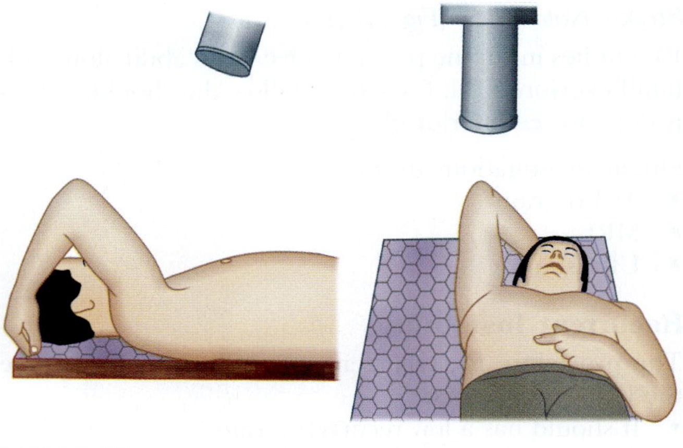

Fig. 23.165: Stryker notch view to see inferior glenoid

Surgical Procedures for Anterior Instability

- Bankart's operation
- Modified Bankart's repair (Montgomery and Jobe, where capsule is reattached to glenoid rim)
- Putti-platt operation (vertical incision on subscapularis and capsule, with double breasting of subscapularis)
- Burkhart and De Beer
- Bristow procedure (coracoid tip osteotomized at base and fixed to glenoid, coracoid tip sutured to anterior portion of scapular neck)
- Magnuson and Stack operation (capsule and subscapularis muscle, attached laterally on humerus)
- O'Brien et al. (capsular shift with incision adjacent to glenoid).

Surgical Procedures for Posterior Instability

- Neer inferior capsular shift procedure,
- Rockwood (capsular shift reconstruction with posterior glenoid osteotomy),
- McLaughlin procedure (transfer of subscapularis tendon into defect),
- Tibone and Bradley (interval made between infraspinatus and teres minor),
- Hawkins and Janda (reversed putti-platt procedure, posterior capsular tendon retensioning procedure).

Bankart's Operation

Subscapularis and shoulder capsule are vertically opened. Lateral leaf of capsule reattached to glenoid rim. Medial leaf of capsule is imbricated and subscapularis is approximated.

Indication: When labrum and capsule are separated from glenoid rim/capsule is thin.

Advantage: Corrects the labral defect and imbricates capsule without internal fixation.

Disadvantage: Technical difficulty.

Traumatic Unidirectional Bankart Surgery (TUBS)

It's a modified bankart repair, by Montgomery and Jobe. Various steps involved are demonstrated in Figures 23.166A to F.

Rehabilitation

Postoperatively

Three weeks: Abduction pillow, passive range of movement.
Three to six weeks: Active range of movement, internal and external rotation.
Six weeks to three months: Active range of movement, shoulder flexion and adduction exercises.
Three to six months: Internal and external rotation, push-ups and chin-ups.

Putti-Platt Operation

The subscapularis and shoulder capsule are incised vertically. The lateral leaf of the capsule is sutured to the capsule and the labrum, the medial leaf is imbricated and the subscapularis is advanced laterally, as shown in Figure 23.167. This produces a substantial barrier against redislocation. No metallic internal fixation is needed. This imbricating procedure rarely is useful when the anterior capsular mechanism is of poor quality or if a large posterior humeral head defect requires, that the surgical procedure used restricts external rotation.

Bristow Procedure (Figs 23.168A to D)

This process is illustrated in Figures 23.168A to D.

McLaughlin Technique for Posterior Shoulder Dislocation

This has been illustrated in Figures 23.169A to D. This technique is involving the following steps:

- Shoulder incised anteriorly through deltopectoral interval

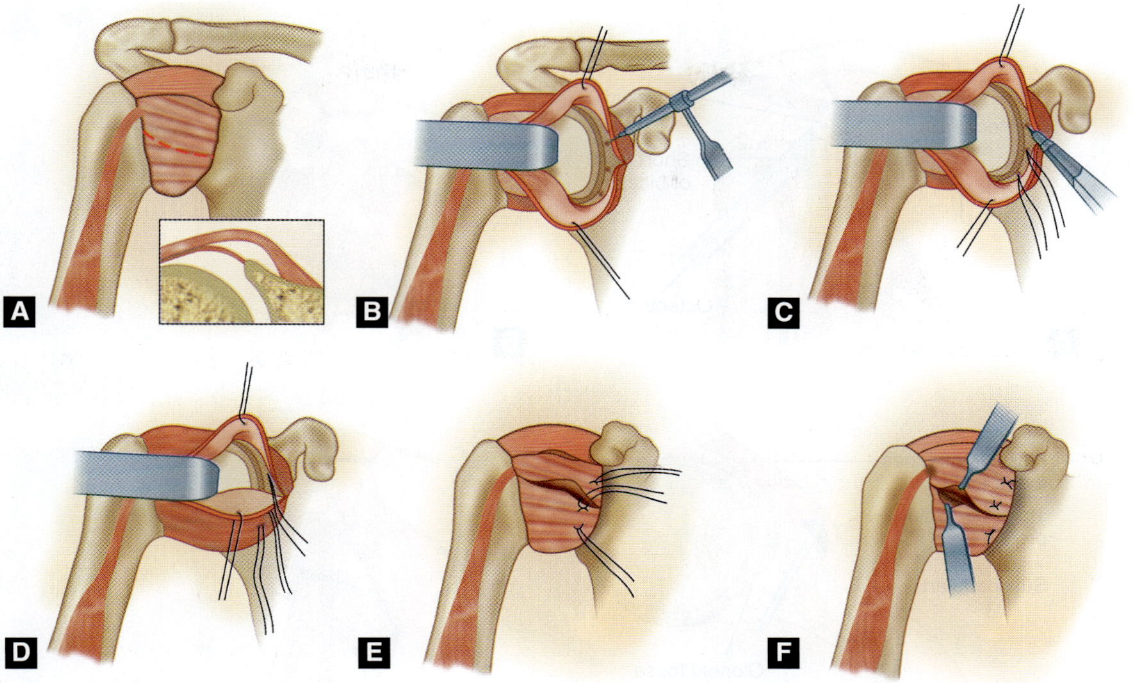

Figs 23.166A to F: (A) Incision 2 cm distal and lateral to coracoid process and inferior to anterior axillary crease; (B) Retract deltoid and cephalic vein laterally and pectoralis major muscle medially; (C) Subscapularis tendon is split at the junction of upper two-third and lower one-third; (D) Horizontal anterior capsulotomy done in line with subscapularis, at 3 O'clock position of glenoid; (E) Stay sutures are taken; (F) Retract the humeral head laterally. Drill holes near glenoid at 3 O', 4 O', 5:30 O' clock, parallel to glenoidal surface. Maintain shoulder in 90º abduction and 60º of external rotation and shift the capsule superiorly

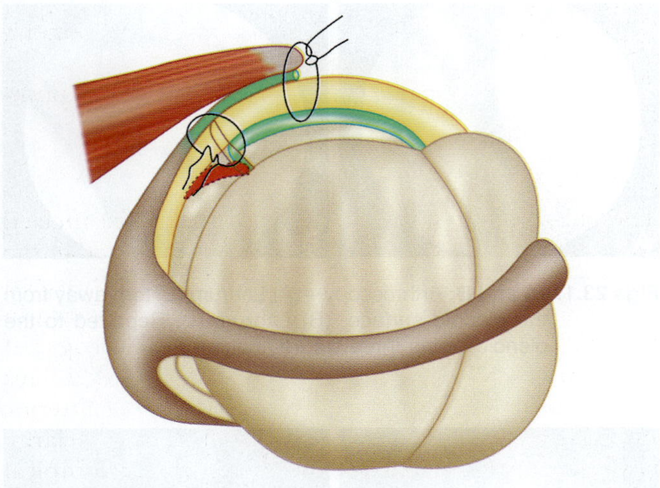

Fig. 23.167: Putti-Platt operation

- Conjoined tendons reflected medially, exposing the subscapularis muscle and transverse inscion is made
- Lesser tuberosity is osteomized, the fragment of lesser tuberosity fill the defect in humeral head
- Debridement of the surface of defect is done in humeral head
- Reattach the subscapularis tendon (medial transportation) to humerus into the depths of defect, by mattress sutures through drill holes in the humeral head.

Arthroscopy

For the most common types of shoulder instability or dislocation, the ligaments at the front of the shoulder, those hold the head in the glenoid socket are torn or loosen from the lip of the glenoid or labrum (Figs 23.170A and 23.171A).

Using special implants called "suture anchors" the surgeon can repair the ligaments and labrum in place and tighten them as necessary. These anchors are buried into the bone and most are made-up of absorbable materials that will disintegrate overtime after the shoulder has healed, as illustrated in the Figures 23.170B and 23.171B.

Acromioclavicular Joint Dislocation

Acromioclavicular (AC) joint as shown in Figure 23.172 is a diarthrodial joint between medial facet of acromion and the lateral (distal) clavicle. It contains intra-articular disk of variable size. Thin capsule of AC is stabilized by the ligaments on all sides. AC ligaments control horizontal

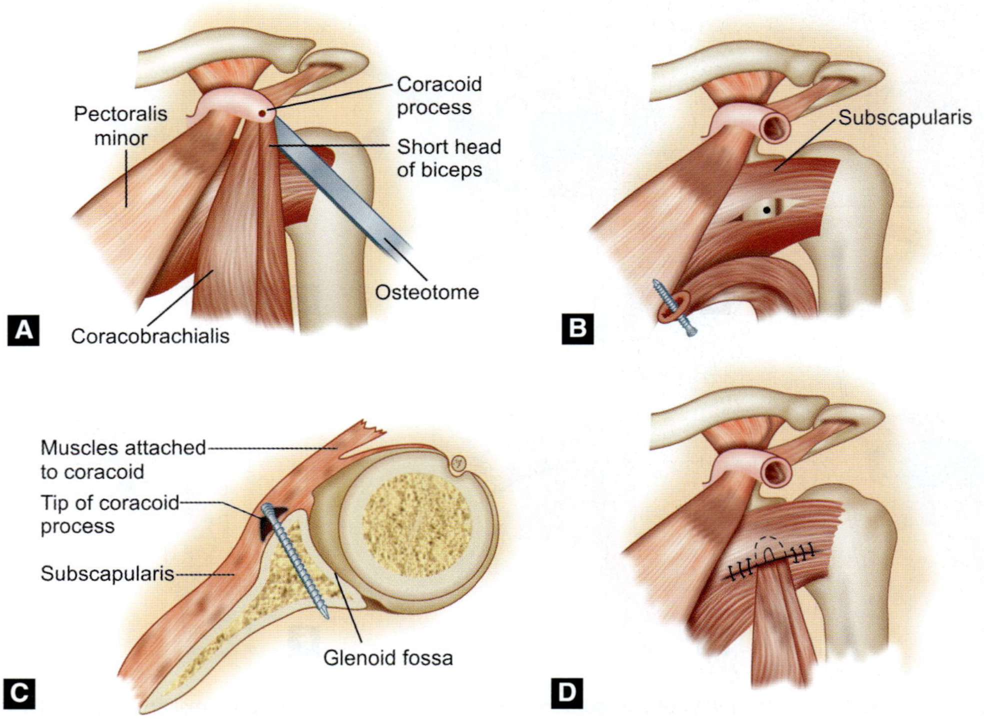

Figs 23.168A to D: Bristow procedure—(A) Detachment of tip of coracoid process; (B) Method of attachment of tip of coracoid to neck of scapula anteriorly; (C) Cross-section through scapula at level of glenoid and humeral head; (D) Bristow procedure completed

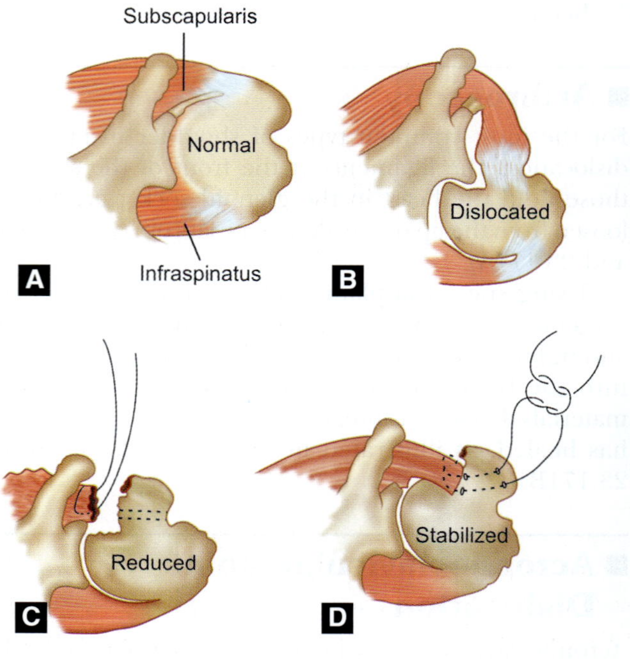

Figs 23.169A to D: McLaughlin technique for posterior shoulder dislocation—(A) Normal shoulder; (B) Shoulder dislocated posteriorly; (C) Reduction of dislocated shoulder; (D) Shoulder stabilized after reduction

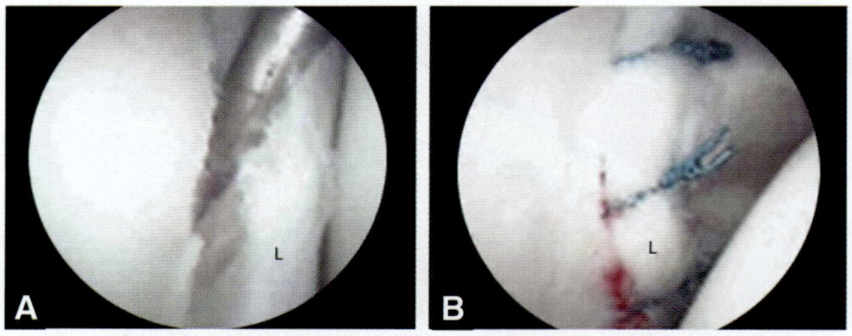

Figs 23.170A and B: Arthroscopy—(A) Labrum (L) torn away from the glenoid surface; (B) Labrum (L) Repaired to the glenoid, using three suture anchors

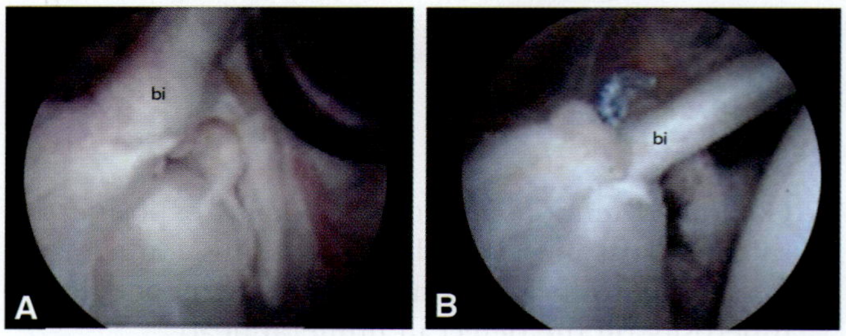

Figs 23.171A and B: (A) Biceps (bi) and labrum torn away from the top of the glenoid; (B) Biceps (bi) and labrum repaired to the labrum using a suture anchor

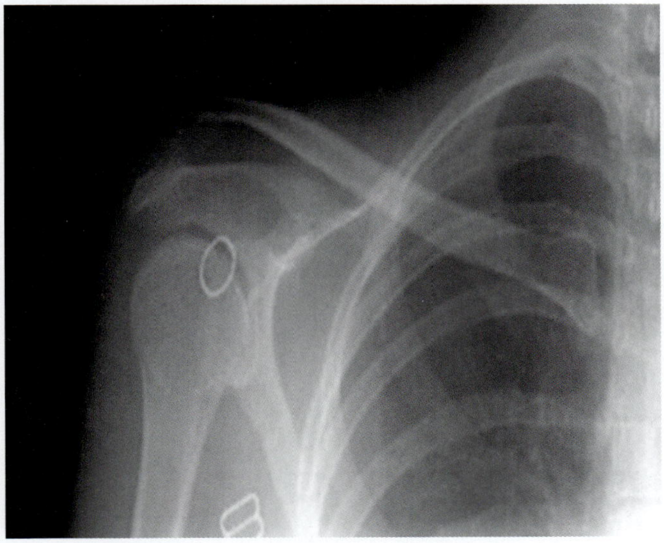

Fig. 23.172: X-ray shoulder shows acromioclavicular joint

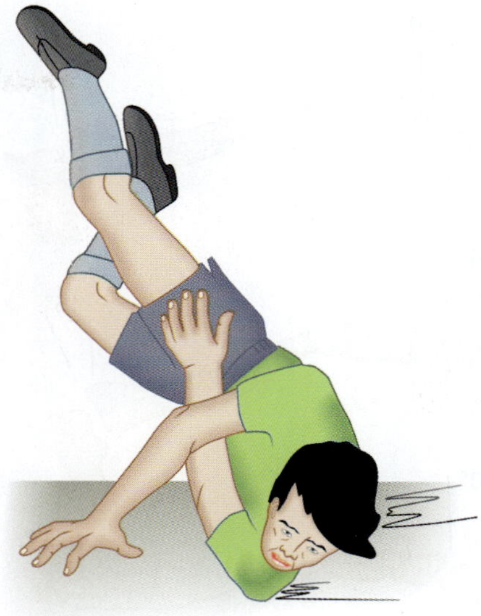

Fig. 23.174: Direct force or a fall on the point of shoulder

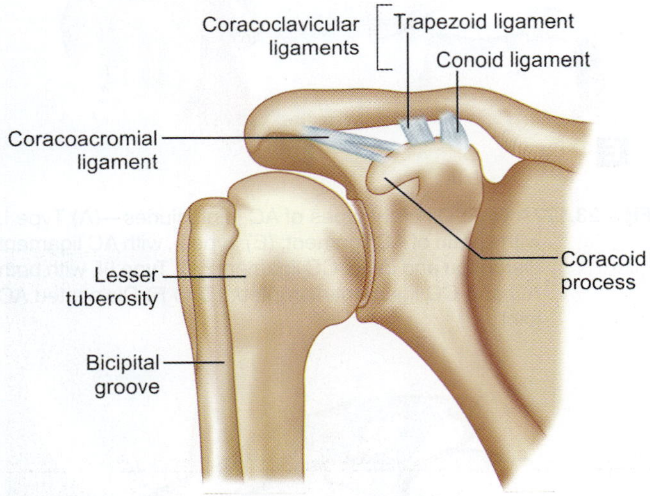

Fig. 23.173: Anatomy of AC joint, showing all surrounding structures

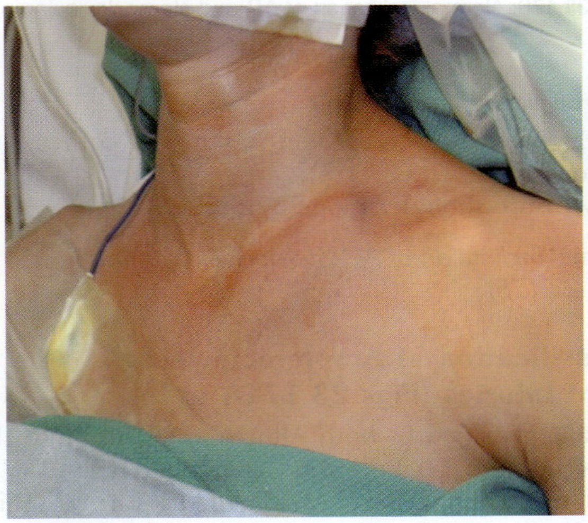

Fig. 23.175: Shoulder inspection in AC joint injury

(anteroposterior) displacement. Superior AC ligament is most important.

Normal Anatomy of AC Joint

Anatomy of AC joint is shown in Figure 23.173.

Mechanism of Injury

- Moderate or high energy traumatic impacts to the shoulder, e.g. fall from height, motor vehicle accident and sports injury
- Blow to the point of the shoulder
- Rarely a direct injury to the clavicle. Direct force onto the superior surface of distal clavicle, with abduction of arm and retraction of scapula, this is shown in Figure 23.174.

Physical Examination

Inspection (Fig. 23.175)

Evaluate deformity and/or displacement. Beware of rare inferior or posterior displacement of distal or medial ends of clavicle. Compare with the opposite side. Find, if there is normal inclination of AC and sternoclavicular joint.

Palpation

- Evaluate pain
- Look for instability with stress.

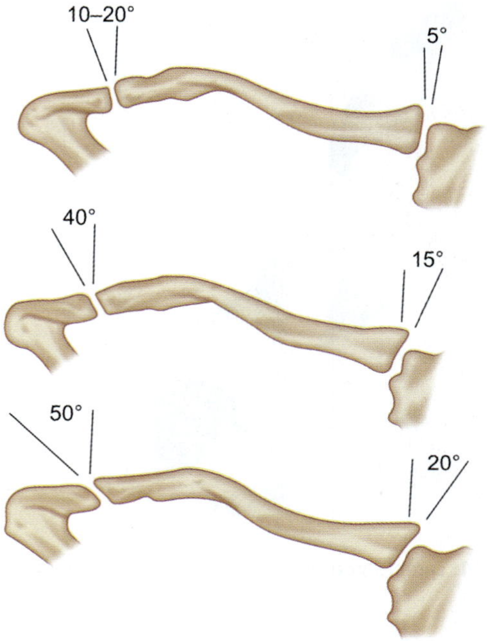

Fig. 23.176: Normal inclination of AC and sternoclavicular joint

Neurovascular Examination

- Evaluate upper extremity's motor and sensory sensation
- Measure shoulder range of motion.

Normal Inclination of AC-Sternoclavicular Joint (Fig. 23.176)

Classification of Acromioclavicular Joint Injuries (Figs 23.177A to F)

Initially classified by both Allman and Tossy into three types (I, II and III). Rockwood later added types IV, V and VI, so that now six types of AC joint injuries are recognized. Classification varies, depending on the degree and the direction of displacement of the distal clavicle.

Type I (Fig. 23.178)

- There is a sprain of acromioclavicular ligament
- AC joint is intact
- Coracoclavicular ligaments is intact
- Deltoid and trapezius muscles are also remain intact.

Type II (Fig. 23.179)

- AC joint disrupted
- Less than 50 percent vertical displacement
- Sprain of the coracoclavicular (CC) ligaments
- CC ligaments intact
- Deltoid and trapezius muscles are also intact

Type III (Fig. 23.180)

- AC ligaments and CC ligaments all disrupted

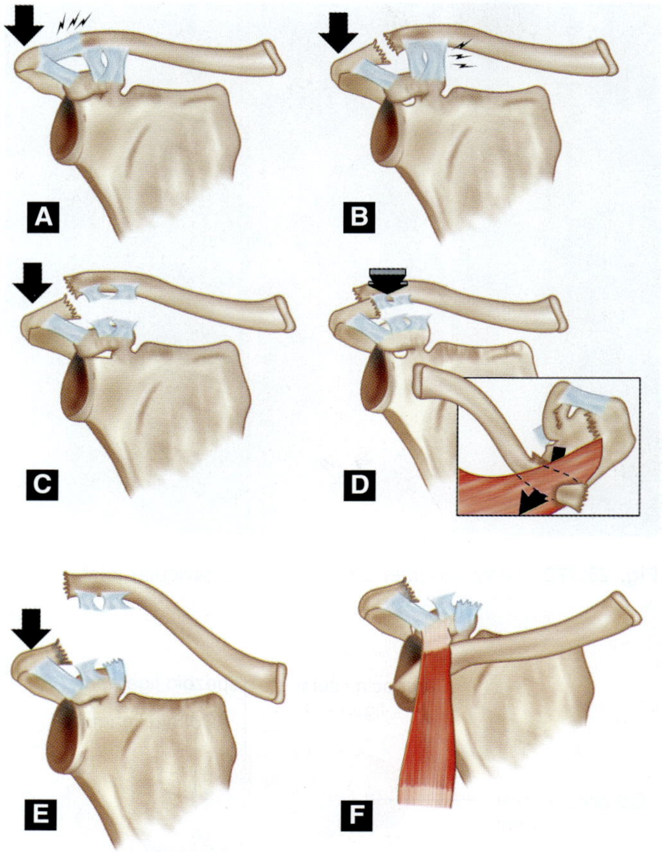

Figs 23.177A to F: Different types of AC joint injuries—(A) Type I, with sprain of AC ligament; (B) Type II, with AC ligament disruption and intact CC ligament; (C) Type III, with both AC and CC ligament disrupted; (D to F) Dislocated AC joint

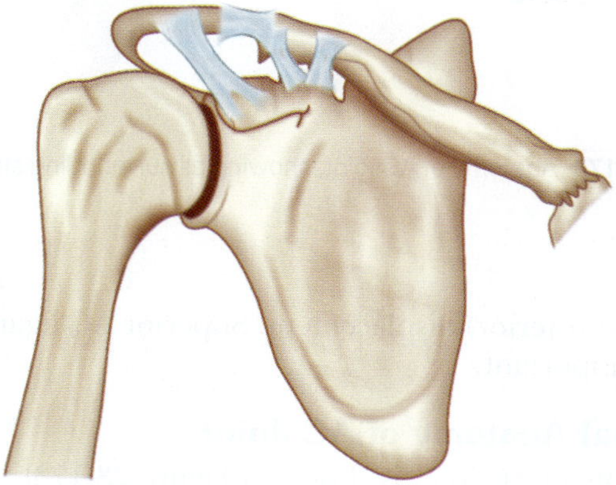

Fig. 23.178: Type I AC joint injury

- AC joint dislocated and the shoulder complex is displaced inferiorly
- CC interspace greater than the normal shoulder (25–100%)
- Deltoid and trapezius muscles usually detached from the distal clavicle.

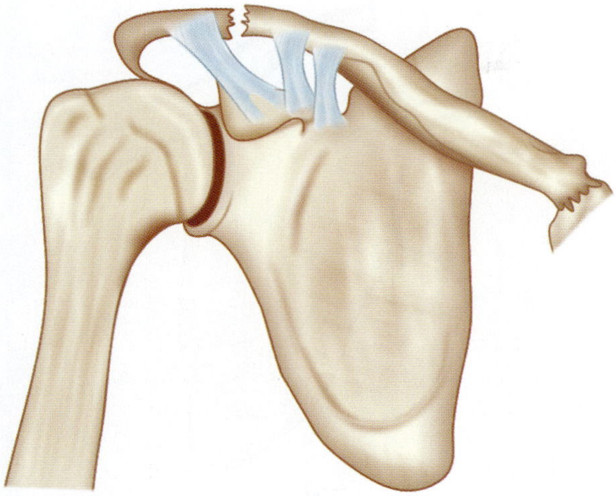

Fig. 23.179: Type II AC joint injury

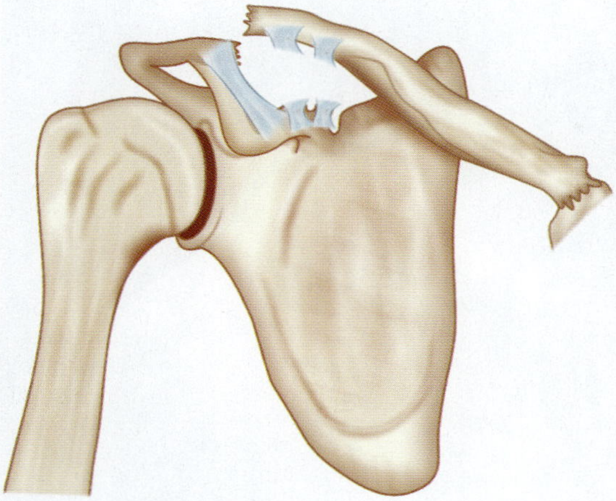

Fig. 23.180: Type III AC joint injury

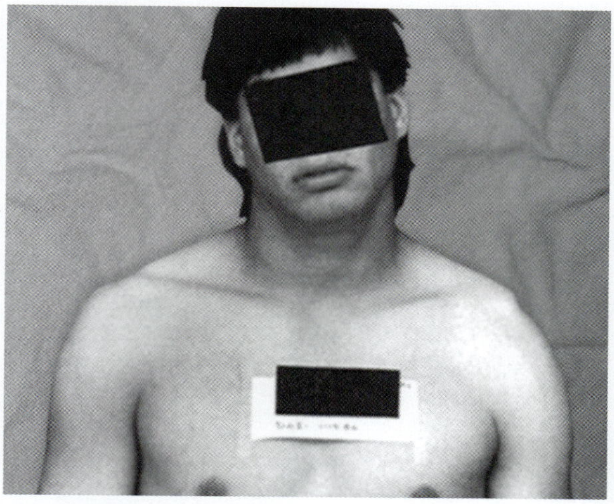

Fig. 23.181: Complete dislocation, Type III variant

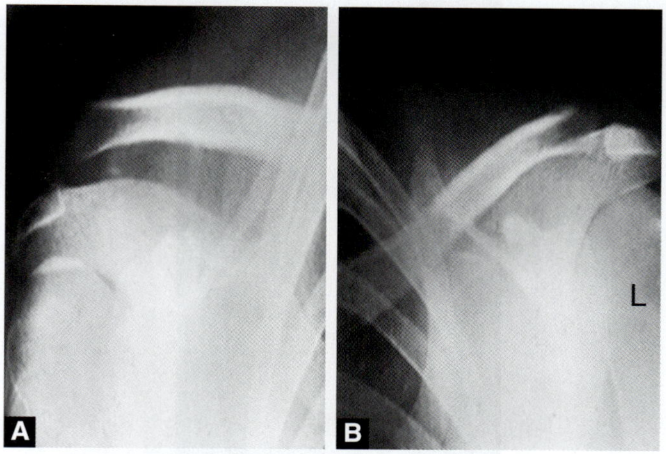

Figs 23.182A and B: Type III injury, X-ray shows increase in the AC joint space

Type III Variants (Figs 23.181 and 23.182)

- Pseudodislocation through an intact periosteal sleeve
- Physeal injury
- Coracoid process fractured.

Type IV (Figs 23.183 to 23.185)

- AC joint dislocated and clavicle displaced posteriorly into or through the trapezius muscle
- AC and CC ligaments are torned
- Deltoid and trapezius muscles are detached from the distal clavicle.

Type V (Figs 23.186 to 23.188)

- AC joint dislocated and there is gross disparity between the clavicle and the scapula
- AC and CC ligaments torned
- Deltoid and trapezius muscles detached from the distal half of clavicle.

Type VI (Figs 23.189 and 23.190)

- AC joint dislocated and clavicle displaced inferior to the acromion or the coracoid process
- AC and CC ligaments torned
- Deltoid and trapezius muscles detached from the distal clavicle.

Stability Provided by Ligaments (Figs 23.191A to C)

- Horizontal stability controlled by AC ligament
- Vertical stability controlled by coracoclavicular ligament.

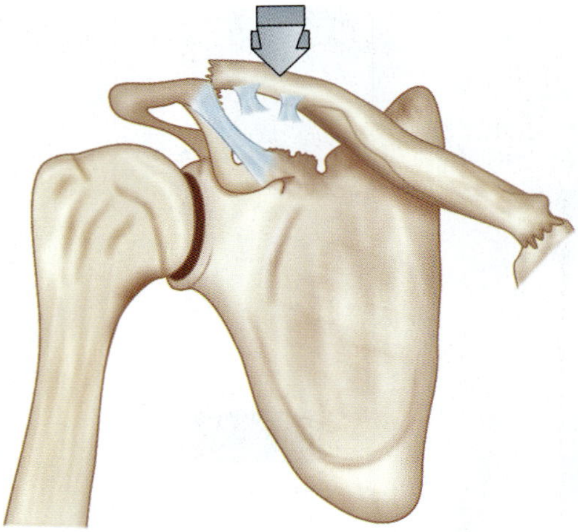

Fig. 23.183: Type IV AC joint injury

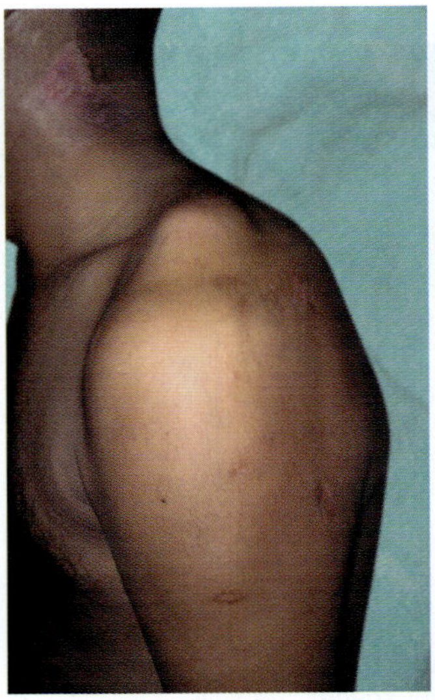

Fig. 23.184: Type IV injury, X-ray shows distal end of clavicle diplaced posteriorly into the trapezius muscle

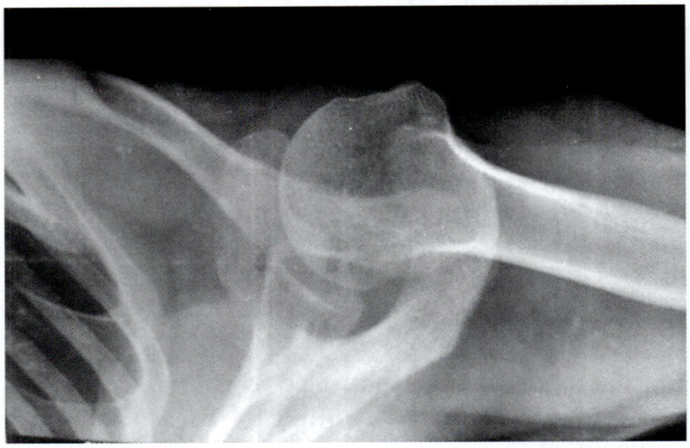

Fig. 23.185: Type IV injury, axillary lateral view

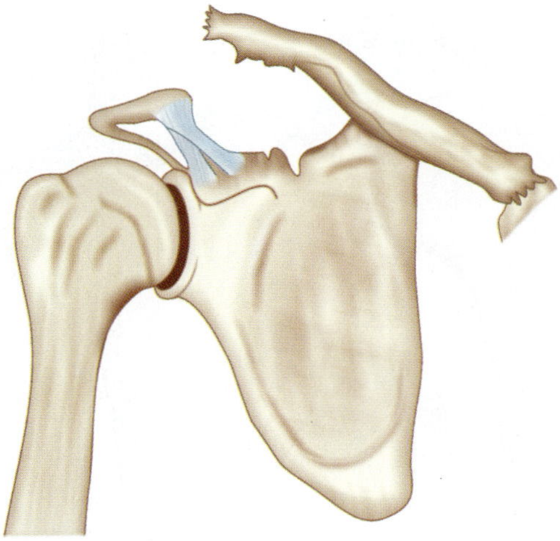

Fig. 23.186: Type V AC joint injury

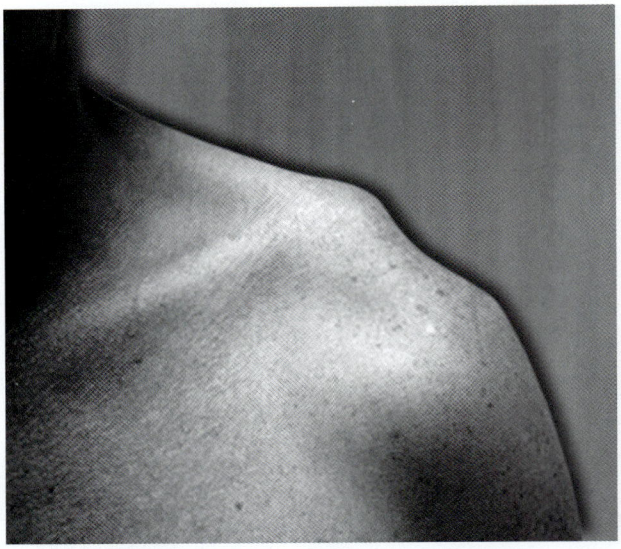

Fig. 23.187: Type V superior displacement of the clavicle

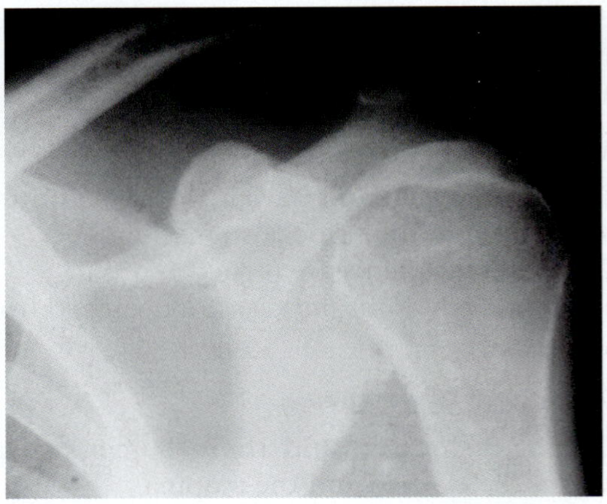

Fig. 23.188: Type V injury, with gross displacement of clavicle from acromion

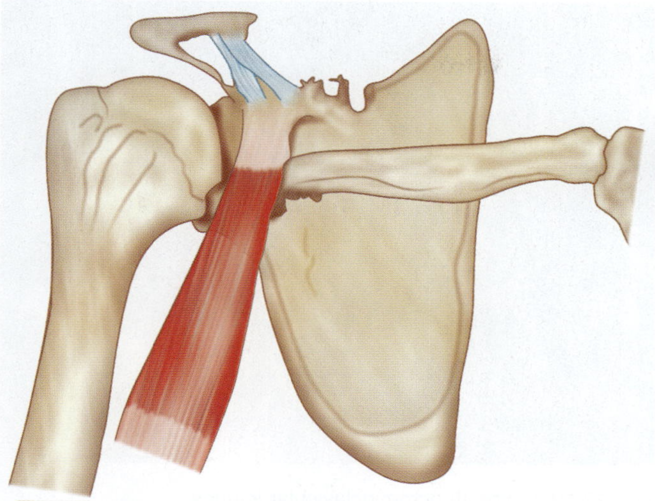

Fig. 23.189: Type VI AC joint injury

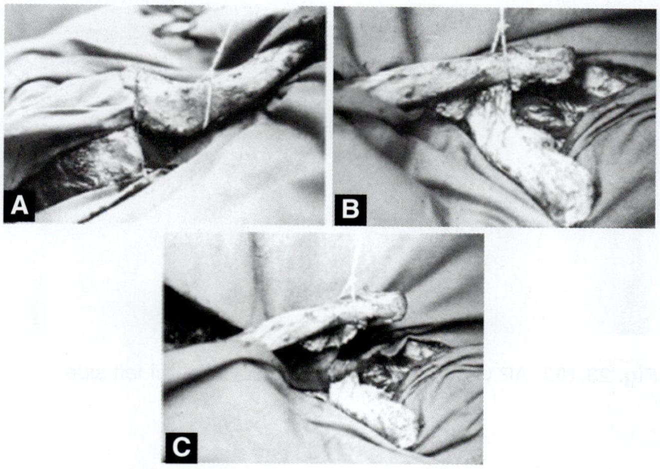

Figs 23.191A to C: The importance of the AC and coracoclavicular ligaments for stability of the AC joint using a fresh cadaver

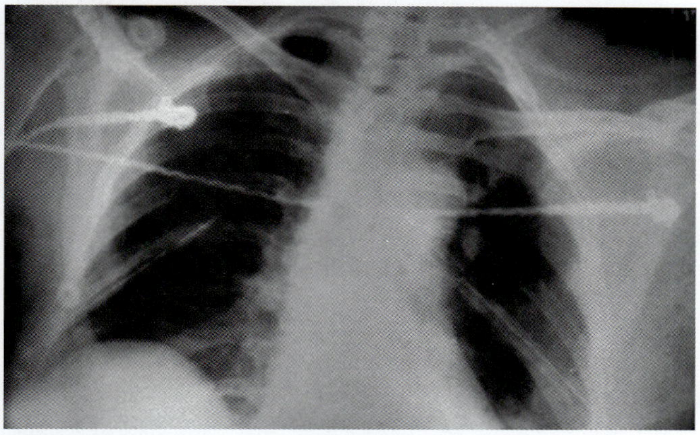

Fig. 23.190: Type VI injury, X-ray showing clavicle in subcoracoid position

Radiographic Evaluation of the AC Joint

Zanca's view (Figs 23.192 and 23.193)

- AP view centered at AC joint with 10° cephalic tilt
- Less voltage than used for AP shoulder.

Stryker notch view (Fig. 23.194)

Stress Views of the Distal Clavicle and AC Joint

- *Rationale*: Stress view, demonstrate instability and differentiate grade III AC separations from partial Grade I and II injuries.
- Performed by having patient hold £10 weight with injured arm.
- Rarely used today, since most AC joint injuries treated in the same manner and management of distal clavicle fractures depends on initial displacement and location of fracture.

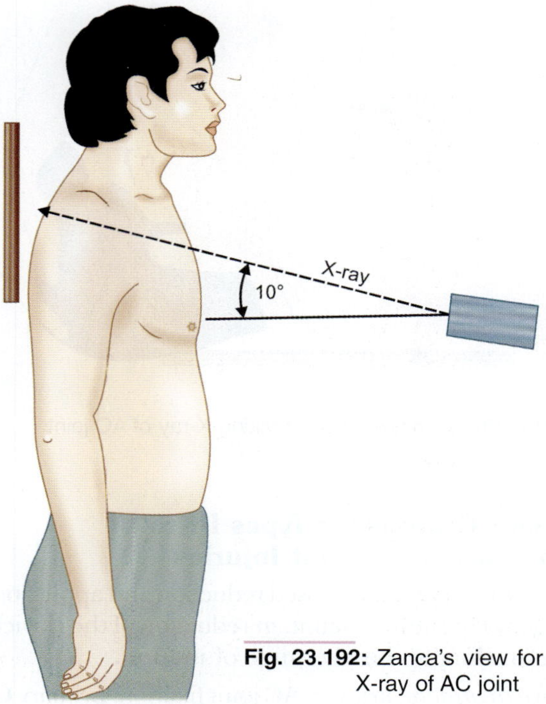

Fig. 23.192: Zanca's view for taking X-ray of AC joint

Treatment Options for Types I and II Acromioclavicular Joint Injuries

Nonoperative: Ice and protection until pain subsides (7–10 days). Return to sports as pain allows (1–2 weeks). No apparent benefit to the use of specialized braces.

Type II operative treatment: Generally reserved only for the patient with chronic pain. Treatment is resection of the distal clavicle and reconstruction of the coracoclavicular ligaments.

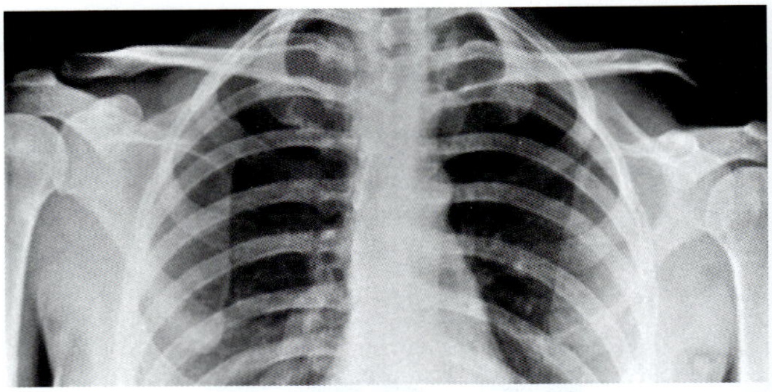

Fig. 23.193: AP view, shows AC joint dislocation of left side

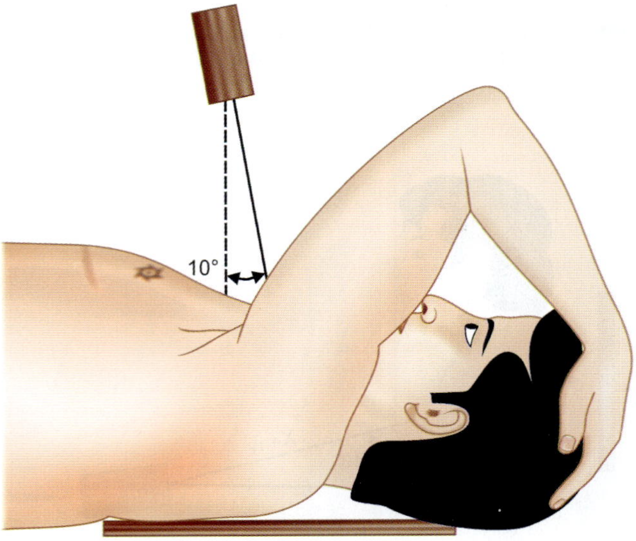

Fig. 23.194: Stryker notch view for taking X-ray of AC joint

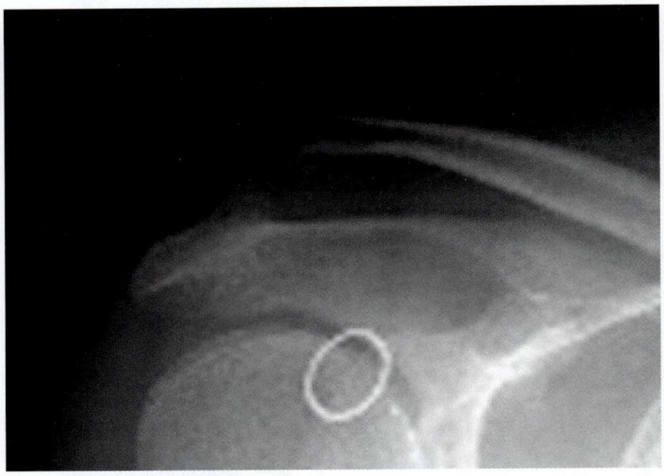

Fig. 23.195: Type III acromioclavicular injuries

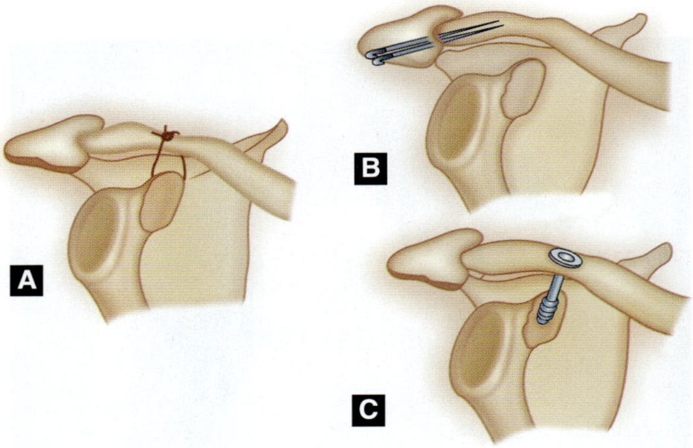

Figs 23.196A to C: Operative procedures for injuries of AC joint—(A) Suture between clavicle and coracoid process; (B) Put K-wires across the AC joint; (C) Lag screw between clavicle and coracoid process

Treatment Options for Types III to VI Acromioclavicular Joint Injuries

Nonoperative treatment: Closed reduction and application of a sling and harness to maintain reduction of the clavicle. Short-term sling and early range of motion.

Operative treatment: Primary AC joint fixation, primary CC ligament fixation, excision of the distal clavicle and dynamic muscle transfers. In type III injuries, need for acute surgical treatment remains very controversial. Most surgeons recommend conservative treatment, except in the throwing athlete or overhead worker. Repair generally, avoided in contact athletes because of the risk of reinjury.

Indications for Acute Surgical Treatment of Acromioclavicular Injuries (Fig. 23.195)

- Type III injuries in highly active patients
- Type IV, V and VI injuries.

Surgical Options for AC Joint Instability

- Coracoid process transfer to distal transfer (dynamic muscle transfer)
- Primary AC joint fixation
- Primary coracoclavicular fixation
- Distal clavicle excision with CC ligament reconstruction.

Operative Procedures for Injuries of AC Joint

Suturing is done between clavicle and coracoid process (Fig. 23.196A). Put K-wires across the AC joint (Fig. 23.196B). Lag screw between clavicle and coracoid process (Fig. 23.196C).

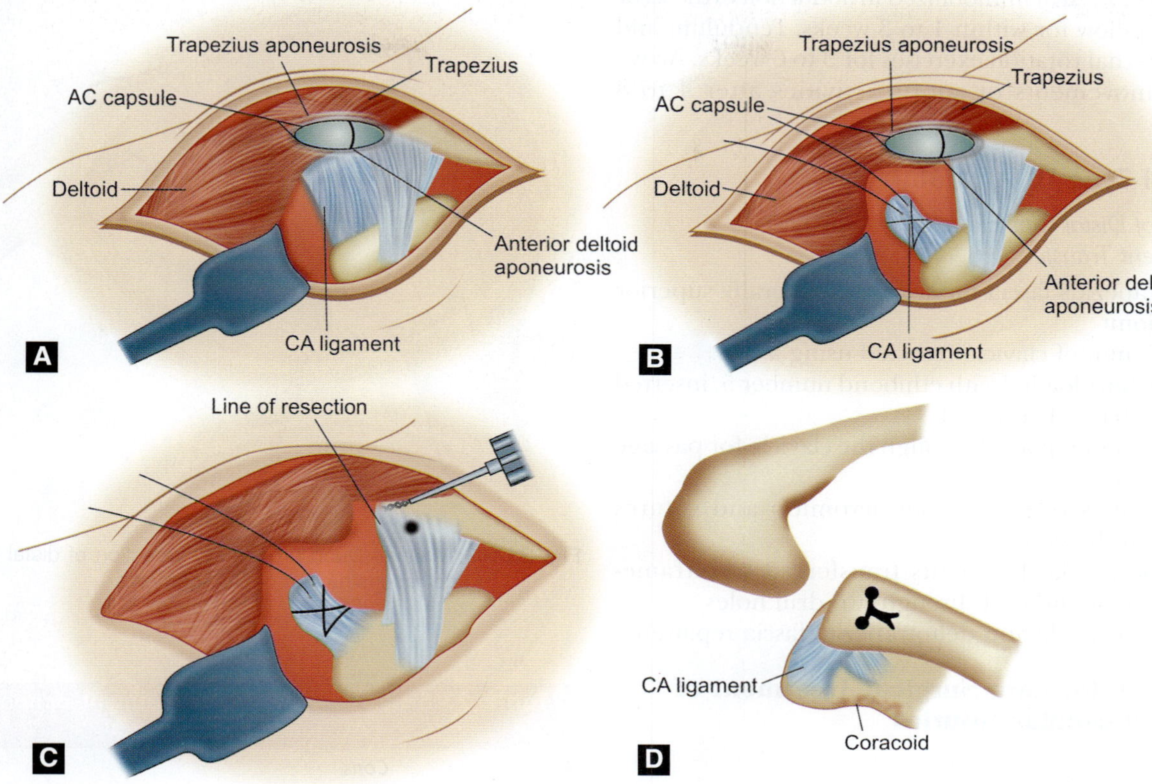

Figs 23.197A to D: Surgical repair of chronic type II AC joint injury—(A and B) Incision on Langer's line medial to AC joint, deltoid muscle is reflected anteriorly and AC joint capsule incised medial to lateral; (C) Drill holes made 5 mm from articular surface and 5 mm of distal end of clavicle is excised. Drill holes placed 2 mm to resection margins; (D) Sutures placed through drill holes, capsule and muscles are then repaired

Surgical Repair of Chronic Type II AC Joint Injury (Figs 23.197A to D)

- *Position:* Back of table, 20° short of vertical position.
- *Capsular flaps*: Small portion of anterior deltoid is reflected from acromion portion, to expose coracoacromial (CA) ligament
- Stay suturing is done on ligament
- Unicortical drill holes placed in distal clavicle (posteriosuperior)
- CA ligament transferred to intramedullary canal.
- Sutures placed through drill holes and tied over the top of clavicle.

Postoperative phase: Arm immobilized in abduction orthosis or abduction pillow for within 1 to 3 weeks. Pendulum and passive external rotation exercises for 3 to 6 weeks. Active range of movements or sports activity after 4 to 8 months.

Operative Stabilization of Type III AC Joint (Fig. 23.198)

- Deltotrapezius fascia incised mediolaterally
- Two holes drilled at the base of coracoid for anchor insertion

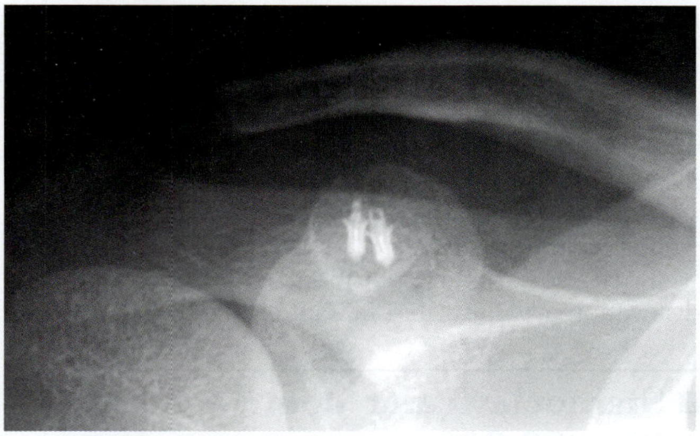

Fig. 23.198: Postoperative X-ray taken after reconstruction, using bone anchors of coracoid

- Sutures inserted at the base of coracoid
- Two drill holes placed through clavicle of passage sutures
- Sutures tied over bony ridges of clavicle to reconstitute coracoclavicular ligament
- Deltotrapezial aponeurosis is repaired

Postoperatively: Arm immobilized in abduction orthosis or abduction pillow for within 1 to 3 weeks. Pendulum and passive external rotation exercises for 3 to 6 weeks. Active range of movements or sports activities after 4 to 8 months.

Repair of Type III AC Joint

Resection of Distal Clavicle and CA Ligament Transfer

- Deltotrapezius fascia incised mediolaterally superior to AC joint
- Distal 5 mm of clavicle resected using a saw
- Two anchors loaded with ethibond number 5, inserted into the base of coracoid
- Two drill holes placed through the clavicle for passage of sutures
- Ligament is released from acromion and sutures placed in the end
- Coracoacromial ligaments transferred to intramedullay canal and tied through two drill holes
- AC joint capsule and deltotrapezial fascia repaired.

Indications for Late Surgical Treatment of Acromioclavicular Injuries

- Pain
- Weakness
- Deformity

Techniques for Late Surgical Treatment of Acromioclavicular Injuries

Reduction of AC joint and repair of AC and CC ligaments. Resection of distal clavicle and reconstruction of CC ligaments (Weaver-Dunn procedure).

Weaver-Dunn Procedure (Fig. 23.199)

- The distal clavicle is excised
- The CA ligament is transferred to the distal clavicle
- The CC ligaments are repaired and/or augmented with a coracoclavicular screw or suture
- Repair of deltotrapezial fascia.

Pros and cons of treatment options of AC joint dislocation are illustrated in Table 23.5.

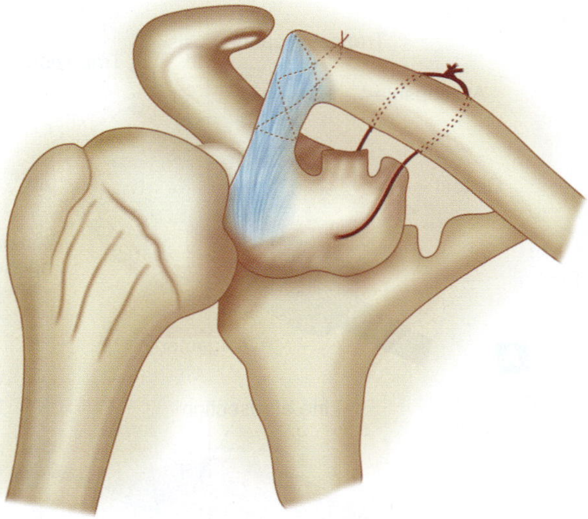

Fig. 23.199: Weaver-Dunn procedure, resection of distal clavicle and reconstruction of CC ligaments

Table 23.5: Pros and cons of treatment options of AC joint dislocation

	Pros	*Cons*
Intra-articular AC fixation	Anatomic reduction	• Hardware failure • Distal clavicel osteolysis
Extra-articular coracoclavicular repair	Superior strength of initial fixation (screw)	• Screw failure • Bone resorption
Ligament reconstruction	• Anatomic repair • No risk of metallic hardware failure	• Less initial fixation strength • Harvest coracoacromial ligament

■ Sternoclavicular Joint (Fig. 23.200)

Anatomy of the Sternoclavicular (SC) Joint

Various structures involved in the joint formation and maintenance of its stability are shown in Figure 23.201. The salient features and accompanied structures of the SC joint are described below:

- Diarthrodial joint
- Saddle shaped
- Poor congruence

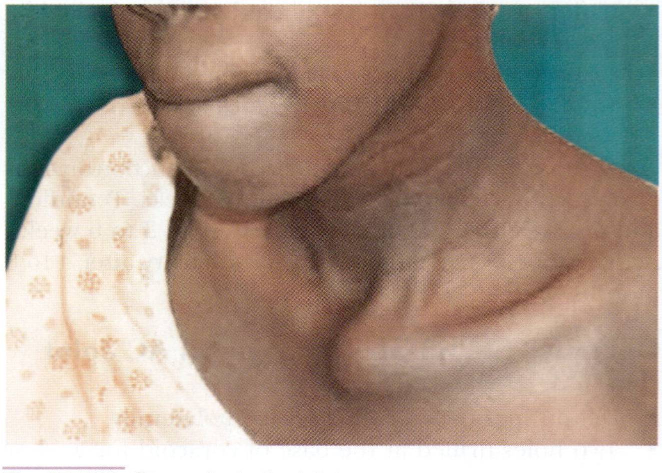

Fig. 23.200: Sternoclavicular joint

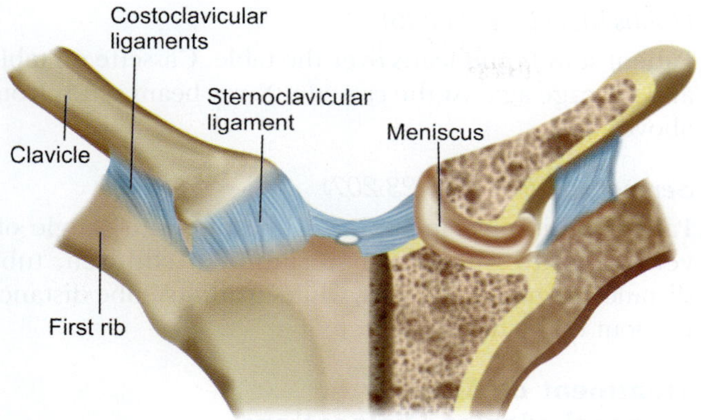

Fig. 23.201: The anatomy of the sternoclavicular joint and accompanying structures

- Intra-articular disk ligament divides SC joint into two separate joint spaces
- Costoclavicular ligament (rhomboid ligament), it is short and strong and consist of an anterior and posterior fasciculus
- Interclavicular ligament connects the superomedial aspects of each clavicle with the capsular ligaments and the upper sternum
- Capsular ligament covers the anterior and posterior aspects of the joint and represents thickenings of the joint capsule. The anterior portion of the ligament is heavier and stronger than the posterior portion.

Epiphysis of the Medial Clavicle

Medial physis: Last of the ossification centers to appear in the body and the last epiphysis to close. Does not ossify until 18 to 20 years of age. Does not unite with the clavicle, until the 23 to 25 years of age.

Anatomical Classification of Injuries of SC Joint (Figs 23.202 and 23.203)

Anterior dislocation: Common, medial end of clavicle displaced anteriorly or anteriosuperiorly with respect to anterior margin of sternum.

Posterior dislocation: Uncommon, clavicle displaced posteriorly with respect to posterior margin of sternum.

Etiological Classification of Injuries to SC Joint

Traumatic Injuries

- *Acute dislocation*: Dislocated sternoclavicular joint, with intra-articular ligaments ruptured.
- *Recurrent dislocation*: If initial dislocation does not heal, mild or moderate forces produce recurrent dislocation.
- *Chronic dislocation*: Original dislocation is unrecognized and irreducible.

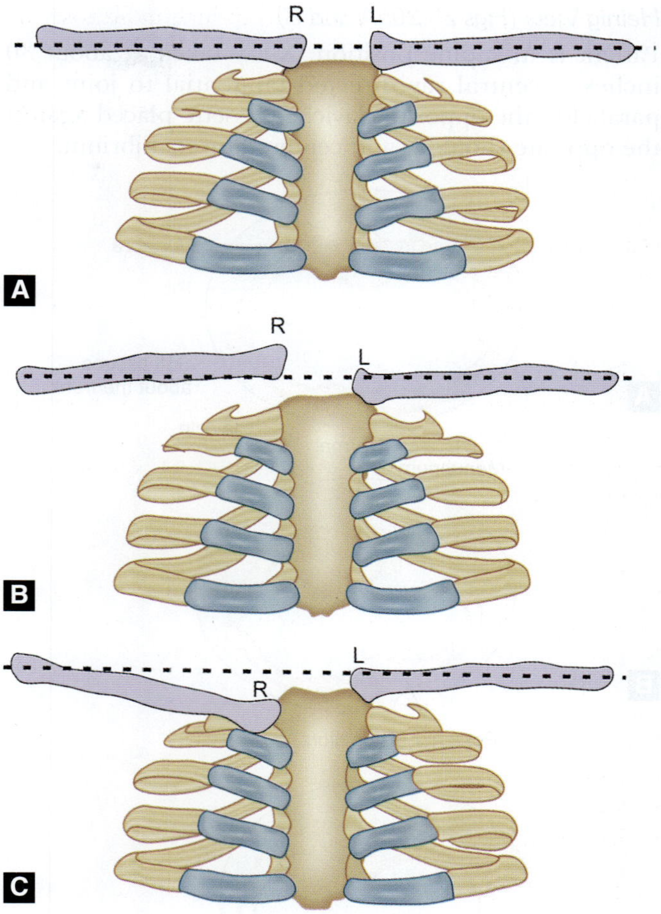

Figs 23.202A to C: Injuries of SC joint—(A) Normal joint; (B) Clavicle right sided (R) dislocated anteriorly; (C) Clavicle right sided; (R) dislocated posteriorly

Atraumatic Injuries

- Spontaneous subluxation or dislocation

Injuries Associated with Sternoclavicular Joint Dislocations (Fig. 23.204)

- Mediastinal compression
- Pneumothorax
- Laceration of the superior vena cava
- Tracheal erosion.

Radiographic Techniques

Radiographic techniques for assessing sternoclavicular injuries include:

- *CT scan:* Best technique for sternoclavicular joint problems
- Tomograms
- MRI
- Ultrasound.

Heinig View (Figs 23.205A and B)

Patient is in supine position. X-ray taken at about 30 inches, a central ray directed tangential to joint and parallel to the opposite clavicle. Cassette placed against the opposite shoulder and centered on manibrium.

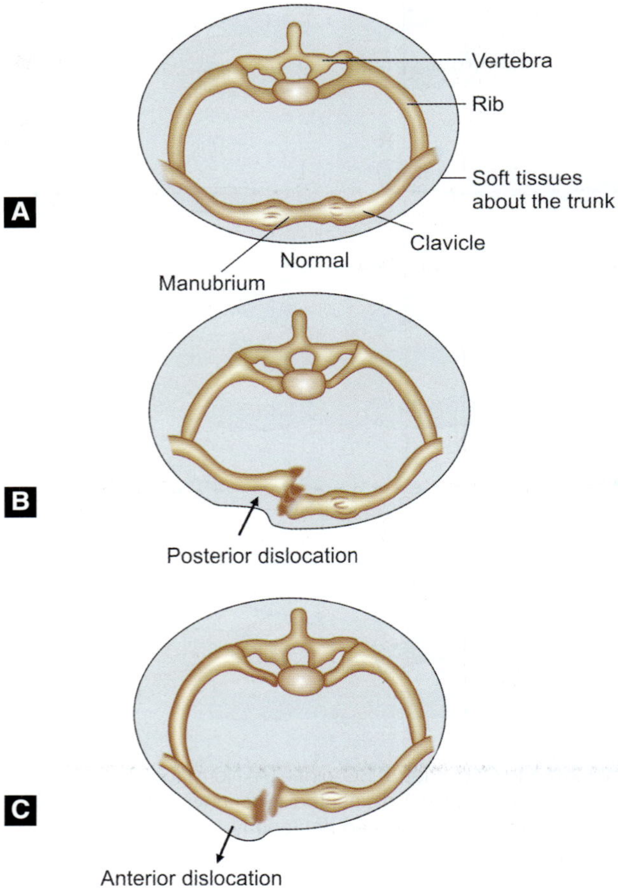

Figs 23.203A to C: Cross-section through thorax, showing injuries of SC joint—(A) Normal joint; (B) Joint dislocated posteriorly; (C) Joint anteriorly dislocated

Hobbs View (Fig. 23.206)

Patient stands and leans over the table. Cassette on table and rib cage against the cassette. X-ray beam sends from above.

Serendipity View (Fig. 23.207)

Patient positioned in supine. Tube tilted 40° angle off vertical and centered on sternum. In children, tube distance is about 45 inches, while in adults, tube distance is about 60 inches.

Treatment of Anterior Sternoclavicular Dislocations

Nonoperative treatment: Analgesics and immobilization are main nonoperative means of treatment. Functional outcomes are usually good.

Closed reduction: Often not much successful. Direct pressure over the medial end of the clavicle may reduce the joint.

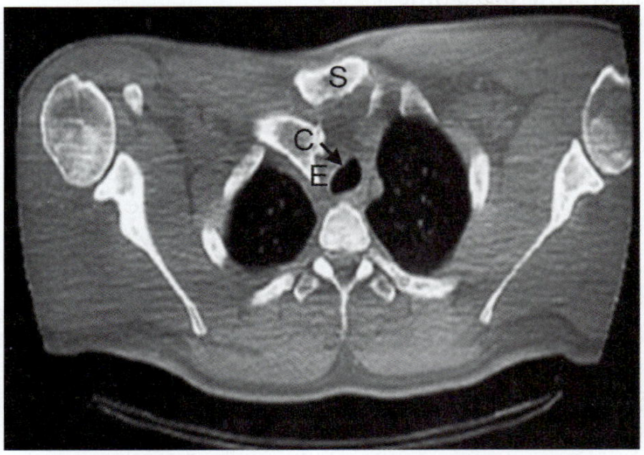

Fig. 23.204: Injuries associated with sternoclavicular joint dislocations—S. Sternum; C. Clavicle; E. Erosion of trachea

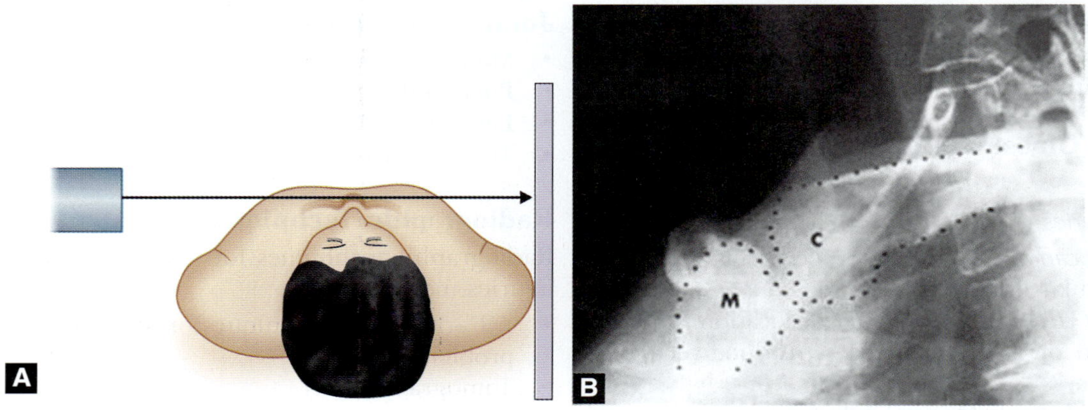

Figs 23.205A and B: Heinig view

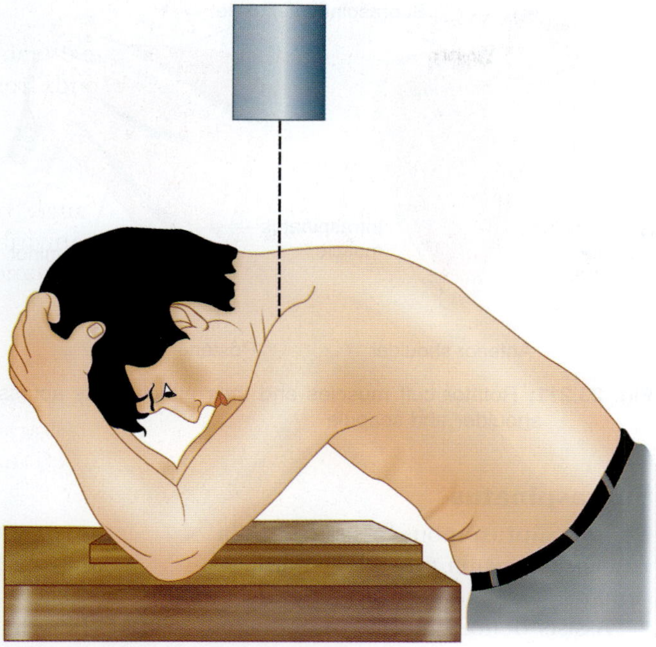

Fig. 23.206: Hobbs view

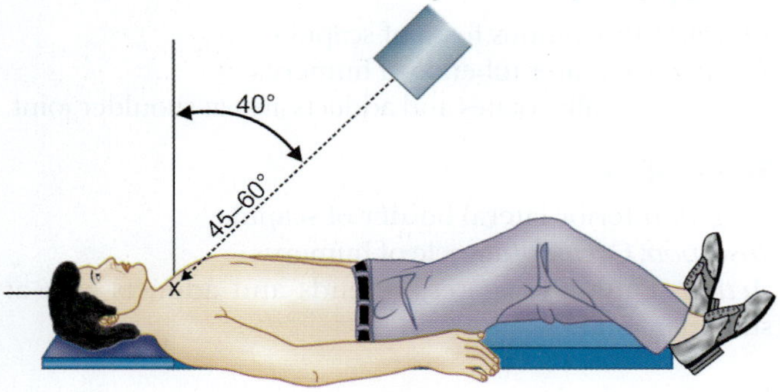

Fig. 23.207: Serendipity view

Treatment of Posterior Sternoclavicular Dislocations

Careful examination of the patient is extremely important to rule out vascular compromise. Consider CT to rule out mediastinal compression. Attempt closed reduction, it is often successful and remains stable.

Closed Reduction Techniques

This has been depicted in Figures 23.208 and 23.209.

Techniques employed are:

- Abduction traction
- Adduction traction
- *Towel clip*: Anterior force applied to clavicle by percutaneously applied towel clip.

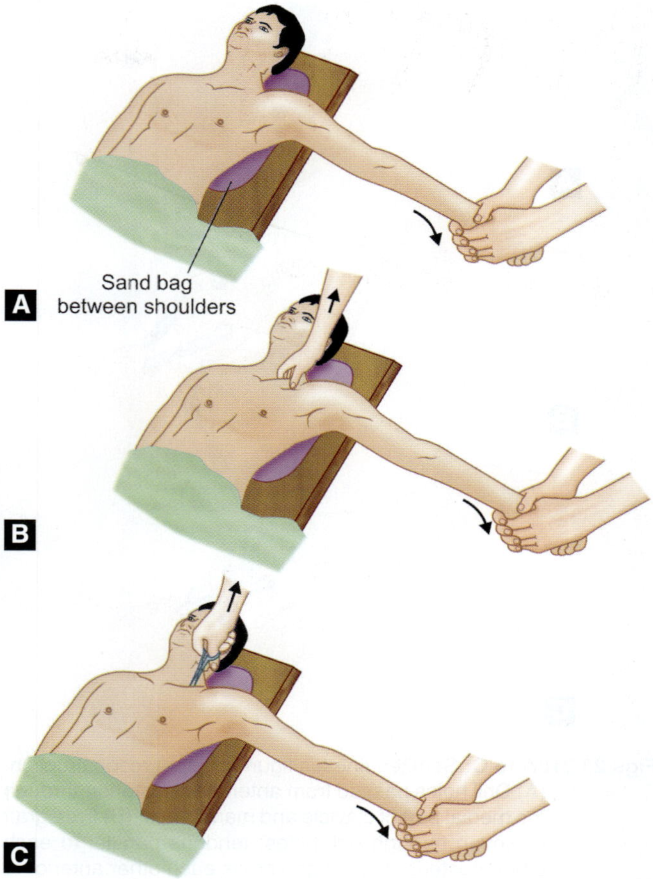

Figs 23.208A to C: Closed reduction technique for dislocated SC joint

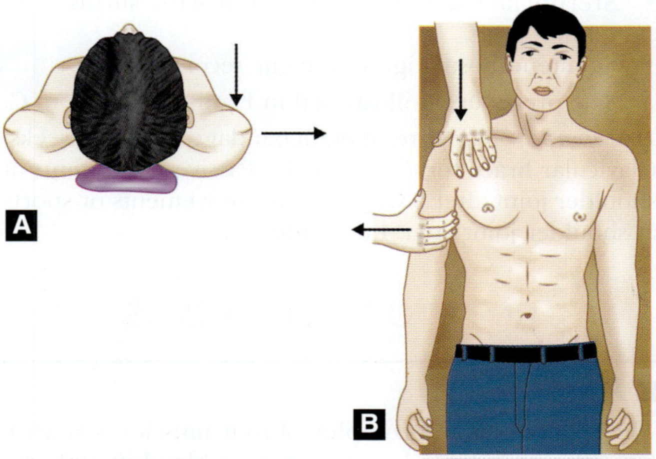

Figs 23.209A and B: Buckerfield-Castle technique for SC joint reduction

Operative Techniques

- *Resection arthroplasty:* May result in instability of remaining clavicle unless stabilization is done. Suggest minimal resection of bone and fixation of medial clavicle to first rib.

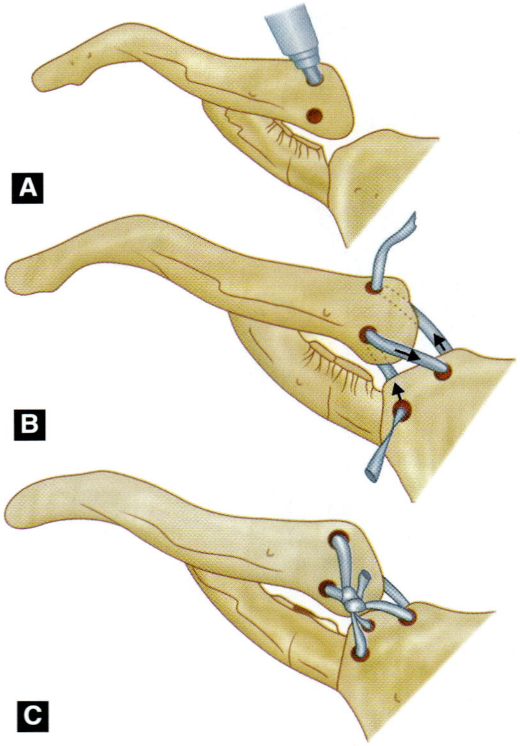

Figs 23.210A to C: Semitendinosus figure-of-eight reconstruction. (A) Drill holes passed from anterior to posterior, through the medial part of clavicle and manubrium; (B) Free graft is woven through drill holes, tendons parallel to each other, posterior to joint and cross each other anterior to the joint; (C) Tendon tied in square knot and is secured with sutures

- Sternoclavicular reconstruction with suture and tendon graft.
- Semitendinosus figure-of-eight reconstruction.

The procedure is illustrated in Figures 23.210A to C.

Postoperatively: Figure-of-eight bandage for 4 to 6 weeks. Clavicular brace for 4 to 6 weeks. Passive movements at shoulder joint after 6 weeks. Active movements or sports at shoulder joint after 4 to 6 months.

ROTATOR CUFF TEARS

Anatomy

The rotator cuff is a complex of four muscles that arise from the scapula and whose tendons blend in with the subjacent capsule, as they attach to the tuberosities of the humerus. The four muscles forming rotator cuff are:

1. Subscapularis
2. Infraspinatus
3. Teres minor
4. Supraspinatus.

Different rotator cuff muscles and their attachments across shoulder and scapula are shown in Figure 23.211.

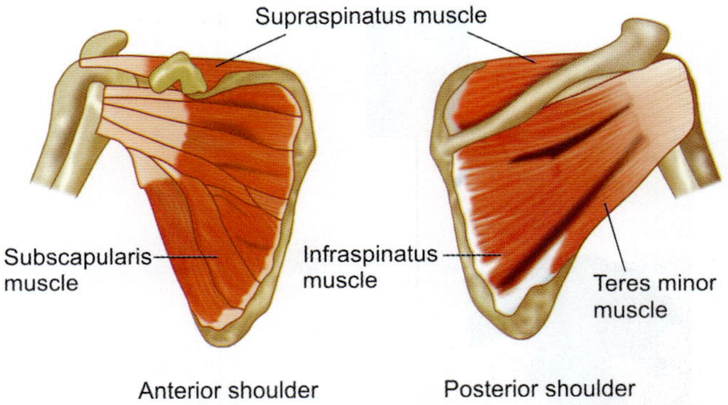

Fig. 23.211: Rotator cuff muscles and their attachments across shoulder and scapula

Supraspinatus

Origin: Supraspinous fossa of scapula
Insertion: Greater tubercle of humerus
Action:

- Assists deltoid muscle in abducting arm at shoulder joint.
- Initiates the first 30 to 60° of abduction at which point the deltoid takes over.

Infraspinatus

Origin: Infraspinous fossa of scapula
Insertion: Greater tubercle of humerus
Action: Laterally rotates and adducts arm at shoulder joint.

Teres Minor

Origin: Inferior lateral border of scapula
Insertion: Greater tubercle of humerus
Action: Laterally rotates, extends and adducts arm at shoulder joint.

Subscapularis

Origin: Subscapular fossa of scapula
Insertion: Lesser tubercle of humerus
Action: Medially rotates arm at shoulder joint.

Functions of Rotator Cuff Muscles

- They compress the head into the glenoid fossa, thereby providing a critical stabilizing mechanism to the shoulder known as concavity compression.
- They rotate the humerus with respect to the scapula.
- They provide muscular balance, a critical function, as illustrated in the Figure 23.212.

Vascularity

They are supplied by a vascular network that received contributions from the anterior humeral circumflex, the subscapular and the suprascapular arteries. The relative undervascularized portion is more proximal to supraspinatus insertion.

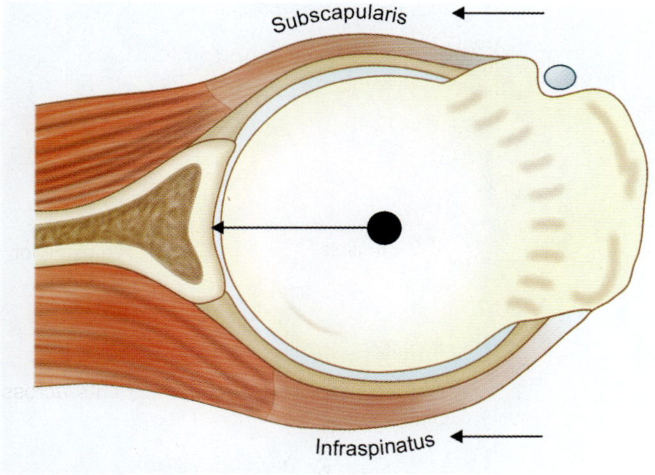

Fig. 23.212: Balancing function of rotator cuff muscles

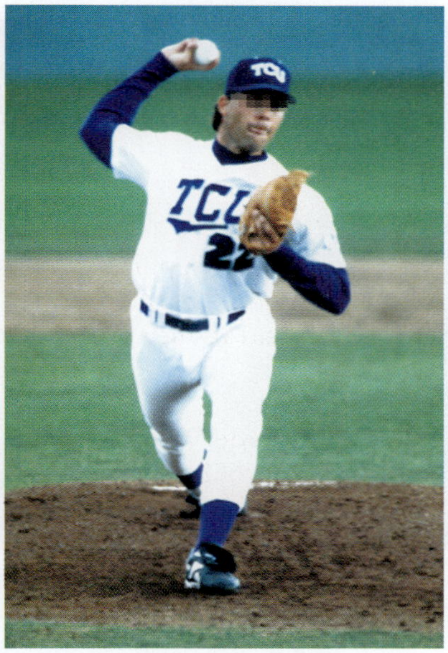

Fig. 23.213: Chronic causes of rotator cuff tear, due to overhead activities as in baseball players

Causes of Injury to Rotator Cuff Muscles

Chronic Tear

Found among people in occupations or sports requiring excessive overhead activity, e.g. painters, baseball pitchers, as depicted in the Figure 23.213. Variations in the shoulder structure causing narrowing under the outer edge of the collarbone.

Acute Tear

Acute or sudden powerful raising of the arm against resistance, often in an attempt to cushion a fall, e.g. heavy weight lifting or a fall on the shoulder. Injury usually

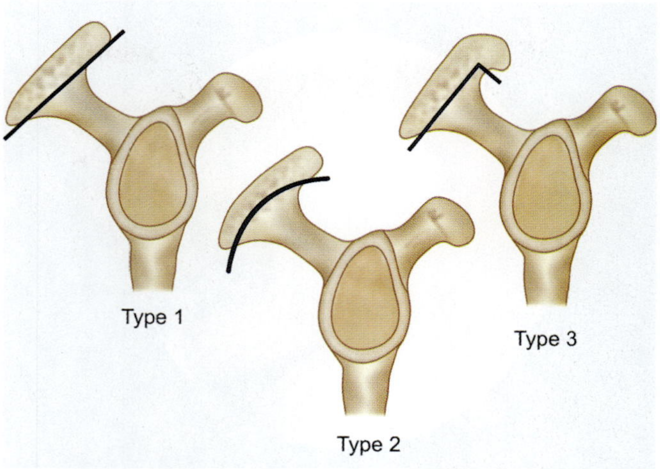

Fig. 23.214: Bigliani and Morrison classification of three types of acromions

associated with a significant amount of force, if person is younger than 30 years of age.

Other Causes

- Age related degeneration
- Compromised microvascular supply.

Outlet Impingement

The rotator cuff is surrounded by the coracoacromial arch, which comprises the supraspinatus outlet and consists of the acromion, coracoacromial ligament and coracoid process.The shape of the acromion has been implicated in rotator cuff pathology.

Bigliani and Morrison Classification

Bigliani and Morrison classified three types of acromions based on cadaveric examination.

- *Type I:* Flat
- *Type II:* Curved
- *Type III:* Hooked

Bigliani noted a significant increase in rotator cuff tears in curved (type II) and hooked (type III) acromions, these are shown in Figure 23.214.

Types of Rotator Cuff Pathology

- Simple tendinitis with swelling and inflammation (more commonly seen in younger patients with robust tissue).
- A partial thickness tear, involving only a portion of the rotator cuff fibers (involving less or more than 50 percent of the depth of the tendon).
- Full thickness tears with complete detachment from its normal insertion (as we often find in the elderly) due to severely degenerated tendons, as shown in Figure 23.215.

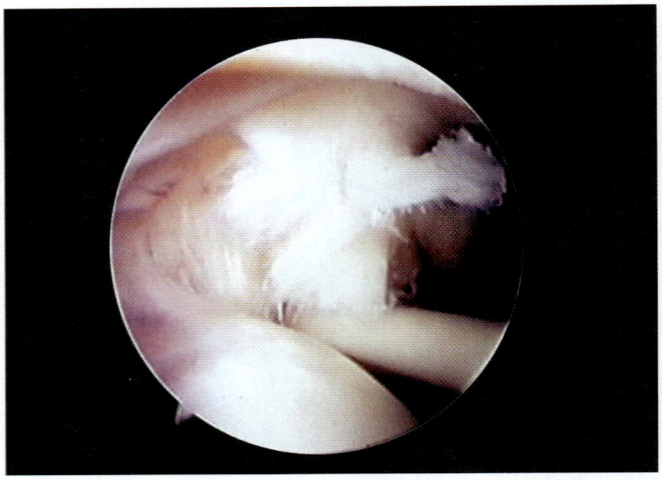

Fig. 23.215: A full thickness tear with complete detachment from its normal insertion

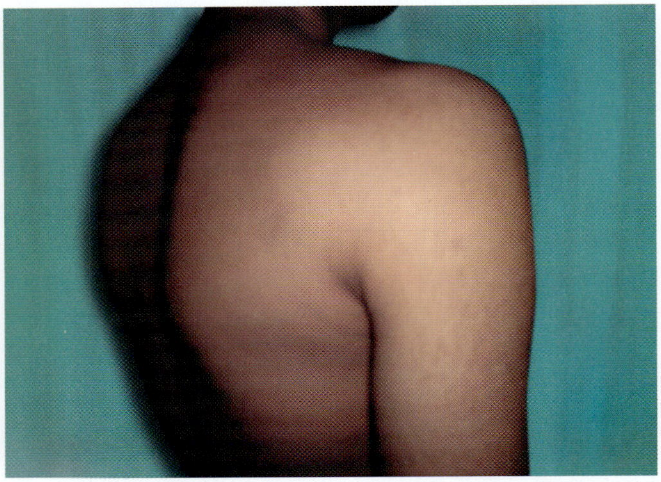

Fig. 23.216: Examination of the affected side of the shoulder

Classification

i. Based on dimensions given by Cofield tears are classified as:
  - *Small tears:* Less than 1 cm
  - *Medium tears:* 1 to less than 3 cm
  - *Large tears:* 3 to less than 5 cm
  - *Massive tears:* 5 cm or larger
  - Ellman presented a classification based on:

ii. Descriptions of location, e.g. articular, bursal and interstitial
  - Grading, like grade 1 for less than 3 mm deep, grade 2 for 3 to 6 mm deep and grade 3 for more than 6 mm deep

iii. Third classification based on tear area (in mm^2).

Clinical Evaluation

- History of trauma, occupation
- Complaints, like pain (location, aggravating factors)
- If there is decrease in sleep?
- Overhead weakness
- Stiffness, catching, popping of joint.

Inspection (Figs 23.216 and 23.217)

The therapist will examine the shoulder, looking for swelling, bruising, muscle wasting, postural issues, etc. It is important that the injured side is compared to the unaffected side at all times.

Palpation (Figs 23.218 and 23.219)

- Tenderness
- Range of motion both active and passive
- Weakness
- Instability
- Roughness or crepitus.

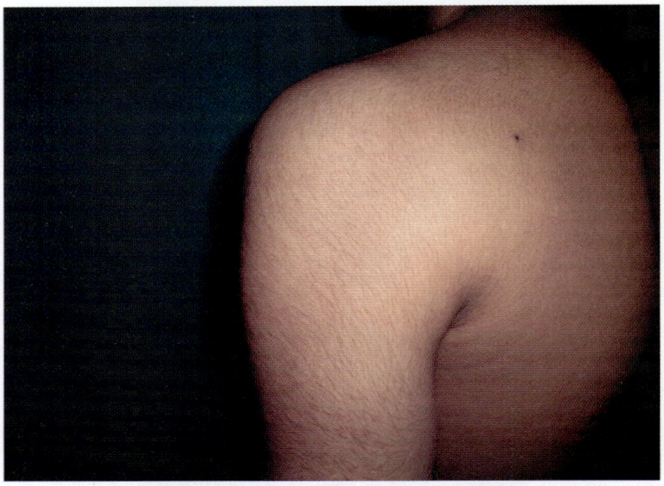

Fig. 23.217: Examination of the unaffected side of the shoulder and compare it with the affected side

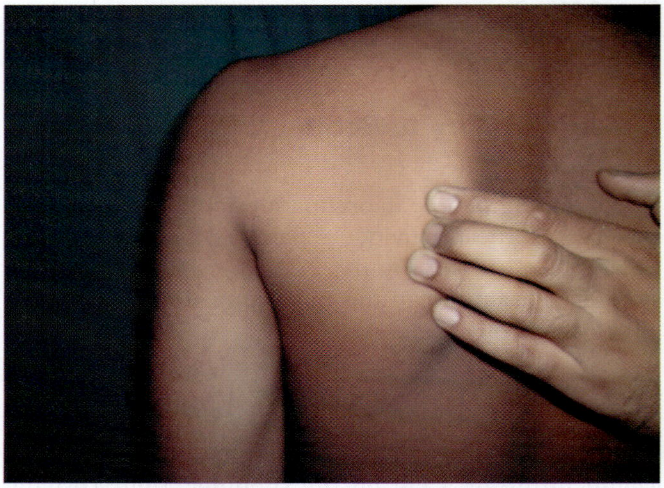

Fig. 23.218: Palpation done to check the roughness

Stiffness

Stiffness may be demonstrable as limitations in internal rotation, with the arm in abduction (measure in degrees from the neutral position) or with reaching up the back (posterior segment reached with the thumb), in cross-body adduction (measure in centimeters from the ipsilateral antecubital fossa to the contralateral acromion or coracoid), in flexion (measure in degrees from the neutral position) or in external rotation (measure in degrees from the neutral position), this is shown in Figures 23.220 and 23.221.

Weakness

Testing for weakness in abduction is done specifically for the supraspinatus tendon, which is the most common tendon that get torn out easily, as illustrated in Figure 23.222.

Subscapularis: Isometric internal rotation of the arm with the elbow flexed to 90° and the hand held posteriorly just off the waist.

Infraspinatus: Isometric external rotation of the arm held at the side in neutral rotation with the elbow flexed to 90°.

Subacromial Roughness

This is demonstrated in Figure 23.223, a test of a patient's passive range of motion of the arm in an abducted position is done and the physician palpates for roughness underneath the acromion.

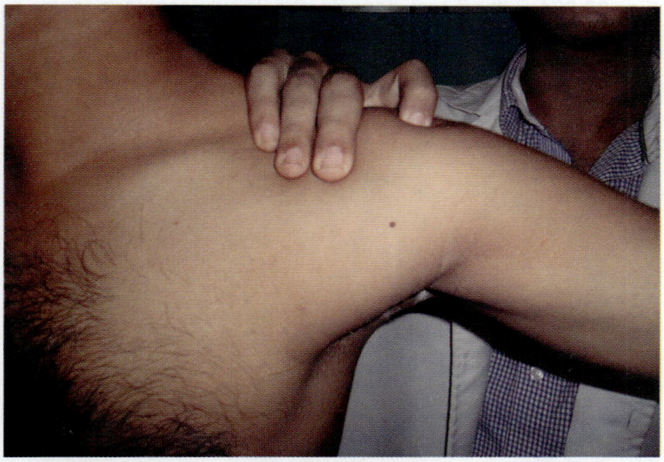

Fig. 23.219: Palpation done to check any crepitus

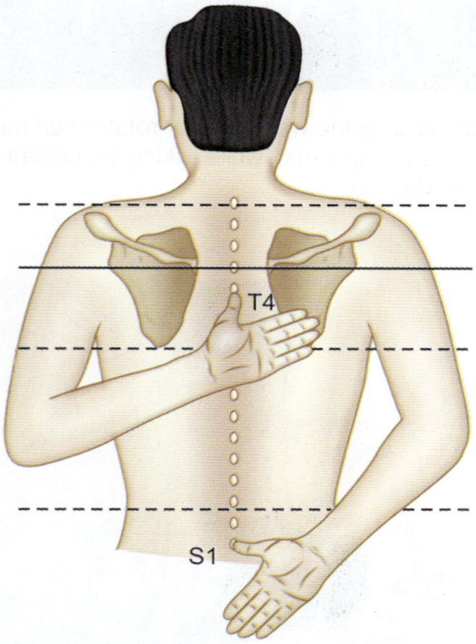

Fig. 23.221: With reaching up the back, measuring the posterior segment reached with the thumb

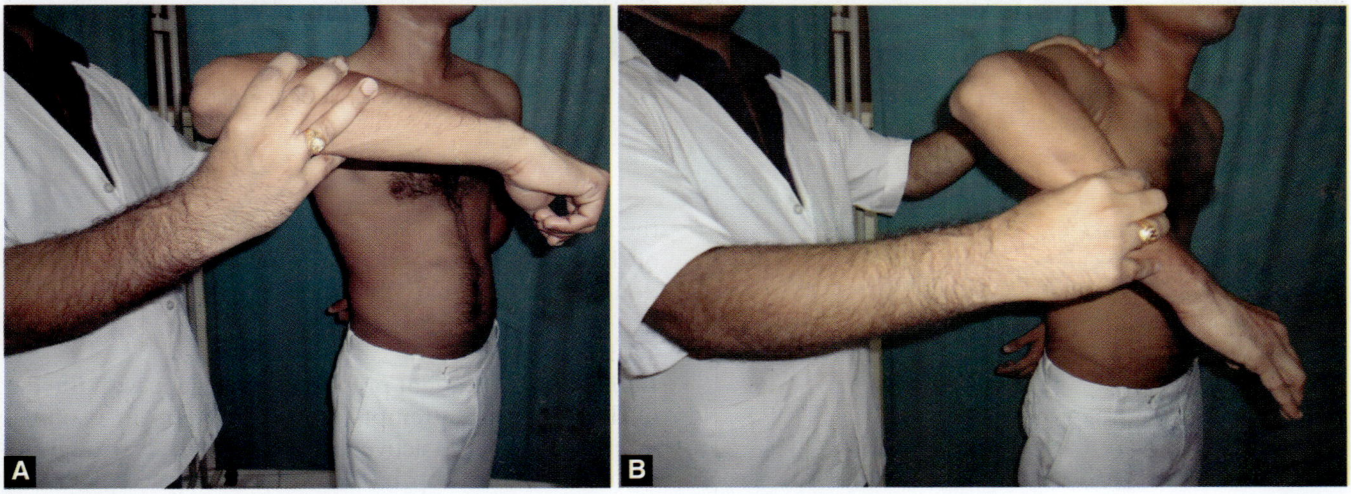

Figs 23.220A and B: Arm is internally rotated, while keeping shoulder in abduction

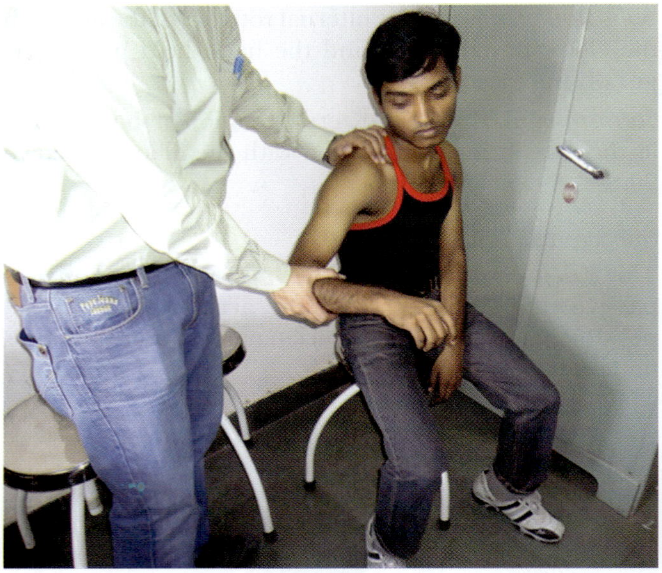

Fig. 23.222: Testing the weakness of rotator cuff muscles (mainly suprascapularis), while asking the patient to do shoulder abduction

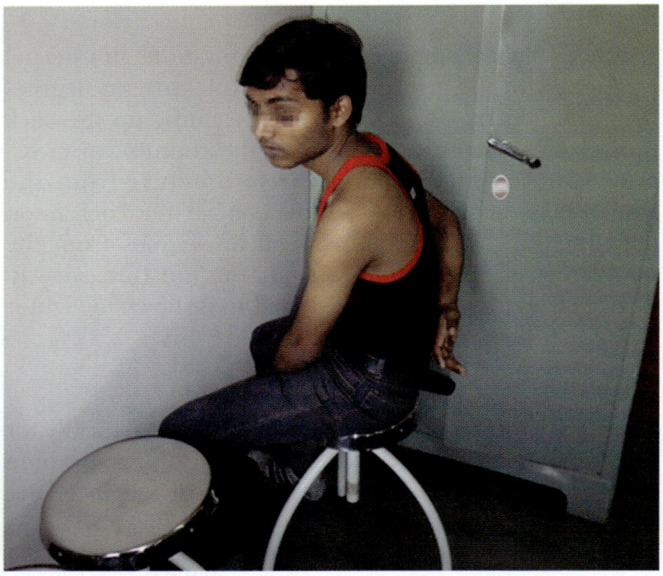

Fig. 23.224: Lift-off test done to check subscapularis injury or weakness

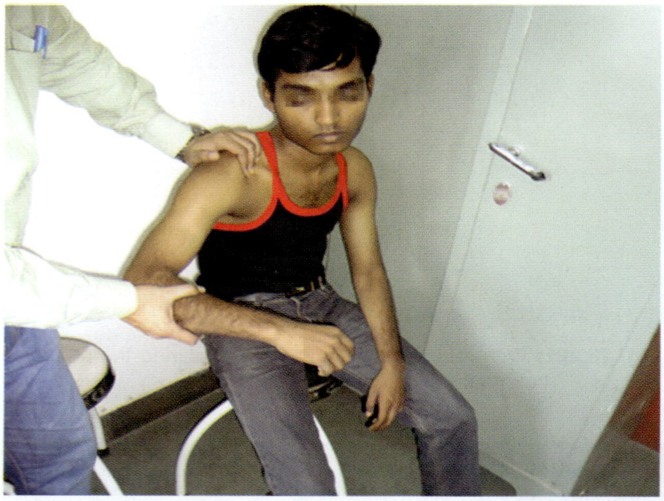

Fig. 23.223: Subacromial roughness is palpated while patient's arm is abducted passively

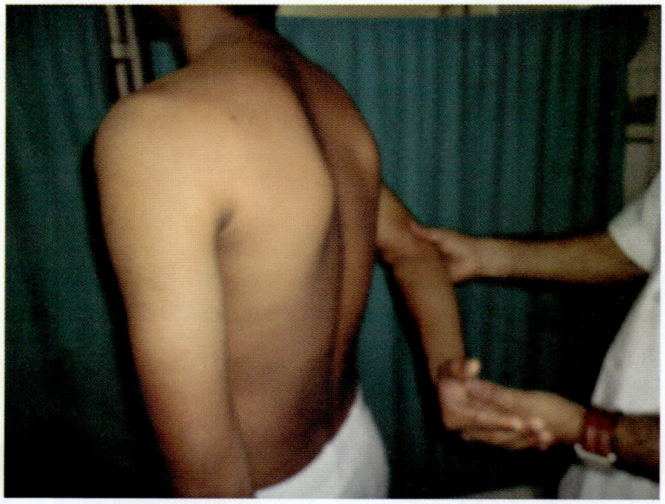

Fig. 23.225: Patient unable to lift off the hand, indicates positive test

Provacative Tests

- Lift-off test
- Belly-press test
- External rotation stress test
- External rotation lag sign
- Drop sign
- Internal rotation lag sign.

Lift-off Test

With the patient seated or standing, the arm is internally rotated, and the dorsum of the hand is placed against the lower back. If the patient is unable to lift the dorsum of the hand off the back, the test is positive. This test is done for subscapularis (Figs 23.224 and 23.225).

Belly-press Test

In this test, the patient presses the abdomen with the flat of the hand and attempts to keep the arm in maximal internal rotation. If active internal rotation is strong, the elbow does not drop backward, meaning it remains in front of the trunk. If the strength of the subscapularis is impaired, maximal internal rotation cannot be

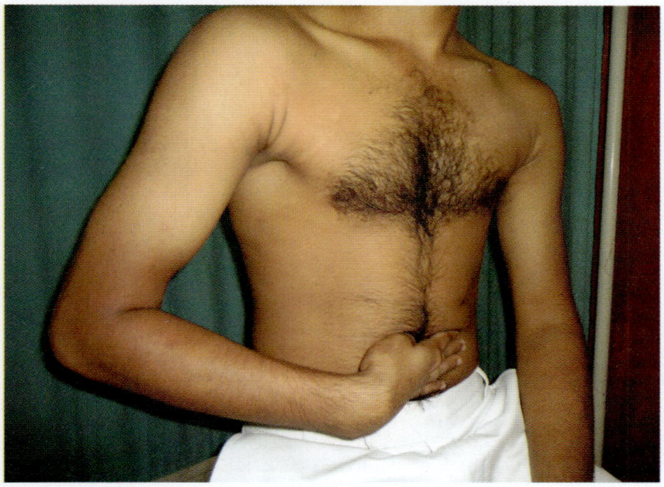

Fig. 23.226: Patient tends to flex the wrist to press against the abdomen, indicates subscapularis muscle being torned

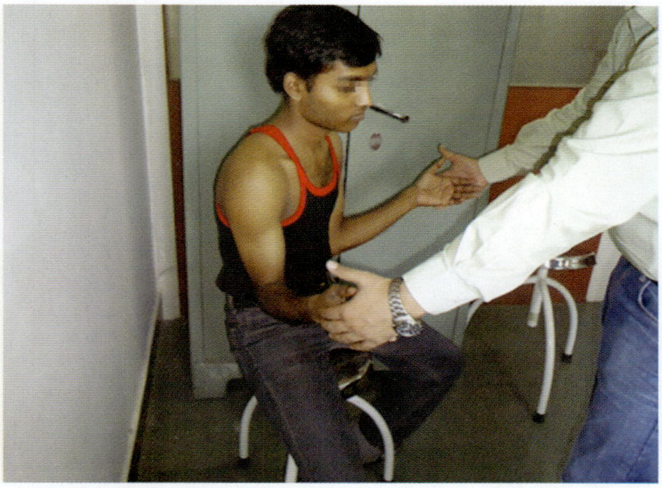

Fig. 23.228: External rotation stress test

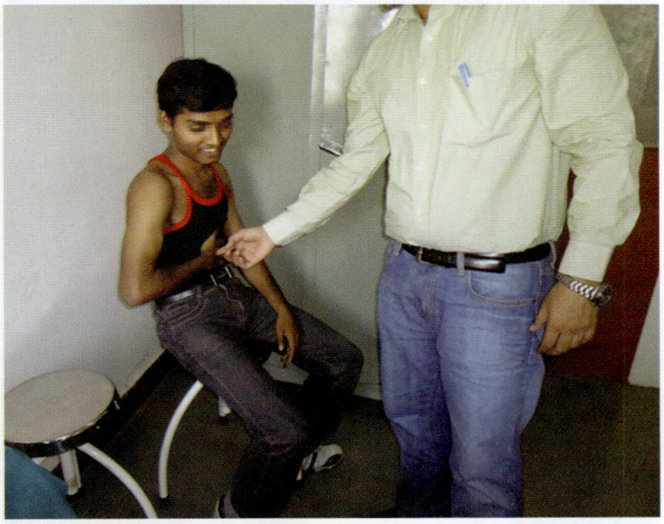

Fig. 23.227: Belly press test done to test the integrity of subscapularis tendon

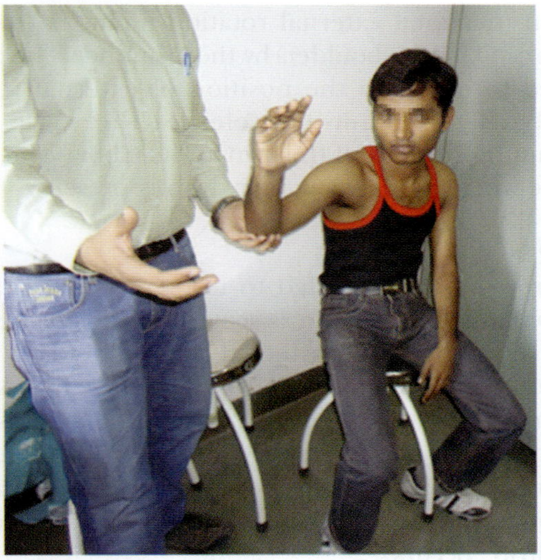

Fig. 23.229: The external rotation lag sign, to test the integrity of the supraspinatus and infraspinatus tendons

maintained, the patient feels the weakness and the elbow drops back behind the trunk. The patient exerts pressure on the abdomen, by extending the shoulder, rather than by internally rotating it. Other investigators have noted that when the subscapularis tendon is torn, patients tend to flex the wrist to press against the abdomen and are unable to hold the elbow forward, as shown in Figures 23.226 and 23.227.

External Rotation Stress Test (Fig. 23.228)

The external rotation stress test is intended to test the integrity of the external rotators of the shoulder, specifically the infraspinatus and the teres minor. With the patient's arms by his or her side in neutral flexion and abduction, the shoulders are externally rotated by 45 to 60°. The examiner applies force against the dorsum of the hands, attempting to rotate the shoulders internally back to neutral, while the patient is asked to resist. Pain and weakness suggest inflammation or tearing of the infraspinatus or the teres minor or both.

External Rotation Lag Sign (Fig. 23.229)

The external rotation lag sign test is designed to test the integrity of the supraspinatus and infraspinatus tendons. The patient is seated with his or her back to the examiner. The elbow is passively flexed to 90° and the shoulder is

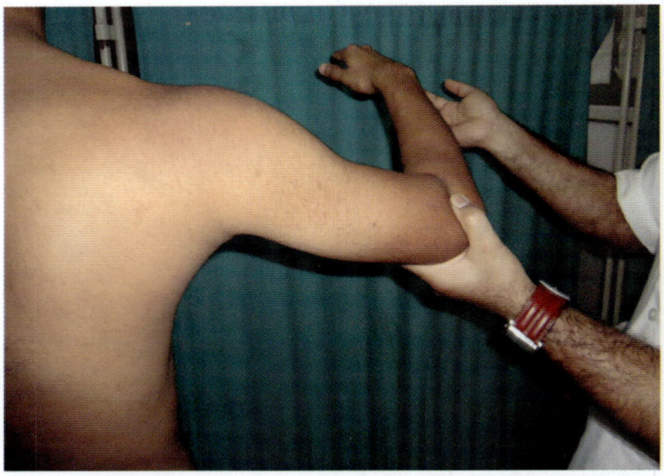

Fig. 23.230: The drop sign to test the integrity of the infraspinatus

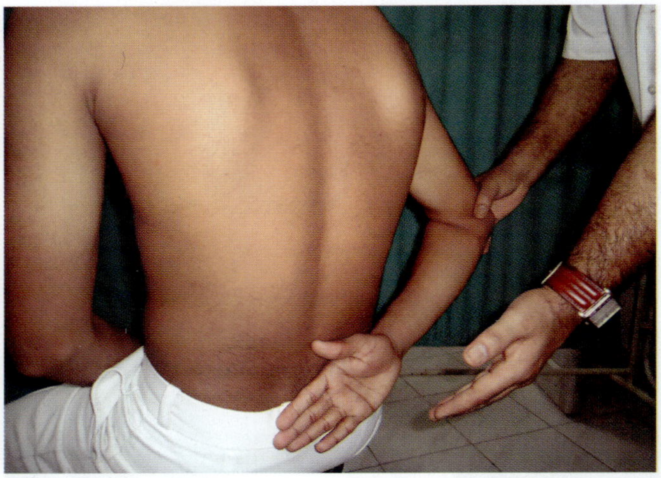

Fig. 23.231: Internal rotation lag sign

held at 20° of elevation and near maximal external rotation (maximal external rotation minus 5°, to avoid elastic recoil in the shoulder) by the examiner. The patient is asked to maintain the position of external rotation actively as the examiner releases the wrist, while maintaining support of the arm at the elbow. The sign is positive when a lag, or angular drop is present.

Drop Sign (Fig. 23.230)

The drop sign is intended to test the integrity of the infraspinatus. The patient is seated with his or her back to the examiner. The affected arm is held at 90° of elevation in the scapular plane and at almost full external rotation with the elbow flexed at 90°. The patient is asked to maintain this position actively as the examiner releases the wrist while supporting the elbow, which is mainly a function of the infraspinatus. The sign is positive if a lag or a "drop" occurs.

Internal Rotation Lag Sign (Fig. 23.231)

The patient is seated with his or her back to the examiner. The affected arm is held by the examiner in almost maximal internal rotation. The elbow is flexed to 90°, and the shoulder is held at 20° of elevation and 20° of extension. The dorsum of the hand is passively lifted away from the lumbar region until almost full internal rotation is reached. The patient is asked to maintain this position actively as the examiner releases the wrist, while maintaining support at the elbow. The sign is positive when a lag occurs.

Differential Diagnosis

- Acromioclavicular arthritis
- Frozen shoulder
- Glenohumeral arthritis
- Herniated cervical disk
- Suprascapular nerve entrapment
- Fracture

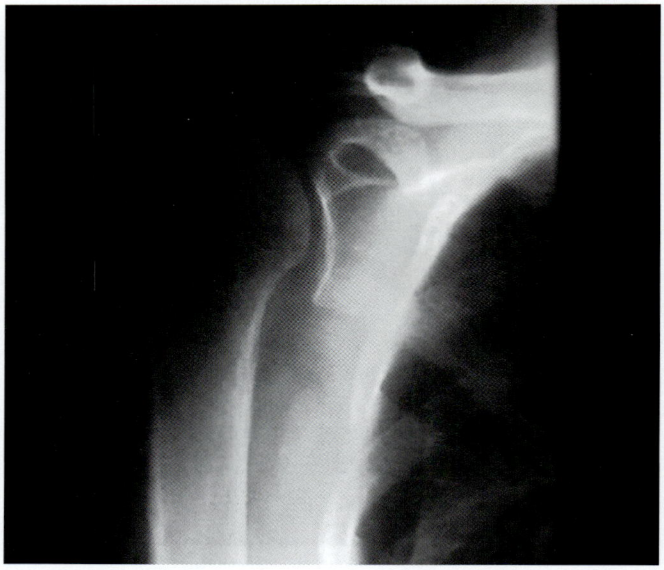

Fig. 23.232: X-ray findings in rotator cuff injuries

Diagnostic Imaging

X-Rays

Reactive changes of the greater tuberosity on the undersurface of the acromion, sourcil or eyebrow and spur is seen, as shown in Figure 23.232. These occur due to failure of the cuff to keep the humeral head centered within the glenoid concavity, thus allowing it to ride higher due to unbalanced action of the deltoid and they rub on each other.

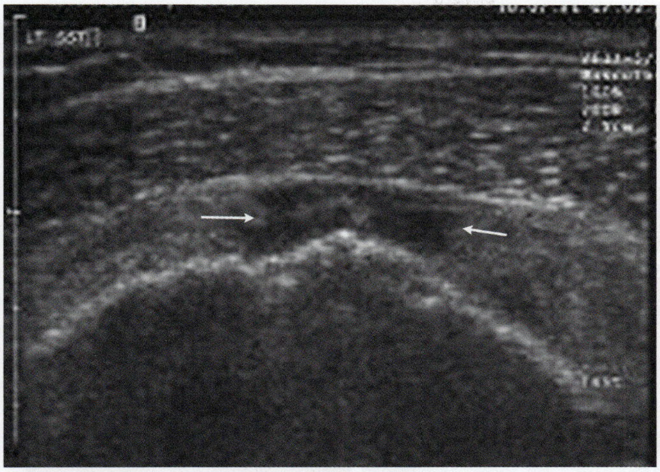

Fig. 23.233: Ultrasound used as a diagnostic technique to investigate about rotator cuff injuries

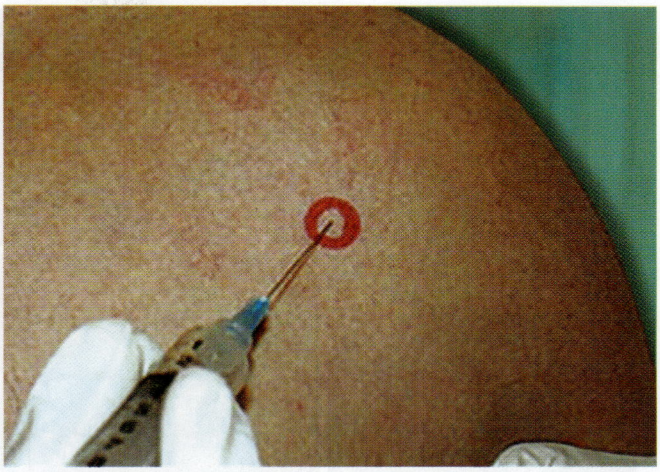

Fig. 23.235: Patient is given subacromial injections

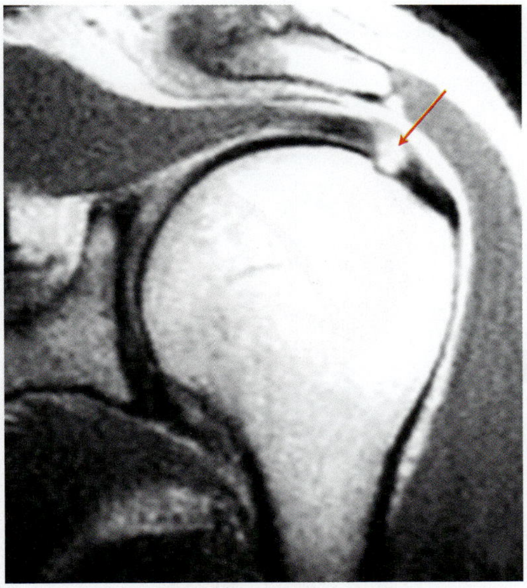

Fig. 23.234: MRI of shoulder showing rotator cuff injuries

High-riding humeral head: Humeral head riding up and out of the normal glenoid concavity due to a loss of the normal compressive forces of the rotator cuff tendons, holding it into the socket.

Other Imaging Studies

- Arthrogram
- Ultrasound (Fig. 23.233)
- Magnetic resonance imaging (MRI) (Fig. 23.234)
- Computed tomography (CT scan)

Treatment

Conservative Treatment

- Rest
- Nonsteroidal anti-inflammatory drugs (NSAIDs)
- Subacromial injections (Fig. 23.235)
- Muscle strengthening exercises.

Surgical Management

- Arthroscopic repair (Figs 23.236A and B)
- Open acromioplasty (Figs 23.237A to D)
- Open rotator cuff repairs
- Tendon transfers
- Humeral head replacement with maintenance of the coracoacromial arch for rotator cuff arthropathy.

Rotator Cuff Repair

McLaughlin technique illustrated in Figures 23.238A and B, sutures are passed through appropriately placed bony holes and cuff edge is drawn deep into trough.

Tendon Transfer

The tendon transfer procedure is illustrated in Figures 23.239 and 23.240.

After Treatment

After standard repair, an abduction pillow, a low profile pillow sling or shoulder immobilizer is worn for 6 weeks. It is removed for assisted exercises in flexion and external rotation to avoid adhesions, disuse atrophy and disruption of the repairs. The repair is weakest at 3 weeks and tendon strength is less than at the time of surgery for the first 3 months after the surgery. Empirically, we advance to isometric external rotation exercises at 6 weeks and at 12 weeks active motion is permitted. Patients are cautioned that overaggressive use of the extremity can lead to disruption of the repair for 6 to 12 months.

Complications

- Failed repairs
- Persistent subacromial impingement

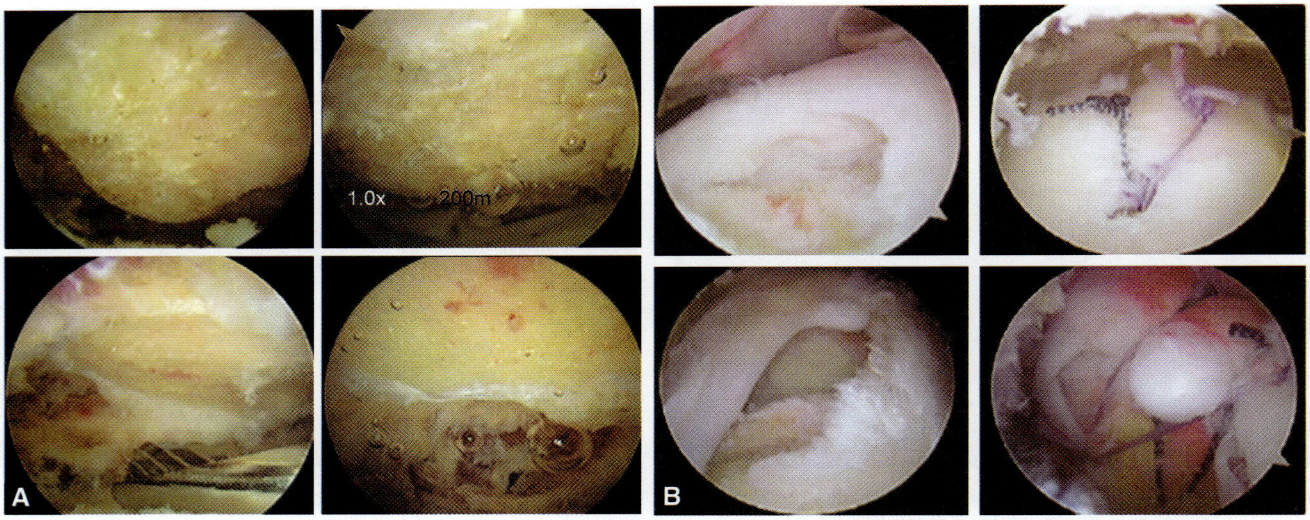

Figs 23.236A and B: Arthroscopic repair

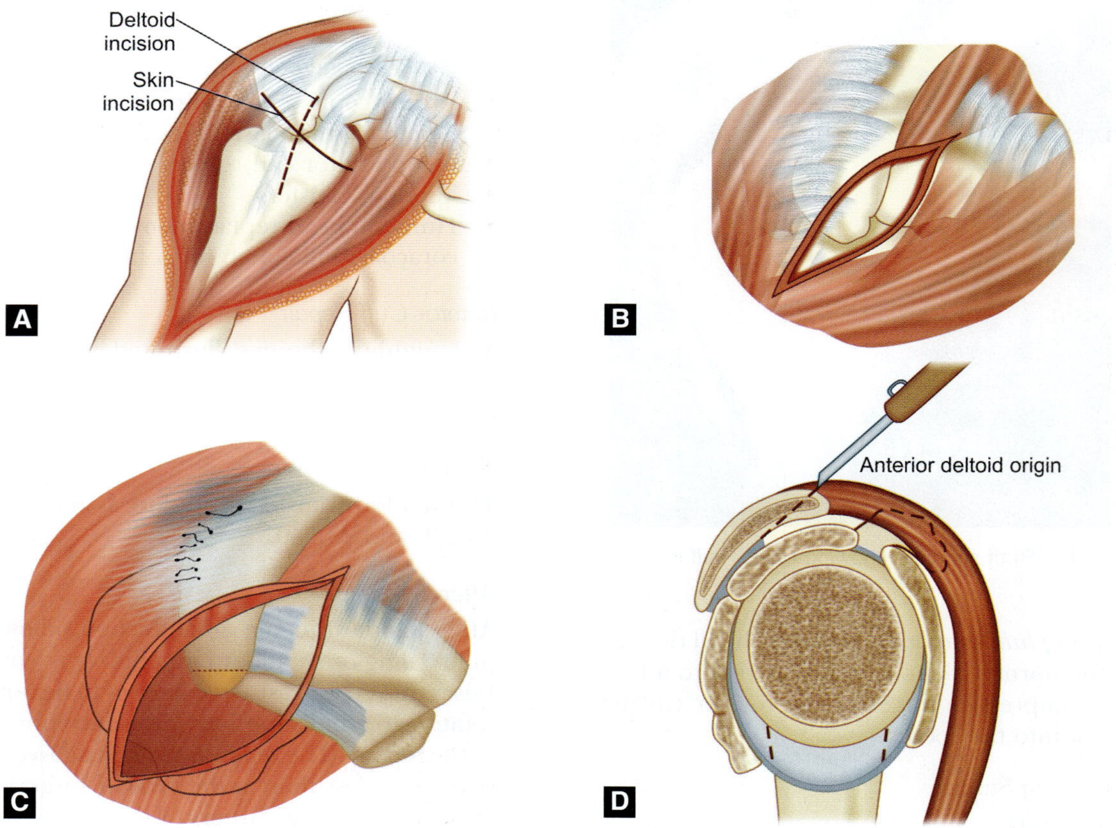

Figs 23.237A to D: Open acromioplastic repair

- Stiffness
- Heterotropic ossification
- Deltoid insufficiency

Calcific Tendinitis (Fig. 23.241)

Calcifying tendinitis of the rotator cuff is a common disorder of unknown etiology in which calcium crystals deposited in a living tendon in the course of reactive calcification usually undergone overtime with spontaneous resorption followed by healing of the tendon. Most commonly supraspinatus tendon is involved. Codman, pointed out that diseases in the supraspinatus tendon tend to occur in a specific area of the tendon, i.e. about half an inch proximal to the insertion. He called this area, *the critical portion.*

Classification

This classification is based on the French Arthroscopic Society:

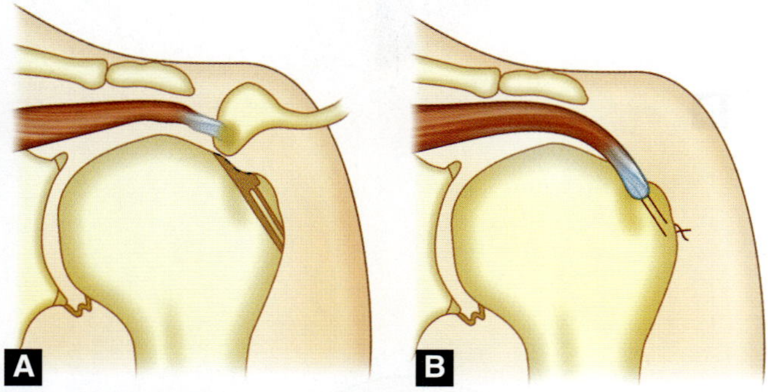

Figs 23.238A and B: McLaughlin technique of rotator cuff repair

Type A: Sharply delineated, dense and homogeneous appearance.

Type B: Sharply delineated, dense and multiple fragments.

Type C: Heterogeneous appearance and fluffy.

Type D: Dystrophic calcifications at the tendon insertion.

Chronological Progression

Phase I: Precalcification stage, the site of predilection for calcification (possibly a site with a diminished blood supply) undergoes fibrocartilaginous metaplasia.

Phase II: Calcification stage, during this stage, calcium is deposited into the matrix vesicles, which are excreted by the cells and coalesce into larger calcium deposits.

Phase III: Postcalcification phase, during this phase, the granulation tissue matures into mature collagen aligned along stress lines with the longitudinal axis of the tendon, reconstituting the tendon.

Clinical Findings

- Pain is most common symptom associated with redness and swelling
- Painful arc of motion
- Range of motion decreased.

Imaging (Fig. 23.242)

Treatment

- Aspiration and needling of calcium deposits
- Excision of calcium deposits, as shown in Figures 23.243A and B.

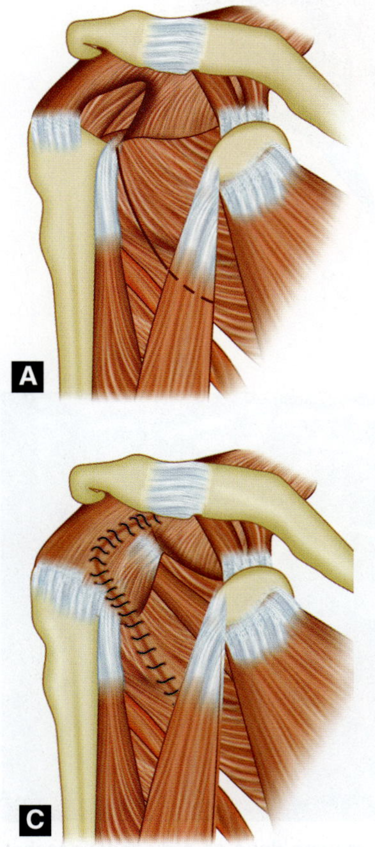

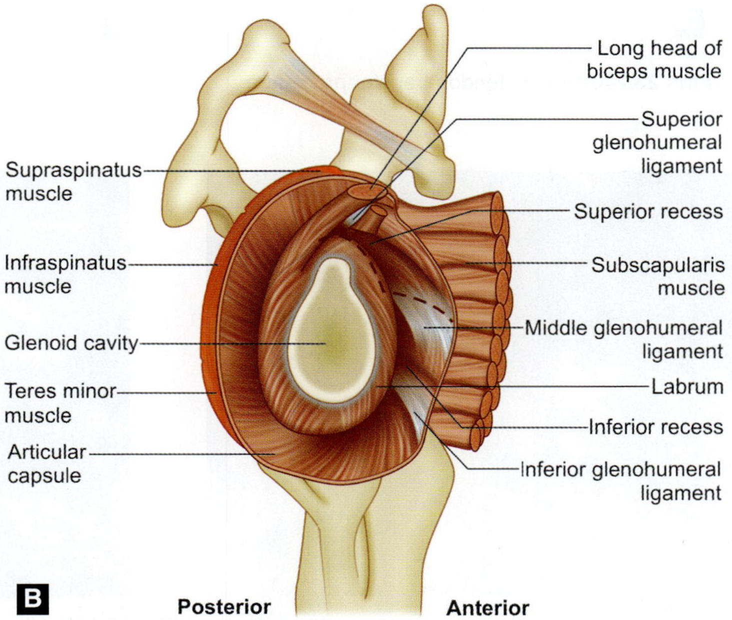

Figs 23.239A to C: Technique or method employed for tendon transfer

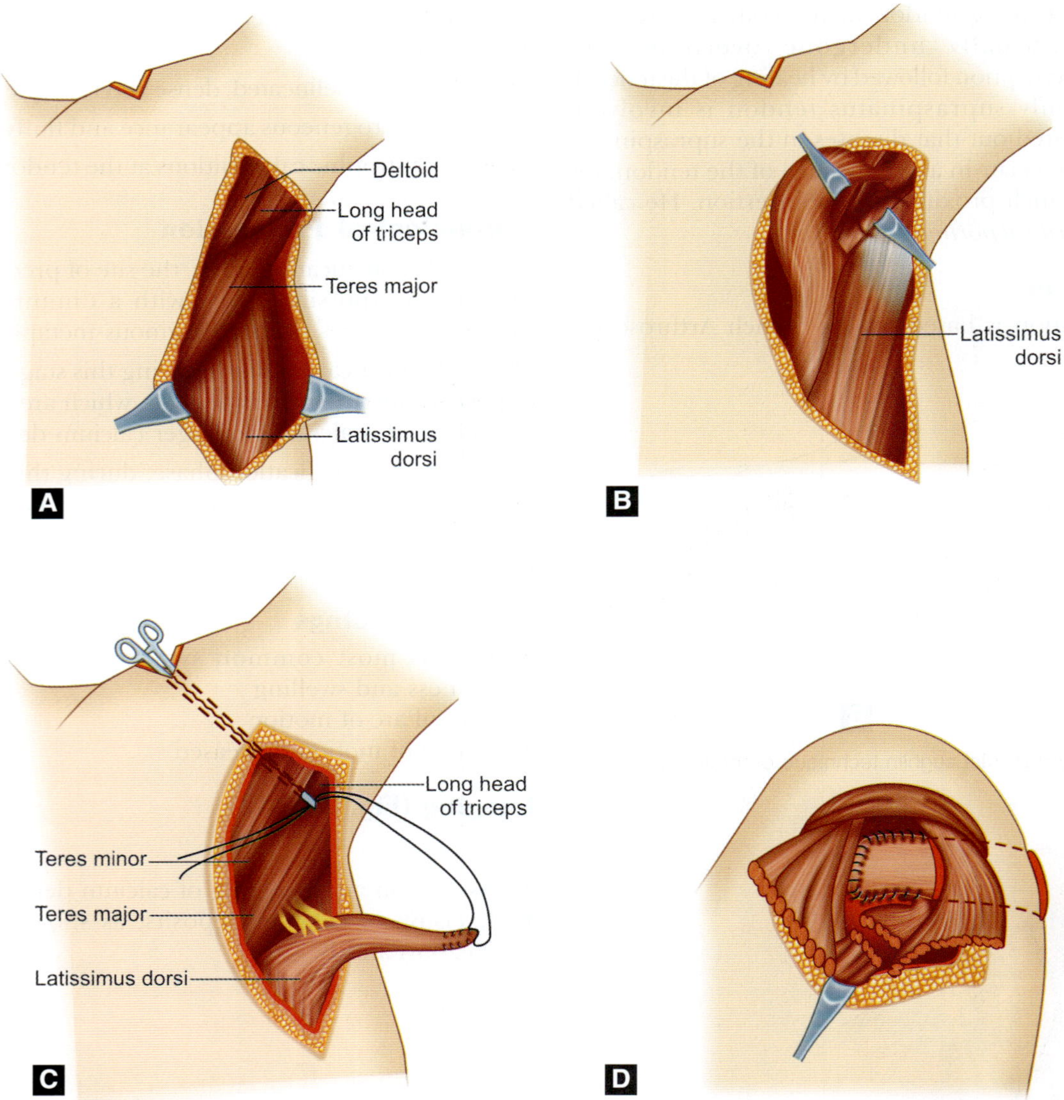

Figs 23.240A to D: Tendon transfer procedure

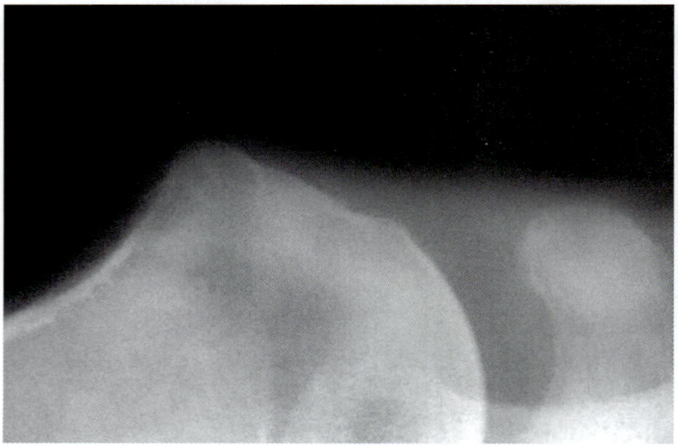

Fig. 23.241: Critical point for calcific tendinitis in supraspinatus

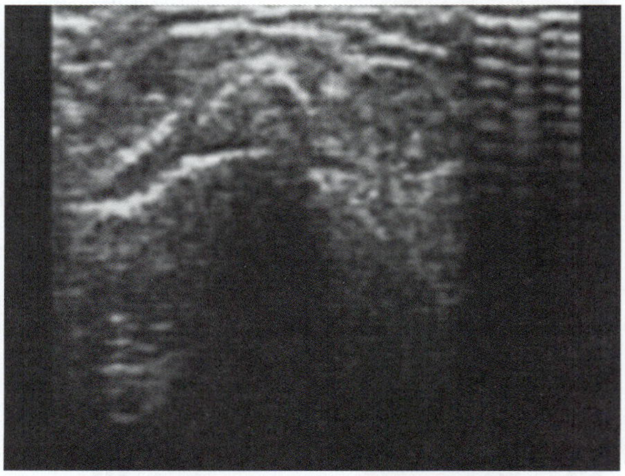

Fig. 23.242: Ultrasound imaging done as a diagnostic technique, to investigate about calcific tendinitis

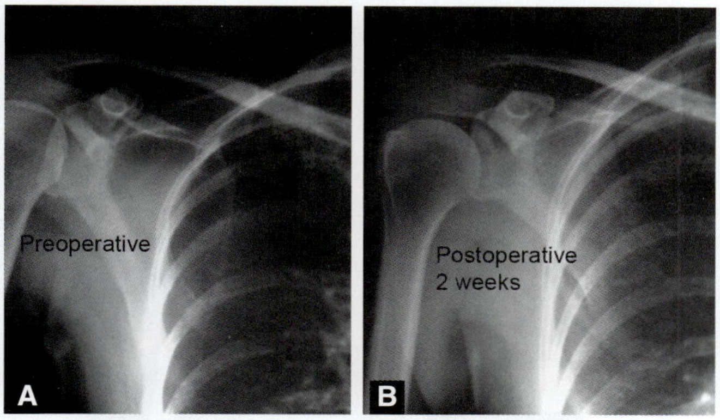

Figs 23.243A and B: Radiographs showing excision of calcium deposits from tendon operatively—(A) Preoperative; (B) Postoperative view

SHOULDER ARTHRODESIS

History

Around the turn of the 20th century, shoulder arthrodesis was a relatively common procedure. Indications at that time were mainly for upper extremity paralysis, due to polio or shoulder joint destruction, caused by tuberculosis. A purely extra-articular technique of shoulder arthrodesis was recommended for tuberculous infection, to prevent invasion from the infected joint. With the advent of antitubercular drugs, this technique became unnecessary. Later, procedures were described that placed various types of bone graft into the beds of the decorticated glenohumeral or acromiohumeral joints or both. Internal fixation is now recommended because external support alone rarely maintains complete fixation of the shoulder. Internal fixation allows better stabilization of contact surfaces and promotes fusion.

In the early 1950s, Charnley introduced the use of external fixation to apply compression across the fusion site. The external fixator was removed at 6 weeks and a spica cast was worn for 3 months. Most studies employing Charney's technique, reported fusion rates greater than 90 percent. External fixation is still useful in certain patients, especially if infection is present or trauma has occurred with significant soft-tissue injury. In 1957, Carroll suggested using a wire loop to connect the glenoid and humeral head, allowing postoperative changing of arm position. In this technique, a 22-gauge wire is routed through the humeral head and the anterosuperior quadrant of the glenoid, exiting the glenoid neck inferior to the coracoid process.

The 1960s saw the introduction of internal fixation for shoulder arthrodesis. Moseley and May described a technique, using internal fixation with two screws. Charnley and Houston described a technique that combined external fixation with internal fixation using screws. Disadvantages of screw fixation are a higher nonunion rate and the need for prolonged spica casting. In 1970, the Association of Orthopedics (AO) group published its technique of plate and screw fixation, to allow mobilization of the patient without a spica cast. Kostuik and Schatzker introduced the use of a second posterior buttress plate and obtained union in all 18 shoulders, they repaired using this technique. In the late 1980s, Richards et al. described a technique using a malleable pelvic reconstruction plate, without bone grafting. Followed by six postoperative weeks of spica casting.

Indications

Indications for glenohumeral arthrodesis are:
- Infection
- Paralytic disorders
- Unreconstructable rotator cuff tears
- Combined insufficiency of rotator cuff and deltoid.
- Failed shoulder arthroplasty
- Arthritic diseases unsuitable for arthroplasty
- Recurrent dislocations
- Neoplastic lesions.

Position (Figs 23.244A to D)

The proper position of the arm at the time of arthrodesis is controversial. In 1974, Rowe recognized the advantages of minimizing abduction and flexion. Cofield and Briggs, found the amount of internal rotation, to be the most important factor in determining the functional success of the operation. Hawkins and Neer, performed a functional analysis in 17 patients, who had shoulder arthrodesis and identified a range of acceptable positions. They recommended 25 to 40° of abduction, 20 to 30° of flexion and 25 to 30° of internal rotation. Abduction can be determined at the time of surgery, by clinically measuring the angle formed by the body and the humerus. This angle or an angle specifically determined preoperatively, can be determined by obtaining an anteroposterior radiographic view, using the spine rather than the border of the scapula as a landmark, as recommended by Ingram and Miller.

Flexion is determined, by observing the angle that the humerus forms with the horizontal plane in a supine patient. After the positions of abduction and flexion have been determined, the elbow is flexed to 90°. The hand is positioned over the ipsilateral area of the chest between the sternum and axilla, so that further flexion of the elbow allows the top of the thumb to touch the chin (Figs 23.245A and B).

Surgical Techniques

When choosing the technique to be used, an attempt at fusion should be made between the acromion and humeral head and the glenohumeral joint. Stable internal

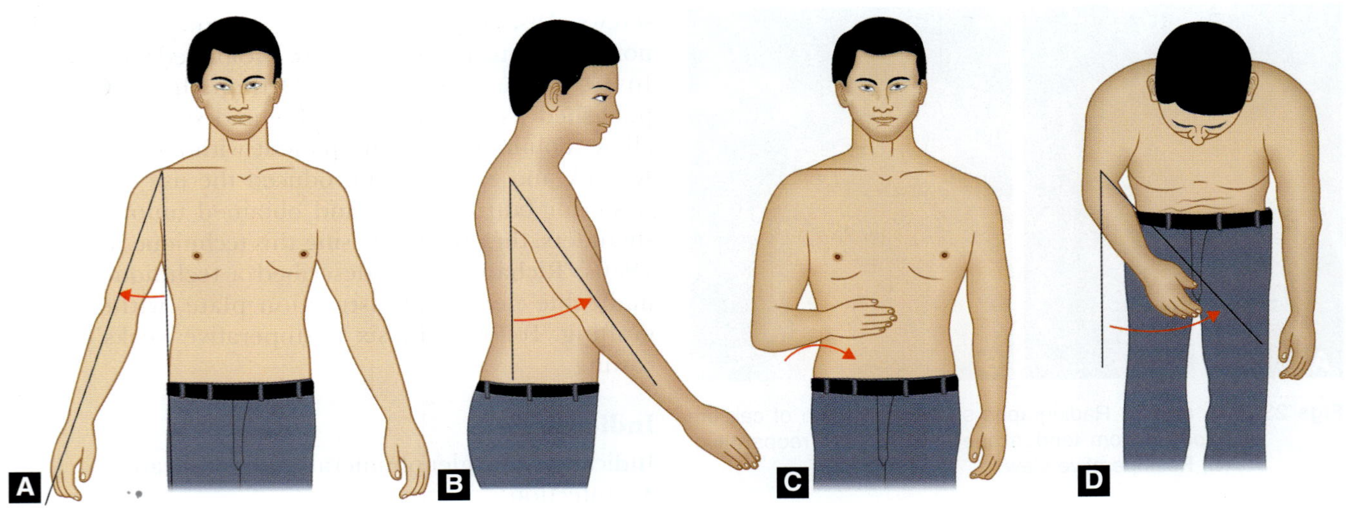

Figs 23.244A to D: Various positions of arm at the time of arthrodesis

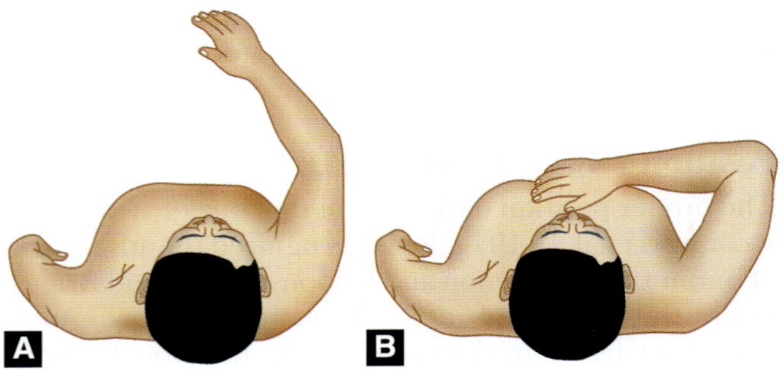

Figs 23.245A and B: Recommended position of limb for shoulder arthrodesis—(A) Arm is abducted and flexed; (B) The hand is positioned over the ipsilateral area of the chest between the sternum and axilla, so that further flexion of the elbow allows the top of the thumb to touch the chin

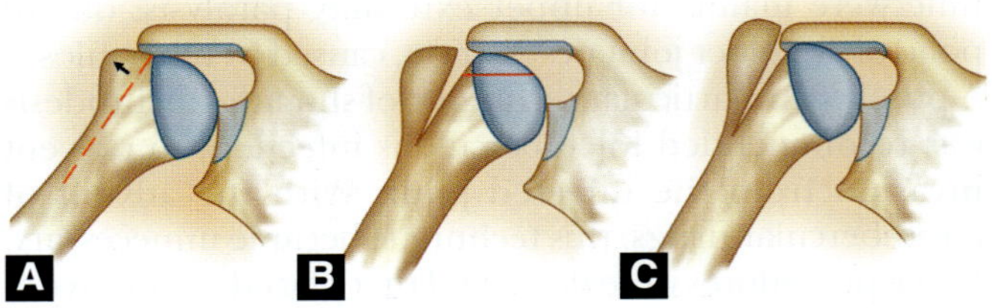

Figs 23.246A to C: Various steps involved in Charnley and Houston technique of compression arthrodesis of shoulder

fixation can reduce the need for bone grafting and external fixation or spica casting.

Methods

- External fixation
- Internal fixation
- Intenal fixation with bone grafting.

External Fixation

Charnley described a procedure to accomplish shoulder arthrodesis, by applying external compression. In 1964, Charnley and Houston modified this technique to allow easier adjustment of arm position. Charnley and Houston technique of compression arthrodesis of shoulder involve following steps:

- First apply the trunk portion of a shoulder spica cast with the patient awake, allow it to harden, then bivalve it and save it for later use. Position the patient in a semireclining or beach chair posture and make a saber cut incision, centered over the lateral border of the acromion.
- Using electrocautery, take down the anterior and lateral deltoid muscle, tag and retract this muscle. Excise the soft tissue from the subacromial space. Denude the upper half of the glenoid fossa of articular cartilage and the undersurface of the acromion to bleeding bone. Remove the articular cartilage from the humeral head and reduce the joint.
- With an osteotome, split off the greater tuberosity and resect enough bone from the humeral head, to allow it to sublux superiorly against the undersurface of the acromion and the superior part of the glenoid fossa. Use the resected bone as graft material around the fusion, this is illustrated in Figures 23.246A to C.
- Insert a 4 mm pin from the posterosuperior aspect of the acromion into the scapular neck deep to the glenoid fossa, as shown in Figure 23.247. Another pin can be placed in the base of the coracoid process.

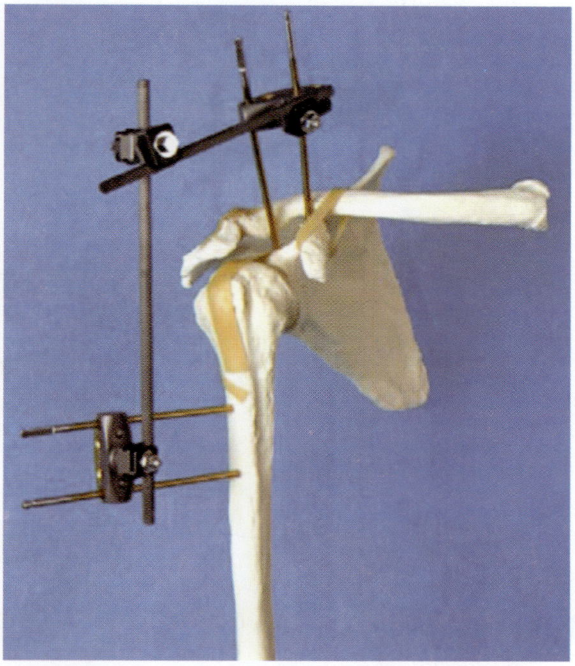

Fig. 23.247: Illustration showing methods employed in inserting a 4 mm pin from the posterosuperior aspect of the acromion into the scapular neck deep to the glenoid fossa

- Insert a second set of similar pins into the surgical neck of the humerus posterolaterally, perpendicular to the shaft of the humerus.
- Construct an external frame of adjustable pin clamps and bars, connect it to the pins for application of compression with the arm in the desired position for arthrodesis. Reattach the deltoid to the acromion and close the wound in layers over a drain. Apply the previously made part of the shoulder spica cast and complete it, incorporating the external fixator.

After Treatment

The pins and external fixator are removed at 5 to 6 weeks and the cast is changed. The second cast is removed at 12 weeks from the time of surgery and the shoulder is examined for stability. Immobilization is continued until the arthrodesis is solid.

Screw Fixation

Cofield described a shoulder fusion technique, using screw fixation through a strap incision that may be extended posteriorly, if needed, as shown in Figure 23.248. The position and number of screws used vary, depending on the indication for arthrodesis and the condition of the bone at the time of surgery, this is demonstrated in Figures 23.249 and 23.250. Advantages of screw overplate fixation include, less soft-tissue dissection, lower infection rate, decreased rate of

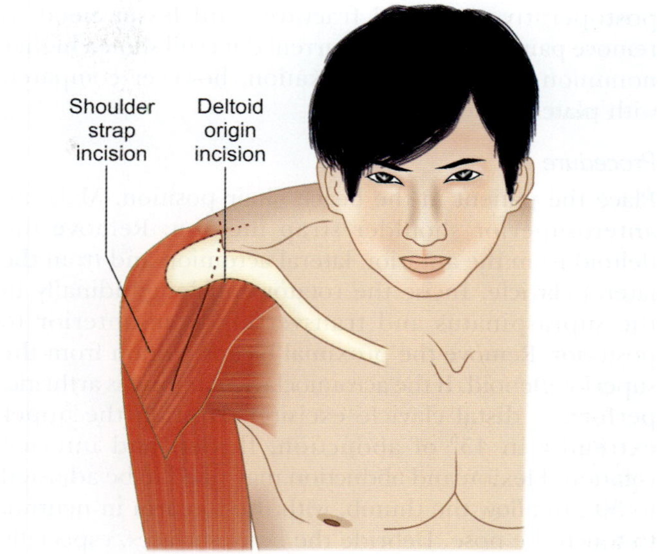

Fig. 23.248: Shoulder fusion technique by screw fixation through a strap incision

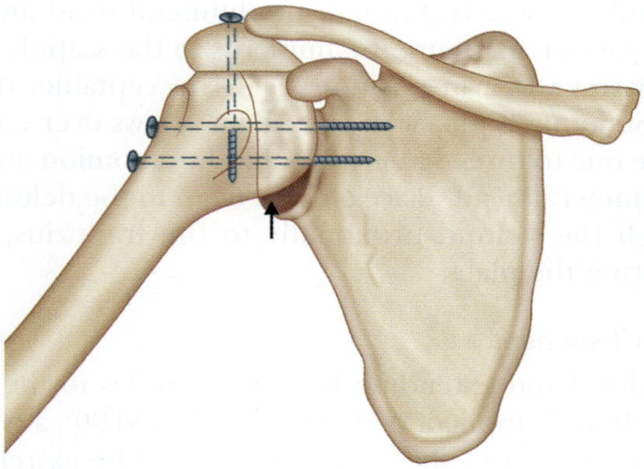

Fig. 23.249: Shoulder arthrodesis with screw fixation

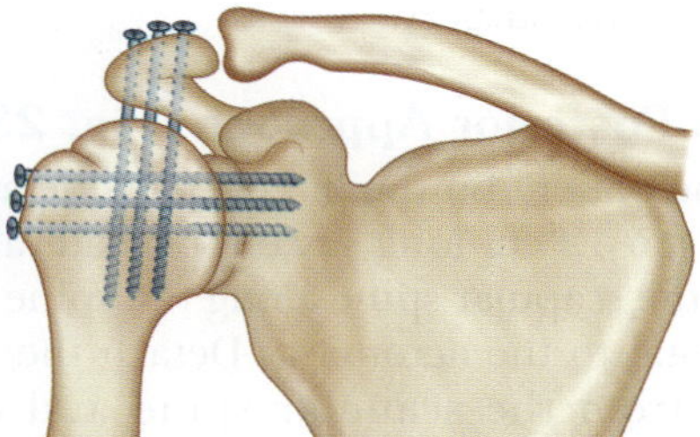

Fig. 23.250: Shoulder arthrodesis with screw fixation. The position and number of screws used vary, depending on the indication for arthrodesis and the condition of the bone at the time of surgery

postoperative humeral fractures and lesser need to remove painful hardware. Current data still show a higher nonunion rate with screw fixation, however compared with plate fixation.

Procedure

Place the patient in the beach chair position. Make an anterosuperior shoulder strap incision. Remove the deltoid from the anterior, lateral acromion and from the lateral clavicle. Incise the rotator cuff longitudinally in the supraspinatus and transversely from anterior to posterior. Remove the proximal biceps tendon from the superior glenoid. If the acromioclavicular joint is arthritic, perform a distal clavicle excision. Position the upper extremity in 45° of abduction, flexion and internal rotation. Flexion and abduction may need to be adjusted to 30°, to allow the thumb, with the forearm in neutral, to touch the nose. Debride the bony surfaces, especially the humeral head, to increase surface contact areas.

Definitive fixation is determined by the indication for arthrodesis and by the status of bone stock. Drill two or three 0.125 inch of Steinmann pins or guidewires for cannulated screws, through the humeral head and into the glenoid, to secure the humerus to the scapula.

Assess the arm position. If it is acceptable, replace the Steinmann pins with cancellous screws over washers. Place one to three screws through the acromion and into the humeral head. Place a drain deep to the deltoid and attach the deltoid proximally to the trapezius, while covering the plate.

After Treatment

A pelvic band extending from the nipples to the pubic symphysis is applied. With the elbow flexed 90°, a cylinder cast is applied to the upper extremity. The extremity is suspended by two wooden struts or a cockup wrist splint is used. At 1 to 2 weeks after surgery, a plastic shoulder spica cast is applied and worn until union is achieved, 12 to 16 weeks after surgery.

Uematsu Posterior Approach (Fig. 23.251)

Position the patient on the unaffected side and make an incision 10 to 12 cm long, extending laterally from the middle of the scapular spine along the spine and ending 2.5 cm, distal to the acromion. Detach the deltoid and trapezius from the scapular spine and expose the supraspinatus and infraspinatus and retract them out of the way.

Make an oblique osteotomy from the lateral third of the scapular spine to the spinoglenoid notch and lateral third of the acromion, without entering the acromioclavicular joint. The osteotomized fragment may be used as a muscle pedicle bone graft, if the deltoid attachment is retained. Otherwise, it may be used as a free graft. Divide the tendinous attachments of the supraspinatus and infraspinatus, about 1.5 cm from their insertions on the greater tuberosity. Remove all articular cartilage from the glenoid fossa, humeral head and decorticate the posterior aspect of the glenoid fossa.

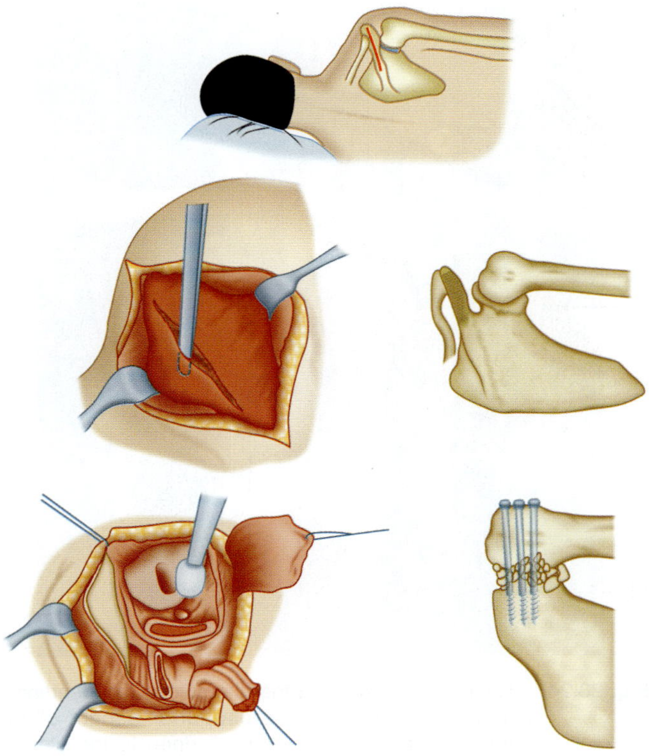

Fig. 23.251: Uematsu posterior approach for shoulder arthrodesis

Position the arm in 20° of abduction, 30° of forward flexion and 40° of internal rotation. This is determined clinically with the arm at the side of the body. Insert three ASIF cancellous screws through the humeral head into the glenoid fossa and scapular neck. Check for stability and use additional screws if necessary. Fix the acromial bone graft posteriorly. Close the wound in layers over a drain, taking care to secure a tight closure of the trapeziodeltoid interval. Apply a sterile dressing and suspend the arm by overhead skin traction.

After Treatment

The dressing is changed and the drain is removed on the second day. With the patient standing, a shoulder spica cast is applied. A cast is worn for 3 months or until union become solid radiographically. Then rehabilitation of the upper extremity is begun.

Tension Band Fixation (Fig. 23.252)

In 1998, Mohammed reported his results of shoulder arthrodesis, using a rush rod, tension band and a muscle pedicle graft through a posterior approach.

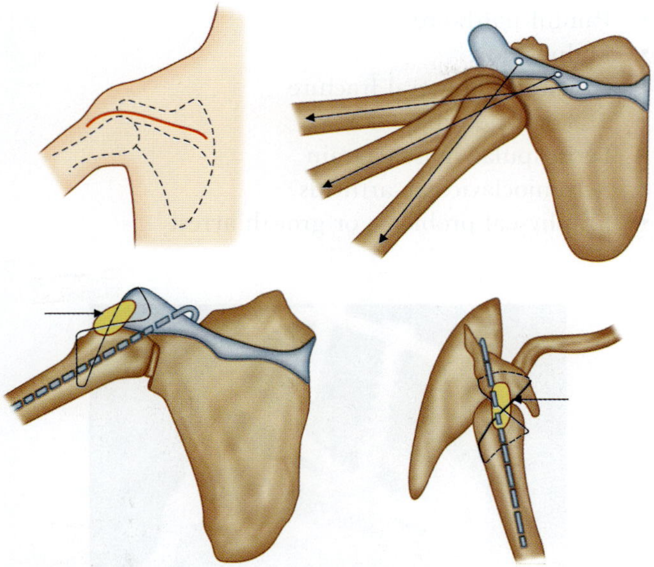

Fig. 23.252: Tension band wiring performed through posterior approach

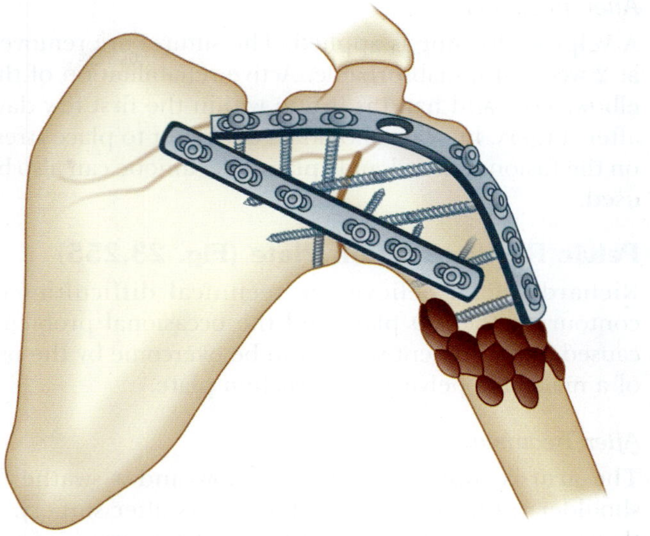

Fig. 23.254: The plate initially fasten with a long cortical screw inserted vertically into the scapular neck and remaining proximal screws into the scapula using standard AO technique

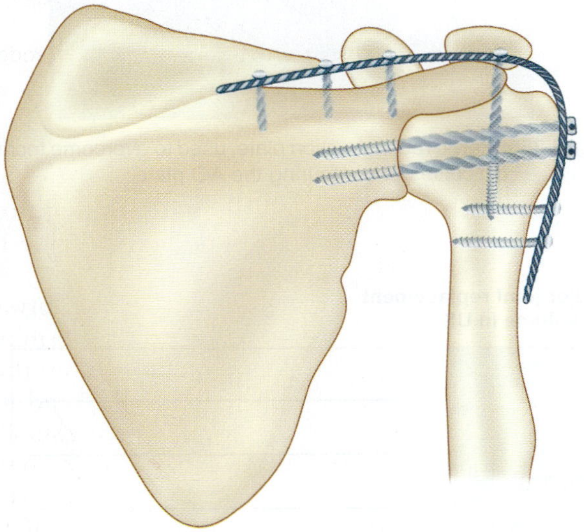

Fig. 23.253: Plate fixation for shoulder arthrodesis

After Treatment

A shoulder spica cast is applied and movement of the wrist and elbow is allowed after 4 to 6 weeks. External support of the shoulder is maintained, until radiographic union is shown, usually at 8 to 10 weeks.

Plate Fixation (Fig. 23.253)

The AO group has described a double plating technique for rigid stabilization in glenohumeral arthrodesis. The disadvantage is the possible need for a second procedure to remove the implants after arthrodesis is solid.

Technique

Place the patient in the lateral decubitus position. Make an incision along the spine of the scapula, over the acromion and along the proximal third of the humerus. Expose the scapular spine, glenoid fossa and proximal third of the humerus. Denude the glenoid fossa and humeral head of all cartilage. Decorticate the undersurface of the acromion and the lateral portion of the humerus for contact with the acromion. An osteotomy of the acromion may be necessary to increase surface contact between the plate and bones. Position the humeral head in the desired position in the glenoid fossa. Use a malleable template, to determine the contour for a standard broad AO plate and contour the plate with bending press and irons. The plate is to lie along the scapular spine, over the acromion and against the proximal third of the humerus.

Fasten the plate initially with a long cortical screw inserted vertically into the scapular neck. Insert the remaining proximal screws into the scapula using standard AO technique, as illustrated in Figure 23.254. Displace the humerus superiorly and medially to lie against the acromion and glenoid fossa in the desired position for arthrodesis. Fix the plate distally, with two screws that pass through it, the humeral head, into the glenoid fossa and scapular neck. Insert at least two more screws to fix the plate to the humerus. If the plate does not achieve complete stability at the arthrodesis site, apply a second plate posteriorly from the scapular spine to the humerus. Apply bone grafts as desired and close the wound in layers over drains.

After Treatment

A Velpeau dressing is applied. The sutures are removed at 2 weeks if nonabsorbable. Active rehabilitation of the elbow, wrist and hand is begun within the first few days after surgery, but care should be taken not to place stress on the fusion site. A double plating technique can also be used.

Pelvic Reconstruction Plate (Fig. 23.255)

Richards et al. believe the technical difficulties of contouring the AO plate and the occasional problems caused by prominent screws can be overcome by the use of a malleable pelvic reconstruction plate.

After Treatment

The arm is supported with a pillow and a swathe. A shoulder spica cast is applied 48 hours after surgery. If there is no radiographic evidence of loosening of the internal fixation device 6 weeks after surgery, the arm is placed in a sling. Only gentle range of motion exercises are allowed, until union is seen on radiograph. Strenuous activity is delayed for at least 16 weeks after surgery.

Complications of Glenohumeral Arthrodesis

- Infection
- Wound hematoma
- Skin slough
- Pressure sores under spica cast
- Pseudarthrosis/nonunion
- Painful hardware
- Malposition
- Ipsilateral humeral fracture
- Traction neuritis
- Periscapular muscle strain
- Acromioclavicular arthritis
- Epiphyseal problems or growth arrest

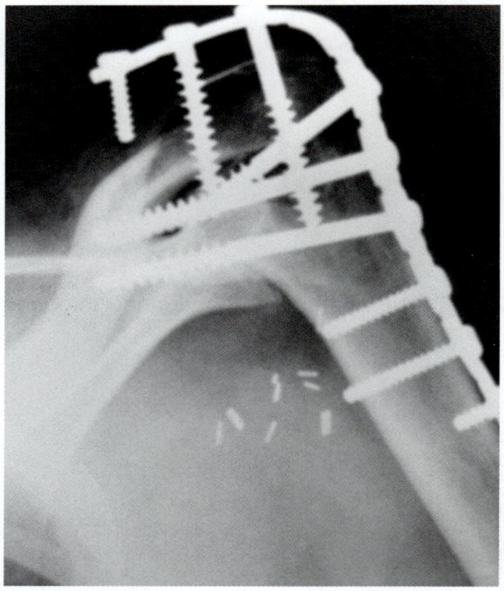

Fig. 23.255: Pelvic reconstruction plate, used to overcome technical difficulties of contouring the AO plate

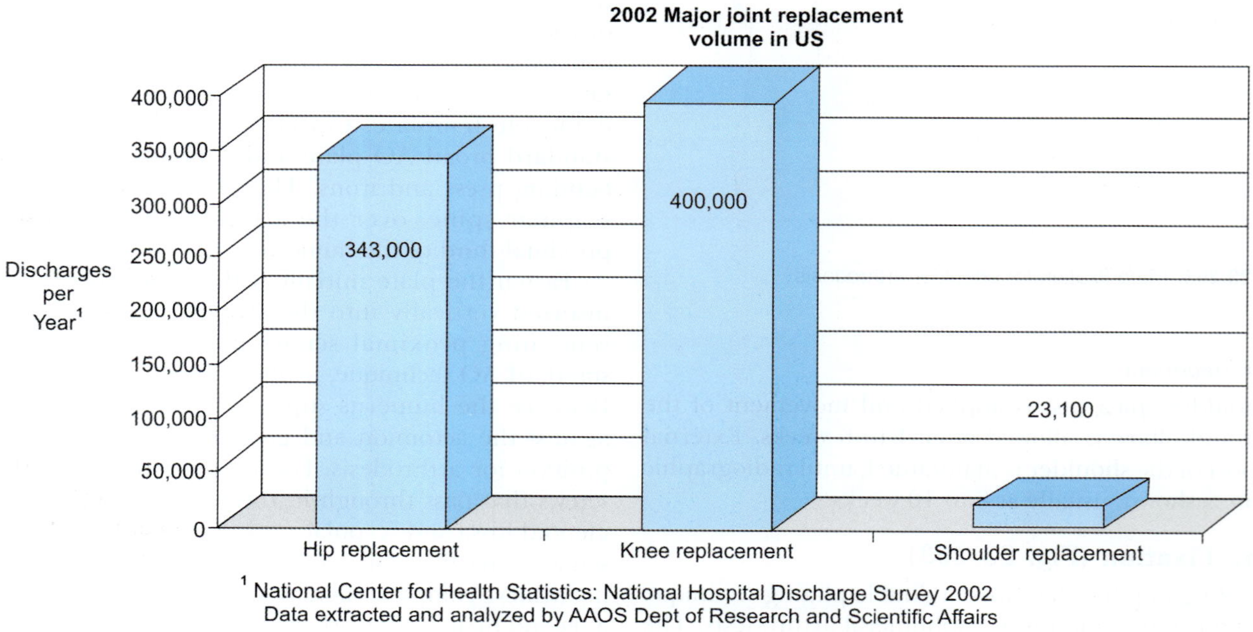

Fig. 23.256: Major joint replacement surgeries in terms of volume

SHOULDER ARTHROPLASTY

Lesions of the shoulder requiring arthroplasty are less common than lesions involving the weight bearing joints of the body, such as hip and knee. A comparison between major joint replacement surgeries in terms of volume is shown in Figure 23.256.

The Shoulder (Fig. 23.257)

- Greatest range of motion (ROM)
- No inherent bony stability
- Relies on soft tissues for stability
- Many injuries involve the soft tissues, e.g. rotator cuff and labrum
- Little glenoid bone stock (Fig. 23.257).

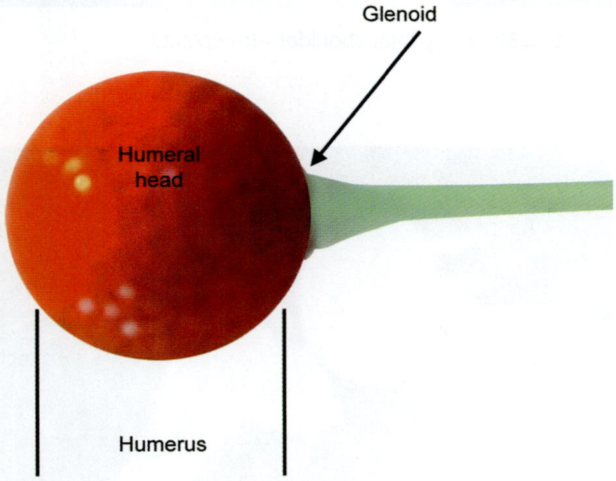

Fig. 23.257: Glenohumeral joint compared to a golf ball on a tea

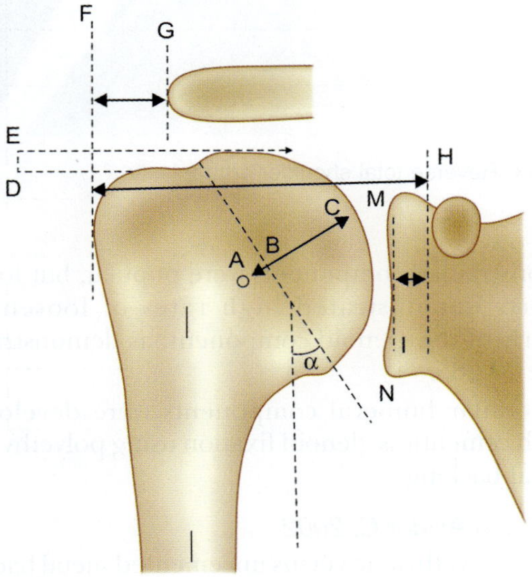

Fig. 23.258: Shoulder joint biomechanics—F–H = Offset; B–C = Head thickness; D–E = 8 mm

Other anatomic variables to consider:

- Glenoid with 2° antiversion to 7° retroversion
- *Humeral offset:* Medially (coronal) of 4 to 14 mm, posteriorly (transverse) of 2 to 10 mm
- Glenoid inclination varies from 7 to 20°
- Humeral head inclination of 30 to 55°
- Humeral head is in 20 to 40° of retroversion
- Axial computed tomography (CT scan) of the glenohumeral joint is a valuable preop planning tool.

Biomechanics (Fig. 23.258)

Top of the humeral head is higher than greater tuberosity, as illustrated in Figure 23.259.

Indications for Shoulder Arthroplasty (Fig. 23.260)

- Osteoarthritis
- Rheumatoid arthritis
- Rotator cuff tear arthropathy
- Avascular necrosis
- Post-traumatic arthritis
- Severe proximal humeral fractures
- Neoplastic lesions.

Choice of Prosthesis

Following points are considered before applying prosthesis:

- Patient's age
- Condition of glenoid surface and bone stock
- Axillary nerve palsy is a relative contraindication to arthroplasty.

Arthroplasty Options

Different arthroplastic techniques are illustrated in Figures 23.261 to 23.263.

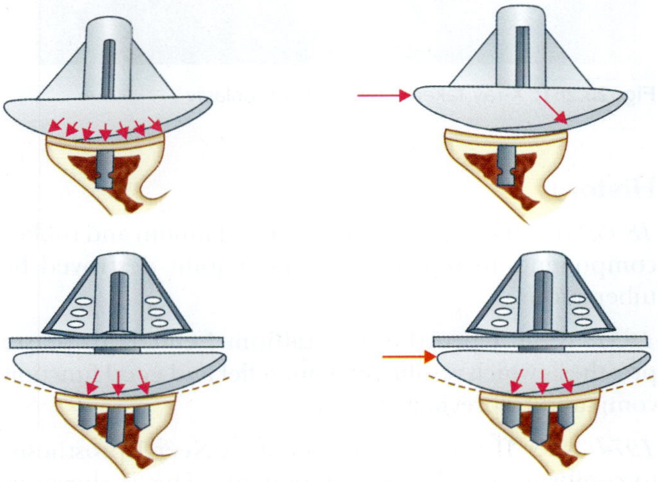

Fig. 23.259: Illustration showing top of the humeral head is higher than greater tuberosity

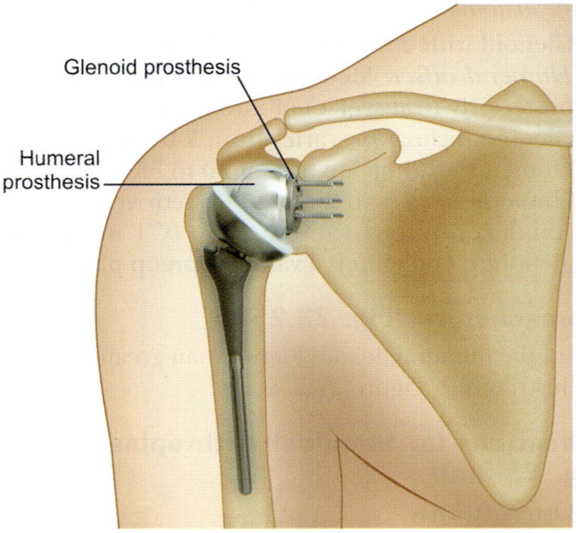

Fig. 23.260: Total shoulder arthroplasty

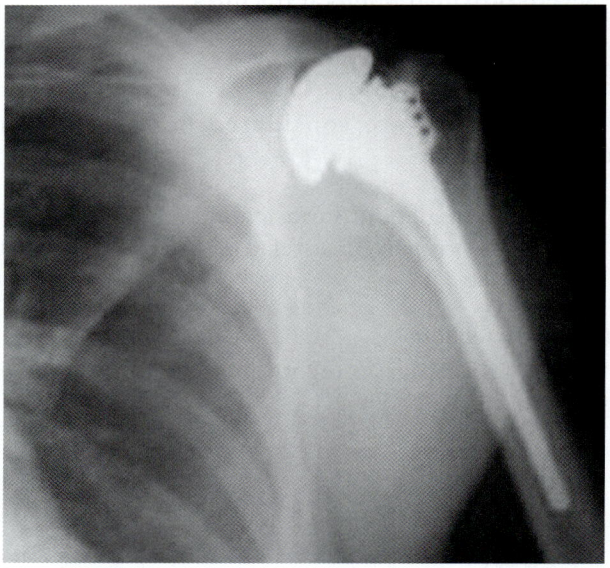

Fig. 23.261: X-ray taken after hemiarthroplasty

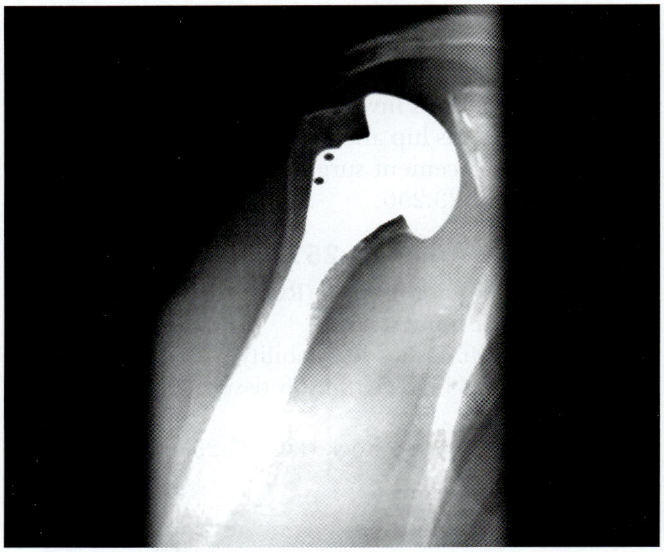

Fig. 23.262: X-ray total shoulder arthroplasty

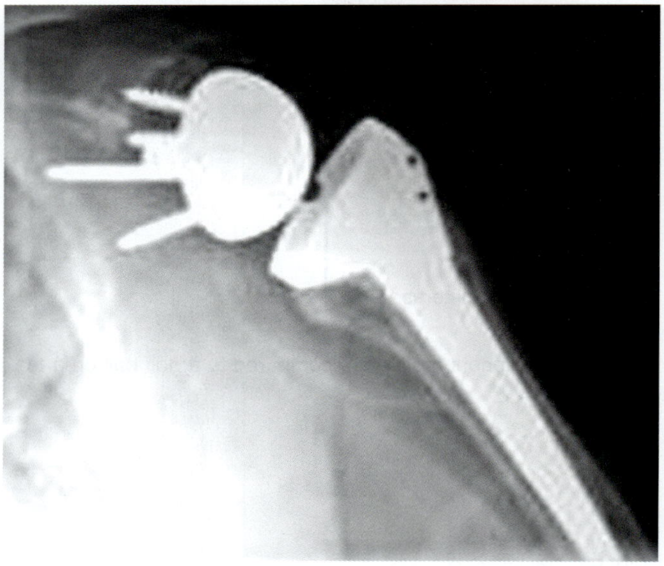

Fig. 23.263: Reverse total shoulder arthroplasty

History

1893: French surgeon Pean inserted platinum and rubber components to replace a shoulder joint destroyed by tuberculosis.

1951: Neer I prosthesis, vitallium hemiarthroplasty prosthesis which resulted in pain relief and good function compared to previous options.

1974: Neer II prosthesis (a modified Neer I prosthesis, to conform to a glenoid component). This is shown in Figure 23.264.

1970: Constrained components were popular, but follow up reports demonstrated high rates of loosening, particularly of the glenoid component, as demonstrated in Figure 23.265.

1980: Modular humeral components were developed along with cementless glenoid fixation using polyethylene on a metal backing.

Boileau P and Avidor C, 2002

Cemented polyethylene versus uncemented metal backed glenoid components in total shoulder arthroplasty: a prospective, double-blind, randomized study.

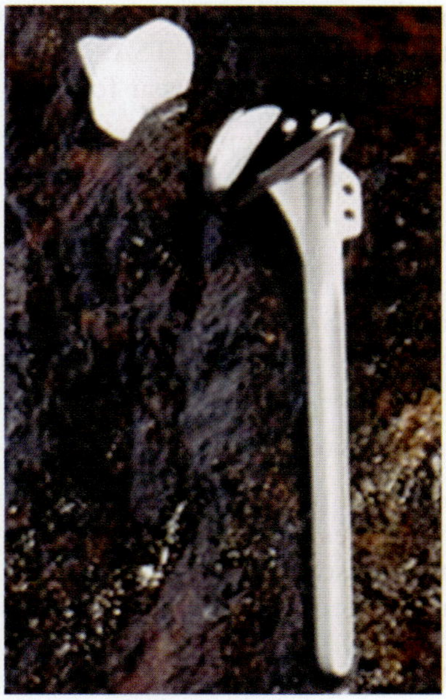

Fig. 23.264: Neer II prosthesis

Fourty shoulders with 3 years follow-up:

Metal-backed: Two percent radiolucent lines, 100 percent progressive, 25 percent loose in 3 years. It is associated with shift and osteolysis.

Cemented: Eighty percent radiolucent lines, 25 percent progressive. None, loose in 3 years.

Source: Boileau P, Avidor C. J Shoulder Elbow Surg. 2002; 11(4):351-9.

Other problems with metal-backed glenoid components are:

- Metal backing increased the thickness of the component and often leads to over stuffing of the joint
- To avoid over stuffing of the joint, the polyethylene thickness had to be reduced, resulting in accelerated polywear and failure
- Polymetal disassociation occurred with unacceptable frequency.

Humeral Components (Table 23.6)

Cemented vs pressfit humeral components: Harris, Jobe and Dai reported less micromotion with proximally cemented stems. Fully cemented stems provide no additional benefit or stability over proximally cemented stems. Sanchez-Sotelo reported a low rate of stem loosening regardless of fixation, but pressfit prosthesis developed more radiolucent lines in the first 4 years.

Need for modularity: Re-establishing normal glenohumeral anatomic relationships is important to ensure optimal results.

Table 23.6: Different humeral components of a prosthesis

Cemented	*Prox porous coated*	*Fully porous coated*
Good for osteopenic bone	Need good bone stock	Need good bone stock
Lower risk of intraoperative fracture	Higher risk of intraoperative fracture	Higher risk of intraoperative fracture
More stress-shielding	Less stress-shielding	Less stress-shielding
Hard to revise	Easier to revise	Hard to revise

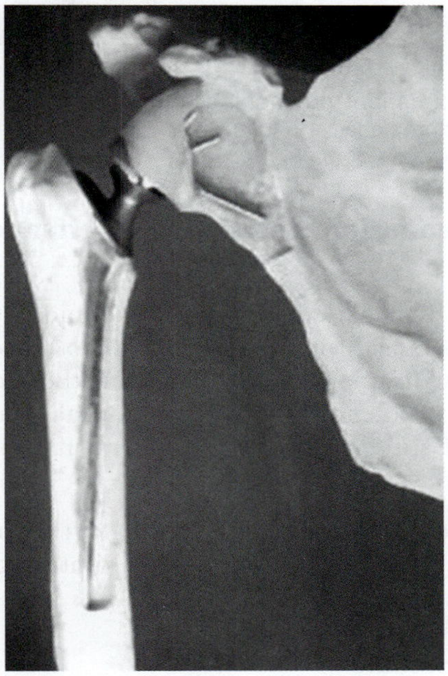

Fig. 23.265: A loosened prosthesis

Contraindications to Shoulder Arthroplasty

- Active or recent shoulder joint infection
- Paralysis with complete loss of rotator cuff and deltoid function
- A neuropathic arthropathy
- Irreparable rotator cuff tear is a relative contraindication to glenoid resurfacing.

Surgical Approach (Fig. 23.266)

Osteoarthritis (OA)

In addition to the universal features of osteoarthritic joints, shoulder can also demonstrate joint space narrowing, cysts, osteophytes, Posterior glenoid erosion, flattening of the humeral head, enlargement of the humeral head and rotator cuff tears are uncommon in OA.

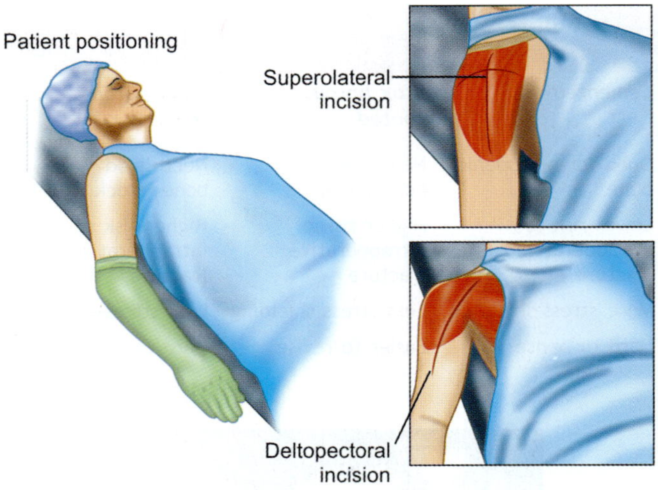

Fig. 23.266: Patient positioning and incisions for shoulder arthroplasty

Recommendation Based on Experience

Neer, 1998

"When the articular surface of the glenoid is good, the results of hemiarthroplasty are similar to those of Total Shoulder Arthroplasty (TSA). Wear on the glenoid has not been a problem, if the articular surface was good at the time of surgery and glenohumeral motion was re-established".

Source: Neer CS II. Replacement arthroplasty for glenohumeral osteoarthritis. J Bone Joint Surg. (AM)

Hemi vs Total Shoulder

- Easy procedure
- Short operating time
- Less risk of instability
- Can be revised to TSA
- Less reliable pain relief
- Progressive glenoid erosion may cause results to deteriorate over time
- Need concentric glenoid
- More consistent pain relief
- Better fulcrum for active motion
- Difficult procedure
- Longer operation room (OR) time
- Polywear can cause loosening of both the components
- More glenoid bone loss.

Recommendations Based on Evidence

Kirkley et al., 2000

Forty-two patients, three surgeons (stratified), one year follow-up, no significant difference in Western Ontario Shoulder Instability Index (WOSI), American Shoulder and Elbow Surgeons Standardized Shoulder Assessment Form (ASES), Diability of Arm Shoulder and Hand questionnaire (DASH) constant score or ROM. Trend towards better pain relief with TSA. Two hemipatients crossed-over to TSA, after one year follow-up.

Source: Kirkley, et al. Replacement arthroplasty for glenohumeral osteoarthritis. J Bone Joint Surg (AM).

Gartsman, 2000

Fifty-one shoulders, average followup of 35 months, show no difference in ASES or UCLA scores. Significantly better pain relief with TSA. Three patients crossed over to TSA by 35 months.

Source: Bryant D, Litchfield R, 2005.

A comparison of pain, strength, range of motion and functional outcomes after hemiarthroplasty and total shoulder arthroplasty in patients with osteoarthritis of the shoulder. A systematic review and meta-analysis is as follows:

Included four randomized controlled trials. On an average, two years followup. TSA resulted in significantly improved UCLA scores, pain relief and increased forward elevation by 13. This meta-analysis concluded that at 2 years of followup, TSA provided a better functional outcome, however the problems of glenoid component loosening in the TSA group and progressive glenoid erosion in the hemi group may affect the eventual long-term outcome. Hence, longer followup is necessary.

Source: Bryant D, Litchfield R. J Bone Joint Surg Am. 2005;87(9):1947-56.

Haines JF et al., 2006

The results of arthroplasty in osteoarthritis of the shoulder:

A prospective study of 124 shoulder arthroplasties for OA (Hemi and TSA), shows similar improvement in pain and function in both the groups, if rotator cuff was intact. Better results with hemi if rotator cuff tear is present. With hemi, revision at mean of 1.5 years for glenoid pain and TSA, revision at mean of 4.5 years for glenoid loosening.

Source: Haines JF et al. J Bone Joint Surg Br. 2006; 88(4):496-501

Technical Issues to Consider

OA tends to result in posterior glenoid wear/erosion, which if accepted, will lead to a retroverted glenoid component. Compensate by anterior reaming or placing the humeral component in lesser retroversion and failure to do so will resulted in posterior instability.

Rheumatoid Arthritis (Fig. 23.267)

Associated abnormalities are:

- Periarticular erosions
- Periarticular osteopenia

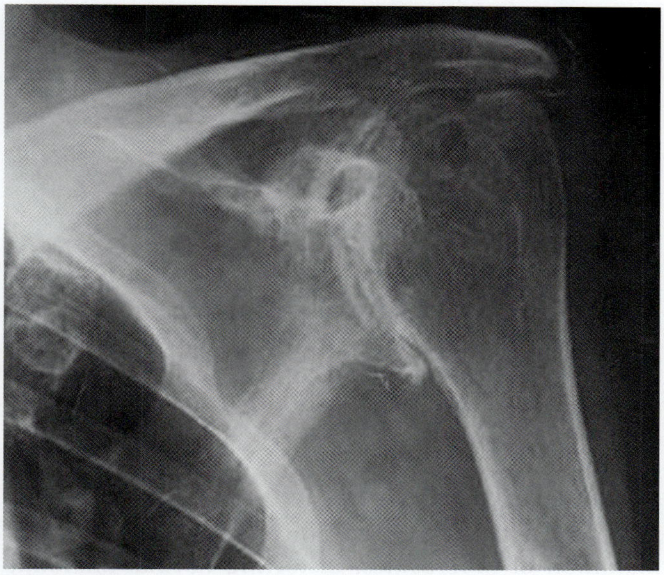

Fig. 23.267: X-ray shows rheumatoid arthritis of shoulder

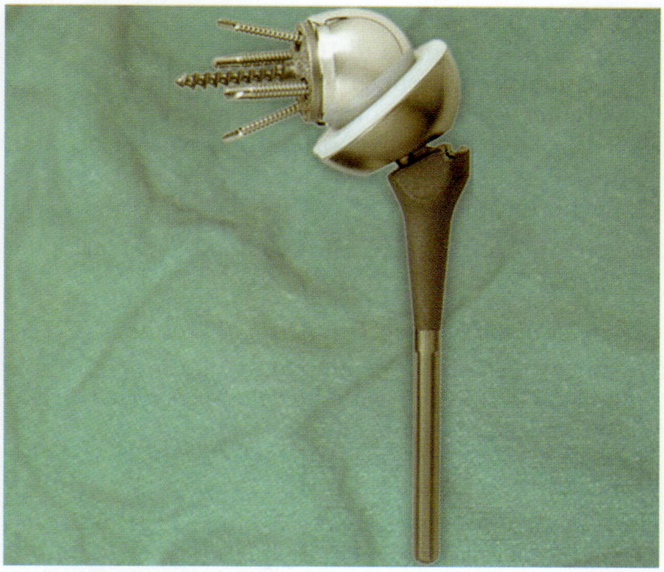

Fig. 23.268: Prosthesis used for reverse total shoulder arthroplasty

- Thin cortices
- Adjacent joint involvement.

Choice of prosthesis/arthroplasty include:

- Cemented short stemmed prosthesis
- Gill, Cofield et al. recommend at least 60 mm between the cement mantles of ipsilateral shoulder and elbow arthroplasties.
- If this cannot be achieved, join both cement mantles together.
- Generally, TSA performed due to destruction of the glenoid articular surface by the disease.
- Glenoid erosion may require bone grafting. However, if glenoid is eroded to the level of the coracoid process, glenoid resurfacing is contraindicated.

Rotator Cuff Arthropathy

Described by Neer, Craig and Fukada in 1983. A distinct form of osteoarthritis associated with a massive chronic rotator cuff tear. Generally, rotator cuff tears occur in less than 10 percent of shoulders with OA. A function of the rotator cuff is to depress the humeral head and keep it centered on the glenoid fossa. Massive rotator cuff tears result in proximal migration of the humeral head. This is a contraindication to glenoid resurfacing, as it results in an eccentric (superior) glenoid loading and early component loosening.

Surgical Options

- Hemiarthroplasty with a large head
- Repair of rotator cuff and TSA
- Reverse TSA.

Outcomes of hemiarthroplasty are:

Rockwood: Eighty-six percent satisfactory results after 4 years.

Zuckerman: Ninty-three percent adequate pain relief and 90 percent had improved function for Activities of Daily Living (ADL's).

Sanches-Sotelo: Seventy-five percent modest improvements in ROM and strength for ADL's. good pain relief.

Field et al. and Sanchez-sotelo reported that, impaired deltoid function and previous subacromial decompression (loss of coracoacromial ligament) were significantly associated with clinical shoulder instability post-hemiarthroplasty.

Reverse Total Shoulder Arthroplasty (Fig. 23.268)

- Lateralizes the center of rotation and places the deltoid at a mechanical advantage
- More inherent stability prevents proximal migration of humeral head, by restoring deltoid lever arm.

Outcomes of the Reverse Total Shoulder Arthroplasty

Frankle M and Siegel S, 2005

The reverse shoulder prosthesis for glenohumeral arthritis is associated with severe rotator cuff deficiency. A minimum 2 years follow-up study of sixty patients.

Different outcomes are illustrated below:

- Average age = 70 years
- Improved ASES scores

- Improved ROM:
  - Flexion: From 55 to 105°
  - Abduction: From 41 to 102°
- Seventeen percent Complication rate
- Seven failures were reported and five out of them revised to new reverse TSA and two revised to hemiarthroplasties.

Source: Frankle M, Siegel S. J Bone Joint Surg Am. 2005; 87(8):1697-705.

Outcomes of the Reverse TSA (Delta III Prosthesis)

Treatment of painful pseudoparesis due to irreparable rotator cuff dysfunction with the delta III reverse ball and socket total shoulder prosthesis.

Werner CM and Glbart M, 2005

Fifty-eight consecutive patients, average age is 68 years. 41 cases were revisions. Follow-up period is of 38 months. Improved constant score, pain reduction and improved ROM are:

- Flexion, from 42 to 100°, abduction, from 43 to 90°
- 50 percent complication rate (including minor)
- If there surgery done, to increase 1° of ROM there is 18 percent reoperation rate
- If a revision surgery is done, there is about 39 percent of reoperation rate
- Reverse total shoulder arthroplasty is hard to revise, as little glenoid bone stock is left once component is removed, this is shown in Figure 23.269.

Source: Werner CM, Glbart M. J Bone Joint Surg Am. 2005;87(7):1476-86.

Osteonecrosis (Fig. 23.270)

Causes

- Corticosteroids
- Alcoholism
- Sickle cell disease
- Lupus
- Idiopathic.

Treatment Options

Usually young patients with adequate bone stock, prefer proximally porous coated, pressfit humeral prosthesis, as it is less stress shielding and is easier to revise, if necessary. Resurface glenoid only in stage V osteonecrosis (glenoid erosion).

Post-traumatic Arthritis

Due to fractures treated conservatively. May have malunion of tuberosities, distorting normal anatomic landmarks. Twelve percent of patients have axillary nerve palsies (Neer). Many have soft tissue contractures and muscle weakness.

Complications

- Instability (1.2%)
- Excessive retro/anteversion
- Head too small
- Head too low (postfracture)
- Subscapularis rupture
- Rotator cuff tear (2%)
- Results in superior migration of humerus and glenoid loosening

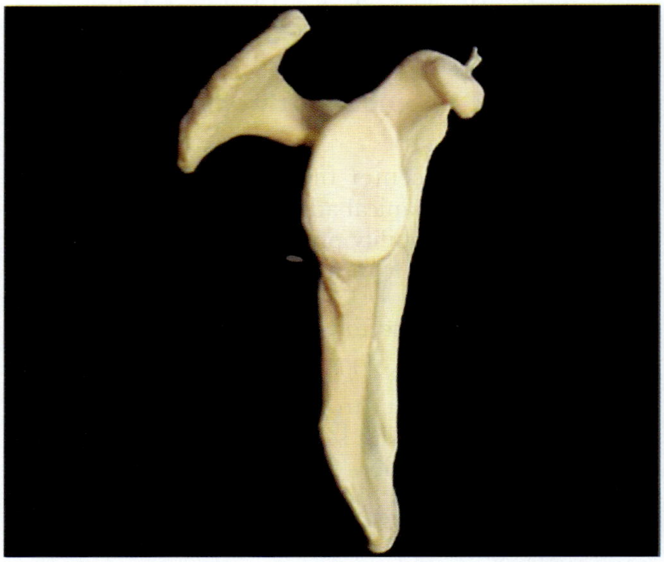

Fig. 23.269: Reduction in glenoid bone stock after reverse total shoulder arthroplasty

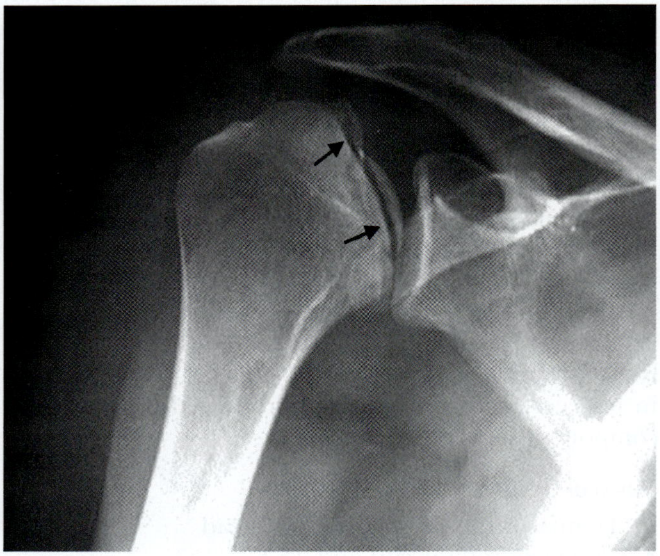

Fig. 23.270: X-ray shows osteonecrosis (arrows)

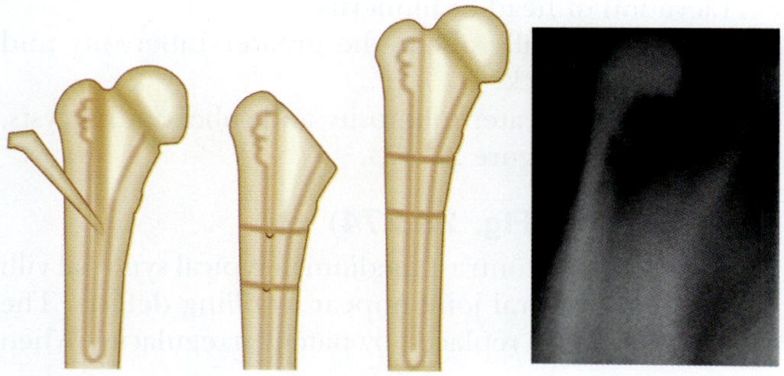

Fig. 23.271: Revision arthroplasty performed with longitudinal osteotomy

- Infection (0.5%), e.g. *Staphylococcus aureus.* Infection is more common after revision surgery
- Heterotopic ossification (10–45%)
  - Common in males
  - Diagnosis of osteoarthritis
  - Low-grade
  - Nonprogressive and does not affect the outcome
- Stiffness
  - Depends on indication for arthroplasty
  - Subscapularis shortening
  - Oversized components
  - Inappropriate rehabilitation
- Periprosthetic fracture
- Intraoperative (1%)
- Postoperative (0.5–2%)
  - Most common in rheumatoid arthritis (RA)
  - Eighty-five percent of patients are women
  - Glenoid fractures are rare
- Axillary nerve injury
  - Rare
  - Higher risk during revision surgery
  - Usually a neuropraxia.

Ultimate Bailouts

- Excision arthroplasty
- Shoulder arthrodesis.

Revision Arthroplasty

Controlled longitudinal osteotomy for removal, revised with long stem prosthesis and cerclage wires, as illustrated in Figure 23.271.

INFLAMMATIONS AROUND SHOULDER

Inflammations around shoulder can be due to following factors:

Autoimmune

- Rheumatoid arthritis
- Seronegative inflammatory arthritis
- Crystalline arthropathies (metabolic), e.g. gout, pseudogout, calcium hydroxyapatite crystal arthritis.

Infective

- Septic arthritis
- Tuberculosis

Rheumatoid Arthritis of Shoulder

Shoulder joint is often involved in approximately 90 percent patients, with longstanding Rheumatoid Arthritis (RA). The pathology extends to subacromial bursa and synovial sheath of biceps tendon. The main destructive entity is inflamed and proliferating synovium.

Three Stages of the Disease

Stage I: Stage of acute synovitis
Stage II: Intermediate stage of synovial proliferation
Stage III: Final stage of destruction.

In early stages, recurring episodes of acute synovial inflammation occur associated with effusions. Eventually, inflammation spreads to subacromial bursa and bicipital sheath. The synovial tissue proliferates and destroys the capsule. Slowly the capsule and surrounding muscles contract producing adduction and internal rotation deformity. In the last stage proliferated synovium forms *pannus* and destroys the articular cartilage, subchondral bone and biceps tendon. The rotator cuff and capsule gets weakened by synovial distension and invasion. The tendon may rupture, but may remain fixed by peritendinous adhesions in the groove.

Clinical Features

Rheumatoid shoulder assumes many forms. Acute inflammation may be limited to glenohumeral joint or it may appear as subacromial bursitis or bicipital tenosynovitis. Pertinent symptoms and findings of individual components of rheumatoid disease of shoulder are as follow:

Synovitis

- Usually occur in early stage
- Pain with temporary limited motion
- Tender anterior joint line
- It is confirmed by aspiration.

Tendinitis of Capsule and Cuff

- Painful weak abduction
- Active abduction limited because of pain, but passive is full
- Local tenderness and supraspinatus atrophy
- Drop arm test is negative.

Rupture of Cuff

- Patient is unable to actively abduct shoulder to 90°, which is almost impossible or very weak
- Drop arm test is positive.

Tenosynovitis of Long Head of Biceps Tendon

- Tenderness over biceps tendon
- Boggy soft tissue mass may be palpable along the tendon
- Yergason's sign positive
- Pain over biceps tendon on passive maximal external rotation.

Rupture of Biceps Tendon (Fig. 23.272)

Usually follows trauma. When rupture is incomplete pain is chronic until the distal end of tendon becomes adherent in its groove. If the rupture is complete tendon separation may occur and the muscle belly is palpable as a prominent mass distally in arm called popeye muscle.

Dislocation of Biceps Tendon from Groove

Groove is empty or tendon may be palpable as slipping on external rotation. Abbott-Saunders test is positive.

Subacromial Bursitis

Aspiration reveals typical fluid and later boggy swelling appears.

Symptoms in Later Stage of Inflammation

- Shoulder is stiff and painful
- Range of active and passive motion are reduced.

X-ray Findings

- These include osteoporosis
- Narrowing of joint space
- Elevation of head of humerus
- Erosions, usually about the greater tuberosity and anatomical neck
- Sclerosis of greater tuberosity and subchondral cysts, as shown in Figure 23.273.

Arthrography (Fig. 23.274)

After injection of contrast medium, a typical synovial villi of the glenohumeral joint appear as filling defects. The capsular outline is replaced by patchy irregularity. When

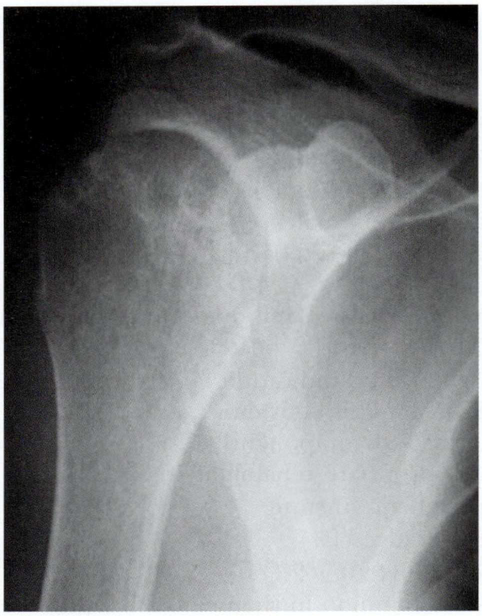

Fig. 23.273: X-ray showing sclerosis of greater tuberosity and subchondral cysts

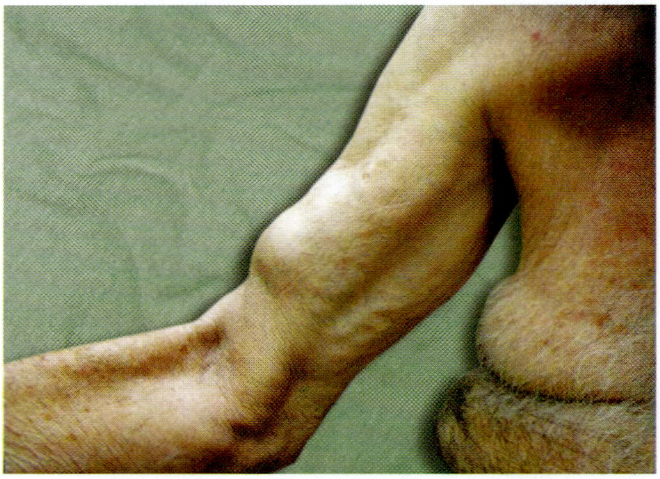

Fig. 23.272: Rupture of biceps tendon: Ruptured muscle belly is palpable as a prominent mass distally in arm called popeye muscle

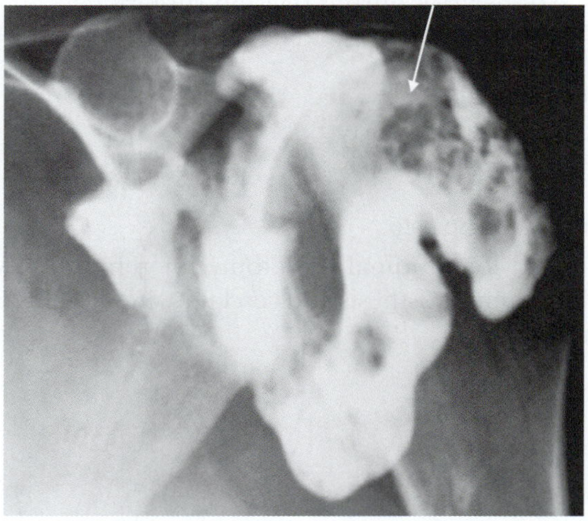

Fig. 23.274: Arthrography done by injecting contrast medium (arrow)

the cuff is ruptured, the dye enters the subacromial space, where the defects of villous synovial hypertrophy are revealed. Normally, the contrast enters the bicipital sheath. When the sheath is obliterated by adhesions, it fills unevenly or not at all. When the capsule is contracted, the shadow of axillary recess is reduced.

MRI

Magnetic resonance imaging (MRI) is useful in delineating the soft tissue component of the disease. The extent of synovial proliferation and joint effusion can be visualized. More importantly, the integrity of the rotator cuff can be determined with pathology, ranging from mild inflammation to full thickness tears.

CT Scan

Bone destruction and alteration in the normal osseous architecture is best evaluated with computed tomography (CT) scan.

Treatment

Initial nonsurgical management of rheumatoid arthritis, affecting the shoulder is appropriate in the early phases of disease with minimal bony destruction. Physical therapy may be helpful in maintaining active and passive motion during acute exacerbations and gradually adding resistive exercises to preserve strength. Limited trials of corticosteroid injections may be useful in reducing the symptoms of acute inflammation unresponsive to oral medications. When the medical line of nonsteroidal anti-inflammatory medications, antimetabolic drugs, steroids and disease modifying drugs has been exhausted, then surgical intervention should be considered.

In patients with joint swelling and pain, but relative preservation of the glenohumeral articular surfaces, bursectomy and synovectomy may be useful. Synovectomy may also help slow disease progression in aggressive cases of synovitis. In addition to synovectomy and bursectomy, a cuff defect must be repaired, the capsule is released, the intra-articular portion of the bicipital tendon is resected and the extra-articular portion is fixed in its groove. For associated acromioclavicolar arthritis, the outer end of clavicle should be resected.

To overcome adduction and internal rotation contracture, subscapularis tendon is lengthened and the adductors (trapezius and rhomboids) are sectioned. Hemiarthroplasty or total shoulder arthroplasty should be considered for patients with severe pain and functional limitation, unresponsive to more conservative modalities. The indications for humeral head replacement are an irreparable rotator cuff tear or inadequate glenoid bone stock, precluding adequate fixation of the polyethylene component. Arthrodesis is rarely indicated, as it completely restricts motion and it appears to encourage deterioration of other joints of the extremity.

■ Septic Arthritis

Septic arthritis of the shoulder is an inflammation of the glenohumeral joint, involving one or more foreign pathogens that cause or are suspected of causing an inflammation. These pathogens can be bacteria, viruses, fungi or parasites. These pathogens can gain access to the joint through a number of different means.

Joint sepsis may be classified according to pathogenesis. There are three basic mechanisms:

1. Hematogenous dissemination
2. Direct inoculation
3. Contiguous spread from adjacent osteomyelitis.

Hematogenous Septic Arthritis

Hematogenous dissemination from another organ systems, such as skin breakdown, urinary system infections or pneumonia are most common. In the shoulder, branches of the suprascapular and subscapular arteries along with the medial and lateral circumflex humeral arteries form an extra capsular arterial ring, which supplies to the proximal humerus. This anastamosis gives off branches, which penetrate the capsule and form an intra-articular synovial ring. This has been termed the transition zone and is located between the synovium and the articular surface.

It is in this area that the arterioles form loop, acutely toward the periphery, causing a low flow state, making the area more susceptible to receptor specific interaction of the pathogen and the cell surface. Spontaneous shoulder sepsis is the result of joint invasion. During the abundance of the synovial vasculature and the absence of a basement membrane between the endothelial cells synovial joints, are more vulnerable to seeding by bacteria. Most patients with hematogenous nongonococcal bacterial arthritis have at least one underlying chronic medical risk factor. These factors may be local, such as prosthetic and metallic implants or systemic, such as cancer, cirrhosis, rheumatoid arthritis and intermittent bacteremic episodes from intravenous drug abuse or indwelling catheters.

Direct Inoculation

Direct inoculation may be traumatic or iatrogenic, e.g. Repeated corticosteroid injections, arthroscopy and open surgical procedures, such as rotator cuff repair and arthroplasty. The existence of foreign bodies in or around the joint, such as nonabsorbable suture, stainless steel, cobalt chrome alloys, methylmethacrylate and polyethylene or devitalized bone from trauma has provided a nidus for adhesion and colonization by the bacteria. This nidus allows a glycocalyx biofilm to be expressed by the bacteria, which contributes to antibiotic resistance and limits the effectiveness of the immune response of the host.

Septic Arthritis from Contiguous Osteomyelitis

Hematogenous osteomyelitis commonly involves the metaphyseal area of rapidly growing long bones. When septic arthritis results from a contiguous infection, such as osteomyelitis, it spreads from the bone to synovium and then to the joint space. This happens most often in infancy, when there is a vascular anastomosis between the epiphysis and the metaphysis. Between the ages of 8 to 18 months, the last vestiges of the nutrient artery system close down at the growth plate, reaching sinusoidal veins and causing a low flow state. The open physis at this point provides an effective barrier to the spread of infection to the joint, by obliterating this vascular anastomosis. All synovial joints contain synovial fluid, which can act as an excellent growth medium for bacteria and have a relative lack of immunologic resistance. Type B synoviocytes are weakly phagocytic.

Bacteriology

Certain organisms, such as *Neisseria gonorrhoeae* and *Staphylococcus aureus (S. aureus)*, seem to have avidity for the synovium, causing septic arthritis out of proportion to their incidence of bacteremia. *S. aureus* is the most common cause of adult, nongonococcal bacterial arthritis, occurring in up to 50 percent of patients.

Gram-negative bacilli have been increasing in incidence, ranging from 5 to 30 percent of all shoulder infections. *Escherichia coli* and *Proteus* species are common infecting gram-negative organisms from the urinary tract and occur in patients, who are not intravenous drug abusers. *Pseudomonas* and *Serratia* are the common organisms in intravenous drug addicts. *Streptococcus pneumoniae* is the most common organism in patients with chronic alcoholism and hypogammaglobulinemia. Polymicrobial infections of the shoulder occur in 5 to 15 percent of patients, often associated with an extra-articular polymicrobial infection or penetrating trauma, especially in immunocompromised patients.

Clinical Features

The typical clinical presentation of shoulder sepsis consists of complaints of pain, warmth, and swelling. Patient may exhibit a prodromal phase of malaise, low grade fever, lethargy, and anorexia before the acute onset. The acute phase usually consists of fever and chills, with severe, incapacitating shoulder pain.

Physical examination reveals local signs of infection, such as erythema, edema, tenderness, increased warmth and limitation in range of motion. Atypical presentation occurs, when there is chronic arthritis, immunocompromised state, extreme age and intravenous drug use or low grade prosthetic joint infection. Previous use of antibiotics as well as corticosteroids or nonsteroidal anti-inflammatory medication, may mask symptoms.

Laboratory Findings

The White Blood Cell (WBC) count may be normal to slightly elevated:

- Raised Erythrocyte Sedimentation Rate (ESR)
- *C reactive protien (CRP):* It has been shown to increase more rapidly than the erythrocyte sedimentation rate and may be of great value in the second, third or fourth day of treatment, to evaluate recovery when the sedimentation rate is still increasing
- Blood cultures
- Joint aspiration and culture
- *Synovial fluid analysis:* On gross examination, the fluid is often thick, yellow, and cloudy
- Leukocyte counts greater than 50,000 WBC per cubic millimeter
- *Glucose levels are decreased:* Levels of 20 to 40 mg per deciliter below the serum level are consistent with pyarthrosis.

Imaging Studies

X-Ray

X-rays in early stages may show joint subluxation or soft tissue swelling, due to either joint effusion or synovial hypertrophy. Later joint space narrowing and marginal erosions appear radiographically.

MRI

MRI gives excellent resolution of soft tissues and fluid collections with an extremely high sensitivity, demonstrating abnormalities within 24 hours. MRI can clearly demonstrate cartilage destruction and small joint effusions as well as intramedullary bone destruction and marrow edema.

CT Scan

Computed tomography (CT) scan can give better bony resolution than either plain radiographs or MRI, clearly depicting subtle bone destruction.

Bone Scan

Technetium 99m (^{99m}Tc) bone scan.

Arthroscopy

Arthroscopy can be a helpful diagnostic as well as therapeutic modality. Arthroscopic examination of a septic joint usually reveals inflamed and friable synovium with fibrinous exudates. Adhesions and loculations of pus may also be present. In addition to visualization of the joint, direct synovial biopsy and culture of multiple sites can be obtained.

Treatment

Prompt recognition, correct diagnosis, joint decompression and an organism specific antibiotic regimen are essential. Initial period of intravenous administration, usually of 3 to 7 days is followed by oral administration. The total duration of antibiotic regimen varies with the pathogen being isolated, the patient's underlying condition and adjuvant medical or surgical procedures. For gonococcal septic arthritis, 7 to 10 days are generally recommended. For streptococci or *Haemophilus* species, 2 to 3 weeks duration is usually adequate. Cases in which more virulent organisms, such as *S. aureus* or gram-negative bacilli are isolated, 4 to 6 weeks course of appropriate antibiotic is required. Immunocompromised patients or those with a slow clinical response will need the full 6 weeks of treatment.

Antibiotic impregnated polymethylmethacrylate: Antibiotic impregnated, Polymethylmethacrylate (PAMMA) has been used in the treatment of infections of the soft tissue and joint arthroplasty as well as osteomyelitis. The main advantage of this treatment is that it allows for a high concentration of antibiotics to be delivered locally, while minimizing the risk of systemic toxicity.

Evacuation and decompression of the joint: The goals of treatment of septic shoulder include sterilization and decompression of the joint with removal of all inflammatory cells, lysosomal, preoteolytic enzymes and fibrinous materials.

Arthroscopy: The diagnostic advantage of arthroscopy is that it allows for direct visualization of the entire joint. Visualization is essential in determining the extent of the disease and enabling tissue biopsy in atypical or challenging cases. The therapeutic advantage of arthroscopy is that the joint can be adequately drained, thoroughly debrided and copiously irrigated. Prognostically, arthroscopic irrigation and drainage reduces hospital stay and allows for early ROM, which may be helpful in preserving joint function.

Tuberculosis of the Shoulder

This is very rare, constituting nearly 1 to 2 percent of skeletal tuberculosis and can start in any of the following sites:

- Glenoid
- Head of humerus
- Synovium (rarely)

Clinical Features

Earlier Stage (Fig. 23.275)

- Painful limitation of abduction and external rotation occur early
- Marked wasting of the deltoid, supraspinatus other muscles
- Common variety is dry type and is called as *caries sicca,* since there is no effusion in the joint.
- Cold abscess formed could present at:
  - Supraspinous fossa
  - Deltoid
  - Biceps.

Late Stage (Fig. 23.276)

- Destruction of the upper end of the humerus and glenoid cavity
- Fibrous ankylosis is the end result.

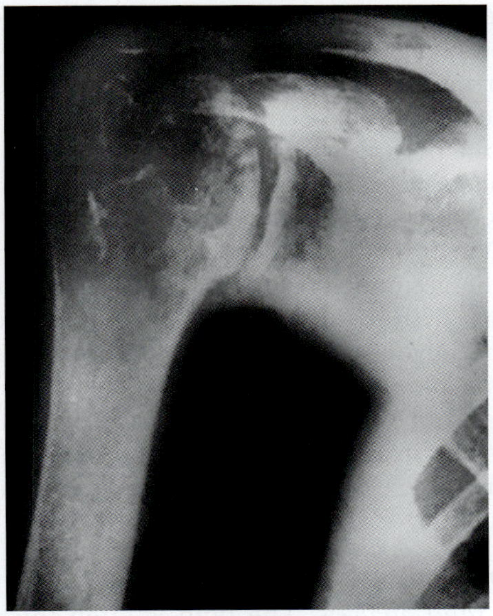

Fig. 23.275: X-ray shows earlier stage of tuberculosis of the shoulder

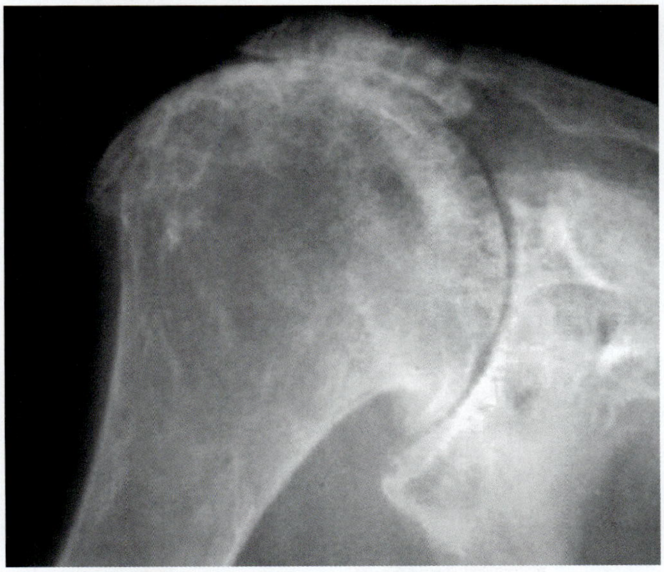

Fig. 23.276: X-ray shows later stage of tuberculosis of the shoulder

Radiology

- Generalized rarefaction
- Articular cartilage erosion
- Cavities in the head of humerus
- Periosteal reaction.

Treatment

Chemotherapy is the mainstay of the treatment. Shoulder immobilization by plaster is done, by keeping shoulder spica in 70 to 90° of abduction, 30° of forward flexion and about 30° of internal rotation, to encourage ankylosis in functional position for 3 months. Arthrodesis in painful ankylosis, recurrence, etc.

■ Bursitis

Subacromial Bursitis (Fig. 23.277)

The subacromial bursa lies under the upper part of the deltoid and extends upwards underneath the acromion process. This bursa serves to reduce friction and to permit the greater tuberosity of the humerus to rotate inwards under the acromion process in movements of abduction and rotation of shoulder.

The inflammation of bursa occurs mostly as a consequence of a lesion, involving neighboring structures. It is not a structure where disease starts, but it limits disease in the adjacent structures, by temporary adhesions causing fixation of parts. The floor of the bursa is more prone towards pathological changes, owing to relative avascularity and inert supraspinatus tendon, which makes it the most vulnerable part.

Clinical Features

Pain in shoulder is felt on abduction and internal rotation. Pain is usually felt at the insertion of deltoid. Pain is severe at night. Tenderness is present over anterior aspect of humeral head. Usually there is a point of tenderness on the greater tuberosity, which starts disappearing under the acromion on abduction (Dawnbarn's sign). X-ray may show calcareous deposits in the supraspinatus tendon and occasional bony spurs.

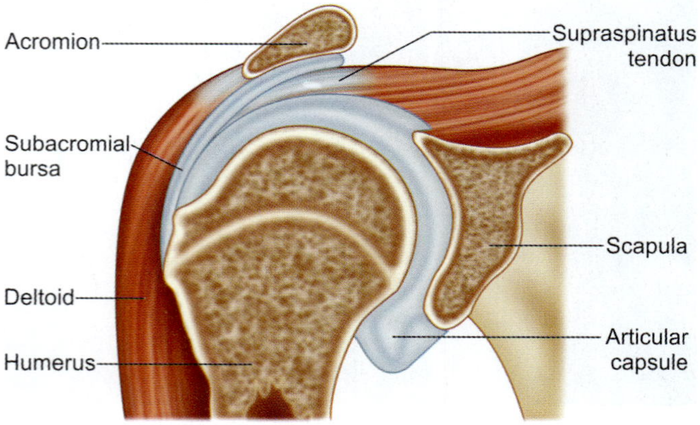

Fig. 23.277: Anatomical position of subacromial bursa

Subcoracoid Bursitis

The sub coracoid bursa is situated between the tip of the coracoid process and the capsule of shoulder joint. It extends up to and even over the lesser tuberosity. Strenuous usage of arm cause irritation of bursa from the pressure of the lesser tuberosity against the coracoid. Patients complain of pain in the region of coracoid. Tenderness is present between coracoid and lesser tuberosity.

In late cases, in which adhesions are present, with marked limitation in lateral rotation and abduction. A diagnostic injection of 5 ml of 1 percent lignocaine with hydrocortisone into this area produces relief from pain.

Treatment

In acute cases rest of shoulder in sling, together with anti-inflammatory drugs over a course of a week. In failed cases injection of 5 ml of 1 percent lignocaine with hydrocortisone into tender bursa is helpful. However, this is contraindicated in infection.

In cases of persistent bursitis, exploration and excision of the inflamed bursa together with the removal of calcified deposits in the supraspinatus tendon.

■ Crystalline Arthritis

Calcium Pyrophosphate Dihydrate (CPPD)

Calcium pyrophosphate dihydrate deposition disease is a disorder of the articular tissues, resulting from the liberation and deposition of calcium pyrophosphate dihydrate crystals. Clinically, two stages of the disorder have been recognized.

- Occurrence of acute attacks of synovitis precipitated by the liberation, accumulation and reactivity from calcium pyrophosphate crystals within the intra-articular space. These are termed as pseudogout, these attacks clinically resembles gout.
- CPPD arthropathy will evolve from repeated attacks and the accumulation of deposits of pyrophosphate crystals within the articular cartilage. Secondary degenerative arthritis will develop, accompanied by chronic pain. A propensity for elderly women is recognized with this form. X-ray shows crystal deposition in articular cartilage of humeral head and progressive deterioration of glenohumeral articulation, as shown in Figure 23.278.

Laboratory Findings

Synovial fluid analysis: The fluid is often thicker than normal and at times turbid, especially in elderly women.

Characteristic rhomboid shaped positively birefringent crystals are identified. Some are intracellular, following engulfment by polymorphonuclear cells, as depicted in Figure 23.279.

Note: Readers are requested to refer Inflammations around elbow for further reading.

■ Gout

Gout is a disease characterized by hyperuricemia and resultant accumulation of sodium urate crystals within tissues and joints. It is the most common inflammatory arthropathy in men older than 40 years of age and its occurrence is at its peak in the fifth decade. It may be the presenting joint in a postoperative flare and in postmenopausal women.

The uric acid crystals are engulfed by macrophages triggering immunological reaction. Mediators of inflammatory response, including chemotactic factors, e.g. lysozymes, collagenase, oxygen radicals and prostaglandins. All these triggering factors are released and cause inflammation. The synovium is stimulated and proliferates, which results in an acute inflammatory cellular infiltrate to rapidly develop. When the joint has been subject to repeated attacks, a local foreign body reaction ensues with the synovium and results in the local resorption of the adjacent cartilage and bone. Radiographically, this is what is seen as the punched out lesions, without an associated bony response.

Clinical Features

- With glenohumeral joint involvement, patients will present with an acute onset of shoulder pain.
- These patients are often obese, men are mostly involved and sometimes found to have ingested excessive alcohol.
- Physical findings of an acute gouty arthritis include, decreased range of motion of the shoulder, overlying warmth, tenderness and perhaps swelling. Occasionally, these patients will have fever.

X-Ray Findings (Fig. 23.280)

Radiographs will show juxta-articular osteopenia and perhaps juxta-articular tophi. Sharply outlined erosions, punched out with sclerotic margins and overhanging edges will be present.

Laboratory Findings

- Elevated serum uric acid levels
- *Synovial fluid analysis (Fig. 23.281):* Presence of monosodium urate crystals, often intracellular and can be visualized with a polarizing microscope. Needle like crystals and are negatively birefringent.

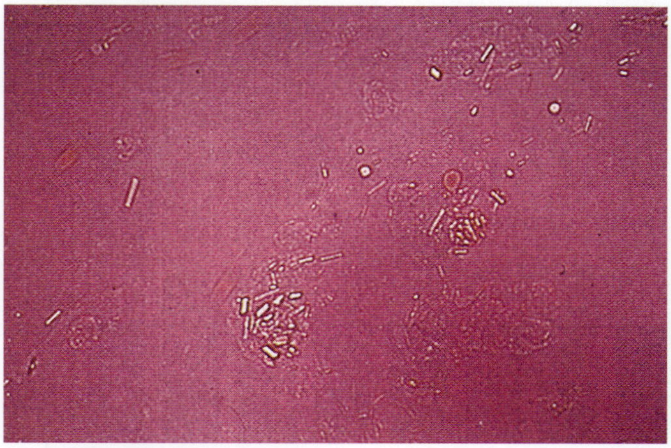

Fig 23.279: Synovial fluid analysis, shows characteristic rhomboid shaped positively birefringent crystals

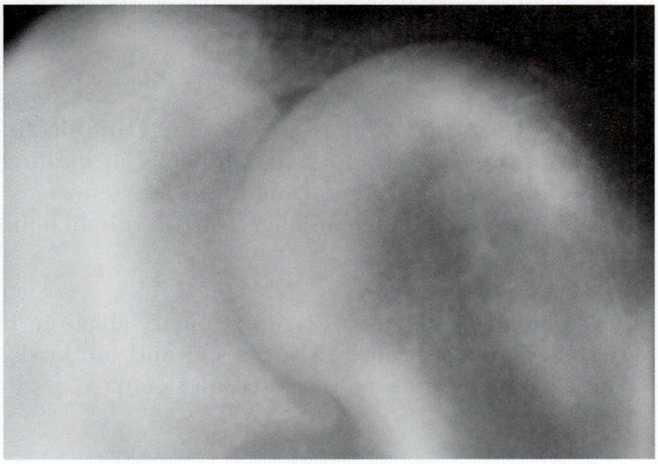

Fig. 23.278: X-ray shows crystal deposition in articular cartilage of humeral head, resulting in deterioration of glenohumeral articulation

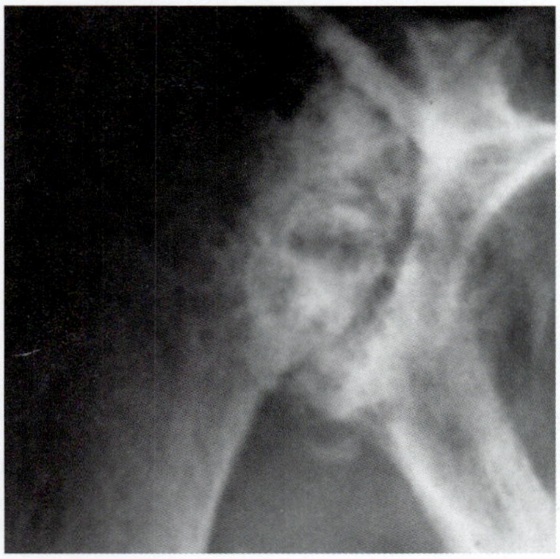

Fig. 23.280: X-ray shows degenerative manifestations of gout

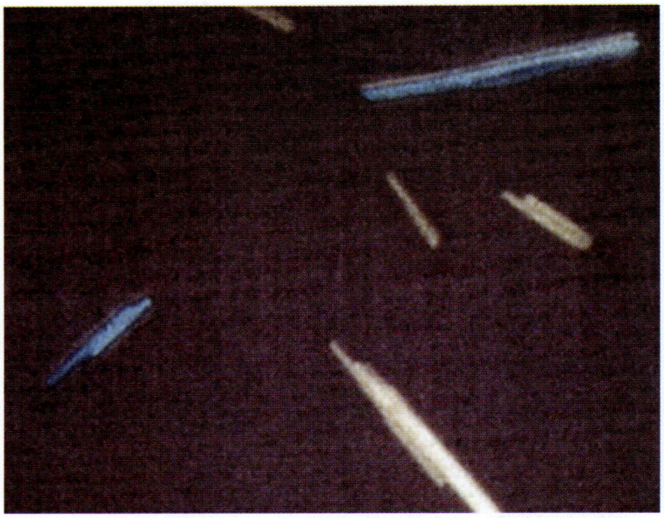

Fig. 23.281: Synovial fluid analysis shows needle like crystals of monosodium urate crystals

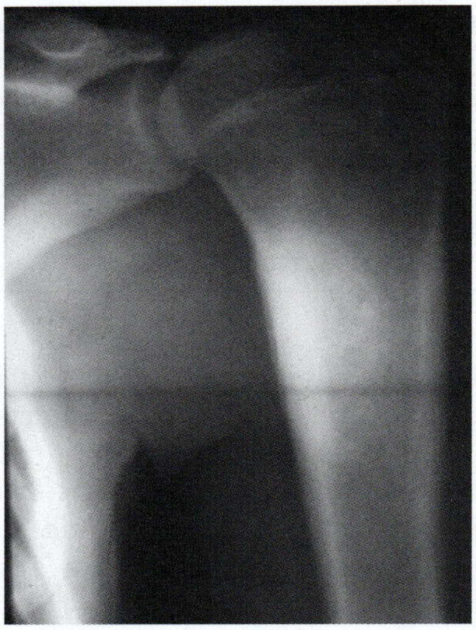

Fig. 23.282: Osteoidosteoma, shows large area of reactive bone surrounding a small, subcentimeter radiolucent nidus

TUMORS AROUND THE SHOULDER

Bone Tumors

- Benign
- Malignant.

Soft Tissue Tumors

- Benign
- Malignant.

Benign Bone Tumors

Benign bone tumors include:

- Osteoidosteoma
- Osteoblastoma
- Osteochondroma
- Chondroblastoma
- Enchondroma
- Unicameral bone cysts
- Aneurasmal bone cyst (ABC)
- Fibrous dysplasia
- Nonossifying fibroma
- Giant cell tumor

Osteoidosteoma

This small benign bone tumor occurs in patients of any age, most commonly in children and young adults. It shows predilection for male sex. Only 10 to 15 percent of cases of osteoid. Osteoma occurs in the shoulder, main site are proximal end of the humerus or glenoid.

Symptoms

Osteoidosteoma typically displays the classic symptom of night pain, which is relieved by salicylates, e.g. aspirin.

Investigations (Fig. 23.282)

Radiographically, it is characterized by a large area of reactive bone, surrounding a small, subcentimeter radiolucent nidus. Technetium bone scan, osteoid-osteoma has impressive increased activity. The central nidus can be visualized as a distinct cortical hole on computed tomography (CT scanning).

Differential Diagnosis

It consists of osteoblastoma, osteomyelitis (Brodie's abscess) and intraosseous ganglion. Histologically, this lucent nidus is a well demarcated, small area of immature and very active osteoblastic tissue.

Treatment

Preoperative localization is an extremely important strategy, to prevent intraoperative difficulty in locating these lesions and thus minimizing local recurrences.

Operative treatment is curettage, with or without bone grafting, e.g.

- En bloc excision
- CT guided percutaneous radiofrequency ablation. It has been introduced as a successful and minimally invasive method of treating osteoidosteomas.

Osteoblastoma

Osteoblastoma is a larger version of osteoidosteoma (giant osteoidosteoma), it is typified by a large lucent area (greater than 2 cm) of osteoblastic tissue, surrounded by a thin, sclerotic and reactive rim of bone.

Incidence: About 10 percent of the total osteoblastoma. It mainly occurs in adults.

Histopathology

- Scattered mitotic figures
- Proliferation of immature plump osteoblasts
- Prominent vascular and stromal tissue component.

Imaging

X-rays (Fig. 23.283): X-rays show radiolucent lesion, which is surrounded by a thin margin of reactive bone, which may have an expanded aneurysmal appearance.

CT scan and MRI: These confirm preoperative diagnosis and help in determining surgical approach.

Angiography is used for staging aggressive tumors.

Bone scan shows intense radioisotope uptake that helps localize the lesion.

Treatment

En bloc marginal excision is the treatment of choice. Active tumors are more likely to recur, if intracapsular resection is performed. Risk of recurrence after marginal excision of aggresive stage third is 30 to 50 percent. Radiation therapy or chemotherapy is not effective.

Osteochondroma

The incidence of cartilaginous tumors in the shoulder is secondary only to those occurring in the pelvis.

Incidence: Solitary osteochondroma or exostosis, is the most common benign tumor of the shoulder, fourth of all exostoses occur in the proximal part of the humerus. It can be found in patients of any age, but it stops growing when skeletal maturity is achieved.

Pathogenesis: It is a developmental abnormality arising from the peripheral growth plate and is typically active and benign lesions during skeletal growth.

Clinical Features

It is usually painless but causes symptoms by pressure on adjacent structures. The cartilaginous cap may impinge adjacent neurovascular structures.

Investigations (Figs 23.284A and B)

The plain radiograph is usually diagnostic, a smooth excrescence of metaphyseal cancellous bone that is confluent and continuous with the normal metaphyseal bone.

Histopathology: Exostoses can appear as pedunculated, stalk-like lesions or sessile lesions. The risk of a secondary chondrosarcoma arising out of an exostosis is approximately 1 percent per lesion, although rates are as high as 10–30 percent in patients with multiple hereditary exostoses.

Secondary chondrosarcoma can arise in adult patients with pain and an enlarging soft tissue mass or intraosseous bony erosions. Evidence of a thickened cartilaginous cap (1 cm) on CT scan, in association with a soft tissue mass, pain or radiographic evidence of malignant degeneration, suggests a secondary chondrosarcoma.

Treatment

Treatment of a solitary exostosis is done, when it is causing mechanical pressure symptoms or for cosmetic purposes

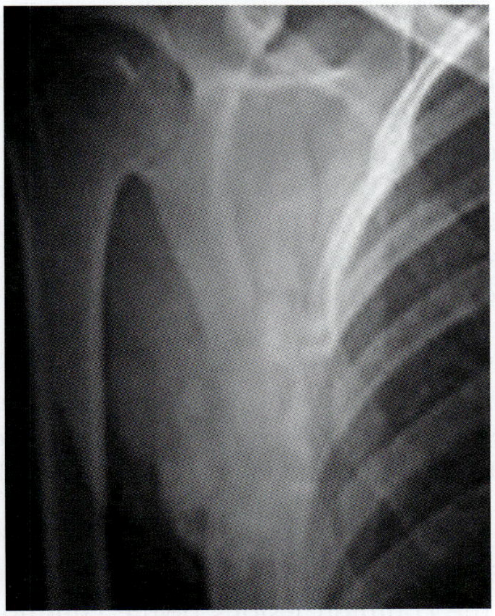

Fig. 23.283: Osteoblastoma shows radiolucent lesion, surrounded by a thin margin of reactive bone, which have an expanded aneurysmal appearance

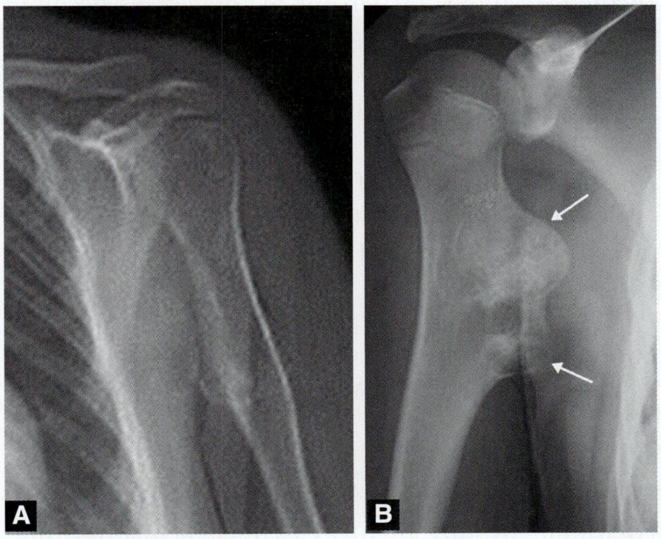

Figs 23.284A and B: Osteochondroma, with smooth excrescence of metaphyseal cancellous bone that continue with the normal metaphyseal bone

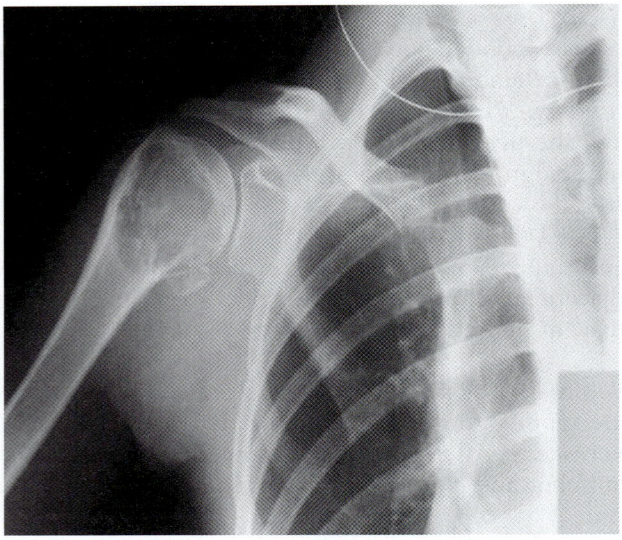

Fig. 23.285: X-ray shows well circumscribed, chondroblastoma lesion, centered in epiphysis with surrounding rim of reactive bone

involves excision of the tumor. Excision should be through the base of the lesion and also the cartilaginous cap should be excised to prevent recurrence. In the sessile form, care should be taken to excise the cartilaginous cap, in order to prevent a recurrence.

Chondroblastoma (Fig. 23.285)

Chondroblastoma is an aggressive benign cartilaginous tumor. Chondroblastoma occur as a round or oval lesion containing fine calcifications, surrounded by a reactive bony margin. It occurs as an active, benign stage II lesion, although it also has a more aggressive stage three form.

Incidence: About 25 percent of total cases occur in humerus.

Site: Most common site is proximal humerus.

Age: Usually occurs in adolescent or young adult with 2:1 male predominence.

Histologically: It consists of aneurysmal tissue, chicken wire calcifications and immature paving stone chondroblasts.

X-ray: Well circumscribed lesion, centered in epiphysis, with surrounding rim of reactive bone are seen. Fifty percent of cases will show calcification.

Differential diagnosis: It has to be differentiated from Giant Cell Tumor (GCT). GCT will not have a rim of sclerotic bone and intralesional calcification. It may have soft tissue component.

Treatment

Treatment usually involves extensive intralesional curettage, which results in a large subchondral defect of the humeral head that requiring bone graft, to prevent subchondral and cartilaginous collapse.

An adjuvant agent, such as hydrogen peroxide or cryotherapy can help to decrease local recurrence rates. Patients need to be followed up in every 6 months for 3 years.

Recurrence occurs in 10 to 20 percent of cases. Benign pulmonary metastasis occur in 1 percent of cases should be treated by resection.

Enchondroma

Enchondroma is a benign lesion of hyaline cartilage. They are common and affects all age groups. It is most commonly found in the small tubular bones of the hand, but also occurs in the proximal end of the humerus in 10 to 15 percent of cases.

Enchondromas are usually solitary, but multiple, typically unilateral (Ollier's disease) or Maffucci's syndrome (enchondromatosis with multiple hemangiomas of skin or viscera or both). Tumors are located on epiphysis, metaphysis and even on the shaft.

Clinical Features

Patient can present with deformities, caused by lack of epiphyseal growth and metaphyseal widening.

It is usually painless. Pain may occur when it is associated with some pathological fracture. When an enchondroma occurs adjacent to a joint, which is symptomatic for degenerative reasons, clinical assessment of bone pain related to the enchondroma may be difficult. It makes the initial evaluation of intraosseous cartilage tumors difficult because intrinsic bone pain is an important symptom, suggesting a low grade malignancy. Thus we have to differentiate from the intraosseous symptom with intra-articular symptom.

Investigation

X-ray (Fig. 23.286)

It shows benign appearing lesion, with intralesional calcification. Calcification described as stippled, punctate or popcorn type. Sometimes erosion and cortex expansion is seen. However, if the deep endosteal erosion involves greater than two-thirds of the total cortex thickness, then it suggests a malignancy. If soft tissue mass is present it indicates chondrosarcoma.

Treatment

The risk of malignant transformation of solitary lesions is extremely small. The risk of malignant transformation is 25 to 30 percent in Ollier's disease and even higher in Maffucci's syndrome.

Unicameral Bone Cysts (UBC)

They are the common lesions of the childhood more consistent with a developmental or reactive lesion than a true tumor.

Age: Occurs in first to second decade of age.

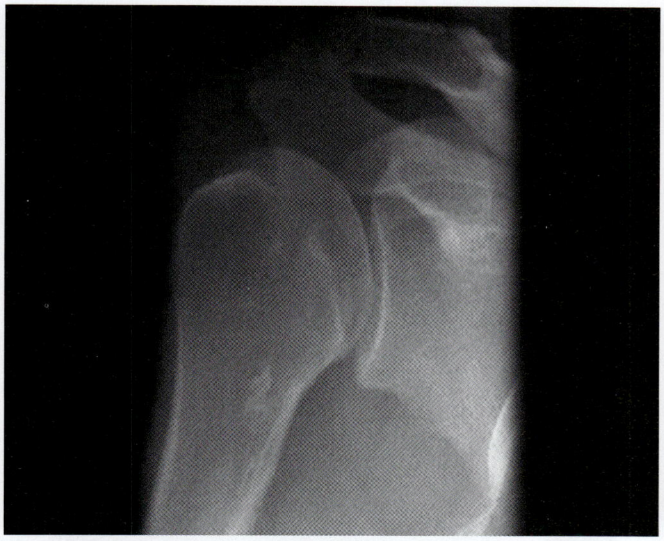

Fig. 23.286: X-ray shows, enchondroma of the shoulder

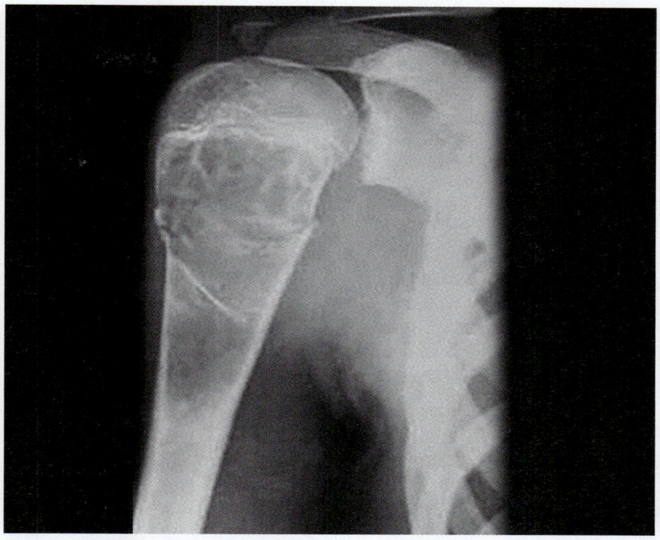

Fig. 23.287: X-ray shows, unicameral bone cysts

Sex: Shows 2:1, male predominance.

Site: Most common in proximal humerus. Lesions are active during the skeletal growth and usually heal spontaneously at maturity.

Clinical Features

Usually asymptomatic unless a pathological fracture has occurred. Two-thirds of patients may present with a pathological fracture. Fracture may stimulate a cyst to heal.

Investigation (Fig. 23.287)

X-ray: Shows centrally located purely lytic lesion well marginated outline.

Cysts may expand concentrically, but it never penetrates the cortex. Occasionally, (20%) thinned cortical fragment fractures and falls into the base of the lesion This fallen fragment sign is pathognomic for unicameral bone cysts with fracture. They are classified as active, when they are within 1 cm of the physis and latent, when they are closer to diaphysis.

Treatment (Figs 23.288A and B)

Small asymptomatic cysts can be treated with observation and serial radiographs. Larger lesions are usually treated with curretage with or without bone grafting and internal fixation. Percutaneous aspiration and injection using either:

- Steroid
- Bone marrow aspirate
- Demeniralized bone matrix
- Calcium sulphate
- Hydroxy appetite crystals high porosity
- Cancellous allografts.

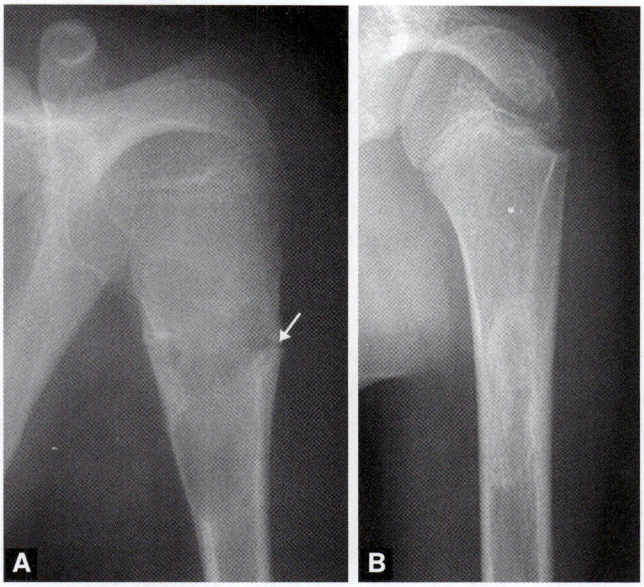

Figs 23.288A and B: (A) Unicameral bone cysts, at the upper end of humerus; (B) Follow-up X-ray after one year treated with aspiration and steroid injection

Aneurysmal Bone Cyst

Aneurysmal bone cyst (ABC) is locally destructive, blood filled reactive lesions of bone and are not to be considered as true neoplasm.

Site: Most commonly occur at proximal humerus.

Age-sex: Before second decade of life with slight female predominance.

Clinical features: Mild to moderate pain present for several weeks to months.

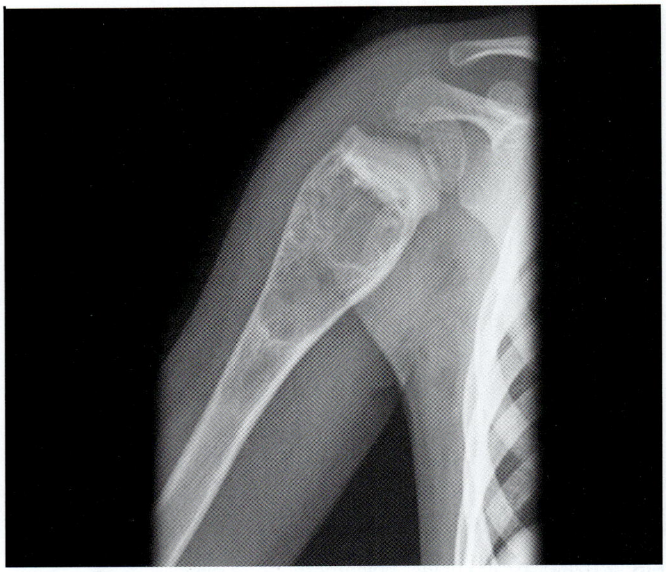

Fig. 23.289: X-ray shows aneurysmal bone cyst, commonly located in metaphysis

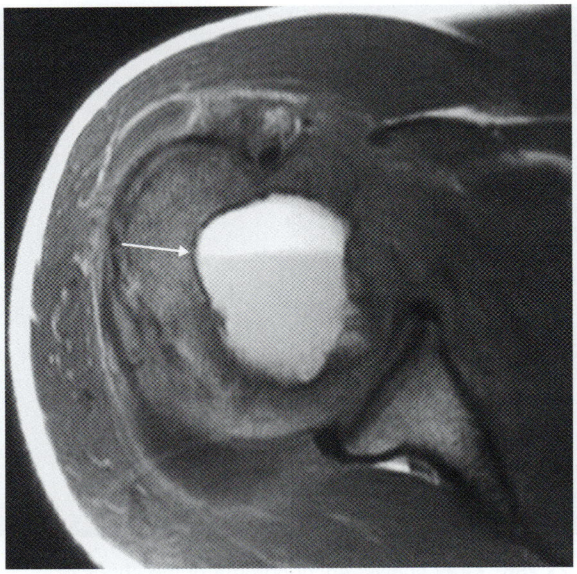

Fig. 23.290: MRI showing double density fluid level

Radiological Investigations (Fig. 23.289)

X-ray: Expansile lytic lesion that elevates periosteum, but remained contained by thin shell of the cortical bone. Most often located in metaphysis.

MRI (Fig. 23.290): Shows multiloculated cavities and fluid levels when differentiating between a UBC and ABC presence of a double density fluid level and intralesional septations indicates ABC.

Histopathology (Fig. 23.291)

It shows hemorrhagic tissue, with cavernous spaces, separated by cellular stroma. The lining of cavitary spaces consists of compressed fibroblasts and histiocytes.

Treatment

Extended curettage with a bone graft substitute is usually advised. The recurrence rate after curettage is 10 to 20 percent. Recurrence can be treated with the same approach as the primary lesions.

Fibrous Dysplasia

Fibrous dysplasia is a congenital dysplasia of bone, may exist in mono-ostotic or polyostotic form that often presents as a painful lesion secondary to pathologic fracture. The hallmark is replacement of normal bone, by fibrous tissue and small woven spicules of bone.
Site: Epiphysis, metaphysis and diaphysis.

Associated abnormalities: Sexual precocity, abnormal skin pigmentation, intramuscular myxoma and thyroid disease.

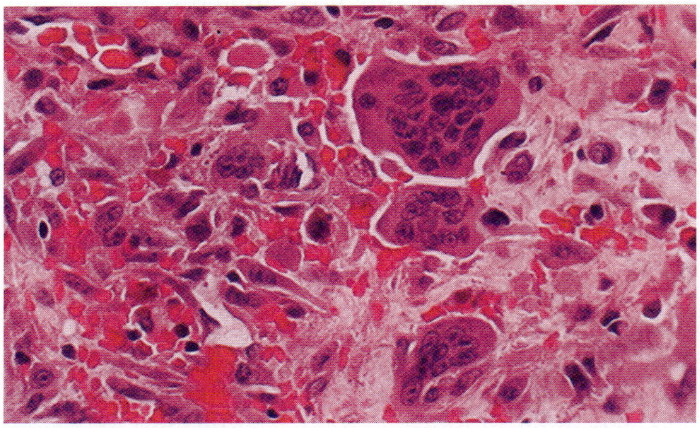

Fig. 23.291: Hemorrhagic tissue, cavernous spaces, fibroblasts and histiocytes seen in aneurysmal bone cyst

Investigations

The typical plain radiograph demonstrates a ground glass density, with cortical thickening, as shown in the Figures 23.292A and B. Bone scan also shows increased activity. Histology shows furnace of dysplastic bone activity.

Treatment

When associated with symptoms or pathologic fracture, diaphyseal involvement usually requires intramedullary fixation rather than bone grafting because cancellous bone graft is consistently consumed by the dysplastic process and is ineffective in resolving the weakened dysplastic bone. Deformities are corrected by osteotomy with internal fixation.

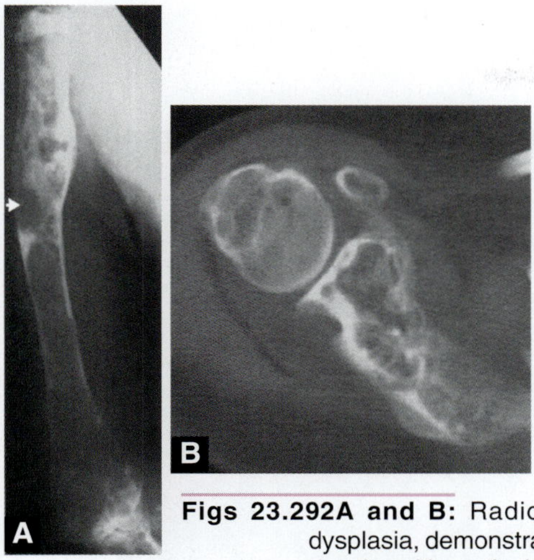

Figs 23.292A and B: Radiograph of fibrous dysplasia, demonstrates a ground glass density with cortical thickening

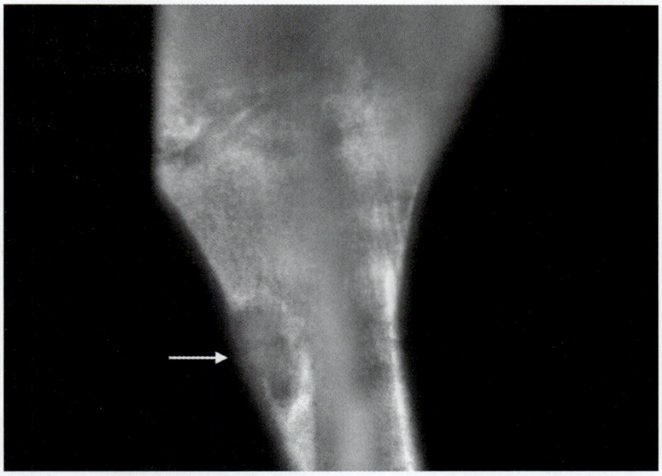

Fig. 23.293: Nonossifying fibroma

Nonossifying Fibroma (Fig. 23.293)

Nonossifying fibroma is a benign fibrous lesion. Radiographically, it is visible as an eccentric and well defined lucent lesion that has a scalloped border abutting the adjacent cortex.

When the lesion is smaller than 4 cm, it may be referred to as a fibrous cortical defect. When lesions are longer than 5 cm or occupying more than half the transverse diameter of the bone, these lesions are at the risk for pathologic fracture. The majority of nonossifying fibromas, heal spontaneously and require no treatment.

Giant Cell Tumor

Giant cell tumor (GCT) of bone is a benign and locally aggressive lesion.

Site: Uncommon in proximal end of the humerus (5%).

Radiological Findings

GCT is a radiolucent, epiphysometaphyseal tumor, which commonly has a distinct bony margin and is associated with extensive subchondral bone erosion. There can be bony expansion, cortical destruction or frank extension of the tumor mass into the soft tissues. Periosteal reaction is uncommon unless there has been a prior pathologic fracture.

Treatment

Treatment alternatives for GCT include:

- Curettage, with or without local adjuvant treatment
- Marginal resection

Local adjuvant therapy used in conjunction with curettage includes, the application of phenol, bone cement (cementation) or liquid nitrogen (cryotherapy). The local recurrence rate after curettage alone is 20 to 30 percent for active lesions and 5 percent after marginal resection.

■ Malignant Bone Tumors

Osteosarcoma

Osteosarcoma is the most common malignant primary bone tumor after myeloma. It is the most common primary sarcoma occurring in the shoulder, followed by Ewing's sarcoma and chondrosarcoma. It has typically developed in the adolescent age group, although a significant percentage of patients are the young adults, usually in third decade of their life.

Clinical Features

- Bone pain
- Night pain
- Pain unrelated to joint motion
- Tender soft tissue mass.

The average duration of symptoms at initial assessment is 3 to 6 months, which reflects the subtle nature of the preliminary symptoms and the need for early recognition of intraosseous pain and night pain, as a warning symptom.

Approximately 10 to 15 percent of all osteosarcomas occur in the proximal part of the humerus, whereas 1 to 2 percent developed in the scapula or clavicle.

The typical X-ray for osteosarcoma has a codman triangle, sunburst or hair on end pattern, with penetration of the adjacent cortex. MRI is gold standard investigation for osteosarcoma, it determines the extent of soft tissue and bony involvement. CT scan determines extent of bony involvement not soft tissue, this is illustrated in Figures 23.294A to E.

Variants of osteosarcoma include, telangiectatic (vascular) osteosarcoma, secondary osteosarcoma (Paget's disease or radiation induced) and various low grade lesions, such as periosteal and parosteal osteosarcoma. The basic histologic criterion for the diagnosis of classic

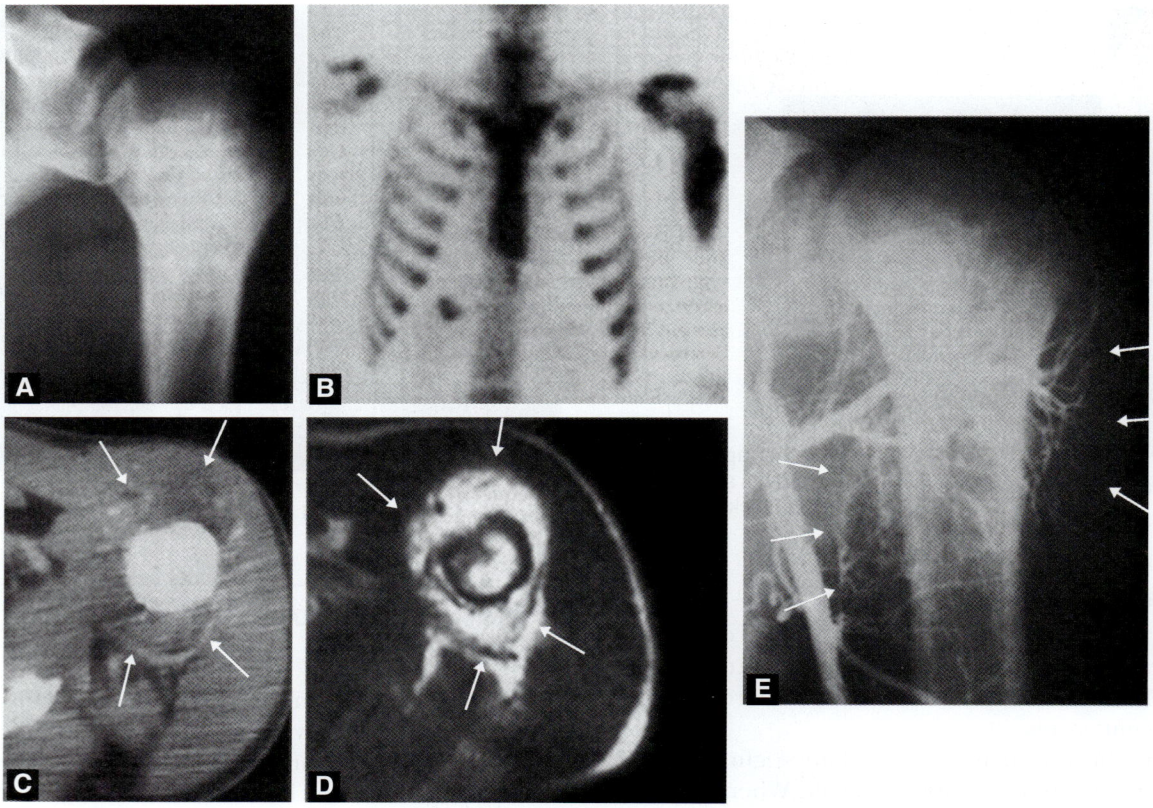

Figs 23.294A to E: (A) X-ray shows osteosarcoma of the proximal end of the humerus, suggests soft tissue involvement; (B) Bone scan shows significant extension proximally and distally in the humerus; (C) CT scan of the same patient does not demonstrate the extent of soft tissue extension (arrows); (D and E) MRI through the same area of the humerus, demonstrating circumferential soft tissue involvement (arrows)

osteosarcoma includes, a malignant stroma producing (spindle cells) tumor or immature neoplastic osteoid.

Classification

It is classified into three types histologically:

- Osteoblastic
- Chondroblastic
- Fibroblastic

Treatment

Currently, treatment for high-grade osteosarcoma consists of:

- Neoadjuvant chemotherapy
- Wide or radical surgery (resection or amputation)
- Adjuvant chemotherapy. It is a radioresistant malignant bone tumor.

Prognosis

The overall survival rate for patients with osteosarcoma at 5 years of follow-up is approximately 70 percent, with appropriate chemotherapy and surgery.

Chondrosarcoma

Chondrosarcoma can develop *de novo*, as a primary chondrosarcoma or it can arise out of a pre-existing benign cartilage lesion, known as secondary chondrosarcoma. Primary chondrosarcoma is more commonly seen in the middle decades of life and its incidence in the shoulder is secondary to that in the pelvis or hip joint. It is the most common primary bone malignancy to arise in the coracoid process.

These tumors are typically manifested as intraosseous lesions with poorly defined margins and faint intrinsic calcifications. Secondary chondrosarcoma, occurs in young adults and accounts for approximately 25 percent of all chondrosarcomas.

X-Ray

X-ray finding are enlarging radiolucent areas within the lesion or endosteal cortical erosions along the cortical margins, as shown in Figures 23.295A and B.

Bone Scan

Technetium bone scans are typically moderately hot.

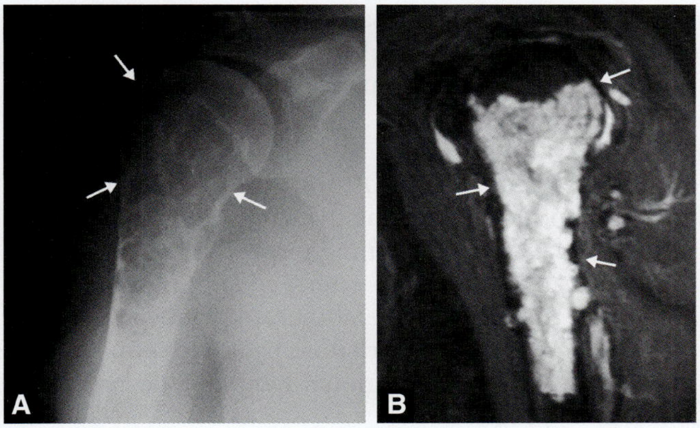

Figs 23.295A and B: (A) The distinct endosteal cortical erosions (arrows), suggest a low-grade chondrosarcoma; (B) Sagittal MRI of the proximal end of the humerus, demonstrating high signal intensity the cartilage and the extent of intraosseous involvement (arrows)

Histopathology: Hypercellularity, pleomorphism and evidence of mitotic activity, such as double nucleated lacunae and cellular atypia. These findings can also be seen in multiple enchondroma.

Treatment

Low-grade chondrosarcomas may be treated surgically with curettage and bone grafting. Whereas, high grade tumors deserve surgical resection and reconstruction of the limb.

Ewing Sarcoma

It is second most common intraosseous malignancy in adolescence. Children are more commonly affected than adults. It is not a common tumor around shoulder.

X-Ray

Mottled-moth eaten appearance, destruction of bone, with both lytic and blastic areas. There is periosteal reactive new bone formation, which may form layers, forming classical onion peel appearance.

MRI

MRI is required to know the extent of bony destruction and soft tissue involvement.

Multiple Myeloma (Figs 23.296A to C)

Multiple myeloma is the most common primary malignancy of bone. It occurs in middle decades of life. The shoulder girdle is involved in 5 to 10 percent of cases. The most common site of involvement is the axial skeleton.

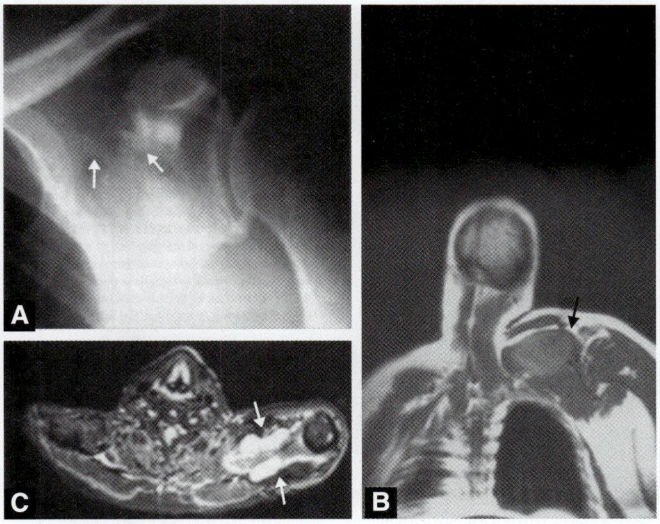

Figs 23.296A to C: (A) X-ray of a 42-year-old man, with left shoulder pain and a lytic scapular lesion (arrows); (B) MRI in the same patient, demonstrates a suprascapular soft tissue mass (arrow); (C) MRI view of the same patient, shows a lesion wrapped anteriorly and posteriorly over the scapula (arrows)

Prognosis

The overall prognosis is poor, newer treatments involving aggressive chemotherapy and plasma cell antibodies offer hope for the future.

Benign Soft Tissue Tumors

Ganglion

It is a common soft tissue tumor that is often confused with other cystic lesions. They are filled with a characteristic gelatinous material. In the shoulder, they are often associated with degenerative conditions or a labral tear. When located in the spinoglenoid notch, a ganglion may produce suprascapular nerve palsy secondary to nerve entrapment.

Lipoma (Fig. 23.297)

Lipomas can occur intramuscularly or within normal fat planes of the axilla or the subscapular planes. They often appear in the anterior part of deltoid as a large, soft, nontender and intramuscular mass. A few lipomas are tender or firm and show history of a change in size.

On MRI or CT scan, a benign lipoma usually has a uniform, fatty consistency.

Hemangioma

Hemangioma, typically appear as an enlarging intramuscular lesions in a child or young adult. They are

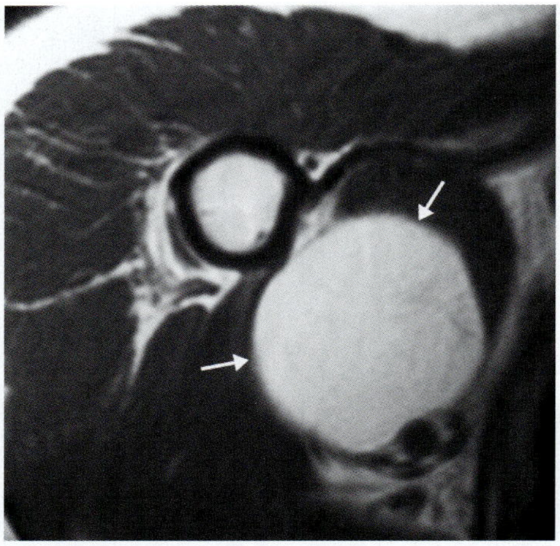

Fig. 23.297: MRI shows a benign lipoma, usually has a uniform fatty consistency

best visualized by MRI and typically have a serpiginous configuration of vessels. If they are intimately involved with a major vessel, they should also be evaluated with an arteriogram. Well localized lesions are more easily resected than the more extensive congenital lesions. Embolization and interferon treatment show, mix results in halting the progression of disease.

Fibromatosis

Fibromatosis (desmoid) is a locally aggressive lesion found in young children, teenagers and young adults. These lesions have a firm consistency on clinical examination and may be associated with osseous erosions or invasion of a neurovascular bundle. Recurrence rate is quite high. Rarely they have pulmonary metastasis.

Malignant Soft Tissue Tumors

Soft Tissue Sarcoma

Upper extrimity is involved in 25 percent of total cases.

Clinical Features

- Firm mass
- Large (5 cm) or enlarging
- Deep or subfascial
- Non tender

The most common soft tissue sarcoma in adults is malignant fibrous histiocytoma, which occurs most often in older adults (50–70 years). Liposarcoma typically occurs in the lower extremities in young adults, as a large lesion, with a histology ranging from low-grade to high-grade or pleomorphic. Synovial sarcoma is a less common lesion associated with faint soft tissue calcifications, a juxta-articular location and a high metastatic rate. Fibrosarcoma, rhabdomyosarcoma, leiomyosarcoma, clear cell sarcoma and epithelioid lesions are other, less common soft tissue malignancies.

Treatment

Regardless of the tissue type, the grade of the lesion and the anatomic location of the primary tumor are the most significant factors determining prognosis and treatment.

Soft-tissue sarcomas of intermediate grade histology are usually treated with chemotherapy. Synovial sarcoma, epithelioid sarcoma, and rhabdomyosarcoma have high incidence (10–20%) of regional lymph node metastasis and a poor prognosis.

BRACHIAL PLEXUS INJURY AND ITS MANAGEMENT

Anatomy

The dorsal and ventral rootlets exit the spinal cord and merge to form the spinal nerves, which leave the intervertebral foramina and quickly divide into dorsal and ventral rami, as shown in Figure 23.298. The origin of brachial plexus is from the ventral rami of C5 through C8 and T1 spinal nerves. Sometimes contributions may originate from, C4 (prefixed) and T2 (postfixed).

Roots (Fig. 23.299)

- The upper roots (C5–C8) descend towards the first rib, whereas the lower T1 root ascend over the first rib to form the brachial plexus

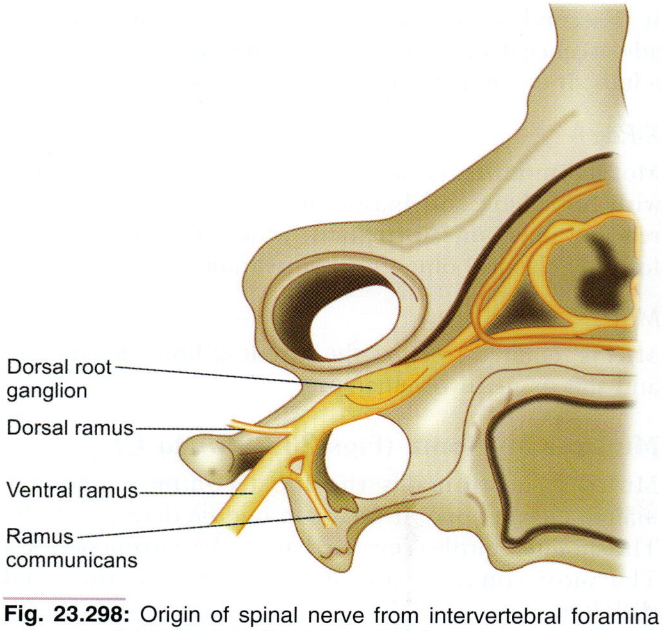

Fig. 23.298: Origin of spinal nerve from intervertebral foramina forming ventral and dorsal rami

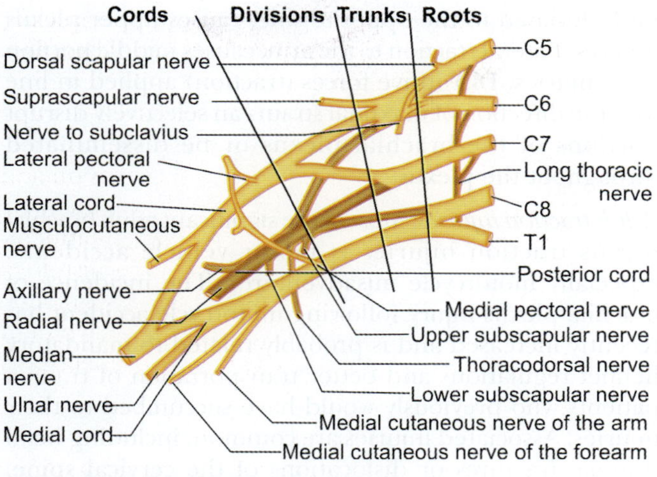

Fig. 23.299: Brachial plexus and its components

- Sympathetic fibers join the nerve roots as they traverse between the scalene muscles
- C5 and C6 receive fibers from the middle sympathetic cervical ganglion and C7–T1, acquire fibers from the cervicothoracic ganglion
- These sympathetic fibers control blood vessel smooth muscle contraction (vasoconstriction) and sweat gland activity.

Trunks (Fig. 23.299)

- The ventral rami of C5 and C6 combine to form the upper trunk
- The C7 ramus continued alone as the middle trunk
- C8 and T1 unite to form the lower trunk
- The trunks are located in the posterior triangle of the neck, enclosed by the posterior border of the sternocleidomastoid muscle, anterior border of the upper trapezius and clavicle.

Divisions and Cords

- Each trunk divides into anterior and posterior divisions and proceeds behind the clavicle
- The divisions then merge into three cords, named in relation to the axillary artery
- The anterior divisions of the upper and middle trunks combine to form the lateral cord
- The anterior division of the inferior trunk continues as the medial cord
- The three posterior divisions converge to form the posterior cord.

Branches

- The cords proceed behind the pectoralis minor muscle into the axilla and divide into two terminal branches
- The lateral cord terminates, as the musculocutaneous nerve and a branch to the median nerve
- The posterior cord divides into the axillary and the radial nerves
- The medial cord continues as the ulnar nerve and a branch to the median nerve
- Several branches arise from the roots, trunks and cords of the brachial plexus.

Branches at the Root Level

- The dorsal scapular nerve arises from C5 and innervates levator scapula and rhomboid muscles.
- The long thoracic nerve arises from C5, C6 and C7 and is supplied to serratus anterior muscle.
- The phrenic nerve arises from C3, C4 and C5 and crosses the anterior scalene muscle to enter the thorax. This nerve may get injured in nerve root injuries, with subsequent hemidiaphragm paralysis.

Branches at the Trunk Level

- The suprascapular nerve arises from the upper trunk and is supplied to supraspinatus and infraspinatus muscles.
- The nerve to the subclavius arises from anterior surface of the upper trunk and innervates subclavius muscle.
- There are no branches from the plexus at the division level.

Branches at the Cord Level

1. *From the lateral cord*: The lateral pectoral nerve arises to innervate the clavicular part of the pectoralis major.
2. *From the posterior cord*: The upper subscapular, thoracodorsal and lower subscapular nerves:
    - The upper subscapular nerve innervates the upper portion of the subscapularis muscle
    - The lower subscapular nerve innervates the lower portion of the subscapularis muscle and teres major muscle
    - The thoracodorsal nerve originates between the upper and lower subscapular nerves, passes behind the axillary artery and supplies the latissimus dorsi muscle.
3. *From the medial cord*: One motor and two sensory branches arises:
    - The medial pectoral nerve innervates pectoralis minor muscle and the sternocostal portion of the pectoralis major muscle
    - The medial brachial and medial antebrachial cutaneous nerves are the only sensory branches to arise directly from the brachial plexus and supply the arm and forearm respectively.

■ Etiology

Brachial plexus injuries can affect a wide range of individuals from newborns to the elderly. Obstetric brachial plexus palsy can occur during passage through the birth canal, whereas adolescent and adult injury may be secondary to domestic violence, vehicular trauma, athletic endeavors or systemic disease:

- Trauma
  - Nonpenetrating (traction)
  - Penetrating, e.g. knife or Gun Shot Wound (GSW)
- Nerve entrapment
  - Thoracic outlet syndrome
- Infection
  - Viral plexopathy (parsonage—Turner syndrome)
- Radiation
  - Fibrosis
  - Malignant degeneration after radiation
- Tumors
  - Primary (schwannomas or neurofibromas)
  - Secondary (pulmonary apices)
- Neuropathies
- Iatrogenic
  - Axillary or scalene anesthesia
  - Surgical biopsy
  - Intraoperative positioning
  - Median sternotomy
  - Inadvertent traction

Nonpenetrating Trauma

- Nonpenetrating trauma is the leading cause of injury to the brachial plexus
- The mechanism of injury in almost all injuries is traction that produces tension across the brachial plexus
- The mechanism by which the traction is produced is variable and may be from:
  - Traction to the extremity
  - Forcible head rotation from the shoulder
  - Direct depression of the shoulder girdle
  - Iatrogenic, malpositioning of the patient on the operation theater (OT) table.

Traction Injuries

With traction injuries, there is a stretch of the nerve beyond the physiological limits that nerve can withstand. There is a direct reduction of intraneural blood flow with increasing strain. A 15 percent elongation will reduce blood flow approximately 80 to 100 percent. Continued elongation will cause overt ischemia and disruption of nerve metabolism. Persisted traction will ultimately disrupt nerve continuity. Traction, therefore can cause nerve injury ranging from a temporary disruption in nerve fiber conduction to functional discontinuity of the nerve fibers and sheath. The upper plexus is taut with the arm dangling at the side and the lower plexus is taut with the arm abducted and elevated.

Traction with the arm forcibly abducted, can causes lower plexus injuries and with the arm adducted and the neck deviated to the opposite side, causes upper plexus injuries. Lateral traction to the arm, causes middle portion (C7) injuries. Disruptive forces (traction) applied in line with the direction of maximal strain can selectively disrupt portions of the brachial plexus or be disseminated throughout the plexus.

Adult traction injuries: Most of the significant adult brachial plexus traction injuries is motor vehicle accidents, especially motorcycle misadventures. The incidence of brachial plexus injury following motorcycle accident has recently increased and is probably related to mandatory helmet regulations and better transportation of trauma patients who previously would have succumbed to their injuries. Associated injuries are common, including head trauma, fractures or dislocations of the cervical spine, shoulder, forearm, and hand.

Minor stretch injuries (burners, stingers) of the plexus are common in contact sports, especially football, because tackling drives the shoulder downward and forcibly flexes the neck toward the contralateral side. The athlete experiences a burning pain and paresthesia that radiates from the supraclavicular area into the arm. Transient weakness and sensory abnormalities are present. The symptoms and signs of these stretch injuries usually resolve spontaneously over a few minutes. However, a cervical spine fracture, dislocation or a severe brachial plexus injury can occur during impact with subsequent quadriplegia or a permanent neurologic deficit. These injuries will have persistent weakness and limited neck motion. Shoulder dislocations are often related to sporting accidents and can produce nerve injuries of the axillary, suprascapular or musculocutaneous nerves. These are usually (80%) temporary lesions that resolve over 4 to 6 months. However, violent high energy trauma can cause disruption of nerve fiber integrity at the time of dislocation.

Obstetric traction injuries: Traction injuries can occur during birth and are associated with difficult deliveries. Traction to the head with forceful tilting from the fixed shoulder (lateral neck flexion) during delivery can stretch the upper plexus. Instrumentation (forceps, vacuum) to after coming head in postmature delivery, as demonstrated in Figures 23.300A to D. Injury can also occur during breech presentation as the lower roots are stretched during hyperabduction of the ipsilateral arm during delivery.

Penetrating Trauma

Penetrating trauma to the brachial plexus is often secondary to gunshot wounds or stabbings. Bullet injuries act as projectile missiles that cause neural injury by means of a blast effect or less commonly direct nerve transection. In contrast, stab wounds transect portions of the plexus or cause vascular injury with secondary nerve compression by expanding hematoma. Most commonly, the upper and

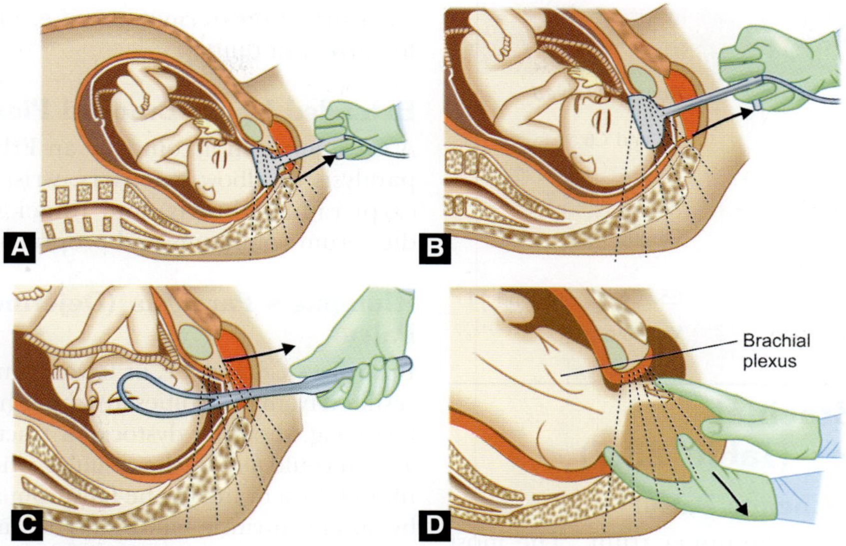

Figs 23.300A to D: Use of instruments for delivery can resulted in injuries to brachial plexus

midplexus are involved, as clavicle protects the lower elements.

Infection

Infection is an uncommon cause of brachial plexopathy and the exact etiology remains obscure. Both viral pathogens and secondary immunologic factors proposed as the possibilities. This brachial neuritis, also known as Parsonage-Turner syndrome, presents with an acute onset of intense pain about the shoulder girdle without antecedent trauma. Weakness of the muscles innervated by the affected nerves develops after the initial pain response. The suprascapular or long thoracic nerve is the most commonly affected. The natural history of brachial neuritis is resolution of the pain followed by improvement in motor function.

Electromyographic abnormalities of the denervated muscles are apparent 3 to 4 weeks after the initial pain response, with positive sharp waves and fibrillation potentials. The treatment is conservative management with observation and serial examinations. However, prolonged recovery time and persistent weakness is not uncommon even years after the brachial neuritis.

■ Classification of Brachial Plexus Injury

The lesion in brachial plexus injury is classified according to the anatomic location and extent of nerve involvement.

Based on Anatomic Location

i. *Supraclavicular lesions:* Affect roots, trunks and divisions
ii. *Infraclavicular lesions:* Affect cords and branches

Supraclavicular Lesions

Supraclavicular lesions can be due to:

- Avulsion injury or
- Ruptures

Avulsion Injury

The supraclavicular injury from traction can disrupt the rootlet connection with the spinal cord and is called an avulsion injury. An avulsion separates the motor cell body in the spinal cord from its axons, but the sensory cell body located in the dorsal root ganglion remains connected to its axons. The motor portion of the nerve, therefore undergoes wallerian degeneration with degradation of the axons and myelin sheaths. The sensory fibers are spared from wallerian degeneration, but have been irrevocably detached from the spinal cord. The injury will cause a clinical motor and sensory loss, whereas electrodiagnostic studies will reveal abnormal motor findings with intact sensory conduction. Rarely, the rupture can affect only the motor or sensory rootlets.

Rupture

The injury interrupting nerve continuity at the trunk level is called a rupture. Ruptures of the plexus separate both motor and sensory cell bodies from their axons and wallerian degeneration occurs across all fibers. Discontinuity by rupture can be treated by various surgical techniques to re-establish nerve continuity, whereas avulsion injuries are irreparable. The diagnosis can be difficult, for traction can cause a combination of rupture and avulsion injuries at different levels, which will complicate accurate diagnosis. Supraclavicular lesions account for most brachial plexus injuries (75% approximately) and are also subdivided into groups according to the pattern of involvement.

Table 23.7: Various patterns and roots involved in brachial plexus injuries	
Pattern	*Roots involved*
Upper brachial plexus (Erb-Duchenne paralysis)	C5 and C6
Extended upper brachial plexus	C5, C6 and C7
Lower brachial plexus (Dejerine-Klumpke's paralysis)	C8 and T1
Total brachial plexus lesion	C5, C6, C7, C8 and T1
Peripheral brachial plexus lesion	Variable

■ Patterns of Brachial Plexus Injuries (Table 23.7)

Erb's Palsy (Erb-Duchenne Palsy)

It involves C5 and C6 or the upper trunk. The most common cause of Erb's Palsy is dystocia. Other causes include pressure on the raised arms during a breech delivery, clavicle fracture in neonates, traumatic fall onto the side of the head and shoulder, as shown in Figure 23.301. The most commonly involved nerves are suprascapular nerve, musculocutaneous nerve and axillary nerve. It is characterized by:

- Loss of elbow flexion
- Weakness of shoulder abduction and external rotation
- Paralysis and atrophy of the deltoid, biceps and brachialis muscles.

The position of the limb in Erb's palsy is characteristic, the arm hangs by the side and is rotated medially and the forearm is extended and pronated, as depicted in Figure 23.302. Sensory deficit is apparent in the corresponding dermatome, i.e. on radial side of the forearm and thumb.

Extended Upper Brachial Plexus Lesion

A C7 injury can accompany an Erb's palsy. In addition paralysis of elbow extensers, wrist extensers (extensor carpi radialis brevis) and finger extensers (extensor digitorum communis and proprius) are also present.

Klumpke's Paralysis (Dejerine-Klumpke's Palsy)

It involves C8 and T1, or lower trunk. The injury can be resulted from difficulties in proper handling during child birth, e.g. shoulder dystocia or traction on the abducted arm. It could also be the result of, when someone catching himself by a branch as he falls from a tree. Characterized by absent intrinsic hand musculature and finger flexors (flexor digitorum profundus and superficialis) with intact shoulder, elbow and wrist function.

Sensory deficit is situated over the ulnar side of the forearm and hand. Involvement of T1 may result in Horner's syndrome, as shown in Figure 23.303, with ptosis, miosis and anhydrosis.

Total Brachial Plexus Lesion

The injury can include the entire plexus (C5, C6, C7, C8 and T1), which causes a flail and anesthetic arm. The brachial plexus may be injured by direct violence, gunshot wounds, by violent traction on the arm or by efforts at reducing a dislocation of the shoulder joint. The amount of paralysis will depend on the amount of injury to the constituent nerves. Supraclavicular lesions can also be

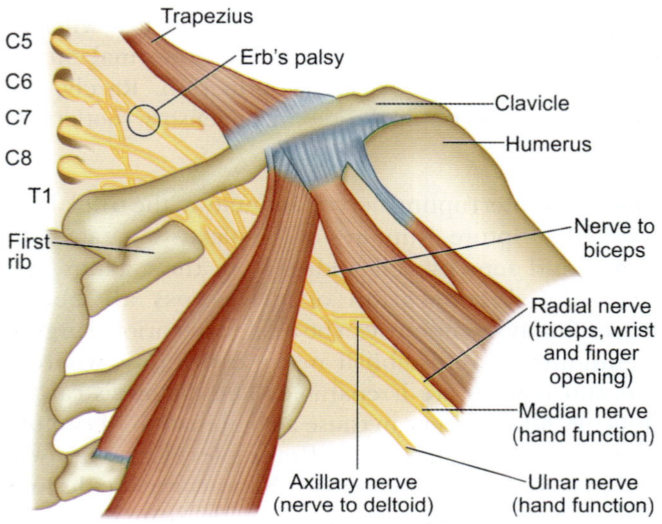

Fig. 23.301: The roots and trunk involved in Erb's palsy

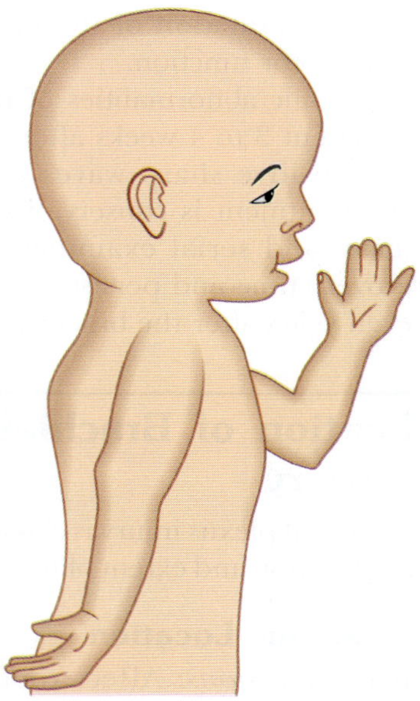

Fig. 23.302: Typical position of the upper limb in Erb's palsy

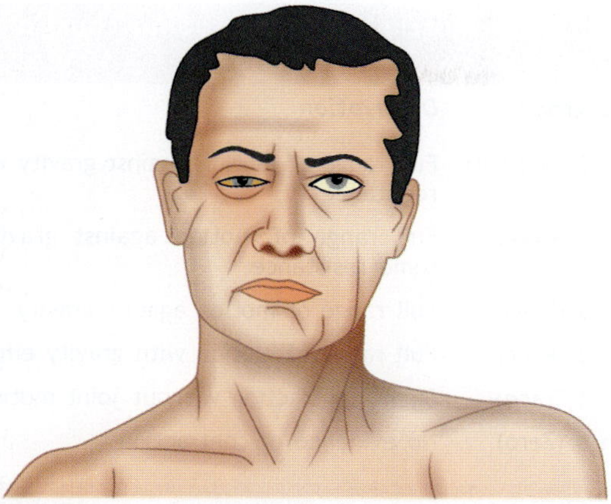

Fig. 23.303: Horner's syndrome due to the injury involving T1 root

isolated to peripheral branches, such as the suprascapular or long thoracic nerve. This can be secondary to trauma, infection and surgical positioning (iatrogenic).

Infraclavicular Lesions

They are less common (25% approximately). Usually, represent stretch injuries from an associated shoulder dislocation or fracture. These injuries represent peripheral nerve lesions of the plexus. The axillary nerve is particularly susceptible to traction because it is securely anchored as it traverses the quadrangular space. However, injury to the musculocutaneous nerve and other elements of the brachial plexus can occur after severe trauma.

Based on Degree of Intraneural Damage

- Neuropraxia
- Axonotmesis
- Neurotmesis

Neuropraxia

Its a segmental demyelination with maintenance of intact nerve fibers and axonal sheath. A temporary conduction block follows, without axonal damage and Wallerian degeneration. Complete recovery occurs over the ensuing days to weeks as remyelinization is completed.

Axonotmesis

It is disruption of nerve fiber integrity with preservation of the axonal sheath and framework. Wallerian degeneration and nerve fiber regeneration are necessary for recovery. The axons distal to the injury degrade from lack of nutrition and loss of blood supply. The regeneration rate is approximately 1 mm per day or 1 inch per month. The distal nerve injuries have a better prognosis because the extent of Wallerian degeneration is decreased and the proximity to the motor endplates is increased.

Neurotmesis

It is disruption of the nerve fiber and axonal sheath. Transection is the classic example of this injury, but severe traction or contusion can produce a similar injury with irreversible intraneural scarring. The prognosis is bleak without surgical resection of the intervening scar and nerve coaptation by direct repair or graft interposition to allow for nerve regeneration. A severe brachial plexus injury often represents a combined lesion, with elements of neuropraxia, axonotmesis and neurotmesis. This combination injury further complicates accurate diagnosis and predictions for recovery.

Evaluation of Brachial Plexus Injury

The clinical evaluation of the patient with a brachial plexus injury begins with a careful history and detailed examination. The examination should include the head, neck, thorax, injured extremity and neurovascular systems. Knowledge of brachial plexus anatomy and concomitant muscle innervation is a prerequisite to accurate diagnosis. Imaging studies and electrodiagnostic tests provide supplemental information to further clarify the extent of injury. The goal of this evaluation is to precisely define the location and extent of nerve injury. This information will direct treatment, which may range from continued observation to prompt surgical intervention.

Adult injury: Usually referred after treatment of any life-threatening injuries.

History taking: Inquiry to the mechanism of injury and degree of energy involved. The force applied (direction, magnitude and duration), position of extremity and concomitant injuries (fractures, dislocations, visceral damage, head trauma and vascular disruptions) are important details. An instantaneous deficit implies nerve laceration, whereas a delayed onset indicates a compressive neuropathy by an expanding hematoma or false aneurysm.

Examination

- The posture of the extremity and the manner by which the patient uses the extremity are important indicators of the segment of the brachial plexus involved.
- Neurological examination shows motor and sensory deficit.
- An inventory of the muscles innervated by the brachial plexus is imperative to accurately define the injury and provides a baseline to assess recovery.

Brachial Plexus Examination Sheet

Muscle tested (both right and left side)

1. Trapezius (C3, C4, Cranial nerve XI)
2. Levator scapula (C3, C4, C5)
3. Rhomboids (C4, C5)
4. Supraspinatus (C5, C6)
5. Infraspinatus (C5, C6)
6. Serratus anterior (C5, C6, C7)
7. Teres major (C5, C6)
8. Subscapularis (C5, C6)
9. Pectoralis major clavicle (C5, C6, C7)
10. Pectoralis major sternocostal (C6, C7, C8, T1)
11. Latissimus dorsi (C6, C7, C8)
12. Biceps and brachialis (C5, C6)
13. Deltoid (C5, C6)
14. Teres minor (C5, C6)
15. Pronator quadratus (C7, C8, T1)
16. Pronator teres (C6, C7)
17. Flexor carpi radialis (C6, C7)
18. Flexor digitorum profundus II, III (C7, C8, T1)
19. Flexor digitorum superficialis (C7, C8, T1)
20. Flexor pollicis longus (C7, C8, T1)
21. Abductor pollicis brevis (C6, C7, C8, T1)
22. Opponens pollicis (C8, T1)
23. Lumbricals (C8, T1)
24. Triceps (C6, C7, C8)
25. Supinator (C5, C6)
26. Brachioradialis (C5, C6)
27. Extensor carpi radialis longus (C6, C7)
28. Extensor carpi radialis brevis (C6, C7, C8)
29. Extensor carpi ulnaris (C7, C8)
30. Extensor digitorum communis (C7, C8)
31. Extensor digiti minimi (C7, C8)
32. Extensor indicis (C7, C8)
33. Extensor pollicis longus (C7, C8)
34. Extensor pollicis brevis (C6, C7)
35. Abductor pollicis longus (C6, C7)
36. Flexor carpi ulnaris (C7, C8, T1)
37. Flexor digitorum prof. IV, V (C7, C8 and T1)
38. Abductor digiti minimi (C8, T1)
39. Abductor pollicis (C8, T1)
40. Opponens digiti (C8, T1)
41. Interossei (C8, T1)

Muscle Grading Chart (Table 23.8)

Careful examination of the muscles innervated by the proximal branches from the brachial plexus will help define the proximity of the plexus lesion to the spinal cord. Disruption of the dorsal rami (paraspinal muscles), dorsal scapular (rhomboids and levator scapulae) and long thoracic (serratus anterior) nerves are suggestive of an avulsion injury.

The presence of a Horner's syndrome results in a drooped eyelid, constricted pupil, sunken globe and sweating deficiency that usually implies an avulsion injury at C8 and T1.

Table 23.8: Muscle strength grading chart and its description

Muscle grade	*Description*
Grade: 5 (Normal)	Full range of motion against gravity with full resistance
Grade: 4 (Good)	Full range of motion against gravity with some resistance
Grade: 3 (Fair)	Full range of motion against gravity
Grade: 2 (Poor)	Full range of motion with gravity eliminated
Grade: 1(Trace)	Slight contraction without joint motion
Grade: 0 (Zero)	No evidence of contraction

Table 23.9: Indicators of avulsion injuries and poor prognosis for recovery

Finding	*Implication*
Denervation of paraspinal muscles	Dorsal rami injury
Denervation of rhomboid muscles	Dorsal scapular (C5) injury
Scapular winging	Long thoracic (C5, C7 and C8) injury
Horner's syndrome	Cervicothoracic sympathetic injury
Absent Tinel's sign	Preganglionic separation from cord
Sensory impairment of neck	Cervical plexus injury
Hemidiaphragm paralysis	Phrenic nerve injury
Cervical transverse process fracture	Avulsion fracture with root injury
Pseudomeningocele	Dura and arachnoid avulsion injury
Anesthesia and intact CV	Dorsal ganglion intact, but avulsion from cord

Indicators of Avulsion Injuries and Poor Prognosis for Recovery (Table 23.9)

Percussion of the supra and infraclavicular plexus is performed. A Tinel's sign is indicative of a postganglionic injury, e.g. rupture. This sign will be absent in a preganglionic lesion, e.g. avulsion because the link to the spinal cord and brain has been disrupted. Postganglionic injuries are further localized by examination of the intermediate and terminal branches. The status of the suprascapular (spinati), thoracodorsal (latissimus dorsi), subscapular (subscapularis and teres major), pectoral (pectoralis major and minor) will further define the injury.

Examination of the pectoralis major muscle is particularly helpful because of its dual segmental innervation from the lateral pectoral (C5, C6 and C7) and medial pectoral (C8 and T1) nerves from the lateral and medial cords respectively. Selective atrophy of the clavicular head (lateral pectoral) or sternocostal head (medial pectoral) facilitates diagnosis, whereas complete atrophy implies a global injury.

A peripheral vascular examination is a fundamental component of the evaluation, for damage to the axillary or subclavian vessels can occur. Decreased or absent peripheral pulses, a delayed neurologic deficit (expanding hematoma) and penetrating trauma warrant arteriography.

■ Obstetric Brachial Plexus Palsy

The history is extremely important. Prenatal, postnatal and birth information should be obtained. Risk factors for an obstetric palsy include a difficult or prolonged delivery, large birth weight, shoulder dystocia, breech presentation and forceps or vacuum extraction. A cesarean delivery does not negate the possibility of brachial plexus injury. In fact, bilateral plexus injuries can occur after cesarean section.

Examination

Difficult, because of lack of cooperation. Observation of the affected extremity often provides valuable information of the underlying pathology. Upper root or trunk injuries (Erb's palsy) and total plexus palsy are common. Isolated lower root or trunk (Klumpke's palsy) injuries are rare in obstetric injuries.

The presence of a Horner's syndrome (ptosis, miosis, enophthalmos and ipsilateral facial anhydrosis) is an important observation that implies proximal avulsion injury of the lower trunk, with disruption of the communicating branch supplying sympathetic fibers to the cervicothoracic ganglion.

Palpation of the clavicle and shoulder girdle may reveal crepitation or abundant callus formation. An acute fracture will inhibit voluntary movement and mimic brachial plexus injuries (pseudoparalysis).

Range of Motion (ROM): A newborn with a brachial plexus injury will have full passive motion, whereas a congenital shoulder dislocation will lack passive motion. Ultrasound may be required to confirm this diagnosis because the newborn humeral head is not calcified.

Assessment of Motor Function

Its a challenging task that requires patience and diligence. The initial goal is to determine the absence or presence of function, as actual grading of muscle strength is impossible.

- *Moro reflex:* The newborn can be aroused by the startle reaction or Moro reflex. This should produce extensor tone in the legs and arms
- The grasp reaction by palmar stimulation should illicit finger flexion. Absence of these primitive reflexes indicates a neurologic problem

Table 23.10: Radiographic findings in injuries to the brachial plexus

Plain X-ray film	*Findings*	*Significance*
Chest	Elevated hemidiaphragm	Phrenic injury, proximal plexus and possible preganglionic avulsion
	First rib fracture	Subclavian or axillary artery injury and lower trunk injury
Cervical spine	Fracture or dislocation	Cervical spine injury
	Transverse process fractured	Preganglionic avulsion injury
Clavile	Fracture	Possible traction injury to plexus or pseudoparalysis
Shoulder	Glenohumeral dislocation	Infraclavicular injury
	Scapulothoracic dissociation	Severe neurovascular injury

- In the infant, a collection of toys, rattles and sweets is necessary to incite movement of the injured extremity
- The effect of gravity can be altered by changing the position of the child to assess weak but functioning muscle
- Sensory function is also difficult to assess, as the only reaction obtained only to some painful stimuli, which will erase any chance of further cooperation.

Imaging Studies

Radiographic Findings (Table 23.10)

Angiography

Angiography is indicated if there is any question of the vascular status of the extremity or integrity of the subclavian or axillary vessels. Penetrating trauma or an expanding hematoma also requires angiography.

Myelography (Figs 23.304A and B)

Myelography is used to define the presence or absence of a pseudomeningocele, a meningeal pouch filled with cerebrospinal fluid that extends through the intervertebral foramen into the paraspinal area. It occurs during root avulsion injury.

Inability to visualize the nerve root on the myelogram further supports the diagnosis of an avulsion injury. However, false-positive psuedomeningocele result has been found in patients in whom the rootlets were intact with isolated dura rupture and false-negative results have been reported during surgical exploration.

Methods recommended to improve the diagnostic accuracy of myelography are to delay the test for 4–6 weeks after injury, to allow for resolution of local swelling and intradural blood clots and also by using computed

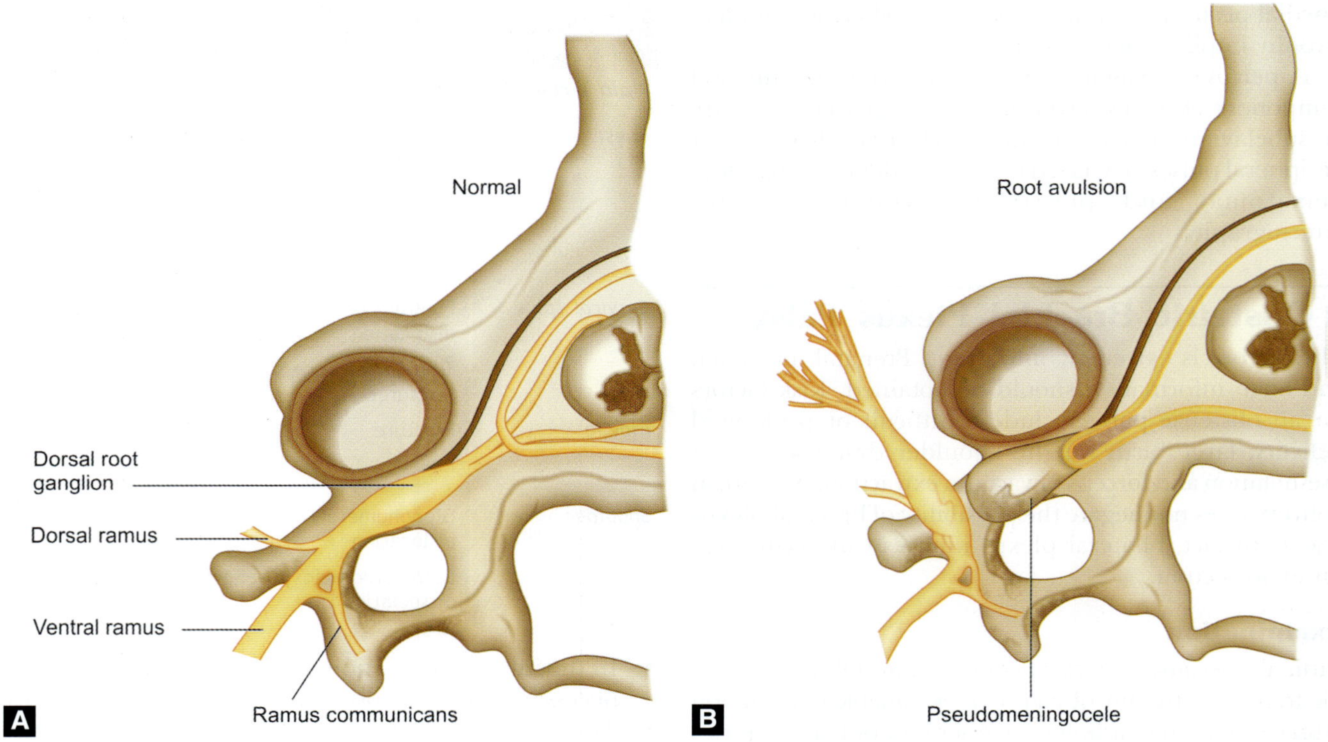

Figs 23.304A and B: Formation of pseudomeningocele, due to root avulsion injury—(A) Normal; (B) Pseudomeningocele, extends through the intervertebral foramen into the paraspinal area after root avulsion injury

tomography (CT myelography) to visualize small pseudomeningoceles.

MRI (Fig. 23.305)

Magnetic resonance imaging has become the primary imaging modality. The MRI provides multiplanar imaging to assess the various components of the brachial plexus. Varying the pulse sequence will provide high resolution images that will facilitate identification of plexus pathology.

MRI offers better evaluation of the trunks and cords, with potential verification of a neuroma by an abnormal signal. MRI is the modality of choice to evaluate neoplasms of the brachial plexus. Diagnosis of root avulsion (pseudomeningocele and nonvisualization of a nerve root) is used with MRI.

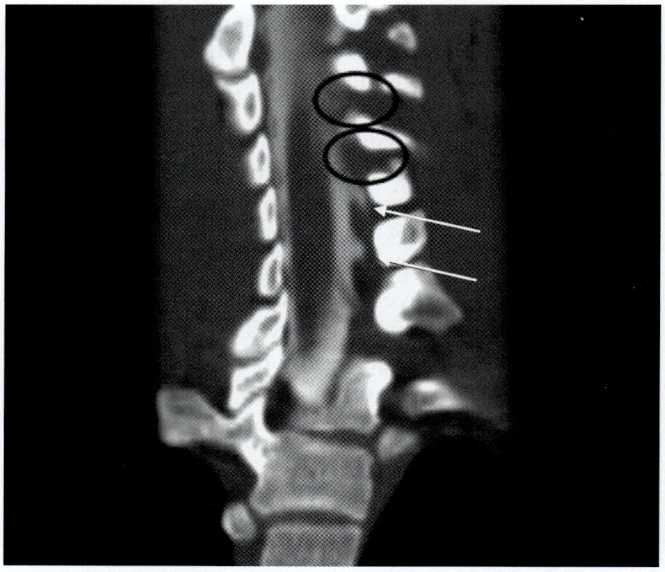

Fig. 23.305: MRI of spine provides multiplanar imaging to assess the various components of the brachial plexus

Electrodiagnostic Studies

Electrodiagnostic testing plays an integral part in the diagnosis and treatment of brachial plexus lesions. Methods employed are:

- Electromyography
- Nerve conduction velocity measurements
- Somatosensory evoked potentials
- Nerve action potentials

Electromyography: Electromyography (EMG) records the electrical activity of muscle fibers at rest and during activation. This signal is recorded by the insertion of EMG needles into the muscle. The normal muscle is silent at rest and active during contraction. A denervated muscle will exhibit spontaneous electrical discharge, i.e.

fibrillations and positive sharp wave, when the EMG needle is inserted. These findings are not present until 2–4 weeks after denervation. A reinnervated muscle will begin to show reinnervation or nascent potentials (polyphasic low amplitude recordings). EMG examination of the muscles innervated by the brachial plexus can provide valuable information about the degree of injury and early recovery.

An EMG evaluation of the more proximal branches from the brachial plexus can help differentiate an avulsion injury from a rupture. For example, fibrillations and positive sharp waves of the paraspinal muscles (innervated by the dorsal rami from the spinal nerve), imply an avulsion injury, whereas preservation of a normal electrical signal suggests a more distal lesion. The EMG is also useful to differentiate the degree of intraneural injury (neuropraxia, axonotmesis and neurotmesis) and to follow the progress after injury. A neuropraxia can be differentiated from a more severe nerve injury by the absence of fibrillation potentials and positive sharp waves. These denervation changes will be present in an axonotmesis or neurotmesis. Serial EMG evaluations can distinguish an axonotmetic lesion by the spontaneous return of nascent units or reinnervation potentials that will precede clinical recovery of function. A neurotmetic injury will not exhibit EMG signs of spontaneous recovery.

Conduction velocity (CV): The conduction velocity is the distance between two sites of stimulation divided by, the time for the nerve action potential to travel from proximal to distal. The integrity of the peripheral nerve is determined by the measurement of the conduction velocity. The motor or sensory latency can be measured depending on the recording of the Compound Motor Action Potential (CMAP) or the Sensory Nerve Action Potential (SNAP). A severed nerve will lose the capability to conduct an action potential distal to the lesion as the nerve degenerates. However, the distal portion of the nerve may be able to conduct for several days after injury until degeneration occurs. Therefore, testing should be delayed for at least 3 weeks to allow time for loss of conduction and denervation changes in muscle.

The status of the SNAP and corresponding sensory nerve conduction velocity is helpful in differentiating preganglionic avulsion injuries from postganglionic lesions. The presence of an intact sensory CV in an anesthetic part of the arm indicates a preganglionic injury, for the sensory nerve is not separated from its cell body (dorsal root ganglion). The CMAP or motor Nerve Conduction Velocity (NCV) is absent in both preganglionic and postganglionic injuries and is not a distinguishing factor.

Somatosensory evoked potentials (SEP): SEPs are electrical responses of the brain and spinal cord to the stimulation of peripheral sensory fibers. Recordings of the conduction from the stimulating electrode to the central nervous system can be useful for the detection of lesions within the sensory system. This technique can be employed to assess conduction across the brachial plexus and during surgery to define irreparable nerve root avulsions. The absence of SEPs recorded over the spinal cord or contralateral sensorimotor cortex on nerve root stimulation indicates a root avulsion and is a contraindication for nerve grafting.

Nerve action potentials (NAPs): NAPs are used intraoperatively to assess lesions in continuity. Stimulating and recording of a nerve proximal and distal to a neuroma can identify the presence or absence of axonal continuity. The presence of NAPs indicates propagation of an action potential along viable nerve fibers. This can help the surgeon decide between neurolysis or excision and interposition grafting.

Treatment

Conservative Treatment

- *A period of immobilization*: For about 3 to 4 weeks to allow the fractures and wounds to heal, to prevent further damage. This is achieved by static splints.
- *Physiotherapy*: After 3 to 4 weeks mobilization of the affected extremity is done in order to prevent contractures.
- *Electrostimulation of paralyzed muscle*: To maintain electrical activity in the paralyzed muscles and also it induces axon regeneration via yet unknown chemotaxis.

Surgical Treatment

Surgical goals: The surgeon should have clear and reasonable surgical goals, which in order of priority are:

- Restoration of elbow flexion
- Restoration of shoulder abduction
- Restoration of sensation to the medial border of the forearm and hand

Depending on the extent of injury, various surgical techniques may be required, including primary neurorrhaphy, neurolysis, nerve grafting and neurotization.

Treatment of avulsion injuries: Currently, there is no surgical treatment to restore nerve rootlet connection (avulsion or intraspinal injuries) with the spinal cord. The current treatment options for avulsion injuries are nerve grafting to other viable proximal stumps or a nerve transfer. Neurotization between the intercostal nerves and the musculocutaneous nerve to restore elbow flexion may be considered.

Treatment of lesions in continuity: Neurolysis is performed for lesions in continuity and the extent of neurolysis will vary with the degree of constricting scar. Epineurotomy may be sufficient in instances of external compression from limited fibrosis, whereas epifascicular epineurectomy may be necessary in an advanced interfascicular compression from fibrosis around the fascicles.

Treatment of lesions without continuity: The initial treatment is to resect the neuroma that forms at the proximal and distal nerve stumps until normal nerve consistency and fascicular anatomy is encountered. The distal stumps are now primed for coaptation with a viable inflow for regeneration of axons. Restoration of continuity can be accomplished by nerve grafting or nerve transfer.

Nerve grafting: Nerve grafting is the placement of intercalary nerve grafts that act as scaffolding for regenerating axons. Nerve grafting is the preferred technique for most lesions with loss of continuity. The interposition of nerve segments link the proximal and distal axons and serve as a conduit to channel, the growing axons to the periphery. The donor nerve is usually the sural nerve from the lower extremity, harvested at the time of brachial plexus exploration. Other potential options are the ipsilateral medial antebrachial cutaneous and superficial radial nerves.

Nerve transfer: Nerve transfer is indicated in avulsion injuries and large or extensive defects of the brachial plexus. The indications for nerve transfer increases as the number of avulsed roots multiplies. This technique involves the connection of an expandable donor motor nerve to provide an axonal source for regeneration of the distal stump. The donor neurons will reinnervate the muscle and function will require voluntary control of the transferred nerve. Similar to a tendon transfer, activation of the donor nerve to achieve function will require a period of training. Involuntary muscle activation may occur, until transformation has taken place.

There are numerous donor nerves available for transfer, including the spinal accessory nerve, cervical plexus, phrenic, intercostal nerves and various portions of the affected plexus (intraplexal transfer).

Oberlin transfer: Transfer of a single fascicle of ulnar nerve to the motor branch of biceps and a fascicle median to the brachialis. Partial transfer of ulnar nerve to the biceps motor branch is made through a longitudinal incision on the anteromedial aspect of the upper arm.

The musculocutaneous nerve is identified after it traverses the coracobrachialis muscle. The biceps motor branch is traced as far proximally as possible and then sectioned. The ulnar nerve is identified at the same level and a longitudinal epineurotomy is done. One ulnar nerve fascicle, carrying motor fibers to the flexor carpi ulnaris (confirmed by electrical stimulation) is minimally dissected, sectioned and coapted to the biceps motor branch with 10-0 nylon sutures. Fascicle of the median nerve that innervated the wrist flexor is identified and coapted with the motor branch to the brachialis, ensuring a tension free nerve anastomosis.

Postoperatively the flexed arm is strapped to the chest for a period of 3 weeks. After that gradually increasing passive exercises are begun. Paralyzed muscles are subjected to electrical stimulation till a grade three power is achieved. After brachial plexus repair and reconstruction, 12 to 18 months are required to determine the extent of neural regeneration. If recovery is considered inadequate, peripheral reconstruction should be considered.

Tendon transfers, around the shoulder that may be considered include:
- Trapezius to deltoid transfer as described by Saha to improve abduction
- Latissimus dorsi transfer to improve external rotation as described by L'Episcopo.

Shoulder arthrodesis, is helpful if active scapulothoracic motion is preserved and has been shown to improve elbow flexion by preventing uncontrolled internal rotation of the shoulder. Shoulder should be fused in only 20° to 30° of abduction because most of these patients rely heavily on arm-trunk prehension.

Operations to restore elbow flexion include transfers of:
- Latissimus dorsi
- Pectoralis major
- Triceps
- Sternocleidomastoid
- Flexor pronator mass.

Restoration of elbow flexion is helpful to the patient, even if the hand is functionless.

Amputation: It is performed rarely. If the patient is certain that the dead weight of a functionless upper extremity is disabling, amputation and prosthetic fitting may be helpful. Amputation should never be performed for pain relief.

Obstetric Brachial Plexus Surgery

Surgery for obstetric lesions is usually performed between 6 and 12 months of age. The obstetric injuries most commonly involve the upper plexus and are usually postganglionic ruptures that can be reconstructed by interposition grafting.

Surgical Methods

Various surgical techniques have been advocated for:
- Root avulsion injuries C5 to T1
- Avulsion of some roots and extraforaminal rupture of other spinal nerves
- Rupture of trunks, cords and individual terminal branches
- Individual nerve injuries.

Root Avulsion of C5 to T1

It can be treated by:

- Conservative treatment
- Nerve transfers

At shoulder: Transfer of 11th cranial nerve (spinal accessory) to suprascapular nerve. Transfer of intercostals nerve to medial pectoral nerve.

At elbow: Transfer of intercostal nerves to musculocutaneous nerve.

For sensation: Sensory rami of intercostal nerves are directed preferentially to the median nerve vesicles, to get sensation in the median nerve supplied area.

Avulsion of Roots and Extraforaminal Rupture of other Spinal Nerves

- *Extraforaminal rupture of C5 and root avulsion of C6 to T1:* Neurotization of suprascapular nerve with 11th cranial nerve. C5 extraforaminal root is sutured to the posterior cord and lateral cord origins. Neurotization of intercostals nerves to middle trunk.
- *Extraforaminal rupture C5, C6 and C7 to T1 root avulsions:* Intraplexial neurotization of avulsed C7 to C6. Connecting lateral cord to the stump of C5. Connecting posterior cord to the stump of C6. Repair the suprascapular nerve with 11th nerve.
- *Extraforaminal rupture C5, C6, C7 and C8, T1 avulsions:* C5 and C6 to be sutured (neurorrhaphy). Avulsed C8 division for medial cord is connected to anteroinferior portion of C7. Avulsed C8 division going to the posterior cord is connected to intercostals nerves. Neurotization of 11th nerve to suprascaplular nerve.

Rupture of Trunks, Cords and Individual Terminal Branches

Upper trunk lesions: Connecting posterior part of C5,C6 to posterior cord. Connecting anterior part of C5,C6 to lateral cord. Repair of suprascapular nerve using 11th nerve (Spinal Accessory) transfer.

Lower trunk lesions: Neurotization of medial cord, ulnar nerve and medial origin of median nerve, using intercostals nerves.

Cord lesions: Cord lesions can be repaired by:

- Direct repair
- Nerve grafting.

Deformities in Long Standing Paralyzed Upper Limb in Brachial Plexus Injury

Shoulder: Adduction, internal rotation deformity with inability to abduct and externally rotate.

Elbow: Fixed flexion deformity

Forearm: Supination deformity

Hand: Claw hand.

Reconstructive Surgeries for Upper Limb

Shoulder

- *Fair bank's procedure*: Superior portion of tendon of pectoralis major is sectioned at its insertion, entire tendon of subscapularis and anterior capsule of shoulder are divided.
- *Sever's procedure:* Tendons of pectoralis major and subscapularis are completely divided without opening the capsule. When coracobrachialis and short head of biceps are contracted, their tendons at coracoids are released.
- *L'Episcopo and Sever operation:* Constitute the first stage. The teres major is transferred posteriorly over the lateral aspect of humerus, where it acts as an external rotator. The latismus dorsi can be similarly transferred.
- *Green's procedure*: Instead of complete division, the tendons of subscapularis and pectoralis major are lengthened to preserve internal rotation. Both latismus dorsi and teres major are rerouted to act as external rotators. Overgrowth of coracoids and acromion are excised. Osteotomy of humerus to correct internal rotation also done.
- *Derotation osteotomy of humerus for posterior torsion/subluxation*: First Sever's operation is done thereby, correcting adduction and internal rotation. This reduces humeral head back into the glenoid. After sufficient immobilization in the corrected position, the humeral head is held in its normal relationship to glenoid, while surgical neck is osteotomized and distal humerus rotated internally. Immobilization continued until union has occurred.
- *Saha's transfer for supraspinatus and infraspinatus*:
  - *For supraspinatus:* Transfer of sternocleidomastoid, Scalenus anterior and scalenus medius is done
  - *For infraspinatus:* Transfer of teres major and latissimus dorsi is done.
- *For deltoid paralysis*:
  - *Lange's procedure*: Insertion of trapezius to humerus using silk sutures
  - *Meyer's procedure*: Used fascia lata instead of silk. But delayed problems of adherence and decreased Range of Motion (ROM) are seen
  - *Saha's procedure*: Transfer trapezius along with part of clavicle and spine of scapula to proximal humerus and fixed with screws

Elbow

Operations to restore active flexor power to elbow include:

- *Steindler's flexoplasty*: Transfer of common flexor origin more proximally.

- *Bunnel's modification of Steindler's flexoplasty:* Common flexor origin transferred proximally and anteriorly.
- *Bunnel's anterior transfer* of triceps to bicipetal tuberosity. When the pectoralis major and triceps as well as the biceps and brachialis are partially weakened, the further two muscles can be transferred to reinforce the flexor muscle of elbow.
- *Correction of elbow deformity*: Removal of radial head should await skeletal maturity. Arthrodesis of elbow at 90° is an alternative when muscles are unavailable for transfer.

Forearm

Correction of Forearm Deformity

- Fixed pronation deformity, generally left alone.
- Fixed supination deformity:
  - Zancolli's transfer for rerouting the biceps
  - Manual osteoclasis and fixing in needed degree of pronation.

Hand

Correction of claw hand deformity can be done by following procedures:

- Restoration of opposition of thumb
- Restoration of adduction of thumb
- Restoration of abduction of index finger
- Restoration of intrinsic function of fingers.

1. *Restoration of opposition of thumb by:*
   - Riordans' technique
   - Brand technique
   - Burkhalter technique
   - Groves and Goldner technique
   - Litter technique
   - Camitz technique.
2. *Restoration of adduction of thumb by:*
   - Royale-Thompson technique
   - Boye's technique
   - Smith technique.
3. *Restoration of abduction of index finger*: This is done by using palmaris brevis, brachioradialis, external carpi radialis brevis muscles.
4. *Restoration of intrinsic function of fingers by:*
   - Bunnel's technique
   - Riordan's technique
   - Zancollis capsulodesis
   - Fowler transfer
   - Brand's transfer of Extensor Carpi Radialis Longus (ECRL)
   - Brand's transfer of extensor carpi radialis brevis (ECRB)
   - Fowler tenodesis.

Table 23.11: The most common sites and causes of compression in thoracic outlet syndrome

Site	*Principal cause*
Superior thoracic outlet	First rib or cervical rib
Scalene interval or triangle	Scalene muscles or fibrous bands
Costoclavicular space	Narrow clavicle-first rib distance
Subcoracoid area	Coracoid process

THORACIC OUTLET SYNDROME

■ Anatomy

The thoracic outlet begins just distal to the intervertebral foramina and extends to the coracoid process as depicted in Figure 23.306. The most common sites of compression in thoracic outlet syndrome (TOS) are:

- The superior thoracic outlet
- The scalene interval or triangle
- The costoclavicular space
- The subcoracoid area.

These sites are enumerated in Table 23.11. This compression can be static or dynamic with dependence on posture and activity.

■ Thoracic Outlet Syndrome

The thoracic outlet syndromes comprise three different clinical pathophysiologic entities.

- Neurologic thoracic outlet syndrome
- Vascular thoracic outlet syndrome
- Thoracic outlet syndrome of pain and sensory symptoms.

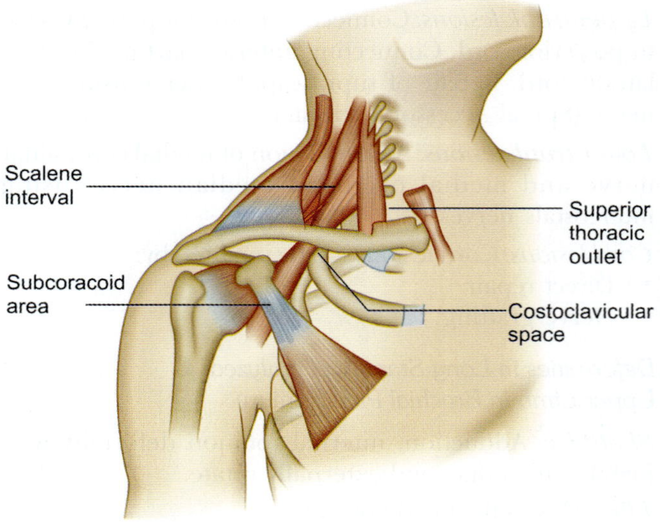

Fig. 23.306: Extent of the thoracic outlet

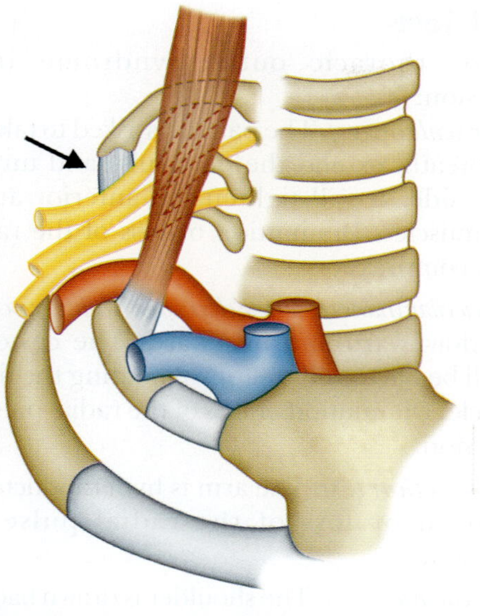

Fig. 23.307: Rudimentary cervical rib (arrow) with a fibrous band extending to the upper surface of the first rib

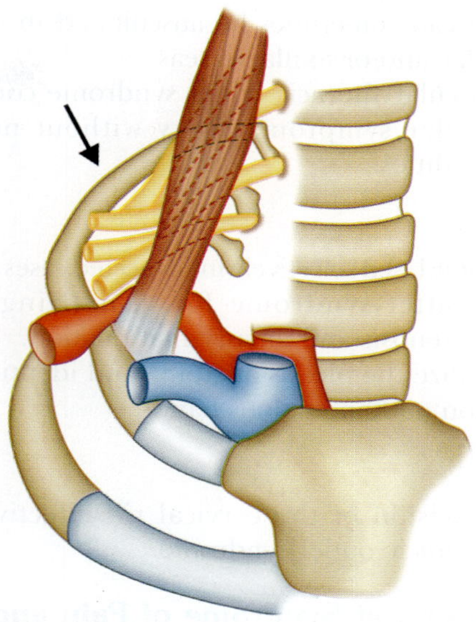

Fig. 23.308: Vascular thoracic outlet syndrome, subclavian artery wedged between the anterior scalene muscle and the cervical rib that causes its compression

Neurologic Thoracic Outlet Syndrome (Fig. 23.307)

Neurologic thoracic outlet syndrome is found mainly in women. It begins to manifest itself as a pain along the medial aspect of the arm and forearm. Paresthesias are found extending into the ulnar border of the hand. Muscle weakness and atrophy occur later. Muscle atrophy is selective for the abductor pollicis brevis and the opponens muscles of the thenar eminence of hand.

Wasting of all the intrinsic muscles of the hand is possible with the progression of the condition. There are no vascular symptoms. Sensory abnormalities are referrable to the lower trunk of the brachial plexus. A well developed cervical or rudimentary cervical rib with a fibrous band extending to the upper surface of the first rib may impinge on the lower trunk of the brachial plexus.

Similarly, anatomic abnormalities of the first rib may stretch and angulate the lower trunk of the brachial plexus. The scalenus anticus syndrome involves hypertrophy of the anterior scalene muscle and compression of the brachial plexus as it passes through the interscalene groove between the anterior and middle scalene muscles. Hyperabduction syndrome or subcoracoid-pectoralis minor syndrome involves compression of the brachial plexus with lateral abduction of the arm to an elevated position. In this position, structures, like the brachial plexus and vasculature are compressed by tension of the pectoralis minor muscle and to a lesser extent, the coracoid process.

Investigations

X-rays will almost uniformly show the characteristic bony abnormality, responsible for the neurologic symptomatology. If a bony abnormality is not seen, then consideration must be given to the presence of fibrous bands, scalenus anticus syndrome or hyperabduction syndrome.

Electrophysiologic studies can differentiate neurologic TOS from carpal tunnel syndrome and ulnar neuropathy. Somato Sensory Evoked Potentials (SSEPs), following stimulation of the ulnar nerve at the wrist, may actually be a more useful technique.

Treatment

Supraclavicular exploration with release of the compressive anatomy is the most satisfactory treatment for neurologic thoracic outlet syndrome. Patient experiences immediate relief of pain.

Vascular Thoracic Outlet Syndrome

In patients with a well developed first rib, the subclavian artery may be angulated over the cervical rib and wedged between the anterior scalene muscle and the cervical rib, as shown in Figure 23.308. The subclavian artery will become narrowed and will develop an area of poststenotic dilation. Thrombus may accumulate in the poststenotic dilation. Its fragments may embolize to the hand. This produces vascular symptomatology.

Clinical Features

- Intermittent blanching of the hands and fingers
- Pulses may be diminished or absent

- A bruit can sometimes be auscultated in the supraclavicular and/or axillary areas
- The vascular thoracic outlet syndrome consists only of vascular symptomatology without neurologic abnormalities.

Diagnosis

Angiography: Used selectively in suspected cases of vascular thoracic outlet syndrome for visualizing a mural thrombus, stenosis and aneurysmal dilation.
MRI: Visualize the plexus anatomy and identify areas of compression and anomalous bands.

Treatment

Surgical excision of the cervical rib effectively treats vascular thoracic outlet syndrome.

Thoracic Outlet Syndrome of Pain and Sensory Symptoms

This is more common, but obscure form of thoracic outlet syndrome, where patients present with less clearly defined symptomatology. Such patients will usually present with a diffuse nagging ache and numbness in the arm. The pain in the arm will be made worse by carrying heavy objects or holding the arm in a particular position. Paresthesias may occur concomitantly with the pain or may be temporally distinct. Paresthesias are usually appreciated in the medial aspect of the arm and forearm and sometimes in the hand.

Pathophysiology

The exact pathophysiology is obscure.Various proposed mechanisms include:
- Compression of the subclavian artery and/or brachial plexus between the lower end of the anterior scalene muscle and the first rib
- Vascular factors, i.e. venous rather than arterial compression
- Costoclavicular syndrome.

How to Differentiate Between Cervical Spondylosis and TOS? (Table 23.12)

Investigations: X-rays, electromyography (EMG), nerve conduction studies, SSEPs and arteriography are usually normal and of limited value.

Table 23.12: Difference between cervical spondylosis and TOS

Maneuver	*TOS*	*Cervical spondylosis*
Drooping/depression of shoulder	Produces symptoms	Relieves of symptoms
Elevation of shoulder	Relieves symptoms	Produces symptoms

Special Tests

Tests for thoracic outlet syndrome indicating compression:
Adson or scalene test: The patient is asked to take and hold a deep breath, extend the neck fully and turn the face into one side. It will tighten the anterior and middle scalene muscles. Diminution or loss of the radial pulse suggests compression.

Costoclavicular maneuver or Eden's test (military position): The back is downward and backward. The costoclavicular space will be narrowed by approximating the first rib and the clavicle. Diminution or loss of the radial pulse suggests compression.

Hyperabduction test: The arm is hyperabducted to 180°. Diminution or loss of the radial pulse suggests compression.

Arm claudication test: The shoulder is drawn backward and upward. The arm is raised horizontally with the elbow flexed to 90°. With excise of hands, pain and numbness indicates compression.

Allen test: The examiner flexes the patient's elbow to 90° while the shoulder is abducted and extended horizontally and rotated laterally. The patient is asked to turn their head away from the tested arm. The radial pulse is palpated and if it disappears as the patient's head is rotated the test is considered positive.

Hallstead test: This test is like the Adson's maneuver, but hear neck is turned to opposite side.

Treatment

- *Physical therapy:* Exercises to counteract and strengthen drooping shoulders have been proposed as a possible treatment.
- First rib resection is often performed in patients with this more obscure but common form of thoracic outlet syndrome.

■ Costoclavicular Syndrome

The costoclavicular syndrome suggests that the subclavian artery and/or the brachial plexus are intermittently compressed between the clavicle and a normal first rib. Patients, who are believed to have costoclavicular syndrome are the women with long necks and drooping shoulders, women with pendulous breasts, patients of new-widow syndrome and women carrying heavy back packs.

Symptomatology has been hypothesized to result from chronic stretching of the brachial plexus. Following symptoms are identified:
- Sense of fullness in the hand and fingers
- Cramping pain in the forearm and hand
- Vague shoulder pain
- Swollen and engorged veins—intermittent

- Shoulder Range of Motion (ROM) is maintained.
- Costoclavicular maneuver and Eden's Test are diagnostic.

■ Cervical Rib Syndrome

There is a congenital overdevelopment (bony or fibrous) of the C7 costal process. It can be unilateral or bilateral and is usually, asymptomatic. Occurs in 1 percent of the population and only 10 percent of those are symptomatic. Pain and paresthesias in the medial forearm and hand is present, which usually relieved by changing position. Patient can have weakness and difficulty with fine motor control. Prolapse of Intervertebral Discs (PIVD) of C4, C5, C6 should be considered as a differential diagnosis for the abnormality.

Treatment

Surgical resection of the cervical rib is performed.

24 Hip Joint

- Anatomy and Biomechanics of Hip Joint
- Developmental Dysplasia of the Hip
- Congenital Coxa Vara
- Acetabular Fractures
- Fractures of the Femoral Neck
- Intertrochanteric Femoral Fractures
- Subtrochanteric Femoral Fractures
- Traumatic Dislocation of Hip
- Infections of Hip Joint
- Tuberculosis of Hip Joint
- Degenerative Osteoarthritis
- Rheumatoid Arthritis of Hip
- Legg-Calve-Perthes Disease
- Tumors Around Hip
- Osteotomies Around the Hip
- Surgical Approaches To Hip

ANATOMY AND BIOMECHANICS OF HIP JOINT

Anatomy of Hip Joint (Fig. 24.1)

Type

Hip joint is ball and socket, variety of synovial joint. The head of femur articulates with the acetabulum of hip bone to form hip joint. It is unique, as it has high degree of stability and mobility.

Articular Surface

Head of the Femur

- Directed medially, upward, slightly forward
- Articulates with acetabulum to form hip joint
- Roughened pit situated just below and behind
- The center of the head is called fovea
- Forms more than half a sphere and is covered with hyaline cartilage except at the fovea capitis.

Neck Shaft Angle (Fig. 24.2)

Neck shaft angle is 120° (115°–145°). The axis of the femoral head and neck forms an angle with the axis of the femoral shaft. It is called the angle of inclination/neck shaft angle. It is smaller in women as compared to men normally owing to the greater width of female pelvis. With normal angle the greater trochanter lies at the level of the center of femoral head.

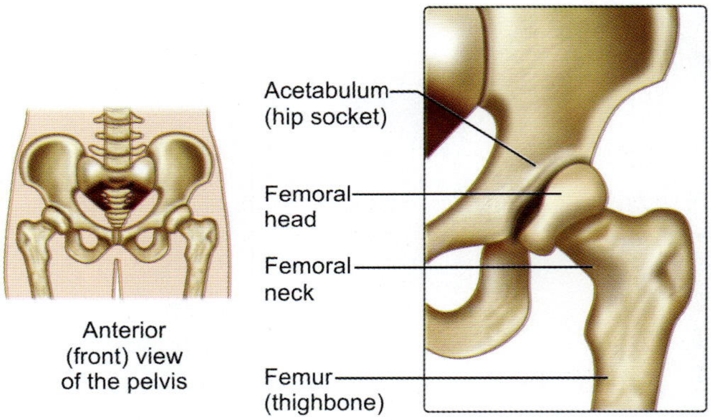

Fig. 24.1: Anatomy of hip joint

Angle of Anteversion (Fig. 24.3)

A line parallel to the posterior femoral condyles and line through the head and neck of the femur normally makes an angle with each other that average 15 to 20° in adults without impairment. It is also called as angle of torsion.

Articular Surface

Acetabulum: It is formed by:

- *Ilium:* It forms the upper 2/5th region
- *Pubis:* It forms the anterior 1/5th region
- *Ischium:* It forms the posterior 2/5th region
- It is deep cup shaped, hemispherical cavity on the lateral aspect of the hip bone
- It is directed laterally, downward and forwards
- Margin of the acetabulum is deficient, this deficiency called as acetabular notch. It is bridged by transverse ligament.

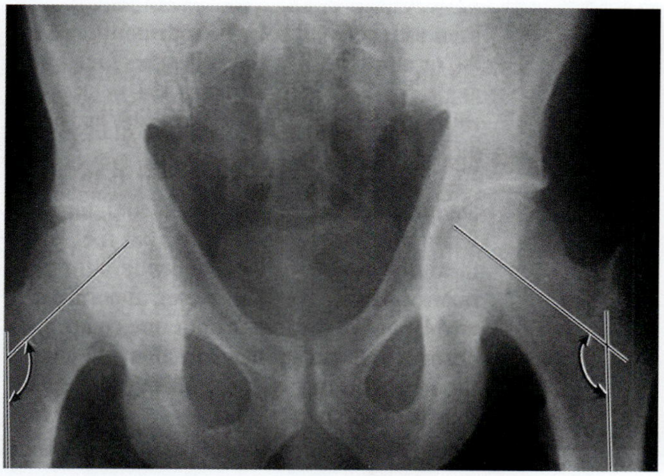

Fig. 24.2: The axis of the femoral head and neck forms an angle with the axis of the femoral shaft called the angle of inclination. In this adult subject without impairments, the angles are slightly less than 130°, with a couple of degrees of variation from side to side

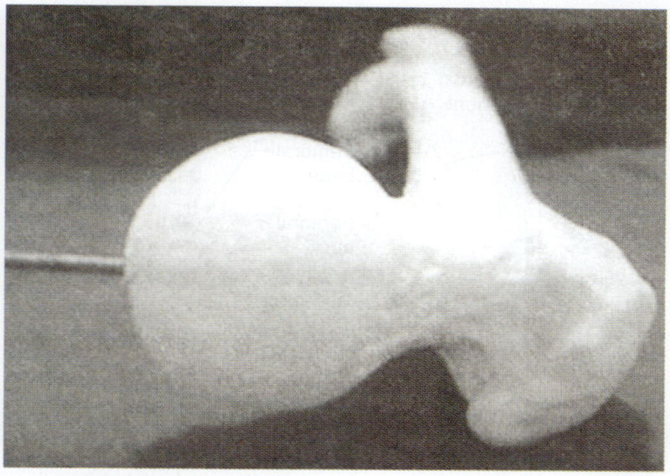

Fig. 24.3: Angle of anteversion

- Nonarticular roughened floor called acetabular fossa, contains mass of fat lined by synovial membrane.
- It also has a horseshoe shaped, lunate articular surface, which is covered by cartilage.

Stability of Hip Joint

Stability of the joint depends on:

- Depth of the acetabulum and narrowing of its mouth by acetabular labrum
- Tension and strength of the ligaments
- Strength of the surrounding muscles
- The length and obliquity of the neck of the femur.

Normal Growth and Development

- Embryologically, the acetabulum and femoral head develop from the same primitive mesenchymal cells.
- Cleft develops in precartilaginous cells at 7th week and this defines both structures
- At 11 weeks hip joint fully formed
- Acetabular growth continues throughout intrauterine life with development of labrum
- At birth femoral head deeply seated in acetabulum by surface tension of synovial fluid and very difficult to dislocate
- In developmental dysplasia of hip, this shape and tension is abnormal in addition to capsular laxity
- The cartilage complex is triradiate directed medially and cup-shaped laterally
- Interposed between ilium above and ischium below and pubis anteriorly
- Acetabular cartilage forms outer 2/3 cavity and the nonarticular medial wall form by triradiate cartilage which is the common physis of these three bones
- Fibrocartilaginous labrum forms at margin of acetabular cartilage and joint capsule inserts just above its rim
- Articular cartilage covers portion articulating with femoral head opposite side is a growth plate with degenerating cells facing towards the pelvic bone it opposes
- Triradiate cartilage is triphalanged with each side of each limb having a growth plate which allows interstitial growth within the cartilage causing expansion of hip joint diameter during growth
- In the infant the greater trochanter, proximal femur and intertrochanteric portion is cartilage
- At 4 to 7 months proximal ossification center appears, which enlarges along cartilaginous anlage, until adult life when only thin layer of articular cartilage persists.
- Experimental studies in humans with unreduced hips suggest the main stimulus for concave shape of the acetabulum is presence of spherical head
- For normal depth of acetabulum to increase several factors play a role
  - Spherical femoral head
  - Normal appositional growth within cartilage
  - Periosteal new bone formation in adjacent pelvic bones
  - Development of three secondary ossification centers
  - Normal growth and development occur through balanced growth of proximal femur, acetabulum, triradiate cartilages and the adjacent bones.

Ligaments (Fig. 24.4)

- Fibrous capsule
- Iliofemoral ligament

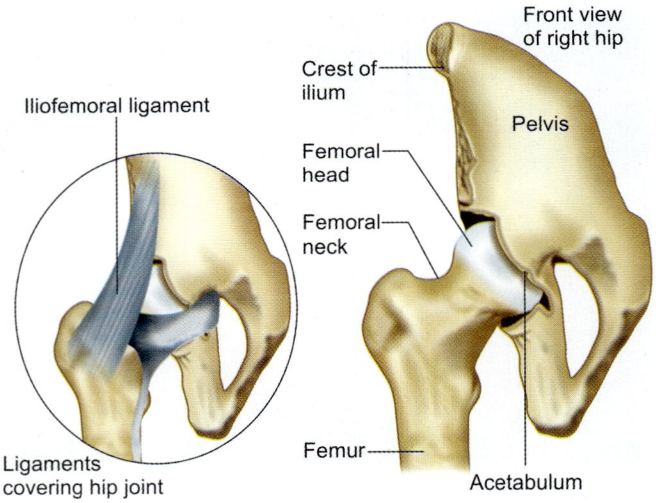

Fig. 24.4: Different ligaments around hip joint

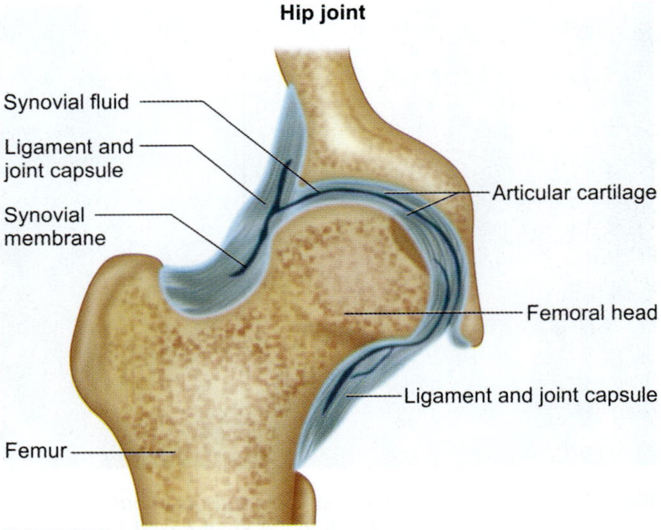

Fig. 24.5: The fibrous capsule of hip joint

- Pubofemoral ligament
- Ischiofemoral ligament
- Ligament of the head of the femur
- Acetabular labrum
- Transverse acetabular ligament.

Fibrous Capsule (Fig. 24.5)

The capsule is attached on the hip bone to the acetabular labrum and on the femur to the inter trochanteric line in front. Anterolaterally the capsule is thick and firmly attached, as this part is subjected to maximum tension in standing posture. The capsule is made of two types of fibers:

- *Outer fibers:* Longitudinal, forms the retinacula, through which passes the blood vessels supplying the head and neck of femur.
- *Inner fibers:* Circular called as zona orbicularis.

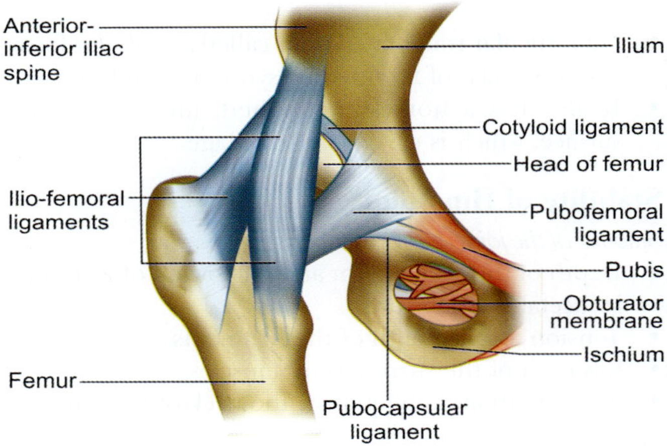

Fig. 24.6: Different ligaments and their attachments around hip joint

Iliofemoral Ligament

- Also called as ligament of "Bigelow"
- It is inverted Y shaped. Is the one of the strongest ligament in the body
- It is the chief stabilizer of hip in standing position.

Pubofemoral Ligament (Fig. 24.6)

Supports the joint inferomedially

Ischiofemoral Ligament

- Is comparatively weak
- Covers the joint posteriorly

Ligament of the Head of the Femur

Also called as round ligament or ligament teres. It is a flat and triangular ligament. The apex is attached to the fovea capitis and the base to the transverse ligament and the margins of the acetabular notch. It transmits arteries to the head of femur from the acetabular branches of the obturator and medial circumflex femoral arteries.

Acetabular Labrum

It is a fibrocartilaginous rim attached to the margins of the acetabulum. It narrows the mouth of acetabulum, this helps in holding the head of femur in position.

Transverse Acetabulum Ligament

It is a part of acetabular labrum, which bridges the acetabular notch. Thus, the notch is converted into a foramen, which transmits acetabular vessels and nerve to the joint.

■ Surface Anatomy: The Anterior Hip Region

Bony Landmarks

- Anterosuperior iliac spine
- Tubercle of the iliac crest at the widest part of pelvis
- Pubic symphysis in the midline anteriorly
- Pubic tubercle about one inch lateral to the symphysis
- The greater trochanter
- A line drawn horizontally from the pubic tubercle passes through femoral head.

Superficial Fascia

It is composed of fatty layer and a deep membranous layer. The later is separated from the deep fascia by loose areolar tissue, but is firmly fused to deep fascia along a horizontal line immediately below the inguinal ligament and to the front of pubis and the pubic arch. Due to this attachment, urinary extravasations from the perineum to the abdomen cannot descend into the thigh.

Fascia Lata

It is thickened deep fascia, covering the thigh. It is attached above at the anterior-superior iliac spine (ASIS), the inguinal ligament, the body of pubic bone, the pubic arch, the ischial tuberosity, the sacrotuberous ligament and as the gluteal fascia attached to sacrum and the iliac crest. It is extremely strong laterally because in between two layers, there runs a broad band of coarse vertical fibers the iliotibial band.

Iliotibial Tract/Band

It is a conjoint aponeurosis of tensor fascia latae and the gluteus maximus and runs distally to insert upon the head of fibula and the anterolateral aspect of tibia. The band is often thickened and contracted in poliomyelitis. Shortening of the band produces a flexion and abduction deformity of the hip because the plane of the band lies lateral and anterior to the axis of hip motion.

Long Saphenous Vein

Courses along the medial aspect of thigh. It receives three tributaries, which accompany the superficial inguinal branches of femoral artery:

i. Superficial external pudendal
ii. Superficial epigastric
iii. Superficial circumflex iliac.

Long saphenous vein (LSV) than passes through an opening in the fascia lata, the fossa ovalies, to reach the femoral vein. This aperture in deep fascia is located one and half inches below and lateral to pubic tubercle, where it is of surgical important in treating femoral hernia and varicose veins.

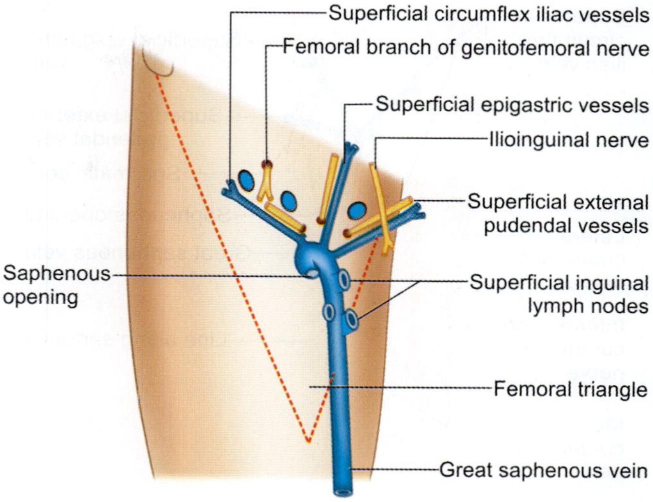

Fig. 24.7: The anterior hip region, showing inguinal lymph glands

Inguinal Lymph Glands

Two groups (superficial and deep), these are shown in Figure 24.7.

1. *Superficial group:*
   - An upper horizontal group, lying below the inguinal ligament and draining the inguinal, lower abdominal and perineal region.
   - The lower group lies about the long saphenous vein and receives superficial lymph vessels from the lower limb.
2. *The deep group:* One to three in numbers, lies on medial side of the femoral vein in the femoral canal and receives the deep lymph vessels of the lower limb, including those draining the popliteal glands. It also drains the pelvic organs and thus becomes painful and swollen in pelvic inflammatory disease.

Cutaneous Nerves (Fig. 24.8)

The lateral, intermediate and the medial cutaneous nerves of thigh (from femoral), supply the lateral, anterior and medial aspect of the thigh, respectively.

- *The lateral femoral cutaneous nerve:* Often arises from the lumbar plexus and enters the thigh beneath the inguinal ligament close to ASIS it is involved in meralgia paresthetica, a condition characterized by sensory deficit along the lateral aspect of thigh.
- *Ilioinguinal nerve:* From lumbar plexus L1, emerges from superficial inguinal ring and supplies not only the scrotum or labium majus, but also the skin of the adjacent aspect of the thigh.
- *Genitofemoral nerve:* From the l plexus at L1 and L2, sends a femoral branch to supply an area immediately below the inguinal ligament.

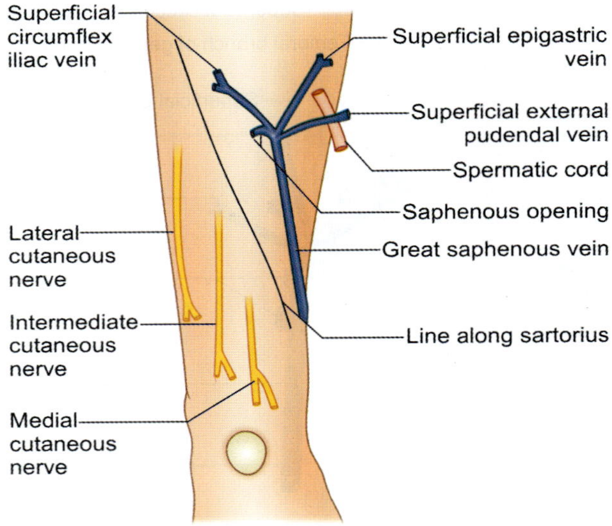

Fig. 24.8: Cutaneous nerves on anterior thigh/hip region

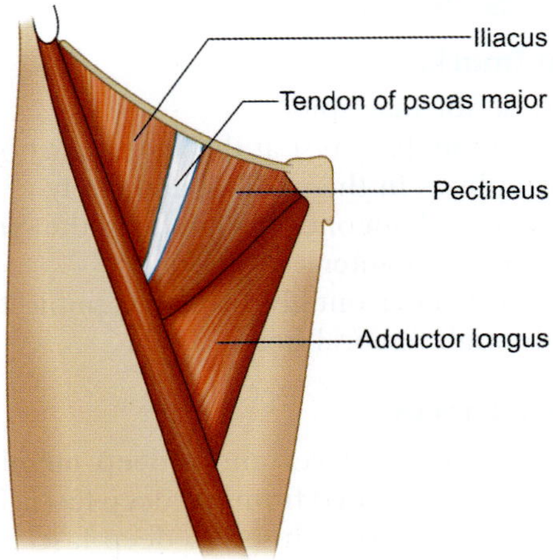

Fig. 24.10: Structures forming the floor of the femoral triangle

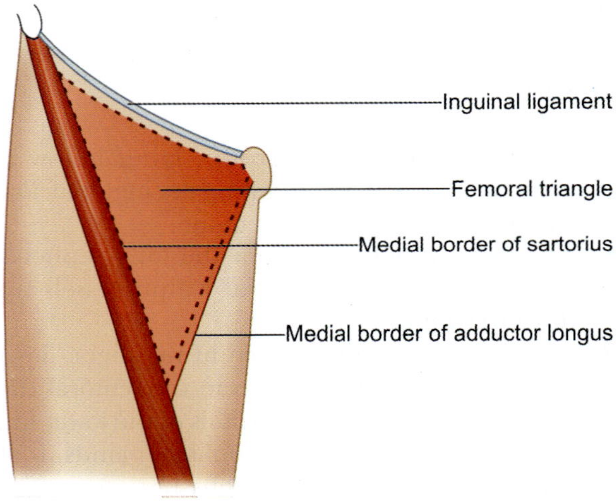

Fig. 24.9: Boundaries of femoral triangle

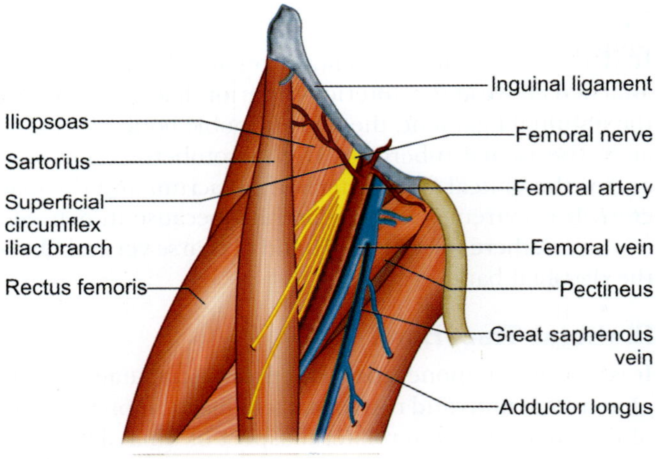

Fig. 24.11: Course of femoral artery on anterior hip region

Scarpa's or Femoral Triangle

- It is a triangular area, bounded above by the inguinal ligament, laterally by medial border if sartorius and medially by medial border of adductor longus, as shown in Figure 24.9.
- Floor of the triangle is formed medially by adductor longus and pectineus and laterally by the iliacus and psoas major, as illustrated in Figure 24.10.
- Roof is formed by: (i) skin, (ii) superficial fascia, containing superior inguinal lymph nodes, femoral branch or genitofemoral nerve, branches of ilioinguinal nerve, superficial branch of femoral artery and accompanying vein and (iii) deep fascia, with saphenous opening and cribriform fascia.
- The head of femur can be localized by determining the midinguinal point of crossing of femoral artery, then measuring one inch distally and laterally.

Blood Supply

- *Femoral artery (Fig. 24.11):* It runs behind the midinguinal point and enters the femoral triangle.
- *Profunda femoral artery:* Arises from lateral aspect of the femoral artery, at or just below the inguinal ligament.
- *Femoral circumflex artery (Fig. 24.12):* It has two branches:
  i. The lateral femoral circumflex artery
  ii. The medial femoral circumflex femoral artery.

  Both these arteries anastomose with each other, with first perforating artery below and the gluteal arteries above, to form the crucial arterial anastomosis of hip.

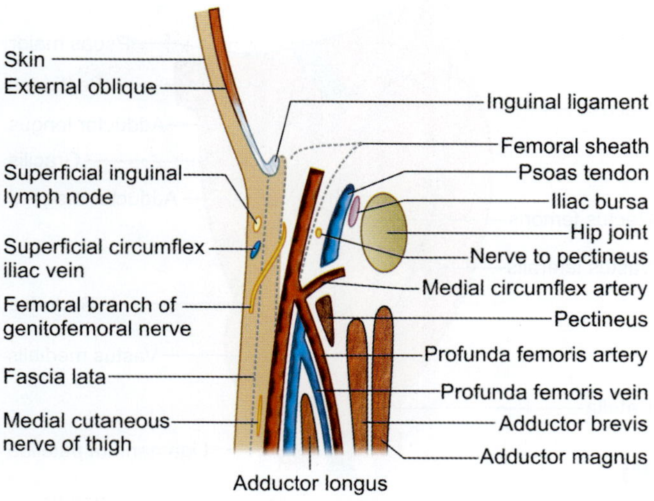

Fig. 24.12: Course of femoral circumflex arteries

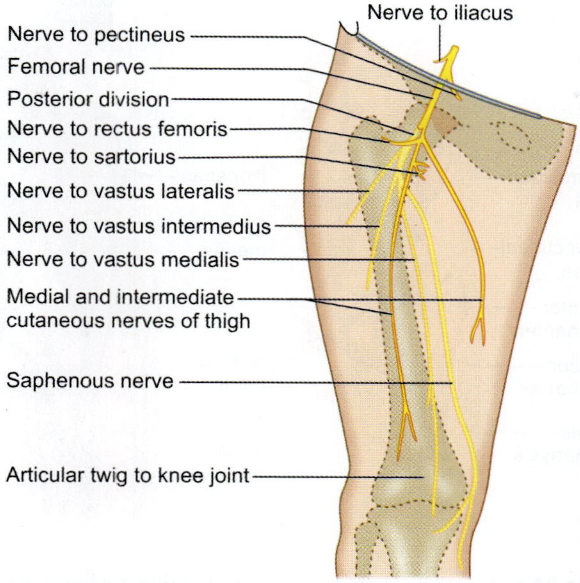

Fig. 24.13: Nerve supply to the anterior hip/thigh region (Branches of the posterior division are shown in interrupted line)

Femoral Vein and Femoral Nerve

1. *Femoral vein:* It begins as an upward continuation of the popliteal vein at the lower end of the adductor canal and ends by becoming continuous with the external iliac vein behind the inguinal ligament.
2. *Femoral nerve (L2, L3, L4):* It enters the thigh just lateral to the femoral artery and breaks up into numerous branches, as shown in Figure 24.13.
   - Its muscular branches, includes those to pectineus, sartorius and the quadriceps.
   - Cutaneous branches are the medial and the intermediate femoral cutaneous and the saphenous nerve.

All the adductors are supplied by obturator nerve, except pectineus, which is supplied by femoral nerve, hence this explains why some adductor power remains after complete obturator neurectomy.

Muscles of Anterior (Extensor Compartment) of Thigh (Figs 24.14A and B)

These are enumerated in the Table 24.1.

- *Sartorius:* Arises by a fibrous origin with inguinal ligament from ASIS.
- *Quadriceps femoris:* So called because it is composed of four parts: (i) rectus femoris, (ii) vastus lateralies, (iii) medialis and (iv) intermedius.
- *Rectus femoris:* Supplied by femoral nerve. It arises by a straight head from the ASIS and by an oblique head from the supra-acetabular rim. It helps in extension of knee and acts as flexors of hip joint.

Muscles of Medial Hip Region (Table 24.2)

Adductor muscles (Figs 24.14A and B)

The muscles are disposed in three layers:

1. The anterior layer is composed of pectineus and the adductor longus
2. The middle layer consist of adductor brevis
3. The posterior layer is adductor magnus, arises mainly from the side of the pubic arch and is inserted along the back of femur.

Psoas Major and Iliacus

Both muscle originates intra-abdominally and enter the thigh behind the inguinal ligament. They are inserted by a common tendon into the lesser troch. The united iliopsoas crosses over the capsule of the hip joint, a bursa innervating between the structures. This bursa often communicates with the joint through an aperture in the capsule and is affected by the same disease process that affect the joint. Infection of the upper lumbar spine particularly TB often develops an exudates, which descends downwards beneath the psoas fascia as an abscess at the hip region.

■ Gluteal Region Bony Landmarks

- The iliac crest
- Anterior-superior iliac spine (ASIS)
- Posterior-superior iliac spine (PSIS)
- Ischial tuberosity
  – A line drawn transversely at the level of ischial tuberosity, crosses the lesser trochanter.

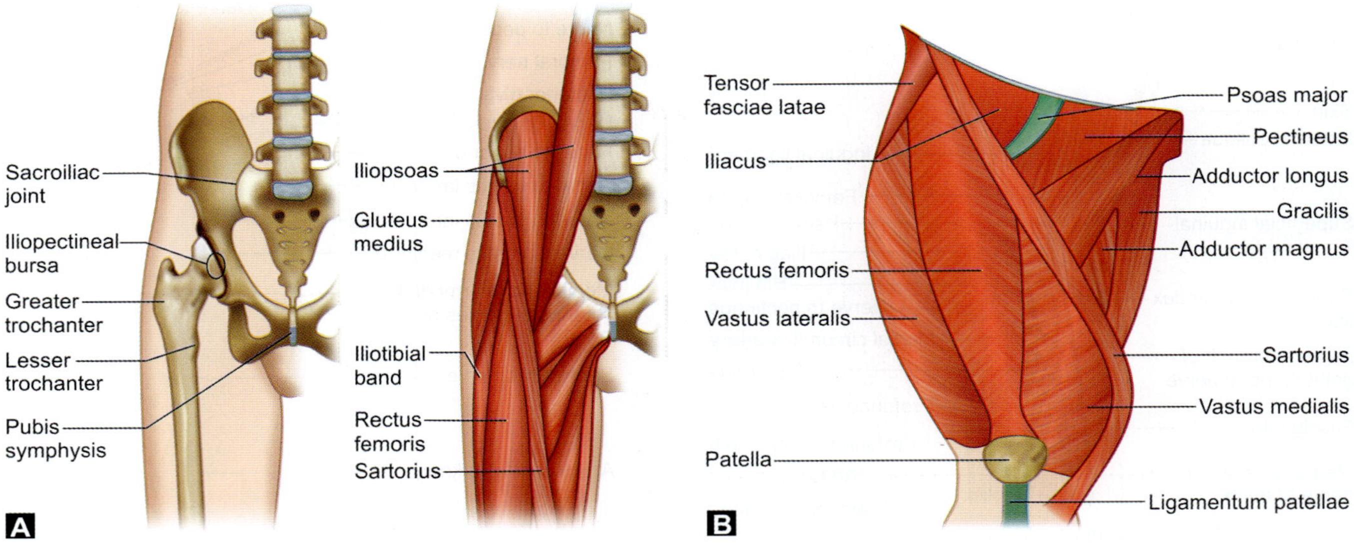

Figs 24.14A and B: (A) Muscles in the anterior extensor compartment of hip; (B) Muscles in the medial compartment of thigh or hip

Table 24.1: Muscles of the anterior or extensor compartment of hip/thigh

Muscle	*Origin from*	*Insertion into*
Sartorius	• Anterior-superior iliac spine • Upper half of the notch below the spine	Upper part of the medial surface of the shaft of the tibia in front of the insertions of the gracilis and the semitendinosus
Quadriceps femoris • *Rectus femoris* Fusiform, superficial fibers bipennate, deep fibers straight	• *Straight head:* From the upper half of the anterior-inferior iliac spine • *Reflected head:* From the groove above the margin of the acetabulum and the capsule of the hip joint	Base of patella
• *Vastus lateralis* Forms large part of quadriceps femoris	The origin is linear The line runs along: • Upper part of intertrochanteric line • Anterior and inferior borders of greater trochanter • Lateral lip of gluteal tuberosity • Upper half of lateral lip of linea aspera	• Lateral part of the base of patella • Upper one-third of the lateral border of patella • Expansion to the capsule of knee joint, tibia and iliotibial tract
• *Vastus medialis*	The origin in linear The line runs along: • Lower part of intertrochanteric line • Spiral line • Medial lip of linea aspera • Upper one-fourth of medial supracondylar line	Medial one-third of the base and upper two-thirds of the medial border of the patella
• *Vastus intermedius*	Upper three-fourths of the anterior and lateral surfaces of the shaft of femur	Base of patella *Note:* The patella is a sesamoid bone in the tendon of the quadriceps femoris. The ligamentum patellae is the actual tendon of the quadriceps femoris, which is inserted to the tibial tuberosity

– A line drawn from a point on the iliac crest a hand breath in front of the PSIS. Directly outward to the tip of the greater trochanter represents the upper border of gluteus maximus muscle.

– By drawing a line from the PSIS to the tip of coccyx, the mid point of this line extends out to the tip of the greater trochanter corresponds to the lower border of the pyriformis muscle.

Table 24.2: Muscles of the medial compartment of thigh

Muscle	Origin form	Insertion into
• *Adductor longus* This is a triangular muscle, forming the medial part of the floor of the femoral triangle. It lies in the plane of the pectinecs	It arises by a narrow, flat tendon from the front of the body of the pubis in the angle between the pubic crest and the pubic symphysis	The linea aspera in middle one-third of the shaft of the femur between the vastus medialis and the adductor brevis and magnus
• *Adductor brevis* The muscle lies behind the pectineus and adductor longus	• The anterior surface of the body of the pubis • Outer surface of the inferior ramus of the pubis between the gracilis and the obturator externus • Outer surface of the ramus of the ischium between the gracilis and the adductor magnus	Line extending from the lesser trochanter to the upper part of the linea aspera, behind the upper part of adductor longus
• *Adductor magnus* This is the largest muscles of this compartment. Because of its double nerve supply, it is called a hybrid muscle	• Inferolateral part of the ischial tuberosity • Ramus of the ischium • Lower part of the inferior ramus of the pubis	• Medial margin of gluteal tuberosity • Linea aspera • Medial supracondylar line • Adductor tubercle
• *Gracilis*	• Medial margin of the lower half of the body of the pubis • Inferior ramus of the pubis • The adjoining part of the ramus of the ischium	Upper part of the medial surface of tibia behind the sartorius and in front of the semitendinosus
• *Pectineus* This is flat, quardrilateral muscle. It forms a part of the floor of the femoral triangle	• pecten pubis • Upper half of the pectineal surface of the superior ramus of the pubis • Fascia covering the pectineus	Line extending from lesser trochanter to the linea aspera

Muscles of Gluteal Region (Table 24.3)

Gluteus Maximus

The deep fascia over this muscle is thin and transparent. It is a thick fibered rhomboid shaped muscle innervated by inferior gluteal nerve. It arises from the PSIS, sacrotuberous ligament, the lower sacrum and coccyx, as shown in Figure 24.15. It passes laterally and distally towards the upper femur, where a portion of its upper fibers insert into the gluteal tuberosity, the remainder ending in a band like aponeurosis, which joins a similar band like aponeurosis of the tensor fascia lata, distal to the greater tuberosity to form the iliotibial tract. Its function is to extend hip joint, its motion is assisted by hamstrings. Many arteries and veins enter the under surface, a muscle splitting incision will cause extensive hemorrhage.

Structures Entering at the Lower Border of Pyriformis

This includes

- Sciatic nerve
- Posterior cutaneous nerve of thigh
- Inferior gluteal nerve and vessels
- Internal pudendal nerve and vessels, which emerges at the lower border of pyriformis.

Structures Entering at the Upper Border of Pyriformis

This includes superior gluteal nerves and vessels.

- *Gluteus medius and minimus:* Fan shaped, arises from most of lateral surface of the ilium and insert into the lateral and anterior aspect of greater trochanter (GT). It functions as abductors of thigh.
- *Tensor fascia lata:* Arises from ASIS and the outer lip of the iliac crest. It is directed downwards and slightly backwards and is continued as iliotibial tract and innervated by superior gluteal nerve.
- *Quadratus femoris:* It appears to be the proximal portion of the adductor magnus. It arises from lateral border of iliotibial tract (IT) and extends laterally to insert into the quadrate tubercle behind the GT. Nerve to qudratus, lies below sciatic nerve.
- *Obturator internus, superior and inferior gamellus:* This muscles occupies interval between the pyriformis and the quadratus. Obturator internus arises from the internal aspect of the innominate bone, makes right angled turn and goes out through lesser sciatic foramen. Its tendon passes across the posterior surface of ischium and the capsule of hip joint to reach up border of the GT. The superior gamellus arises from ischial spine and the inferior gamellus, from the ischial tuberosity. Both are inserted adjacent to ischial tuberosity. They are the lateral rotators of thigh.

Table 24.3: Muscles of the gluteal region

Muscle	*Origin*	*Insertion into*	*Nerve supply*
• *Gluteus maximus* This is a large, quadrilateral powerful muscle covering mainly the posterior surface of pelvis	• Outer slope of the dorsal segment of iliac crest • Posterior gluteal line • Posterior part of gluteal surface of ilium behind the posterior gluteal line • Aponeurosis of erector spinae • Dorsal surface of lower part of sacrum • Side of coccyx • Sacrotuberous ligament • Fascia covering gluteus maximus	• The deep fibers of the lower part of the muscle are inserted into the gluteal tuberosity • The greater part of the muscle is inserted into the iliotibial tract	Inferior gluteal nerve (L5, S1, S2)
• *Gluteus medius* It is fan-shaped, and covers the lateral surface of the pelvis and hip	Gluteal surface of ilium between the anterior and posterior gluteal lines	The greater trochanter of femur, on oblique ridge on the lateral surface. The ridge runs downwards and forwards	Superior gluteal nerve (L4, L5, S1)
• *Gluteus minimus* It is fan-shaped, and is covered by the gluteus medius	Gluteal surface of ilium between the anterior and inferior gluteal lines	Greater trochanter of femur, on a ridge on the lateral part of the anterior surface	Superior gluteal nerve (L4, L5, S1)
• *Piriformis* Lies below and parallel to the posterior border of the gluteus medius	It arises within the pelvis form: • Pelvic surface of the middle three digitations • Upper margin of the greater sciatic notch and the adjoining areas of the sacroiliac joint and of the sacrotuberous ligament	The rounded tendon is inserted into the apex of the greater trochanter of the femur	Ventral rami of S1, S2
• *Gemellus superior* Small muscle lying along the upper border of the tendon of the obturator internus	Posterior surface of the ischial spine and upper part of lesser sciatic notch	Blends with tendon of obturator internus, and gets inserted into medial surface of greater trochanter of femur	Nerve to obturator internus (L5, S1, S2)
• *Gemellus inferior* Small muscle lying along the lower border of the tendon of the obturator internus	Upper part of the ischial tuberosity and lower part of lesser sciatic notch	Same as above	Nerve to quadratus femoris (L4, L5, S1)
• *Obturator internus* Fan-shaped, flattened belly lies in pelvis and the tendon in the gluteal region	• Pelvic surface of obturator membrane • Pelvic surface of the body of the ischium, ischial tuberosity, ischiopubic rami, and ilium below the pelvic brim • Obturator fascia	The tendon of the obturator internus leaves the pelvis through the lesser sciatic foramen. Here it bends at a right angle around the lesser sciatic notch and runs laterally to be inserted into the medial surface of the greater trochanter of the femur	Nerve to obturator internus (L5, S1, S2)
• *Quadratus femoris* Quadrilateral muscle lying between inferior gemellus and adductor magnus	Upper part of the outer border of ischial tuberosity	Quadrate tubercle and the area below it	Nerve to quadratus femoris (L4, L5, S1)
• *Obturator externus* Triangular in shape, covers the outer surface of the anterior wall of the pelvis	• Outer surface of obturator membrane • Outer surface of the bony margins of obturator foramen	The muscle ends in a tendon which runs upwards and laterally behind the neck of the femur to reach the gluteal region where it is inserted into trochanteric fossa (on medial side of the greater trochanter)	Posterior division of obturator nerve (L2, L3, L4)
• *Tensor fasciae latae* Lies between the gluteal region and the front of the thigh	Anterior 5 cm of the outer lip of the iliac crest up to the tubercle	Iliotibial tract 3.5 cm below the level of greater trochanter	Superior gluteal nerve, (L4, L5, S1)

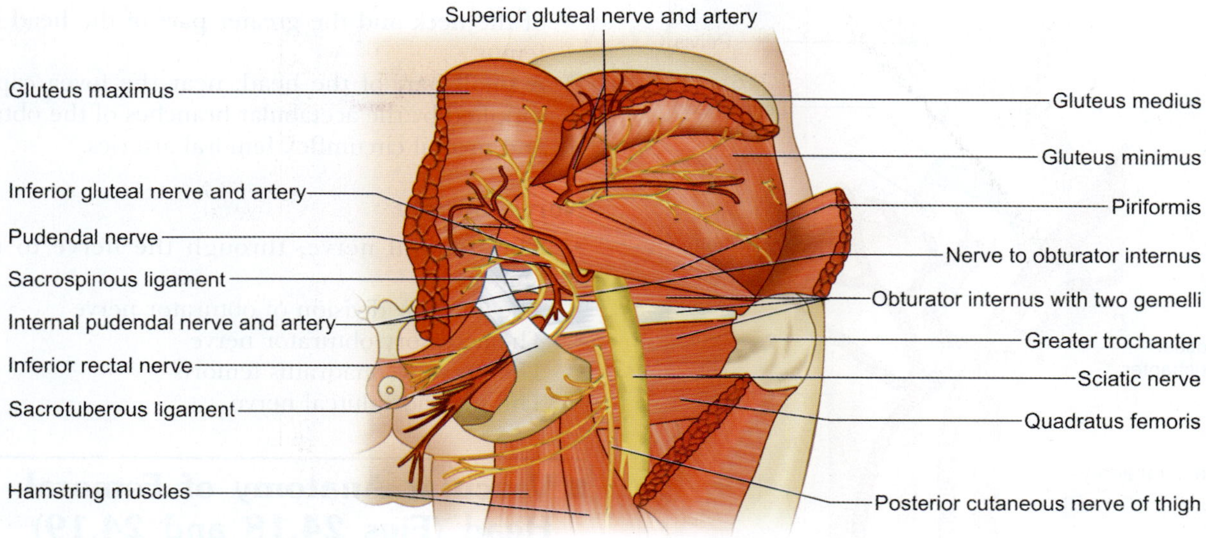

Fig. 24.15: Gluteus maximus muscle, its origin, blood supply, nerves and surrounding structures

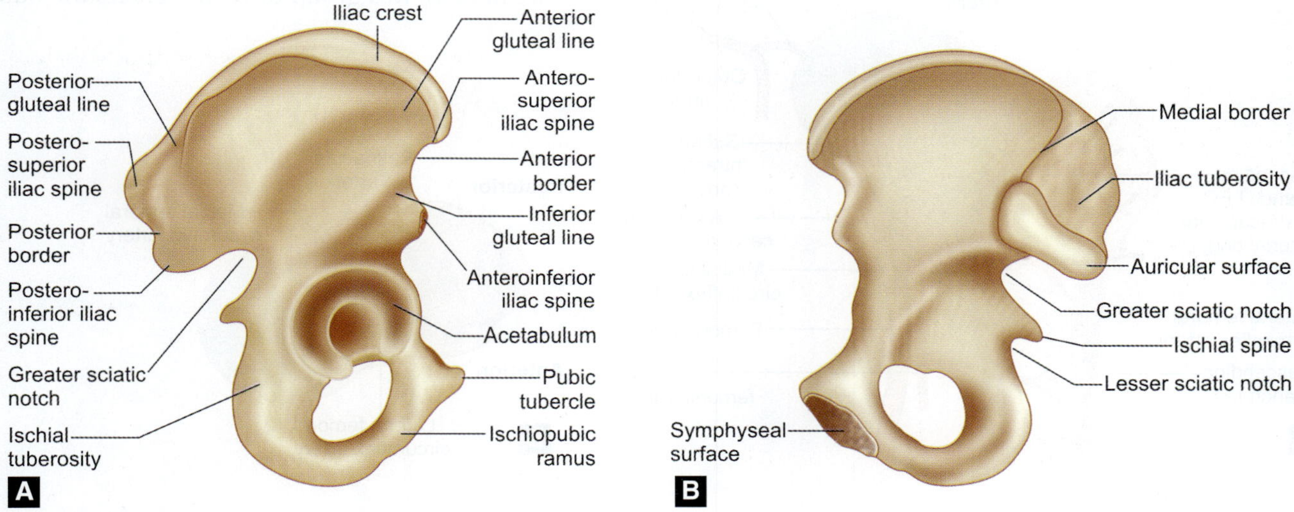

Figs 24.16A and B: Anatomy of bony pelvis

■ Bony Pelvis (Figs 24.16A and B)

It is composed of three main parts:

- Ilium
- Ischium
- Pubis

These three parts meet in a cup shaped cavity called as acetabulum, which receives the femoral head.

Ilium: It is a large flat fan shaped bone, lies above the acetabulum. It is crest is subcutaneous and during the growth period is surmounted by an apophysis. Ossification of the apophysis takes place in a line extending along the entire length of the crest. Completion of this line of ossification, coincides with termination of longitudinal growth. This sign is utilized in management of scoliosis of idiopathic type.

■ Blood Supply and Nerve Supply of Hip Joint

Blood Supply (Fig. 24.17)

- The hip is supplied by obturator artery, two circumflex femoral and two gluteal arteries.
- The median and lateral circumflex femoral arteries form an arterial circle around the capsular attachment on the neck of femur. Retinacular arteries arises from this circle and supply the intracapsular part

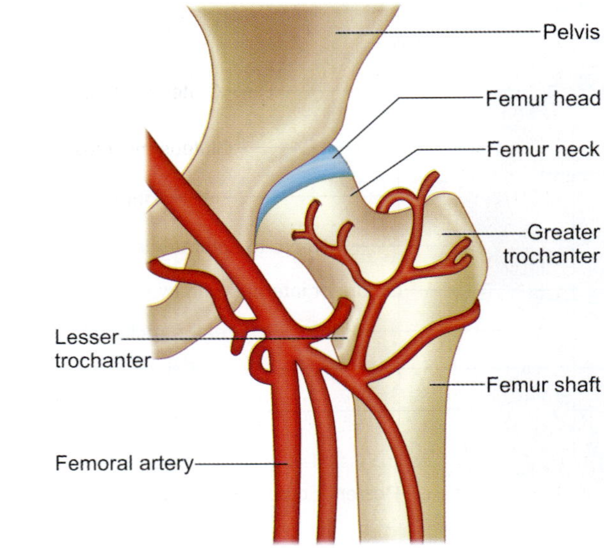

Fig. 24.17: Course of femoral artery around hip

of the neck and the greater part of the head of the femur.

- A small part of the head, near the fovea capitis is supplied by the acetabular branches of the obturator and medial circumflex femoral arteries.

Nerve Supply

- The femoral nerve, through the nerve to rectus femoris
- The anterior division of obturator nerve
- The accessory obturator nerve
- The nerve to quadratus femoris
- The superior gluteal nerve.

■ Vascular Anatomy of Femoral Head (Figs 24.18 and 24.19)

- *Growth period:* At birth nutrition of femoral head is derived from three sources.
  1. Lateral epiphyseal (from medial femoral circumflex), this group of vessels enters the outer

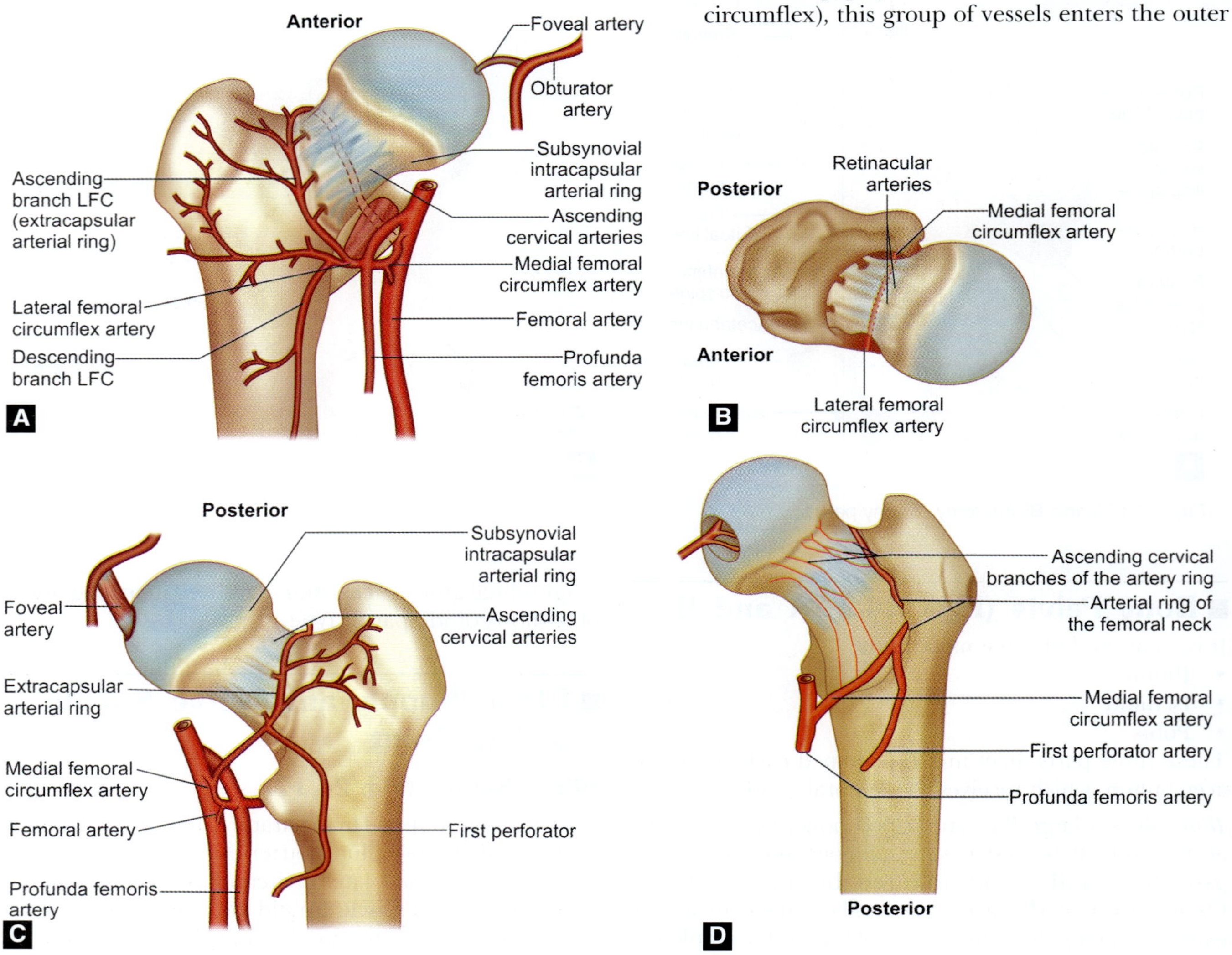

Figs 24.18A to D: Blood Supply to femoral head

part of the femoral head in the region of the trochanteric notch and advances horizontally towards the center of the head.

2. Metaphyseal, from medial femoral circumflex, this series of straight vessels ascends vertically through the cartilaginous head.
3. Ligamentum teres vessels, from acetabular branch of obturator, these vessel barely supply a superficial portion of the femoral head.

Delay in ossification of the epiphysis commonly observed in CDH could be explained by capsular stretching obliterating the lateral epiphyseal vessels, while the metaphyseal vessels remains intact. After four months of age, the ascending metaphyseal vessels decrease in number, hence the main vascular supply at this time is through the lateral epiphyseal arteries. Obstruction of these vessel, theoretically produce the picture of Legg-Perthes disease.

After 7 years of age, the vessels from ligamentum teres penetrates more deeply and join the lateral epiphyseal vessels, in supplying the head. The cartilaginous epiphyseal plate constitute a barrier to metaphyseal blood flow, until epiphyseal fusion takes place. Vascularity of the metaphysis is profuse during puberty in the period immediately preceding fusion. Hence, when reducing an old slipped epiphysis by open operation, it is advisable to perforate the epiphyseal plate, to allow ready access of metaphyseal vessels into the head.

- *Adult period:* The lateral epiphyseal arteries anastomose with the medial epiphyseal artery, which enters the fovea capitis. These cross the epiphysis horizontally and send branches mainly towards the articular margin. The main source of blood supply to the femoral head is through the lateral epiphyseal arteries, originating from the medial femoral circumflex. It is important to note that the intrinsic vascular tree remains patent with advancing age. Blood supply of femoral head is illustrated in Flow chart 24.1.

Flow chart 24.1: Blood supply of femoral head

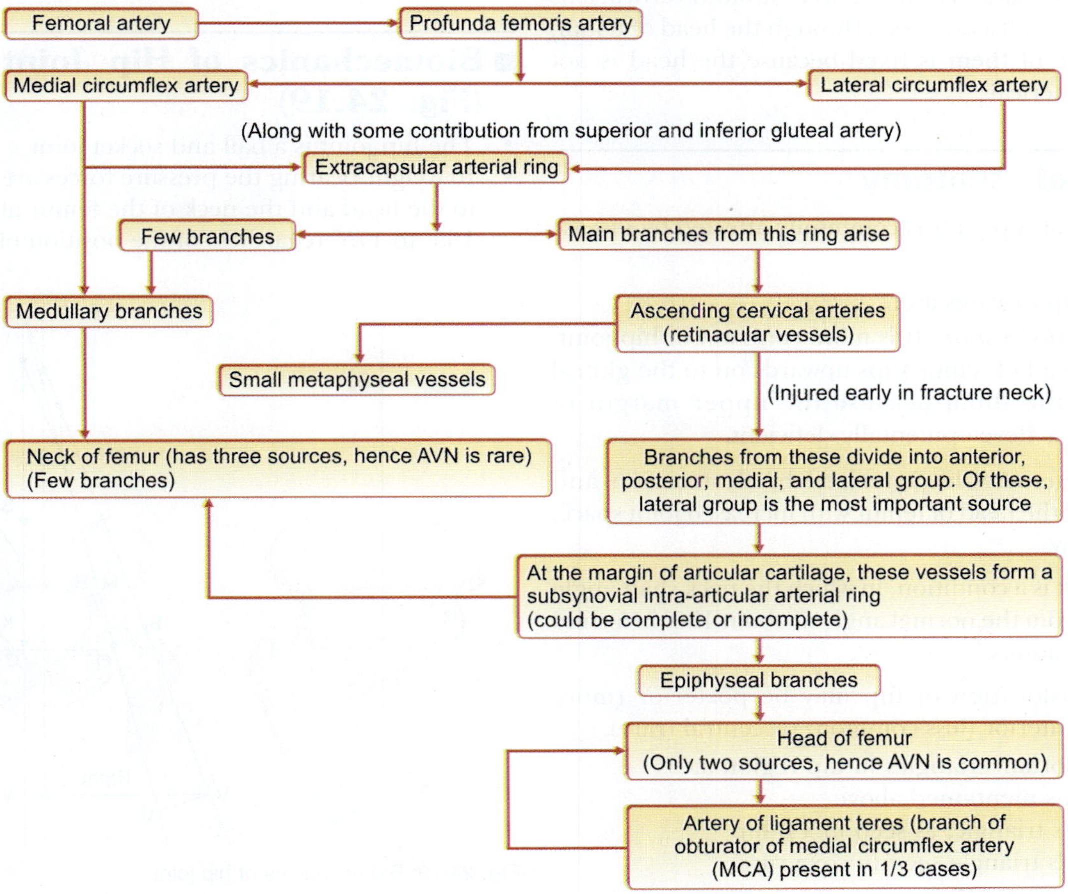

Table 24.4: Movements around hip joint and muscles carrying out those movements and their nerve supply

Movements	*Axis*	*Range of motion*	*Prime mover*	*Nerve supply*	*Assisted by*
Flexion	Transverse axis	0° to 120°	Psoas major	L 2-3	Rectus femoris sartorius, pectineus TFL Adductor longus, brevis and magnus
Extension	Transverse axis	0° to 5°-20°	Gluteus maximus and hamstrings	Inferior gluteal nerve sciatic nerve	
Abduction	AP axis	0°to 40°	Gluteus medius	Superior gluteal nerve (L4,5,S1)	Tensor fascia lata, sartorius, gluteus minimus and maximus
Adduction	AP axis	0°to 25°	Adductor longus, Magnus brevis	Obturator nerve (L3,4) and femoral nerve (L2,3,4)	Pectineus and gracillis
External rotation	Vertical axis	0°to 45°	Obturator externus. Internus, quadratus femoris, superior and inferior gamelli	S1,2,3,4, L5, S	Sartorius and long head of biceps femoris, pyriformis
Internal rotation	Vertical axis	0°to35°-45°	Gluteus minimus and TFL	Superior gluteal nerve	Gluteus medius

Movements Around Hip (Table 24.4)

- Flexion and extension occur around a transverse axis
- Abduction and adduction around anteroposterior axis
- Medial and lateral rotation occur around vertical axis
- In general, all axes passes through the head of femur, but none of them is fixed because the head is not quite spherical.

Clinical Anatomy

The region of hip joint is commonly affected by disease or injury.

Common hip diseases are:

Congenital dislocation: It is more common in hip joint. Here, the head of femur slips upwards on to the gluteal surface of the ilium because the upper margin of acetabulum is developmentally deficient.

Perthe's disease: Characterized by destruction and flattening of the head of femur with increased joint space, seen in X-ray.

Coxa vara: It is a condition, in which the neck shaft angle is reduced from the normal angle of about 150° in a child and 127° in adults.

Injuries: Dislocation of hip may be posterior (more common), anterior (less common) or central (rare).

Various important triangles in hip region are:

- Scarpas as mentioned above
- Babcock's triangle, as seen in TB hip
- Fairbank's triangle seen in coxa vara

Hip diseases show an interesting pattern

- Below 5 years of age: CDH and TB
- 5 to 10 years: Perthe's disease
- 10 to 20 years: Coxa vara
- Above 40 years: Osteoarthritis.

Biomechanics of Hip Joint (Fig. 24.19)

- The hip joint is a ball and socket joint
- In weight-bearing the pressure forces are transmitted to the head and the neck of the femur at an angle of 165° to 175° regardless of the position of pelvis.

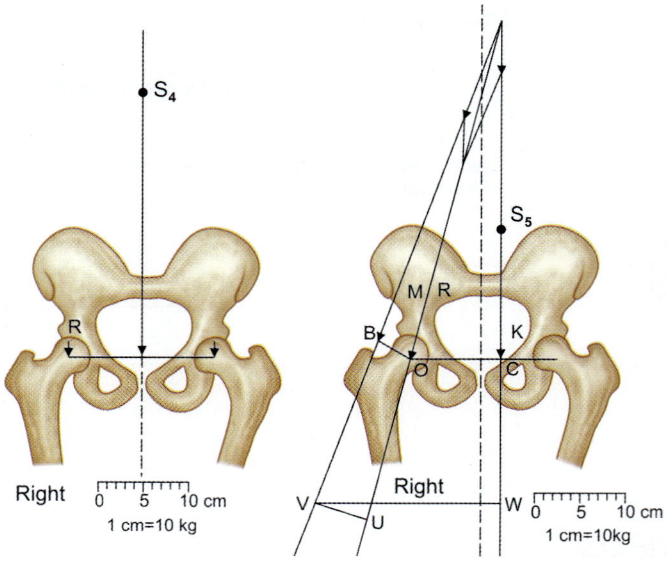

Fig. 24.19: Biomechanics of hip joint

- The plane of force coincides with the strongly developed trabeculae, which lie in the medial portion of femoral neck and extends upwards through the superomedial aspect of the femoral head.
- When the weight of the body above the lower extremities rests equally on two normal hip joints, the static force on each hip is one half of or less than one-third the total body weight.
- The left lower extremity is lifted, as in swing phase of walking, the weight of the left lower extremity is added to that of the body weight and the center of gravity normally in the median sagittal plane is displaced to the left.
- The abductor muscles exert a counter balancing force to maintain equilibrium. The pressure exerted on the head of the right hip is the sum of these two forces, as shown in Figure 24.20.
- The pressure exerted on the head of the right femur is the sum of these two forces. Each force is related to the relative length of the levers, as shown in Figure 24.21.
- If the abductor lever (B to O) is one-third that of the lever arm from the head to the center of gravity (O to C), the downward pull of the abductors must be three times the force of gravity to maintain balance, therefore the total pressure on the head is four times the superimposed weight.
- The longer the abductor lever (i.e. the more laterally placed insertion of the abductors), the less the ratio bet the levers, less the abduction force required to maintain balance and the less the pressure force upon the femoral head, as illustrated in Figure 24.22.

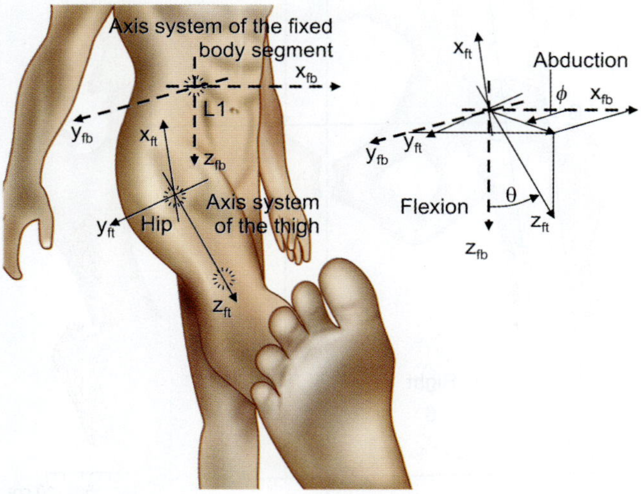

Fig. 24.20: The abductor muscles acting to counter balance force, exerted on the head of hip to maintain equilibrium

■ Clinical Applications (Figs 24.23 and 24.24)

- When hip is in valgus, the short abductor lever arm requires tremendous abduction pull on the hip and the resultant pressure on the head may be as much as seven or eight times the supported weight.
- To reduce the pressure and pain, the patient lists the trunk towards the hip and displaces the center of gravity in that direction. Consequently, less pull on the abductors is required and the force on the femoral head is reduced. This is characteristic waddle and limp of coxa valga, a means of relieving stress on the hip.

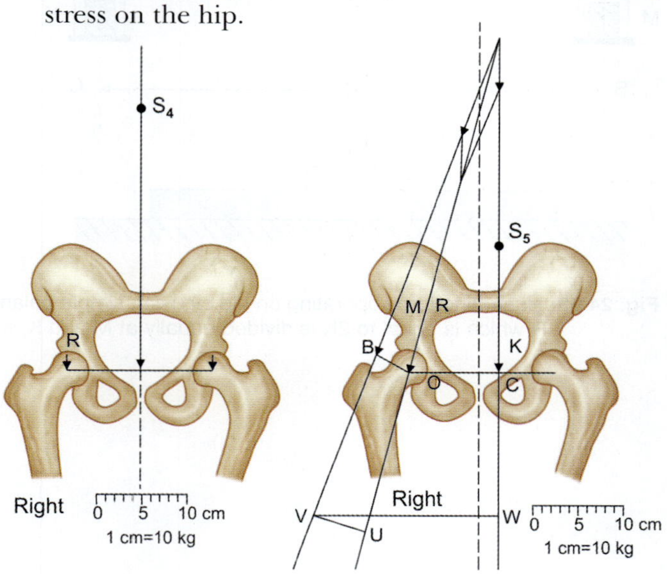

Fig. 24.21: Forces acting on the head of the femur

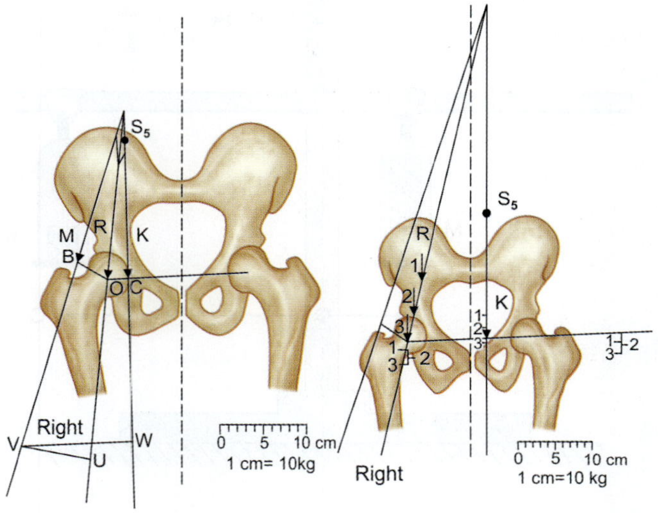

Fig. 24.22: Abductor lever arm and force ratio required to maintain balance

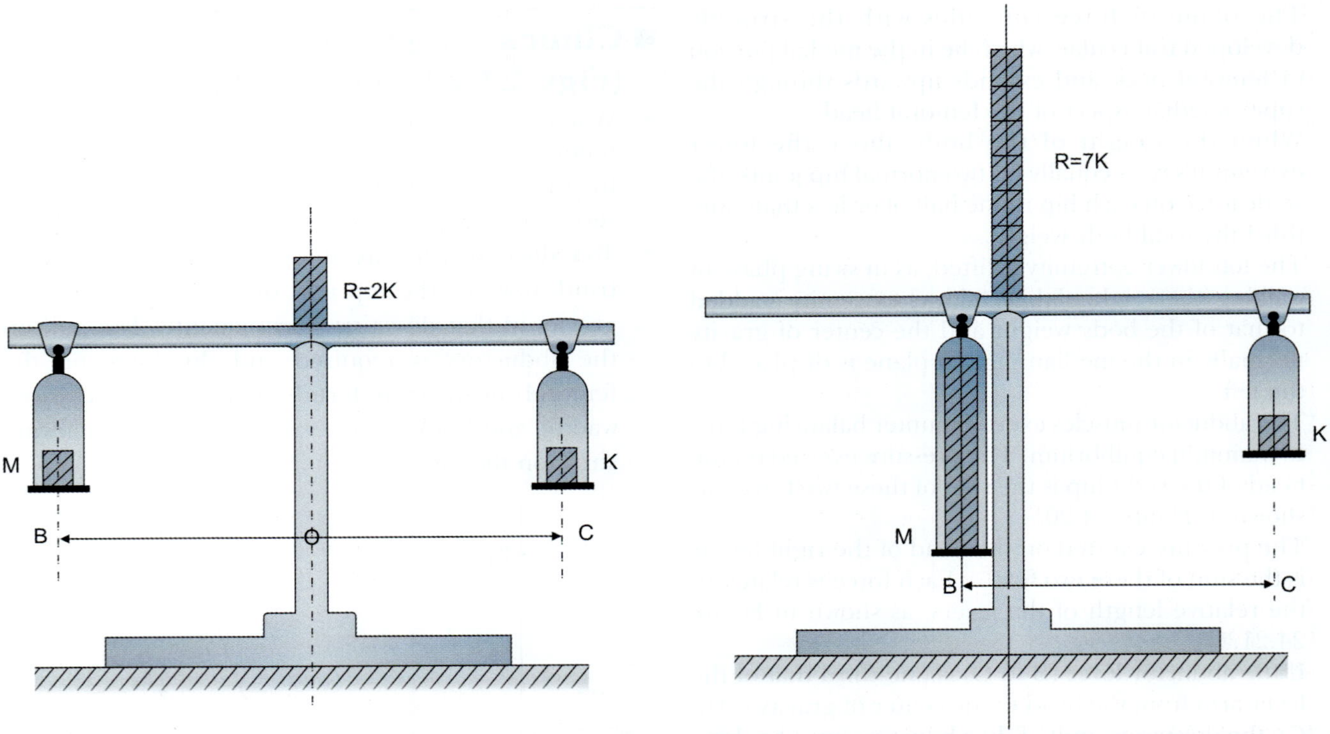

Fig. 24.23: Illustrating force operating on hip by using simple balance—R. Vector, K. Body weight, M. Muscle force. Superimpose weight R which is equal to 2K is divided equally at M and K, a balancing condition

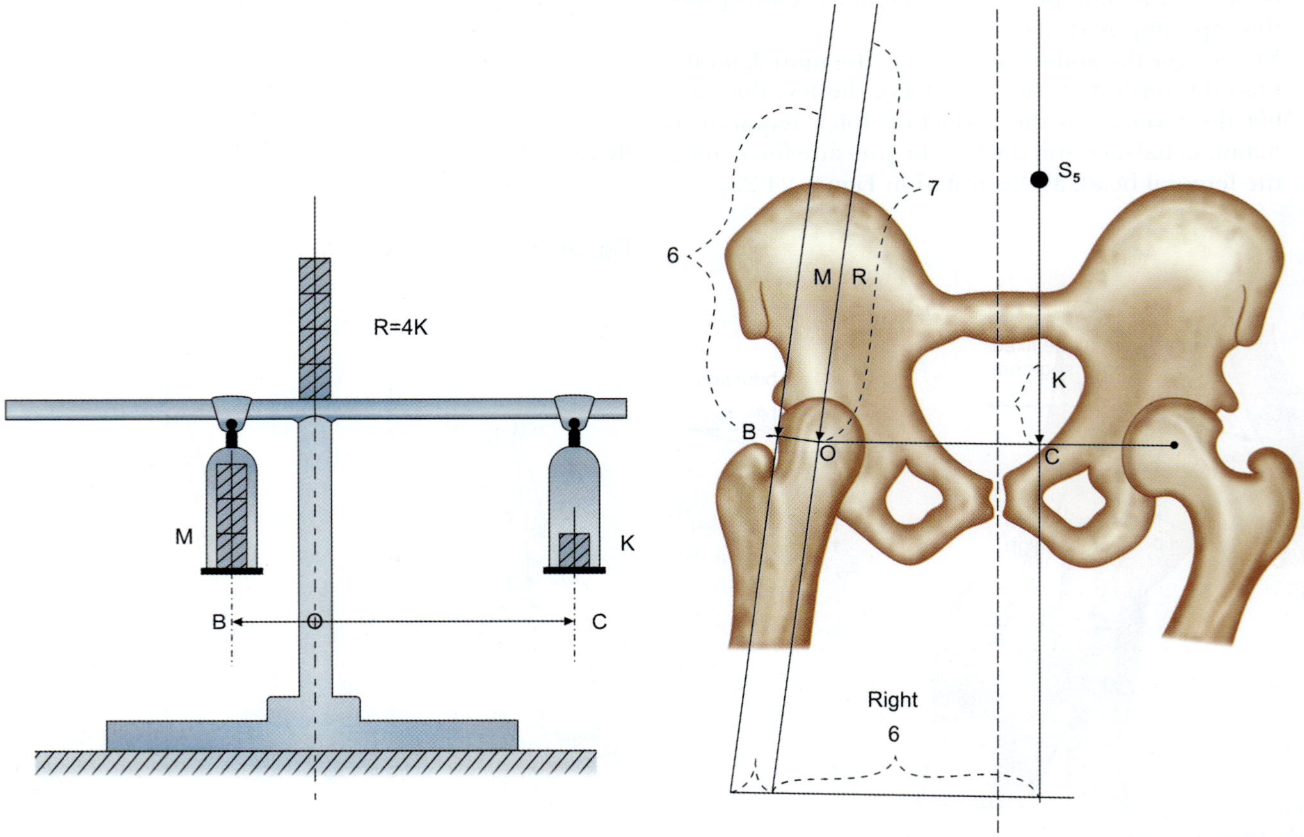

Fig. 24.24: Forces on valgus hip. The pull of abductor at B is at the end of an abnormally short liver arm,B to O,which is only one sixth of O to C. The pull downward at B must be six times K in order to maintain equilibrium when left foot raised. The total pressure on stationary right hip is seven times K

- The secondary strain on the lumbar spine caused by this lateral lurching produces backache and increased pressure on the femoral head increases degeneration.
- The use of a cane in the opposite hand, by working through the long lever arm can reduce static force on the hip in multiples of pressure force exerted downward on the cane.
- The normal length of femoral neck should be preserved wherever possible, particularly in prosthetic replacement operations. Maintenance of an adequate abductor lever will lessen pressure and enable the prosthesis to withstand stresses for a longer period of time.
- When abductor paralysis exists, equilibrium cannot be attained. The individual shifts laterally and displaces the center of gravity over the affected hip, so that forces are minimal and vertical. During the growth period, the epiphyseal plate tends to remain perpendicular to these forces and consequently shifts to a horizontal position. The result is a coxa valga deformity. Similar mechanism is operative in valgus associated with congenital dislocation of hip.
- In subluxated hip, the greater trochanter is closer to the fulcrum point. The force acts only along the upper border of the acetabulum.
- An adduction osteotomy, to create a varus deformity will produce these effects, the trochanter will be displaced a greater distance from the pelvis, thereby reducing the load on the femoral head and the line of force will be made to act on the center about a large acetabular area. Relief of pain and fatigue is accomplished.

DEVELOPMENTAL DYSPLASIA OF THE HIP

■ Introduction

It was previously known as congenital dislocation of the hip, implying a condition that existed at birth. It is a developmental defect and encompasses embryonic, fetal and infantile periods. It includes congenital dislocation and developmental hip problems, including subluxation, dislocation and dysplasia. Normal growth and development occurs during this defect. Embryologically, the acetabulum and femoral head develop from the same primitive mesenchymal cells. Cleft develops in precartilaginous cells at 7th week and this defines both structures. On 11th week hip joint is fully formed and acetabular growth continues throughout intrauterine life with development of labrum. By birth, femoral head is deeply seated in acetabulum by surface tension of synovial fluid and is very difficult to dislocate. In developmental dysplasia of hip, this shape and tension is abnormal in addition to capsular laxity. The cartilage complex is 3D with triradiate shape medially and cup-shape laterally, interposed between ilium above and ischium below and pubis anteriorly.

Acetabular cartilage forms outer 2/3 cavity and the nonarticular medial wall is formed by triradiate cartilage, which is the common physis of these three bones. Fibrocartilaginous labrum forms at margin of acetabular cartilage and joint capsule inserts just above its rim. Articular cartilage covers portion articulating with femoral head and opposite side is a growth plate with degenerating cells, facing towards the pelvic bone it opposes. Triradiate cartilage is triphalanged with each side of each limb having a growth plate, which allows interstitial growth within the cartilage causing expansion of hip joint diameter during growth. In the infant the greater trochanter, proximal femur and intertrochanteric portion is cartilage. Within 5 to 7 months proximal ossification center appears, which enlarges along cartilaginous anlage until adult life, when only thin layer of articular cartilage persists. Experimental studies in humans with unreduced hips suggest the main stimulus for concave shape of the acetabulum is presence of spherical head. To increase normal depth of acetabulum, several factors play a role, they are as follows:

- Spherical femoral head
- Normal appositional growth within cartilage
- Periosteal new bone formation in adjacent pelvic bones
- Development of three secondary ossification centers
- Normal growth and development occur through balanced growth of proximal femur, acetabulum and triradiate cartilages and the adjacent bones, as shown in Figures 24.25 and 24.26.

Developmental dysplasia of the hip is the spectrum of disorders of development of the hip that present in different form at different ages. The common etiology is excessive laxity of the hip capsule, which fails to maintain the femoral head within the acetabulum, as shown in Figure 24.27. The syndrome in the newborn consists of instability of the hip, such that the femoral head can be displaced partially (subluxated) or fully (dislocated) from the acetabulum by an examiner.

Epidemiology

- 1 in 100 newborns examined, have evidence of instability (positive Barlow or Ortolani)
- 1 in 1000 live births true dislocation
- Most detectable at birth in nursery
- Barlow stated that 60 percent stabilize in 1st week and 88 percent stabilize in first two months without treatment, remaining 12 percent are true dislocations.

Etiology

- Genetic and ethnic

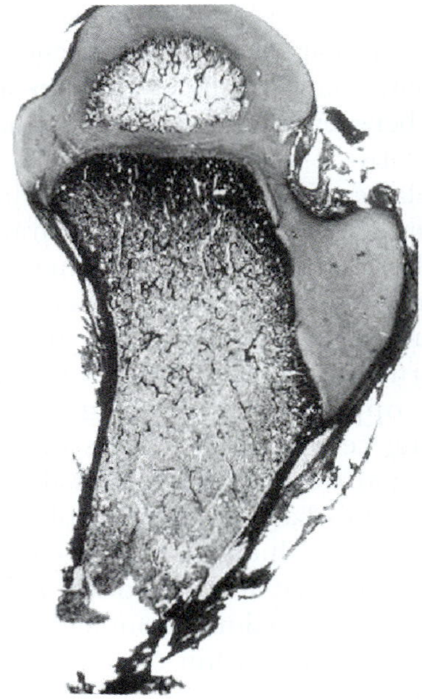

Fig. 24.25: Normally grown proximal femur

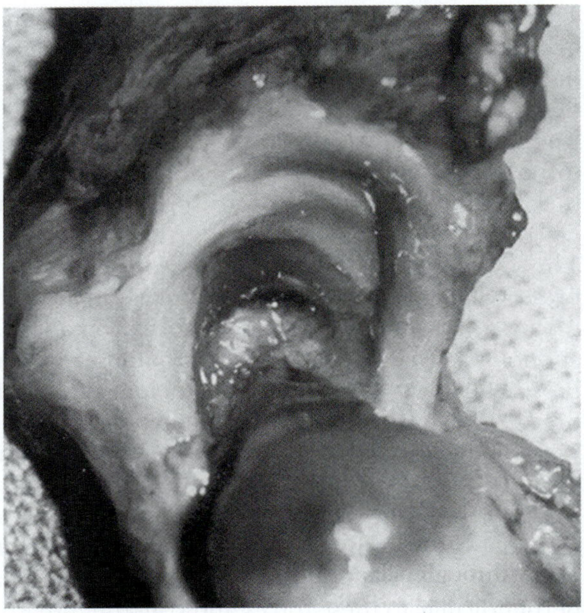

Fig. 24.27: Due to excessive laxity of hip capsule, it is unable to maintain the femoral head within the acetabulum

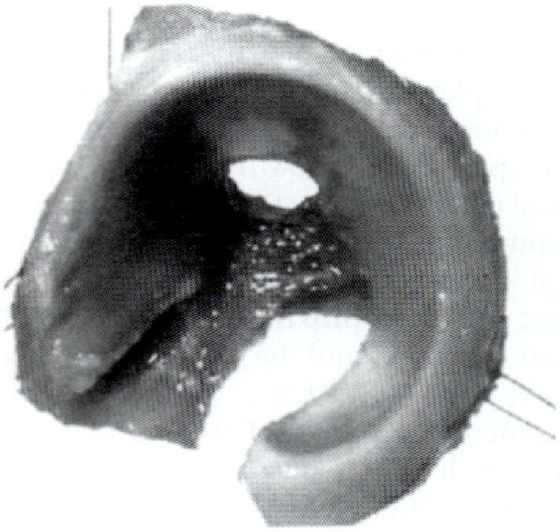

Fig. 24.26: Normally grown acetabulum, triradiate cartilages and the adjacent bones

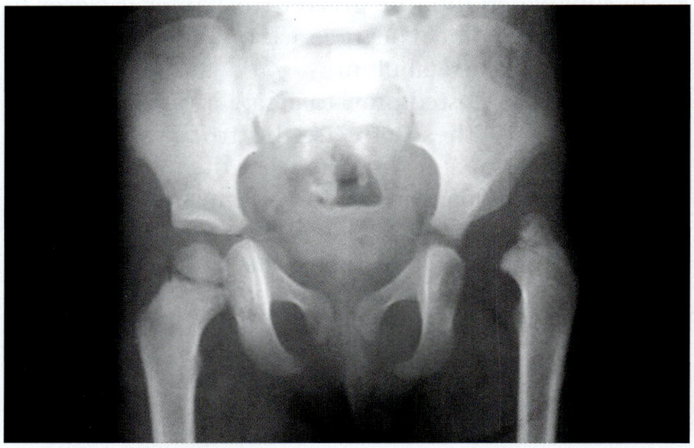

Fig. 24.28: Shallow acetabulum with steep sloping roof in CDH of hip joint

- Increased native Americans but very low in southern Chinese and Africans
- Positive family history 12 to 33 percent
- Uncommon in India and some Asian countries because of cultural practice
- *Hormonal theory:* It may occur due to maternal relaxin hormone, crossing placental barrier and leading to joint laxity and dislocation in female fetus.
- *Mechanical theory:* Intrauterine factors that are involved are:
  - Breech position
  - Oligohydramnios
  - Neuromuscular conditions like myelomeningocele
- *Germ plasma theory:* Teratologic dislocation of the hip are dislocated before birth, having limited range of motion and are not reducible on examination associated with myelodysplasias and arthrogyroposis.

Pathophysiology

- Shallow acetabulum with steep sloping roof (Fig. 24.28)
- Hypertrophy of ligamentum teres occurs
- Stretched capsule of hip joint
- Limbus (fibrocartilagenous labrum) folded into the acetabular cavity
- Femoral head is dislocated upwards and laterally

- Epiphysis is small and ossifies late
- Femoral neck is excessively anteverted.

Capsule

- Capsule could show hour glass constriction, one containing head and other containing acetabulum.
- Constriction is produced by iliopsoas and the ligamentum teres passes through this constriction and it is hypertrophied.

Muscles

- *Pelvifemoral group:* Adductors, sartorius, gracilis, rectus femoris, hamstrings, tensor fascia lata are shortened and they prevent the reduction of head.
- *Pelvitrochanteric group:* Obturator, quadrates femoris and ilio-psoas are elongated and the psoas forms an obstacle to reduction.
- *Gluteal muscles:* They show little organic change but power is diminished.

Physical Examination

- *Ortolani test* (Fig. 24.29): Hip flexion and abduction is done, trochanter is elevated and femoral head glides into acetabulum.
- *Barlow test* (Fig. 24.30): It is a provocative test where hip is flexed and adducted and head is palpated to exit the acetabulum partially or completely over a rim.

Diagnosis

Galeazzi's Sign (Fig. 24.31)

- Flex both hips and one side shows apparent femoral shortening
- Asymmetry gluteal, thigh or labial folds
- Limblength inequality
- Waddling gait and hyperlordosis in bilateral cases.

Radiological Diagnosis

X-rays (Figs 24.32 to 24.34)

- Perkins line, vertical line at outer border of acetabulum
- *Hilgenreiner's line*: Horizontal line at triradiate cartilage
- *Shenton's line*: It is smooth curve between inferior border of neck of femur and superior margin of obturator foramen, as shown in Figures 24.34A and B.
- Acetabular index (Fig. 24.32)
- Center edge (CE) angle of Wiberg (Fig. 24.33).

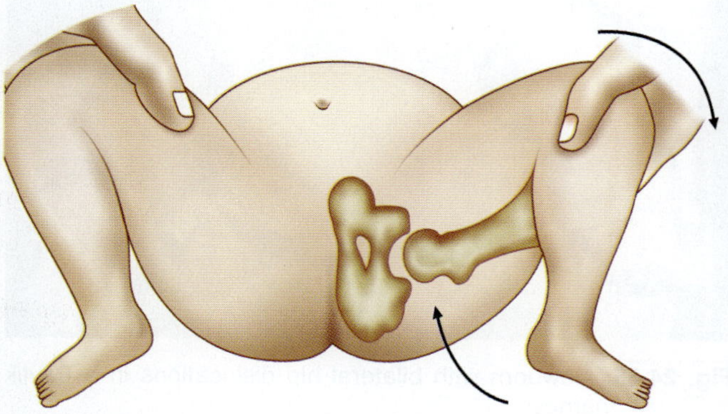

Fig. 24.29: Ortolani's test

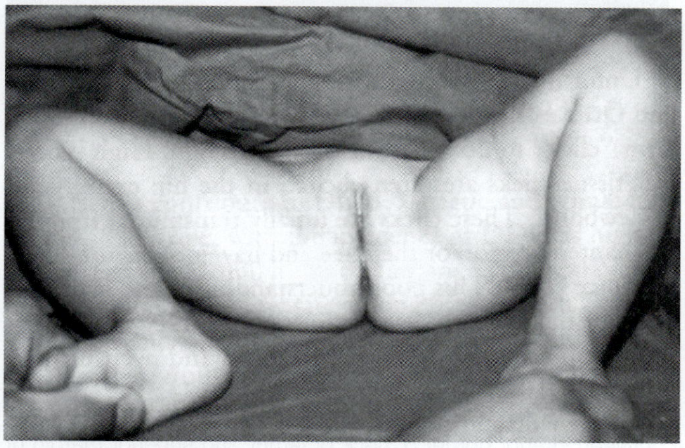

Fig. 24.30: Barlow's test

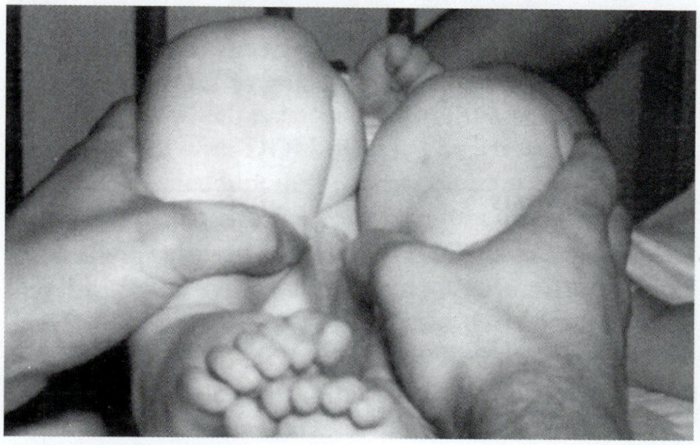

Fig. 24.31: Galeazzi's sign

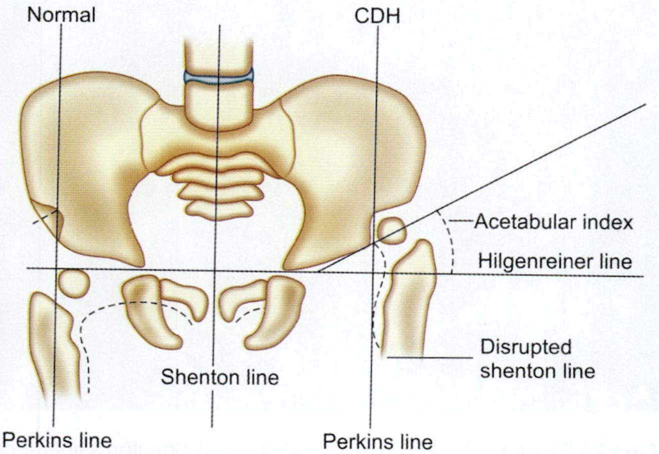

Fig. 24.32: Acetabular index

Graff's Ultrasound Classification

- *Type 1:* Normal hip
- *Type 2:* Immature or somewhat abnormal
- *Type 3:* Hips are subluxated
- *Type 4:* Hips are dislocated

Treatment of Hip Dislocation

Zero to Six Months

- Goal is to obtain reduction and maintain reduction, to provide optimal environment for femoral head and acetabular development.
- *Lovell and Winter's:* Treatment is initiated immediately on diagnosis.
- *American Academy of Orthopedic Surgeons (AAOS):* Subluxation often corrects after three weeks and may be observed without treatment. If persists on clinical examination or USG beyond three weeks, then treatment indicated. Actual dislocation diagnosed at birth treatment should be immediate.
- *Pavlik harness:* The most common device for treatment of developmental displasia of the hip (DDH) in newborn is Pavlik harness, as illustrated in Figure 24.35. It prevents hip extension and adduction, but allows flexion and abduction, which lead to reduction and stabilization. Success rate is 95 percent if maintained full time six weeks. Chest strap at nipple line. Shoulder straps set to hold cross strap at this level. Anterior strap flexes hip 100° to 110°. Posterior strap prevents adduction and allow comfortable abduction. Safe zone is defined as the arc of abduction and adduction that is between redislocation and comfortable unforced abduction. Indications include, presence of reducible hip and femoral head directed towards triradiate cartilage on X-ray. It is followed by weekly intervals, by clinical examination and USG for

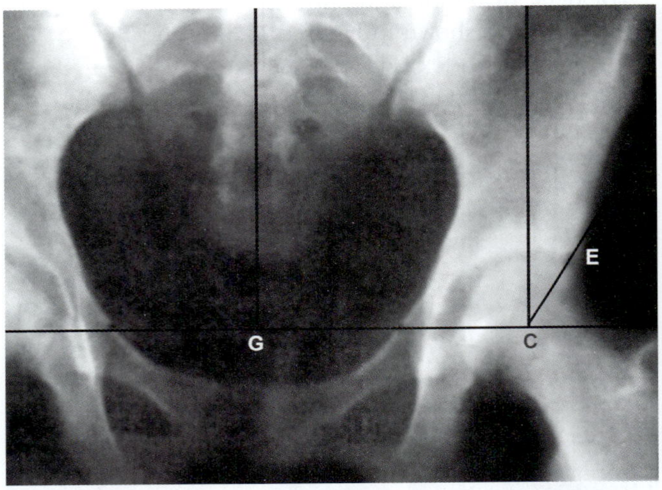

Fig. 24.33: X-ray showing center edge (CE) angle of Wiberg

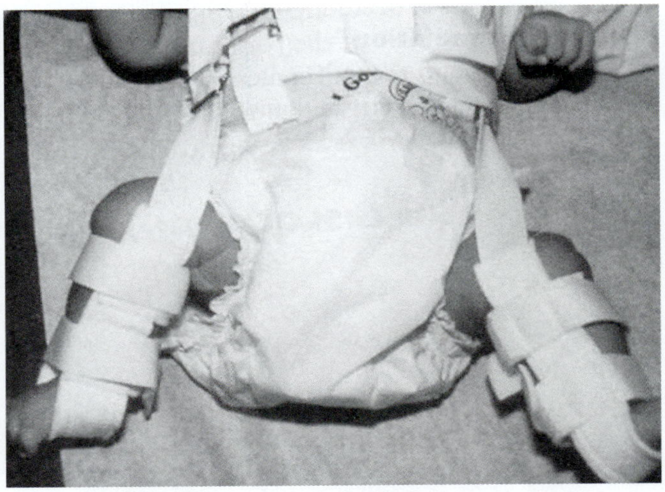

Fig. 24.35: Newborn with bilateral hip dislocations in a Pavlik harness

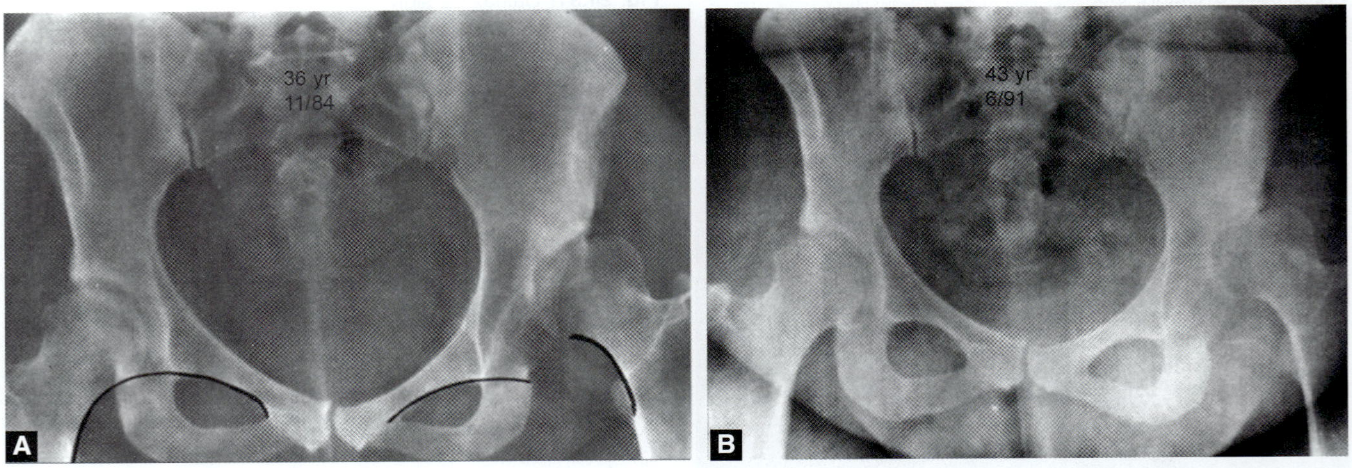

Figs 24.34A and B: X-ray showing CDH—(A) Shenton's line, a curve between inferior border of neck of femur and superior margin of obturator foramen; (B) X-ray of pelvis and hip joint

two weeks, if not reduced other methods pursued. Once successfully reduced, harness continued for children age at stability more than three months. Worn full time for half interval, if stability continues and then weaned off. End of weaning process, X-ray pelvis obtained and if normal discontinue harness.
- *von Rosen splint,* shown in Figure 24.36.

Complications

- *Failure*: Poor compliance, inaccurate position and persistence of inadequate treatment, greater than 2 to 3 weeks.
- Femoral nerve compression to hyperflexion
- Inferior dislocation
- Skin breakdown
- Avascular necrosis (AVN).

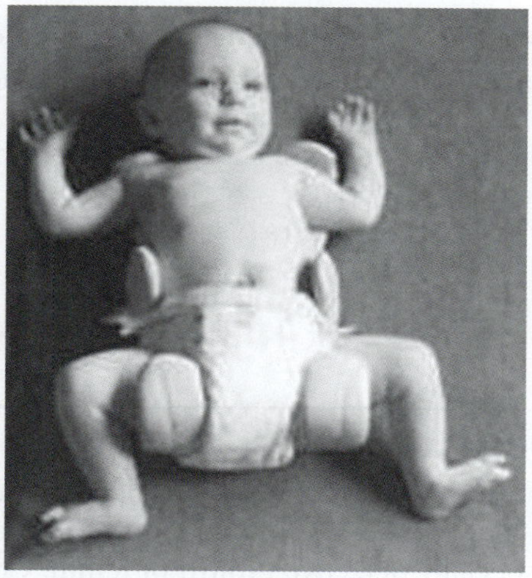

Fig. 24.36: von Rosen splint

At Six to Eighteen Months

- Closed reduction and spica cast immobilization recommended.
- Traction is controversial with theoretical benefit of gradual stretching of soft tissues, impeding reduction and neurovascular bundles to decrease AVN.
- Skin traction preferred, however may vary with surgeon. Usually 1 to 2 weeks. Scientific evidence supporting this is lacking.
- Traction give may include Bryant's traction, this is shown in Figures 24.37A and B.
- Reduction maintained in spica cast well molded to greater trochanter, to prevent redislocation. Hip-spica reduction is shown in Figures 24.38A and B.
- Human position of hyperflexion and limited abduction preferred.
- Avoid forced abduction with internal rotation, as increased incidence of proximal femoral growth disturbance.

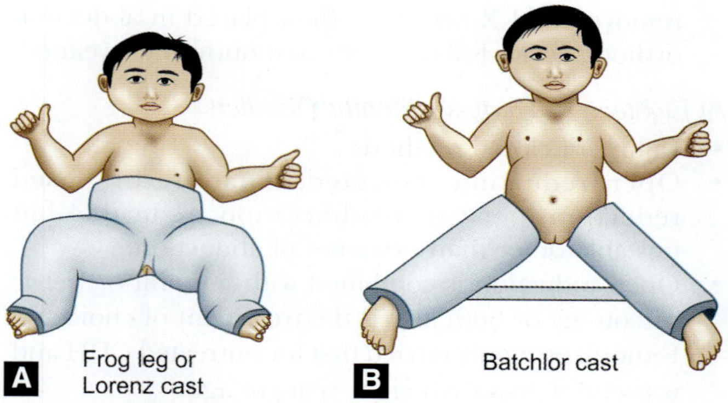

Figs 24.38A and B: Reduction maintained in spica cast or hip-spica

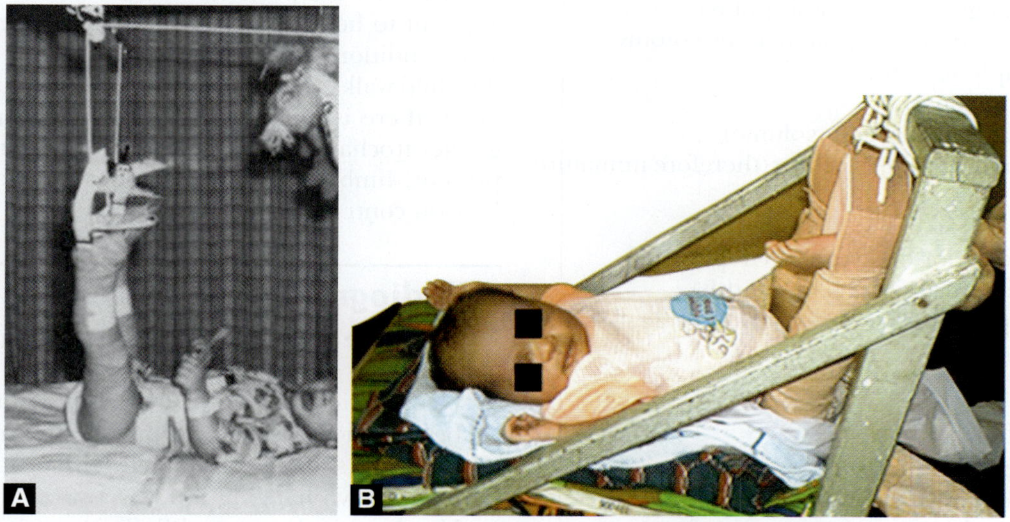

Figs 24.37A and B: (A) Position of limb, while giving Bryant's traction; (B) Showing a child with CDH, given Bryant's traction

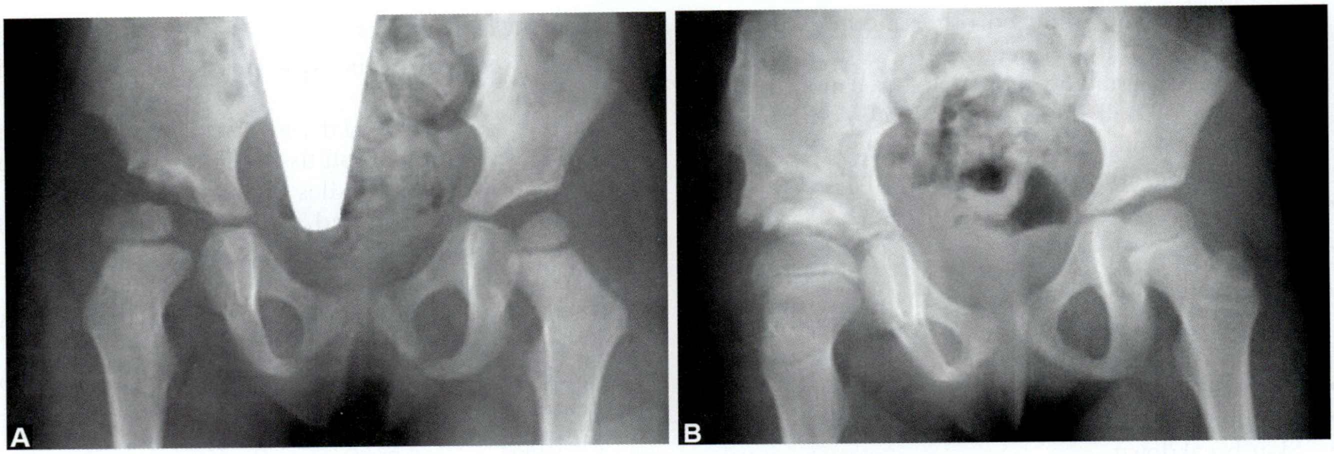

Figs 24.39A and B: Salter osteotomy in CDH—(A) Preoperative X-ray; (B) Postoperative X-ray

- Cast in place for six weeks then repeat CT scan, to confirm reduction.
- Casting continued for three months, at which point removed and X-ray done, then placed in abduction orthotic device full time for two months then weaned.

At Eighteen to Thirty-six Months (Toddlers)

- Failure of closed methods
- Open reduction indicated, if failure of closed reduction, persistent subluxation, reducible but unstable other than extremes of abduction.
- Open reduction is combined with femoral or pelvic osteotomy or both and is the treatment of choice.
- Femoral ostetomy is tried first for untreated CDH and is useful in less than eight years of age.

Osteotomies for CDH

- Redirectional
  - Salter (hinges on symphysis pubis)
  - Sutherland double innominate osteotomy
  - Steel (triple osteotomy)
  - Ganz (rotational)
- Acetabuloplasties (decrease volume)
  - Hinge on triradiate cartilage (therefore immature patients)
  - Pemberton
  - Dega (posterior coverage in CP patients)
- Salter's osteotomy (Figs 24.39A and B)
- Pemberton pericapsular osteotomy (Figs 24.40A and B)
- Chiari osteotomy

At Three to Eight Years of Child

- Open reduction is treatment of choice
- Usually followed with femoral shortening
- If necessary pelvic osteotomy may be done

At Eight to Eighteen Years (Juvenile and Young Adults)

- Femoral and pelvic osteotomy should be done. This is shown in Figures 24.41A and B.
- Total hip replacement should be thought, when osteoarthritis develops
- Rarely arthrodesis occurs.

CONGENITAL COXA VARA

Introduction

Coxa vara may be a primary congenital deformity occurring alone or in association with other congenital defects, especially defective growth of femur. Congenital coxa vara also sometimes described as cervical or infantile coxa vara is characterized in radiograph according to Fairbank, by the presence of a triangular piece of neck adjacent to head being separated from the rest of bone. The condition is bilateral. The symptoms appear when the child walks. The patient is small in stature and limps. Often there is pain and stiffness. On examination, the greater trochanter is at higher level, shortening of limb is present, limb is in rotation and abduction is limited. Flexion contracture may also present.

Radiographic Features

- The angle of neck is reduced to somewhat below right angle.
- Neck varies in length, but is short and may even become nonexistent and may be fragmented. Often the neck shows a prolonged lower extremity, which forms down hanging hip.
- Head is translucent and fluffy in appearance

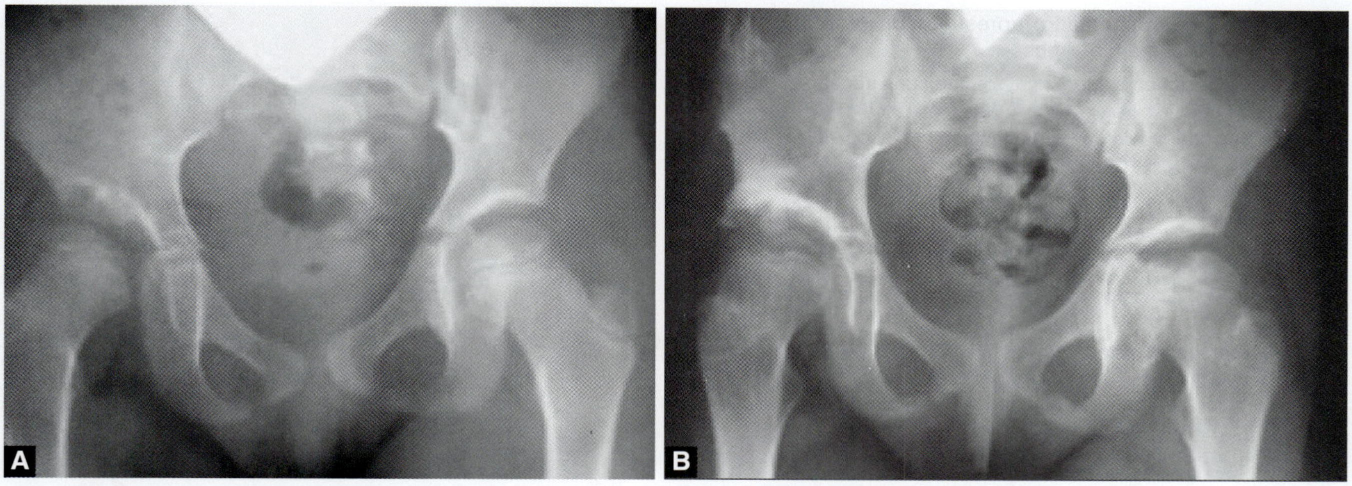

Figs 24.40A and B: Pemberton pericapsular osteotomy procedure for carrying out pemberton pericapsular osteotomy; (A and B) X-rays taken before and after performing osteotomy

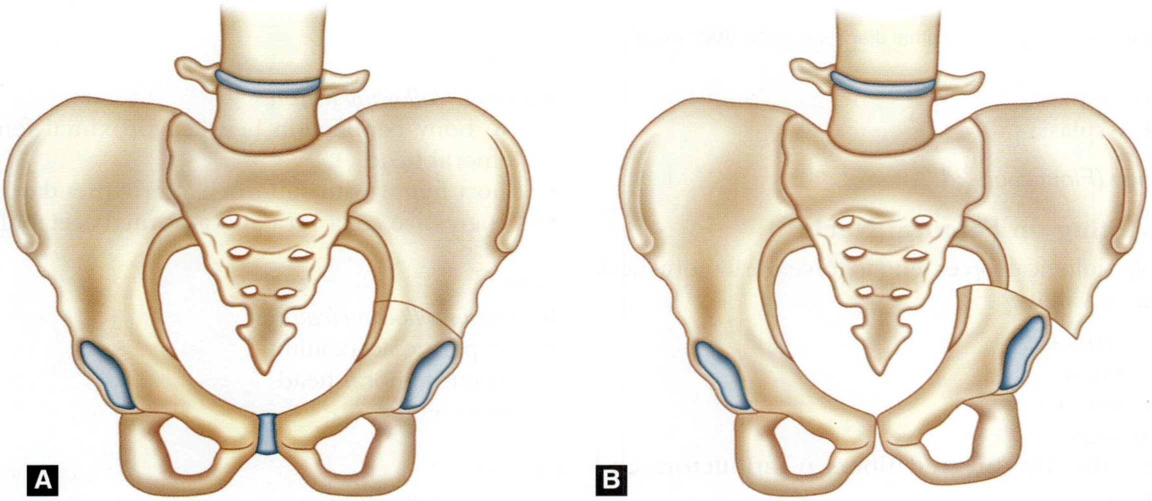

Figs 24.41A and B: Femoral and pelvic osteotomy

- There is fragment of bone, which is triangular in shape, occupying the lower part of the neck close to head, bounded by two clear bands transversing the neck and forming the inverted "V".

Treatment

Angulation osteotomy of Dickson type is done at the level of intertrochanteric region. In this, wedge shape area of bone is removed and vertical epiphysis becomes horizontal in shape and relives the shearing stress and reduces the varus deformity.

Proximal Femoral Focal Deficiency

In proximal femoral focal deficiency (PFFD), congenital shortening of the femur occurs. Incidence is 1 per 50,000 live birth. Dysgenesis of proximal portion of the femur occurs, with partial skeletal defect in the proximal femur, with unstable hip joint and shortening of femur.

Other associated anomalies are:

- Fibular hemimelia
- Agenesis of cruciate ligaments of the knee
- Club foot
- Congenital heart anomalies

Flow chart 24.2: Schematic representation of embryological development of limbs

Gestational age 32 days: Limb buds appears
↓
Mesoderm laid down in a fashion proximodistal fashion
↓
Completed 10 days later
↓
5th week : Individual muscles differentiate
↓
7th week : Ossification of bones
↓
4-7 weeks of gestation:
Teratogenic factors may disturb normal development
↓
Transplantation before nerve growth may lead to normal development
↓
One common cartilage precursor
↓
Cleft formation to form ilium and proximal femoral components
↓
Ossification center appearance
↓
Femoral head: 1st year of life ← → Greater trochanter: 4th year of life
↓
Thus two separate areas of growth
↓
Determines: Length of proximal diaphysis,neck shaft angle

- Spinal dysplasia
- Facial dysplasia

Embryology (Flow chart 24.2)

Forces Acting on Femoral Neck

Certain physiological forces tend to force the femoral neck into varus or valgus.

Factors for varus are
- Body weight
- Rectus femoris
- Hamstrings
- Longitudinally directed fibers of adductors and abductors

The opposing valgus forces are
- Horizontally directed external rotators
- Adductors.

Classifications of PFFD

- Aitken's classification
- Pappa's classification
- Kalamchi classification

Aitken's Classification (Fig. 24.42)

Class A
- Congenital short femur is present with:
  - Bowing
  - Coxa vara
- Normal acetabulum is present along with absence of femoral neck.

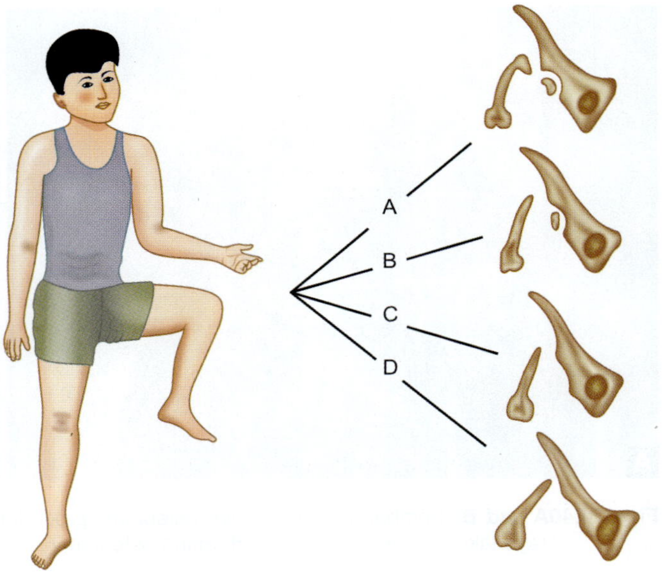

Fig. 24.42: Schematic representation of the four radiographic subclasses of proximal femoral focal deficiency

Class B

It contains following features
- No bony connection between proximal femur and femoral head
- Short femur with sub-trochanteric pseudarthrosis
- Progressive coxa vara and a normal acetabulum

Class C

It contains following features
- Dysplastic acetabulum
- Absent femoral head
- Short femur.

Class D

It contains following features
- Acetabulum and femoral head is totally absent
- Proximal femur is extremely short and pointed.

Pappa's Classification

Class I (Fig. 24.43)
- *Femoral-pelvic abnormalities*
  - Femur absent, ischiopubic bone structures underdeveloped and deficient
  - Lack of acetabular development.
- Associated abnormalities: Fibula absent
- Treatment objectives: Prosthetic management.

Class II (Aitken D, Fig. 24.44)
- *Femoral-pelvic abnormalities*
  - Femoral shortening (70–90%)
  - Femoral head is absent
  - Ischiopubic bone structures delayed in ossification

Pappa's classification

Class I

Femoral-pelvic abnormalities	Femur absent ischiopubic bone structures underdeveloped acetabular structure under developed
Associated abnormalities	Fibula absent
Treatment objectives	Prosthetic management

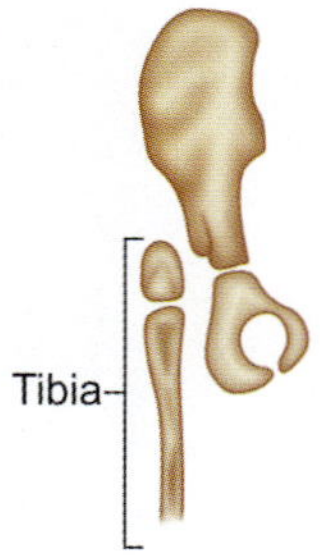

Fig. 24.43: Class I type of proximal femoral deficiency

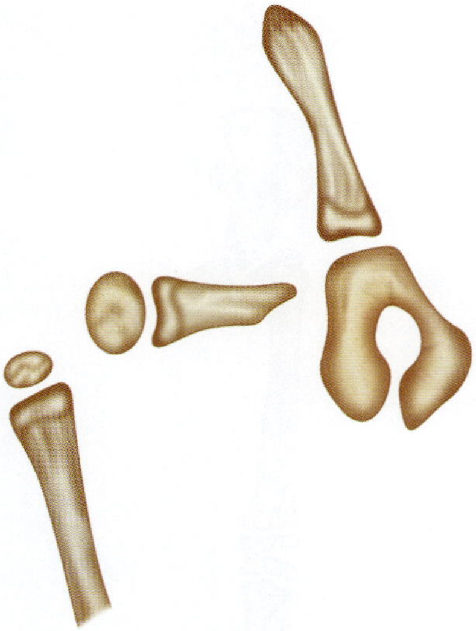

Fig. 24.44: Class II (Aitken D) type of proximal femoral deficiency

- *Associated abnormalities:* Tibia shortened, fibula, foot, knee and ankle joint abnormal
- *Treatment objectives:* Pelvic femoral stability through prosthetic management.

Class III (Aitken B, Fig. 24.45)

- *Femoral-pelvic abnormalities*
  - Femoral shortening (45–80%)
  - No osseus connection between femoral shaft and head
  - Femoral head ossification delayed
  - Acetabulum may be absent
  - Femoral condyles maldeveloped
- *Associated abnormalities*
  - Tibia shortened (0–40%)
  - Fibula shortened (5–100%)

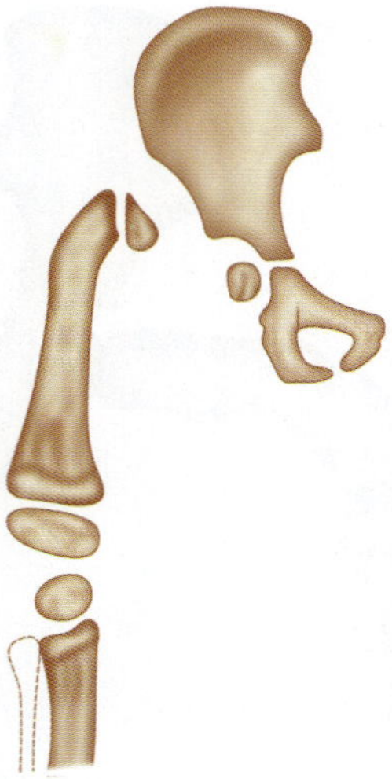

Fig. 24.45: Class III (Aitken B) type of proximal femoral deficiency

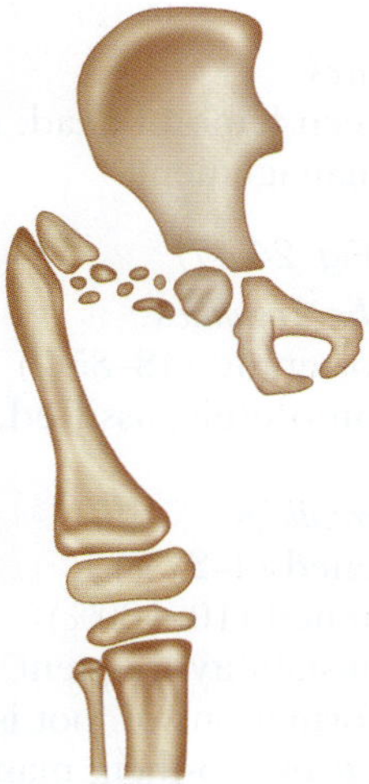

Fig. 24.46: Class IV (Aitken) type of proximal femoral deficiency

  - Patella absent or small and high riding
  - Knee joint instability common
  - Foot malformed
- *Treatment objectives:* Prosthetic management.

Class IV (Aitken A, Fig. 24.46)

- *Femoral-pelvic abnormalities*
  - Femoral shortening (40–67%)
  - Femoral head and shaft joined by irregular calcification in fibrocartilaginous matrix
- *Associated abnormalities*
  - Tibia shortened (0–20%)
  - Fibula shortened (4–60%)
  - Knee joint instability frequent
  - Foot malformed with infrequent malformations

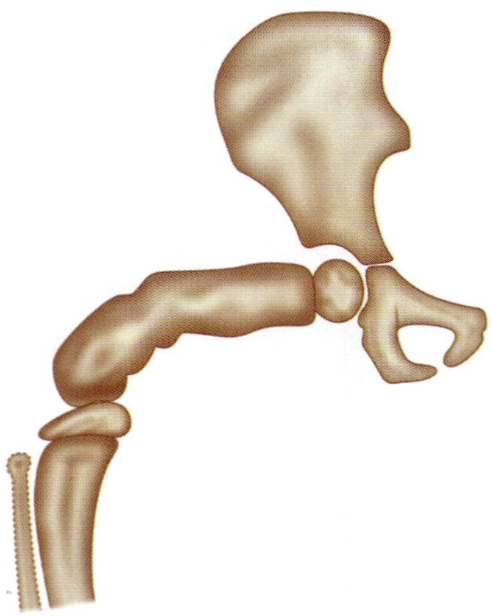

Fig. 24.47: Class V (Aitken A) type of proximal femoral deficiency

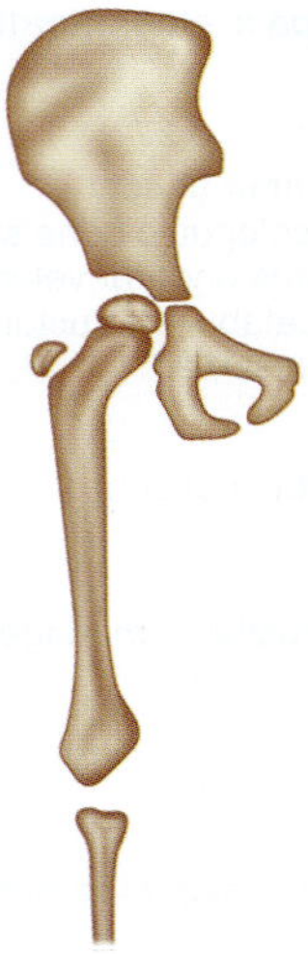

Fig. 24.48: Class VI type of proximal femoral deficiency

- *Treatment objectives*
  - Union between femoral head, neck and shaft
  - Prosthetic management

Class V (Aitken A, Fig. 24.47)

- *Femoral-pelvic abnormalities*
  - Femoral shortening (48–85%)
  - Femur incompletely ossified, hypoplastic and irregular
- *Associated abnormalities*
  - Tibia shortened (4–27%)
  - Fibula shortened (10–100%)
  - Knee joint instability frequent
  - Severe malformations of foot is common
- *Treatment objectives:* Prosthetic management

Class VI (Fig. 24.48)

- *Femoral-pelvic abnormalities*
  - Femoral shortening (30–60%)
  - Distal femur short, irregular and hypoplastic
  - Irregular distal femoral diaphysis
- *Associated abnormalities*
  - Single bone, lower leg
  - Patella absent
  - Foot malformed
- *Treatment objectives:* Prosthetic management

Class VII (Fig. 24.49)

- *Femoral-pelvic abnormalities*
  - Femoral shortening (10–50%)
  - Coxa vara
  - Hypoplastic femur
  - Proximal femoral diaphysis irregular with thickened cortex
  - Lateral femoral condyle deficiency common
  - Valgus distal femur

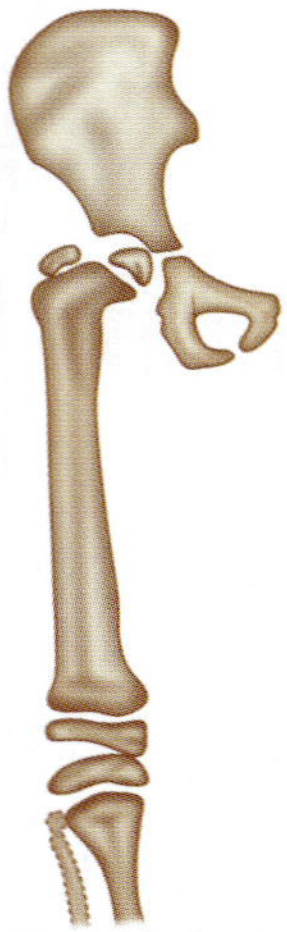

Fig. 24.49: Class VII type of proximal femoral deficiency

- *Associated abnormalities*
  - Tibia shortened (<10–24%)
  - Fibula shortened (<10–100%)
  - Lateral high riding patella is common.

Class VIII (Fig. 24.50)

- *Femoral pelvic abnormalities*
  - Femoral shortening (10–41%)
  - Femoral-pelvic abnormalities
  - Coxa valga
  - Hypoplastic femur
  - Femoral head and neck smaller
  - Proximal femoral physis horizontal
  - Abnormality of femoral condyled common, with associated boing of shaft and valgus of distal femur.

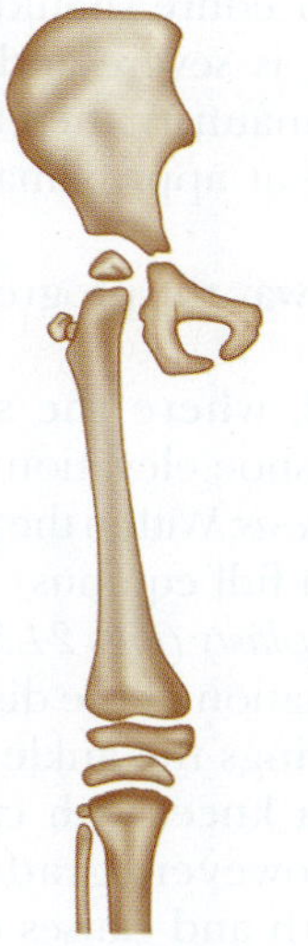

Fig. 24.50: Class VIII type of proximal femoral deficiency

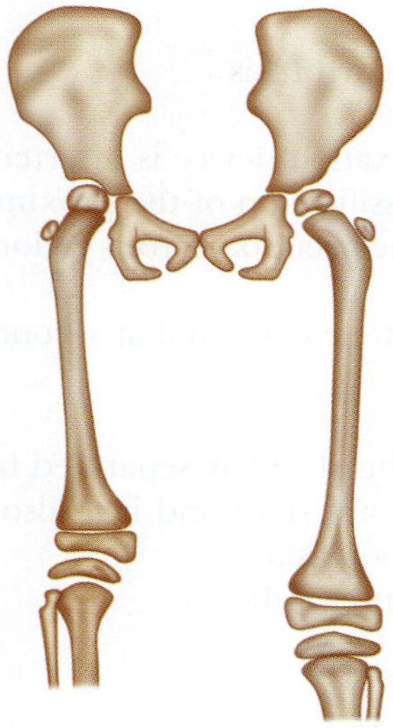

Fig. 24.51: Class IX type of proximal femoral deficiency

- *Associated abnormalities*
  - Tibia shortened (0–36%)
  - Fibula shortened (0–100%)
  - Lateral and high riding patella is common
  - Foot malformed
- *Treatment objectives*
  - Extremity length equality
  - Improved alignment of
    a. proximal and
    b. distal femur

Class IX (Fig. 24.51)

- *Femoral-pelvic abnormalities*
  - Femoral shortening (6–20%)
  - Hypoplastic femur
- *Associated abnormalities*
  - Tibia shortened (0–15%)
  - Fibula shortened (3–30%)
  - Additional ipsilateral and contralateral malformations are common
- *Treatment objectives:* Extremity length equality

Kalamchi Classification

He developed a simple classification scheme, which is as follows:

- *Group I:* Short femur and intact hip joint
- *Group II:* Short femur and coxa vara of hip
- *Group III:* Short femur well developed acetabulum and femoral head
- *Group IV:* Absent hip joint and dysplastic femoral segment
- *Group V:* Total absence of the femur.

■ Treatment

Proximal femoral focal deficiency (PFFD) presents multiple problems of management, depending upon the degree of various elements of the deformity including:

- Instability of the hip
- Malrotation
- Inadequate proximal musculature
- Inequality of the leg length

Instability of the Hip

This could be due to iliofemoral maldevelopment and muscle inadequacy. In milder forms, coxa vara leads to proximal displacement of greater trochanter, due to abductor insufficiency and lurching gait. In moderate type, pseudoarthrosis adds to instability. In severe type, failure of joint formation leads to slip femoral head proximally. When acetabulum can be identified on roentgenogram, cartilaginous head and neck, although not visible, are already present. Allow spontaneous ossification of the head and neck and bony bridging across the pseudoarthrosis, to take place. For reducing the degree of coxa vara, bone graft is placed across pseudarthrosis into the femoral head and neck. Before this, presence of proximal element of the femur should be confirmed by arthrography. This surgical procedure is not generally accepted. Moreover, spontaneous ossification, although delayed, generally takes place and the coxa vara deformity can be dealt with later.

In Type 1 or 2 Deformity

Coxa vara is corrected and held with a fixation device. This should be done at an early age.

In Type 3

- Excise pseudoarthrosis
- Correct varus
- Single unit fixation device is inserted alternatively
- Encourage ossification of the proximal femur
- Healing of the pseudoarthrosis is done by inserting a bone graft
- Coxa vara can be corrected at second operation.

In Type 4

- Hypoplastic head widely separated from the tapered
- Sclerotic femoral shaft and it is also associated with muscular hypoplasia
- Results are unrewarding.

In Type 5

- Acetabulum absent
- Reconstruction is not possible.

Malrotation and Inadequate Proximal Musculature

- Hip usually has a fixed flexion and external rotation contracture
- Flexion to 90° and abduction to 30° is functionally useful
- Gluteal muscles are usually good, whereas quadriceps is hypoplastic
- On active flexion of hip, contraction of sartorius can be demonstrated. Its action is to draw the limb into "sitting tailor" position. Consequently, despite the hip flexion contracture, function is good and treatment for this not required.

Leg Length Inequality

Generally femur is 20 to 40 percent of normal length. When lower limb inequality is mild, epiphysiodesis or leg lengthening procedure should be done. Usually, the femoral shortening is severe and progressive and may exceed 12 inches at maturity, therefore foot of the affected leg will come to lie at approximately the same level as the normal knee.

In the following way the progressive deformity should be handled:

- In young child, where the shortening is not yet severe, hence a shoe elevation is sufficient
- *Extension prosthesis*: Within the prosthesis, foot is placed on a platform in full equinus
- *Van Nes rotationplasty (Figs 24.52A to E):* Arthrodesis of the knee and rotation of the distal portion of the limb through 180° brings the ankle into a position, where it functions as a knee, with calf muscle acting as a quadriceps. However, gradual derotation takes place with growth and causes difficulty with fitting a functional prosthesis.
- *Syme's amputation:* This provides an excellent end bearing stump, allowing ready fitting of a prosthesis at an early age, when the child quickly adapts to the prosthesis
- *Arthrodesis of the knee:* Provides a single skeletal lever so that available muscle can act more efficiently across the hip joint.

The procedure of choice

- Early syme's amputation, as soon as walking is established and an end bearing prosthesis.
- With the growth, thigh-to-leg disproportion increases, hence arthrodesis of the knee is done.

■ Slipped Capital Femoral Epiphysis

Slip capital femoral epiphysis (SCFE) is a disorder in which capital femoral epiphysis is displaced from the

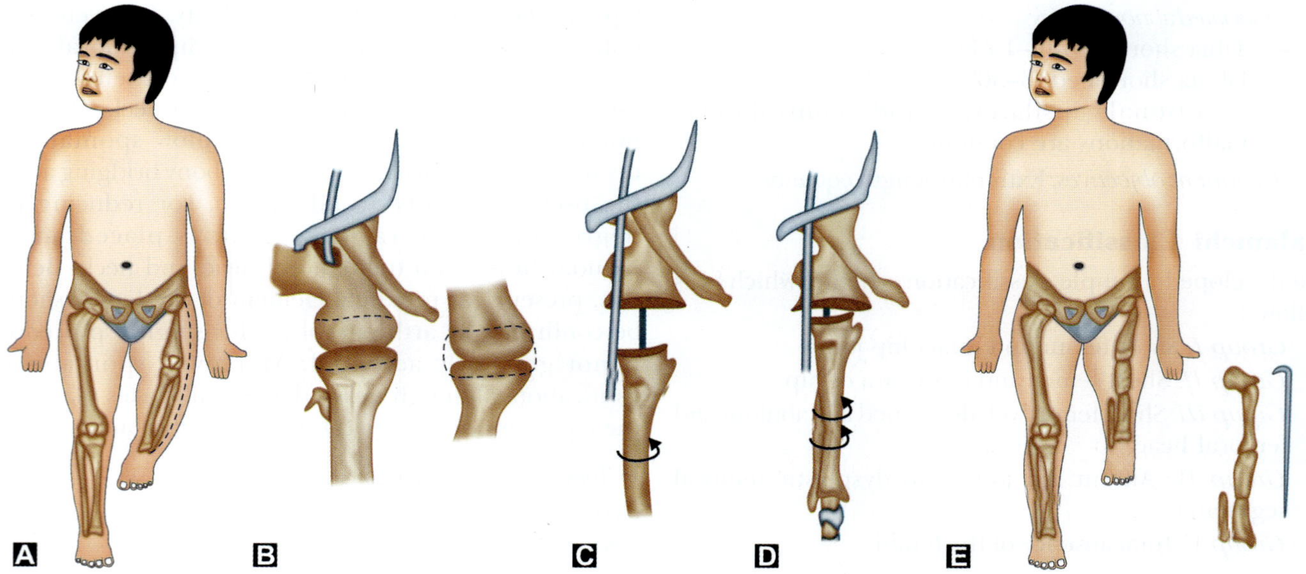

Figs 24.52A to E: Van Nes rotationplasty

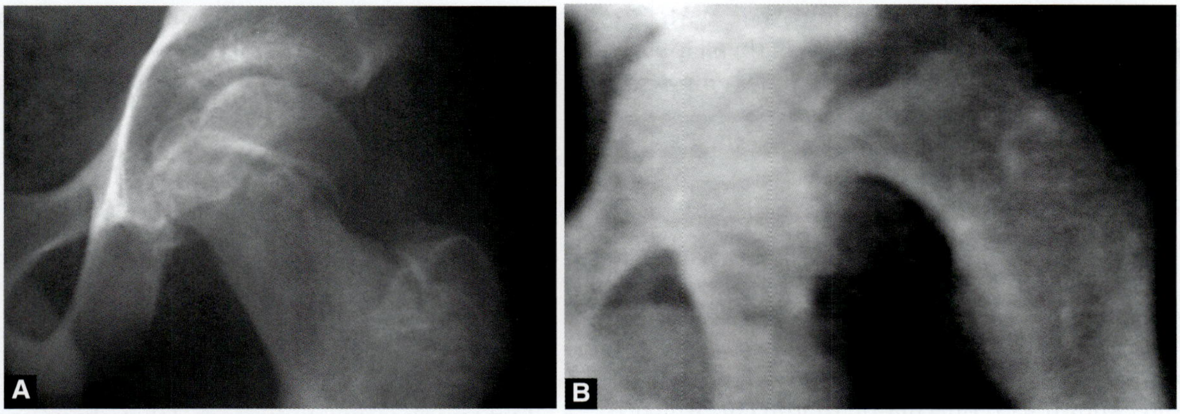

Figs 24.53A and B: (A) Slip capital femoral epiphysis; (B) SCFE, where capital femoral epiphysis is displaced from the metaphysis through the physeal plate

metaphysis through the physeal plate. Slip capital femoral epiphysis (SCFE) is actually a misnomer in that the head is held in the acetabulum by the ligamentum teres and thus it is actually the neck that comes upward and outwards, while the head remains posterior and downward in the acetabulum. A varus relation exists between the head and neck, but occasionally the slip is into valgus, with head displaced superiorly and posteriorly in relation to the neck, as shown in Figures 24.53A and B.

Incidence

- Every 2 in 100,000 so, the rate is 0.002 percent
- Boys (10–16 years)
- Girls (10–14 years)
- Male to female ratio is 2.5:1
- Blacks are suffering more than white people
- Five percent of sufferers having their parents have or had SCFE
- Left hip is twice as often affected as right hip
- Mostly bilateral
- Seventeen to thirty-seven percent in adolescents
- Fifty percent are simultaneous and 50 percent are sequential
- In younger child (physically or chronologically), the greater risk of subsequent bilateral involvement.
- A contralateral slip will usually present within two years
- Twenty percent are bilateral at time of presentation, as shown in Figure 24.54.

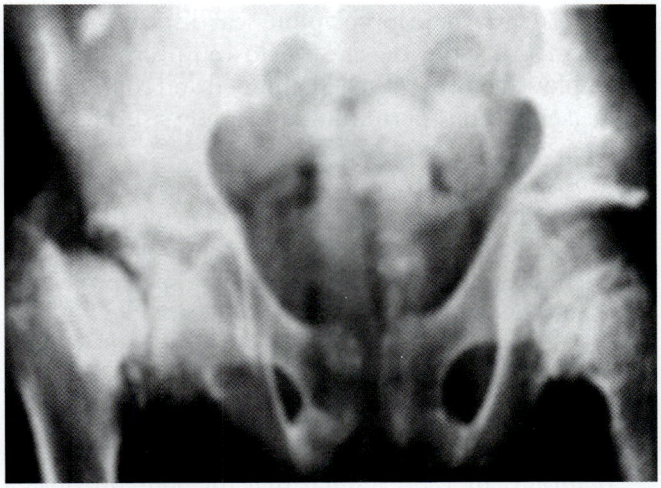

Fig. 24.54: Slip capital femoral epiphysis, generally have bilateral presentation

Etiology

- Unknown
- Hormonal theory
- Although the softening is due to a failure of maturation of cartilage into bone, analysis of evidence seems to suggest that it is the result of a hormonal imbalance.
- *Siberberg and Sibelberg:* In 1949 has observed with experiments in animals, by administration of hyperestrogen, to weaken or change in epiphyseal plate.
- Duthie and Barker, in 1955 by cortisone.
- *Harris:* In 1950 has showed GH increased thickness of epiphyseal plates, which required less force to slip and estrogen led to thinner required more force with experiments in rats.
- Unfortunately, there are no human studies to support any theory for hormonal basis for slipping.
- *Burrows:* In his careful survey of 100 cases found that a quarter of boys and two-thirds of girls, showed evidence of some endocrine defect, quite apart from those who are unusually fat.
- Moreover, although line of separation is at the usual level at the junction is at the metaphysis with epiphyseal cartilage, epiphysis in its backward and

downward displacement does not carry with it a triangular fragment from the margin of the diaphysis, over which it is displaced as it does in other epiphyseal injuries.

Traumatic Theory

- There is no doubt that trauma and static influences are both important factors development of SCFE
- *Key:* In 1930 pointed out that pathological conditions may be neither in the bone nor in the epiphyseal cartilage, but in the periosteum of femoral neck, in childhood periosteum is thick and thrown into ridges or folds known as retinacula of Weitbrecht, which is the chief factors in holding the head in place. In adolescence this periosteum begins to atrophy and to approach the adult type, thus producing weakness at epiphyseal line. Moreover, coxa vara gives a history of rapid growth prior to epiphyseal displacement and during this period the periosteum crossing the epiphyseal line is stretched, thinned and consequently weakened, thus permitting the epiphysis to be easily separated.
- *Fairbank:* Pointed out that the epiphysis is set obliquely on the neck and faces upwards and medially. This setting, somewhat insecure as a means of supporting the body weight is strengthened by a spur projecting from the lower half of the metaphysis.
- *Haas:* In 1948 showed, once the periosteum has been stripped off the humeral epiphysis of rats, the middle zone of epiphyseal plate will slip when a shearing stress is applied.
- *Walmsley:* In 1938 showed that the spur provides a natural ledge, on which the epiphysis rests. Occasionally the spur ossifies from a separate secondary center, which may remain isolated from the rest of metaphysis by a strip of cartilage till puberty. This increase in amount of cartilage weakens the neck in proportion to the body weight, while the inadequacy of the spur, increased occasionally by fragmentation of its center, allows the epiphysis to slide downwards.

Proven Associations

- Hypothyroidism
- Renal disease (renal osteodystrophy)
- Hypogonadism or hypopituitarism
- Secondary to mechanical disturbances
- Increased retroversion ≥ increase force on epiphysis
- Obesity
- Secondary to biochemical abnormality in cartilage collagen
- Sometimes adults men suffering from Simmond's disease
- Hypopituitarism resulting from intracranial tumor
- Affected boys may have excessively fat with hypopituitarism of French type, i.e. undeveloped testis and absence of pubic hair and axillary hair.

Pathology

Synovium Shows

- Synovitis with hypertrophy
- Hyperplasia of synovial cells
- Villus formation
- Increased vascularity
- Round cell infiltration
- Light microscopic studies reveal that physis is widened and irregular, sometimes reaching 12 mm in width. In SCFE hypertrophic zone may constitute up to 80 percent of the physis width
- Slip occurs through the zone of cell hypertrophy, with occasional extension into the calcifying cartilage.

Symptomatology

Idiopathic

- Onset is gradual
- Patient gets tired easily after walking or standing
- Pain is confined to hip, but usually radiates down to lower thigh and knee, relieved by rest in early stage. It is also accompanied by limping
- Limitation of abduction
- Affected leg gradually becomes shorter and smaller. Movements are restricted and leg may be in full external rotation.

Traumatic

- History of trauma (fall or blow on hip) and is very trivial
- Dull ache associated with little disability in the hip, although occasionally pain is severe and it prevents from being able to walk.

Physical Signs

At Early Stage

- Pain
- Waddling gait
- Body sway over affected side
- Pelvis on sound side tends to drop when weight borne on affected extremity.

On Standing

- Leg rotated laterally, abducted and pelvis tilted on affected side
- Slight scoliosis towards affected side is present lumber and in sound side thoracic buttock atrophied and gluteal fold lower than normal side.

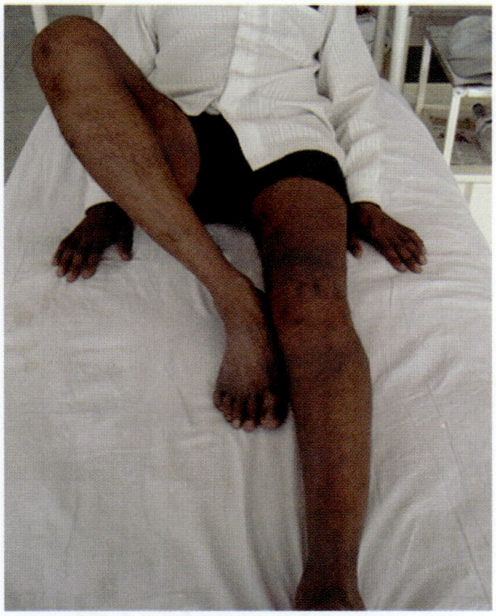

Fig. 24.55: Position of the leg in recumbent position

On Recumbent Position (Fig. 24.55)

- *Position of leg:* Lateral rotation and slight abduction. Flexion is limited up to 80° or 90° and as thigh is flexed, it rotates laterally.
- *Axis deviation:* Adduction and lateral rotation are free, but abduction, medial rotation and extension are greatly restricted.

Radiological Findings (Figs 24.56A to C)

X-rays

- AP view
- True lateral view
- Frog leg lateral view–Lauwenstein view (Fig. 24.56C)

Preslipping Stage

- Minimal slipping, indicated by the absence of normal shoulder on the upper aspect of neck and head, i.e. *Trethowan's sign*, as shown in Figures 24.57A and B. A line drawn from superior surface of the neck will pass above the femoral head rather than it passing through 20 percent of the head normally.
- Lateral view shows slightest backward displacement.
- *Billing's lateral view of hip (Fig. 24.58):* An accurate measurement of epiphyseal slip can be obtained, with patient lying in supine on X-ray table and the knee in 90° of flexion. The hip is allowed to fall into a position of external rotation and abduction. The knee is supported to bring the shaft of the femur to a position of 25° of elevation, while the height of malleolus is adjusted.
- *Interpretation:* The neck axis is indicated by relatively straight anterior border of distal half of femoral neck and shaft axis by anterior border of upper third of femoral shaft line, connecting anterior and posterior margins of epiphysis define epiphyseal plane.

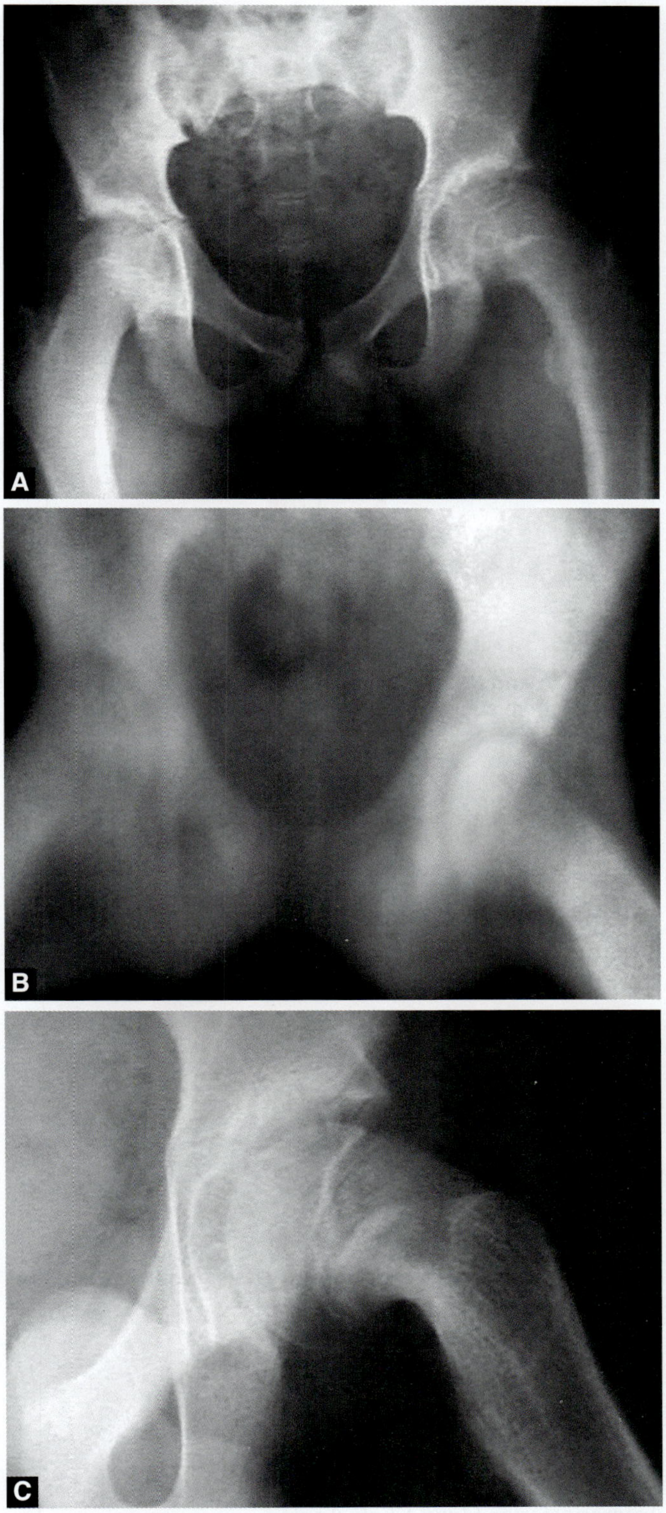

Figs 24.56A to C: Lateral view showing slipped capital femoral epiphysis

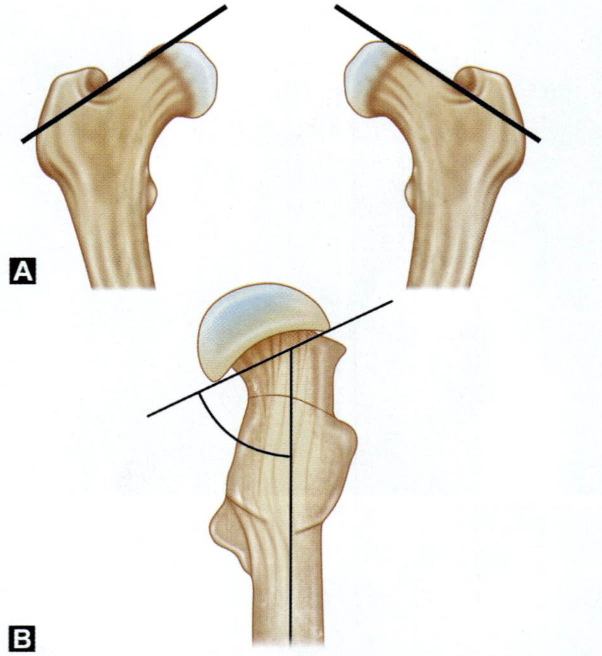

Figs 24.57A and B: Trethowan's sign. (A) Lateral view; (B) A view from above

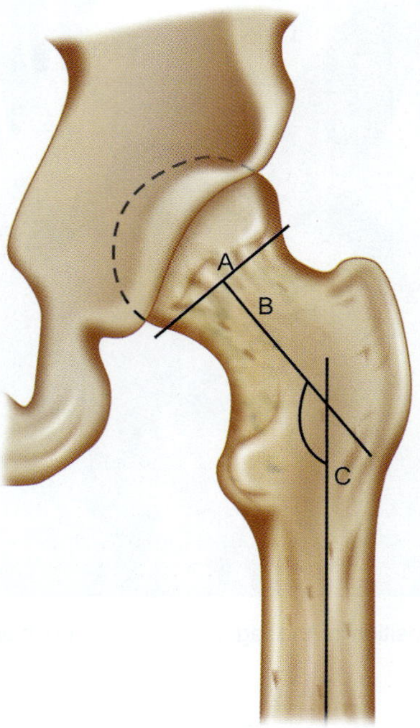

Fig. 24.59: The angle form between this two line is anteroposterior head shaft angle (normal 145°)—A. Line drawn across the base of epiphysis connecting both superior and inferior margins of epiphysis; B. Another line drawn perpendicular to it; C. A straight line drawn over shaft of femur joining the perpendicular line

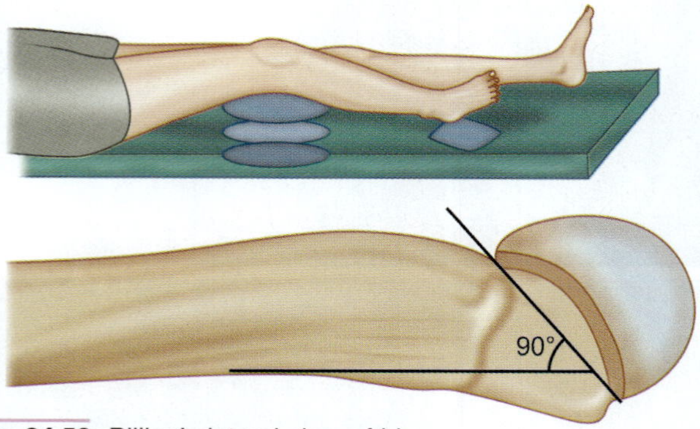

Fig. 24.58: Billing's lateral view of hip

Early Radiographic Sign

- *Lateral view:* Cup shaped epiphysis. No longer fitting into cup surface of metaphysic.
- *AP view:* Decrease in depth.

Late Radiographic Sign

AP view: Epiphysis lie well below its normal level with backwards rotation.

Anteroposterior Head Shaft Angle

- Line drawn across the base of epiphysis connecting both superior and inferior margins of epiphysis.
- Another line drawn perpendicular to it.
- A straight line drawn over shaft of femur joining the perpendicular line.
- The angle form between this two line is anteroposterior head shaft angle (normal 145°), as shown in Figure 24.59.
- This angle difference between the two side represents the amount of correction needed on the anterior surface of femur.
- Frog leg lateral head shaft angle, as shown in Figure 24.60.
- Lines are drawn in the same fashion. In both normal and affected side angle is determined (normal range 0°–25°).
- The difference of retroversion between affected and normal side determine the lateral wedge to be removed, to correct the posterior angulation.

Severity

It can be seen in radiograph and classified by maximal anatomic displacement, either on AP or lateral view.

- *Minimal slip:* Maximal displacement is less than one-third the diameter of the neck.
- *Moderate slip:* Greater than 1 cm of displacement, but less than half the diameter of the neck.
- *Severe slip:* Displacement more than 50 percent diameter of the neck.

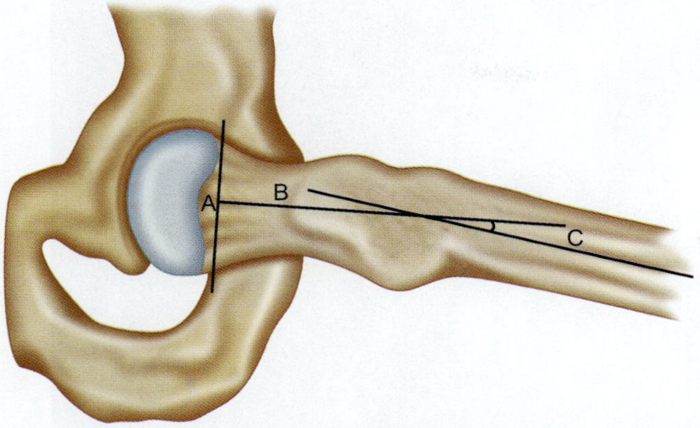

Fig. 24.60: Frog leg lateral head shaft angle—A. Line drawn across the base of epiphysis connecting both superior and inferior margins of epiphysis; B. Another line drawn perpendicular to it; C. A straight line drawn over shaft of femur joining the perpendicular line

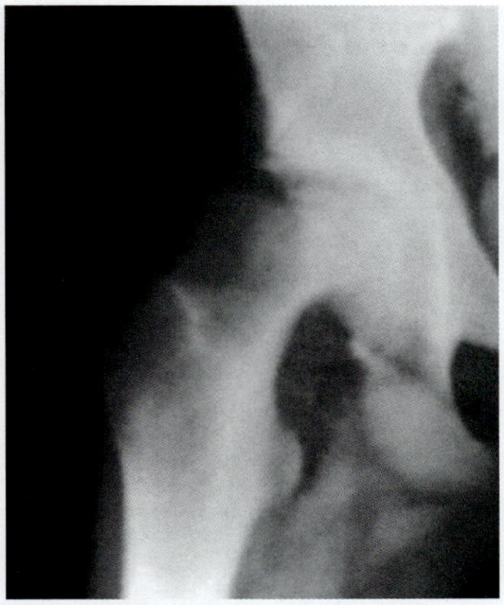

Fig. 24.61: Acute SCFE

Other Investigations

Computed Tomography Scan

Findings: Computed tomography (CT) is a sensitive method for measuring the degree of tilt and detecting disease, it can help in defining whether growth plate is open.

Magnetic Resonance Imaging

Findings: The earliest way to detect SCFE is by using magnetic resonance tomography. With MRI, early marrow edema and slippage can be demonstrated. MRI can be considered in patients for whom the clinical suspicion of SCFE is high and in whom the radiographs appear normal. MRI can be considered for follow-up imaging of the contralateral hip.

Ultrasound

Ultrasonographic findings are rarely specific and the sensitivity of sonography is unknown. Hip effusions of blood often have been reported and are suggestive of fracture.

Classification (Fig. 24.61)

Traditional Classification by Dunn

- Acute < 3 weeks of symptoms
- Chronic > 3 weeks of symptoms
- Acute on chronic > 3 weeks of symptoms and sudden exacerbation.

Newer Classification by Loder (Figs 24.62A and B)

- *Unstable:* Ambulation is impossible, with or without crutches
- *Stable:* Ambulation is possible with or without crutches.

Surgical Treatment

Goals

- Prevent further slipping
- Close the growth plate
- Safely restore normal anatomy
- Reduction or osteotomy

Treatment Options

- Pin *in situ*
- Reduction and pinning
- Bone peg epiphysiodesis
- Osteotomy
- Reconstruction by arthroplasty and arthrodesis
- Each technique has proponents and opponents and the choice of treatment, must be individualized for each child, depending on age, type of slip and severity of displacement.

Pinning in situ (Figs 24.63 and 24.64)

- Internal fixation with single cannulated screws or pins (Moore or Knowles). Screws are extremely effective for stable SCFE
- There is decreased complications compared to multiple pins (pin protrusion and chondrolysis), however its use is controversial in the unstable SCFE.
- Some advocate two screws, while others have excellent results with single screw. No biomechanical benefit found with two screws
- The fixation device must enter the epiphysis perpendicular to physeal plate of femoral head and must cross it, but well short of subchondral cortex.

Reduction

- It is very controversial, becoming timely

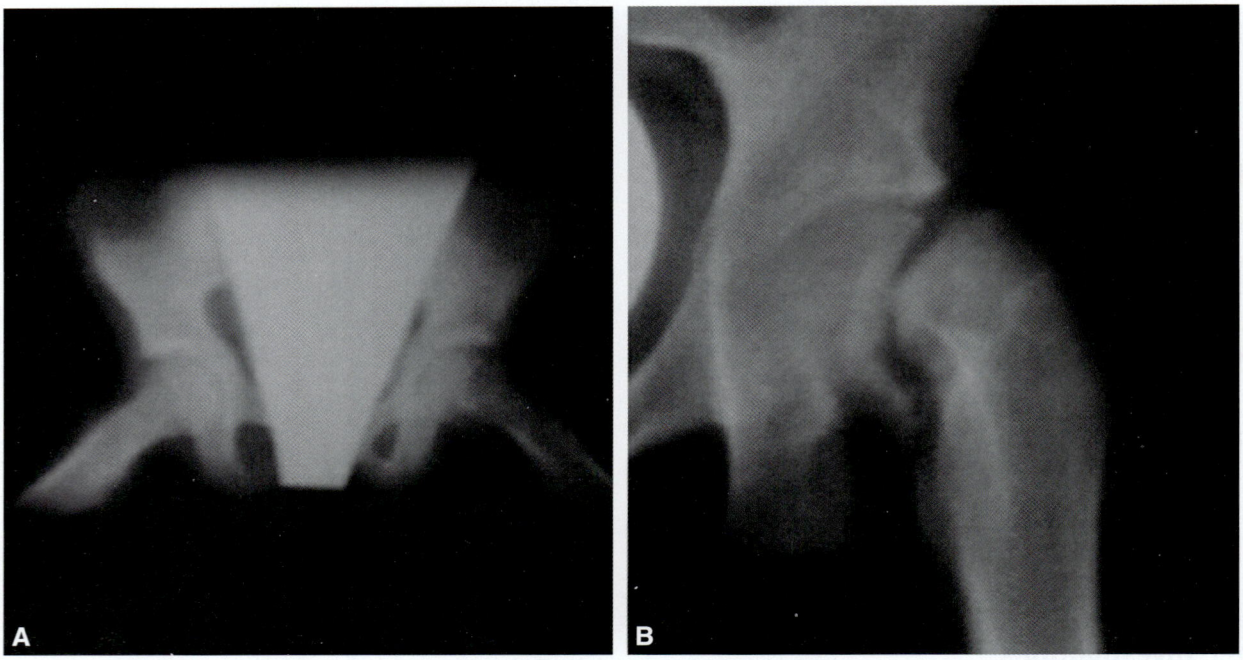

Figs 24.62A and B: (A) Frog leg view; (B) AP view showing SCFE

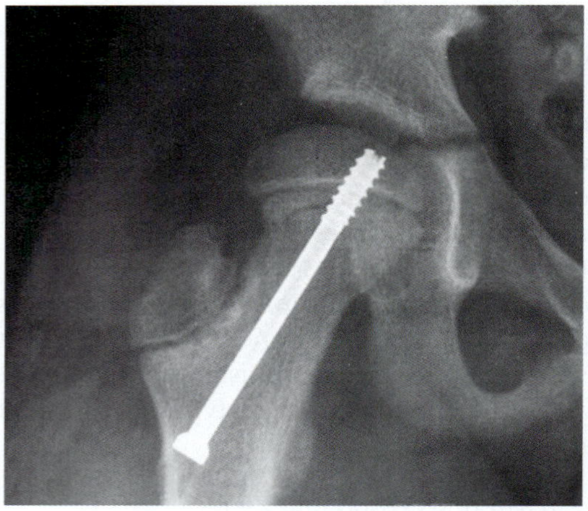

Fig. 24.63: Internal fixation, with single cannulated screws in SCFE

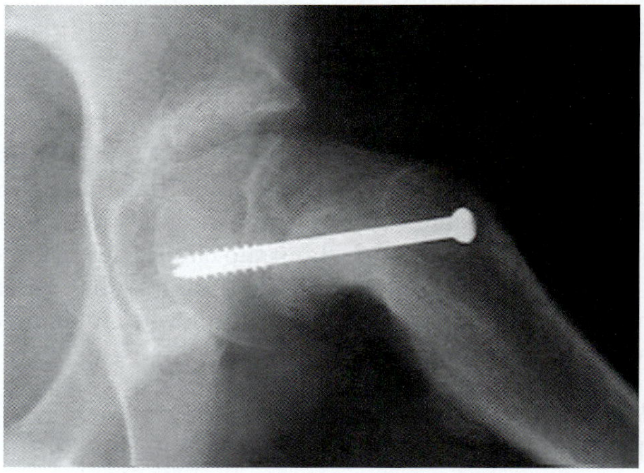

Fig. 24.64: Screw fixation in case of stable SCFC

- Reduction gives poor results especially in a chronic SCFE
- Necessity
  - In mild cases, not required
  - Moderate, probably not required
  - Unstable, severe slips
- Can make pinning technically easier

Bone Peg Epiphysiodesis (Fig. 24.65)

Advantages

- Popularity increased after complication followed after pin or screw penetration into joint.
- Rapid physeal closure and low incidence of complication.
- Useful in moderate or severe slips.

Disadvantages

- Need longer operating time, increased blood loss, longer hospitilization and rehabilitation.
- Bad results in mild acute and chronic slips.

Osteotomy (Fig. 24.66)

Indication

- Moderately or severely displaced chronic slips

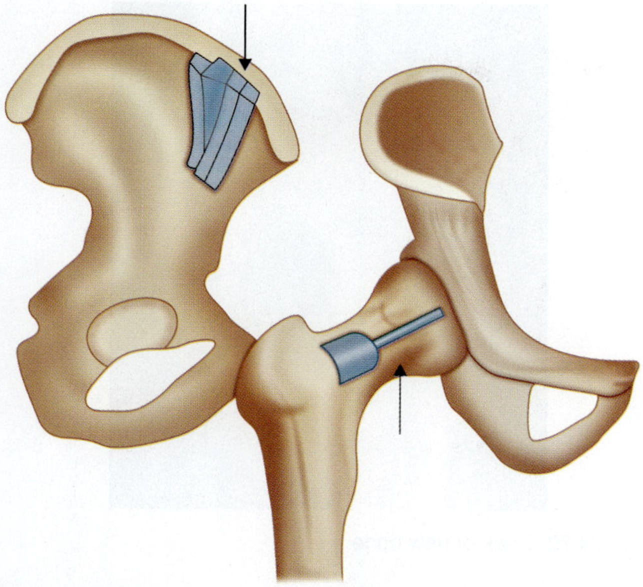

Fig. 24.65: Bone peg epiphysiodesis

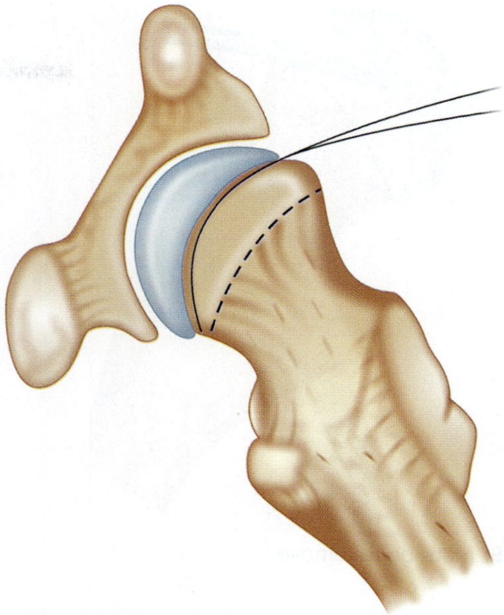

Fig. 24.67: Osteotomy made distal to physis

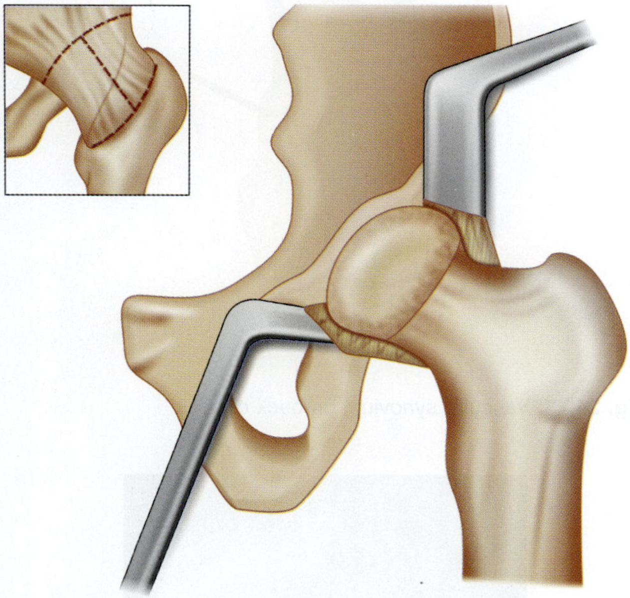

Fig. 24.66: Cuneiform osteotomy of femoral neck, joint capsule incised longitudinally

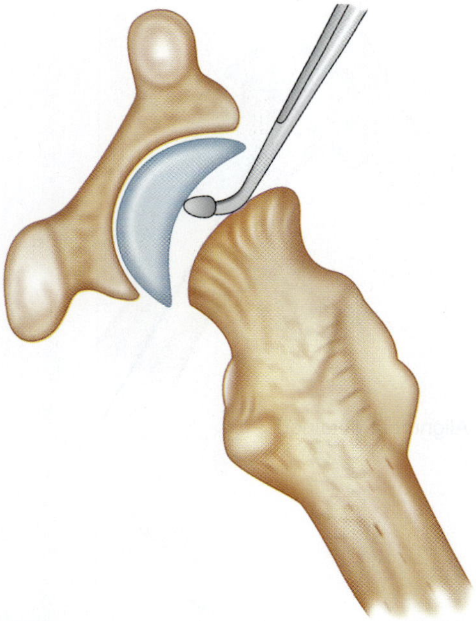

Fig. 24.68: Wedge of bone removed

- Malunion of a chronic slip in poor position
- Femoral neck osteotomies.

Cuneiform osteotomy of femoral neck by Fish (Figs 24.66 to 26.71).

Cuneiform osteotomy of femoral neck by Duun (Figs 24.72 to 24.76).

Compensatory basilar osteotomy of femoral neck by Kramer (Figs 24.77 to 24.79).

Cross osteotomy of head (Fig. 24.80)

Extracapsular base of neck osteotomy by Abraham (Figs 24.81 to 24.84).

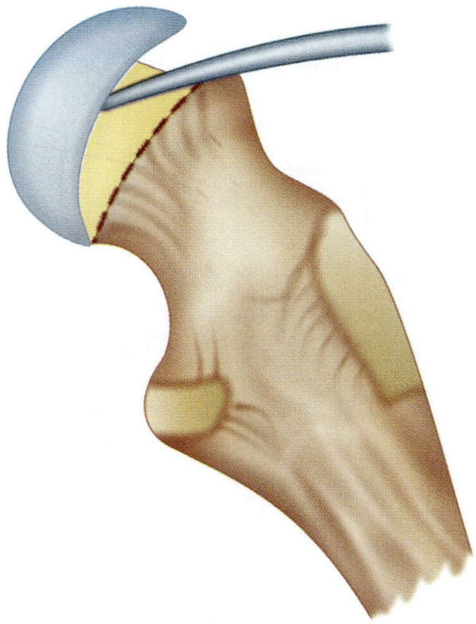

Fig. 24.69: More bone remove

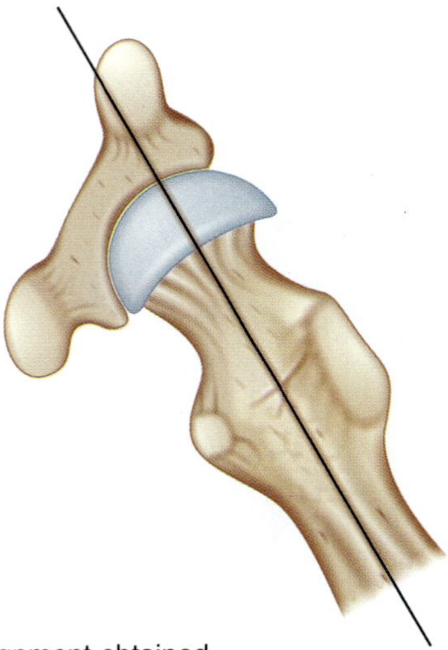

Fig. 24.70: Alignment obtained

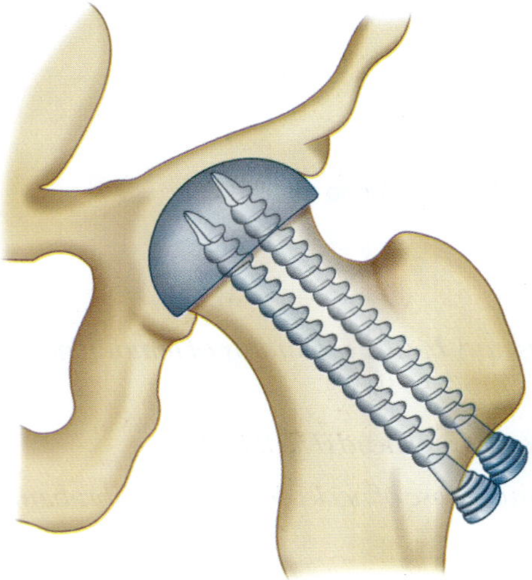

Fig. 24.71: Epiphysis fixed with pins

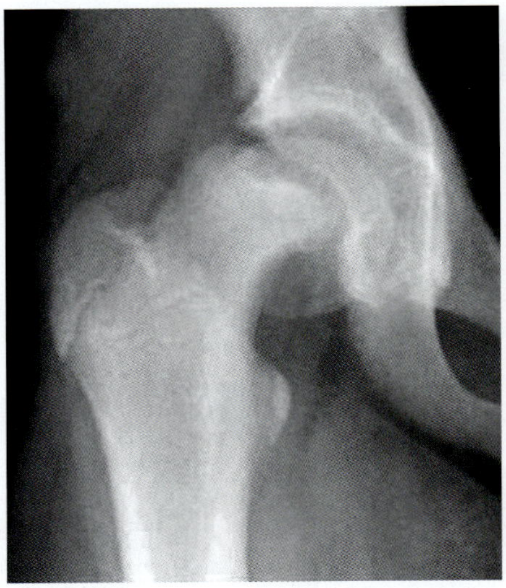

Fig. 24.72: Beak of new bone

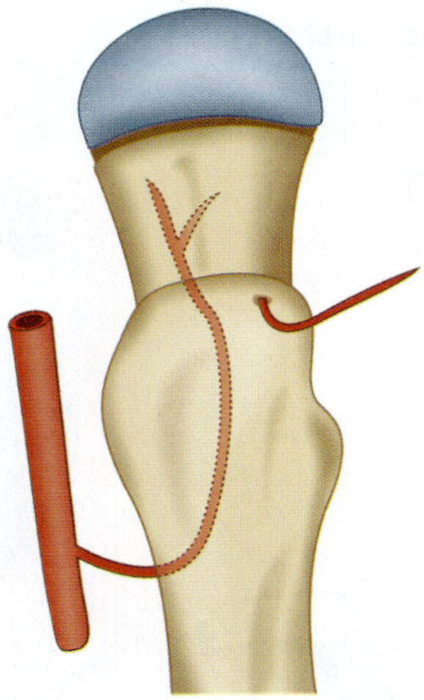

Fig. 24.73: Vascular synovium on back of neck

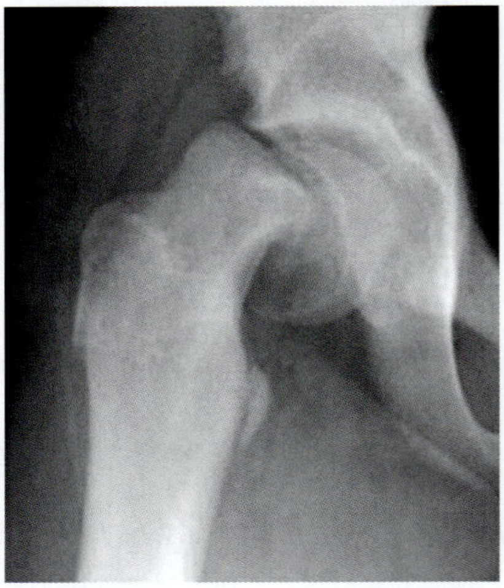

Fig. 24.74: Incision in synovium and head detached, preserve blood supply and exposing beak of new bone

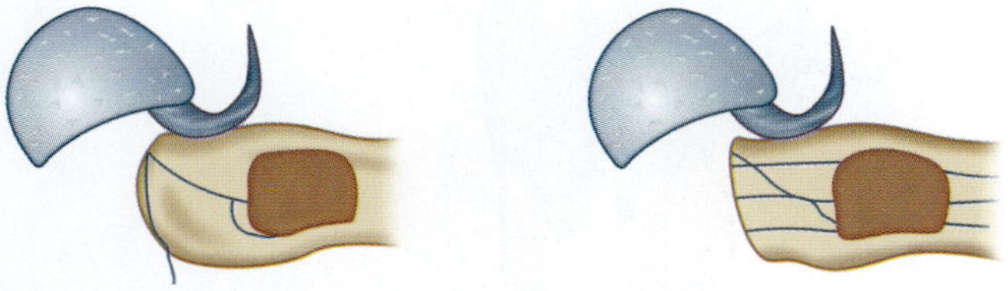

Fig. 24.75: Beak removed and threaded pins inserted

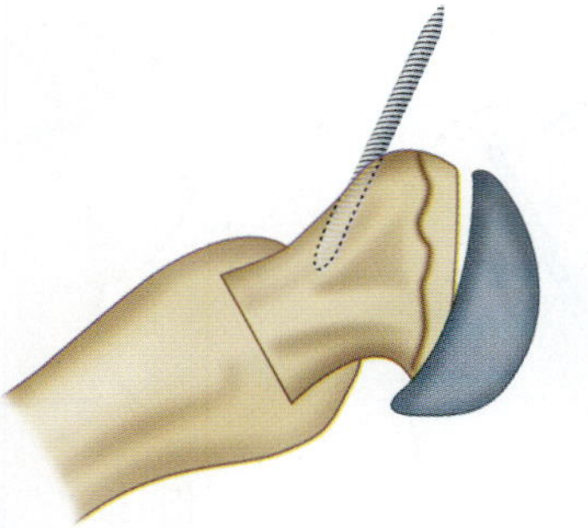

Fig. 24.78: Steinmann pin inserted into femoral neck

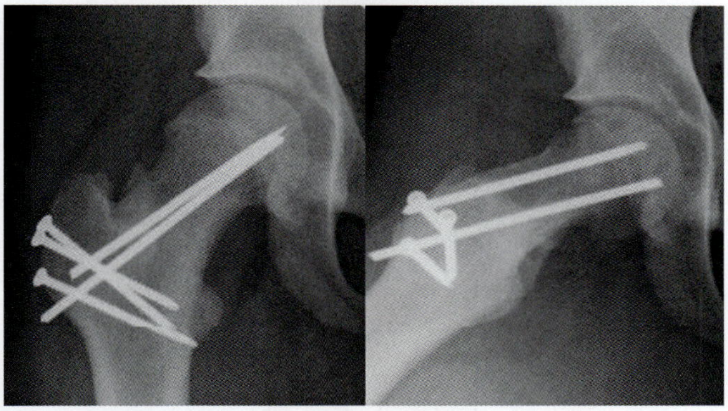

Fig. 24.76: Head square on neck and deformity is reduced

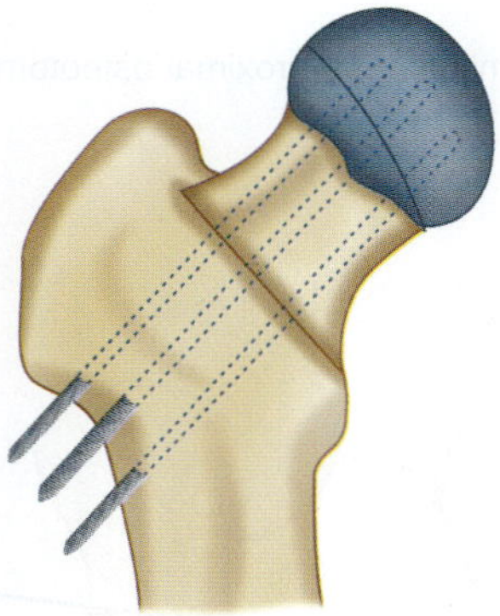

Fig. 24.79: Osteotomy closed and pins inserted from outer cortex of shaft through neck

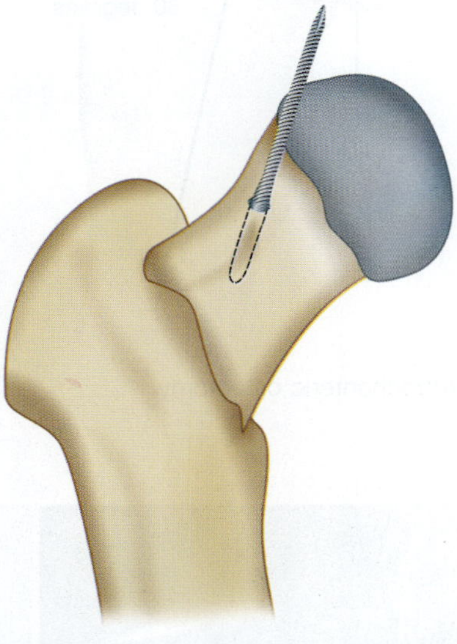

Fig. 24.77: Widest part of wedge in line with widest part of slip

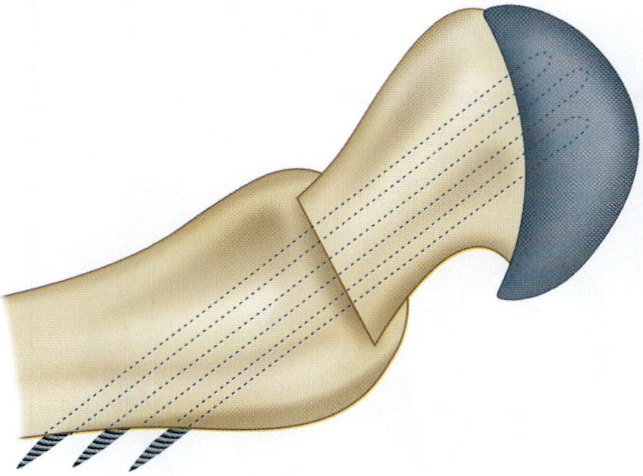

Fig. 24.80: Pins fix osteotomy and cross physis, prevent further slip

Intertrochanteric Osteotomy (Figs 24.85 and 24.86)

Slip capital femoral epiphysis (SCFE), when chronically slipped and united in poor position, a trochanteric osteotomy to produce an opposite deformity may be indicated.

Biplane Wedge Osteotomy by Southwick

- Transverse line drawn on anterior and lateral surface of bone.
- At level of lesser trochanter, junction of lateral and anterior surface identified.

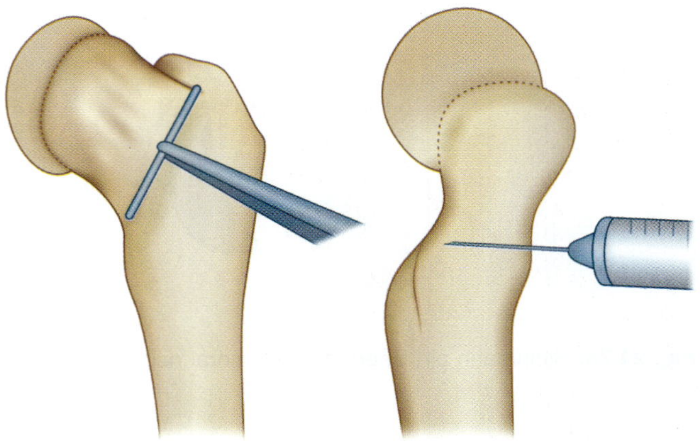

Fig. 24.81: Determination of proximal osteotomy cut

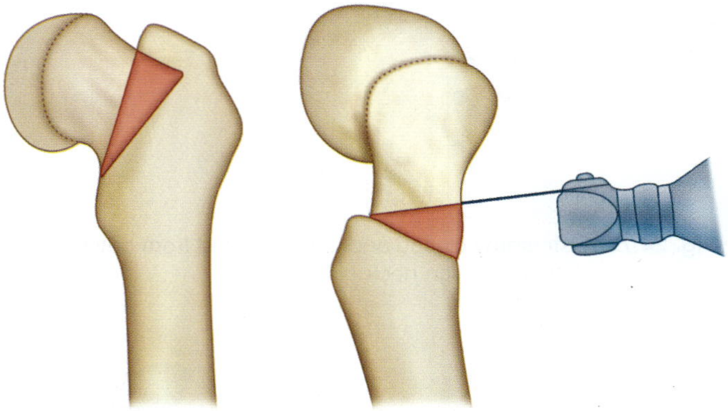

Fig. 24.82: Osteotomy cut made

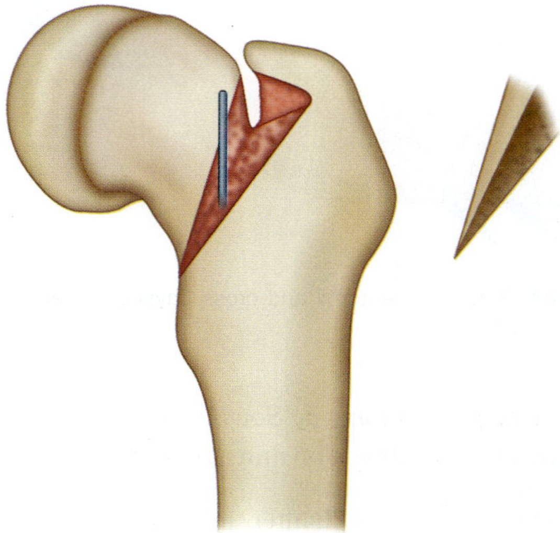

Fig. 24.83: Removal of bony wedge

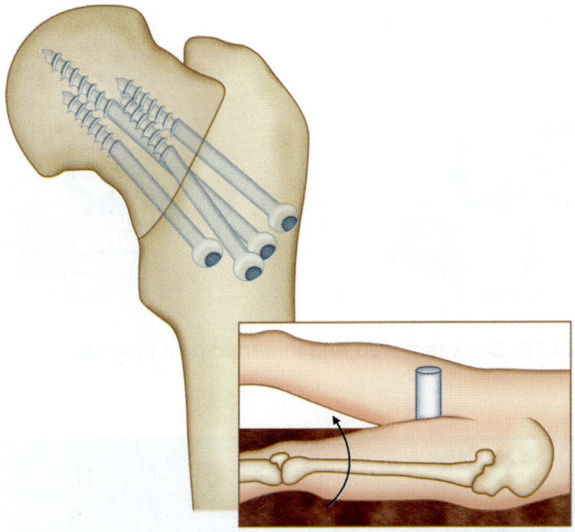

Fig. 24.84: Fixation with cannulated screw

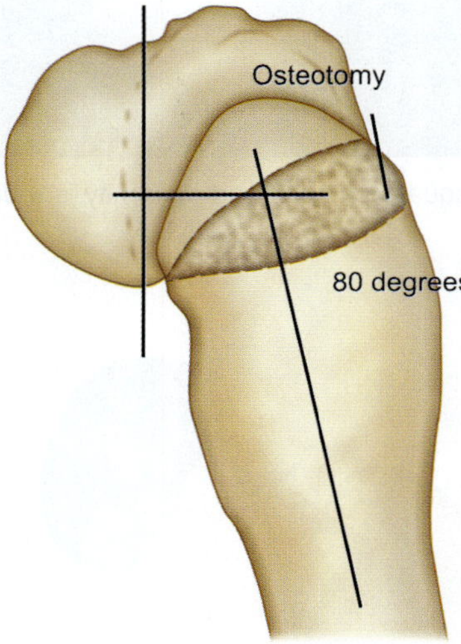

Fig. 24.85: Intertrochanteric osteotomy

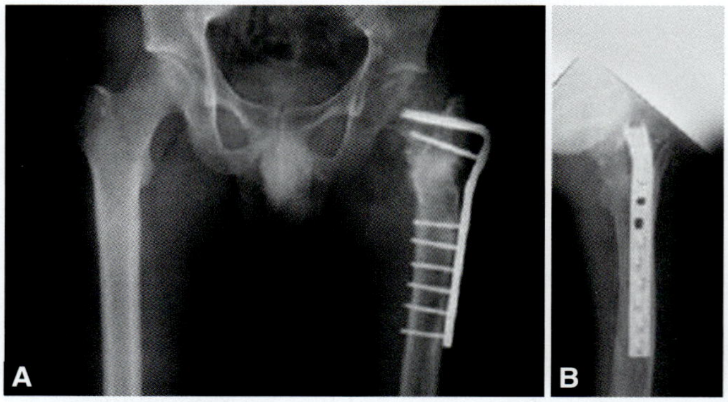

Figs 24.86A and B: After osteotomy

■ Complications

AVN

Etiology

- Single most repeatable finding is reduction.
- *Stable SCFE:* Iatrogenic with reduction
- Unstable SCFE
  - More likely the result of slip, not reduction
  - Immediate reduction and fixation vs traction prior to fixation to reduce AVN
  - One screw vs two
  - Role of pretreatment bone scan
- Chondrolysis associations
  - Five to seven percent of SCFE
  - Increased incidence in more severe slips
  - Increased with spica casts
  - Pin penetration.

Chondrolysis

Diagnosis

- *Clinical:* Pain out of proportion to SCFE severity
- *Radiographic:*
  - Increased joint space narrowing 50 percent
  - Persistent juxta-articular osteoporosis
  - Subchondral errosion of femoral head/acetabulum
- *Bone scan:* Marked periarticular uptake.

Treatment

- Remove protruding pins
- Rest and NWB
- NSAID.

ACETABULAR FRACTURES

Acetabular fractures generally are caused by high energy trauma and associated injuries are common. Treatment should follow advanced trauma life support (ALTS) protocol with management of acetabular fractures appropriately integrated. The patient is placed in skeletal traction to maintain reduction, while the other acute injuries are treated. In general, operative treatment should not be considered emergency, except, in open fracture management. Fracture associated with irreducible dislocation of hip, to prevent avascular necrosis. In general, operative treatment should not be considered emergency, except, in open fracture management and fracture associated with irreducible dislocation of hip to prevent avascular necrosis.

■ Anatomy

Letournel and Judet, described the acetabulum as being composed of two columns in the shape of an inverted Y. These columns support the articular surface of the acetabulum. The columns are connected to the sacroiliac joint by a thick strut of bone, the sciatic buttress, as shown in Figures 24.87A and B.

Anterior column: It is formed by:

- Bone of the iliac crest
- Iliac spines
- Anterior half of the acetabulum
- Pubis (Fig. 24.88).

Posterior column: It is composed of:

- Ischium
- Ischial spine
- Posterior half of the acetabulum
- Dense bone forming the sciatic notch, as shown in Figure 24.88
- *Dome of the acetabulum:* It is the weight-bearing portion of the articular surface that supports the femoral head, as shown in Figure 24.89.

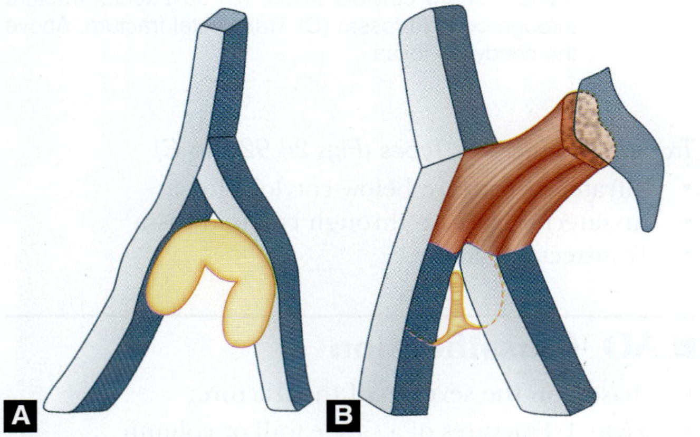

Figs 24.87A and B: Acetabular columns supporting articular surfaces of the acetabulum, with sciatic buttress

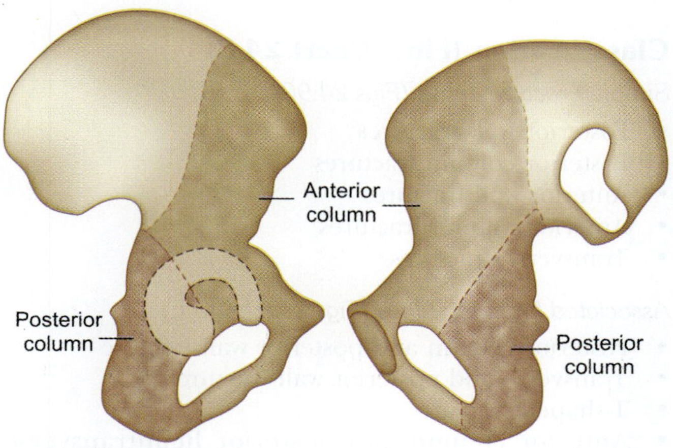

Fig. 24.88: Anterior and posterior columns around acetabulum

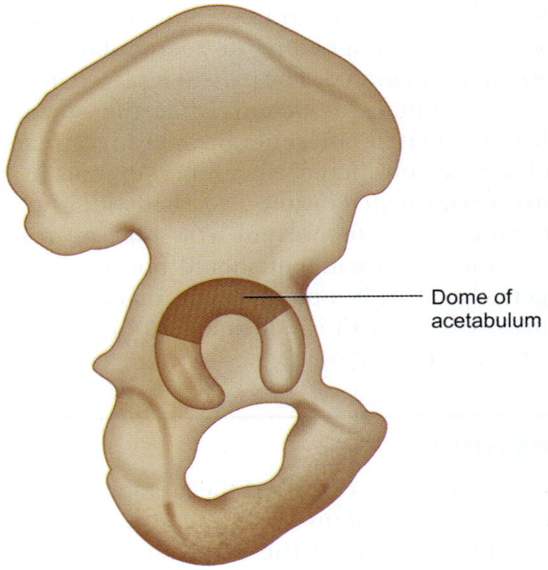

Fig. 24.89: Dome of the acetabulum (gray surface)

Flow chart 24.3: Letournel and Judet classification of acetabular fracture

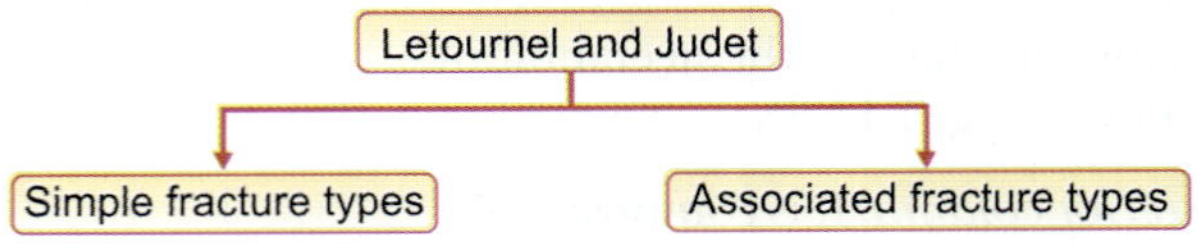

The column concept is used in

- Classification of these fractures
- Fracture patterns
- Operative approaches
- Internal fixation.
- Anatomical restoration of the dome with concentric reduction of the femoral head is the goal in both nonoperative and operative management.

Classification (Flow Chart 24.3)

Simple Fracture Types (Figs 24.90A to E)

- Posterior wall fractures
- Posterior column fractures
- Anterior wall fractures
- Anterior column fractures
- Transverse fractures

Associated Fracture Types (Figs 24.91A to E)

- Posterior column and posterior wall fracture
- Transverse and posterior wall fracture
- T-shaped fracture
- Anterior column and posterior hemitransverse fracture
- Complete both column fracture.

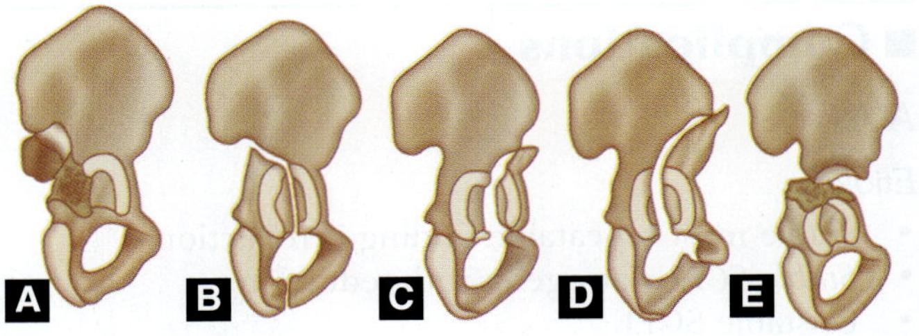

Figs 24.90A to E: Simple fracture type of acetabular fracture—(A) Posterior wall fractures; (B) Posterior column fractures; (C) Anterior wall fractures; (D) Anterior column fractures; (E) Transverse fractures

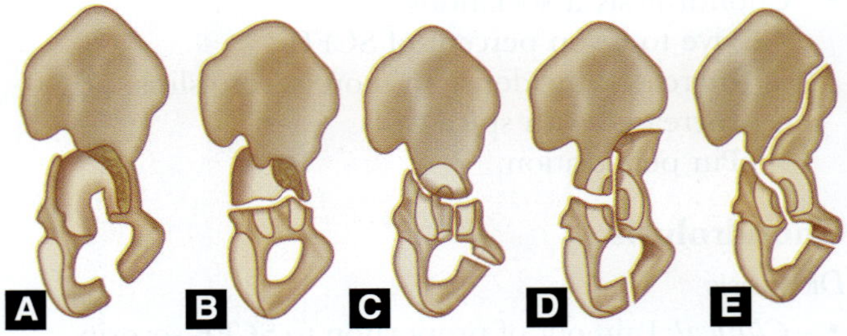

Figs 24.91A to E: Associated fractures types of acetabular fracture—(A) Posterior column and posterior wall fracture; (B) Transverse and posterior wall fracture; (C) T-shaped fracture; (D) Anterior column and posterior hemitransverse fracture; (E) Complete both column fracture

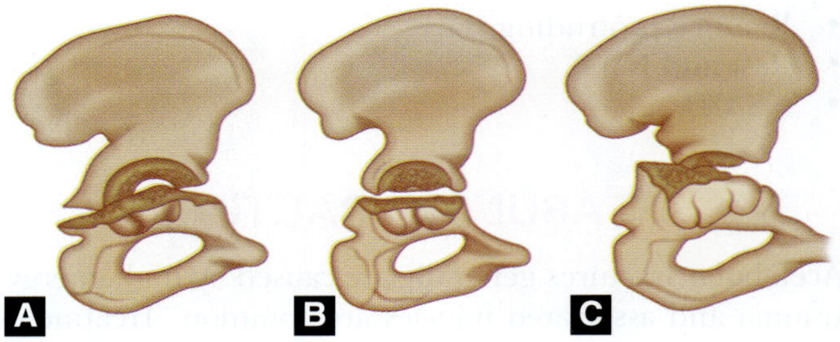

Figs 24.92A to C: Transverse fractures types—(A) Infratectal fracture below cotyloid fossa; (B) Juxtatectal fracture through cotyloid fossa; (C) Transtectal fracture. Above the condyloid fossa

Transverse Fractures Types (Figs 24.92A to C)

- Infratectal fracture below cotyloid fossa
- Juxtatectal fracture through cotyloid fossa
- Transtectal fracture.

■ AO Classification

It is based on the severity of the fracture:

- *Type A:* Fractures of a single wall or column
- *Type B:* Fractures of both anterior and posterior columns

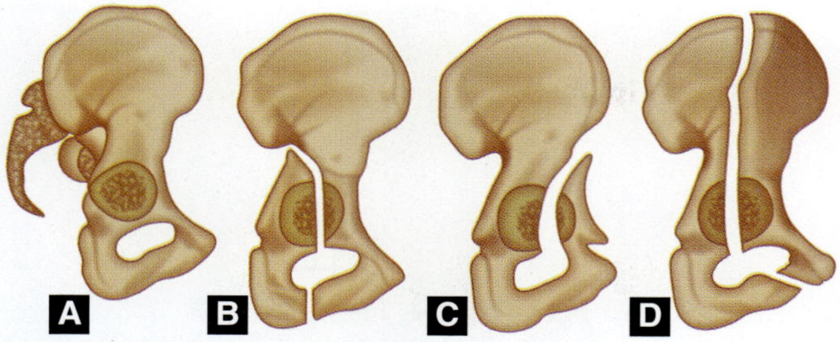

Figs 24.93A to D: Type A fractures—(A) Posterior wall fracture; (B) Posterior column fracture; (C) Anterior wall fracture; (D) Anterior column fracture

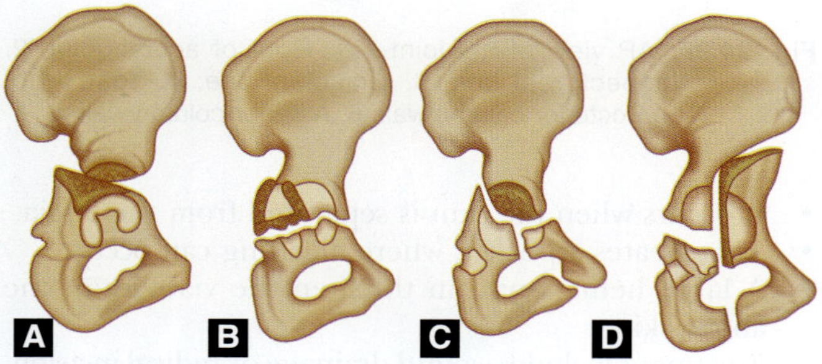

Figs 24.94A to D: Type B fractures—(A) Transverse fracture; (B) Transverse and posterior wall fracture; (C) T-shaped fracture; (D) Anterior wall/column and posterior hemitransverse fracture

- *Type C:* Fractures of both columns, but all articular segments are detached from the remaining segment of intact ilium
- Each type has subtypes 1, 2, 3 depending on the characteristics of the fracture.

Type A fractures (Figs 24.93A to D)
- Posterior wall fracture
- Posterior column fracture
- Anterior wall fracture
- Anterior column fracture.

Type B fractures (Figs 24.94A to D)
- Transverse fracture
- Transverse and posterior wall fracture
- T-shaped fracture.

Type C fractures (Figs 24.95A to C)
- Anterior wall/column and posterior hemitransverse fracture
- ACF extending of iliac crest
- ACF extending to anterior border ilium
- Fractures enters sacroiliac joint.

Tiles Classification

Tile proposed adding qualifiers, i.e. the factors that affect the prognosis of the injury to the AO classification. These include:

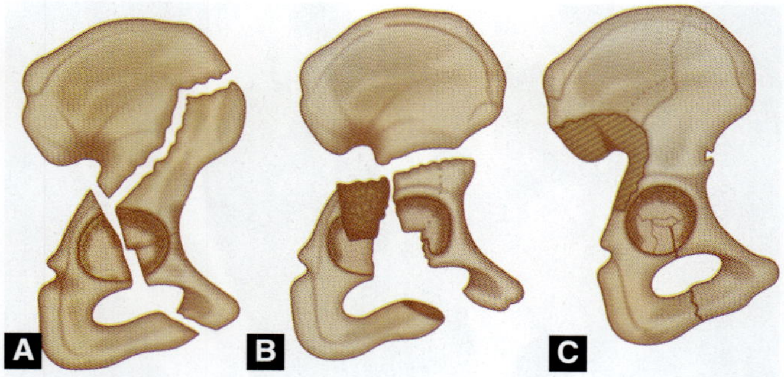

Figs 24.95A to C: Type C fractures—(A) ACF extending to iliac crest; (B) ACF extending to anterior border of ilium; (C) Fractures enters sacroiliac joint

- Femoral head subluxation or dislocation
- Acetabular or femoral articular surface damage
- Intra-articular fragments
- Non-displaced fractures.

Central Fracture Dislocation (Figs 24.96A and B)

There are two types of central fracture dislocation:

Group I: Fracture with an intact weight-bearing articular surface. It is caused due to forces along the femur and direct forces to the trochanter.

Group II: Acetabulum is reduced to bag of bones. It is caused by direct injury to the trochanter or pelvis.

Mechanism of Injury (Table 24.5)

Acetabular fractures are generally caused by high energy trauma. These fractures occur as force is transmitted from the femur to the pelvis via femoral head. The fracture pattern depends on:
- Position of the hip at the time of injury
- Direction of the impact
- Magnitude of the impact
- Strength of the bone, as in osteoporotic bones, there may be low energy trauma.

Clinical Picture

- Acetabular fractures are usually associated with other injuries
- Treatment should follow advanced trauma life support (ATLS) protocol with management of acetabular fractures appropriately integrated.
- The patient is placed in skeletal traction to maintain reduction, while the other acute injuries are treated.
- Any neurological and vascular injuries should be looked for.

Morel-Lavallee Lesion
- It may occur in both pelvic and acetabulur fractures with a shear component to the injury.

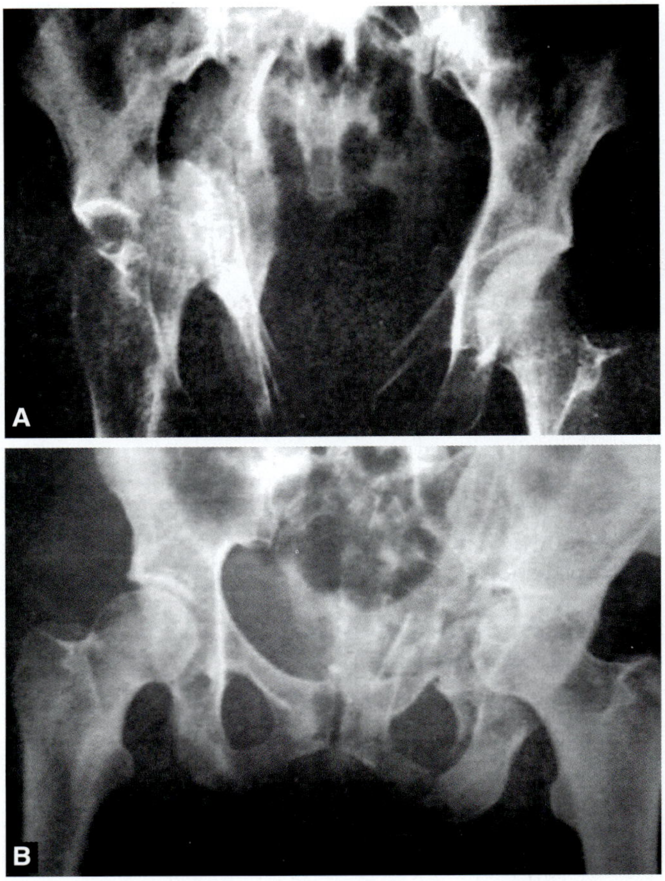

Figs 24.96A and B: Central fracture dislocation of acetabulum—(A) Group I fracture, with an intact weight-bearing articular surface; (B) Group II, acetabulum is reduced to bag of bones, caused by direct injury to the trochanter and pelvis

Table 24.5: Mechanism of injury and fracture pattern, force and position of hip during injury

Force	*Hip abduction*	*Hip rotation*	*Fracture pattern*
Along axis of femoral neck	Neutral	Neutral	Anterior column and posterior hemitransverse
	Neutral	25° ER	Anterior column
	Neutral	50° ER	Anterior wall
	Neutral	20° IR	T-shaped
	Neutral	50° IR	Posterior column
	Adduction	20° IR	Transtectal transverse
	Abduction	20° IR	Juxta/infratectal transverse
Along axis of femoral shaft (hip flexed 90°)	Neutral	Any	Posterior wall
	Abduction	Any	Transverse and posterior wall
	Adduction	Any	Posterior hip dislocation
Along axis of femoral shaft (hip extended)	Neutral	Any	Posterosuperior fracture of posterior wall
	Abduction	Any	Transtectal transverse

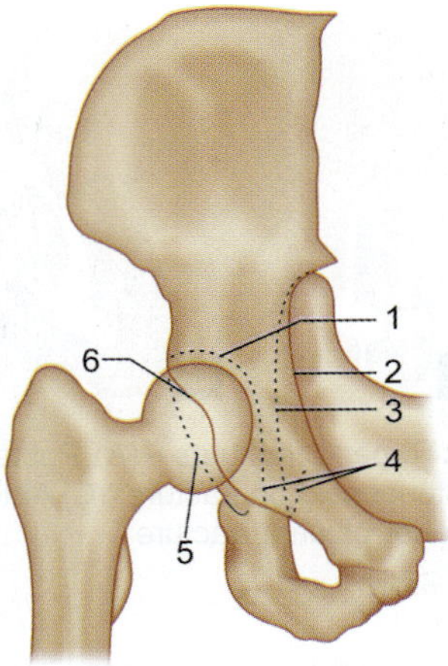

Fig. 24.97: AP view of hip joint— 1. Roof of acetabulum; 2. Iliopectoreal line; 3. Ilioischial line; 4. Tear drop; 5. Posterior column/wall; 6. Anterior column/wall

- It occurs when the skin is separated from the fascia.
- This creates a pocket, where bleeding can occur
- A large hematoma can threaten the viability of the above skin.
- Treatment includes wound drainage or radical incision.

Radiological Evaluation

The views to be taken are:
- Anteroposterior view
- Judet views
- *Iliac oblique*: The pelvis is rotated 45° with unaffected side up
- *Obturator oblique*: The pelvis is rotated 45°, with the injured side up. A proper view will show the coccyx centered over femoral head
- *Pelvic inlet view*: It is obtained by 40° caudocranial projection
- *Pelvic outlet view*: It is obtained by 40° craniocephalic projection.

Anteroposterior View (Fig. 24.97)

- *Iliopectinal line:* Anterior column
- *Ilioischial line:* Posterior column
- *Tear drop:* Relation of columns tear
- Roof of acetabulum
- Anterior column/wall
- Posterior column/wall

Iliac Oblique View

Figure 24.98 shows iliac oblique view.

Obturator Oblique View (Fig. 24.99)

- Roof arc measurements (Matta). It is done to quantify acetabular dome after fracture, as shown in Figures 24.100A to C.
  - Medial roof arc measured on AP view
  - Anterior roof arc measured on obturator oblique view

– *Posterior roof arc measurement on iliac oblique view:* It is measured by drawing a vertical line through the center of femoral head and second line through center of the head to the location of fracture at the articular surface. If the measurements in a displaced fractures are less than 45°, operative treatment is indicated.

Spur Sign (Figs 24.101A and B)

- It is demonstrated on obturator iliac view
- Pathogonomic of both column fracture
- It represents the remaining portion of ilium still attached to sacrum and is seen projected lateral to medially displaced acetabulum.

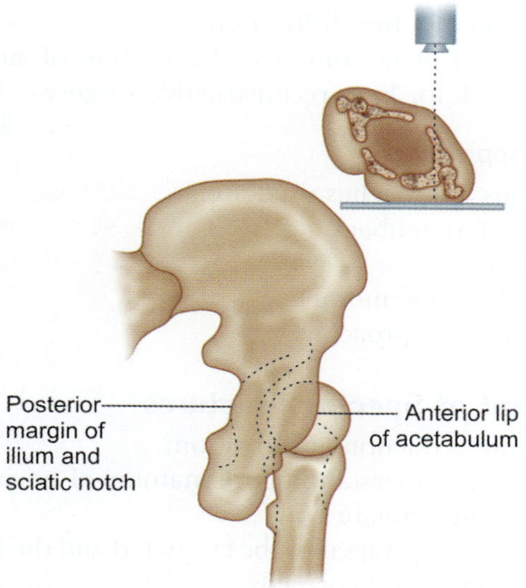

Fig. 24.98: Iliac oblique view

Inlet and Outlet Views (Figs 24.102 and 24.103)

- These views are not mandatory for acetabular fractures
- These can be done, to diagnose and characterize concurrent injuries to the pelvic ring.

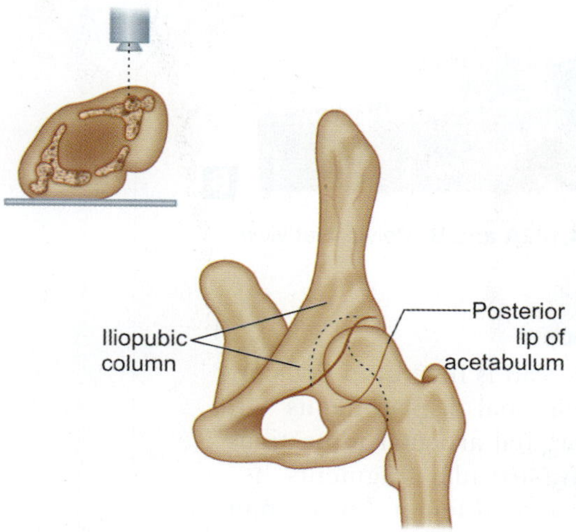

Fig. 24.99: Obturator oblique view

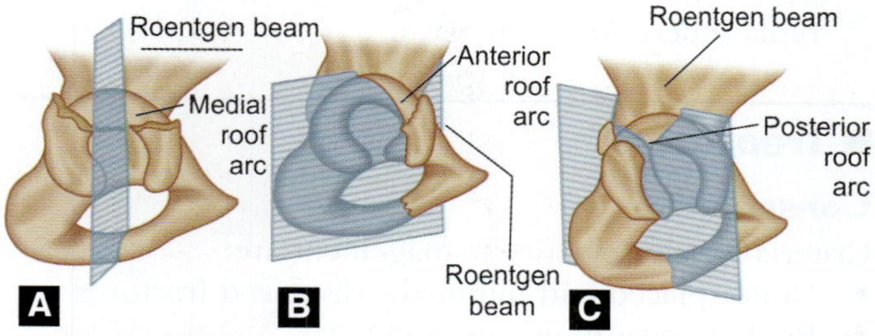

Figs 24.100A to C: (A) Medial roof arc measurement on AP; (B) Anterior roof arc on obturator oblique view; (C) Posterior roof arc measurement on iliac oblique view

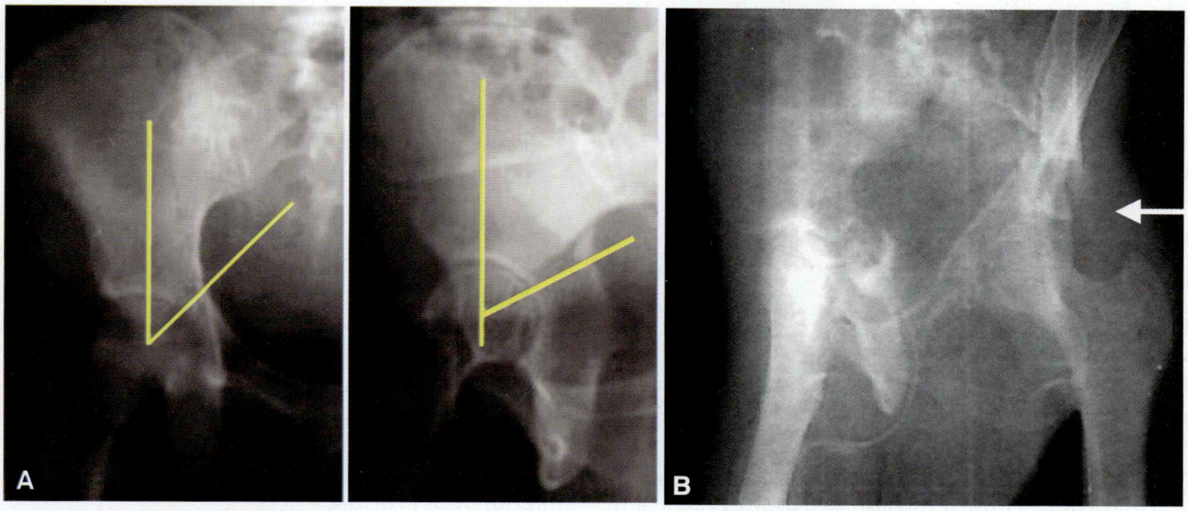

Figs 24.101A and B: Spur sign

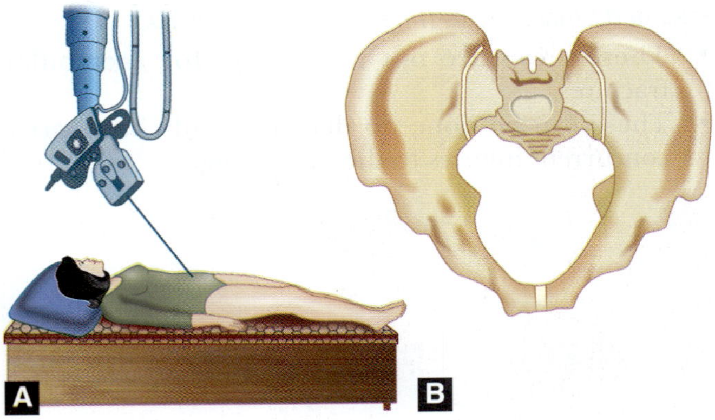

Figs 24.102A and B: Pelvic inlet view

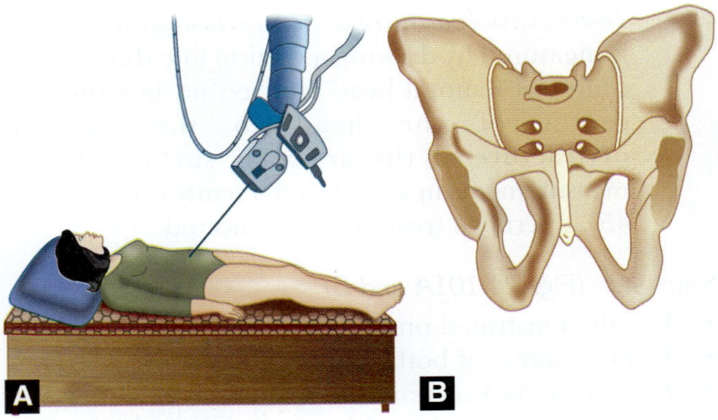

Figs 24.103A and B: Pelvic outlet view

CT Scan

- CT scan is helpful in detecting
- Rotational displacements
- Marginal articular impactions
- Intra-articular fragments
- Associated femoral head injuries
- Accurate assessment of size of a posterior wall fragment
- 3D CT is helpful for understanding the relationship between multiple sites of injury, but is not a replacement for plain X-ray.

Treatment

Conservative

Criteria for conservative management are:

- Nondisplaced and minimally displaced fractures
- Roof arc measurements >45°
- No femoral head subluxation on three X-rays, taken without traction
- Fractures with displacement, but the region of the joint involved is unimportant prognostically
- Secondary congruence in both column fractures
- No fracture involvement in cranial 10 mm of joint on CT (CT subchondral arc)
- For posterior wall fractures, <40 percent of width of wall on CT
- Medical contraindication to surgery
- Local soft tissue problems.

Operative

Criteria for operative treatment are:

- Roof arc measurements >45°
- Subluxation of femoral head from a displaced acetabular fracture noted on any of three standard views
- >50 percent involvement of the articular surface of posterior wall or clinical instability with hip flexion to 90° in posterior wall fractures
- Incarcerated fragments in acetabulum after closed reduction of a hip dislocation
- Prevention of nonunion and retention of sufficient bone stock for later reconstructive surgery.

Surgical Approaches

The various approaches used are:

- Kocher-Langenbeck
- Ilioinguinal
- Extended iliofemoral
- Combined approaches.

Treatment of Specific Fractures

For accurate reduction and fixation:

- Thorough understanding of anatomy of normal and injured innominate bone.
- Preoperative X-rays must be evaluated and the fracture pattern classified correctly.
- The presence and number of free articular fragments and areas of marginal impaction must be identified.

Posterior Wall Fractures (Fig. 24.104)

- Most common of the acetabular fractures
- Treated through Kocher-Langenbeck approach
- Patient is positioned in either prone or lateral position
- Fixation is done by using lag screws and reconstruction plate placed from the ischium over the retroacetabular surface onto the lateral ilium.

Posterior Column Fracture

- Relatively uncommon fractures
- Kocher-Langenbeck is used
- Rotational deformity is corrected with a shanz in ischium to control rotation.
- Fixation is done with lag screw combined with a contoured reconstruction plate along the posterior column, as shown in Figure 24.105.

Anterior Wall Fracture

- Isolated anterior wall fractures are uncommon

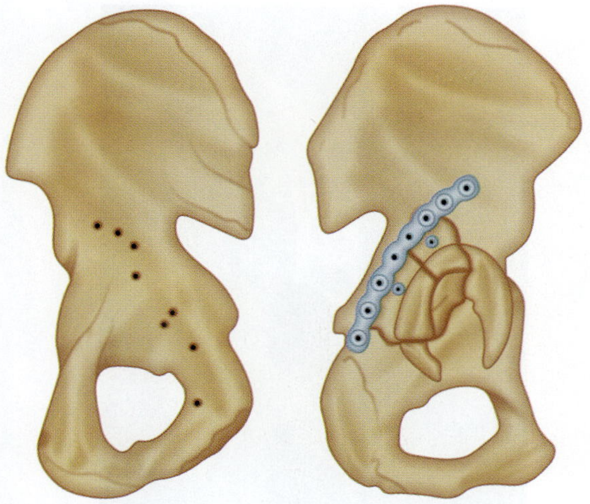

Fig. 24.104: Fixation of posterior wall fracture, using lag screws and reconstruction plate

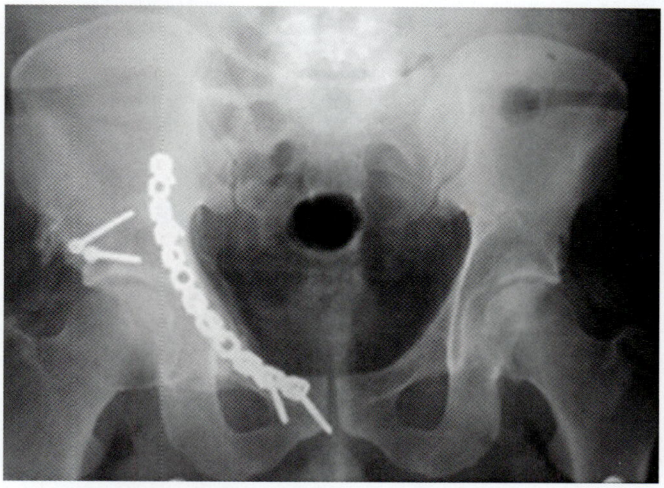

Fig. 24.106: Anterior wall fracture fixation with a buttress plate from iliac fossa to superior ramus

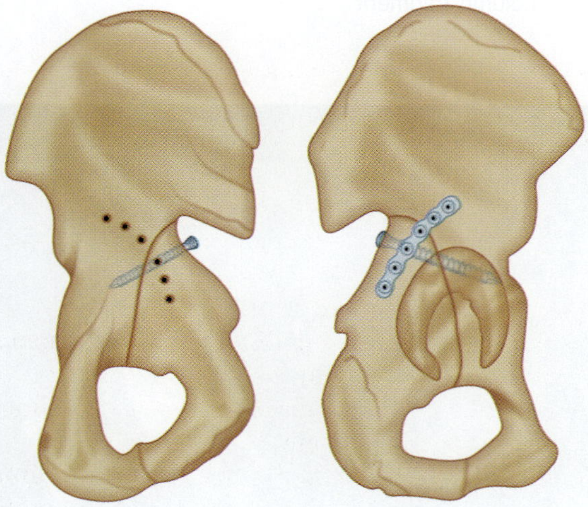

Fig. 24.105: Posterior column fracture repair, with lag screw combined with a contoured reconstruction plate

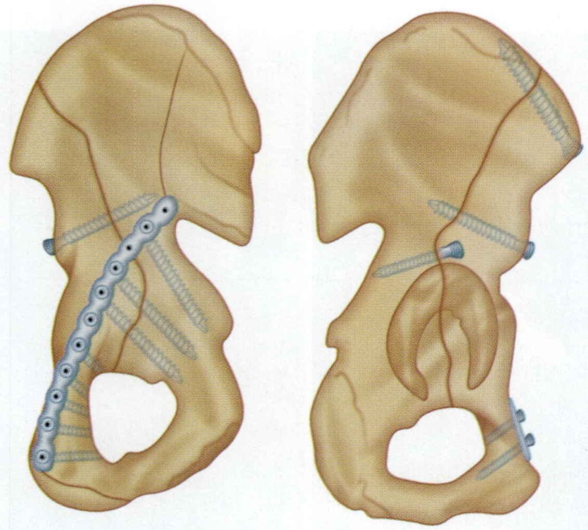

Fig. 24.107: Anterior column fracture, fixed with a contoured plate along the pelvic brim and several lag screws

- They are sometimes associated with anterior hip dislocation
- Ilioinguinal or iliofemoral approaches are used for its reduction
- Fractures are fixed with a buttress plate from iliac fossa to superior ramus, as shown in Figure 24.106
- Interfragmentary screws are also used.

Anterior Column Fractures

- These fractures are approached through ilioinguinal or iliofemoral approach.
- They are fixed with a contoured plate along the pelvic brim and several lag screws are placed between inner and outer tables of innominate bone, as illustrated in Figure 24.107.

Transverse Fractures

- Posterior, ilioinguinal or combined approach
- Posterior fixation, by buttress plate along posterior column with anterior fixation with 3.5 mm lag screw from above the acetabulum
- Anterior fixation, by contoured plate along the pelvic brim with lag screw directed down the posterior column, as shown in Figures 24.108 and 24.109.

Posterior Column and Posterior Wall

- Kocher-Langenbeck approach with or without trochanteric osteotomy.
- Column fracture is reduced first and a short reconstruction plate is placed posteriorly along posterior edge of column.

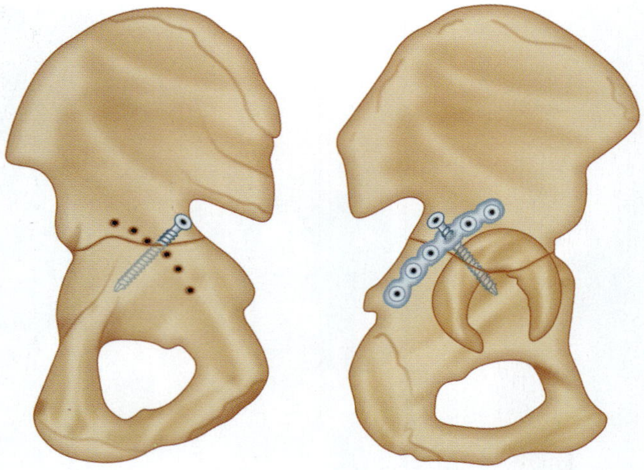

Fig. 24.108: Anterior fixation, by contoured plate along the pelvic brim with lag screw directed down the posterior column

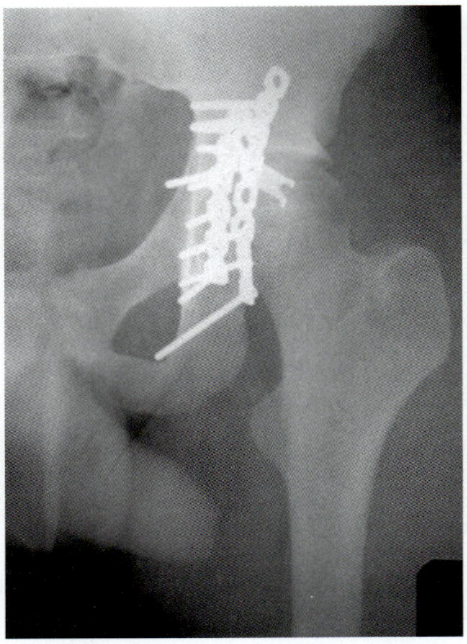

Fig. 24.110: A separate plate is used for fixing posterior wall and column fragment

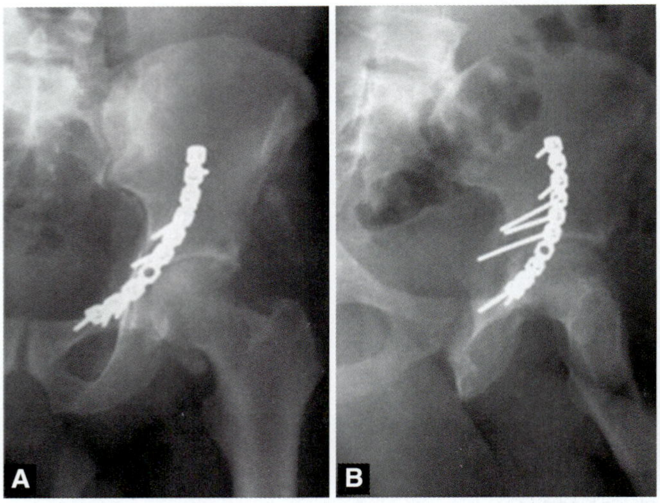

Figs 24.109A and B: X-ray showing the transverse fracture fixation

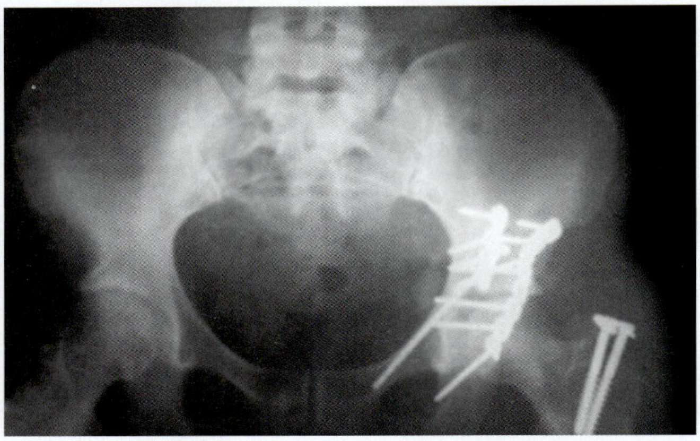

Fig. 24.111: Combined approach used for fixing transverse and posterior wall fracture

- A separate plate is used for wall fragment and screws through this plate, secure rotational reduction of posterior column, as shown in Figure 24.110.

Transverse Fracture and Posterior Wall

Combined approach is necessary, as the posterior wall fragment requires a posterior exposure, but anterior part of the transverse fracture is difficult to reduce through this approach. Fixation is variable depending on the specific fractures, as shown in Figure 24.111.

T-type and Anterior Column Posterior Hemitransverse Fractures

These two patterns can be treated by ilioinguinal approach. If both the anterior and posterior components of fracture are significantly displaced then combined approach is required. Fixation is done with a contoured plate placed along the pelvic brim with lag screws extending into either posterior/anterior column, as shown in Figure 24.112.

Both Column Fractures

These fractures can be treated through an anterior ilioinguinal approach, but a posterior apporach is required for sacroiliac joint involvement, a significant posterior wall fracture or intra-articular comminution. Reduction begins from most proximal part of fracture and proceeds towards joint. Fixation varies according to fracture pattern, as shown in Figure 24.113.

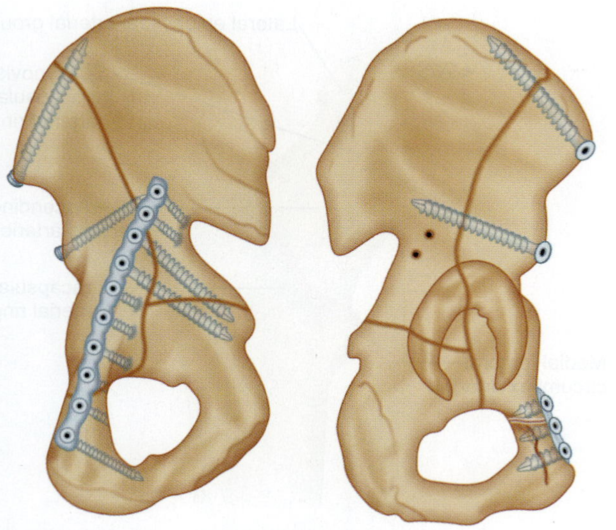

Fig. 24.112: T-type and anterior column posterior hemitransverse fractures reduction by ilioinguinal approach

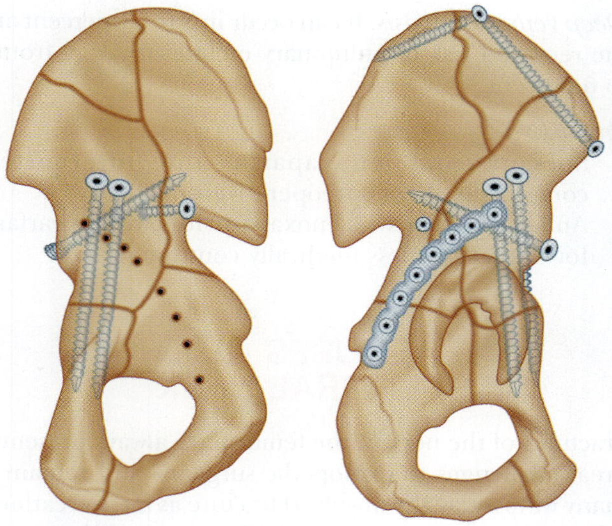

Fig. 24.113: Both column fracture reduction by ilioinguinal approach

Central Fracture Dislocation

Group I: Conservative treatment include traction applied in two planes, (1) Longitudinal traction to leg by Hamilton Russell, using a tibial Steinmann's pin, (2) Lateral traction, to correct central displacement of femoral head.

Operative treatment: Posterior approach is taken. Reduction is maintained, by a small four hole plate screwed into adjacent parts of iliac and ischial components.

Group II: *Conservative:* These fractures are better left in displaced portion or pulled out as far as longitudinal traction permits.

Postoperative Management

- Closed suction drain for two days
- Antibiotics for 5 days
- Passive motion of hip on second day
- Touch down ambulation with crutches on fourth day and progression depending on other injuries
- Minimal weight-bearing for eight weeks, for simple fractures and 12 weeks, in others.

Complications

- Post-traumatic arthritis
- Avascular necrosis of femoral head
- Infection
- Sciatic nerve palsies
- Heterotopic ossification
- Deep vein thrombosis

Post-traumatic arthritis: The incidence is about 17 percent. Imperfect reduction increases the chances of arthritis. Both column and transverse-posterior wall fractures have worse results than associated types: due to imperfect reduction. Even after perfect reduction, the rate of arthritis is about 10 percent. Primary total hip replacement (THR) can be done for a comminuted, incongruous both column fracture. Secondary THR has been done for post-traumatic arthritis, though loosening and revision rates for cemented acetabular sockets, is a common problem.

Avascular necrosis: More frequent in fractures associated with posterior dislocation. The rate after dislocation is about 7.5 percent. It is roentographically apparent within 2 years in most patients. Avascular necrosis (AVN) of posterior wall can be caused by the injury or by excessive exposure, as the only blood supply is the injured posterior capsule of the hip.

Infection: It occurs in 1 to 5 percent of cases. Factors which increase the risk of infection are:

- Suprapubic catheter in ilioinguinal approach
- Morel-Lavalle lesion

Sciatic nerve palsies: Due to initial injury, incidence is 10 to 15 percent. Due to surgery, incidence is 2 to 6 percent. It is more often associated with:

- Posterior fracture pattern
- Kocher-Langenbeck approach
- Extensile exposures.

Heterotopic ossification: Occurs in about 14 to 50 percent patients. More common after extensile or Kocher-Langenbeck approaches.

Prophylaxis

- *Indomethacin:* 25 mg TDS for 4 to 6 weeks.
- *Radiation:* One time dose of 700 cGy in patients, in whom indomethacin is contraindicated.

Deep vein thrombosis: It can occur in 8 to 61 percent and the reported risk of pulmonary embolism range from 2 to 6 percent.

Prophylaxis

- Subcutaneous enoxaparin and intermittent compression boots preoperatively.
- Anticoagulation, with enoxaparin followed by warfarin for 6 weeks, unless medically contraindicated.

FRACTURES OF THE FEMORAL NECK

Fractures of the neck of the femur have always presented great challenges to orthopedic surgeons and remain in many ways today the unsolved fracture as far as treatment and results are concerned. With life expectancy increasing with each decade, our society is becoming increasingly an active geriatric society, with significant numbers of hospitalized and nursing home patients with femoral neck fractures and their sequel.

Fracture Fixation

Femoral neck fractures in young patients usually are caused by high-energy trauma and often are associated with multiple injuries and high rates of osteonecrosis and nonunion. Results after this injury apparently depend on:

- The extent of the injury, such as the amount of displacement, the amount of comminution and whether the circulation has been disturbed.
- The adequacy of the reduction
- The adequacy of fixation.

Even when nondisplaced, there is no assurance that a fracture of the femoral neck will attain an excellent result. Early anatomical reduction, compression of the fracture and rigid internal fixation are used to promote union, but the surgeon probably has less control over osteonecrosis because the blood supply to the femoral head after femoral neck fracture is quite precarious. Crock described the blood supply to the proximal end of the femur, dividing it into three major groups:

- An extracapsular arterial ring located at the base of the femoral neck,
- Ascending cervical branches of the arterial ring on the surface of the femoral neck
- Arteries of the ligamentum teres, as shown in Figure 24.114.

The extracapsular arterial ring is formed posteriorly, by a large branch of the medial femoral circumflex artery and anteriorly by a branch from the lateral femoral circumflex artery. The ascending cervical branches or retinacular vessels ascend on the surface of the femoral neck in anterior, posterior, medial and lateral groups,

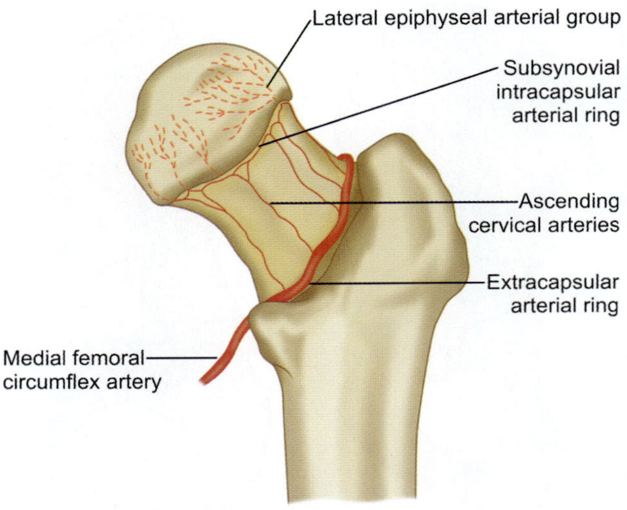

Fig. 24.114: Arteries of the ligamentum teres

the lateral vessels are the most important. Their proximity to the surface of the femoral neck makes them vulnerable to injury in femoral neck fractures. As the articular margin of the femoral head is approached by the ascending cervical vessels, a second less distinct ring of vessels is formed, referred by Chung as the subsynovial intra-articular arterial ring. It is from this ring of vessels that vessels penetrate the head and are referred to as the epiphyseal arteries, the most important being the lateral epiphyseal arterial group supplying the lateral weight-bearing portion of the femoral head. These epiphyseal vessels are joined by inferior metaphyseal vessels and vessels from the ligamentum teres.

Nonunion

Femoral neck fractures usually are entirely intracapsular and common to all intracapsular fractures, the synovial fluid bathing. The fracture may interfere with the healing process because the femoral neck essentially has no periosteal layer, all healing must be endosteal. Angiogenic-inhibiting factors in synovial fluid also can inhibit fracture repair. These factors, along with the precarious blood supply to the femoral head, make healing unpredictable and nonunions fairly frequent. With anatomical reduction and stable fixation, the incidence of nonunion should be acceptably low.

Osteonecrosis

As with nonunion, the development of osteonecrosis correlates with the extent of initial trauma and the displacement of the fracture, with some question concerning the tamponading effect of the intracapsular hematoma. Urgent, gentle reduction and fixation of these fractures should be done, especially in younger patients. They suggested that prompt reduction of the displacement possibly may open some of the retinacular vessels that are temporarily closed by kinking or stretching and rigid fixation may permit re-establishment of some vascular continuity that otherwise might not be preserved, if reduction and fixation are delayed. In the meta-analysis of Damany et al. however there was no statistically significant difference in osteonecrosis rates in fractures treated early (<12 hours) compared with fractures treated late (>12 hours) or in fractures treated with open reduction compared with closed reduction. Radiographic evidence of osteonecrosis does not always indicate a poor functional result and the late effects of osteonecrosis may take many years to develop. Some scientists showed that intracapsular pressures after femoral neck fractures are higher in nondisplaced fractures than in displaced fractures and Harper, Barnes and Gregg showed increased intraosseous pressure within the femoral head after intracapsular femoral neck fractures. Joint aspiration lowered the intraosseous pressure and increased the pulse pressure within the femoral head. They and others recommended routine aspiration or capsulotomy, to decompress this increased intracapsular pressure. No study to date has conclusively shown a decreased rate of osteonecrosis with routine capsulotomy or hip aspiration. We do not routinely decompress the hip joint by aspiration or capsulotomy in geriatric patients, but we may decompress the hip capsule in younger patients.

The method of fracture fixation can have an effect on the rate of osteonecrosis and nonunion with femoral neck fractures. The use of a single large compression hip screw for fixation of femoral neck fractures was shown by Madsen et al. and Christie et al. to result in lower rates of union for intracapsular fractures. In some intracapsular femoral neck fractures at the base of the femoral neck and in severely comminuted femoral neck fractures, however multiple pin fixations is not ideal because of the lack of an adequate posteromedial buttress. For these fractures, the use of a hip compression screw with side plate is indicated, usually with the addition of a supplemental antirotation screw, a short barrel and possibly a lateral buttress plate, if the fracture extends into lateral cortex. The adequacy of reduction attained with displaced femoral neck fractures has been shown to affect the rates of nonunion and osteonecrosis. Garden originally described his alignment index, as a guide to adequacy of a given reduction. On the anteroposterior view, the angle between the central compressive trabeculae within the femoral head and the medial cortex of the femur is measured. According to Garden, this angle is normally 160°, as shown in Figure 24.115. On the lateral view, the major trabeculae are in the same axis as the axis of the femoral neck or lie at an angle of 180°. Garden showed higher rates of union and lower rates of osteonecrosis, if the compressive trabeculae of the femoral head were aligned with the medial cortex of the femur on the anteroposterior view between an angle of 155° and 180°. On the lateral view, he described an acceptable reduction to be within the same range of 155 to 180°, although he strived to correct the entire anterior angulation, this is illustrated in Figure 24.116. He found that osteonecrosis was universal, when in the anteroposterior view, fractures were reduced with an alignment index of less than 150° or more than 185°, implicating angular and rotational malunion in the incidence of osteonecrosis. Other authors, such as Smyth and Shah, reported similar findings.

Multiple methods have been used to determine preoperatively the vascularity of the femoral head in femoral neck fractures. To date, bone scans have failed

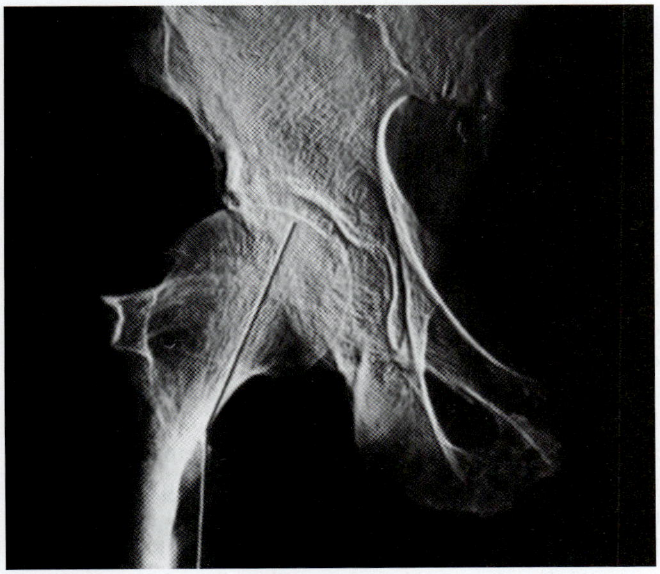

Fig. 24.115: The angle between the central compressive trabeculae, within the femoral head and the medial cortex of the femur is measured

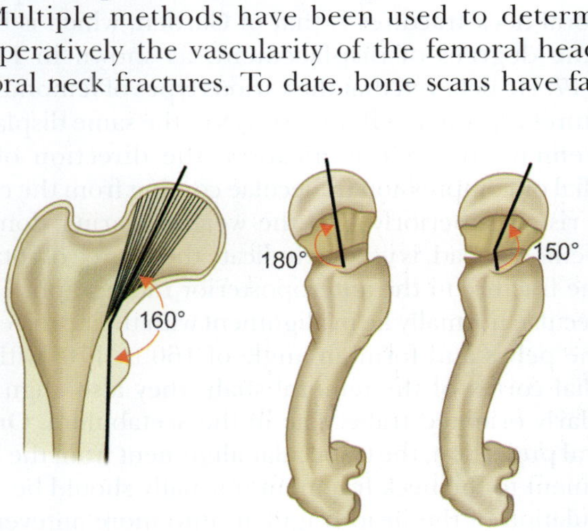

Fig. 24.116: On the lateral view, an acceptable reduction to be within the same range of 155–180°

to show adequate sensitivity or specificity to have useful predictive value. Speer et al. found no evidence of osteonecrosis within the first 48 hours after displaced fracture on standard T1 and T2 weighted MRI. They hypothesized that the fatty marrow within the femoral head was relatively resistant to the anoxic insult, with fat cell death occurring over 2 to 5 days and that this fatty marrow was responsible for the normal signal seen within the femoral head on MRI. A postoperative bone scan has been shown to correlate with eventual rates of nonunion and osteonecrosis in femoral neck fractures. Scientists showed that bone scans performed within 2 weeks of operative treatment were able to determine the healing course in 306 fractures (uneventful healing, hardware failure, nonunion and osteonecrosis) with a prognostic accuracy. The patients were followed, until fracture union until conversion to hip arthroplasty or for 2 years. Of these patients, some healed and had no evidence of osteonecrosis. Thirteen patients eventually had arthroplasty for osteonecrosis, nonunion or both.

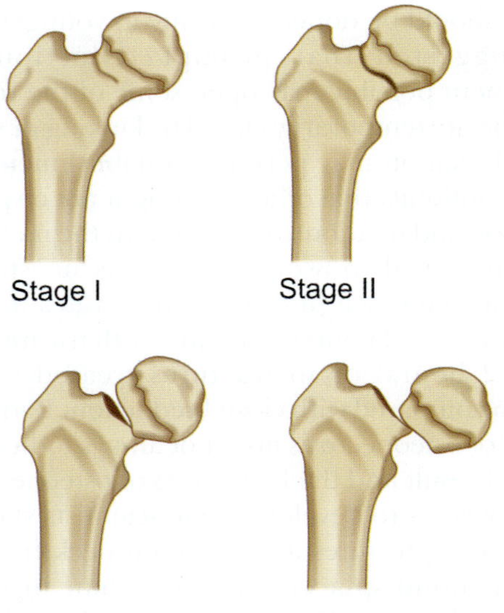

Fig. 24.117: Common classification of displaced femoral neck fractures, by Garden

■ Classification

Various classifications have been described for fractures of the femoral neck. Structurally, there are:

- impacted fractures,
- nondisplaced fractures and
- displaced fractures.

  Causatively, in addition to fractures resulting from trauma without other complicating conditions, there are:
  - stress fractures
  - pathological fractures
  - postirradiation fractures.

The latter three are discussed separately in this chapter. The most common classification of displaced femoral neck fractures is that of Garden, which is based on the degrees of displacement, as shown in Figure 24.117. He believed that the various types of femoral neck fractures represent different stages of the same displacing movement. In his classification, the direction of the medial or compression trabeculae coming from the calcar and rising superiorly into the weight-bearing dome of the femoral head, is used to indicate the degree of rotation of the fracture in the anteroposterior radiograph. These trabeculae normally lie in alignment with their projections in the pelvis and form an angle of 160 to 170° with the medial cortex of the femoral shaft, they also align with similarly oriented trabeculae in the acetabulum. On the lateral projection, the trabecular alignment from the head fragment to the neck fragment normally should be 180°. Angulation of the head fragment into more anteversion or retroversion would affect the alignment of these trabeculae.

Stage I: In Garden stage I fractures, the fracture is incomplete, with the head tilted in a posterolateral direction. Practically speaking, this is an impacted fracture.

Stage II: Garden stage II fractures are complete, but undisplaced.

Stage III: Garden stage III fractures are complete and partially displaced, as judged by the direction of the trabecular stream in the head fragment, but the two fragments remain in contact with each other.

Stage IV: In Garden stage IV fractures, the fragments are completely displaced and the trabeculae of the femoral head realign themselves with the trabeculae within the acetabulum.

Although Garden's classification system is the most commonly used, it has been difficult to apply without significant interobserver variability. The distinction between displaced and nondisplaced fractures (stages I and II compared with stages III and IV) was much more consistent and was thought by many to be the only reliable distinction.

In the AO classification system, as shown in Figure 24.118 fractures of the femoral neck are classified as subcapital with no or minimal displacement (type B1), transcervical (type B2) or displaced subcapital fractures (type B3). Each of these types is identified further. Type B1 fractures may be impacted in valgus of 15° or more (type B1.1), impacted in valgus of less than 15° (type B1.2) or nonimpacted (type B1.3). Transcervical (type B2)

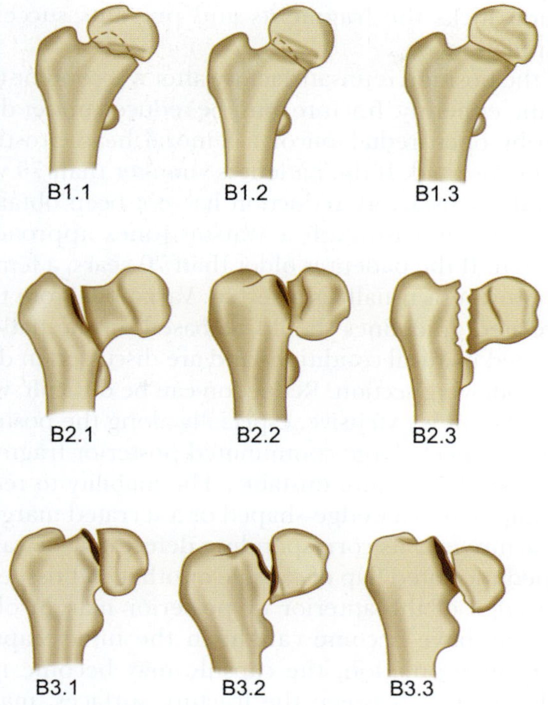

Fig. 24.118: AO classification of femoral neck fracture

fractures may be basicervical (type B2.1), midcervical with adduction (type B2.2) or midcervical with shear (type B2.3). Displaced subcapital fractures (type B3) may be moderately displaced in varus and external rotation (type B3.1), moderately displaced with vertical translation and external rotation (type B3.2) or markedly displaced (type B3.3). Type B3 fractures have the worst prognosis.

Whichever classification system is used, impacted fractures must be distinguished from nondisplaced fractures of the neck of the femur. Impacted fracture surfaces are crushed together or invaginated, so that the trabeculae and usually the cortex of the neck are pushed into the soft trabecular bone of the head. This impaction imparts a significant amount of stability at the fracture site and suggests a conservative or nonoperative approach. In nondisplaced fractures of the femoral neck (Garden stage II), there is no impaction and no inherent stability and almost all subsequently displace, if not internally fixed. Rates of nonunion and osteonecrosis for nondisplaced fractures are low, when these fractures are treated with multiple screw fixation. Many different devices have been devised for internal fixation of femoral neck fractures, but currently two are commonly used:

- Multiple cannulated screws and
- Collapsible compression screw and side plate combinations that are typically used with an additional antirotation screw.

The following principles of preoperative preparation, reduction of the fracture, fluoroscopic control, surgical exposure and insertion of internal fixation are common to many of the techniques. Fixation with cannulated screws usually is adequate for most femoral neck fractures. In a review of femoral neck fractures in young patients, Kyle determined that the most consistently good results were obtained with anatomical reduction and fixation with some form of multiple screw fixations. Scientists have found a distinct correlation between fixation with screws and the strength of the lateral cortex. Based on their studies, they concluded that if the lateral cortex does not provide sufficient stability to prevent toggling of the screws and reduction of torsional forces, complications and nonunions occur more frequently. We most often use cannulated screws for fixation of femoral neck fractures. If osteopenia or comminution of the lateral cortex is severe, we infrequently use a compression hip screw with a small side plate and accessory screws, as advocated by scientists to control rotational forces around the lag screw further. If satisfactory reduction cannot be obtained by closed methods, open reduction is indicated. Satisfactory reduction should be evaluated by the Garden alignment index.

Treatment

We prefer manipulation and closed reduction of femoral neck fractures and perform open reduction, only when anatomical closed reduction is not attainable and the patient is not a good candidate for a hemiarthroplasty with a femoral head prosthesis.

Closed Reduction

Whitman described a method that involves traction on the limb in extension, internal rotation in extension and abduction, and abduction and internal rotation. We usually have success with this method. With the patient supine on the fracture table, the normal extremity is tied to the footplate.

The fractured extremity is tied to the other footplate in an externally rotated position. With the extremity externally rotated, it is abducted approximately 20° and enough traction is applied to regain slightly more than normal length. The extremity is internally rotated, until the patella is internally rotated 20 to 30°. Scientists described a technique of manipulation with the hip in flexion that we have found satisfactory, when the Whitman technique is unsuccessful. In his technique, the affected limb is flexed at the hip to 90° and the thigh is slightly internally rotated, traction is applied in line with the femur. The limb is circumducted into abduction, maintaining the internal rotation and is brought down to table level in extension. Scientists evaluated the reduction with a "heel-palm" test, in which the patient's heel is placed in the palm of the surgeon's outstretched hand. If reduction is complete, the limb does not externally rotate spontaneously. The foot is tied to the footplate with the extremity in only 15 to 20° of abduction, neutral flexion and extension and firm internal rotation of approximately 20°. This position usually places the head, neck and trochanter on a horizontal plane. The position is verified, by image intensification in the anteroposterior and lateral planes.

Evaluation of Reduction (Fig. 24.119)

On the lateral fluoroscopic view, only the slightest variation from the anatomical position is permissible. On the anteroposterior view, anatomical position or a slight valgus relationship of the head and neck is acceptable. Garden proposed an index for acceptable reduction, using the trabecular pattern alignment, as viewed in the anteroposterior and lateral radiographic planes. On the anteroposterior view, the angle formed by the central axis of the medial trabecular system in the head fragment and the medial cortex of the femoral shaft should measure no less than 160° and no more than 180°. An angle less than 160° denotes an unacceptable varus reduction and an angle more than 180° indicates severe valgus, which has been shown to increase the risk of osteonecrosis and degenerative changes within the joint caused by hip joint incongruity. On the lateral view, Garden's alignment index should be within 20° of the normal 180° straight line along the neck. If the femoral head is anteverted or retroverted and this angle is less than 150°, an unstable, nonanatomical reduction is present and remanipulation should be considered. Any variation from these rigid requirements demands that the hip be remanipulated. If remanipulation is necessary, the limb first must be brought into full external rotation because the internally rotated position locks the fragments and prevents successful manipulation.

If the position is unsatisfactory after a second or third attempt, either the fracture must be reduced under direct vision by open reduction or a femoral head prosthesis must be inserted. If the patient is younger than 70 years old and a satisfactory reduction has not been obtained, open reduction through a Watson-Jones approach is preferred. If the patient is older than 70 years, a femoral head prosthesis usually is inserted. Variations from these age-related guidelines should be based on the patient's associated medical conditions and are discussed in detail in the following section. Reduction can be difficult, when comminution is extensive, especially along the posterior part of the neck; large comminuted posterior fragments may make the fracture unstable. The inability to reduce by manipulation a wedge-shaped or a serrated margin of the fracture into its corresponding defect may be caused by a pedunculated flap of capsule or other soft tissue or a sharp edge of the anterior or posterior margin of the neck may have become caught in the intact capsule. During manipulation, the capsule may become more tightly impaled between the fracture surfaces, making proper apposition impossible. As already stated, an accurate reduction is an absolute requirement for internal fixation, if it is not obtained, internal fixation should not proceed further.

Open Reduction and Internal Fixation (Figs 24.120A to F)

Patient positioning and draping after fracture reduction are performed in a similar manner to that described for internal fixation of intertrochanteric fracture. If open reduction is performed, the usual lateral incision is extended proximally and anteriorly, as in a Watson-Jones

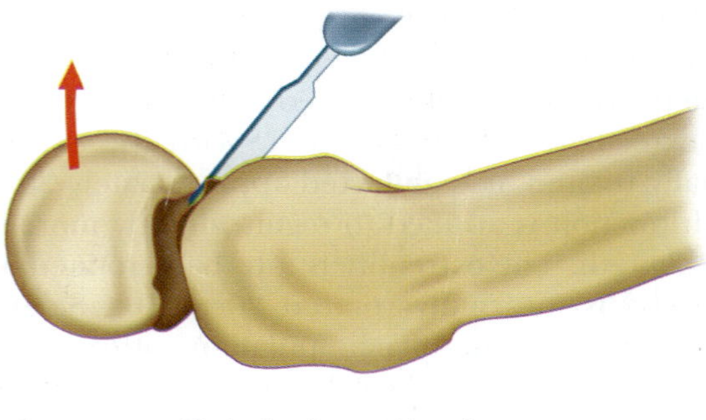

Fig. 24.119: An osteotome or elevator inserted into the anterior aspect of the fracture can be used to manipulate the femoral head fragment

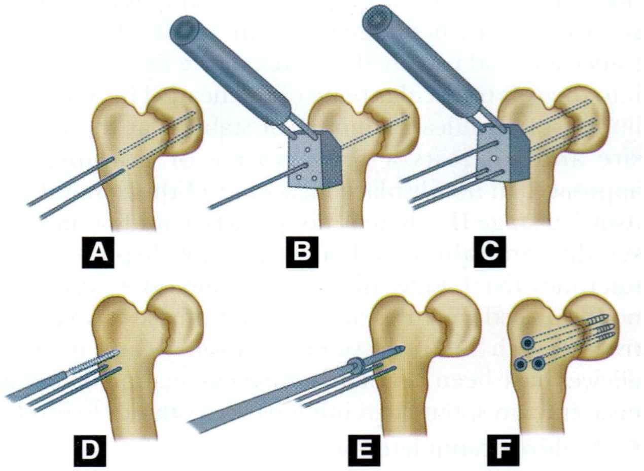

Figs 24.120A to F: Open reduction and internal fixation after reduction guide pins are inserted for provisional fixation. The fracture can then be fixed definitively with three screws

approach. The capsule is opened and the fracture is reduced under direct vision. Open reduction in this manner is not an easy surgical exercise. If the extremity is kept in the extended position in traction, the exposure to the femoral neck through the anterior capsule can be extremely difficult because of the tightness of the anterior and anterolateral thigh and hip muscles in this position. The femoral head is largely covered and within the acetabulum is difficult to manipulate and the fracture is not easily aligned, even with it exposed and visible. Flexing the hip 20° or 30° greatly aids in the exposure and reduction. An osteotome or elevator inserted into the anterior aspect of the fracture can be used to manipulate the femoral head fragment, as shown in Figure 24.119. When the fracture has been satisfactorily reduced, guide pins are inserted for provisional fixation and views with the image intensifier are obtained to check their position. The fracture can be fixed definitively with three screws.

Some surgeons have suggested open reduction through a posterior approach, but we have had no experience with this approach. The reason for nonanatomical reduction often involves comminution of the posterior femoral neck and advocates of the posterior approach have suggested that this is the most direct route to obtain anatomical reduction. If a posterior approach is used for open reduction, further damage to the most important vascular supply to the femoral head, traversing the posterior femoral neck through its retinaculum and the lateral epiphyseal arterial group is a distinct risk. Many authors have evaluated the number of screws and the configuration in the neck for the greatest degree of stability. The usual number of screws recommended is three to four and the location and arrangement of the screws in the neck should be as recommended by Booth et al. in the calcar and more peripheral positions. Screws positioned along the posterior femoral neck may resist retroversion forces, as screws along the calcar resist varus forces.

■ After Treatment

The patient is allowed to sit on the day after surgery. Ambulation with a walker is allowed as soon as possible. Weight-bearing varies depending on the stability of the fracture construct (quality of the bone, reduction and screw fixation), but there is evidence that with adequately fixed fractures, at least partial weight-bearing can be allowed immediately in most patients with no increased incidence of hardware failure. Scientists analyzed weight bearing after femoral neck intertrochanteric hip fractures and found that patients allowed to bear weight, as tolerated voluntarily, which will limit the amount of weight, they apply to their fractured hip and increase the weight gradually as the fracture heals. We encourage our patients to ambulate with "protected" weight-bearing and try to not let a strict nonweight-bearing status restrict the patient's rehabilitation. Many of these patients become unable to ambulate at all, if weight bearing is restricted, so we usually err on the side of allowing weight to be applied to the hip, rather than have the patient be in bed or a chair for a prolonged time. The patient is encouraged to bear full weight by 6 to 8 weeks.

Fixation with a Compression Hip Screw and Plate

Although current literature reviews indicate poorer results after fixation of femoral neck fractures with hip compression screws alone than after multiple screw fixation, if the bone is osteoporotic or the lateral cortex is comminuted, the use of a side plate and accessory screws. The technique is the same as that described for intertrochanteric fractures, with the addition of accessory screws inserted through the femoral neck into the head before insertion of the large lag screw. The function of the accessory screws is to prevent rotation of the neck, while inserting the large lag screw into the hard bone in the femoral head. These screws should be left in place to resist torsional deformation of the femoral neck fracture further.

Prosthetic Replacement for Recent Femoral Neck Fractures

For displaced fractures of the femoral neck, reduction, compression and rigid internal fixation are required, if union is to be predictable because nonunion and osteonecrosis develop frequently after internal fixation of displaced femoral neck fractures, many surgeons recommend primary prosthetic replacement, as an alternative in elderly ambulatory patients. Although, the use of a prosthesis avoids nonunion and osteonecrosis, it also may be followed by complications. Their study showed a higher rate of revision in patients older than 80 years treated with internal fixation of a displaced femoral neck fracture compared with patients, who were treated with hemiarthroplasty. There was no difference, however in the revision rates of nondisplaced fractures treated by internal fixation or hemiarthroplasty in this age group. In patients 65 to 80 years old, regardless of the amount of displacement, no difference was noted in revision rates after hemiarthroplasty or internal fixation. These authors noted a significantly higher mortality rate associated with internal fixation than with hemiarthroplasty for patients in this age group.

Complications, revision rates and other outcomes were the same regardless of whether, a unipolar or bipolar prosthesis was use and whether an anterior or posterior approach for hemiarthroplasty was used in patients 65 to 80 years old. After the first month, there were no differences in the cumulative mortality rates between the two groups. Increased blood loss, longer operative times and greater infection and mortality rates occurred, however with arthroplasty. Several authors have listed the advantages and disadvantages of and the indications for prosthetic replacement for recent displaced fractures of the femoral neck and no two totally agree. The advantages and disadvantages can be summarized as in Tables 24.6 and 24.7.

Based on the relative advantages and disadvantages, various authors have proposed indications for prosthetic replacement and internal fixation for displaced intracapsular fractures. Many indications for the use of a prosthesis are controversial, some of the indication are enumerated in the Tables 24.8 and 24.9. A treatment algorithm based on our treatment preferences: closed reduction and internal fixation (CRIF); not applicable (NA) then ORIF.

Table 24.6: Advantages of prosthetic replacement

1. Prosthetic replacement allows immediate weight-bearing to return elderly patients to activity and help avoid complications of recumbency and inactivity.
   - When the concept of prosthetic replacement was first introduced, this perhaps was the most important advantage.
   - As patients with internal fixation devices are more aggressively mobilized than in the past, and most are allowed at least partial immediate weight-bearing, this advantage is less distinct than previously thought.
2. As a primary procedure, prosthetic replacement eliminates osteonecrosis and nonunion as complications of femoral neck fractures.
   - There still is no completely reliable way of identifying femoral heads with a significantly damaged blood supply before definitive surgery.
   - Developing technology may allow definitive preoperative identification of these avascular femoral heads and provide useful information in making the decision between prosthetic replacement and internal fixation.
3. Prosthetic replacement of displaced femoral neck fractures reduces the incidence of reoperation compared with internal fixation.

   This argument applies only to elderly individuals with a limited life expectancy because the cumulative rate of reoperation for prosthetic replacement increases with time.

Table 24.7: The recognized disadvantages of using a prosthesis in a fresh femoral neck fracture

1. After the femoral head and neck have been discarded in favor of a metal implant, salvage procedures become complicated if there is mechanical failure or infection.
   - The use of a prosthesis for most fractures of the femoral neck ignores the fact that at least two-thirds of patients treated by internal fixation have functional hips that last the remainder of their lifetimes.
   - *It is appropriate to remember Boyd and Salvatore's comment:* "The sacrifice of the head and neck and replacement by a metallic foreign substance is not the answer for the majority of patients; in over half, the best available material is in the acetabulum, and its indiscriminate removal should be avoided."
2. The operation for inserting a prosthesis generally is considered to be more extensive than that required for an uncomplicated internal fixation procedure.
   - Larger exposure is required, and blood loss is greater. Many authors have reported slightly higher perioperative mortality rates for patients treated with prosthetic replacement than for patients treated with internal fixation. This finding has a definite selection bias, however, because patients undergoing hemiarthroplasty tend to be more elderly and have more medical comorbidities.

Selection of a Prosthesis

With the development of bipolar endoprostheses, the use of fixed head endoprostheses has declined. Although, the Austin-Moore prosthesis has produced excellent results, thigh pain and protrusioacetabuli in younger patients have been associated with this device. Revision to a total hip arthroplasty also is difficult and the complication rate is much higher when an Austin-Moore prosthesis has been used. We still use the Austin-Moore prosthesis on rare occasions, but only in patients with extremely limited ambulation and short life expectancy. Modern low cost femoral stems, with modular unipolar or bipolar femoral heads are currently in use that allows revision to a total hip arthroplasty, often without revision of the femoral component. They also allow some adjustment of the prosthetic femoral neck length for stability and offset considerations. For active patients in whom a prosthesis is indicated, we prefer a cemented or cementless total hip femoral component with a bipolar or unipolar head attachment.

Bipolar vs Unipolar

- The complications of persistent pain and protrusio acetabuli with unipolar hemiarthroplasties have led many surgeons to choose a bipolar system.
- Studies suggest that the current generation of bipolar hemiarthroplasties have a lower incidence of protrusio acetabuli than do earlier designs.

Table 24.8: Relative indications for hemiarthroplasty

1. *Advanced physiological age:* Advanced age alone is not a true indication for a prosthesis, although some local and systemic diseases that occur in older patients, especially if they occur in combination, might be. Prosthetic replacement probably should be reserved for patients 70 years old or older with a life expectancy of no more than 10 to 15 years. Some definite exceptions to this statement are mentioned later.
2. *Fracture-dislocation of the hip in an older patient:* If the fracture involves the superior weight-bearing surface of the head (Pipkin type II; the Pipkin classification system is discussed in the section on dislocation and fracture-dislocation of the hip), the insertion of a prosthesis is preferable to closed treatment or open reduction of the fragment. If a substantial fragment of the inferior part of the head is fractured (Pipkin type I), the dislocation should be reduced promptly and, if the head fragment is not caught in the joint, treated closed;
   - If necessary, open reduction of the hip can be performed, and the fragment can be removed. Such treatment results in a good hip if the superior weight bearing surface of the head is intact.

Table 24.9: Stronger indications for hemiarthroplasty

1. A fracture that cannot be satisfactorily reduced or fixed with stability, especially with posterior comminution.
2. Femoral neck fractures that lose fixation several weeks after operation.
3. *Some pre-existing lesions of the hip:* In patients with pre-existing lesions, an arthroplasty already may have been indicated and the fracture merely makes the decision immediate
   - Patients with osteonecrosis of the head of the femur from unknown causes, from irradiation, or from a previous dislocation and patients with severe rheumatoid or degenerative arthritis of the hip probably would have a better hip after insertion of a prosthesis than before the fracture.
   - In one study of rheumatoid patients, Strömqvist, Kelly, and Lidgren reported a 95 percent rate of loss of reduction or superior segmental collapse compared with 50 percent in a matched nonrheumatoid group most of these patients are candidates for total hip arthroplasty rather than femoral head replacement.
4. *Malignancy:* A malignancy may be an indication for the insertion of a prosthesis. A patient with a short life expectancy, whether the fracture is pathological or primarily the result of trauma, is best treated with a prosthesis.
   - If the fracture is pathological, the insertion of a prosthesis offers not only a good solution, but also an opportunity to perform an open biopsy and to establish a definite diagnosis.
   - In pathological fractures, supplementing the fixation with methylmethacrylate usually provides sufficient stability.
5. *Neurological disorders:* Patients subject to uncontrolled epileptic seizures and patients with severe uncontrolled parkinsonism are treated better with a primary prosthesis. Many of these disorders are controllable, however, and the indication may not always be absolute.
6. Old, undiagnosed fractures of the femoral neck. Occasionally, a fracture of the femoral neck goes undiscovered for several weeks. Sometimes multiple injuries may delay treatment of a fractured femoral neck even after its diagnosis.
   - An untreated, unreduced, and unimpacted fracture of the femoral neck that is more than 3 weeks old should have a primary prosthesis, other things being equal.
   - Before the use of prostheses, we saw many patients with fractures of the femoral neck 3 weeks old that healed satisfactorily with nothing more than reduction and rigid internal fixation.
   - The odds for favorable results decline, however, with the passage of time after a displaced fracture.
7. Fracture of the neck of the femur with complete dislocation of the femoral head. This lesion is rare and is best treated by primary prosthetic replacement because osteonecrosis of the head is certain under these circumstances.
8. A patient who probably cannot withstand two operations. If a patient's general condition prohibits a second operation, a primary prosthesis is justified. In patients who have unstable multiple medical problems, we occasionally perform a closed reduction with percutaneous multiple screw fixation using intravenous sedation and generous amounts of local lidocaine infiltration anesthesia.
9. Patients with psychoses or mental deterioration. Elderly patients with fractures of the femoral neck often already have Alzheimer disease, and protected weight bearing in such patients may be unreliable, with immediate unprotected weight bearing resulting in possible loss of fixation, especially in severely comminuted fractures. A primary prosthesis may be justified in these circumstances.

- Some authors have found, however that the motion of the inner bearing surface may not last and that all bipolar hips functionally become unipolar implants.

Cemented vs Cementless

- Emery et al. found significantly better pain relief after cemented. Thompson hemiarthroplasties than after the use of uncemented Austin-Moore prostheses.
- This also has been our experience and we cement many endoprostheses used for femoral neck fractures.
- We use contemporary cement techniques that include distal femoral canal occlusion, pulsatile lavage of the canal and meticulous drying of the canal before cement insertion with a cement gun, avoiding significant cement pressurization.
- As many patients have compromised cardiopulmonary reserve and a recent long bone fracture, we avoid the further metabolic insult of cement pressurization.
- If uncemented hemiarthroplasty is done for femoral neck fracture, we prefer to use a proximally porous textured total hip style stem, rather than a nonporous "press-fit"type stem.
- The lack of biological fixation of the nontextured stem inserted without cement may cause long-term thigh pain.

Total Hip Arthroplasty

Primary total hip arthroplasty is indicated in patients with significant pre-existing joint destruction caused by rheumatoid disease, osteonecrosis or osteoarthritis. The clinical results and survivorship of primary hip arthroplasty in this setting have varied from excellent to poor. There seems to be a definite increased risk of dislocation in this population compared with the risk after purely elective total hip arthroplasty. Scientists, reported their results after total hip arthroplasty for femoral neck fractures and noted that although results were good, the complication rate was higher than those reported in other studies of hemiarthroplasties. We rarely perform total hip arthroplasty for a femoral neck fracture.

Surgical Approaches

We most frequently use a posterior approach for the insertion of femoral head prostheses after acute fractures of the neck of the femur. Numerous authors recommend a more anterior approach, such as a Hardinge approach because complications, especially infection and prosthetic dislocation occur more frequently, when a posterior approach is used. Advocates of an anterior approach state that infection and dislocation are infrequent with that approach because of the greater distance of the anterior incision from the perineum and the absence of an incision through the strong posterior capsule. Unquestionably, getting these elderly patients out of bed to a sitting position places considerable stress on the posterior capsule and posterior approaches can make the hip more vulnerable to dislocation. We occasionally use an anterior approach in patients with bowel incontinence, in unreliable patients, who are likely to violate the standard total hip range-of-motion precautions and in patients, who are spastic and tend to flex and adduct their hips in household ambulation. An adductor tenotomy may be indicated in this last group of patients. Patients with Parkinson disease have been identified, as being at risk for posterior dislocation. Failures after internal fixation of fractures of the hip can be caused by:

- infection
- loss of fixation
- nonunion or
- osteonecrosis.

Infection after internal fixation of intertrochanteric fractures or fractures of the femoral neck is serious and usually leads to significant compromise of hip function. Many patients have diseases, such as diabetes or infections of other organ systems, which have been shown to retard fracture repair. Incisions for hip surgery are near the perineum and are easily contaminated. Intraoperative wound contamination from wide exposure and prolonged operating time and postoperative hematomas are other factors. Disoriented patients sometimes remove the postoperative dressing and directly contaminate the wound. Adding to the problem is the fact that many infections are not evident, until after the patient has been discharged and the patient may not exhibit the classic signs and symptoms of an infection. Even when none of the cardinal signs and symptoms of infection, such as fever, chills, redness or drainage are present, an infection should be suspected, if a patient complains of persistent pain, especially if motion is painful, if the sedimentation rate is elevated, if the joint space is progressively becoming more narrow on radiographs, if there is progressive loss of bone density around the head, neck or acetabulum or if there is any sign of loosening of the internal fixation appliance. Aspiration of the hip joint may allow early diagnosis. Organisms normally considered to be contaminants or nonpathogens may produce infections that appear late. Superficial infections usually appear within the first 1 to 2 weeks after surgery and usually respond to drainage and antibiotics. Early deep infections generally produce all the cardinal signs and symptoms of an acute infection and demand aggressive early treatment with wide drainage and the appropriate antibiotics. If the infection involves the hip joint in a patient with a femoral neck fracture, the internal fixation usually should be removed, only if it is unstable, however control of the infection takes precedence over further efforts to obtain union of the fracture.

In many patients, femoral head resection is required because the head becomes a sequestrum. If an intertrochanteric or subtrochanteric fracture becomes infected, it should be widely drained. The internal fixation device is left in place, however if it is still providing rigid fixation of the fracture and the joint is not involved. The infection may continue in a subacute or chronic form, as long as the device remains in place, but union of the fracture can occur despite this. The fixation device can be removed after union and the infection usually can be cleared. Late deep infections without joint involvement should be managed in a similar manner with drainage and appropriate antibiotics, leaving the fixation device in place, if fracture healing is incomplete or removing it, if the fracture has united.

Stress Fractures of the Femoral Neck

Stress fractures of the femoral neck can occur in young, vigorous individuals with unaccustomed strenuous activity, such as athletics, running or marching long distances. In elderly individuals, they can occur because of one of the metabolic disorders of bone. Frequently, routine anteroposterior and lateral radiographs initially are normal with the diagnosis confirmed by bone scan or MRI.

Femoral neck stress fractures have been classified according to the location of the fracture in the femoral neck.

Type I: Lateral fractures, often referred to as tension fractures, are more unstable and prone to displacement. We recommend internal fixation with multiple screws for this fracture.

Type II: Medial compression fractures, can be treated nonoperatively with rest followed by a period of protected weight bearing. Radiographs should be made at multiple intervals to confirm progression toward union without displacement. If a patient cannot comply with activity restriction, internal fixation is recommended.

Type III: Fractures, are displaced and require closed or open reduction with screw fixation or hemiarthroplasty, depending on the patient's age and medical circumstances.

Pathological Fractures of the Femoral Neck

The proximal end of the femur is a common location for the spread of metastatic disease. Pathological fracture in this area is commonly the presenting symptom that leads to and establishes the diagnosis of malignancy. Pathological fractures or impending pathological fractures in the subtrochanteric and intertrochanteric region should be fixed internally, using techniques and devices discussed in the previous sections. In addition to internal fixation, the bulk of the tumor at the pathological site can be removed and fixation supplemented with polymethylmethacrylate (PMMA). We prefer to use a cephalomedullary reconstruction nail for pathological fractures of the intertrochanteric and subtrochanteric regions and to stabilize the entire femur prophylactically, with or without PMMA. Depending on the aggressiveness of the tumor, fractures so treated may heal. Pathological fractures arising from metastatic disease in the femoral head and neck usually are best treated by removal of the head and neck and replacement with a femoral head prosthesis. The prosthesis should be secured in the medullary canal with PMMA.

Postirradiation Fractures of the Femoral Neck

If a patient has received radiation therapy for pelvic malignancy months or years before sustaining a fracture of the femoral neck, the surgeon should try to determine whether the fracture is pathological and the result of irradiation, whether it is a pathological fracture arising from a metastatic lesion or an extension of the primary tumor or whether it is a simple fracture totally attributable to trauma. Clinical signs and symptoms suggesting irradiation, as the cause of fracture are prodromal pain localized to the hip or radiating to the knee, followed by a gradually increasing limp and disability, as might occur with a slipped femoral epiphysis. Although, the patient is able to walk, coxa vara deformity may have already occurred. Some scientists described the radiographic characteristics as:

- The fracture is subcapital or high in the neck
- Before the fracture occurs, an irregular transverse line of increased density is the only evidence that fracture is impending
- Scattered areas of increased translucency sometimes may be seen in the femoral neck
- Characteristically, there is a coxa vara deformity, as in an adduction fracture
- Rotation or angulation of the head is slight on the anteroposterior and lateral view
- After the fracture heals, considerable sclerosis can be seen at the fracture and in the adjacent bone.

The fracture is preceded by a loss of trabecular bulk and the blood supply is not obliterated and is not responsible for the bony changes; the meager blood supply of the femoral head can be increased by radiation therapy, unless intensive direct irradiation has produced complete cellular destruction. They recommended early internal fixation, without manipulation of the fragments. They found that these fractures heal well, often with "skillful neglect" as the treatment that many heal in less time than average and that the usual complications of nonunion and osteonecrosis of the femoral head probably are less common than after fractures that occur purely from trauma. Internal fixation was used when the fracture continued to displace or when separation of the fragments already existed. Only in the old and markedly displaced fractures was a major reconstructive procedure necessary.

Table 24.10: Indications for inserting prosthesis instead of using internal fixation for pathological fractures
1. If the fracture is the result of irradiation and has been present for some time, efforts to correct the deformity and preserve the head usually fail. Fractures with minimal deformity and of recent onset should be fixed internally
2. If the patient's life expectancy is uncertain because of an aggressive malignancy, this fact favors a method that would provide early function and ambulation The stages of the primary malignancy must be considered; the presence of multiple metastatic lesions or a life expectancy of only a few weeks or months would favor the use of a prosthesis.

In deciding whether to insert a prosthesis instead of using internal fixation for a pathological fracture of the femoral neck, this is illustrated in Table 24.10.

Fractures of the Femoral Neck with Ipsilateral Femoral Shaft Fractures

Fracture of the femoral neck with ipsilateral femoral shaft fracture is an unusual segmental fracture of the femur that initially was reported by Delaney and Street, as an incidental finding during intramedullary nailing of a femoral fracture. Approximately 19 percent of ipsilateral femoral neck fractures are discovered late or during treatment of femoral shaft fractures. Fractures of the femoral shaft can occur in combination with subtrochanteric fractures, intertrochanteric fractures, nondisplaced femoral neck fractures or displaced femoral neck fractures. Shaft fractures with displaced femoral neck fractures, as expected have the worst prognosis. More than 60 different methods have been advocated in the literature for treatment of this rare injury. This is a better prognosis than usually is seen for femoral neck fractures, and it is attributed to the fact that most of the energy, causing the fractures is dissipated to the femoral shaft, with less resultant displacement of the femoral neck fracture. Any patient sustaining high-energy trauma should be thoroughly examined with a radiographic survey of the femoral neck area, to rule out this combination of injuries. We routinely re-examine the femoral neck under fluoroscopy after all intramedullary nailings of the femur. The best treatment of these fractures is controversial.

Considering the greater significance of failure of femoral neck fractures in young patients, most authors emphasize making the fracture of the femoral neck a greater priority. Some authors now recommend femoral neck fixation with screws and an intercondylar retrograde femoral nail. The use of a hip compression screw and long side plate also has been reported. The Russell-Taylor reconstruction nail was designed specifically for this injury. It allows fixation by two self-compressing lag screws in the femoral head, for control of torsional forces around the femoral neck, in conjunction with a cephalomedullary nail. In a series of 30 consecutive femoral neck and shaft fractures treated with Russell-Taylor reconstruction nails, Azar and Russell reported one femoral neck nonunion and one patient who developed osteonecrosis. We advocate anatomical reduction of femoral neck fractures before stabilization with the implant.

Many new cephalomedullary implants with a reconstruction mode are now available. We currently use the Trigen nail in the Recon mode or a retrograde intramedullary nail with cannulated screws placed into the femoral neck proximal to the nail to treat these injuries. Although, we have had good results with closed reduction of the shaft after preliminary neck fixation and insertion of a reconstruction nail, the technique requires careful and constant imaging of the femoral neck fracture, to ensure no displacement occurs during nailing. Two screws must be used for femoral head fixation, and the threads must be placed well into the head for adequate stability of the femoral neck portion. When an undetected femoral neck fracture is found after conventional intramedullary nailing of a femoral shaft fracture, the nail should be left in place and cannulated screws should be inserted from the lateral shaft of the femur, anterior to the femoral nail, into the middle of the femoral head to fix the femoral neck fracture.

INTERTROCHANTERIC FEMORAL FRACTURES

Most intertrochanteric femoral fractures occur in patients older than 70 years old. It includes fractures from the extracapsular part of the neck to a point 5 cm distal to the lesser trochanter.

Classification

Boyd and Griffin classified fractures in the peritrochanteric area of the femur into four types. Their classification, which included fractures from the extracapsular part of the neck to a point 5 cm distal to the lesser trochanter, follows. These are shown in Figure 24.121.

Type I: Fractures that extend along the intertrochanteric line from the greater to the lesser trochanter. Reduction usually is simple and is maintained with little difficulty. Results generally are satisfactory.

Type II: Comminuted fractures, the main fracture being along the intertrochanteric line, but with multiple fractures in the cortex. Reduction of these fractures is more difficult because the comminution can vary from slight to extreme. A particularly deceptive form is the fracture, in which an anteroposterior linear intertrochanteric fracture occurs, as in type 1, but with an additional fracture in the coronal plane, which can be seen on the lateral radiograph.

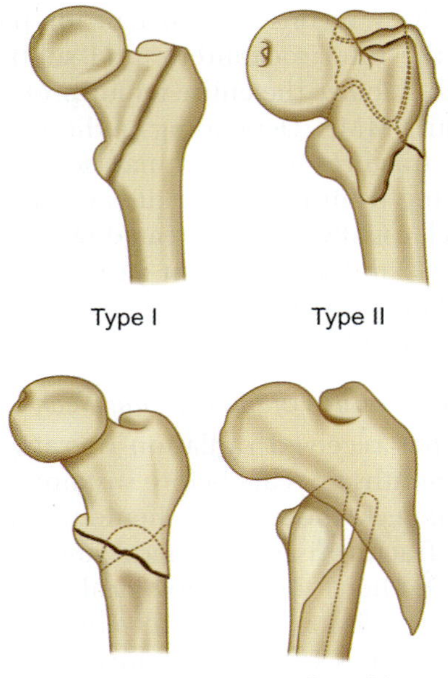

Fig. 24.121: Classification of intertrochanteric femoral fractures

Type III: Fractures that are basically subtrochanteric with at least one fracture passing across the proximal end of the shaft just distal to or at the lesser trochanter. Varying degrees of comminution are associated. These fractures usually are more difficult to reduce and result in more complications at operation and during convalescence.

Type IV: Fractures of the trochanteric region and the proximal shaft, with fracture in at least two planes, one of which usually is the sagittal plane and may be difficult to see on routine anteroposterior radiographs. If open reduction and internal fixation are used, two-plane fixation is required because of the spiral, oblique or butterfly fracture of the shaft.

The most difficult types to manage are types III and IV, which are accounted for only about one-third of the trochanteric fractures in Boyd and Griffin's series. Evans devised a widely used classification system based on the division of fractures into stable and unstable groups, as shown in Figure 24.122. He divided unstable fractures further into those, in which stability could be restored by anatomical or near-anatomical reduction and those in which anatomical reduction would not create stability. In an Evans type I fracture, the fracture line extends upward and outward from the lesser trochanter. In type II, reverse obliquity fracture, the major fracture line extends outward and downward from the lesser trochanter. Type II fractures have a tendency toward medial displacement

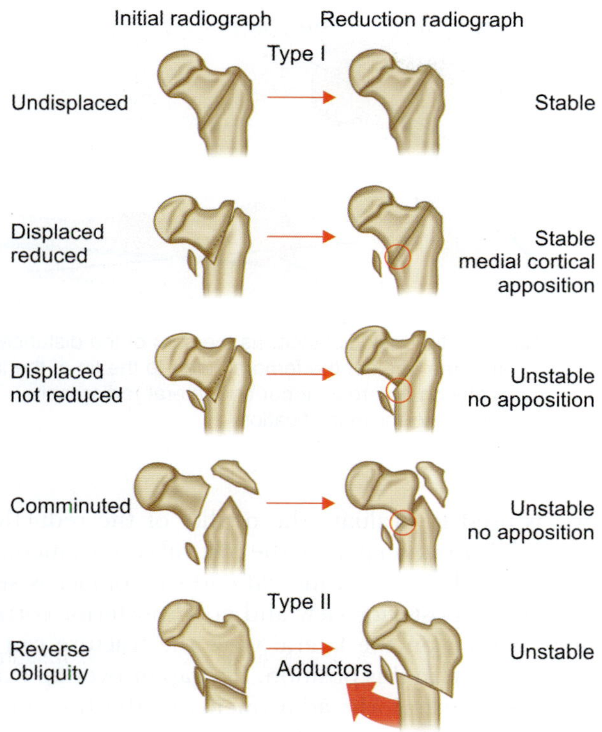

Fig. 24.122: Evans classification system based on the division of fractures into stable and unstable groups

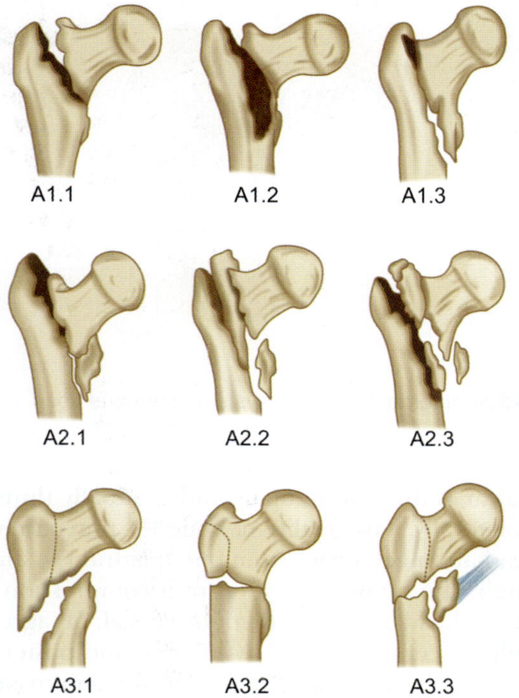

Fig. 24.123: AO classification of trochanteric fractures

of the femoral shaft because of the pull of the adductor muscles.

The AO group classified trochanteric fractures as described in Figure 24.123. A1 fractures are uncomminuted, A2 fractures have increasing comminution and A3 fractures have subtrochanteric extensions or reverse obliquity. AO fractures A1.1 through A2.1 are commonly described as stable and fractures A2.2 through A3.3, usually are unstable. The orientation of the trabeculae is along the lines of stress, with thicker trabeculae coming from the calcar and passing superiorly into the weight-bearing dome of the femoral head, as shown in Figure 24.123.

Nonoperative Treatment

Closed methods of treatment of intertrochanteric fractures have largely been abandoned.

Rigid internal fixation of intertrochanteric fractures with early mobilization of the patient should be considered standard treatment. Medical complications after internal fixation are fewer and less serious than complications after nonoperative treatment. Only comfortable nonambulatory patients or patients with brief life expectancies should be treated nonoperatively.

Operative Treatment

One goal of operative treatment is strong, stable fixation of the fracture fragments. Scientists listed the following variables, as those that determine the strength of the fracture fragment-implant assembly:

- Bone quality
- Fragment geometry
- Reduction
- Implant design
- Implant placement

Of these five elements of stable fixation, the surgeon can control only the quality of the reduction and the choice of implant and its placement. As most patients with intertrochanteric fractures have considerable osteopenia, with the quality of bone for the purchase of fixation within the femoral head and neck less than desirable, it is important that the internal fixation device be placed in that part of the head and neck where the quality of bone is best. A scientist described the internal trabecular system of the femoral head, as illustrated in the Figure 24.124. The orientation of the trabeculae is along the lines of stress, with thicker trabeculae coming from the calcar and passing superiorly into the weight-bearing dome of the femoral head. Smaller trabeculae extend from the inferior region of the foveal area across the head and the superior portion of the femoral neck and into the trochanter and to the lateral cortex. The calcar is a dense, vertical plate of bone extending from the posteromedial portion of the femoral shaft under the lesser trochanter and radiating laterally to the greater trochanter, reinforcing the femoral neck posteroinferiorly.

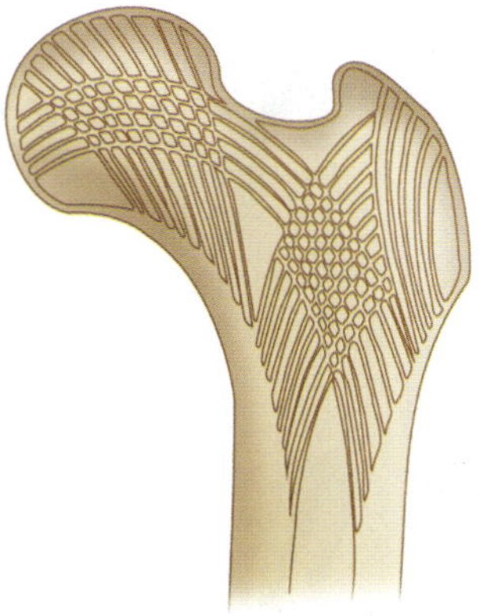

Fig. 24.124: Internal trabecular system of femoral head

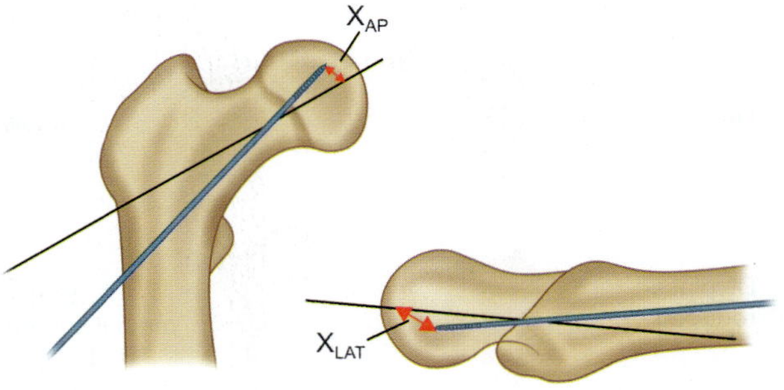

Fig. 24.125: The tip-apex distance, as the sum of the distances from the apex of the femoral head to the tip of the lag screw on anteroposterior and lateral radiographs, correcting for magnification

The calcar is thickest medially and gradually thins, as it passes laterally. The quality of bone for purchase within the head and neck varies from one quadrant to another. Although, the optimal position of a compression screw within the head and neck is controversial, all agree that it should be central or slightly inferior and posterior.

The bone of poorest quality is in the anterosuperior aspect of the head and neck. Optimal positioning of the device is controlled by the surgeon. A scientist described the tip-apex distance, as the sum of the distances from the apex of the femoral head to the tip of the lag screw on anteroposterior and lateral radiographs, correcting for magnification. Scientists have found that, if this sum was less than 25 mm, there were no failures caused by cutting out of the lag screw, as depicted in Figure 24.125. Scientists showed that the tip-apex distance also is crucial, when using intramedullary nails and compression hip screws to prevent cutout and loss of reduction.

It is important before treatment to distinguish by radiographs, whether the intertrochanteric fracture is stable or unstable based on fracture geometry and whether reduction can restore cortical contact medially and posteriorly. The status of the lesser trochanter is important in evaluating the stability of the reduction. If the lesser trochanter is displaced with a large fragment, a significant cortical defect is present posteromedially, and the fracture geometry indicates a potentially unstable reduction. The surgeon should carefully inspect the radiographs for this defect or palpate this region to feel for a defect. If the defect is seen on preoperative radiographs, the decision may be made to change internal fixation devices from a plate to an intramedullary device. Reduction can be done by open or closed means, with either method, the objective is a stable reduction, whether anatomical or nonanatomical.

Usually, closed reduction by manipulation should be attempted initially. In most fractures, an anatomical reduction with posteromedial apposition is possible. Fluoroscopy, with good-quality anteroposterior and lateral views, is used to evaluate the quality of the reduction, with special attention paid to the cortical contact medially and posteriorly. If good medial cortical contact is seen on the anteroposterior view and good posterior cortical contact is seen on the lateral view, the fracture can be internally fixed in this position. If a gap or overlap exists medially or posteriorly, adjustments in the traction or rotation may correct the reduction to a stable anatomical position. Frequently, in comminuted fractures, the distal shaft fragment sags posteriorly and may be difficult to correct by closed manipulation. In such cases, open anatomical reduction should be considered and the posterior sag may be corrected by lifting up with a hip skid under the fracture by an assistant. This position may need to be maintained during internal fixation to prevent recurrence of the deformity. In an *in vitro*, biomechanical study of posterior sag of 30° or more in two-part intertro chanteric fractures, scientists found no significant difference in construct strength or stability. If necessary, an open anatomical reduction of the medial and posterior cortical support usually can be accomplished by applying a bone-holding forceps across the fracture in an anteroposterior plane while adjusting the traction and rotation.

When an anatomically stable reduction has been achieved, a compression hip screw or other device can be used to secure the reduction. In rare cases, if the fracture is severely comminuted, anatomical reduction even by open means is difficult, if not impossible. In such circumstances, it may be wise to accept the nonanatomical, but stable reduction obtained by medial displacement techniques; however, a reduction that is nonanatomical and unstable should not be accepted. Stable fractures are treated by internal fixation after anatomical reduction. Unstable fractures usually can be treated by anatomical reduction, with the use of a collapsible fixation device, such as a hip compression screw or cephalomedullary nail. Such collapsible internal fixation devices permit the proximal fragment, to collapse or settle onto the fixation

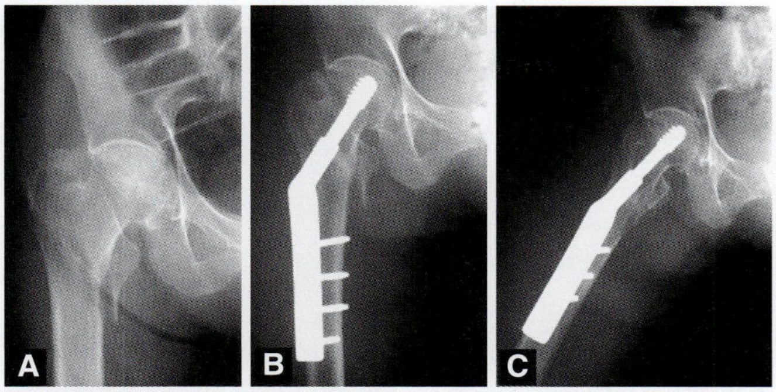

Figs 24.126A to C: Unstable fractures treated by anatomical reduction, with the use of a collapsible fixation device, such as a hip compression screw or cephalomedullary nail

device, seeking its own position of stability, with the shaft usually displacing medially, as shown in Figures 24.126A to C. Enlarged width to improve purchase in soft bone. We routinely use prophylactic antibiotics in the perioperative. Some authors have suggested that unstable trochanteric fractures in patients with severely osteoporotic bone are best thought of as pathological fractures and that the use of PMMA, to augment the fixation can improve stability in these patients. They recommended PMMA augmentation for unstable trochanteric fractures in elderly patients with severe osteoporosis, for whom no better form of fixation is available and the bone is too porotic to hold a screw. Some orthopedic manufacturers have introduced "super lag" screws that have screw threads of an period. Generally, a first generation cephalosporin is administered immediately before surgery and is continued for 24 hours after surgery. Some form of prophylactic anticoagulation therapy also is indicated, such as ultra-low-molecular-weight heparin (enoxaparin) or warfarin (Coumadin), however these are associated with complications of bleeding and postoperative hematomas. As of yet, there is no ideal prophylaxis for thromboembolism in these patients. Physical therapy is essential for successful restoration of mobility. The goal of physical therapy is a return to prefracture ambulation and overall function. Age younger than 85 years and the absence of multiple comorbid conditions correlated with the resumption of prefracture ambulatory status. We routinely have patients ambulating the day after surgery. When stable fixation has been achieved, as is our goal, we allow weight bearing as tolerated or full weight-bearing immediately. In this population, patients often do not have the upper body strength or balance to be less than full weight-bearing.

Implant Selection

Two broad categories of internal fixation devices are commonly used for intertrochanteric femoral fractures, sliding compression hip screws with side plate assemblies, as shown in Figure 24.127 and intramedullary fixation devices, shown in Figures 24.128A and B. Sliding hip screws, include traditional compression hip screws that provide compression in the intertrochanteric plane and compression plates that provide additional compression axially, as depicted in Figure 24.129. The intramedullary compression-type screw may be short and end in the diaphyseal femur or long and end in the supracondylar region.

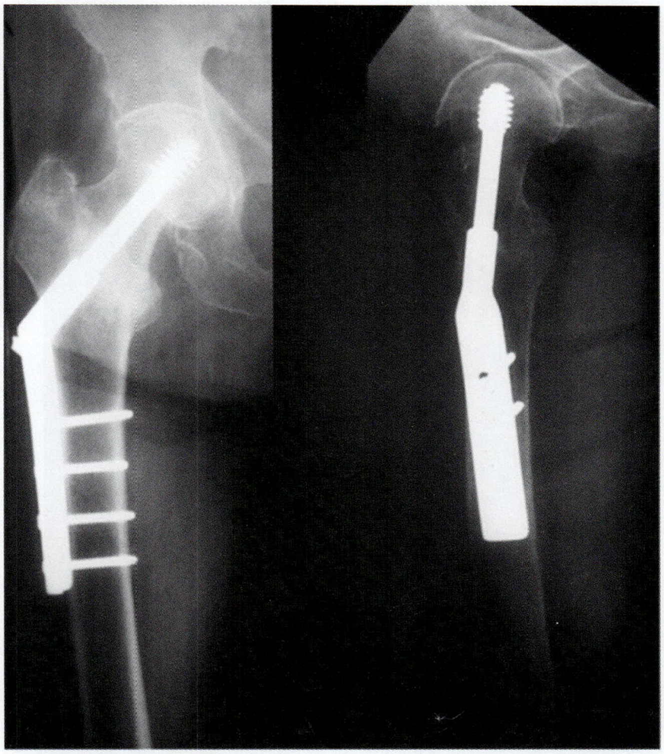

Fig. 24.127: Intertrochanteric femoral fractures treatment, using sliding compression hip screws with side plate assemblies

The preferred type of device is controversial. Intramedullary nails have a biomechanical and biological advantage over standard compression hip screws. Intramedullary nails can be inserted with less exposure of the fracture and less blood loss, although they require more fluoroscopic exposure and have been associated with fracture comminution. Biomechanically, nails allow for stable anatomical fixation of more comminuted fractures, without shortening the abductor moment arm or changing the proximal femoral anatomy. These devices provide fracture stability by virtue of allowing the lateral aspect of the head and neck, to come to rest against the nail in the medullary canal. Due to complication, we prefer the longer version of these implants, which extends to the supracondylar region of the femur, as shown in Figure 24.130. Intramedullary nails seem to have some advantage in unstable fractures, especially fractures with

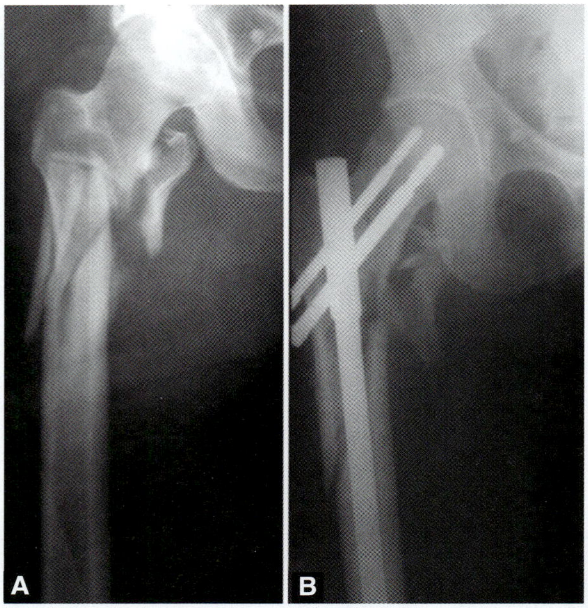

Figs 24.128A and B: Intertrochanteric femoral fractures treatment, using intramedullary fixation devices

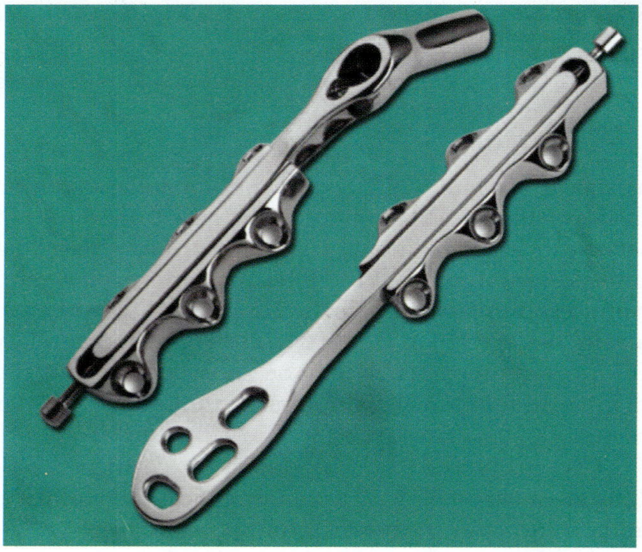

Fig. 24.129: Sliding hip screws, include traditional compression hip screws that provide compression in the intertrochanteric plane and compression plates that provide additional compression axially

reverse obliquity and subtrochanteric extension that cannot be treated easily with standard hip compression screws institution. Stable fractures (AO A1.1 through A2.1) may be treated by either devices, but the literature does not support the routine use of intramedullary nails in stable fractures because of concerns over the added complexity of the procedure and added expense of the intramedullary implants.

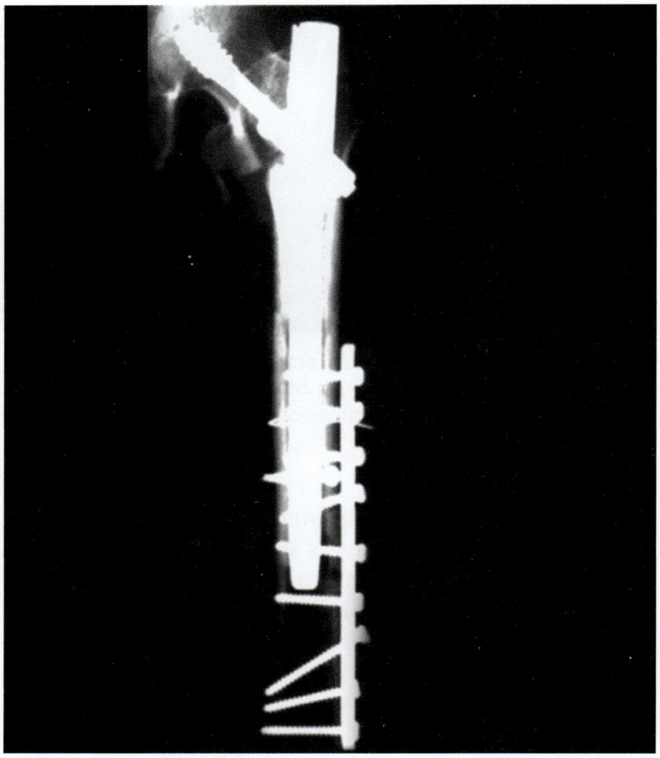

Fig. 24.130: Intramedullary nails

Fixation with Sliding Compression Hip Screw Devices

Sliding compression screw assemblies were introduced, to allow compression of some intertrochanteric fractures. The depth to which the lag screw fixation is inserted into the head is crucial for maximal purchase on the proximal fragment; the screw should be inserted to within 1 cm of the subchondral bone. The optimal angle between the barrel and the side plate of a hip compression screw is controversial. Many authors have argued that 150° plates are preferable because the angle of the lag screw more closely parallels the compressive forces within the femoral neck. Theoretically, this should lead to less binding of the screw within the barrel of the side plate and less chance of failure of the implant from bending. In clinical studies, however no difference has been found in the compression ability of 135° hip compression screws and 150° devices. Plate fracture secondary to failure in a bending mode has been reported only rarely in true intertrochanteric fractures. More problematic is the placement of 150° lag screws in the center of the femoral head because they tend toward superior placement within the head, leading to a higher chance of screw cutout. Due to the 135° devices are easily placed and because their clinical results are similar to those for the 150° plates, the higher angle plates are only rarely indicated for extremely valgus femoral necks and more distal fractures.

In the past, with fixation devices that did not allow collapse, medial displacement osteotomy was performed more frequently. They found that in four-part intertrochanteric fractures, anatomical reduction with the sliding hip screw, regardless of the presence of a posteromedial fragment, provided significantly higher compression across the calcar region and significantly lower tensile strain on the side plate than did medial displacement osteotomy. Scientists compared unstable intertrochanteric fractures treated with anatomical reduction and a hip compression screw with fractures treated with medial displacement osteotomy and found no significant differences in eventual healing or walking ability, although surgery time and blood loss were higher in the osteotomy group. These researchers concluded that there was no advantage to medial displacement osteotomy in these fractures. A short-barrel side plate often is needed with this technique, to prevent impingement of the compression screw against the barrel in the neck of the femur with this configuration. Disadvantages include a larger plate profile and the possibility of mechanical failure of the angle-locking mechanism. This aids in resisting lateral sliding of the proximal fragment and maintaining an anatomical reduction, as illustrated in Figure 24.131. The current version of this device, allows for sliding of the screw in the barrel and is applied on top of a compression hip screw. This technique adds to surgical time, blood loss and amount of dissection needed to apply the device. The two barrels and screws are inserted in the head of the femur and all screws are

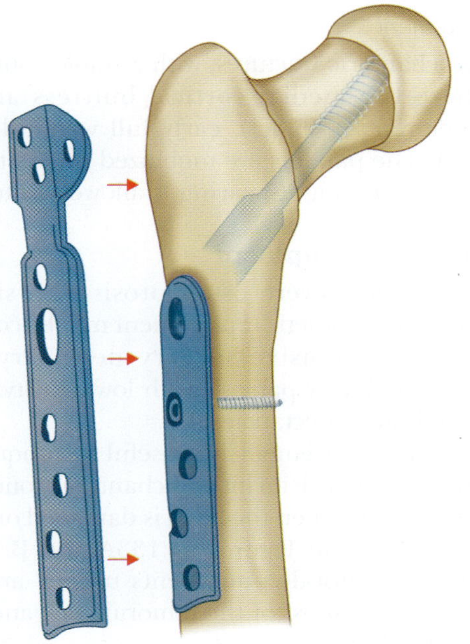

Fig. 24.131: Reduction with a hip compression screw and medial displacement osteotomy. A short-barrel side plate often is needed with this technique, to prevent impingement of the compression screw against the barrel in the neck of the femur with this configuration

inserted percutaneously. We have limited experience with these devices and the literature has not supported their widespread use.

Compression Hip Screw Fixation of an Intertrochanteric Hip Fracture

The techniques for hip screw insertion are similar for all devices. The technique described next is for the Richards classic compression screw.

After Treatment

The patient is mobilized the day after surgery and active exercises of the upper and lower extremities are begun. Depending on the patient's condition and the stability of the internal fixation, weight-bearing to tolerance is begun using a walker.

Biaxial Compression Plate Fixation

Medoff modified the standard compression hip screw, recognizing the need for axial compression until stability is obtained, especially in intertrochanteric fractures with a significant subtrochanteric component. His modification includes the traditional proximal screw in a barrel, a two-part sliding plate and a distally positioned compression screw, to compress the proximal femoral fracture fragment to the shaft in the subtrochanteric region.

The plate that is applied to the lateral part of the femur is in two parts, with the barrel and proximal part sliding into a slot on the distal part that is fixed to the femur with oblique screws. It usually is recommended for unstable intertrochanteric fractures and subtrochanteric fractures. The Medoff plate comes in two versions: six-hole and four-hole plates. The six-hole plate has an axial compression screw at the end of the plate and a proximal blocking screw, to prevent barrel back-out in highly comminuted fractures and to provide for more axial and anatomical compression.

Intertrochanteric Osteotomy

Emphasizing that restoration of medial continuity is essential to successful internal fixation of three-part and four-part intertrochanteric fractures, as shown in Figure 24.132. More recent studies have indicated, however that anatomical reduction allows greater load sharing, by the bone than does medial displacement osteotomy and that with sliding hip compression screw devices, stability is not improved by osteotomy. Knowledge of these techniques is still occasionally useful in some extremely comminuted fractures, in which anatomical reduction is not feasible.

Fixation with Intramedullary Devices

Intramedullary devices have at least theoretical advantages over open reduction procedures in that the surgical procedure for insertion is much less extensive,

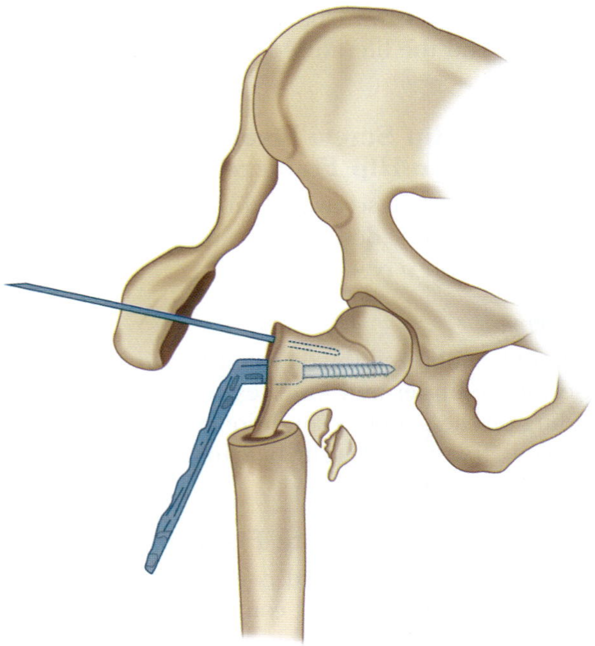

Fig. 24.132: Intertrochanteric osteotomy

the fracture is not opened, and the operating time and blood loss may be lessened. With the fixation device within the medullary canal, the bending moment on it is considerably less than on standard compression screw and side plate devices. Cephalomedullary nails, such as the Gamma nail, the intramedullary hip screw and interlocking intramedullary nails inserted in the Recon mode, have been used for fixation of unstable intertrochanteric fractures. These devices are centromedullary nails with proximal fixation into the femoral head by nails, screws or blades.

The Gamma nail and intramedullary hip screw began, as shorter nails than reconstruction nails, with the device ending within the diaphysis of the femur. This allows relatively reliable targeting of the distal interlocking screws through a proximally attached insertion guide.

Changes in the angle of the nail and a smaller diameter have decreased the incidence of this complication, but because there is still a risk of late fracture and because this patient population is at risk for further falls, we advocate the use of long intramedullary nails that end at the supracondylar region of the femur. Unless, there is extensive comminution that increases the risk for shortening, or unless the medullary canal is unusually large increasing the risk for late malrotation, we usually do not lock the distal ends of these long nails when used for intertrochanteric fractures.

The literature on these devices and our experience are limited. These devices seem to have some benefit in reverse obliquity intertrochanteric fractures and in fractures with subtrochanteric extension, but not for routine, stable intertrochanteric hip fractures. The technique for intramedullary hip screw placement is similar to the Gamma nail technique and is useful in the treatment of unstable peritrochanteric fractures, reverse obliquity fractures and subtrochanteric fractures. The intramedullary hip screw nail is cannulated with a 4° mediolateral bend, to allow for insertion through the greater trochanter. It is used with a standard Richards AMBI/Classic lag screw (½-inch thread diameter) and compression screw. A sleeve over the lag screw is used to prevent rotation, while allowing the lag screw to slide. The long nail is designed for subtrochanteric fractures, femoral reconstruction after tumor resection, prophylactic nailing of impending pathological fractures and leg-length discrepancies after femoral fracture. The nail has a distal diameter of 10 mm and is available in lengths of 34 cm, 38 cm and 42 cm and angles of 130° and 135°. A slight bend in the nail conforms to the natural bow of the femoral shaft and the 10° of anteversion, matches the angle of the femoral head in relation to the shaft of the femur. Distal locking is accomplished with 4.5 mm locking screws. The long nail has a proximal diameter of 17.5 mm. The operation is performed on a standard fracture table and requires the use of an image intensifier, which produces images in two planes. Anteroposterior and lateral views of the proximal one half of the femur should be obtained preoperatively or fluoroscopically, at the time of surgery. Severe deformities of the femoral canal or excessive anterior bowing may preclude the use of an intramedullary device.

After Treatment

In peritrochanteric fractures, with a stable configuration (i.e. where the medial cortical buttress and lesser trochanter remain intact), early full weight-bearing is permitted. The patients are mobilized the first day after surgery and full weight-bearing is allowed as tolerated.

Prosthetic Arthroplasty

In patients with severe osteoporosis with significant comminution, prosthetic replacement may be considered, however the extensive surgery necessary may be unjustified in elderly patients with low activity demands and limited life expectancies.

Prosthetic replacement is a useful technique for the occasional patient with an intertrochanteric nonunion and failure of fixation, when the head is damaged or the bone is poor, as shown in Figures 24.133A and B. In calcar replacement, femoral components usually are needed because of loss of most of the femoral neck and possibly the lesser trochanter.

Salvage Procedures

If there is a nonunion or loss of fixation of an intertrochanteric fracture and the articular cartilage of the

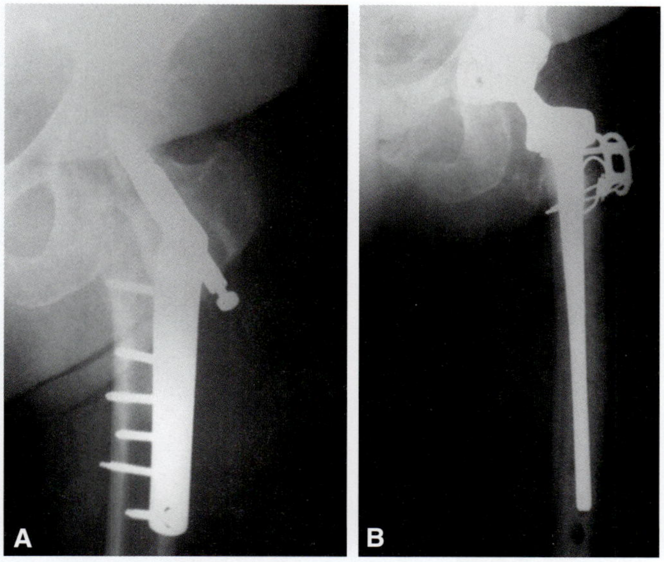

Figs 24.133A and B: Prosthetic replacement for intertrochanteric nonunion and failure of fixation

head has not been damaged by the implant, the hip may be saved by revising the internal fixation and bone grafting the fracture. In a series of 20 patients (mean age 58 years) by Haidukewych and Berry, 11 patients had secondary hip fixation with an angled blade plate, five had a dynamic hip screw, three had a condylar screw and one had a cephalomedullary nail. Bone grafting was used in all patients and 19 of the 20 healed. We usually change from intramedullary to extramedullary forms of fixation (or vice versa).

SUBTROCHANTERIC FEMORAL FRACTURES

Some scientists called attention to subtrochanteric fractures, as a variant of peritrochanteric fractures and noted their higher incidence of unsatisfactory results after operative treatment. Since that time, subtrochanteric fractures have been variously defined, but most authors limit the term to fractures between the lesser trochanter and the isthmus of the diaphysis. They have a bimodal age distribution and different mechanisms of injury. Older patients typically sustain low-velocity trauma, whereas in younger patients these fractures commonly result from high-energy trauma and often are associated with other fractures and injuries. Restoration of femoral length and rotation and correction of femoral head and neck angulation to restore adequate abductor tension and strength are essential, to restoring maximal ambulatory capacity.

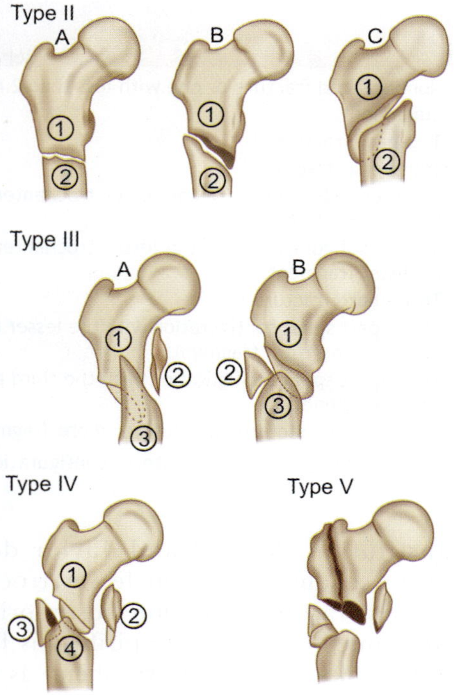

Fig. 24.134: Seinsheimer, classification of femoral subchondral fractures

Classification

The introduction of various classification systems gives some insight into the evolution of treatment options and indicates the uncertainty regarding the treatment and prognosis of this complex fracture. Boyd and Griffin in their classification of trochanteric fractures, included subtrochanteric elements in types III and IV. According to Fielding's classification of subtrochanteric fractures, a type I fracture is at the level of the lesser trochanter, a type II fracture is 2.5 to 5 cm below the lesser trochanter and a type III fracture is 5 to 7.5 cm below the lesser trochanter. Transverse fractures fit this classification well, but oblique and comminuted fractures may involve more than one of the levels described and should be classified according to, where the major portion of the fracture occurs. Traditionally, fractures at the upper level have a better prognosis for union than fractures at the lower level. Seinsheimer, developed the following classification system based on the number of fragments and the location and configuration of the fracture lines, as shown in Figure 24.134 and Table 24.11.

With the development of modern reconstruction nails, also known as second-generation intramedullary nails, the classification schemes of Fielding and Seinsheimer have become less useful because they do not separate fractures according to the different treatment methods.

Table 24.11: Seinsheimer, classification system for femoral subchondral fractures

Type I:	Nondisplaced fracture or one with less than 2 mm of displacement
Type II:	Two-part fracture
Type IIA:	Transverse fracture
Type IIB:	Spiral configuration with the lesser trochanter attached to proximal fragment
Type IIC:	Spiral configuration with the lesser trochanter attached to distal fragment
Type III:	Three-part fracture
Type IIIA:	Three-part spiral configuration with the lesser trochanter a part of the third fragment
Type IIIB:	Three-part spiral configuration with the third part a butterfly fragment
Type IV:	Comminuted fracture with four or more fragments
Type V:	Subtrochanteric-intertrochanteric configuration

At this institution, Russell and Taylor devised a classification scheme based on lesser trochanteric continuity and fracture extension posteriorly on the greater trochanter involving the piriformis fossa, the major two variables influencing treatment, as shown in Figure 24.135.

Type I fractures do not extend into the piriformis fossa, whereas type II fractures do involve the piriformis fossa, in the past, the most commonly used nail entry portal. In type IA fractures, the lesser trochanter is intact and in type IB fractures, the lesser trochanter is fractured. In type IA fractures, comminution and fracture lines extend from below the lesser trochanter to the femoral isthmus, any degree of comminution may be present in this area, including bicortical comminution. Type IB fractures have fracture lines and comminution, involving the area of the lesser trochanter to the isthmus (see Figure Type IIA fractures extend from the lesser trochanter to the isthmus, with extension into the piriformis fossa, as detected on lateral radiographs, but significant comminution or major fracture of the lesser trochanter is not present). In type IIB fractures, the fracture extends into the piriformis fossa with significant comminution of the medial femoral cortex and loss of continuity of the lesser trochanter. In type I fractures, closed intramedullary nailing has the advantage of minimizing vascular compromise of the fracture fragments. In type II fractures, the extension into the piriformis fossa complicates closed nailing techniques. In type IA and IIA fractures, the lesser trochanter is intact, making medial stability more likely. Plate fixation may be the device of choice. With the development of nails that are placed through a trochanteric portal, it is even more likely that the nail's entry portal will be fractured. For this reason, careful attention to surgical technique is necessary, to avoid further comminution of the fracture or inadvertently displacing the fracture during nail insertion.

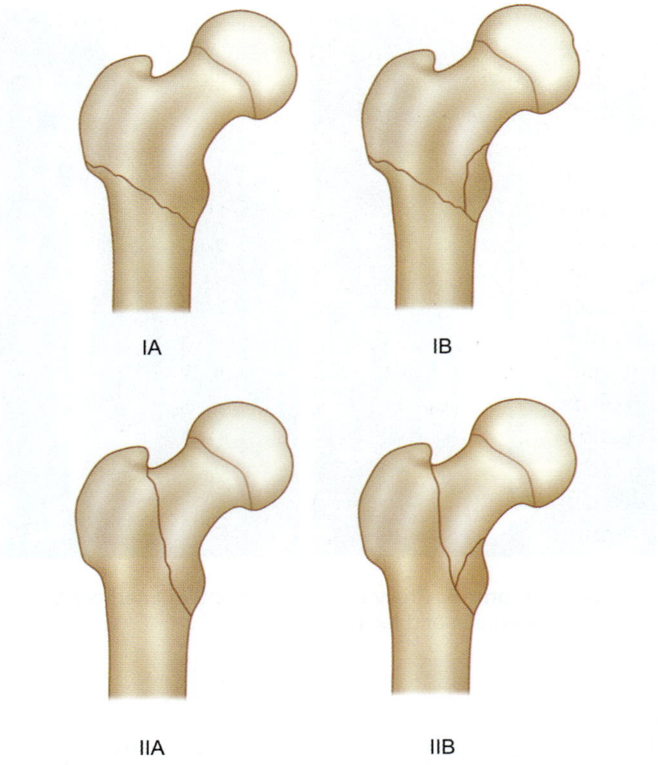

Fig. 24.135: Russell and Taylor classification of femoral subchondral fractures

Treatment

Treatment methods for subtrochanteric fractures have included nonoperative methods, such as traction techniques, which yielded variable results. Plate and screw fixation of subtrochanteric fractures is still advocated by many authors, especially for fractures with intertrochanteric extension, such as Russell-Taylor types IIA and IIB fractures. In this group, all fractures united and there were no deep infections. Compression hip screws have been a popular method of internal fixation for subtrochanteric fractures. They credit at least a portion of their good results, to the approach that preserves the fracture's vascularity. Advantages of intramedullary devices also include retained blood supply to bone fragments, less operative blood loss and less disruption of the fracture environment. Modern reconstruction nails have greatly improved the outcome and ease of treatment of subtrochanteric fractures. The first modern cephalomedullary reconstruction nail, the Russell-Taylor reconstruction nail is a closed-section, stainless steel nail with proximal interlocking screws that extend into the femoral head and distal interlocking screws similar to standard first-generation interlocking nails. In the original series of patients treated with this device, 59 subtrochanteric fractures all healed uneventfully without the need for bone grafting, auxiliary fixation, immobilization, or nail dynamization (removal of the distal locking screws to allow fracture impaction in cases of delayed union).

Short cephalomedullary nails, principally the Gamma nail and similar devices, including the intramedullary hip screw have been used for high subtrochanteric fractures and for intertrochanteric fractures with subtrochanteric extension. A potential complication of these devices is late femoral fracture at the tip of the device, this does not occur with nails that extend well into the distal metaphysis of the femur. For this reason, we usually do not use short intramedullary devices. Before the development of closed-section interlocking reconstruction nails, complex subtrochanteric fractures were treated at our institution with compression hip screws and side plates with bone grafting, if the medial cortex was comminuted. Difficulty often was encountered, when comminution was extensive. Cephalomedullary interlocking nailing allows length and rotational control, even when the lesser trochanter is not intact. Involvement of the piriformis fossa, the entry portal for the device, does not contraindicate its use, but does increase the technical difficulty of placement. The choice of treatment of subtrochanteric fractures depends on several factors.

- When the greater and lesser trochanters are intact, conventional interlocking intramedullary nailing may be indicated.
- In fractures with extension into the lesser trochanter, the Russell-Taylor reconstruction nail, inserted with closed techniques is our treatment of choice.
- Plate and screw fixation probably is best used for fractures in patients with pre-existing deformities of the proximal femur, previous implants or Russell-Taylor type IIA fractures.
- Pathological fractures of the subtrochanteric area are best treated with reconstruction nails, which allow stabilization of the entire femur.
- In general, our treatment recommendations are based on the involvement of the piriformis fossa or greater trochanter, as the usual entry portals for nails.
- Regular interlocking intramedullary nails can be used for fixation of most femoral fractures between the distal fifth of the femur and a point just distal to the lesser trochanter.
- We prefer a cephalomedullary reconstruction nail, for fractures with extension into the lesser trochanter (Russell-Taylor type IB), as shown in Figures 24.136A and B.

Russell-Taylor types IIA and IIB fractures can be treated with reconstruction nails, although the technique becomes more demanding, as shown in Figures 24.137A to C. Closed techniques, with image intensifier guidance can be used. Determination of the proper entry portal is more difficult, improper positioning of the nail can occur,

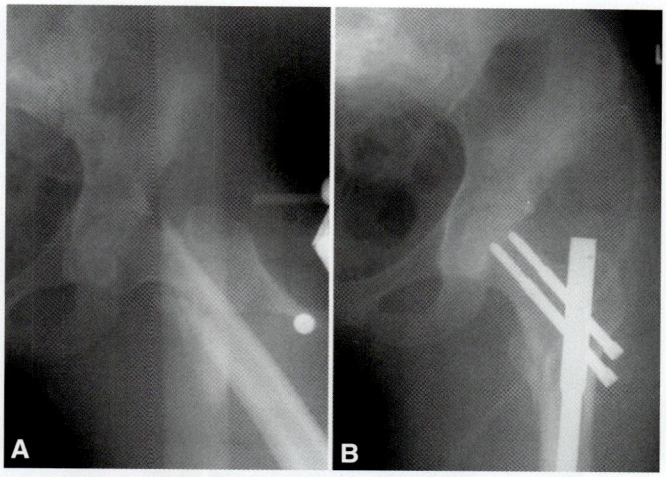

Figs 24.136A and B: Intramedullary nailing: Cephalomedullary reconstruction nail for fractures with extension into the lesser trochanter

if the guidewire or nail, itself slips posteriorly in the comminution around the trochanteric or piriformis fossa entry portal, stabilization of the posterior fragment may be inadequate and nail placement lateral to the correct portal predisposes to varus deformity at the fracture. In a series of 61 unstable subtrochanteric fractures treated at this clinic with Russell-Taylor reconstruction nails, 12 displayed extension of the fracture into the piriformis fossa (Russell-Taylor types IIA and IIB). Careful attention to proper guidewire positioning, allowed successful nail placement in all 12 fractures. Type II fractures, with involvement of the piriformis fossa, can also be fixed with a hip compression screw or Medoff plate and an indirect reduction technique. For type IIB fractures, autogenous bone grafting should be considered at the time of fixation of the fracture if the fracture is opened.

Fixation with an Interlocking Reconstruction Nail

Care must be taken, however to avoid the same complications that occur with nailing of any fracture, in which the entry portal is involved in the fracture site, displacement of the fracture and the nail not being contained within the bone. In subtrochanteric fractures, there is a tendency for the nail to fall posteriorly out of the femur proximally, if the greater trochanter is comminuted and a portal is placed there. The TriGen nail has replaced the Russell-Taylor nail at our clinic, as the cephalomedullary nail of choice in subtrochanteric fractures. It is a titanium closed-section nail that has a 5° lateral proximal bow, to make use of a trochanteric entry portal. Two holes in the nail allow two 6.4 mm, titanium, and partially threaded locking screws, to be inserted into the femoral head. The angle between the shaft of the nail and the proximal locking screws is 135°. Lengths

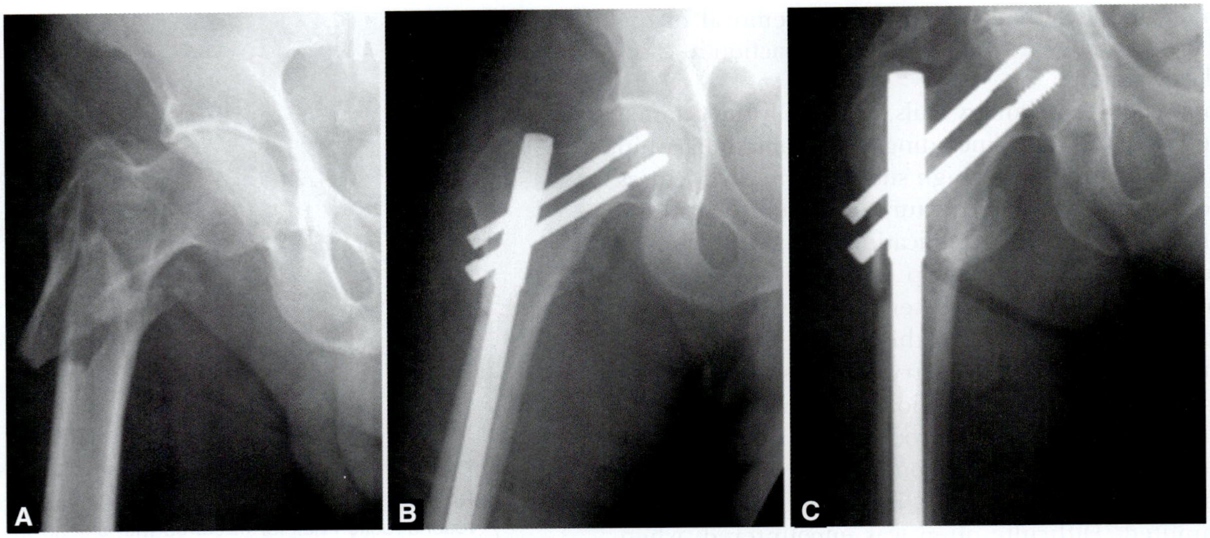

Figs 24.137A to C: Reconstruction nailing in Russell-Taylor types IIA and IIB fractures

range from 30 to 50 cm and the nail comes in 10 mm, 11.5 mm and 13 mm diameters.

After Treatment

The patient is allowed to ambulate partial weight bearing, with crutches the day after surgery. Progressive weight-bearing is based on radiographic evidence of callus formation.

Fixation with Hip Compression Screw and Side Plate

Biomechanical and clinical studies have indicated that Russell-Taylor type II subtrochanteric fractures can be fixed adequately with a hip compression screw and side plate combination.

Newer systems have improved fatigue characteristics and loss of fixation usually occurs from cutout of the screw from the femoral head, rather than from fracture of the plate, as occurred with older designs. For subtrochanteric fractures, detailed preoperative planning is essential. Lag screw fixation of major fragments should be planned carefully, to avoid placing the screws in areas that would be compromised by plate application. We use an AO femoral distractor and the indirect reduction technique described by Kinast et al. After provisional reduction has been obtained and is held with Kirschner wires, the hip compression screw is inserted in the standard manner. At least four screws should engage both cortices in the distal fragment. Lag screws can be used through the plate, but screw fixation in the proximal fragment, prevents the compression screw from obtaining some dynamization. The hip compression screw device used should prevent rotation of the lag screw in the barrel. If medial dissection is necessary, autogenous iliac bone grafting should be used. In a similar way, the Medoff plate can be used, especially if the comminution does not extend distally down the shaft of the femur.

Indirect Reduction and Fixation with a 95° Condylar Plate

Some scientists compared their results of open reduction and blade plate fixation of subtrochanteric fractures with indirect reduction and fixation.

After Treatment

After treatment is similar to that for hip compression screw fixation of intertrochanteric fractures. Generally, the medial buttress is not completely restored and only touch-down weight bearing is allowed, until signs of early fracture healing are present at 6 to 8 weeks. Full weight-bearing, usually is delayed for up to 3 months after surgery.

TRAUMATIC DISLOCATION OF HIP

■ Introduction

Hip dislocations were once a rarity and have become increasingly common due to increased number of automobile accidents and high speed transportation. Traumatic dislocation of hip joint, include pure hip dislocation, dislocation with fracture femoral neck and dislocations with fracture of acetabulum.

Joint Contact Area (Fig. 24.138)

Throughout ROM:
- Fourty percent of femoral head is in contact with acetabular articular cartilage.
- Ten percent of femoral head is in contact with labrum.

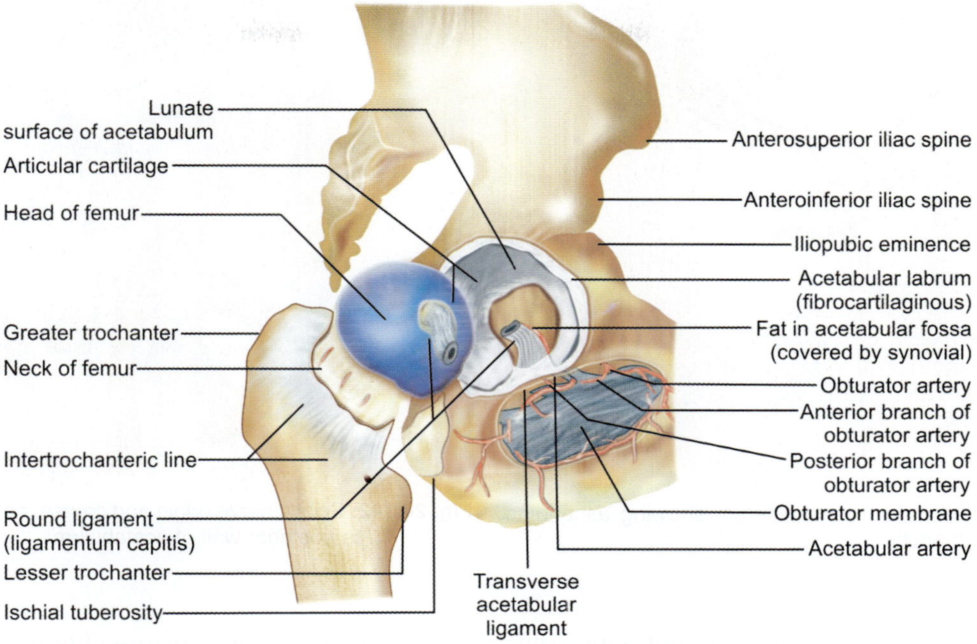

Fig. 24.138: Hip joint opened lateral view, showing joint contact areas

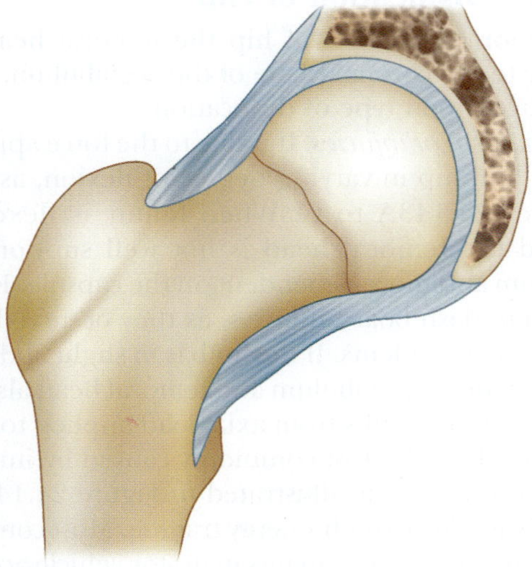

Fig. 24.139: Hip joint capsule

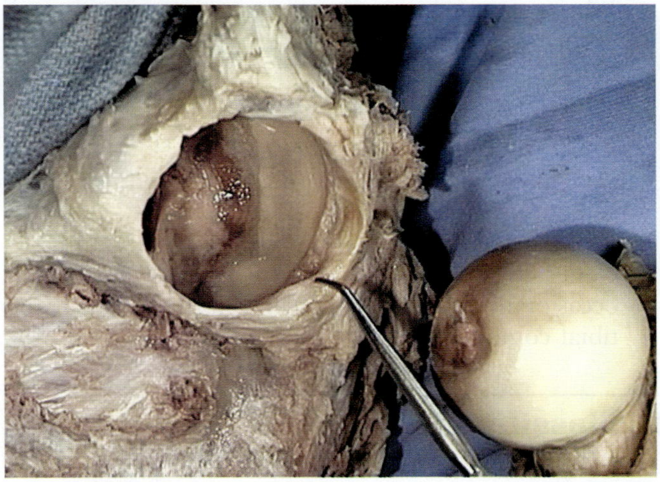

Fig. 24.140: Opened hip joint with acetabular labrum

Hip Joint Capsule (Fig. 24.139)

Extends from intertrochanteric ridge of proximal femur to bony perimeter of acetabulum. It has several thick bands of fibrous tissue:

Iliofemoral Ligament

- Upside-down "Y"
- Blocks hip extension
- Allows muscle relaxation with standing.

Acetabular Labrum (Fig. 24.140)

- Strong fibrous ring
- Increases femoral head coverage
- Contributes to hip joint stability.

Blood Supply to Femoral Head (See Figs 24.18A to C)

Artery of Ligamentum Teres

- Most important in children

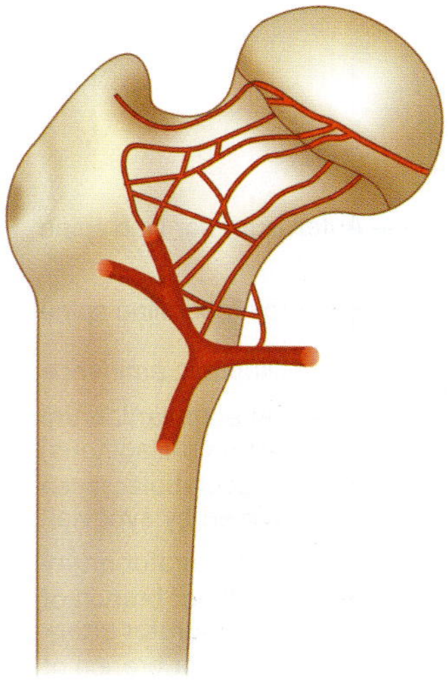

Fig. 24.141: Arteries of ligamentum teres, showing ascending cervical branches

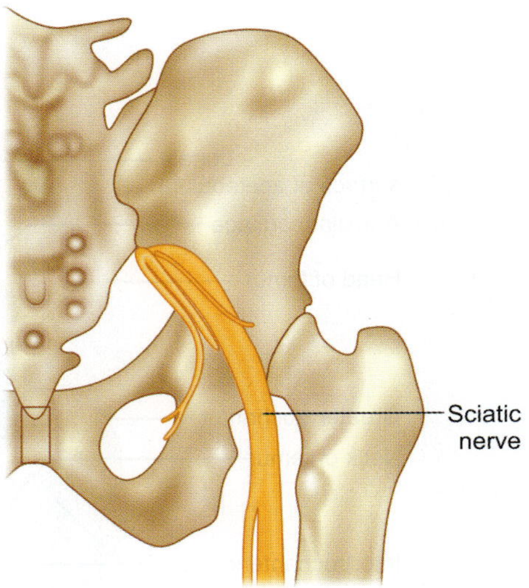

Fig. 24.142: Sciatic nerve origin and course, as it passes posterior to posterior wall of acetabulum

- Its contribution decreases with age and is probably insignificant in elderly patients
- *Ascending cervical branches (Fig. 24.141):* Arise from ring at base of neck. Ring is formed by branches of medial and lateral circumflex femoral arteries. Penetrate capsule near its femoral attachment and ascend along neck. Perforate bone just distal to articular cartilage. It is highly susceptible to injury with hip dislocation.

Sciatic Nerve (Fig. 24.142)

- It is formed from roots of L4 to S3.
- Peroneal and tibial components differentiate early, sometimes as proximal as in pelvis.
- Passes posterior to posterior wall of acetabulum.
- Generally, passes inferior to piriformis muscle, but occasionally the piriformis will split the peroneal and tibial components.

Classification of Hip Dislocation

I. Congenital
II. Acquired
  a. Traumatic
  b. Pathological, e.g. tubercular arthritis and pyogenic arthritis
  c. Paralytic, e.g. poliomyelitis and cerebral palsy

Classification of traumatic dislocation hip:

I. Simple dislocations
  a. Posterior dislocation
  b. Anterior dislocation
II. Fracture dislocations
  a. Associated with fracture of acetabular rim
  b. Associated with fracture of femoral head
  c. Associated with fracture of femoral neck
  d. Associated with fracture of femur
  e. Central fracture dislocation

Posterior Dislocation of Hip

In posterior dislocation of hip the femoral head rests posterior to the coronal plane of the acetabulum. This is the most common type of dislocation.

Mechanism of injuries: It is due to the force applied to the knee and hip in varying degree of flexion, as shown in Figures 24.143A to C. When femur is flexed and adducted the femoral head is not well supported by acetabulum and more dependent on the capsule. Funsten called them dash board injuries, as they occurred in the motor vehicle accidents. If the limb is in slight abduction, fracture of rim of acetabulum and femoral head also takes place. Generally results from axial load applied to femur, while hip is flexed. Most commonly caused by impact of dashboard on knee, as illustrated in Figure 24.144. It is almost always due to high-energy trauma. Most commonly involve unrestrained occupants in motor vehicle accidents (MVAs). It can also occur in pedestrian-MVAs, falls from heights, industrial accidents and sporting injuries.

Pathoanatomy of Dislocations

In posterior dislocation, capsule is torn either directly or inferoposteriorly depending upon the amount of flexion at the time of injury. "Y" ligament is generally intact. Capsule is sripped from its acetabular attachment. In anterior dislocation, psoas acts as a fulcrum and the capsule is disrupted anteriorly and inferiorly. Femoral vessels may be injured.

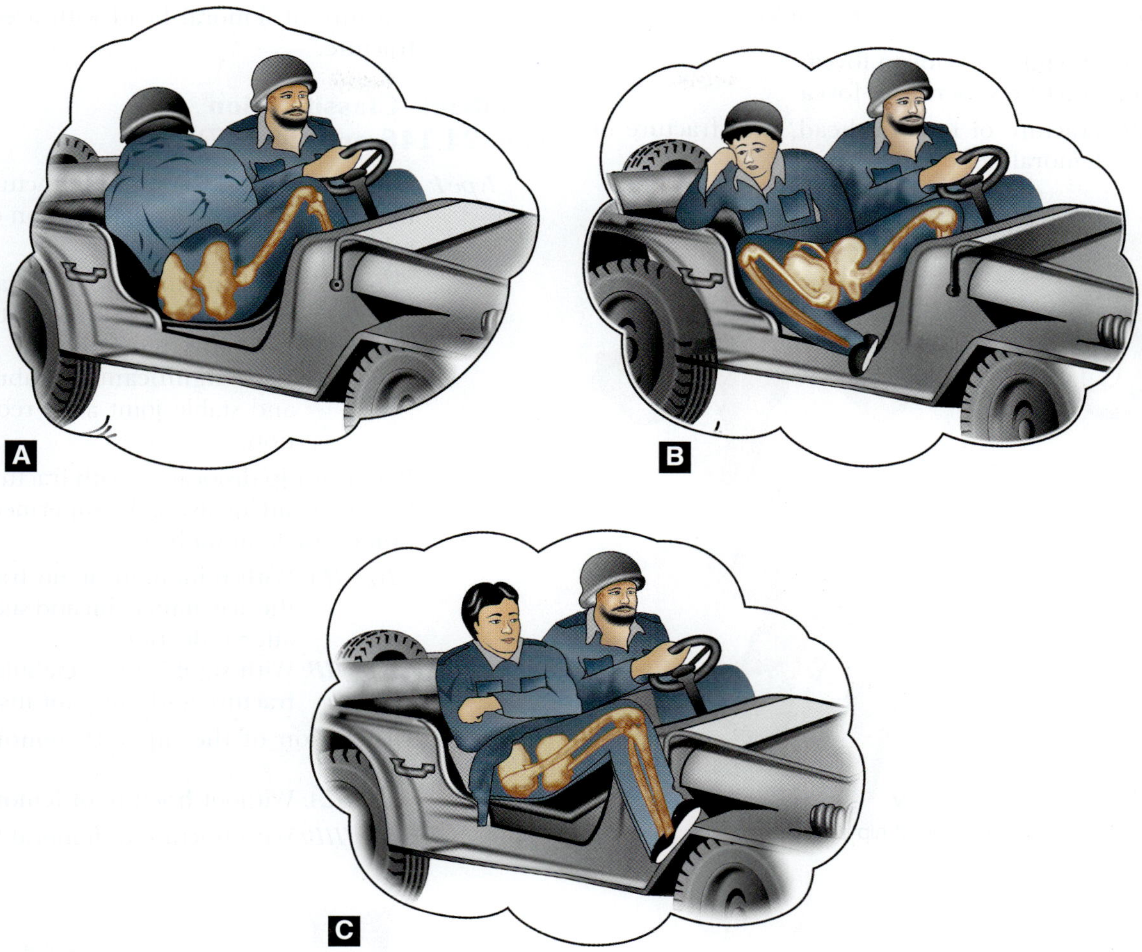

Figs 24.143A to C: Different mechanisms of posterior hip dislocation

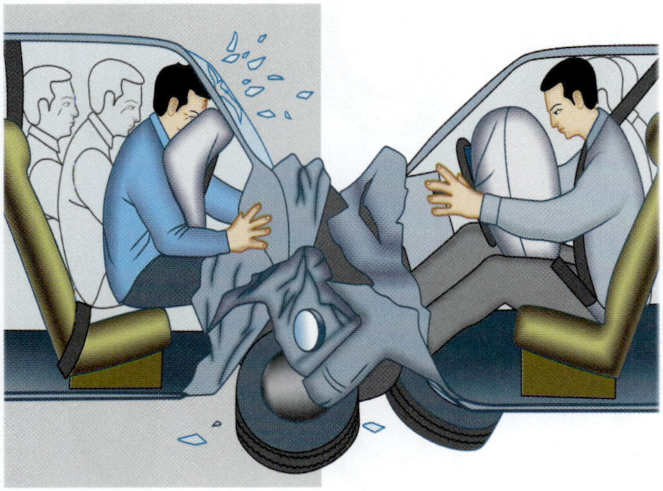

Fig. 24.144: MVA with resulted axial load on the hip and by the impact of dashboard on knee, causing posterior hip dislocation

Effect of Dislocation on Femoral Head Circulation

- When capsule tears, ascending cervical branches are torn or stretched.
- Artery of ligamentum teres is torn.
- Some ascending cervical branches may remain kinked or compressed, until the hip is reduced.
- Thus, early reduction of the dislocated hip can improve blood flow to femoral head.

Thomas and Epstein classification of hip dislocations (Most well-known)

Type I: Pure dislocation with atmost a small posterior wall fragment.

Type II: Dislocation with large posterior wall fragment.

Type III: Dislocation with comminuted posterior wall.

Type IV: Dislocation with "acetabular floor" fracture (probably transverse and posterior wall acetabulum fracture-dislocation).

Type V: Dislocation with femoral head fracture.

Pipkin Classification (Fig. 24.145)

Type I: Fracture inferior to fovea
Type II: Fracture superior to fovea
Type III: Fracture of femoral head, with fracture of femoral neck

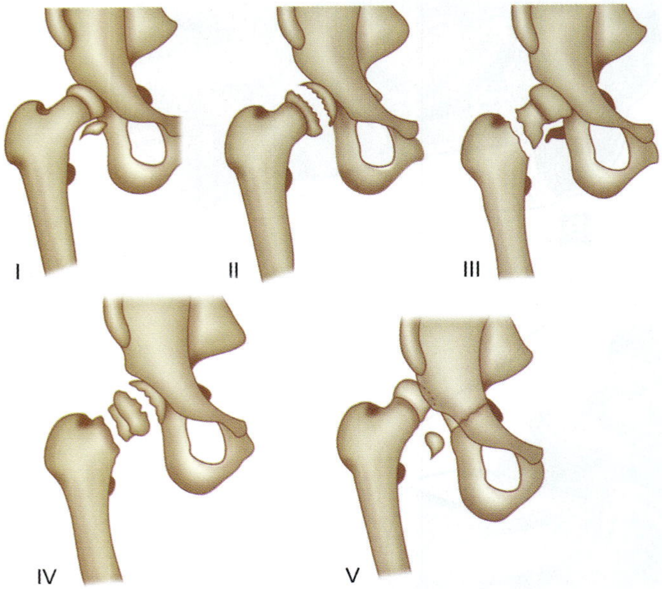

Fig. 24.145: Pipkin classification of hip dislocation

Type IV: Fracture of femoral head with acetabulum fracture.

Brumback Classification (Figs 24.146 and 24.147)

Type I: Posterior hip dislocation with fracture of the involving the inferomedial portion of femoral head.
- *Type IA:* With minimum or no fracture of the acetabular rim and stable hip joint after reduction.
- *Type IB:* With significant acetabular rim and stable joint after reconstruction.

Type II: Posterior hip dislocation with fracture of the femoral head involving the supermedial portion of the femoral head
- *Type IIA:* With minimum or no fracture of the acetabular rim and stable joint after reduction.
- *Type IIB:* With significant acetabular fracture and hip joint instability.

Type III: Dislocation of the hip with femoral neck fracture
- *Type IIIA:* Without fracture of femoral head
- *Type IIIB:* With fracture of femoral head

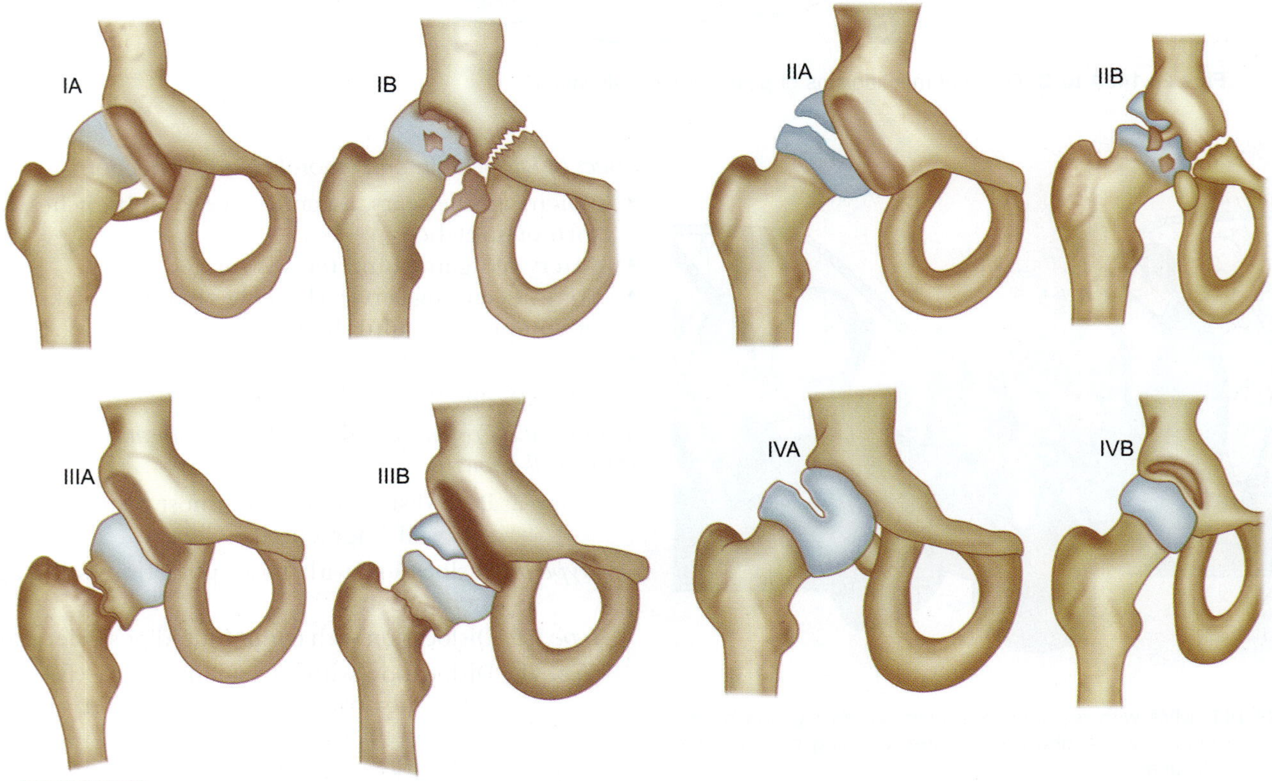

Fig. 24.146: Brumback classification of hip dislocation

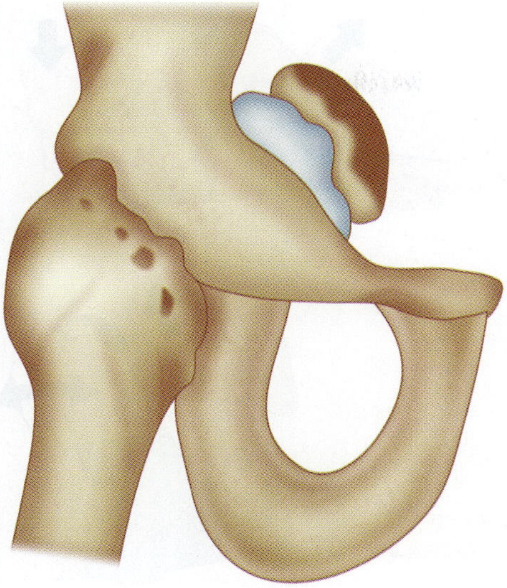

Fig. 24.147: Brumback classification of hip dislocation—Type V central fracture dislocation of hip

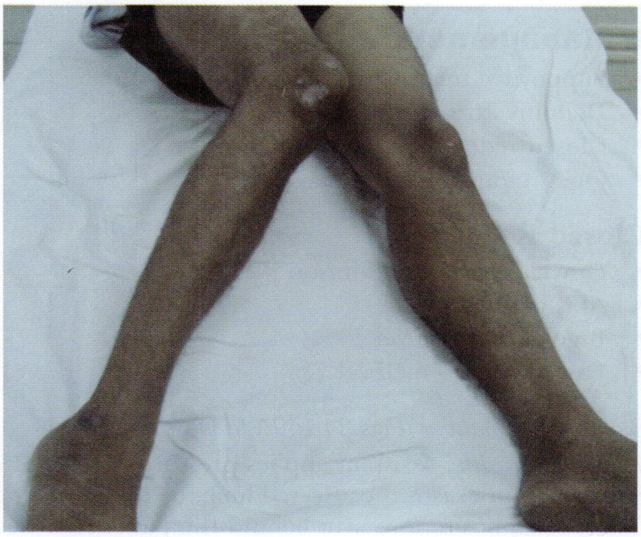

Fig. 24.148: Posterior dislocation—Hip flexed, internally rotated and adducted

Type IV: Anterior dislocation of femoral head

Type IVA: *Indentation type:* Depression of the superolateral surface of the femoral head

Type IVB: *Transchondral type:* Osteocartilaginous fracture of the weight-bearing surface of the femoral head.

Type V: Central fracture dislocation of the hip with femoral head fracture.

Stewart and Milford Classification

Type I: Simple dislocation without fracture

Type II: Dislocation with one or more rim fragments, but with sufficient socket to ensure stability after reduction

Type III: Dislocation with fracture of the rim producing gross instability

Type IV: Dislocation with fracture of the head and neck of femur.

Evaluation

History

- Significant trauma, usually MVA.
- Awake, alert patients have severe pain in hip region.

Physical Examination

Classical appearance of posterior dislocation of hip, as shown in Figure 24.148.

Unclassical presentation (posture) if

- Femoral head or neck fracture
- Femoral shaft fracture
- Obtunded patient.

Signs and Symptoms

- Pain on palpation of hip
- Pain with attempted motion of hip
- Possible neurological impairment
- Vascular sign of narath positive
- Femoral head can be palpated in the gluteal region
- Associated ligamentous injury to the ipsilateral knee
- Fracture of the head of femur, femora shaft and acetabulum
- Sciatic nerve injury
- Patient might be in shock.

Investigations

X-rays: These include:

- AP X-ray
- Oblique lateral view of pelvis
- Posterior oblique view
- Full length femur.

X-ray findings

- Loss of congruence of femoral head with roof of acetabulum
- Head will appear smaller than the contralateral head
- Overlapping of the head with the acetabulum
- Lesser trochanter lies apparent and neck seen due to internal rotation
- Break in shentons line.

CT scan to delineate fracture fragments size and location—Routine lab investigations.

■ Management

- Supportive treatment, e.g. treat shock
- Definitive treatment
- Closed reduction
- Open reduction

Closed Reduction

- Gravity method of Stimson
- Allis maneuver
- Bigelow's maneuver
- East baltimore method

Bigelow's Maneuver (Figs 24.149A to D)

Patient is supine: Assistant applies pressure to the ASIS. Surgeon then grasps the affected limb, by the ankle and places hisopposite fore arm behind the patient's flexed knee.

Longitudinal traction is then applied in the direction of the deformity, followed by the flexion of hip to 90° or greater, while mantaining it in an adduction internally rotated position. This relaxes the "Y" ligament. Femur head comes near the posterior inferior rim of acetabulum. While continuing the traction femoral head is relocated in the acetabulum, by combination of abduction, external rotation and extension of hip.

Gravity Method of Stimson (Fig. 24.150)

Associated injuries prevented, using method. Patient is positioned in prone. Assistant stabilizes pelvis. Involved hip and knee flexed 90°. Grasp knee, just distal to flexed knee. Apply longitudinal force and gentle internal and external rotation.

Allis Maneuver (Figs 24.151A to D)

Patient is supine. Pelvis is stabilized, by assistant applying pressure to ASIS. Surgeon apply longitudinal traction in line of deformity, followed by flexion of the hip to 90°, while continuing traction. Internal and external rotation of hip is then performed until reduction is achieved. Limb is then brought to neutral position.

East Baltimore Lift

Patient is placed supine. Patient's leg is flexed so that the hip and the knee are in 90°. Surgeon places his arm, which is closest to the patient's head under the proximal calf of the patient. Cradling the leg in his elbow, with his hand resting on the shoulder of his assistant. His other hand grasps the patient's ankle. The assistant's arm passes under the proximal calf of the patient and rests on the surgeon shoulder. Surgeon and assistant squat slightly with knees bend. Then they straighten up together to apply traction to the hip without straining their backs. The surgeon rotates the leg and the ankle and the second assistant stabilizes the pelvis.

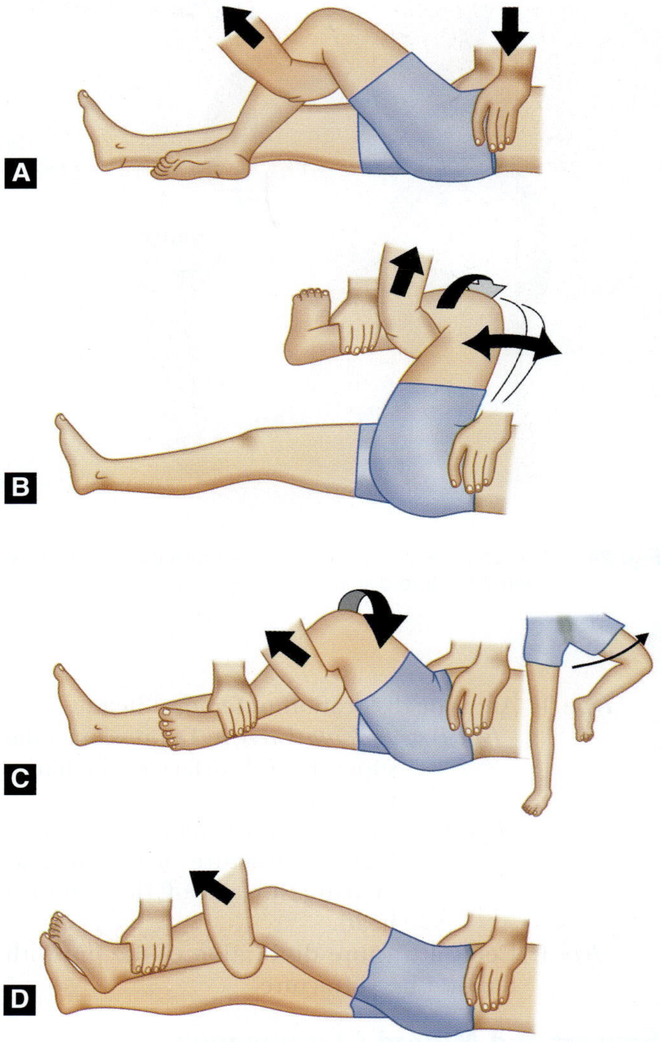

Figs 24.149A to D: Different steps of Bigelow's maneuver of closed reduction

Management After Closed Reduction

After closed reduction light skin or skeletal traction is recommended to provide comfort and allow capsular healing. Traction prevents recurrent dislocation, by keeping it in extension abduction and external rotation. Traction is maintained until hip is pain free and good range of motion achieved. Time of weight-bearing is controversial. Stuck and valerian recommended nonweight-bearing for 6 to 12 weeks. Stewart recommended weight-bearing 2 to 4 weeks after reduction.

Open Reduction

Indications of Open Reduction

- If closed reduction is not possible after one or two attempts
- Button holing of the femoral head through casule

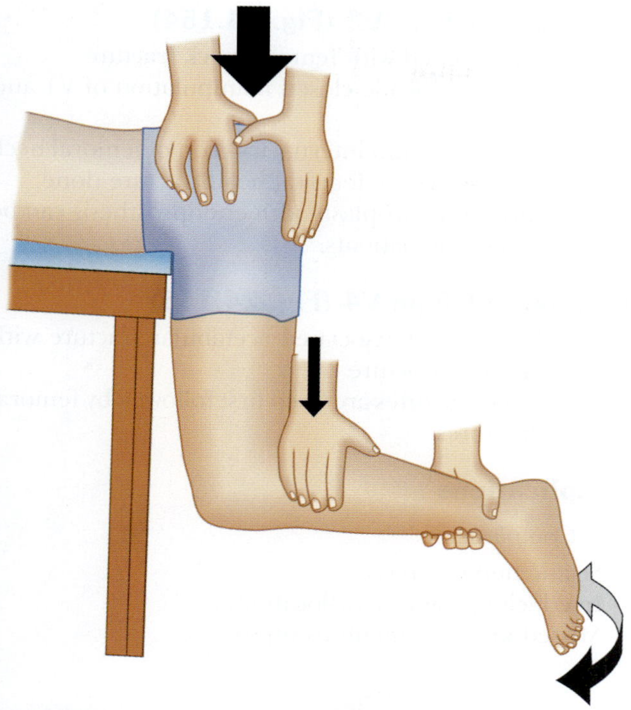

Fig. 24.150: Gravity method of Stimson for reduction

- Displacement of piriformis muscle across the acetabulum
- Concentric reduction is prevented by invested acetabular labrum
- Presence of osteochondral loose bodies with in the acetabulum.

Three approaches have been described:

- Anterior approach (Smith Petersons anterior iliofemoral approach)
- Posterior approach (osborne)
- Posterolateral approach (Kocher-Langenback)

Posterior approach is superior to anterior approach because most offending structure are more easily reached through the posterior approach. Anterior approach has more chances of avascular necrosis, as posterior retinacular vessels are damaged during dislocation and this approach damages the remaining anterior vascular supply.

After Treatment

Thomas or bucks traction is given, to immobilize the hip when reduction is stable. Active exercises and physical therapy advocated by 3 to 10 days. Weight-bearing is gradually resumed after 3 to 4 weeks.

Treatment of Type II, III and IV Dislocation

Primary closed reduction, dislocation with acetabular fracture should be reduced, as quick as possible. If fails, open reduction is done to prevent further damage to femoral head.

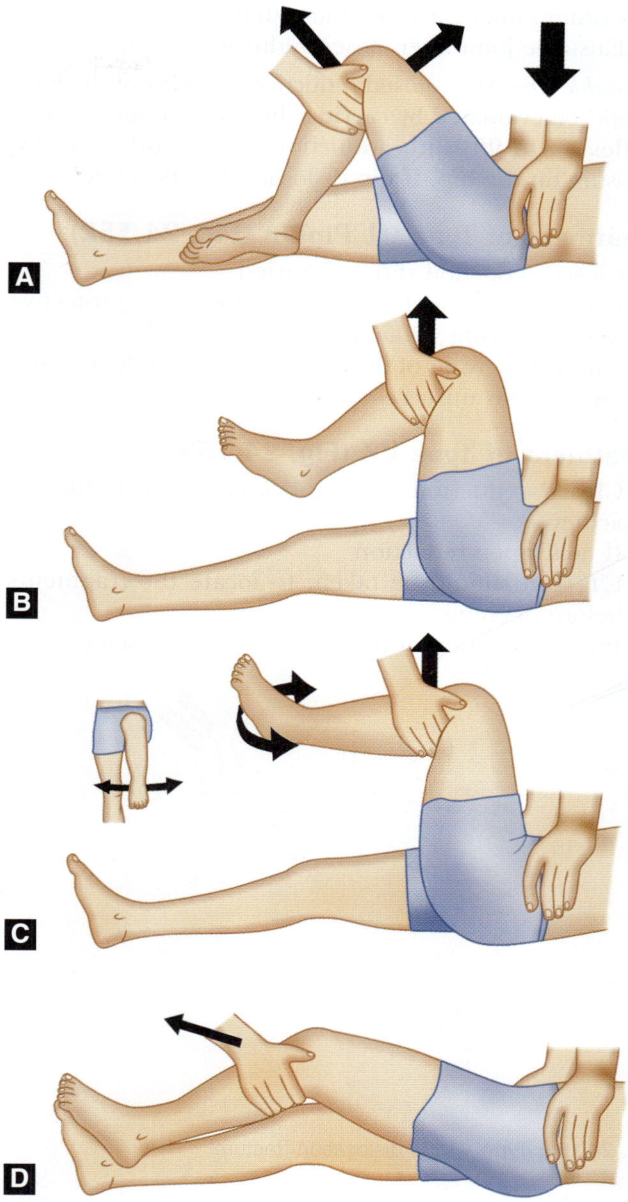

Figs 24.151A to D: Allis maneuver of reduction

Primary Open Reduction

Indications of primary open reduction:

- Large posterior hip fragment that did not get reduced on closed method
- Presence of fracture bone fragments in the acetabulum
- Fracture of the femoral head prevented reduction
- Displaced posterior rim fracture associated with sciatic nerve palsy

- Communited fracture of acetabulum
- Unstable joint after closed reduction.

Unstable hip: After closed reduction, stability of the joint should be evaluated by carring the hip through a range of flexion to 90° with adduction to 20° and posterior pressure on the hip. If hip dislocates it is unstable.

Treatment of Type V1 Pipkin (Fig. 24.152)

- Closed reduction should be tried
- If reduced, 6 weeks traction followed by protective weight-bearing walking is recommended
- Surgical excision of fragments is done, only if closed reduction is unsuccessful.

Treatment of Type V2 (Fig. 24.153)

- Closed reduction tried and anatomical reduction achieved
- If fails, open reduction
- CT scan should be taken, to locate the fragments before opening
- Internal fixation of fragments, by hebert screw.

Treatment of Type V3 (Fig. 24.154)

- This is associated with femoral neck fracture
- Usually occurs, while closed manipulation of V1 and V2
- Open reduction and internal fixation of femoral neck fracture followed by femoral head fracture done
- Alternatively arthroplasty with endoprosthesis can be done in elderly patients.

Treatment of Type V4 (Fig. 24.155)

- In this there are associated acetabular fracture with femoral head fracture
- Acetabular fractures are fixed first followed by femoral head fractures.

Complications

Early Complications

- Sciatic nerve peresis
- Irreducile posterior dislocation
- Missed knee ligamentous injury

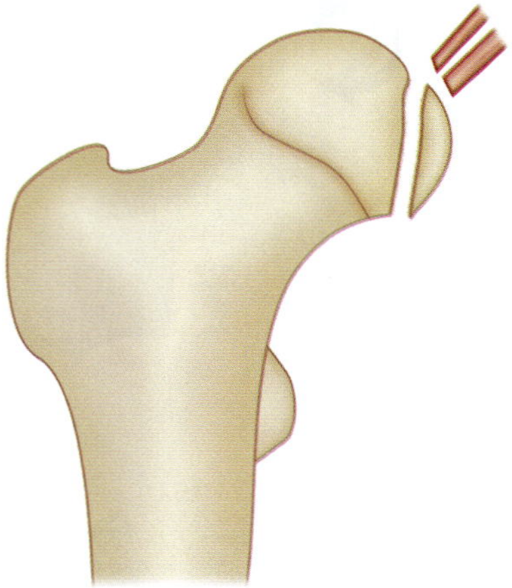

Fig. 24.152: Type V1 hip dislocation-fracture

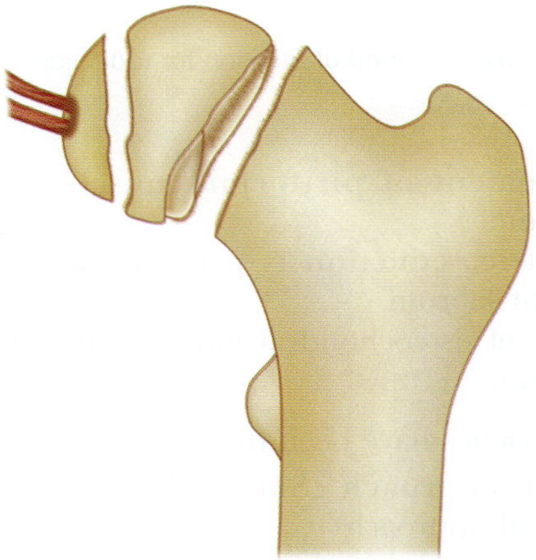

Fig. 24.154: Type V3 hip dislocation-fracture

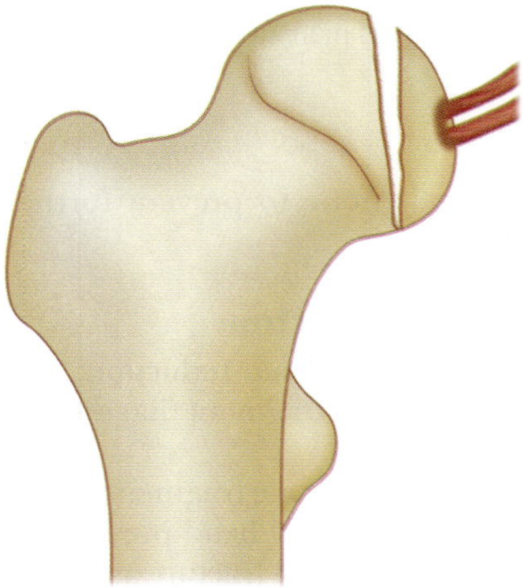

Fig. 24.153: Type V2 hip dislocation-fracture

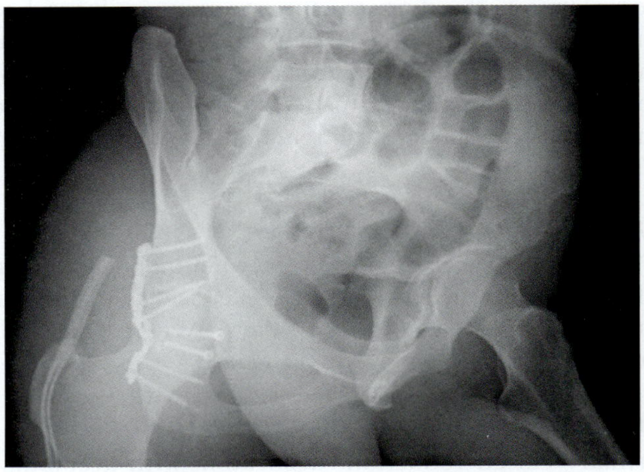

Fig. 24.155: Acetabular reconstruction with head fixation

Late Complications

- Recurrent posterior dislocation
- Myositis ossificans
- Avascular necrosis
- Post-traumatic arthritis
- Unreduced posterior fracture
- Heterotrophic calcification
- Malunion

Sciatic Nerve Paresis

Sciatic nerve paresis are two types:

1. *Prereduction paresis:* Commonly peroneal component is involved. Eight to nineteen percent patients present with this complications. There is a direct contusion and ischemia of sciatic nerve takes place. Sixty to seventy percent recover partially or completely. Management, include patients with simple dislocation reduction of the disloction. In patients, with associated fracture of posterior lip decompression is corrected with ORIF.
2. *Postreduction paresis:* Surgical exploration is indicated, to check if the nerve has been trapped in the joint. Thomas splint should not be used because the ring of the splint draws the nerve tighter. If complaints of pain and paresthesia present, the hip should be extended and the knee flexed, in order to reduce the nerve stress.

Rehabilitation, after sciatic nerve injury include

- A well padded short leg plaster cast with tibial pin, maintains the foot in position and prevents pressure ulcers.
- After open reduction, to relieve pressure on nerve is done. Care should be taken to avoid fixed flexion deformity.
- Periodic electromyograms and physical examination after every three weeks should be done.
- If permanent sciatic paralysis foot-drop splint and walking callipers for good function should be given.
- If common peroneal is paralyzed, transfer of tibialis posterior tendon through interosseus membrane with tripple arthrodesis can be done.

Recurrent Posterior Dislocations

It occurs in 0.3 to 1.2 percent of all dislocated hips. Two theories have been given:

- Build up of the hydrostatic pressure in the joint cavity, owing to a one way valve in the posterior capsule forced the head of femur across the acetabular rim.
- Repeated injury and a chronically intoxicated state a shallow acetabulum, deficient posterior rim and a massive soft tissue injury.

Causes

- Acetabular or femoral dysplasia
- Acetabular fracture
- Joint infection
- Paralysis
- Generalized ligamentous relaxation
- Massive soft tissue damage
- Delayed reduction of hip
- Inadequate reduction of the previously dislocated hip.

Management

- Combined CT with arthrography should be done, to locate the tear in the capsule
- Tear are usually anterior with anterior dislocation and posterior with posterior dislocation.

Various Procedures

- Posterior bone block and innominate osteotomy
- Plication of the enlarged capsule and posterior muscles including quadratus femoris and gemelli.
- Transfer of the piriformis tendon over the posterior capsule for posterior dislocation.
- Transfer of iliopsoas for anterior dislocation.
- Modified bankarts type repair throught the postero-lateral approach for post-traumatic posterior recurrent dislocation of hip.

■ Anterior Dislocation

It consists of 10 to 15 percent of traumatic dislocations of hip. In anterior dislocation of hip, the femoral head rests anterior to the coronal plane of the actebulum.

Classification

Modified Epstein Classification

Type I: Superior pubic/subspinous
- *Type IA:* No associated fractures
- *Type IB:* Associated fractures of head and neck of femur
- *Type IC:* Associated fracture of acetabulum

Type II: Inferior obturator/perineal dislocation
- *Type IIA:* No associated fracture
- *Type IIB:* Associated fracture of head and neck femur
- *Type IIC:* Associated fracture of acetabulum.

Mechanism of Injury

Occurs in automobile accidents, when knee strikes the dashboard with the thigh abducted. In fall from a height, or secondary to a blow to the back of the patient, while in squatted position. The neck of the femur or the greater trochanter impinges on the rim of the acetabulum and thereby levers the head of the femur, out of the acetabulum through a tear in the anterior hip capsule. The degree of flexion determines, whether a superior or inferior type of dislocation.

Clinical Diagnosis

- Attitude of limb is flexion or extension, abduction and external rotation
- Extremity is slighly short in superior type and long in inferior type
- In superior dislocations the femoral head is palpable in the vicinity of ASIS and is palpable in the groin in the pubic type.
- In inferior type, fullness in palpable in the region of the obturator foramen.
- Extreme abduction with external rotation of hip.
- Anterior hip capsule is torn or avulsed.
- Femoral head is levered out anteriorly
- Inferior type of dislocation, results from simultaneous hip abduction and external rotation, whereas superior type dislocation results from hip abduction, external rotation and hip extension.
- The mechanism of bilateral anterior dislocation is with the pelvis fixed both the legs are froced into flexion, abduction and external rotation.
- Anterior dislocation is usually associated with femoral head fractures
- Anterior dislocation with femoral neck fracture is rare.

Investigations

X-rays

- AP X-ray
- Oblique lateral view of pelvis
- Posterior oblique view
- Full length femur
- CT scan, to delineate fracture fragments size and location
- Routine lab investigations.

Management

Early diagnosis and prompt closed reduction under general anesthesia (GA) are the treatment of choice, however certain dislocations require open reduction, if hip cannot be reduced in GA. Gravity method of Stimson, is primarily used for posterior dislocation of hip. In inferior obturator type of dislocation reduction can be achieved by this method, whereas superior dislocation of the pubic type, in which the hip presents in extension are not amenable to the procedures.

Reverse Bigelow's Maneuver

The position of the patient is partial flexion and abduction. Two methods of reduction are indicated:

- First is the lifting method, in which a firm jerk is applied to the flexed thigh. This method often results in reduction except in pubic dislocations.
- If the lifting method fails, the second method is used, in which the hip is adducted sharply, internally rotated and extended. Complication of this method is fracture of the femoral neck.

Allis's Maneuver

Assistant stabilizes the pelvis, by holding at the ASIS. Longitudinal traction is applied in the line with the axis of the femur and the hip is slightly flexed. Then gently adduct and internally rotate the femur, to achieve the reduction.

Open Reduction

If a large area of weight-bearing surface of the femoral head is fractured, from the superior and the anterolateral aspects, then open reduction and internal fixation is done, using Watson Jone approach and Smith Petersons technique.

Postreduction Management

It includes traction angles from 8 days to 4 to 6 weeks. Controlled range of motion is instituted during this time, to aid nutrition of articular cartilage. Avoid extremes of abductions and external rotation, to avoid redislocation.

Complications

- *Neurovascular compromise:* Direct pressure on the femoral artery, vein or nerve resulting in distal neurovascular compromise in pubic or subspinous dislocation.
- *Irreducibility:* Obstruction to the closed reduction, include bone locking in the obturator foramen and interposition of the tissues, including the rectus femoris, iliopsoas muscle and anterior hip capsule.
- *Recurrent dislocation:* Inadequate immobilization during the postoperative reduction.

■ Chronic Unreduced Hip Dislocations

Dislocation more than 3 months is considered to be chronic. They can be either:

- Anterior dislocation
- Posterior dislocation

Chronic Anterior Hip Dislocation

- It is rare
- Surgical treatment is done, by intertrochanteric osteotomy. It is done to correct the deformity and improve body mechanics and balance. Two methods are used to perform intertrochanteric osteotomy:

- Aggarwal and Singh method
- Modified girdelstone arthroplasty by Nagi

Aggarwal and Singh method: This is usually followed, in which gibsons approach is taken. Femur is divided along the line joining the greater trochanter and the lesser trochanter. Limb is then adducted extended and internally rotated. Patient is given skin traction for 6 weeks to prevent rotational deformity. Crutch walking at 6 weeks and full weight bearing walking at 3 to 4 months.

Nagi method: In this method the femoral neck is exposed by the Smith Petersons or the Watson and jones approach. Subcapital osteotomy is performed, attemptying to leave as much neck as possible without disturbing the femoral head. By manipulating the leg, the cut femoral neck is displaced into the acetabulum. Postoperatively 5 kg traction is maintained for 6 weeks. Nonweight-bearing walking by 6 weeks and gradual weight-bearing started at 3 months.

Comparison

Nagi method is easier to do, THR after this operation as the anatomy of the proximal femur is undisturbed, while Aggarwal and Singh method is more stable, fixed hip can be achieved.

Chronic Posterior Hip Dislocation

- More common
- Two main causes are:
  - Fracture of the femoral head or acetabular rim and
  - Avascular necrosis.

Treatment of Type I

Gupta method: Tibial pin traction is given for 18 kg weight. Patient is kept in sedation and muscle relaxation during traction. By fifth day, usually femoral head is at or below the level of acetabulum. Limb is then abducted every 4th day and weight reduced by 3.6 kg. After head is reduced in acetabulum, 7 kg weight traction maintained for next 2 weeks. Nonweight-bearing at 4 weeks and weight-bearing at 3 months.

Treatment of Type II, III, IV

- Skeletal traction
- Open reduction and fixation of the fracture fragments
- In young patients arthrodesis, if come with complications as avascular necrosis.

Central Acetabular Fracture Dislocation

In this type fracture disocation, involving the medial acetabular wall or the superior weight-bearing dome of the acetabulum is present, with or without associated control displacement of the head of the femur. It occurs in all adult age groups. It is now considered as fracture of the acetabulum.

INFECTIONS OF HIP JOINT

■ Pyogenic Arthritis

It is a purulent infection of the joint cavity, due to pyogenic organisms and productive of purulent exudates. It is also known as septic arthritis and suppurative arthritis. It is more common in childhood and the ratio of the pyogenic arthritis in adult, as compared to the children's is 1:1.5. Infant and young children's hip are more commonly involved. Multiple joint involvement occur in 5 percent of cases and 75 percent of the cases occur in children under 5 years of age, as shown in Figures 24.156 and 24.157.

Etiology

Common organisms: These include, *Staphylococcus aureus* most common, pneumococci, gonococci, *E. coli* and *H. influenzae* (account for the most of the cases between 6 months to 2 years of age).

Susceptible group

- Infants and neonates
- Elderly patients with pre-existing joint diseases
- Immunocompromised patients.

Route of infections: Route of infection is divided into three types:

- *Hematogenous spread:* Infection is usually in GIT, urinary tract, teeth, tonsil, pneumonia
- *Direct extension:* Spread from local abcess, osteomyelitis or infected compound fracture
- Direct implantation of bacteria through puncture wound.

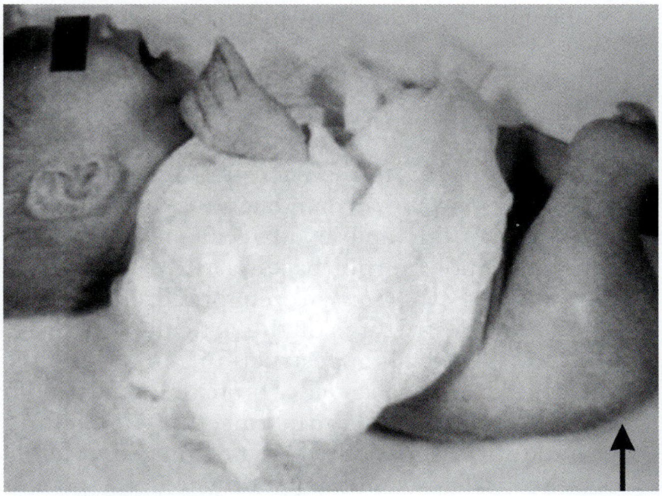

Fig. 24.156: Pyogenic arthritis of hip in an infant

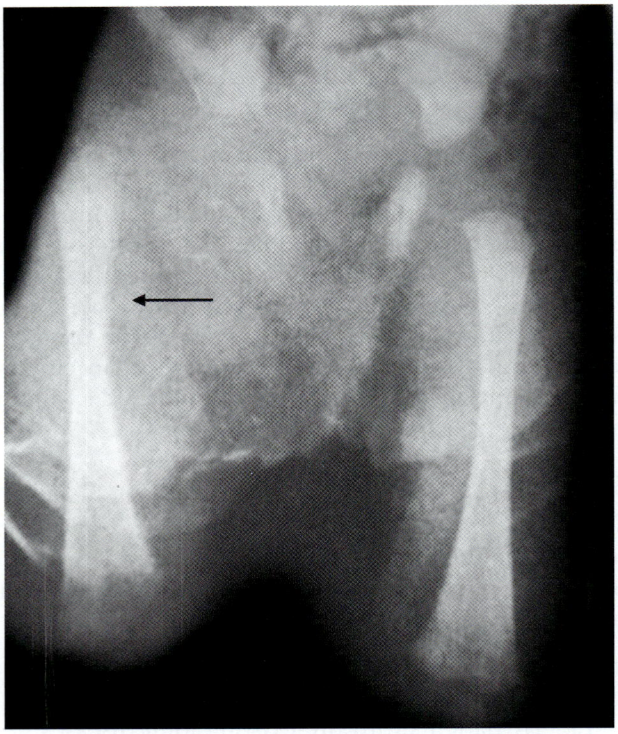

Fig. 24.157: X-ray showing pyogenic hip arthritis in infant

Pathology

The reaction of the joint is determined by the virulance of the organisms and the resistance of the individuals, in any case there is exudation of the fluid in the joint cavity. It will be serous, seropurulent or may frankly purulent.

- *Serous type:* Joint is distended with clear serous fluid, with dilatation of vessels of synovial membrane and capsule. The effusion may subside or may recur or it may become seropurulent or actually purulent.
- *Serofibrinous arthritis:* In this the synovial membrane is not only hyperemic, but inflamed so the joint is covered with serofibrinous exudate and cavity filled with cloudy fluid with large number of polymorphs and large mononuclear cell. Organisms present in the joint fluid.
- *Purulent arthritis:* Most severe type of arthritis. In this, most of the joint and surrounding structure are quickly involved, considerable exudate in the joint cavity containing polymorph, bacteria, RBC and fibrin. Capsule and synovium are engorged edematous. There is a destruction of the articular cartilage. Mechanism, causing destruction; enzymes, like plasmin, kinase, collagenase, protease, cathepsins B and D and prostaglandin raised. Encroaching granulation from synovia, synovium completely detached to lie free in the joint cavity in the pool of pus. Thus, bone are exposed, infection may spread and causes osteomyelitis, which lead to sequestration, suppuration and necrosis. Intra-articular ligaments may destroyed and finally capsule is perforated and pus escaping from the joint, to form an extra-articular or periarticular abscess and at the end results complete resolution, dislocation, absorption of head and ankylosis.

Clinical Feature

Serous Type (Acute Synovitis)

- Tense painful swelling of the joint
- Local rise of temperature
- Severe tenderness in the joint
- Muscle spasm present.

Serofibrinous Type

- Joint is exquisitely tender and swollen
- High fever and night pain occur
- Movement are severly restricted
- Muscle spasm.

Suppurative Type

- It is most severe form of disease
- In the early stages, symptoms are those of the acute synovitis
- In this patient feel extremely ill and joint is more painful and limb wastes rapidly.

Investigations

- Total count is raise, with polymorphonuclear leukocyte
- ESR raised
- CPR elevated
- Blood culture may be positive
- Joint aspirate examine for the culture and sensitivity, gram stain-cocci or bacilli, glucose is low, but protein are high and its turbid appearance
- *Radiograph:* In the early stage showes increase joint space and the soft tissue shadow
- In the later stage show osteoporosis, cartilage destruction, decreased joint space, bone necrosis, epiphyseal premature closure and fibrous or bony ankylosis is present, as shown in Figures 24.158A and B
- Ultrasound, it detect joint effusion
- Isotope bone scan are performed, to distinguish cellulitis, septic arthritis and osteomyelitis.

Differential Diagnosis

- Acute rheumatism and rheumatoid arthritis
- Acute osteomyelitis
- Acute (non-supperative) arthritis

Complications

- Joint stiffness
- Joint instability-subluxation dislocation

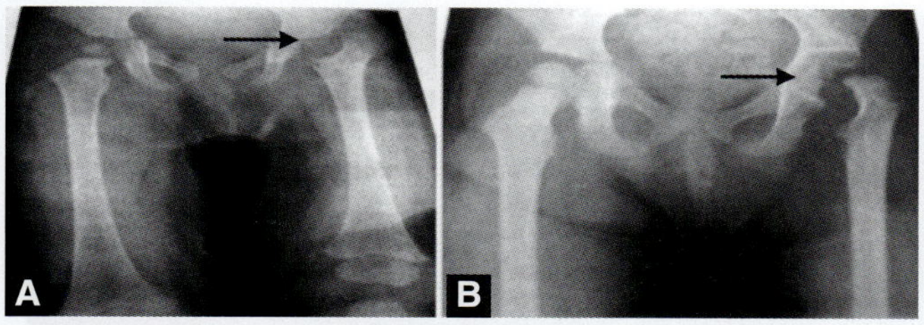

Figs 24.158A and B: Later stage of pyogenic arthritis, show osteoporosis, cartilage destruction, decreased joint space, bone necrosis, epiphyseal premature closure and fibrous or bony ankylosis is present—(A) Arrow showing destruction of fomoral head; (B) Arrow showing involvement of acetabulum

- Arthritis
- Epiphyseal growth disturbance
- Ankylosis-cartilagenous, fibrous and bony
- Amyloidosis
- Pelvic abscess
- Chronic osteomyelitis

Treatment

Principles of treatment are
- Early diagnosis
- Antibiotics required for 4 to 6 weeks and used higher antibiotics
- Immobilized and give rest to joint by splintage or light traction and hip should be in abduction to prevent dislocation
- Removal of pus and decompression to prevent cartilage destruction.

Treatment Consists of Bed Rest
- *Antibiotic:* Intravenous cloxacillin and ampicillin is given as soon as sample of blood and synovial fluid collected for culture and antibiotic must be given for 3 to 6 weeks.
- *Immobilization:* Relieved the pain and spread of the infection and it is achieved by light skin traction CR splintage with compression bandage, with hip in abduction and it is continue till patient is pain free.
- *Joint decompression:* It reduces the intra-articular tension, also prevent avascular necrosis of femoral head and also subluxation or dislocation of hip.
- *Aspiration of hip joint:* In the children, anterior aspiration technique is used and in adult posterior aspiration technique used.
- *Posterior drainage:* Ober technique is used and done by taking the Moore's approach.
- *Anterior drainage:* It is done, by taking the Smith Peterson approach
- Lateral drainage
- Medial drainage
- *Arthroscopic lavage:* A recent advance technique.

Acute Infective Arthritis of Infants (Tom Smith's Arthritis)

It is a pyogenic arthritis or septic infection of the joint in small infants below one year of the age. Smith was the first to describe septic arthritis in neonate and infants.

Etiology

Secondary to neighboring bone lesion, i.e. from metaphysis to epiphysis because vessels from metaphysis penetrate the growth plate, up to the age of one and half year. Joint may be infected through the blood stream, usually from the infected umbilicus, oronasal infection, respiratory tract infection, etc. Proteolytic enzymes derived from leukocytes and bacteria cause cartilage destruction. The most common organism is *S. aureus* followed by *Streptococcus,* influenza, *Pneumococcus, E.coli,* etc.

Pathology

Infection start in synovial membrane lining the joint. This rapidly inflamed and edematous and from it surface it poured out synovial fluid, plasma and leukocyte. Filling the joint with turbid exudates, containing a large number of polymorphonucler leukocyte and fibrin. If the infection is severe mesothelium lining of the synovial membrane is destroyed and its place is taken by mass of the granulation tissue. Articular cartilage is also involved and lead to impairment of joint function.

Clinical Feature

- Child is very ill, toxic, high grade fever and irritable
- Joint is swollen, painfull and hot
- Movement of the limb are painful
- Hip may be flexed, abducted and slightely externally rotated
- Sometimes extensive fluctuant absess may be present in the thigh or buttocks
- Sometimes, when child may be brought month later the limb is shortened and child has unstable hip gait. The joint is hypermobile.

Differential Diagnosis

- Acute rheumatic fever
- Tuberculous arthritis
- Traumatic synovitis
- Hemophilic arthritis

Investigation

- Total count is raised and polymorphonuclear leukocyte is present
- Blood for culture demostrates septicemia
- Aspiration of the joint fluid, establishes diagnosis
- *X-rays:* First sign is swelling due to joint effusion and edema of soft tissue.

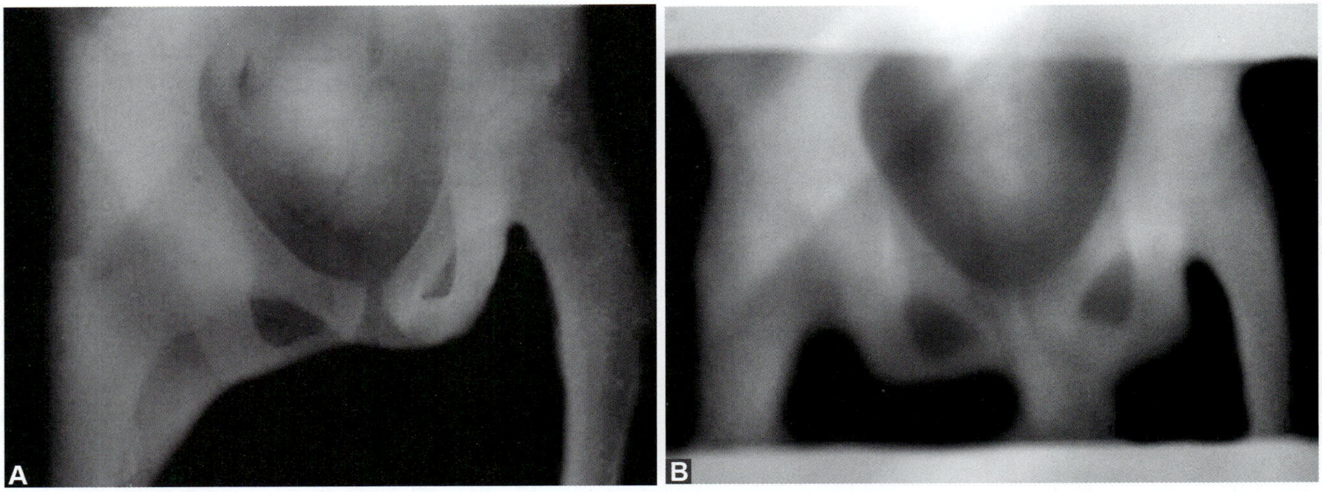

Figs 24.159A and B: Sequelae of Tom Smith arthritis

Radiographs (Figs 24.159A and B)

Classification

I. Eyre-Brook classification:

Type 1: Recovery occur with coxa magna.

Type 2: Destruction or severe damage to the capital epiphysis with the femoral neck remaining in the acetabulum or a deformed femoral head in valgus or varus.

Type 3: Destruction or severe damage to the growth plate.

Type 4: Destruction of the capital epiphysis with dislocation or severe subluxation of hip.

II. Choi's classification:

Type 1: Deformity involved transient ischemia of the epiphysis, with or without mild coxa magna, and these hips did not need reconstruction.

Type 2: Deformity included deformity of the epiphysis, physis and metaphysis and these hip needed an operation to prevent subluxation; the goal of operation included improvement in acetabular coverage.

Type 3: Deformity involved malalignment of femoral neck with extreme anteversion or retroversion or with a pseudoarthrosis of femoral neck that needs realignment osteotomy of proximal part of femur or bone grafting for pseudoarthrosis.

Type 4: Deformity, which included severe limb length discrepancy and incompetent articulation of hip needs operation such as pemberton osteotomy, trochantric arthroplasty, arthrodesis and lengthening of ipsilateral tibia.

III. *Johari's classification* (Table 24.12)

Table 24.12: Johari's classification of Tom Smith arthritis

Group I:	Loss of CFE/neck, metaphyseal spike present—sable
Group II:	Loss of CEF and neck—unstable
Group IIIA:	Dislocation, CFE present—unstable
Group IIIB:	Subluxation, CFE present—unstable
Group IV:	Articular incongruity, AVN, coxa magna, breva, trochanteric overgrowth—stable
Group V:	Pseudarthrosis of neck of femur—stable/unstable

This is also shown in Figures 24.160A to F.

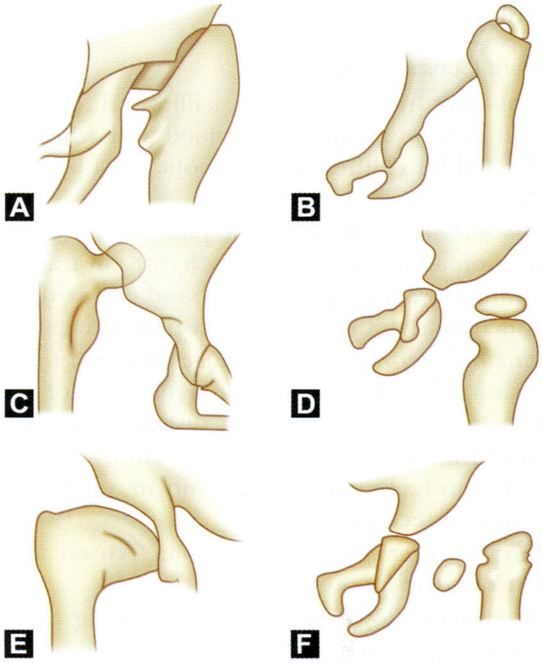

Figs 24.160A to F: Johari's classification of Tom Smith arthritis. (A) Group I arthritis; (B) Group II; (C) Group IIIA; (D) Group IIIB; (E) Group IV; (F) Group V arthritis

Radiology and Diagnosis of Sequelae

- Ossification of the head and neck is delayed and translucency persists
- On X-ray, telescopic sign is positive
- Differential diagnosis, with positive telescopic sign:
  - Dislocation of hip
  - Pseudoarthrosis of the neck of femur
  - Complete destruction of the head and neck
  - On X-ray telescopic sign is negative, then head may be osteoporotic, avascular necrosis and may partially destroyed.

Treatment

Type I: Lesion, with no instability or significant deformity should be simply kept under observation, with the use of the abduction plaster cast or brace.

Type II: Sequelae, with a deformed coxa vara or valga may need treatment initially with the orthosis. If there is dislocation or severe coxa valga or vara, then femoral or pelvis osteotomy needed.

Type III: Sequelae, the pseudoarthrosis and nonunion may be treated with subtrochantric osteotomy, with bone grafting and internal fixation with lag screw.

Type IV: Lesion, reconstructive surgeries done.

Operation to Stabilize the Hip

- Arthrodesis
- Pelvic osteotomy
- High femoral osteotomy
- Trochantric arthroplasty combined with proximal femoral osteotomy
- Harmon or L-Episcopo reconstruction
- *To correct deformities:* Flexion and adduction contracture is treated, by an adductor tenotomy and hip is ankylosed in flexion and adduction, then it is treated by intertrochantric osteotomy.
- Operation to equalized leg length, this is done only after all reconstructive operation are done.

TUBERCULOSIS OF HIP JOINT

Introduction

Tuberculous disease of the hip is very common. The frequency of the involvement is next to spinal tuberculosis. In long series, it is 15 percent of total skeletal TB and age group affected is first three decades of life.

Pathology (Fig. 24.161)

The initial focus of the tuberculosis lesion may start in acetabular roof, epiphyses, metaphyseal region (Babcock's triangle), greater trochanter and rarely in synovial membrane.

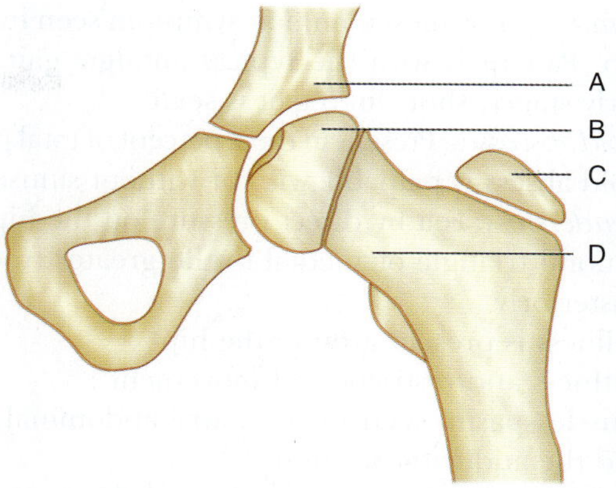

Fig. 24.161: Main foci of tuberculosis lesions—A. Roof of acetabulum; B. Epiphysis; C. Greater trochanter; D. Babcock's triangle

Acetabular Roof

- The joint involvement is late
- Mild symptoms are seen
- No extensive destruction of acetabular roof is seen.

Greater Trochanter

- Overlying bursa is involved
- Joint involvement is late.

Epiphyses and Metaphyseal Region

- As intracapsular early involvement of joint
- Both are rapidly distructive.

Synovium

- Involvement of the synovium is very rare
- Early joint involvement seen

May form cold abscesses, which may penetrate the joint and inferior weak part of capsule or rarely on the acetabular floor and from this it is perforated and present in femoral triangle, inguinal region, medial, lateral or posterior aspect of thigh, ischiorectal fossa or pelvis and lower part of thigh knee because of spread along neurovascular bundle.

In the acetabular roof, psoas abscess and pelvic abscess are there. If it is above urogenital diaphragm then, it will track above inguinal ligament. If it is below urogenital diaphragm, then will track into ischiorectal fossa.

Clinical Features

- *Night cries:* Patient wakes up from sleep during night because of pain. Pain is because of the relaxation of protective muscle spasm there is irritation of eroded cartilage gives rise to pain
- *Pain:* Pain is more towards the end of the day and it is referred to the medial aspect of the thigh and knee

- *Limping:* It is most common symptom seen in the TB hip. Patient is with the typical antalgic gait (this is early stage), short limb gait is seen
- *Cold abscesses:* Present in the 8 percent of total patients. Cold absess is palpable with or without sinuses
- *Tenderness:* Felt by direct pressure on the hip in the femoral triangle or medial to the greater trochanter posteriorly
- Fullness is present around the hip
- Stiffness and restriction of movement
- Muscle spasm, seen in the lower abdominal muscle and the adductor of thigh
- Pathological subluxation and the dislocation hip
- Constutional symptoms, loss of weight, loss of appetite, low grade fever and cough.

Stage I (Tuberculous Synovitis)

- In the early disease of the hip joint due to the juxta articular osseous lesion, causing the irritable hip
- Joint held in position of maximum capacity, i.e. flexion, abduction and external rotation leading to apparent shortening
- No true shortening
- Only the movement are painful and limited.

Stage II (Early Arthritis) (Fig. 24.162)

- Actual destruction or damage to articular cartilage
- Local signs become more prominent because of spasm of adductor and flexors
- Assume deformity of flexion, adduction and internal rotation
- True shortening of less than 1 cm
- Appreciable muscle wasting
- Restriction of movement in all direction due to pain and muscle spasm.
- *X-ray shows*
  - Osteoporosis of bone
  - Slight diminution of joint space
  - Erosions of articular cartilage margins.

Stage III (Advanced Arthritis)

- Further advancement of destruction
- Flexion, adduction and internal rotation deformities will pronounced
- Restriction of movement
- Apparent as well as true shortening
- Gross restriction of femoral head and acetabulum
- Muscle wasting
- Capsule is further destroyed and thickened and contracted.

Stage IV (Advanced Arthritis with Subluxation/ Dislocation)

- Further destruction of femoral head, acetabulum, capsule and upper end of femur is displaced upwards and dorsally, in wondering or migrating acetabulum.
- Shentons arc is broken
- Destruction of capsule may leads to frank pathological posterior dislocation of femoral head
- Movements are increased as compared to previous stages
- X-ray showing wandering acetabulum, as shown in Figure 24.163.
- Other X-ray findings (Fig. 24.164):
  - Gross osteoporosis of bone
  - Destroyed head and acetabulum
  - Mostly posterior dislocation, rarely protrusio acetabuli can occur
  - Shentons line broken
  - Morter and Pestle appearance

In certain cases of tuberculous arthritis (stage 2, 3 and 4), the hip may not assume the classical triple deformity of flexion, adduction and internal rotation, instead the deformity may be that of flexion, abduction and external rotation with the lateral aspect of thigh of the diseased hip resting on bed. This is due to adaptation of latter posture for relief of pain or due to destruction in iliofemoral "Y" ligament by tuberculous process.

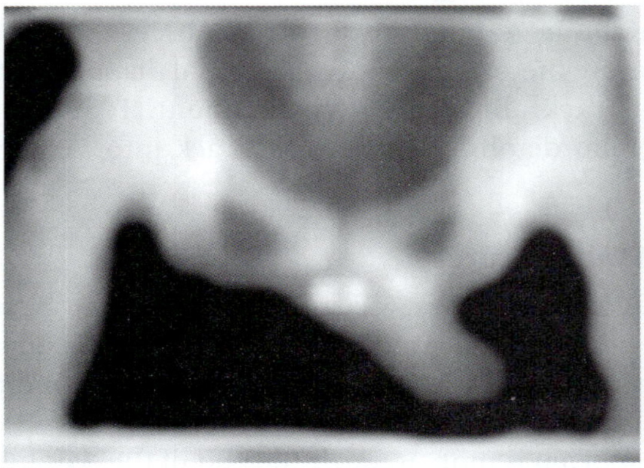

Fig. 24.162: Stage II early tubercular arthritis

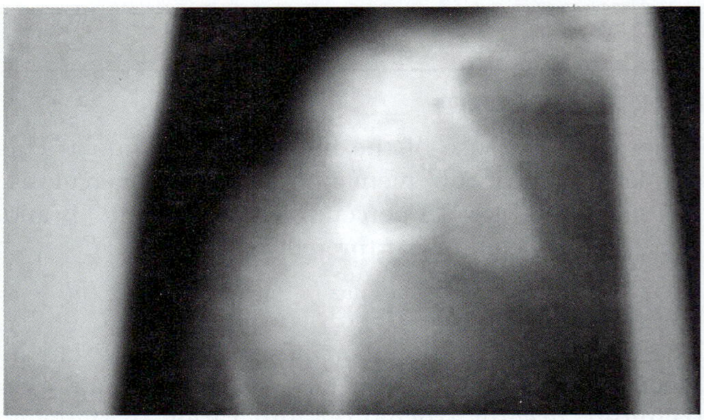

Fig. 24.163: X-ray showing wandering acetabulum in advanced tubercular arthritis

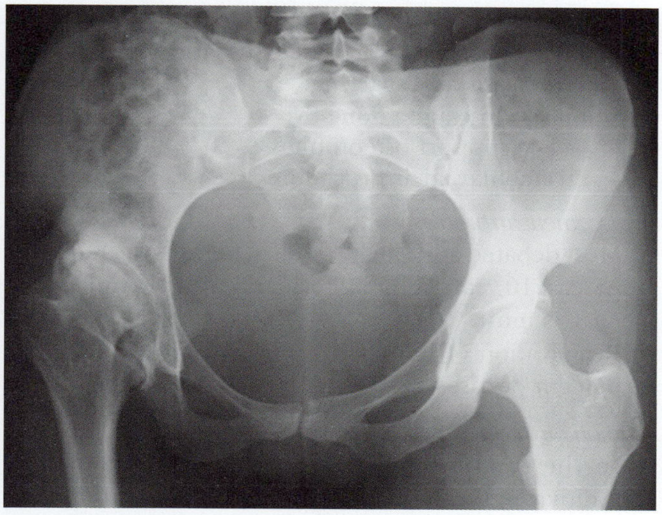

Fig. 24.164: Stage IV (advanced arthritis with subluxation/dislocation)

Radiological Classification

Shanmugasundaram (1980), C for child and A for adult

- Normal appearance (C)
- Traveling acetabulum (C, A)
- Perthes' type (C)
- Dislocated hip (C)
- Protrusion acetabuli (C, A)
- Atrophic type (A)
- Morter and Pestle type (C, A).

Investigation

- Hemoglobin (Hb percent)
- ESR, raised in active stage
- Mountax test (in children), indicates an active infection and sensitization of child to *Mycobacterium* infection
- TB ELISA (usually in gram titer, is active)
- X-ray hip AP and lateral and X-ray chest PA veiw
- Biopsy and histopathological examination.

■ Treatment

General

- Good nutrition diet
- Fresh air
- Rest
- Analgesics
- Proper positioning of limb
- Maintainance of good hygine
- Traction

Advantages of Traction

- Gives rest to the part
- Relieves muscle spasm and pain
- Prevents subluxation and dislocation, by keeping leg in abduction
- Maintains joint space and keep the articular surface away.

Chemotherapy—Antitubercular Treatment (ATT)

For First 4 Months

- Isoniazid 300 mg/kg body weight
- Rifampicin 450 mg/kg body weight
- Ethambutol 1200 mg/kg body weight

For Second 4 Months

- Isoniazid 300 mg/kg body weight
- Pyrazinamide 1500 mg/kg body weight

For Third 4 Months

- Isoniazid 300 mg/kg body weight
- Rifampicin 450 mg/kg body weight

For Fourth 4 Months

- Isoniazid 300 mg/kg body weight
- These are the triple regime.

Management of cold abscess: Any palpable cold abscess may be aspirated with instillation of streptomycin with or without isoniazid.

Surgical Treatment

Indications for surgery are

- If response to the conservative treatment is not favorable
- Patient presenting with sound ankylosis in bad position
- Mobility at hip joint.

Synovectomy and Debridement

Indications

- Synovitis
- Early arthritis
- In addition to synovectomy; removal of loose bodies/rice body, debris, pannus covering articular cartilage, loose articular cartilage and careful curettage of osseous juxta-articular foci can be performed.

Complications

- AVN
- SCFE in children
- Fracture of femoral neck and acetabulum
- Secondary infections

Osteotomy

Indications

- Sound ankylosis in bad position, require upper femoral corrective osteotomy.

- Unsound ankylosis in bad position becomes an osseous fusion, by a high femoral corrective osteotomy.
- Can be done at any age.
- Ideal site is as near as possible to the deformed joint.

Arthrodesis

- Done in adult patients
- Can be done in active as well as healed stage
- Failure of conservative treatment
- Recurrence of pain and deformity
- Certain destructive lesion, e.g. the formation of the sequestra in head or neck of femur or in acetabulum.

Methods

- Intra-articular
- Extra-articular
- Combined (panarticular)
- In extra-articular methods
  - Iliofemoral arthrodesis (Hibb's) in abduction deformity
  - Ischiofemoral arthrodesis (Brittain's technique) in adduction deformity.

Disadvantage of arthrodesis: Activity not possible after arthrodesis are

- Bending
- Sitting cross leg
- Squatting
- Sports and running
- Bicycling.

Complications of arthrodesis

- Early development of degenerative arthritis of
  - Lumbosacral spine
  - Ipsilateral knee
  - Contralateral hip
- Increased energy expenditure of ambulation.

Girdlestone's Excision Arthroplasty

- Girdlestone's excision arthroplasty can safely carried out in healed or active disease after completion of growth potential of hip.
- This procedure provides mobile and painless hip joint, with control of infection and correction of deformity.
- Excision of:
  - Femoral head and neck
  - Proximal part of trochanter
  - Acetabular rim
- Safely done in healed/active disease after completion of growth potential.
- Procedure provides painless, mobile hip joint with control of infection and correction deformity.
- Postoperative skeletal traction in abduction for minimum 3 months minimizes shortening and gross instability. Instability will be minimized due to maturation and contractures of soft tissues around hip.

Disadvantages

- Relative unstable joint, when disease heals without much fibrosis and scarring.
- Stabilization can be done by:
  - Pelvic support osteotomies
  - Acetabular shelf procedure

Replacement arthroplasty

- Most debated and can be done in highly selected cases
- At least 10 years, after last evidence of active infections
- ATT is must
- Reactivation of infection is noted in about 10 to 30 percent of cases.

Amniotic arthroplasty

- In the treatment of tuberculous arthritis of hip, multilayered cap of amniotic membrane was used.
- Vishwakarma (1986) stated that of the out 28 patients, 25 showed good range of painless movement and stable joint.

Recent Advance Techniques in Management of Tuberculosis of Hip Joint

- Amniotic arthroplasty for tuberculosis of hip
- Charnley low friction arthroplasty in tuberculosis of hip
- Gene therapy in tuberculosis of hip
- Interpositional arthroplasties
- Total hip replacement.

Gene therapy in tuberculosis of hip: Impressive advances, in our knowledge of the molecular genetic basis of skeletal disorders and fracture healing, have led to the development of novel therapeutics based on ectopic expression of one or more genes in patient cells that can influence repair or regenerative processes in bone. Gene therapy is an attractive new approach to the treatment of bone disorders. Orthopedics has become one of the most promising areas of research into gene therapy. This is because many potential orthopedic targets for gene therapy, unlike traditional targets, such as cancer and severe genetic disorders, neither present difficult delivery problems nor require prolonged periods of gene expression. Gene therapy offers new possibilities for the clinical management of orthopedic conditions that are difficult to treat by traditional surgical or medical means. Impaired bone healing, need for extensive bone formation, cartilage repair and metabolic bone diseases are all conditions, where alterations of the signaling peptides involved may provide cure or improvement. Several preclinical studies have shown that gene transfer technology has the ability to deliver osteogenic molecules, to precise anatomical locations at therapeutic levels for sustained periods of time. Both *in vivo* and *ex vivo* transduction of cells, can induce bone formation at ectopic and orthotopic sites. Genetic engineering of adult stem cells from various sources with osteogenic genes has led to enhanced fracture repair, spinal fusion and rapid healing of bone defects in animal models. Although, still a relatively immature field, proof-of-principle for enhanced bone formation through skeletal gene therapy has already been established. The challenge now is to more precisely define optimal cellular targets and therapeutic genes and to develop safe and efficient ways to deliver therapeutic genes to target cells. Skeletal gene therapy can have an enormous impact on patient care. The next 5 years will present us with unparalleled opportunities to develop more effective therapeutic strategies and overcome obstacles, presented by current gene transfer technologies.

DEGENERATIVE OSTEOARTHRITIS

■ Introduction

It is characterized by degenerative changes in articular cartilage of diarthrodial joints and subsequent new bone formation at the articular margins. The term osteoarthritis was coined by John Spendon. However, it is misnomer and the right term is osteoarthrosis or degenerative joint disease. Pathologically, it may be defined as a condition of synovial joints characterized by:

- Focal loss of articular hyaline cartilage, as shown in Figure 24.165.
- Simultaneous proliferation of new bone, with remodeling of joint contour. This is illustrated in Figure 24.166.

Incidence: By the age of 40 years, about 40 percent of population has radiological sign of osteoarthrosis of major weight-bearing joints (knee, hip). Fifty percent of these will be symptomatic.

Risk Factors

- Age
- Female sex
- Race
- Genetic factors
- Major joint trauma
- Repetitive stress
- Obesity
- Congenital development defects
- Metabolic endocrine disorders

Etiology

Age: Process begins in second decade of life and by 50 to 65 of age 80 percent have radiological evidence of disease, as shown in Figure 24.167.

Sex: Female > male

Obesity: Twice as prevalent in obese.

Occupation: With physical activities involving repetitive use of particular joints over period of time.

Mechanical factors: Mechanical stress, gross anatomical damage, subtle mechanical derangement (IDK-long standing), joint hypermobility and direct articular cartilage damage.

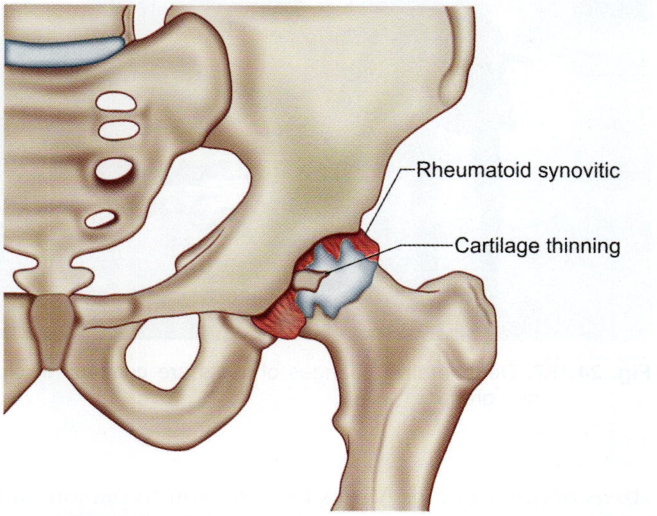

Fig. 24.165: Degenerative changes in articular cartilage, with focal loss of articular hyaline cartilage

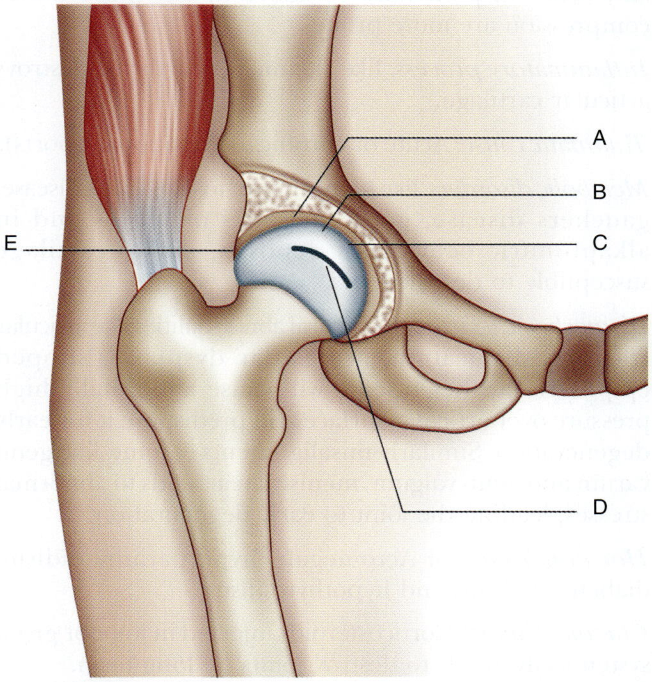

Fig. 24.166: Proliferation of new bone and remodeling of joint contour, with focal degenerative changes—A. Proliferation of new bone; B. Remodeling of joint contour; C. Head of femur; D. Articular surface of femur; E. Defect in articular surface

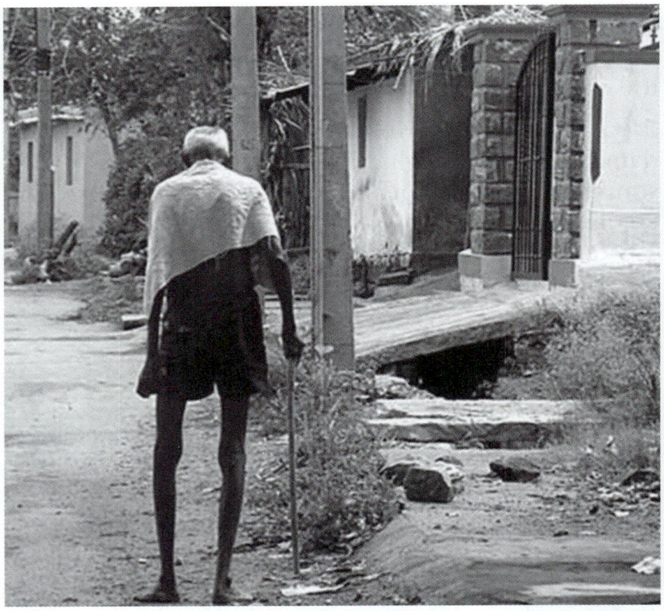

Fig. 24.167: Degenerative changes of joints are common in old age group

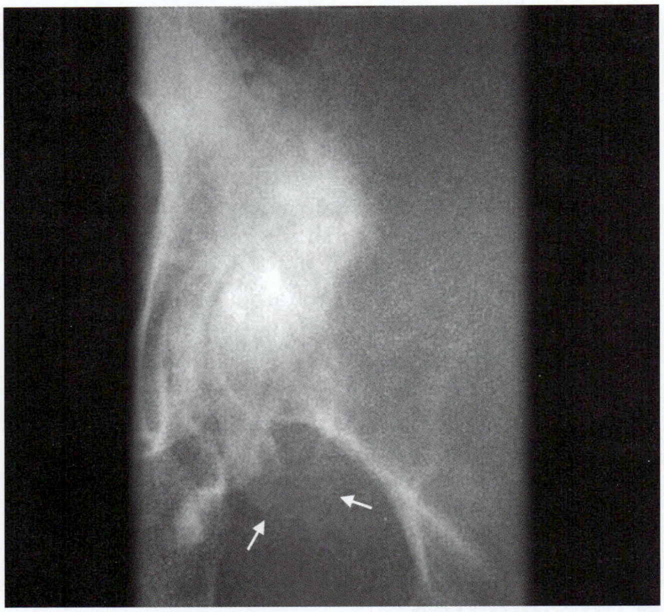

Fig. 24.168: X-ray showing subchondral sclerosis of hip joint. Arrows showing osteophytes

Areas of involvement: Varies from person to person and from joint to joint. In female DIP and first MCP is most commonly involved. In males hip are most commonly involved. In females knees are most commonly involved. Any synovial joint may be affected, but those under compression are more prone.

Inflammatory process, like rheumatoid arthritis destroys articular cartilage.

Traumatic cause: Acute or chronic (occupational, sports).

Metabolic disorders, like hemochromatosis, wilsons disease, gauchers disease, gouty deposits of urates and in alkaptonuric ochronosis deposits, makes cartilage susceptible to destruction.

Biomechanical factors: Structural abnormalities like articular fracture, dislocation, acetabular dysplasia, slipped epiphysis, perthes disease will cause abnormally high pressure over articular surface and predispose it for early degeneration. Similarly misalignments of joint, like genu varum and genu valgum, meniscal tear leads to abnormal stresses, leading the joint to early degeneration.

Hormonal effects: Acromegaly, hyperparathyroidism, diabetes mellitus and hypothyroidism.

Chemical injury: Corticosteroids injected in joint or given systemically, tends to destroy joints on long-term.

Repeated intrasynovial hemorrhage: Iron and blood pigments, alters physical and chemical properties of cartilage and causes its early degeneration, e.g. hemophilic arthritis.

Pathophysiology

The primary lesion consists of degeneration of hyaline cartilage. As a result, the cartilage is easily and rapidly eroded, until ultimately the bone matrix is exposed. The erosion of the cartilage is not uniform, so relatively at first area of bone are exposed in a patchy fashion and there are intervening islands of relatively normal cartilage. The perichondrium and the cartilage round the periphery of the joint are stimulated into activity and as a result, the nonarticular areas of the bones are elevated above the remainder of the surface and project circumferentially, to give the appearance known as "lipping".

Formation of osteophytes: These cartilagenous outgrowth ossifies to form osteophyte. Local periosteal new bone formation, particularly around capsular attachment also leads to osteophyte formation.

Synovitis and capsulitis: Detached cartilagenous flakes, which lies freely in the joint cavity are readily absorbed by synovial membrane and leads to synovitis followed by fibrosis. Proteoglycans leaks from damaged articular cartilage, produces irritation to synovial membrane and capsule, which undergoes hyperplasia.

Subchondral sclerosis: Proliferation of blood vessels along the subchondral bone leads to osteoporosis initially, followed by invasion of larger blood vessels, leading to subchondral sclerosis, as shown in Figure 24.168.

Formation of subchondral cyst: Edema of subchondral bone marrow, followed by formation of mucinous fatty marrow

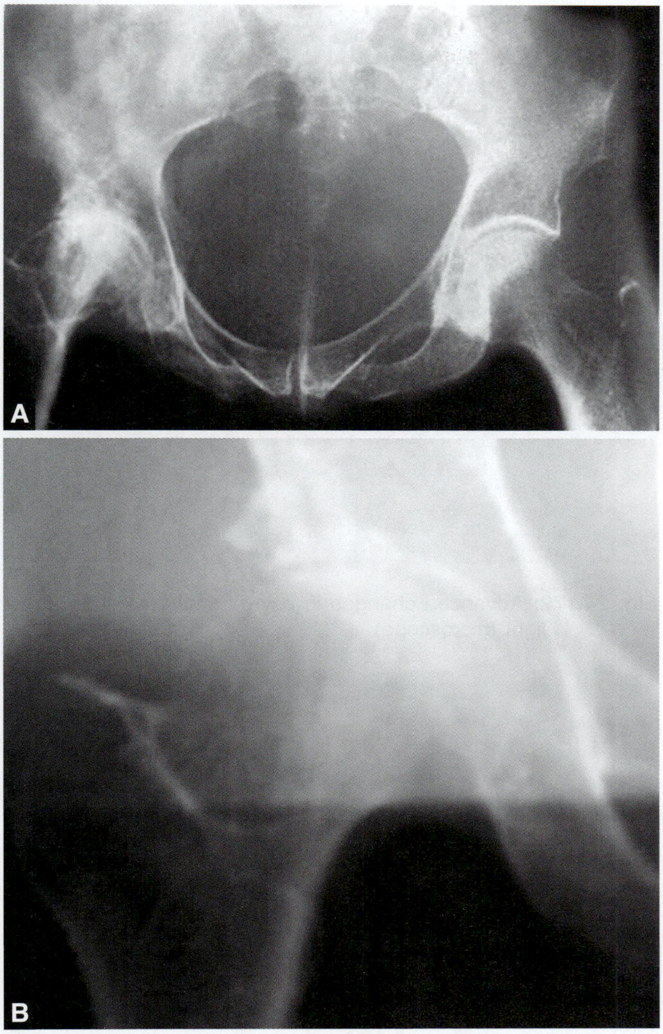

Figs 24.169A and B: Progression of osteoarthritis of the hip over period of time. There is narrowing of joint space, early cyst formation and early thickening of the both femoral head and acetabulum

with dilatation of surrounding sinusoids, leads to cyst formation. There is mucoid secretion within the center of this area and the expansion of the cyst cavities, by osteoclastic resorption of bony trabeculae. Surrounding this, there is some osteoblastic response and a sclerotic wall is formed. Other theories are that these cysts arise from herniation of synovial fluid through cracks within the denuded subchondral bone plate, as shown in Figures 24.169A and B.

Formation of loose bodies: The synovial membrane and capsule are involved in the late stages and are the site of inflammation and adhesions. The synovial tags or polypi are insinuated into the joint and when very exuberant the process is referred to as "lipoma arborescens". Occasionally, cartilage formation occurs in these tags and they are liable to be broken off into the joint, when they form loose bodies.

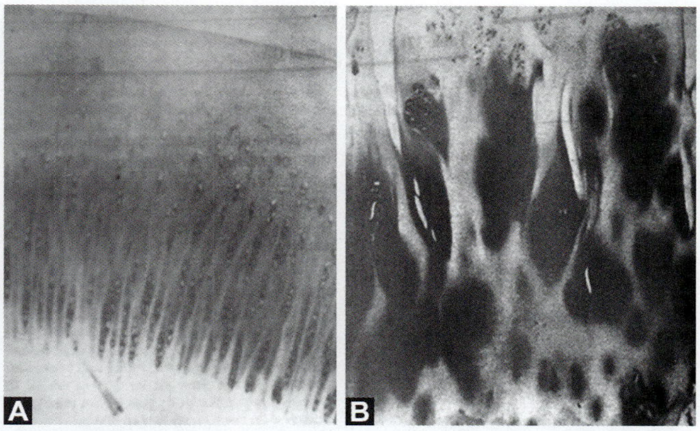

Figs 24.170A and B: Early changes in osteoarthritis (as seen under light microscope)

Eburnation: The exposed bone ends of the articular surface are subjected to considerable friction, in consequence the bone trabeculae in the immediate neighborhood fracture and repair and the marrow space are obliterated. The change involves only a thin layer abutting on the joint and when the surface of this layer gradually becomes more and more smooth and polished, as a result of the continual rubbing, the process is known as eburnation. An osteoarthritic joint rarely, if ever, becomes completely ankylosed, in contrast to the rheumatoid form, in which ankylosis is frequent. Nevertheless, the gross peripheral proliferation and the presence of osteophytic outgrowths and dense capsular fibrosis may impede the free movements of the joint and even simulate a degree of fusion which does not, in fact, exist.

Stages of Osteoarthritis as Seen under Light Microscopy

Early (Figs 24.170A and B)

- Surface irregularities or fibrillation with small clefts not extending beyond superficial zone
- Slight hypercellularity
- Minimal loss of mucopolysaccharides.

Moderately Advanced (Fig. 24.171)

- More extensive loss of surface
- Clefts extending into middle zone and occasionally into calcified zone
- Loss of mucopolysacchrides, extend into middle zone
- Hypercellularity in clusters of cells or chondrocyte clones.

Advanced Changes (Fig. 24.172)

- Thickness of cartilage reduced
- Clefts may extend down to subchondral bone

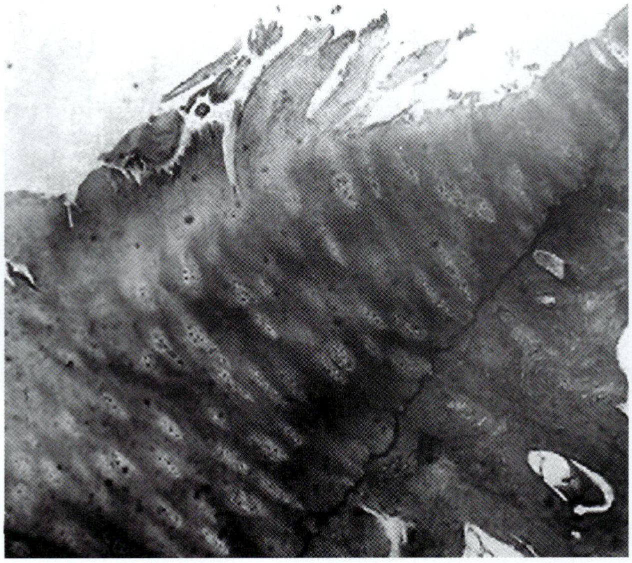

Fig. 24.171: Moderately advanced changes in osteoarthritis (as seen under light microscope)

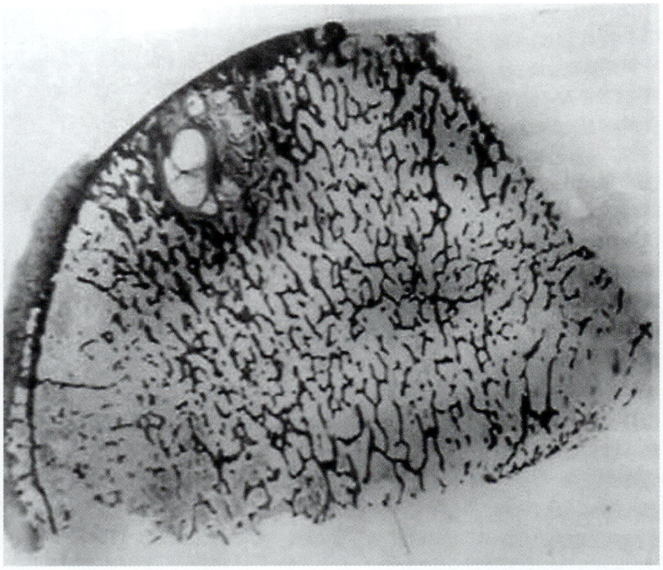

Fig. 24.172: Advanced changes in osteoarthritis (as seen under light microscope)

- Mucopolysaccharides markedly reduced through entire thickness of cartilage
- In some areas, complete loss of cartilage with exposure of thick and eburnated subchondral bone.

Sites of Osteoarthritis

Figure 24.173 shows different sites of osteoarthritis.

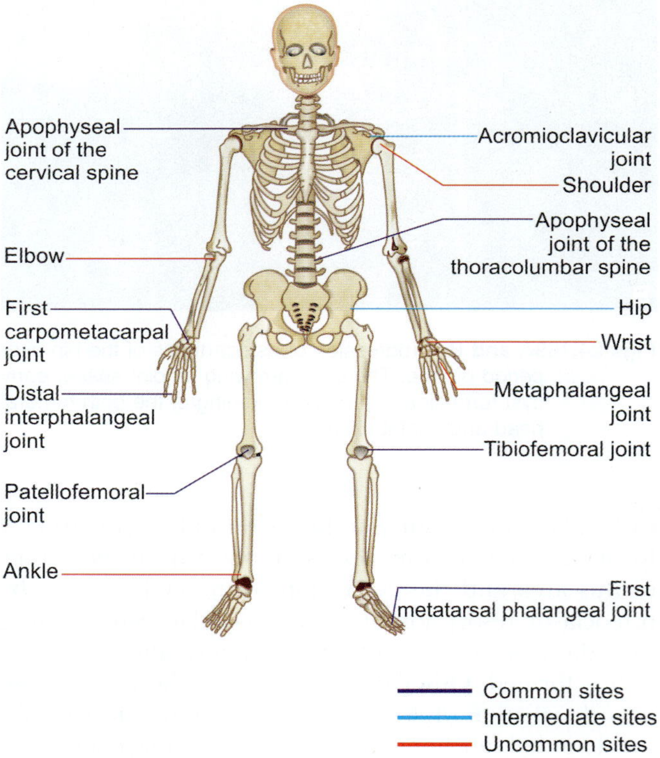

Fig. 24.173: Different sites of osteoarthritis

Osteoarthritis of Hip (Figs 24.174A to C)

- Familiarly called as malum coxa senilis
- Most commonly targets the superior aspects of the joint.
- Often unilateral at presentation, often progresses with superolateral migration of the femoral head and has a poor prognosis.
- The less common central (medial) OA, shows more central cartilage loss and is largely confined to women.
- It is often bilateral at presentation, may associate with nodal generalized OA, uncommonly progresses with axial femoral migration and has a better prognosis.

Classification

Primary OA of Hip

- This is idiopathic and forms 50 percent of the osteoarthritis of the hip
- In this variety, the exact cause is not known and the causative factors suspected are increased anteversion and the trabecular microfracture, causing stiffening of the subchondral bone.

Secondary OA of Hip

Following factors are responsible:

- Incongruity of the articular surface, e.g. trauma, perthes, CDH, slipped epiphysis, etc.

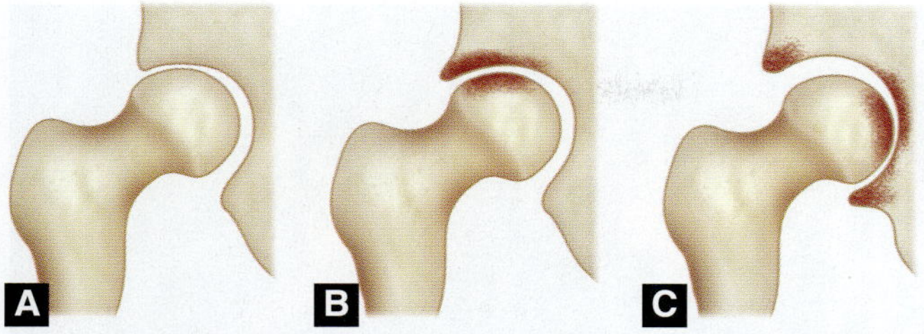

Figs 24.174A to C: Osteoarthritis of hip, often unilateral at presentation and progresses with superolateral migration of the femoral head

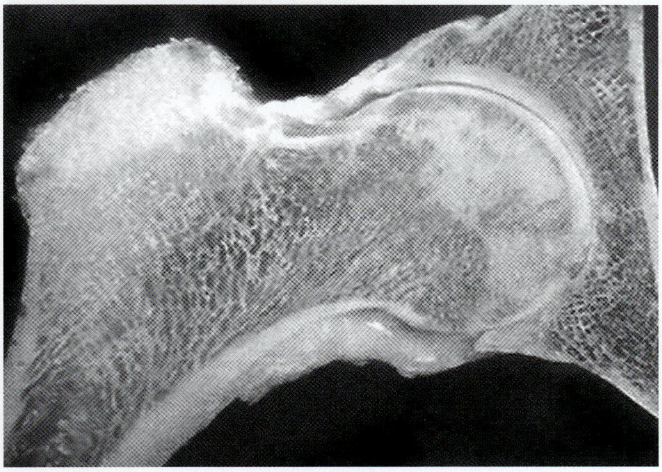

Fig. 24.175: Pathological changes in OA of hip

- Instability of the hip, e.g. subluxation.
- Concentration of pressure load, e.g. coxa vara, anteversion.
- Direct injury, e.g. infection, trauma, etc.
- Constitutional cause, e.g. obesity, hyperthyroidism, etc.
- Bone diseases, like AVN, rheumatoid arthritis, etc.

Pathology (Fig. 24.175)

The earliest change in OA begins in the hyaline cartilage. Harrison believed that this is not at the summit of the femoral head of the femur (i.e. at the main pressure area), but at the non-pressure area of the lower part of the head, which is opposite to the acetabulum without an articular lining. He said that use and compression are necessary, to maintain the nutrition of the articular cartilage. The intermittent pumping action of alternate pressure and rest forces the synovial fluid into the cartilage. Hence, where pressure is absent, nutrition is likely to be absent and degeneration occurs more readily. The immediate reaction of the cartilage is proliferation of the subchondral blood vessels, which is interpreted as an attempt to bring about repair. Calcification and ossification take place in the deeper layers of the cartilage, then the blood vessels enter this calcified cartilage and further calcification takes place ahead of them. In nonpressure areas, this process continues indefinitely, the vessels spread outwards, preceded by a vanguard of calcification capped with a layer of fibrocartilage, this gradually increasing the size of the bone to form osteophytes. In vascular zone, beneath the pressure area cysts are formed and these cysts always communicate with the joint through small openings. The cyst increases in size from the intermittent pressure of the synovial fluid. At the late stage the hyperemic bone, no longer protected by its coverings of articular cartilage, decreases in height as a result of successive trabecular fractures. Areas of hyperemia, as well as venous stasis are seen and cause the severe, constant night pain in late disease. In response to the progressive breakdown of articular cartilage with loss of matrix proteoglycan and collagen and death of chondrocytes, there is response in the residual tissue of cellular division and increased glycosaminoglycan synthesis. In any event the repair response of the cartilage is never sufficient to effect repair. Thus inevitable gradual progression of the disease occurs.

Synovial Membrane and Capsule (Figs 24.176A and B)

As matrix proteoglycan begins to leak out of the damaged articular cartilage, it produces direct irritation and inflammation of the synovial membrane, which undergoes hyperplasia of the lining layer and hyperemia. With the progressive accumulation of more cartilage and late bone debris the inflammation persists and inflammatory cells are seen in the subsynovial tissue. With the hyperplasia, the synovium is thrown into folds and villi though these are never so profuse, as in rheumatoid arthritis. Fragments of cartilage and bone are engulfed by the synovial membrane and are seen in the subintima. Metaplasia of the synovium may occur with the point of attachment to the articular margins. These pedunculated masses may break off into the joint to form loose bodies or "joint mice". Loose fragments of cartilage and bone from the degenerating articular surface or from osteophytes may also remain free in the joint, giving rise to symptoms of "locking". The underlying capsule also becomes involved by the inflammatory process. As fibrosis commences in the synovium and capsule, the latter becomes thickened and shortened with resultant reduction in joint movements.

Clinical Features

- *Pain:* Often described as a deep ache and is localized to the involved joint. Typically, the pain of OA is aggravated by joint use and relieved by rest, but as disease progresses, it may become persistent.
- Stiffness of the hip joint
- Muscle spasm

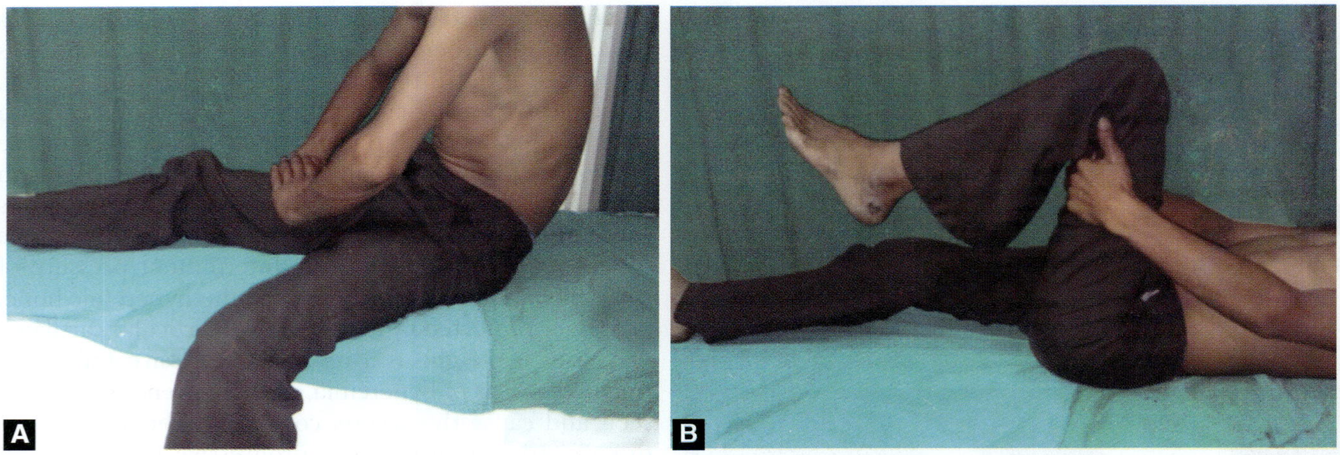

Figs 24.176A and B: Affect of inflammatory changes on synovial membrane and joint capsule

- Restriction of terminal movements
- Deformity-thigh is flexed, adducted and externally rotated
- Shortening leading to limp, while walking
- Disturbed sleep.

Physical Examination

- Localized tenderness and bony or soft tissue swelling
- Bony crepitus are palpable, sometimes audible, coarse crepitus (rough articular surface)
- Joint line tenderness or periarticular tenderness
- Synovial effusions, if present are usually not large
- Palpation may reveal some warmth over the joint
- Periarticular muscle atrophy may be due to disuse or to reflex inhibition of muscle contraction
- In advanced stages of OA, there may be gross deformity, bony hypertrophy, subluxation and marked loss of joint motion.

Deformity in OA Hip

In 80 percent there is adduction, external rotation and flexion deformity with joint space narrowing, cysts and sclerosis in the superior segment of the femoral head and acetabulum. There is a somewhat valgus position of the femoral neck and a bony buttress develops on the inferior aspects of the neck. In 10 percent there is external rotation of the femur but the leg is in neutral of slightly abducted. The radiological changes are seen mostly in the medial segment of the joint and there is a varus deformity of the femoral neck. In further 10 percent, there is concentric loss of cartilage space on the radiographs and the deformity is of flexion and slight abduction. The appearance may be similar to those of rheumatoid arthritis, except that there is hypertrophy of bone rather than atrophy of subchondral bone.

Investigations

- Routine investigations in primary OA are usually in normal limits.
- Analysis of synovial fluid reveals mild leukocytosis, with a predominance of mononuclear cells
- Other investigations are depending upon the predisposing factors, if present
- Radiographs of both the hips
- Ultrasound, arthroscopy and MRI have limited role.

Radiology (Fig. 24.177)

Stage I: Hyperemia with periarticular osteoporosis.
Stage II: Reduction in joint space.
Stage III: Osteophytes formation, with subchondral sclerocystic changes.
Stage IV: Complete loss of joint space with or without subluxation.

Differential Diagnosis

The diagnosis of chronic arthritis is seldom difficult, unless pain and swelling are limited to one joint. When the onset is acute, gout, pseudogout, rheumatic fever and infective arthritis have first to be considered. In the younger people, it may be necessary to distinguish between rheumatoid arthritis, gouty diasthesis, gonococcal arthritis and tuberculosis.

Laboratory and radiological differentiation in RA and OA illustrated in Table 24.13.

Treatment Options

- Medications
- Injections
- Physical therapy
- Weight loss

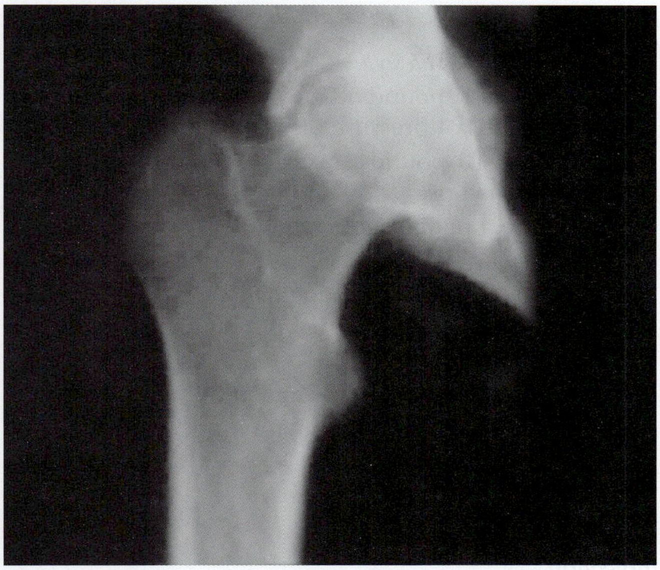

Fig. 24.177: Radiographs showing OA of hip

Table 24.13: Laboratory differentiation in rheumatoid arthritis and osteoarthritis

	Rheumatoid arthritis	*Osteoarthritis*
Agglutination reactions	Positive in over 50% of typical cases	Never definitely positive
Sedimentation rate	Usually greatly increased; tends to return to normal as patient improves	Normal or only slightly increased
Roentgeno-graphic appearances	*Early:* Osteoporosis, periarticular swelling, and joint effusion *Late:* Narrowing of joint space, bone destruction, ankylosis, and deformities	*Early:* No osteoporosis; slight lipping at joint margins *Late:* Marked lipping, osteophytes narrowing of joint space deformation of articular bone ends

- Nutrition consult
- Surgery

Conservative

- Rest
- Active and passive range of motion
- Abstinence from weight-bearing
- Vertical load reduction
- Traction
- Physical therapy
- Orthotics
- Heat therapy
- Graduated exercise
- Drug therapy

Drug Therapy

- NSAIDs
- Chondrosynthesis drugs
- Chondroprotective and disease modifying drugs
- Antioxidants vitamins
- Antioxidants minerals
- Semi-invasive treatment

NSAIDs

Diclofenac and aceclofenac: These drugs produces their anti-inflammatory and analgesic effect, by inhibiting cyclo-oxygenase and thus preventing production of prostaglandins from arachidonic acid. In addition aceclofenac, has shown some stimulatory effects on cartilage matrix synthesis, that may be linked to ability of drug to inhibit IL-1 activity.

Chondrosynthetic Drugs

Glucosamine: Rejoint is the sulfate derivative of amino monosaccharide glucosamine, a normal constituent glucosaminoglycan in the cartilage. Given orally in the dose of 1500 mg daily in divided doses for long periods, it is claimed to slow down the progression of OA.

Chondroitin

- Nonspecific slow acting chondroprotective, but helps in chondrosynthesis.
- Supplement action of glucosamine.
- Inhibits proinflammatory prostaglandin/leukotrienes.
- Inhibit hyaluronidase enzyme, e.g. breakdown HA molecule and viscosity of synovial fluid.

Chondroprotective and Disease Modifying Drugs

- Inhibit pain by inhibiting synthesis of cytokines.
- Improves mobility, by stimulating the production of collagen II and proteoglycan.
- Reduces stiffness, by stimulating the production of Hyalurons.

Others

- Antioxidant vitamins, e.g. vitamin C, E, beta-carotene.
- Antioxidant minerals, e.g. selenium, Mn, Zn.

Newer drugs

- Diacerein
- Dosage 50 mg twice daily
- Inhibits the production of IL-1
- Also inhibits the secretion of other enzymes involved in cartilage destruction, like myeloperoxidase, β-glucuronidase and elastase.

Semi-invasive Treatment Corticosteroids

a. *Intra-articular cortisone*
   - Temporary relief
   - Satisfying and lasting in mild and moderate cases.
   - When there is no response to conservative treatment in acute inflammatory phase.
   - In case of severe OA, there is pain in pericapsular site (outside joint)—Pes anserinus and biceps. Local steroid, shows good result:

  - Risk of joint infection
  - Hypopigmentation
  - Subcutaneous atrophy
  - Osteonecrosis
- Repeated—Long acting depot preparation.

b. *Intra-articular injection of hyaluronic acid*
It includes viscosupplementation therapy:
- Safe and effective
- Pain, improves joints function for months
- Five injections, weekly.

Physical Therapy

- Flexibility
- Strength
- Walking pattern
- Leg length
- Shoes
- Weight
- Lifestyle
- Goals

I. *Flexibility (Figs 24.178 and 24.179)*

II. *Strength (Figs 24.180A to C)*
- Slow
- Rhythmic
- Light resistance
- 30 min/day
- 6 days/week

III. *Walking patten and shoes (Figs 24.181A and B)*

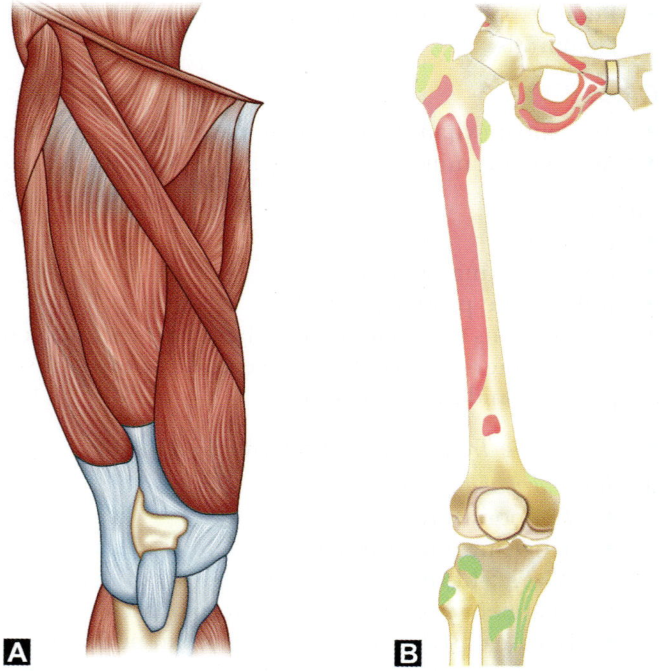

Figs 24.178A and B: Musculature around hip joint

IV. *Leg length (Figs 24.182A and B)*

V. *Body weight and lifestyle*
- For every 1 pound of body weight you lose, it takes 3 pounds of pressure off your hips
- Losing 10 pounds, takes 30 pounds of pressure off your hips
- Create a manageable schedule
- Alternate heavy tasks with light tasks
- Change positions frequently
- Plan rest breaks during your activities
- Apply heat and/or cold
- Heat, increases blood circulation
- Cold, decreases inflammation and pain
- 15 minutes maximum

Operative Treatment

Indication

- Pain unrelieved by conservative treatment
- Limitation of movements
- Flexion adduction deformity, with pelvic tilt and distortion of the lumbar spine.

Surgical Options

- Synovectomy
- Arthroscopic lavage with debridement
- Osteotomies
- Arthrodesis
- Arthroplasties

Arthroscopy

- Joint clean-up
- Symptom relief
- Fifty to ninty percent for cartilage tears of socket
- Limited benefit for arthritis.

Arthrodesis (Figs 24.183 and 24.184)

- Usually Watson Jones arthrodesis is performed
- Hip is exposed through a Smith Petersen approach
- The head and the acetabulum are thoroughly denuded
- The nail is inserted through the neck and the head, so that 1 inch of the nail engages in the pelvis
- A bone graft removed from the ilium is inserted through a slot in the superior acetabular rim and fixed by a screw to the neck, as shown in Figure 24.182.

Osteotomies

- Correction of mechanical malalignment
- Brings into contact nondamaged articular surface, hence reducing friction and pain
- Alters weight-bearing and joint reaction forces
- Decongests venous stasis and venous hypertension in metaphyseal trabecular bone.

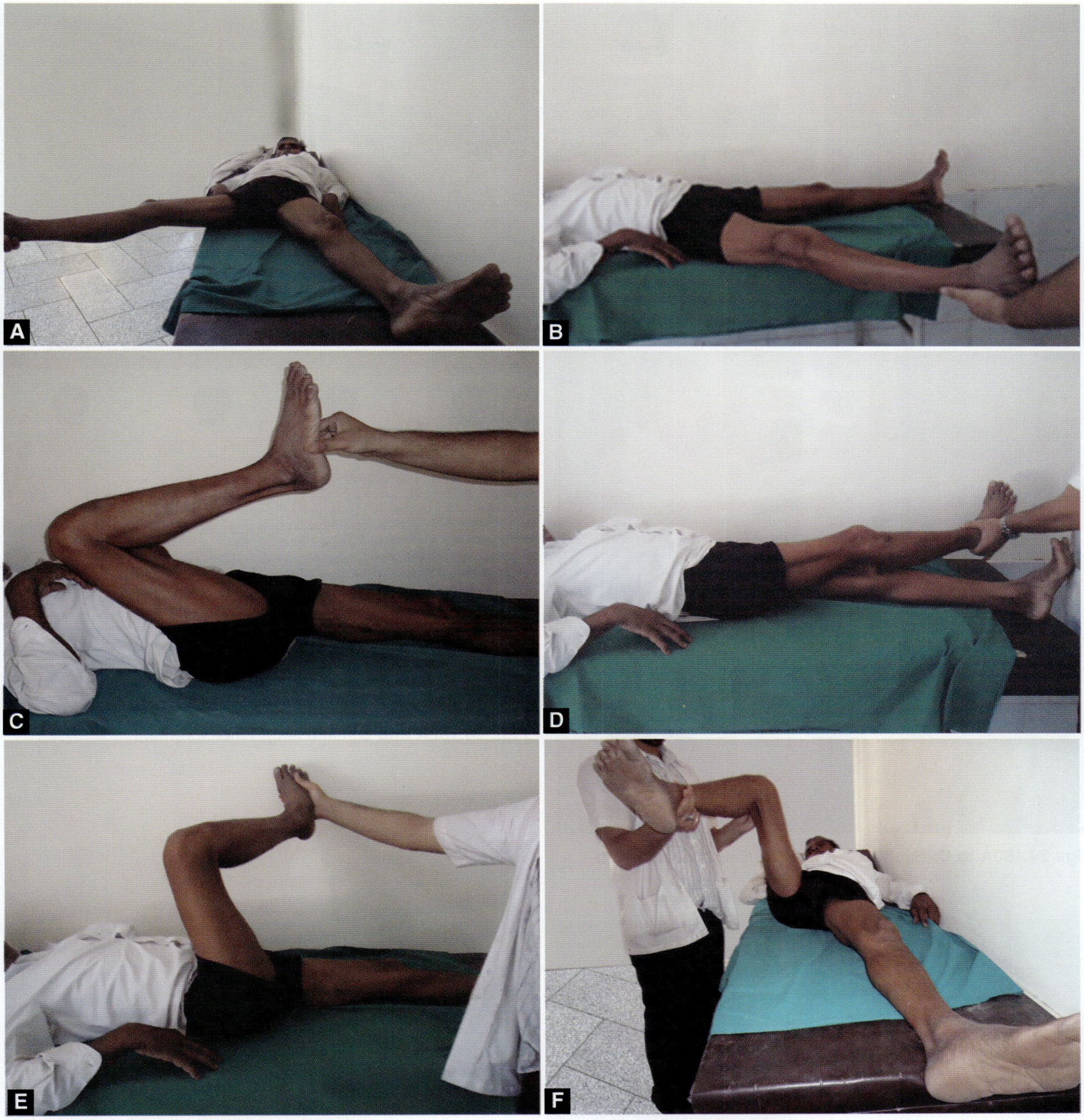

Figs 24.179A to F: Lower limb flexibility exercises

Intertrochanteric osteotomy (Fig. 24.185): Intertrochanteric osteotomy for the relief of pain in an OA hip was introduced by McMurray, which is based on principle of providing pelvic support through the shaft of femur. Pain was relieved because of the altered thrust of weight-bearing and rotation of the femoral head, which brought an unaffected portion of the femoral articular cartilage in contact with the acetabulum. It requires displacement of the distal femoral fragments beneath the inferior acetabular rim.

Pauwel's varus osteotomy (Figs 24.186 and 24.187): The clinical indications for varus osteotmy, according to Blount, are hips with painless, adequate abduction and

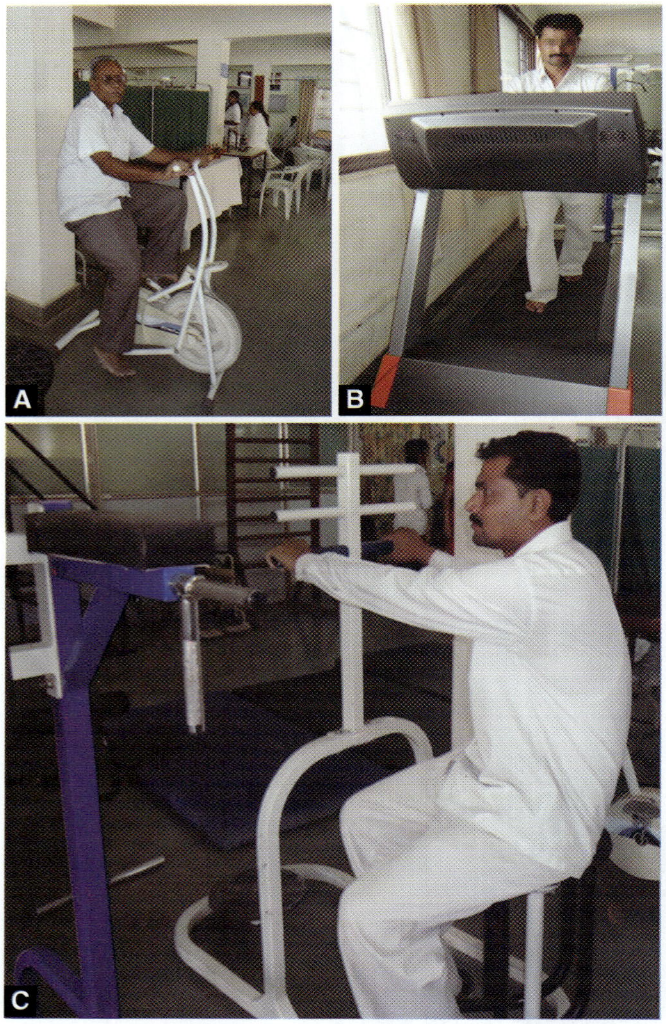

Figs 24.180A to C: Strength building exercises of lower limb

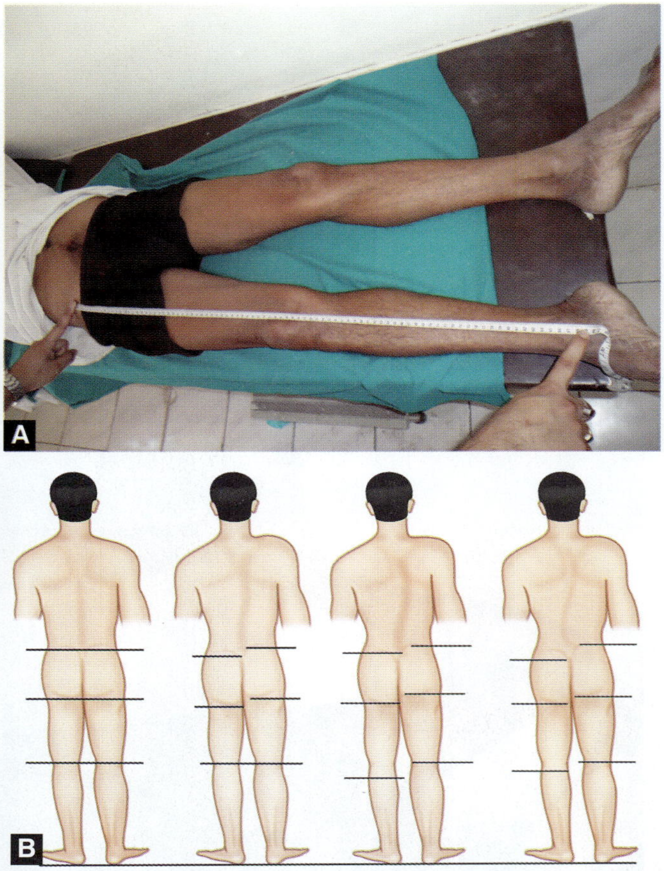

Figs 24.182A and B: Limb length measurement

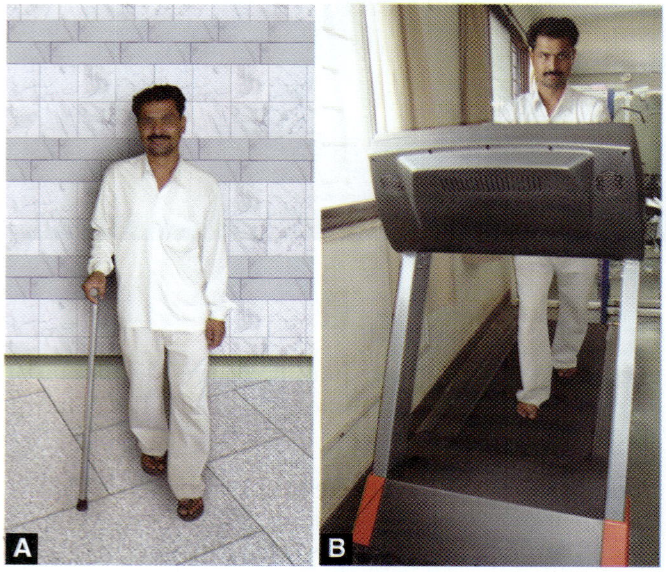

Figs 24.181A and B: Walking pattern

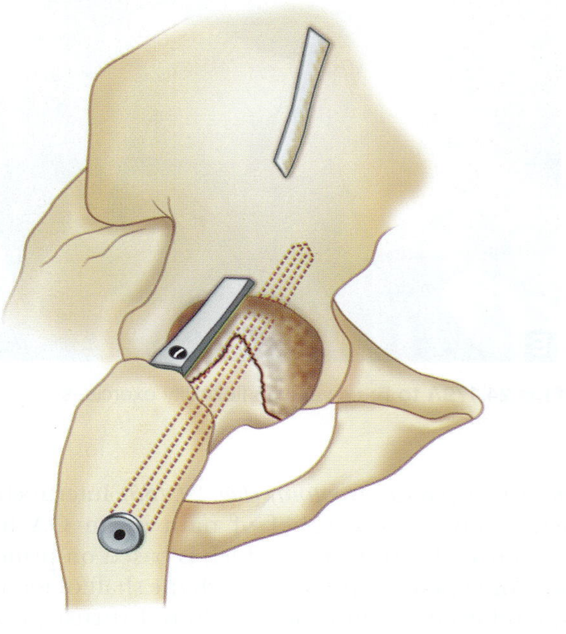

Fig. 24.183: Hip arthrodesis: A bone graft removed from the ilium is inserted through a slot in the superior acetabular rim and fixed by a screw to the neck

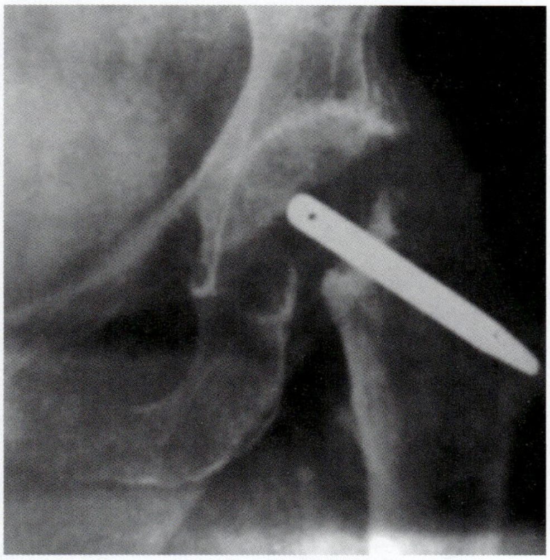

Fig. 24.184: Hip prosthesis, Judet type. Roentgenographic appearance. This was the forerunner of the modern hip prosthesis. The head was composed of acrylic. Breakage and loosening were frequent

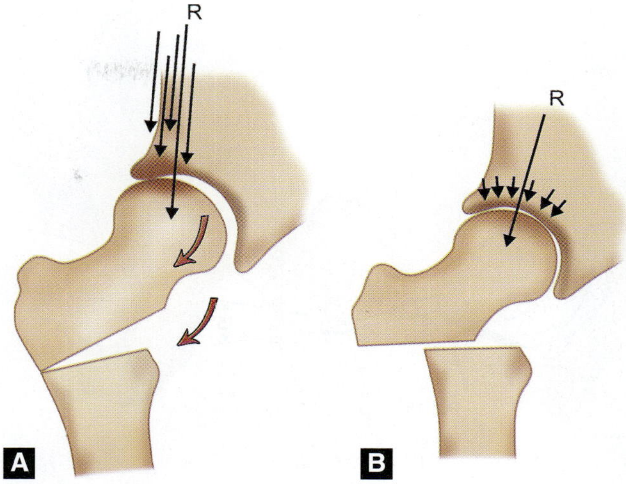

Figs 24.186A and B: Pauwel's varus osteotomy. Arrow forces directed acetabulum to head of femur

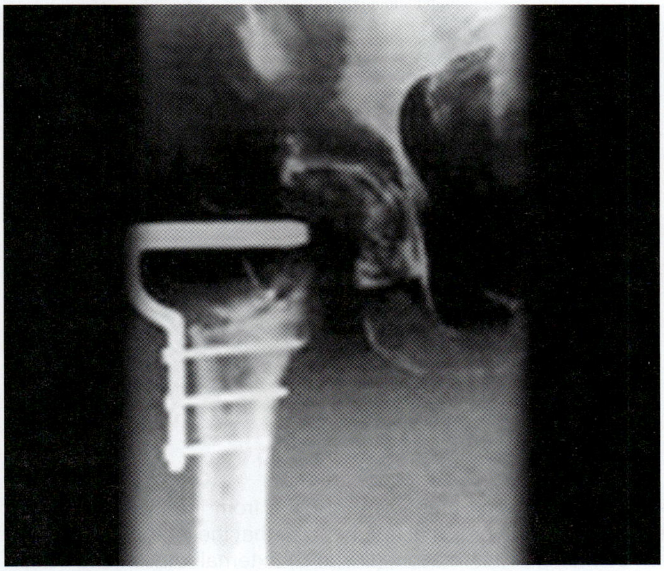

Fig. 24.185: Intertrochanteric osteotomy for pain relief

limited painful adduction, an antalgic gait and apparent lengthening. Varus osteotomy consists of resecting a segment of bone from the intertrochanteric area, with its base directed medially. The wedge must be removed from the proximal fragment, so that the level of transection of the distal shaft fragment lies transverse and therefore, will not interfere with rotation. External rotation and flexion deformity are corrected, by rotating the extremity inward, with the base of the wedge extended towards the posterior aspect to permit anterior angulation.

Valgus osteotomy (Figs 24.188 and 24.189): An abduction (valgus) osteotomy is indicated for the OA hip in patient who walks with a Trendelenburg Lurch and has an adduction deformity and in whom further abduction is not possible, adduction is limited and painful and repositioning of the femoral head within the acetabulum is demonstrable on the roentgenogram, when the hip is adducted. Wedge of bone is resected laterally. Insertion of nail plate forms an angle with outer aspect of shaft. Shaft has been abducted, fragment ends were approximated and compression device is in place. Compression is applied and first screws are inserted.

Arthroplasty

- Interposition (cup) arthroplasty
- Excision arthroplasty
- Total replacement arthroplasty

Total Hip Replacement (THR) (Figs 24.190 and 24.191)

- Uncemented THR
- Cemented THR
- Surface replacement

Indications

- The procedure is effective in the treatment of severe osteoarthritis, primary or secondary to trauma, congenital dysplasia, protrusio acetabulae, avascular necrosis, local benign neoplasm and metabolic disease.
- The patient should be over 60 years of age, because the durability and long-term biological effects of the component and cement materials are not yet established. (exceptionally, the procedure may be done

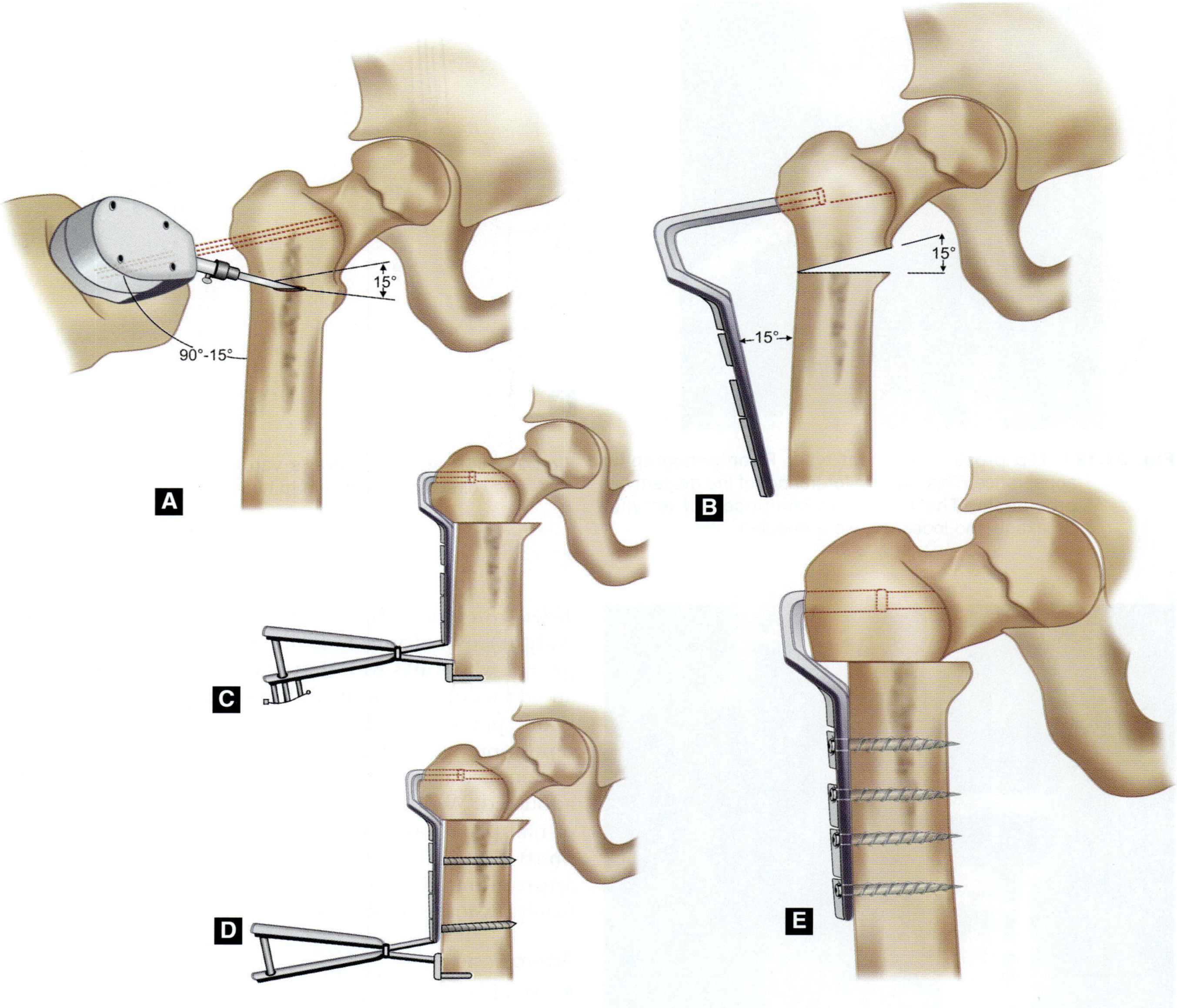

Figs 24.187A to E: Different steps in performing varus osteotomy—(A to C) Resecting a segment of bone from the intertrochanteric area, with its base directed medially. The wedge must be removed from the proximal fragment, so that the level of transection of the distal shaft fragment lies transverse and therefore, will not interfere with rotation; (D and E) External rotation and flexion deformity are corrected by rotating the extremity inward, with the base of the wedge extended towards the posterior aspect to permit anterior angulation

in younger patients, especially with bilateral hip disease).

- If the previous operations (e.g. prosthesis, cup arthroplasty, osteotomy) was unsuccessful, infection as a cause of failure must be ruled out, prior to total hip replacement. In doubtful cases, the hardware must be removed and cultures obtained before total hip replacement at a later date.
- In bilateral cases, the interval between two operations should be less than 3 months.

Contraindications

- When the infection is recent or remote
- When the person is under 60 years of age, especially when the alternative surgery is available
- When pain is not severe.

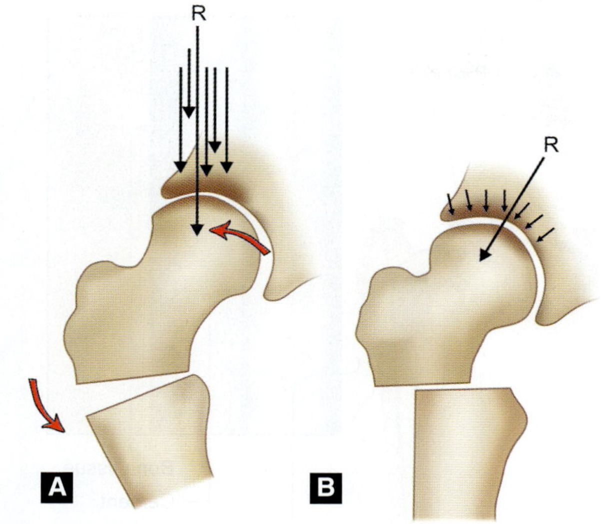

Figs 24.188A and B: An abduction (valgus) osteotomy

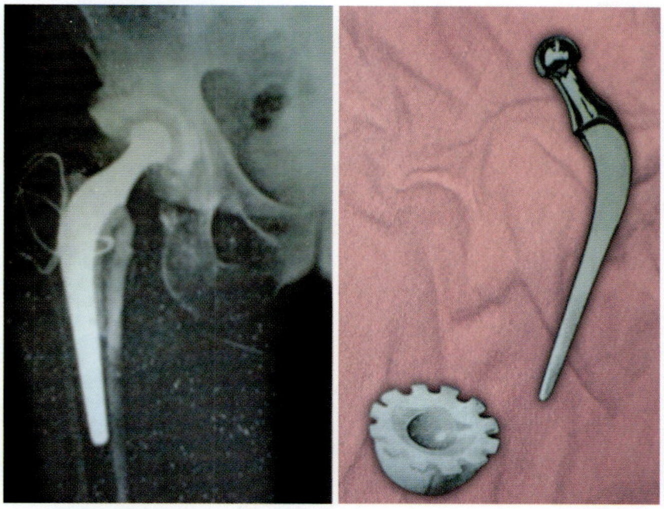

Fig. 24.190: Cemented THR with hip prosthesis

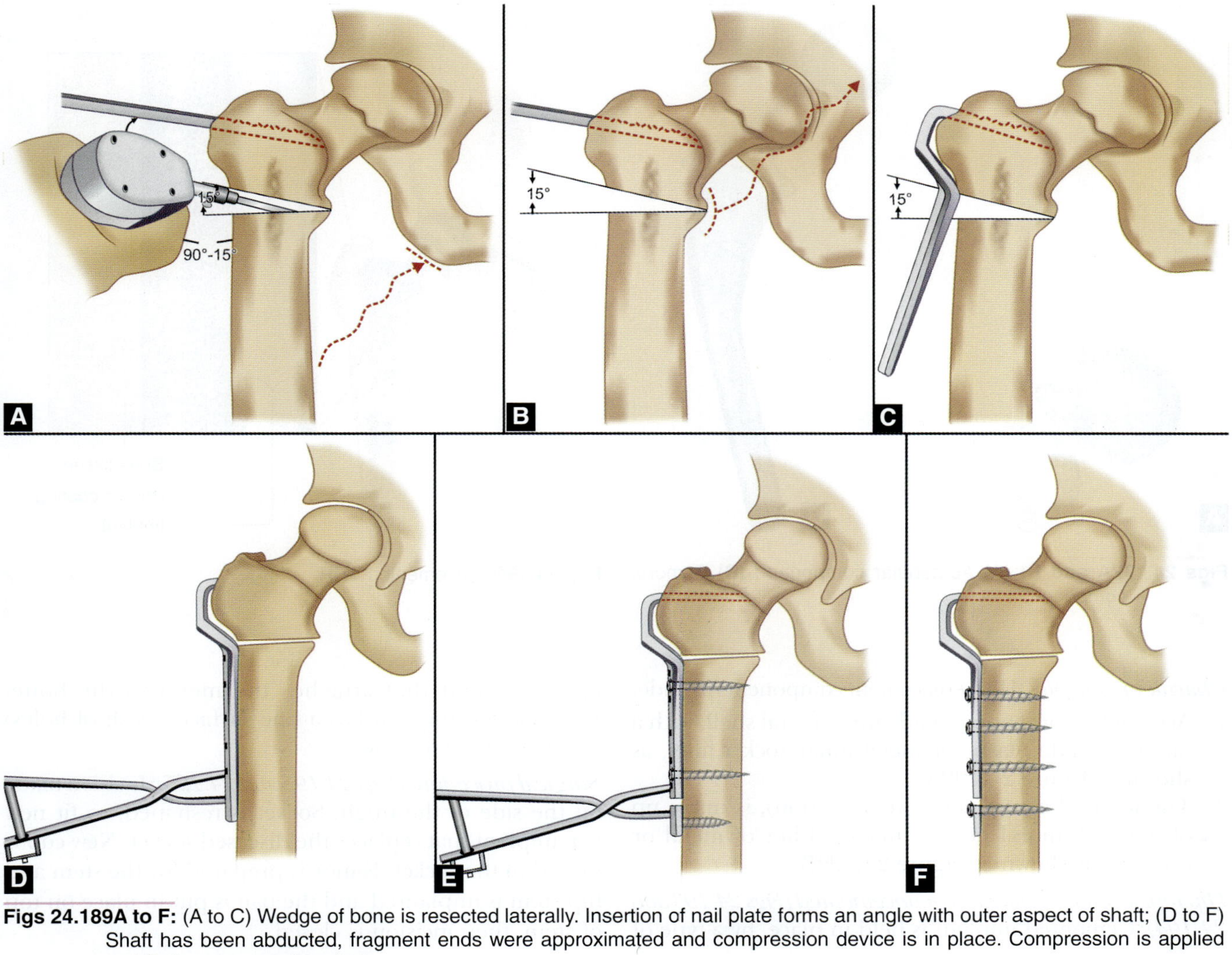

Figs 24.189A to F: (A to C) Wedge of bone is resected laterally. Insertion of nail plate forms an angle with outer aspect of shaft; (D to F) Shaft has been abducted, fragment ends were approximated and compression device is in place. Compression is applied and first screws are inserted

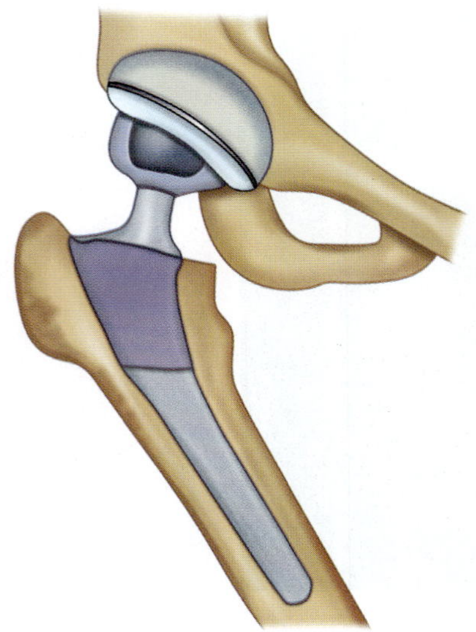

Fig. 24.191: Uncemented total hip replacement

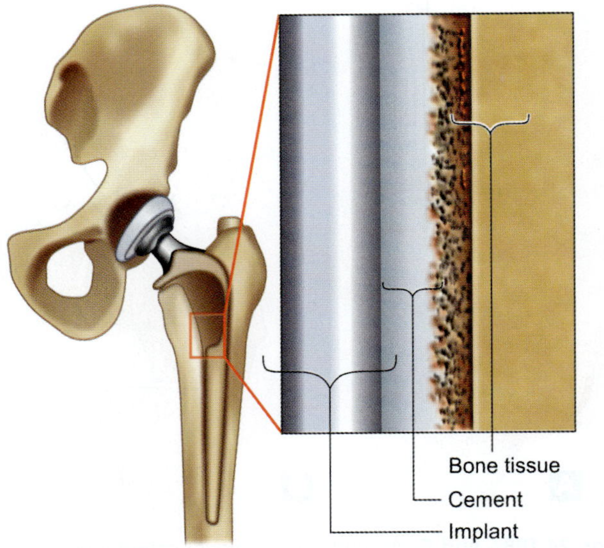

Fig. 24.193: Cemented hip replacement

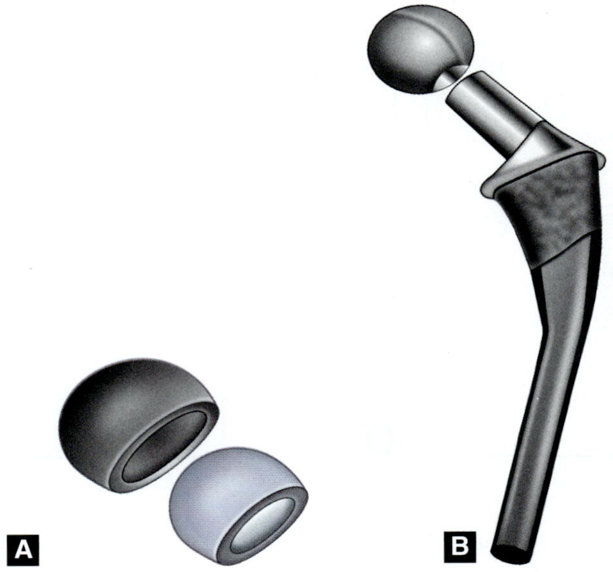

Figs 24.192A and B: (A) Acetabular component; (B) Femoral component

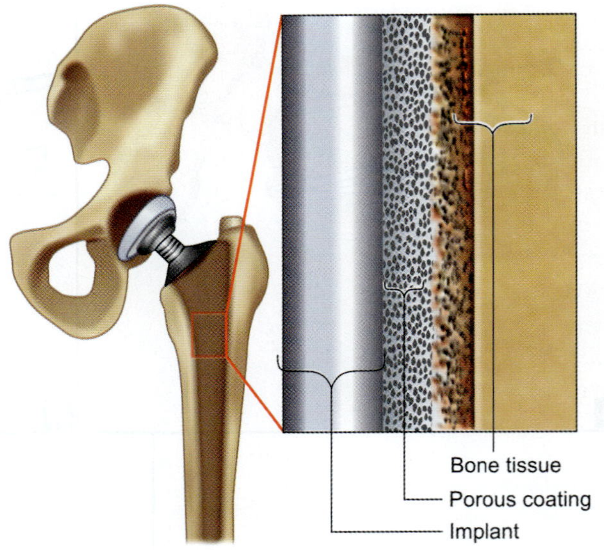

Fig. 24.194: Uncemented THR

Charnley principles: Hip replacement components include:

1. Acetabular component made up of metal shell, with a medical grade plastic or metal inner socket liner, as shown in Figure 24.192A.
2. The femoral component (stem portion), is made up of metal. Femoral head is made, either of metal or ceramic, as shown in Figure 24.192B.

Hip replacement: cemented or uncemented (Figs 24.193 and 24.194): Cemented implant is held in place, by a type of epoxy cement that attaches the metal to the bone. Uncemented implant has a fine surface (mesh of holes) allowing tissue to grow.

Surgical procedure (Figs 24.195 and 24.196): Incision made on the side of the thigh. Socket is reshaped, to fit new cup implant that replaces the diseased socket. New cup is placed in the socket. Femur is prepared for the stem and hip stem is implanted and the ball is put in place on top of stem, then incision is closed.

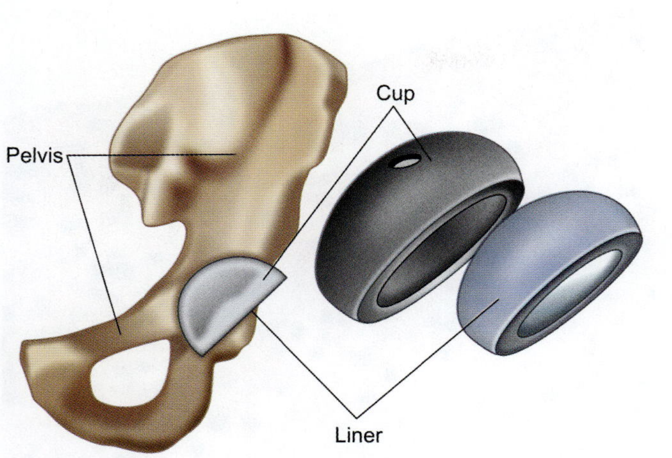

Fig. 24.195: Incision made on the side of the thigh. Socket is reshaped, to fit new cup implant that replaces the diseased socket

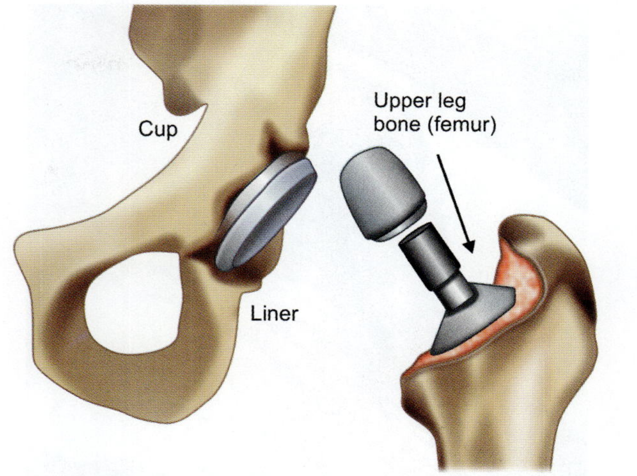

Fig. 24.196: New cup is placed in the socket. Femur is prepared for the stem and hip stem is implanted and the ball is put in place on top of stem, then incision is closed

RHEUMATOID ARTHRITIS OF HIP

Introduction

Rheumatoid arthritis is a chronic inflammatory systemic disease of young or middle aged adults, characterized by destructive and proliferative changes in synovial membrane, periarticular structures, skeletal muscle and perineural sheaths. Eventually, joints are destroyed, ankylosed and deformed. Rheumatoid arthritis (RA) is a systemic inflammatory disorder that mainly affects the diarthrodial joint. The clinical course of the disorder is extremely variable, ranging from mild, self limiting arthritis to rapidly progressive multisystem inflammation with profound morbidity and mortality. The small joints of the fingers and toes are the first to be affected. As the disease progresses, it tends to spread to involve the wrists, elbows, shoulders, knees, ankles, subtalar and midtarsal joints.

Etiology

- Cause remains unknown
- Might be manifestation of the response to an infectious agent in a genetically susceptible host. Possible causative agents are: *Mycoplasma, Epstein-Barr virus* (EBV), *Cytomegalovirus*, *Parvovirus* and *Rubella virus*.
- Environmental trigger, e.g. smoking
- Genetic traits, e.g. $HLADR_4$ and DR_1.

Epidemiology

- RA has a high prevalence in the Indian population (around 0.75%)

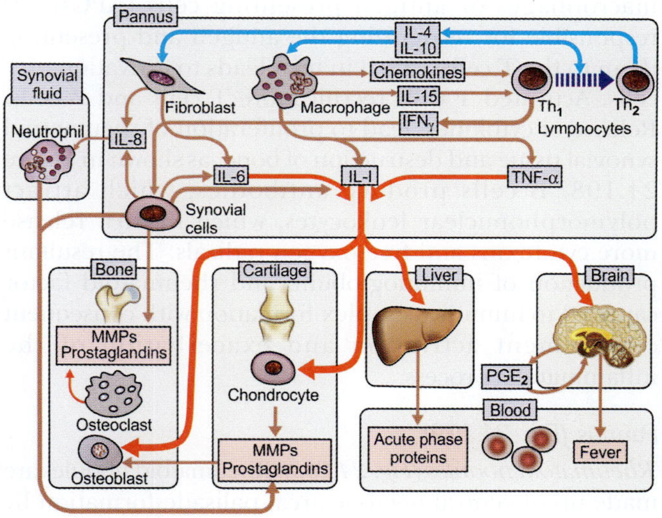

Fig. 24.197: Pathogenesis of RA of hip

- Thus projected population of at least 7 million patients.
- Male:female ratio is 1:3
- The peak age of onset is in the fourth decade in females and slightly later in males.
- 40 to 60 percent with advance RA will
  - Survive 5 years or less following diagnosis
  - Die 10 to 15 years earlier than expected.

Pathogenesis (Fig. 24.197)

In RA, the immune system loses its ability to recognize synovial tissue, as self-tissue and thus, attacks the synovial tissue and causes inflammation and destruction. The

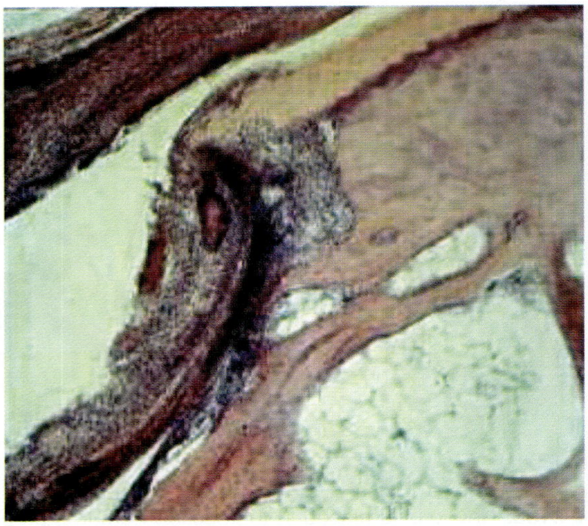

Fig. 24.198: Rheumatoid synovial tissue

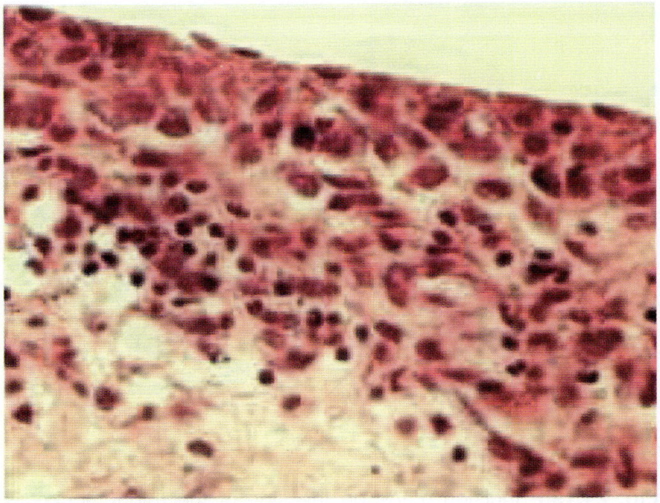

Fig. 24.199: Pannus: Thickened synovium with lymphocytic infiltrate and neovascularization

macrophages or antigen presenting cells (APCs) are responsible for recognizing the antigen and presenting them to the T cells, which in turn leads to activation of T cells. Activated T cells recruit more T cells and B cells. Release of cytokines, lead to proliferation of rheumatoid synovial tissue and destruction of bone, as shown in Figure 24.198. B cells produce antibodies, which attract polymorphonuclear leukocytes, which in turn release more cytotoxins and free oxygen radicals. The resultant production of immunoglobulin and rheumatoid factor can lead to immune complex formation with consequent complement activation and exacerbation of the inflammatory process.

Pannus (Fig. 24.199)

Rheumatoid nodules (Fig. 24.200): Rheumatoid nodules are made up of central necrotic area, palisade formation by mononuclear cells, round cell infiltration and fibrous capsule.

Clinical Features

- Joint swelling
- Pain/stiffness (commonly in morning and lasting for more than 1 hour) and pain on motion
- Tenderness
- Weakness
- Deformity
- Fatigue
- Malaise
- Fever
- Weight loss
- Depression

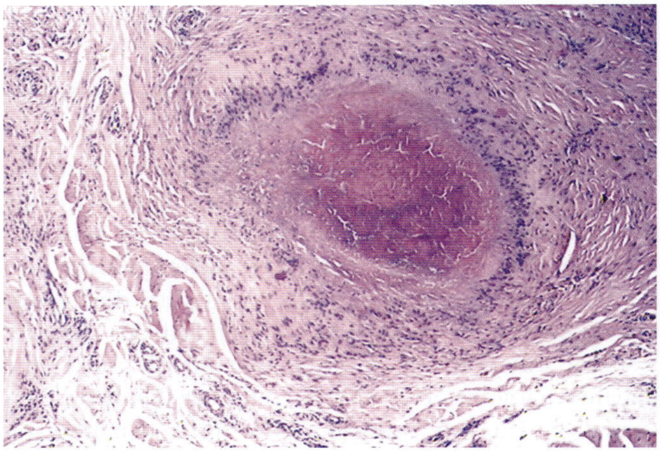

Fig. 24.200: Rheumatoid nodules formation in RA

Extra-articular manifestations (Table 24.14)

Table 24.14: Extra-articular manifestation of RA

Organ system	*Involvement*
Skin	Rheumatoid nodules
Ocular	Episcleritis and scleritis
Cardiac	Pericarditis and myocarditis
Pulmonary	Nodules and pleural effusion
Neurological	Neuropathy and cervical cord compression
Lymphatic	Splenomegaly
Musculoskeletal	Muscle wasting and tenosynovitis
Hematologic	Anemia and thrombocytosis
Vascular	Vasculitis

Diagnosis

- Laboratory findings
- Serologic tests
- Roentgenographic findings.

Laboratory Findings

- ESR is elevated particularly during active stage
- During periods of remission ESR continues increase, but to a lesser extent
- Hypochromic normocytic anemia is frequently associated.

Serologic Tests

- *RA factor:* Serum from patient contains a substance of unknown composition—RA factor.
  Rheumatoid factor: Most common autoantibody in RA and detected in 70 to 80 percent of RA patients. RA factor does not have a predictive value for diagnosis, but has a good predictive value for poorer outcome. Their presence in joints is believed to contribute to the inflammatory reaction. RA factor in presence of gamma globulin is capable of agglutinating certain strains of streptococci, sensitized sheep cells and latex particles. A convenient lab procedure uses a standard suspension of latex particles in a solution of gamma globulins.
- *Latex fixation test on serum*
  - *Latex suspension:* Unknown serum and gamma globulin
  - *Agglutination occurs:* Serum contains, adequate amount of RA factor.
  - *No agglutination:* Serum contains inadequate amount of RA factor.
  - If there is no agglutination then second more sensitive test must be performed.
- *The inhibition test*
  - Rheumatoid serum of known high agglutinating activity, unknown euglobulin and standard gamma globulin latex suspension
  - This test uses characteristics of euglobulin from unknown serum
  - Euglobulin from normal serum neutralizes the rheumatoid factor, thereby inhibiting agglutination
  - Euglobulin of rheumatoid serum has no effect on the rheumatoid factor and agglutination proceeds unhindered
  - The inhibition test is very sensitive. It is likely to be positive, even when the rheumatoid factor is present in minute amounts. When an unknown serum shows negative latex fixation test and positive inhibition test, the arthritis may be a part of rheumatoid spondylitis or a lupus erythmatosus.

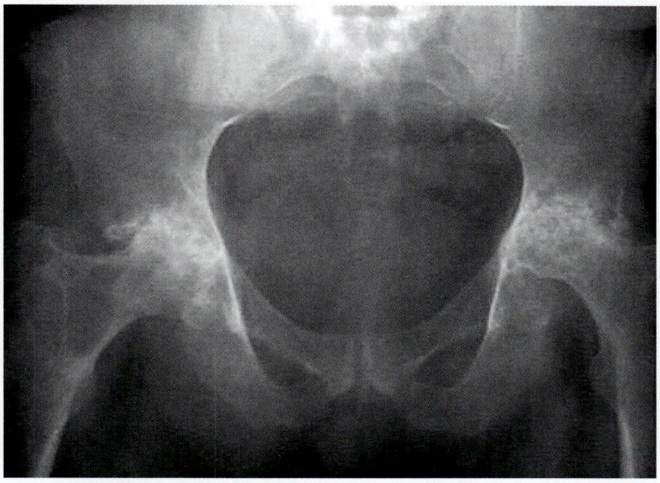

Fig. 24.201: X-ray showing pathological changes in hip due to RA

Roentgenographic Findings (Fig. 24.201)

Early changes: Osteoporosis, periarticular swelling and joint effusion.

Late changes: Narrowing of joint space, bone destruction, ankylosis and deformities.

Criteria for Diagnosis

- Morning stiffness
- Pain on motion or tenderness in atleast one joint
- Swelling (soft tissue thickening or fluid; not bony outgrowth alone) in at least one joint continuously for not less than 6 weeks
- Swelling of at least one other joint
- Symmetrical joint swelling
- Subcutaneous nodules
- X-ray changes typical of rheumatoid arthritis
- Positive latex fixation test
- Poor mucin clot
- Characteristic histologic changes in synovial membrane
- Characteristic histologic changes in nodules.

Classic: Any seven criteria for at least 6 weeks.

Definite: Any five criteria for at least 6 weeks.

Probable: Any three criteria for at least 4 weeks.

American College of Rheumatology (ACR) Clinical Classification Criteria for Rheumatoid Arthritis

This is based on history, physical examination, laboratory and radiographic findings, as shown in Table 24.15.

ACR Classification Criteria for Determining Progression of Rheumatoid Arthritis (Flow chart 24.4)

Table 24.15: American College of Rheumatology (ACR) clinical classification criteria for RA of the following must be present with 1 through 4 present a minimum of 6 weeks

Morning stiffness ≥ 1 hour
• Arthritis of 3 or more of the following joints: Right or left PIP, MCP, wrist, elbow, knee, ankle, and MTP joints - Arthritis of wrist, MCP, or PIP joint - Symmetric involvement of joints
• Rheumatoid nodules over bony prominences, or extensor surfaces, or in juxta-articular regions - Positive serum rheumatoid factor
• Radiographic changes including erosions or bony decalcification localized in or adjacent to the involved joints

■ American College of Rheumatology Classification Criteria for Determining Clinical Remission in Rheumatoid Arthritis

Five or more of the following present at least two consecutive months:

- Morning stiffness less than 15 minutes
- No fatigue
- No joint pain
- No joint tenderness or pain on motion
- No soft tissue swelling in joints or tendon sheaths
- ESR (Westergren method) less than 30 mm/hour for a female or 20 mm/hour for a male.

American College of Rheumatology Classification Criteria of Functional Status in Rheumatoid Arthritis

Class I: Completely able to perform usual activities of daily living (self-care, vocational and avocational).

Class II: Able to perform usual self-care and vocational activities, but limited in avocational activities.

Class III: Able to perform usual self-care activities, but limited in vocational and avocational activities.

Class IV: Limited ability to perform usual self-care, vocational and avocational activities.

Treatment

The goals of the therapy of RA are:

- Relief of pain
- Reduction of inflammation
- Maintenance of function, this is illustrated in Flow chart 24.5.

Treatment of RA can be divided into three modes:

i. Conservative
ii. Surgical
iii. Rehabilitation

Conservative Treatment

Rest: Complete bedrest

Removal of foci of infection: Teeth, tonsils, sinuses and pelvic organs are investigated and infections are eliminated.

Nutritious diet: A diet high in calories and high in vitamins is essential.

Transfusions and hematinics: These are continually necessary during entire course of disease.

Flow chart 24.4: American College of Rheumatology criteria for determining progression of RA

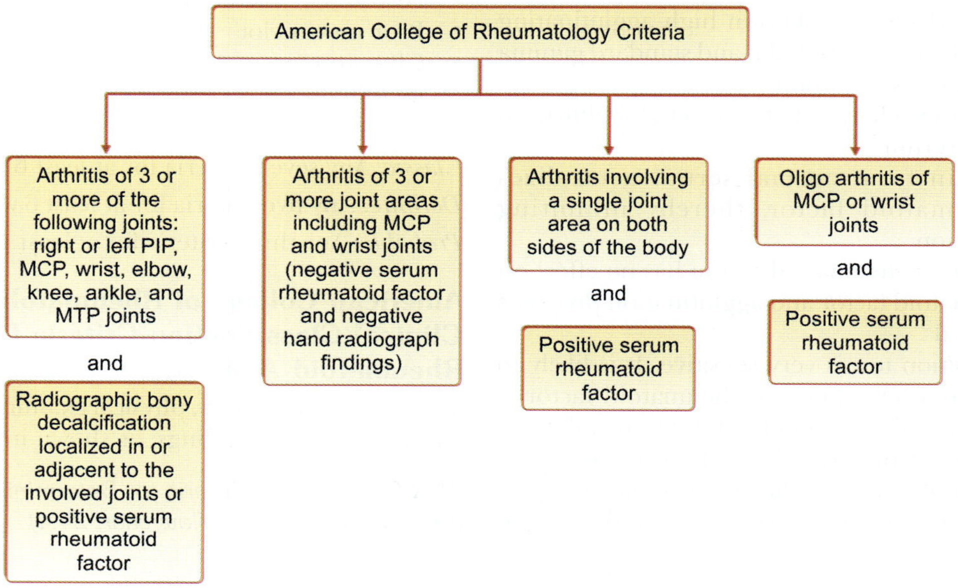

Flow chart 24.5: Treatment goals in RA pyramid of the rapeutic options in rheumatoid arthritis

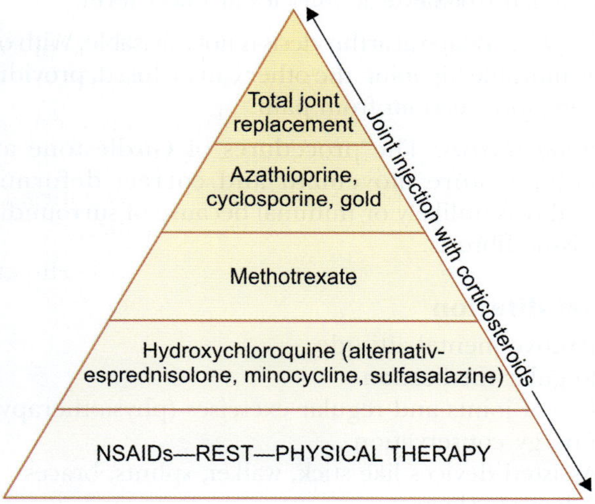

Hormones: Combination of estrogen and androgen are given for their anabolic effect, to bone structure.

Dilute HCl: It is given to combat achlorhydria that leads to anemia.

Splinting: Inflammed joint is immobilized in plaster splint, to relieve pain and reduce inflammation and the position of function is desirable in event that ankylosis occurs.

Position of rest for inflammed hip

- 5° of flexion, 5° of abduction and neutral rotation.
- *Cortisone:* 17-hydroxy-11-dehydrocorticosterone

Synthetic steroids: Prednisone, prednisolone, triamcinolone and dexamethasone.

ACTH: Stimulates adrenal cortex to produce more of compound E and F. It is injected in daily dose of 100 mg.

Salicylates: These are anti-inflammatory, analgesic and antipyretic compounds. These are the drugs of choice for RA. Most common and most effective is acetyl salicyclic acid (aspirin, ASA). Around 10 to 15 gm, 300 mg tablets in four divided doses are given.

NSAIDs

a. *Sulindac:* 400 mg/day
b. *Naproxen:* 250 to 500 mg BD orally
c. *Tolmetin:* 1200 mg/day in three divided doses
d. *Ibuprofen:* 300 mg, 400 mg, 600 mg, 3 to 4 times/day half hour before or 2 to 3 hours after meals
e. *Piroxicam:* 20 mg/day orally
f. *Indomethacin:* 25 mg doses QID
g. *Phenylbutazone:* 300 to 600 mg/day in divided doses, if there is no response for one week, then abandon the drug and if there is adequate response then reduce the dose to less than 400 mg/day.
h. *Gold salts:* Gold sodium thiomalate (myochrysine)
   - *Procedure:* It is given deep intramuscular
   - *Dosage:* First injection of 10 mg dose is given for the first week followed by 25 mg dose, second weeks followed by 50 mg dose and third weeks. 50 mg dose is repeated weekly for 4 to 5 months, until total of 1 g of dose is given. With each dose 10 ml of 10 percent calcium is given, to decrease the possibility of reaction. Another course, given after 6 to 12 months or after remission
   - Change of symptoms is expected after 6 to 15 weeks. If there is no improvement after 5 months, then abandon the drug
   - Sensitivity test to be done. Toxic reactions that can occur are:
     - Pruritis
     - Stomatitis
     - Diarrhea
     - Microscopic hematuria
     - Albuminuria
     - Granulocytopenia
     - Thrombocytopenia
     - Every 2 weeks a complete blood count and platelet count is done
     - The reduction of hemoglobin, leucocytes, platelets and tendency to eosinophilia are danger signals
     - In case of toxic reactions British-Anti-Lewisite (BAL), dimercaprol is given
   - *Contraindications:* Hepatic or renal damage and blood dyscrasias.
i. *Combined cortisone and gold therapy:* Has a little advantage over gold therapy alone.
j. *Manipulation:* Gentle prolonged traction and gradual spontaneous correction by active motion.
k. *X-ray treatment:* More useful in RA of spine.
l. *Relief of muscle spasm:* Drugs most commonly used for this are:
   - Myanesin
   - Carisoprodol
   - Diazepam
m. *Aspiration:* It is done, when there is recurrent effusion that causes pain.
n. *Hydrocortisone injections*
   - When only one or two large joints involved.
   - Compound injected intra-articularly.
   - Reduces inflammation and eliminates pain.
   - Constitutional effects are avoided.
   - *Dose:* 1ml of suspension.
o. *Intra-articular irradiation:*
   Radioactive colloidal gold injected into the joint.
p. *Special drugs:*
   - *Antimalarial compounds:*
     - Chloroquine
     - Hydroxychloroquine

- *Immunosuppresive agents*
  - Azathioprine
  - Penicillamine
  - Cyclophosphamide
- *Protozoacides*
  - Clotrimazole
  - Copper sulfate

Surgical Treatment

- Hip is generally involved at a late stage of severe generalized disease
- Multiple joint involvement of both lower extremities is the rule
- Flexion contractures of hips and knees are common
- The objectives are relief of pain, provision of increased motion and maintainence of stability.

Surgical options
- Synovectomy
- Total hip replacement
- Arthroplasty of Smith Peterson
- Arthrodesis
- Pseudoarthrosis

Synovectomy: Role of synovectomy is to remove large bulk of diseased tissue, so that drugs can have a effect on the joint.

Total hip replacement: Complete prosthetic replacement, using both acetabular and femoral components is the ideal procedure. Procedure is generally reserved for adult at middle age and beyond. Done preferably before the advanced destructive stage of disease.

Arthroplasty of Smith Peterson: A vitallium mold (65% cobalt, 30% chromium and 5% molybdenum) is interposed, the articular surfaces become lined with smooth glistening fibrocartilage and the underlining bone becomes more firm.

Reankylosis is less likely than when other interposing material, such as fascia lata is used. Recurrence of stiffness and deformity is greater in rheumatoid arthritis than in degenerative, but some useful motion is gained, permitting ambulation with canes and sitting on high chairs. Rarely the femoral head and neck within the cup may undergo resorption, subluxation or dislocation.

Technical principals for arthroplasty: Enlarge the acetabulum, consistent with stability of mold and neck. Excise the entire capsule and diseased synovial tissue. Replace the blood lost. Coagulate raw bone surfaces after reshaping, to prevent new bone formation. Adapt modifications to rheumatoid arthritis, to gain more mobility inspite of marked ankylosis.

a. *Whiteman reconstruction:* Remove head, reshape neck, displace greater trochanter downward, before interposing cup.

b. *Colonna:* Remove head and neck, reshape trochanter, which forms new articulating surface, detach and reattach trochanteric muscles at lower level.

Arthrodesis: Bilateral arthrodesis is not advisable. With one freely movable hip joint, the other can be fused, providing stability and freedom from pain.

Pseudoarthrosis: The procedures of Girdlestone and Batchlor restore movement and correct deformity. Instability is unlikely or minimal because of surrounding soft tissue fibrosis.

Rehabilitation

- Positive mental attitude
- Regular medication
- Use of joints and regular exercises (physiotherapy)
- Energy conservation
- Assisted devices like stick, walker, splints, braces
- Adequate sleep
- *Massage:* Myofacial and centrifugal
- Relaxation techniques
- Modification in daily activities, like use of western toilets, bath aids, railings, longe handle broomsticks and mop to clean the floors.

LEGG-CALVE-PERTHES DISEASE

Introduction

Legg-Calve-Perthes disease (also known as perthes, osteochondritis deformans juvenilis and coxa plana) is a self limiting, affection of the hip occurring in children characterized by aseptic necrosis of the whole or part of the femoral head produced by interruption of its blood supply, followed by subchondral fracture, revascularization and repair of dead bone.

History

1909 Waldenstrom, was the first to describe the condition and mistakenly ascribed it as tuberculosis of hip.

1910 Legg and Calve and Perthes, describe the condition independently.

1913 Perthes, gave a precise description of the disease and recognized its ischemic nature.

1922 Waldenstrom, correctly interpreted and described the stages of the disease.

Incidence

- Disorder of the hip in young children
- Usually ages 4 to 8 years
- As early as 2 years, as late as teens
- Boys:girls ratio is 4 to 5:1

- Bilateral 10 to 12 percent
- No evidence of inheritance
- It is rare in blacks, Indians and Polynesians, with higher incidence seen in whites and eskimos.

Predisposing Factors

- *Age:* Predominately affected are children between the ages of 3 and 12 with peak at 6 years of age
- *Sex:* Male have more predilection with ratio of 4:1
- Either hip may be affected. Bilateral cases are rare with about 15 percent of incidence
- *Genetic factor:* The disease is found to be familial in 6 percent—4 percent of cases. It occurred more often in later born children particularly the third to sixth child
- A higher than normal incidence of minor congenital genitourinary anomalies, such as renal abnormalities, inguinal hernia or undescended testicles is seen in children with perthes disease
- *Abnormal growth and development:* The bone age of children with perthes disease is typically lower than their chronological age by 1 to 3 years. The affected child are smaller in all dimensions (except head circumference), with disproportionately smaller distal segment of the extremities
- *Environmental factors:* Although, the effect of environment on the incidence of the disorder is unclear, a high percentage of involved children come from low socioeconomic groups, whether this reflect dieatry or environmental influence or combination thereof is certain
- *Regional factor:* The disease occurs predominately in asians, eskimos and whites, have a higher incidence of the disease, whereas Australians, American, Indians and blacks have lower incidence.

Etiology

- Perthes disease is produced by impairment of the blood supply to the femoral head
- Multiple episodes of infarction are required to produce the pathological defect of perthes disease
- The exact cause of interruption of blood supply remains obscure
- Numerous theories/hypothesis speculating on the pathogenesis of the disease have been proposed.

Trueta hypothesis: This hypothesis is based on the variation of vascular pattern of femoral capital epiphysis with advancing growth. After 8 years, the foveolar arteries of the ligamentum teres contribute blood supply to femoral head and with lateral epiphyseal again provide double source of blood and the incidence of disease begins to decline at this age. Thus, trueta postulated that the solitary blood supply between the age 4 to 8 years, make this group vulnerable to ischemic necrosis.

Caffeys hypothesis: According to caffey, the radiological features of perthes are more consistent with an avascular necrosis, resulting from intraepiphyseal compression of blood supply to ossification center. The increased density of the necrotic bone is at first, a result of compression of femoral head by the acetabular roof and later by newly formed bone superimpozed on yet unresorbed old necrotic bone.

Other theories: Increased intra-articular pressure and tampanode compression of the retinacular vessels around the femoral neck and a casual relationship between acute transient synovitis and perthes have been postulated. Kleinman and Black reported increased blood viscosity in perthes patients. The venous drainage have been disturbed in perthes, due to increased intravenous pressure. Patient with perthes disease have low levels of somatomedin C.

Pathogenesis

Loss of blood supply produces AVN of the epiphyseal ossification center, followed by resorption of dead bone and replacement with newly formed immature bone. The process is described in stages.

Incipient or synovitis stage (Fig. 24.202)

- Last 1 to 3 weeks
- Synovium is swollen, hyperemic and edematous.
- Joint fluid is increased and absence of inflammatory cells.

Stage of AVN (Fig. 24.203)

- AVN involves portion of ossific nucleus situated anteriorly
- Amorphous debries fills the marrow spaces
- Trabeculaes are crushed into minute fragments and compressed into a compact bone accounting for increased density on radiograph

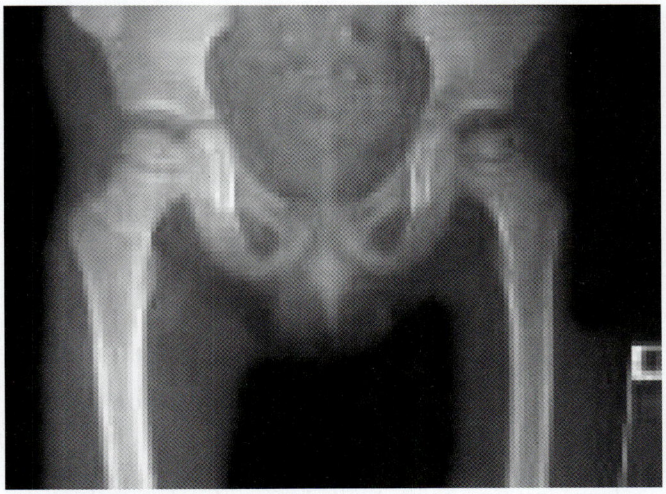

Fig. 24.202: Incipient or synovitis stage

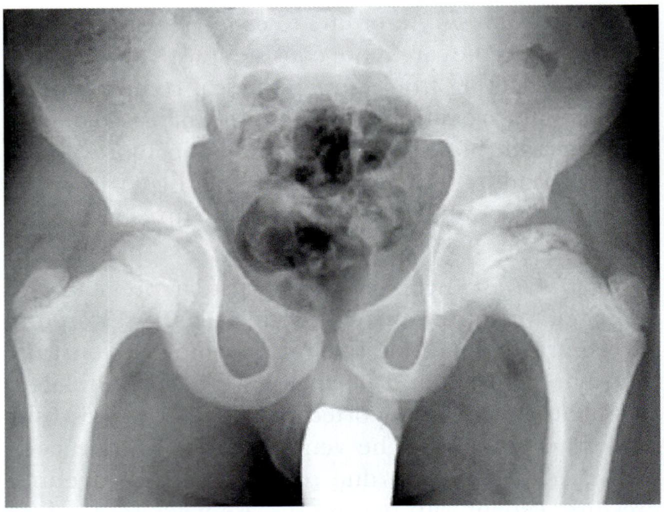

Fig. 24.203: Stage of AVN

- The increased opacity is contrasted
- Marked demineralization of adjacent metaphysic, as a result of hypervascularity, constitutes preparation for invasion of vascular connective tissue towards necrotic bone
- The cartilage is viable, nutrition is derived from synovial fluid
- Stage last 6 months to one year.

Stage of Fragmentation or Regeneration

- Necrotic bone resorbed and replaced by viable bone
- Radiographic fragmented appearance results many tonge-like roads of vessels, appear to come from ligamentum teres periosteum and metaphysis
- Subchondral fractures of necrotic bone, multiple minute trabecular fragments compressed together
- Cartilage remains normal
- The countor of the newly formed soft bone develops in response to the external forces
- Stage extents over 2 to 3 years.

Healed or Residual Stage

- Formation of normal bone, alongside replacing slowly resorbing bone
- Newly formed bone is immature, formed of slender trabeculae and easily compressed together with necrotic fragments
- The compression is limited to anterior portion of head, creating a cup shaped defect seen on frog leg view
- Defect appears cystic
- The ossific nucleus assumes a mushroom shaped countor
- *Appearance of greater trochanter:* It becomes strikingly large in some cases. Since longitudinal growth of the femoral neck may cease completely at 12 to 14 years of age, whereas growth of the greater trochanter continues until 17 to 18 years, a discrepancy in growth and the greater trochanter may result. The elevation impairs the power of pelvitrochanteric abductor muscles, manifested by positive Trendelenburg sign, as shown in Figure 24.204.

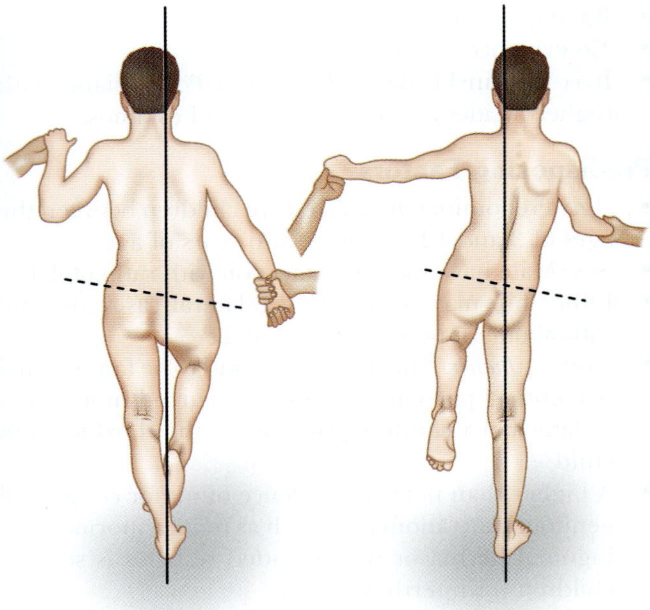

Fig. 24.204: Trendelenburg sign

Clinical Features

Symptoms

- Most children present with mild and intermittent pain in the thigh or a limb or both
- The onset of pain may be acute or insidious
- The classical presentation is described as a "painles limb" the child limps, but does not complain of discomfort
- Pain is aggravated by movement of hip and relieved by rest
- History of trauma usually a mild is present.

Examination

- Antalgic gait
- Proximal thigh atrophy
- Muscle spasm, secondary to irritable hip
- Limitation of abduction and internal rotation
- FFD is present
- Axis deviation is present due to central collapse
- Differential rotation
- Trendelenburg test positive with free abduction and adduction range.

Imaging

- AP pelvis
- Frog leg lateral
- Ultrasonography
- Bone scan
- Arthrography
- MRI role is undefined

Radiographic Studies (Fig. 24.205)

- Increased head socket distance (Waldenstrom's sign)
- Bulging of the joint capsule
- Rarefaction or rounding of the lateral margin of metaphysis (Gage' sign)
- A strip, shaped subcortical area ventrolaterally in the epiphysis
- Rarefaction in the lateral outline of the epiphysis close to the epiphyseal plate
- Band shaped osteoporosis in the metaphysis close to epiphyseal plate
- Translucent area in the medial metaphyseal zone
- Changes in roof on the acetabulum,
- The capital epiphysis smaller than in the unaffected hip but shape and structure of the epiphysis normal

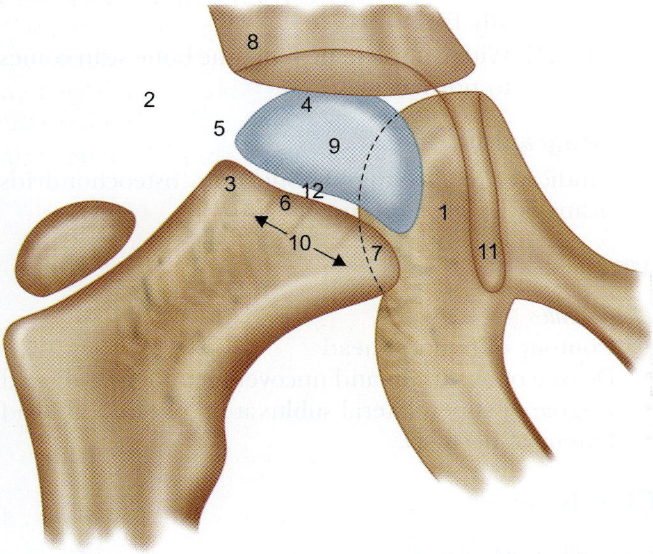

Fig. 24.205: 1. Increased head socket distance (Waldenstrom's sign); 2. Bulging of the joint capsule; 3. Rarefaction or rounding of the lateral margin of metaphysis (Gage' sign); 4. A strip, shaped subcortical area ventrolaterally in the epiphysis; 5. Rarefaction in the lateral outline of the epiphysis close to the epiphyseal plate; 6. Band shaped osteoporosis in the metaphysis close to epiphyseal plate; 7. Translucent area in the medial metaphyseal zone; 8. Changes in roof on the acetabulum; 9. The capital epiphysis smaller than in the unaffected hip but shape and structure of the epiphysis normal; 10. Enlargement of neck of femur; 11. The tear shaped phenomenon, widening of Kohler's tear-shaped figure; 12. Thickening of epiphyseal plate

- Enlargement of neck of femur
- The tear shaped phenomenon, widening of Kohler's tear-shaped figure
- Thickening of epiphyseal plate.

Radiographic Stages

Four Waldenstrom stages have identified:

- Initial stage
- Fragmentation stage
- Reossification stage
- Healed stage

Initial Stage (Figs 24.206A and B)

Early radiographic signs are:

- Failure of femoral ossification to grow
- Widening of medial joint space
- "Crescent sign"
- Irregular physeal plate
- Blurry/radiolucent metaphysis

Fragmentation Stage (Figs 24.207A and B)

- Bony epiphysis begins to fragment
- Areas of increased lucency and density
- Evidence of repair aspects of disease

Reossification Stage (Figs 24.208A and B)

- Normal bone density returns
- Alterations in shape of femoral head and neck evident

Healed Stage

- Left with residual deformity from disease and repair process
- Differs from AVN following fracture or dislocation.

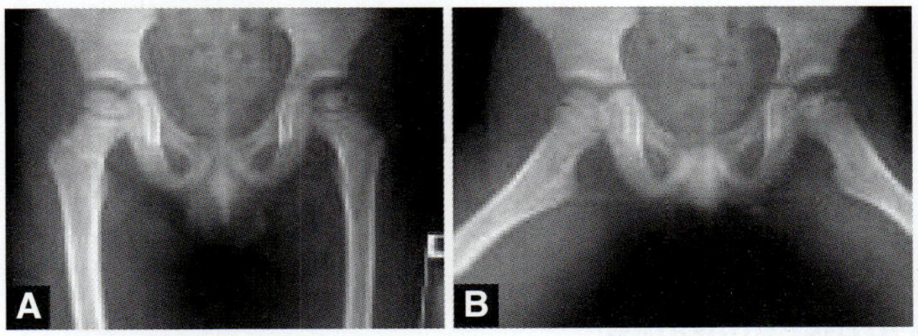

Figs 24.206A and B: Initial stage or early radiographic signs

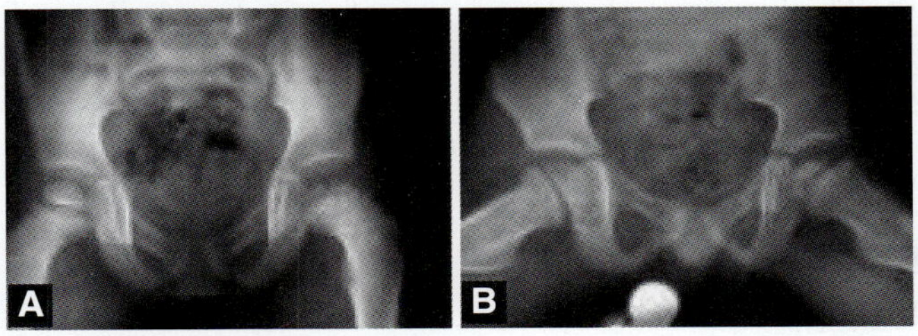

Figs 24.207A and B: Fragmentation stage

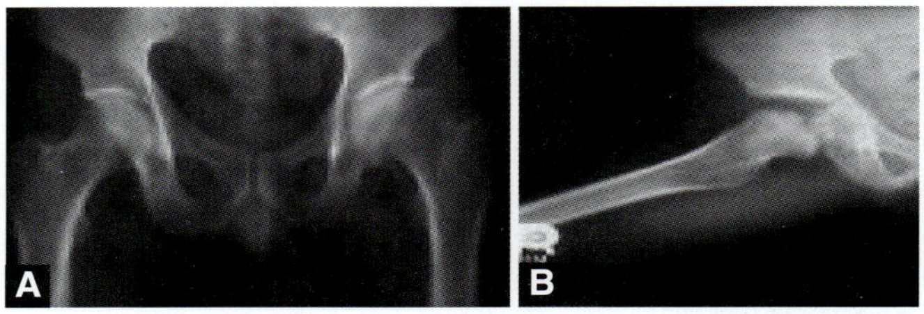

Figs 24.208A and B: Radiographical findings in reossification stage of RA

- "Head at risk sign"
  - A transradiant "V" on the lateral side of epiphysis, formed by small osteoporotic segment, which is seen on the anteroposterior X-ray
  - Calcification lateral to epiphysis
  - Lateral subluxation of the femoral head, measured as an increase in the width of the inferomedial joint space
  - A horizontal epiphyseal line seen in AP view
  - Diffuse metaphyseal changes.
- Extensive involvement of EOC
- Child over 6 years of age
- Early closure of the epiphyseal plate
- Stage of disease advanced, when first seen
- Female patient invariably has group 3 or 4
- When any two of the first five signs listed above are found, a head at risk is said to exist. Catteralls head at risk signs (poor prognosis)
  - *Clinically*
    a. Progressive loss of movement
    b. Adduction contracture
    c. Heavy child
  - *Radiological*
    a. Lateral subluxation of head (head partially uncovered) most important
    b. Whole of head involved
    c. Calcification lateral to epiphysis
    d. Metaphyseal cysts
    e. Gage sign
    f. Horizontal physis

Ultrasonography

- Effusion of hip (which when persistent should make one suspicion of Perthes)
- Thickening and enlargement of articular cartilage of the epiphysis.
- Lateral and anterior uncoverage of head and flattening of femoral head.
- Irregularity and deformation of bony epiphysis.

Bone Scan

During the course of Perthes disease bone scan shows following stages:

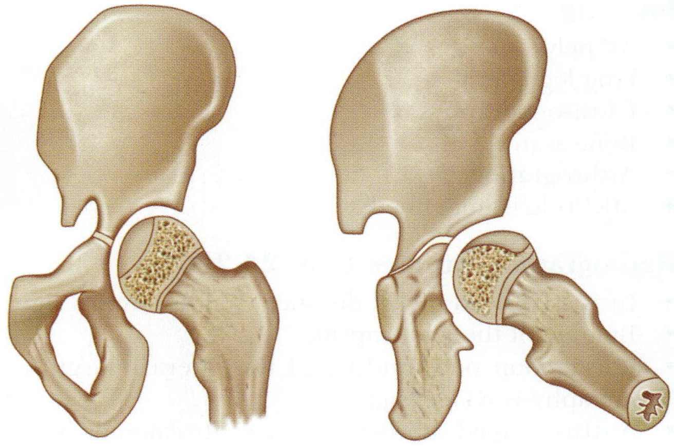

Fig. 24.209: Stage I of Catteralls classification

Stage I: The whole ossific nucleus appears avascular.

Stage II: When revascularization takes place by recanalization, a lateral column is seen on the bone scan, this is a good prognostic sign.

Stage III: The anterolateral part of epiphysis gradually fills.

Stage IV: With complete healing, the bone scan comes to normal.

Arthrography

It is indicated to in hinged abduction, osteochondritis dessicans or a torn labrum.

MRI

Demostrates

- Contour of femoral head
- Degree of extrusion and uncoverage of femoral head
- Degree of superolateral subluxation of femoral head
- Extent of necrosis.

Classification

Catteralls Classification

Stage I: Anteromedial portion head involved and no collapse, metaphyseal changes do not occur and the epiphyseal plate is not involved. Heal without sequeale. This is shown in Figure 24.209.

Stage II: There is a fragmentation of involved segment. The involved segment shows increased density and uninvolved pillars of normal bone prevent significant collapse. Regeneration without much loss of height and the end result is good. Metaphyseal reaction localized, as shown in Figure 24.210.

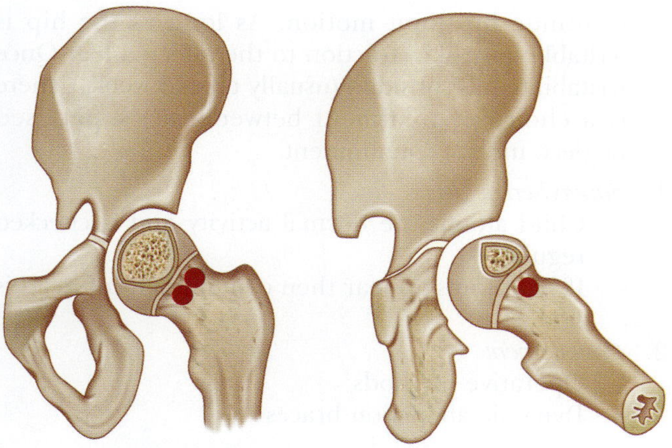

Fig. 24.210: Stage II of Catteralls classification

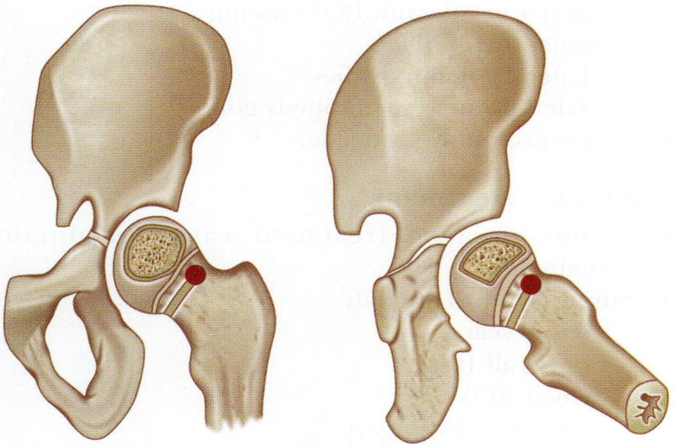

Fig. 24.211: Stage III of Catteralls classification

Stage III: More of the head involved. Shows head within head. The metaphysis is diffusely involved. Broad neck and the epiphyseal plate is unprotected. Results are poor. This is illustrated in Figure 24.211.

Stage IV: Whole is involved and sever collapse occurs early. Metaphyseal changes are extensive. Epiphyseal plate involved, abnormal growth present, like coxa magna, coxa breva, coxa vara and coxa valga, as shown in Figure 24.212.

Herrings Classification (Lateral Pillar Classification)

Group A: There is no collapse of the lateral pillar.

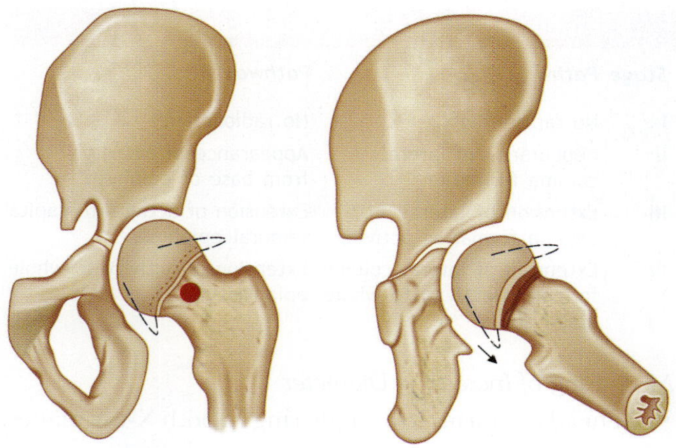

Fig. 24.212: Stage IV of Catteralls classification

Group B: Lateral pillar margins, has more than 50 percent of original height.

Group C: Collapse of lateral pillar more than 50 percent.

Salter-Thompson

Stage A: Lateral portion of femoral epiphysis present, same as catterall 1st and 2nd stages (less than 50% head involved).

Stage B: Lateral portion of femoral capital epiphysis absent, same as catterall 3rd and 4th stages (more than 50% head involved, lateral margin of epiphysis protects from stress).

Ponsetti Classification

- Those with 50 percent less involved head
- Those with more than 50 percent of involved head
- *Deformities at maturity*
  - Coxa magna—enlarged head
  - Hanging rope sign, characteristic of old perthes
  - Coxa brevis, short neck and overgrowth of trochanter, as a result of premature femoral neck physeal growth arrest
  - *Coxa irregularis:* Collapse and lateral extrusion of the femoral head, forming a groove under the lateral edge of acetabulum
  - Osteochondritis dessicans.

Stulberg Classification of the End Result

Class 1: Completely normal

Class 2: Spherical less than 2 mm coxa magna, with short neck

Class 3: Elliptical greater than 2 mm, but not flat.

Class 4: Flat femoral head and acetabulum.

Class 5: Flat femoral head and round acetabulum.

Table 24.16: Conway classification of RA

Stage	Pathway A	Pathway B
I	No radioactivity	No radioactivity
II	Appearance of lateral column formation	Appearance of activity from base of epiphysis
III	Extension of lateral column formation activity	Extension of activity to capital femoral epiphysis
IV	Extension of lateral column formation activity to whole epiphysis	Extension of activity to whole epiphysis

Mose-Ring of Increasing Diameter

- If head conforms to a single ring in both X-ray planes, good prognosis.
- If head varies from perfect circle by no more than 2 mm, fair result.
- If head varies by more than 2 mm in any plane, poor result.

Conway Classification (Table 24.16)

It is based on nuclear scanning (Scintigraphy). This is illustrated in Figure 24.213.

Treatment

Principles of treatment:

- Preserve normal femoral acetabular congruity
- Containment of head
- Eliminate or reduce load bearing
- Encourage weight bearing in abduction

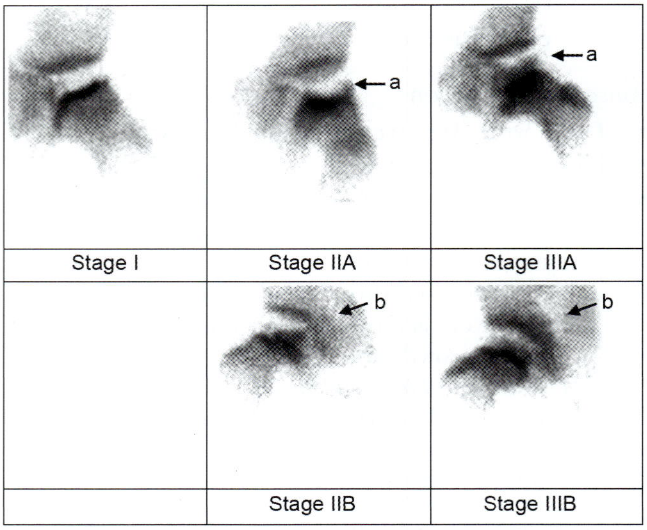

Fig. 24.213: Scintigraphic stages of Conway classification of LCP. Stage I (total avascularity of proximal femoral epiphysis) is observed at initial stage of disease. Appearance of lateral column formation, a. characterizes a pathway (stages IIA and IIIA). In b pathway, as neovascularization progresses, extension of activity from metaphysis is observed (stages IIB and IIIB), without lateral column formation b

- Continue hip joint motion. As long as the hip is irritable, give skin traction to the affected leg. Once irritability has subsided (usually takes 3 weeks), there is a choice of treatment between: (1) supervised neglect and (2) containment.

1. *Supervised neglect*
   - Child attains the normal activity and is checked regularly.
   - If symptoms appear then containment of head is done.
2. *Containment*
   - Operative methods
   - Dynamic abduction braces

Conservative treatment

- Broomstick plaster or scottish rite abduction brace (Figs 24.214)
- Newington childrens ambulatory brace (Fig. 24.215)

Nonoperative Treatment

- *Check serial radiographs*
  Q3 and 4 mostly with ROM testing
- *Continue bracing until*
  - Lateral column ossifies
  - Sclerotic areas in epiphysis gone
- Cast/brace uninvolved side.

Operative Treatment

- If nonoperative treatment cannot maintain containment
- Surgically ideal patient:
  - 6 to 9 years
  - Catterall II-III
  - Good ROM
  - <12 months surgery
  - In collapsing phase

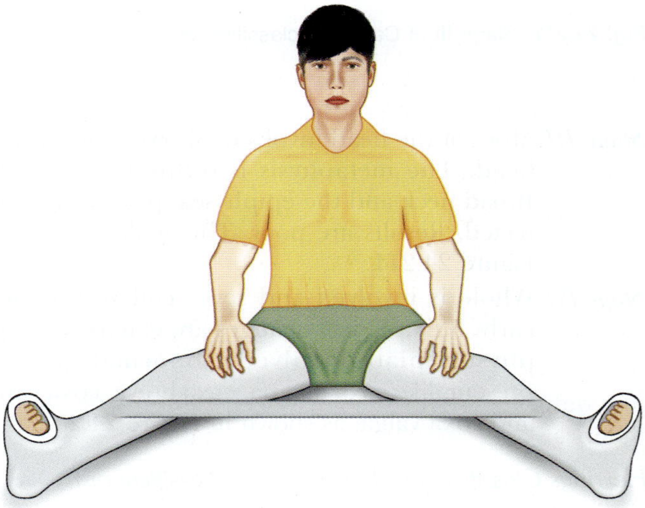

Fig. 24.214: Broomstick plaster or scottish rite abduction brace

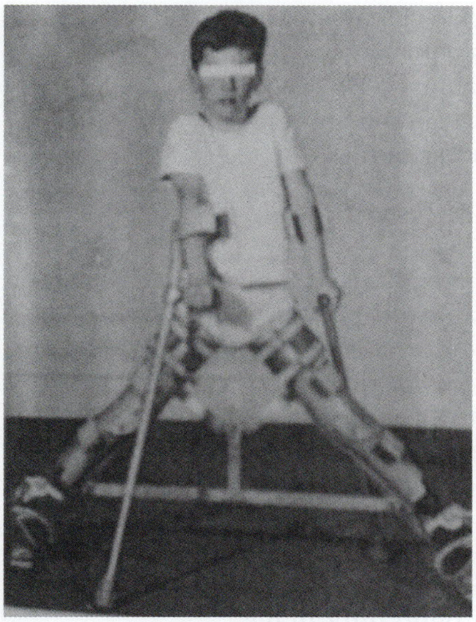

Fig. 24.215: Newingtons children's ambulatory brace

Benjamin Joseph's criteria for containment surgery in late onset perthes disease (in children of age 7 to 12 years)

Stage I: Containment surgery indicated
Stage II: Containment surgery indicated
Stage III: Containment surgery not indicated
Stage IV: Containment surgery not indicated

The concept of containment with weight-bearing: Although, others had previously recommended immobilization of the hip in wide abduction combined with complete bedrest, Petrie and Bitenc were the first to propose the position of wide abduction for the purpose of diminishing abduction forces on the femoral head, while permitting full weight-bearing. The efficacy of the concept of containment of the femoral head was demonstrated in experimental investigation of avascular necrosis of the femoral head in young pigs by Salter et al. Subsequently, Lloyd-Roberts et al. concluded that methods of early treatment, either surgical or non-surgical that do not include the concept of containment, seem to be of little value in Legg-Perthes disease.

Basic premises concerning treatment: Children, who acquire Legg-Perthes disease are not systemically ill. They have only a local disease. From humanitarian point of view, treatment should interfere, as little as possible with the child's normal psychological and physical development. Legg-Perthes disease is a self-healing process. Therefore, the only justification for treatment is the prevention of femoral head deformity and secondary degenerative arthritis. The decision concerning the need for the treatment of a given child, should be based on a knowledge of the prognosis for that particular child. Lloyd-Roberts et al. made an important contribution, in emphasizing that no children with Group-I involvement and relatively few with Group-II involvement, require any treatment whatsoever. All forms of the treatment should be based on a sound understanding of the underlying pathogenesis of the disease.

Basic principles of all forms of treatment: Obtain and maintain a full or almost full range of motion of the hip joint. Obtain and maintain containment of the femoral head in the position of weight-bearing, by preventing or correcting subluxation of the hip. Provided these two principles have been achieved, then and only then encourage full weight-bearing, on the involved hip (a turnabout from the principle of nonweight-bearing that prevailed during the first five decades, following the original description of the disease).

Classification of currently acceptable forms of management

- Observation only
- Intermittent symptomatic treatment (temporary), brief periods of traction, slings and springs or crutches (with or without a Snyder sling or Salter stirrup)
- Definitive early treatment (to prevent deformity)
  A. Non-surgical
    a. Abduction casts (Petrie and Bitenc)
    b. Abduction orthoses (Toronto, Newington, New Orleans, Atlanta, and others)
  B. Surgical
    – Femoral osteotomy
      a. Varus (Soeur and de Racker)
      b. Rotation (Axer)
      c. Combined varus and rotation (Somerville, Lloyd-Roberts et al. and Catterall)
    – Innominate osteotomy (Salter et al.) combined with adductor tenotomy and illopsoas release.
- Late surgical treatment (to correct existing deformity)
  A. Muscle release and arthrotomy, followed by abduction casts
  B. Partial excision of the femoral head
    i. Peripheral cheilectomy (Garceau et al.)
    ii. Central (loose fragment of osteochondritis dissecans)
  C. Abduction (valgus) osteotomy of the femur (Salter et al. and Catterall)
  D. Distal and lateral transfer of the greater trochanter
- Late surgical treatment (for secondary degenerative arthritis)
  A. Femoral osteotomy
  B. Arthrodesis
  C. Arthroplasties including prosthetic joint replacement.

Definitive early surgical treatment (to prevent deformity)

Indications

- Involvement of more than half of the femoral head (Catterall groups III and IV or Salter group B)
- Age at onset for more than 6 years (possibly more than 5 years in girls)
- Loss of containment of femoral head-that is, subluxation of femoral head in the position of weight-bearing.

Prerequisites

- A full or almost full range of motion at hip joint (which may necessitate traction or slings and springs to overcome irritability of the hip or even surgical release of the adductor muscles, to overcome contractures, followed by abductor casts for a few weeks or longer)
- A round or almost round femoral head and hence, reasonable congruity of the hip joint in abduction (which may have to be established by an arthrogram, if there has been significant resorption of the femoral head).

Contraindications

- Lack of a good indication (because the child does not need surgical treatment)
- Lack of the prerequisites (because the child cannot be helped by such surgical treatment).

Surgical Options

- Pelvic osteotomies, like Salter, Chiari and Shelf.
- Varus derotation osteotomy
- Late stages, valgus extension osteotomy and cheilectomy
- Arthodesis should be preserved for patient, with severe deformity and done after skeletal maturity.

Prognosis

- Sixty percent of children do well without treatment
- Age is key prognostic factor:
  - <6 years, shows good outcome regardless of treatment
  - Six to eight years, not always good results, with just containment
  - >9 years, containment option is questionable, poorer prognosis and significant residual defect
- Flat femoral head incongruent with acetabulum, have worst prognosis
- Do not treat in reossification stage (>15 months).

Differential Diagnosis

- Important to rule out infectious etiology (septic arthritis and toxic synovitis)
- *Others*
  - Chondrolysis
  - Neoplasm
  - Juvenile rheumatoid arthritis
  - Sickle cell anemia
  - Osteomyelitis
  - Traumatic AVN
  - Lymphoma
  - Medication

Late Effects or Sequelae of Legg-Calves-Perthes

- Coxa magna
- Coxa irregularis, irregular head formation
- Physeal arrest patterns
- Osteochondritis dessicans
- Coxa breva, due to relative overgrowth of greater trochanter and short femoral head
- Hinged abduction of the hip
- Osteoarthritis

TUMORS AROUND HIP

Tumors around hip can be:

- Benign
- Malignant

Benign Tumors around Hip

I. Bone forming tumors
  - Osteoid osteoma
  - Osteoblastoma

II. Cartilaginous tumors
  - Osteochondroma
  - Chondroma (enchondroma and periosteal chondroma)
  - Multiple enchondromatosis (Ollier disease)

III. Fibrous lesions
  - Fibrous cortical defect
  - Benign fibrous histiocytoma
  - Fibrous dysplasia
  - Desmoplastic fibroma
  - Giant cell reaction (giant cell reparative granuloma)

IV. Cystic lesions
  - Unicameral cyst
  - Aneurysmal bone cyst

V. Miscellaneous
  - Neural tumors
  - Osteochondromatosis
  - Synovioma
  - Pigmented villonodular synovitis

Malignant Tumors around Hip

- Chondrosarcomas
- Osteosarcomas
- Chordomas
- Metastatic tumors
- Multiple myeloma
- Lymphoma

Table 24.17: Enneking's system of staging

I-A	G1, T1, M0	Low grade, intracompartmental, no metastasis
I-B	G1, T2, M0	Low grade, extracompartmental, no metastasis
II-A	G2, T1, M0	High grade, intracompartmental, no metastasis
II-B	G2, T2, M0	High grade, extracompartmental, no metastasis
III-A	G1 or G2, T1, M1	Any grade, intracompartmental, metastasis
III-B	G1 or G2, T2, M1	Any grade, extracompartmental, metastasis

Tumors Classification

WHO Classification

I. Lichtenstein classification of primary bone tumors
II. Classification of bone tumors (Briston university)
III. ABC classification by Charles Price
IV. Ennekings system of staging

Enneking's System of Staging (Table 24.17)

1. Based on degree of anaplasia, it is divided into two types
   a. G1–low grade
   b. G2–high grade
2. Based on the tumor location
   - Intracompartmental (T1)
   - Extracompartmental (T2)
3. Based on metastasis
   - Absent (m0)
   - Present (m1)

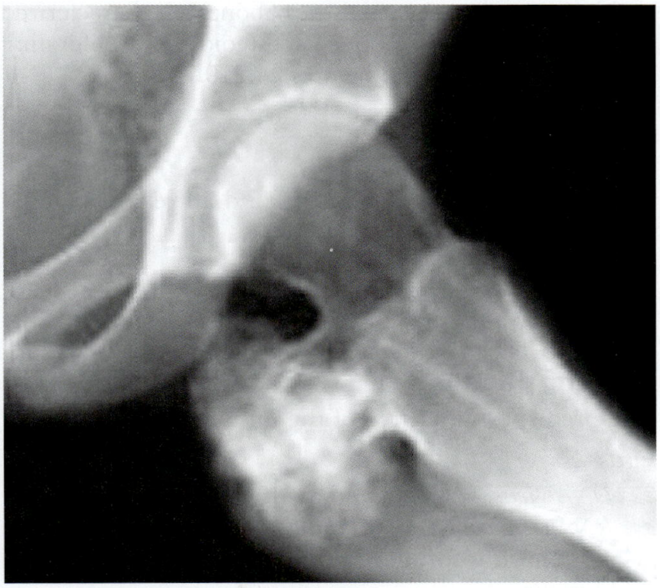

Fig. 24.216: Osteochondroma of hip

Commonly found tumors around hip are

- Osteochondroma
- Osteosarcoma
- Chondrosarcoma
- Multiple enchondromatosis (Ollier's disease)
- Aneurysmal bone cyst
- Unicameral bone cyst
- Fibrous dysplasia
- Chondroma

Osteochondroma

It is most common benign bone tumor. It accounts for 20 to 50 percent of benign bone tumors and 10 to 15 percent of all bone tumors. Approximately, 15 percent of patients with osteochondromas have multiple lesions. It is an offshoot from the spongy bone tissue covered with a cartilaginous cap, as shown in Figure 24.216.

Age: Common during the growth period.

Sex: Male preponderance (male/female ratio 1.5:1).

Area: Sites of tendinous attachments and metaphysis of femur around hip.

Theory of Histogenesis

Exact cause is not known. Cambium layer of periosteum retains throughout life its ability to form cartilage and bone, due to perverted activity of periosteum that it reverts to its role as "perichodrium". At point of tendinous insertion, there are focal accumulation of embryonic connective tissue.

Clinical Features

Symptoms: Usually symptomless. Patient may complain of pain, swelling, bursitis, malignant change, fracture, neuropathies, etc. may developed.

Signs

- Firm non-tender swelling fixed to bone around the joints
- An inflammed bursa causes tenderness and local warmth
- Decreased joint movements and tumor causing mechanical block.

Roentgenographic Findings (Figs 24.217 and 24.218)

Osteochondromas are of two types:
1. Stalked
2. Broad based or sessile

Sessile lesions cover a wide area and as a result cause metaphyseal widening or a "trumpet shaped deformity" on X-ray.

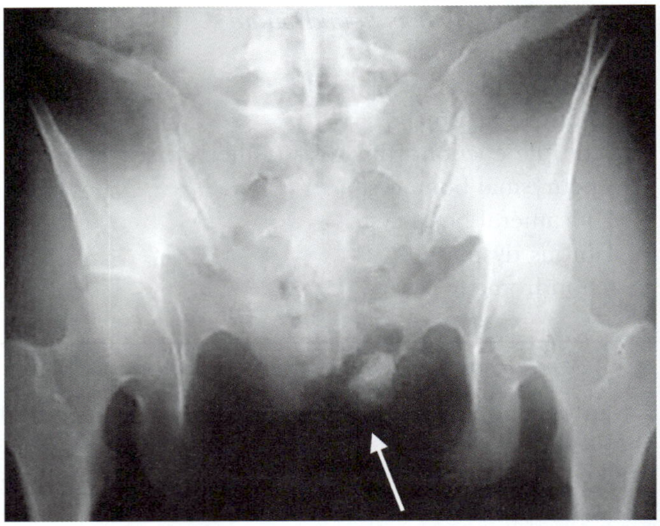

Fig. 24.217: X-ray PBH-AP showing osteochondroma of pelvis. Arrows showing osteosarcoma of pelvis

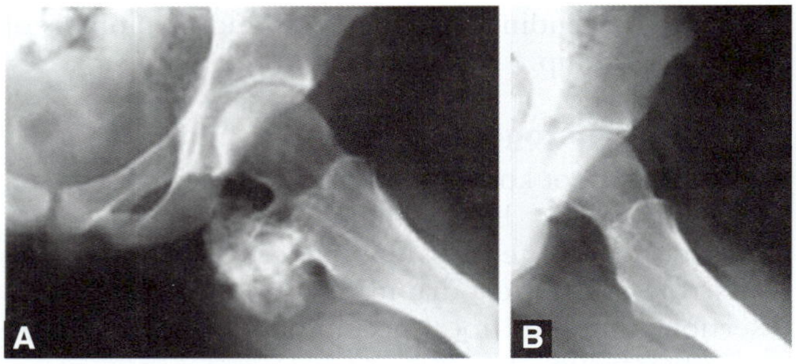

Figs 24.218A and B: Osteochondroma of hip: Sessile lesions cover a wide area and as a result cause metaphyseal widening or a "trumpet shaped deformity"—(A) Preoperative roentgenogram; (B) After excision of lesion

Treatment

Usually it requires no treatment. Surgical treatment excision should consist of an en bloc resection is indicated when:

- Joint interference
- Painful bursitis
- Fracture of the bony stalk
- Malignant change
- Pressure on the neighboring vessels/nerves

Prognosis: The risk of malignant transformation to chondrosarcoma in hereditary multiple osteochondromatosis is unknown, but may be 25 to 30 percent compared to approximately 1 percent for a solitary osteochondromas.

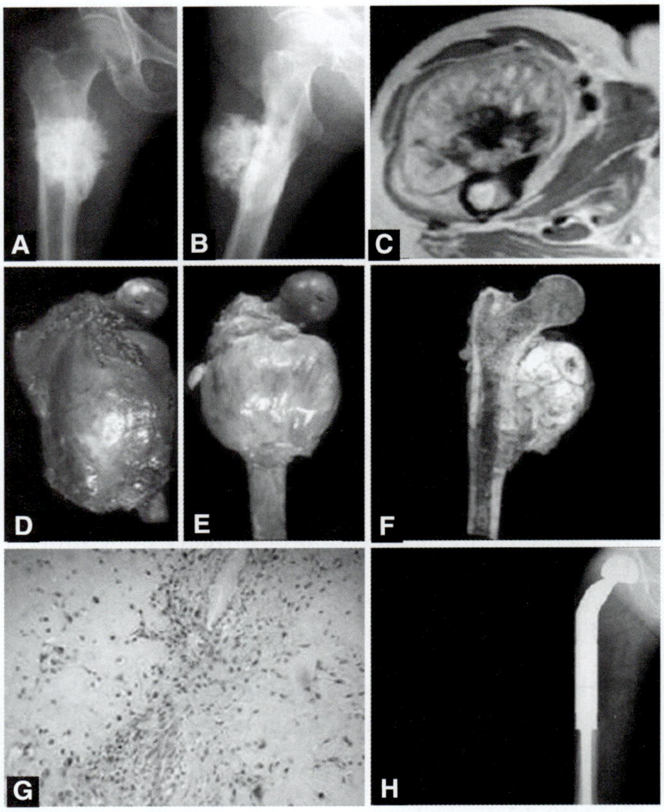

Figs 24.219A to H: (A) to (F) Different stages of osteosarcoma of hip; (G) Histological findings; (H) Prosthetic replacement of the hip

Osteosarcoma

It is a malignant primary bone tumor, arising from multipotent mesenchymal tissue of bone. It is characterized by direct formation of bone or osteoid, by proliferating tumor cells, as shown in Figures 24.219A to H.

Incidence

- Common malignant tumor
- Occurs in young, between 10 and 20 years of age.

Sites (Fig. 24.220)

- Metaphysis of long bones
- Proximal one-third of femur.

Exciting Factors

The predisposing factors of the tumors are:

Virus

- *DNA virus:* Polyoma and SV-40 virus
- *RNA virus:* Harvey and moloney sarcoma virus. These are known to produce tumors in animals and not in humans.

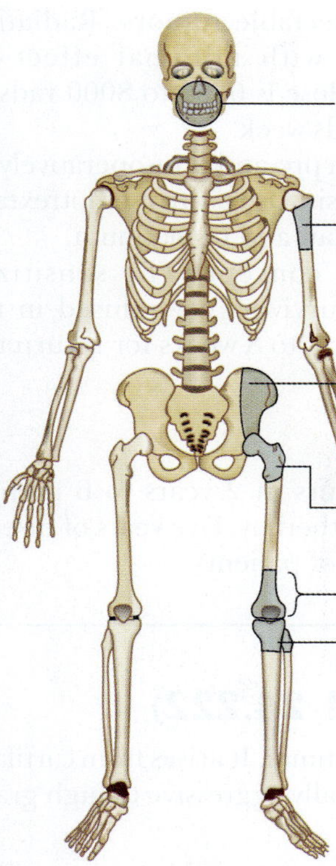

Fig. 24.220: Distribution of osteosarcoma in body

Radiation

A dose of 2000 rads, can set malignancy in the bone.

Chemicals

Beryllium compounds and methylcholanthrene.

Clinical Features

- Pain is the initial and dominating symptom
- Bony swelling appears after some week
- Swelling progressively increases in size.

General Examination

- General health deteriorates with anemia, loss of weight and cachexia
- Patient develops pulmonary symptoms due to secondaries.

On examination

- Swelling is fusiform
- Skin is stretched, shiny and vascular, with prominent veins
- Swelling is warm to touch and show pulsation, if tumor is highly vascular
- It is firm to hard in consistency
- In late stages, tumor fungates.

Classification of Osteosarcoma

Primary osteosarcomas

- Conventional
  - Osteoblastic
  - Chondroblastic
  - Fibroblastic
  - Small cell
  - Telangiectatic
- Surface (juxtacortical) osteosarcoma
  - Parosteal osteosarcoma
  - Periosteal osteosarcoma
  - High grade surface osteosarcoma

Secondary osteosarcoma

- Post irradiation
- Pagets sarcoma
- Solitary/multiple osteochondromatosis
- Bone infarction
- Chronic osteomyelities
- *Miscellaneous:* GCT, fibrous dysplasia, chondroblastoma and osteoblastoma.

Rare osteosarcoma

- Li fraumeni syndrome
- Osteosarcoma of the jaw
- Multicentric osteosarcoma.

Pathology

Grossly: It is a large tumor with areas of distruction gives an appearance of leg of mutton. Consistency ranges from hard to soft. Color of tumor could be white, if fibroblastic; yellowish white, if osteoblastic and bluish, if cartilaginous. At the areas of rapid growth, there are areas of cavitation, necrotic foci and hemorrhages. Sun-ray appearance seen is due to the bone diposition along the vessels. Codmans triangle is the reactive bone formation parallel to the bone.

Histology

- Small spindle cells with hyperchromatic nuclei
- Shape may be round, cuboidal and columnar
- Cells are pleomorphic in nature
- Giant cells are often present
- Matrix may be myxomatous, cartilaginous or osseous.
- Areas of hemorrhages may be present.

Radiological Features

Tumor arises from metaphyseal region of the bone either centrally or from cortex. Mottled area of rarefaction, with areas of osteosclerosis. When it extends beyond the cortex, the periosteum is raised and there is new bone formation in lines at right angle to the cortex this cause sun-ray appearance on X-ray. Codmans triangle is seen at the junction of normal bone and tumor area it is a reactive new bone formation subperiosteally, ghost shadow and CXR may show secondaries in chest.

Treatment

The aim of treatment is to confirm the diagnosis and to evaluate the spread and to execute adequate treatment. Confirmation of diagnosis is done clinically, histologically, radiologically and laboratory findings. Evaluation of the spread of the tumors is done. Lung is common area of metastasis CXR should be done. CT and MRI will detect the extent of tumor and soft tissue involvement. Bone scan will detect skip lesions.

Surgery

- Early and radical ablation is the surgery of choice.
- Limb salvage, if no joint involved
- En block resection of proximal femur
- Reconstruction–bipolar with long stem, combined with allograft
- Amputation remains the mainstay. Level of amputation is upper end femur-hind quarter amputation and hip disarticulation.

Newer Techniques

- Limb salvage, with tumor endoprosthesis.
- Juxta-articular-intraepiphyseal resection and biological reconstruction.
- *Megavoltage radiotherapy:* Radiation is given preoperatively, to decrease the viable cells that get disseminated into bloodstream. It is a useful adjuvant in the treatment of resectable tumors. Radiation destroys tumor cells, with minimal effect on uninvolved parts. Total dose is 6000 to 8000 rads or 230 rads/day or 1000 rads/week.
- *Chemotherapy:* It is given pre-and post-operatively, to control the micrometastasis. Drugs are methotrextate, citrovorum factor, endoxan and cisplatinum.
- *Immunotherapy:* New concept. The sensitized lymphocytes from the survivors are infused in the patient. Follow-up, every 6 to 8 weeks for recurrence and metastasis.

Prognosis

Without therapy, death occurs in 2 years to 6 months and with surgery and chemotherapy. Five years of disease free life, seen in 70 percent of patients.

■ Chondrosarcoma (Figs 24.221 and 24.222)

It is malignant slow growing tumor. It arises from cartilage cell. It ranges from being locally aggressive to high grade malignancy.

Incidence: Second in frequency to osteosarcoma.

Site: Common are proximal femur.

Sex: Males commonly affect then females (male/female ratio 1.5:1).

Location: Long bone from diaphyseal-metaphyseal region.

Age: Twenty to sixty years of age.

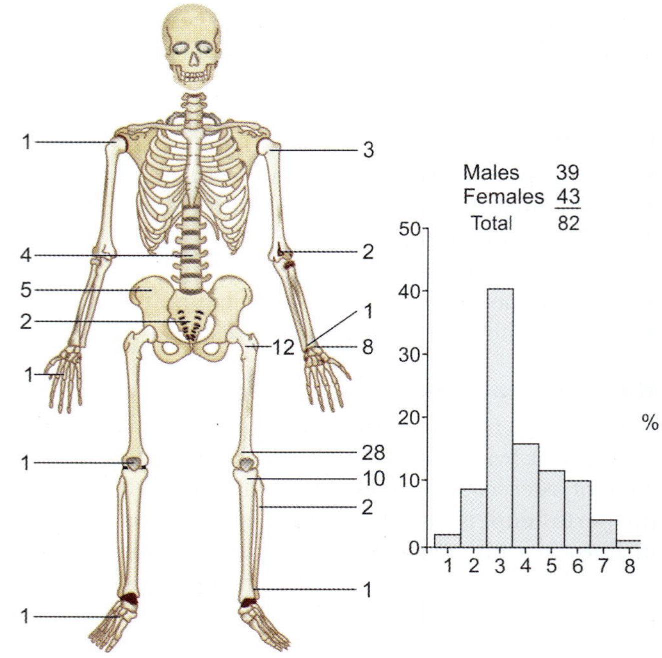

Fig. 24.221: Distribution of skeletal chondrosarcoma

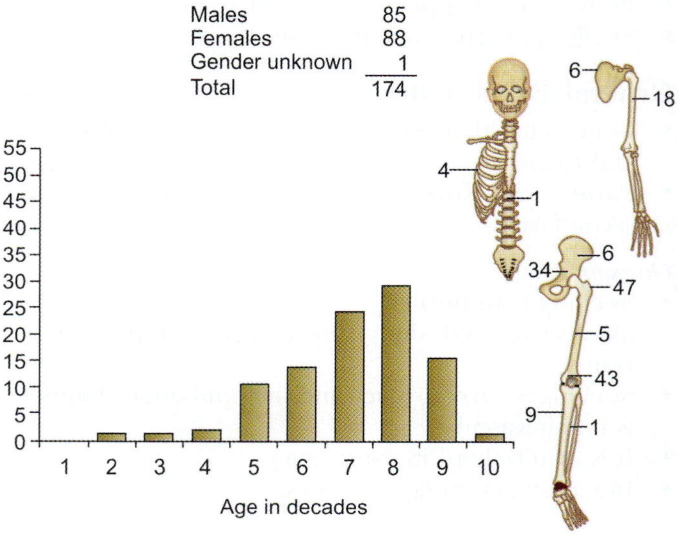

Fig. 24.222: Distribution of dedifferentiated chondrosarcoma

Classification

Primary

- Central (medullary) type
- Juxta-cortical (peri/parosteal)
- Clear cell chondrosarcoma
- Mesenchymal chondrosarcoma
- Dedifferentiated chondrosarcoma

Secondary

Arising from pre-existing benign condition, like exostosis or multiple enchondroma.

Pathology

Macroscopically

- Tumor is lobulated appears as white or bluish mass
- Firm in consistency
- Areas of myxomatous degeneration and softening
- Irregular patchy areas of calcification seen microscopically
- Masses of cartilage cell with more than one nucleus, hyperchromatic.

Histologically

Tumor is graded as:

- *Grade 1:* Low grade
- *Grade 2:* Intermidiate grade
- *Grade 3:* High grade

Clinical Features

- Pelvic tumors present with urinary frequency or obstruction or may masquerade as "groin muscle pulls".
- Patient complains of swelling with history of dull aching pain.
- Swelling is hard in consistency with lobulated surface.
- Grows very slowly and may causes mechanical restriction of joint movements.

Radiological Features (Fig. 24.223)

Central Tumors

- Central lytic lesion, with calcification gives fluffy, cotton wool, popcorn or breadcrumb appearance.
- It invades the soft tissue little or no periosteal reaction.

Peripheral Tumors (Fig. 24.224)

Very large tumors and central part is calcified.

Treatment

- Surgery is the treatment of choice
- Low and medium grade, requires wide excision, e.g. hind quarter for pelvic girdle
- High grade lesion, requires radical excision and chemotherapy
- *Palliative radiotherapy:* If tumor is present in inaccessible area.

Prognosis

- Poor in axial skeleton and proximal bone tumors
- Childhood and young adults
- Cytologically, suggesting high grade malignancy or secondary chondrosarcoma.
- Survival time after treatment is 10 years.

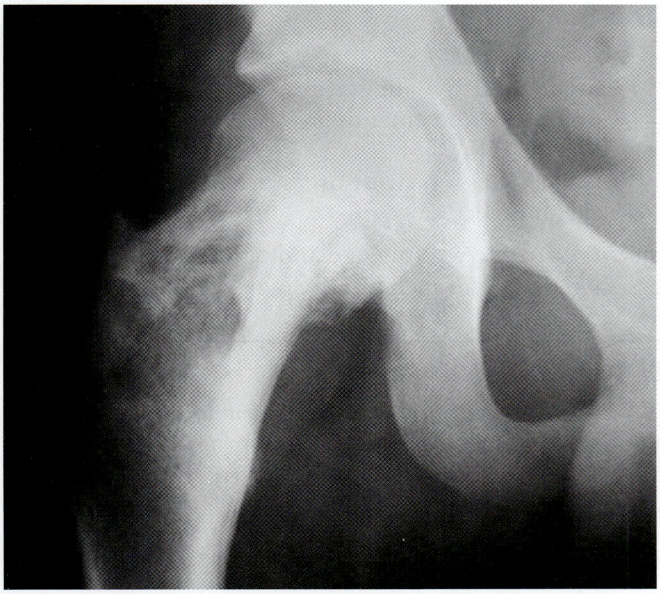

Fig. 24.223: Radiograph showing chondrosarcoma

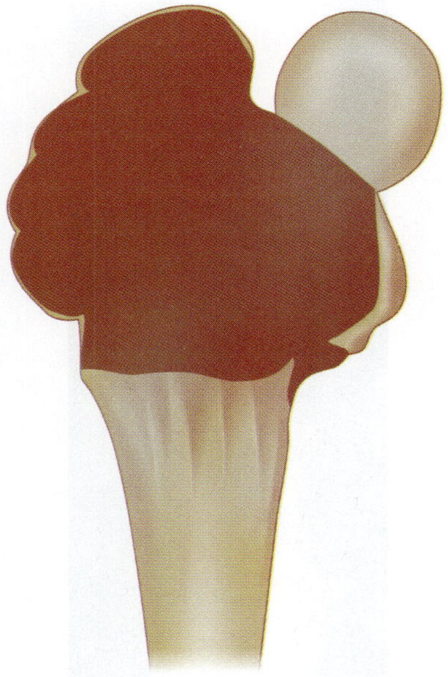

Fig. 24.224: Chondrosarcoma of hip

Multiple Enchondromatosis (Ollier's Disease)

It is a rare disease, in which many cartilaginous tumors appear in both the large and small tubular bones and in the flat bones. It is caused by failure of normal endochondral ossification, as shown in Figure 24.225.

Age: 25 to 40 years.

Site: Located in the epiphysis and the adjacent parts of the metaphysis and shaft and many bones or only a few may be affected.

Deformities resulting from the tumors include
- Shortening caused by lack of epiphyseal growth
- Broadening of the metaphysis
- Bowing of the long bones
- Multiple lesions of the small bones of the hand may cause considerable disability
- An occasional lesion has the characteristics of both fibrous dysplasia and enchondromatosis.

When associated with hemangiomas of the overlying soft tissues, the disease is known as Maffucci syndrome. The individual lesions are quite similar to solitary enchondromas, but often the cellular changes are more bizarre, they have a definite tendency to become malignant. The diagnosis of enchondroma is made on roentgenogram.

Treatment

If malignant transformation is suspected, open surgical biopsy is mandatory. Although, the individual lesions are usually not treated, the more obvious deformities can be corrected by osteotomy.

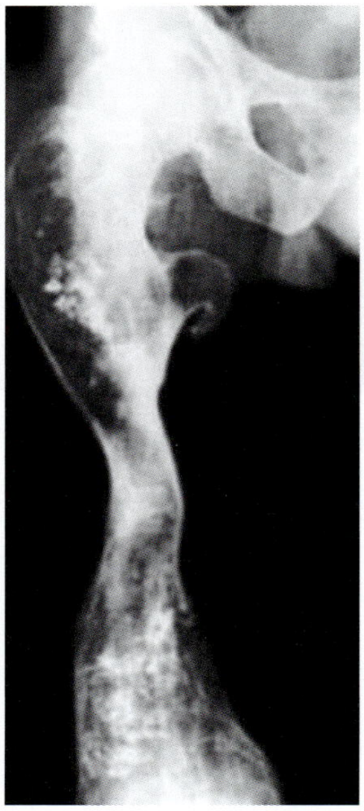

Fig. 24.225: Multiple enchondromatosis (Ollier's disease)

Aneurysmal Bone Cyst

Aneurysmal bone cysts is benign cystic lesion of bone, composed of blood filled spaces separated by connective tissue septa containing fibroblast, osteoclast–type giant cells and reactive woven bone. Benign solitary and expansible, an erosive lesion of bone. ABC can be a tumor of undefined neoplastic nature.

Incidence: One percent of benign bone lesion.

Age: Most frequent in children (85 percent cases<20 years old).

Sex: Female to male ratio is 2:1.

Radiological Classification of Juxtaphyseal Aneurysmal Bone Cyst (Campanacci's Classification)

Type I: Cyst in middle with little or no expansion.
Type II: Lesion substitutes the whole bone segment.
Type III: Eccentric interosseous lesion with little or no expansion.
Type IV: Subperiosteal cyst and superficial erosion of cortex.
Type V: Periosteum eroded and expansion into soft tissue.

I. Primary lesion (*de novo*)
   - *Incidence:* 70 percent of ABC's
   - *Cause:* Trauma or vascular disturbances.

II. Secondary with precursor lesion
   - *Incidence:* 30 percent
   - *Cause:* Common precursor lesion is GCT 19 to 39 percent
   - *Other precursor lesion:* Osteoblastoma, fibroma, chondroblastoma, osteosarcoma and UBC.

Treatment

Recommended surgeries
- Curettage with bone grafting
- Curettage with cementing
- Cryosurgery
- En bloc excision, with or without reconstruction of skeletal defect.

Local recurrence: Young age and open growth plates are associated with an increased risk of local recurrence.

Unicameral Cyst

Thin walled cavity in metaphysis of long bone closely adjacent to the growth plate and migrate away from it, as it matures. Pathological fracture are common. Rarely affect epiphyseal growth plate.

Etiology

- Unknown
- Popular theory–local trauma

- Local venous congestion
- Increase in intraosseous pressure
- Reactive bone resorption
- Cyst fluid—Prostaglandin IL and IB
- Bone resorption.

Types

I. Active cyst
  - Under 10 years
  - Fills most of the metaphysis
  - Thin bony wall
  - Continue to enlarge
  - Pathological fractures

II. Passive cyst
  - Over 12 years
  - Separated from growth plate
  - Thick bony wall
  - Cease to expand
  - *Age:* Fifty percent lesion in less than 10 years, 40 percent in 10 to 20 years. At proximal end femur in adolescent and adult, with mean age of 20.
  - *Sex:* Male to female ratio is 2:1
  - *Location:* Always in metaphysis of upper end femur (40% cases) and less common sites is ilium.

Pathology

Gross area of fusiform expansion and periosteum lifts away.

Underlying tissue: Egg shell thin, semitranslucent, bluish and easily penetrated.

Cavity: Single chamber containing yellow fluid. Following a healed fracture cavity, divided by fibro-osseous septe.

Microscopic: The connective tissue composed of fibroblasts lying on vascular collagenous tissue containing multinucleated giant cells, foam cells containing hemosiderin, lipids and cholesterol crystals.

Clinical Features

- Asymptomatic, until trivial trauma
- Local aching pain, due to fracture through cyst wall
- Local swelling and tenderness
- Intermittent limp in weight-bearing bones
- Pathological fractures (50% cases)
- Infarction of the thinned cortex (25% cases)
- Displacement of the cyst down the shaft
- Growth disturbances
- Coxa vara deformity in proximal femoral region
- Shortening and overgrowth.

Diagnosis (Figs 24.226A to F)

- X-ray
  - Large, well localized, radiolucent, expansile defect in metaphysis. Regional cortex attenuated.

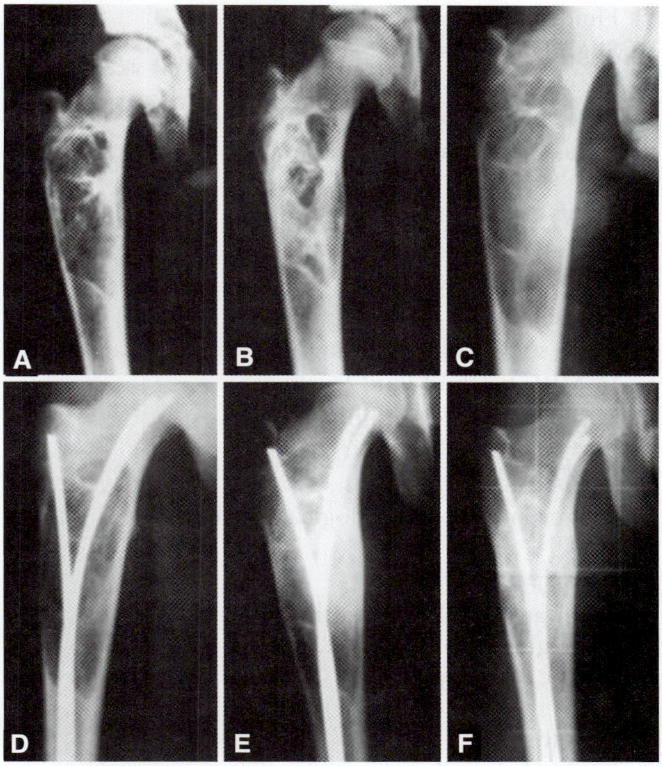

Figs 24.226A to F: (A) Solitary bone cyst in femur of 7-year-old child; (B) After three infiltrations of methylprednisolone; (C) Recurrence of cyst after five infiltrations; (D) After nailing with three ender nails because of large size of cyst; (E) One month after operation; (F) Eight months after operation, remodeling of bone tissue is evident

  - Pseudoloculated form, following a fracture healing
  - Fallen leaf sign, fragment of cortex in the cyst
  - In proximal femur, cyst in subcapital area of neck, calcar is preserved.
- *CT scan:* Only useful if lesion in pelvis.
- *MRI:* Not useful, as it demonstrates only fluid signals.
- *Bone scan:* Light peripheral uptake with cold center.
- *Fluid aspiration:* Aspiration of fluid and injection of radio-opaque substance. Aspirated fluid shows increased level of PG E2.
- Open biopsy and cytology.

Differential Diagnosis

- Eosinophilic granuloma
- Enchondroma
- Fibrous dysplasia
- Giant cell tumor
- Aneurysmal bone cyst

Simple Bone Cyst

- Minimal pain unless fracture

- Fluid filled cavity
- Slightly expansile
- X-ray shows few loculations
- MRI shows prominent fluid-fluid levels
- It has membranous lining

Aneurysmal Bone Cyst

- Aching pain without fracture
- Blood filled cavity
- Very expansile
- X-ray shows many loculations
- In MRI, no fluid-fluid levels
- Mesenchymal tissue lining.

Treatment

Goal: Prevention of pathological fracture.

Modalities

I. Curettage and bone grafting
  - High recurrence rate
  - For active cyst (50%)
  - For passive cyst (10%)

II. Steroids
  - *Methyl-prednisolone:* 80 to 200 mg in fused in cavity
  - Unpredictable response
  - Failure in weight bearing bones
  - *Autologous bone marrow injection:* Unsatisfactory response (F Lokeiec et al.)
  - *Multiple drill holes:* Unpredictable response (T Shinozaki et al.)

Fibrous Dysplasia

It is a skeletal developmental anomaly of the bone-forming mesenchyme that manifests as a defect in osteoblastic differentiation and maturation. Thus, leading to replacement of normal marrow and cancellous bone, by immature bone and fibrous stroma. It is a uncommon benign disorder characterized by a tumor, like proliferation of fibro-osseous tissue. Etiology is unknown.

Types

- Monostotic—confined to one bone
- Polyostotic—multiple bone involvement

Age: Disease of childhood may progress beyond puberty and through adulthood

Sex: Equal distribution.

Location

- Monostotic form (70 to 80%)—Femur (23%)
- Polyostotic form (20 to 30%)—Femur (91%), pelvis (78%), then long bones of lower limb and metaphysical.

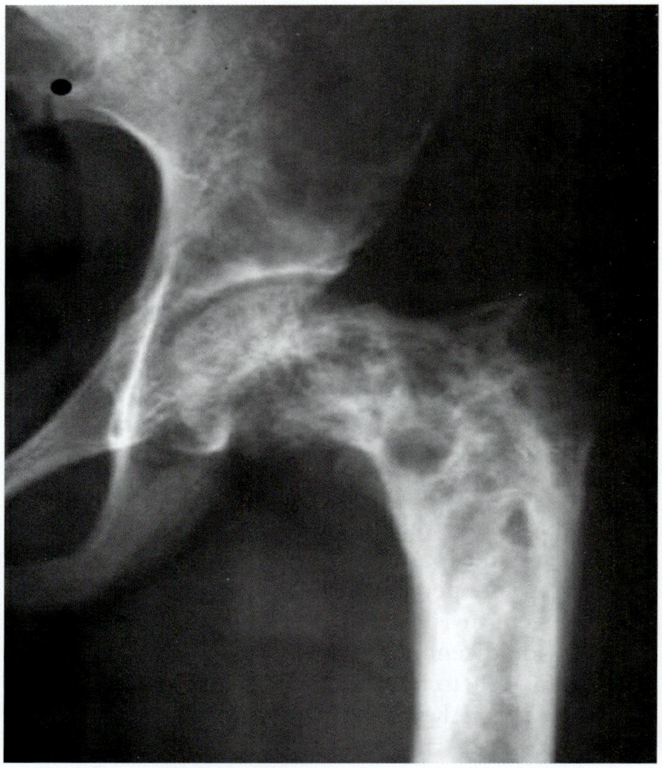

Fig. 24.227: Gross pathological appearance in fibrous dysplasia, with Shepherd Crook deformity

Pathology

Gross appearance: Bony structure is replaced by avascular fibrous tissues, in which thin trabaculae are formed. Gross appearance shows bony irregularity and bent appearance. Cortex is thin and bulged outward. Tissues are reddish gray and tough fibrous. Pathological fractures are undisplaced, usually heal readily with deformity. Shepheard Crook deformity is present, as shown in Figure 24.227.

Microscopic appearance: Dense, mature, collagenase tissues with fibrous bone trabaculae. Fibroblast are elongated and placed in linear or whorled intersecting bundles. Trabaculae appear as Chinese letter or alphabet soup fashion. Classic lesion, in which bone develops by metaplasia, absence of osteoblast and giant cells are sparse.

Clinical Feature

- Early childhood
- Mild and asymptomatic
- Onset of symptoms >10 years
- Limp, pain in leg and fracture
- Females show abnormal vaginal bleeding
- Bending deformity in weight-bearing bones
- Shepherd Crook deformity

- Skull show hyperostosis at the base and is asymetrical
- Café-eu-late spots in polyostotic
- Sexual precocity in females
- *McCune-Albright syndrome*
  - Polyostotic fibrous dysplasia
  - Pigmentation
  - Sexual precocity in female.

Diagnosis

Laboratory findings: Normal

- Serum calcium
- Serum phosphorus
- Serum alkaline phosphatase raised in severe conditions.

Radiological Findings

- *X-ray*
  - Localized, well circumscribed lesion in shaft
  - Ground glass appearance
  - Cystic or multilocular
  - Cortex—thinned and expanded
  - Skull—hyperostotic formation at base
- *Bone scan*
  - Active lesion—increased uptake
  - Inactive lesion—decreased uptake
- *CT scan:* To evaluate extent of bone involvement
- *MRI:* To find sarcomatous changes
- *Biopsy:* It is confirmatory.

Differential Diagnosis

- Hyperparathyroidism
- Osteogenesis imperfecta
- Neurofibromatosis
- Paget's disease

Management

Medical: Biphosphonate (Fosamax)

- 35 mg weekly for children
- 70 mg weekly for adults
- Long-term therapy for symptomatic and large lesions.

Postoperative

- IV biphosphonate including zolendronic acid, symptomatic or critical lesions, monthly for 3 to 6 months.

Surgical (Figs 24.228A to C)

- Curettage—high rate of local recurrence
- Curettage and bone grafting, preferably in nonweight-bearing bones
- Curettage with cortical bone grafting and implant fixation in weight-bearing bones
- In proximal femur, rigid intramedullary fixation, with strongest possible device.

Radiotherapy

Contraindicated: Increased risk of sarcomatous changes.

Prognosis

- *Mono-ostotic:* Excellent, if the bone can be strengthened
- *Polyostotic:* Several operative procedures, to achieve bone strength and correct deformity
- *Malignant degeneration:* Extremely rare.

■ Chondroma

Including enchondroma and periosteal chondromas. It is a benign tumor of mature hyaline cartilage (chondromas), are usually located centrally in bone and

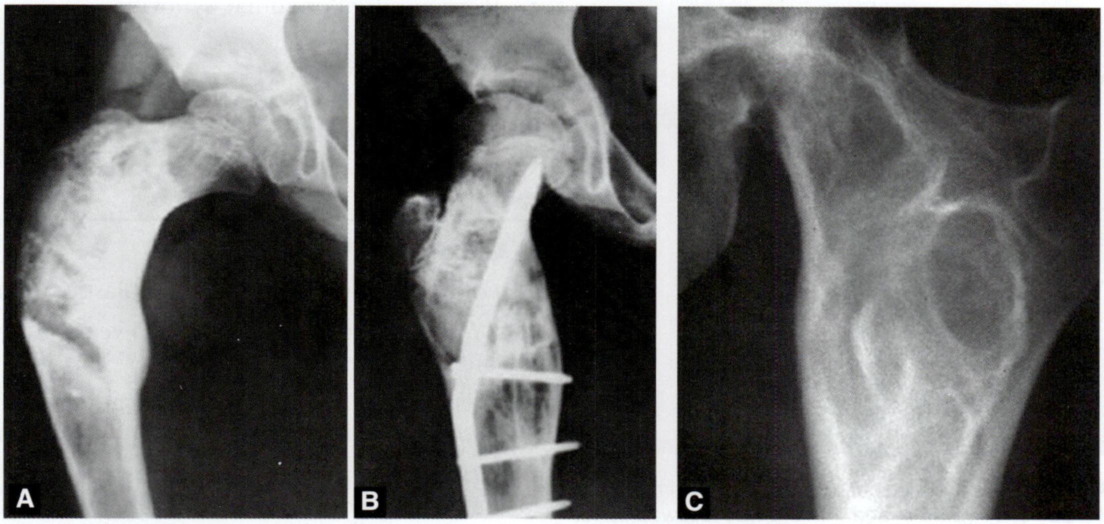

Figs 24.228A to C: Fibrous dysplasia—(A and B) Shepherd's Crook deformity; (B) Deformity has been corrected by osteotomy and cystic lesion has been filled with grafts

are known as enchondromas. Less frequently they are located sub-periosteally and are known as juxtacortical or sub-periosteal chondromas.

Age: Occur during the second, third and fourth decades of life.

Site: Most common sites of manifestations include:

- Metaphysis is usually involved.
- Enchondroma, the most frequent tumor of bone in the hand, rarely exhibits aggressive behavior and is sometimes referred to as cartilaginous hamartoma.
- The long bones of the extremities are involved less frequently, but enchondromas of the humerus and femur are not rare.
- Vertebral involvement has been reported.

Symptoms

- Often are nonspecific and some lesions being discovered incidentally, during an unrelated roentgenographic examination.
- Usually the tumor is found after a pathological fracture.
- Pain is an ominous symptom and suggests that the tumor is growing and may be malignant.

Roentgenographic Findings (Figs 24.229A to C)

- It depends on the location and extent of calcification of the tumor.
- A central lesion in a small tubular bone of the hand or foot, usually appears as a well circumscribed area of rarefaction, most frequently diaphyseal, cortex around it may be expanded.
- A juxtacortical lesion is eccentric and is located beneath the periosteum in a well-defined cortical defect.

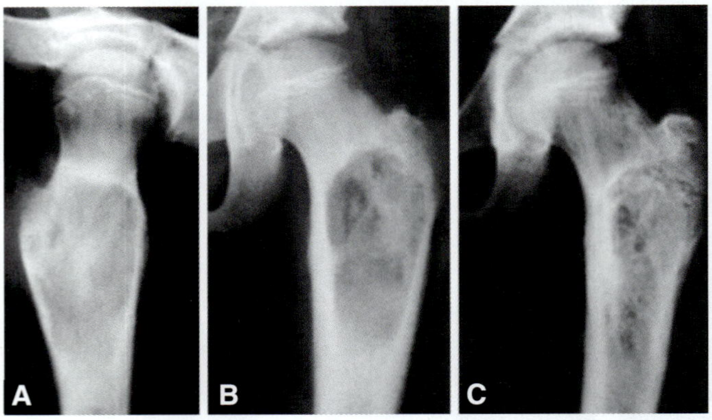

Figs 24.229A to C: X-rays showing enchondroma in proximal femur of a boy of 11 years of age. Patient was followed up for 15 years, after curettage of enchondroma and there was no evidence of recurrence found

- Small flocculent foci of calcification are often seen within the tumor and in a long bone, the tumor may be highly calcified and radiopaque.

Pathology

The differentiation of benign from malignant cartilaginous tumors is one of the most difficult problems in bone pathology. All available tissue must be examined and even then the diagnosis may depend more on the clinical and roentgenographic features, than on the microscopic changes. Juxtacortical chondromas and enchondromas of the hands may be quite cellular and contain many atypical cells and still be benign. Conversely, enchondromas of long bones often appear benign microscopically, but tend to recur after removal. Some uncalcified enchondromas, may mimic a variety of lytic lesions, both clinically and on roentgenograms and the heavily calcified enchondromas of long bones may resemble bone infarcts or so called bone islands.

Treatment

- Curettage is done and the wall is cauterized if the tumor is small
- Surgery done in cases of large tumors is excision and removal of capsule, to prevent recurrence
- Radical resection done for tumors of long bones and pelvis.

Less commonly tumors found around hip are

- Osteoid osteoma
- Giant cell tumor
- Chordoma
- Metastatic tumors
- Multiple myeloma
- Osteochondromatosis
- Synovioma
- Pigmented villonodular synovitis
- Lymphoma
- Fibrous cortical defect
- Benign fibrous histiocytoma
- Neural tumors
- Desmoplastic fibroma.

■ Osteoid Osteoma

Osteoid osteoma is a benign osteoblastic tumor.

Sex: Young adults between 10 to 25 years of age. Male to female ratio is 2:1.

Age: Found in the first-three decades of life, but an occasional lesion has been reported in older patients.

Location: The proximal femur is the most common location. Osteoid osteoma is found in the diaphysis or the metaphysis of the proximal end of the bone more often than the distal end.

Incidence: Approximately, 10 percent of benign bone tumors. Five percent are subperiosteal, 5 percent of sciatica are due to osteoid osteoma.

Pathology

Vascular mesenchymal type of connective tissue stroma, with proliferating fibroblasts and osteoblasts surrounds abundant pink staining osteoid tissue. Osteoid forms irregular branching network, surrounding the poorly formed tissue at the center of lesion is marked bony proliferation. Marrow is fibrous, cartilage is never found.

Clinical Features

- The typical patient has pain that is worse at night and relieved by aspirin (aspirin tumor)
- The person may limp
- When the lesion is near a joint, swelling, stiffness and contracture may occur
- When in a vertebra, scoliosis may occur. Occasionally, osteoid osteoma occurs with minimal pain
- In children, overgrowth and angular deformities may occur
- Systemic symptoms are absent.

Radiographic Findings (Fig. 24.230)

- Small rarefied lesions <2 cm in diameter in cortex, subcortical or subperiosteal regions
- Surrounded by thick sclerotic bone
- Small dense center of ossification—Nidus
- CT/MRI useful to identify and localize the lesion
- A bone scan is helpful in detecting small lesions that may be overlooked on roentgenograms
- The "double-density sign", which is a focal area of increased activity with a second smaller area of increased uptake superimposed on it is said to be diagnostic of osteoid osteoma.

Treatment

Conservative: Rest to the part and analgesics (aspirin).

Surgical

- To effect a cure, the entire nidus must be removed
- Block resection of the nidus; however if the lesion is in cortical bone, this method increases the risk of subsequent fracture (Figs 24.231A and B)
- An alternative method suggested by Johnston, is to shave the reactive bone with a sharp osteotome, until the nidus is encountered then curet the exposed nidus
- CT-guided percutaneous resection, allows precise localization and removal of the nidus through a small access without the need for removal of an excessive amount of bone
- Percutaneous radiofrequency ablation of osteoid osteomas and believe their results are equivalent to operative excision

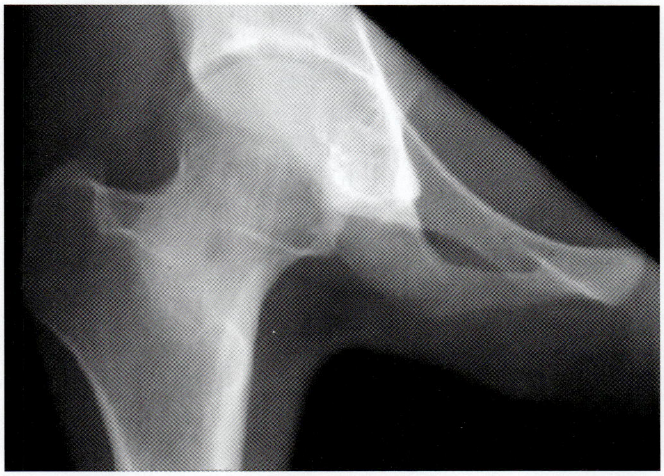

Fig. 24.230: Osteoid osteoma of hip

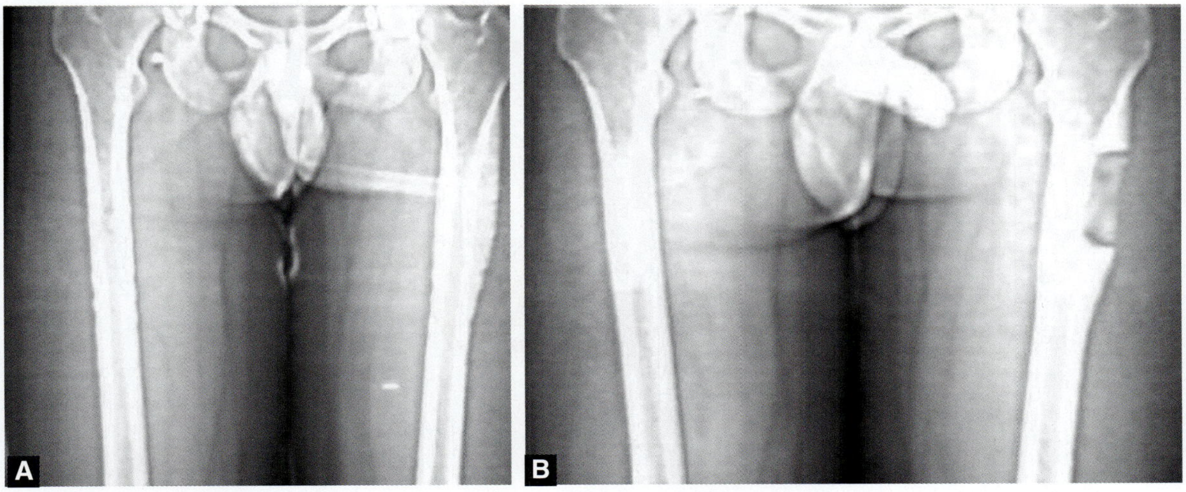

Figs 24.231A and B: Osteoid osteoma (preoperative and postoperative)

- For rare intra-articular situations, arthroscopically assisted excision
- MRI guided cryotreatment.

Recurrence and Malignancy

- After complete removal of tumor along with nidus recurrence is very rare.
- No malignant change has ever been documented.

■ Giant Cell Tumor

Benign giant cell tumor is an osteolytic tumor, arising from the epiphysis and is common in young adults. Though, it is benign it is locally malignant.

Sex: The male to female ratio is 1.5:1.

Age: It is common between 15 and 35 years of age (80 percent occur in more than 20 years of age and the average age group is 35 years).

Sites: It is shown in Figure 24.232:

- Giant cell tumor may occur in the sacrum
- Upper end of femur.

Pathology

Grossly, the tumor consist of ragged, friable and bleeding tissue filled with old or fresh blood clot, with various sized cysts and cavities. Color varies from red and brown. Epiphyseal end of the bone is distorted. Tumor extension in the joint cavity is usually not seen and there is no evidence of periosteal reaction.

Microscopically, the tumor is encompassed, by a fibrous capsule at the periphery. Presence of abundant tumor giant cells, are quiet characteristic. These cells are characterized by their larger size, multiple nuclei more than 150 in number, which are distributed throughout the cell. Appearance of spindle cell, indicate malignant potential.

Histological Grading (Jaffe's Criterion)

Grade I: Presence of characteristic stromal cell, Little intercellular collagen and spindle are adjacent to the necrotic tissue.

Grade II: Random distribution of giant cell are seen among the stromal cells.

Grade III: Nuclei of giant cell are indentical to those of the stromal cells.

Clinical Features

- The course of the tumor is chronic.
- Unlike osteogenic sarcoma, pain is not the presenting feature but trauma is the patient complains of swelling, which is situated on one side of the bone.
- Skin over the tumor is stretched, but there are no dialated vein.
- Tenderness is moderate or absent egg shell crackling sensation may be present or absent.

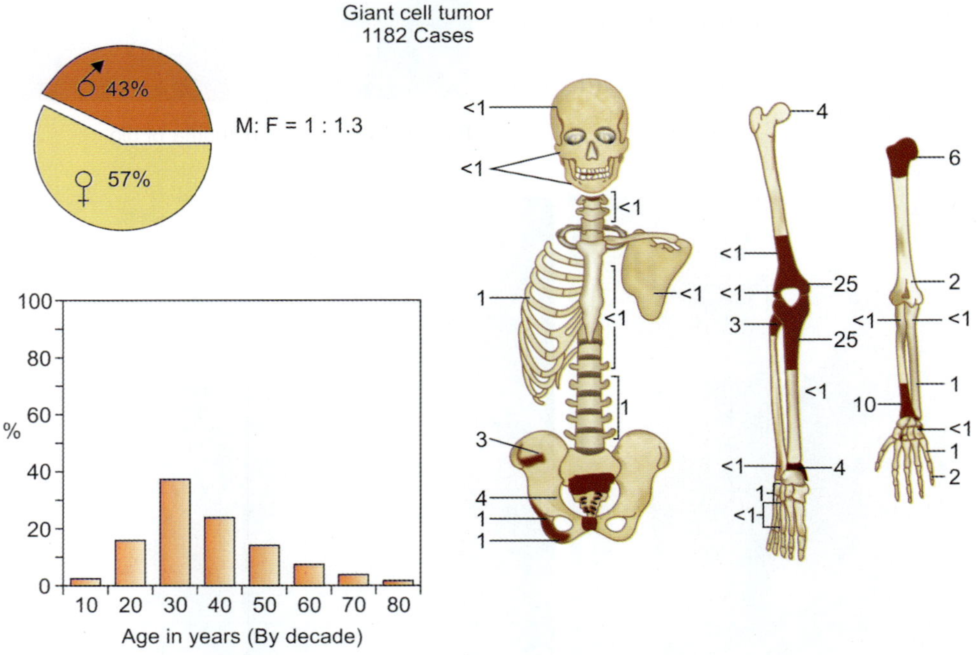

Fig. 24.232: Common site of occurrence of GCT

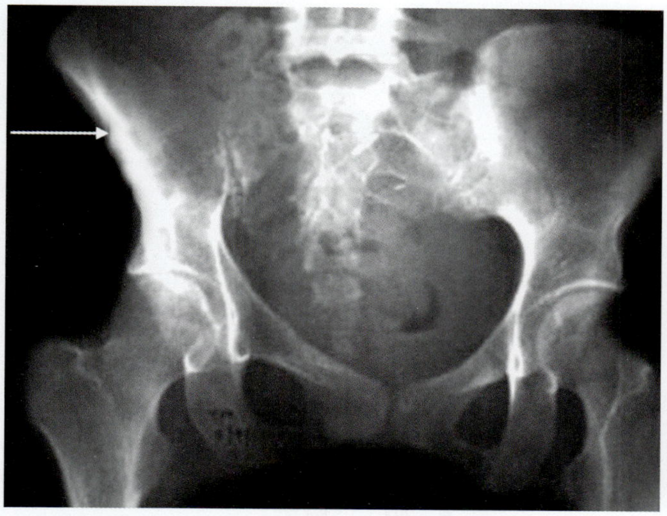

Fig. 24.233: X-ray showing GCT of hip, arrow showing GCT

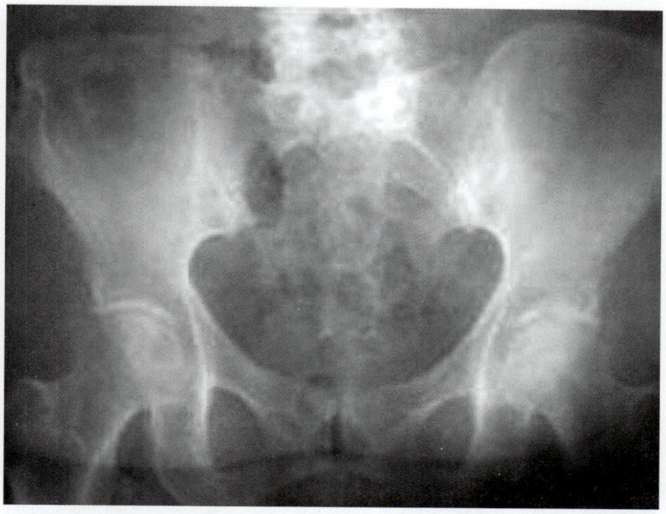

Fig. 24.234: Chondroma of hip

- Invasion in the joint is rare and joint effusion is rare.
- Pathological fracture is a late feature.

Radiology (Fig. 24.233)

- An osteolytic area is seen near the epiphysis
- The cortex is thin and expanded
- There is no periosteal new bone formation
- Thin septa of bone transverse the interior of bone and gives it soap bubble appearance.
- The cortex may be disrupted in late stages
- Joint extension is rare.

Companacci's Radiographic Grading

Grade 1: Cystic lesion
Grade 2: Cortex is thin, but not perforated
Grade 3: Cortex is perforated, with extension in the soft tissue.

Enneking's Staging of Benign GCT

Stage 1 (Latent)

- Incidence is 10 to 15 percent
- Discovered accidentally
- No symptoms
- Pathological fractures may be present

Stage 2 (active)

- Incidence is 70 percent
- Symptomatic
- Pathological fracture may be present
- Benign.

Stage 3 (aggressive)

- Incidence is 10 to 15 percent
- Symptomatic rapidly growing
- Benign
- Cortex is perforated

Treatment

- Intralesional excision by "extended" curettage is the treatment of choice.
- Curettage and bone grafting
- En bloc resection
- Curettage and acrylic bone cementation
- Curettage and cryosurgery
- Arthodesis
- Arthoplasty.
- Radiotherapy

■ Chordoma

Chordoma is a rare malignant neoplasm that arises from notochord remnants, as shown in Figure 24.234. Chordomas account for 1 to 4 percent of all bone tumors. The ratio of male to female is 2:1. Chordoma is the most common primary malignancy of the sacrum. Over 50 percent of chordomas arise in the sacrococcygeal area, peak incidence for sacrococcygeal chordomas occurs in the fifth through seventh decades. Most series demonstrate a marked male predominance (as high as 3:1), especially for sacrococcygeal tumors.

Clinical Features

- Sacrococcygeal tumors often present as low back pain, with no characteristic pattern or time course.
- Bowel and bladder dysfunction.
- Presacral tumors can sometimes be palpated on rectal examination.
- Sacral tumors are often large at presentation, as a large volume of tumor can be accommodated within the pelvis.

X-rays: On plain X-ray, chordomas appear as a solitary mid-line lesion with bony destruction. There is often an

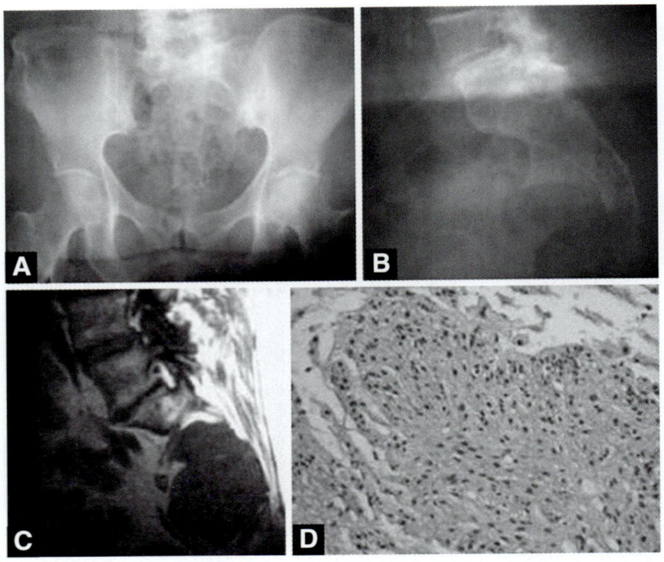

Figs 24.235A to D: Anteroposterior (A) and lateral (B) views of sacrum of patient with sacrococcygeal chordoma. This lesion could easily be missed because of overlying bowel gas. (C) MRI clearly demonstrates lesion. (D) Typical microscopic appearance of chordoma. Cells with abundant vacuolated cytoplasm (physaliferous cells) are arranged in cords with mucinous background

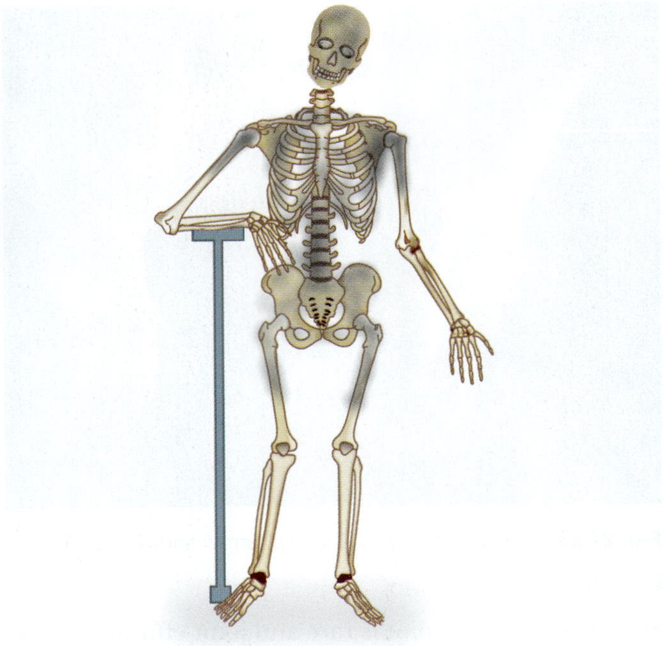

Fig. 24.236: Sites of frequent metastasis to the skeleton (gray highlighted area) commonly involves pelvis and proximal end of femur

accompanying soft tissue mass. Approximately, half of the time focal calcifications are present.

CT and MRI scans help demonstrate the soft tissue component, calcifications and epidural extension. MRI is helpful in identifying local recurrences.

Bone scan: Chordomas have reduced uptake on bone scan.

Examination (Figs 24.235A to D)

On gross examination chordomas are soft, blue-gray, lobulated tumors.

There are gelatinous translucent areas and often a capsule is present.

The lesion often tracks along nerve roots in the sacral plexus or out the sciatic notch in planes of least resistance.

Under the Microscope

The chordomas are characterized by lobules and fibrous septa. The malignant cell has eosinophilic cytoplasm. Prominent vacuoles of mucus push the nuclei to the side, resulting in "physaliferous" cells from the Greek word for bubble or drop.

Treatment

The treatment of chordomas is difficult. Wide surgical excision is desirable, but rarely feasible based on the anatomic location of the tumor. With sacrococcygeal tumors, sexual function and sphincter control may be compromised after surgery. Radiation is used, if complete resection is impossible. Chordomas metastasize to lymph nodes, lungs, liver and bone. Chemotherapy can be used for late stage disease.

■ Metastatic Tumors of Bones

These are cancerous tumors originating in the other organs and involving the skeletal structures of the body. Bones may be involved by:
- direct invasion,
- blood-borne metastasis and
- very rarely, through the lymphatics.

Incidence: 27 to 70 Percent

Tendency percentage wise:
- Carcinoma breast (73%)
- Lung (32%)
- Kidney (24%)
- Rectum (13%)
- Stomach (11%)

Sites: Sites of frequent metastasis to the skeleton are shown in Figure 24.236.

Clinical Features

- Adult and middle age patient
- Pain, pathological fracture or anemia. Pathological fractures are frequent in femur.

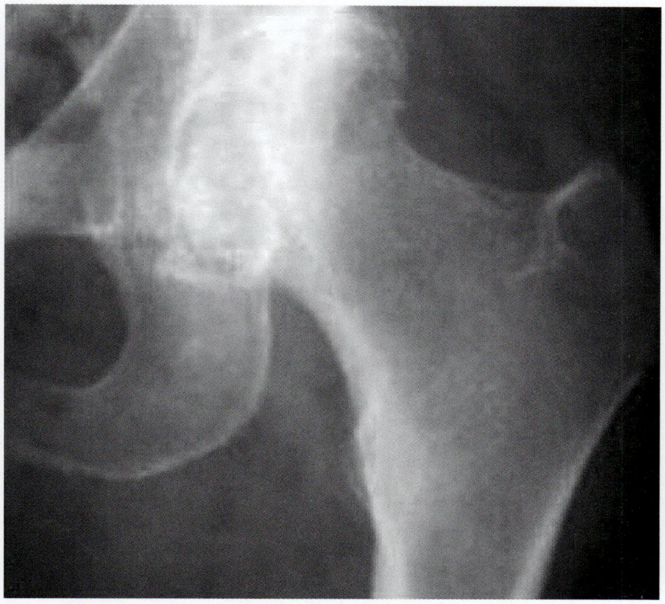

Fig. 24.237 X-ray showing malignant osteoblastic and osteolytic tumors of hip

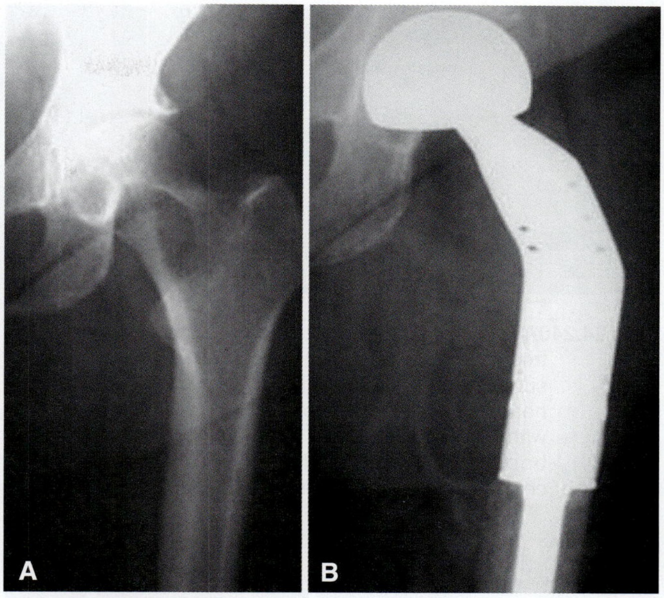

Figs 24.238A and B: (A) X-ray showing malignant tumor of hip; (B) Tumor excision followed by prosthesis implantation

Laboratory Diagnosis

- Blood picture show anemia, thrombocytopenia, leukocytosis or leukopenia, eosinophilia, etc.
- Alkaline phosphatase has increased
- Acid phosphatase increased in cancer of prostrate.

Investigation

- *Radiology* (Fig. 24.237)
  - Osteolytic and osteoblastic variety
  - Periosteal reaction and mottled or marble appearance
- Bone scan
- Fine needle biopsy.

Treatment (Figs 24.238 to 24.241)

- Radiotherapy 3000 rads to 4000 rads for 3 to 4 weeks
- *Surgery:* Internal fixation with acrylic cement for pathological fractures
- Hormone therapy
- Radioisotope therapy
- Chemotherapy
- Radiofrequency ablation.

■ Multiple Myeloma

Malignant tumor arising from plasma cell of reticuloendothelial cell of bone marrow. It can occur as a solitary plasmocytoma, multiple myeloma or generalized myelomatosis. This is shown in Figures 24.242A to D.

Incidence: Accounts for 45 percent of total malignant tumors.

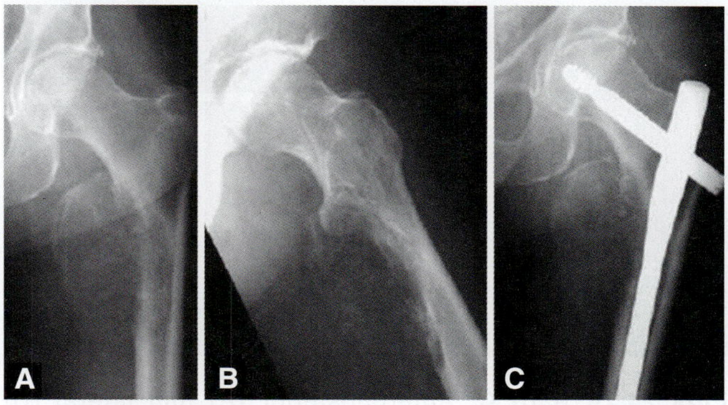

Figs 24.239A to C: Anteroposterior (A) and lateral; (B) roentgenograms of left hip of a 44-year-old man, with metastatic bladder cancer; (C) Anteroposterior view after prophylactic fixation with long gamma nail

Age: Fifty to eighty years of age. Males are commonly affected (male to female ratio is 2:1).

Site: Proximal femur and pelvis.

Pathology

Grossly

- Tumor is dark red in color
- Soft in consistency and lies within medulla
- The cortex is thin and broken.

Microscopically

- Consist of round cells with eccentrically placed nucleus with nucleolus.

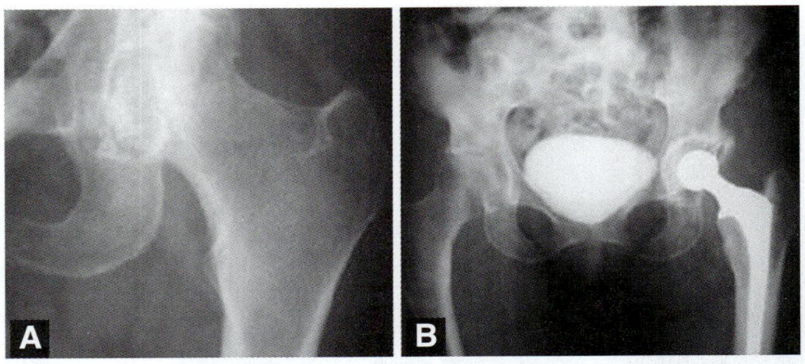

Figs 24.240A and B: (A) Anteroposterior view of left hip of patient treated with radiation for metastatic breast cancer. She subsequently, developed avascular necrosis of femoral head; (B) Anteroposterior view of pelvis after treatment with cemented total hip arthroplasty. As the bone had been irradiated, both femoral and acetabular components were cemented

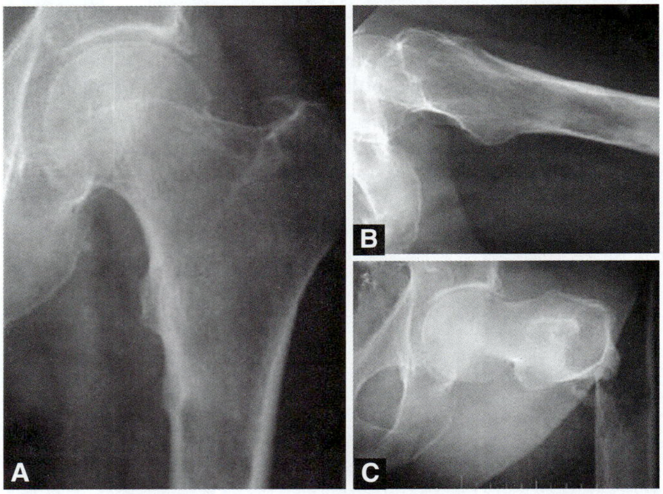

Figs 24.241A to C: Anteroposterior (A) and lateral (B) roentgenograms of proximal femur of 82-year-old man, with metastatic kidney cancer reveal multiple lytic lesions. Patient failed to respond to radiation treatment. Prophylactic internal fixation was scheduled, however operation was cancelled because patient was considered medically unstable for surgery; (C) Anteroposterior view of left hip of same patient several weeks later after sustaining pathological fracture. Surgery is now more difficult and patient has experienced greater morbidity

- Chromatin is sparsed and is arranged in spokes of wheel fashion.
- Perinuclear halo typical of plasma cell not seen in multiple myeloma.

Associated Pathology

- Interstitial fibrosis in the kidney
- Nodules in the lungs
- Amylodosis may occur.

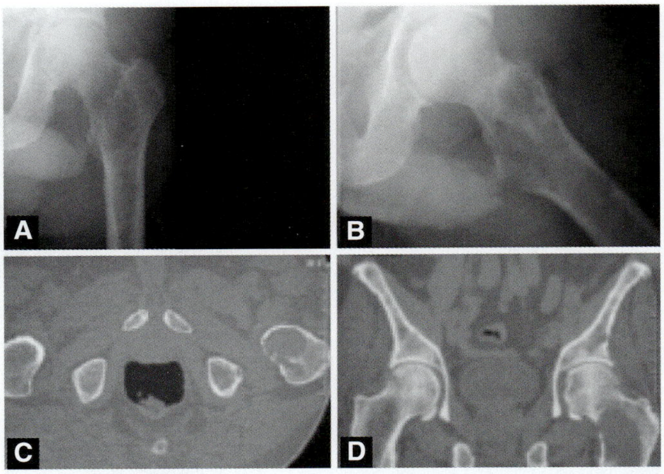

Figs 24.242A to D: Anteroposterior (A) and lateral (B) roentgenograms of proximal femur of 61-year-old man with multiple myeloma demonstrate multiple lytic lesions; (C) and (D) CT better demonstrates extent of lesions and need for prophylactic fixation

Clinical Features

General Examination

Patient becomes severly anemic, loses weight and becomes cachetic. In the late stage patient develops hyperazotemia, uremic syndrome, hypercalcemia, hyperuremic syndrome and hemorrhagic diasthesis.

Sign and Symptoms

- Generalized bone pain and pain in back.
- Pain may be intermittent, but later become intense.
- In the early stages, there are hardly any clinical symptoms.
- Late stages patient complains of soft tissue swelling and sign of pathological fracture.
- Tumor is chronic and tubular block due to protein cast may be seen causing renal failure (myeloma kidney).

Investigation

- *Radiological features*
  - Affected bone shows diffuse osteoporosis or lytic lesion.
  - Punched out lesion in the pelvis; skull bones; ribs.
- *Laboratory findings*
  - Low Hb%
  - High ESR
  - Increased total protein A/G ratio reversed
  - Increased serum calcium
  - Low to normal alkaline phosphatase
  - Urine Bence-Jones protein are found in 30 percent of patient

- *Serum electrophoresis:* Abnormal spike of gamma globulin in 90 percent of cases
- *Sternal puncture:* Myeloma cell may be seen
- Bone biopsy
- Bone scan
- Open biopsy
- Alpha-2 microglobulin tumor marker.

Treatment

- Chemotherapy is the mainstay of the treatment
- Drugs used are melphalan, cyclophosphamide, vincristine and steroids.
- High dose of vincristine, doxorubicin and dexamethasone (VDD) is new and better alternative. Tumor is radiosensitive and localized lesions are treated with radiation for pain relief.

Surgery

- In case of pathological fractures
- Decompression of cords in neurological involvement.

Prognosis

- Disease is widespread and fatal
- Death in 3 to 5 years.

Complications

- Pathological fractures of rib
- Spinal cord or nerve root compression
- Renal failure
- Severe infection
- Amylodosis.

Osteochondromatosis (Fig. 24.243)

Osteochondromatosis can be (1) Hereditary multiple osteocartilagenous exostoses (HMOCE) and (2) Hereditary multiple exostoses (HME). HMOCE is a rare, autosomal dominant condition, where an genetic error of bone growth results in the formation of multiple osteochondromas. The condition can range from a mild nuisance to a very severe, disabling and even potentially deadly problem, depending on the number and location of the lesions. HMOCE is an autosomal dominant condition. The condition is genetically heterogeneous and it has been linked to three loci including 8*q*24.1 (EXT1), 11*p*11-12 (EXT2) and 19*p* (EXT3). EXT1 and EXT2 are proposed tumor supressor genes, which may be lost in HMOCE, resulting in the growth of the lesions. The condition can lead to both sessile and pedunculated lesions.

Occurrence: The lesions may occur on different bones or on the same bone and symptoms present in the first decade of life.

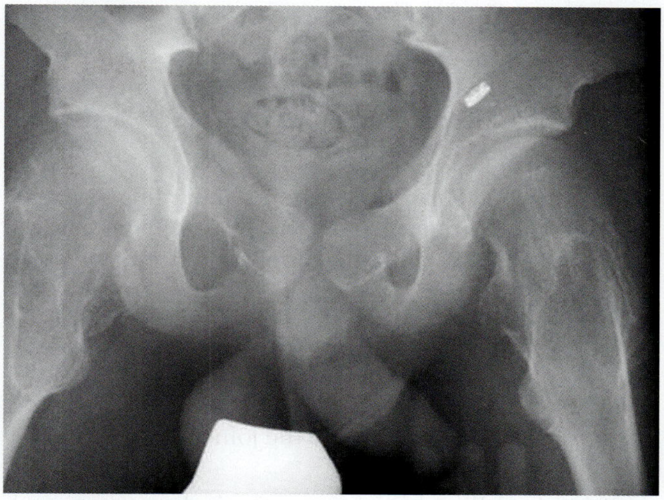

Fig. 24.243: Osteochondromatosis of hip

Clinical Features

Patients may have short stature. Limb-length discrepancies. The lesions cluster at the metaphyseal ends of the bones near the joint and may lead to loss of motion, hip dysplasia, joint subluxation, nerve compression, vascular pseudoaneurysm, cord compression and pain. The risk of malignant transformation to chondrosarcoma in hereditary multiple osteochondromatosis is unknown, but may be 25 to 30 percent compared to approximately one percent for a solitary osteochondromas. The risk of malignant degeneration increases as the number and size of the osteochondromas increases. Large deep osteochondromas, often located on the pelvis or the spine, where malignant transformation, may be more likely and much more difficult to treat.

Treatment

Surgical removal of troublesome lesions or lesions, which appear to possess malignant potential is associated with a good outcome. Significant angular deformities of the lower limb can be reduced or eliminated with realignment procedures, which should improve function and reduce pain. Early surgical corrections of deformities has been advocated to improve function. Indications for surgical removal include persistant pain, functional impairment, joint subluxation, neuropraxia and others.

Synovioma

The synovioma (synovial sarcoma, synovial sarcomesothelioma, cancerous synovial tumor) is a slow growing malignant tumor occurring in juxtaposition to and often attached to synovial tissue, but almost invariably lies outside the joint.

Pathology

Grossly, the tumor is sharply circumscribed, rounded and lobulated. As it grows, it compresses the surrounding tissue, which becomes attenuated to form a pseudo-capsule.

Microscopically: Three basic patterns, indicating a synovial origin are formation of tissue spaces, formation of cell tufts. Epithelia, like cells on a supporting stroma of tissue.

Clinical Features

Age: Young adults 25 to 40 years.

Site: Lower extremity.

Position: In soft tissue, outside the joint.

Symptoms:
- Painful swelling begins in periarticular or peritend-inous site
- Increases slowly, large swelling with severe pain
- Swelling is firm or soft, moderately tender.

Course: Very slow, metastasizes eventually to lungs.

Roentgenographic Findings

- Soft tissue technique reveals a rounded and lobulated shadow
- Stippling is observed, if tumor contains small areas of calcification.

Prognosis and Treatment
- Tumor is slow growing and metastasizes late
- Local excision is inadequate
- Radical amputation is indicated.

Pigmented Villonodular Synovitis

Pigmented villonodular synovitis (PVNS) is a locally aggressive synovial tumor. There are two forms of PVNS: (1) diffuse and (2) nodular. PVNS occur in the hips.

Incidence: PVNS has the highest prevalence during the third and fourth decades and it affects males and females equally.

Signs/symptoms: It presents as a painless or mildly painful joint with swelling. Mechanical interference cause stiffness, locking, limitation of motion and snapping sensations at times.

On aspiration: Thick orange brown fluid containing cholesterol in large amounts is pathognomonic. Hemosiderin is also present.

Radiological appearance of PVNS depends on the location. Bone erosion or cysts will be present in tighter joints, like the hip. The joint space is usually preserved and there may be an effusion.

CT scan is able to pick up the hemosiderin and demonstrates the extent of the synovial involvement as well as bone erosion and cysts. Hemosiderin appears as low or absent signal on both T1 and T2 weighted images.

Pathology: On gross examination, the diffuse form of PVNS is a tanned mass of villi and folds of synovium. The lesion may be sessile or have several pedunculated nodules. Bony invasion through the joint capsule is possible. The local form of PVNS is a pedunculated firm nodule.

Treatment: Treatment of PVNS is surgical excision. Recurrences are common due to the difficulty of complete surgical excision. Hence, radiotherapy has been recommended.

■ Lymphoma

Lymphoma may involve bone primarily or secondarily.

Occurrence: Lymphoma can occur at any age, but becomes more common in the sixth and seventh decades of life.

Sex: The male to female ratio is approximately 1.5:1.

Location: The femur is the most common bone involved, followed by the pelvis.

Signs/Symptoms: Most patients complain of localized pain or swelling.

Roentgenographically: Lymphoma usually appears as an ill-defined area of bone destruction, frequently diaphyseal and often has a permeative appearance. The cortex may be thickened, but a periosteal reaction rarely is seen.

Microscopically, osseous lymphomas are composed of a mixture of both large and small lymphoid cells with both cleaved and non-cleaved nuclei. A discussion on the classification of lymphomas is beyond the scope of this text.

Prognosis: Patients with primary lymphoma of bone have a better prognosis (approximately 55 percent, 5 years survival) than those with systemic disease (less than 25% and 5 years survival).

Treatment: The primary treatment of lymphoma is chemotherapy. Local control usually is attained with radiation treatment. Surgical intervention is therefore rarely needed, but may be indicated for treatment of impending or actual pathological fractures.

■ Benign Fibrous Histiocytoma

Fibrous histiocytoma was first described by Dahlin in 1978. This lesion occurs most frequently in the soft tissues and is less common in bone. Although, it is histologically similar to that of nonossifying fibroma, it is a much more aggressive tumor in its biological behavior and roentgenographic characteristics. Unlike, nonossifying fibroma, which usually is an eccentric metaphyseal lesion, benign fibrous histiocytoma may occur in the diaphysis or epiphysis of long bones or in the pelvis. It is further distinguished by its occurrence in older patients between the ages of 30 and 40 years. Roentgenographically, benign fibrous histiocytoma is a well-defined, lytic, expanding lesion with little periosteal reaction. Bone scans usually are mildly positive. Unlike, nonossifying fibroma, this lesion is considered a true neoplasm.

Treatment: Due to its tendency for local recurrence (persistence), aggressive curettage or when feasible, wide excision is necessary.

■ Fibrous Cortical Defect

Fibrous cortical defects, although classified as bone tumors are probably developmental abnormalities and are believed to occur in as many as 35 percent of children. Generally, these lesions occur in the metaphyseal region of long bones in individuals between the ages of 2 and 20 years and occur predominantly in males. Approximately, 40 percent are found in the femur, although some occur in the ilium.

On plain roentgenograms, a fibrous cortical defect appears as a circular or oval, eccentrically located radiolucent area, near the physis of a long bone. The margins of the defect are smooth or lobulated with a well-defined thin rim of sclerosis. Computed tomography (CT) may be useful, especially if the diagnosis is uncertain.

Histologically the defect is filled with spindle-shaped cells distributed in a whorled or storiform pattern. There is fibroblastic proliferation with high cellularity. Multiple fibrous cortical defects occur in approximately 50 percent of patients. Usually they are bilateral and symmetrical. Five percent of patients with multiple fibrous cortical defects also have neurofibromatosis. Several authors have suggested stress or trauma as a cause. Regardless, the defects resolve without treatment, the disappearance perhaps being the result of physiological remodeling of bone.

■ Neural Tumors

Neurogenous tumors of bone are quite rare, but definite neurilemomas have been described. On roentgenograms they are seen as discrete lytic lesions. Their microscopic appearance is similar to that of neurilemomas of soft tissue. Neurofibromas also develop in bone, especially in von Recklinghausen disease. A variety of other musculoskeletal abnormalities not necessarily related to the presence of discrete neurofibromas may be found, such as hypertrophy of parts, kyphoscoliosis, congenital bowing of bones, and congenital pseudarthrosis of bones.

■ Desmoplastic Fibroma

Desmoplastic fibroma is a rare, densely collagenized tumor of fibrous tissue histologically similar to the soft tissue desmoid tumors.

Sex: Males and females are affected with nearly equal frequency.

Age: The lesion has been seen in patients as young as 8 years of age and as old as 80.

Location: The long tubular bones are involved most often, but involvement of the pelvis has been reported.

Clinical findings: Include pain late in the clinical course and swelling. It may present as an effusion if near a joint. The roentgenograms reveal a lytic defect centrally located and usually well circumscribed. Plain X-ray shows an osteolytic, expansile, medullary lesion with well defined sclerotic margins. The oval tumor is often found in the metaphysic, aligned with the long axis of the bone. There is usually thinned cortex and the fine intralesional trabeculae give a lobulated appearance that is described as "soap-bubbly". Microscopically; it is hypocellular and fibroblastic and contains much collagen and few mitoses.

Treatment: This tumor does not metastasize, but local recurrence or persistence is common. Wide local resection is the preferred surgical treatment, since persistence after curettage occurs in 40 to 66 percent of patients. One study has recommended "aggressive curettage" as a surgical option. Radiotherapy is not recommended because of the increased risk of sarcomatous change. Tamoxifen and indomethacin have been reported to reduce the size of soft tissue desmoid tumors and may be useful as adjuvants in the bony counterpart.

OSTEOTOMIES AROUND THE HIP

■ Introduction

With the advent of arthroplasty, numbers of osteotomies around hip have decreased, but they can still be used in pediatric and healthy young patients, who have a longer life expectancy.

Indications

Children

- Developmental dysplasia of hip (DDH)
- Slipped capital femoral epiphysis
- Legg-Calve-Perthes disease.

Adults

- Osteoarthritis
- Nonunion fracture neck femur
- Osteonecrosis.

■ Developmental Dysplasia of Hip

These can be divided according to the age group of the child.
Toddler: 18 to 36 months of age
Juvenile: 3 to 8 years
Adult: More than 8 years.

Toddler (18–36 Months)

Femoral Derotation Osteotomy

Proximal femoral derotation or varus osteotomy is indicated in subluxation or dysplasia of the hip, when reorientation can stabilize a reduction, resolve mild subluxation or stimulate remodeling of the joint. Often, it is used to achieve a congruent joint in the weight-bearing position after closed or open reduction, to allow a child of walking age to ambulate with less risk of subluxation. When acetabular dysplasia persists after reduction, femoral osteotomy can stimulate remodeling of the acetabulum, if done by 5 years of age. The usual deformity of the femur in congenital hip dysplasia is excessive anteversion. This contributes to anterolateral subluxation in the weight-bearing position and encourages superolateral subluxation in the sitting position. Femoral derotation alone is generally sufficient to correct the deformity. Internal fixation is necessary for femoral osteotomy. Rigid fixation with a small plate (for derotation alone) or a pediatric blade plate (for a varus osteotomy in an older child) is advocated. The perineum will appear wide, until the child grows and that a limp may persist for 2 to 3 months, but will eventually disappear. The osteotomy is done at the intertrochanteric or subtrochanteric region and a medial wedge removed for varus positioning, followed by derotation of the distal fragment and application of the plate.

Juvenile (3–8 Years)

Treatment osteotomies can be divided into: (1) pelvic osteotomies and (2) femoral osteotomies. The pelvic osteotomies include:

- Osteotomy of the innominate bone–Salter's
- Acetabuloplasty–Pemberton
- Osteotomies that free the acetabulum
- Steel, Dega, Tonnis, Tachdjian
- Periacetabular osteotomy–Ganz (bernese)
- Shelf operation–Staheli
- Innominate osteotomy with medial displacement of the acetabulum–Chiari

A. *Salter's osteotomy (Figs 24.244A and B):* It is designed to limit anterolateral subluxation, by improving coverage in this area. The Salter osteotomy, as it goes completely through the pelvis, allows anterior and lateral rotation of the acetabulum through an axis, formed by the sciatic notch and the pubic symphysis, as illustrated in Figure 24.244A. The osteotomy is held open anterolaterally, by a wedge of bone and thus the roof of the acetabulum is shifted more anteriorly and laterally, as shown in Figure 24.244B. It is contraindicated in patients with non-concentric hips or severe dysplasia.

B. *Pemberton osteotomy (Fig. 24.245):* It is an incomplete pericapsular osteotomy of the ilium that hinges the anterolateral acetabular roof on the flexible triradiate cartilage for correction. This actually changes the configuration of the acetabulum and introduces joint incongruence that must be corrected by remodeling during growth. It is indicated, when there is an elongated, dysplastic acetabulum, but it is most effectively done in children younger than 8 years, as there is still flexibility in the triradiate cartilage and growth remains for remodeling of the joint surfaces. Wedge of bone is impacted into the open osteotomy site.

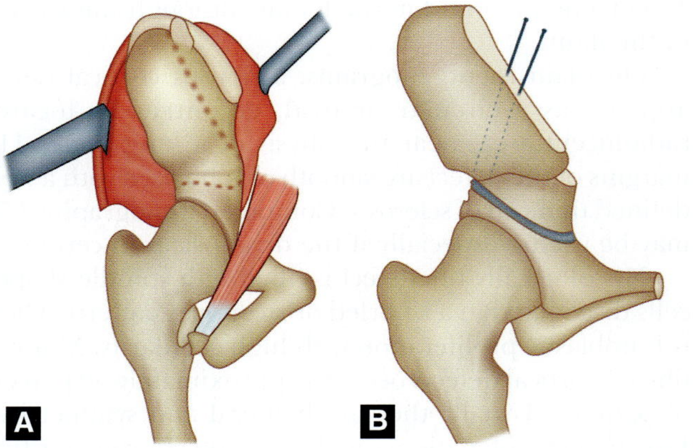

Figs 24.244A and B: Salter's osteotomy—(A) In the pelvis, it allows anterior and lateral rotation of the acetabulum through an axis, formed by the sciatic notch and the pubic symphysis; (B) The osteotomy is held open anterolaterally, by a wedge of bone and thus the roof of the acetabulum is shifted more anteriorly and laterally

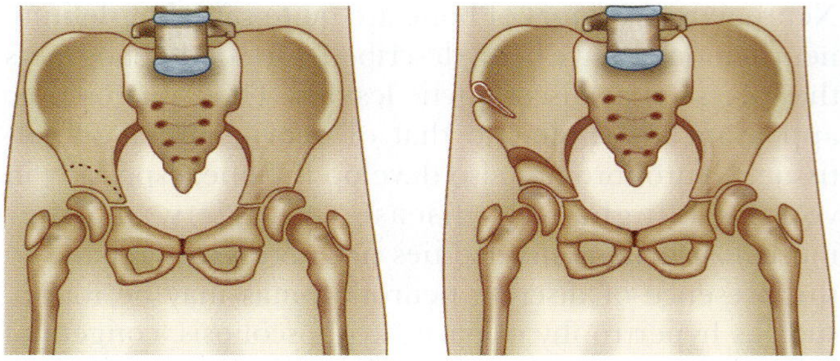

Fig. 24.245: Pemberton osteotomy

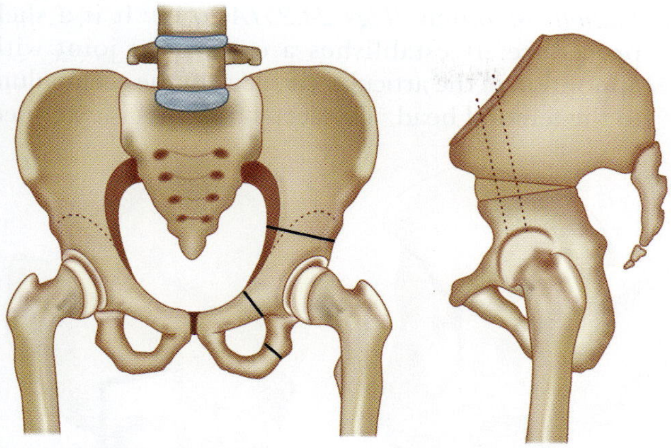

Fig. 24.246: Osteotomies that free the acetabulum

C. *Osteotomies that free the acetabulum (Fig. 24.246):* These osteotomies free part of the pelvis, creating a movable segment of bone that includes the acetabulum. They are indicated in patients with residual dysplasia and subluxation, in whom remodeling of the acetabulum is not possible. These surgeries place the articular cartilage over the femoral head.
   - *Steel (triple innominate) osteotomy:* In this, the ischium, the superior pubic ramus and the ilium, superior to the acetabulum are all divided and the acetabulum is repositioned and stabilized by a bone graft and metal pins.
   - *Eppright (dial) osteotomy:* The entire acetabulum superiorly, posteriorly, inferiorly and anteriorly is freed and a single segment of bone is redirected to cover the femoral head.

   Steel makes the pubic cut through an inguinal incision and the ischial cut through the buttock. Tönnis uses a posterior gluteal approach for the ischial cut. He felt that redirection should emphasize more lateral and less anterior coverage of the hip than advocated by salter or steel. Tachdjian performs the ischial cut anteromedially through a subinguinal incision between the adductor magnus and obturator externus, as shown in Figures 24.247A to C.

D. *Dega osteotomy (Figs 24.248A to D):* It is a transiliacosteotomy for treatment of residual acetabular dysplasia. It involves osteotomy of the anterior and middle portions of the inner cortex of the ilium, leaving an intact hinge posteriorly, consisting of the intact posteromedial iliac cortex and sciatic notch.

E. *Periacetabular osteotomies–Ganz (bernese) osteotomy (Figs 24.249 and 24.250):* It is a triplanar periacetabular osteotomy for adults, with dysplastic hips that require correction of congruency and containment to the femoral head. It redirects the position of the acetabulum, to reduce sheer forces and decrease compressive forces on the articular cartilage. The quantity of cartilage that already exists is rotated into a more favorable position. The advantages are:
   - Only one approach is used
   - Large amount of correction can be obtained

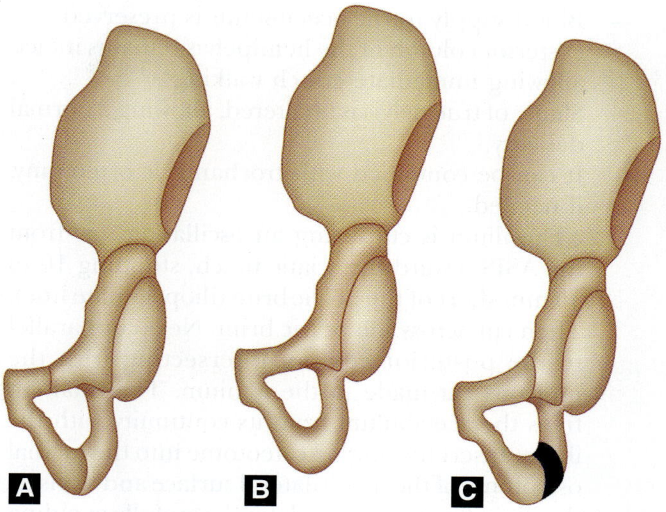

Figs 24.247A to C: Tachdjian ostetomy, where the ischial cut is made anteromedially, through a subinguinal incision between the adductor magnus and obturator externus

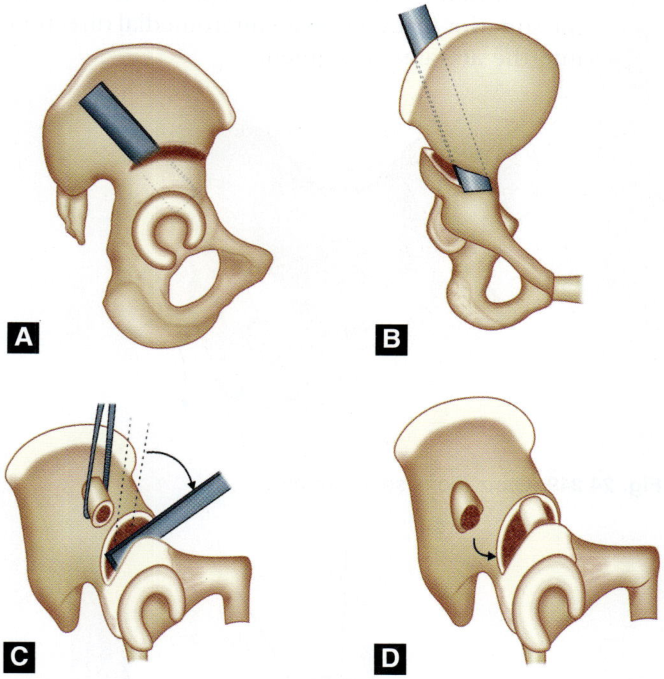

Figs 24.248A to D: Dega osteotomy—(A) and (B) Osteotomy of the anterior and middle portions of the inner cortex of the ilium, leaving an intact hinge posteriorly; (C) Osteotomy site is leaving open to accept bone graft; (D) Second graft inserted more posteriorly

- Blood supply to the acetabulum is preserved
- Posterior column of the hemipelvis remains intact, allowing immediate crutch walking
- Shape of true pelvis is unaltered, allowing a normal delivery
- It can be combined with trochanteric osteotomy, if needed.

The ilium is cut, using an oscillating saw from the ASIS toward the sciatic notch, stopping 10 to 15 mm short of the pelvic brim (iliopectinate line). Then cut across the pelvic brim. Next cut parallel to the posterior column intersecting with the previous cut made in the ischium. The final cut frees the acetabulum from its continuity with the ilium. Insert the angled osteotome into the medial osteotomy of the quadrilateral surface and transect the ilium from medial to lateral, carefully avoiding the hip joint. Reorient the acetabulum fragment, to improve both lateral and anterior coverage of the femoral head. Fix the osteotomy by inserting three or four AO 4.5 or 3.5 mm pelvic screws from the superior iliac crest in an inferomedial direction into the acetabular segment.

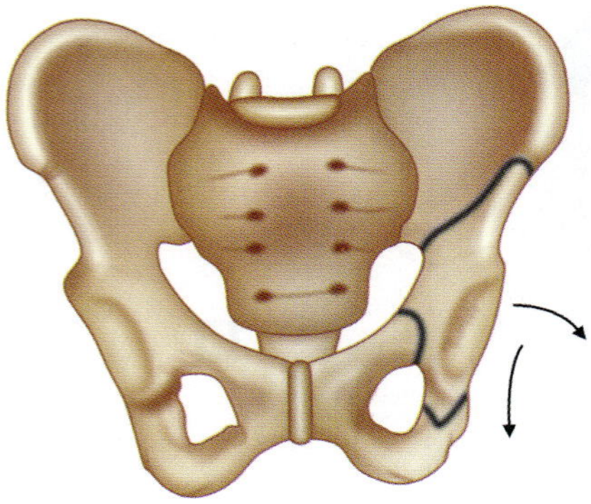

Fig. 24.249: Ganz (bernese) osteotomy

F. *Staheli osteotomy (Figs 24.251A to C):* It is a shelf procedure. It establishes a congruous joint with apposition of the articular cartilage of the acetabulum to the femoral head. The acetabular roof is extended

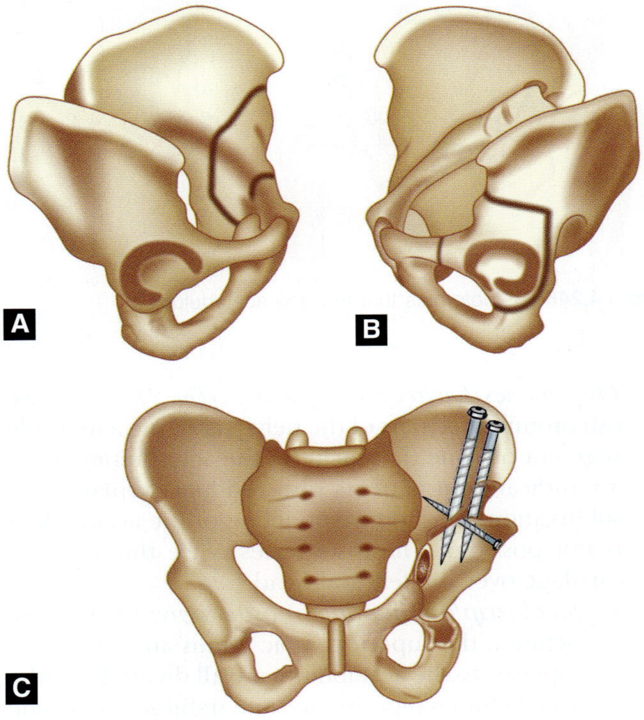

Figs 24.250A to C: (A) The ilium is cut, using an oscillating saw from the ASIS toward the sciatic notch, stopping 10 to 15 mm short of the pelvic brim (iliopectinate line); (B) Then cut across the pelvic brim. Next cut parallel to the posterior column intersecting with the previous cut made in the ischium. The final cut frees the acetabulum from its continuity with the ilium; (C) Fix the osteotomy, by inserting three or four AO 4.5 or 3.5 mm pelvic screws from the superior iliac crest in an inferomedial direction into the acetabular segment

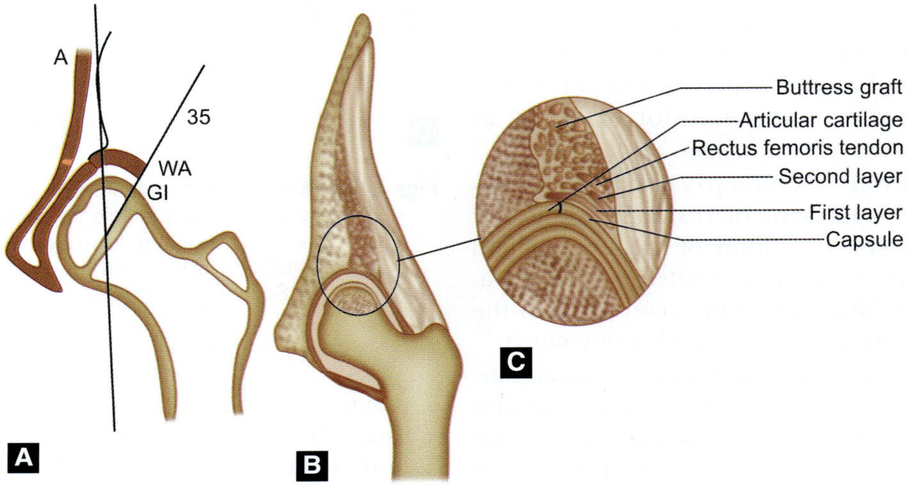

Figs 24.251A to C: Staheli osteotomy

laterally, posteriorly or anteriorly, by a graft or by turning the acetabular roof and part of the lateral cortex of the ilium over the femoral head.

G. *Chiari osteotomy (Figs 24.252A and B):* It is an innominate osteotomy, with medial displacement of the acetabulum. It is an modified shelf operation that places the femoral head beneath a surface of bone and joint capsule and corrects pathological lateral displacement of the femur. The osteotomy is made at the level of the acetabulum and femur are displaced medially. The inferior surface of the proximal fragment forms a roof over the femoral head.

Adults (More than 8 Years)

- *Lorenz bifurcation osteotomy (Figs 24.253A to C):* It is an oblique osteotomy below the level of lesser trochanter. The proximal end of the distal fragment is displaced into the acetabulum. The distal end of the proximal fragment abuts against the side of the shaft.
- *Schanz low-subtrochanteric osteotomy:* The osteotomy of the femur is done at the level of the tuber ischii. The distal fragment is abducted, internally rotated and extended. The angle at the osteotomy site points medially, abutting against the pelvis and the angle anteriorly corrects the lumbar lordosis. The proximal fragments adduction increases the efficiency of the abductors. Downward inclination of the pelvis and abduction of the limb produces apparent lengthening.
- *Hass osteotomy:* It is done below the level of the lesser trochanter. The lesser trochanter becomes displaced in the acetabulum, as the proximal fragment is adducted.

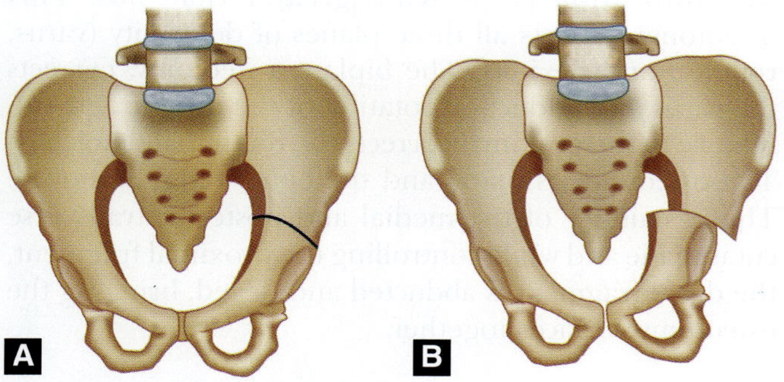

Figs 24.252A and B: Chiari osteotomy

Slipped Capital Femoral Epiphysis

- *Proximal femoral osteotomy:*
  - *Physeal osteotomy:* Dunn procedure and cuneiform osteotomy (fish procedure).
- *Basilar neck osteotomy:* Intracapsular osteotomy (Kramer technique), extracapsular osteotomy (Barmada/Abraham technique)
- *Intertrochanteric osteotomy:* Biplane trochanteric osteotomy (Southwick technique).

Dunn's Procedure (Figs 24.254A to C)

Indication for this procedure is a chronic slipped capital femoral epiphysis (SCFE) of more than one-third the diameter of the physis or an acute-on-chronic SCFE, radiographically demonstrated by the presence of new bone along the posterior aspect of the metaphysis. After achieving reduction, two osteotomies are done. The first is in the long axis of the neck to remove the bony beak. The second is to shorten the neck a few millimeters.

Cuneiform Osteotomy (Fish) (Figs 24.255A and B)

The indication is an SCFE greater than 30° with an open physis. The osteotomy is made at the metaphyseal region, by removing small pieces of bone with a sharp osteotome and mallet. Further removal of the physeal cartilage with a curet and then reduction of the epiphysis on the metaphysis is carried out. After reduction of the epiphysis, it is fixed with three or four threaded pins.

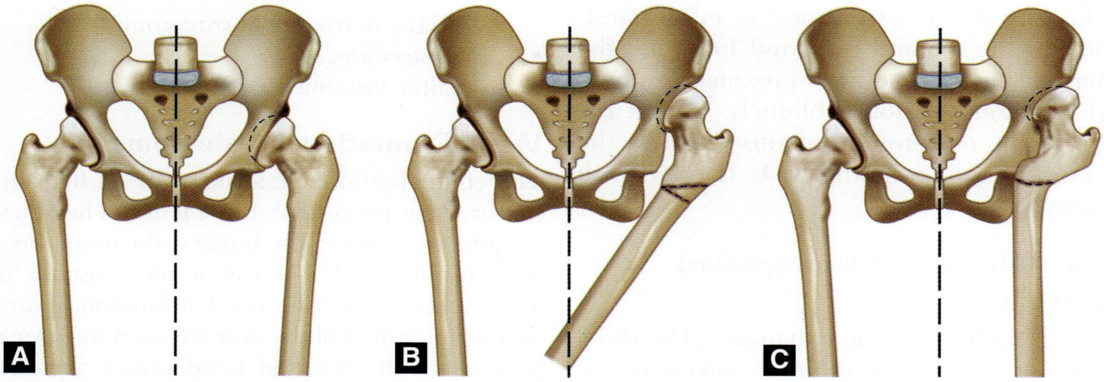

Figs 24.253A to C: Lorenz bifurcation osteotomy

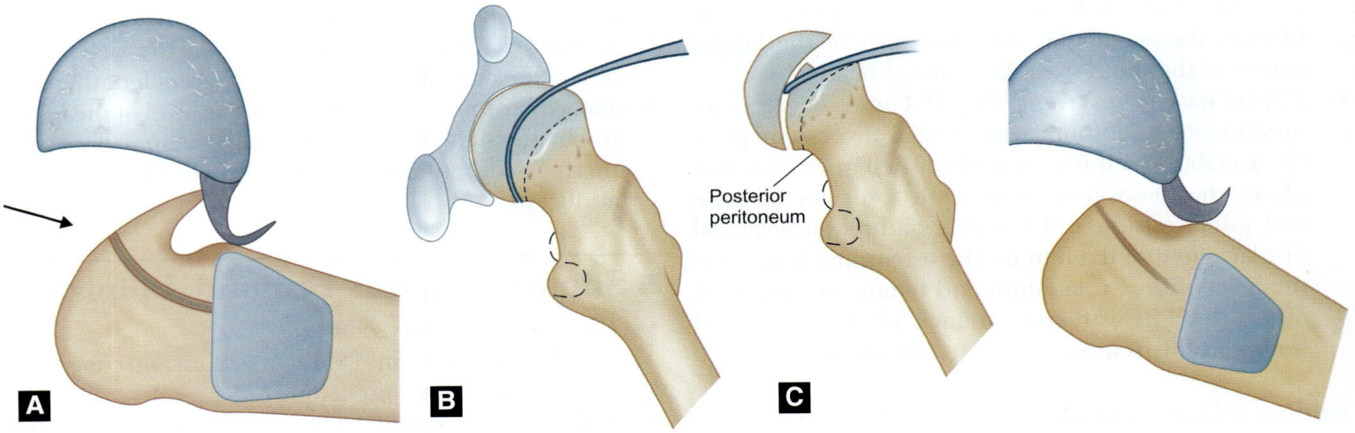

Figs 24.254A to C: Dunn's procedure—(A) After achieving reduction, osteotomy is done in the long axis of the neck to remove the bony beak; (B) and (C) Second osteotomy is done to shorten the neck a few millimeters

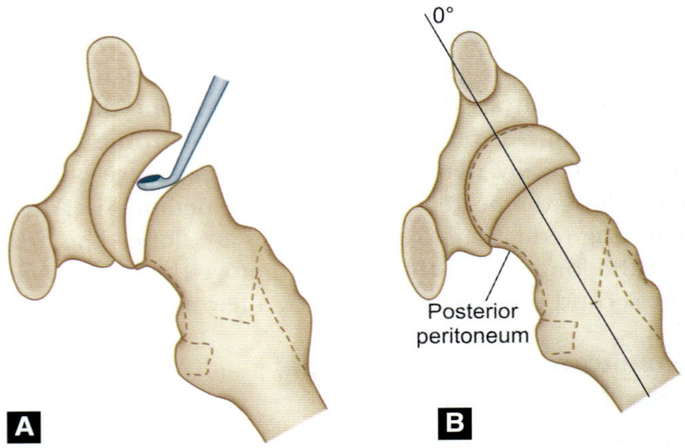

Figs 24.255A and B: Cuneiform osteotomy (Fish)

Kramers Technique

Indications are an SCFE greater than 40°, on either the AP or the lateral radiographic view. The widest part of the wedge is removed in line with the widest portion of the slipped epiphysis, in the anterior and superior aspects of the neck. The distal osteotomy is made first, perpendicular to the femoral neck and following the anterior intertrochanteric line from proximal to distal. The second osteotomy is done obliquely, so that the cutting edge of the osteotome remains distal to the posterior retinacular blood supply. It is fixed with Steinmann pins.

Barmada and Abraham (Extracapsular) (Figs 24.256A to C)

The indication is an SCFE greater than 50°. The distal osteotomy starts at the base of the neck inferiorly and extends obliquely along the intertrochanteric line to the greater trochanter. The proximal osteotomy starts at the same position distally and extends proximally, so that a proximally based triangle is formed. The lower extremity is internally rotated and abducted to close the osteotomy site and is fixed with three to four screws.

Biplane Trochanteric Osteotomy (Southwick Technique) (Figs 24.257A to C)

The indication is an SCFE greater than 30°. This osteotomy corrects all three planes of deformity (varus, rotation and flexion). The biplane osteotomy, corrects the varus and adduction-rotation of the distal fragment, relative to the proximal corrects the rotational deformity. The osteotomy is made and the bone wedge removed. The remainder of the medial and posterior transverse cut is made and while controlling the proximal fragment, the distal fragment is abducted and flexed, bringing the osteotomy surfaces together.

■ Legg-Calvé-Perthes Disease

- *Femoral osteotomy:*
  - Varus derotational osteotomy
  - Valgus derotational osteotomy
- *Pelvic osteotomy:*
  - Salter innominate osteotomy.

Varus Derotational Osteotomy

The child should have at least 30° of hip abduction to perform this procedure. If the femoral head levers out of the joint with abduction (hinge abduction), this osteotomy is contraindicated. The osteotomy is usually performed at the subtrochanteric level. The amount of varus is based on the amount of abduction required to cover the lateral portion of the femoral head under the acetabulum. Fixation is done with one of the blade plates or screw plate devices specifically designed for children, as shown

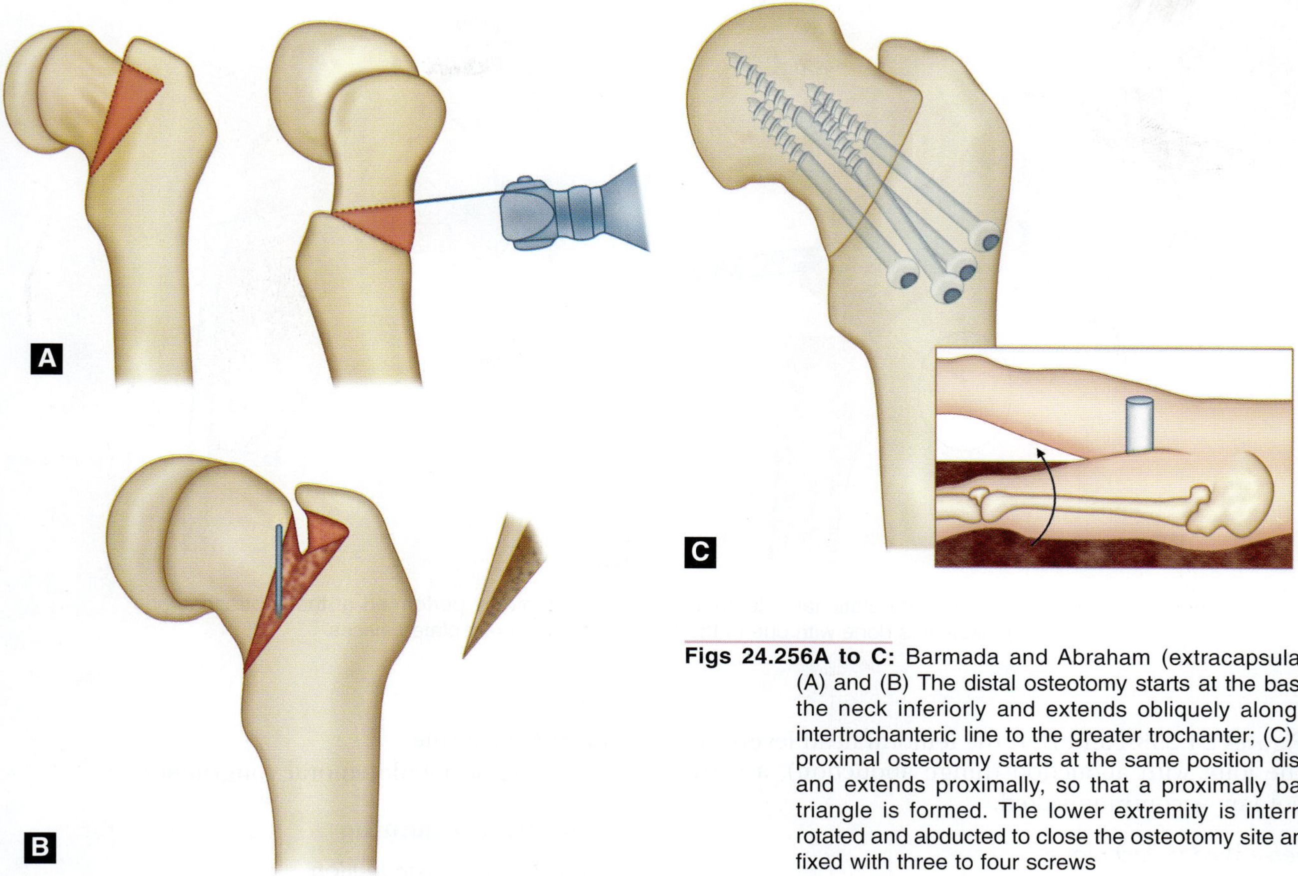

Figs 24.256A to C: Barmada and Abraham (extracapsular)—(A) and (B) The distal osteotomy starts at the base of the neck inferiorly and extends obliquely along the intertrochanteric line to the greater trochanter; (C) The proximal osteotomy starts at the same position distally and extends proximally, so that a proximally based triangle is formed. The lower extremity is internally rotated and abducted to close the osteotomy site and is fixed with three to four screws

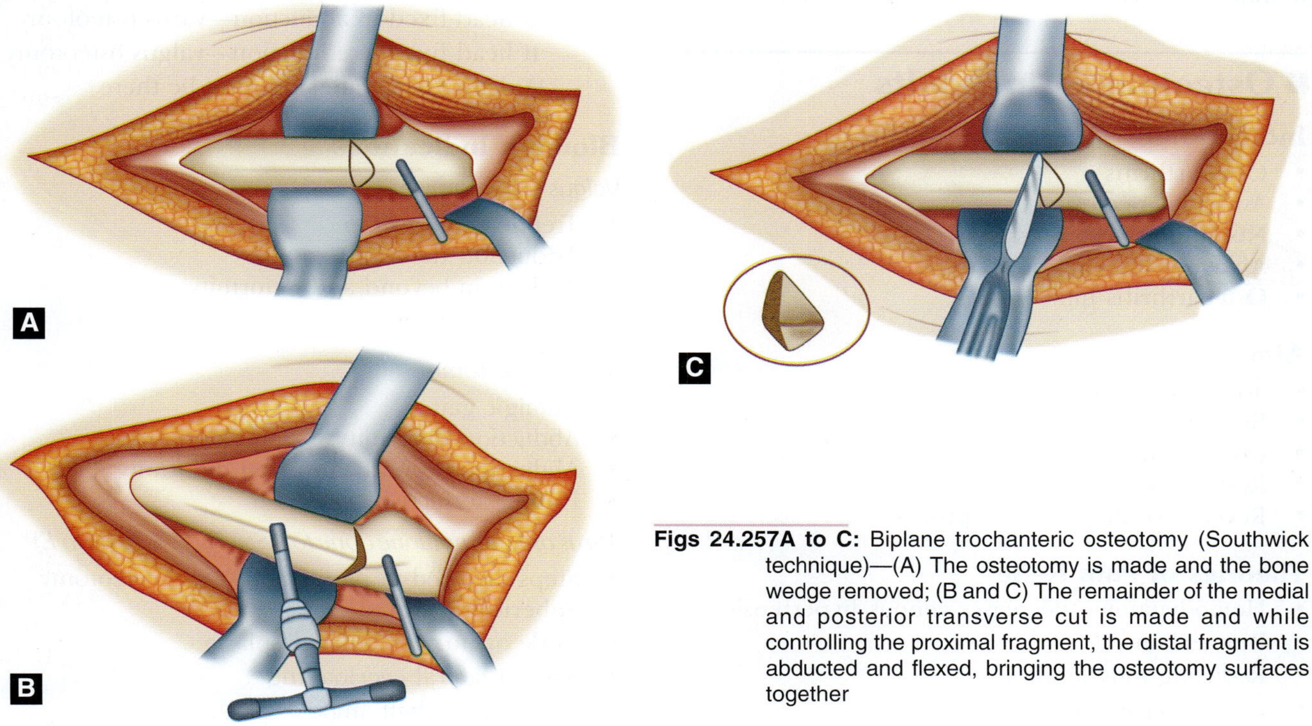

Figs 24.257A to C: Biplane trochanteric osteotomy (Southwick technique)—(A) The osteotomy is made and the bone wedge removed; (B and C) The remainder of the medial and posterior transverse cut is made and while controlling the proximal fragment, the distal fragment is abducted and flexed, bringing the osteotomy surfaces together

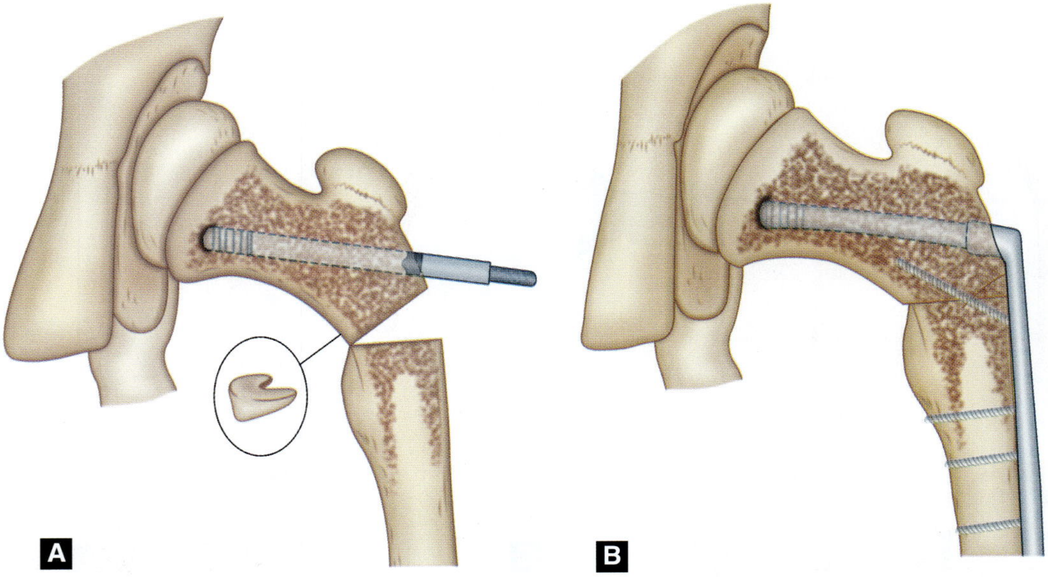

Figs 24.258A and B: Varus derotational osteotomy—(A) The osteotomy performed at the subtrochanteric level; (B) Fixation is done with one of the blade plates or screw plate devices

in Figures 24.258A and B. If the femoral head levers out of the joint with abduction (hinge abduction), a varus osteotomy is contraindicated.

Reverse Wedge Technique

Removal of wedge one half of calculated height medially and inserting laterally and fixation with pre-bend plate. Advantage are: (1) shortening minimized and (2) minimum wedge. POP (hip spica) applied for 6 to 8 weeks.

Osteotomies in Adults

Indications

- Osteoarthritis
- Avascular necrosis
- Non-union neck femur
- Ankylosis after septic arthritis
- Osteoarthritis hip.

Aim

- To relieve pain
- Restoration of motion
- Correction of deformity
- Restoration of stability
- Reversal of degenerative process.

Theories of Pain Relief

- Hemodynamic—decreases venous hypertension
- Biomechanical
- Reducing muscle force
- Displacing fulcrum
- Relaxing capsule
- Restoring acetabulofemoral congruency.

Preoperative Planning

Detailed Physical Examination

- Preoperative X-rays—standing AP and lateral
- Hip in maximum abduction and adduction
  - If adduction is restricted—adductor tenotomy
  - If head fixed in abduction—varus osteotomy
  - If head fixed in adduction—valgus osteotomy
  - At least 70° free flexion must be there.

Blount's Indications

Valgus Osteotomy

- Trendelenburg limp
- Adduction deformity
- Adduction beyond add deformity
- Painful abduction.

Varus Osteotomy

- Antalgic gait
- Abduction deformity
- Abduction beyond abduction deformity
- Painful adduction.

Varus osteotomy alone done for (See Figs 24.187A to E)

- Steps involved in performing varus osteotomy
- Spherical head
- Little or no acetabular dysplasia
- Sign of lateral overloading
- Valgus neck shaft angle > 135°.

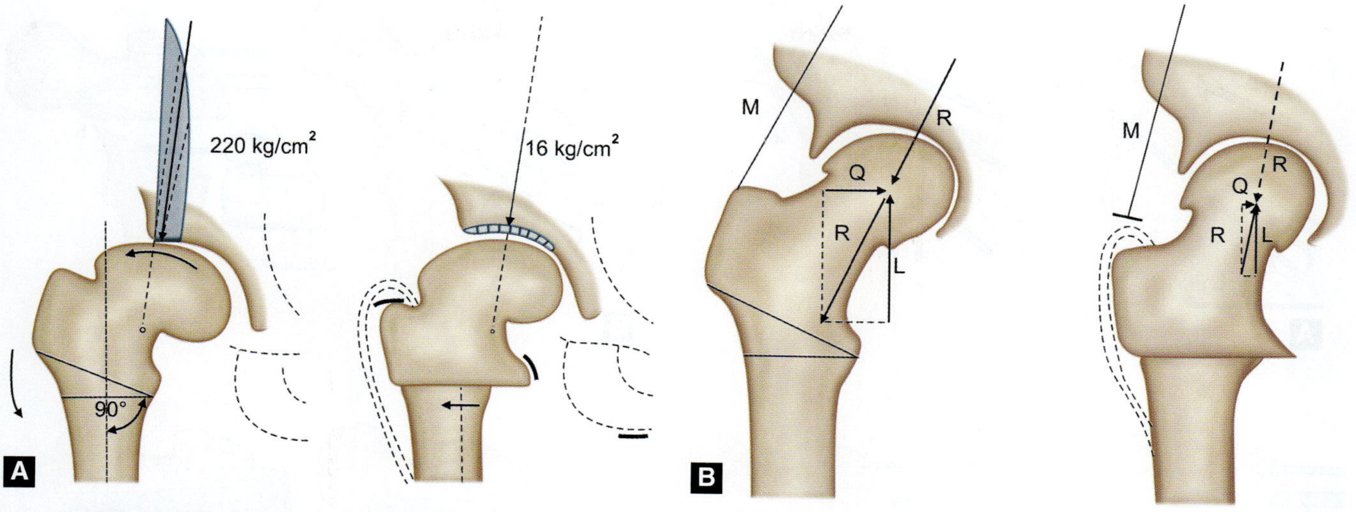

Figs 24.259A and B: Steps involved in valgus osteotomy

Valgus osteotomy alone (Figs 24.259A and B)

- In patients greater than 50 years with OA hip dysplasia to delay THR
- Patient in sixth decade with medial head osteophyte and subchondral sclerosis in lateral roof
- Seventh decade with OA for pain relief, whom THR is contraindicated
- Protrusive OA.

Pauwel's Type 1 Varus

- Medially based wedge
- Abduction lever arm increased
- Relaxes abductors, psoas and adductors
- Extension obtained by taking wedge posteriorly.

Disadvantages

- Shortening
- Trendelenburg gait
- Prominence of greater trochanter.

Pauwel's Type 2 Valgus (See Figs 24.189A to F)

- Steps involved in the correction of Pauwel's type 2 valgus
- Acetabular dysplasia, with femoral head uncovered anterolaterally
- Extension added by taking wedge posteriorly
- Increase weight-bearing area of femoral head, but no muscle relaxation.

Complication

- Nonunion
- Unpredictable results.

Müller Technique (Figs 24.260A to D)

- Lateral approach
- Medially based wedge taken from proximal fragment
- Fixed with compression blade plate
- Müllers modification—short wedge taken medially and placed laterally.

Contraindications

- Free flexion <50
- Rheumatoid arthritis
- AVN stage III and IV
- Fixed adduction deformity for varus and fixed abduction deformity for valgus
- Fixed external rotation deformity >25°
- Knock knee for valgus.

Blount's Displacement Osteotomy (Figs 24.261A to D)

- Just proximal to lesser trochanter
- Oblique direction
- Angle of osteotomy decided from preoperative X-ray
- Lateral approach, distal fragment displaced medially
- Blade plate
- Postoperative crutch walking after few days
- Weight-bearing after solid union

McMurray Osteotomy

- Severe OA with large hypertrophic loose spurs on head preventing rotation into valgus\varus, so that adduction or abduction gets fixed
- Nonunion fracture of Neck of Femur (NoF)

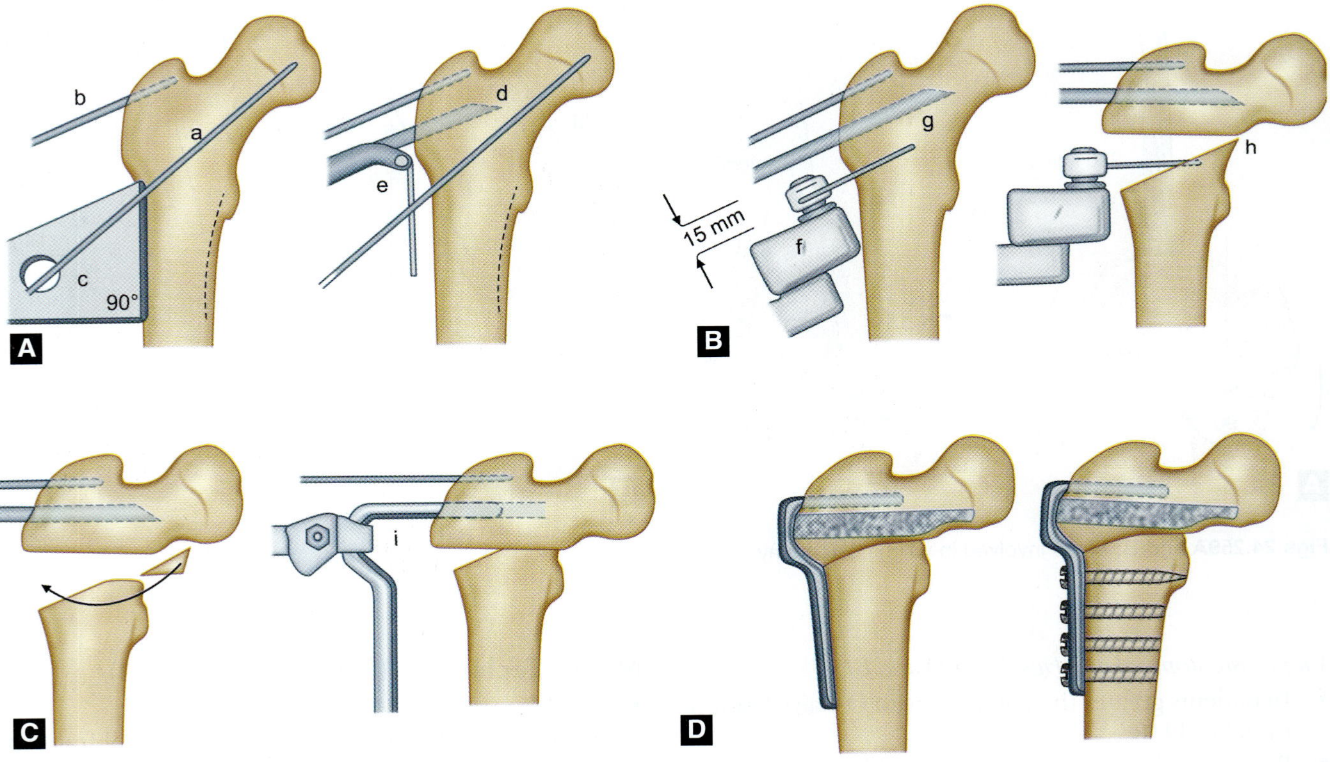

Figs 24.260A to D: Steps involved in performing Müller's technique

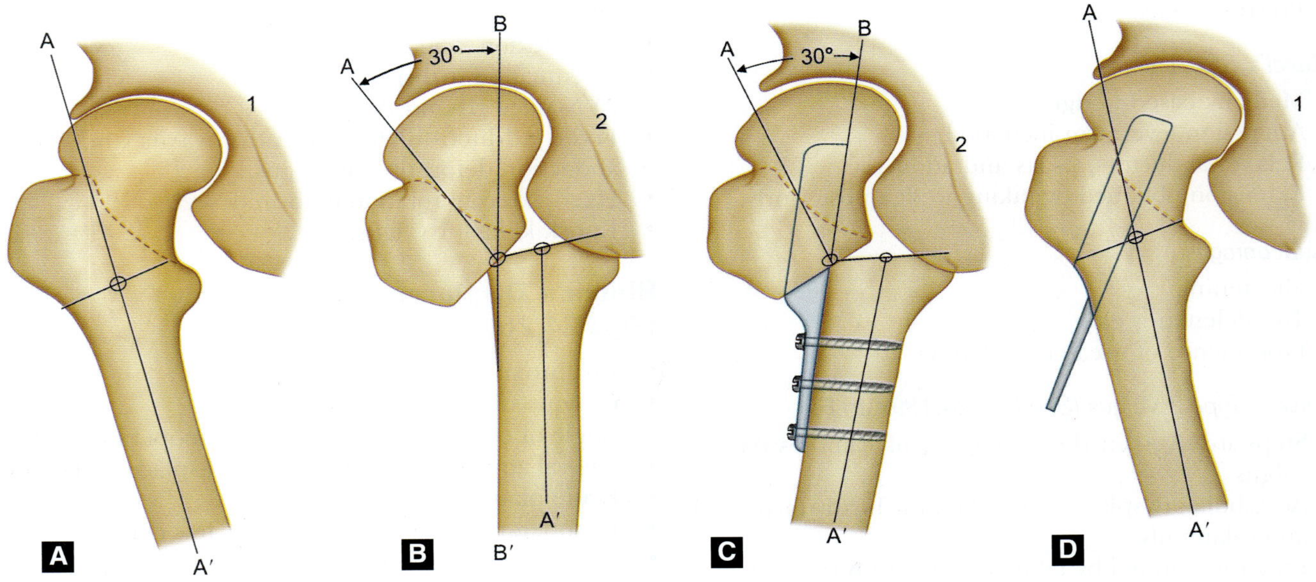

Figs 24.261A to D: Blount's displacement osteotomy

- Neither increase nor decrease weight bearing surface of femur
- Done to relieve pain in patient who are not suitable for THR
- *Principle:* Preliminary traction and adductor tenotomy. Oblique osteotomy from lower border of lateral aspect of shaft below lesser trochanter to a level above lesser trochanter medially, as shown in Figure 24.262. Shaft

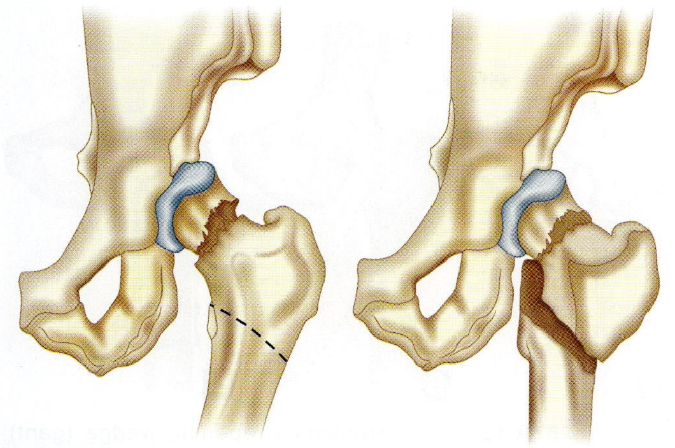

Fig. 24.262: McMurray osteotomy

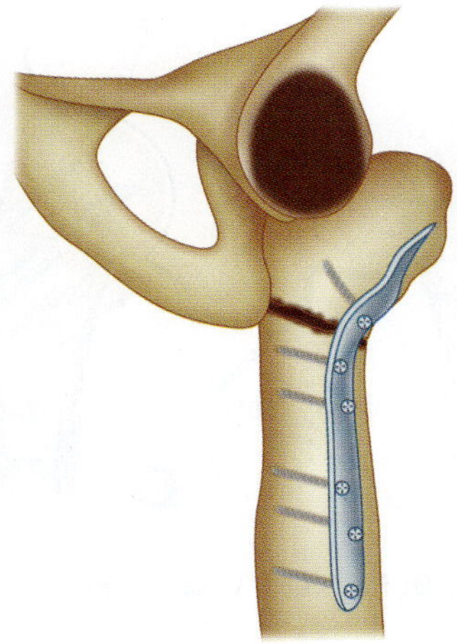

Fig. 24.263: Milch-Bachelor osteotomy

displaced medially, in nonunion completely displaced distal fragment is under head, in OA only only 20° displaced. POP–spica applied for 2 weeks
- *Disadvantage:* Instability and shortening.

Milch-Bachelor Osteotomy (Fig. 24.263)

It is a salvage osteotomy. Indications are:
- OA for pain relief
- Old unreduced dislocation with pain and instabilty
- Combination of girdle stone and schanz.

Disadvantage: Instability, weak muscular control, prolonged period of traction and bedrest.

Advantage: Lengthening, bony support, lever arm more, correct lordosis and rotation deformity.

Smith Peterson approach
- Level at tuber ischii
- Ci–opposite hip ankylosed in abduction.

Avascular Necrosis (AVN) Femoral Head

Aim

- Reposition of necrotic anterosuperior part of femoral head into nonweight-bearing portion
- Femoral head and neck segment rotated anteriorly, so weight-bearing on posterior articular surface, which is not involved
- Useful in stage I and II
- Postoperative degenerative change in stage III.

Transtrochanteric Rotational Osteotomy (Sujioka) (Figs 24.264A and B)

- Preoperative lateral view of femoral head, with patient supine, hip flexed 90°, abducted, neutral rotation intact area greater than one-third of articular surface.

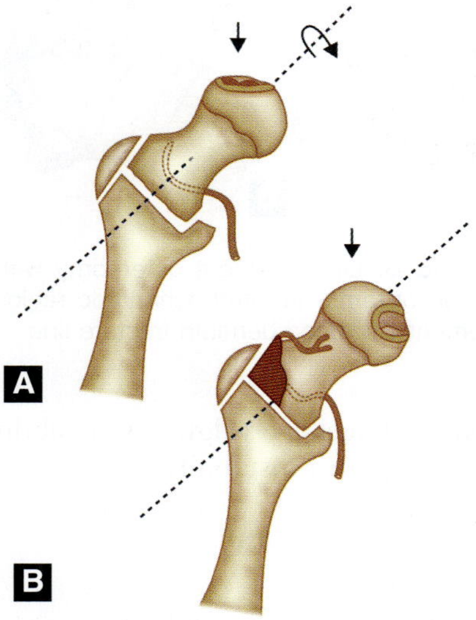

Figs 24.264A and B: Transtrochanteric rotational osteotomy (Sujioka), arrow showing direction of rotation to change the weight bearing area

- Technically demanding procedure with fairly high complication rates.

Technique: Capsule cut near rim of acetabulum. Transtrochanteric osteotomy is done 10 mm distal to inter trochanteric line. Leave lesser trochanter with distal fragment and head rotated 45° to 90°. Postoperative skin traction given for 3 weeks, weight-bearing for 8 weeks and crutches for a year.

Nonunion Fracture of Neck of Femur

- Children, adults <60 years with viable neck
- *Principle:* Weight-bearing shifted medially and shearing force at fracture site becomes horizontal.

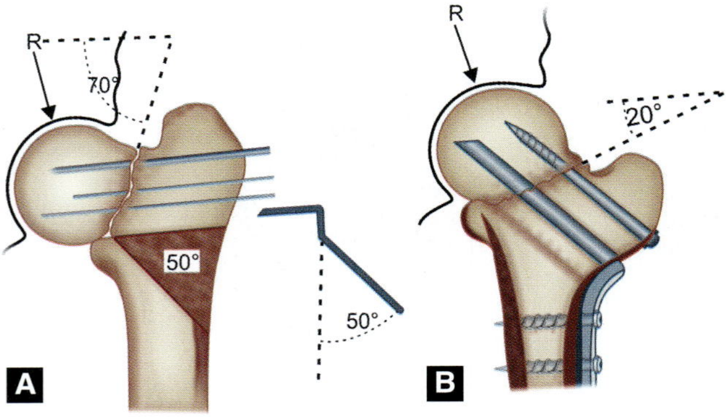

Figs 24.265A and B: Pauwel's "y" osteotomy

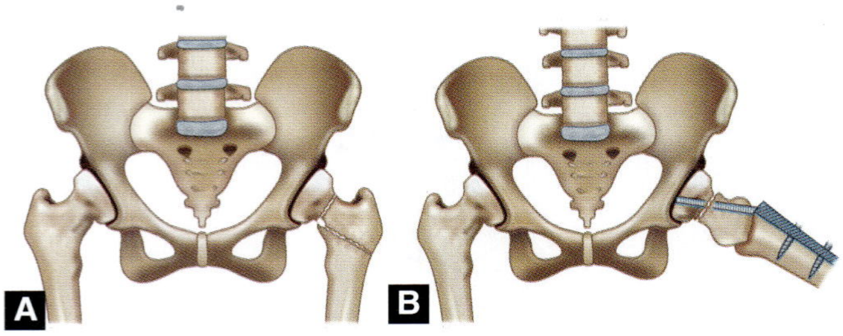

Figs 24.266A and B: Displacement osteotomy with horizontal section of femur in intertrochanteric region and distal fragment displaced beneath fracture line

- *Disadvantage:* Excessive valgus, short abductor lever arm, shortening and instability.

Pauwel's "Y" Osteotomy (Figs 24.265A and B)

- Produce valgus neck shaft angle
- Vascular proximal end of shaft displaced medially to bridge nonunion site
- Prerequisite—viable head
- *Indication:* Nonunion fracture of NOF with absorption of neck and proximal displacement of distal fragment.
- *Dickson high geometric:* Osteotomy below greater trochanter, distal fragment is abducted to 60° and fixed with blade plate.
- *Puttis osteotomy:* Nonunion transcervical fracture.
- Displacement osteotomy with horizontal section of femur in intertrochanteric region and distal fragment displaced beneath fracture line, as shown in Figures 24.266A and B.

■ Septic Arthritis Ankylosed Hip

Ankylosis in unsound position treated by intertrochanteric osteotomy, as illustrated in Figures 24.267A to C.

- *Transverse opening wedge (Gant):* Level of osteotomy is proximal to lesser trochanter. It is a very simple procedure, cause limb lengthening. Nonunion in adults are common and is usually unstable initially.

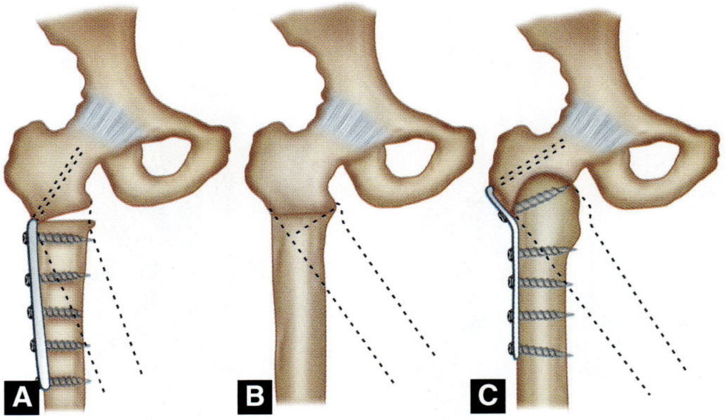

Figs 24.267A to C: (A) Transverse opening wedge (gant); (B) Whitman closing wedge; (C) Brackett ball and socket technique

- *Whitman closing wedge:* It is a stable, shortening osteotomy. Lateral based wedge osteotomy procedure.
- *Brackett ball and socket*
  - Stability without shortening
  - Extensive dissection
  - In biplane deformities difficult to perform.

SURGICAL APPROACHES TO HIP

Surgical approaches to the hip may be classified as:

A. Anterior
B. Anterolateral
C. Posterolateral
D. Lateral
E. Posterior
F. Medial

■ Anterior Approach (Figs 24.268 to 24.273)

Smith Peterson approach improved and revived interest in the anterior iliofemoral approach and now it used often and gives safe access to the hip joint and ilium. It exploits the internervous plane between the sartorius (femoral nerve) and tensor fasciae latae (superior gluteal nerve) to penetrate the outer layer of the joint musculature.

Anterior approach by two techniques:

1. Smith Peterson
2. Somerville.

Smith Peterson Approach

Position of patient: Place the patient supine on operating table. If the approach is to be used for pelvic osteotomy

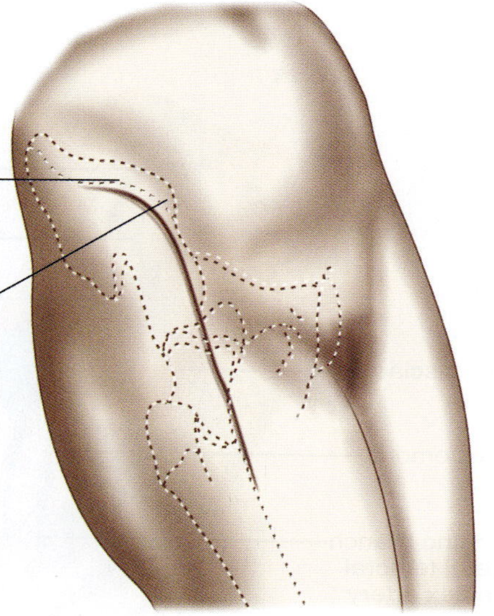

Fig. 24.268: Make a long incision at the middle of the iliac crest. Carry it anteriorly to the anterosuperior iliac spine and then distally and slightly laterally 10 to 12 cm

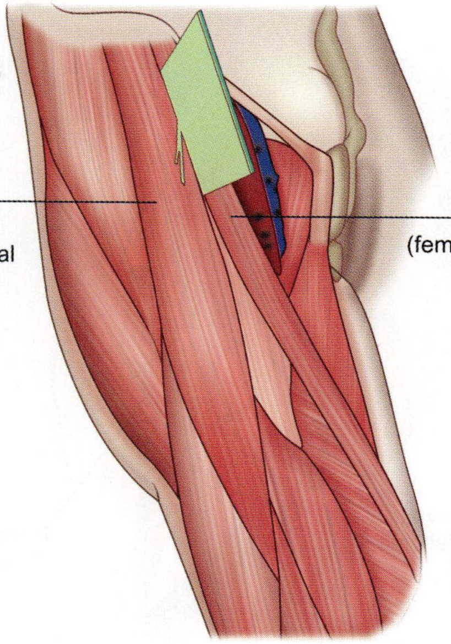

Fig. 24.269: Superficial plane of incision

then place sand bag under the affected buttocks, to push the hemipelvis forward.

Landmarks and Incision

Landmarks: The anterosuperior iliac spine is subcutaneous and easily palpable in thin patients. In obese patients it is covered by adipose tissue and is more difficult to find. You can locate it most easily, if you bring your thumbs up from beneath the bony protuberance.

Incision: Make a long incision at the middle of the iliac crest or for a larger exposure, as far posteriorly on the crest as desired. Carry it anteriorly to the anterosuperior iliac spine and then distally and slightly laterally 10 to 12 cm, as shown in Figure 24.268.

Internervous Planes

Two internervous planes are used:
1. Superficial internervous plane
2. Deep internervous plane.

Superficial plane: Superficial plane lies between the sartorius (femoral nerve) and tensor fasciae latae (superior gluteal nerve), as shown in Figure 24.269.

Deep internervous plane: It lies between the rectus femoris (femoral nerve) and the gluteus medius (superior gluteal nerve), as shown in Figure 24.270.

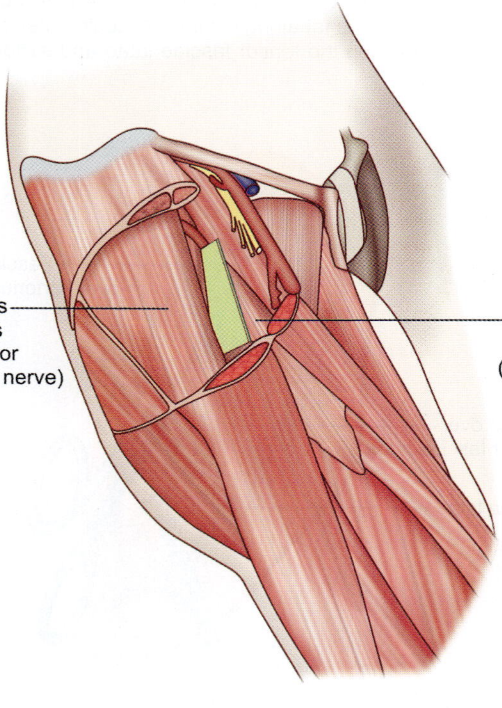

Fig. 24.270: Deep intravenous plane

Superficial Surgical Dissection (Figs 24.271 to 24.273)

Externally rotate the leg to stretch the sartorius muscle, making it more prominent. Identify the gap between the tensor fasciae latae and sartorius by palpation. With scissors carefully dissect down through the subcutaneous fat along the intermuscular interval. Avoid cutting the lateral femoral cutaneous nerve, which pierces the deep fascia of the thigh close to the intermuscular interval. Incise the deep fasciae on the medial side of the tensor

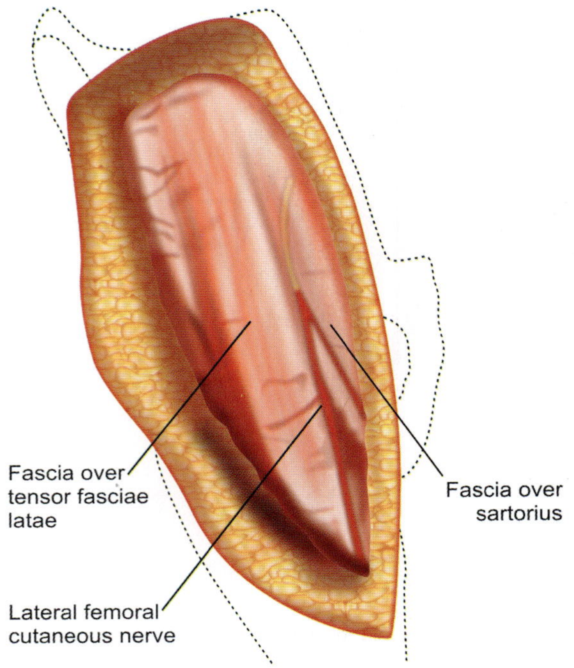

Fig. 24.271: With scissors carefully dissect down through the subcutaneous fat along the intermuscular interval in the gap between the tensor fasciae latae and sartorius

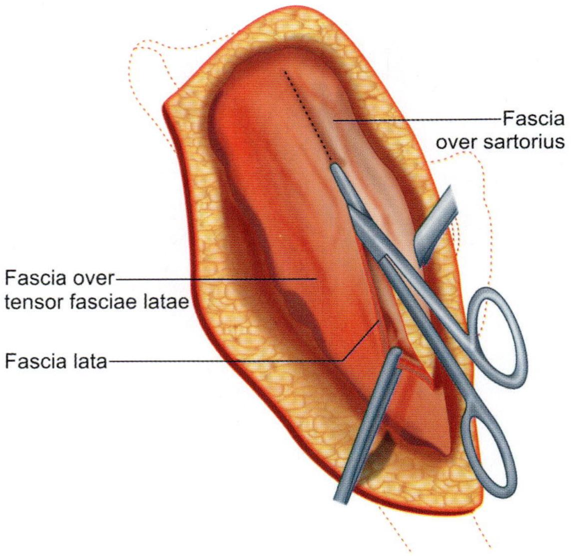

Fig. 24.272: Incise the deep fascia on the medial side of the tensor fasciae latae

fascia latae. Retract the sartorius upward and medially and the tensor fasciae latae downward and laterally. Detach the iliac origin of the tensor fasciae latae to

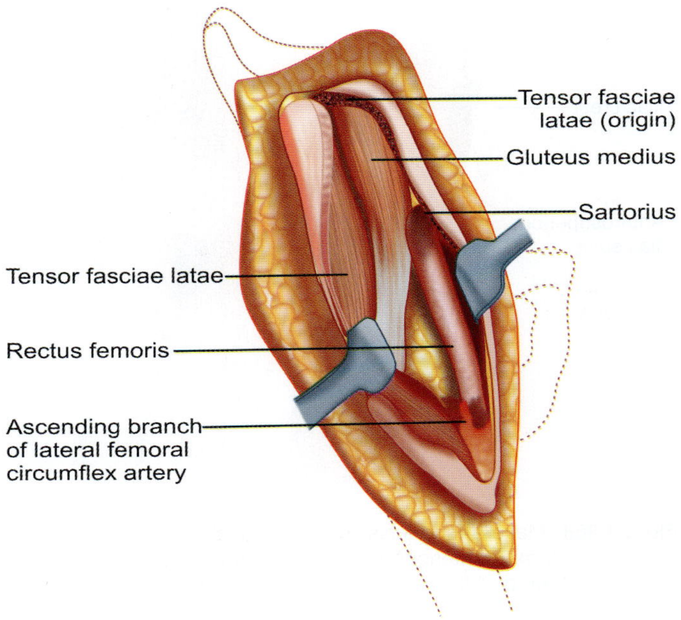

Fig. 24.273: Retract the sartorius upward and medially and the tensor fascia latae downward and laterally. Detach the iliac origin of the tensor fascia latae to develop the internervous plane

develop the internervous plane. The large ascending branch of the lateral femoral circumflex artery crosses the gap between the two muscles below the anterosuperior iliac spine. It must be ligated or coagulated.

Deep Surgical Dissection (Figs 24.274 to 24.276)

Retracting the tensor fasciae latae and the sartorius brings you onto two muscles of the deep layer of the hip musculature, the rectus femoris (femoral nerve) and gluteal medius (superior gluteal nerve), as shown in Figure 24.274. The rectus femoris originate from two heads, the direct head from the anteroinferior iliac spine and the reflected head from the superior lip of the acetabulum. The reflected head also takes origin from the anterior capsule of the hip joint. If you have difficulty in identifying the plane between the rectus femoris and the gluteus medius, palpate the femoral artery. The femoral pulse is well medial to the intermuscular interval, if you dissect near it, you are out of plane. Detach the rectus femoris from both its origin and retract it medially. Retract gluteus medius laterally. Capsule of the hip joint is now exposed. Inferomedially, you can see the iliopsoas, as it approaches the lesser trochanter, retract it medially. Iliopsoas is often partly attached to the inferior aspect of the hip joint capsule and must be release from it. Inferolaterally, the

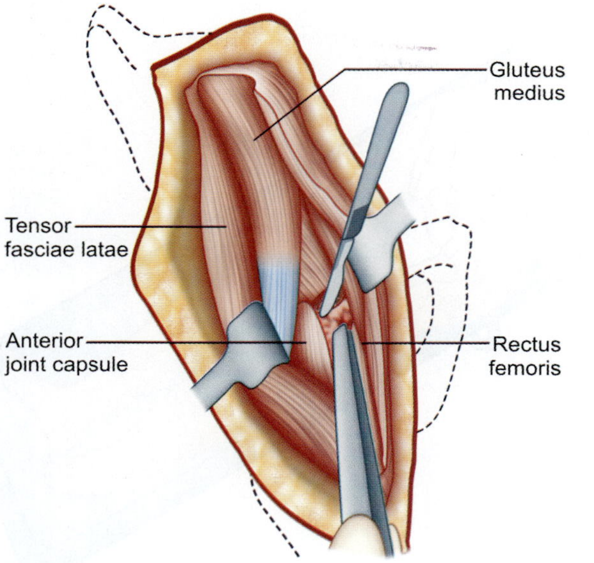

Fig. 24.274: Retracting the tensor fasciae latae and the sartorius brings you onto two muscles of the deep layer of the hip musculature, the rectus femoris (femoral nerve) and gluteal medius (superior gluteal nerve)

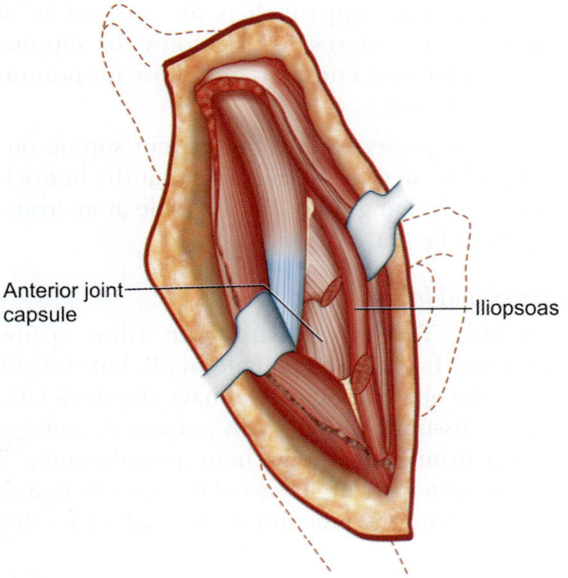

Fig. 24.275: Detach the rectus femoris from both its origin and retract it medially. Retract gluteus medius laterally

shaft of the femur lies under cover of the vastus lateralis. Adduct and fully externally rotate the leg, to put the capsule on stretch, define the capsule with blunt dissection. Incise the hip joint capsule as surgery requires, with either a longitudinal or T-shaped capsular incision. Dislocate the hip by external rotation after the capsulotomy.

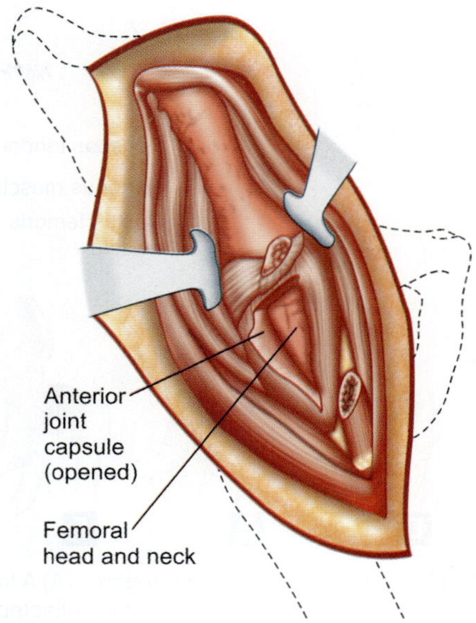

Fig. 24.276: Incise the hip joint capsule as surgery requires, with either a longitudinal or T-shaped capsular incision. Dislocate the hip by external rotation after the capsulotomy

Somerville Approach (Figs 24.277A to F)

Somerville described anterior approach using the transverse bikini incision, for irreducible congenital dislocation of the hip in a young child. This approach allows sufficient exposure of the ilium. For dislocated hip, the following sequential steps must be performed, psoas tenotomy, complete medial capsulotomy, including transverse acetabular ligament, excision of hypertrophied ligamentum teres and reduction of femoral head into the true acetabulum. Place the sandbag beneath the affected hip. Make the straight skin incision, beginning anteriorly inferior and medial to the anterosuperior iliac spine and coursing obliquely superiorly and posteriorly to the middle of iliac crest.

Deepen the incision and expose crest. Then reflect the abductor muscle subperiosteally from the iliac wing distally to the capsule of the joint. Increase the exposure of the capsule by separating tensor fasciae latae from the sartorius for about 2.5 cm inferior to the anterosuperior spine. Next expose the reflected head of the rectus femoris and separate it from the acetabulum and capsule, leaving straight head attached to the anteroinferior spine, as shown Figure 24.277B. The head may be detached to increase exposure. Near the acetabular rim make a small incision in the capsule and extend it anteriorly to a point deep to the rectus and posteriorly to the posterosuperior margin of the joint, as shown in Figure 24.277C. Exert enough traction on the limb to distract the cartilage of the femoral head from that of the acetabulum about 0.7 cm. Examine the inside of the acetabulum visually, as

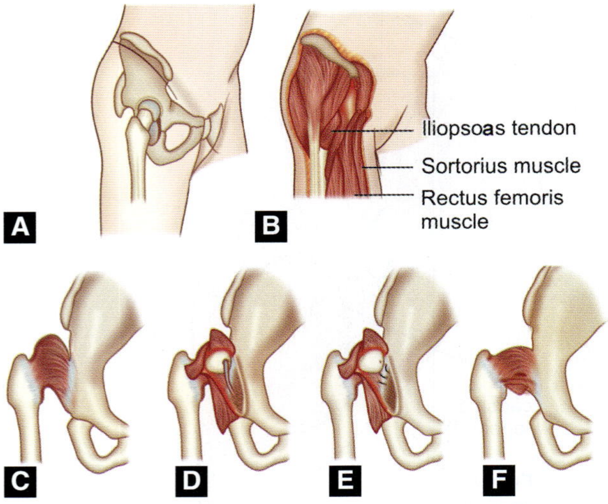

Figs 24.277A to F: Somerville anterior approach—(A) A transverse bikini incision made; (B) Expose the reflected head of the rectus femoris and separate it from the acetabulum and capsule, leaving straight head attached to the anteroinferior spine; (C) Near the acetabular rim make a small incision in the capsule and extend it anteriorly to a point deep to the rectus and posteriorly to the posterosuperior margin of the joint; (D) Exert enough traction on the limb to distract the cartilage of the femoral head from that of the acetabulum about 0.7cm and examine the inside of the acetabulum visually; (E) Radial incision in acetabular labrum and removal of all tissue of all tissue from depth of true acetabulum; (F) Capsulorraphy after excision of redundant capsule

illustrated in Figure 24.277D. If no inverted limbus seen, insert a blunt hook and palpate the joint for free edge of an inverted limbus. If one is found, place the tip of the hook deep to the limbus and force it through its base and then separate from its periphery that part of the limbus lying anterior to the hook come out. Then with Kocher forceps, grasp the limbus by the end thus freed and excise it with strong curved scissor or make radial T-shaped incision to evert the limb and allow reduction of femoral head as illustrated in Figure 24.277E. Reduce the head into the acetabulum by abducting the thigh 30° and internally rotating it. Hold the joint in this position and close the capsule, as depicted in Figure 24.277F. Reattach the muscle to the iliac crest, close the skin and apply the spica cast.

■ Anterolateral Approach (Figs 24.278 to 24.281)

Smith Petersen described a modification of the anterior iliofemoral approach that he used for the open reduction and the internal fixation of the fracture of the femoral neck. This approach retains the advantage of the anterior iliofemoral approach, but expose the trochanteric region

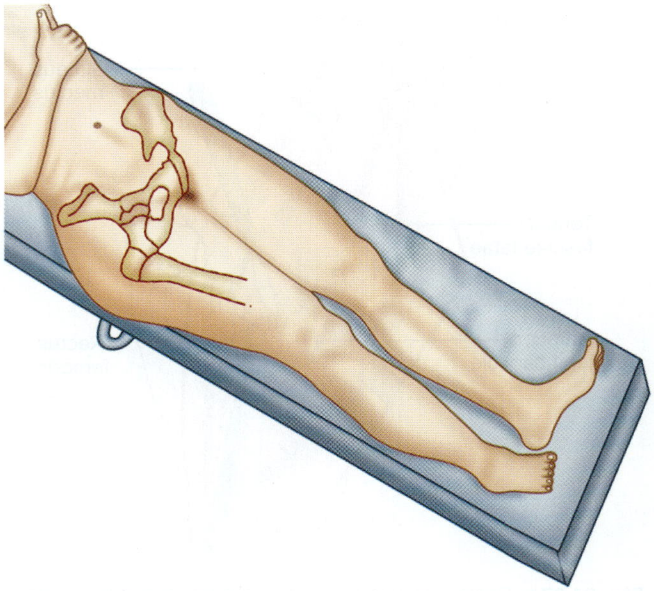

Fig. 24.278: Anterolateral surgical approach

laterally. This makes aligning a fracture or osteotomy of the femoral neck and inserting pins or nail under direct vision easier. This approach is also useful in such reconstructive procedures, as osteotomy for slipping of the proximal femoral epiphysis and those for non-union of the femoral neck.

Position of the patient: Place the patient supine on the operating table, so close to the edge that the buttocks of the affected side hang over. Tilt the table away from you as the patient lie flat.

Landmarks and Incision

Landmarks: The anterosuperior iliac spine is subcutaneous. It is easy to palpate in all, but difficult to palpate in the obese patient, who have the thick layer of the adipose tissue covering it. To palpate it, bring your thumbs up from beneath the bony protuberance. The greater trochanter is a large mass of the bone that projects up and back from the junction of the shaft of the femur and its neck.

Incision: Make the skin incision along the anterior third of the iliac crest and then along the anterior border of the tensor fascia latae muscle, curve it posteriorly across the insertion of this muscle into the iliotibial band in the subtrochanteric region (usually at a point 8 to 10 cm below the base of the greater trochanter) and end it there.

Anterolateral Surgical Approach

- Incise the fascia along the anterior border of the tensor fascia latae muscle. Identify and protect the lateral femoral cutaneous nerve, as illustrated in Figure 24.279.

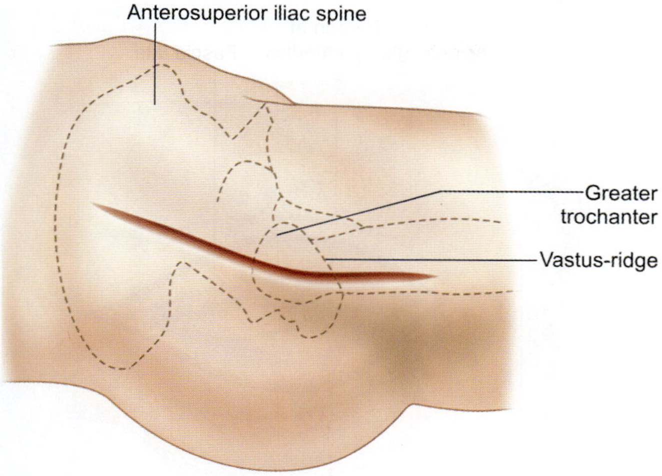

Fig. 24.279: Incise the fascia along the anterior border of the tensor fascia latae muscle

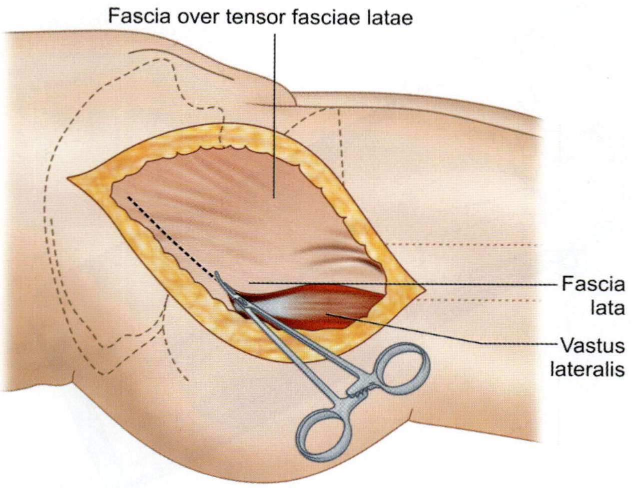

Fig. 24.280: Next cleanly incise the muscle attachment to the lateral aspect of the ilium along the iliac crest to make the periosteum easier

- Next cleanly incise the muscle attachment to the lateral aspect of the ilium, along the iliac crest to make the periosteum elevation easier. Reflect it as continuous structure, without fraying distally to the superior margin of the acetabulum, as shown in Figure 24.280.
- Then divide the muscle attachment between the anterosuperior iliac spine and the acetabular labrum. The flap thus, reflected consist of the tensor fascia latae, the gluteal minimus and the anterior part of the gluteus medius, this is illustrated in Figure 24.281.
- Inferiorly carry the fascial incision across the insertion of the tensor fascia latae into the iliotibial band and expose the lateral part of the rectus femoris and anterior part of the vastus lateralis muscle.
- Begin the capsular incision on the inferior aspect of the capsule just lateral to the acetabular labrum from this poit extend it proximally, parallel with the acetabular labrum to the superior aspect of the capsule and then curved it laterally continuing on beyond the capsule to the base of the greater trochanter.
- This incision divides that part of the reflected head of the rectus femoris that blend into capsule inferior to its insertion into the superior margin of the acetabulum. By reflecting it with the capsule, flap is inforced and repair is thus made easier.

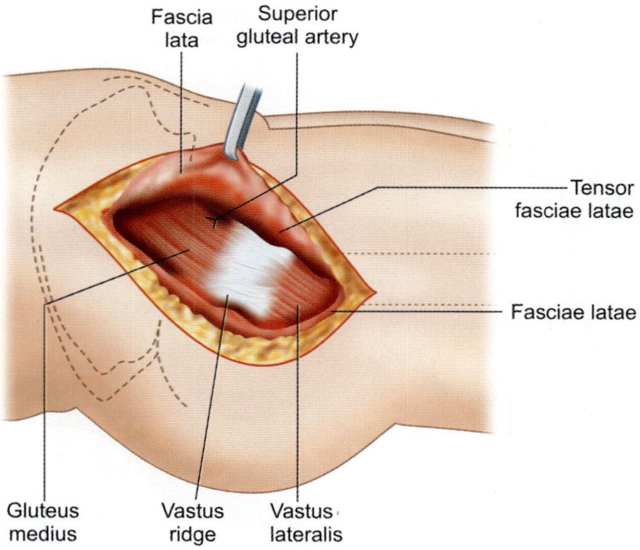

Fig. 24.281: Divide the muscle attachment between the anterosuperior iliac spine and the acetabular labrum. The flap thus, reflected consist of the tensor fascia latae, the gluteal minimus and the anterior part of the gluteus medius

■ Lateral Approach (Figs 24.282 to 24.284)

Lateral approach or transgluteal approach is described by the Wastson Jones, Harris, Macfarland and Osborne, Hardinge, McLauchlan and Hay.

Position of the patient: Place the patient supine on the operating table, with the greater trochanter at the edge of the table. This allow the buttocks muscle and gluteal fat to fall posteriorly away from the operating table.

Landmarks and Incision

Landmarks: Palpate the anterosuperior iliac spine upward from below. Palpate the lateral aspect of the greater trochanter and below that the line of the femur that feel like a resistance against the examining hand.

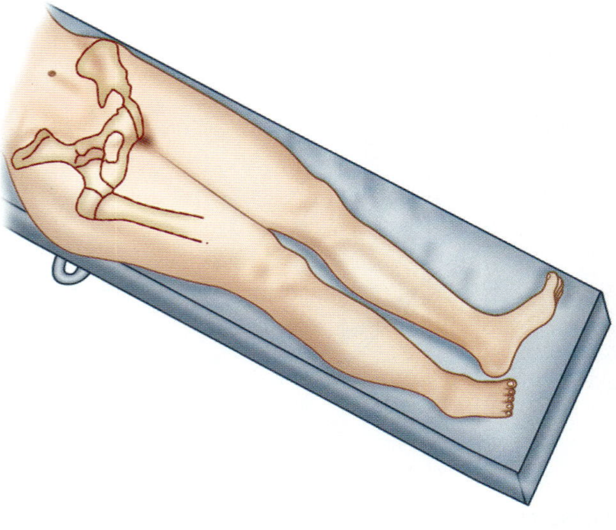

Fig 24.282: Position of the patient for lateral surgical approach

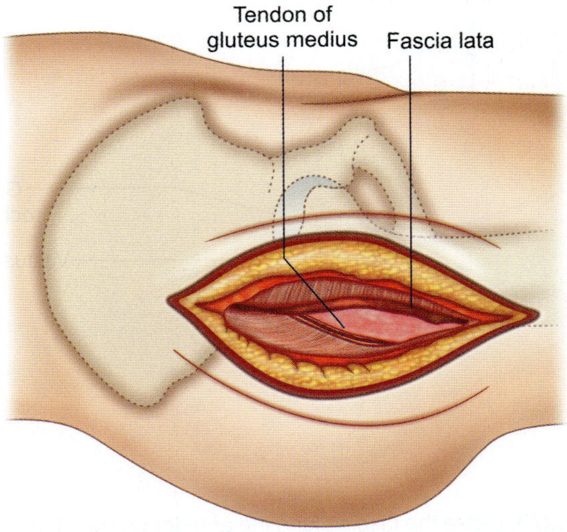

Fig. 24.284: Superficial surgical dissection in lateral approach, vastus lateralis and gluteus medius are now exposed

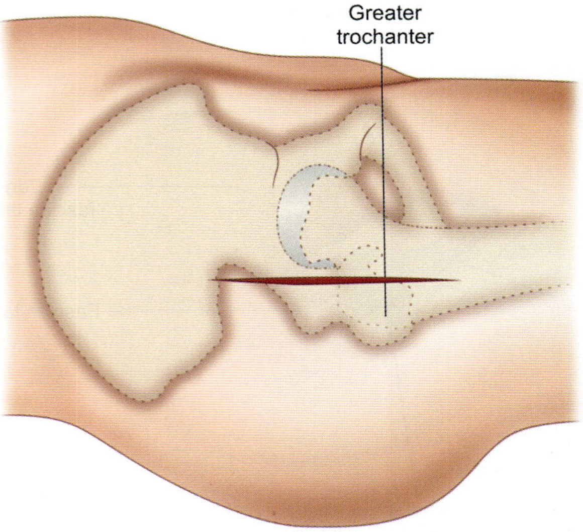

Fig. 24.283: Incision line for lateral approach, a longitudinal incision is made that passes over the center of the tip of the greater trochanter and extends down the line of the shaft of the femur for approximately 8 cm

Incision: Begin the incision 5 cm above the tip of the greater trochanter. Make a longitudinal incision that passes over the center of the tip of the greater trochanter and extends down the line of the shaft of the femur for approximately 8 cm.

Internervous plane: There is no true internervous plane. The fiber of the gluteus medius muscle are split in their own line distal to the point, where the superior gluteal nerve supplies the muscle. The vastus lateralis muscle is also split in its own line lateral to the point, where it is supplied by the femoral nerve.

Superficial Surgical Dissection

- Incise the fat and underlying deep fascia in line with the skin incision
- Retract the cut edge of the fascia to pull the tensor fascia latae anteriorly and the gluteus maximus posteriorly
- Detach any fiber of the gluteus medius that attach to the deep surface of this fascia by sharp dissection
- The vastus lateralis and gluteus medius are now exposed, as shown in Figure 24.284.

Deep Surgical Dissection (Figs 24.285 to 24.289)

- Split the fiber of the gluteus medius muscle in the direction of their fiber beginning in the middle of the trochanter
- Do not go more than 3 cm above the upper border of the trochanter because more proximal dissection may damage branches of the superior gluteal nerve
- Split the fiber of the vastus lateralis muscle overlying the lateral aspect of the base of the greater trochanter
- Next, develop an anterior flap that consists of the anterior part of the gluteus medius muscle with the underlying gluteus minimus and anterior part of the vastus lateralis
- You will need to detach the muscles from greater trochanter, either by sharp dissection or by lifting off a small flake of bone, as illustrated in Figure 24.285
- Continue developing this anterior flap, following the contour of the bone onto the femoral neck, until the anterior hip joint capsule is fully exposed

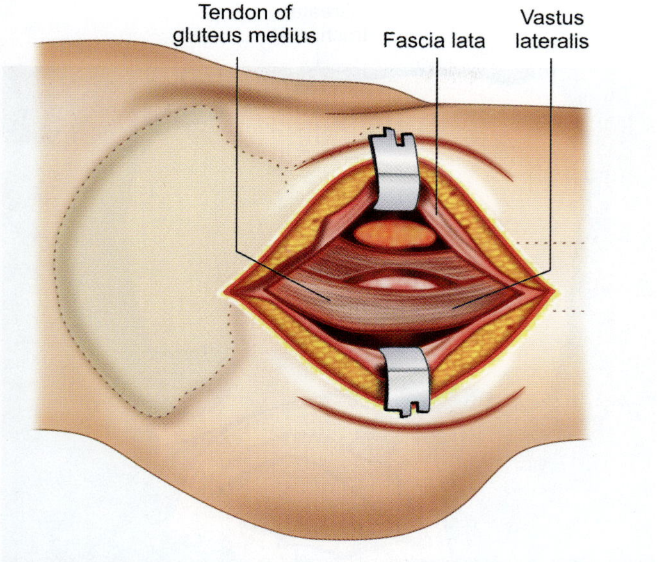

Fig. 24.285: Deep surgical dissection detaches the muscle from greater trochanter, either by sharp dissection or by lifting off a small flake of bone

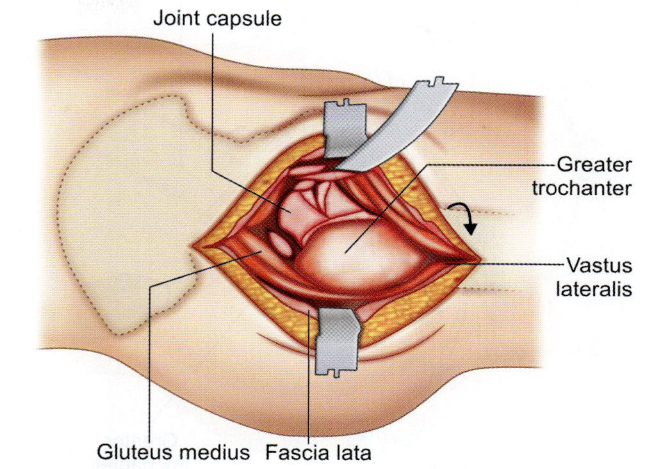

Fig. 24.287: Enter the capsule using a longitudinal T-shaped incision

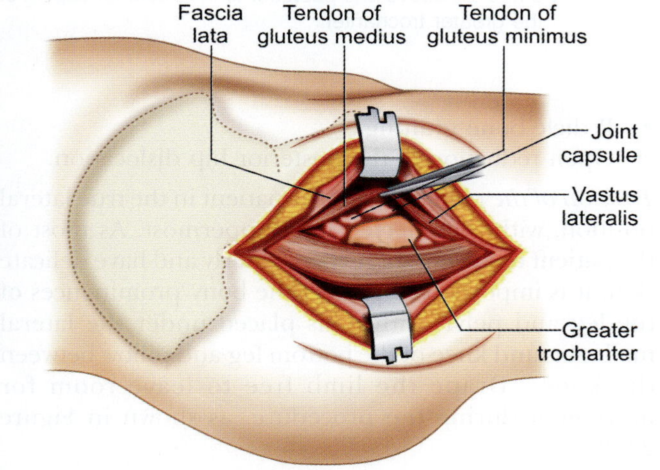

Fig. 24.286: Detach the insertion of the gluteus minimus tendon to the anterior part of the greater trochanter

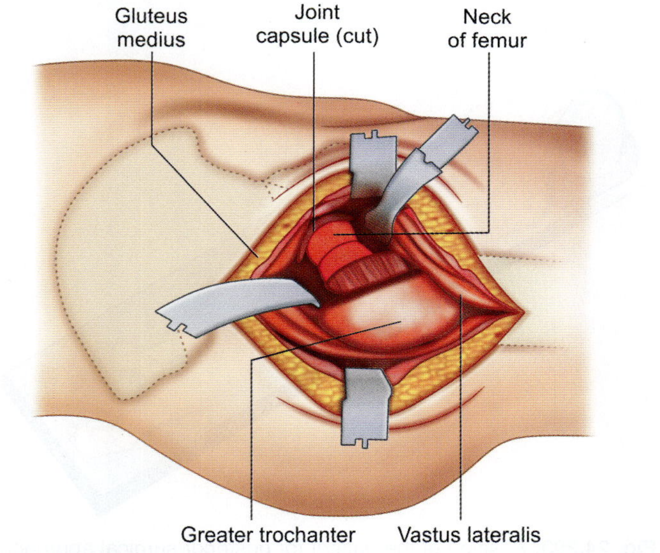

Fig. 24.288: Osteotomize the femoral neck

- You need to detach the insertion of the gluteus minimus tendon to the anterior part of the greater trochanter
- Enter the capsule using a longitudinal T-shaped incision
- Osteotomize the femoral neck
- Extract the femoral head using a cork screw
- Complete the exposure of the acetabulum, by inserting appropriate retractors around the acetabulum.

Dangers

Nerves: The superior gluteal nerve runs between the gluteal medius and minimus muscle approximately 3 to 5 cm above the upper border of the greater trochanter. More proximal dissection may cut this nerve or may produce the traction injury. The femoral nerve the most lateral structure in the anterior neurovascular bundle of the thigh is vulnerable to inappropriately placed retractor. Anterior retractor should placed strictly on the bone of the anterior aspect of the acetabulum.

Vessels: The femoral artery and nerve are also vulnerable to inappropriately placed anterior retractor. The transverse branch of the lateral circumflex artery of the thigh is cut as the vastus lateralis is mobilized and it must be cauterized during the approach.

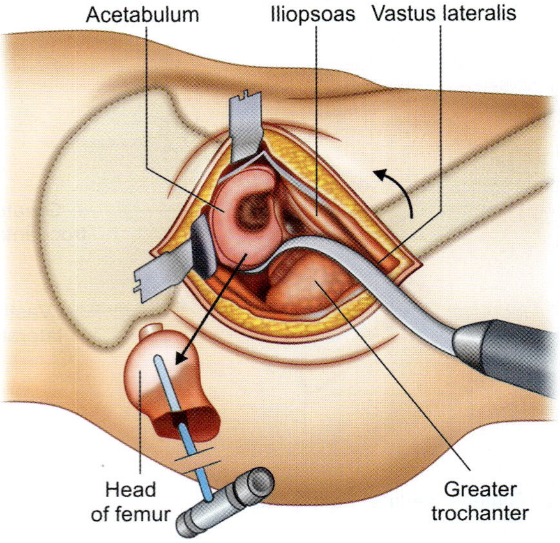

Fig. 24.289: Complete the exposure of the acetabulum, by inserting appropriate retractors around the acetabulum

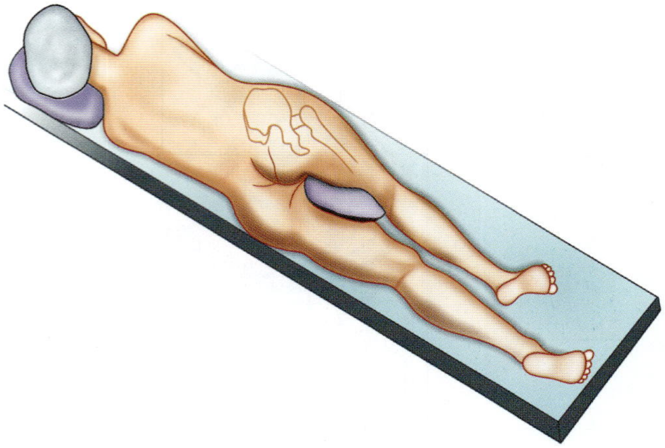

Fig. 24.290: Position of the patient for posterior surgical approach

■ Posterior Approach (Figs 24.290 to 24.292)

Posterior approach is the most common and practical of those used to expose the hip joint and popularized by Moore. It is also called the southern approach. The uses of the posterior approach are as follows:

- Hemiarthroplasty
- Total hip replacement
- Open reduction and internal fixation of posterior acetabular fracture
- Dependent drainage of hip sepsis
- Removal of loose bodies from the hip joint

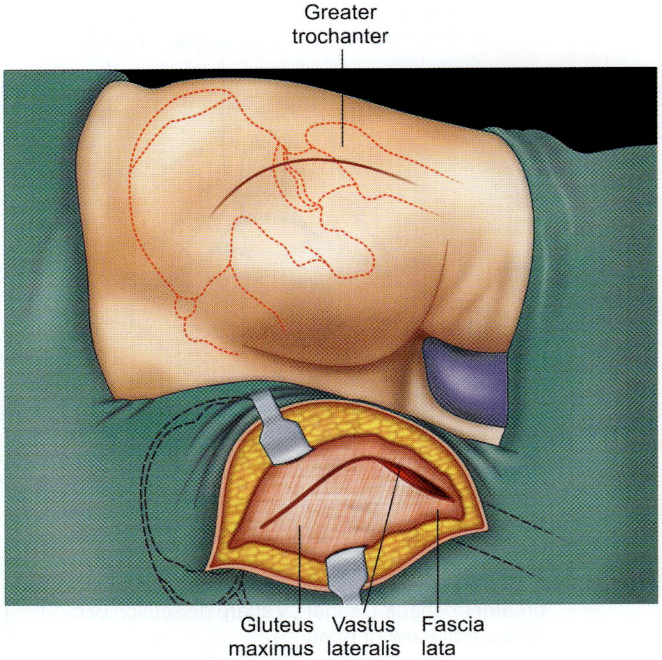

Fig. 24.291: Incision for posterior surgical approach begins some 6 to 8 cm above and posterior to the posterior aspect of the greater trochanter

- Pedicle bone grafting
- Open reduction of the posterior hip dislocation.

Position of the patient: Place the patient in the true lateral position, with the affected limb uppermost. As most of the patient requiring surgery are elderly and have delicate skin, it is important to protect the bony prominences of the leg and pelvis with pads placed under the lateral malleolus and knee of the bottom leg and pillow between the knees. Drape the limb free to leave room for movement during the procedure, as shown in Figure 24.290.

Landmarks and Incision

Landmarks: Palpate in detail the grater trochanter on the outer aspect of the thigh. The posterior edge of the trochanter is more superficial than the anterior and lateral portions and as such it is easier to palpate.

Incision: Make a 10 to 15 cm curved incision centered on the posterior aspect of the greater trochanter. Begin your incision some 6 to 8 cm above and posterior to the posterior aspect of the greater trochanter. The part of the incision that runs from this point to the posterior aspect of the trochanter is in line with the fiber of the gluteus maximus, as illustrated in Figures 24.291 and 24.292.

Internervous plane: There is no true internervous plane in this approach. However, gluteus maximus, which is split

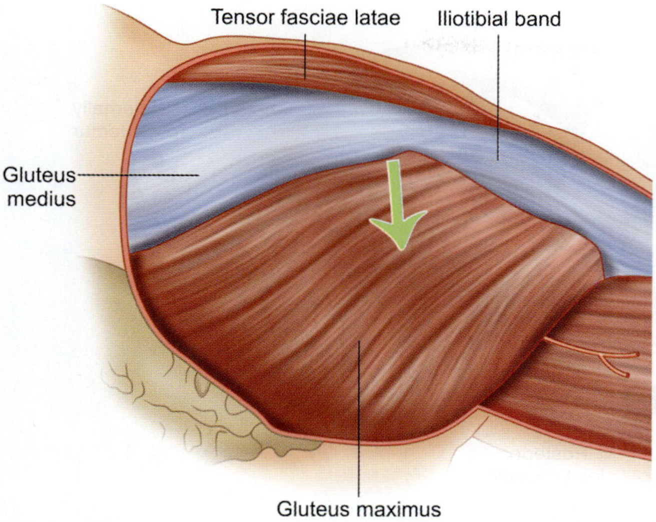

Fig. 24.292: The part of the incision runs from this point to the posterior aspect of the trochanter is in line with the fiber of the gluteus maximus, arrow showing line of gluteus maximus fibers

in the line of its fibers, is not significantly denervated because it receives its nerve supply well medial to the split.

Superficial Surgical Dissection

- Incise the fascia lata on the lateral aspect of the femur to uncover the vastus lateralis
- Lengthen the fascial incision superiorly in line with the skin incision and split the fibers of the gluteus maximus by blunt dissection, as shown in Figure 24.293
- The gluteus maximus received its blood supply from the superior and inferior gluteal arteries, which enter the deep surface of the muscle
- In addition to the arterial bleeding venous bleeding must be anticipated
- If you split the muscle gently, you may be able to pick up, coagulate and cut the crossing vessels before they are stretched and avulsed by blunt dissection of the split.

Deep Surgical Dissection (Figs 24.294 to 24.297)

- Retract the fibers of the split gluteus maximus and the deep fascia of the thigh
- Underneath is the posterolateral aspect of the hip joint, still covered by short external rotators muscles, which attach to the upper part of the posterolateral aspect of the femur
- Remember that the sciatic nerve leave the pelvis through the greater sciatic notch and runs down the back of the thigh on the short external rotator muscle

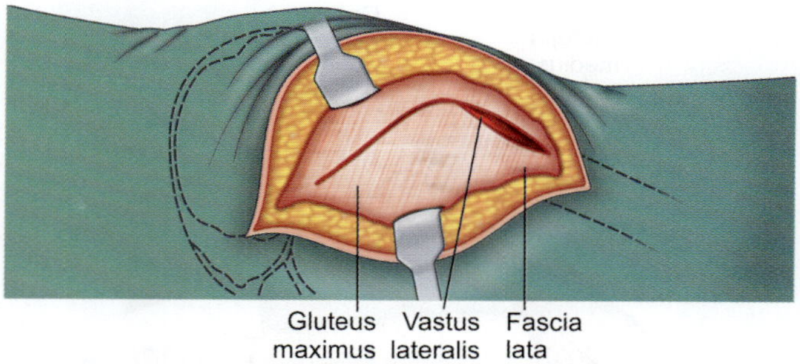

Fig. 24.293: Lengthen the fascial incision superiorly in line with the skin incision and split the fibers of the gluteus maximus by blunt dissection

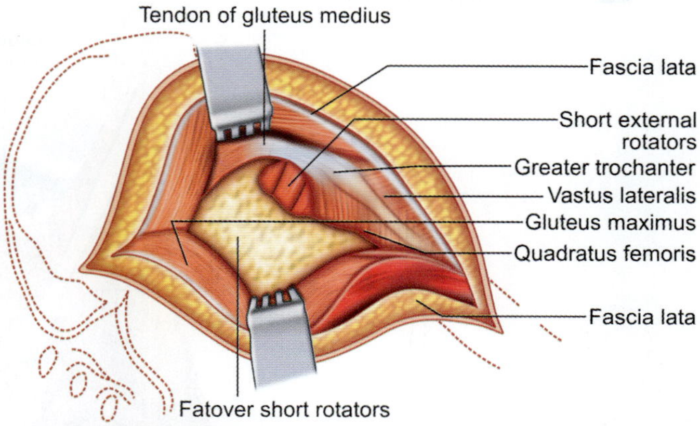

Fig. 24.294: Retract the fibers of the split gluteus maximus and the deep fascia of the thigh

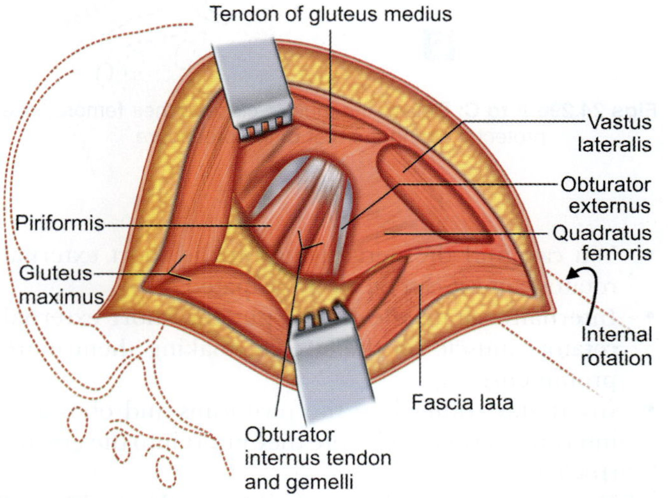

Fig. 24.295: Underneath is the posterolateral aspect of the hip joint, still covered by short external rotators muscles, which attach to the upper part of the posterolateral aspect of the femur

- The nerve crosses obturator internus, two gamelli and the quadratus femoris before disappearing beneath the femoral attachment of the gluteus maximus muscle

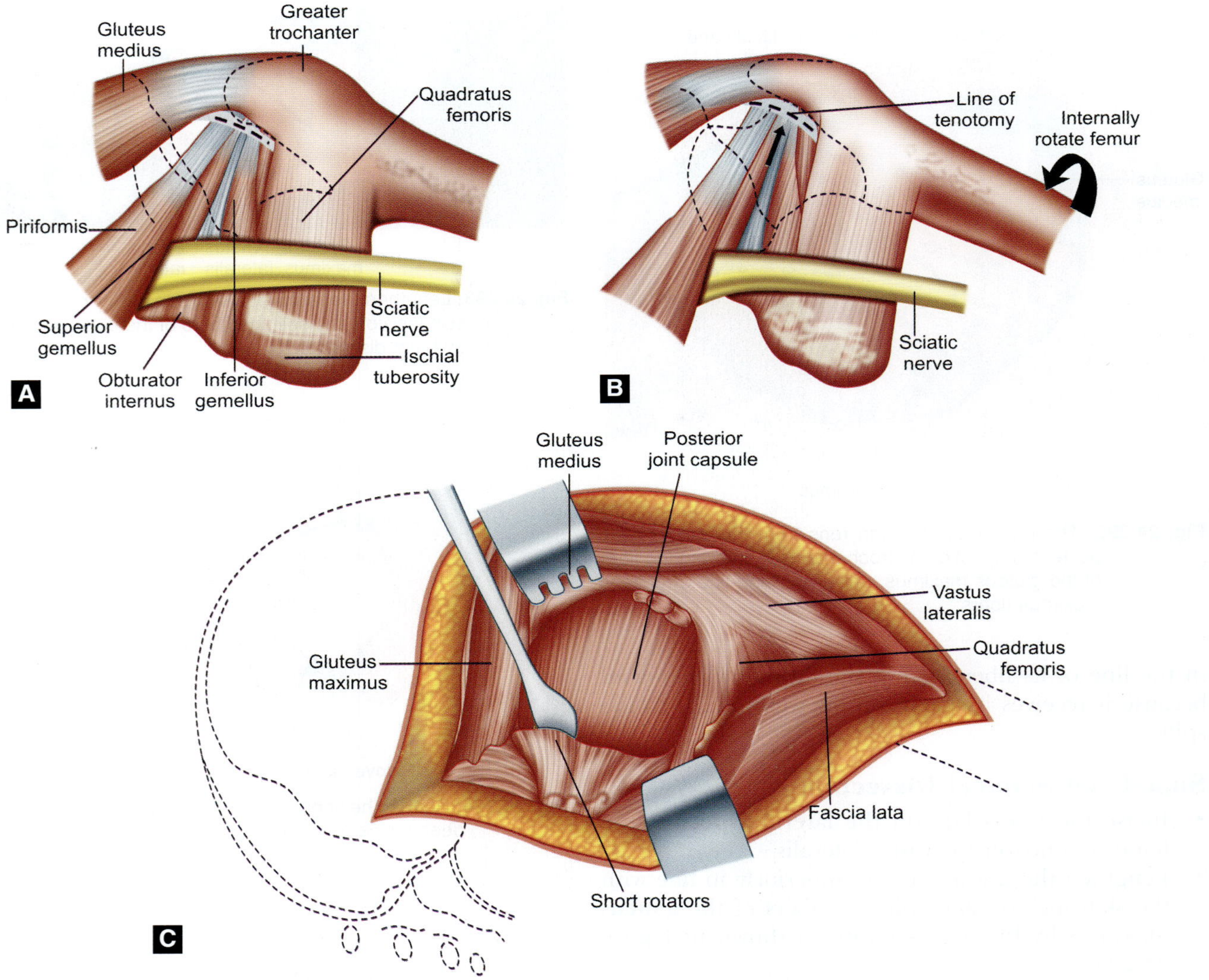

Figs 24.296 A to C: Detach the muscle close to their femoral insertion and reflect them backward, laying them over the sciatic nerve to protect it during the rest of the procedure

- You can find the nerve lying on the short external rotators and it can be easily palpated
- Internally rotate the hip to put the short external rotators muscle on the stretch (making them more prominent)
- Insert stay suture into the piriformis and obturator internus tendon just before they insert into the greater trochanter
- Detach the muscle close to their femoral insertion and reflect them backward, laying them over the sciatic nerve to protect it during the rest of the procedure, as shown in Figures 24.296A to C
- The posterior aspect of the hip joint capsule is now fully exposed
- The joint capsule can be incised with a longitudinal or T-shaped incision

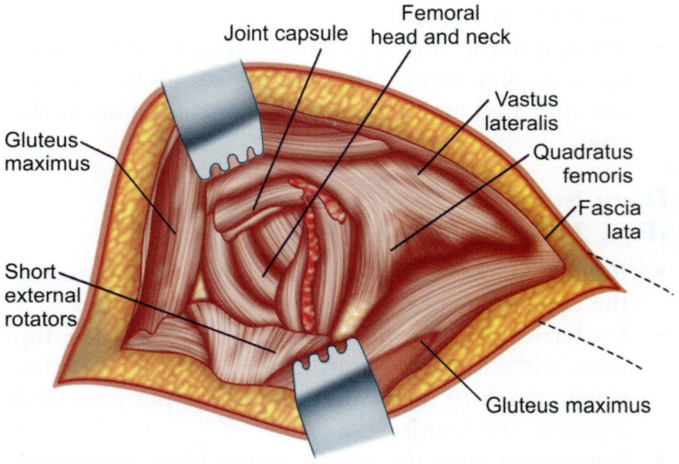

Fig. 24.297: Posterior joint capsulotomy exposed the femoral head and neck

- Dislocation of the hip is achieved by internal rotation after capsulotomy
- Posterior joint capsulotomy will have exposed the femoral head and neck.

■ Medial Approach (Figs 24.298 to 24.300)

The medial approach attributed to Ludloff was originally designed for surgery on flexed, abducted and externally rotated hips. The uses of the medial approach in open reduction of congenital dislocation of the hip, include biopsy and treatment of the tumors of the inferior portion of the femoral neck, in release of the psoas muscle and obturator neurectomy.

Position of the patient (Fig. 24.298): Place the patient supine on the operating table with affected hip flexed, abducted and externally rotated.

Landmarks and Incision

Landmarks: Palpate the adductor longus from the medial side of the thigh and follow it up to its origin at the pelvis in the angle between the pubic crest and symphysis. With your finger anchored on the greater trochanter, move your thumb along the inguinal creases medially and obliquely downward until you can feel the pubic tubercle.

Incision: Make a longitudinal incision on the medial side of the thigh, starting at a point 3 cm below the pubic tubercle. The incision runs down over the adductor longus, as shown in Figure 24.299.

Internervous plane: The superficial dissection does not exploit an internervous plane, since both the adductor longus and gracilis are innervated by the anterior division of the obturator nerve. The plane nevertheless safe for the dissection, both muscles receive their nerve supplies proximal to the dissection. More deeply, the plane of the dissection lies between the adductor brevis and adductor magnus. The adductor brevis is supplied by the anterior branch of the obturator nerve. The adductor magnus has two nerve supplies—its adductor portion is supplies by the posterior division of the obturator nerve and its ischial portion is supplied by the tibial part of sciatic nerve.

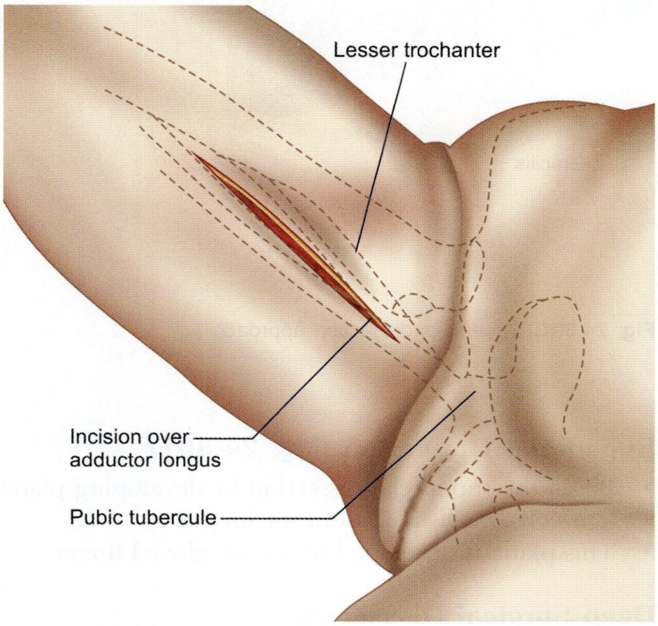

Fig. 24.299: A longitudinal incision is made on the medial side of the thigh, starting at a point 3 cm below the pubic tubercle. The incision runs down over the adductor longus

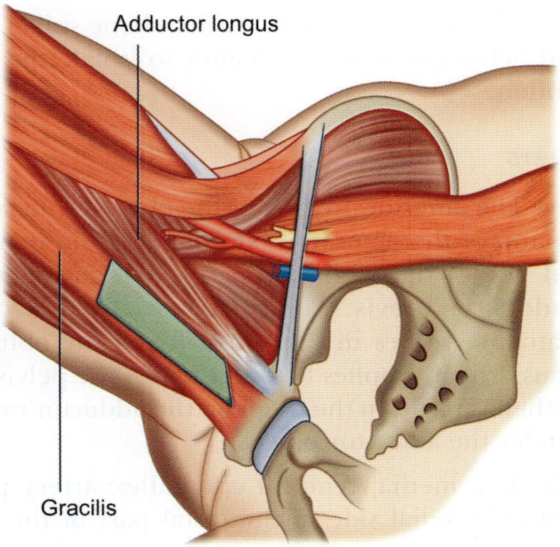

Fig. 24.300: The plane of the dissection lies between the adductor brevis and adductor magnus

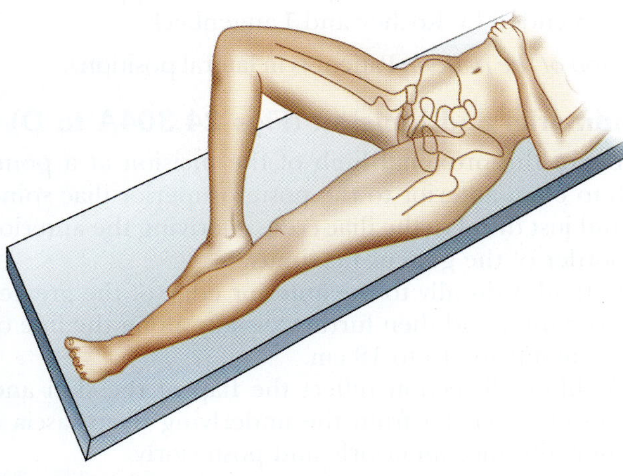

Fig. 24.298: Patient's position in medial surgical approach

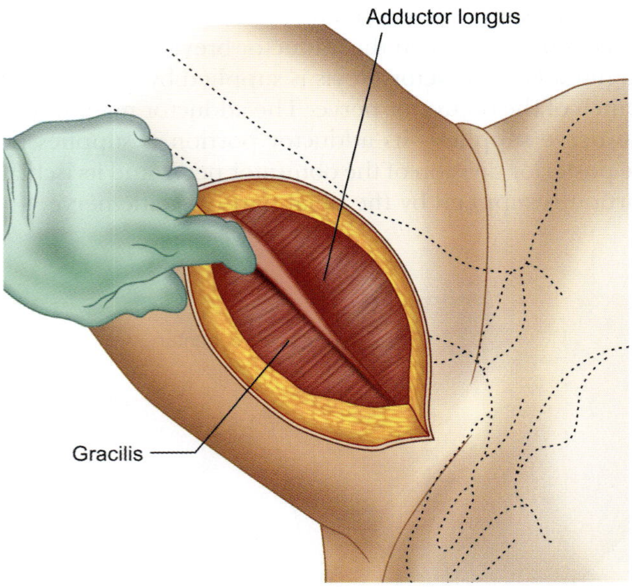

Fig. 24.301: Superficial dissection approach

Superficial Dissection (Fig. 24.301)

- Begin the superficial dissection by developing plane between gracilis and adductor longus
- This plane is developed with your gloved finger.

Deep Surgical Dissection (Figs 24.302A and B)

- Continue the dissection in the interval between the adductor brevis and the adductor magnus, until you feel the trochanter on the floor of the wound
- Try to protect the posterior division of the obturator nerve
- Place the narrow retractor (such as bone spike) above and below the lesser trochanter to isolate the psoas tendon.

Dangers

Nerves: The anterior division of the obturator nerve lies on the top of the obturator externus and run down the medial side of the thigh between the adductor longus and adductor brevis. The posterior division of the obturator nerve lies in the substance of the obturator externus, which supplies before it leaves the pelvis. The nerve then runs down the thigh on the adductor magnus and under the adductor brevis.

Vessels: The medial femoral circumflex artery passes around the medial side of the distal part of the psoas tendon.

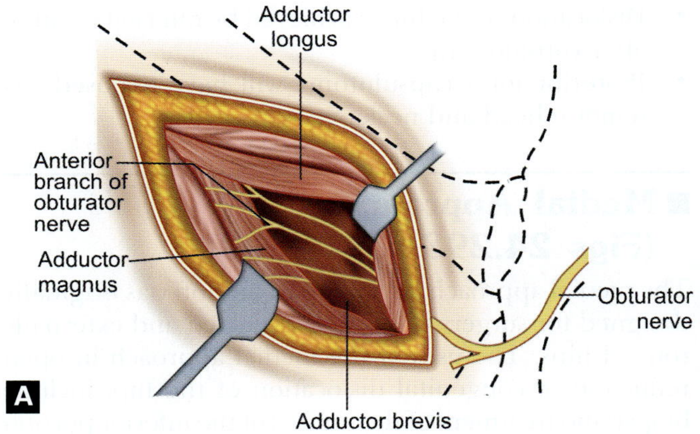

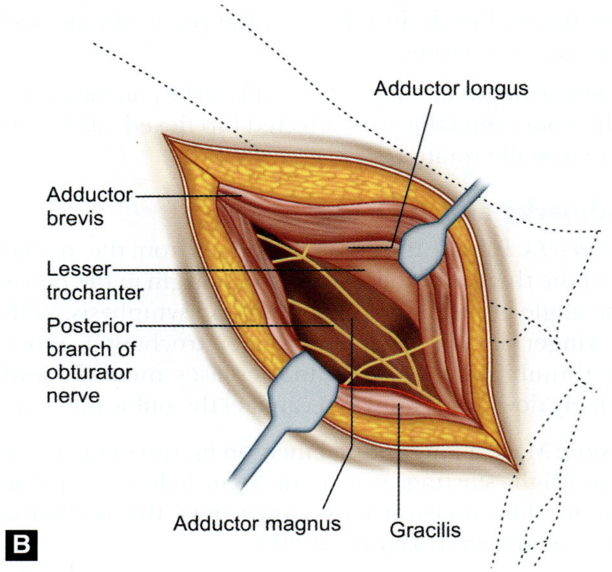

Figs 24.302A and B: Deep surgical dissection approach

■ Posterolateral Approach (Figs 24.303 to 24.305)

Gibson first described the posterolateral approach and recommended by Kocher and Langenbeck.

Position of the patient: Patient is in lateral position.

Landmarks and Incision (Figs 24.304A to D)

- Begin the proximal limb of the incision at a point 6 to 8 cm anterior to the posterosuperior iliac spine and just distal to the iliac crest, overlying the anterior border of the gluteus maximus
- Extend it distally to the anterior edge of the greater trochanter and then further distally along the line of the femur for 15 to 18 cm.
- By blunt dissection reflect the flap of the skin and subcutaneous fat from the underlying deep fascia a short distance anteriorly and posteriorly.

- Then incise iliotibial band in line with its fiber, beginning at the distal end of the wound and extending proximally to the greater trochanter.

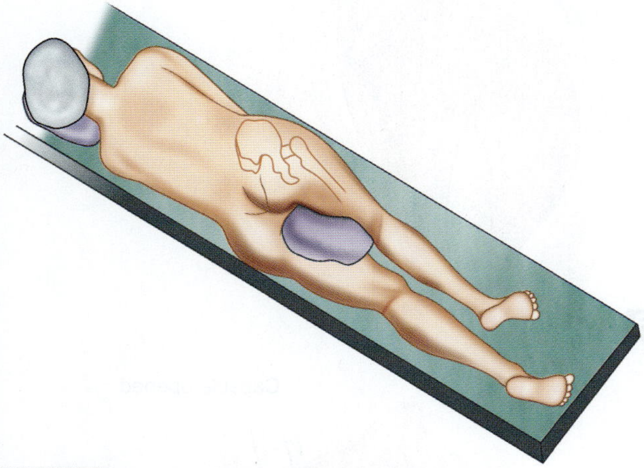

Fig. 24.303: Position of the patient in posterolateral surgical approach

- Next, abduct the thigh, insert the gloved finger through the proximal end of the incision in the band, locate by palpation the sulcus at the anterior border of the gluteus maximus muscle and extend the incision proximally along this sulcus.
- Then adduct the thigh, reflect the anterior and posterior masses and expose the greater trochanter and the muscles that insert into it.
- Next, separate the posterior border of the gluteus medius muscle from the adjacent pyriformis tendon by blunt dissection.
- Divide the gluteus medius and minimus muscles at their insertion, but leave enough of their tendon attached to the greater trochanter to permit easy closure of the wound.
- Reflect these muscle anteriorly
- The anterior and superior parts of the joint capsule can now be seen
- Incise the capsule superiorly in the axis of the femoral neck from the acetabulum to the

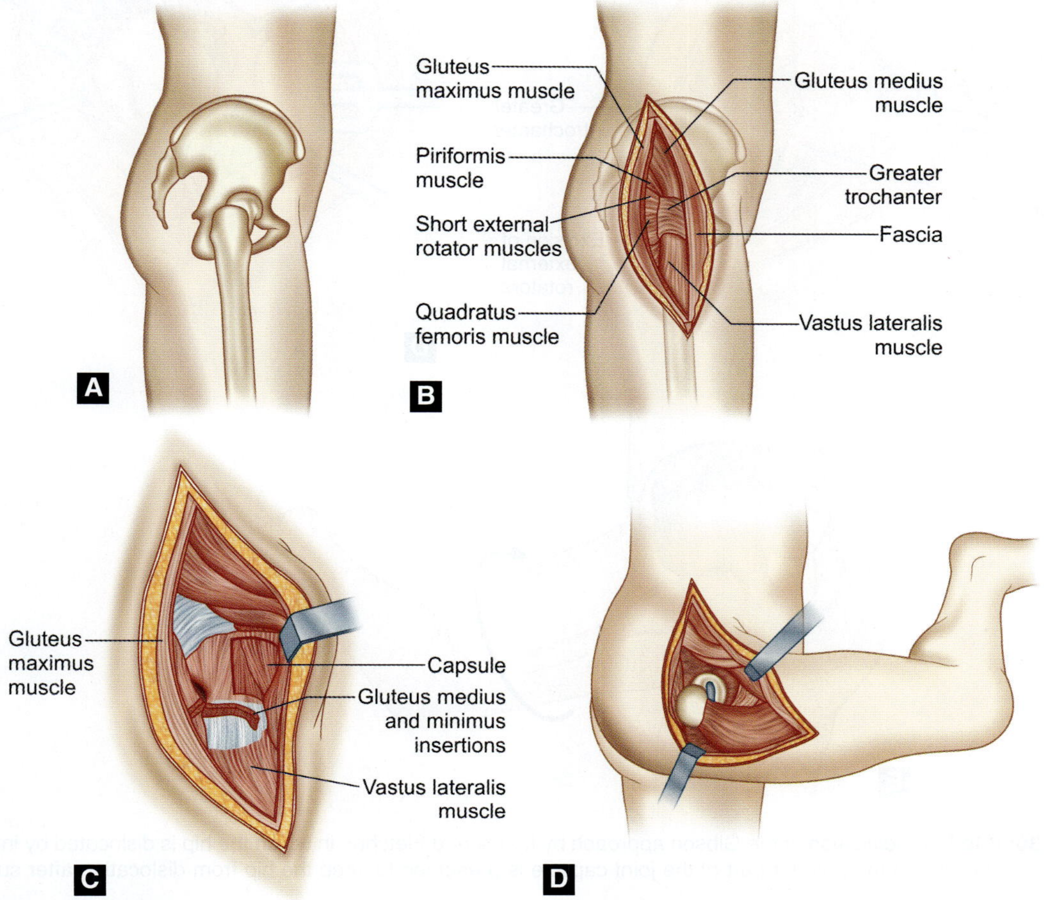

Figs 24.304A to D: Gibson posterolateral approach to hip joint—(A) Skin incision; (B) Anterior and posterior muscle masses have been retracted to expose greater trochanter and muscles that insert into it; (C) Gluteus medius and minimus have been near their insertion into greater trochanter and retracted incision in capsule is shown; (D) Hip joint has been dislocated by flexing, abducting and externally rotating thigh

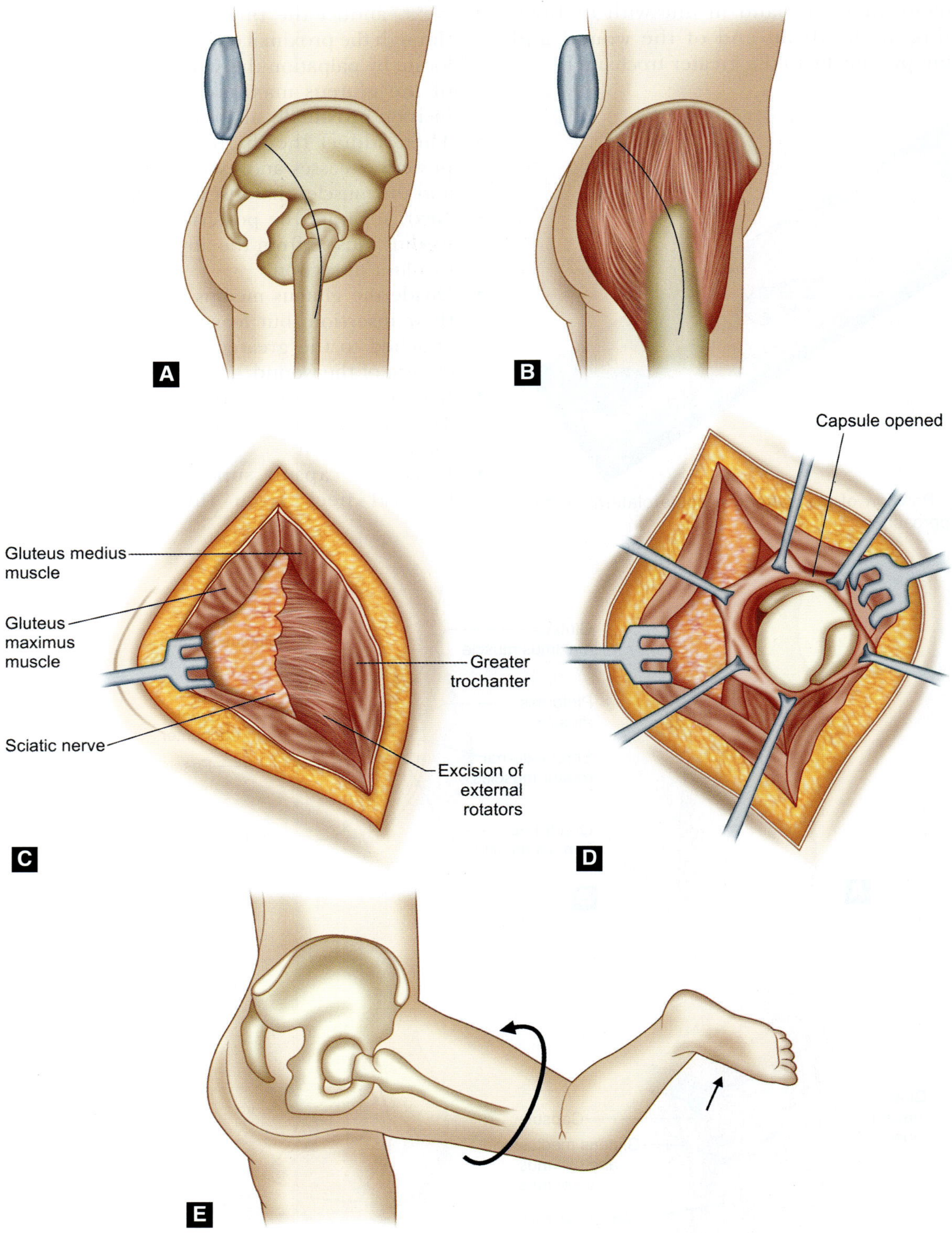

Figs 24.305A to E: Modification of the Gibson approach by Marcy and Fletcher, in which the hip is dislocated by internal rotation and the anterior part of the joint capsule is preserved to keep the hip from dislocating after surgery

intertrochantric line; incise as much of the capsule as desired along the joint line anteriorly and along the anterior intertrochantric line laterally

- The hip can now be dislocated by flexing the hip and knee and abducting and externally rotating the thigh
- Figures 24.305A to E, shows a modification of the Gibson approach by Marcy and Fletcher, in which the hip is dislocated by internal rotation and the anterior part of the joint capsule is preserved to keep the hip from dislocating after surgery.

Bibliography

1. Acar A, Turhan V, Diktas H, et al. A case of brucellosis complicated with endocarditis, pyelonephritis, sacroileitis and thyroiditis. Mikrobiyol Bul. 2009;43(1):141-5.
2. Aleto T, Ritter MA, Berend ME. Case report: superficial femoral artery injury resulting from cerclage wiring during revision THA. Clin Orthop Relat Res. 2008;466(3): 749-53.
3. Banas B, Kowalczyk B. A strategy of rehabilitation in children with proximal femoral focal deficiency treated with modified Van Nes rotationplasty. Chir Narzadow Ruchu Ortop Pol. 2006;71(4):313-5.
4. Bernaerts A, Pouillon M, De Ridder K, et al. Value of magnetic resonance imaging in early assessment of proximal femoral focal deficiency (PFFD). JBR-BTR. 2006; 89(6):325-7.
5. Chan WC, Veraitch O, Radford W, et al. Chronic lymphoedema complicated by septic arthritis of the hip. Br J Dermatol. 2009;160(5):1130-2.
6. Engell V, Bach A, Davidsen M, Møller-Madsen B. Purulent coxitis in 8-year-old boy caused by *Salmonella enteritidis*. Ugeskr Laeger. 2009;171(18):1515-6.
7. Ergin H, Semerci CN, Bican M, et al. A case with proximal femoral focal deficiency (PFFD) and fibular A/hypoplasia (FA/H) associated with urogenital anomalies. Turk J Pediatr. 2006;48(4):380-2.
8. Gérard R, Stindel E, Dardenne G, et al. Greater trochanter displacements after Charnley'strochanterotomy, during passive hip movements: a real-time 3D cadaveric approach. Surg Radiol Anat. 2009;31(8):605-13.
9. Jain A, Pradhan S, Jain S, et al. Fatal intraoperative pulmonary embolism in a child-a case report. Paediatr Anaesth 2009;19(3):286-7.
10. Janmohammadi N, Roushan MR. False negative serological tests may lead to misdiagnosis and mismanagement in osteoarticular brucellosis. Trop Doct 2009;39(2):88-90.
11. Kesson AM, Bellemore MC, O'Mara TJ, et al. Scedosporium prolificans osteomyelitis in an immunocompetent child treated with a novel agent, hexadecylphospocholine (miltefosine), in combination with terbinafine and voriconazole: a case report. Clin Infect Dis. 2009;48(9): 1257-61.
12. Mont MA, McGrath MS, Ulrich SD, et al. Metal-on-metal total hip resurfacing arthroplasty in the presence of extra-articular deformities or implants. J Bone Joint Surg Am. 2008;90 (Suppl 3):45-51.
13. Muñoz-Mahamud E, Casanova L, Font L, et al. Septic arthritis of the hip caused by nontyphi Salmonella after urinary tract infection. Am J Emerg Med. 2009;27(3): 373. e5-373.e8.
14. Oh KY, Frias AE, Byrne JL, et al. Unilateral short femur-what does this mean? Report of 3 cases. Ultrasound Q. 2008;24(2):89-92.
15. Peltola H, Pääkkönen M, Kallio P, et al. Prospective, randomized trial of 10 days versus 30 days of antimicrobial treatment, including a short-term course of parenteral therapy, for childhood septic arthritis. Osteomyelitis-Septic Arthritis (OM-SA) Study Group. Clin Infect Dis. 2009; 48(9):1201-10.
16. Philippot R, Delangle F, Verdot FX, et al. Femoral deficiency reconstruction using a hydroxyapatite-coated locked modular stem. A series of 43 total hip revisions. Orthop Traumatol Surg Res. 2009;95(2):119-26 (Epub 2009 Mar 17).
17. Pollard TC, Gwilym SE, Carr AJ. The assessment of early osteoarthritis. J Bone Joint Surg Br. 2008;90(4):411-21 (Review).
18. Ramseier LE, Exner GU. Lengthening of proximal femoral focal deficiency using a hybrid fixation with inclusion of the knee joint. Orthopade. 2007;36(6):582, 584-7.
19. Roux N, Pieters S. Prosthetic management 56 years after rotationplasty due to proximal femoral focal deficiency (PFFD). Prosthet Orthot Int. 2007;31(3):313-20.
20. Rutz E, Brunner R. Septic arthritis of the hip–current concepts. Hip Int. 2009;19 (Suppl 6):S9-12.
21. Salavati M. Proximal femoral focal deficiency (PFFD) in a young Doberman pinscher. J Small Anim Pract. 2008; 49(9):486.
22. Sulaiman AR, Nawaz H, Munajat I, et al. Proximal femoral focal deficiency as a manifestation of Antley-Bixler syndrome: a case report. J Orthop Surg (Hong-Kong). 2007;15(1):84-6.
23. Tamaki Y, Takakubo Y, Goto K, et al. Increased expression of toll-like receptors in aseptic loose periprosthetic tissues and septic synovial membranes around total hip implants. J Rheumatol 2009;36(3):598-608 (Epub 2009 Feb 4).
24. Togrul E, Ozkan C, Kalacý A, et al. New Technique of Subtrochanteric Shortening in Total Hip Arthroplasty for Crowe Types 3 to 4 Dysplasia of the Hip Using Endosteal Bone Pegs. J Arthroplasty. 2010;25(3):465-70 (Epub 2009 Jul 4).
25. Turan H, Serefhanoglu K, Karadeli E, et al. A case of brucellosis with abscess of the iliacus muscle, olecranon bursitis, and sacroiliitis. Int J Infect Dis. 2009;13(6):e485-7 (Epub 2009 Apr 24).
26. Volpon JB, Batista LC, Shimano MM, et al. Tension band wire fixation for valgusosteotomies of the proximal femur: a biomechanical study of three configurations of fixation. ClinBiomech (Bristol, Avon). 2008;23(4):395-401 (Epub 2008 Jan 9).
27. Westberry DE, Davids JR. Proximal focal femoral deficiency (PFFD): management options and controversies. Hip Int. 2009;19 (Suppl 6):18-25 (Review).
28. Wirth T. Spondyloepiphyseal and metaphyseal dysplasia. Orthopade. 2008;37(1):8-16 (Review).

25 Knee

- Synovial Chondromatosis
- Knee Joint Examination
- Congenital Anomalies Around the Knee Joint
- Deformities Around Knee
- Dislocation of Patella
- Fractures Around the Knee Joint
- Meniscal Injuries
- Cruciate Ligament Injuries
- Osteochondritis, Chondromalacia Patella and Synovial Chondromatosis
- Tumors Around Knee
- Synovial Fluid Examination

SYNOVIAL CHONDROMATOSIS

Knee Joint

Gross anatomy of a knee joint and its accompanying structures are shown in Figures 25.1 and 25.2.

Introduction

Type of Joint

The knee is a complex, compound, condyloid variety of a synovial joint. It comprises of:

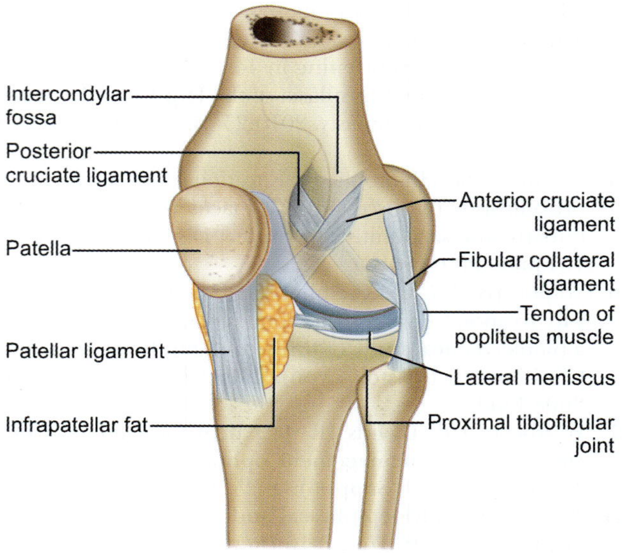

Fig. 25.1: Gross anatomy of knee joint

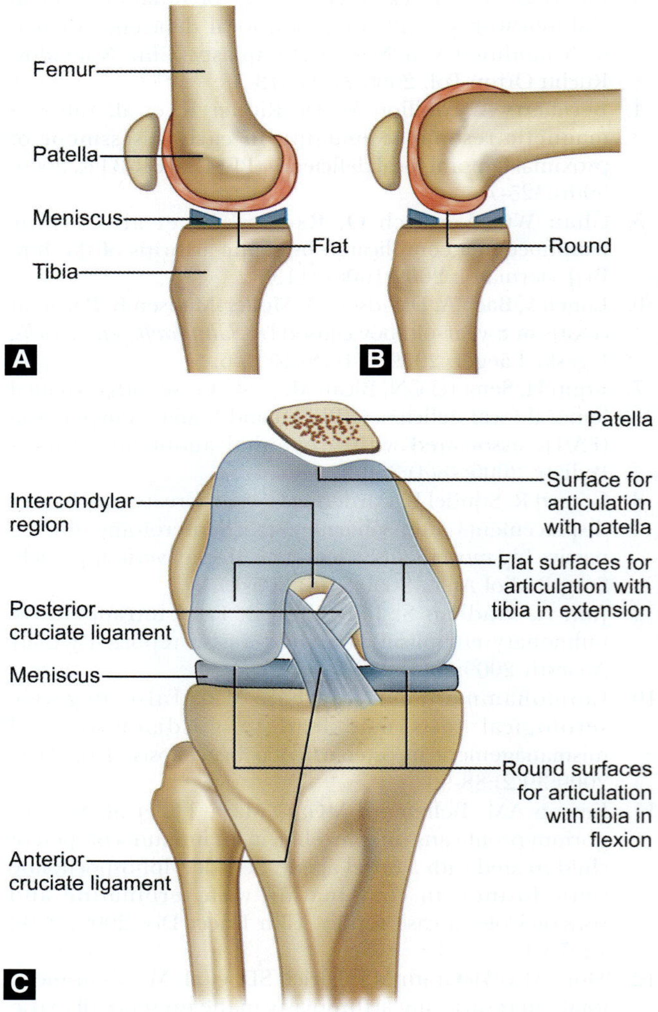

Figs 25.2A to C: Knee joint—(A) Bony component of a knee joint; (B) Femur moving over tibia; (C) Articular surfaces and ligaments of knee joint

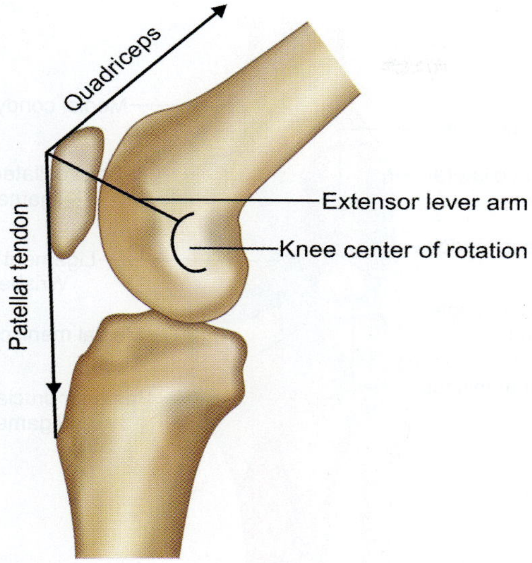

Fig. 25.3: Patella helps in lengthening the extensor lever arm, by displacing force vectors of quadriceps and patellar tendons away from center of rotation of knee

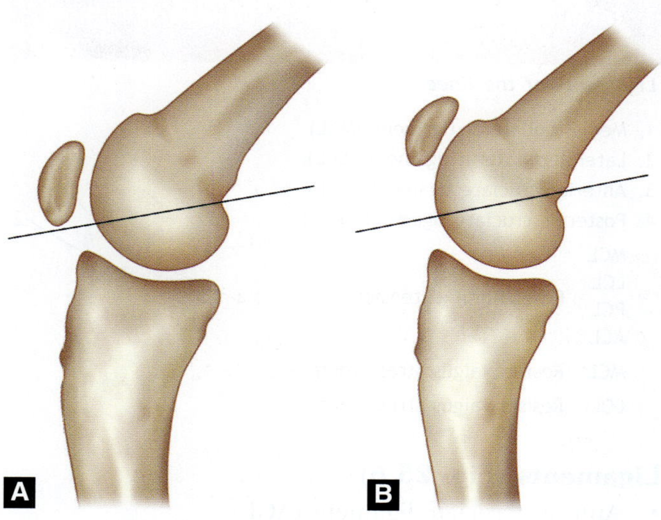

Figs 25.4A and B: Blumensaat's line—(A) Normal patella; (B) Patella alta

- *The femoropatellar joint*: Articulation between femur and patella.
- *The femorotibial joint*: Articulation between femur and tibia, which is weight-bearing.

Articular Surfaces

The articular surfaces are covered by hyaline cartilage. The major surfaces include: The two femoral condyles and the adjacent surfaces of the superior aspect of the tibial condyles.

Patella (Fig. 25.3)

Patella is a sesamoid bone of the quadriceps muscle. Its primary function is to lengthen the extensor lever arm, by displacing force vectors of quadriceps and patella tendons away from center of rotation of knee. The inferior articular surface of the patella contacts the trochlea in 20° of knee flexion. The mid portion, articulates with the trochlea at 60° and the superior portion at 90° of flexion. In extreme flexion, beyond 120° the patella articulates only medially and laterally with the condyles and the quadriceps tendon articulates with the trochlea.

Geometry

Blumensaat's Line (Figs 25.4A and B)

- The lower border of patella normally lies at a line projected forward from the intercondylar notch at 30° of flexion.
- In patella alta, the lower edge of the patella lies well above this line.

Q-Angle (Fig. 25.5)

It was described by Hvid and is defined as an angle between the extended anatomical axis of the femur and

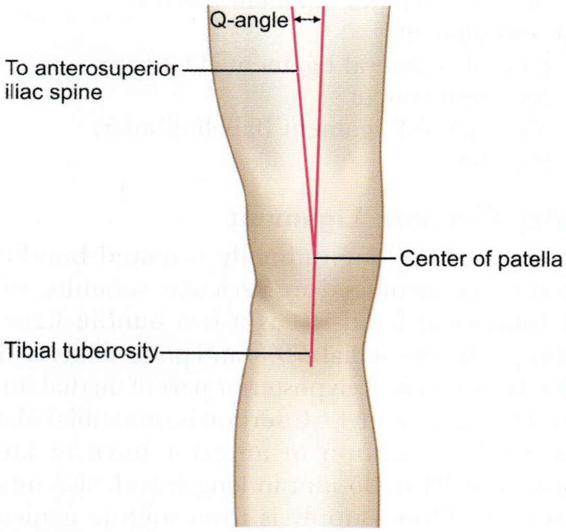

Fig. 25.5: Q-angle and landmarks forming this angle

line between the center of patella and tibial tubercle. It determines the divergence of quadriceps from the vertical (20° or more lateral displacement of patella).

Muscles Acting on Knee Joint

The principal muscles acting on the knee are:

Extensor: Quadriceps femoris

Flexors: Hamstrings assisted by gracilis, gastrocnemius and sartorius.

Medial rotator: Popliteus (unscrews the knee).

Ligaments of the Knee

Various ligaments and their functions are enumerated in Table 25.1.

Table 25.1: Various ligaments of knee and their function

Ligaments of the Knee	
1. Medial collateral ligament (MCL)	
2. Lateral collateral ligament (LCL)	
3. Anterior cruciate ligament (ACL)	
4. Posterior cruciate ligament (PCL)	
MCL LCL PCL ACL	Resist/limit extension
MCL	Resists valgus stress/force
LCL	Resists valgus stress/force

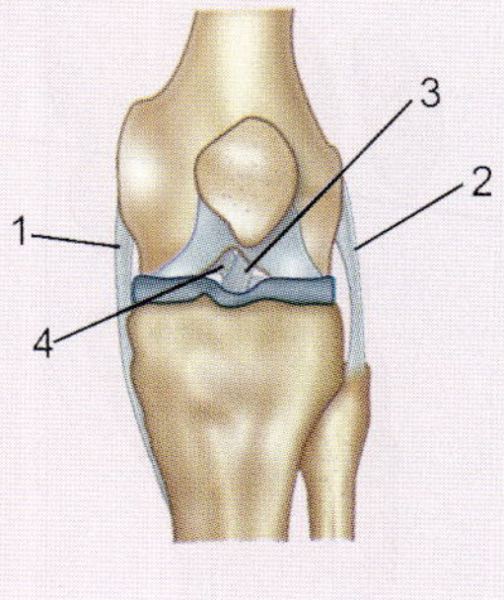

Ligaments (Fig. 25.6)

- Anterior cruciate ligament (ACL)
- Posterior cruciate ligament (PCL)
- Medial ligaments
  - Capsular ligaments
  - Posterior oblique ligament
  - Medial collateral ligament (MCL)
- Lateral ligaments
  - Lateral collateral ligament (LCL)
  - Arcuate ligament
  - Short lateral ligament (fabellofibular)
  - Popliteus

Anterior Cruciate Ligament

It is composed of longitudinally oriented bundles of collagen tissue, arranged in fascicular subunits, within larger functional bands. It is a two bundle ligament consisting of anteromedial (70%) and posterolateral (30%) bundles. Its origin is from posterior part of medial surface of lateral femoral condyle. Insertion is onto tibial plateau medial to the insertion of anterior horn of lateral meniscus. It is 31 to 35 mm in length and 31.3 mm^2 in cross section. Blood supply is from middle geniculate artery, which pierces the posterior capsule. Nerve innervation is by posterior articular nerve, a branch of tibial nerve.

Functions

It is the primary restraint to the anterior tibial displacement. The anteromedial band is tight in flexion, providing the primary restraint, whereas the posterolateral bundle is tight in extension. The posterolateral bundle, provides the principal resistance for hyperextension. In addition it has a proprioceptive function.

Posterior Cruciate Ligament

It is composed of two major parts:

1. A large anterior portion forms the bulk.
2. A small posterior portion that runs obliquely to the back of tibia (thus the reason for double bundle repair).

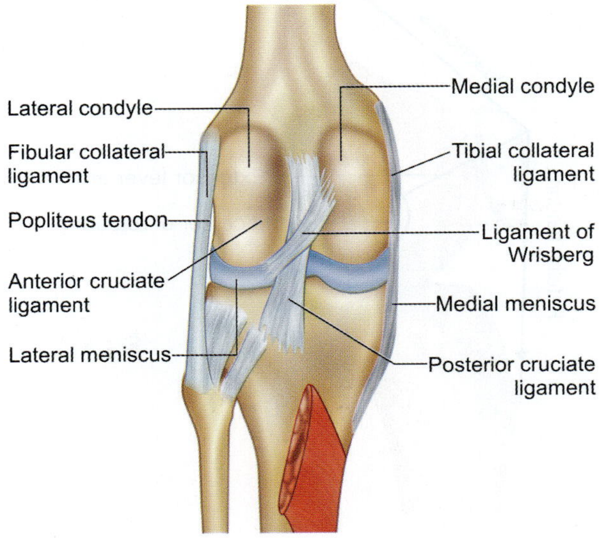

Fig. 25.6: Various ligaments of knee joint and their attachments

Origin is from the posterior part of the lateral surface of medial condyle. Insertion is in the depression behind and below the intra-articular portion of tibia and a slip to the posterior horn of lateral meniscus. It is more vertically than obliquely oriented and is the axis around which the rotation of knee occurs.

Functions

- It provides resistance to the posterior translation of tibia on the femur.
- It guides the 'screw home' mechanism of internal rotation of femur, during terminal extension of knee.
- It acts as a check for hyperextension, only if the anterior cruciate ligament is ruptured.

Capsular Ligaments (Fig. 25.7)

The medial capsule of the knee forms a composite of three groups of capsular ligaments:

- Anterior portion is the anterior capsule, which extends distally from the quadriceps aponeurosis. It is taut, when knee is flexed and relaxed, when knee is extended
- The middle portion is the deep layer of the MCL and its origin is medial epicondyle of femur, anterior to the attachment of MCL and inserted to the medial meniscus. It holds the meniscus firmly to the femur
- Posterior portion, embraces the posterior surface of the medial femoral condyle. When the knee is extended, it is taut and is lax, when knee is flexed.

Posterior Oblique Ligament (Figs 25.8 and 25.9)

The posteromedial capsule is reinforced by three oblique thickenings having common origin from the adductor tubercle and are:

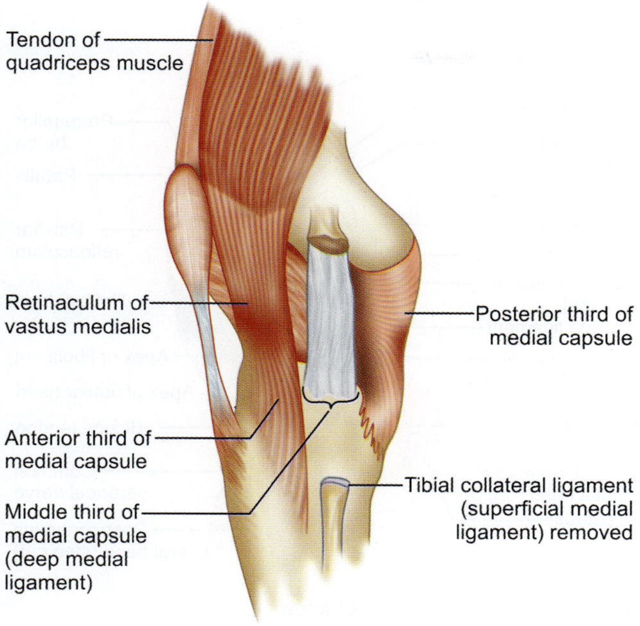

Fig. 25.7: Ligaments around knee

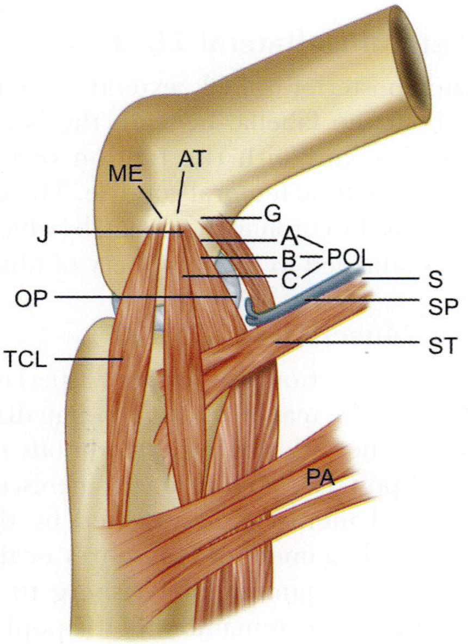

Fig. 25.8: Posterior oblique ligament—A. Superior or capsular arm of posterior oblique ligament (POL); AT. Adductor tubercle; B. Central or tibial arm of posterior oblique ligament; C. Superficial arm of posterior oblique ligament; J. Common ligament of origin of posterior oblique ligament; ME. Medial epicondyle; OP. Oblique popliteal ligament; PA. Pes anserinus; S. Common tendon of semimembranosus; SP. Portion of semimembranosus tendon that becomes oblique popliteal ligament; ST. Portion of semimembranosus tendon that goes to posteromedial corner of tibia; TCL. tibial collateral ligament; G. Gastrocnemius muscle

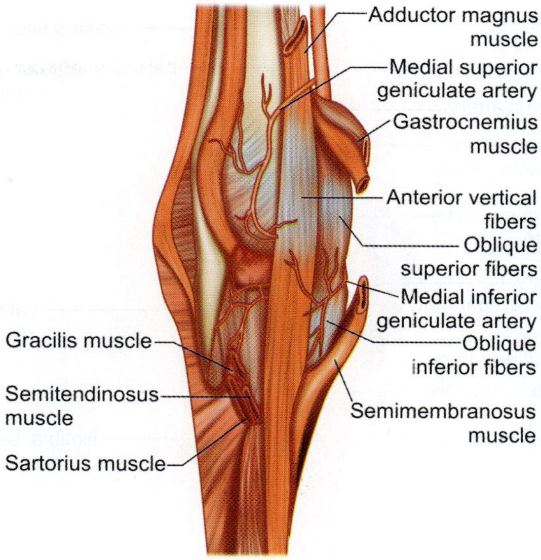

Fig. 25.9: Medial (tibial) collateral ligament

Central arm: A strong central arm passing to the posteromedial edge of the tibia, which is firmly fixed to the medial meniscus.

Superior arm: Superior arm extending outwards within the capsule to blend with the oblique popliteal ligament

Inferior arm: Inferior arm, which attaches to the sheath covering semimembranosus and the tibia. Its function is to augment the stabilizing effect of MCL.

The posterior capsule, must be relaxed by flexion of knee, before applying valgus stress in isolated rupture of MCL. Valgus stress test is positive, in extension, indicates MCL and posterior capsule injury. Valgus stress test positive, only in flexion, indicates only MCL injury.

Medial Collateral Ligament (Tibial)

It is a strong flat membranous band and is a main stabilizer of the medial aspect of the knee. It is 8 to 10 cm in length. Origin from medial epicondyle of femur. Insertion is inferior to the medial surface of tibia 4 to 5 cm below to the tibial articular surface. Anterior fibers extend vertically and parallel and the posterior fibers, follow the oblique course towards the posterior capsule.

In complete extension, both the fibers are taut and prevent the hyperextension of knee joint. In flexion, the anterior long fibers remain taut and oblique fibers are relaxed, restraining abduction of tibia in all positions. In full extension the oblique portion restrains, posterior gliding of tibia on femur and prevents external rotation of tibia.

Lateral Ligaments

Comprises of three parts:

Anterior third: Anterior third, consists of capsular ligament: Extending laterally and backward, from the patellar

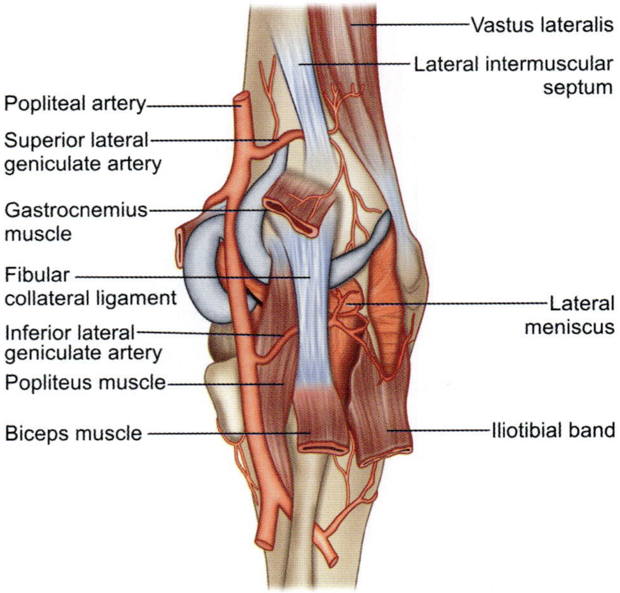

Fig. 25.10: Lateral collateral ligament (fibular)

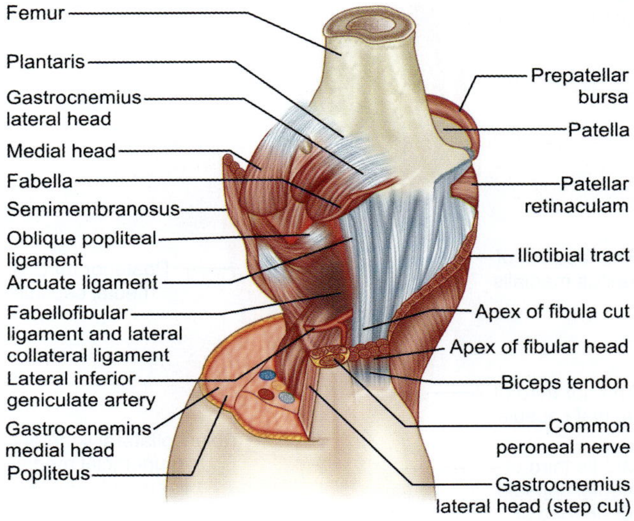

Fig. 25.11: Lateral ligaments of knee

tendon to the anterior border of iliotibial band. It is reinforced by distal retinacule of the quadriceps expansion.

Middle third: Middle third, composed of iliotibial band and capsular ligament deep to it. It is the major lateral support of the knee in about 30° of flexion. The iliotibial band, passes posterior to the center of rotation, when the knee is flexed and it restrains forward displacement and internal rotation of tibia from full extension to 45° of flexion.

Posterior third: Posterior third, includes the ligaments, which are collectively called as the 'arcuate complex'. This includes:

- Lateral collateral ligament
- Arcuate ligament
- Short lateral collateral ligament (fabellofibular ligament)
- Popliteus muscle

Lateral Collateral Ligament (Fibular) (Fig. 25.10)

It is a strong round band, attaching above to the lateral femoral epicondyle and below to the head of fibula. It is separated from the lateral meniscus by popliteal tendon. Distally, the tendon of biceps is inserted into the head of the fibula, divided into two parts, to enclose the ligament from which it is separated by the bursa.

Arcuate Ligament (Fig. 25.11)

It is a thick capsular segment, passing from the head of fibula to the posterolateral aspect of the lateral femoral condyle. The lateral limb is strong and is attached to femoral condyle and popliteus tendon. The weaker medial limb curves over the popliteus and is attached to the posterior arch of lateral meniscus. Its function is to stabilize the lateral tibial condyle against posterior displacement, during hyperextension.

Short Lateral Collateral Ligament

It is situated posterior to LCL, extends from the fibula to a point about the fabella, beneath the lateral head of gastrocnemius and with the tendon of popliteus, it attaches to the lateral femoral condyle. The deep layer is thin and forms the coronary ligament, by which the lateral meniscus is attached to the periphery of tibia.

Popliteus Muscle (Fig. 25.12)

The popliteus arises from the posterior aspect of tibia above the soleal line. The major superior and medial portion of muscle is attached, through the tendinous fibers to the periphery of posterior arch of lateral meniscus.

The lateral meniscus is attached by the anterior meniscofemoral ligament of Humphrey or the posterior meniscofemoral ligament of Wrisberg to the medial femoral condyle. The remainder of the popliteus muscle converges, to form a tendon and attaches to the outer aspect of lateral femoral condyle, as shown in Figures 25.13A and B.

Humphrey Ligament

Also known as anterior meniscofemoral ligament, is less than one-third the diameter of the PCL. It arises from the posterior horn of the lateral meniscus, runs anterior to the PCL and inserts at the distal edge of the femoral PCL. Its attachment may be confused for the PCL, during

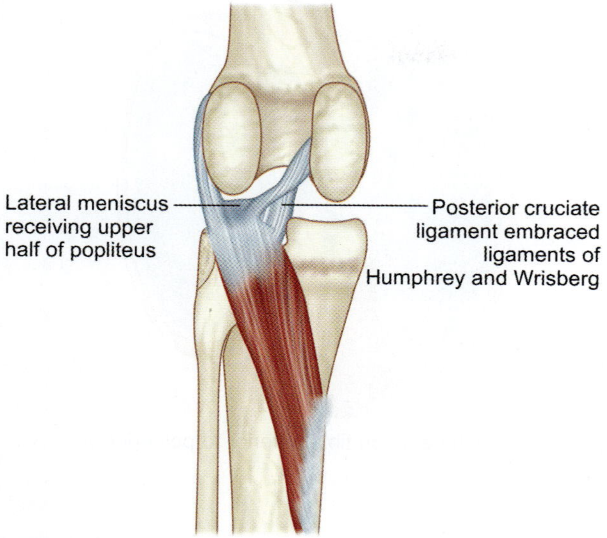

Fig. 25.12: Popliteus muscle

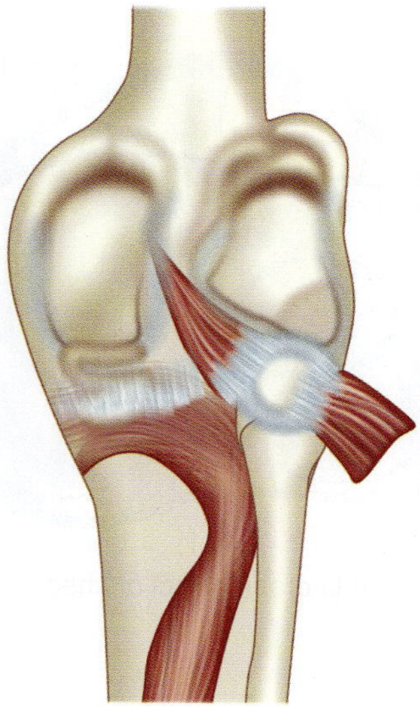

Fig. 25.14: Wrisberg's ligament

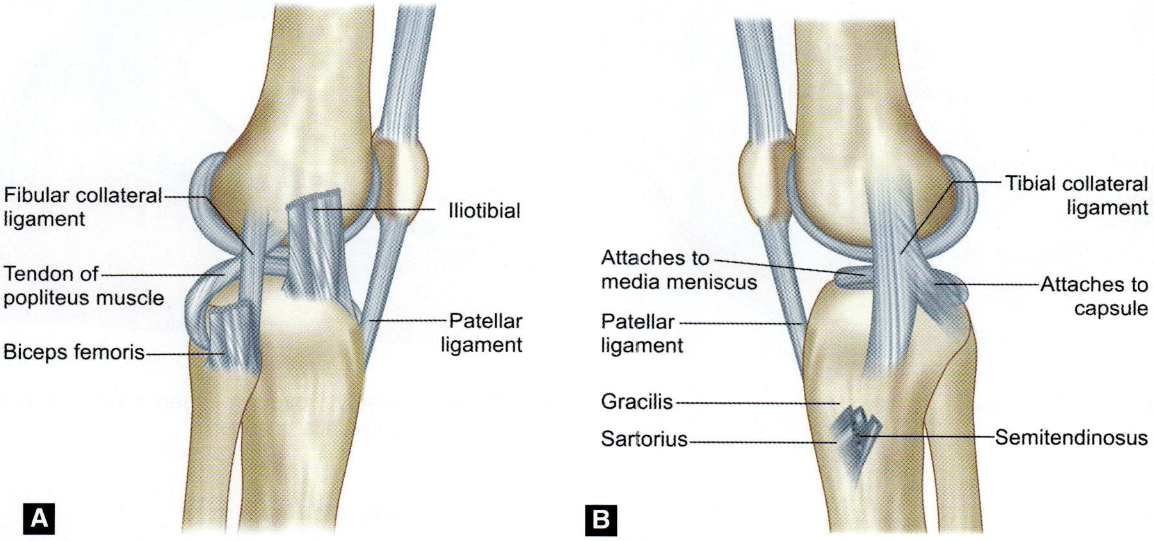

Figs 25.13A and B: (A) Lateral meniscal attachments; (B) Medial meniscus attachments

arthroscopy. In this situation, tug on the ligament, while observing for motion of the lateral meniscus.

Wrisberg's Ligament (Fig. 25.14)

Also known as posterior meniscofemoral ligament, usually larger than ligament of Humphrey (up to 1.5 the diameter of the PCL), extends from the posterior horn of lateral meniscus to medial femoral condyle.

Menisci (Figs 25.15 and 25.16)

Two menisci, which are fibrocartilaginous C-shaped cartilages are:

- Medial meniscus
- Lateral meniscus
- The menisci improve the congruency between femoral and tibial condyles and act as shock absorbers.

Characteristics Features

- Semilunar cartilage
- Wedge shaped
- Fibrocartilaginous
- Triangular on cross section (CS)
- Cover half to two-thirds of surface
- Laterally shorter, small "O" shaped
- Medially longer "C" shaped

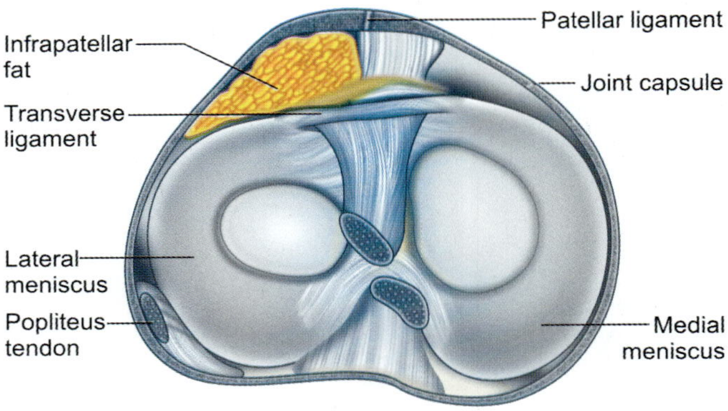

Fig. 25.15: Medial and lateral menisci of knee

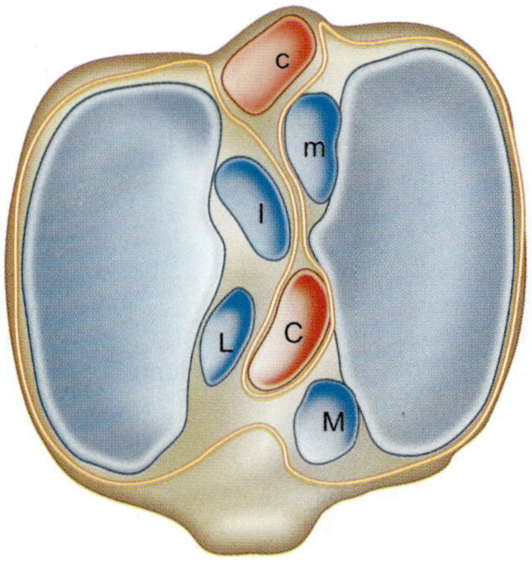

Fig. 25.17: Attachments on tibia anterior to posterior

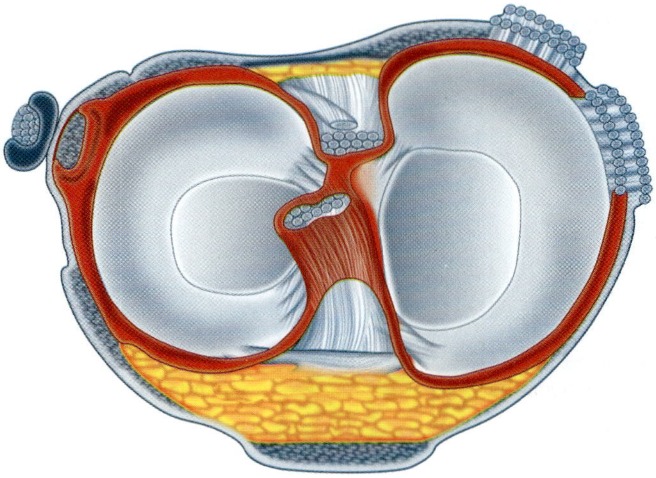

Fig. 25.16: Menisci of knee

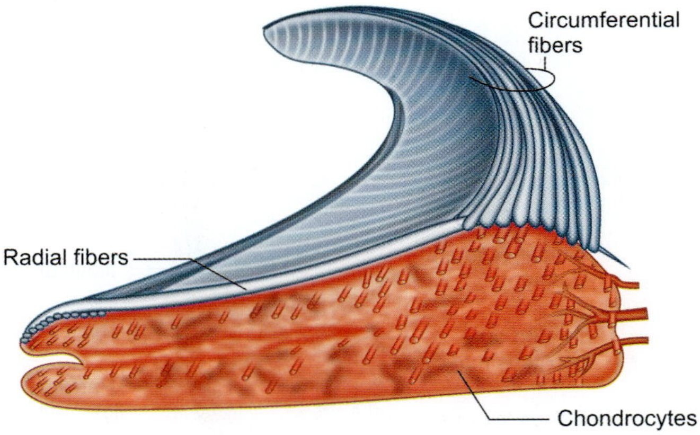

Fig. 25.18: Densely woven collagen arranged in radial and circumferential manner

Attachments

Anterior to posterior: This has been shown in Figure 25.17 and can be summarized as follows:

M : Medial meniscus anterior horn
C : Anterior cruciate ligament
L : Lateral meniscus anterior horn
l : Lateral meniscus posterior horn
m : Medial meniscus posterior horn
c : Posterior cruciate ligament

Structure

Composed of densely woven collagen fibers (Fig. 25.18)

Blood Supply

- Largely avascular, except in periphery, from medial and lateral geniculate arteries
- *Vascular zones*: White on white, white on red and red on red are shown in Figure 25.19.

Meniscal Healing and Repair

The vascular supply to the meniscus determines its potential for repair. The experimental findings and clinical observations of Arnoczky et al. demonstrated that the peripheral meniscal blood supply is capable of producing a reparative response, similar to that observed in other connective tissues. Perimeniscal capillary plexus, which supplies the peripheral 10 to 25 percent of the menisci.

Regenerative power: Peripheral vascular areas (red on red) of meniscus have got some regenerative capacity. Hence, total menisectomy is not preferred nowadays.

Functions

- Fillers of vacant joint
- Act as a secondary stabilizer
- Lubrication and nutrition
- Shock absorption
- Deepening the cavity

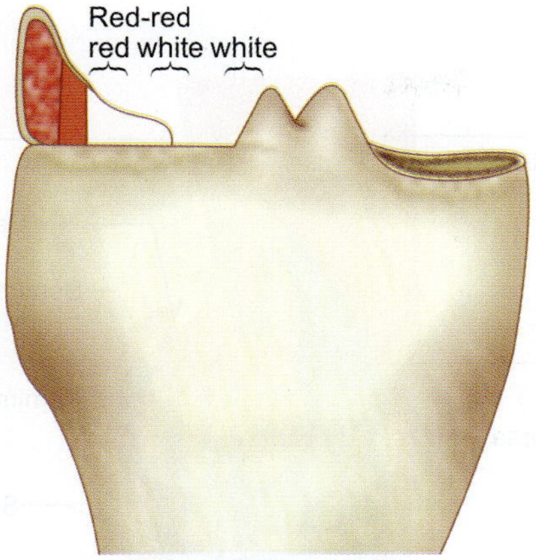

Fig. 25.19: Vascular zones of meniscal blood supply

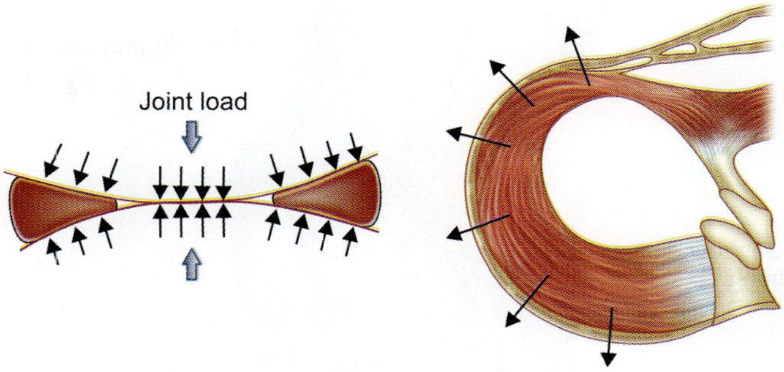

Fig. 25.20: Load bearing function of menisci

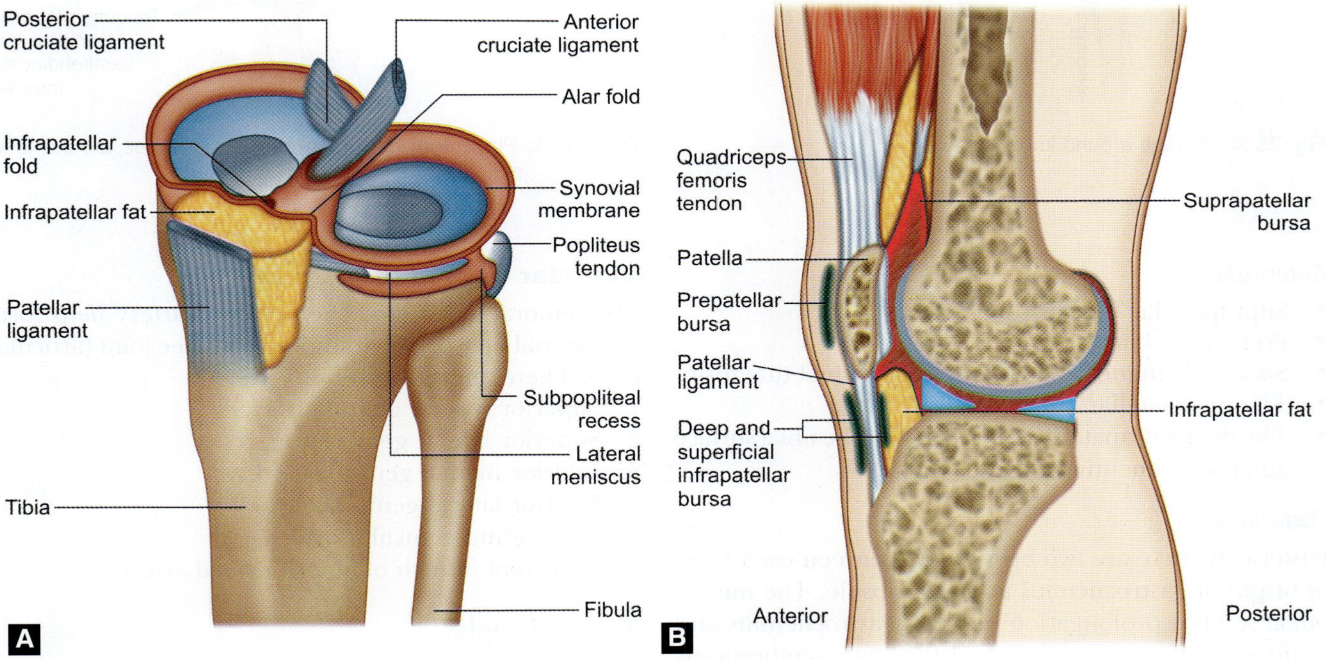

Figs 25.21A and B: Synovial membrane attached to margins of articular surfaces and margines of menisci

- The menisci, improves the congruency between femoral and tibial condyles
- Role in shock absorption
- *Load bearing function*: 40 to 60 percent load is on meniscus. Lateral meniscus bear greater weight than medial (Fig. 25.20).

■ Synovial Membrane

Attached to the margins of the articular surfaces and to the superior and inferior outer margins of the menisci (Figs 25.21A and B). It forms two pouches to provide low friction surfaces for the movement of tendons.

■ Subpopliteal Recess Suprapatellar Bursa (Figs 25.22 and 25.23)

Bursae

There are numerous bursae in the vicinity of the knee in relation to the attachments of various muscles and ligaments.

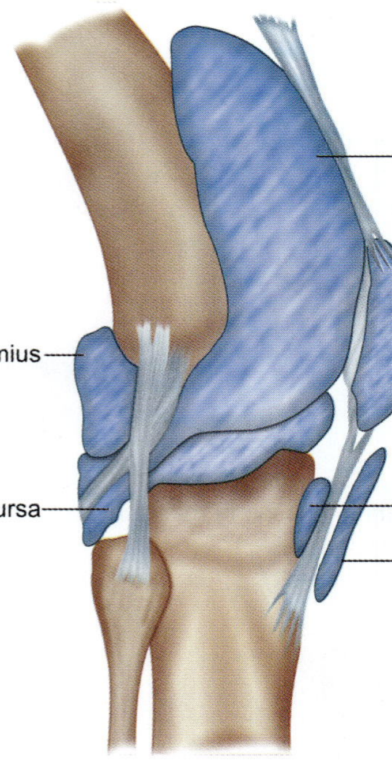

Fig. 25.22: Bursae around knee joint

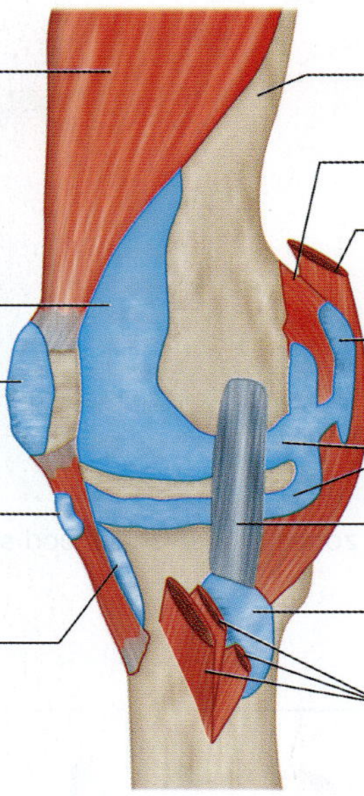

Fig. 25.23: Placement of bursae beneath muscles around knee joint

Anteriorly

- Suprapatellar bursa
- Prepatellar bursa
- Small subcutaneous bursa infront of tibial tuberosity
- The infrapatellar bursa
- The deep infrapatellar bursa between the tibial surface and the ligamentum patella.

Posteriorly

Posteriorly there are two bursae one between each head of origin of gastrocnemius and the capsule. The medial bursa sends a prolongation between gastrocnemius and semimembranosus and is called the semimembranosus bursa.

Medially

Anserine bursa separates the tendons of sartorius, gracilis and semimembranosus from the medial collateral ligament. Two bursae seperating the tendon of semimembranosus from the medial collateral ligament medially and the head of tibia laterally.

Laterally

One between biceps tendon and the lateral collateral ligament. One between the lateral collateral ligament and popliteus tendon and one between popliteus tendon and lateral condyle of femur.

Vascular Supply (Fig. 25.24)

The femoral artery and the popliteal artery help form the arterial network surrounding the knee joint (articular rete). There are six main branches:

1. Superior medial genicular artery
2. Superior lateral genicular artery
3. Inferior medial genicular artery
4. Inferior lateral genicular artery
5. Descending genicular artery
6. Recurrent branch of anterior tibial artery.

Nerve Supply

The knee joint is innervated, by branches from the obturator, femoral, tibial and common fibular nerves.

Cutaneous Nerves

- Anterior division of the lateral cutaneous nerve of thigh.
- Intermediate cutaneous nerve of thigh.
- Anterior and posterior divisions of the medial cutaneous nerve of thigh.

Saphenous Nerve

- Posterior cutaneous nerve of thigh.
- Posterior cutaneous nerve of calf.
- Lateral cutaneous nerve of calf (from peroneal).
- Anastomotic peroneal nerve of the leg (from peroneal).

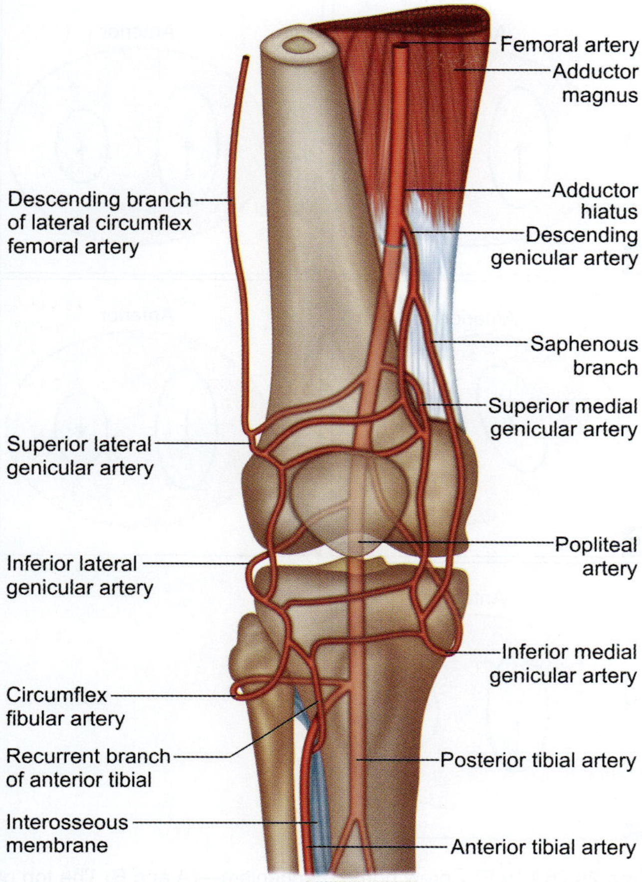

Fig. 25.24: Vascular supply around knee joint

- The infrapatellar branch of the saphenous nerve is divided most frequently, causing anesthesia about the tibial tubercle.

Knee Biomechanics

Introduction

- Mechanical and anatomical axis
- Instant center of rotation of knee
- ROM of knee joint
- Axis of motion
- Tibiofemoral arthrokinematics
- The 'screw-home' mechanism
- Ligamentous forces
- Knee stabilizers
- Normal kinetics of a step/gait

Mechanical Axis and Anatomical Axis (Fig. 25.25)

Instant center of rotation of knee and knee angles required performing activities of daily living (ADL's) are shown in Tables 25.2 and 25.3.

Frankel and Burstein introduced the concept of instant centers of motion. Mechanical and anatomical axis of lower limb, extend from center of femoral head to the center of ankle joint and passes near the center of knee joint. It is in 3° of valgus from vertical axis of body. Anatomical axis of femur is in 6° of valgus from mechanical axis of lower limb and 9° of valgus from vertical axis of the body Anatomical axis of tibia lies in 2 to 3° of varus from the vertical axis.

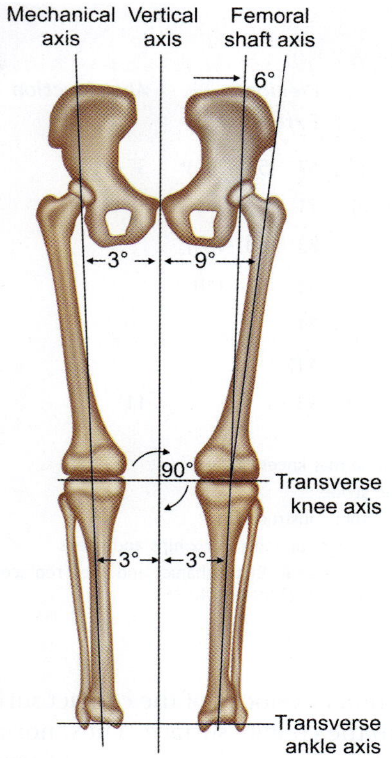

Fig. 25.25: Mechanical and anatomical axis of the knee joint

Table 25.2: Instant center of rotation of knee joint during lower limb movements

During knee extension	
Open chain	*Closed chain*
Tibia glides anteriorly on femur	Femur glides posteriorly on tibia
From 20° knee flexion to full extension	
Tibia rotates externally	Femur rotates internally on stable tibia
During knee flexion	
Open chain	*Closed chain*
Tibia glides posteriorly on femur	Femur glides anteriorly on tibia
From full knee extension to 20° flexion	
Tibia rotates internally	Femur rotates externally on stable tibia

They also showed that the axis, about which flexion/extension occurs shift backward in relation to tibia with increasing flexion. The least resistance to motion occurs

Table 25.3: Knee motion requirements for activities of daily living (ADL)

Type of ADL	Flexion/ Extension	Ab-Adduction	Rotation
Walking (swing)	67° (54°-79°)*	3°+11°†	7° + 8° = 15
Walking (stance)	21° (8°-29°)		
Stairs	83° (60°-98°)		
Sitting	93° (69°-110°)		
Lifting (1) ‡	71°		
Lifting (2)§	117°		
Components for ADL	93°	11°	13°

* Ranges in 44 normal knees
† Total for one stride
‡ Lifting (1)—without instruction
§ Lifting (2)—with instruction to flex hips and knees
Kettelkamp DB, Nasca R. Biomechanics and knee replacement arthroplasty. Orthop 1973;94:8-14.

in the direction of velocity of the contact surface, when it is tangent to the contact surface. Thus, normally for any selected instant center, the direction of velocity will be tangent to the contact surface. By marking a succession of instant centers for every few degrees, the normal pathway of instant centers can be mapped out.

ROM of Knee Joint

- *Flexion and extension:* 15 to 140°
- *Varus and valgus:* 6 to 8° in extension
- *Internal and external rotation:* 25 to 30° in flexion.

Tibiofemoral Arthrokinematics

The Screw-Home Mechanism (Figs 25.26A to E)

Rotation between the tibia and femur occurs automatically between full extension (0°) and 20° of knee flexion.

During knee extension, the tibia glides anteriorly on the femur. During the last 20° of knee extension, anterior tibial glide persists on the tibia medial condyle, because its articular surface is longer in that dimension than the lateral condyle. Prologed anterior glide, on the medial side produces external tibial rotation, the screw-home mechanism.

The screw-home mechanism reverses during knee flexion. When the knee begins to flex from a position of full extension, posterior tibial glide begins first on the longer medial condyle. Between 0° extension and 20° of flexion, posterior glide on the medial side produces relative tibial internal rotation, a 'reversal of the screw-home' mechanism.

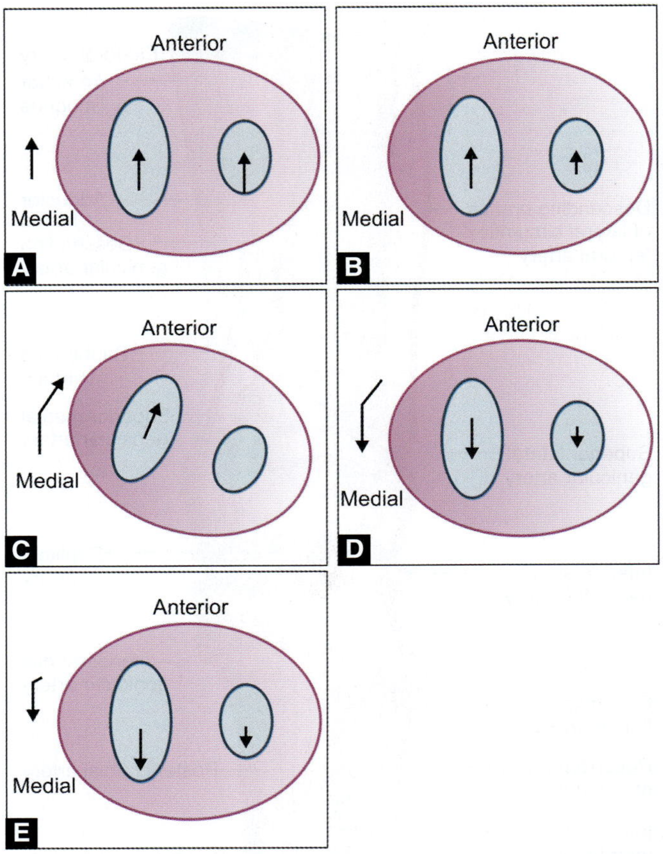

Figs 25.26A to E: Screw home mechanism—(A and B) The top of the right tibial plateau, as we look down on it, during knee motion; (C) On extension, the tibia glides anteriorly on the femur; (D and E) Last 20° of knee extension, anterior tibial glide persists on the tibia medial condyle

Ligamentous Structure Responsible for Tibial Glide

Tibial glides are produce by ligamentous forces, operating at different knee ROM. These are summarized below:

i. *During knee flexion*: Tibia rolls posteriorly, elongating ACL. ACL pull on tibia, causes it to glide posteriorly.
ii. *During knee extension*: Tibia rolls anteriorly, elongating PCL. PCL pull on tibia, causes it to glide anteriorly.

Stability Around Knee

Knee stability is provided by muscles and ligament which act as:

I. *Intrinsic stabilizers,* e.g. cruciate ligaments and menisci.
II. *Extrinsic stabilizers,* including:
   - Static stabilizers, e.g.
     - Capsule and capsular ligament
     - Extracapsular ligament
   - Dynamic stabilizers, which include:

– Musculotendinous units and their aponeurosis, but the protective reflexes act too slowly to prevent many injuries.

■ Compartmentization of Knee Joint

Hughston and Slocum divided the knee vertically in a sagittal plane, into various compartments and describe various structures within those compartments:

- *Medial compartment:* Medial compartment can be further divided into following parts:
  - *Anterior third*: It is made of thin capsule, which tightens in flexion and is reinforced by quadriceps.
  - *Middle third:* It is the capsular ligament and supported superficially, by medial collateral ligament.
  - *Posterior third:* The capsule is thickened and it is called the posterior oblique ligament and is supported by the semimembranosus tendon. Dynamic support is also from the pes anserinus and gastrocnemius muscles.

Supporting Structures

Medial collateral ligament (MCL): It provides primary valgus restraint (57–78% restraining moment of knee). Its femoral attachment fans out around axis of rotation. It is lax in flexion.

Muscles–semimembranosis (Expansion): Internally rotates tibia on femur. Tenses posterior/medial capsular structures, which are lax in knee flexion. It acts with ACL.

- *Lateral compartment*
  - *Anterior third:* There is a thin capsule anteriorly.
  - *Middle third:* The capsule is strengthened by the lateral capsular ligament and is reinforced by the iliotibial tract.
  - *Posterior third:* It is the arcuate complex, made up of the collateral ligament, arcuate ligament and aponeurotic tendon of popliteus. Dynamic support is from biceps femoris, popliteus and gastrocnemius muscles.

Lateral collateral ligament (LCL): Primary varus restraint. It is lax in flexion. Biceps femoris passes it and blends with insertion and maintains the tension.

Muscle–biceps femoris: Flexor (with semimembranosus and pes anserinus). Externally rotates tibia and tenses lateral collateral ligament (LCL). It is also considered as a dynamic assistor of PCL.

Flexible Half Sleeves (Posterior Halves of Knee)

Nicholas introduced the concept of flexible half sleeves, which encases the posterior halves of the femur and tibia and prevent the hyperextension.

These are:

Medial quadruple complex: Structures present under this complex are semimembranosis, oblique popliteal ligament, medial collateral ligament and tendon of pes anserinus.

Lateral quadruple complex: Iliotibial tract, lateral collateral ligament, popliteus tendon and biceps tendon, including arcuate ligament.

Central quadruple complex: Expansion of capsule into the joint, including both cruciates and menisci.

Cruciates

Anterior Cruciate Ligament (ACL)

Primary static restraint to anterior displacement of tibia, tense in extension, lax in flexion, as shown in Figures 25.27A and B.

Posterior Cruciate Ligament (PCL) (Figs 25.28A to C)

Primary restraint to posterior displacement of tibia. Relaxed in extension, tense in flexion. Restraint to varus/valgus forces. Resists rotation, specially internal rotation of tibia on femur, as shown in Figure 25.29.

Kinetics of Gait

Gait Cycle

Normal gait can be divided into different phases, which are illustrated as follows:

Just prior to heel strike: Maximum extension and maximum external rotation

Heel strike: Maximum valgus

Flat foot: Flexion and internal rotation progress

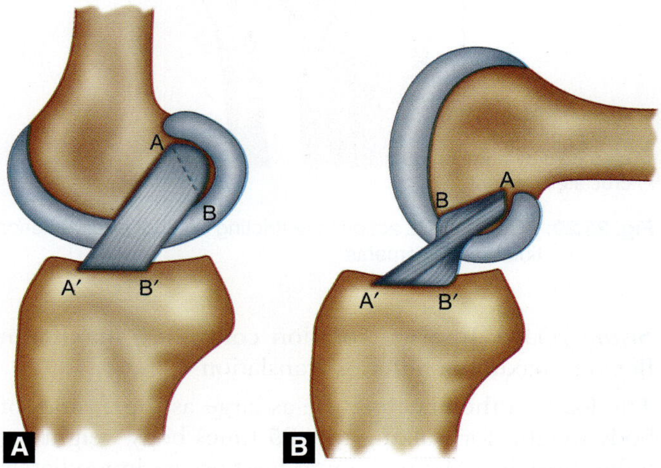

Figs 25.27A and B: (A) ACL tense in knee extension; (B) Lax during flexion

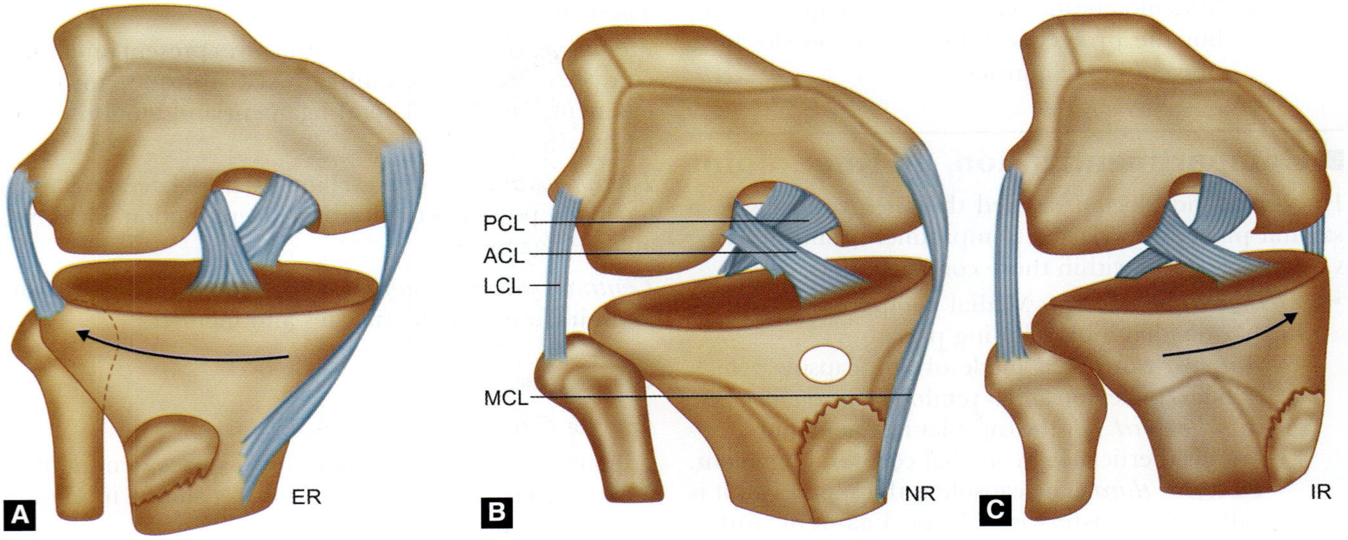

Figs 25.28A to C: Action of PCL during knee movements

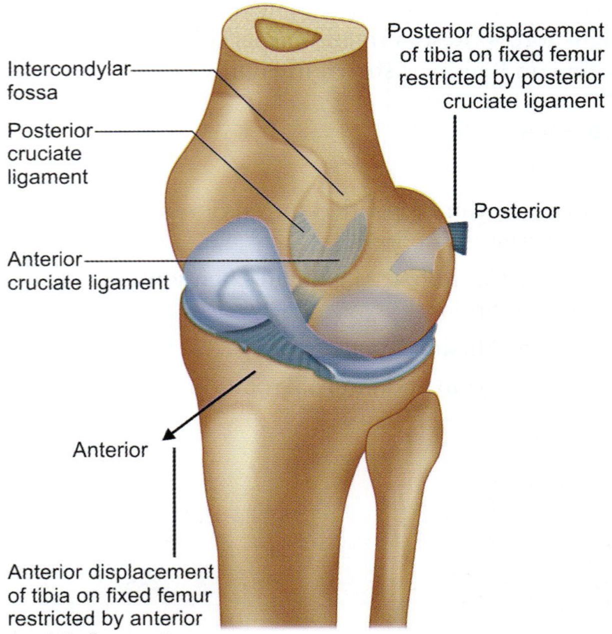

Fig. 25.29: ACL and PCL action in restricting anterior and posterior tibial displacements

Swing phase: Internal rotation continues, maximum flexion, maximum anterior translation

The load on the knee may be as large as three times of body weight, for walking to 4.25 times body weight for going upstairs. The maximum load occurs immediately after heel strike and shortly after heel off. The greater portion of load is transmitted by the medial compartment (25% greater), but the center of joint pressure ossilates between medial and lateral compartments. A 10° of varus/valgus deformity will double the load in affected compartment. At 30° of flexion, it is two times of body weight. Loading and the contact area is 12 cm^2, with the meniscus intact but only 3.5 cm^2 without meniscus.

KNEE JOINT EXAMINATION

Goals

Take a standardized, evidence based history and physical examination of patients with knee injuries. An important reason for achieving these skills is to provide patients with correct and timely diagnosis, therefore giving them a greater chance of restoring normal pain-free use of their limb.

Assessing a Knee

Components of the assessment include:
- Focused history
- Attentive physical examination
- Thoughtfully ordered test or studies

History

Complaints in knee:
- Pain
- Swelling
- Instability
- History of trauma
- Deformity
- Restricted range of motion (ROM)
  a. Pain assessment
    – Pain site, i.e. on medial, lateral, anterior and posterior aspects of knee

- Onset, whether acute or chronic
- Duration
- Aggravating factors, e.g. activities involving change in position, stairs climbing and kneeling.
- Relieving factors, e.g. ice, medications, crutches and radiation.

b. Swelling
  - Duration
  - Mode of onset
  - Progress of swelling
  - Site

c. Associated symptoms
d. History of trauma
e. Mechanism of injury

   Following questions need to be answered, while deciding mechanism of injury.
   - If it was contact or noncontact injury?
   - If contact, what part of the knee was contacted?
   - Anterior blow?
   - Valgus force?
   - Varus force?
   - Was foot of affected knee planted on the ground?

f. Injury associated events
   - Swelling after injury (immediate vs delayed)
   - Catching or locking
   - Buckling/instability (giving way)

g. *Deformity:* Associated history of trauma present since birth.
h. Restricted ROM
i. Prerequisites

   Both the knees must be examined simultaneously for comparative study. Pelvis to toes should be exposed. Examine in various positions as and when required.

Knee Examination

It includes examination of following:
- Gait
- Attitude
- Inspection
- Palpation
- Movements
- Measurements
- Special tests
- Neurovascular assessment

Gait

Antalgic gait: Seen in painful conditions

Waddaling gait: Varus deformity

Charlie Chaplin gait: Seen in external tibial torsion

Stiff knee gait: Affected knee swings outwards.

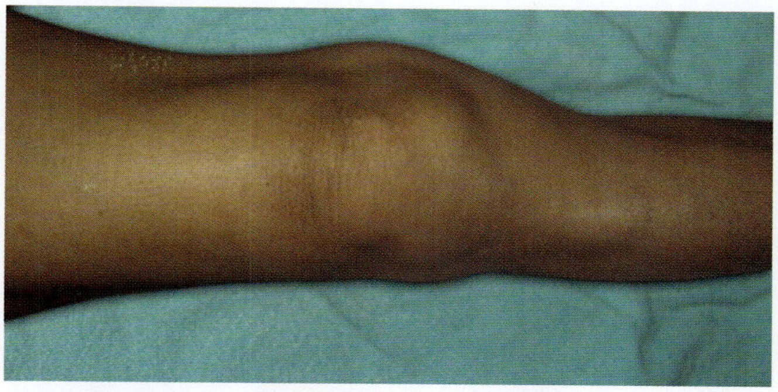

Fig. 25.30: Inspection of knee joint

Attitude

It is the position of the limb in relation to the rest of the body. The position in which patient is comfortable in keeping the limb.

Inspection (Fig. 25.30)

From Front

Swelling: Swelling confined to the limits of synovial cavity and suprapatellar pouch, can be due to:
- Effusion
- Hemarthrosis
- Pyoarthrosis
- Space occupying lesion in joint

  Swelling extending beyond the limits of joint cavity can be due to:
  - Infection
  - Tumor
  - Major injury.

Lumps: Note the presence of localized swellings prepatellar bursitis, infrapatellar bursitis, meniscus cyst, exostosis, etc. (Fig. 25.31).

Discoloration: Any bruising, which suggest trauma to the superficial tissues or knee ligaments.

Skin marks: Look for scar marks and sinuses.

From Side
- Normal contour
- Vastus lateralis bulge
- Iliotibial band
- Biceps femoris bulge
- Fibular neck depression.

From Behind
- Contour of back of thigh
- Popliteal fossa
- Prominent hamstrings
- Varicosity
- Swelling
- Visible pulsations

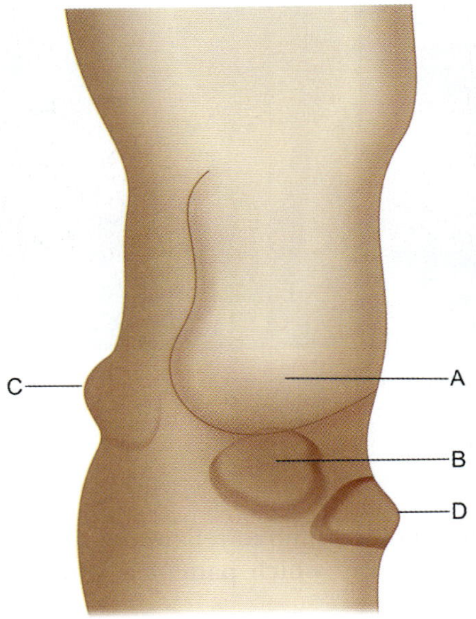

Figs 25.31: Knee joint inspection (from front)—A. Prepatellar bursitis; B. Infrapatellar bursitis; C. Meniscal cyst; D. Exostosis

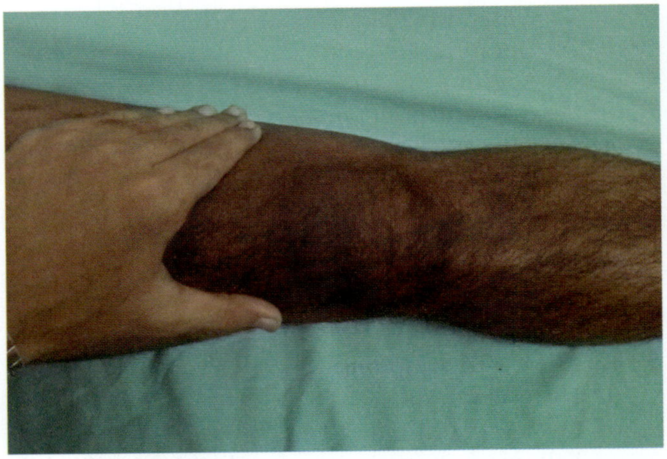

Fig. 25.32: Squeezing the suprapatellar pouch towards the knee joint

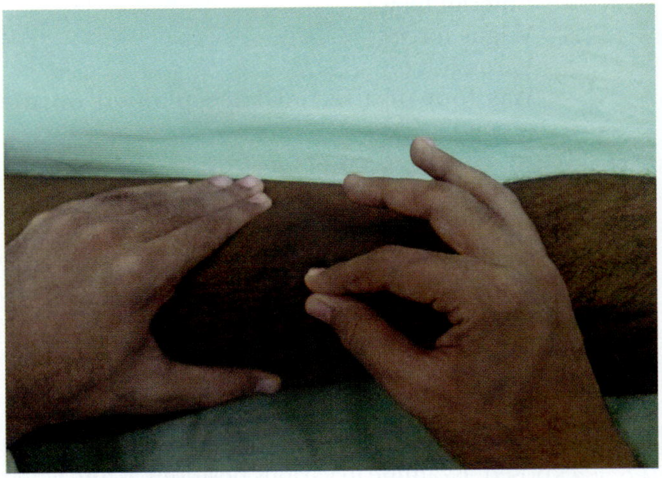

Fig. 25.33: Patellar tap test

Palpation

While palpating, look for the following:

- *Temperature:* It is felt by the back of the hand and is compared to that of the normal side.
- *Tenderness:* Joint line, includes both anterior and posterior joint line.
- Swelling
- Synovial membrane
- Joint line
- Popliteal fossa
- Patella and patellofemoral joint
- Muscles.

Swelling and Effusion

Size, shape, temperature, surface, edge, consistency, skin over the swelling, etc. should be noted. For effusion, following tests can be done:

- *Fullness of infrapatellar fossa:* Done if fluid quantity is small. Compress the fossa, the fluid is displaced but slowly refills after release of pressure.
- *Patellar tap (Figs 25.32 and 25.33):* Extend the knee fully (cannot be done if fixed flexion deformity (FFD) of knee is present). Squeeze the suprapatellar pouch towards the knee joint and give a jerk posteriorly, with the tips of thumb and index finger. The patella displaces the fluid and then again bounces back producing the tap.
- *Cross fluctuation test (Fig. 25.34):* Put the thumb and index finger of one hand on both sides of the infrapatellar fossa. Push the fluid by the thumb and index finger of opposite hand placed over the suprapatellar pouch and feel for the fluctuation. Useful for a larger effusion and fat knee. With thumb on one side of joint and fingers on other compress the knee to empty the hollows at the side of joint. With the other hand force fluid from suprapatellar pouch, distally in to the knee. Force of fluid transmitted is picked by compressing hand.
- *Fluid displacement:* Useful for minimal effusion. Evacuate suprapatellar pouch, then stroke the medial side of the joint to displace any excess fluid in the main joint cavity to the lateral side of joint. Similarly other side is be tested. Excess fluid will move across the joint and distend other side.

Palpation of a Bursa

- Consistency
- Mobility
- Translucency

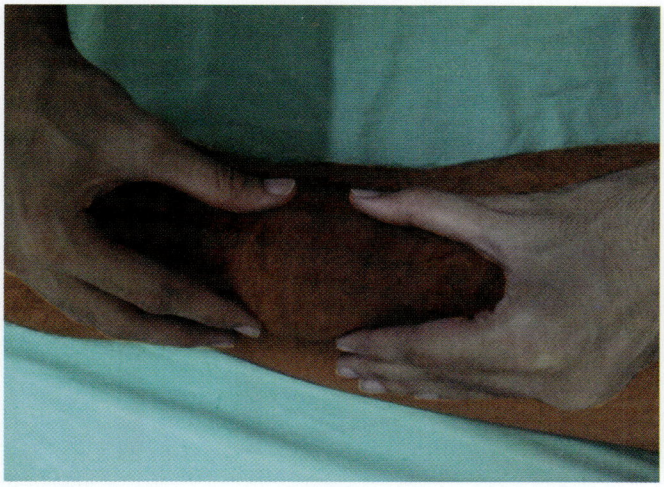

Fig. 25.34: Cross fluctuation test

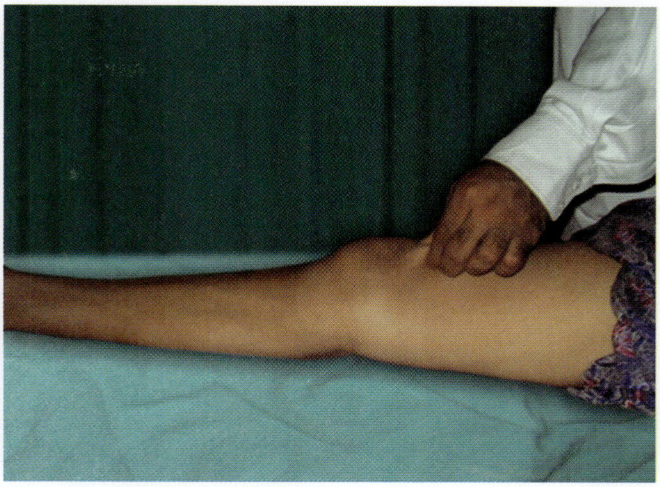

Fig. 25.35: Testing synovial thickening

- Relationship with the tendon. This is done by making the appropriate tendon taut.
- Swelling in the popliteal fossa should be examined for expansile pulsations.

Synovial Thickening (Fig. 25.35)

- Pick up the skin and relaxed quadriceps tendon to assess the thickness of synovial membrane in suprapatellar pouch
- It is thickened in RA and vilonodular synovitis.

Joint Line

Knee joint line should be palpated for its sharpness, tenderness or presence of any cysts.

Popliteal Fossa Inspection

Patient prone and knee is flexed. Look for any changes in:

- Knee joint
- Popliteal artery
- Areolar tissue
- Vein
- Nerves
- Tendons

Patella and Patellofemoral Joint (Fig. 25.36)

Tenderness: Palpate the patella and its margins for tenderness.

Mobility: Move patella up and down and from side to side with relaxed quadriceps. Move the patella proximally and distally, at the same time, pressing it down hard against femoral condyle. Pain is produced in chondromalacia patella and retropatellar arthritis.

Patellar grind test: It is done by applying pressure to the patella and manually displacing it medially, laterally,

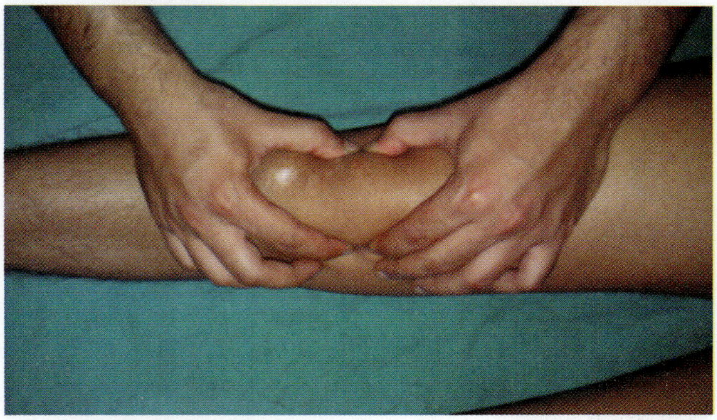

Fig. 25.36: Checking the mobility of the patella

superiorly and inferiorly in the trochlear groove. Test produces anterior knee pain, when patellofemoral pathologies are present.

Muscles

All the muscles around knees are palpated look for the wasting.

Bony Palpation

- *Femoral condyles*: Anteroinferior, lateral and medial portions are palpated, while flexing the knee gradually.
- *Tibial condyles*: Palpate articular surfaces anterolaterally and anteromedially, with knee in 90° of flexion.

Range of Motion

- *Extension:* Flexion 0 to 135°
- Describe loss of degrees of extension, e.g. 5° of FFD *Flexion (Figs 25.37 and 25.38):* Measure the range of

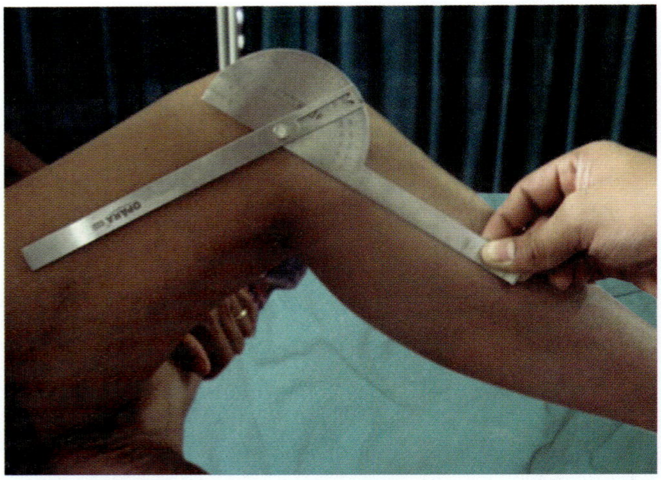

Fig. 25.37: Knee flexion ROM measured, using goniometer

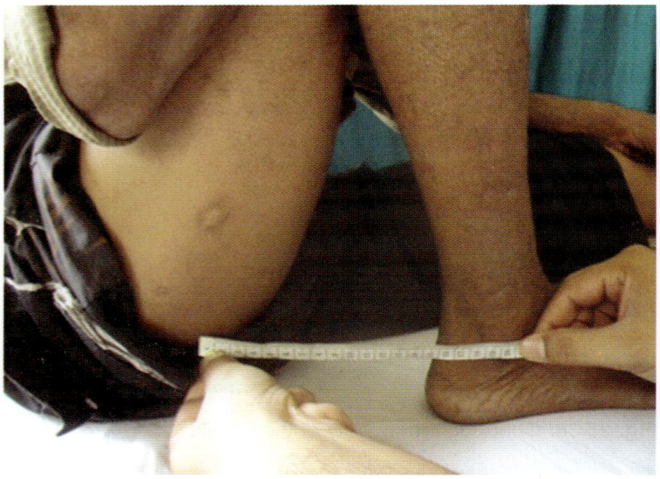

Fig. 25.38: Measurement of heel to buttock distance

flexion in degrees starting from zero position of normal full extension. Flexion of 135° is regarded as normal. Compare the two sides. Measure the heel to buttock distance with the leg fully flexed (1cm equals to 1.5°), as shown in Figure 25.38.

Extension (Fig. 25.39): Ask the patient to stand up from the squatting position. Note whether he is able to stand straight with the knee in full extension. Ask patient to sit on the edge of the couch and to extend the legs fully. Full extension is recorded as 0°. Loss of full extension is recorded, as knee lacks x° of extension. Examine the patient in prone position, fully relaxed, with legs hanging over the edge of table. Loss of extension should be obvious from the position of heels, as shown in Figure 25.40. A springy block to full extension is suggestive of bucket handle tear. A rigid block is seen in arthritic condition.

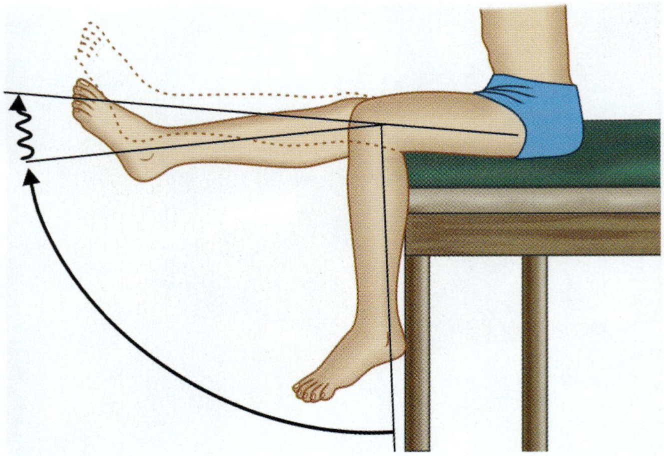

Fig. 25.39: Knee extension ROM

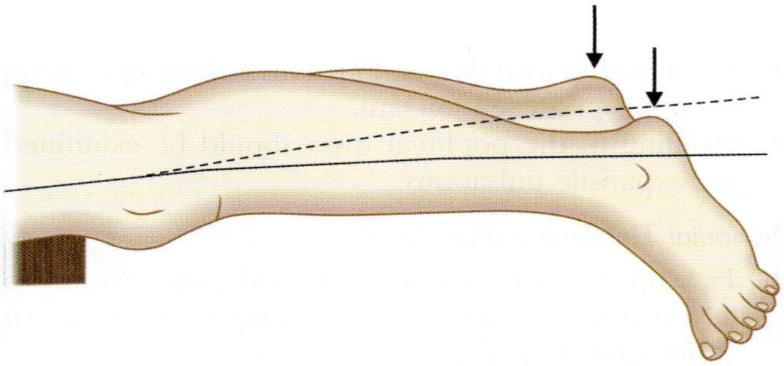

Fig. 25.40: Loss of extension measured from the level of heel (arrows)

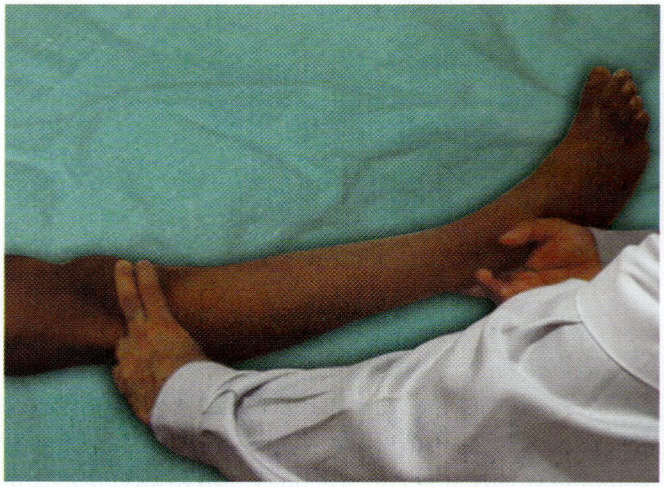

Fig. 25.41: Rotation of knee

Hyperextension (Figs 25.41 and 25.42): This is present, if knee extends beyond the point when tibia and femur are in line. If present look for other signs of joint laxity. It is seen most frequently seen in girls and is associated with

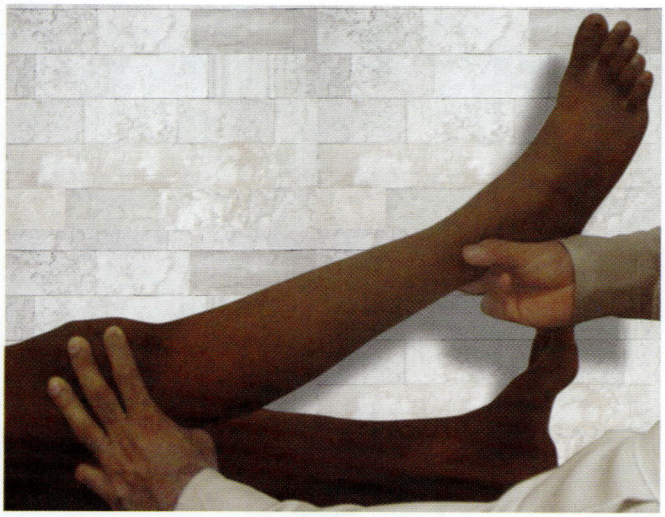

Fig. 25.42: Excess angulation beyond 0° of normal extension or knee hyperextension

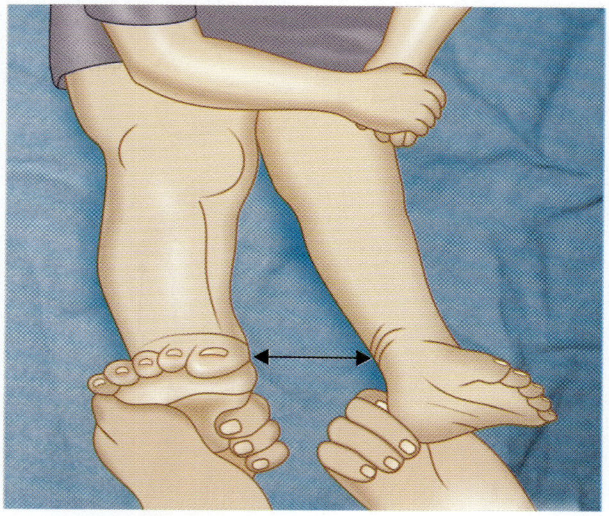

Fig. 25.44: Measuring intermalleolar gap (arrow)

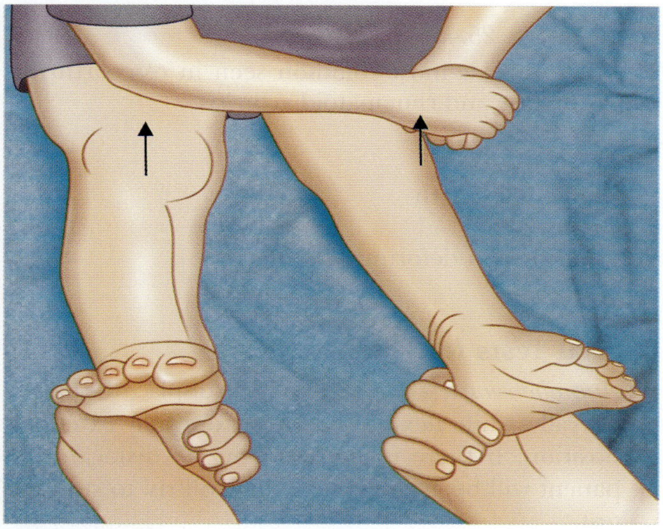

Fig. 25.43: Genu valgum—checking for unilateral or bilateral genu valgum

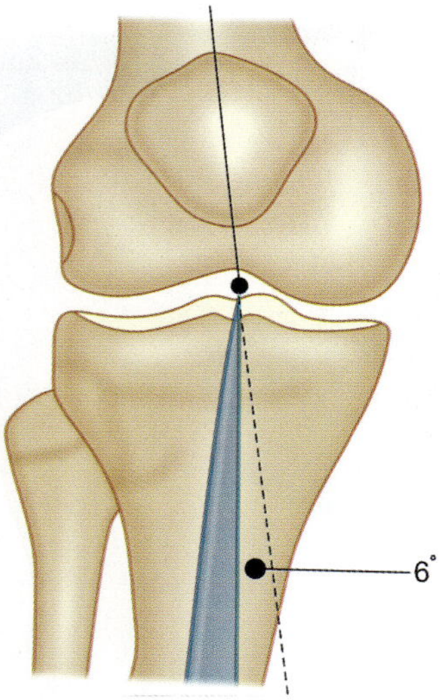

Fig. 25.45: Genu valgum measured by angle formed by tibial and femoral shaft in adult

high patella (patella alta), chondromalacia patella and recurrent dislocation of patella.

Internal and external rotation: Place your hand on the patient's thigh just above the knee to stabilize the femur. Grasp his heel, with your free hand and rotate the tibia. At the same time palpated the tibial tubercle to ensure that it is moving. Normally, approximately 10° of rotatory motion on each side.

Genu Valgum

In Children (Figs 25.43 and 25.44)

- Unilateral or bilateral (Fig. 25.43)
- It is measured by intermalleolar gap (Fig. 25.44). Grasp the child by ankle and rotate the legs, until patellae are vertical. Now bring the legs together to touch lightly at knees and measure the gap between the malleoli. Normally they both should touch. In 10 to 16 years of age group, less than 8 cm in females and less than 4 cm in male is regarded as normal.

In Adults (Fig. 25.45)

It is measured, by angle formed by tibial and femoral shaft. Normal angle is approximately 6° in adult. In adults, the deformity is seen most often in association with RA. It is also common in teen age girls.

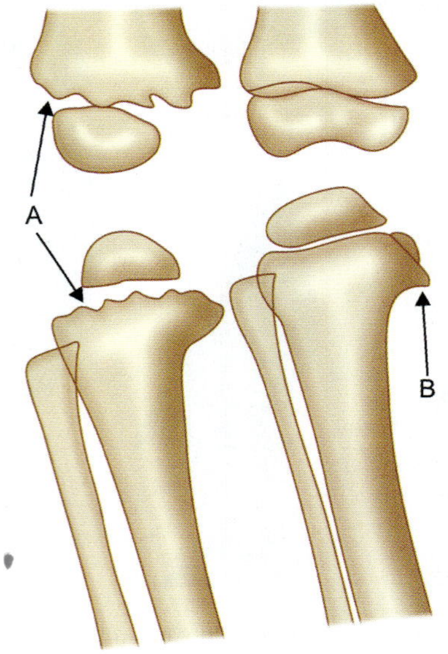

Fig. 25.46: Genu varum

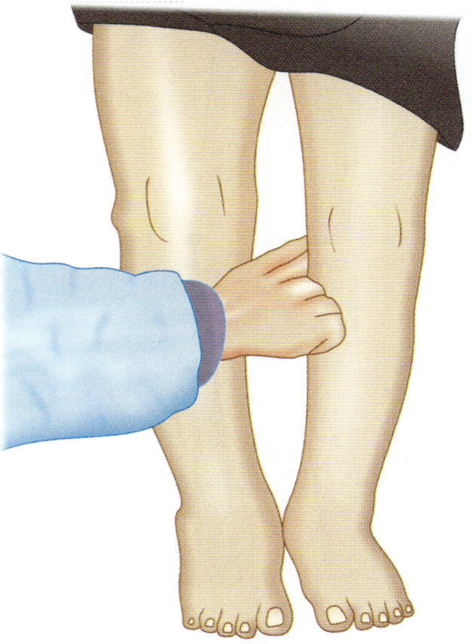

Fig. 25.47: Genu varum in children is measured by finding distance between the knees, using the fingers as a guage

Genu Varum (Figs 25.46 and 25.47)

In Children

Measure the distance between the knees, using the fingers as a guage as shown in Figure 25.47. Patient should be weight-bearing and both patella should face forwards to counter any effect of hip rotation. In 10 to 16 years of age group less than 4 cm in female less than 5 cm in males is normal. In tibia vara note sharply down turned medial metapyseal border. Radiological varus is normal till child is 18 months old.

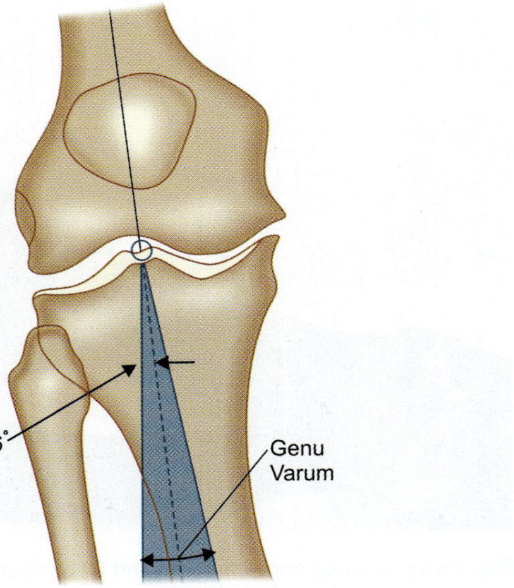

Fig. 25.48: Measurement of genu varum in adults

In Adults (Fig. 25.48)

The deformity is most common seen in osteoarthritis, pagets disease and rhuematoid arthritis.

Measurements

- Segmental length
- Girth
- Fixed flexion deformity
- Q angle.

Special Tests for Patella

- *Apprehension test (Fig. 25.49):* Try to displace the patella laterally, while flexing the knee from fully extended position. If there is any tendency to dislocate the patient will be apprehensive and will try to stop the test.
- *Dynamic patellar tracking:* Position examiner standing in front of the seated patient, while patient slowly extends the knee. Positive 'j' sign (slight lateral subluxation of patella as the knee approaches full extension) indicates maltracking. Patella should move superiorly rather than laterally.
- *Patellar tilt test (Fig. 25.50):* Patient positioned in extended knee. The examiner's fingers are placed along the medial side of patella with the thumb hooked on the lateral aspect. Inability to raise the lateral facet to the horizontal plane, indicates the excessive lateral retinacular tightness.

Special Test for Effusion

- Patellar tap
- Fluid displacement

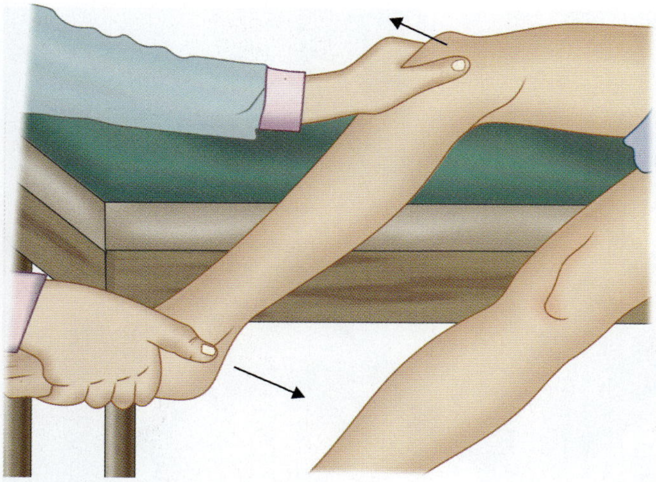

Fig. 25.49: Apprehension test

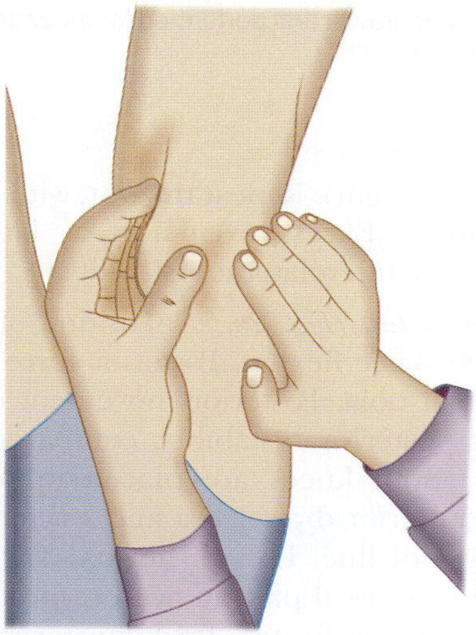

Fig. 25.50: Patellar tilt test

- Cross fluctuation
- Transillumination

Patellar tap test: Milk the synovial fluid out of the suprapatellar pouch, with the index and thumb from 15 cm above upper border of patella. Place the tips of thumb and three fingers of free hand on the patella and jerk it towards femur. A click as the patella strikes the condyles, indicates the presence of effusion.

False negative: Too slight, too tense, loculated and thick fluid.

■ Stability Tests

Unidirectional

- Varus and valgus test in extension and 30° flexion
- Anterior and posterior drawer test

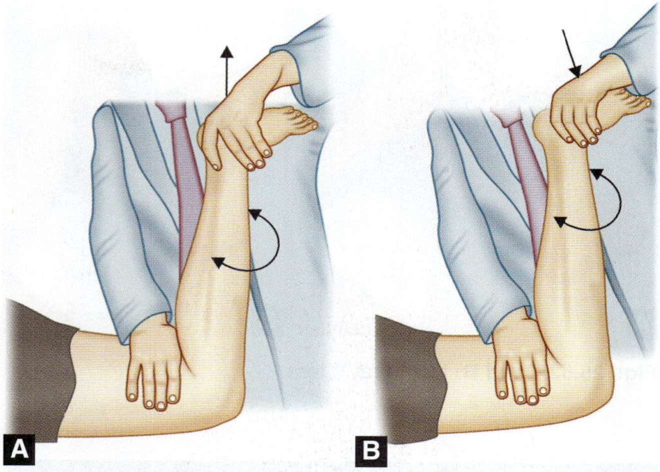

Figs 25.51A and B: Apley's grinding test—(A) Extending the knee after, internally rotating, any limitation or pain is noted; (B) Sharp pain, on pressing the limb along the axis of limb and externally rotating the foot, indicates medial meniscus tear and pain on internal rotation, indicates lateral meniscus tear

- Lachman's test
- Quadriceps active test.

Rotatory Instability

- Slocum rotatory drawer test
- Lateral pivot shift test
- Jerk test
- Jerk test for Houghston and Losee
- Flexion rotation drawer test
- External rotation recurvatum test
- Reverse pivot shift test
- Tibial external rotation test
- Posterolateral drawer test
- Bounce home test
- Wilson test.

Tests for Meniscus Injury

- Apley's grinding
- McMurray's test.

Tests for Ligaments Injury

- Anterior drawer test
- Posterior drawer test
- Lachman test
- Valgus stress test
- Varus stress test
- Active quadriceps test.

Apley's grinding test (Figs 25.51A and B): Patient lying prone. Grasp the foot, externally rotate it and flex the knee, then rotate foot internally and extend knee. Any limitation of rotation or pain is noted. Then press the limb along the axis of limb and externally rotate foot. Sharp pain,

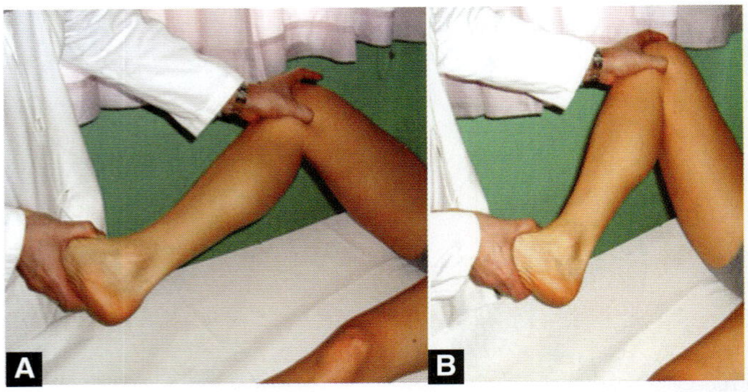

Figs 25.52A and B: McMurray's test

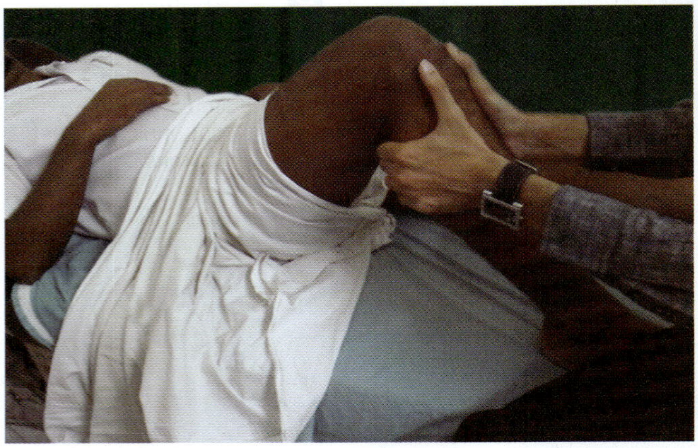

Fig. 25.53: Anterior drawer test performed for testing anteromedial instability

indicates medial meniscus tear. Lateral meniscus is tested by foot internally rotated.

McMurray's test (Figs 25.52A and B): Patient is positioned in supine. Put thumb and index finger along the joint line. Flex and abduct the knee and externally rotate the foot. Now extend the joint, a click associated with sharp pain, indicates medial meniscus tear. A click occurring between complete flexion of the knee and 90° is from posterior peripheral tear. A click occurring in greater degree of extension, suggests a tear in the middle and anterior portion of meniscus. For lateral meniscus, repeat the test with leg adducted and foot internally rotated.

Anterior drawer test (Fig. 25.53): Position of the patient is supine lying, hip flexed to 45° and knee to 90°. Steady foot, by sitting close to it. Grasp the leg firmly, with thumbs on tibial tubercle and jerk the leg towards you. Look the tibial movement on femur. Movement of tibia 6 to 8 mm greater than that of opposite knee, indicates a torn of anterior cruciate ligament (ACL). Repeat test with foot in 30° of external rotation. Excess excursion of medial tibial condyle, suggests anteromedial instability

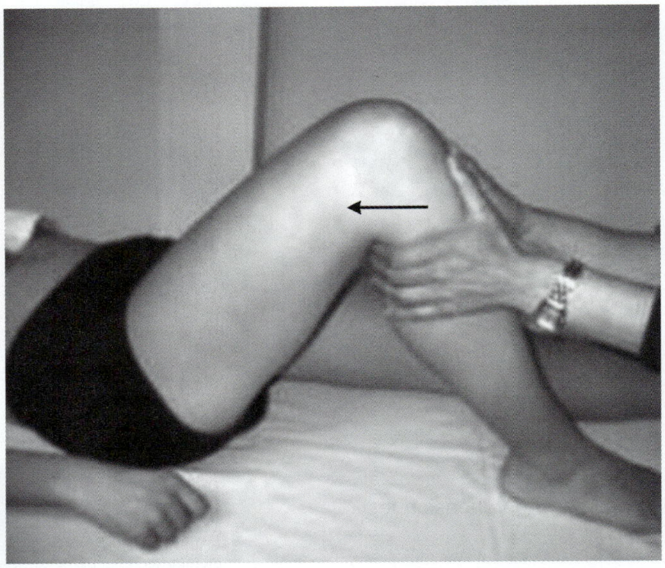

Fig. 25.54: Posterior drawer test performed for measuring posterior instability

(ACL, medial ligament). Repeat the test, with foot in 30° internal rotation. Excess excursion of lateral tibial condyle, suggests anterolateral instability.

Posterior drawer test (Fig. 25.54): Position of patient is supine with 90° knee flexion. Posterior force is applied on the proximal tibia. Posterior movement of tibia on femur, shows posterior instability, compared with the normal tibia. Both knees are placed in position to perform the posterior drawer test and a thumb on both anteromedial joint line. Loss of normal 1 cm anterior step of the medial tibial plateau, with respect to medial femoral condyle, indicates torn posterior cruciate ligament (PCL).

Gravity test: Hip and knee flexed to 90°. While the heels of each extremity are supported in examiner's hand. By sitting on the side of the patient, note that tibia sags visibly posteriorly from the effects of gravity, suggestive of PCL tear.

Lachman test (Fig. 25.55): Patient positioned in supine. Test can be useful in swollen and painful knee. It is more sensitive test for ACL, because both the fibers of ACL are relaxed in 15° of flexion. Knee is flexed to 15°, femur is stabilized, with one hand and the other tries to lift the tibia forwards with thumb over anteromedial joint margin. When lifting force is applied, anterior translation of tibia is palpated by thumb. Anterior translation, indicates positive test, confirm ACL tear. In fatty patient the test is done with patient in prone position. Encircle tibia with both hands, put index finger and thumb in joint line. Flex the knee to 20°. Push the tibia forwards. Anterior translation of tibia is noted.

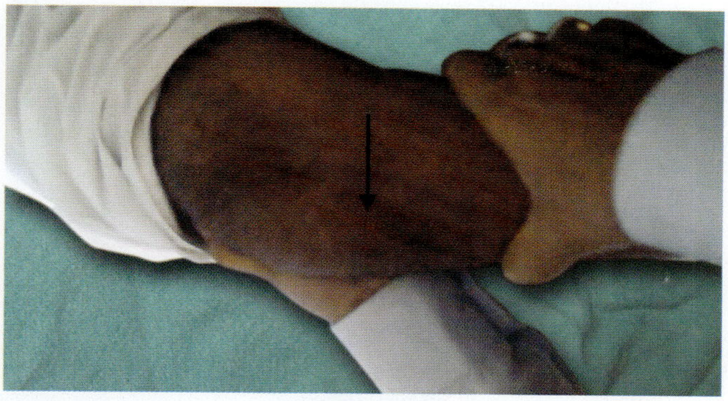

Fig. 25.55: Lachman test—testing the anterior cruciate ligament

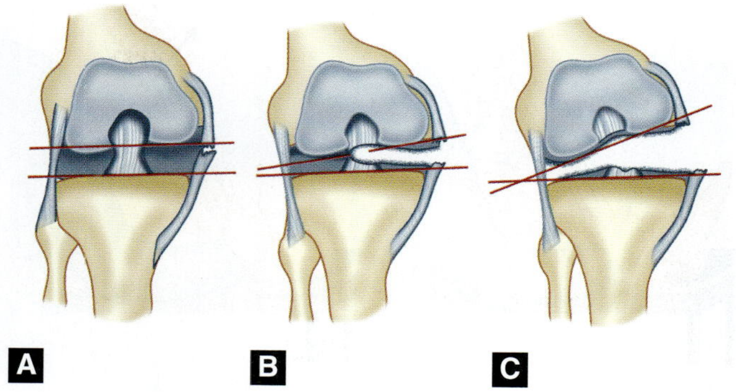

Figs 25.57A to C: Forces acting on the knee joint on performing valgus stress test

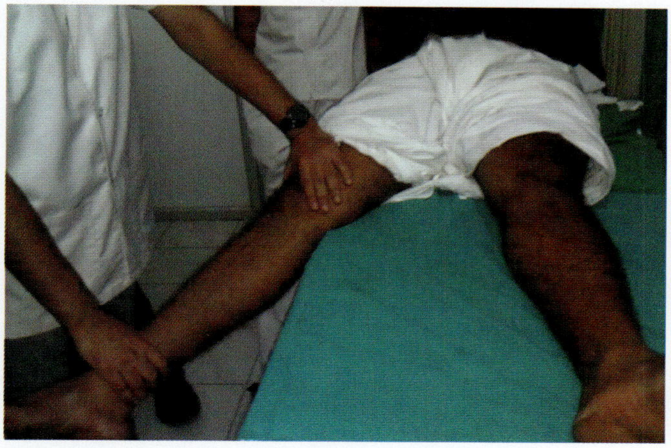

Fig. 25.56: Valgus stress test

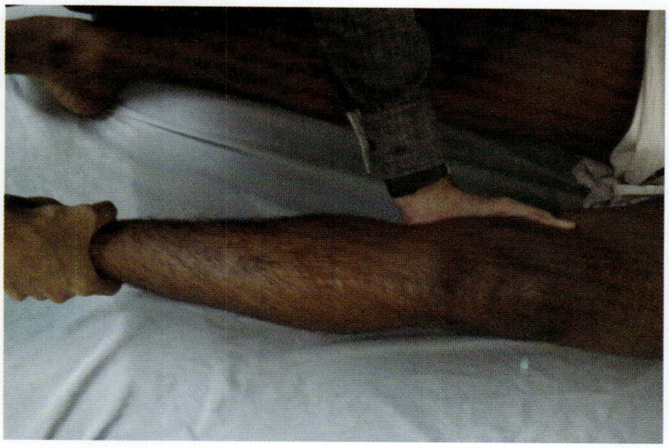

Fig. 25.58: Varus stress test

Valgus stress test (Fig. 25.56): Position is supine lying. Limb is abducted and knee is flexed to 30°. Place one hand over the lateral surface of knee, while supporting the ankle with other hand. Gentle abduction is applied, while the hand at the ankle, externally rotates the leg. The test is repeated several times in this position up to producing mild pain. The knee is brought into full extension and valgus stressing is repeated. Positive test, indicates medial ligaments instability. Tear confined to tibial collateral ligament, while posterior corner and posterior capsule are intact. Valgus stress applied to knee will not cause medial opening. This is possible only when knee is flexed about 30° to relaxes posterior capsule, thereby eliminating lateral stabilizing action, as shown in Figures 25.57A to C. If knee shows medial opening in extension, involvement of cruciate ligament is possibility, even no significant drawer sign can be elicited. If valgus instability extend across to lateral side, in both flexion and extension, then both cruciates are torn.

Varus stress test (Fig. 25.58): Attempt to produce varus deformity, by placing one hand on the medial side of joint and force the ankle medially. Carry the test in 30° flexion and full extension. If there is varus instability in extension and flexion, it will suggest the tear of PCL and lateral ligament complex.

Quadriceps active test (Fig. 25.59): Position of the patient is supine and relaxed. Limb is supported with the knee flexed to 90°. Gentle quadriceps contraction is done, to shift the tibia without extending the knee. Normally, patellar ligament is oriented slightly posterior. In PCL rupture, tibia sags into posterior subluxation and patellar ligament is directed anteriorly (2 mm or more).

Slocum anterior rotary drawer test: The degree of anterior displacement of the tibia on the femur is noted in 15° of internal rotation, 30° of external rotation and neutral rotation. A positive anterior drawer in neutral tibial rotation, that is attenuated, when the test is done on 30° of external rotation and reduced in 15° of internal rotation, indicates anteromedial instability.

Jerk test of Hughston and Losee (Fig. 25.60): Patient kept in supine position and knee flexed to 90°, tibia is rotated

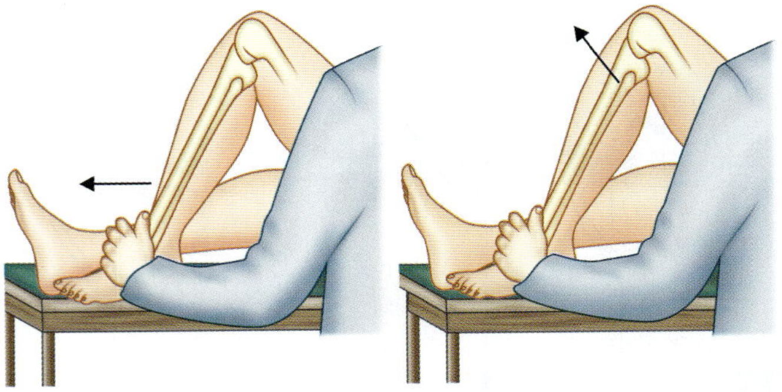

Fig. 25.59: Quadriceps active test

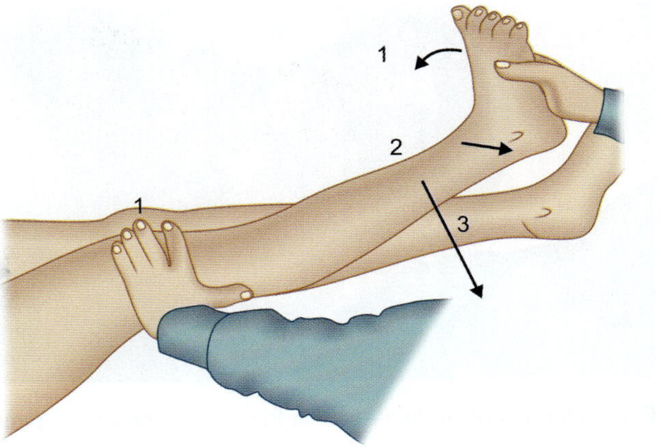

Fig. 25.61: Pivot shift test

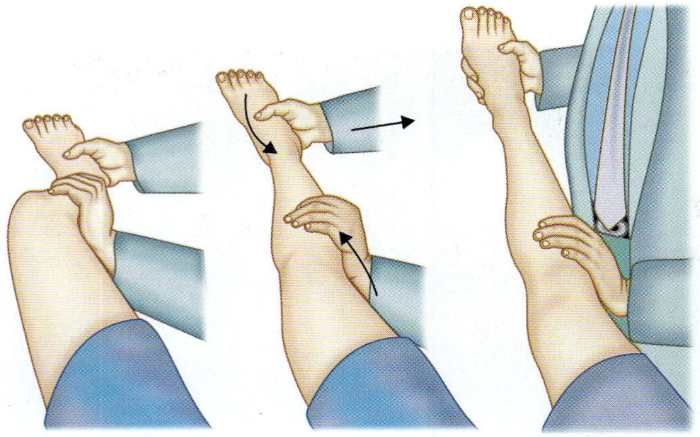

Fig. 25.60: Jerk test of Hughston and Losee

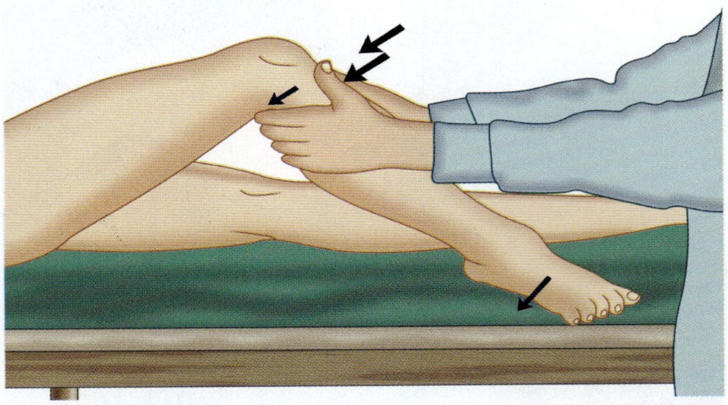

Fig. 25.62: Posterior lateral drawer test

internally. When the right knee is examined, the foot is grasped with the right hand, valgus stress is exerted towards the proximal end of tibia with the left hand. The knee is extended gradually, maintaining the internal rotation and valgus. Tibia spontaneously subluxates forward in the form of sudden jerk at 30° of flexion.

Pivot shift test or macintosh test (Fig. 25.61): Fully extend the knee. While holding the foot in internal rotation, apply valgus test. If the instability is present, tibia will be in subluxated position. Now flex the knee. Reduction should occur at 30°, with obvious jerks. This is positive test, indicates ACL abnormality.

Posterior lateral drawer test (Fig. 25.62): The knee should be flexed to little less than 90° and foot placed in external rotation. Apply back pressure on tibia. Excessive travel on lateral side, is indicative of posterolateral instability (PCL and lateral ligament complex injury).

Flexion rotation drawer test (Figs 25.63A and B): It test ACL in two planes, AP plane and femoral rotation. The result may be positive, when other test for ACL are negative. It combines features of Lachman test and Hughston pivot shift test. With patient supine and knee in full extension, leg is lifted upwards, with the femur allowed to fall back and rotate extenally. This results in anterolateral tibial subluxation, as the starting position for the test. While the knee is flexed and the tibia moves backward and the femur rotates internally, causing the joint to reduce, when the test result is positive. Mild valgus stress and anteior pressure on the upper calf applied by the examiner's hand, can be done to elicit a positive test result.

External rotation recurvatum test (Fig. 25.64): With the patient in supine position, stand at the end of examination couch. Lift the legs by great toes. The test is positive if knee falls into external rotation, varus or recurvatum.

Tibial external rotation test: When an injured knee is tested for posterolateral instability, external rotation of tibia over femur is measured at both 30° and 90° of knee flexion. The medial border of the foot, in its neutral position is used as reference point for external rotation. The degree of external rotation of the foot is measured, relative to the axis of the femur and is compared with the opposite leg. External rotation is measured noting the foot thigh angle. A 10° difference in external rotations between knees

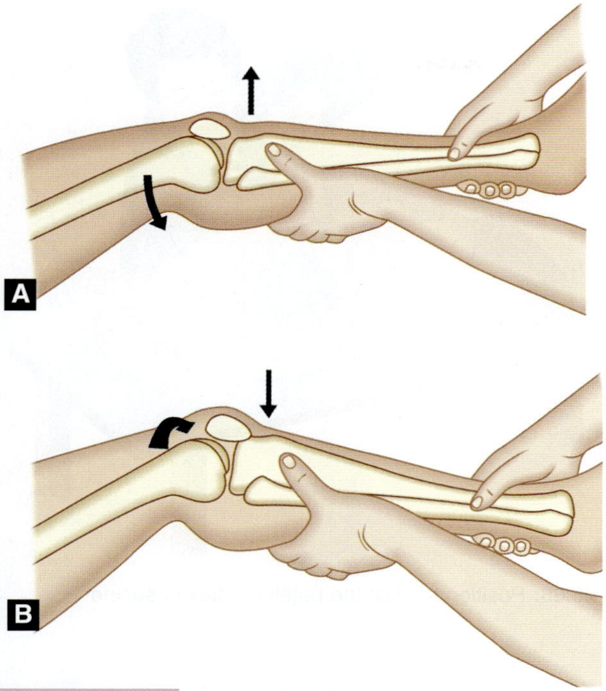

Figs 25.63A and B: Flexion rotation drawer test

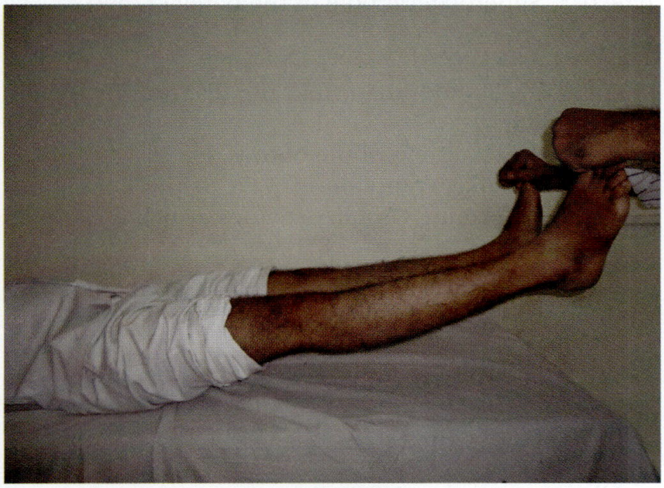

Fig. 25.64: External rotation recurvatum test

is pathological. More than a 10° increase in external rotation, compared with that of the contralateral side at 30° of knee flexion, but not at 90°, indicates an isolated injury to the posterolateral corner. An increase in external rotation, of more than 10° compared with that on the contralateral side at both 30° and 90° of knee flexion, indicates injury of both the posterior cruciate ligament and the posterolateral corner.

Bounce home test (Fig. 25.65): This test is designed to evaluate a lack of full knee extension, secondary to torn meniscus, a loose body or an intracapsular joint swelling. With the patient supine on the table, cup his heel in your palm and bend his knee into full extension. Now passively extend knee, the knee should extend completely or bounce home into extension, with sharp end point. However, if knee falls short, rubbery resistances to further extension, suggesting a meniscus tear.

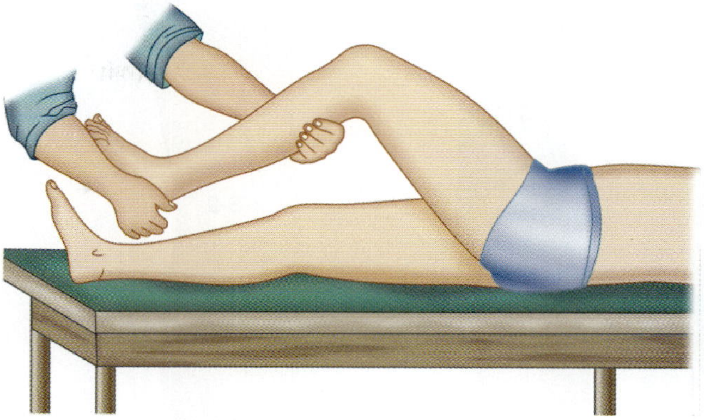

Fig. 25.65: Bounce home test

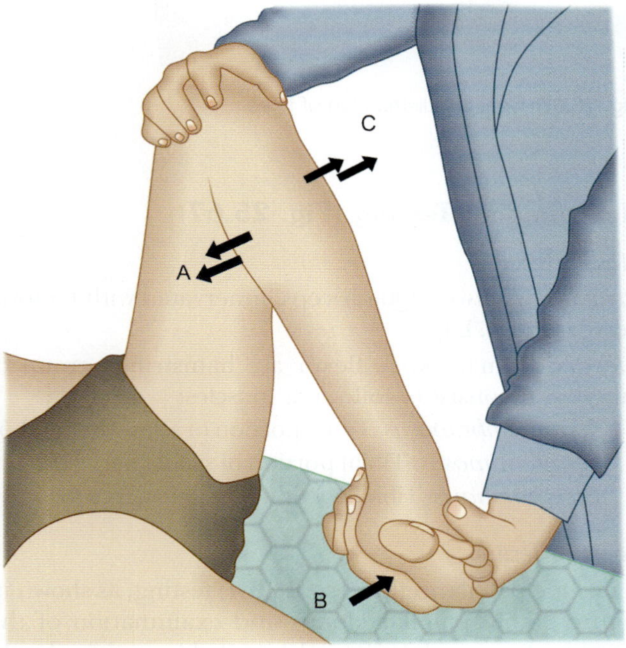

Fig. 25.66: Wilson's test—A. Flexion with internal rotation of knee; B. Extending the knee; C. Pain relieved on externally rotating the knee

Wilson's test (Fig. 25.66): The aim is to cause pressure between ACL and lateral aspect of medial femoral condyle. Flex the knee and internally rotate the foot. Now extend the knee fully. If pain occurs in full extension and is relieved by external rotation of foot. This is for suspected osteochondritis dessicans.

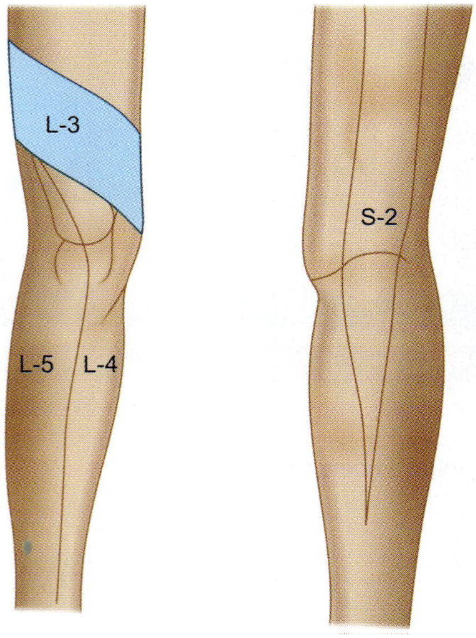

Fig. 25.67: Sensory distribution of knee

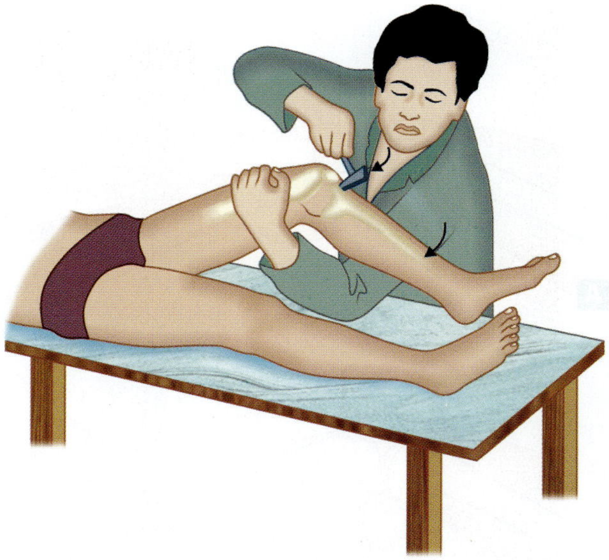

Fig. 25.68: Position to elicit the patellar reflex in supine

Neurological Testing (Fig. 25.67)

Muscle Testing

Primary extensors: Quadriceps, innervated with femoral nerve (L2, L3, L4)

Flexors: Primary knee flexor are hamstrings group of muscles. It consist of following muscles:

- *Semimembranosus:* Tibial portion of sciatic nerve (L5)
- *Semitendinosus*: Tibial portion of sciatic nerve (L5)
- *Biceps femoris*: Tibial portion of sciatic nerve (S1).

Sensory Testing

It include patellar reflex (L2, L3, L4) testing, as shown in Figure 25.68, patellar clonus and examination of the opposite knee and ipsilateral hip. Ankle testing should also be performed.

CONGENITAL ANOMALIES AROUND THE KNEE JOINT

■ Bipartite Patella

Patella normally forms from one ossification center. Sometimes, however ossification occurs from more than two centers, but ultimately they fuse to form one single bone. Failure of fusion of the bones leads to bi or tripartite patellae. Fibrous union of the separately ossified bones keep them bound together.

Classification or Saupe's Classification

Saupe had classified bipartite patellae on the basis of the position of their occurrence as follows:

Type I: Inferior pole of the patella (5%). (Sinding-Lanssen-Johnson syndrome)

Type II: Lateral margins of the patella (20%).

Type III: Superolateral pole of the patella (75%).

Clinical Features

- Generally asymptomatic and the diagnosis is usually incidental.
- *Trauma:* Separation of the fibrous union.
- The child may complain of pain in the knee joint, while performing certain activities, which include:
  - Squatting
  - Stair climbing
  - Activities that load the patellofemoral joint.

Investigations

- *X-rays (Figs 25.69 and 25.70):* It include anteroposterior (AP), lateral and skyline views (squatting).
- Technetium bone scan
- Ultrasonography (USG)
- Magnetic resonance imaging (MRI) (Fig. 25.71).

Treatment Modalities

Treatment options include:

- *Incidental finding:* Leave alone, i.e. no treatment is required.
- *Post-traumatic separation:* Treatment is required.

Initial Treatment

- Reduce activities
- Analgesics
- Knee immobilization in ankle-knee cylindrical casts or braces for 3 to 4 weeks.
- If above interventions fail, surgery might be required.

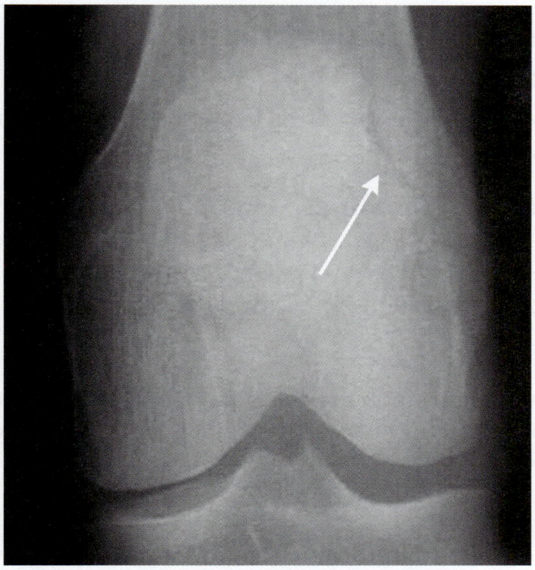

Fig. 25.69: X-ray knee (AP view) showing bipartite patella (arrow)

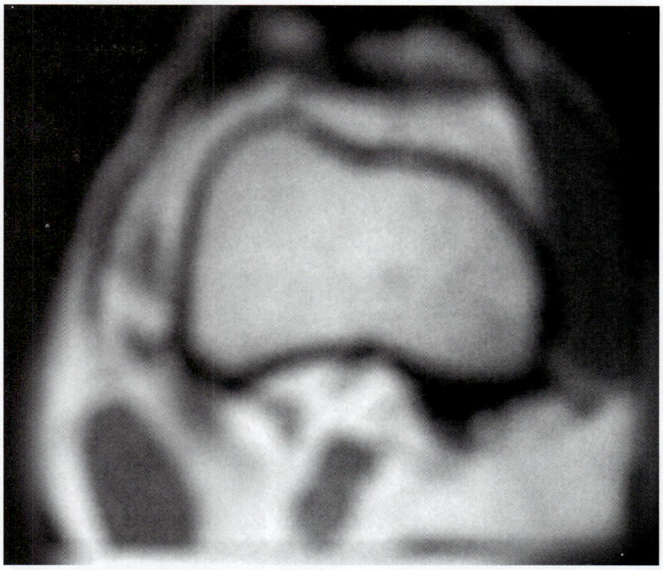

Fig. 25.71: MRI of knee joint, showing bipartite patella

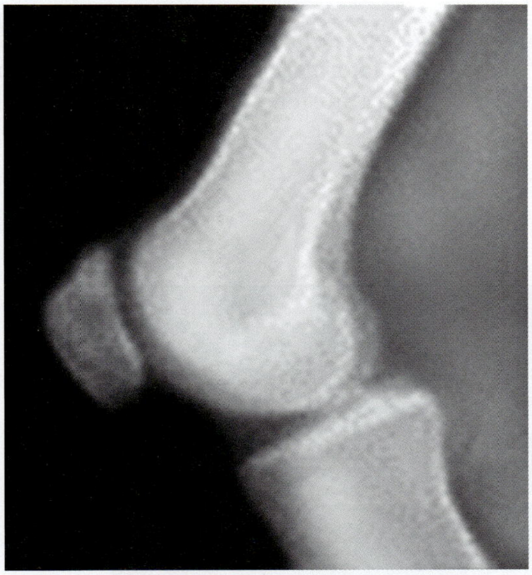

Fig. 25.70: X-ray knee, lateral-skyline view

Surgical Interventions

- Small fragments excision
- *Mori's procedure:* Lateral release done in painful bipartite patella.
- *Ogata's procedure:* It includes following steps:
  - Vastus lateralis is freed from the fragments subperiosteally.
  - Continuity of the insertion of the lateralis tendon to the remainder of the patella is maintained.
  - Unstable fragments removed and stable are left *in situ.*

Congenital Dislocation of Patella

Patella is dislocated at birth. It is mainly familial and generally bilateral. Mostly associated with arthrogryposis multiplex congenital and Down's syndrome.

Pathology

There is an abnormality of the quadriceps mechanism. Vastus lateralis may be abnormal or severely contracted. Patella is dislocated laterally and attached to the anterior aspect of the iliotibial band.

Factors Contributing to Patellar Dislocation

- Genu valgum
- Shallow lateral femoral condyle
- Elongated patellar tendon (high riding patella)
- Deficient vastus medialis
- External tibial torsion or lateral insertion of the patellar tendon
- Deformed patella
- Shallow patellar groove on the femur
- Medial capsular laxity
- Abnormal attachment of the iliotibial tract on patella
- Genu recervatum
- Patellar hypoplasia.

Classification of Patellar Dislocation

Eilert classify patellar dislocations in two types:

1. Congenital or fixed lateral dislocation
2. Obligatory dislocation of the patella

Clinical Features

- Fixed flexion contracture of the knee and an apparent valgus deformity are the key findings
- *Palpation:* Tiny dislocated patella can be felt just lateral to lateral femoral condyle. Intercondylar notch feels empty
- *Range of Motion (ROM):* Extension is restricted
- Patella is irreducible.

Investigations

Investigation done by X-rays (Figs 25.72A and B), MRI and USG.

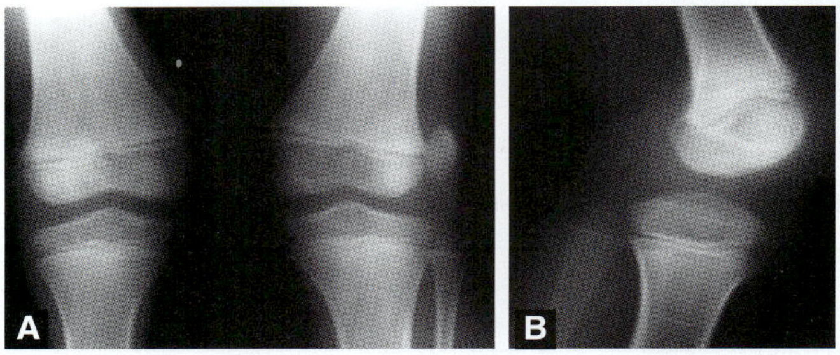

Figs 25.72A and B: X-rays showing congenital dislocation of left patella in 5 years old boy—(A) Anteroposterior view shows fixed lateral dislocation; (B) On lateral view, patella appears absent because of superimposed femoral condyles

■ Lateral Dislocation of Bilateral Patellae

This could be the result of hypoplastic lateral femoral condyle.

Treatment Modalities (Figs 25.73A to C)

If left untreated, loss of extension in gait and progressive valgus deformity of the knee occur. Treatment vary with the age and includes following procedures:

For 6 Months Child

- Quadriceps mobilized and patella released laterally.
- Patellar tendon insertion detatched and reinserted medially.

Older Children

- Medial restraint (semitendinosus transfer) surgery also known as Galleazzi's procedure.
- *Stanisavljevic procedure:* Entire quadriceps is elevated subperiosteally from the femur and rotated medially. Fascia lata excised and used as graft to cover the lateral defect.
- *Langenskiold procedure:* Given by Beaty, Gao, Lee, et al. It includes lateral release, medial plication and patellar tendon transfer.

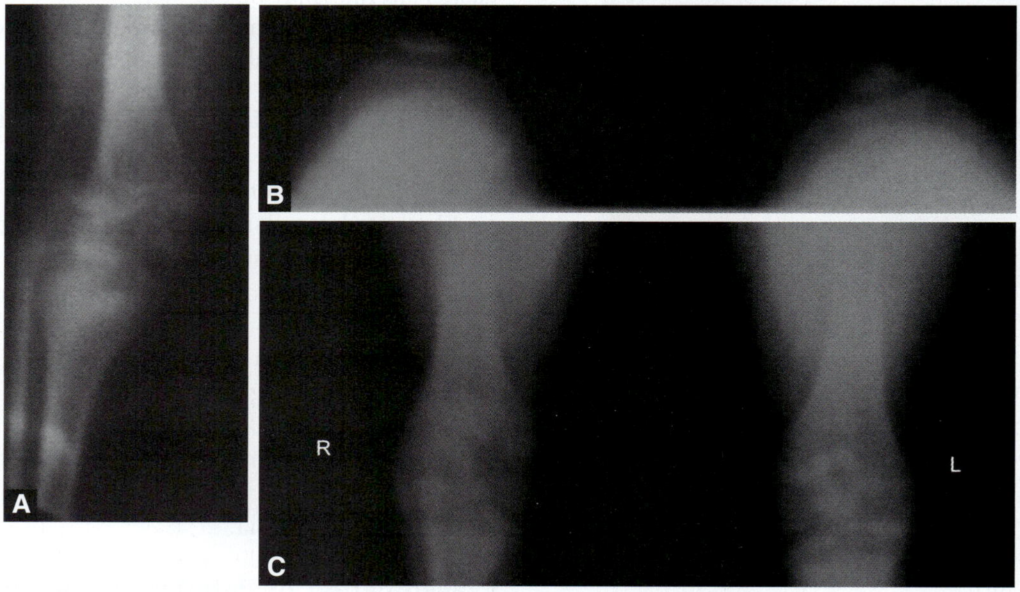

Figs 25.73A to C: Preoperative and postoperative radiographs for dislocated patella—(A) Preoperative radiograph, showing complete lateral dislocation of the patella; (B and C) Postoperative radiographs showing correction

■ Discoid Lateral Meniscus

Also known as snapping or popping knee. It was first described in the late nineteenth century. The normal configuration of a meniscus is a matured crescent moon, whereas, a discoid meniscusis thickened and having shape of very early crescent moon. The discoid shape results in membrane barrier, which prevents normal contact between the articular surfaces of the knee and cause mechanical deformation. Incidence of associated discoid medial meniscus is about 0.3 percent.

Classification of Discoid Lateral Meniscus

Watanabe described three types of discoid lateral meniscus (DLM):

Type I: *Wrisberg ligament type (least common):* It lacks an attachment to stabilize the posterior horn to the tibia. It may also be of normal shape rather than discoid. The only attachment of the posterior horn is to the Wrisberg or meniscofemoral ligament (quadripedal animals), produces an unstable or hypermobile lateral meniscus.

Type II: *Complete type (truly discoid):* Thickened lateral meniscus with normal peripheral attachments. Generally asymptomatic.

Type III: *Incomplete type (Figs 25.74A and B):* Smaller and does not fit the lateral compartment.

Ross' theory (Fig. 25.75): DLM is formed from fibrocartilage, which is laid down in the mesenchyme that normally disappears in the process of joint formation.

Clinical Features

- Patients present with combination of pain, giving way, effusion and clicking or snapping knee.
- *On examination*
  - Palpable snapping on knee flexion and extension.
  - Bulge on lateral joint line, which disappears on knee flexion and extension movements.
  - Lateral joint line tenderness.
  - With torn discoid meniscus, knee is locked and extension is restricted.

Investigations

X-ray Findings (Fig. 25.76)

- Widening of the lateral joint line
- Flattening of the lateral femoral condyle
- Cupping of the lateral aspect of tibial plateau.

MRI (Figs 25.77 to 25.79)

MRI is the modality of choice to evaluate a discoid meniscus before surgery.

Double Contrast Arthrography Obsolete Method

Arthroscopy (Figs 25.80 and 25.81)

Arthroscopic appearance of a complete discoid lateral meniscus. The probe is showing the medial extent of the lateral meniscus, which completely covers the lateral tibial plateau. Arthroscopic photograph following saucerization of a discoid lateral meniscus. The edge of a horizontal tear, which traversed the meniscus, can be observed.

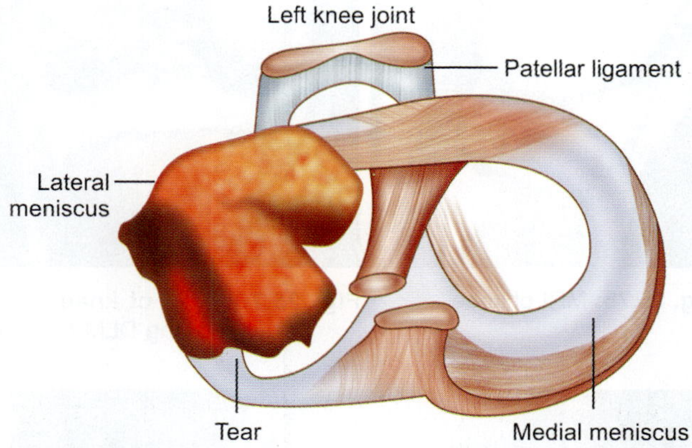

Fig. 25.75: Intra-articular structures of knee joint with both menisci

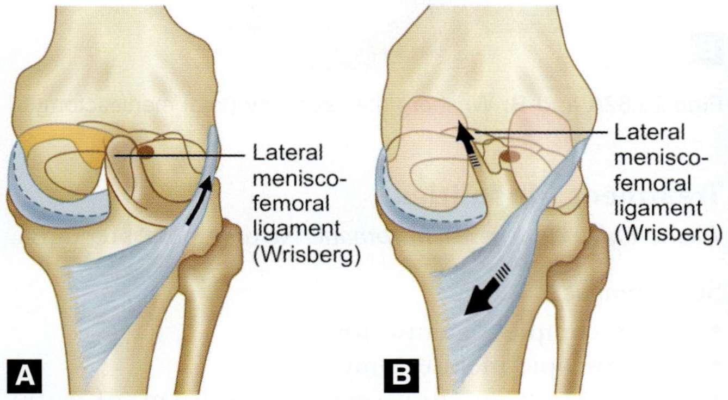

Figs 25.74A and B: Type III, discoid lateral meniscus

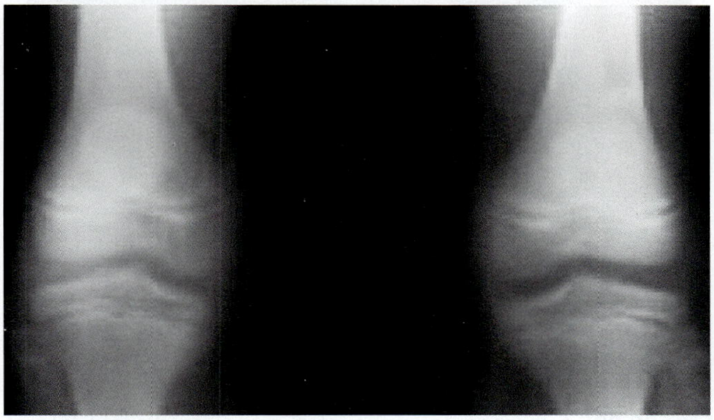

Fig. 25.76: X-ray of knee joint with DLM

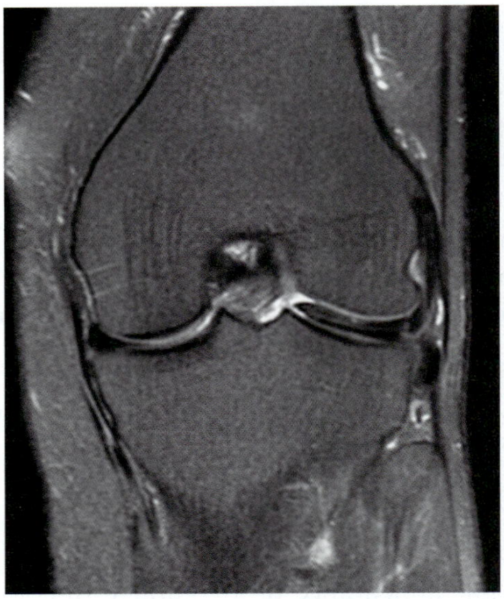

Fig. 25.77: MRI of knee joint, showing discoid lateral meniscus

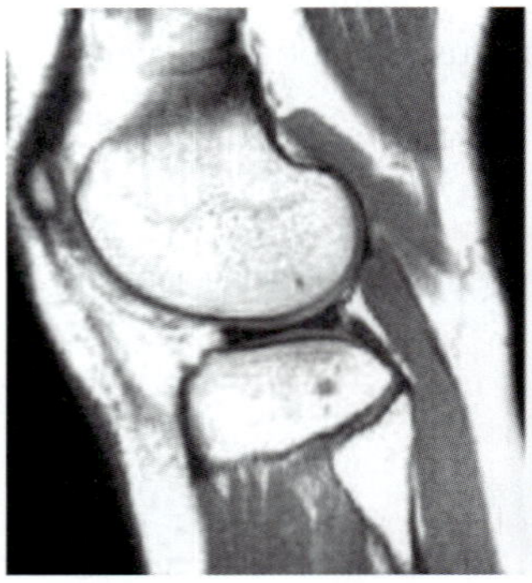

Fig. 25.78: MRI of knee

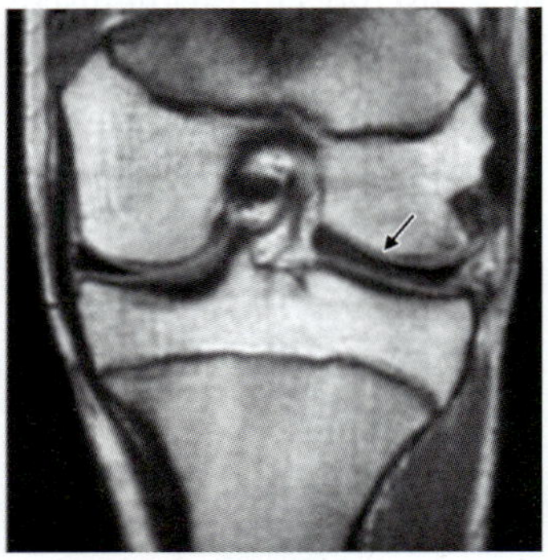

Fig. 25.79: MRI of knee joint, showing DLM (arrow)

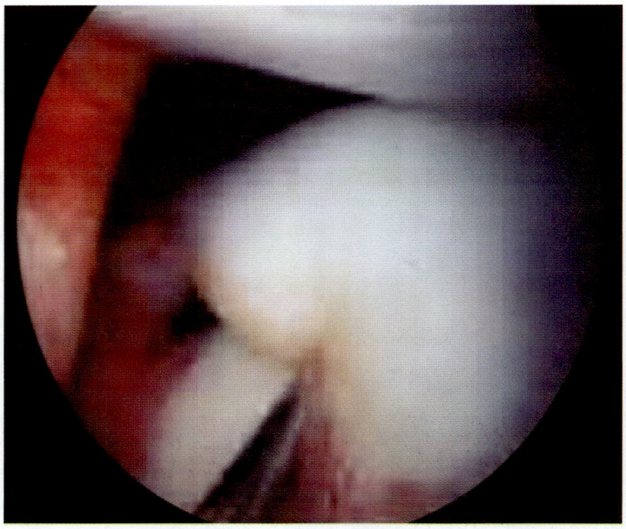

Fig. 25.80: Arthroscopic image of a complete discoid lateral meniscus, showing medial extent of the lateral meniscus

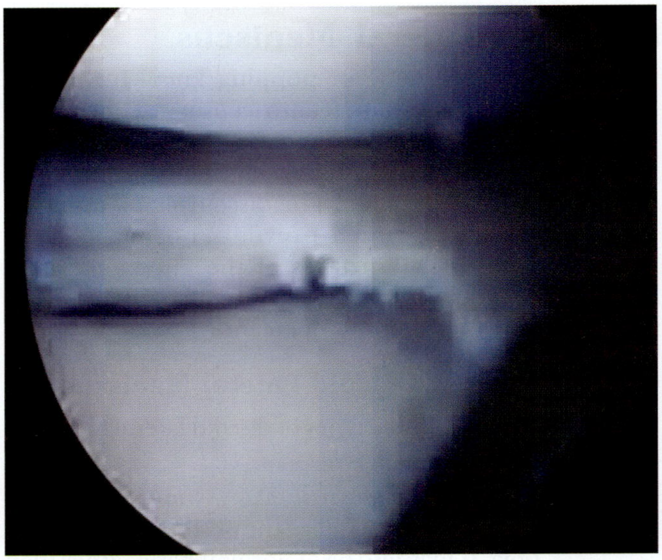

Fig. 25.81: Arthroscopic image showing, the edge of a horizontal tear of lateral discoid meniscus, which traversed the meniscus

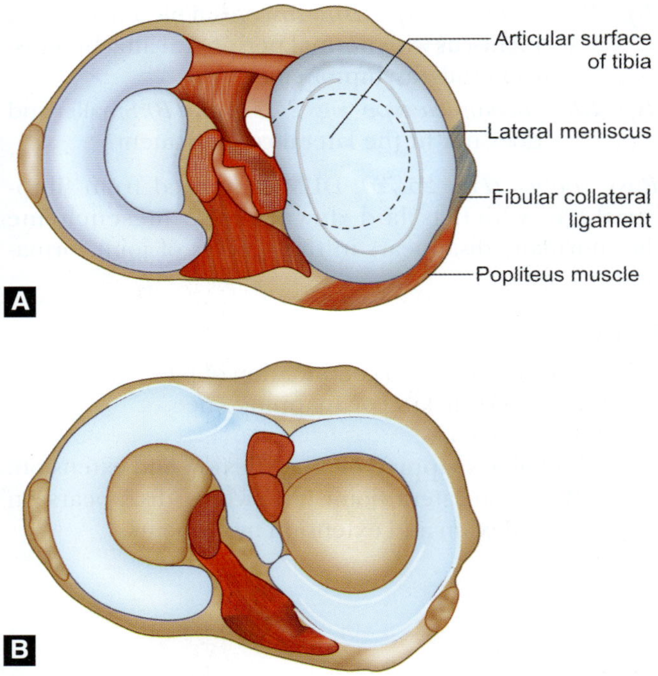

Figs 25.82A and B: Wrisberg menisectomy (total menisectomy)

Treatment Modalities

Incidental finding or asymptomatic: No treatment is required.

Symptomatic

- Open complete menisectomy
- Arthroscopic menisectomy
- Wrisberg type menisectomy, a form of total menisectomy, as shown in Figures 25.82A and B.

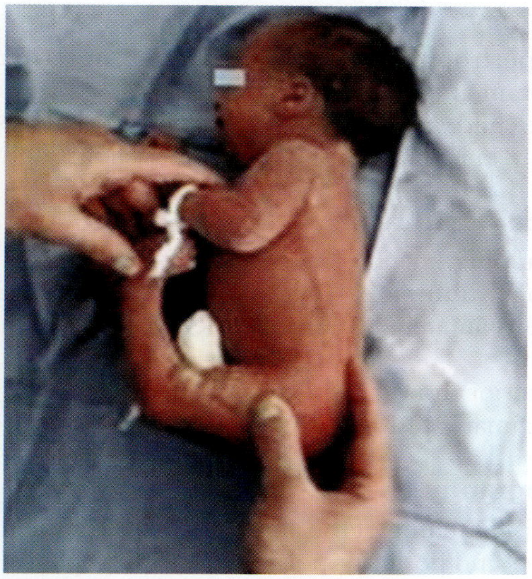

Fig. 25.83: Illustration showing congenital dislocation of knee in a fetus

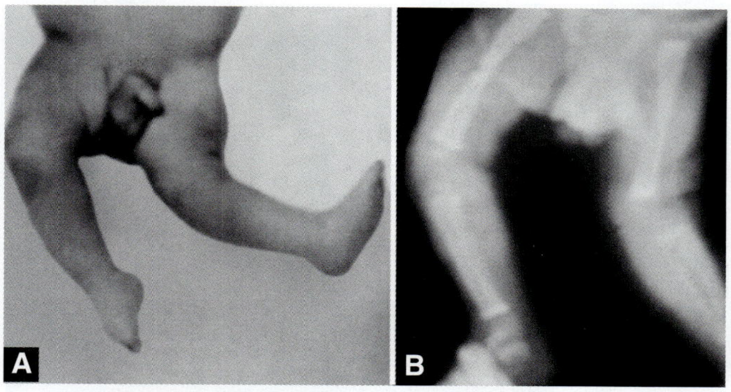

Figs 25.84A and B: Congenitally dislocated knee

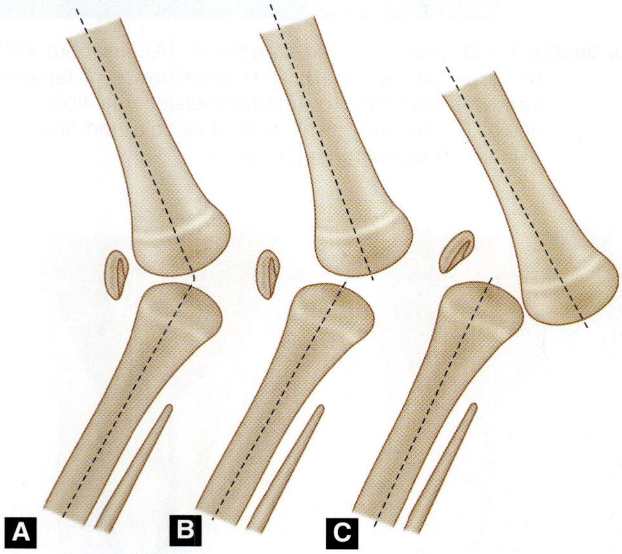

Figs 25.85A to C: Grading for dislocation of knee, depending on the pathology—(A) Congenital hyperextension; (B) Subluxation of knee; (C) Dislocation of knee

Congenital Dislocation of the Knee Joint (Fig. 25.83)

Described by Chasseur (1812) and Chatelain (1822). Shattock described, abnormal fetal position during pregnancy. Kate described, congenital absence of the cruciate ligaments and fibrosis of the quadriceps. Congenital dislocation of the knee joint may be associated with abnormalities, e.g. Larsen's syndrome, myelodysplasia, Ehler's-Danlos syndrome, Streeter's syndrome and arthrogryposis, as shown in Figures 25.84A and B.

Pathology

- Anterior capsule of the knee joint and quadriceps are contracted.
- Intra-articular adhesions, hypoplasia and absence of patella.
- Fibrosis and lack of bulk of vastus lateralis
- Suprapatellar pouch obliterated by adherent quadriceps tendon and patella is displaced laterally.

Grading (Figs 25.85A to C)

Grade I: Congenital hyperextension

Grade II: Congenital hyperextension with anterior subluxation of the tibia on the femur

Grade III (Figs 25.86A to C): Congenital hyperextension, with anterior dislocation of tibia on the femur.

Investigations

Radiographic Findings

- Hypoplasia of the intercondylar eminence of the tibia.
- Hypoplasia of tibial plateau
- Abnormal femoral condyles
- Patellar hypoplasia
- Patellar elongation
- Femoral hypoplasia
- Proximal tibial bowing
- Genu valgus
- Absent patella and proximal fibula.

Treatment Modalities

Nonoperative

- Manipulation with manual traction and relocation.
- Long leg cast with knee in as much flexion as possible.

Operative (Figs 25.87A and B) (Curtis and Fischer Procedure)

- Capsular release and quadriceps lengthening for correction.
- Long leg cast for three months followed by long knee brace for three years.

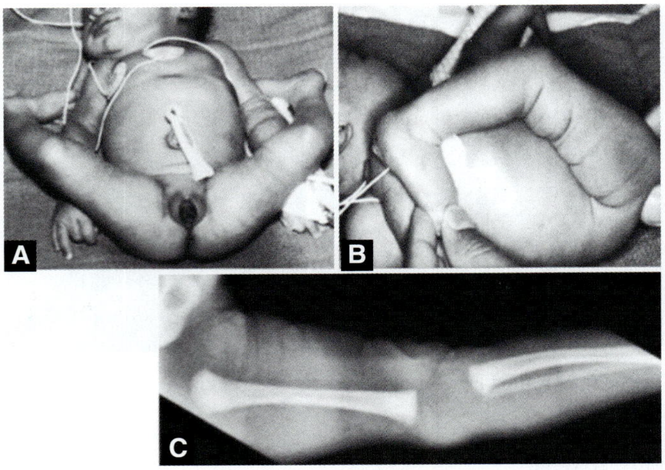

Figs 25.86A to C: Grade III knee dislocation. (A) Newborn with bilateral dislocation; (B) Note prominence of femoral condyles posterior to anteriorly dislocated tibia and fibula; (C) Anterior displacement of tibia and fibula is evident on lateral roentgenogram

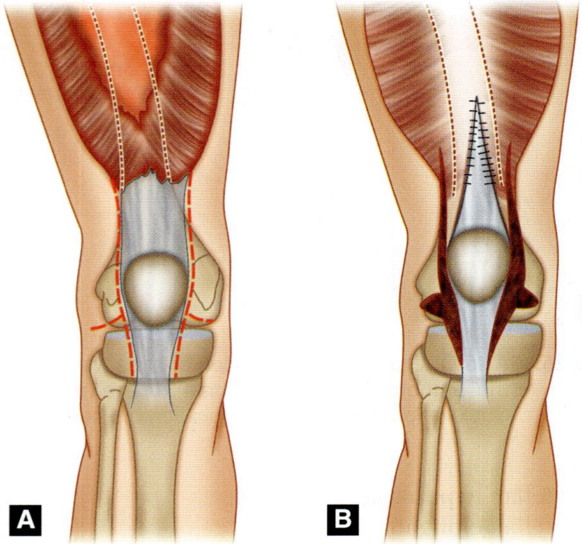

Figs 25.87A and B: Curtis and Fischer procedure for congenital dislocation of knee—(A) Lines of incision to release anterior capsule medially and laterally as well as medial and lateral retinaculum of quadriceps mechanism; (B) Correction after soft tissue release and lengthening of rectus femoris muscle

■ Congenital Tibiofemoral Subluxation

Also known as congenital snapping knee. Anterior subluxation of tibia on the femur on knee extension and reduction on knee flexion. Associated abnormalities include, Larsen's syndrome, Catel-Manzke syndrome, congenital short tibia, etc.

Pathology

- Hypertrophy of the iliotibial tract, intermuscular septum and biceps femoris.
- The child walks, with knee flexed to avoid subluxation.
- With, knee in extension the tibia is subluxated.

Clinical Features

- Snapping knee.
- Tibia subluxates forward on knee extension at approximately 30° of knee flexion, with an audible snap
- Anterior drawer test is positive
- Lachman's test is positive

Radiography

There is flattening of the anterior portion of the femoral condyles and posterior portion of the tibial plateau.

Treatment Modalities

Curtis and Fischer Procedure

Release with sectioning of the iliotibial band and distal portion of the intermuscular septum. Release of insertion of biceps tendon and suture it to the vastus lateralis.

DEFORMITIES AROUND KNEE

■ Deformity of Knee

- Genu valgum or knock knee
- Genu varum or bowleg
- Genu recurvatum or hyperextented knee
- Triple deformities
- Flexion deformity
- Bony structures may become deformed, about the knee as a result the femur or the tibia deviates in the corresponding direction.

■ Genu Varum (Fig. 25.88)

Genu varum is also known as bowleg, consists of outward angulations of the knee joint, the longitudinal axis of the femur and the tibia deviating medially. The deformity involves the tibia alone or femur or both the tibia and fibula.

Causes of Genu Varum

Unilateral Genu Varum

- *Trauma*: Traumatic causes of genu varum includes:
  - Physeal injuries
  - Malunited fracture
  - Ligaments injuries
  - Hemophilic arthritis

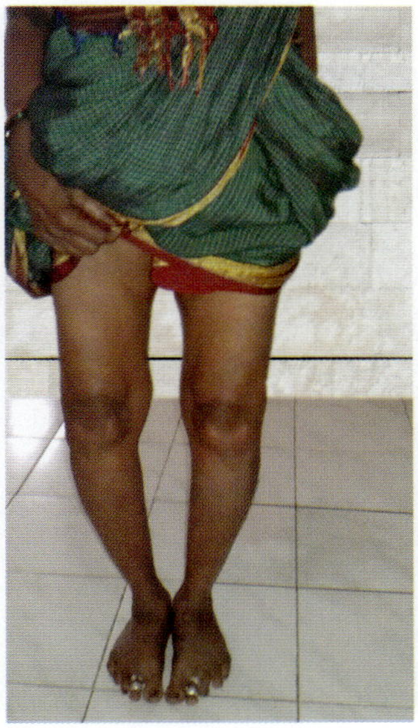

Fig. 25.88: Genu varum of knee

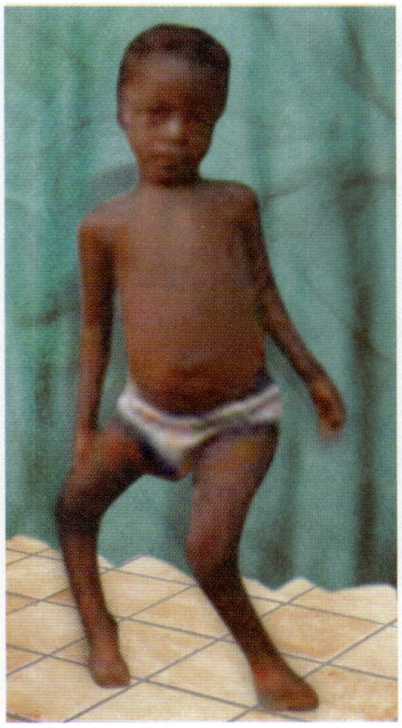

Fig. 25.89: Wind sweep deformity of knee

- *Infection*
  - Osteomyelitis
  - Septic arthritis
- *Tumor*
  - Affecting lower end of femur and upper end of tibia
- *Osteoarthritis*, degenerative disorders.

Bilateral Genu Varum

- *Physiological:* Very common in children of years or less
- *Idiopathic:* It can be due to metabolic and nutritional disturbances, e.g. vitamin D deficiency (ricket), vitamin D resistant rickets, renal osteodystrophy, and hypophosphatasia.
- *Other causes*
  - Blount's disease or tibia vara
  - Osteochondrosis of the upper tibial epiphyseal plate.
  - *Skeletal fluorosis:* This is due to high intake of endemic fluoride in the drinking water from birth
  - Osteogenesis imperfecta, developmental disturbances
  - Paget's disease
  - Skeletal dysplasia
  - Metaphyseal
  - Chondrodysplasia
  - Achondroplasia
  - Enchondromatosis
  - Endocrine disorder
  - Thyroid disorder

Wind Sweep Deformity (Fig. 25.89)

It is a deformity, where both the knee joint are affected. One knee goes in varus and another in valgus.

Causes

- Rickets
- Hemophilic arthritis.

Clinical Examination

Patient sits at the edge of the couch with both legs extended as shown in Figure 25.90. In neutral position of the limb, hold the ankles from behind. Try to approximate both malleoli so that they just touch each other as demonstrated in Figure 25.91. Normally, they touch before the inner surfaces of the knees come together. Rather, there should be on an average 0.5 cm gap between the medial surfaces of the knees. If the gap is more (10–16 years of age group less than 4 cm in females and less than 5 cm in male is regarded as normal) deformity is genu varum. For unilateral genu varus, the distance between the center of the medial surface of medial condyle and central plumb line of the body is measured.

Knee Flexion Test (Fig. 25.92)

This is done to assess, whether the cause of deformity lies in femur or tibia. The procedure for carrying out knee flexion test is as follows:

- Ask the patient to sit in squatting position. If deformity completely disappears, the total fault lies in the lower femur as demonstrated.

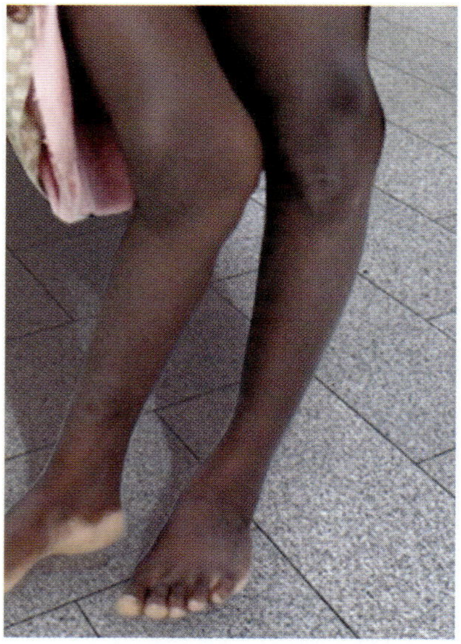

Fig. 25.90: Clinical examination for wind sweep deformity of knee: Patient's legs are kept in extended position

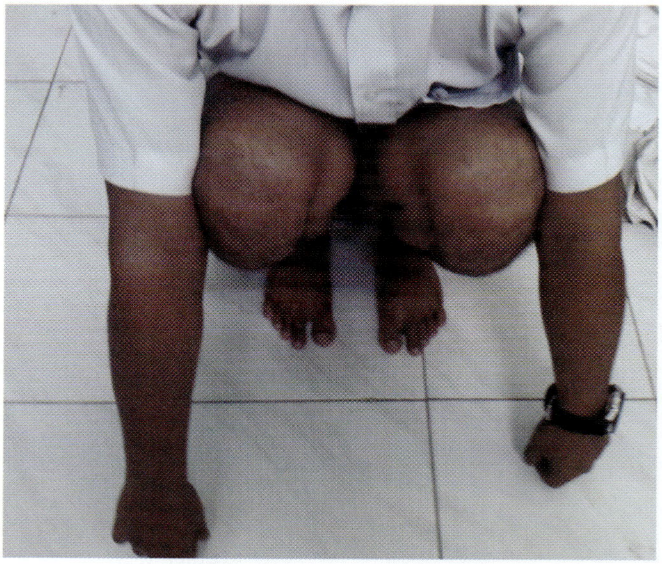

Fig. 25.92: Knee flexion test to assess, the origin (femur or tibia) of deformity

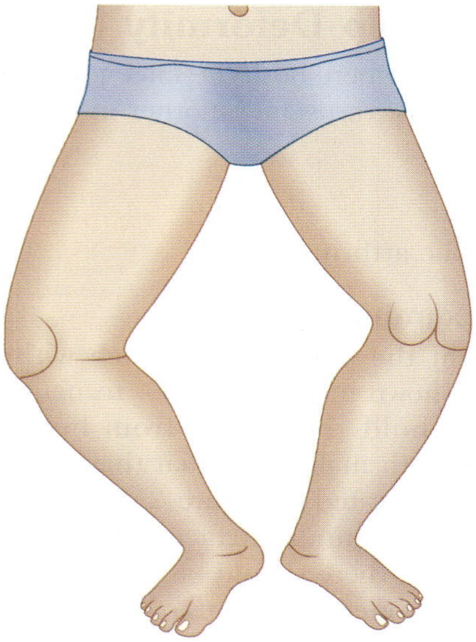

Fig. 25.91: Clinical examination for wind sweep deformity of knee: Both malleoli are approximated so that they touch each other

- If it disappears partially or does not disappear, the fault will be in the tibia or both components (Fig. 25.92).

Investigations

- Routine blood investigation
- Investigate the underlying cause
- X-rays done (usually weight bearing)
- MRI
- CT scan.

Treatment

To treat the underlying cause for which the deformity occurs, such as:

- Adequate supplementation of vitamin D and exposure in sunlight as in rickets.
- Disease modifying antirheumatic drugs (DMARD's) for rheumatoid
- Anti-tuberculosis treatment (ATT) in tuberculosis.
- Drinking water, supplied with fluoride less than 0.5 ppm and improvement of calcium nutrition, which provides protection against the toxic effects of fluoride as in skeletal fluorosis.

However, brace, splint, traction and casting are useful in correcting mild deformity. Whereas, in severe deformities surgery has to be done. There are several surgeries done to correct the knee deformities according to the severity and the types of the disease.

Treatment of Physiological Genu Varum

- Periodic observation
- Examination and follow-up
- Education and reassurance of the parents as in physiological genu varum and valgum that it corrects with growth after three years of age and most of the time required no treatment.
- However, in rare cases of uncorrected physiologic genu varum of about greater than 11°, surgeries are indicated.
- Surgeries performed include:
  - Proximal tibial hemiepiphyseal stapling
  - Proximal tibial hemiepiphysiodesis
  - Osteotomy.

Surgeries Performed in Varus Deformities

Distal Femur

- Valgus osteotomy
- Closing wedge
- Opening wedge
- Callotasis
- Lateral hemiepiphysiodesis
- Lateral hemiepiphyseal stapling
- Percutaneous epiphysiodesis.

Proximal Tibia

- Valgus osteotomy (including derotation and diaphyseal fibular osteomy)
  - Closing wedge
  - Opening wedge
  - Dome
  - Oblique
  - Callotasis
- Lateral hemiepiphyseal stapling (Fig. 25.93)
- Lateral hemiepiphysiodesis
- Percutaneous epiphysiodesis
- Total knee replacement.

Proximal Tibial Hemiepiphyseal Stapling

- Temporary retardation of growth in the lateral aspect of the proximal tibial epiphysis with staples is an effective method for correction of persistent physiologic genu varum.
- If the deformity is severe or there is limited remaining growth, a combined lateral stapling of the distal femoral and the proximal tibial epiphyses may need to be performed.

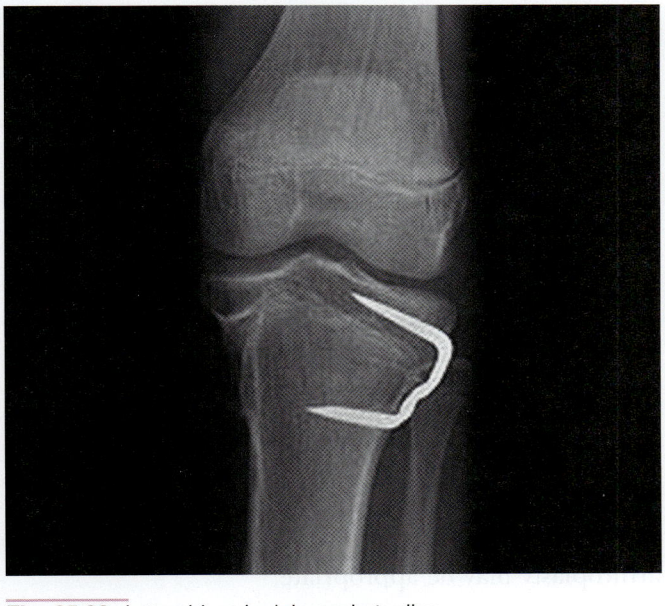

Fig. 25.93: Lateral hemiepiphyseal stapling

- This procedure will not correct any co-existent medial tibial torsion.

Epiphysiodesis

Phemister, described epiphysiodesis in 1933, and his original technique with minor modifications, has been widely used for limb length equalization. Most authors recommend epiphysiodesis, when 2 to 5 cm of shortening is required. Menelaus and others, recommended epiphysiodesis for discrepancies of up to 8 to 10 cm to avoid the complications of limb lengthening. Phemister removed a rectangular piece of the lateral cortex on either side of the epiphysis and reinserted it in a reversed position.

White developed special hollow chisels to remove a square block of bone and curetted the physeal cartilage deep in the hole before replacing the bone blocks in a reversed position. A newer technique of epiphysiodesis, involves the use of percutaneous instrumentation to obliterate the physis through small, cosmetically pleasing incisions. Experimental evidence reported by Canale et al. and Ogilvie, indicate that the physis can be effectively obliterated by this technique. Angled currets can be used instead of high speed burrs, to scrape the epiphyseal cartilage. Metaizeau et al. describe a technique for percutaneous epiphysiodesis using transphyseal screws (PETS).

Proximal Tibial Hemiphysiodesis

- Per-cutaneous closure of the lateral aspect of the proximal tibial epiphysis can be effective in correcting persistent physiologic genu varum in adolescents.
- The indications are essentially the same as for stapling.
- However, once complete correction has been achieved, a second procedure may be necessary on the medial side to prevent overcorrection.
- The proximal fibular epiphysis is usually closed concomitantly. This procedure will not correct any medial tibial torsion.

The indications for surgical treatment in infantile tibia vara include:

- Age 4 years or less
- Failure of orthotic management
- Langenskiöld grade III or higher.

Proximal tibial valgus osteotomy with fibular diaphyseal osteotomy is usually the procedure of choice. Perform an anterior compartment fasciotomy concomitantly (Figs 25.94A to C).

High Tibial Osteotomy

- Coventry stated that normally there is valgus alignment of 5 to 8 degrees in the tibio-femoral angle as measured on roentgenograms taken in the weight-bearing position.

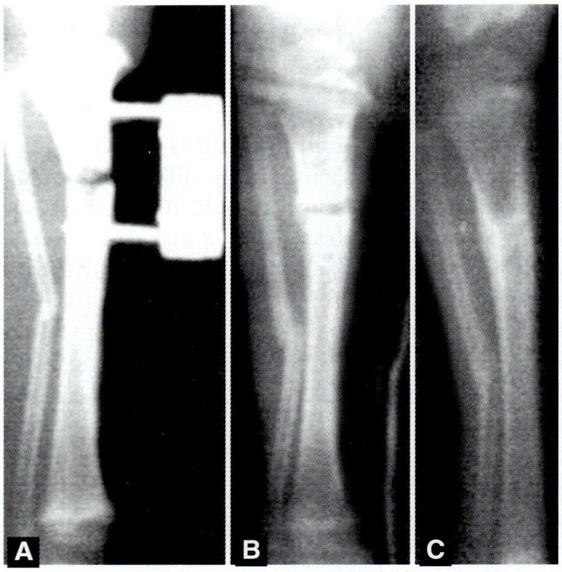

Figs 25.94A to C: Proximal tibial valgus osteotomy with fibular diaphyseal osteotomy

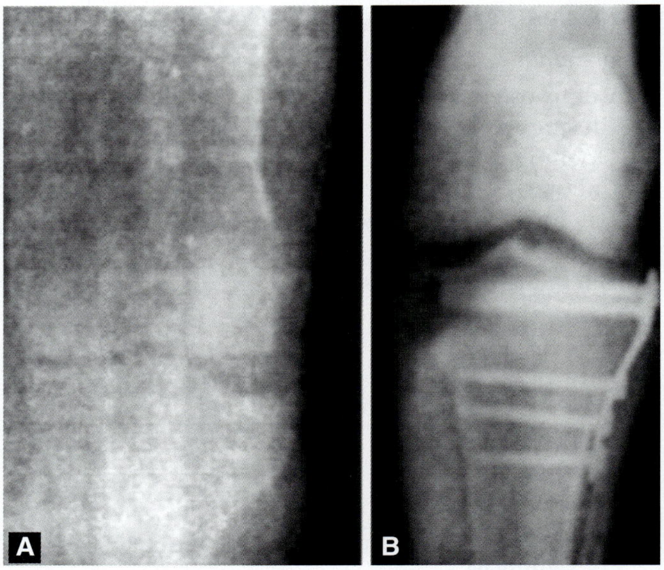

Figs 25.95A and B: Closing wedge osteotomy

- The amount of correction of the arthritic knee needed to achieve a normal angle is calculated, and an additional 3 to 5 degrees of overcorrection is added to achieve approximately 10 degrees of valgus.
- With a varus deformity the only limitation in the amount of correction from a valgus osteotomy is the size of the bone wedge that can be taken proximal to the patellar tendon.

The indications for proximal tibial osteotomy are:

- Pain and disability resulting from osteoarthritis that significantly interfere with employment or recreation.
- Evidence on weight-bearing roentgenograms of degenerative arthritis that is confined to one compartment with a corresponding varus or valgus deformity.
- The ability of the patient to use crutches after the operation and the possession of sufficient muscle strength and motivation to carry out a rehabilitation program.
- Good vascular status without serious arterial insufficiency or large varicosities.

Coventry described a closing wedge osteotomy made proximal to the tibial tuberosity (Figs 25.95A and B)

- To correct a varus deformity coventry recommended a lateral approach.
- The advantages of this osteotomy are that:
  - It is made near the deformity, that is, the knee
  - It is made through cancellous bone, which heals rapidly
  - It permits the fragments to be held firmly in position by one or two staples
  - It permits exploration of the knee through the same incision. After this operation the danger of delayed union or nonunion is slight, and prolonged immobilization in a cast is unnecessary.

Hernigou, described a medial opening wedge tibial osteotomy, which they believed is more precise and allows more exact correction than does a lateral closing wedge osteotomy.

Morrey recommended opening wedge osteotomy if the involved extremity is 2 mm or more shorter than the contralateral extremity.

Opening wedge osteotomy also may be indicated in patients with laxity of the medial collateral ligament or combined anterior cruciate ligament deficiency.

Distal Femoral Osteotomy (Figs 25.96A and B)

- Is usually done if the deformity lies in the femur.
- Valgus osteotomy to correct varus deformity is performed through lateral approach.
- Coventry recommended supracondylar femoral varus osteotomy if the varus deformity is more than 12 degrees or if the joint surface tilt of the tibia is more than 10 degrees.

Total Knee Arthroplasty

If the entire knee joint is involved with osteoarthritis that causes incapacitating pain and disability, total knee arthroplasty may be appropriate.

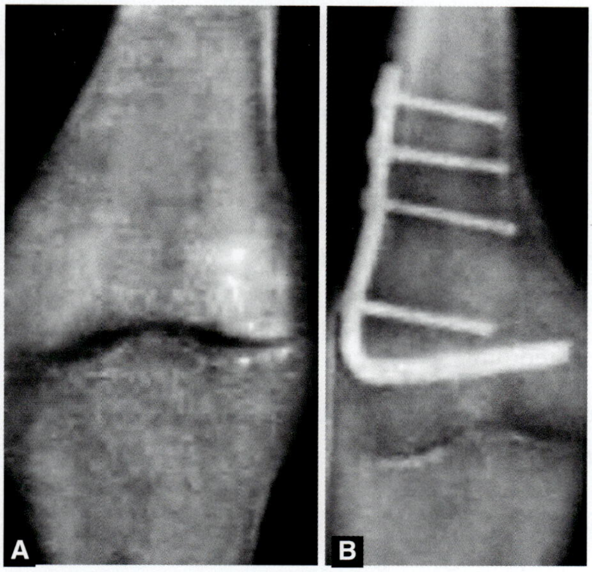

Figs 25.96A and B: Distal femoral osteotomy

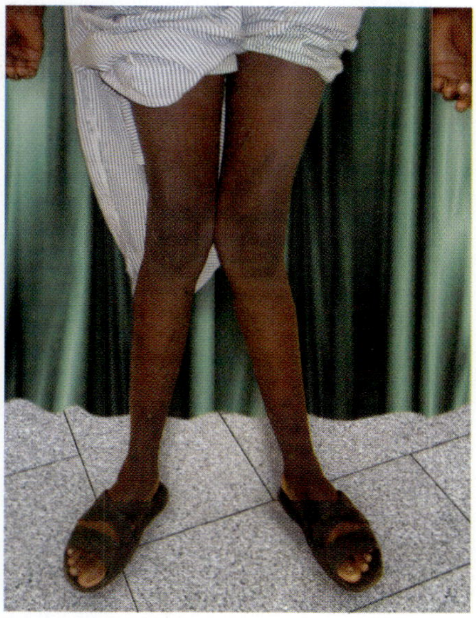

Fig. 25.97: Genu valgum of knee

Genu Valgum (Fig. 25.97)

It is also known as knock knee, consists of medial angulation of the knee and outward deviation of the longitudinal axis of both tibia and femur. In advanced cases, the distal end of femur and tibia are rotated externally. By the pull of the biceps femoris and tensor fascia, femoris and distal shaft of tibia develops a compensatory internal torsion. With subsequent growth, the medial condyle assumes larger proportion than lateral and articular surface lies at an oblique angle. The quadriceps extensor mechanism crosses the joint over the lateral aspect, where the patella tends to subluxate or dislocate outward. On the lateral side, the soft tissue structures, including the biceps, the iliotibial band and peroneal nerve are shortened. On medial side, the soft tissue structures are elongated. The medial collateral ligament is stretched and remains lax, causing instability of the joint.

Causes of Genu Valgum

Unilateral

- *Trauma*: Traumatic causes of genu valgum includes:
  - Physeal injuries
  - Malunited fracture
  - Ligaments injuries
  - Hemophilic arthritis
- *Infection*
  - Osteomyelitis
  - Septic arthritis
- *Tumor*
  - Affecting lower end of femur and upper end of tibia
- *Osteoarthritis,* degenerative disorders.

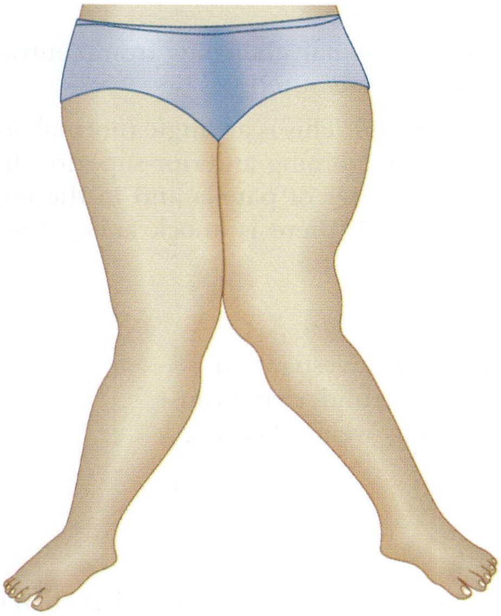

Fig. 25.98: Clinical examination of genu valgum, with knees approximated and gap observed between malleoli

Clinical Examination

Patient sits at the edge of the couch with both legs extended, See Figure 25.43. In neutral position of the limb, hold the ankles from behind. Try to approximate both knee, so that they just touch each other, as demonstrated in Figure 25.98. Normally, both knee and malleoli should touch, but in knock knee, there is a gap between both malleoli (10–16 years of age group, less than 8 cm in female and less than 4 cm in male is regarded as normal). This gap is measured. For unilateral valgus,

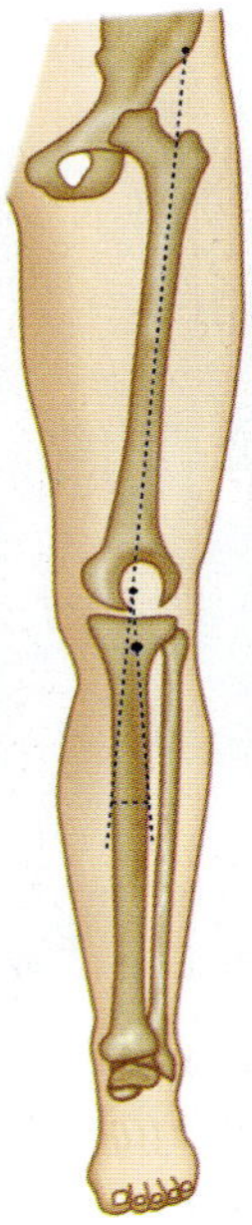

Fig. 25.99: Measurement of Q-angle

the deviation of medial malleolus from central plumb line of the body is measured.

Q-angle (Fig. 25.99): This is an angle (normal angle is of 11°) between a line joining anterior-superior iliac spine (ASIS) with the center of patella and in the line of the patellar ligament. If there is knock knee, this angle is increased.

Investigations

- Routine blood investigation
- Investigate the underlying cause
- X-rays, usually weight-bearing
- MRI
- CT scan

Treatment

Drinking water, supplied with fluoride less than 0.5 ppm and improvement of calcium nutrition, provide protection against the toxic effects of fluoride as in skeletal fluorosis. However, brace, splint, traction and casting are useful in correcting mild deformity. Whereas, in severe deformities surgery has to be done. There are several surgeries done to correct the knee deformities according to the severity and types of the disease. To treat the underlying cause due to which the deformity has occurred, such as adequate supplementation of vitamin D and exposure in sunlight as in rickets. DMARD's for rheumatoid and ATT in tuberculosis are recommended.

Treatment of Physiological Genu Valgum

- Periodic observation
- Examination and follow-up
- Education and reassurance of the parents as in physiological genu varum and valgum, that it corrects with growth after three years of age and most of the time required no treatment.
- However in rare cases of uncorrected physiologic genu valgum of greater than 20° or more than 10 cm separation between malleoli surgeries are indicated.

Surgeries Performed Include

- Medial physeal stapling
- Medial physeal hemiepiphysiodesis
- Osteotomy

Surgeries Performed in Valgus Deformities

Distal Femur

- Varus osteotomy
  - Closing wedge
  - Opening wedge
  - Callotasis
- Medial hemiepiphysiodesis
- Medial hemiepiphyseal stapling
- Percutaneous epiphysiodesis

Proximal Tibia

- Varus osteotomy (including derotation and diaphyseal fibular osteotomy)
  - Closing wedge
  - Opening wedge
  - Dome
  - Oblique
  - Callotasis
- Medial hemiepiphyseal stapling
- Medial hemiepiphysiodesis
- Percutaneous epiphysiodesis
- Total knee replacement.

Medial Physeal Stapling of the Distal Femur or Proximal Tibia (Fig. 25.100)

Retardation of growth about the medial aspect of the distal femur or proximal tibia by medial physeal stapling is a relatively easy. It is a reliable method of correcting a genu valgum deformity, if there is sufficient remaining growth to produce satisfactory alignment. If the deformity is pronounced or there is an insufficient remaining skeletal growth, a combined stapling of the medial aspect of the distal femoral and the proximal tibial physis may be necessary.

Medial Hemiepiphysiodesis of the Distal Femur or Proximal Tibia

Hemiepiphysiodesis of the medial aspect of the distal femur or proximal tibia has been proposed, as a method for gradual correction of genu valgum deformity. However, because of the variability in the data, necessary to make these determinations, a second operative

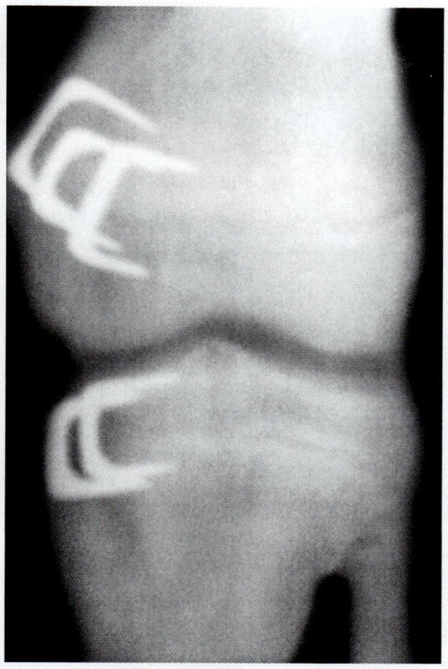

Fig. 25.100: Medial physeal stapling of the distal femur or proximal tibia

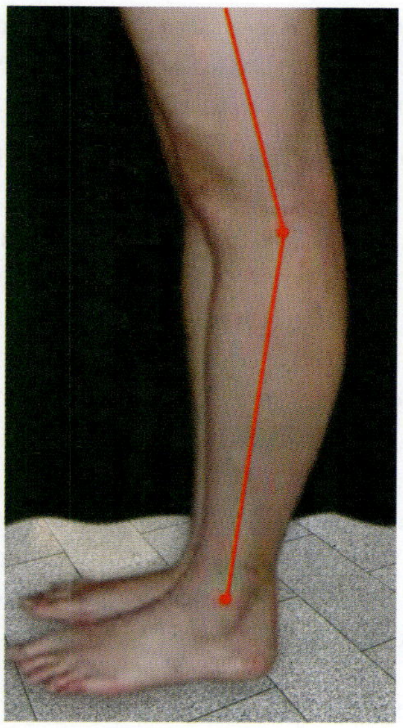

Fig. 25.101: Genu recurvatum

procedure is often required to close the remaining lateral portion of the epiphysis. Rotational bone blocks, as described by Phemister, were once popular. However, the percutaneous techniques of epiphysiodesis using curet, drills, burrs or a combination of these are now preferred. These are as accurate and much more cosmetic than the open bone graft epiphysiodesis techniques. Although this technique is most commonly used for lower extremity length discrepancies, it can also be used successfully in the correction of persistent angular deformities, such as genu valgum and genu varum.

Genu Recurvatum (Fig. 25.101)

In this there is a backward bowing or hyperextension of the knee. There is retarded activity of anterior portion of lower femur or upper tibial epiphyseal plate. The posterior portion of the condyles grows larger in contrast with anterior portion and the articular surfaces are correspondingly inclined in the forward direction (femur inclined forward and upward, while tibia inclined forward and downward in relation to the longitudinal axis of the shaft).

Clinical Features

- Knee fixed in hyperextension with varying degrees of subluxation or dislocation
- Forward movement of tibia on femoral condyles
- Skin over the anterior aspect of joint shows several transverse creases
- Patella is small or absent and always located proximally or laterally
- On posterior aspect both femoral condyles and hamstrings (as tense cords) are palpable.

Causes

Congenital: It includes congenital dislocation of knee, which can be due to following reasons:

- *Traumatic developmental:* This is most common and is due to malposition *in utero*. Legs may be caught by the chin or axilla with the knees extended and uterine compression may prevent them from assuming the usual flexed position
- *A primary embryonic defect:* Usually accompanied by other defects, such as hare lip, cardiac defect, spina bifida, congenital dislocation of hip (CDH), etc.
- Quadriceps contracture or congenital absence or hypoplastic anterior collateral ligament (ACL).
- Post injection contracture
- Arthrogryposis multiplex congenital, a congenital neuromuscular disorder
- Equinus deformity of foot, e.g. congenital talipes equinovarus (CTEV), throws knee into hyperextension.

Trauma

- Physeal injury
- Malunited fracture
- *Ligament's laxity:* This is due to prolonged traction and hyperextension of knee in plaster.

Neuromuscular Disorder

- *Poliomyelitis:* Muscular imbalance, e.g. paralyzed quadriceps or contracture.
- *Charcot's disease:* Disease of central nervous system (CNS), with destructive arthropathy arising from loss of pain, common cause is neurosyphilis.

Metabolic disorder*, e.g. Rickets, due to hypotonia*
Inflammatory, e.g. rheumatoid arthritis, overstretching of the ligaments following chronic or recurrent synovitis.

Extra-articular ankylosis in extension: After fracture of the femur or extensive soft tissue wounds of the anterior aspect of the thigh, scarring or fibrosis of all or a part of the quadriceps mechanism can result in extra-articular ankylosis in extension. Nicoll, emphasized that this deformity may be due to one or more of the following:

- Fibrosis of the vastus medialis scarring down the rectus femoris to the femur in suprapatellar pouch and proximally.
- Adhesions between the patella and femoral condyles.
- Fibrosis and shortening of the lateral expansions of the vasti and their adherance to the femoral condyles.
- Actual shortening of the rectus femoris muscle.

Investigations

- Routine blood investigation
- Investigate the underlying cause
- X-rays, usually weight bearing
- MRI
- CT scan.

Treatment

To treat the underlying cause due to which the deformity has occurred. However, brace, splint, traction and casting are useful in correcting mild deformity. Whereas, in severe deformities surgery has to be done. There are several surgeries done to correct the knee deformities according to the severity and types of the disease.

Surgeries Performed in Genu Recurvatum

- Close wedge osteotomy of proximal tibia
- Soft tissue operation (Triple tenodesis)
- The operation consists of three parts
  - Proximal advancement of posterior capsule of the knee with the joint flexed to 20°.
  - Construction of a check reins in the midline
  - Posteriorly, using tendons of semitendinosus and gracilis
  - Creation of two diagonal straps posteriorly
  - Using the biceps tendon and the anterior half of iliotibial band.
- Thomson's quadriceps plasty
- *Kullman and Leonart's surgery:* Proximal release of rectus femoris in isolated contracture of rectus femoris
- Arthrodesis.

■ Triple Deformity of Knee

It is described as in flexed position of the knee, tibia subluxates posteriorly and laterally. Tibia also rotates laterally over the femoral condyle, as shown in Figures 25.102 and 25.103. Gradually, the leg also goes in valgus, therefore although it has been identified as triple subluxation, actually it is a "quadruple deformity complex".

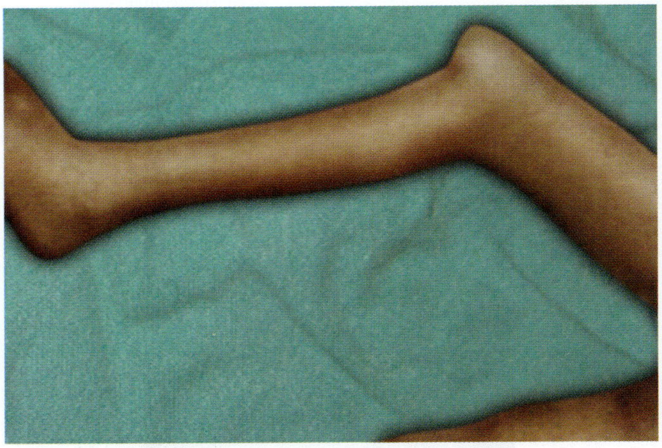

Fig. 25.102: Triple deformity of knee

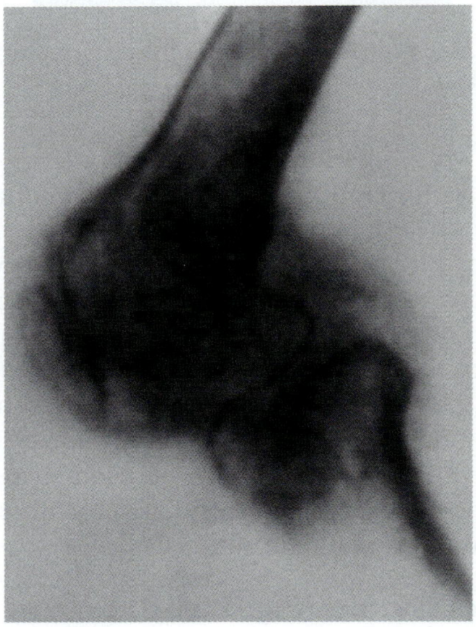

Fig. 25.103: Triple deformity of knee with flexed knee, posteriorly subluxated and laterally rotated tibia

Causes

- *Trauma*
  - Physeal injuries
  - Ligaments injuries
- *Infection*
  - Osteomyelitis
  - Tuberculosis
- *Tumor*
  - Affecting lower end of femur and upper end of tibia

- *Inflammatory disorder*
  - Rheumatoid arthritis
  - Hemophilic arthritis
- *Neuromuscular disorder*
  - Poliomyelitis.

Pathodynamics

The deformed position, allows further mechanical benefit to hamstrings, specially the biceps and iliotibial band, which now become the main flexors of joint. While lying down patient tries to keep the hip in external rotation, till the outer part of the knee rest on a support or couch. In this position gravity assisted contraction of the iliotibial band (IT band) helps in outer subluxation of the tibiofibular component. Taking further advantages, the IT band and bicep femoris contracts further and therefore fibulotibial component rotates laterally.

Above deforming forces pull the leg outwards, i.e. in valgus. The flexed attitude of the knee joint is a protective position and position of rest, therefore in any painful condition, there is early tendency of spasm of the hamstrings. This position, allows enough of posterior space in knee joint for collection of blood or exudates. The posterior capsule starts contracting with this flexed attitude.

Investigations

- Routine blood investigation
- Investigate the underlying cause
- X-rays, usually weight bearing
- MRI
- CT scan.

Treatment

To treat the underlying cause due to which the deformity has occured. However, brace, splint, traction and casting are useful in correcting mild deformity. Whereas, in severe deformities surgery has to be done. There are several surgeries done to correct the knee deformities according to the severity and types of the disease.

Surgeries for Triple Deformity

- Quadriceps plasty is usually done in contracture.
- Proximal tibial osteotomy is usually done, when the deformity lies in the tibia.
- Supracondylar osteotomy of femur is usually done, when the deformity lies in femur.
- Arthrodesis is done in young adults with marked destruction of joints.
- Total knee replacement is done with marked destruction of joints.

Flexion Deformity

Flexion deformity or loss of extension is the protective attitude of the knee joint and position of rest. Flexion up to 20° is common at birth and generally improves spontaneously.

Causes

- *Tumor:* Affecting lower end of femur and upper end of tibia.
- *Degenerative disorders*, e.g. osteoarthritis
- *Neuromuscular disorder*, e.g. poliomyelitis
- *Extra-articular ankylosis in flexion:* Fibrosis and contracture of retropatellar fat pad due to trauma by any surgical procedure and associated structures, that prevent the normal superior and inferior excursion of the patella and hence the extensor mechanism.
- Intra-articular ankylosis in flexion
- *Trauma:* Includes
  - Physeal injuries
  - Malunited fracture
  - Ligaments injuries
- Infection
  - Osteomyelitis
  - Tuberculosis
  - Pyogenic arthritis
- Inflammatory disorder
  - Rheumatoid arthritis
  - Hemophilic arthritis
  - Crystal induced arthritis.

Investigations

- Routine blood investigation
- Investigate the underlying cause
- X-rays, usually weight-bearing
- MRI
- CT scan.

Treatment

To treat the underlying cause due to which the deformity occurs. However, brace, splint, traction and casting are useful in correcting mild deformity. Whereas, in severe deformities surgery has to be done. There are several surgeries done, to correct the knee deformities according to the severity and types of the disease.

Surgeries Performed in Flexion Deformity

- Flexion deformities up to 20° at birth, generally improves spontaneously.
- Flexion deformities greater than 20° in neonates, serial casting is done.
- Flexion deformities greater than three years of age, surgeries are performed. These includes following surgeries:
  - Release of hamstring tendon at knee
  - Posterior capsulotomy of the knee, usually done to achieve full correction.
  - Supracondylar osteotomy is infrequently done in child, approaching skeletal maturity.

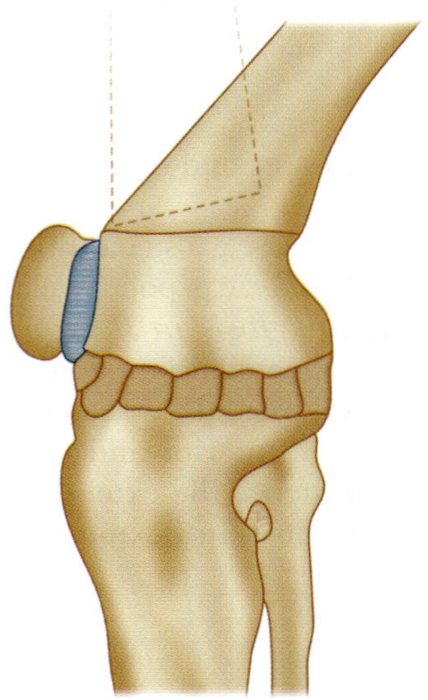

Fig. 25.104: Surgeries performed in ankylosis of knee

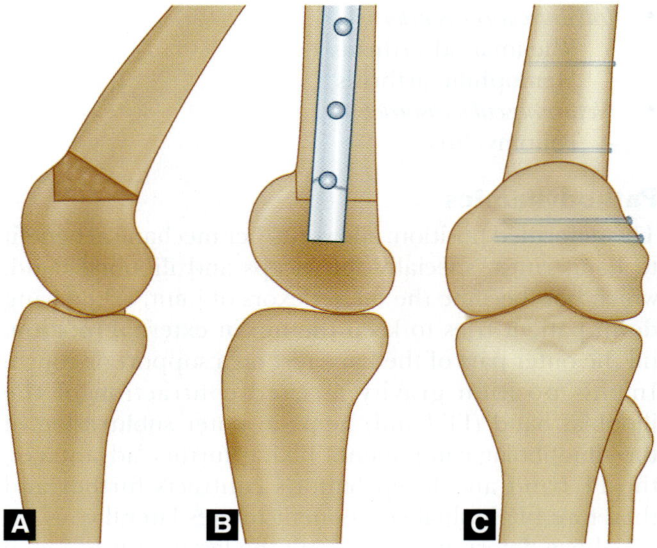

Figs 25.106A to C: Supracondylar controlled rotational osteotomy of femur

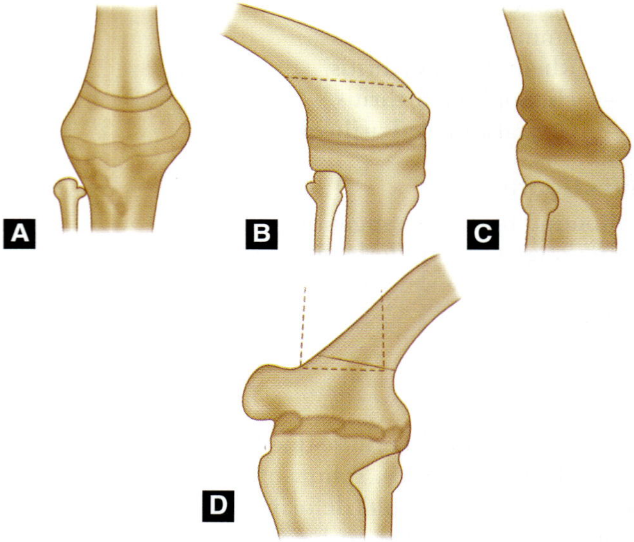

Figs 25.105A to D: Thompson's V-osteotomy of femur

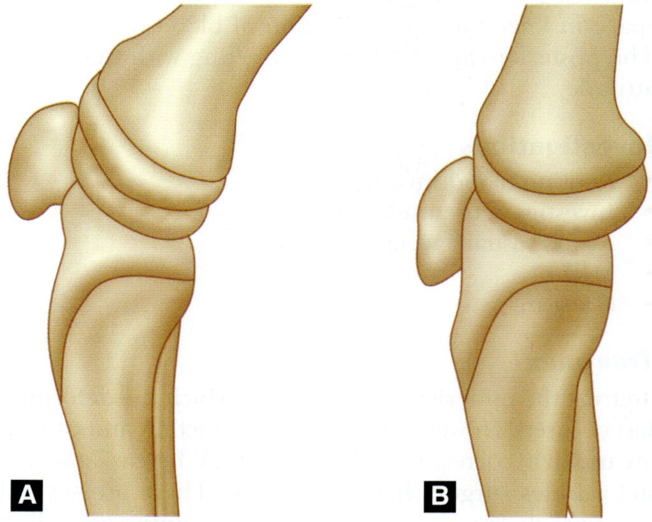

Figs 25.107A and B: Intra-articular osteotomy

Surgeries Performed in Ankylosis of Knee (Fig. 25.104)

Transverse Supracondylar Osteotomy of Femur

Transverse supracondylar osteotomy of femur, usually done when deformity is not severe but the joint is unsuitable for manipulation or soft tissue release. Thompson's V-osteotomy of femur is shown in Figures 25.105A to D.

Supracondylar Controlled Rotational Osteotomy of Femur (Figs 25.106A to C)

Supracondylar controlled rotational osteotomy of femur. It is indicated, when functional range of flexion remains beyond the flexion contracture.

Intra-Articular Osteotomy (Figs 25.107A and B)

Cuneiform Intra-articular Osteotomy (Fig. 25.108).

It is done in intra-articular osseous ankylosis.

DISLOCATION OF PATELLA

Introduction

Normal anatomy of patellofemoral joint and patella are shown in Figures 25.109 and 25.110.

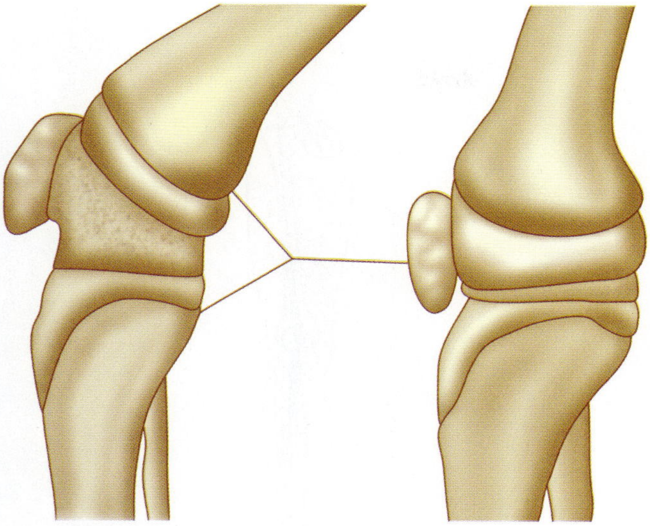

Fig. 25.108: Cuneiform intra-articular osteotomy

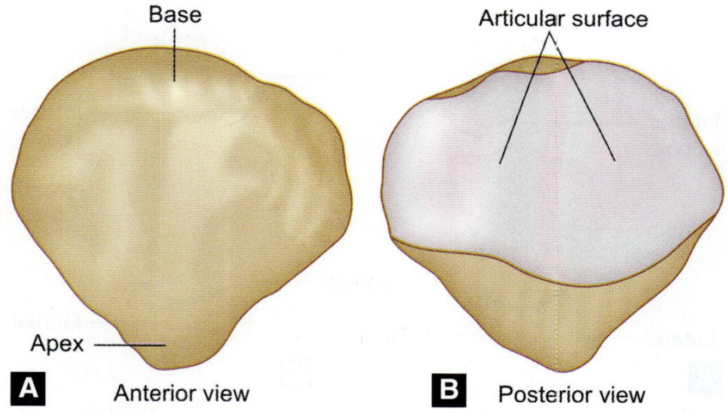

Figs 25.110A and B: Patella bone—(A) Anterior view; (B) Posterior view

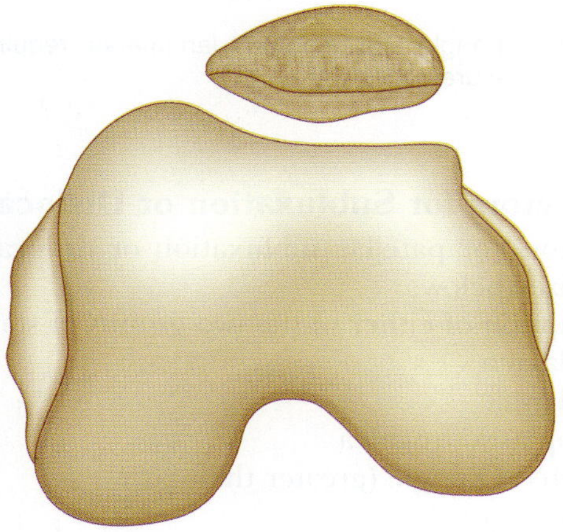

Fig. 25.109: Normal anatomy of patellofemoral joint

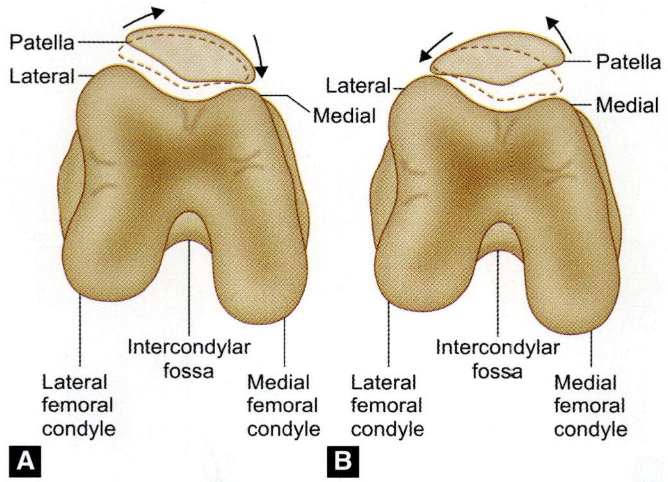

Figs 25.111A and B: Patellar tilting movements—(A) Medial patellar tilting; (B) Lateral patellar tilting

■ Biomechanics

Patella increases the mechanical advantage of extensor muscles. It increases functional lever arm of quadriceps. As knee starts to come into extension, patellar contribution increases until 45° of flexion, at which patella lengthens lever arm by 30 percent, it then decreases with more extension.

Contact Areas

Maximum contact area at 45°: Both the central ridge and the medial and lateral facets are in contact with the sulcus.

Odd facet: Contacts the femur only at maximum flexion. Important biomechanical function

- Transmission of tensile forces
- Increasing extension lever arm

Movements of Patella

- Patellar tilts (Figs 25.111A and B)
- Patellar rotations (Figs 25.112A and B)
- Patellar shifts (Figs 25.113A and B)

The Q-Angle (Fig. 25.114)

Constraints to Dislocation

Constraints for patellar dislocation can be divided into various headings:

- *Bony constraints:* Lateral border of trochlea
- *Soft tissue constraints:* It can be active or passive
  - Active, e.g. vastus medialis obliquus (VMO)
  - Passive, e.g. medial patellofemoral ligament and medial retinaculum.

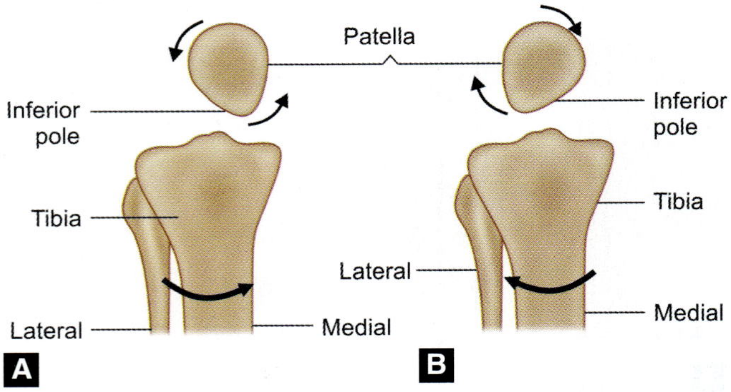

Figs 25.112A and B: Patellar rotational movements—(A) Medial rotation; (B) Lateral rotation

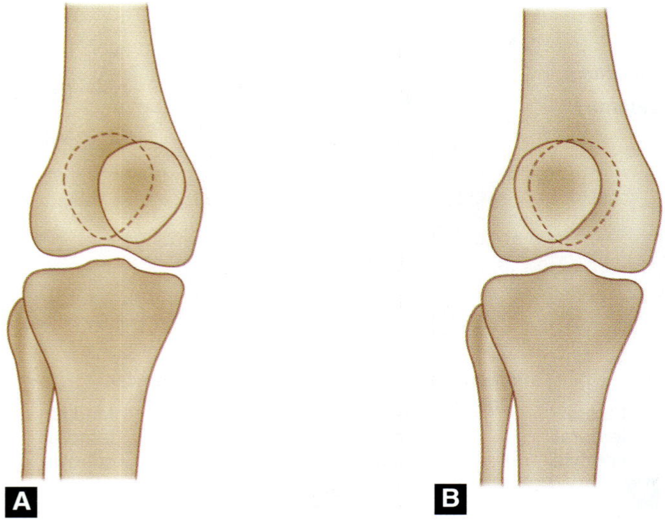

Figs 25.113A and B: Patellar shifts—(A) Medial shift; (B) Lateral shift

Stabilizers of Patellofemoral Joint

Static Stabilizers

These provide fixed inhibition to lateral translation of the patella and most notably include:

- Medial patellofemoral ligament (MPFL)
- Medial meniscopatellar ligament (MMPL)
- Medial patellotibial ligament (MPTL)

Dynamic Stabilizers

These are muscular structures and are primarily the quadriceps group, the VMO muscle. Adductor magnus should also be noted with this group because the distal fibers of the VMO often attach to the adductor magnus tendon.

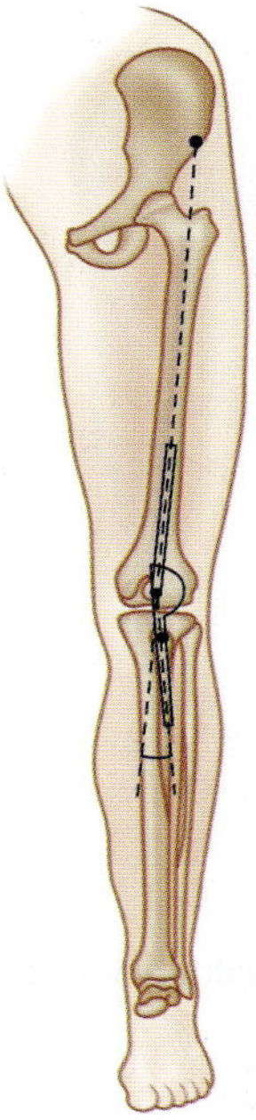

Fig. 25.114: Q-angle and important landmarks, required for its measurement

Risk Factors for Subluxation or Dislocation

Risk factors for patellar subluxation or dislocation are summarized below:

- Disruption of either of the two groups of stabilizers
- Patella alta
- Patellar tilt
- Hypoplastic trochlea
- Elevated Q-angle (greater than 20°)
- Genu valgum
- Increased femoral anteversion
- Coxa valga
- Excess foot pronation
- Lateral tibial tubercle
- External tibial torsion
- Family history of dislocation

The Pathogenesis of Patellar Dislocation

Patellar dislocation is the most common during dancing or throwing a basketball. Here, the feet are planted, the knees are only slightly flexed and the entire torso pivots. The patella is not engaged in trochlea and dislocates.

Types of Patellar Dislocation

- Congenital
- Persistent dislocation
- Obligatory dislocation
- Acquired/adult dislocation
- Acute dislocation
- Traumatic

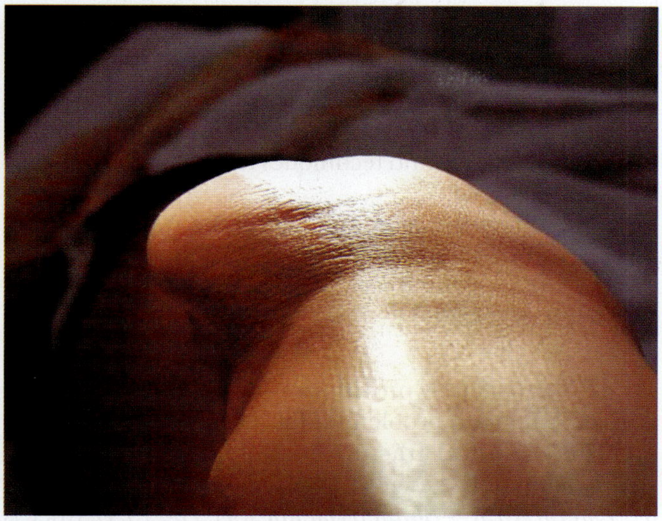

Fig. 25.115: Patient with a chronic patellar dislocation

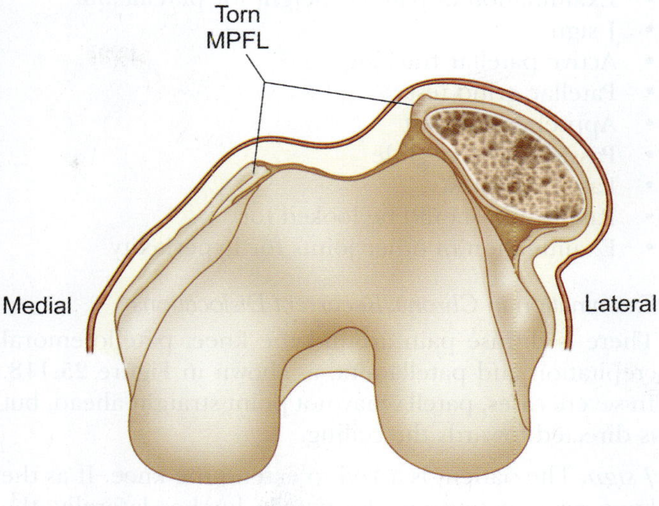

Fig. 25.116: A classic patellar dislocation

- Chronic dislocation (Fig. 25.115)
- Recurrent dislocation
- Habitual dislocation
- Acute patellar dislocation
- Superior patellar dislocation
- Medial patellar dislocation

Acute Dislocation

It is common in athletes. More common in males (male to female ratio is 3:1). The younger the age at which dislocation first occurs, more are the chances of developing recurrent patellar dislocation. It is also associated with stretching of medial soft tissues, e.g. medial patello-femoral ligament and medial retinaculum. Medial structures are torn in sudden and violent dislocation. Articular surface of patella may be damaged. Lateral femoral condyle may be damaged and a loose body can be created, which can be of variable size. A classic patellar dislocation and are form of patellar dislocation are shown in Figures 25.116 and 25.117.

Medial Patellar Dislocation

It is a rare entity, possible in subjects who have undergone any form of patellar realignment. Have a hypoplastic medial femoral condyle and a flat trochlea.

Recurrent and Habitual Patellar Dislocation

Occur sporadically and unpredictably. In most cases, the articular surface of the patella remains in contact with the femur, albeit not the trochlea. Rarely, it may be the result of shortened quadriceps mechanism (Quadriceps contracture). Habitual dislocation is the one which dislocates as a rule, every time the patient flexes the knee.

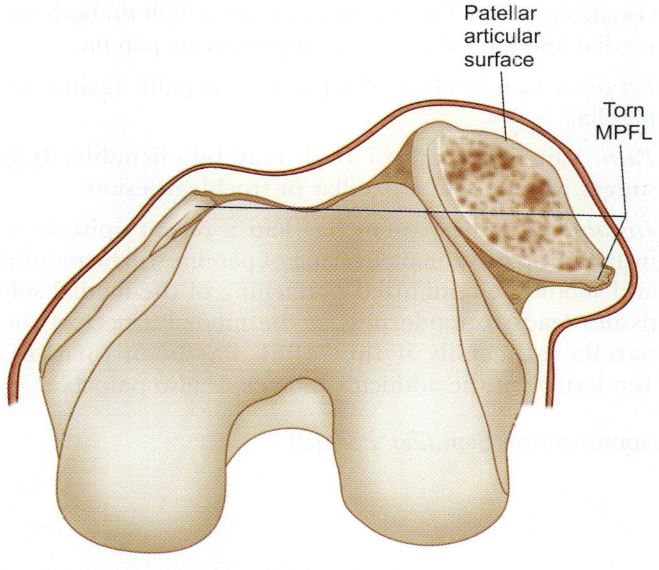

Fig. 25.117: A rare type of patellar dislocation

History: Symptoms may be acute in onset. It may also manifest as a slowly progressive sensation of anterior knee pain with increased physical activity.

Clinical Examination

Examination in Acute Dislocation

- Tenderness in knee on anterior aspect
- Rise of local temperature
- Swelling
- Crepitus
- Effusion

- Examination of patellar height for patella alta
- J sign
- Active patellar tracking
- Patellar grind test
- Apprehension test
- Passive patellar glide
- Patellar tilt test
- Patella alta should be looked for
- Examination of other joints for hyperlaxity

Examination in Chronic/Recurrent Dislocations

There is diffuse pain around the knee, patellofemoral crepitation and patella alta, as shown in Figure 25.118. In severe cases, patella may not point straight ahead, but is directed towards the ceiling.

J sign: The patient is asked to extend the knee. If as the knee nears extension, the patella lurches laterally, the patient is said to exhibit the J sign. It indicates, lateral patellar tracking. It indicates significant bony or soft tissue pathology or both, at the origin of trochlea. This can be visualized well, if the examiner places a digit on both the medial and lateral aspects of the superior patella.

Crepitus: Can be elicited by placing the palm against the patella.

Pain: Pain, grinding or both may be elicitable. It is suggestive of either a patellar or trochlear lesion.

Instability: If the patient has had a recent episode of instability, passive maneuvering of patella, will be painful and should be minimized. Stretching of the medial soft tissues leads to tenderness at the medial aspect of the patella, especially if the MPFL has been torn off. Tenderness at the adductor tubercle is also palpable.

Apprehension Sign (Fig. 25.119)

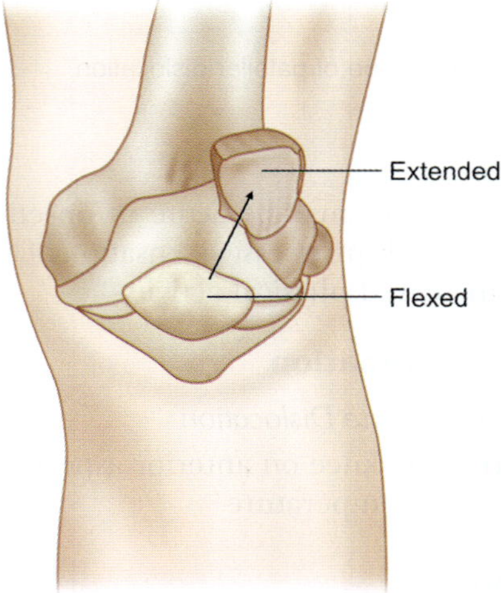

Fig. 25.118: Position of patella in patella alta

Investigations

- Radiographs
- CT scan
- MRI scan.

Radiography: Views and techniques for taking radiographs include:

- Plain anteroposterior and lateral X-rays
- Hughston's tangential view/infrapatellar view
- Laurin's tangential view
- Merchant's view
- Skyline view.

i. *AP X-rays:* Rarely provides any information regarding patellofemoral problems. May reveal bipartite patella. Osteochondral fracture may be diagnosed at the medial patellar edge.

ii. *Lateral X-ray—Blumensaat line (See Fig. 25.4):* Knee is flexed to 30°. A line extending through intercondylar notch, should just touch lower pole of patella. A patella lying above this line is termed as patella alta. Lateral X-ray, crossing sign is shown in Figure 25.120. Lateral X-ray, showing various patellar heights are illustrated in Figures 25.121A to D.

iii. *Blackburne peel ratio:* Ratio of length of articular surface of patella to the length measured from articular surface of tibia to inferior pole of patella. Normal ratio is 0.54-1.06.

iv. *Patellar height:* Assess the position of patella relative to the trochlea in sagittal plane. This is called patellar height.

v. The Insall-Salvati ratio

vi. Blackburne peel ratio

vii. *Measurements of patellofemoral congruence:* This is illustrated in Figures 25.122 and 25.123.

a. *Angle MSL:* Sulcus angle (average value ranges from 137° ± 6°)

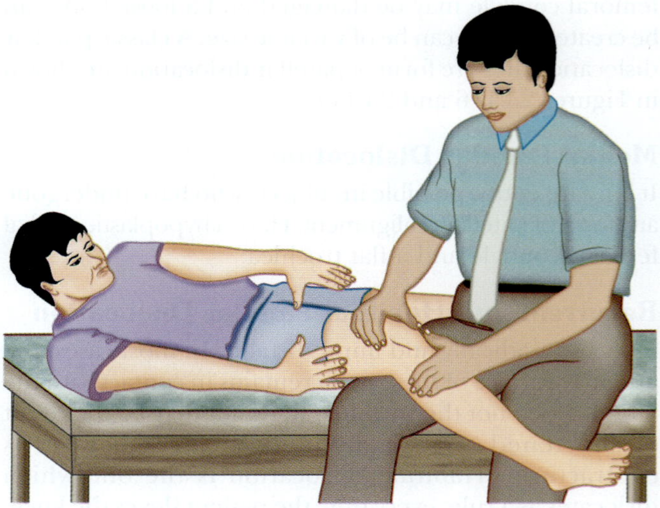

Fig. 25.119: Apprehension sign seen in patellar dislocation

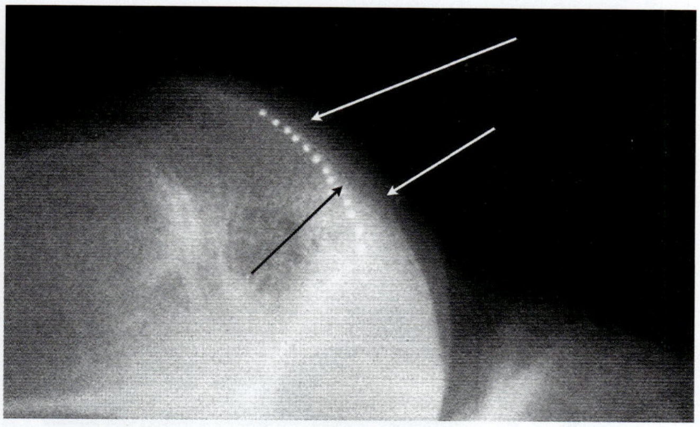

Fig. 25.120: Lateral X-ray (crossing sign)

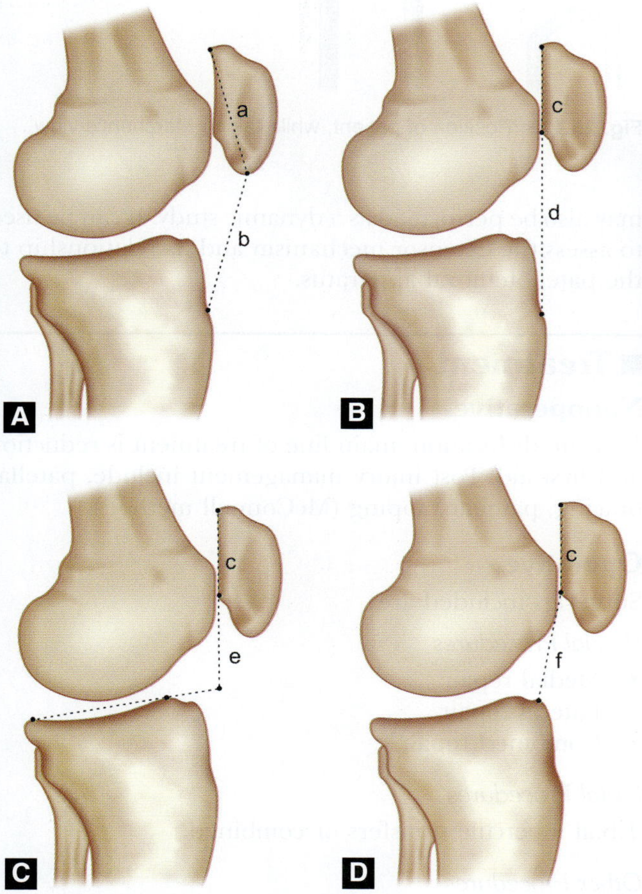

Figs 25.121A to D: Various techniques to measure patellar heights

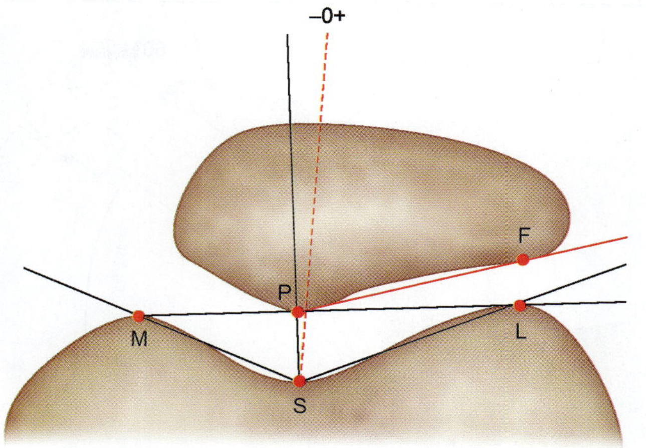

Fig. 25.122: Measuring patellofemoral congruence—F. Facet; L. Lateral condyle; M. Medial condyle; P. Patellar ridge; S. Sulcus

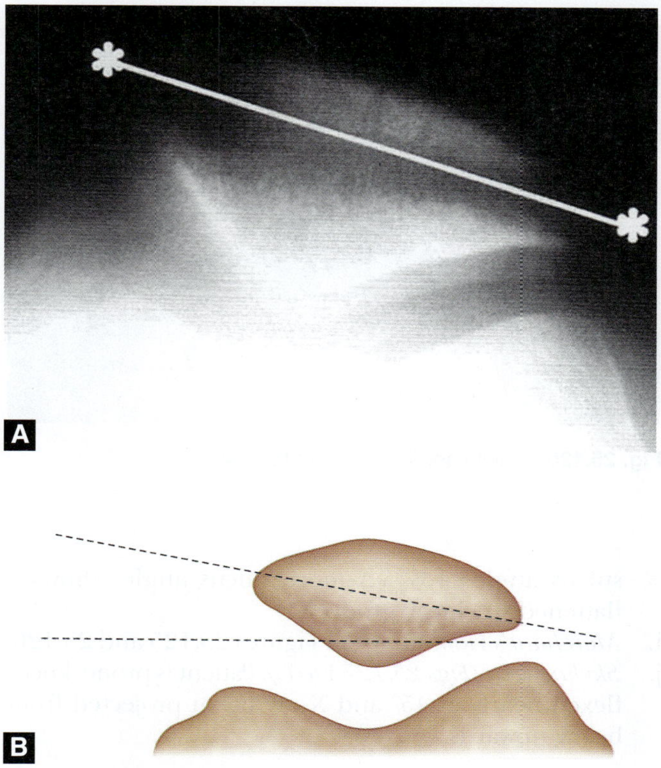

Figs 25.123A and B: Tilt angle of patella

b. *Line SO:* Zero reference line, bisecting sulcus angle.
c. *Anle PSO:* Congruence angle (average value ranges 8° ± 6°)
d. *Line PF:* Lateral facet
e. *Line ML:* Horizontal line on X-ray
f. *Angle FPL:* Patellofemoral angle (should diverge laterally)
g. *Tilt angle (Figs 25.123A and B):* A line is drawn across the medial and lateral borders of patella. The angle between the line and any horizontal line drawn on the X-ray forms the h. Tilt Angle. Normal value is less than 5°. Values more than 10° frankly abnormal.
h. *Hughston's tangential view/infrapatellar view (Fig. 25.124):* Patient is prone, with knees flexed 55°-60°,

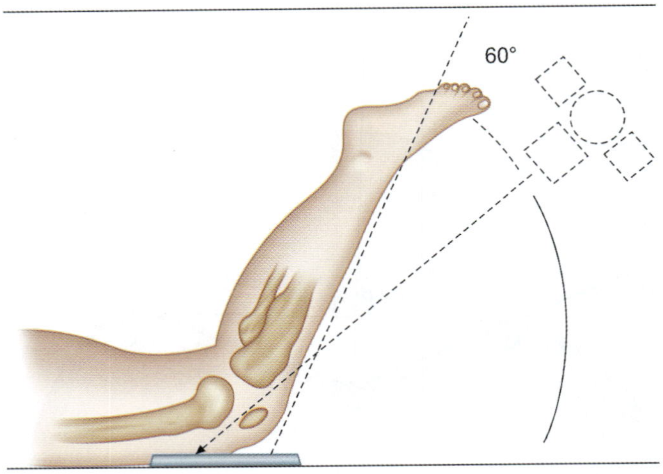

Fig. 25.124: Position of patient is prone, with knees flexed 55°-60° and sulcus angle nearly equal to 137°, while taking Hughston's tangential view/ infrapatellar view

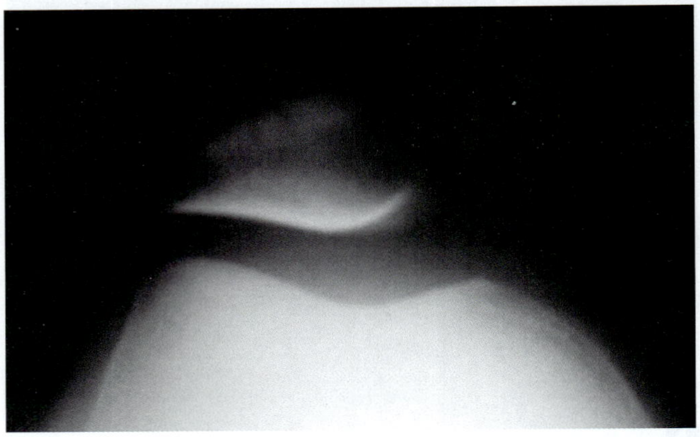

Fig. 25.125: Patella seen in Merchant's view

sulcus angle~137°. A more sulcus angle, shows a flattened trochlear groove

i. *Merchant's view,* shown in Figures 25.125 and 25.126
j. *Skyline view (Figs 25.127A to C):* Patient is prone, knees flexed nearly at 45° and X-ray beam projected from below upwards.

CT/MRI

CT and MRI scans have advantages over plain radiography because these are capable of imaging soft tissues. CT and MRI scan can provide axial views of patellofemoral joint, with knee in extended or slightly flexed position, which is not possible with plain X-rays, used to evaluate the trochlea-tubercle distance. This is the horizontal distance in a vertical plane between the intercondylar notch and the tibial tubercle. Measurements of 15 mm or more indicate malalignment. CT and MRI

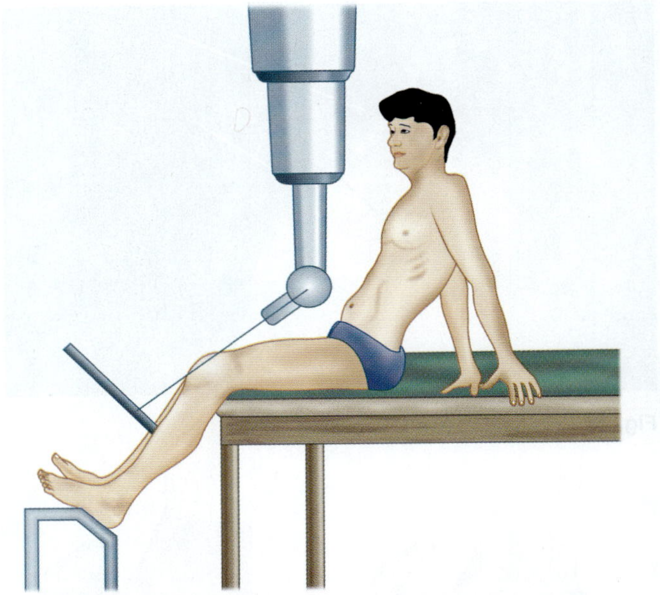

Fig. 25.126: Position of patient, while taking Merchant's view

may also be performed as a dynamic study. It can be used to assess the extensor mechanism and its relationship to the patellofemoral apparatus.

■ Treatment

Nonoperative

In acute dislocation, main line of treatment is reduction and first aid. Post injury management include, patellar bracing, patellar tapping (McConnell method).

Operative

Surgeries included are:

Proxial Procedures

- Medial repair
- Lateral repair
- Combined repair.

Distal Procedures

Tibial tubercule transfers or combined.

Other Procedures

- Tracheoplasty
- Osteotomy
- Arthroscopic debridement
- Patellectomy.

Acute or Urgent Treatment

Acute phase management should apply the "PRICE" principle:

P : Protection of the injured joint
R : Relative rest

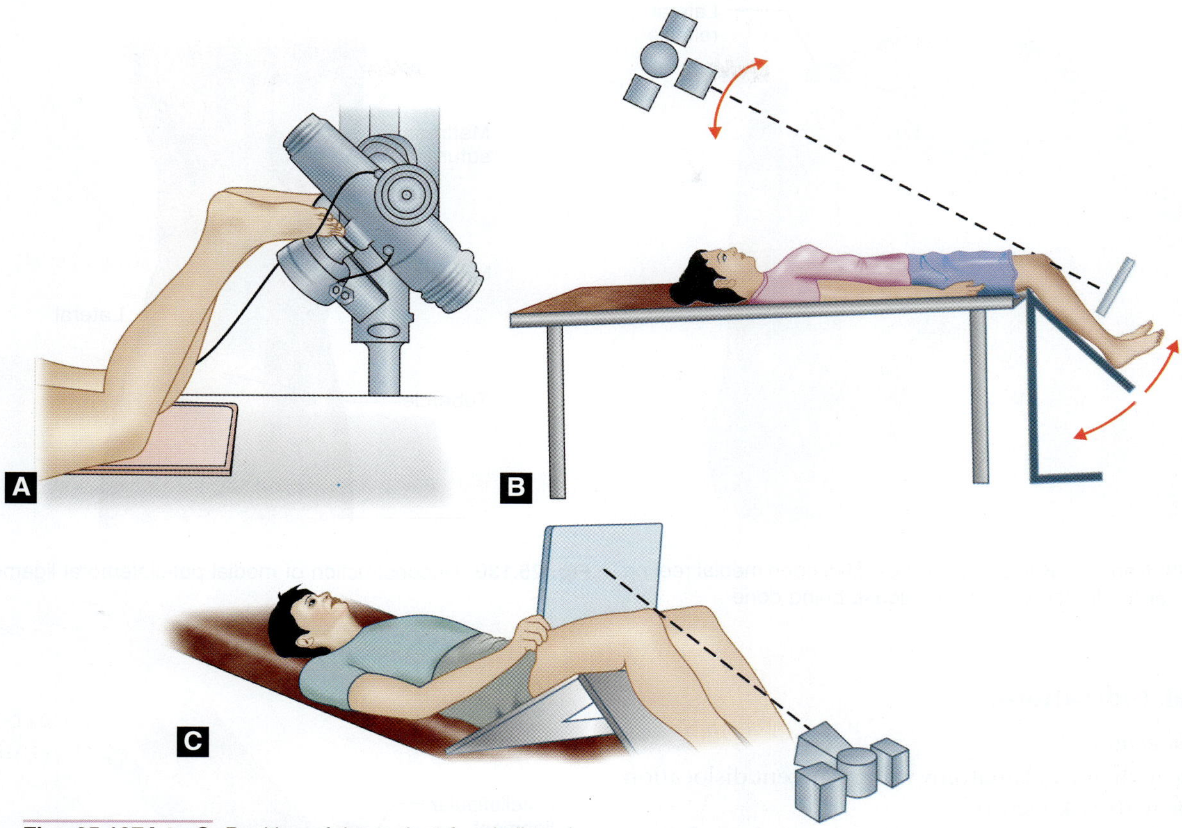

Figs 25.127A to C: Position of the patient for skyline view

I : Ice
C : Compression
E : Elevation to control inflammation.

A reduction may need to be carried out. It can be performed in different forms of dislocations as stated:

In classical dislocation: Slowly extend the knee to maximal extent possible, while pushing medially on the patella.

In turtle-type dislocation: Do not push medially on the patella. The lateral border of patella must be pushed down, while medial border is simultaneously pushed up. Then gradually extend the knee with medial pressure to relocate the patella.

In superior dislocation: Patella must be elevated over the superior osteophyte, responsible for dislocation.

Post-injury Management

- Patellar bracing
- Patellar taping (McConnell method).

Patellar bracing (Fig. 25.128): The goal of bracing is to restore proper alignment. This occurs by mechanical inhibition of lateral patellar motion, with a patellar buttress. Primary benefit may be psychological in nature.

Patellar taping (McConnells' method): Restore proper alignment and control pain.

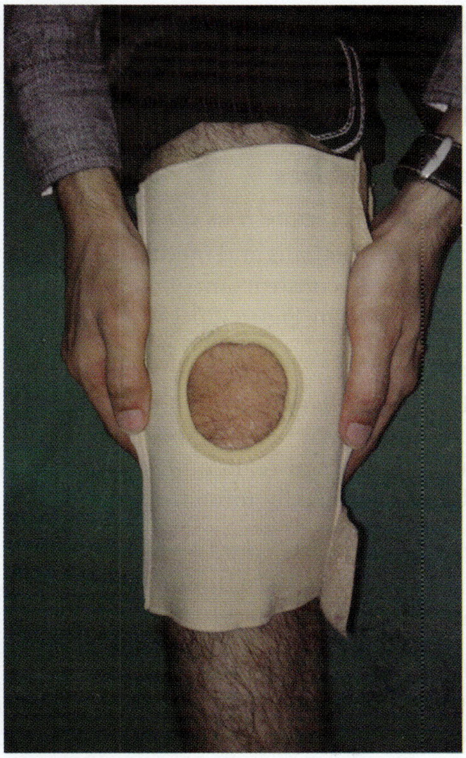

Fig. 25.128: Patellar bracing done, to provide proper alignment

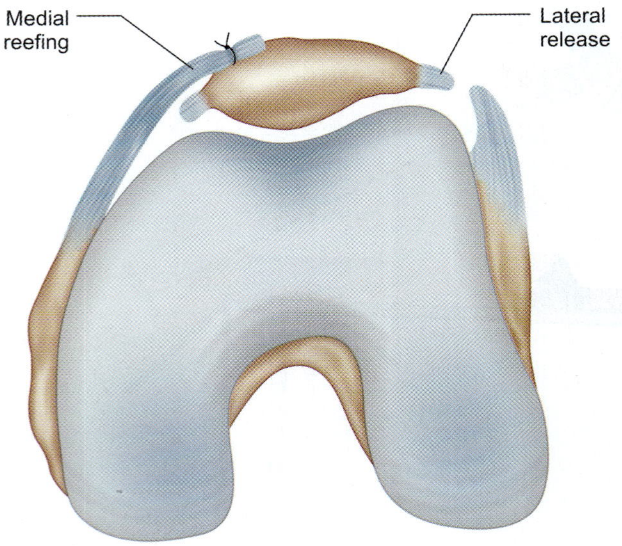

Fig. 25.129: Nam and Karzel procedure—Mini open medial reefing and arthroscopic lateral release being done

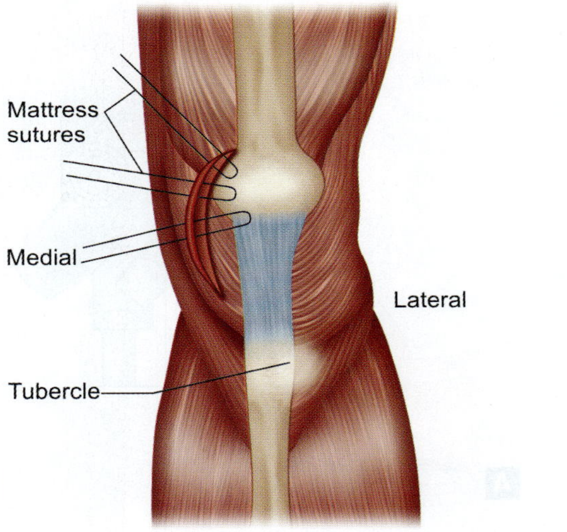

Fig. 25.130: Reconstruction of medial patellofemoral ligament

Surgical Indications

Patient Selection

- Those with normal anatomy with recurrent dislocation
- Those with risk factors
- Osteochondral fracture of lateral femoral condyle
- Age less than 14 years
- Athlete
- Palpable vastus medialis defect
- Evidence of dysplasia
- Family history
- Patella alta.

Proximal Procedures

Nam and Karzel Procedure (Fig. 25.129)

Reefing of vastus medialis and medial retinaculum, using mattress sutures. Reconstruction of medial patellofemoral ligament, as shown in Figure 25.130.

Indications

- Instability secondary to medial laxity, with or without trochlear dysplasia.
- Fine tuning of distal realignment procedures.
- Instability in skeletally immature patients.

Avikainen and Nikku Procedure

Reconstruction of medial patellofemoral ligament, as shown in Figures 25.131 to 25.133.

Muneta Technique (Fig. 25.134)

Used for chronic instability with Q-angle less than 20° or a damaged MPFL with semitendinosus graft. Incision at medial edge of patella. Medial structure of patella consists of three layers. Presynovial fatty layer is between second and deepest layer.

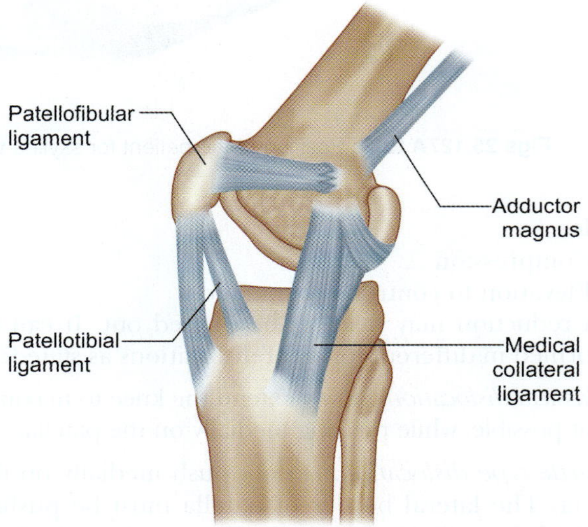

Fig. 25.131: Avikainen and Nikku procedure—MPFL detached from medial femoral epicondyle after acute patellar dislocation

Roux Goldwaith Procedure (Fig. 25.135)

It involves splitting the patellar tendon and medializing the lateral half. A 93 percent success rate is reported.

Distal Procedures

Tibial Tubercle Transfers (Figs 25.136A and B)

a. *Transfer done medially:* By Elmslie-Trillat, include:
   – Lateral retinacular release

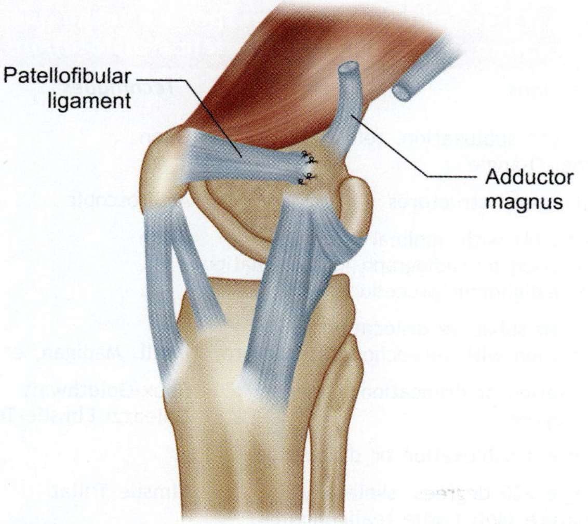

Fig. 25.132: MPFL with firm edge of vastus medialis obliquus muscle is reinserted into periosteum of medial femoral epicondyle and adductor magnus tendon is harvested

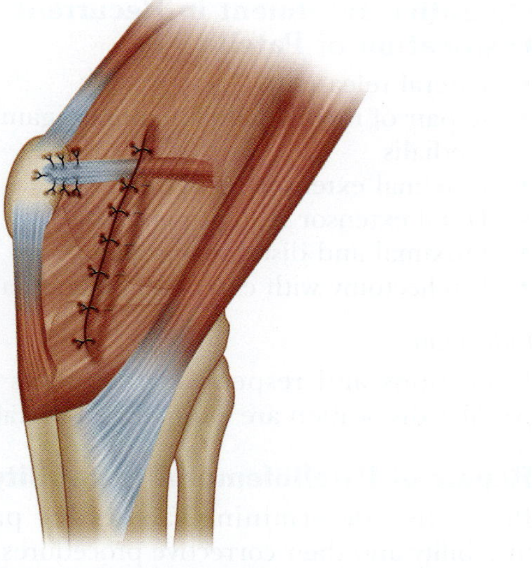

Fig. 25.133: Adductor magnus tendon fixed near medial border of patella and retinaculum is duplicated

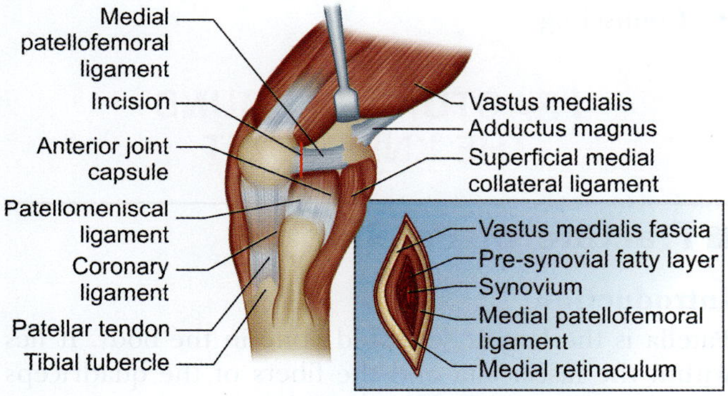

Fig. 25.134: Muneta technique

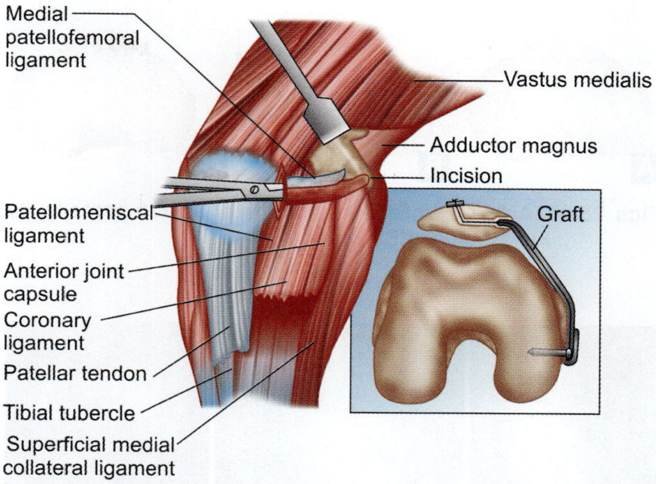

Fig. 25.135: Roux Goldwaith procedure

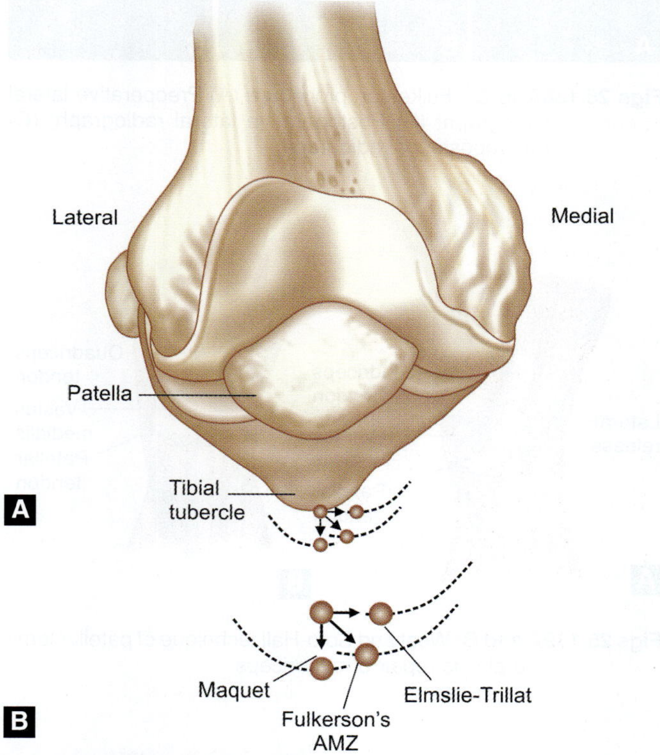

Figs 25.136A and B: Tibial tubercle transfer performed by various procedures—(A) Tibial tubercle shown (view from above); (B) Type of transfers, involving different procedures

- Medial retinacular plication
- Medial transfer of tibial tuberosity

b. *Anteromedially:* Fulkerson's AMZ (Anteromedialization)
   - Fulkerson and Brown (Figs 25.137 and 25.138)

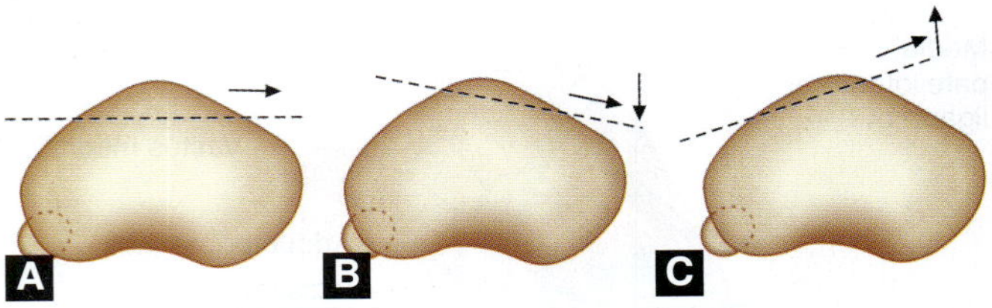

Figs 25.137A to C: Oblique osteotomy of tibial tuberosity, by Fulkerson and Brown

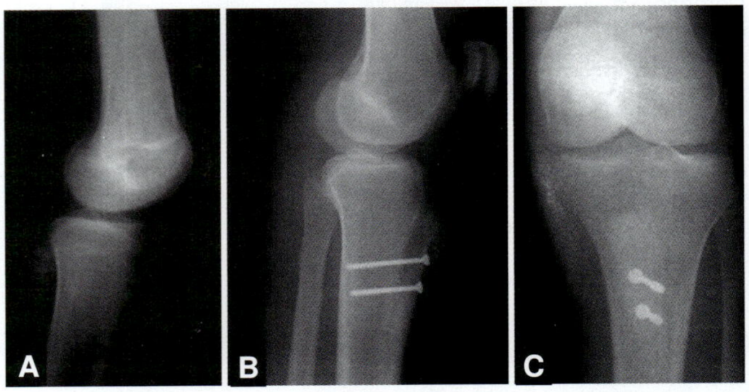

Figs 25.138A to C: Fulkerson procedure (A) Preoperative lateral radiograph; (B) Postoperative lateral radiograph; (C) Anteroposterior radiograph

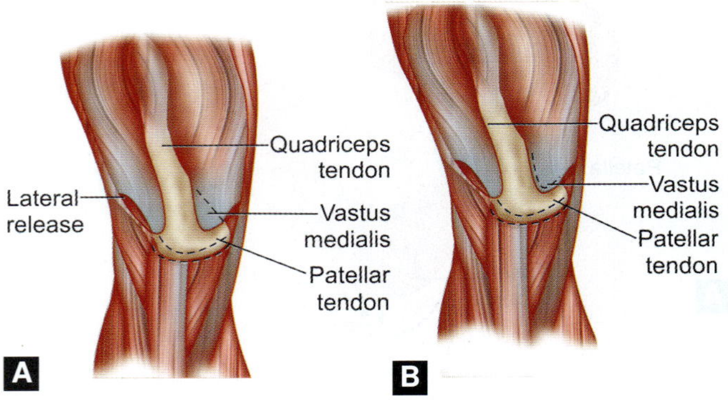

Figs 25.139A and B: West and Soto-Hall technique of patellectomy and plastic repair of quadriceps

Fulkerson Procedure

West and Soto-Hall Technique (Figs 25.139A and B)

Patellectomy and plastic repair of quadriceps. This is performed by putting a U incision over the anterior aspect of patella and a similar U incision over the quadriceps. Patella is excised. Quadriceps and anterior capsule is advanced distally. Vastus medialis insertion is freed in V shaped fashion and sutured, to cover the defect caused by patellectomy.

Table 25.4: Indications and respective technique of treatments for recurrent patellar dislocation

Indications	*Techniques*
Recurrent subluxation, relatively normal Q-angle	Open
Tight lateral structures	Arthroscopic
Lateral tilt with minimal lateral subluxation on radiograph in combination with realignment procedure	Open
Acute or subacute dislocation in association with osteochondral fracture	Insall, Madigan, et al.
Subluxation or dislocation, Q-angle <20 degrees	Roux-Goldthwait Galeazzi Elmslie-Trillat
Recurrent subluxation or dislocation	
Q-angle >20 degrees, skeletally immature (soft-tissue realignment)	Elmslie-Trillat
Q-angle >20 degrees, skeletally mature	
Recurrent dislocations, skeletally mature, Q-angle approaching 20 degrees	Hughston, modified Elmslie-Trillat
Skeletally mature, salvage procedure	West and Soto-Hall

Operative Treatment in Recurrent Dislocation of Patella

- Lateral release
- Repair of medial patellofemoral ligament and vastus medialis
- Proximal extensor realignment
- Distal extensor realignment
- Proximal and distal realignment
- Patellectomy with extensor realignment.

Indication

Indications and respective treatments for recurrent patellar dislocation are enumerated in Table 25.4.

Repair of Patellofemoral Instability

Respective determining factors for patellofemoral instability and their corrective procedures are illustrated in Table 25.5.

Postoperative Treatment

- Physiotherapy
- Counseling

FRACTURES AROUND THE KNEE JOINT

■ Fracture of Patella

Introduction

Patella is the largest sesamoid bone in the body. It lies within the fascia lata and the fibers of the quadriceps tendon. Center of ossification arises at 2 to 3 years of

Table 25.5: Determining factors and corrective procedures of patellofemoral instability	
Determining factors	***Procedure***
• Lateral pain, lateral tilt, mild lateral subluxation, tight lateral structures, Q-angle and Insall index within normal limits	• Arthroscopic lateral release
• Acute dislocation with associated osteochondral fragment or high-level athlete at end of season	• Arthroscope and repair of MPFL and medial retinaculum
• Recurrent instability, deficient medial structures, Q-angle <20 degrees, ATT-TS<15 mm	• MPFL reconstruction
• Recurrence with Insall index <1.2 and Q-angle >20 degrees, ATT-TS >15 mm	• Modified Elmslie-Trillat medial tuberosity transfer, arthroscopic evaluation, lateral release if tightness prevents patellar centering, arthroscopic plication for mild laxity of MPFL
• Recurrence with Insall index >1.2	• Lateral release with distalization and medialization of tibial tuberosity (Simmons procedure)
• Recurrence with grade 3 or grade 4 chondromalacia	• Oblique Fulkerson-type osteotomy leaving at least two-thirds of posteromedial cortex intact
• Recurrence in immature patient	• Proximal realignment

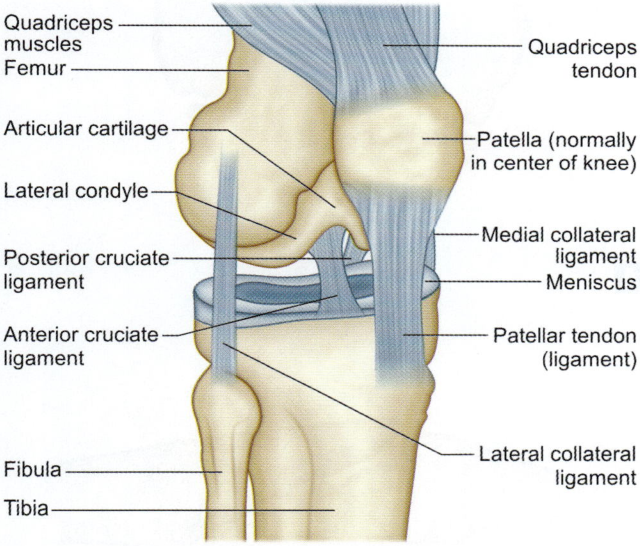

Fig. 25.140: Patellar attachments and surrounding structures

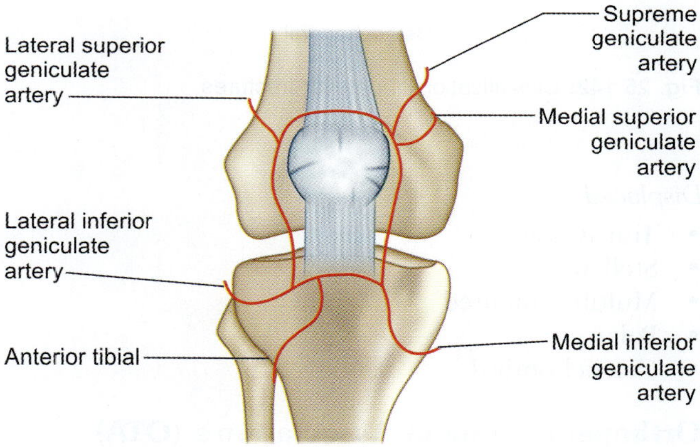

Fig. 25.141: Blood supply of patella

age. The patellofemoral joint is exposed to the highest contact stress of any weight-bearing joint. Therefore, any aberration in its anatomy or alignment may lead to symptomatic degenerative changes. Biomechanics of the patella and the extensor mechanism are important. The main function of the extensor mechanism is to keep the body erect and overcome the force of gravity.

Gross Anatomy (Fig. 25.140)

Arterial Blood Supply of the Patella (Fig. 25.141)

Functions of the patella

- Increase the mechanical advantage of the quadriceps tendon
- Provide protection to the femoral condyles
- Supplement the nourishment of the articular cartilage
- Maximum tensile forces across the quadriceps tendon are 3200 N
- Maximum tensile forces across the patella are 2800 N
- In trained athletes these forces can be up to 6000 N
- Patellofemoral contact stresses are about 2 to 10 N/mm^2

Classification of Patellar Fractures (Fig. 25.142)

Nondisplaced

- Transverse
- Stellate
- Vertical

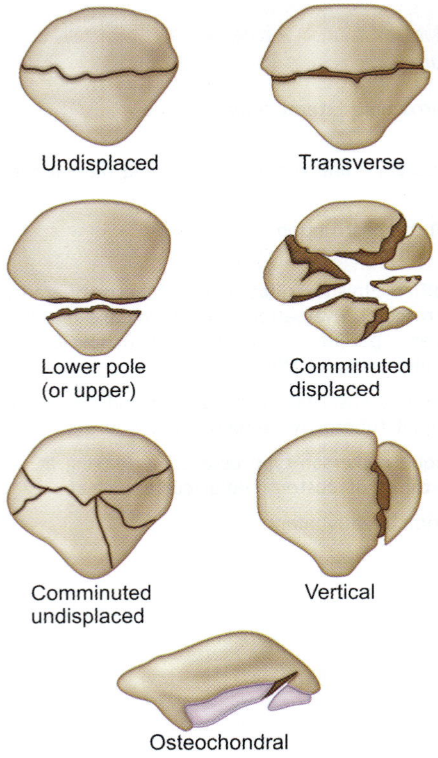

Fig. 25.142: Classification of patellar fractures

Displaced

- Transverse
- Stellate
- Multifragmented
- Polar
- Osteochondral

Orthopedic Trauma Association's (OTA) Classification of Patellar Fractures

Patella Extra-articular (Fig. 25.143)

It can further divided into two types:

i. Avulsion (Fig. 25.144A)
ii. Isolated body (Fig. 25.144B)
  - Simple
  - Multifragmentary

Partial Articular

Extensor mechanism remains intact. These can further be classified into following types:

- Vertical and lateral fracture, which can be:
  - Simple (Figs 25.145A and B)
  - Multifragmentary (Figs 25.146A and B)
- Vertical and medial
  - Simple (Figs 25.147A and B)
  - Multifragmentary (Figs 25.148A and B)
- Multifragmentary stellate (Fig. 25.149).

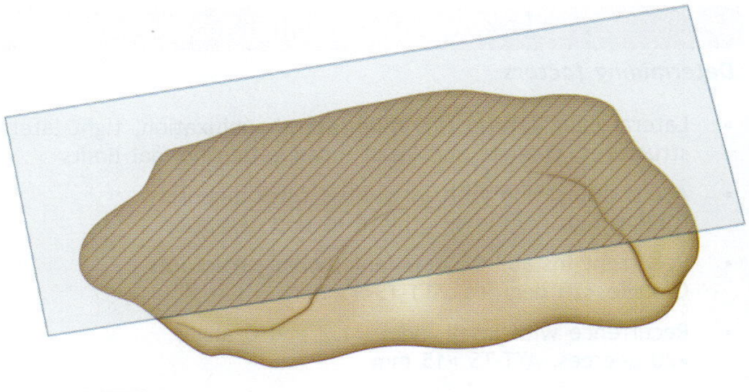

Fig. 25.143: Extra-articular patellar fracture

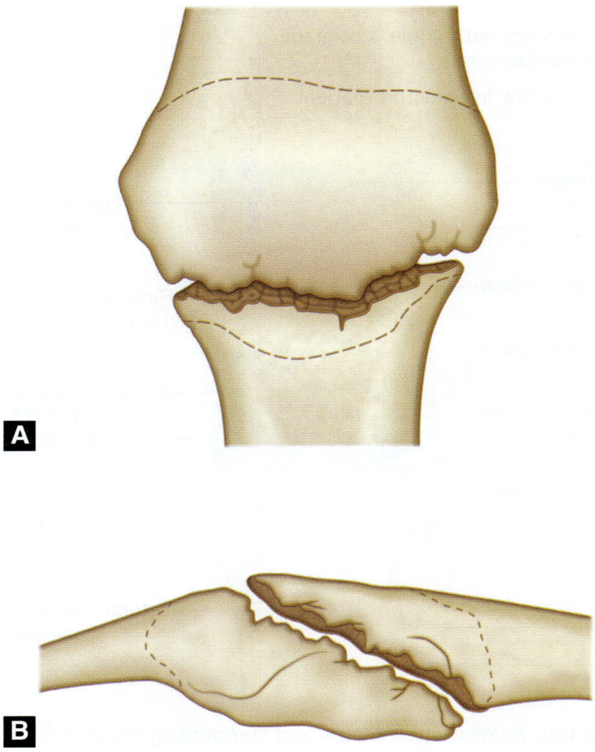

Figs 25.144A and B: Types of extra-articular patellar fractures—(A) Avulsion fracture; (B) Isolated fracture

Complete Articular (Fig. 25.150)

There is a disrupted extensor mechanism. It can be further classified as:

a. Transverse, which can be further divided, based on the part of patella involved.
  - Middle (Fig. 25.151)
  - Proximal (Fig. 25.152)
  - Distal (Fig. 25.153)
b. Transverse with second fragment
  - Middle (Fig. 25.154)
  - Proximal (Fig. 25.155)
  - Distal (Fig. 25.156)

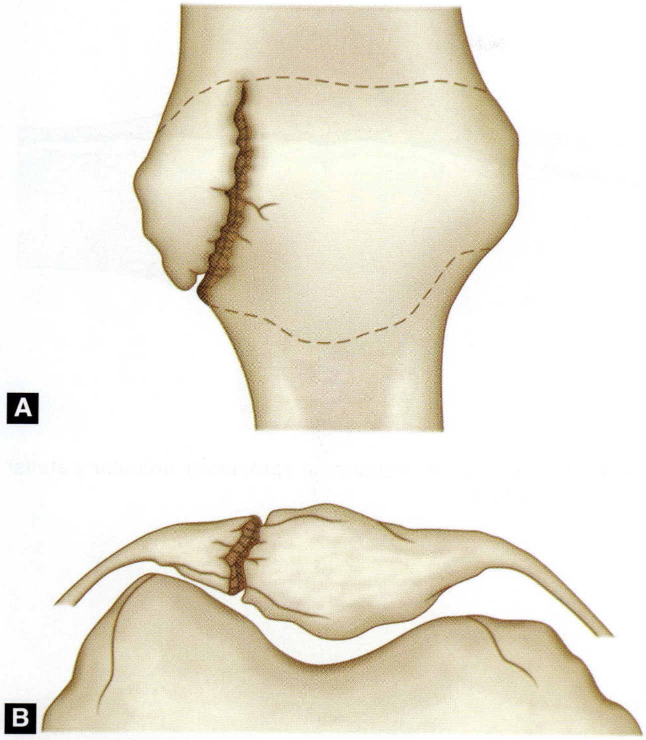

Figs 25.145A and B: Partial articular patellar fracture—simple vertical lateral fracture

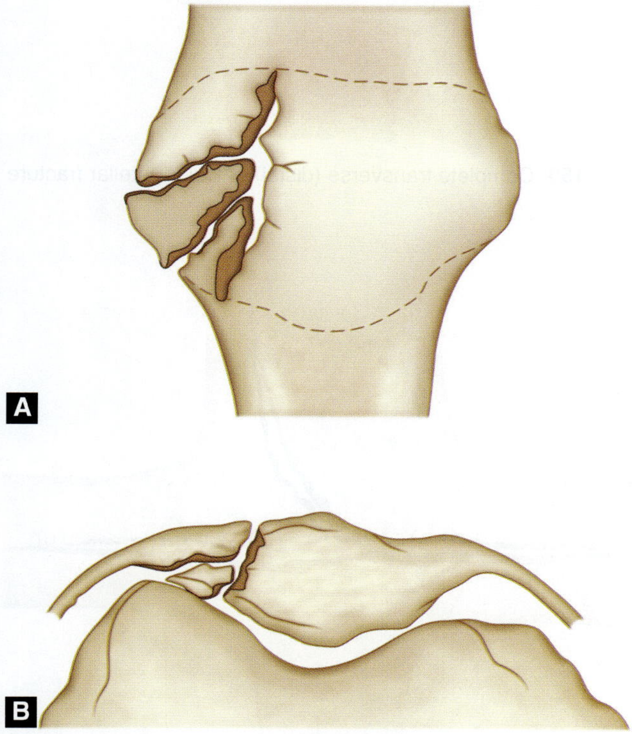

Figs 25.146A and B: Multifragmentary, vertical and lateral, partial articular patellar fracture

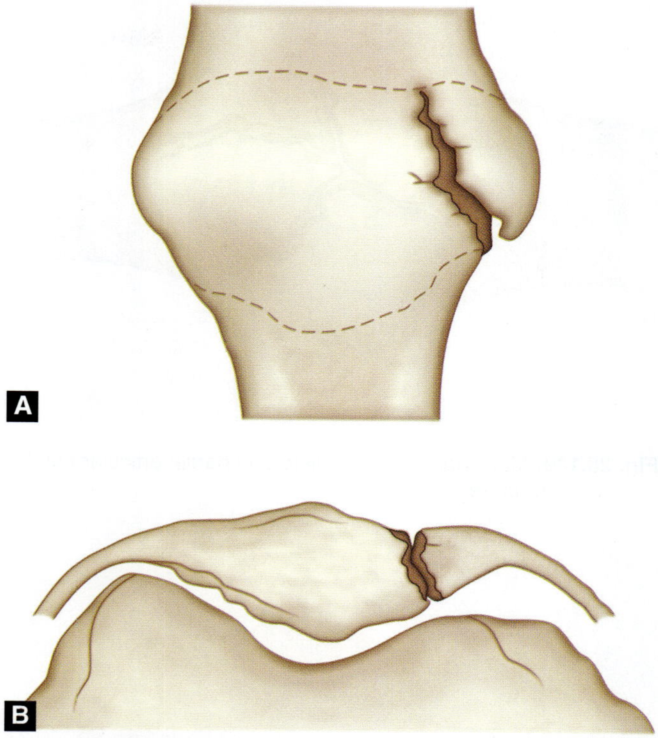

Figs 25.147A and B: Partial articular patellar fracture—simple vertical and medial fracture

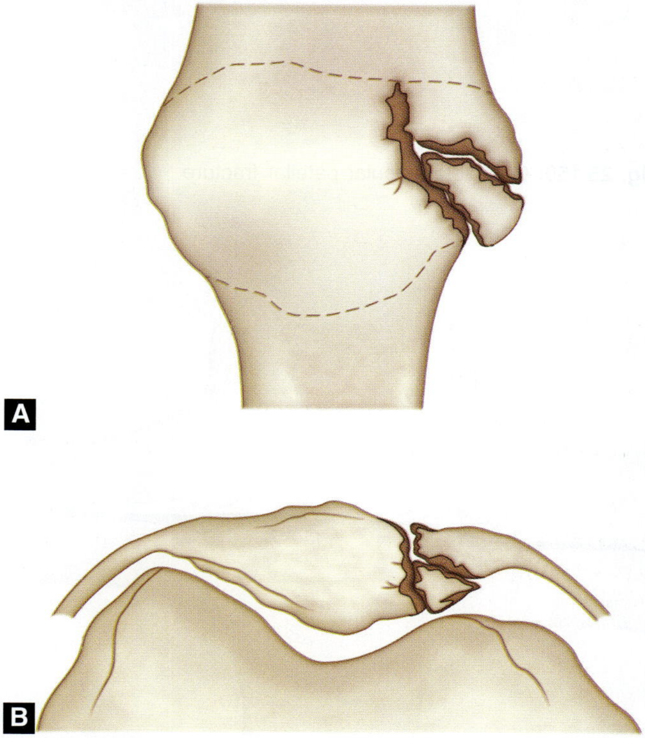

Figs 25.148A and B: Multifragmentary, vertical and medial, partial articular patellar fracture

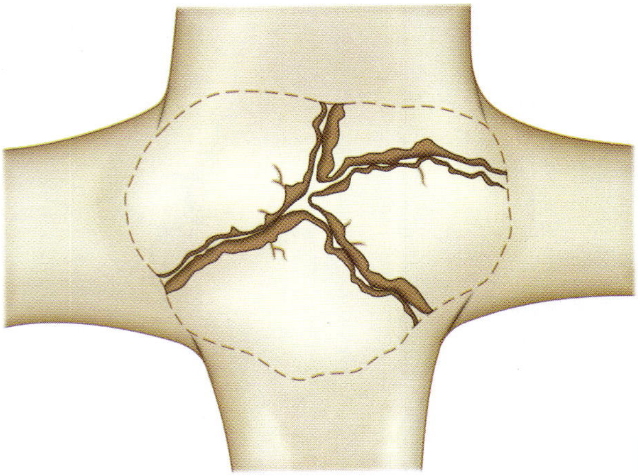

Fig. 25.149: Multifragmentary, stellate and partial articular patellar fracture

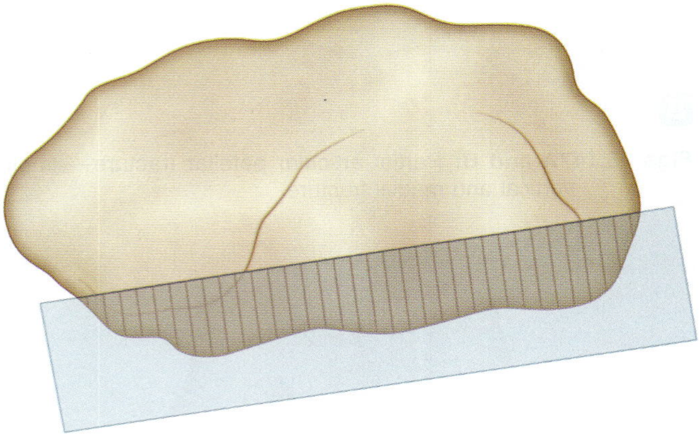

Fig. 25.150: Complete articular patellar fracture

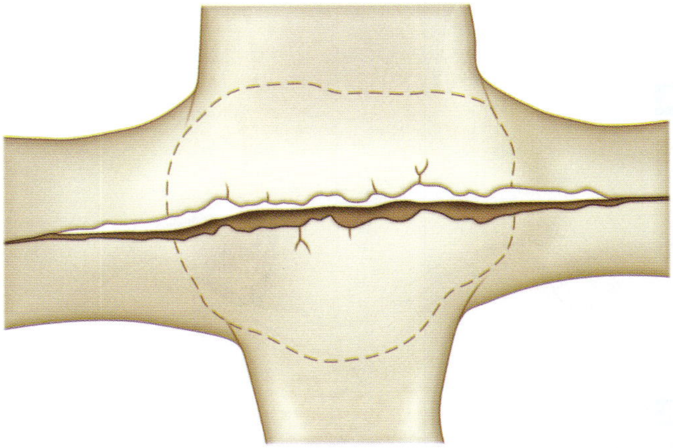

Fig. 25.151: Complete transverse (middle) articular patellar fracture

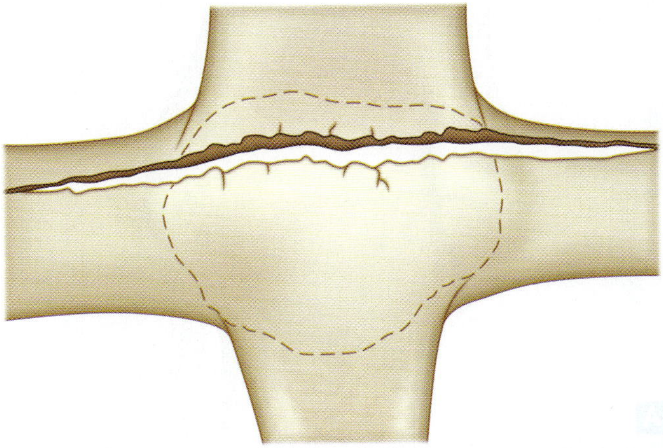

Fig. 25.152: Complete transverse (proximal) articular patellar fracture

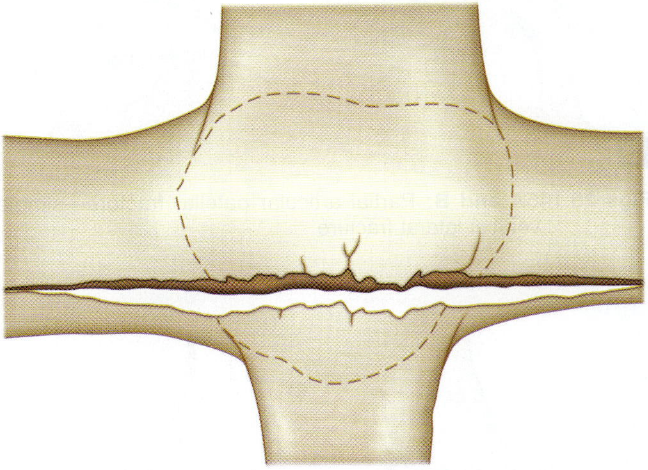

Fig. 25.153: Complete transverse (distal) articular patellar fracture

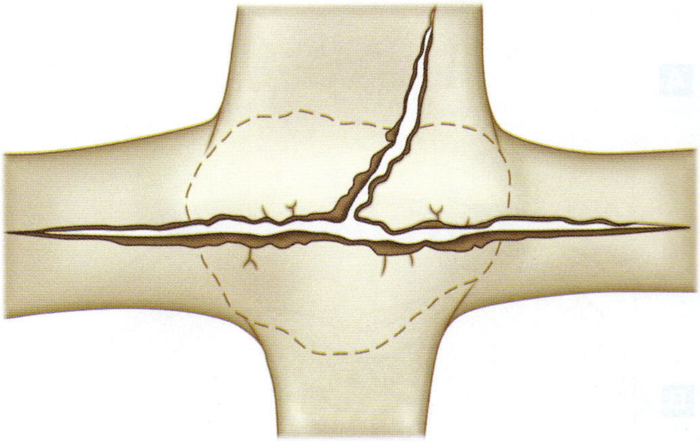

Fig. 25.154: Complete transverse (middle with second fragment) articular patellar fracture

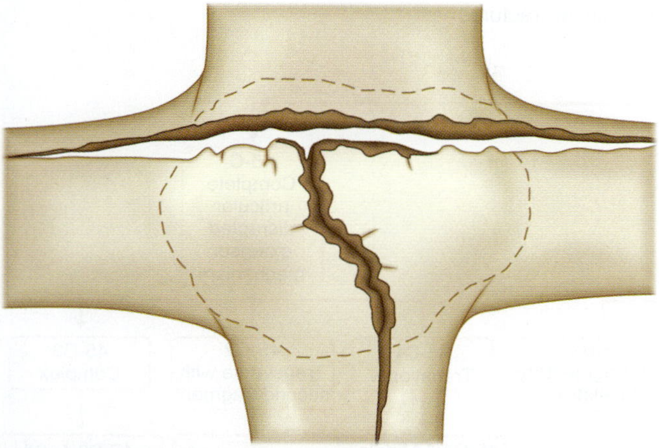

Fig. 25.155: Complete transverse (proximal with second fragment) articular patellar fracture

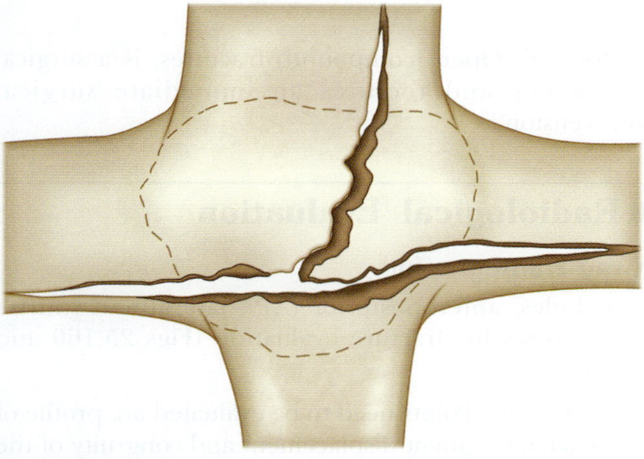

Fig. 25.156: Complete transverse (proximal with second fragment) articular patellar fracture

c. Complex
   - Up to three fracture fragments, as shown in Figure 25.157.
   - More than three fracture fragments, as illustrated in Figure 25.158.
   - Nonreconstructible (Fig. 25.159)

OTA classification of patellar fractures, can be summarized in Flow chart 25.1.

Mechanisms of Injury

Direct injuries: There is direct blow to the patella, e.g.
- Dashboard injuries
- Fall from height on the patella.

It can be associated with:
- Hip dislocation
- Ipsilateral femoral neck or shaft fracture
- Distal femur fracture
- Proximal tibia fracture.

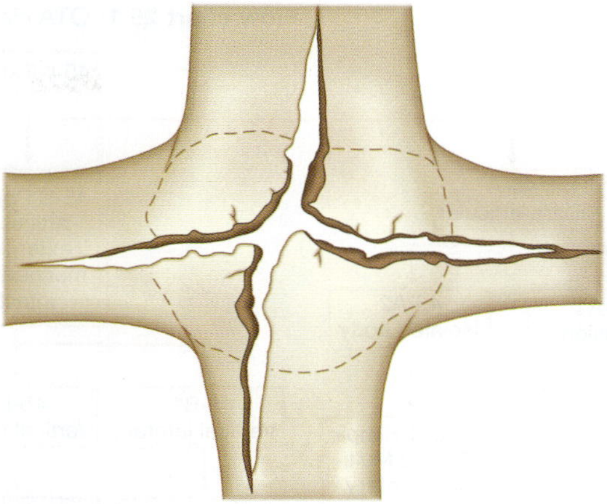

Fig. 25.157: Complete articular patellar fracture, complex form, with up to three fracture sites

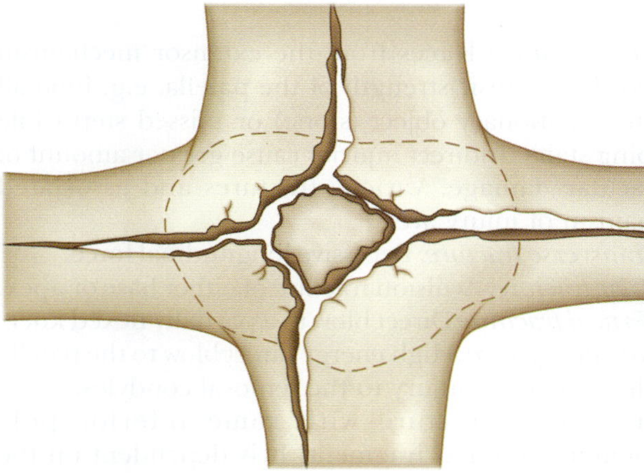

Fig. 25.158: Complete articular patellar fracture, complex form, with more than three fracture sites

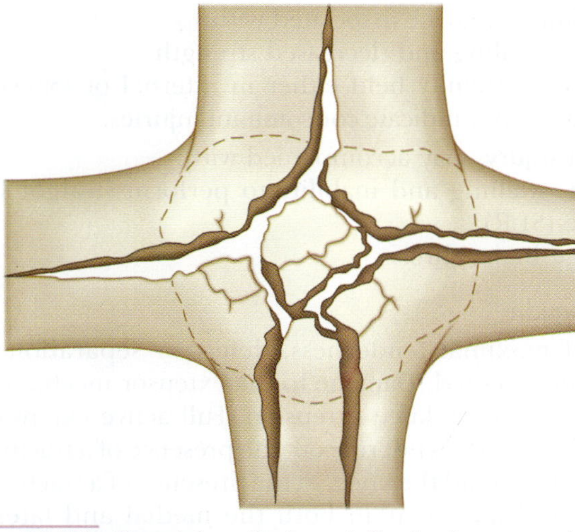

Fig. 25.159: Complete articular patellar fracture, complex form, nonreconstructible

Flow chart 25.1: OTA classification of patellar fractures

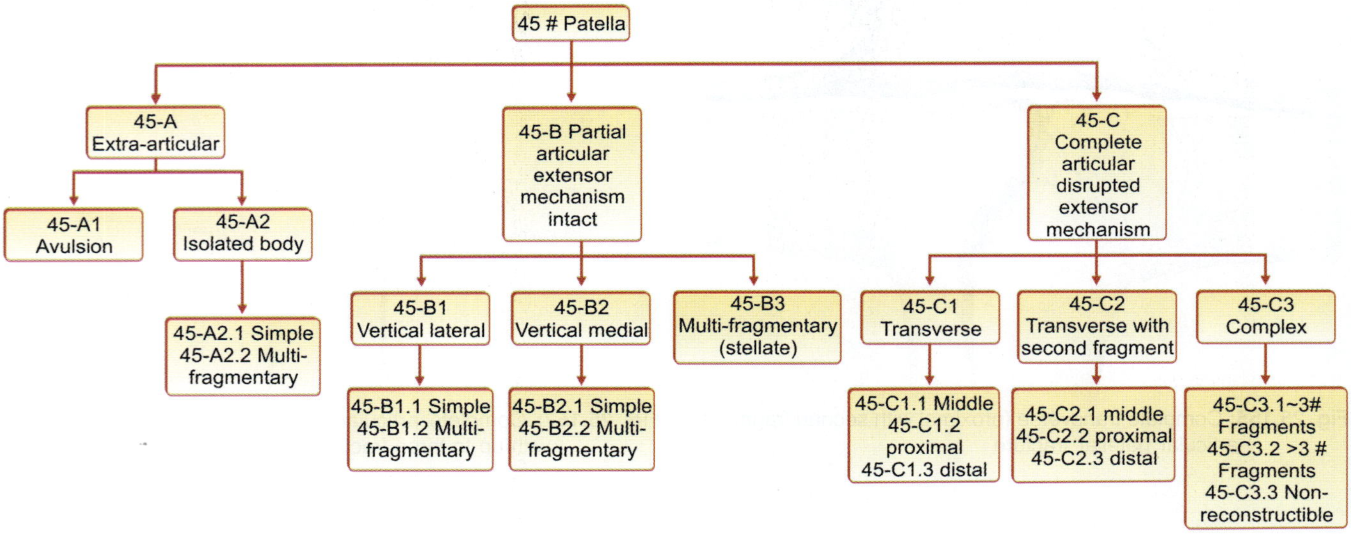

Indirect injuries: Forces from the extensor mechanism exceed the intrinsic strength of the patella, e.g. football kick to a stationary object (stone) or missed step while climbing stairs. Indirect injuries cause greater amount of retinacular damage. Various fractures and associated mechanism of injury are:

- *Transverse fracture:* Excessive longitudinal force.
- *Polar fracture:* Avulsion fracture of either base or apex.
- *Vertical fracture:* Direct blow to a partially flexed knee.
- *Stellate fracture:* High energy direct blow to the patella with associated injury to the femoral condyles.
- Transverse fracture with some inferior pole communition and fragment: It is dependent on the amount of damage to the quadriceps retinaculum.

Clinically

On Inspection

Direct injury, may be associated with:

- Pain, swelling and decreased strength
- Lower extremity held either in internal or external rotation may indicate concomitant injuries.

Indirect injury, may accompanied with:

- Pain, swelling and inability to perform straight leg raise (SLR).
- Large hemarthrosis.

On Palpation

Point of maximal tenderness, defect or separation of fragments is noted. Damage to the extensor mechanism is tested by active knee extension. Full active extension against gravity does not rule out the presence of a fracture. Inability to extend the knee, in the presence of a fractured patella, indicates tear in both the medial and lateral retinaculi. To rule out open fractures, saline load test is performed. Open (compound) fractures, is a surgical emergency and requires an immediate surgical intervention.

■ Radiological Evaluation

X-ray Radiography

It includes, anteroposterior (AP), lateral and sunrise (axial) views for fracture evaluation (Figs 25.160 and 25.161).

Lateral X-rays: Points need to be evaluated are profile of the patella, fragment displacement and congruity of the articular surface. Low riding patella (patella baja), indicates quadriceps tendon rupture. High riding patella (patella alta), indicates patellar tendon rupture.

Method of Insall and Salvati (Fig. 25.162)

It uses the ratio of the greatest diagonal length of patellar to the length of patellar tendon. Normal knee ratio is equal to 1:1. Ratio greater than 0.8, indicates high riding patella or patellar tendon rupture.

Other Radiological Features

Patella should lie in the midline of the femoral sulcus. Patellar height (greater than 2 cm), based on the inferior pole of the patella, which is normally located above a line parallel, with the distal femoral condyle weight-bearing surface, as shown in Figure 25.163.

Proximal pole of the patella should lie below the anterior surface of the femoral shaft with knee flexed to 90°, as shown in Figure 25.164. Lateral X-ray, showing pattern of patellar fracture, communition and separation is illustrated in Figure 25.165.

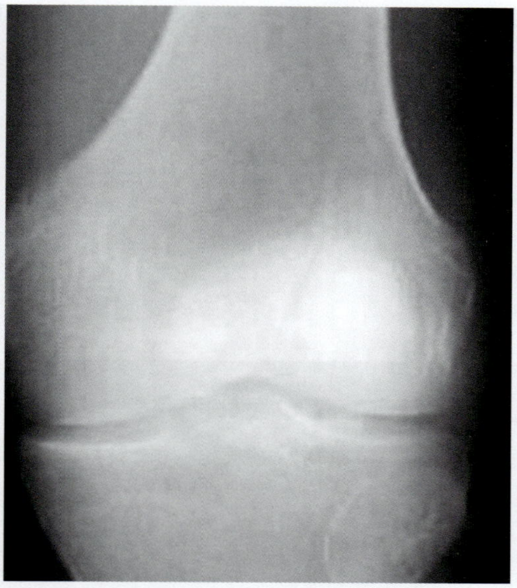

Fig. 25.160: X-ray knee AP view

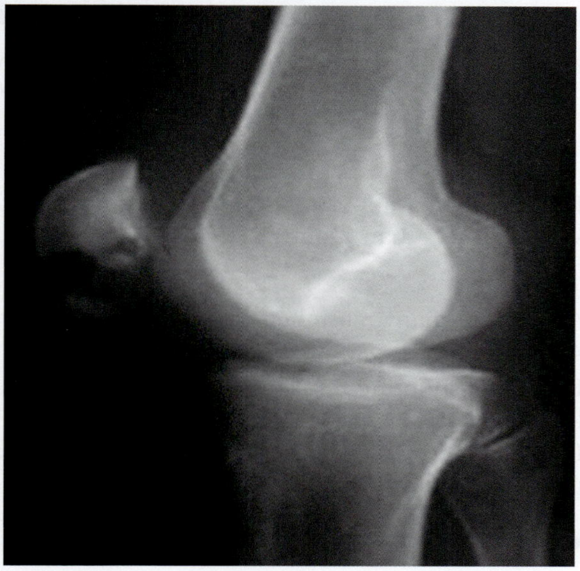

Fig. 25.161: X-ray knee lateral view

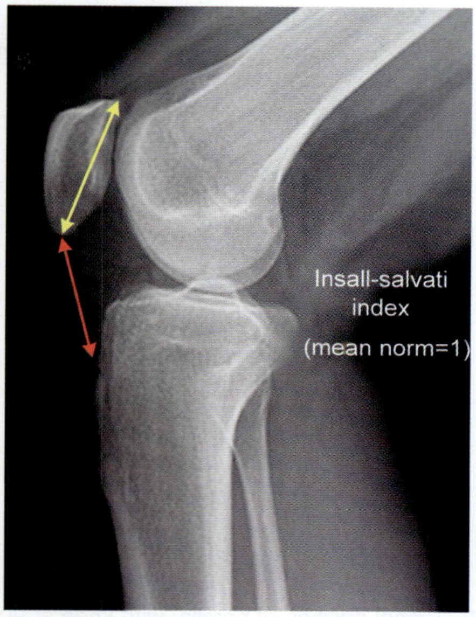

Fig. 25.162: Method of Insall and Salvati for assessing the height of patella

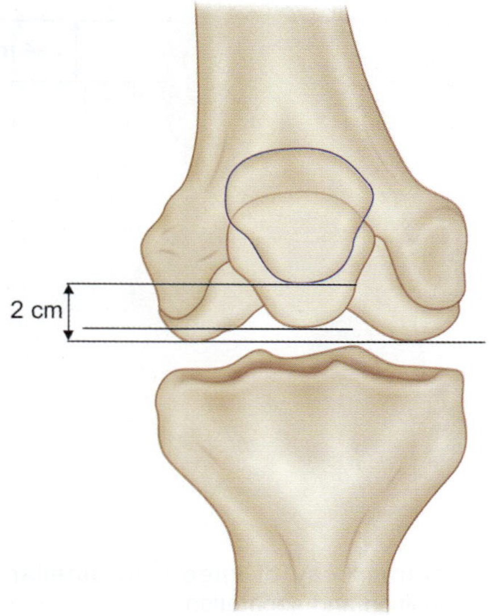

Fig. 25.163: Normal patellar height with respect to distal femoral condyles

Axial or Sunrise View (Figs 25.166A and B)

This is used to detect vertical fracture line displacement and osteochondral defects.

Other Modalities

- Computed tomography (CT scan)
- MRI
- Arthrography
- Standard tomography
- Bone scanning, done to rule out stress fracture.

History of Treatment Modalities

1800: Malgaigne, percutaneous bone clamps.

1887: Sir Hector Cameron (Glasgow, Scotland), first open reduction and fixation using silver threads.

1924: Thompson, partial excision of patella.

Mid 1900: Brooke, Hey-Groves and Watson-Jones, advocated total excision of the patella.

1950: Pauwel, anterior tension band wiring techniques.

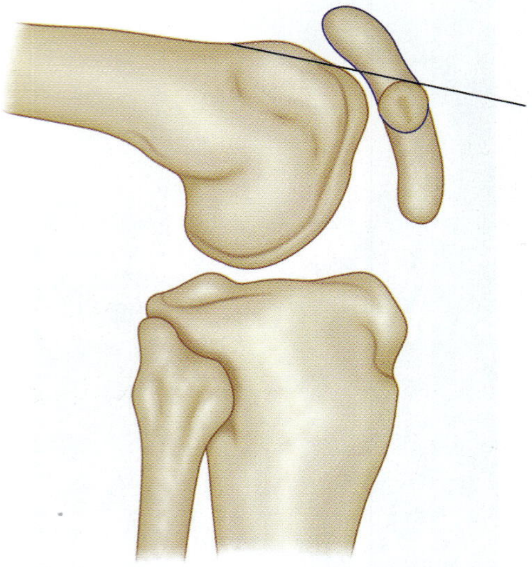

Fig. 25.164: Normal position of patella, with knee at 90° flexion

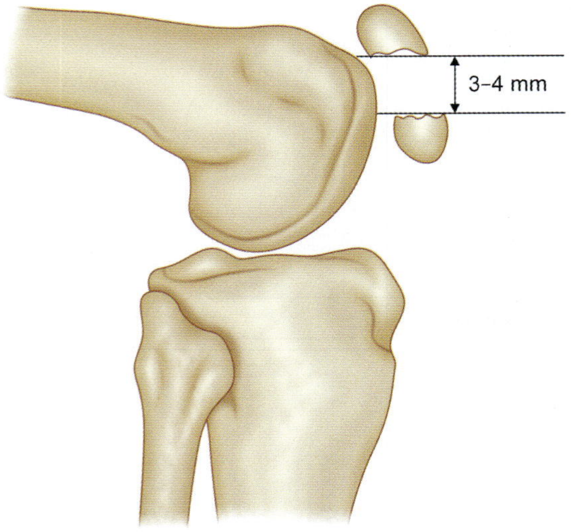

Fig. 25.165: Lateral X-ray of knee with patellar fracture, communition and separation

Current Treatment Options

Operative Treatment

- Tension band wiring techniques
- Partial patellectomy
- Partial patellectomy with tension band wiring
- Total patellar excision or patellectomy

Nonoperative Treatment

Indications

- Nondisplaced fracture, with an intact extensor mechanism.
- Transverse, stellate and vertical fracture.

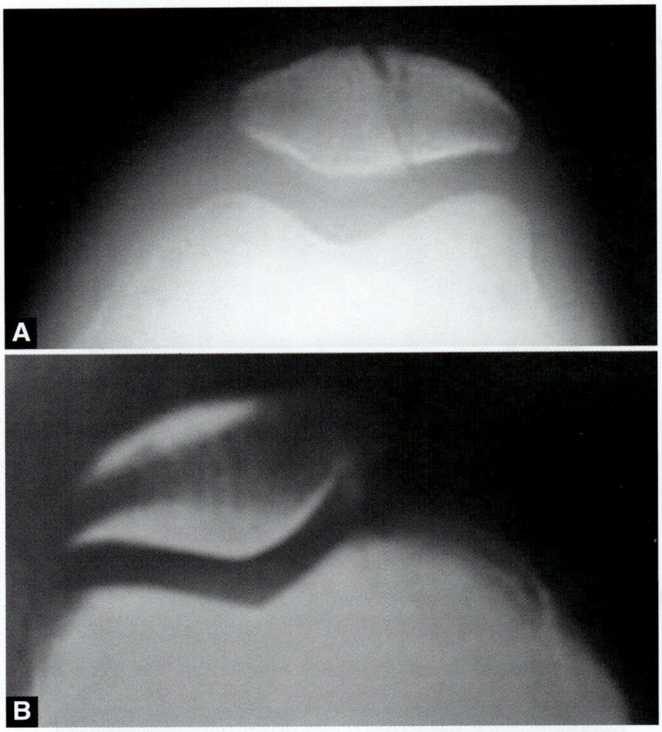

Figs 25.166A and B: Sunrise view—(A) Patellar fracture with vertical fracture line; (B) Patellar fracture with osteochondral defects

- Fragment separation less than 3 mm and articular stepoff of less than 2 mm.

Modalities

- Aspiration of any tense hematoma
- Application of ice and limb elevation
- Extension splinting for 4 to 6 weeks with cylinder or long leg cast.
- Hinged knee or range of motion (ROM) brace locked in extension during ambulation.

Mechanics of Fixation (Figs 25.167A and B)

Surgical Modalities

- Circumferential wire loop fixation (Martin's)
- Wire loop fixation through both fragments (Magnuson's), as shown in Figures 25.168A to C.

Modified Tension Band Wiring (Figs 25.169 to 25.171)

Schauwecker method of compression wiring of patella, using supplemental screws for comminuted fracture. Comminuted fragments are transformed with screws into bifragmental fracture.

Modified tension band internal fixation, using two anterior wire loops and two longitudinally directed Kirschner wires, as demonstrated in Figures 25.172A to C.

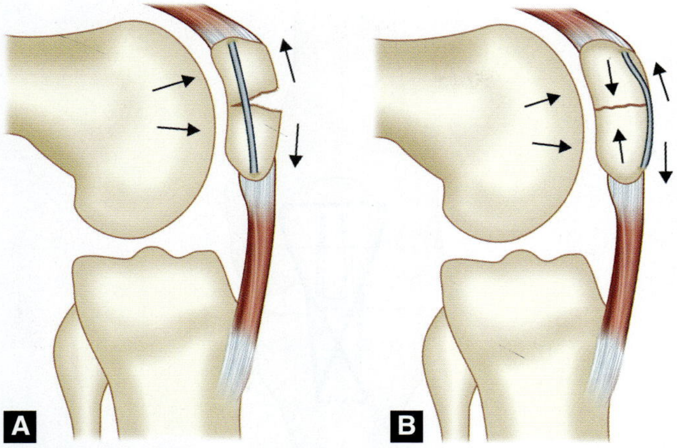

Figs 25.167A and B: (A) Inappropriate position of the tension band wire causes separation of fragments on the tension side of the patella during knee flexion; (B) Correct placement of the tension band wire for fixation of transverse patellar fractures neutralizes the tension side of the patella and on subsequent flexion of the knee, exerts compressive forces across the fracture at the joint surface

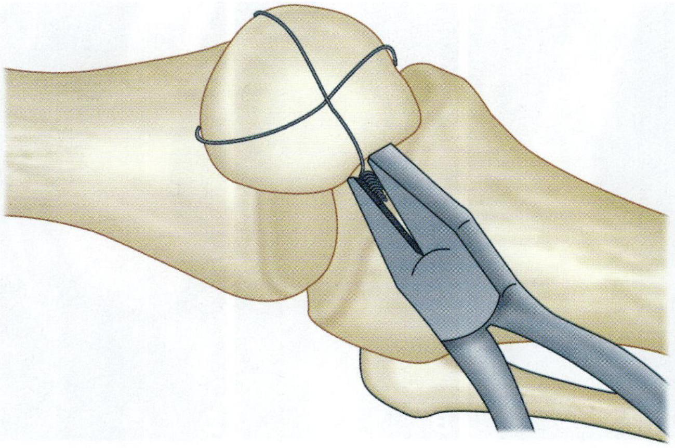

Fig. 25.169: Tension band wiring

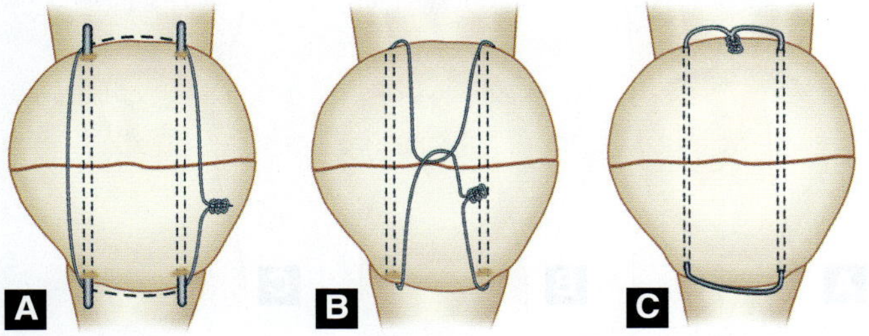

Figs 25.168A to C: (A) Modified tension band; (B) Lotke LAB wiring; (C) Magnuson wiring

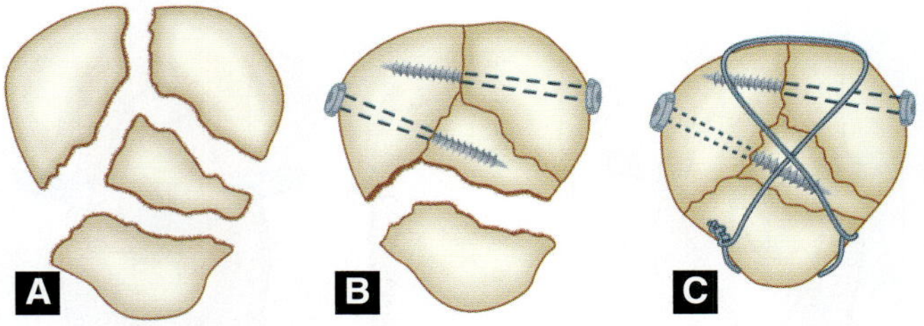

Figs 25.170A to C: Schauwecker method of compression wiring of patella for comminuted fracture—(A) Comminuted fracture; (B) Fracture is transformed, with screws into bifragmental fracture;(C) Using supplemental screws for comminuted fracture

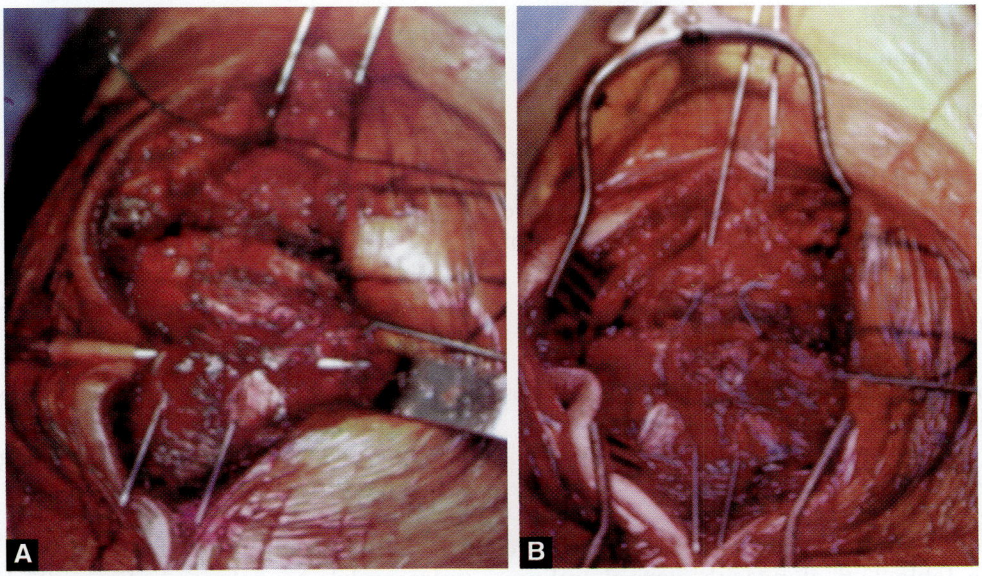

Figs 25.171A and B: Modified tension band wiring surgery being performed (Schauwecker method)

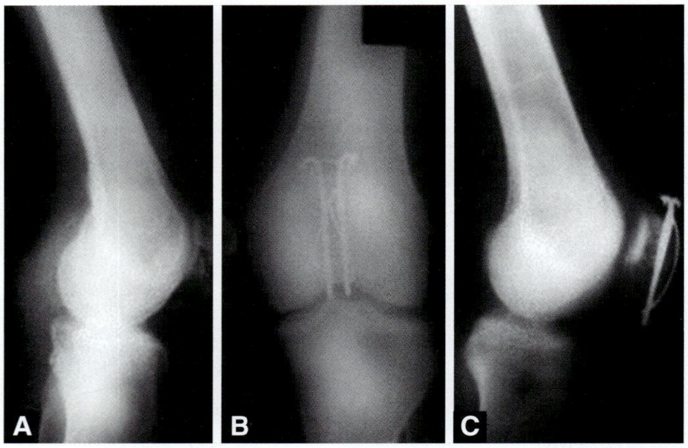

Figs 25.172A to C: Modified tension band wiring—(A) Displaced transverse fracture of patella; (B and C) Postoperative roentgenograms, showing modified tension band internal fixation using two anterior wire loops and two longitudinally directed Kirschner wires

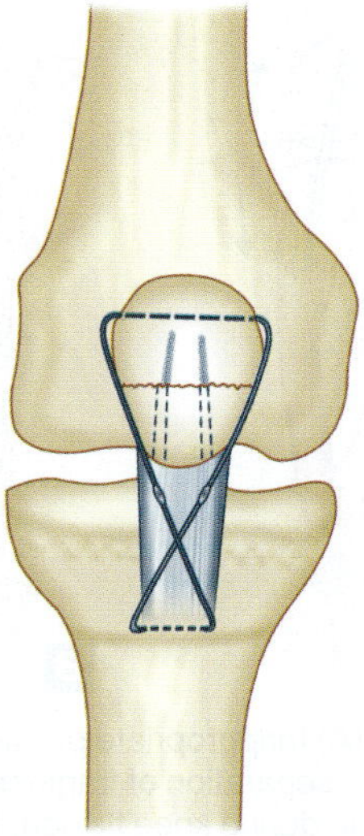

Fig. 25.174: Perry's patellectomy for patellar fracture reduction

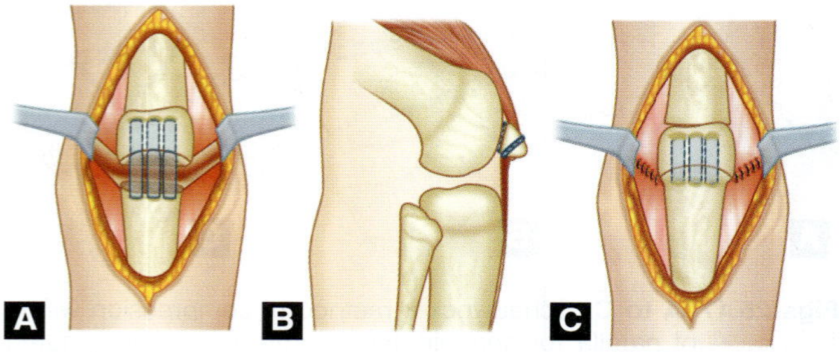

Figs 25.173A to C: (A) Retained fragment is approximated to tendon with large nonabsorbable sutures; (B) Drill holes are oriented to reattach tendon close to the articular surface; (C) Quadriceps expansions are completely repaired

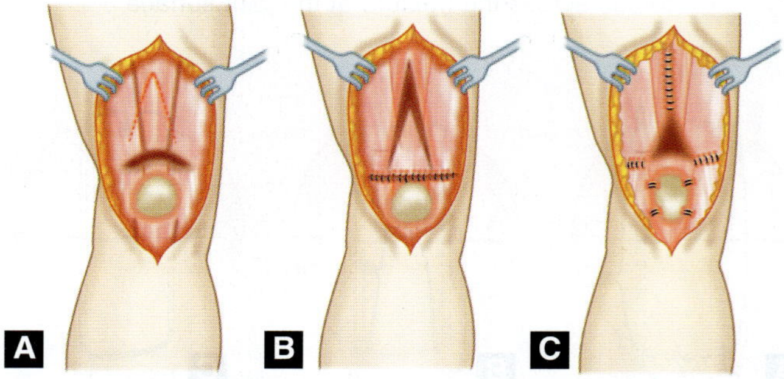

Figs 25.175A to C: Total patellectomy—Quadriceps tendon repair of codivilla

Partial Patellectomy

This method is illustrated in Figures 25.173A to C.

Perry's Patellectomy (Fig. 25.174)

After reduction and internal fixation of patellar fracture, two cables are inserted through transverse holes, drilled in tibial tubercle and proximal pole of patella. They are crossed anteriorly to patellar ligament to form figure of eight and are crimped to each other.

Total Patellectomy (Quadriceps Tendon Repair of Codivilla)

Codivilla tendon lengthening and repair of quadriceps tendon, this is illustrated in Figures 25.175A to C.

Fixation of Osteochondral Fractures (Figs 25.176A to C)

The treatment options for various patellar fractures are illustrated in the Table 25.6, along with surgical outlines for different fractures, in Figures 25.177A to D.

General Surgical Outlines (Figs 25.177A to D)

Complications

- Infections
- Loss of fixation or refractures
- Symptomatic retained hardware
- Delayed union or nonunion
- Post-traumatic osteoarthritis
- Knee stiffness or loss of motion.

■ Fractures of the Distal Femur

Introduction

Fractures of the distal femur are complex injuries, which can be difficult to manage. These serious injuries have the potential to produce significant long-term disability. Those fractures, that involve the distal 15 cm of the femur, including the distal femoral metaphysis (supracondylar) and the articular surface of the distal femur (intracondylar), as shown in Figure 25.178.

Incidence: It accounts for 7 percent of all femoral fractures.

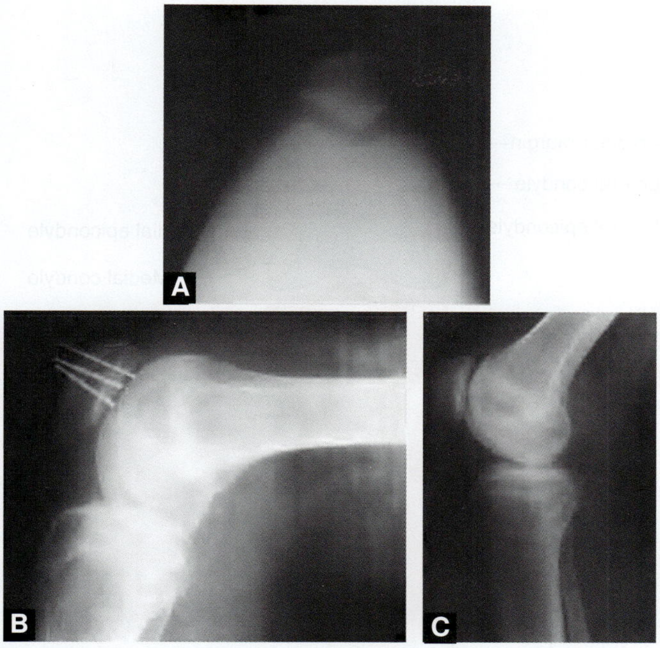

Figs 25.176A to C: (A) Fourteen years old patient, who sustained dislocation of patella with large osteochondral fracture. Osteochondral fragment was not appreciated in roentgenograms but was noted arthroscopically; (B) After open reduction and internal fixation, using Kirschner wires. Wires did not penetrate articular cartilage; (C) Six months postoperatively with Kirschner wires removed

Table 25.6: Patellar fracture treatment options

	Indications	*Treatment*
Nondisplaced		
Transverse	Fragment separation <3 mm	Cylinder cast
Stellate	Articular displacement <2 mm	Range-of-motion brace
Vertical	Intact extensor mechanism	
Displaced		
Transverse	Fragment separation >3 mm Articular displacement >2 mm Disrupted extensor mechanism	MATB Lag screws LAB
Stellate		MATB cerclage MATB, LAB
Comminuted		MATB cerclage, MATB, LAB, partial patellectomy, Patellectomy
Polar		
Proximal		Lag screw
Distal		Partial patellectomy
Osteochondral		Loose body repair/ removal

MATB: Modified anterior tension band; LAB: Longitudinal anterior band

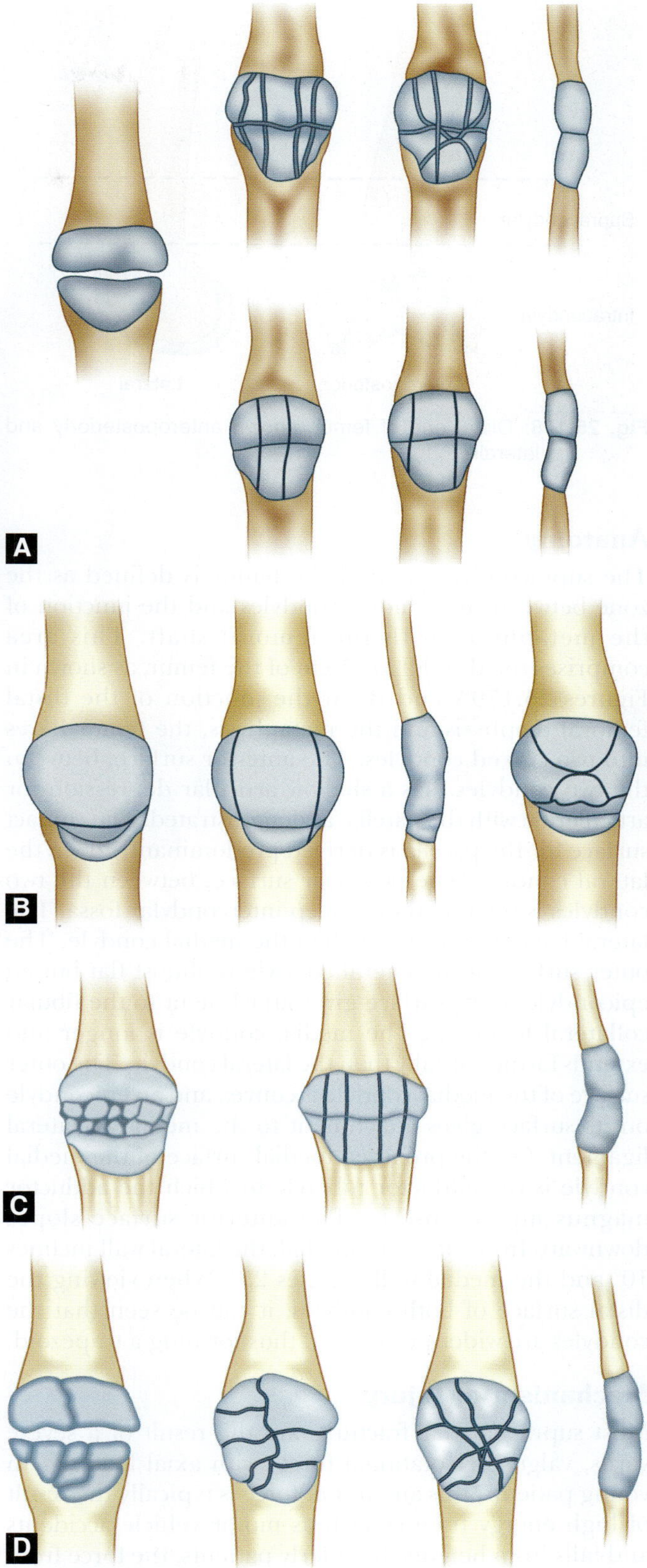

Figs 25.177A to D: (A) Surgical outline for a transverse patellar fracture; (B) Surgical outline for a polar patellar fracture; (C) Surgical outline for a multifragmented patellar fracture; (D) Surgical outline for a comminuted patellar fracture

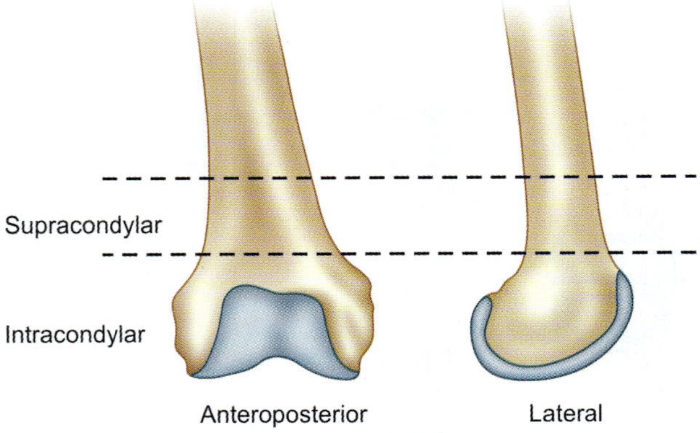

Fig. 25.178: Distal end of femur, shown anteroposteriorly and laterally

Anatomy

The supracondylar area of the femur is defined as the zone between the femoral condyles and the junction of the metaphysis, with the femoral shaft. This area comprises the distal 9 to 15 cm of the femur, as shown in Figures 25.179A and B. At the junction of the distal femoral diaphysis and the metaphysis, the femur flares into two curved condyles. The anterior surface, between the two condyles, has a shallow articular depression for articulation with the patella, as demonstrated. The contact surface for the patella is derived predominantly from the lateral condyle. The posterior surface, between the two condyles is separated by a deep intercondylar fossa. The lateral condyle is broader than the medial condyle. The outer surface of the lateral condyle is almost flat but an epicondyle on its surface gives attachment to the fibular collateral ligament. The medial condyle is longer and extends farther distally than the lateral condyle. The outer surface of the medial condyle is convex and an epicondyle on its surface gives attachment to the medial collateral ligament. On the proximal medial surface of the medial condyle is the adductor tubercle to which the adductor magnus muscle inserts. The anterior surface slopes downward from lateral to medial, the lateral wall inclines 10° and the medial wall inclines 25°. When viewing the distal surface of both condyles, it can be seen that the condyles are wider posteriorly, thus forming a trapezoid.

Mechanism of Injury

Most supracondylar fractures are the result of a severe varus, valgus or rotational force, with axial loading. In young patients, this amount of force is typically the result of high energy trauma such as motor vehicle accidents and falls from heights. In elderly patients, the force from a minor slip and fall on a flexed knee may be sufficient to produce these fractures.

After fracture, the deformities observed are usually those of femoral shortening, apex posterior angulation

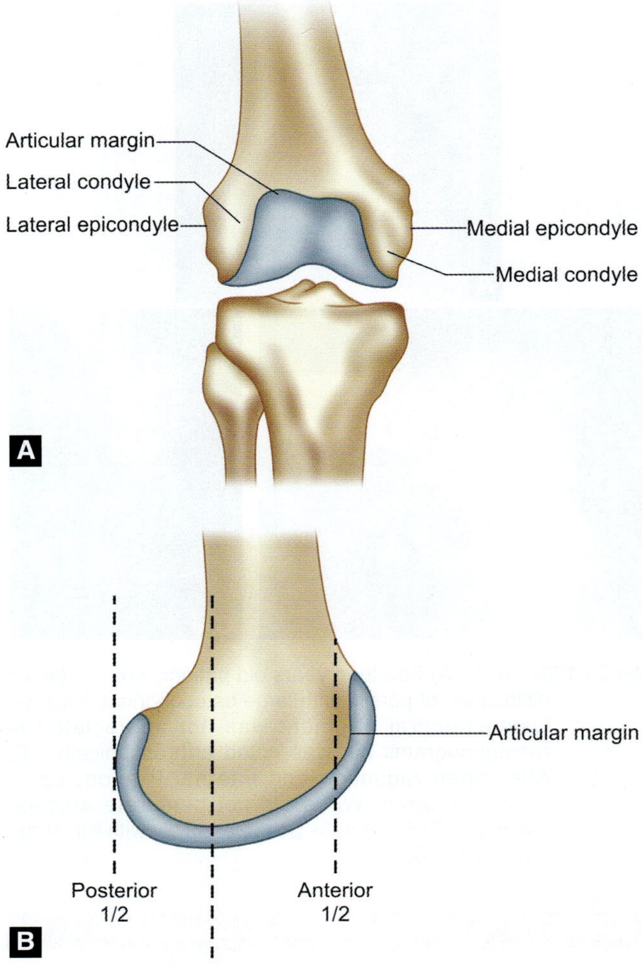

Figs 25.179A and B: Anatomy of distal femur—(A) Anterior view; (B) Lateral view. The shaft of the femur is aligned with the anterior half of the lateral condyle

and posterior displacement of the distal fragment. These deforming forces are produced by the quadriceps, hamstring and gastrocnemius muscles, as shown in Figure 25.180. Varus deformity may result from the pull of the adductor muscles. If an intercondylar fracture is present, there will often be rotational malalignment of the condyles (with resulting joint incongruity) because of the separate attachments of the gastrocnemius muscles to each condyle.

Associated Injuries and Complications

The axial and bending loads applied to the femur in the production of a supracondylar fracture, may produce additional injuries to the same extremity. Physical examination and radiographic assessment must assess the possible presence of a fracture to the acetabulum, the femoral neck and the femoral shaft. Varus or valgus force applied to the knee joint, may result in an associated ligament injury to the knee and it has been reported in

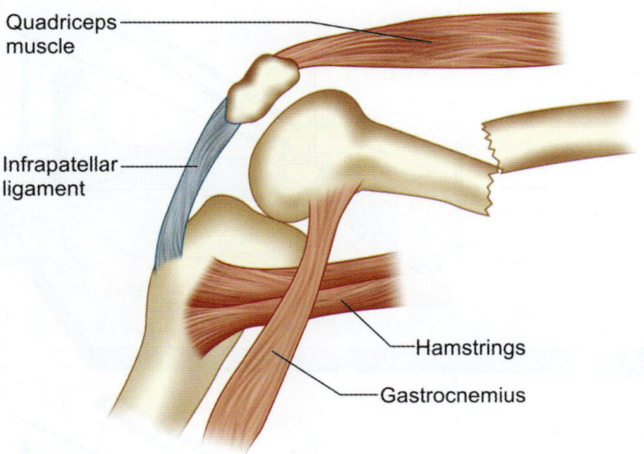

Fig. 25.180: Deforming forces, produced by the quadriceps, hamstring and gastrocnemius muscles after femoral fracture

up to 20 percent of cases. Alternatively, the same force may produce fractures of the tibial plateau or shaft. Open fractures occur in 5 to 10 percent of all supracondylar fractures. The most common site for the open wound is over the anterior thigh proximal to the patella and as a result patients frequently have some damage to the distal quadriceps muscle or tendon.

Diagnosis

Physical Examination

Supracondylar fractures of the femur are often the result of a high energy trauma. Therefore, a complete evaluation of the whole patient should be performed. The presence of other injuries to the same extremity needs to be ruled out, with particular attention to the hip and the leg below the fracture site. The vascular supply to the limb should be assessed, by examining for the presence of a pulse at the popliteal and distal tibial arteries. Motor and sensory function to the leg and foot must be assessed.

Inspection usually shows swelling and deformity around the distal femur and knee. The presence of an open wound in the case of open fractures should be identified. Although manipulation of the injured limb, demonstrates motion and crepitus, this maneuver causes unnecessary pain and should be precluded by the radiographic evaluation. As a part of and immediately after the physical examination, the injured extremity should be gently realigned (if necessary) and splinted before radiographic evaluation.

Classification

A good classification system for supracondylar fractures of the distal femur must have following characteristics features:

- Distinguish among the many possible injuries to this area, including extra-articular, intra-articular and isolated condylar lesions.
- Allow different surgeons, consistently and reliably to grade a fracture pattern into one of the classification groups.
- Assist in deciding the optimal method of treatment for the injury.
- Correlate with the findings of outcome analysis, to allow estimation of prognosis for each injury pattern.

OTA Classification

This system separates supracondylar fractures of the femur into three general types. OTA classification of distal femur fractures. The three types are further subdivided into three groups, as shown in Figures 25.181A to C.

Type A1: Simple (two parts)
Type A2: Metaphyseal wedge
Type A3: Metaphyseal complex (comminuted)
Type B1: Lateral condyle (fracture in the sagittal plane)
Type B2: Medial condyle (fracture in the sagittal plane)
Type B3: Frontal (fracture in the coronal plane)
Type C1: Articular simple and metaphyseal simple ('T' or 'Y' fracture pattern)
Type C2: Articular simple and metaphyseal multifragmentary
Type C3: Multifragmentary articular (Hoffa's fracture)

Radiographic Evaluation

Routine radiographic evaluation of the distal femur and knee, includes standard anteroposterior (AP) and lateral radiographs. Radiographs of the pelvis, the ipsilateral hip and the complete femoral shaft should also be obtained to rule out the presence of associated injuries. Complex intra-articular fractures of the supracondylar area, may be visualized better with additional 45° oblique radiographs. Gentle application of manual traction to the distal extremity, may also help in obtaining a radiograph, which can be more easily interpreted. Both techniques may be helpful to avoid, missing an undisplaced or minimally displaced intercondylar fracture, an injury that is easily missed on cursory assessment of only plain radiographs.

CT Scan

Complex intra-articular fractures and osteochondral lesions, may require additional imaging, with plain or computed tomography, to assist in completing the diagnostic assessment and preoperative planning.

Treatment Alternatives

Nonoperative Treatment

Indications for the nonoperative treatment are ennumerated in Table 25.7.

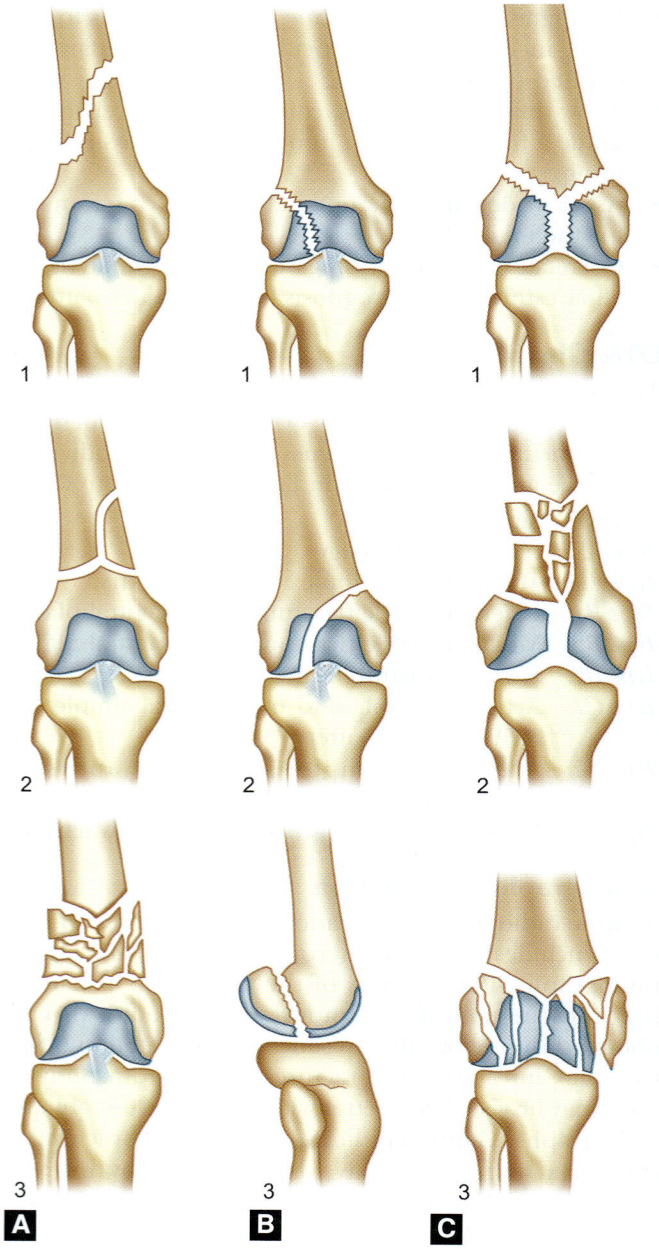

Figs 25.181A to C: OTA classification of the supracondylar fracture of distal femur

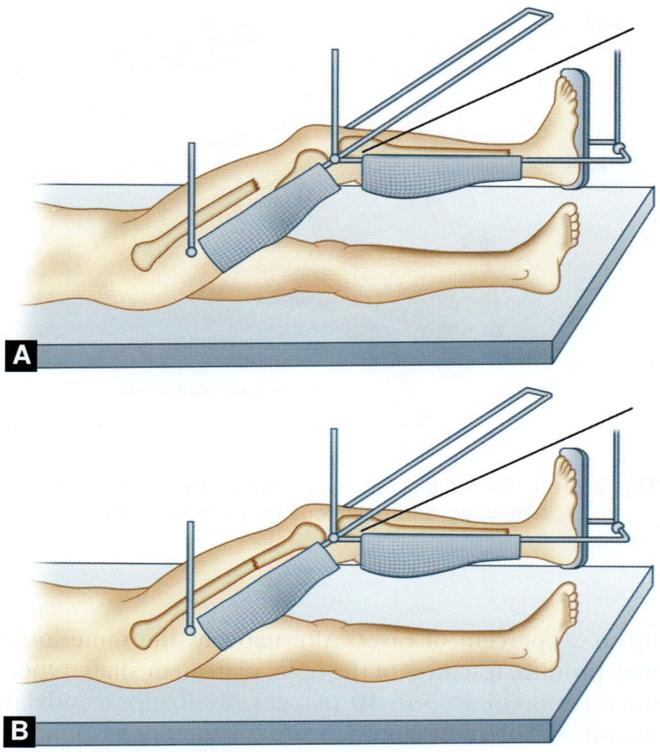

Figs 25.182A and B: Skeletal traction given for 6 to 12 weeks in case of displaced unstable fracture—(A) Displaced fractured segment; (B) Fracture reduce due to skeletal traction

Table 25.7: Indications for nonoperative treatment of supracondylar fracture of distal femur
• Patient factors Medical contraindications to operative treatment Nonambulatory patient (e.g. paraplegia, quadriplegia)
• Fracture factors Undisplaced fracture Impacted stable fracture Unreconstructable fracture Severe osteopenia
• Surgeon factors Lack of experience in operative treatment Unavailability of appropriate instrumentation or facilities

In stable, undisplaced or impacted fractures, immediate mobilization of the patient in a hinged knee brace, with restricted weight-bearing, can be undertaken. Careful radiographic followup is needed to ensure maintenance of position. In displaced, unstable fractures, nonoperative treatment, entails a 6 to 12 weeks period of skeletal traction, as shown in Figures 25.182A and B, followed by bracing. A traction pin is placed in the proximal tibia and the limb is supported on a Thomas splint with a Pearson knee attachment or on a Böhler Braun frame. One then applies 10-15 kg of traction, in line with the thigh segment. The degree of knee flexion is adjusted and the apex of the break in the limb support is positioned to be at the level of the fracture, to overcome the deforming forces.

Radiographs are obtained, and appropriate adjustments in weight and positioning are made, as demonstrated in Figures 25.183A and B. A two pin technique, with a further pin in the distal femur has been recommended for fractures not reducing with just the proximal tibial pin. In supracondylar fractures and those intracondylar fractures, with relatively undisplaced intra-articular components, a single distal femoral pin, for the application of traction is an option. To overcome the muscular forces, tending to extend the distal fracture,

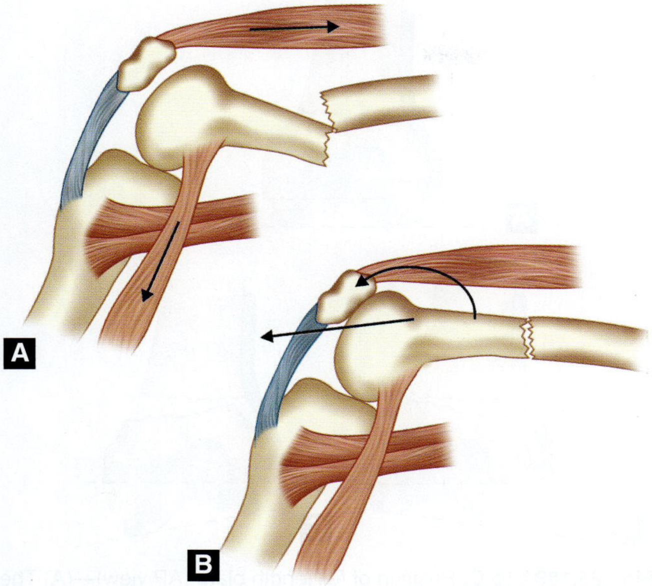

Figs 25.183A and B: Appropriate adjustments in weight and positioning done, while applying skeletal traction

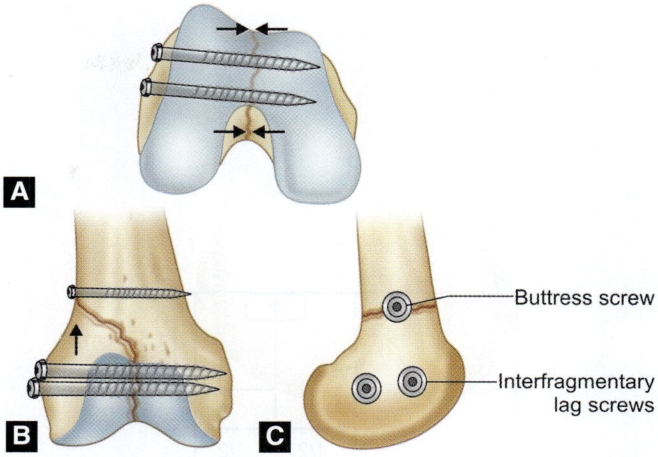

Figs 25.184A to C: Bicondylar fractures, with interfragmental screws

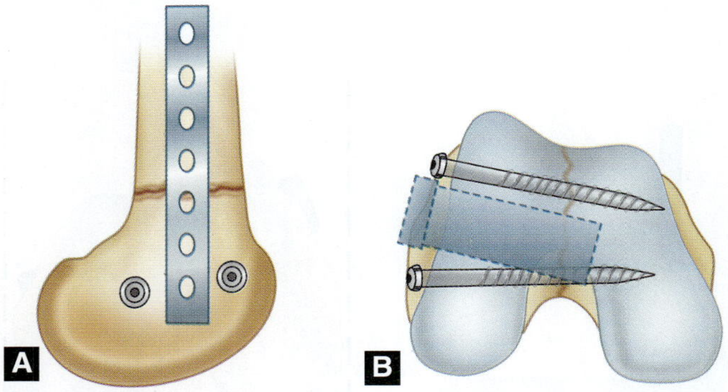

Figs 25.185A and B: The interfragmental screws are placed in a convergent pattern and slightly more proximal to allow for the anticipated plate fixation

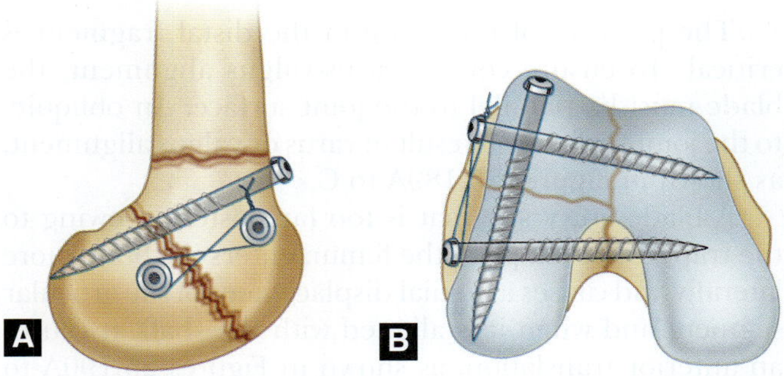

Figs 25.186A and B: A figure of eight wire, placed around the heads of the interfragmental screws, to help to stabilize Hoffa's fracture

the pin should be placed anteriorly in the distal femur. Weekly radiographs are required initially to ensure maintenance of satisfactory alignment. As healing progresses, the knee mobility can be liberated, with the conversion to Neufeld type traction, which tries to prevent permanent knee stiffness. Once the healing is advanced, traction is discontinued and the injured limb is braced to allow protected mobilization. With one tibial pin traction, moving the Pearson knee attachment proximally, so the apex of the leg support is at the level of the fracture, allows for correction of the typical extension posterior displacement deformity.

Operative Treatment and Timing

Operative treatment is indicated for all patients, with distal fractures other than for those situations outlined earlier in the nonoperative section. In bicondylar fractures, the interfragmental screws are placed in a convergent pattern and slightly more proximal to allow for the anticipated plate fixation, as shown in Figures 25.184 to 25.186. In type C3 fractures, with a coronal split (Hoffa's fracture) of the lateral condyle, a figure of eight wire can be placed around the heads of the interfragmental screws, to help to stabilize Hoffa's fracture. An anteroposterior interfragmental screw can also be used, either extra-articularly, as shown here or countersunk into the articular surface, if necessary.

Plates—95° Blade Plate

The center of the blade insertion site is 1.5 to 2 cm from the distal articular surface and in the middle of the anterior half of the longest sagittal diameter of the lateral femoral condyle, as shown in Figures 25.187 and 25.188.

A blade of the length of the full breadth of the distal femur on an anteroposterior radiograph will protrude medially because of the trapezoidal shape of the distal femur.

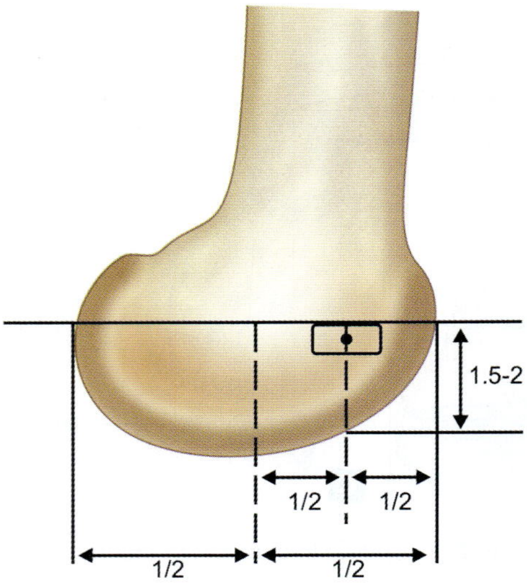

Fig. 25.187: Blade insertion site of the lateral femoral condyle

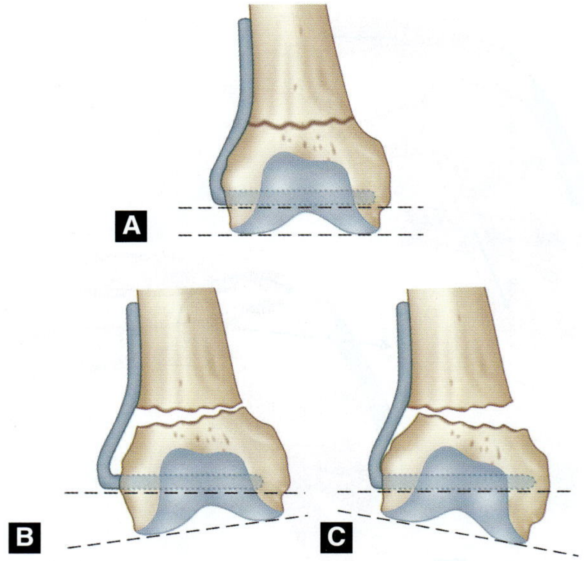

Figs 25.189A to C: Position of full length plate (AP view)—(A) The blade parallel to the joint surface; (B) Varus alignment; (C) Valgus alignment

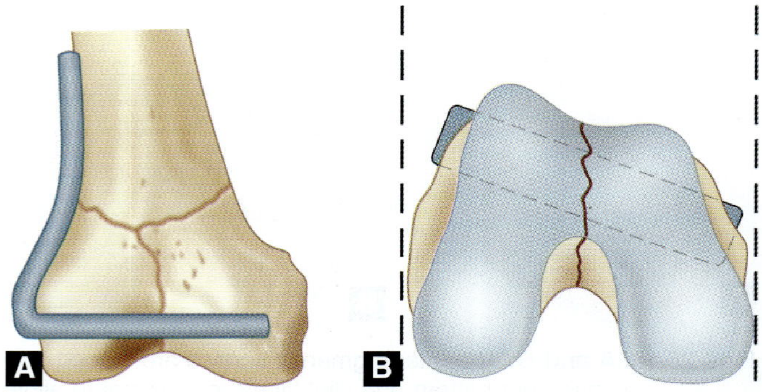

Figs 25.188A and B: 90° blade plate fixation. (A) AP view; (B) Shown from below (intra-articular)

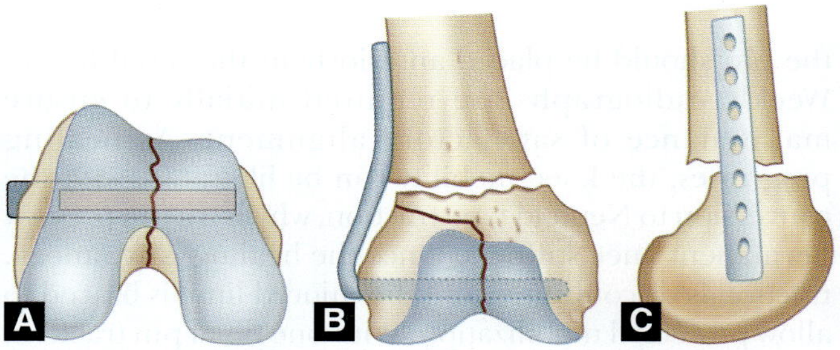

Figs 25.190A to C: Blade entry site position—(A) Blade entry site is too far posterior; (B) It enters the bone more laterally and causes a medial displacement of the articular segment; (C) When aligned with the shaft, causes anterior translation

The position of the blade in the distal fragment is critical. To ensure correct varus-valgus alignment, the blade must be parallel to the joint surface. An obliquity to the joint surface will result in varus or valgus alignment, as shown in Figures 25.189A to C.

A blade entry site that is too far posterior, owing to the trapezoidal shape of the femur, enters the bone more laterally and causes a medial displacement of the articular segment and when it is aligned with the shaft, it causes an anterior translation, as shown in Figures 25.190A to C. A blade that is not perpendicular to the axis of the distal femur will result in extension or flexion deformity. This is illustrated in Figures 25.191A and B.

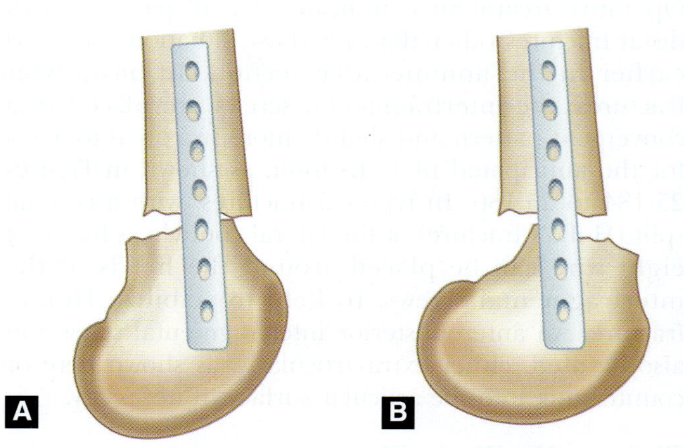

Figs 25.191A and B: Deformities caused with nonperpendicular position of the blade with the axis of distal femur—(A) Extension deformity; (B) Flexion deformity

Dynamic Condylar Screw (Fig. 25.192)

The dynamic condylar screw is a contoured side plate of variable length with a barrel at 95° to the long axis of the plate, which accepts a lag screw of variable length. The two are coupled by a compression screw. The entry site of the dynamic condylar screw as shown in Figures 25.193A

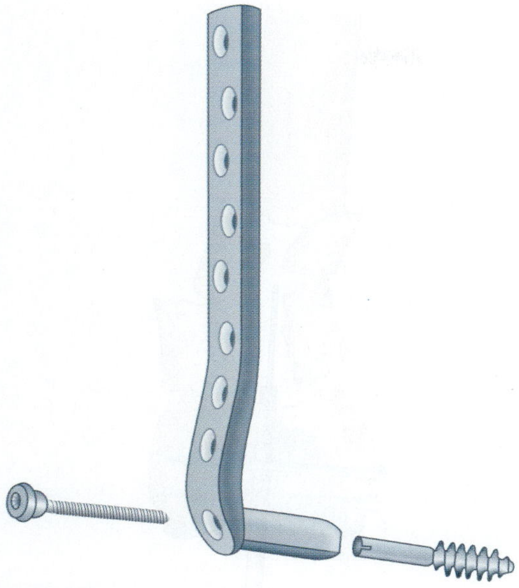

Fig. 25.192: Dynamic condylar screw

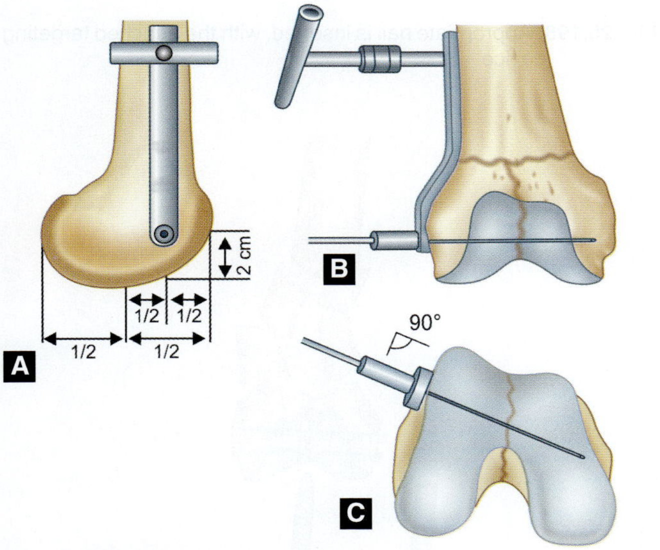

Figs 25.193A to C: (A) The entry site of the dynamic condylar screw; (B) K-wire is placed, parallel to the distal articular surface at screw entry point; (C) K-wire is placed perpendicular to the lateral face of the condyle

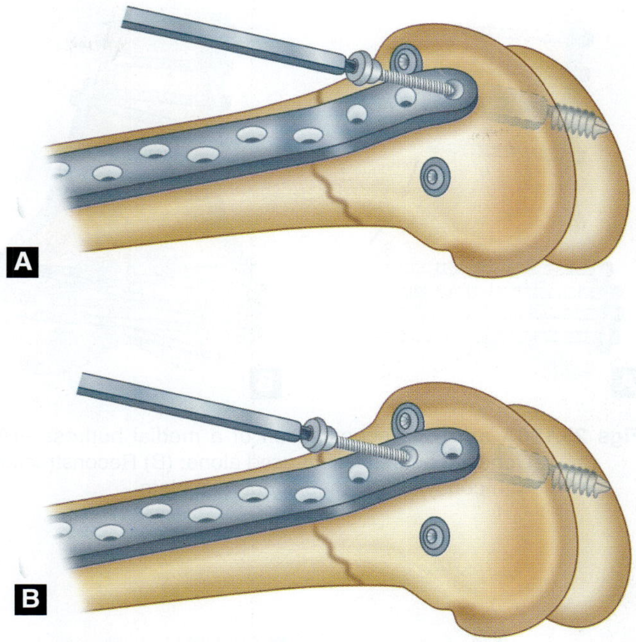

Figs 25.194A and B: (A) Interfragmental compression applied with this screw; (B) Screw placed into the hole adjacent to the barrel

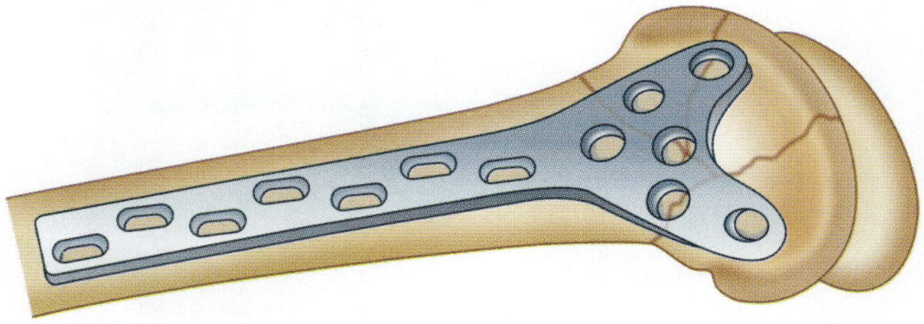

Fig. 25.195: Condylar buttress plate, with multiple points of fixation

to C, is in the middle of the anterior half of the lateral femoral condyle, 2 cm from the distal articular surface. A Kirschner wire (K-wire) is placed at this point parallel to the distal articular surface and perpendicular to the lateral face of the condyle. The K-wire is advanced to the medial cortex, with care taken to avoid penetration because this will result in too long a screw and potentially irritating symptoms.

Insertion of the compression screw links the plate and the lag screw. In the case of an intracondylar fracture, further interfragmental compression can be achieved with this screw. A screw is placed into the hole adjacent to the barrel. This fixes the position of the plate relative to the distal fragment, as shown in Figures 25.194A and B.

Condylar Buttress Plate (Fig. 25.195)

The condylar buttress plate allows multiple points of fixation in the distal femur. It is not symmetric and is therefore side specific. With reconstitution of a medial buttress as shown in Figures 25.196A and B, the condylar buttress plate can be used alone. If the medial distal femur cannot be reconstituted, a medial buttress plate should be considered.

Retrograde Locked Intramedullary Nails (Fig. 25.197)

The entry point for retrograde nailing is at the point, at which the center of the medullary canal projects onto the intracondylar notch on anteroposterior and lateral

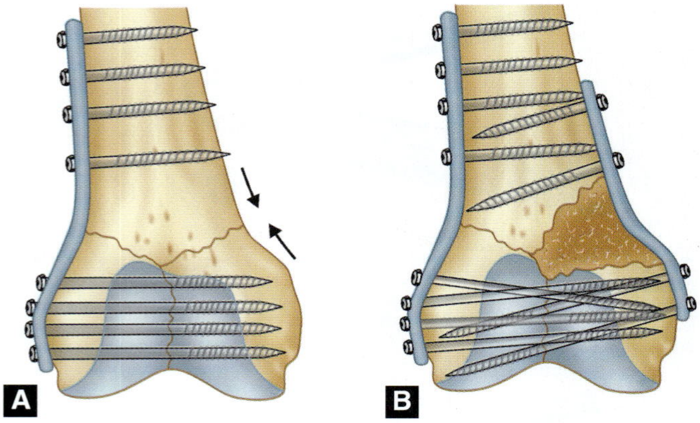

Figs 25.196A and B: Reconstitution of a medial buttress—(A) Condylar buttress plate used alone; (B) Reconstruction with condylar and medial buttress plate

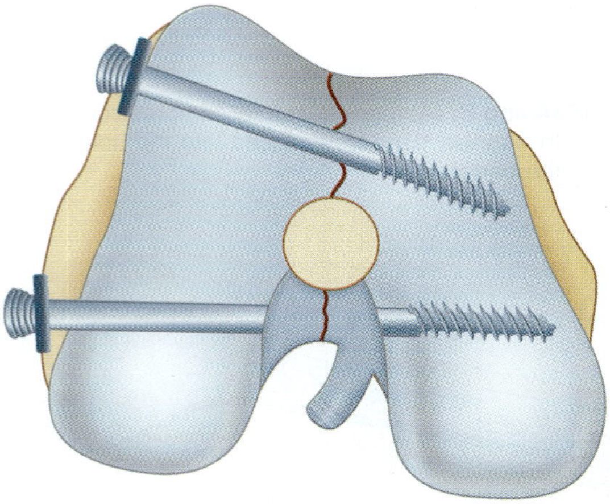

Fig. 25.197: Retrograde locked intramedullary nails

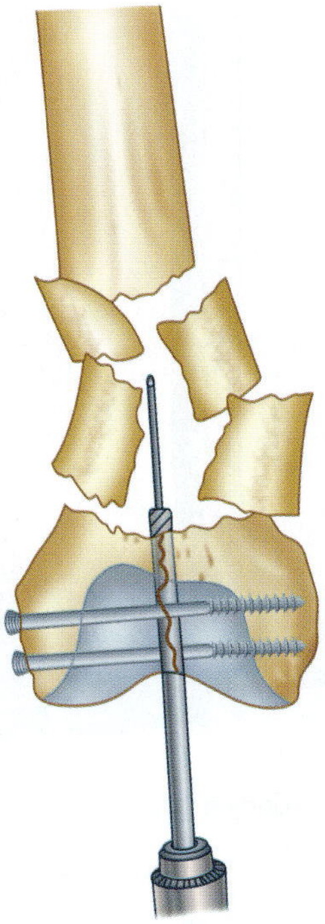

Fig. 25.198: Appropriate nail is inserted, with the attached targeting device

views. It lies just anterior to the posterior cruciate attachment to the femur, at the margin of the patellofemoral articular surface.

Preparation of the Nail Entry Point (Figs 25.198 to 25.201)

An awl may be used or a guidewire may be placed and overdrilled. The appropriate nail is inserted, with the attached targeting device. Care taken, to keep the nail aligned with the distal fragment. With the nail fully seated, the end slightly countersunk, locking screws are placed into the distal fragment with the aid of the nail mounted targeting device. At least two distal locking screws should be used. With the nail now firmly attached to the distal segment, length and rotational alignment can be adjusted. Once satisfactory alignment is achieved, the nail is locked to the proximal segment. The fracture is now grossly realigned.

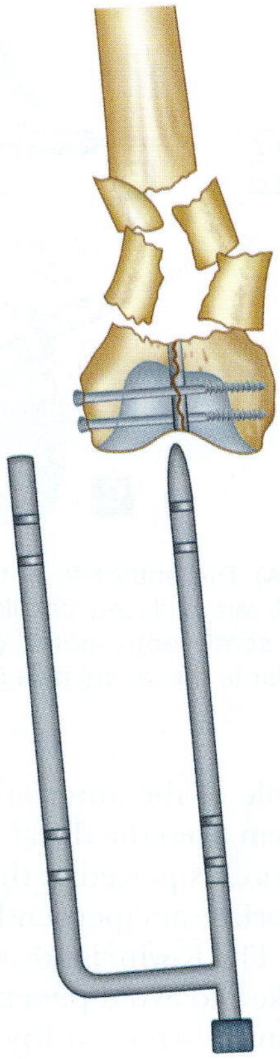

Fig. 25.199: Locking screws are placed into the distal fragment, with the aid of the nail mounted targeting device

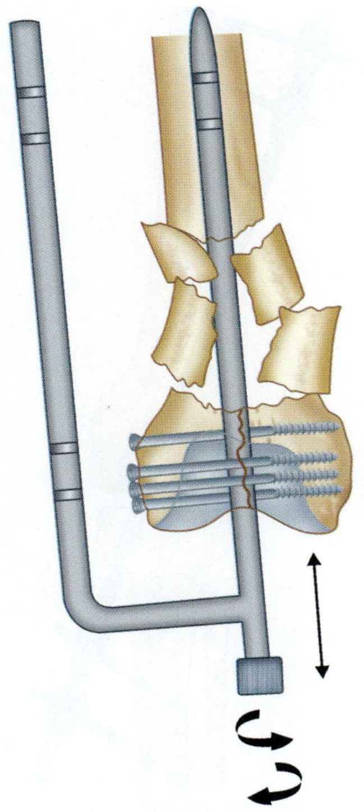

Fig. 25.200: Length and rotational alignment adjusted

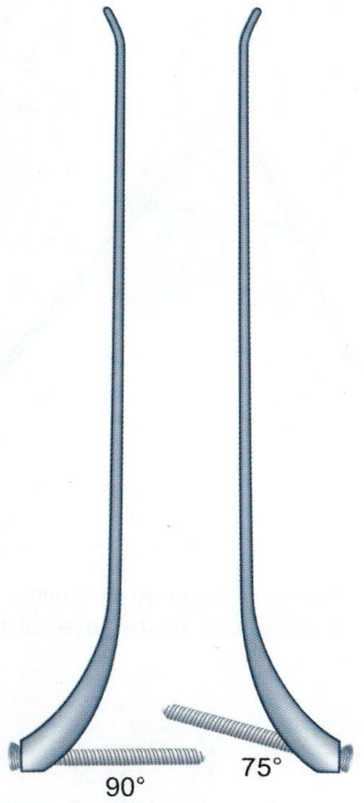

Fig. 25.202: Zickel supracondylar device

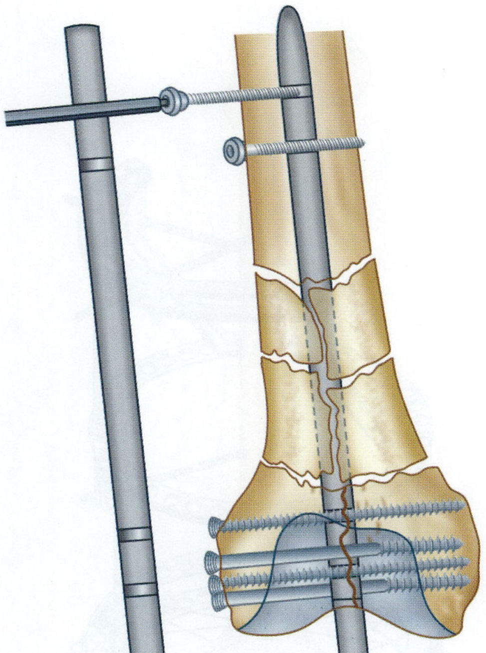

Fig. 25.201: Nail locked to the proximal segment

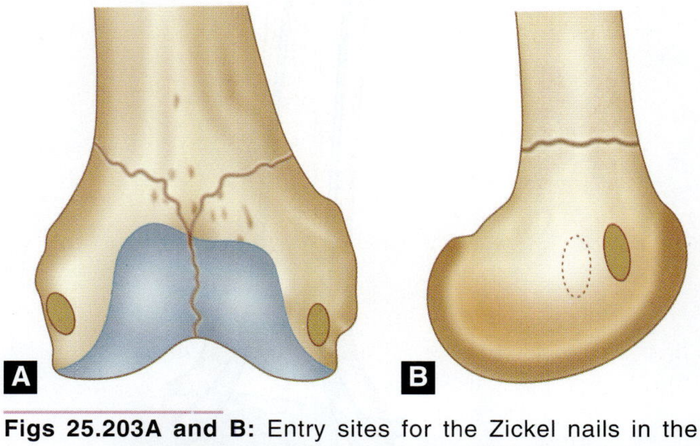

Figs 25.203A and B: Entry sites for the Zickel nails in the epicondylar areas—(A) AP view; (B) Lateral view

Zickel Supracondylar Device (Fig. 25.202)

The entry points for the Zickel nails are in the epicondylar areas just adjacent to the articular surface, in line with the medullary canal from a lateral view. The medial entry site is slightly more posterior to the lateral site. After opening of the entry sites with a curved awl, both nails are advanced to the level of the metaphyseal fracture, as illustrated in Figures 25.203 and 25.204. With alternating tapping, the nails are advanced while the reduction is maintained. The nails are locked in place with screws, with predrilling as necessary. This is demonstrated in Figure 25.205.

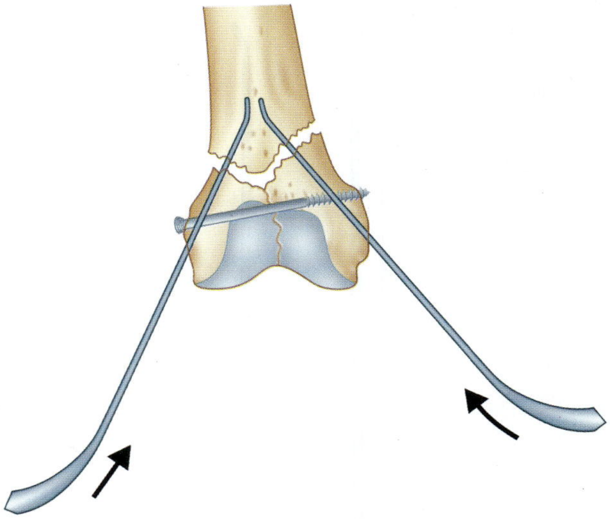

Fig. 25.204: After opening of the entry sites with a curved awl, both nails are advanced to the level of the metaphyseal fracture

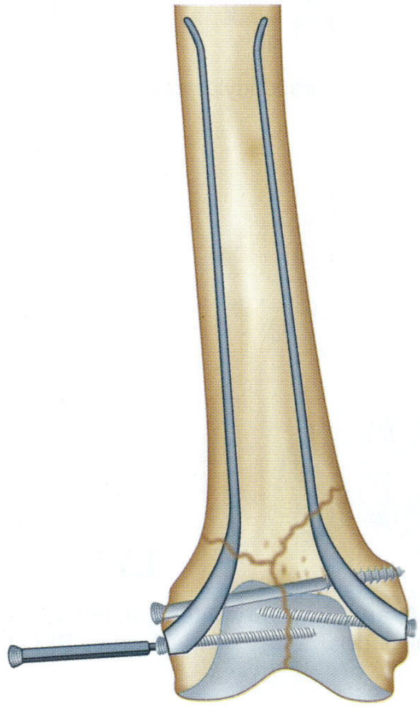

Fig. 25.205: Nails locked with screws

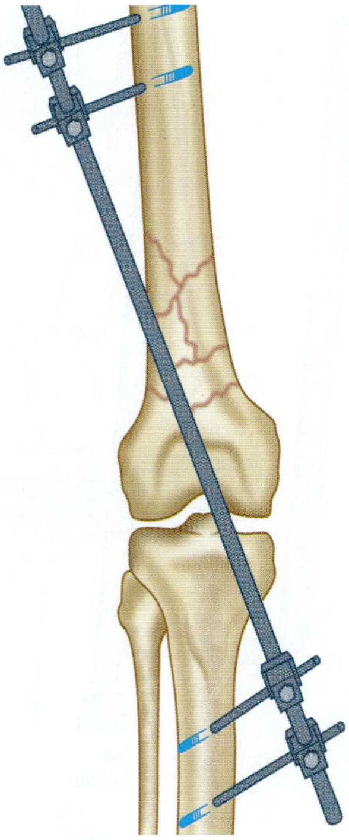

Fig. 25.206: External fixator with half pins placed percutaneously

External Fixation (Figs 25.206 and 25.207)

A spanning external fixator with half-pins placed percutaneously, anterolaterally into the femur and anteriorly in the proximal tibia. The pins should be placed, well outside the zone of planned definitive fixation. One possibility of hybrid external fixation of a distal femur fracture using crossed olive wires for interfragmental compression of the intracondylar component of the fracture, as shown in Figure 25.207.

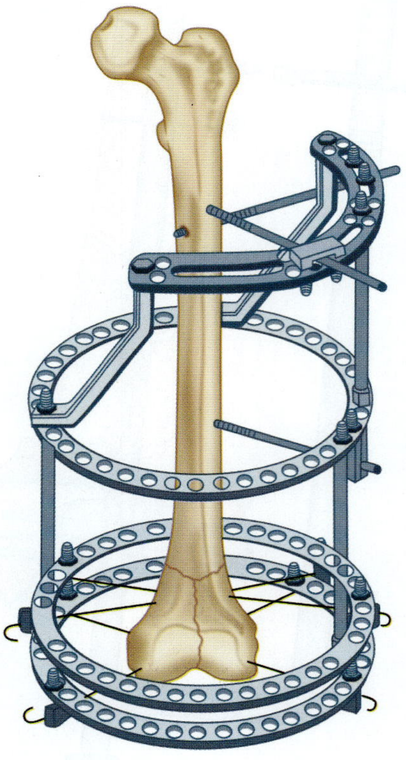

Fig. 25.207: External fixator, with crossed olive wires for interfragmental compression of the intracondylar fracture

Table 25.8: Treatment options for specific fracture types				
Fracture type	***Potential reduction techniques***		***Potential fixation devices***	
A1	Open direct, open indirect, or closed		95-degree blade plate, condylar screw, LCDCP, antegrade IM nail, retrograde IM nail	
A2	Open indirect, or closed		95-degree blade plate, condylar screw, LCDCP, antegrade IM nail, retrograde IM nail	
A3	Open indirect or closed		95-degree blade plate, condylar screw, LCDCP, antegrade IM nail or retrograde IM nail	
B1	Open direct		Interfragmentary lag screws with or without screw or buttress plate	
B2	Open direct		Interfragmentary lag screws with or without buttress screw or buttress plate	
B3	Open direct		Interfragmentary lag screws	
Fracture type	***Intra-articular component***	***Extra-articular component***	***Intra-articular component***	***Extra-articular component***
C1	Open direct	Open indirect or closed	Interfragmentary lag screws	95-degree blade plate, condylar screw, antegrade or retrograde IM nail
C2	Open direct	Open indirect or closed	Interfragmentary lag screws	95-degree blade plate, condylar screw, antegrade or retrograde IM nail
C3	Open direct	Open indirect or closed	Interfragmentary lag screws	95-degree blade plate, condylar screw, condylar buttress plate retrograde nail

IM: Intramedullary; LCDCP: Limited contact dynamic compression plate

Treatment Options for Different Fracture Types

Various treatment options, for specific fracture type are outlined in Table 25.8, as follows:

Type A Fractures (Extra-articular) (Figs 25.208 to 25.210)

Type A1 distal femur fracture, can be fixed with direct open reduction and internal fixation, with interfragmentary lag screws and a dynamic condylar screw. When interlocking intramedullary nailing (antegrade or retrograde) is used, for fixation of distal femoral fractures, at least two interlocking screws must be used in the distal fragment to control angulation in the sagittal plane.

Type B Fractures (Unicondylar) (Figs 25.211 to 25.217)

Computed tomography scan demonstrating better definition of the medial femoral condyle fragment, as shown in Figures 25.216A and B.

Postoperative films after open reduction and internal fixation with 6.5 mm lag screws inserted just adjacent to the articular surface anteriorly and directed posteriorly. This is shown in Figures 25.217A and B.

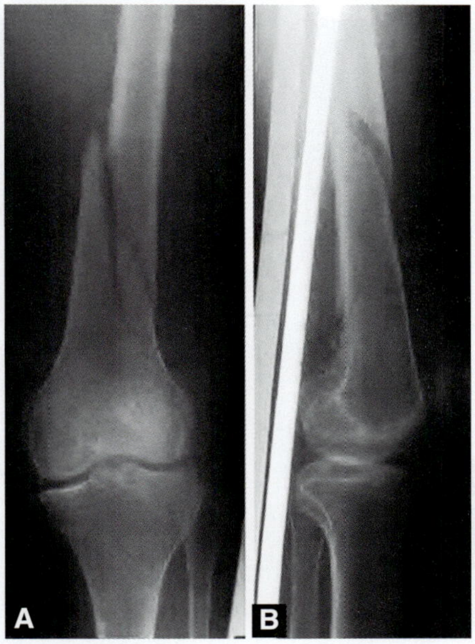

Figs 25.208A and B: Type A1 distal femur fracture—(A) AP view; (B) Lateral view

Type C Fractures (Complete Articular) (Figs 25.218A and B)

The principles used for extra-articular and unicondylar intra-articular fractures of the distal femur are combined, when managing the more complex complete articular fractures. The first step is anatomic reconstruction of articular surface as shown in Figures 25.219A and B, using the techniques described for intra-articular fractures and is of prime importance. The second step is equally important and involves, reduction and fixation of the extra-articular component of the fracture, by using the same techniques, described for treating type A fractures.

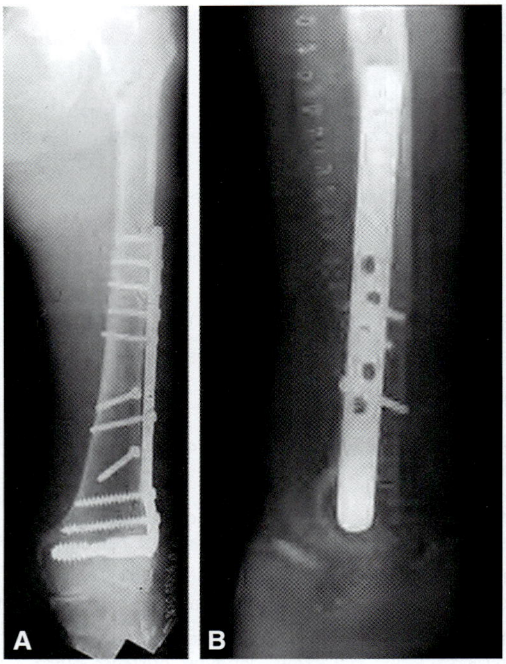

Figs 25.209A and B: Direct open reduction and internal fixation with interfragmentary lag screws and a dynamic condylar screw

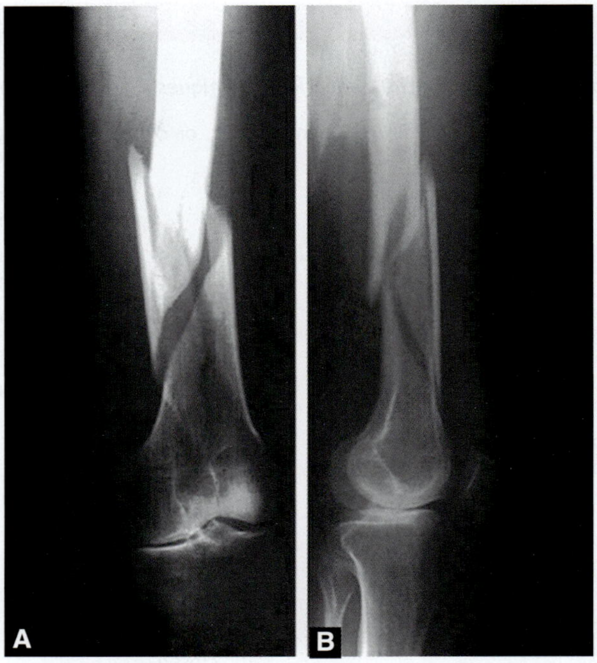

Figs 25.211A and B: Type A3 distal femur fracture— (A) AP radiograph; (B) Lateral radiograph

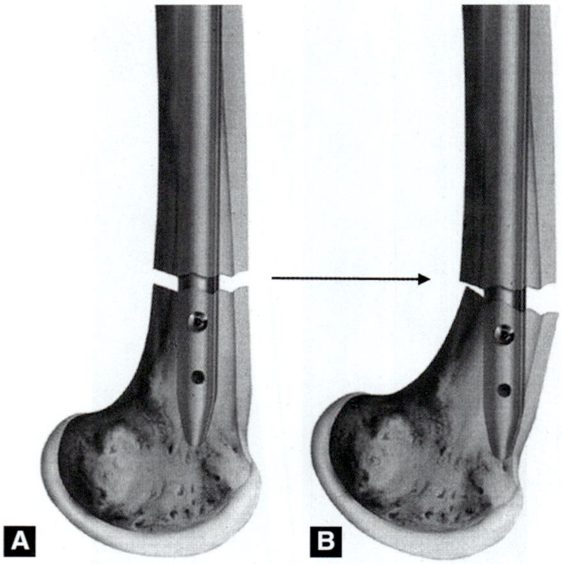

Figs 25.210A and B: (A) Type A distal femur fracture fixed with intramedullary nailing; (B) Postoperative films after closed reduction and static locked reamed antegrade intramedullary nailing

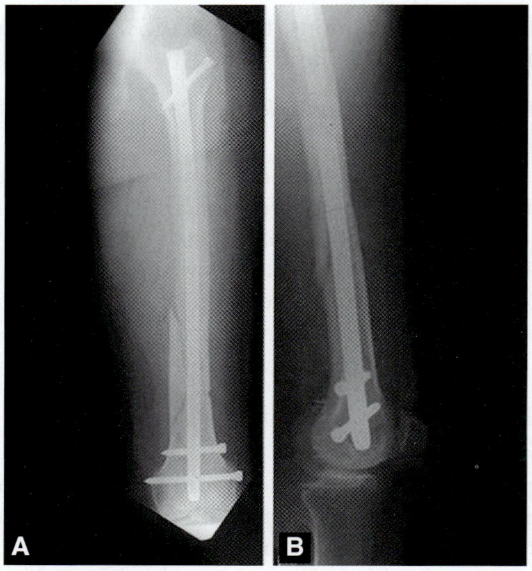

Figs 25.212A and B: Postoperative radiograph after anterograde intramedullary locked nailing for distal femur type A3 fracture

Postoperative films after open reduction and internal fixation, with lag screw fixation of the articular component and indirect reduction and bridge plate fixation, using a dynamic condylar screw for the extra-articular component of the fracture. Progression to healing, as shown in Figures 25.220A and B.

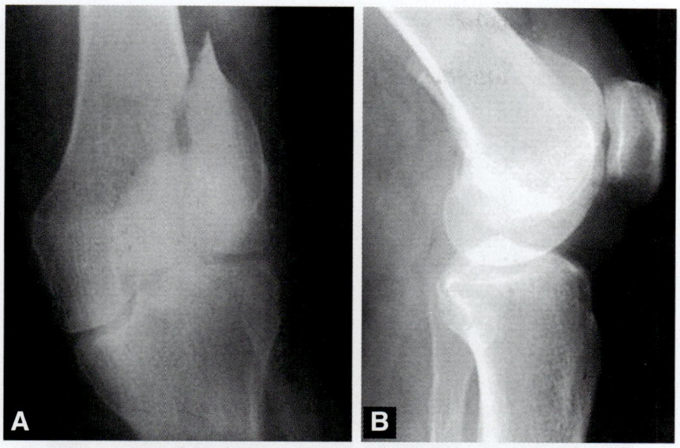

Figs 25.213A and B: X-ray AP and lateral views showing a type B1 distal femur fracture

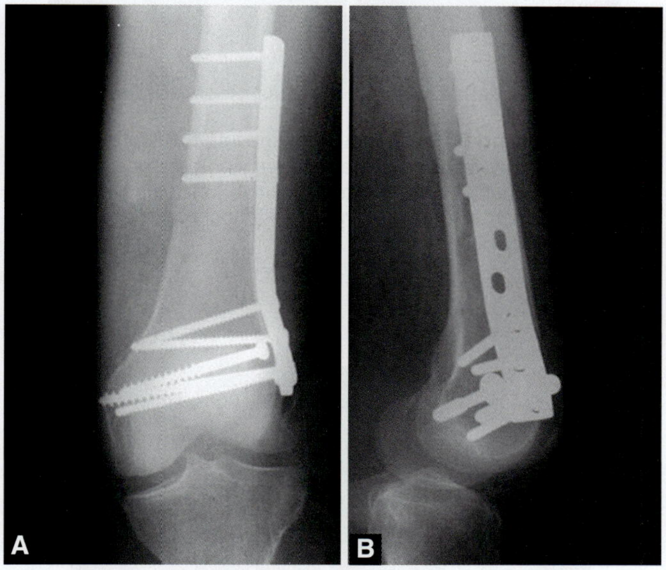

Figs 25.214A and B: X-ray AP and lateral views showing a postoperative type B1 distal femur fracture fixed with plate and multiple screws

Type C2 Distal Femur Fracture (Figs 25.221A and B)

Postoperative films after percutaneous fixation of the articular component and closed reduction and static locked reamed antegrade nailing of the extra-articular component of the fracture, shown in Figures 25.222A and B.

Type C3 Distal Femur Fracture (Figs 25.223 and 25.224)

Postoperative films after open reduction and internal fixation, with lag screw fixation of the articular components and a dynamic condylar screw. A 27 years old man, sustained multiple injuries including this grade IIIA open Association for Osteosynthesis/Association for the Study

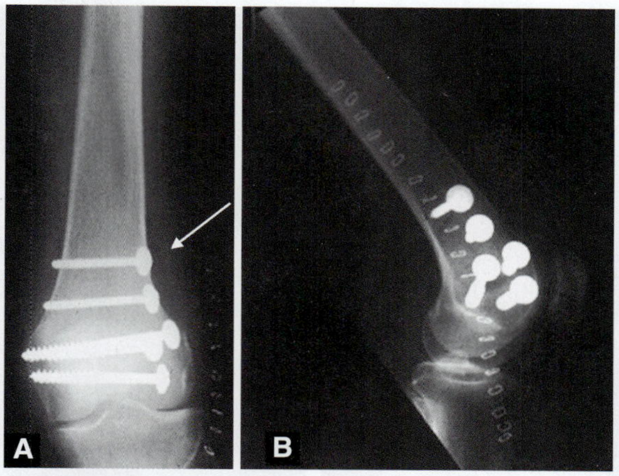

Figs 25.215A and B: In strong bone, a buttress screw (arrow) may be used instead of a buttress plate

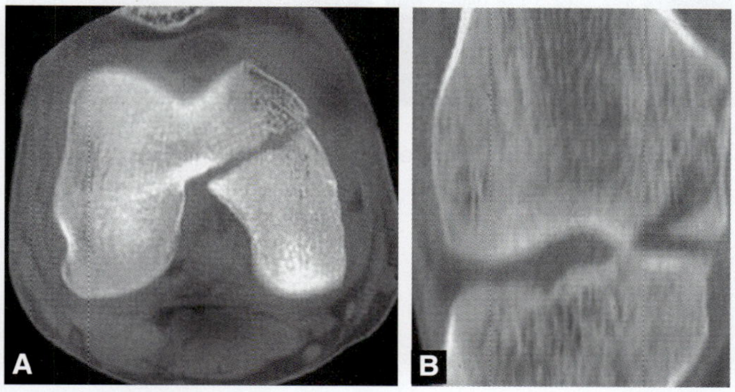

Figs 25.216A and B: CT scan, showing medial femoral condyle fragment

of Internal Fixation (AO/ASIF) C2 supracondylar femur fracture, X-ray shown in Figures 25.225A and B. Extensive comminution led to the use of a lateral condylar buttress plate. To increase stability and to prevent varus deformity, a medial plate and iliac crest bone graft were used, as demonstrated in Figures 25.225 and 25.226.

Early Complications

- *Vascular complications:* One has to be particularly careful to recognize the proximity of the popliteal artery, as it winds from medial to posterior, close to the bone. Arterial injury, especially the more subtle intimal tear, if not recognized and treated promptly, can have disastrous complications.
- *Infection:* Infection is not common, except in open fractures, in which the rate can approach 20 percent. In closed clean fractures, the rate should be about 1 percent, but it rises in patients, with associated vascular injuries or multiple injuries and in immunocompromised patients. In most of these fractures, the surgical approach or the fracture pattern, compromises the integrity of the knee joint.

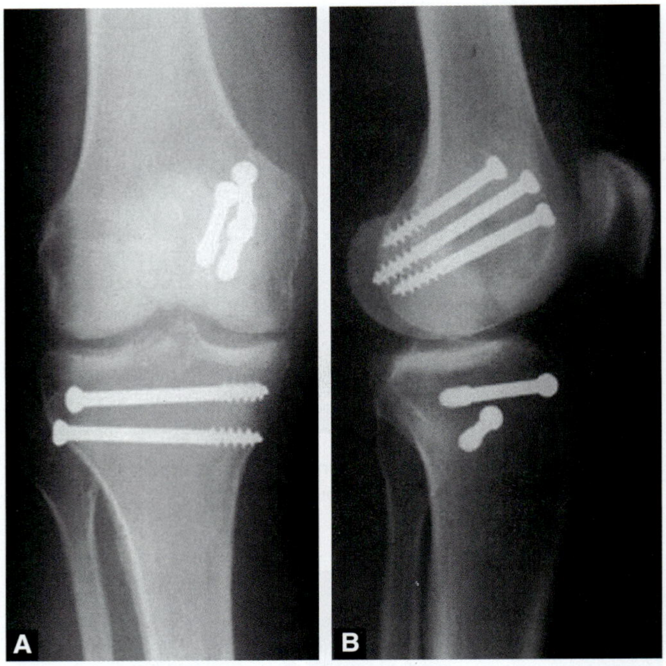

Figs 25.217A and B: Open reduction and internal fixation with 6.5 mm lag screws

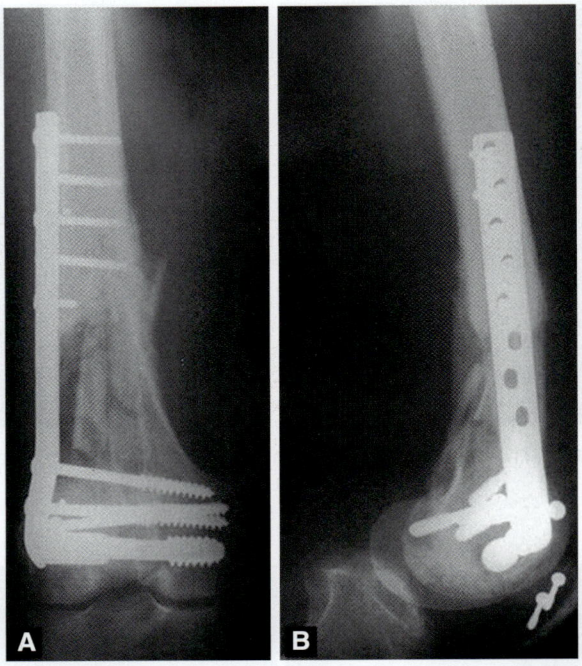

Figs 25.219A and B: Open reduction and internal fixation, with lag screw fixation of the articular component and indirect reduction and bridge plate fixation, using a dynamic condylar screw for the extra-articular component of the fracture

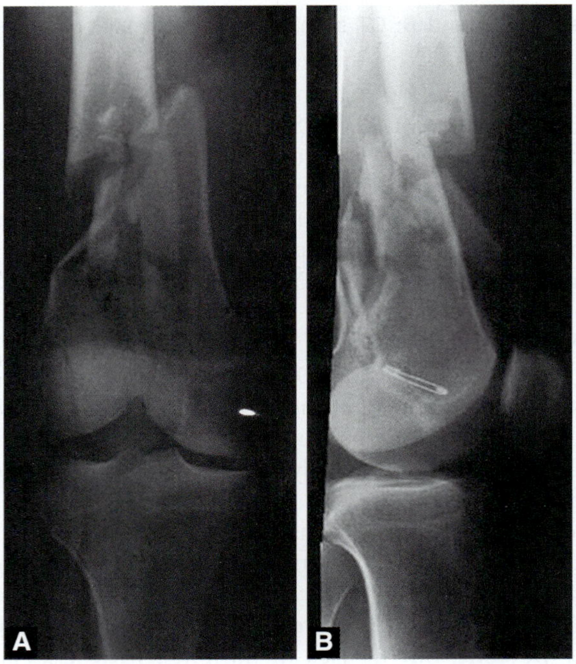

Figs 25.218A and B: Type C fracture (complete articular)

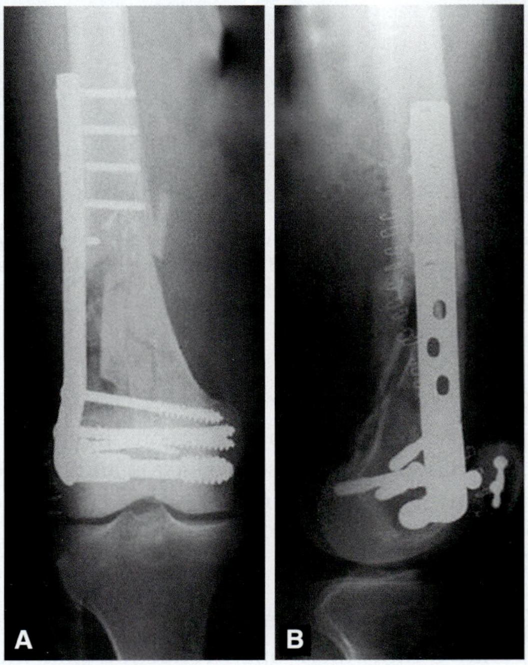

Figs 25.220A and B: Healing after reconstruction

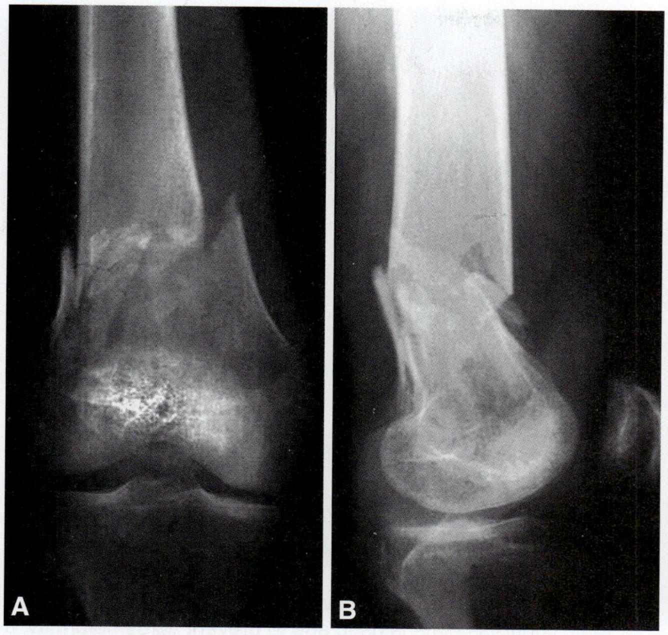

Figs 25.221A and B: Type C2 distal femur fracture— (A) AP view; (B) Lateral view

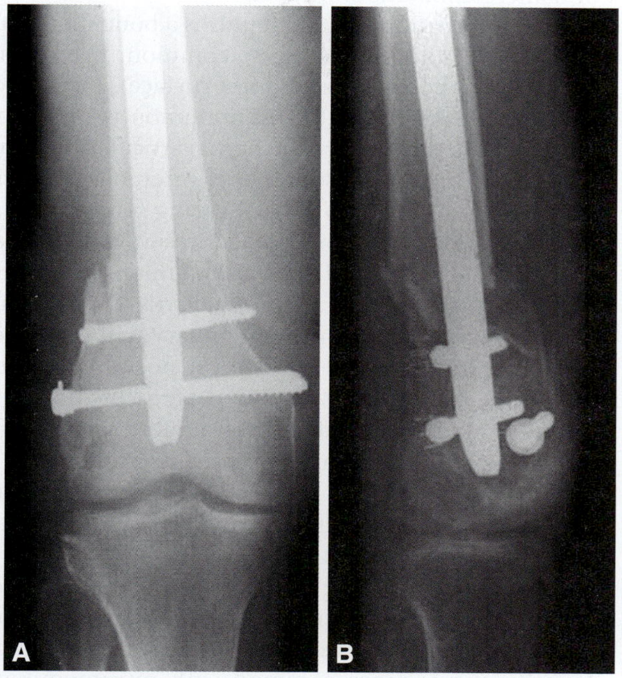

Figs 25.222A and B: Percutaneous fixation of the articular component, closed reduction and static locked reamed, antegrade nailing of the extra-articular component of the fracture

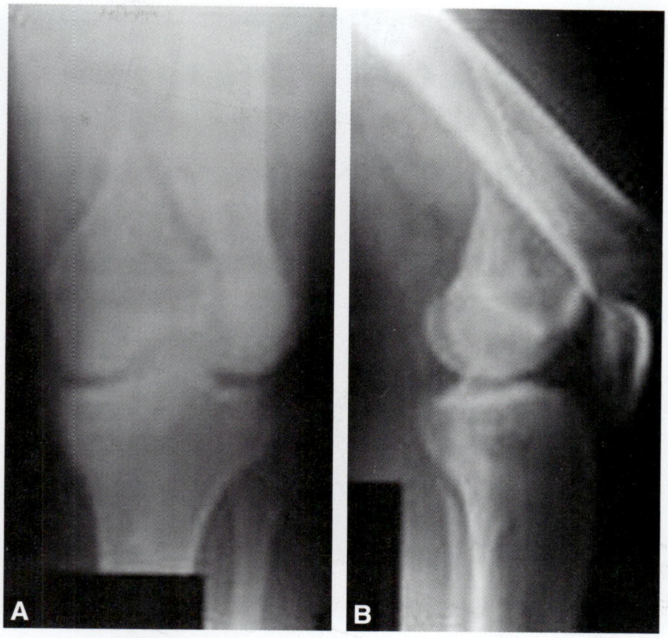

Figs 25.223A and B: Type C3 distal femur fracture

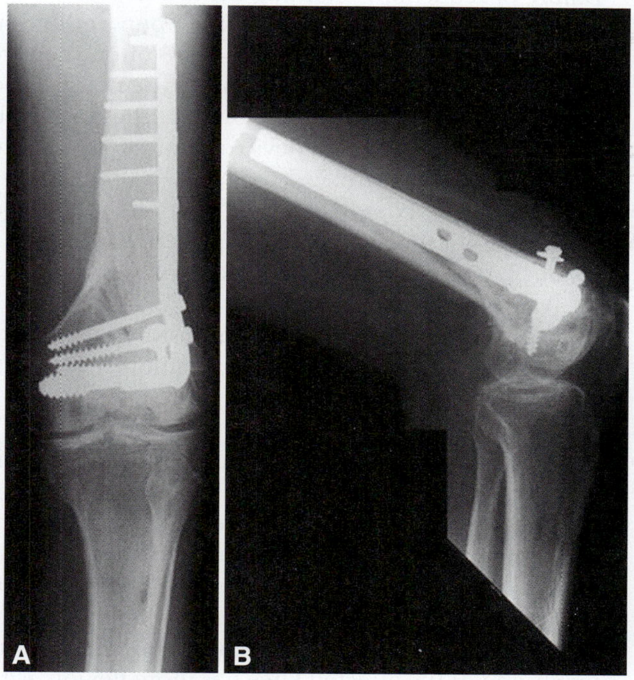

Figs 25.224A and B: Open reduction and internal fixation, with lag screw fixation of the articular components and a dynamic condylar screw

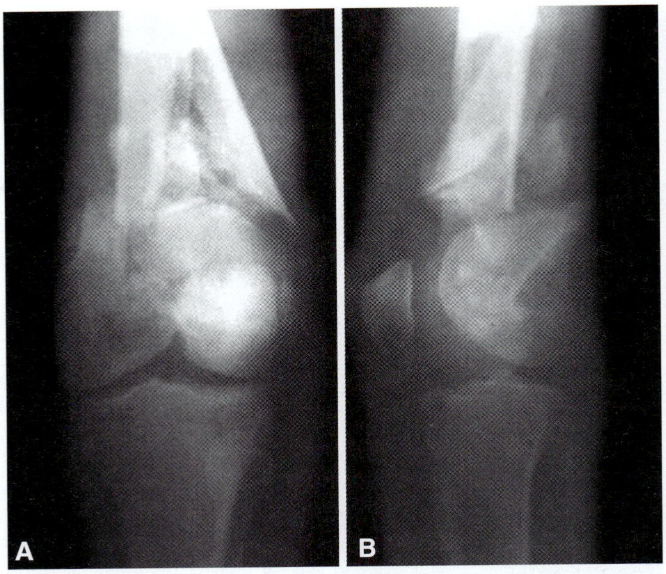

Figs 25.225A and B: Type C2 supracondylar femur fracture

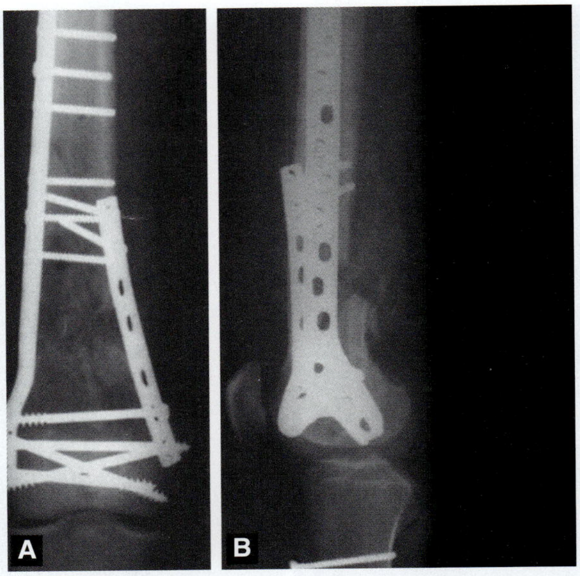

Figs 25.226A and B: For extensive comminution a lateral condylar buttress plate is used and to prevent varus deformity, a medial plate and iliac crest bone graft were used

Therefore, infections should be considered to involve septic arthritis of the knee.

- *Failure of reduction:* Attaining the reduction of distal femoral fractures, even with full open reduction techniques, can be difficult and more often than we would like, the main distal fragments are not in good relation to the main proximal ones. If the fracture is comminuted, the fixation device will often be put into an unreduced fracture.
- *Early failure of fixation:* Internal fixation in the distal femur can fail shortly, after it is applied. It is usually a result of, one of the following factors:
  - Poor bone stock
  - Poor patient compliance with postoperative care
  - Poor surgical planning and execution.

Late Complications

- *Knee stiffness:* Knee stiffness in one form or another, is a not too uncommon sequel of having a fracture of the femur into or just above the knee. The patient may have a fixed flexion deformity, limited range of flexion or both. Knee stiffness can have intra-articular and extra-articular components. It is often difficult to tell preoperatively, which of the components is the major one. If the affected knee has more flexion, with the hip flexed, then the quadriceps (rectus at least) plays a role. In the postoperative period, we use a continuous passive motion machine and epidural analgesia until we are sure, that the patient can maintain a relatively painless range of motion on his or her own. Post-hospital physical therapy and frequent physician followup are necessary.
- *Late infection:* Late infection can be in the form of, osteomyelitis, chronic septic arthritis, infected nonunion or some combination of these.
- *Nonunion:* Fortunately, the femur is a bone that heals readily and nonunion is not so common. Even more fortunately, the epiphyseal (joint surface) portions of the bone heal frequently and nonunion is rare. The exceptions to this rule are the partial articular fractures (type B fractures). These fractures often have vertical fracture lines subject to high shearing forces.
- *Malunion:* Malunions occur, as a result of failure of reduction or failure of fixation. Malunion most often occurs, with the distal fragment in varus. Distal femur fractures fixed with an intramedullary nail is placed, while the patient is in the lateral position. If they develop a malunion, it leads to valgus of the distal fragment. Flexion of the distal fragment seems to be more common, when the fracture is treated with a nail and extension of the distal fragment is more common, when it is treated with a plate or blade plate. Rotation can occur with either technique, but it is usually of greater magnitude, when a nail is used. Malunion in shortening is more common than in lengthening, but both situations are possible. Again, lengthening is more common with intramedullary techniques.
- *Painful internal fixation:* Painful internal fixation is so common after internal fixation of distal femur, that it is as much a necessary evil as a complication. Screws that are too long and protrude out the medial side are particularly troublesome for the patient. These should be avoided in the index operation. When

present, these devices can be removed and replaced or left out, depending on the stage of fracture healing.

- *Post-traumatic osteoarthrosis:* Post-traumatic arthrosis may accompany any intra-articular fracture. It can also occur in extra-articular fractures, which are held in malalignment, particularly varus. Prevention of this complication, at least for many years, is theoretically possible, by anatomic reduction of the distal femoral joint surface, correct alignment and maintenance of knee motion.

MENISCAL INJURIES

The term internal derangement was coined in 1784 by William Hey. It is now loosely applied to a variety of intra-articular and extra-articular disturbances, usually of traumatic origin, that interfere with the function of the joint. Knee joint, showing menisci is illustrated in Figure 25.227.

Functions of the Menisci

- Act as joint filler compensating for the gross incongruity between femoral and tibial articulating surfaces
- Prevent capsular and synovial impingement during flexion and extention movements
- Believed to have a joint lubricating function, helping to distribute synovial fluid throughout the joint and aiding the nutrition of the articular cartilage
- Contribute to stability in all planes by deepening the cavity of the tibial articulating surface, but are especially important rotary stabilizers
- Essential for the smooth transmission from a pure hinge to a gliding or rotary motion as the knee moves from flexion to extension.

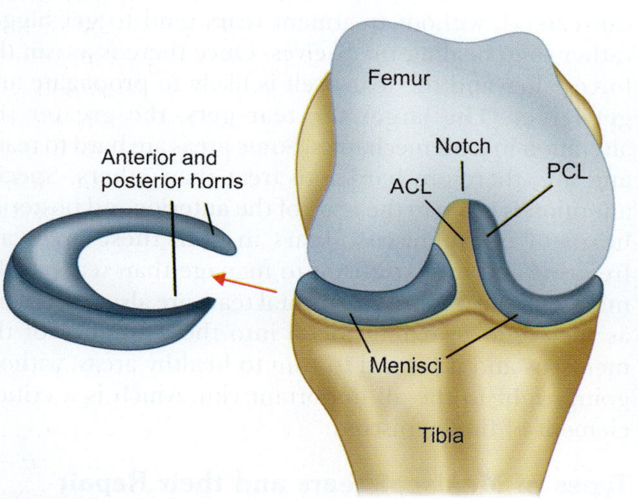

Fig. 25.227: Knee joint showing menisci

Functional Anatomy (Fig. 25.228)

The two menisci differ in shape and mobility. The lateral meniscus is more "O" shaped and is highly mobile, able to slide forwards and backwards with knee movement. The popliteus tendon, passing along one edge, which breaks the attachment to the capsule of the joint, adds to the mobility. The medial meniscus is larger and more "C" shaped and is tightly bound to the capsular structures and to the medial collateral ligament (MCL) along the outer rim. It moves very little with the movement of the knee. It is this inflexibility which leads to the medial meniscus being torn more frequently than the lateral meniscus. The lateral meniscus can move and absorb impact while the medial meniscus will simply tear.

Classification of Meniscal Tears

It can either be:

Primary: Due to damage during a knee injury.

Secondary: Due to consequence of another problem inside the knee.

Compound: Other structures are damaged at the same time.

Primary Tear

In a primary tear, there is usually a twisting force with significant torque, e.g. a footballer kicking a ball at an angle will have his full weight transmitted through one knee via the meniscus.

Secondary Tear

There is usually no directly associated injury. Degenerate tears occur in association with arthritic disorders, where there are destructive chemical substances being released into the joint cavity. The joint surface and the menisci undergo destructive alteration and start to break down and fragments.

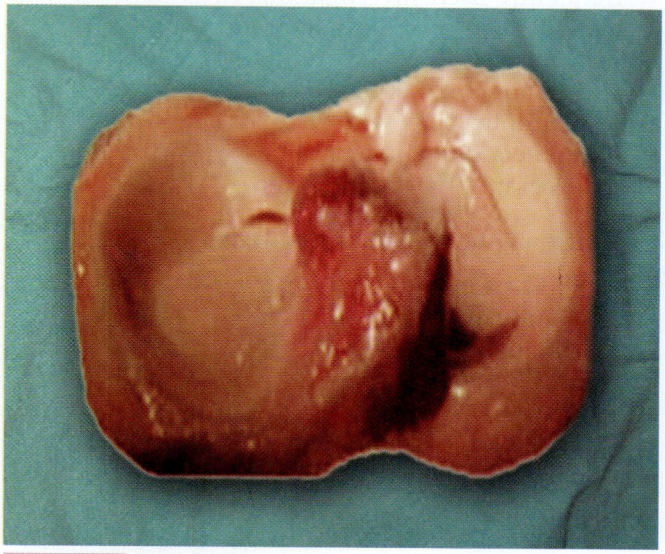

Fig. 25.228: Knee menisci

Compound Tear

Where the meniscus is torn in association with other injuries, the injury may not be simply due to torque. Anything that allows the femur to slip abnormally forward or backward in relation to the tibia may cause some of the forces to be transmitted to the meniscus and result in a meniscus tear. Injuries may include cruciate tears, cruciate and collateral tears and dislocation of the knee.

Mechanism of Injury

The patient gives history of a twisting injury to the knee while the joint was flexed. The leg is firmly fixed to the ground while the thigh is violently rotated. Most commonly, the leg, in relation to the thigh, is rotated externally and abducted.

Diagnosis

History

Often there is a history of twisting injury, followed by swelling of the knee and joint line pain. Commonly the injury occurs in the planted knee. There may be episodes of locking.

Examination

Clinical tests, which may be performed to assess a possible meniscal tear, are:

- McMurray's test
- Apley's grinding test
- Squat test or Waddling test
- The Salli's test.

Special Investigations

- X-rays are largely unhelpful in diagnosing meniscal tears.
- Magnetic resonance imaging (MRI), is one of the most frequently used investigations these days to help identify the type and extent of the tear.
- Arthroscopy
- Ultrasonography
- Scintigraphy
- Computed tomography (CT)
- Arthrography.

Classification of Meniscus Tears

O'connor Classification

- Longitudinal tears
- Horizontal tears
- Oblique tears
- Radial tears
- Variations, which include flap tears, complex tears and degenerative meniscal tears.

Smillie (1978) Classification

- Longitudinal tears
- Peripheral detachments (10%)
- Complete (23%)
- Segmental, either anterior or posterior
- Horizontal tears, anterior, posterior or middle
- Cystic degeneration (12%)
- Congenital abnormalities (5%)
- Degenerative lesions.

Treatment

I. *Conservative*

II. *Operative*

Repair: Inside out technique or outside in technique.
Meniscectomy: Partial meniscectomy, subtotal meniscectomy and total meniscectomy.
Fibrin clot: Meniscal replacement or meniscal transplant.

Conservative Management

Groin to ankle cylinder cast or knee immobilizer for 4–6 weeks. Walking with crutches, with touch down weight bearing, when patient gains active control of extremity in cast. Isometric exercise program to strengthen quadriceps, hamstrings and calf muscles.

Anatomy Issues

A number of issues affect which meniscus tears more frequently and how well different tears heal.

Blood supply: Blood supply is poor on the inner aspect. The blood supply to the structure is from a network of small blood vessels, which penetrate from the wide outer rim. Here, the blood supply is rich and healing is facilitated. In this area tears are referred to as red on red. On the inner sharper rim, however, blood vessels do not penetrate at all. The cells of the meniscus are dependent on any nourishment they can get from the joint fluid. Tears here do not heal. In this area tears are referred to as white on white, as shown in See Figure 25.19.

Tears in between these two regions are referred to as red on white. They may heal but not necessarily. Tears can extend, without treatment tears tend to get bigger rather than healing themselves. Once there is a tear, the forces alter and the tear itself is likely to propagate and get larger. The larger the tear gets, the greater the alteration in joint mechanics. Some areas are hard to reach and are, therefore harder to treat than others. Special attention is given to the tears of the anterior and posterior horns of the meniscus. Tears in both these areas are frequent and more difficult to manage than tears in the middle of the wedge. Horizontal tears are also a problem, as they tend to extend deep into the substance of the meniscus and it is hard to trim to healthy areas, without going right to the all important rim, which is a critical element of the meniscus.

Types of Meniscal Tears and their Repair

The meniscal damage may simply be frayed edge, seen as ragged fronds on the sharp edge of the meniscus, as

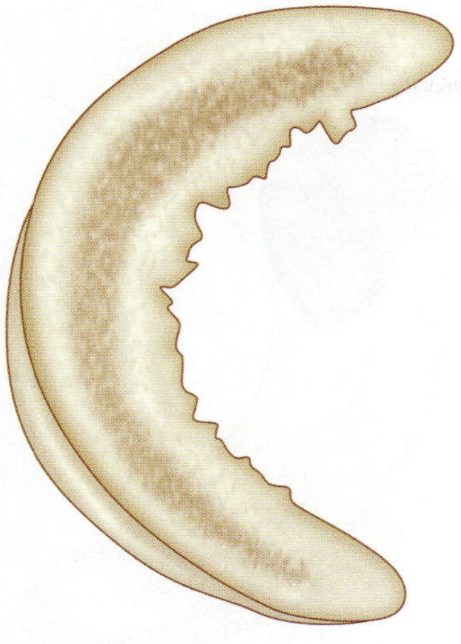

Fig. 25.229: Meniscal damage seen as ragged fronds on the sharp edge of the meniscus

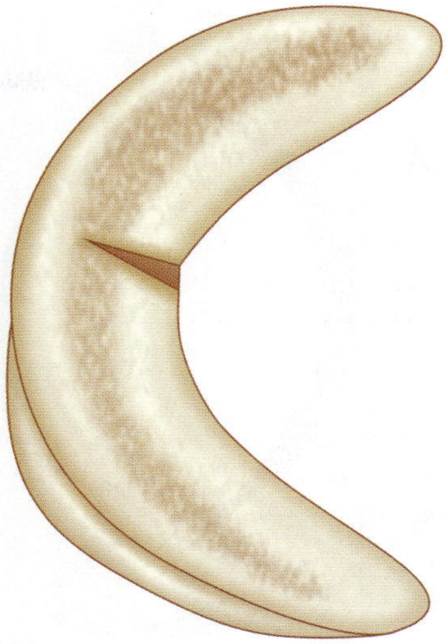

Fig. 25.230: Radial tear

illustrated in Figure 25.229. A frayed inner meniscal rim, seen frequently, is usually of little consequence. The area is trimmed away to tide it up and prevent enzyme release from the area. The degenerate meniscus is more problematic, which refers to when the whole meniscus undergoes internal change and simply collapses in a ragged fashion. The shock absorber function is grossly impaired and the cartilage at the ends of the femur and tibia become stressed and arthritis can ensues. A sharp split from the medial rim towards the lateral rim (across the radius) is known as a radial tear, as shown in Figure 25.230.

This is amenable to suturing, but the inner part may not heal because of poor blood supply in that area, so some trimming may be done. Still it is worth trying to get the outer part to heal, as this part is most important to the meniscus. A neglected radial tear, usually an oblique one may try to heal itself and round off into a rounded beak like a parrot's beak, the parrot beak tear and (Fig. 25.231) this can catch the joint. A circumferential tear extends along the length of the meniscus (along the circumference). Such a tear changes the biomechanics of the knee and may propogate and prevent healing. These types of tears may not go through the full depth of the meniscus, but if they do, they are called bucket handle tears. Bucket handle tears in the white on white, as shown in Figure 25.232 area are usually removed surgically as they do not heal, while tears in the white on red area may be sutured and almost certainly we must try to preserve red on red, which may even heal by themselves.

A horizontal split in the body of the meniscus is called a horizontal cleavage tear. The tear usually begins, quite hidden from view in the inner aspect of the body of the meniscus, although it may be evident on an MRI scan, as

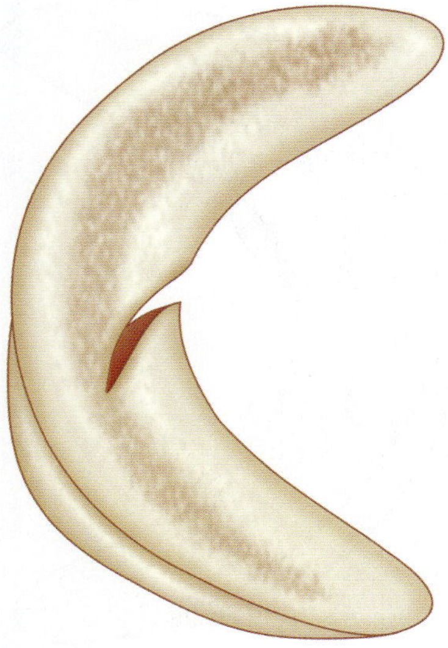

Fig. 25.231: Parrot beak tear

illustrated in Figure 25.233. It most likely starts after a minor injury, followed by a degenerative process, which starts in the damaged area. Regardless the thing burrows away in the inside, splitting the meniscus into top and the bottom sections. Eventually the tear breaks out at the inner aspect and reveals itself. The flap tear is also horizontal, but at the surface of the meniscus rather than in the middle. The flap tends to flick over from time to time causing symptoms, as illustrated in Figure 25.234. The tear is fairly easily dealt with. The flap section is simply trimmed away. There is sufficient body of the meniscus to heal the defect and provide shock absorption to the knee.

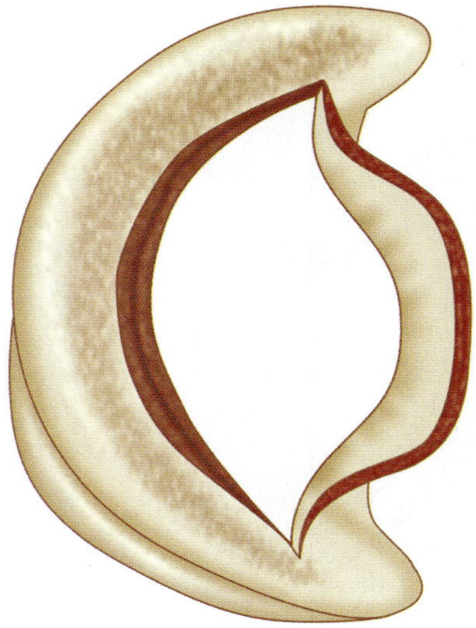

Fig. 25.232: Bucket handle tears of menisci

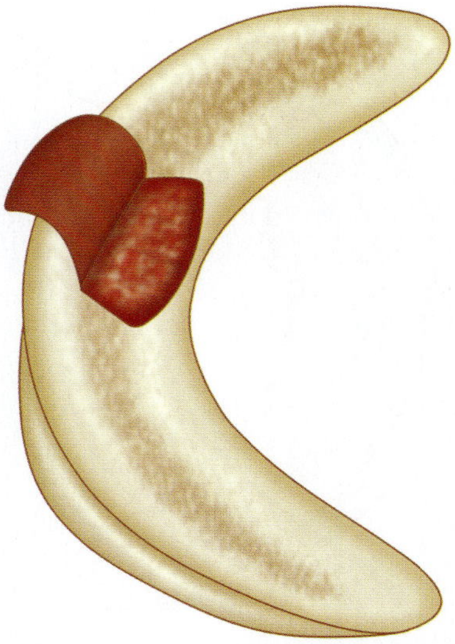

Fig. 25.234: The flap tear shown at the surface of the meniscus

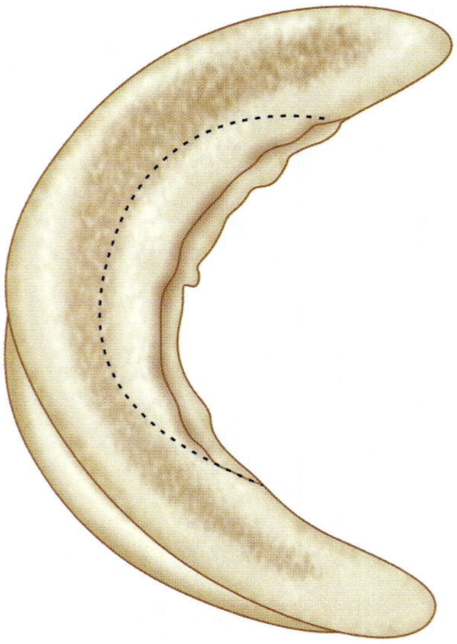

Fig. 25.233: A horizontal split in the body of the meniscus or a horizontal cleavage tear

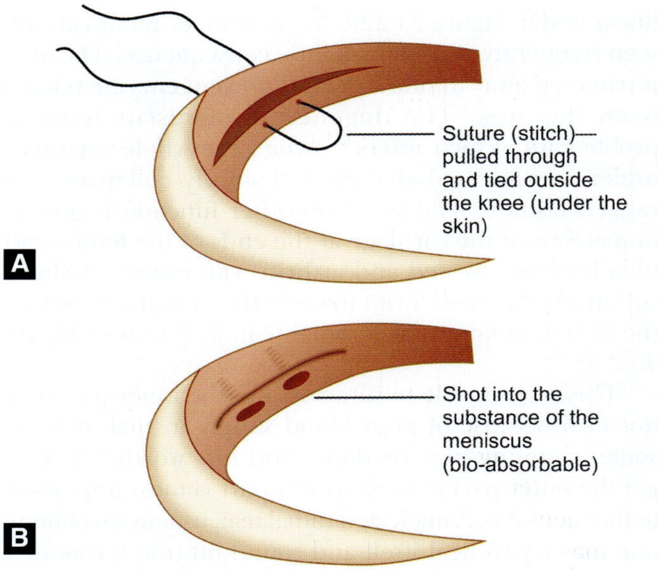

Figs 25.235A and B: Meniscal tear repair—(A) Meniscal sutures; (B) Meniscal arrows

Operative Treatment or Repair of Meniscal Tears (Figs 25.235A and B)

Meniscal Sutures

Suturing is a fairly coarse but effective procedure and can be done arthroscopically. The suture ties are usually threaded out through the joint and the knots are buried just under the skin.

Meniscal Arrows

Little half inch long harpoons, just a millimeter wide, which are knocked or shot into the tear to hold the two surfaces together via the barbs. These are also bioabsorbable.

T-Fixing

This is similar to the harpoons but T shaped rather than harpoon shaped.

Meniscectomy

It can be of following type:

- Partial meniscectomy
- Subtotal meniscectomy
- Total meniscectomy
- Meniscectomy and arthritis

a. *Partial meniscectomy:* Only the loose unstable meniscal fragments are excised. A stable and balanced peripheral rim of healthy meniscal tissue is preserved. Done in bucket handle tears, flap tears and oblique tears.

b. *Subtotal meniscectomy:* Requires excision of portion of the peripheral rim of meniscus. Most of the anterior horn and portion of middle-third of meniscus are not resected. Done in complex or degenerative tears of posterior horns of either meniscus.
c. *Total meniscectomy:* Total removal of meniscus is done, if it is detached from the peripheral meniscosynovial attachment and when there is intrameniscal damage and if the tears are extensive. There is a regenerated meniscus formed, which is fibrocartilagenous and unsuited to mechanical stresses.
d. *Meniscectomy and arthritis:* One big issue about complete meniscectomy is that it is a one way ticket to arthritis. Removal of the all important meniscal rim causes the following consequences:
   - Shock absorption is lost forever.
   - As the spacer on one side of the joint is missing, more forces are transmitted through that side of the joint.
   - The joint surfaces of the femur and tibia are going to become stressed, softened and eventually break down and there will be arthritic pain.

The leg may demonstrate bow-leggedness or knock knees, due to the collapse of the joint on one side (compartment). The knee may seem to thrust outwards, with each step further stressing the joint (lateral thrust). The bone may attempt to heal itself causing bony outgrowths (osteophytes). These may form at the joint line or in the notch, where the cruciate ligaments reside. Eventually the cruciate ligaments may become incompetent and rupture.

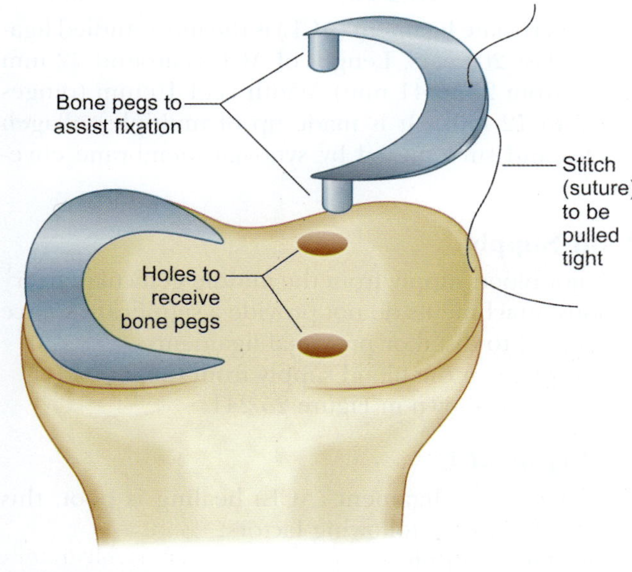

Fig. 25.236: Meniscal transplantation

Meniscal Transplant (Fig. 25.236)

There are two different meniscus replacement procedures:

a. *Meniscal allograft (meniscus transplant):* In this procedure, a cadaver (donor) meniscus is put in place to replace the patient's meniscus.
b. *Meniscal prosthesis or scaffold:* In this a synthetic meniscus (collagen meniscus) is used as a scaffold for the body to replace the meniscus. There are some centers trying the technique of growing the patient's own cells into a scaffold of artificial material, with a view of transplanting that living scaffold to replace the meniscus of patient, with less likelihood of misfit, rejection or infection.

Discoid Meniscus (Fig. 25.237)

It is a developmental anomaly, which happens, when a person is born with a flat round disk for a meniscus, instead of a C shaped wedge. Quite often discoid menisci may be symptomatic, commonly beginning in childhood, clicking or clunking of the knee in certain positions, giving way pain. They can tear like any other meniscus and cause locking and joint line pain. Surgery for a symptomatic discoid meniscus, usually involves, trimming it to approximately the shape of a normal meniscus.

Calcification of Meniscus

Calcification of menisci has been shown in Figure 25.238.

Types of Meniscal Calcification

Primary Type

- Seen in patients with advanced age afflicted with degenerative arthritis.

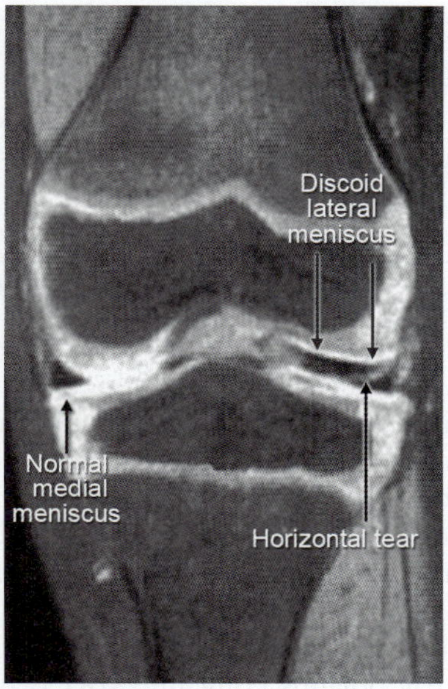

Fig. 25.237: Discoid meniscal anomaly of lateral meniscus (arrows)

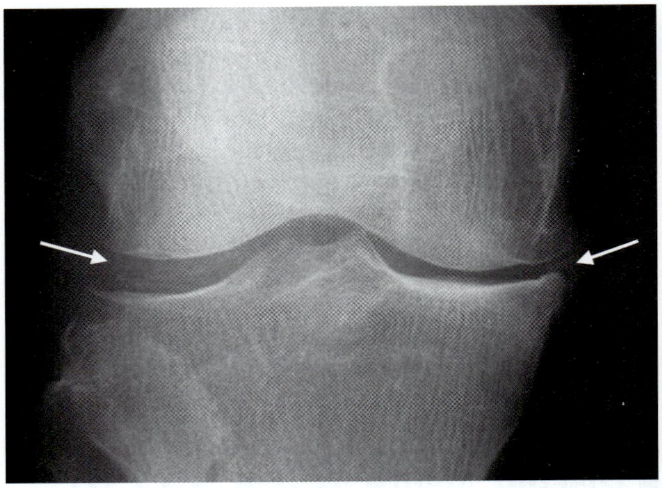

Fig. 25.238: X-ray shows calcification of menisci

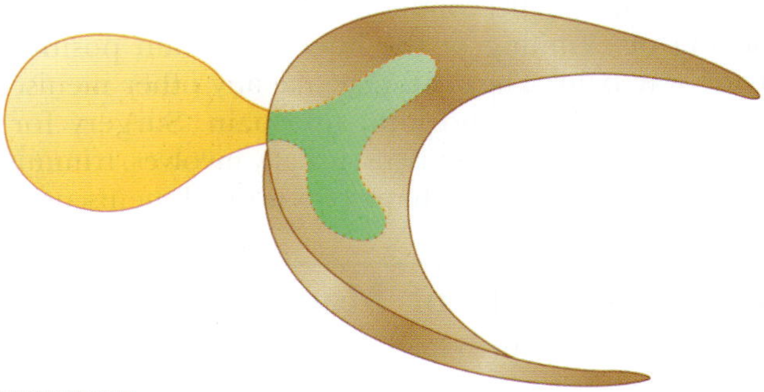

Fig. 25.239: Meniscal cyst

- Also seen in pseudogout, chondrocalcinosis, ankylosing spondylosis, etc.
- X-ray shows calcified menisci as transversely disposed white lines in tibiofemoral interval.

Secondary Type

- Seen in younger people with torn meniscus.
- There is a vague deposit in region of posterior horn, which requires removal.

■ Meniscal Cysts (Fig. 25.239)

These are the defects, which generally originates from a tear within a meniscus. May be degenerative or developmental in origin. Fibrous tissue sac filled with fluid under pressure, may herniate into capsular tissues on the joint line, producing a painful lump, which can sometimes be reduced by pressing on it. May be medial or lateral, commonly associated with horizontal cleavage tear.

Diagnosis

Although, fairly obvious clinically. MRI is quite helpful to clinch the diagnosis.

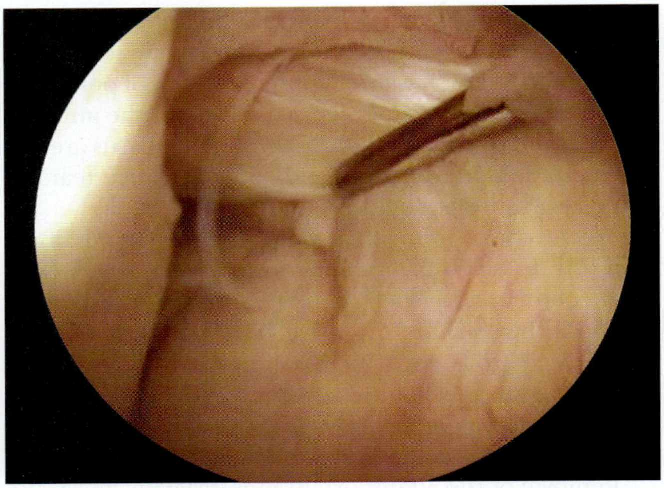

Fig. 25.240: Arthroscopic view of ACL

Management

Arthroscopic surgery is done to exclude the presence of horizontal cleavage tear. If found, the tear is cleaned out and the cyst decompressed from within the meniscus. A partial meniscectomy may be performed. If there is no horizontal cleavage tear, the cyst may be approached from outside of the knee and decompressed. Any other meniscal rim problem can be dealt during surgery.

CRUCIATE LIGAMENT INJURIES

■ Anterior Cruciate Ligament

Anatomy (Fig. 25.240)

Anterior cruciate ligament (ACL) is the most studied ligament in last 20 years. Length of ACL is around 32 mm (ranges from 25 to 41 mm). Width is of 10 mm (ranges from 7 to 12 mm). It is made up of multiple collagen fascicles and surrounded by synovial membrane envelope.

Blood Supply

- Major blood supply from the middle genicular artery
- Bony attachments do not provide a significant source of blood to distal or proximal ligaments
- Also receiven the blood supply from the fat pad

This has been shown in Figure 25.241.

Healing of ACL

Anterior cruciate ligament (ACL) healing is poor, this could be due to the following factors:

- Poor blood supply
- Synovial fluid inhibition

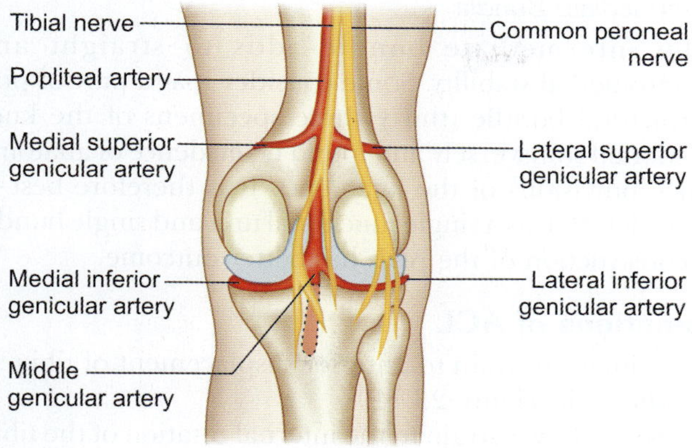

Fig. 25.241: Blood supply to ACL (posterior view)

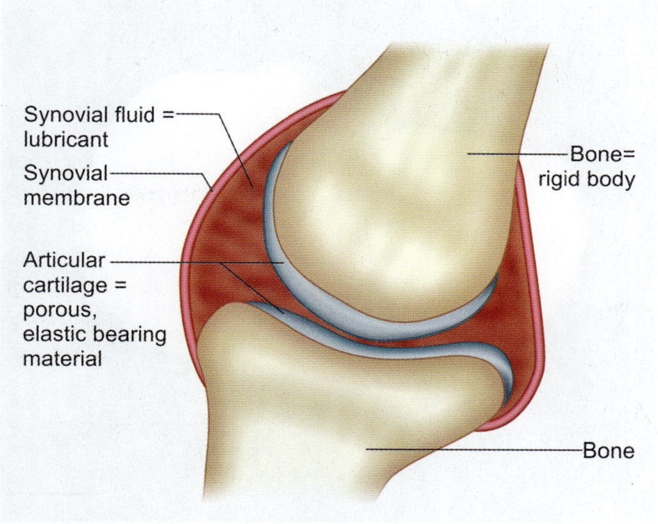

Fig. 25.242: Components of knee joint

- There are excessive mechanical stresses which hamper healing process. Different components of knee are shown in Figure 25.242.

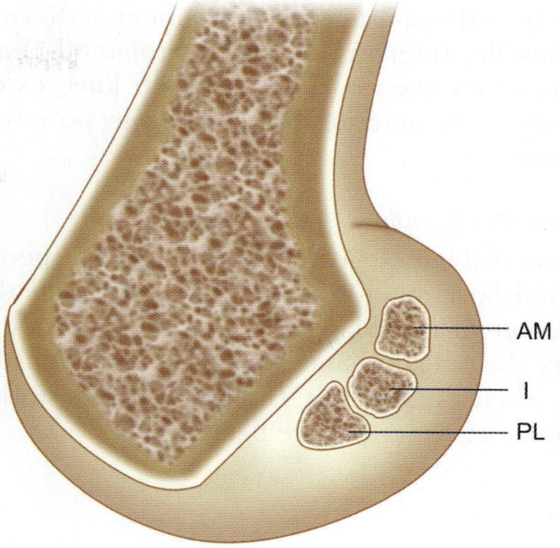

Fig. 25.243: Femoral attachment of ACL—AM. Anteromedial; PL. Posterolateral; I. Intermediate

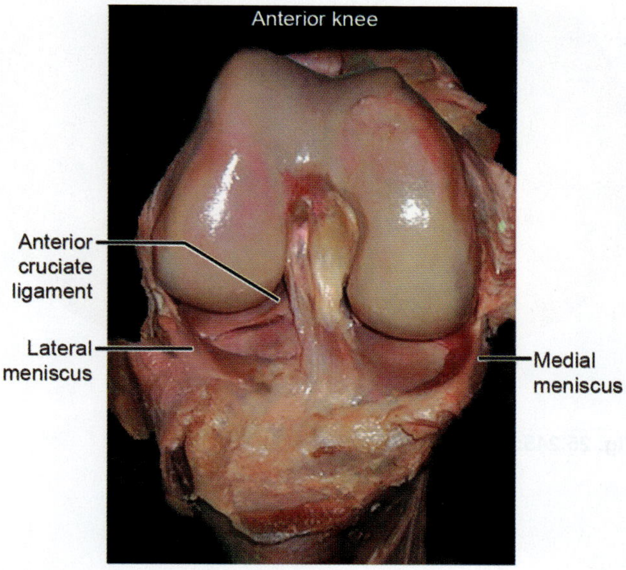

Fig. 25.244: Femoral attachment of ACL

Femoral Attachment (Fig. 25.243)

Anterior cruciate ligament (ACL) arises from the posteromedial corner of medial aspect of lateral femoral condyle in the intercondylar notch, as shown in Figure 25.244. Femoral attachment of ACL is on posterior part of medial surface of lateral condyle well posterior to longitudinal axis of the femoral shaft.

Tibial Attachment (Figs 25.245 to 25.247)

Tibial attachment of ACL is in a fossa in front of and lateral to anterior spine. A rather wide area from 11 mm in width to 17 mm in AP direction (marked red in Figure 25.244). Anterior fibers go forward to the level of transverse meniscal ligament and inserts into the interspinous area of the tibia, as demonstrated in Figure 25.245.

Bundles of ACL (Figs 25.248A and B)

Anterior cruciate ligament is composed of two principal parts

- Small anteromedial band
- A larger bulky posterolateral portion. Anteromedial bundle tight in flexion and posterolateral bundle tight in extension.

Posterolateral Bundle

Represents posterior directed fibers, with its attachment just lateral to midline of the intercondylar eminence and slightly lateral to most lateral attachment of the intermediate bundle. Interruption of posterolateral bundle of ACL increases external rotation. With knee extended, resistance to the anterior drawer test is by posterolateral bulky portion.

Anteromedial Bundle

Anteromedial bundle inserts on the medial aspect of the intercondylar eminence of the tibia and forms the medial corner of the triangle. Anteromedial band is the primary check against anterior translation of tibia on the femur, when the anterior Drawer test is performed in usual manner with the knee flexed.

Intermediate Bundle

The intermediate bundle adds to straight and anteromedial stability. Some consider it as a part of posterolateral bundle (thirty three specimens of the knee sectioned transversely and found no evidence of anatomical subdivisions of the ligament). It is therefore best to consider ACL as a single functional unit and single bundle reconstruction of the ACL has better outcome.

Functions of ACL

- Primary restrain to anterior displacement of tibia, as shown in Figure 25.249.
- Secondary restrain to the internal rotation of the tibia.
- It has minor role in restraining varus valgus.

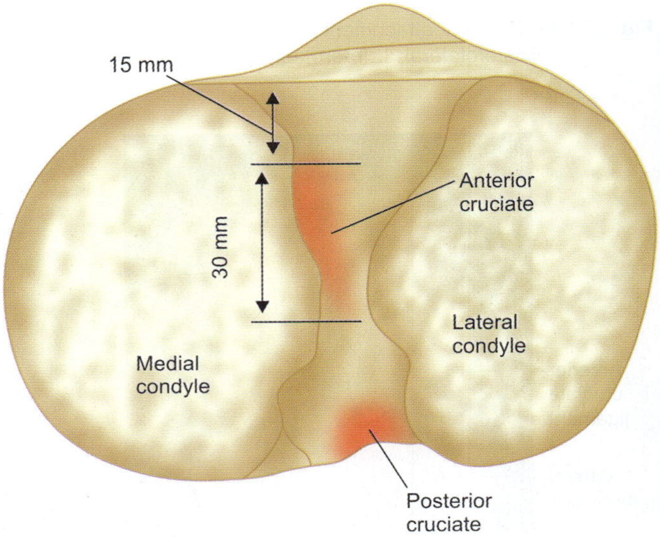

Fig. 25.245: Tibial attachment of ACL

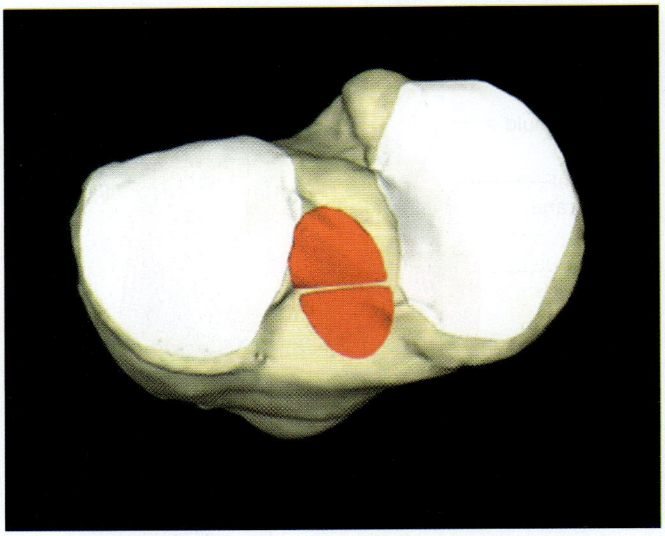

Fig. 25.247: Area of ACL attachment in tibial fossa (shown with red mark in AP direction)

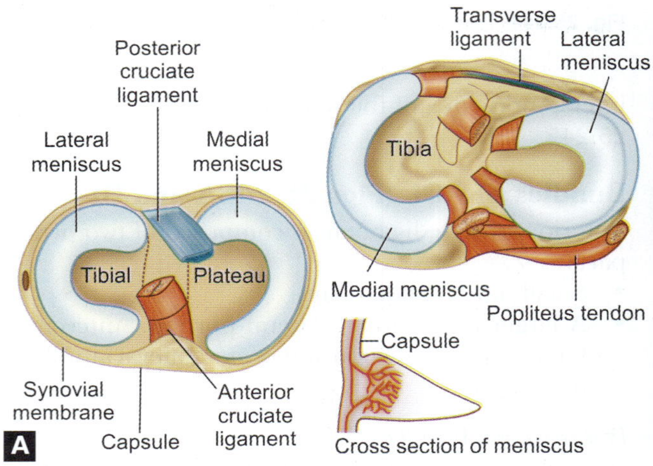

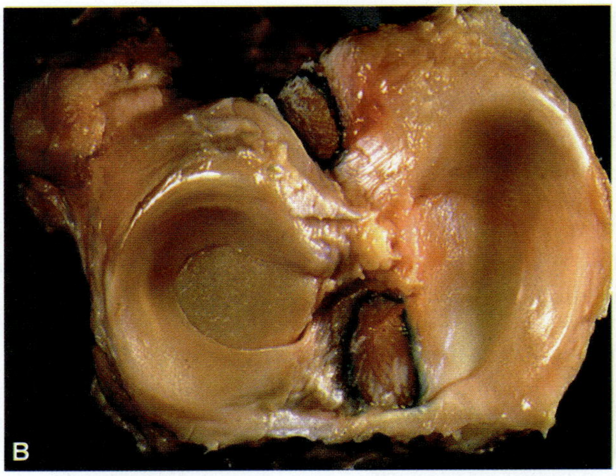

Figs 25.246A and B: Articulate surface of tibia, showing tibial attachment of ACL and other structures

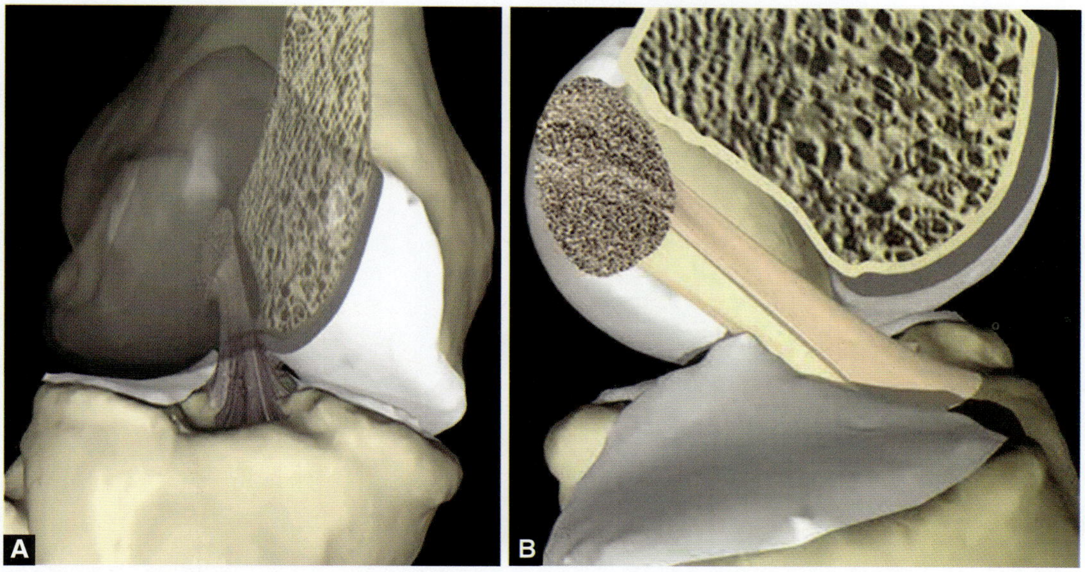

Figs 25.248A and B: Bundles of ACL—(A) Anteromedial bundle of ACL; (B) Posterolateral bundle

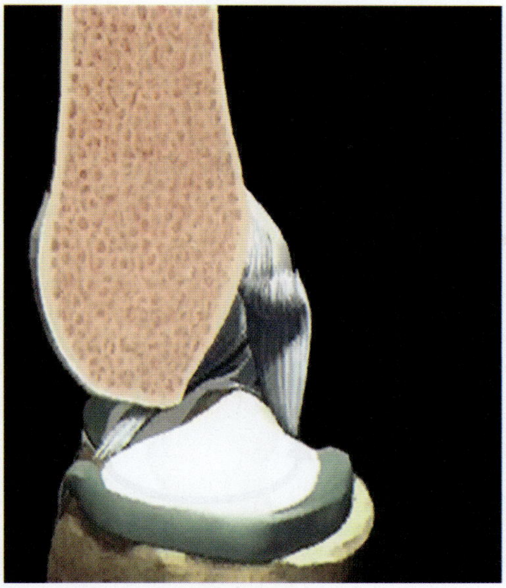

Fig. 25.249: ACL as a primary restrain to anterior displacement of tibia

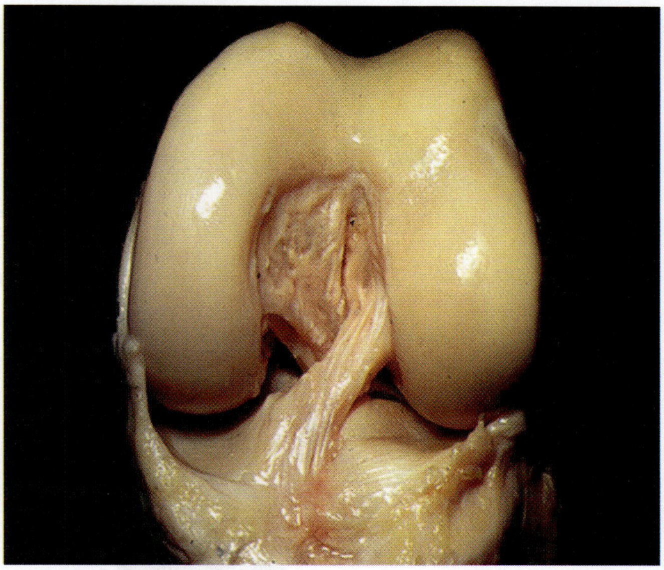

Fig. 25.250: Intercondylar notch with intact ACL

Length and Isometricity

Length of the ACL fibers vary with the degree of flexion

In 90° flexion, length of anteromedial bundle increases 3.3 mm, length of posterolateral bundle decreases by 1.5 mm, therefore the ideal isometric attachment points can not be found during ACL reconstruction.

Intercondylar Notch (Fig. 25.250)

Width

- Anteriorly: 1.8 cm
- Posteriorly: 2.2 cm.

Height

- Proximal: 1.8 cm
- Distal: 1.3 cm
- Maximum: 2.4 cm
- Narrow notch has increase incidence of ACL tear.

Mode of Injury (Figs 25.251 to 25.254)

The classic history of a person sustaining an isolated ACL injury, consists of a noncontact deceleration mechanism, usually occurring with a sudden stopping, cutting or jumping maneuver. The majority of ACL injuries are

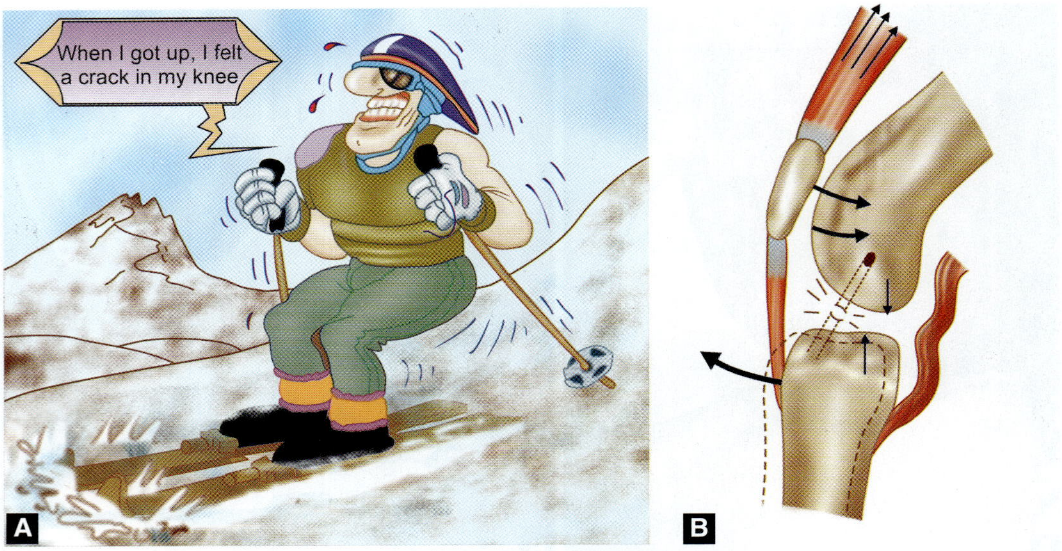

Figs 25.251A and B: ACL injuries in sports like skiing, occurs predominating in noncontact injuries—(A) Muscular contraction in well-developed skiers is sufficient to rupture the ACL due to the sling shot effect; (B) Mechanism of injury in skiers shown as sling shot effect. In addition, there is a lack of coordination in the antagonist hamstring muscles

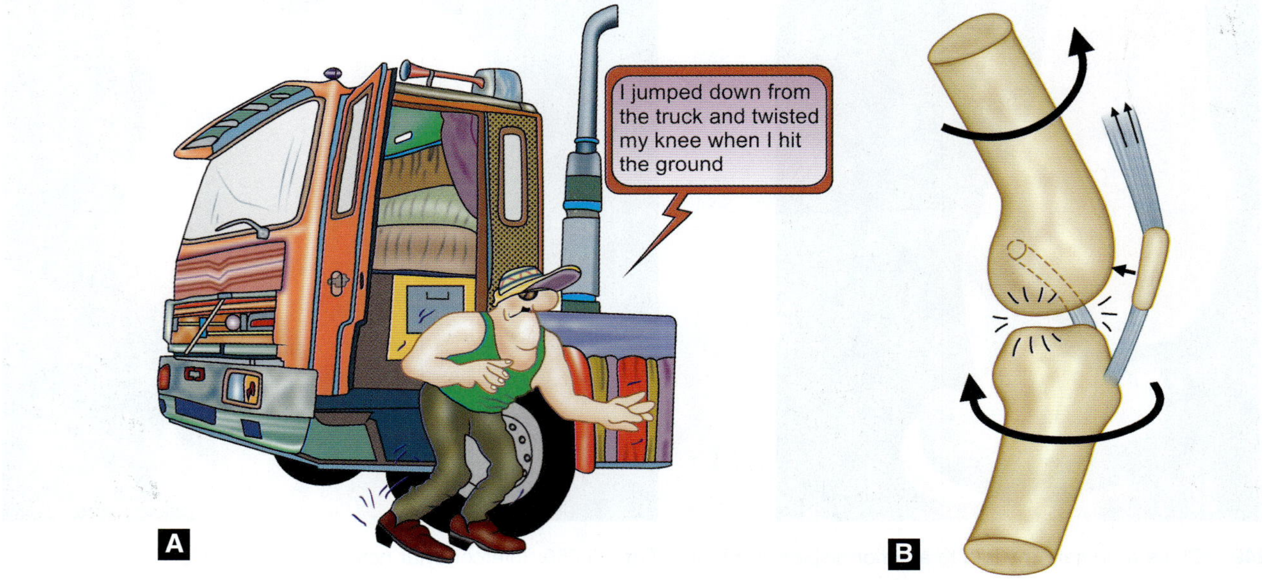

Figs 25.252A and B: (A) ACL injury due to twisting of knee in jumping from bus (height); (B) Mechanism of injury shown, while jumping from height, ACL tear occurs with contraction of the quadriceps muscle, which is an antagonist of the ACL

sustained in sports activities, with basketball, soccer and skiing predominating in noncontact injuries, as shown in Figures 25.251A and B. Contact injuries are frequently described in football players.

Clinical Features

Clinical evaluation should begin with a thorough history and the mechanism of injury is obtained from the patient or any witnesses to the injury. Most ACL injuries are the result of noncontact and rotational forces. Valgus/external rotation, hyperextension and deceleration mechanisms are commonly described. A pop or snap is usually felt or heard and the patient may describe a hyperextension injury. The patient is able to continue activity and within a few hours the knee swells considerably, secondary to hemarthrosisonset of a knee joint effusion within a few

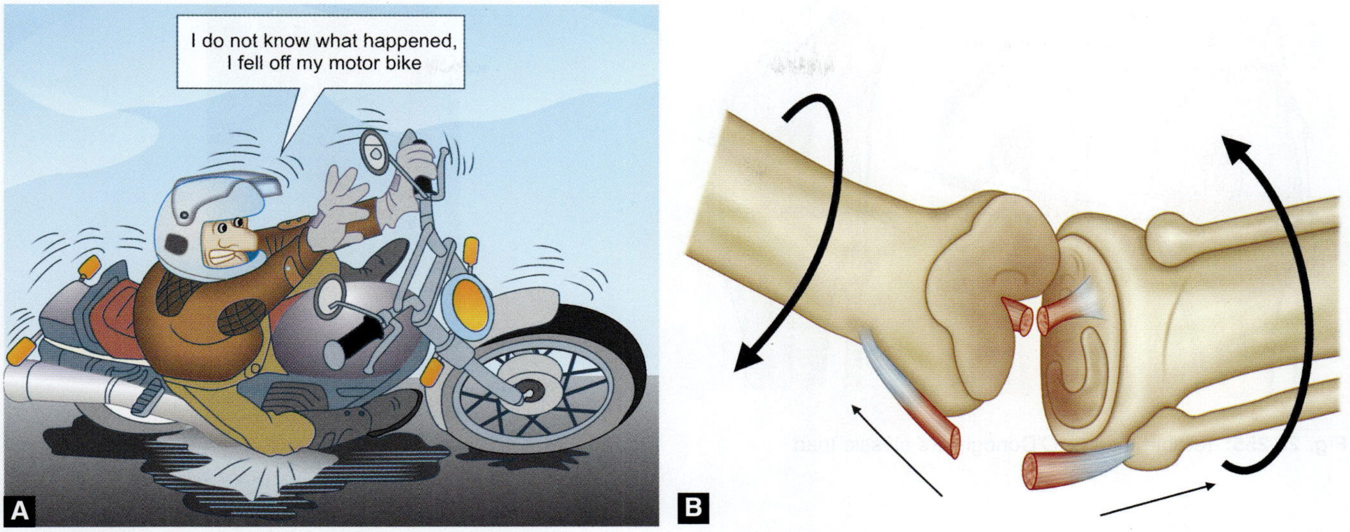

Figs 25.253A and B: (A) ACL tear due to motorcycle injury; (B) Mechanism by which a ligament injury may occur in forced movement provoked by a forced position of knee. Here, the knee is in flexion-varus-internal rotation, aggravated by gravity and the weight of the motor cycle

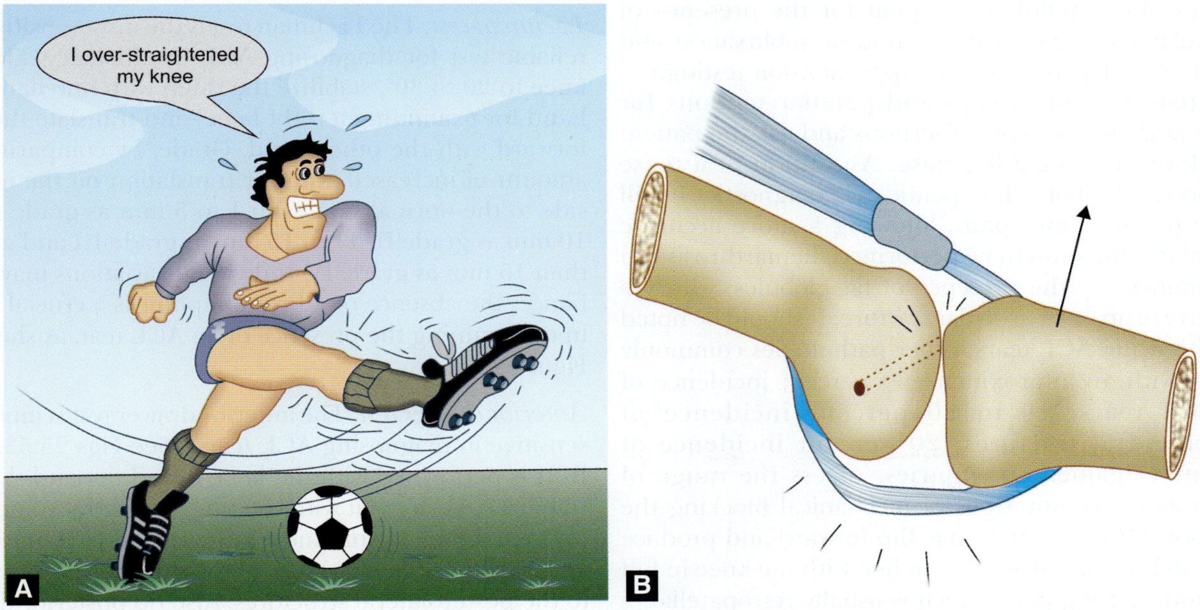

Figs 25.254A and B: (A) ACL tear, while playing football; (B) A mechanism of ACL rupture with or without rupture of the posteromedial and posterolateral structures in hyperextension. The ACL abuts against the intercondylar notch, which acts like the bridge of a stringed instrument against a tight string

hours of injury. Complaints are geared toward a feeling of instability or giving way. Patient is symptomatic with pain and giving way of the knee. Occasionally a second traumatic event or a giving way episode results in a meniscal tear that causes mechanical symptoms, such as locking or catching in the knee. Contact injuries are more likely to result in multiligament injuries, as is seen with terrible triad or O'Donoghue's classic triad, in which a direct blow valgus load on the knee results in injury to the ACL, medial collateral ligament (MCL) and medial meniscus.

Terrible triad (Fig. 25.255): The first restraint to be rupture in valgus is the MCL, followed by the posteromedial corner—the ACL, PCL and lateral arcuate complex.

Physical Examination

Ideally, examine the knee shortly after the injury, before swelling and pain prevent an accurate diagnosis. Examine

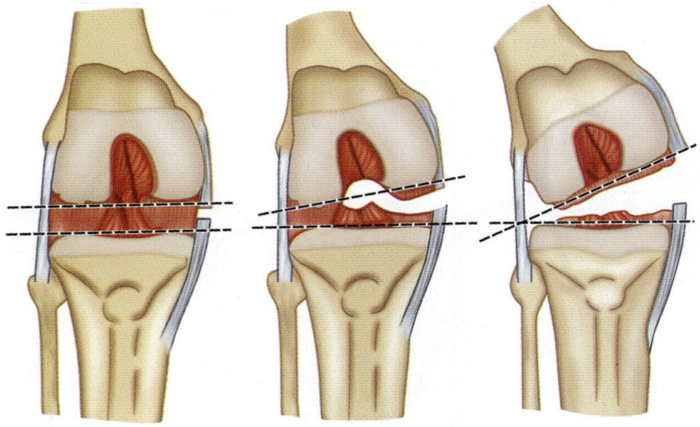

Fig. 25.255: Terrible triad or O'Donoghue's classic triad

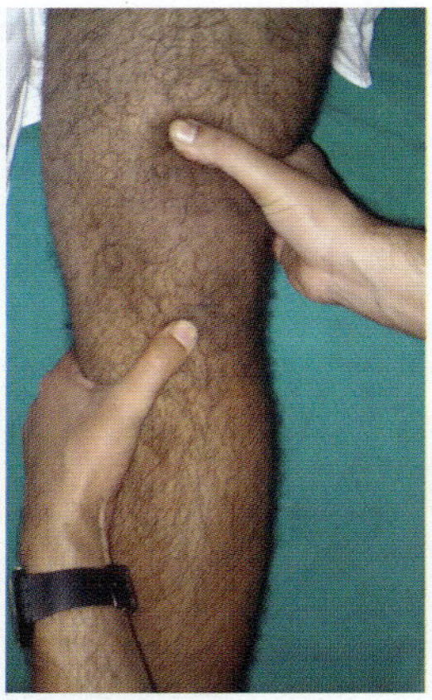

Fig. 25.256: Lachman test

the opposite leg to serve as a baseline for comparison. First inspect the injured leg for abrasions, contusions, ecchymoses and the presence of an effusion. Next, palpate for point tenderness to evaluate associated injuries. Examine the patellofemoral joint for the presence of retinacular tearing or a dislocation or subluxation and perform patellar mobility and apprehension testing.

Palpate the quadriceps and patellar tendons for defects at their respective insertions and ask the patient to perform a straight-leg raise. Aspiration of a tense effusion can be both therapeutic and diagnostic. It will relieve pressure and pain, allowing a more accurate physical examination to be performed, hemarthrosis can be examined for the presence of fat globules, which is indicative of an intra-articular fracture. It should be noted that with acute ACL tears, other pathologies commonly coexist, with an approximate 60 percent incidence of meniscal tears, 10 to 20 percent incidence of osteochondral fractures, 20 percent incidence of associated ligamentous injuries. Assess the range of motion and note any signs of mechanical blocking the distal portion of the ACL may flip forward and produce a block in the anterolateral joint line with the knee in full extension, causing pain, which is usually retropatellar.

Percentage of ACL Tears

Out of all ACL tears mid-substance tears are most common and account for 80 percent of cases, tear at tibial end is rear and account for 3 percent of total cases— tear at femoral end 17 percent.

Pathology of ACL Tears

If ACL injury is less then 3 weeks old, it is acute ACL tear. If injury is more then 3 weeks old, it is chronic ACL tear.

Special Tests for ACL Injury

- Anterior drawer test
- Lachman test
- Rotary Test
- Slocum anterior drawer test
- Jerk test for Houghston and Losee
- Pivot shift test.

Lachman test: The Lachman test is the most sensitive and reliable test for diagnosing ACL insufficiency. Flex the knee to 20 to 30°, stabilize the thigh with one hand (left hand for examining a right knee) and translate the tibia forward with the other hand. Grade, by comparing the amount of increased anterior translation on the injured side to the normal side, with 1 to 5 mm as grade I, 6 to 10 mm as grade II, 11 to 15 mm as grade III and greater than 15 mm as grade IV. Individual variations may exist; hence, the absence of a firm endpoint is a crucial factor in determining the presence of an ACL tear, as shown in Figure 25.256.

Anterior drawer test: The anterior drawer test is much less sensitive in diagnosing ACL tears, (See Figs 25.53A and B. It is performed with the knee flexed 90° and the foot stabilized. Perform it with the tibia in neutral rotation as well as in both internal and external rotation, as increased anterior translation in external rotation may signify injury to the posterolateral structures. Also do posterior drawer testing, as what may seem to be increased anterior translation from a reduced position may actually be reduction of the tibia from a posteriorly subluxated position.

Pivot-shift test: Pivot-shift testing is the most important physical examination maneuver performed, as this phenomenon is pathognomonic for ACL deficiency. Method is to place the hip in slight abduction and flexion and the knee in full extension with the tibia externally rotated, apply a valgus load and flex the knee. This method is chosen because it results in fewer false-negative examinations. The pivot-shift will occur in 15° to 30° of flexion. It represents a reduction of the anteriorly subluxated tibia on the femur, as the knee is moved from extension to flexion. This reduction is the result of the iliotibial band, moving from an anterior position relative to the center of the knee to a posterior position, contributing to the reduction. In examining a right knee, palpate the joint line with your left hand, to ensure that what is being perceived is reduction of the anterior subluxated tibia, rather than posterior subluxation of a reduced tibia, as can be seen with PCL injuries. Causes of false-negative results include a displaced bucket-handle meniscal tear, a complete tear of the MCL and a previous lateral extra-articular tenodesis of the iliotibial band, as shown in Figure 25.257. Grade the examination, as:

- A glide (1 +)
- Jump sensation (2 +)
- Transient lock (3 +).

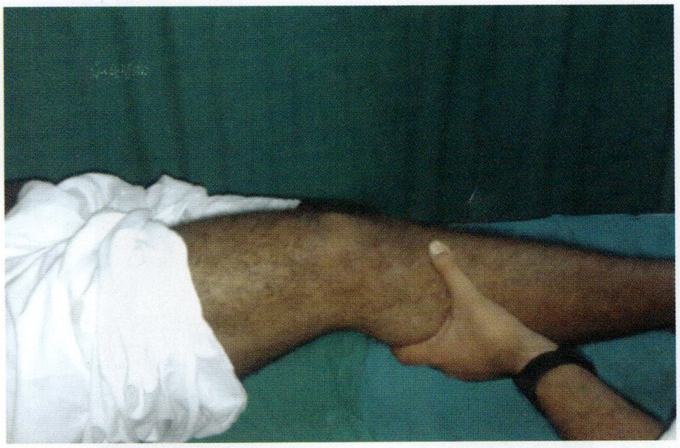

Fig. 25.257: Pivot-shift testing

Hughston's Classification

- *ACL tear:* From femoral site, mid-substance and tibial site
- *With lateral meniscus tear:* Anterior horn, middle body and posterior horn
- *Tibial plateau defect:* Less than 2 mm, 2 to 4 mm and greater than 4 mm defect and OCD
- Collateral ligament injury
- Associated with posterolateral complex injury.

O'Connoly's Classification

It is the same classification as Hughstun's classification, except there is no tibial plateau defect and OCD.

Classification for Tibial Avulsion of ACL

Given by Meyers and Mckeever

Type I: Undisplaced avulsion

Type II: Avulsion with 50 percent contact

Type III: More than 50 percent displaced

Type IV: Type III and rotation.

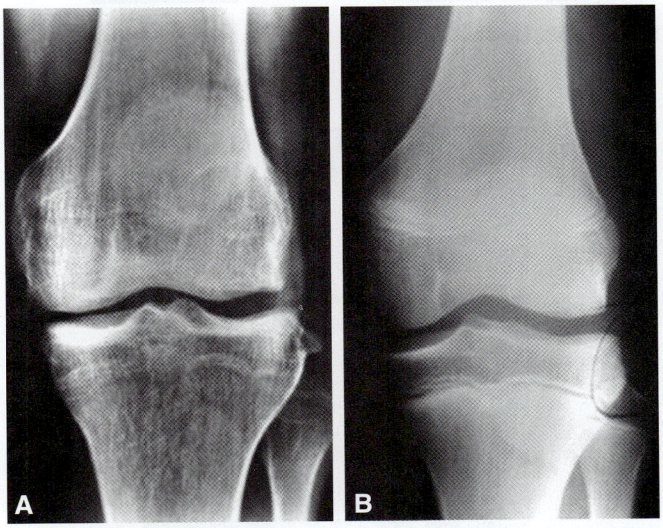

Figs 25.258A and B: X-rays of knee joint. (A) AP view; (B) 45° PA view

Routine Radiographs (Figs 25.258 to 25.260)

Weight-bearing AP, lateral and 45° PA views, as well as a merchant view of the patellofemoral joint. Anteroposterior radiographs of a skeletally mature right knee with chronic ACL insufficiency. A healed Segond fracture is noted by the bony spur on the lateral tibial plateau's lateral cortex, proximal to the fibula. Anteroposterior radiograph of a skeletally immature individual with a painful traumatic effusion. The X-ray reveals a lateral capsular avulsion, indicative of an injury to the ACL.

Notch View (Fig. 25.259)

Notch width index is the ratio of width of intercondylar notch to width of distal femur at level of popliteal groove (arrow). Ruler must be parallel to joint line. Narrowest portion of notch, at level of ruler is to be measured.

Stress View (Fig. 25.260)

Anteroposterior views are taken with varus and valgus stress applied on the knee. Opening of medial and lateral compartment spaces are noted suggesting ligament injury.

MRI (Fig. 25.261)

The addition of magnetic resonance imaging (MRI), though quite sensitive and specific for detection of ACL disruption and meniscal pathology as well as bone bruises, frequently does not change the treatment plan and adds cost to the care of the patient. The MRI was an excellent tool to detect meniscal tears that required surgery, but it was not sensitive or accurate in detecting partial-thickness meniscal lesions and stable full-thickness lesions.

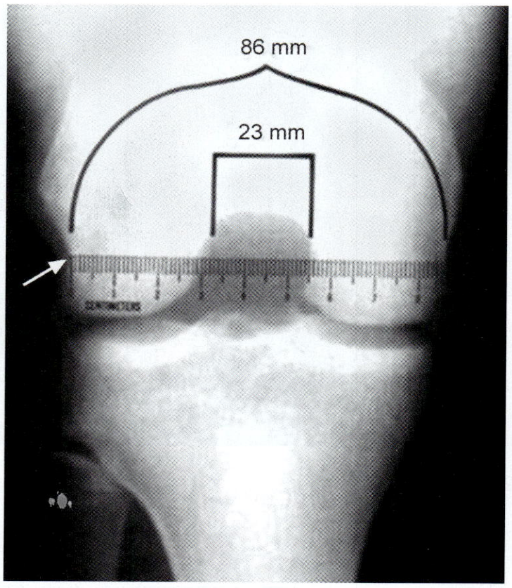

Fig. 25.259: Notch view

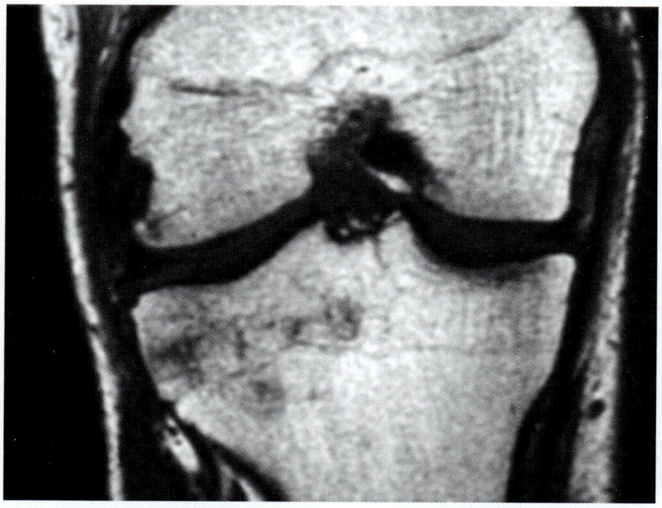

Fig. 25.261: MRI for detecting ACL tear

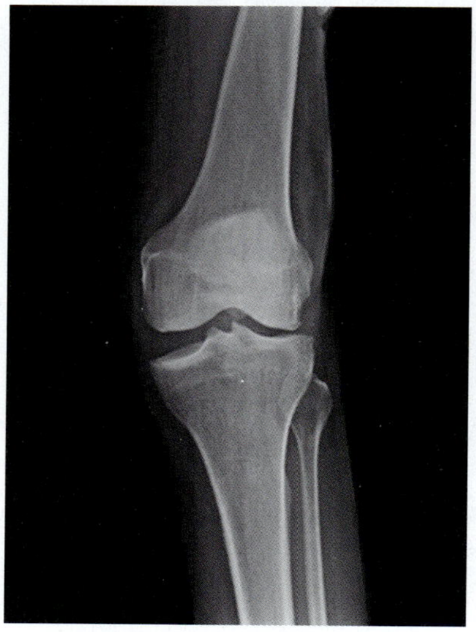

Fig. 25.260: Varus stress view showing increased joint compartment with valgus stress applied

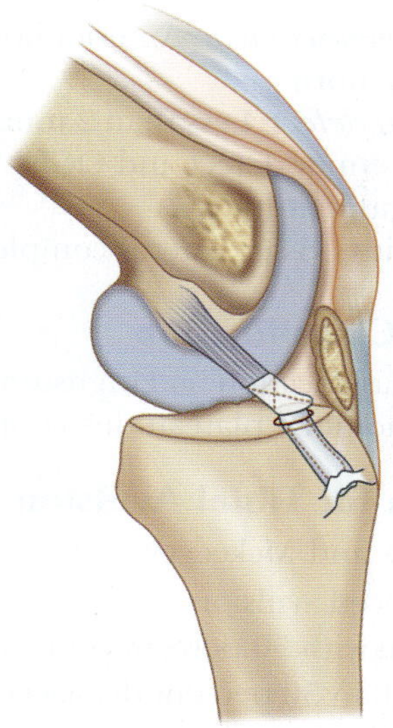

Fig. 25.262: Fixation of the avulsed piece done by clear crater placement of fragment under tension and screw fixation

CT/Bone Scan

Imaging modalities, such as knee arthrogram, CT scan and bone scanning have little place in the evaluation of the ACL-injured patient.

Treatment Options

- ACL avulsions are best treatment with ORIF.
- Nonoperative treatment only in case of undisplaced fracture, with cast in 20° flexion.
- Type II and III need internal fixation.
- Fifty percent cases have partial ACL tear.
- Arthoscopic treatment
- Surgical repair of ACL depends on acute or chronic tear. In acute cases reconstruction is done
- In ACL deficit, knee graft fixation with augmentation is required.

Surgical Treatment (Fig. 25.262)

Fixation of the avulsed piece done by either screw or by sutures anteromedial incision and arthrotomy, clear crater placement of fragment under tension and screw fixation, as shown in Figure 25.263. When fragment is small and screw is not possible, Bunnel suture passed through ACL and sutured through drill holes in tibia, as shown in Figure 25.264. Various pros and cons of graft selection are given in Table 25.9.

Endoscopic Bone-Patellar Tendon-Bone Autograft Technique

Positioning and Arthroscopic Set-up

Perform a thorough examination under anesthesia, including Lachman, anterior and posterior drawer, varus/valgus and pivot-shift testing. Evaluate external rotation at 30° and 90° of flexion, to assess for posterolateral instability and compare findings to the contralateral knee.

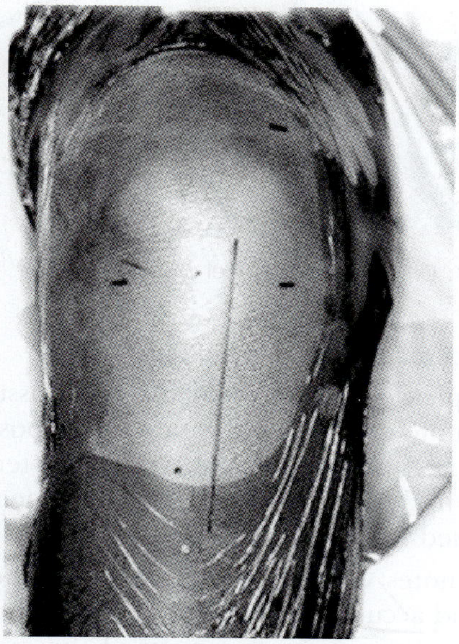

Fig. 25.263: Various portals with skin incision marked

Diagnostic Arthroscopy

Diagnostic arthroscopy consists of evaluation of the suprapatellar pouch, patellofemoral joint, medial and lateral gutters, medial and lateral compartments and the intercondylar notch. Pay particular attention to the menisci, which must be carefully evaluated for the presence of tears. Make all attempts to repair full-thickness longitudinal and bucket-handle tears, generally using an inside-out technique. Partial thickness tears and

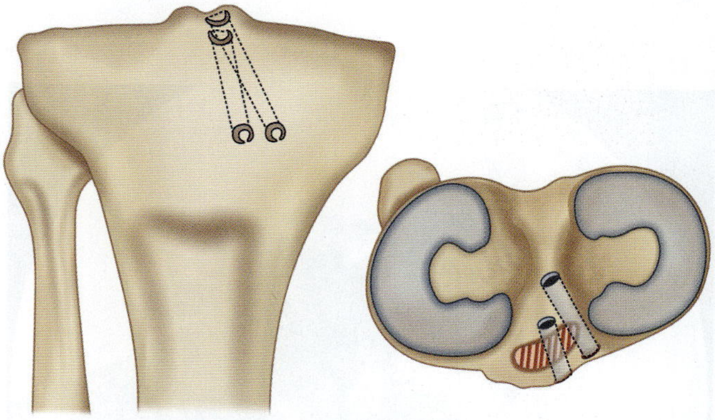

Fig. 25.264: Bunnel suture passed through ACL and sutured through drill holes in tibia

Table 25.9: Pros and cons of graft selection

Graft	*Pros*	*Cons*	*Relative indications and contraindications*
Bone-patellar tendon-bone autograft	Strength Bony fixation Easily harvested Excellent track record	Donor site morbidity Patellar tendinitis Kneeling pain Patella fracture or tendon rupture (rare)	Ind Patient desiring early return to sport Con Patellar instability or tendinitis Occupation requiring prolonged kneeling Narrow (<25 mm) tendon
Bone-patellar tendon-bone allograft	Readily available sources Bony fixation No graft harvest morbidity Faster surgery Smaller incisions No graft sizing difficulties	Possible disease transmission Longer graft incorporation time	Ind Older patient desiring no graft site morbidity and minimal loss of work time Con Younger patient desiring early return to sport
Semitendinosus and gracilis	Small incision Minimal donor site pain Multibundled structure Larger surface area for graft incorporation	Soft tissue fixation Longer graft-to-bone incorporation time Hamstring weakness Can be difficult to harvest Few studies using newer fixation techniques	Ind Pre-existing patellofemoral disease or occupation requiring kneeling Con Inferior result in females (52, 91)
Quadriceps tendon	Small incision Possibly less donor site morbidity strong and large graft	No track record Bony fixation on one side only	Ind Patient desiring autograft tissue with minimal donor site morbidity Con Quadriceps tendinitis or patellofemoral disease

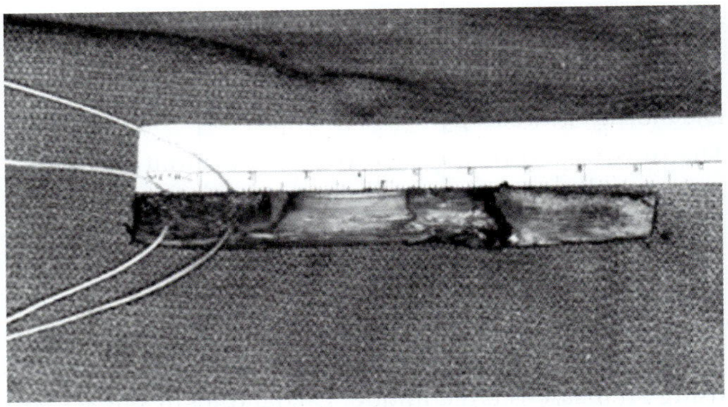

Fig. 25.265: Harvested tendon

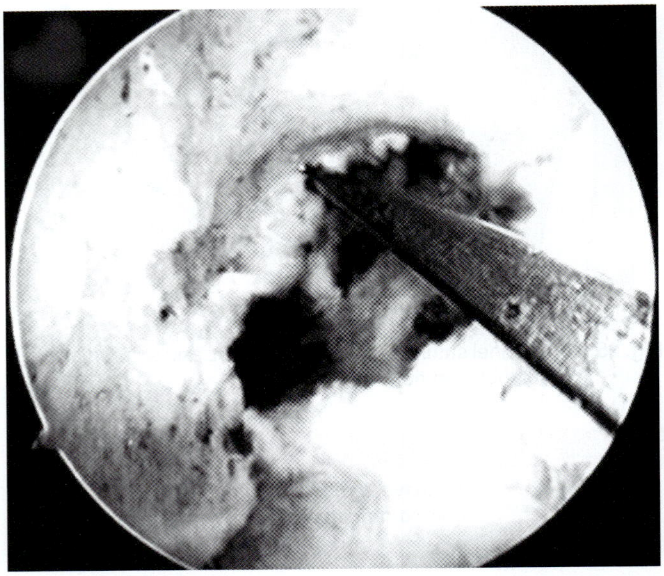

Fig. 25.266: Graft preparation

small tears less than 1 cm that are stable to probing will left alone. Carefully note and grade all articular cartilage injuries.

Visualize the intercondylar notch for evidence of the torn ACL, a long tibial ACL stump scarred to the PCL or roof "vertical strut" sign or failure of the ACL to extend to its normal femoral attachment "empty lateral wall" sign.

Graft Harvest

See Figure 25.265.

Graft Preparation (Fig. 25.266)

Photograph of the harvested tendon. Place two fracture, five ticron sutures in the tibial bone plug and mark the distal cortical surface of the tibial plug with the marking pen. Mark the tendo-osseous junction of the femoral bone plug as well. Bone plugs are approximately 25 mm long, with a tendon length of 42 mm.

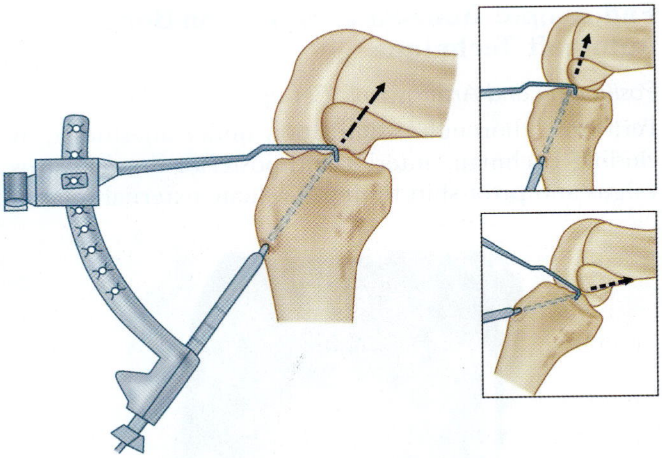

Fig. 25. 267: Different tibial tunnel placements

Notch Preparation and Notchplasty

Arthroscopic view of a right knee. All soft tissue has been cleared out, to ensure visualization of the posterior edge of the notch. A probe is placed over the posterior edge of the femur in the 'over-the-top' position The notchplasty is performed for two purposes.

- It promotes visualization of the 'over-the-top' position and accurate placement of the femoral tunnel
- It helps prevent impingement of the graft with the knee in full extension.

Tibial Tunnel Placement (Fig. 25.267)

A well-placed tunnel will allow for proper endoscopic placement of the femoral tunnel. A tunnel that is too steep (inset B) will preferentially place the femoral tunnel too far anteriorly, whereas a tibial tunnel that is flat (inset C) will tend to place the femoral tunnel too posterior, risking posterior cortical violation. Minor variances may be treated with appropriate flexion of the knee before placement of the "over-the-top" guide and femoral guide pin.

Femoral Socket Placement (Fig. 25.268)

Illustration of a right knee with the "over-the-top" guide placed through the tibial tunnel.

Graft Placement and Fixation (Fig. 25.269)

Use a two-pronged pusher, to guide the graft up the tibial tunnel. Remove the pusher from the tunnel before the tibial bone plug enters its tunnel or the pusher will be difficult to remove. Anteroposterior and lateral views of a right knee, after ACL reconstruction with an endoscopic technique, as shown in Figures 25.270A and B. The lateral view demonstrates proper posterior placement of the femoral tunnel with parallel screw placement. The tibial tunnel enters the joint in the midpoint of the tibial plateau, and the tibial screw is parallel to its bone plug. The AP view confirms parallel screw placement and placement of the femoral socket at the 11 o'clock position.

Endoscopic Hamstring Tendon Technique

The semitendinosus and gracilis tendons have been used effectively in ACL reconstruction for many years. Numerous methods can be used to reconstruct the ACL and the tendons can be folded to produce double, triple or quadruple-stranded graft constructs. Various means of fixation are available, such as suture-post fixation, screws with spiked washers, barbed staple, soft tissue interference screws (both titanium and bioabsorbable), endoscopically placed buttons and cross-pin fixation. Combinations of these techniques are generally used.

Graft Harvest

The semitendinosus and gracilis tendons lie deep to the sartorial fascia, as shown in Figure 25.271. The tendons coalesce at their insertions distally and are more distinct as one palpates posteromedially. The gracilis is proximal to the semitendinosus, and the saphenous nerve crosses the gracilis at the posteromedial joint line. A consistent semitendinosus fascial band arises 7 to 9 cm proximal to the tendon's tibial insertion and inserts into the medial gastrocnemius fascia.

Careful attention is essential, when passing the tendon stripper over the semitendinosus tendon, as illustrated in Figure 25.272. The head of the stripper must pass beneath a fascial sling of the semimembranosus muscle or premature cutting of the semitendinosus will occur.

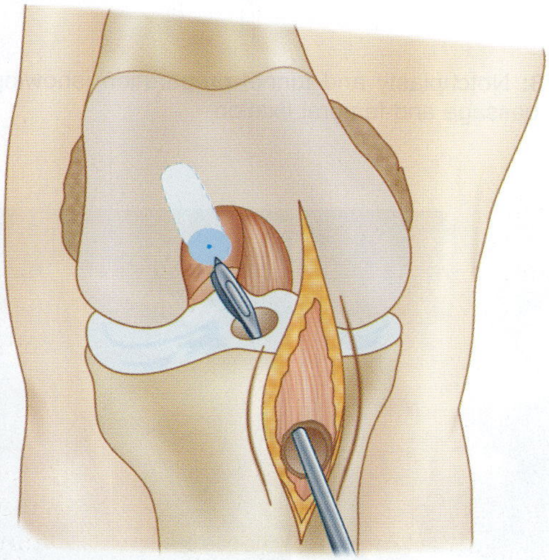

Fig. 25.268: Femoral socket placement

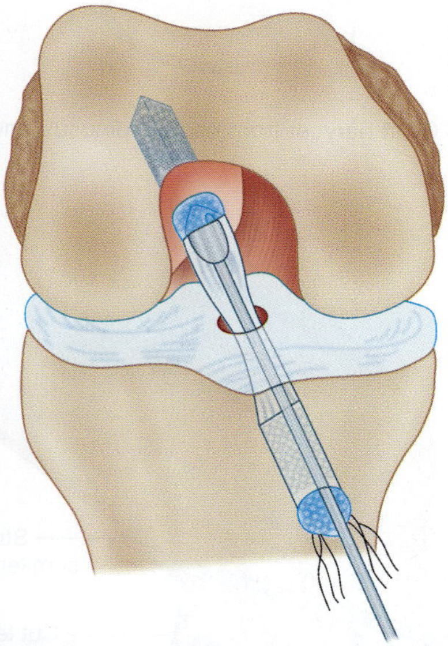

Fig. 25.269: Graft placement and fixation

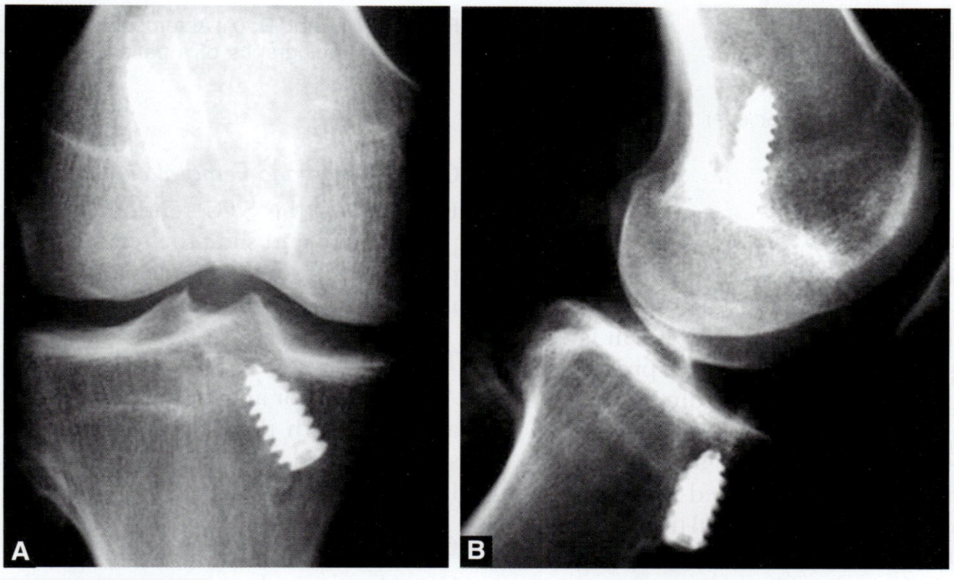

Figs 25.270A and B: X-rays taken after ACL reconstruction—(A) AP view; (B) Lateral view

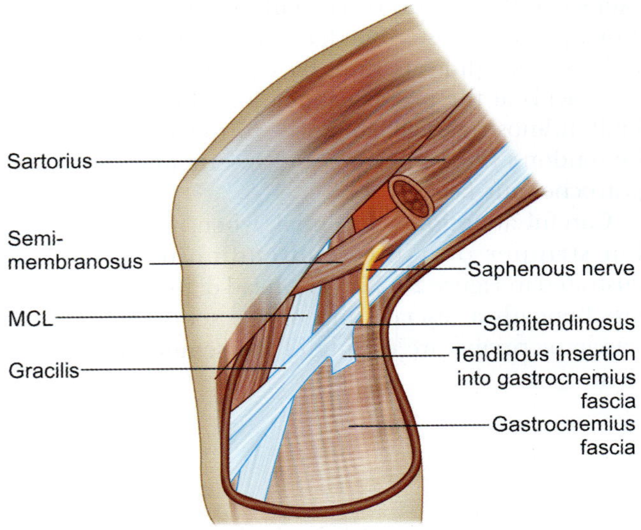

Fig. 25.271: Graft harvest from semitendinosus and gracilis

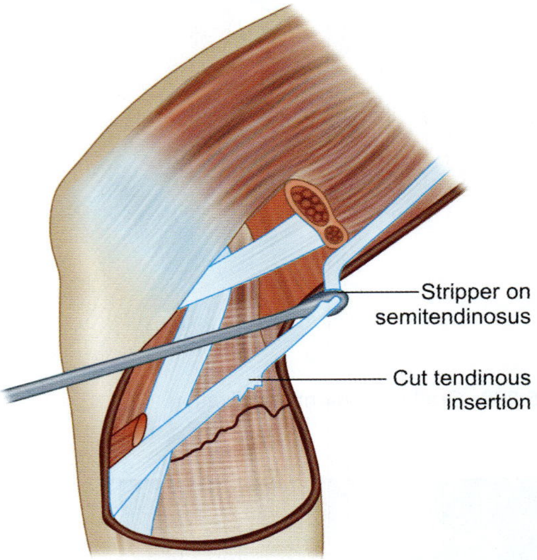

Fig. 25.272: Passing tendon stripper over the semitendinosus tendon for graft harvesting

Graft Preparation

Remove all muscle tissue from both tendons and trim any fascial slips. Place identical baseball stitches on the proximal ends of the tendons. Because 20 cm is usually more than enough tendon length, the thin proximal ends of the tendons may be trimmed accordingly.

Notchplasty and Tunnel Preparation (Fig. 25.273)

A minimal notchplasty should be used for visualization purposes only. Steps to prepare the tibial tunnel and femoral socket are identical to those of the bone to bone (BTB) reconstructive technique described above.

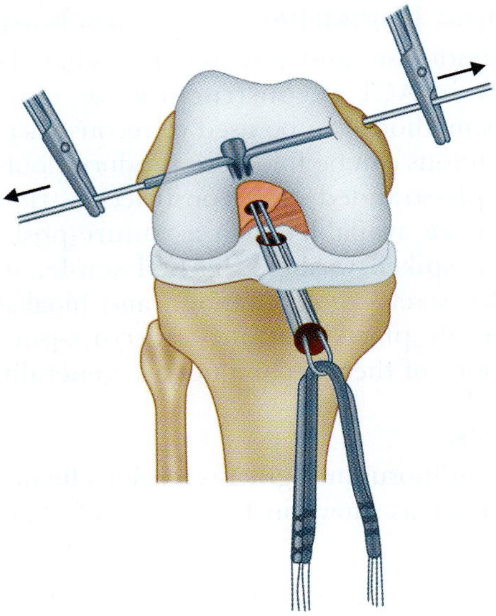

Fig. 25.273: Notchplasty and tunnel preparation, showing graft passage and femoral fixation

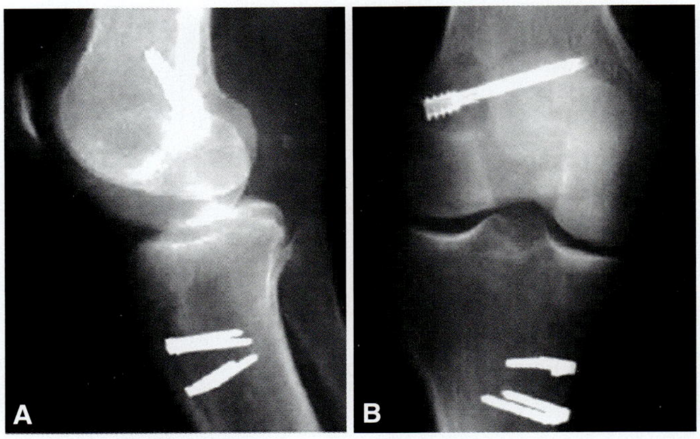

Figs 25.274A and B: (A) Anteroposterior; (B) Lateral postoperative radiographs of a patient, with the TransFix device in place

Graft Passage and Femoral Fixation

Evenly loop the STG tendons around the loop of the passing wire and slide the tendons into their tunnels, by pulling evenly on the medial and lateral ends of the passing wire, as shown in Figure 25.273.

Tibial Fixation (Figs 25.274A and B)

Anteroposterior and lateral postoperative radiographs of a patient, with the TransFix device in place. The tibial side was fixed with two barbed staples in a belt-buckle fashion.

Complications of Surgery

Complications of surgery are shown in Table 25.10.

Table 25.10: Complication and pitfalls of ACL reconstruction and their treatment

Problem	*Incidence*	*Cause*	*Solution*
Anterior knee pain (108)	10-20%	Flexion contracture Donor site morbidity Immobilization	Obtain symmetric knee hyperextension Bone graft patellar defect Early motion
Patellar tendinitis (108)	20% in first year; race afterwards	Donor site morbidity Open-chain rehab	Closed-chain exercises Activity modification
Patella baja	Rare	Immobilization Acute surgery	Accelerated rehab Surgery when full ROM obtained Loosely close tendon defect in flexion (11,12)
Patella fracture	0.35-1.8%	Poor graft harvest Trauma	Careful graft harvest (see above) ORIF (19,28)
Distal femur fracture	Rare	Proximal femoral tunnel in two-incision technique Multiple passes from passing pin in endoscopic technique	Proper orientation of femoral tunnel ORIF (18, 19)
Patella tendon rupture	Rare	Weak remaining tendon trauma	Triangular tibial plug Repair with augmentation (21,47)
Dropped graft	Rare	Poor technique	Soak in 4% chlorhexidine gluconate for 30 min, followed by 30 min soake in triple Abx solution (46) Alternative graft source
Graft laceration during screw placement	Rare	Poor visualization Recessed graft	Graft protector Reverse graft, free bone plug with screw on tibial side (78)
Posterior wall fracture	Rare	Inadequate flexion during socket reaming	Convert to two incision technique (23)
Bone plug fracture	Rare	Inadequate bone plug recession Convergent screw placement	Flip graft, fix tibial side with sutures through tendon fixed to post (± Bioscrew)
Traction suture laceration by screw	Rare	Suture through cortical surface	Sutures through cancellous surface Multiple sutures at different orientations Thin (22G) wire through bone plug
Short hamstring harvesting	1-5%	Poor technique	Shorter femoral socket Tibial fixation with sutures over post Loop only longer graft (cannot do with TransFix) Fix with bioabsorbable screws Use suture and button on femur
Graft impingement	Rare	Improper tibial tunnel placement	Proper planning Increase notchplasty and wallplasty

Postoperative Rehabilitation

The goal of rehabilitation after anterior cruciate ligament surgery is to restore normal joint motion and strength while protecting the ligament graft, this is illustrated in Table 25.11.

■ Posterior Cruciate Ligament Injury

Anatomy of Posterior Cruciate Ligament (Fig. 25.275)

- Intra-articular
- Extrasynovial
- Synovial tissue reflected from posterior capsule.
- Blends distally with posterior capsule and periosteum.
- Average length is 38 mm
- Average width is 13 mm

Femoral Attachment (Figs 25.276 and 25.277)

The posterior cruciate ligament (PCL) attaches proximally to the posterior part of the lateral surface of the medial condyle.

Tibial Attachment

PCL Orientation (Figs 25.278A and B)

- Vertical in coronal plane
- 30° to 45° forward in sagittal plane

Table 25.11: ACL reconstruction rehabilitation checklist

0-2 Weeks

Goals

- Full knee extension ROM
- 90 degrees knee flexion ROM
- Strong QS/SLR without extensor lag
- Emphasize normal gait pattern
- Patellar mobilizations
- Passive extension ROM (emphasize FULL extension)
- Passive, active, and active-assisted ROM knee flexion
- Prone/standing hamstring curls
- QS/SLR all planes (emphasize SLR without extensor lag)
- Electrical stimulation for muscle re-education if poor quadriceps strength
- Begin proprioceptive training (weight shifting BAPS board)
- Edema control
- Partial weight-bearing 50 to 75 percent with crutches or weight-bearing to tolerance with knee immobilizer

2-4 Weeks

Goals

- ROM 0 degrees extension to 120 degrees flexion
- Full weight-bearing without crutches when able to ambulate without limp
- Progress ROM to 120 degrees by 4 weeks
- Progress SLR with weights
- *Bike for ROM:* Begin low resistance program when ROM adequate
- Full weight-bearing without crutches when good quadriceps control and ambulating without limp
- Begin at 2 weeks double leg quarter squats and shuttle squats; progress to single leg
- Begin at 2 weeks leg press (double leg) with light weight and high repetition; progress to single leg
- Lateral step-up (2-4 inches) when able to perform single leg quarter squat
- Wall sits (tibia vertical)
- Hip machine and Hamsting machine when able to perform SLR with 10 pounds. Treadmill with emphasis on normal gait
- Knee extension 90 to 60 degrees with submaximal manual resistance by therapist
- Hip machine and harmstring machine when able to perform SLR with 10 pounds
- Treadmill with emphasis on normal gait
- Knee extension 90 to 60 degrees with submaximal manual resistance by therapist

4-6 Weeks

- Progress to full ROM by 6 weeks
- Begin isokinetic hamstring work at 6 weeks
- Stairmaster (forward/retro)
- Progress closed chain exercises
- Begin high speed isokinetic quadriceps work in 90 to 40 degree range at 6 weeks
- Begin multidirectional lunges at 6 weeks

8-10 Weeks

- Progress above exercises
- Progress isokinetic work
- Begin fitter, slide board, and slow-form running with sport-cord

12-14 Weeks

- Initiate full range knee extension exercises, light weight and high repetition
- Lateral sport-cord drills
- Initiate jogging program if quadriceps strength 65 percent or better
- Initiate light polymetric program if quadriceps strength 65 percent or better, no effusion, full ROM, and knee stable

16-18 Weeks

- Isokinetic strength test for quadriceps and hamstrings
- Progress polymetric program
- Agility training and sport-specific training

5-6 Months

- Retest quadriceps if necessary
- Return to sports determined by physician

Abbreviation: ROM. Range of motion; QS. Quandriceps strengthening; SLR. Straight leg raise

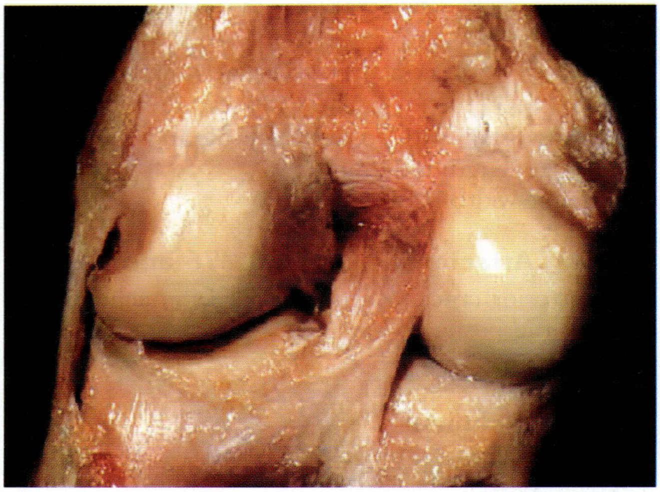

Fig. 25.275: Anatomy of PCL

- It has double the strength of ACL
- Meniscofemoral ligament (Fig. 25.279)

Important Component of PCL Complex

They connect posterior horn of lateral meniscus to the lateral aspect of medial femoral condyle adjacent to origin of PCL

Types

- Ligament of Humphrey
- Ligament of Wrisberg.

Blood Supply and Innervation (Fig. 25.280)

Major blood supply is from the middle genicular artery. PCL is attached posteriorly to the joint capsule, which also contribute to the blood supply. PCL receives its innervation from tibial nerve.

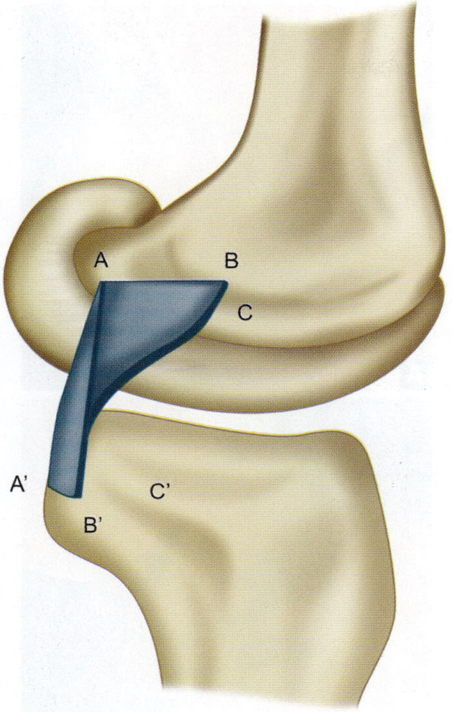

Fig. 25.276: Femoral attachments of ACL. A, B and C denoting attachment of PCL on posterior part of the lateral surface of the medial condyle

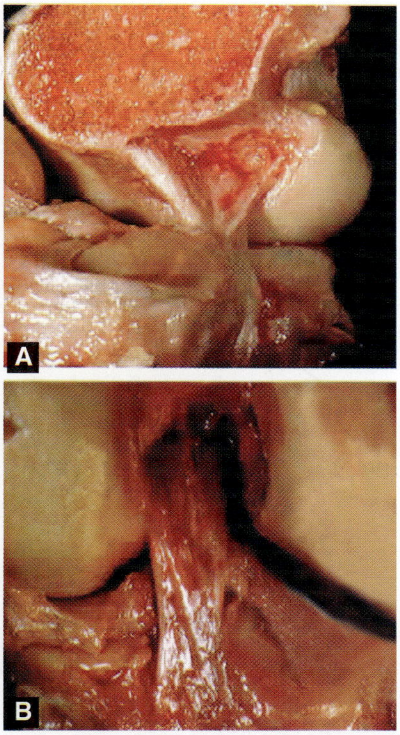

Figs 25.278A and B: PCL orientation—(A) Coronal plane; (B) Sagittal plane

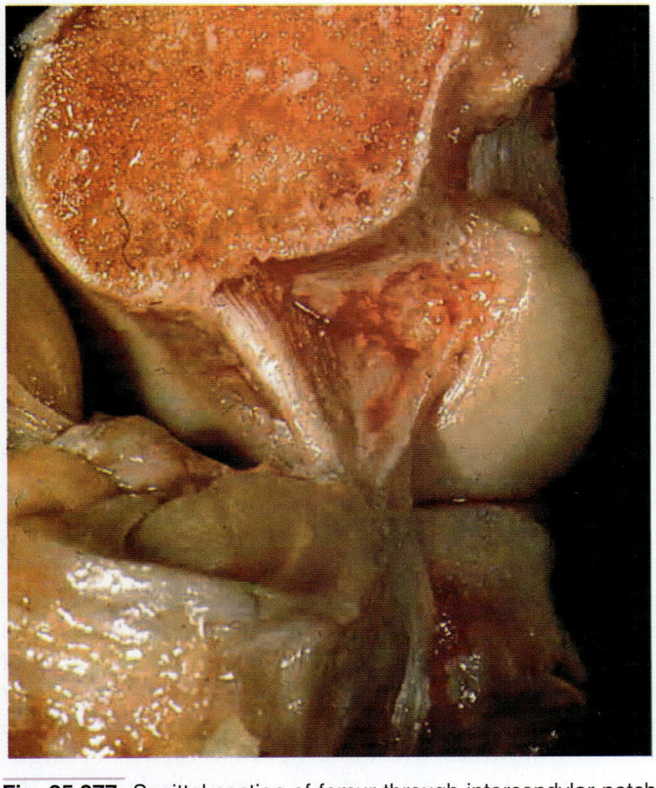

Fig. 25.277: Sagittal section of femur through intercondylar notch showing PCL insertion on medial condyle

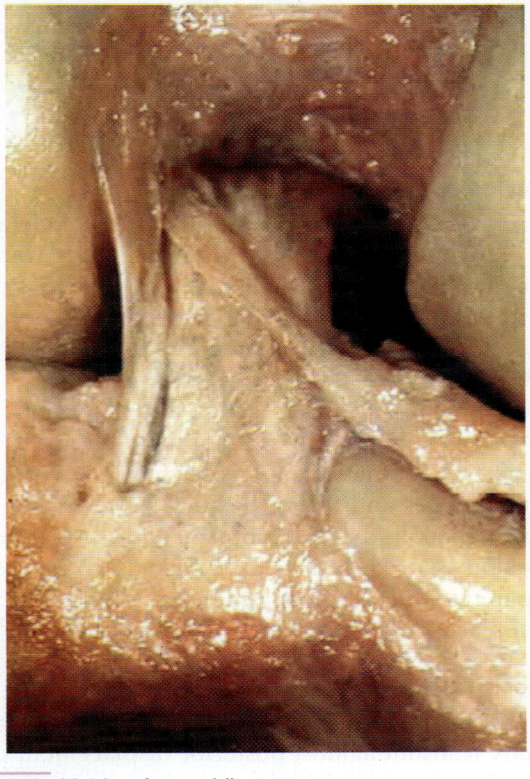

Fig. 25.279: Meniscofemoral ligament

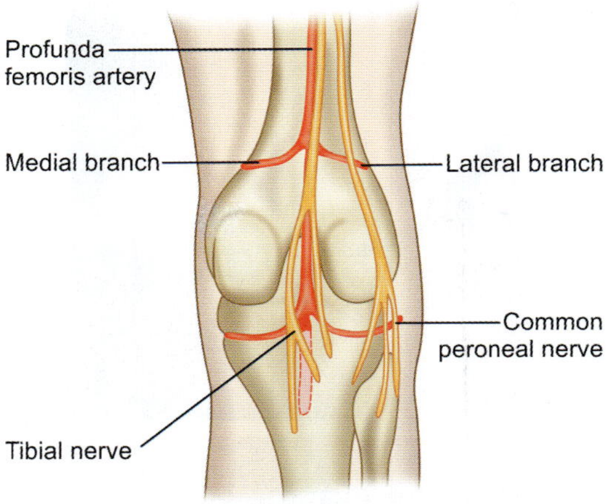

Fig. 25.280: Blood supply and innervation of PCL

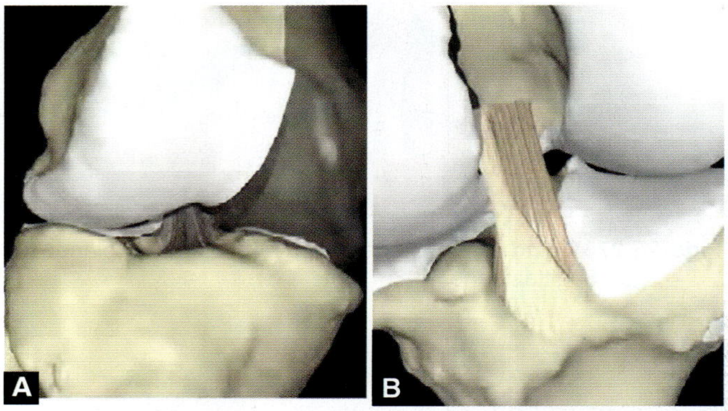

Figs 25.281A and B: Bundles of PCL—(A) Anterolateral bundle; (B) Posteromedial bundle

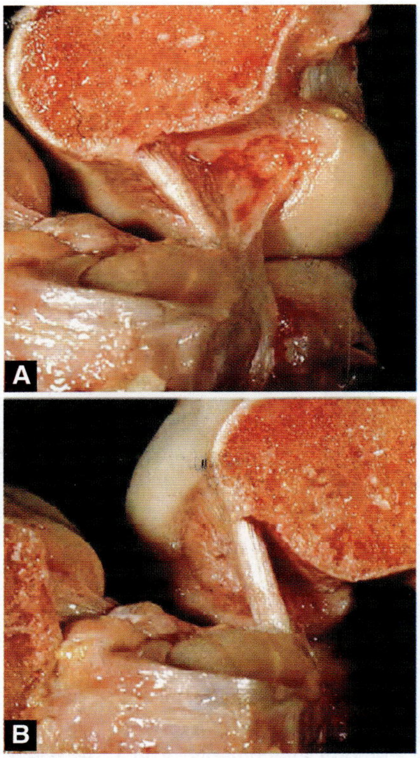

Figs 25.282A and B: Constrain effect by PCL—(A) Anterior fibers, taut in flexion and extension; (B) Posterior (oblique) fibers, taut in extension

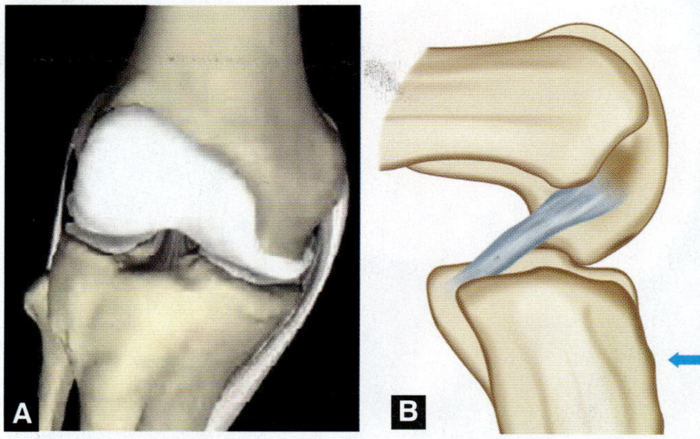

Figs 25.283A and B: PCL as primary restraint against posterior displacement of tibia on the femur

Bundles of PCL

Two sets of nonseparate fibers with anterior fibers being bulk of ligament, as shown in Figures 25.281A and B are anterolateral and posteromedial. Anterolateral is larger than posteromedial bundle.

Constrain Effect (Figs 25.282A and B)

- Anterior fibers, taut in flexion and extension
- Posterior (oblique) fibers, taut in extension.

The PCL isometric zone is narrow. Native PCL has function at 30° and 90° of flexion. A two-strand reconstruction that fills the PCL footprint and allows tightening in flexion is predicted to have increased success rates compared to the traditional single-bundle reconstruction that replaces the anterolateral bundle only.

Function of PCL (Figs 25.283A and B)

The PCL is the major stabilizer of the knee. It provides primary restraint against posterior displacement of tibia on the femur. It acts as a check to hyperextension, only when ACL is ruptured. However, the posterior fibers of the PCL prevent hyperextension. It acts as a secondary restrain to internal tibial rotation during flexion, by winding around the anterior cruciate ligament. In terminal knee extension, the PCL and ACL, with the guidance of the menisci, help externally rotate the tibia to its correct position in relation to the femur (screw home mechanism). Stabilizes the knee against varus or valgus angulation. There is a relation between the PCL and the posterolateral structures of the knee.

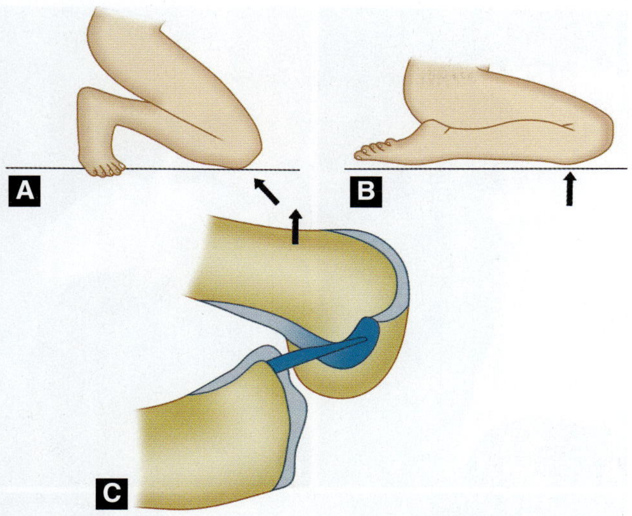

Figs 25.284A to C: PCL injury caused by striking of the flexed tibia on the dashboard in a motor vehicle accident

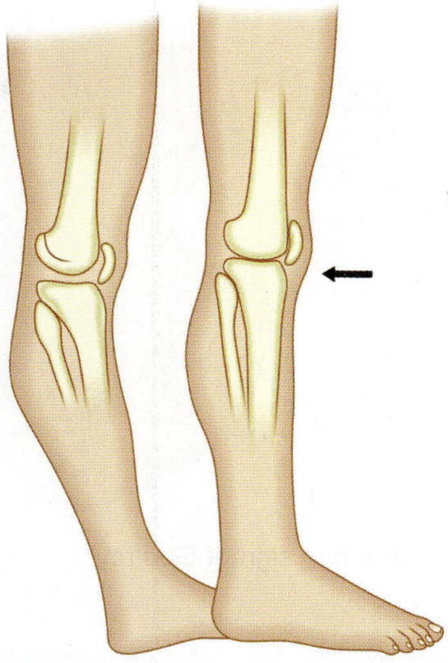

Fig. 25.285: Injury to the PLC results from a blow to the anteromedial proximal tibia, most commonly with the knee in extension

Mode of Injury (Figs 25.284 and 25.285)

As with the anterior cruciate ligament, isolated tears of the posterior cruciate ligament are relatively rare, as a rule ruptures of this ligament are associated with medial or lateral compartment disruptions, especially the latter. Clinically, however isolated tears of the posterior cruciate ligament can be caused by a fall on the flexed knee or striking of the flexed tibia on the dashboard in a motor vehicle accident. Such a mechanism (the upper tibia driven posteriorly with the knee flexed) may produce posterior cruciate ligament disruption as the only clinically detectable instability. Injury to the PLC often results from a blow to the anteromedial proximal tibia, most commonly with the knee in extension, as shown in Figure 25.285.

The result is a varus and rotational moment about the knee. Hyperextension alone or combined with external rotation and knee extension have also been implicated in noncontact injuries to the PLC. These isolated posterior cruciate ligament disruptions can be difficult to diagnose acutely, unless a fragment of bone is avulsed from the posterior tibial insertion and is noted on roentgenograms.

Clinical Features

Acute injury to the PCL may often be missed for several reasons. Often the athlete is unaware of having sustained a significant injury, because many patients have a full range of motion with very little hemarthrosis. Often it is only the posterior drawer test that causes any pain. The presence of a contusion over the proximal anterior tibia may be very helpful in suggesting injury to the PCL. Pain, aching during activity and effusion may be the result of articular cartilage degeneration, which often begins several years before roentgenographic changes are evident.

Posterior cruciate ligament insufficiency consider the problem of functional instability and few emphasize the potential for early degenerative arthritis. The importance of noting the relationship of the proximal tibia to the femur when the knee is flexed to 90° cannot be overemphasized. When the PCL is intact, flexion of the knee to 90° results in the anterior proximal tibia being positioned approximately 1 cm anterior to the distal femoral condyles referred to as a normal anterior step off.

Loss of this normal anterior step off signifies injury to the PCL. The importance of detecting this posterior subluxation has been emphasized by Clancy et al. who state that it is best viewed from the side with the knee flexed to 90°. This posterior subluxation of the proximal tibia with the knee flexed to 90° is also known as the posterior sag sign of Godfrey, as shown in Figure 25.286.

Physical Examination

Posterior Drawer Test (Fig. 25.287)

The true direction of translation of the tibia often is missed. The examiner frequently does not realize that the tibia is starting in a posteriorly subluxed position. The confusion can be prevented by placing both knees in the drawer position (hips flexed 45° and knees flexed 90°), with the examiner's thumbs being placed on the anteromedial joint line of each knee. Normally, there should be 5 to 10 mm of anterior offset of the tibia, relative to the medial femoral condyle. With a posterior cruciate ligament injury, this anterior offset is lost and the tibia appears flush with the femoral condyle, as shown in Figures 25.288A to C.

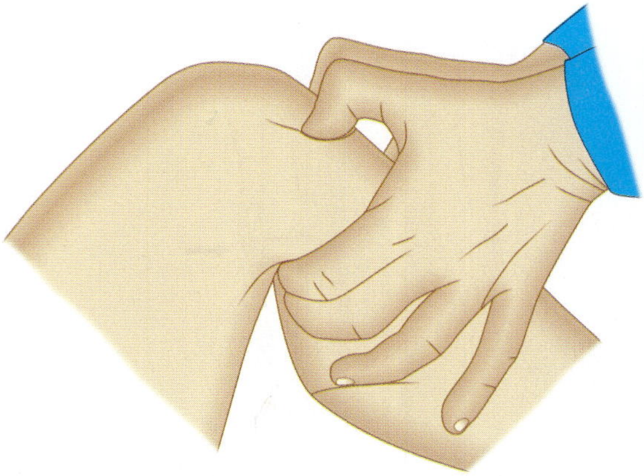

Fig. 25.286: Posterior sag sign of Godfrey

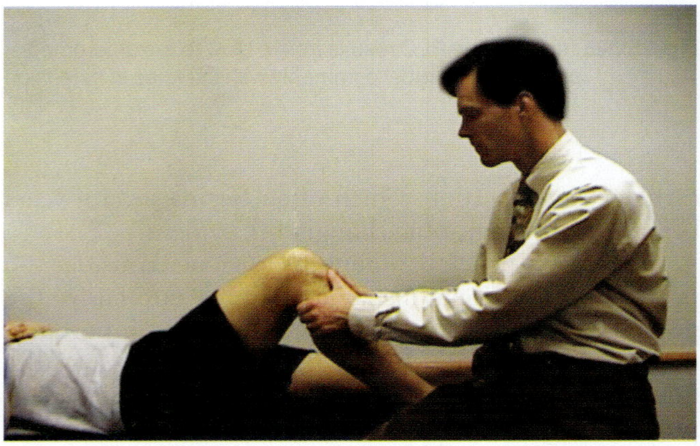

Fig. 25.287: Examiner performing posterior drawer test

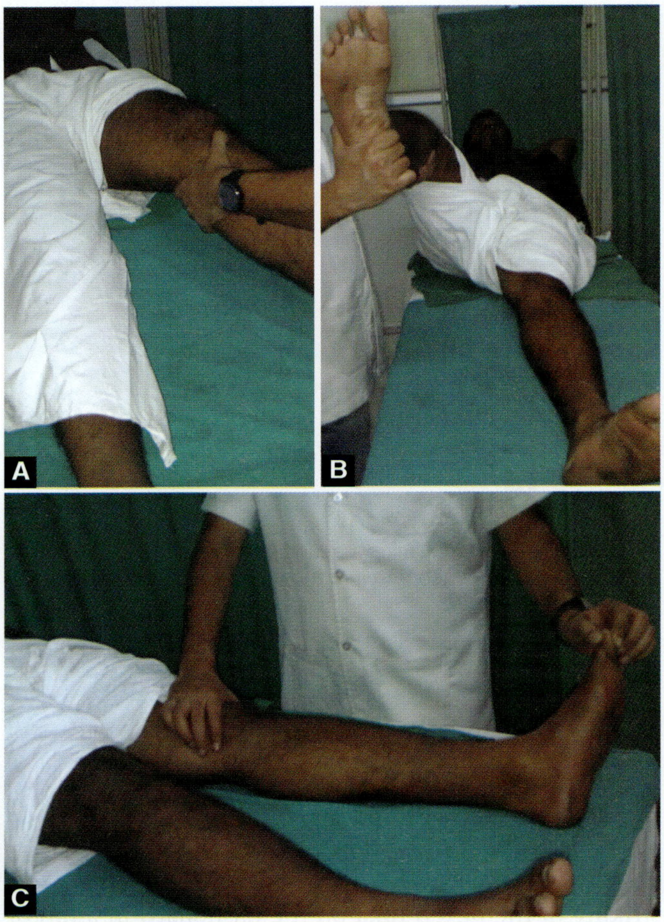

Figs 25.288A to C: Grading of PCL injury

Posterior drawer testing/grading: It includes method of grading the posterior drawer test.

1. This test is graded with respect to the opposite knee. Loss of the normal anterior tibial step off compared with the opposite side, but with the proximal tibial eminence, remaining anterior to the distal femur is considered to be a 1 + posterior drawer.
2. When the proximal tibial eminence can be translated posteriorly to the point, where it is flush with the distal femoral condyles, the posterior drawer is graded 2 +. It is thought to signify complete disruption of the PCL.
3. Translation of the proximal tibial eminence posterior to the distal femoral condyles is considered to be grade 3 + and is thought to signify complete PCL disruption and usually posterolateral ligamentous injury as well. This test, however has been reported to be positive in as few as 10 percent to as many as 76 percent of patients with acute PCL disruptions.

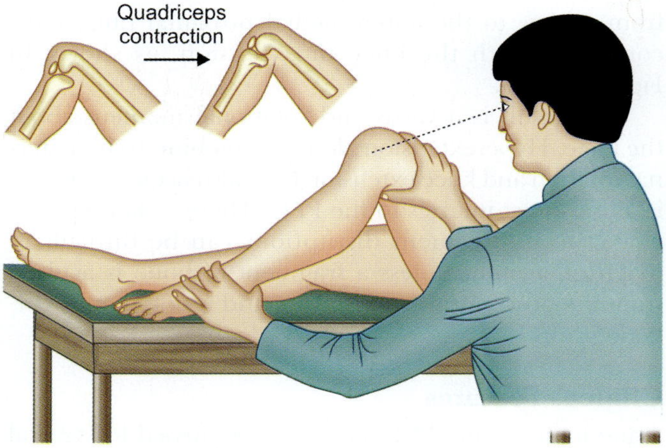

Fig. 25.289: Quadriceps active drawer test

Quadriceps Active Drawer Test (Fig. 25.289)

Due to the presence of muscle spasm, which has been shown to limit the effectiveness of the posterior drawer test in the acute setting, Daniel et al. introduced the quadriceps active drawer test to detect PCL injury. This test is based on the biomechanical relationship between the line of action of the patellar tendon and the resultant quadriceps muscle force. In an intact knee, the line of action of the patellar tendon tends to pull the proximal tibia anterior at low knee-flexion angles. At high knee-flexion angles, the PCL causes the femur to roll back on the proximal tibia and the line of action of the patellar tendon therefore, tends to pull the proximal tibia posterior. The quadriceps-active drawer is performed with the subject relaxed in the supine position, with the knee flexed 70 to 90°. The examiner stabilizes the patient's foot on the table and then asks the patient to slide the foot distally on the table. In the normal knee, the patellar tendon line of action will be directed posteriorly and this quadriceps contraction will not cause any anterior translation of the proximal tibia. In the patient with deficiency of the PCL, however the posterior sag of the proximal tibia results in the line of action of the patellar tendon being directed anteriorly and this quadriceps contraction evokes a notable anterior translation of the proximal tibia.

Rule out injury to the posterolateral structures by the 'dial test', in which external rotation of the tibia at 30° and 90° of knee flexion is compared to that on the opposite side, as shown in Figures 25.290A to C. More than 10° of increased external rotation at 30° is indicative of a posterolateral corner injury and more than 10° of increased external rotation present at 90°, indicates an injury to the posterior cruciate ligament as well.

Routine Radiographs (Fig. 25.291)

Standard anteroposterior, lateral, tunnel and axial patellofemoral views, usually taken in the case of acute PCL injury, often are not diagnostic. The lateral radiograph may show an avulsion of the PCL from its tibial insertion, but this is a relatively uncommon injury. In cases of chronic PCL insufficiency, radiographs may show evidence of arthrosis of the medial and patellofemoral articulations. Lateral radiograph of the knee demonstrating avulsion of the insertion of the PCL from the tibia. Stress roentgenography assists in the diagnosis of the posterior cruciate ligament injuries and a lateral roentgenogram taken of each knee in 70° of flexion. Increased posterior translation of 8 mm or more in stress roentgenograms is indicative of complete rupture.

Magnetic Resonance Imaging (Figs 25.292A and B)

Magnetic resonance imaging (MRI) has greatly increased the accuracy, with which acute ligamentous injuries of the knee may be detected and correctly diagnosed and has allowed the detection of other associated injuries to the menisci, cartilage and subchondral bone. Not only can MRI confirm suspected injury to the PCL, it can also determine the site of injury to the ligament. MRI may show a lesion in continuity of the PCL.

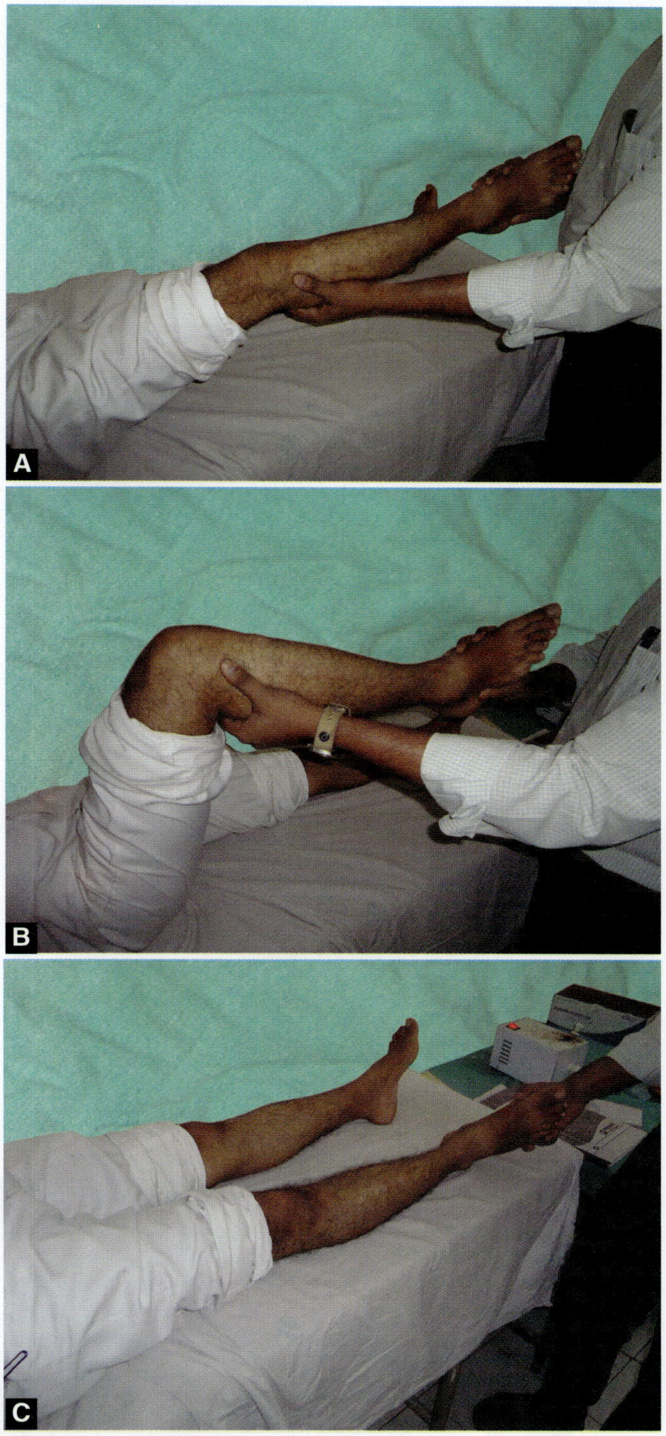

Figs 25.290A to C: Ruling out injury to the posterolateral structures by the 'dial test'

Bone Scan

A bone scan may be helpful in evaluating the progress of a patient with pain and isolated PCL insufficiency. Serial bone scanning may allow early diagnosis of changes of the articular cartilage in the patient, who is being treated nonsurgically.

Treatment

The treatment of the knee with a PCL injury is controversial. Recommendations have been made for both surgical and nonsurgical management, treatment plan is shown in Flow chart 25.2.

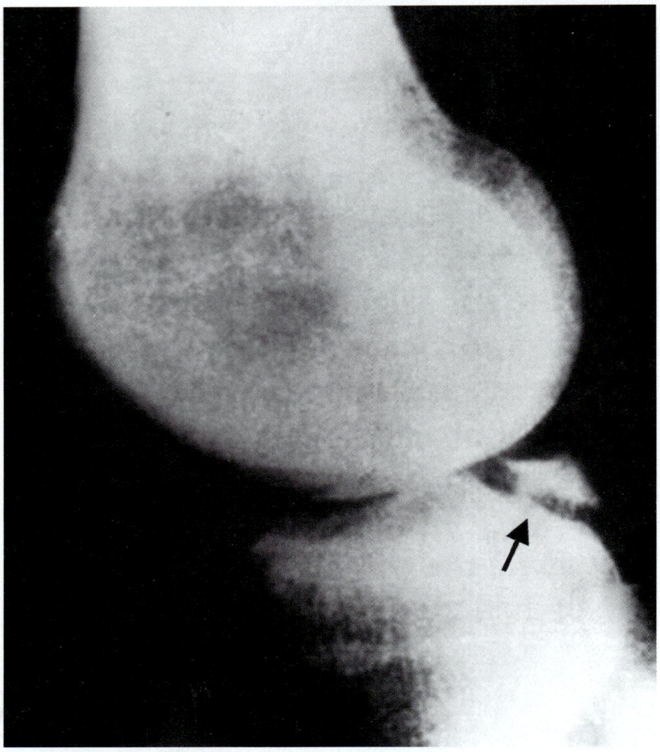

Fig. 25.291: Stress roentgenography to detect PCL tear

Nonoperative Treatment

The commonly quoted criteria for nonoperative treatment include:

- A posterior drawer of less than 10 mm with the tibia in neutral rotation (posterior drawer excursion decreases with internal rotation of the tibia on the femur).
- Less than 5° of abnormal rotary laxity (specifically, abnormal external rotation of the tibia with the knee flexed 30°, indicating posterolateral instability).
- No significant valgus-varus abnormal laxity (no associated significant ligamentous injury).

When the PCL is torn, the patella and patellar tendon take on a more prominent role in the prevention of posterior tibial translation. Also, the increased posterior tibial sag that occurs in the PCL deficient knee, shortens the moment arm of the quadriceps, decreasing its mechanical advantage. Therefore, nonoperative

Flow chart 25.2: Recommendations for both surgical and nonsurgical management

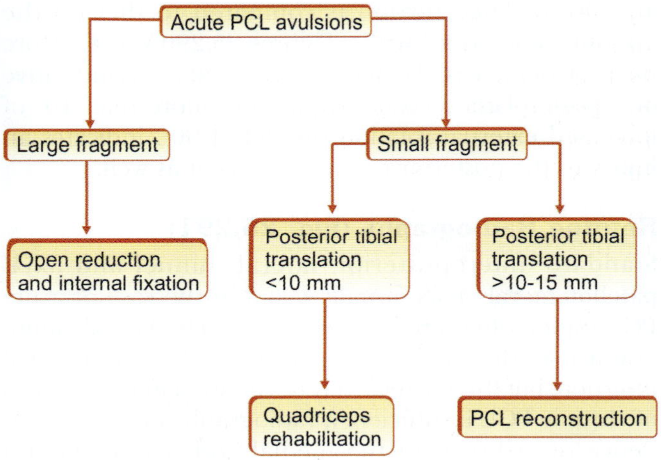

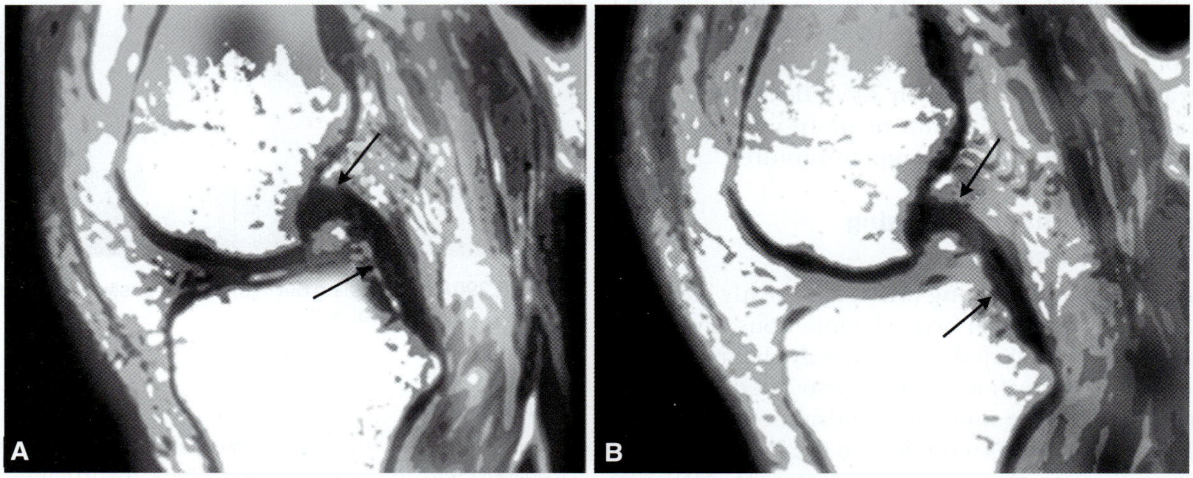

Figs 25.292A and B: Proton-dense sagittal image—(A) T2-weighted sagittal image; (B) An extensive tear involving the proximal and distal portion of the PCL (Arrows)

management of PCL injuries should emphasize quadriceps strengthening, as a key component of the rehabilitation program.

In grade I PCL injuries, a cylindrical cast is given with knee in 10 to 15° of flexion with anterior translation of tibia and gagging the popliteal region with pads, in order to avoid the posterior sagging of tibia. Cast given for 6 to 8 weeks.

Treat undisplaced fractures with immobilization of the knee in extension, using the intact collateral ligaments to help prevent posterior sag. The rehabilitation program employed for the patient with PCL injury involves three phases:

- A maximum protection phase, which is used during the first 2 weeks following injury
- A moderate protection phase, used from week 4 to 6 weeks after injury
- A minimal protection phase, used 6 to 8 weeks after injury.

Surgical Management (Figs 25.293 to 25.295)

Patients with injury to another major knee ligament, in addition to the PCL as well as those with isolated PCL injuries, who continue to have pain or instability, despite use of the above rehabilitation program for at least 3 months, require evaluation for surgical reconstruction.

Avulsion fractures of the tibial insertion of the PCL: The surgical procedure is shown in Figures 25.294 and 25.295.

Reconstruction of PCL, using patellar tendon V graft (Figs 25.296 and 25.297)

Reconstruction of posterior cruciate ligament (using bone-patellar tendon or bone or tendo calcaneus-bone grafts) (Figs 25.297A to C)

Olecranization of patella: This is done to prevent posterior sag of tibia on femur, which would stress graft, as shown in Figure 25.298.

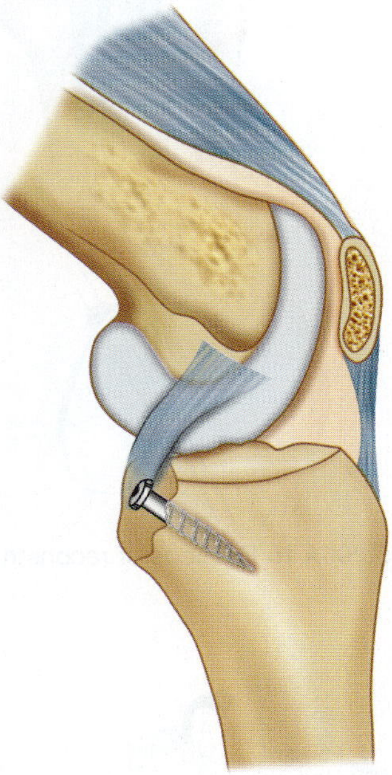

Fig. 25.294: Surgical fixation of avulsion fractures of the tibial insertion of the PCL

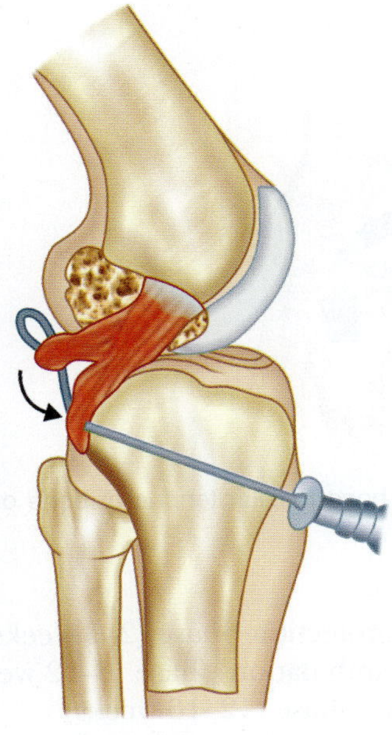

Fig. 25.293: Surgical reconstruction of PCL

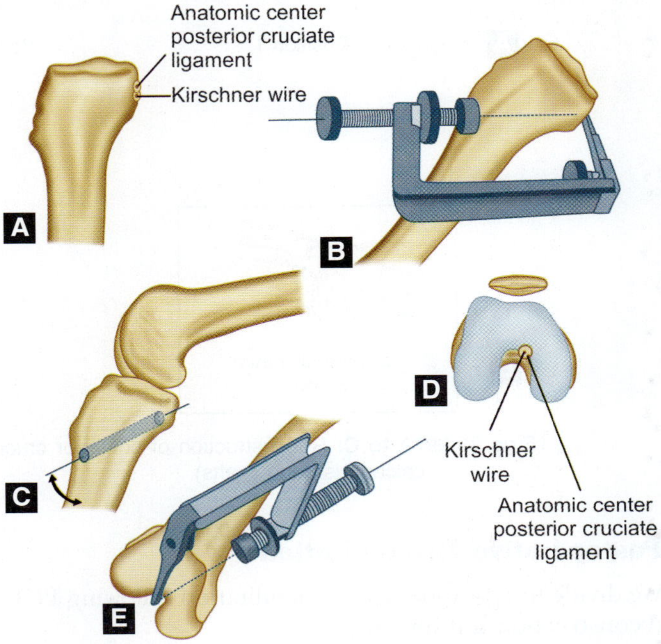

Figs 25.295A to E: Steps of surgical fixation of avulsion fractures of the tibial insertion of the PCL

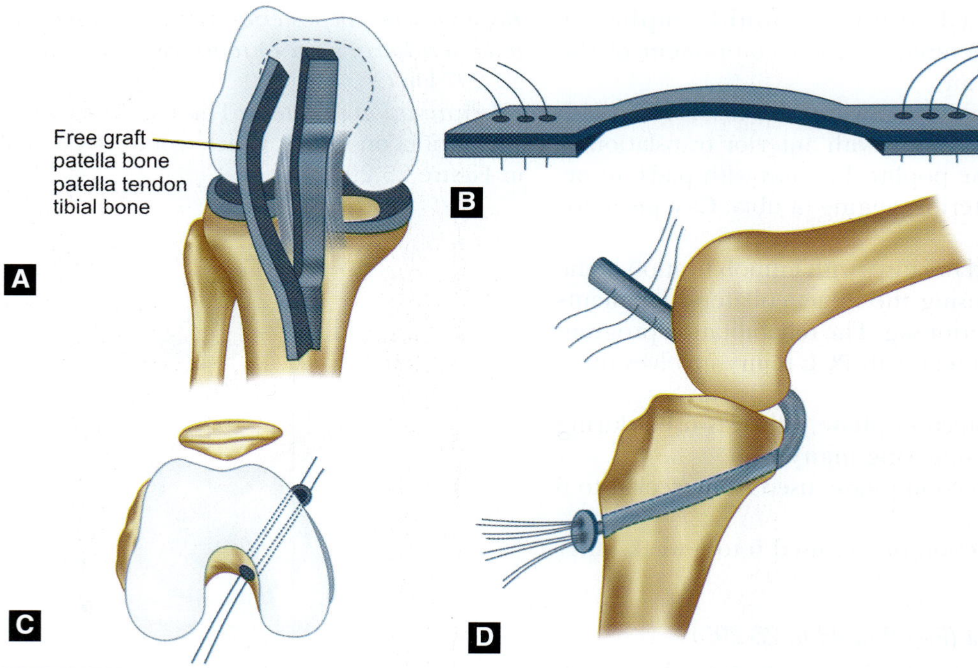

Figs 25.296A to D: Steps of reconstruction of PCL, using patellar tendon 'V' graft

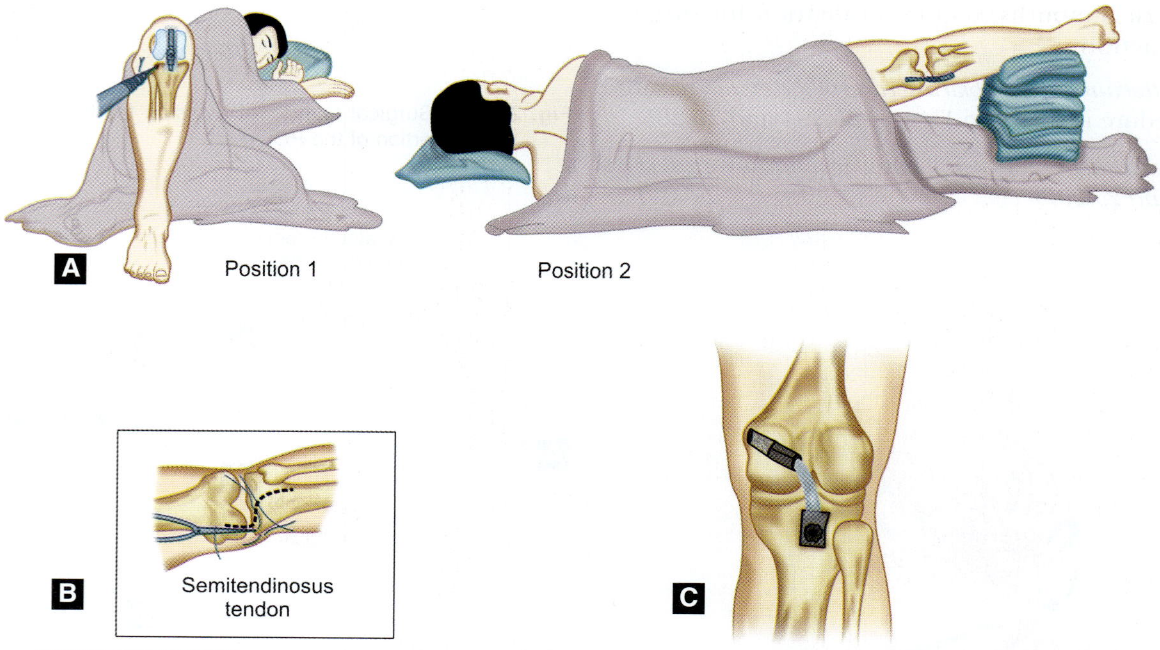

Figs 25.297A to C: Reconstruction of posterior cruciate ligament (using bone-patellar tendon or bone or tendo calcaneus-bone grafts)

Postoperative Rehabilitation

We divide the postoperative rehabilitation following PCL reconstruction into five phases:

- Immediate postoperative phase (first 2 weeks after surgery)
- Maximum protection phase (2–6 weeks)
- Controlled ambulation phase (6–12 weeks)
- Light activity phase (12–16 weeks)
- Return-to-activity phase (16–24 weeks)

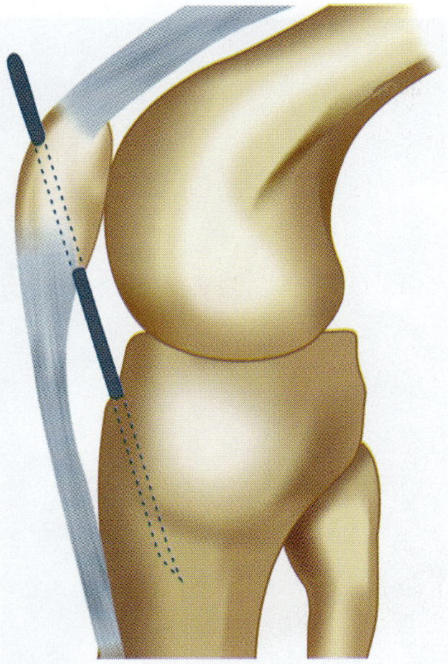

Fig. 25.298: Olecranization of patella

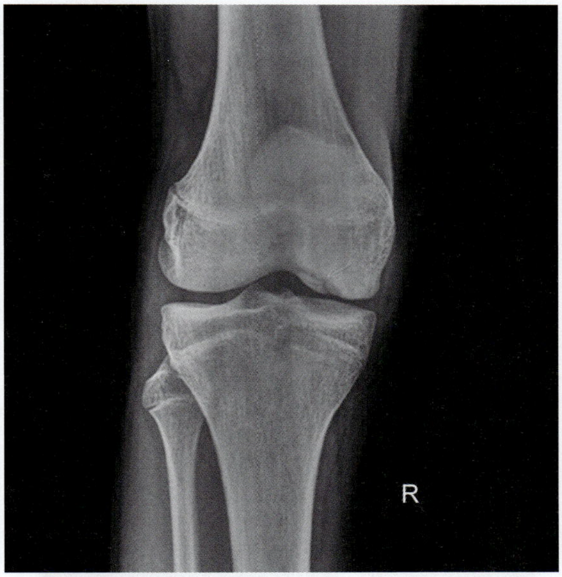

Fig. 25.299: Osteochondritis

Immediate postoperative phase: In the immediate postoperative phase, encourage the patient to bear 50 percent of weight as tolerated, using two crutches and to perform ankle and hip exercises and knee extensions from 60°-0°.

Maximum protection phase: During the maximum protection phase, proceed with full weight-bearing, multiangle quad isometrics at 60°, 40° and 20° leg press and squats from 0°-60° and well-leg bicycling. By 4 weeks, range of motion should be to 90° and bicycling can be encouraged for range of motion and endurance. Begin pool exercises at 5th week.

Controlled ambulation phase: The controlledambulation phase aims to increase quadriceps strength by initiating swimming, closed-kinetic-chain rehabilitation, and a stretching program. By week 12, begin lateral step-ups, cycling for endurance (30 minutes), hamstring curls from 0° to 60° with low weight and a walking program.

Light activity phase: The lightactivity phase continues with the above exercises and allows a light running program.

Return-to-activity phase: By 5 to 6 months after the surgery, the patient can return to sports activities.

OSTEOCHONDRITIS, CHONDROMALACIA PATELLA AND SYNOVIAL CHONDROMATOSIS

■ Osteochondritis

Also called as osteochondrosis. It is shown in Figure 25.299. It is a condition, in which there is compression, fragmentation or separation of small segment of articular cartilage and bone. Affected area shows, features of ischemic necrosis, including death of bone cells in the osteoarticular fragment, reactive vascularity and osteogenesis in the surrounding bone.

Types

- Crushing osteochondritis
- Splitting osteochondritis
- Pulling osteochondritis (tractio apophysitis).

Crushing Osteochondritis

It is usually seen in adolescence. Characterized by spontaneous necrosis of the ossific nucleus in a long bone epiphysis or one of the cuboidal bones of the wrist or foot.

Pathological Changes

These are same as those in other forms of osteonecrosis, i.e. bone death, fragmentation, distortion of the necrotic segment or reactive new bone formation around the ischemic trabeculae.

Examples

- Freiberg's disease of second metatarsal bone, as shown in Figure 25.300
- Kohler's disease of the navicular bone, as shown in Figures 25.301A and B
- Kienbock's disease of the carpal lunate, as shown in Figure 25.302
- Panner's disease of the capitulum.

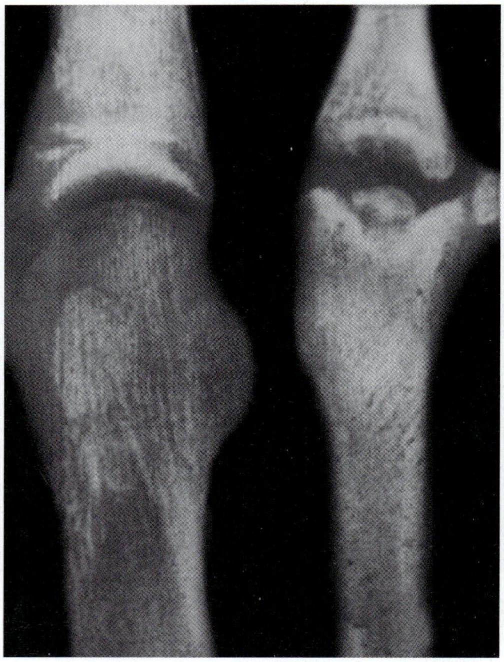

Fig. 25.300: Freiberg's disease of second metatarsal bone

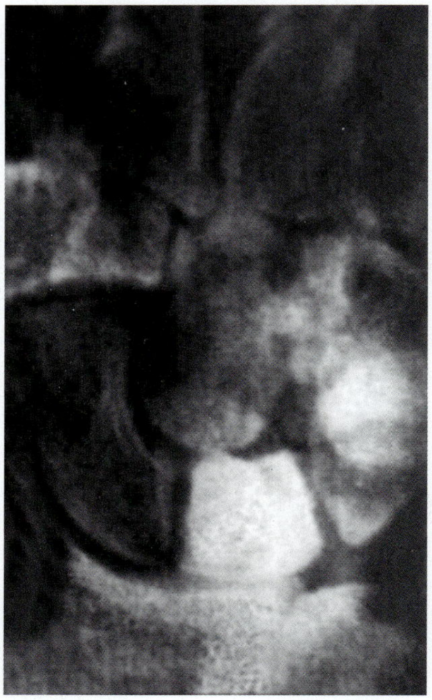

Fig. 25.302: Kienbock's disease of the carpal lunate

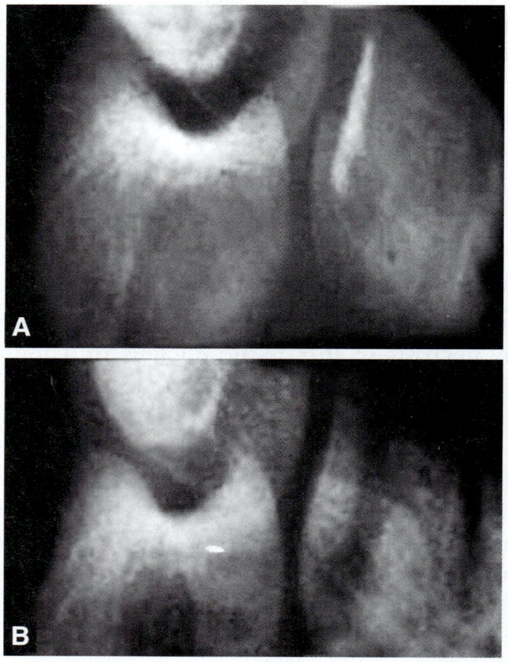

Figs 25.301A and B: Kohler's disease of the navicular bone

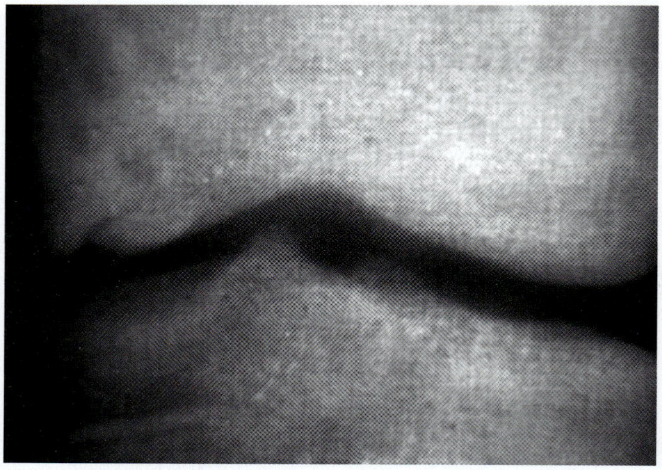

Fig. 25.303: Lateral surface of medial femoral condyle in the knee

Splitting Osteochondritis

Also called as osteochondritis dissecans. A small segment of articular cartilage and the subjacent bone may separate as an avascular fragment. Occurs typically in young adults, usually men are affected.

Location

Affects particular sites:

- Lateral surface of medial femoral condyle in the knee and lateral condyle (Fig. 25.303)
- Humeral capitulum (Fig. 25.304)
- Anteromedial corner of the talus in the ankle, as shown in Figure 25.305
- Patella (posterior aspect in the lower medial quadrant) (Fig. 25.306)
- Superomedial part of the femoral head
- First metatarsal head.

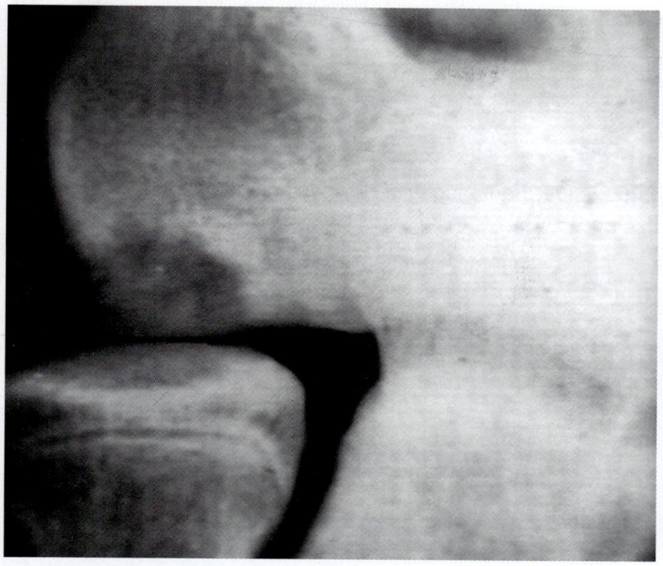

Fig. 25.304: Humeral capitulum

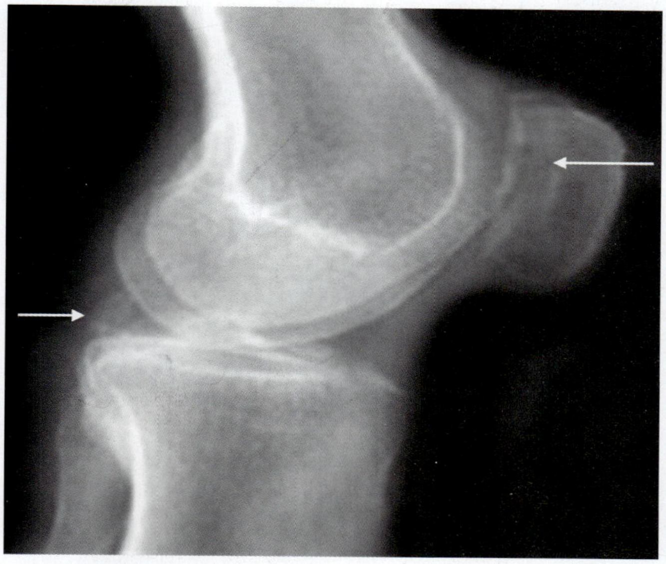

Fig. 25.306: Patella

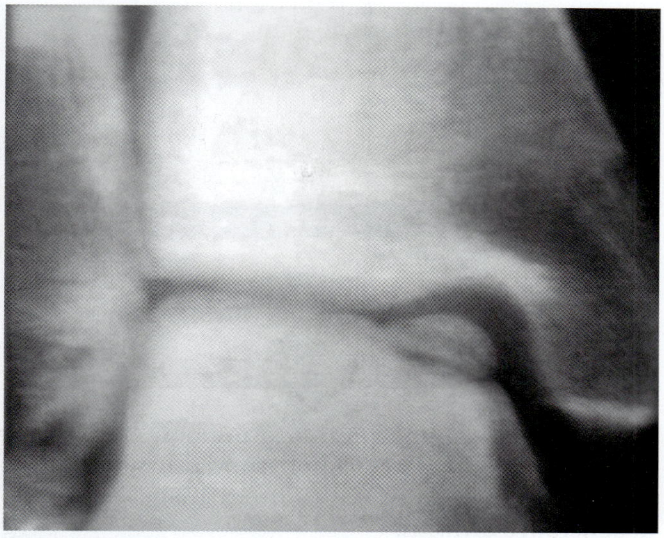

Fig. 25.305: Anteromedial corner of the talus in the ankle

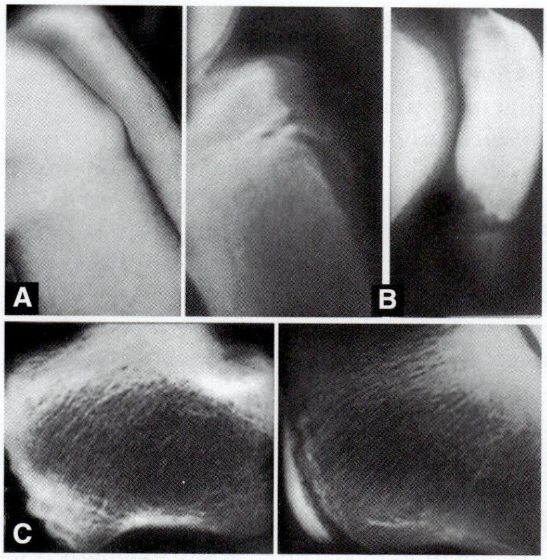

Figs 25.307A to C: Larsen Johannson disease of patella

Pulling Osteochondritis

Also called as traction apophysitis. It is seen in:

- The tibial tuberosity (Osgood-Schlatters disease)
- Calcaneal apophysis (Sever's disease)
- Larsen Johansson disease of patella, as shown in Figures 25.307A to C.

■ Osteochondritis Dissecans (Fig. 25.308)

Introduction

Defined as a condition of unknown etiology, occurring in children and adolescents. Characterized by the development of a small segment of necrotic subchondral bone in a joint. It results from, loss of blood supply to an area of bone beneath the cartilaginous surface of the joint.

In 1558, Ambroise Paré, removed loose bodies from a knee joint.

In 1870, Paget described 'quiet necrosis', within the knee.

In 1887, Koing, coined the term 'osteochondritis dissecans'. He proposed, this condition was caused by spontaneous necrosis due to trauma. Knee joint is most commonly affected. Other joints such as, the hip, ankle, elbow and patella are infrequently involved.

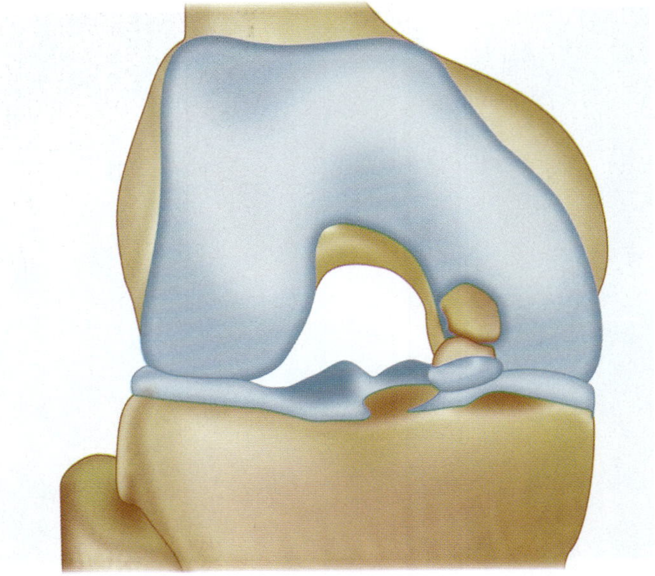

Fig. 25.308: Osteochondritis dissecans (OCD)

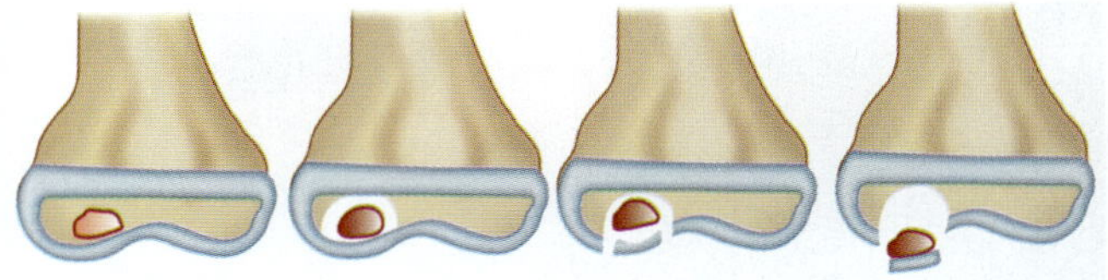

Fig. 25.309: Four stages of development of OCD

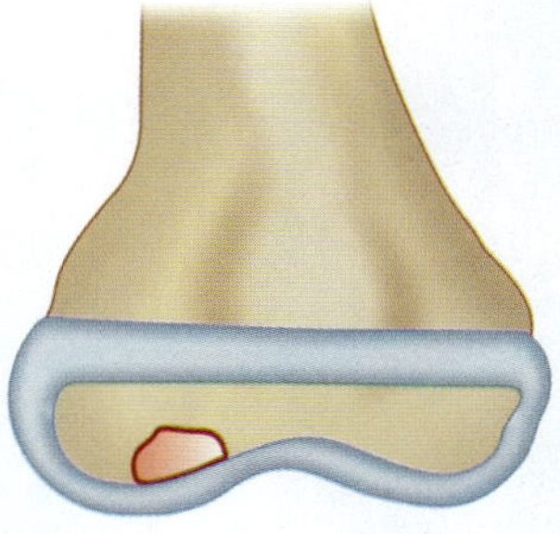

Fig. 25.310: Stage I of OCD

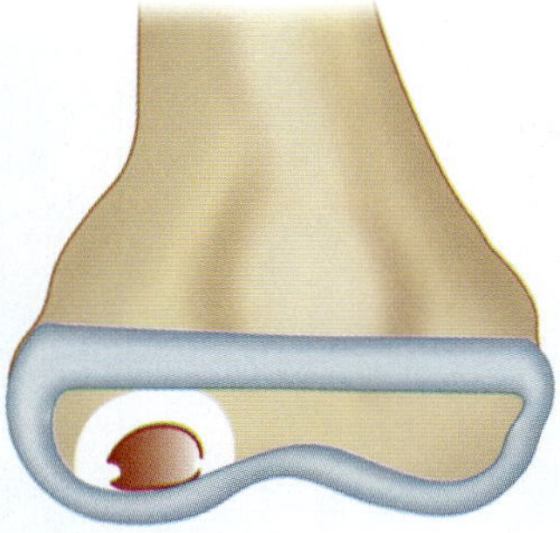

Fig. 25.311: Stage II of OCD

Etiology

- Unknown
- Exogenous trauma
- *Endogenous trauma:* As impact from the tibial spine can occur, with violent internal rotation of the tibia
- Ischemia, by thrombus or embolus
- Abnormal ossification within the physis
- Constitutional or genetic predisposition
- Combination of above.

Incidence

Sex ratio: Male to female (2:1)

Age: Children and adolescents (10–20 years). Knee joint, most commonly affected (75%).

Site: Lateral surface of medial femoral condyle (85%), near the attachment of posterior cruciate ligament (PCL). 20–30 percent may be bilateral.

Other sites: Patella (posterior aspect, in the lower medial quadrant). Anteromedial corner of the talus in the ankle. Superomedial part of femoral head, humeral capitulum and the first metatarsal head.

Pathogenesis

The picture is one of aseptic necrosis. Repitative trauma deprived of a small fragment of its blood supply. Osteocyte begins to degenerate and marrow elements are transformed to amorphous debris. Capillaries invades the necrotic area. New bone replaces necrotic bone by creeping substitution. Overlying cartilage remains viable, as it receives its nutition from synovial fluid. Continuous motion, causes cartilage to disintegrate and the fragment is extruded out of in the joint. It forms loose body, which remains attach by a pedicle of synovial tissue. The residual cavity get filled with fibrocartilage leading to degenerative arthritis.

Pathophysiology (Fig. 25.309)

Once a lesion is present, it typically progresses through four stages unless appropriately treated.

Stage I: Consists of a small area of compression of subchondral bone, as shown in Figure 25.310.

Stage II: Consists of a partially detached osteochondral fragment. A radiograph of the bone may reveal a well-circumscribed area of sclerotic subchondral bone separated from the remainder of the epiphysis by a radiolucent line. This is shown in Figure 25.311.

Stage III: Lesions are the most common and consist of a completely detached fragment that remains within the underlying crater bed, as demonstrated in Figure 25.312.

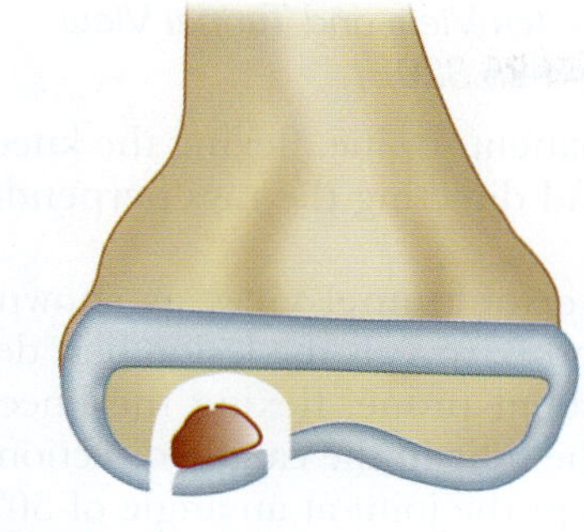

Fig. 25.312: Stage III of OCD

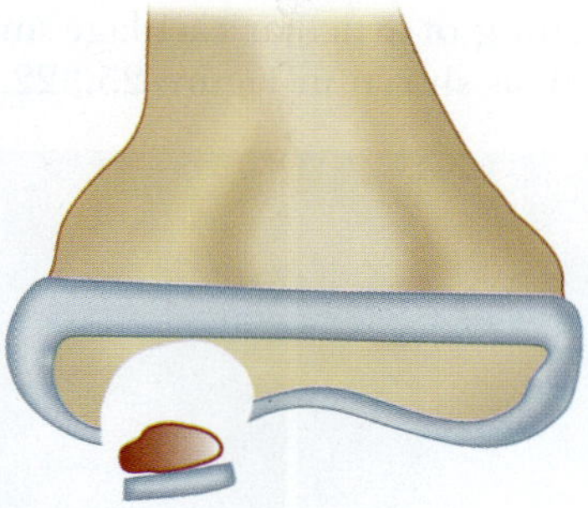

Fig. 25.313: Stage IV of OCD

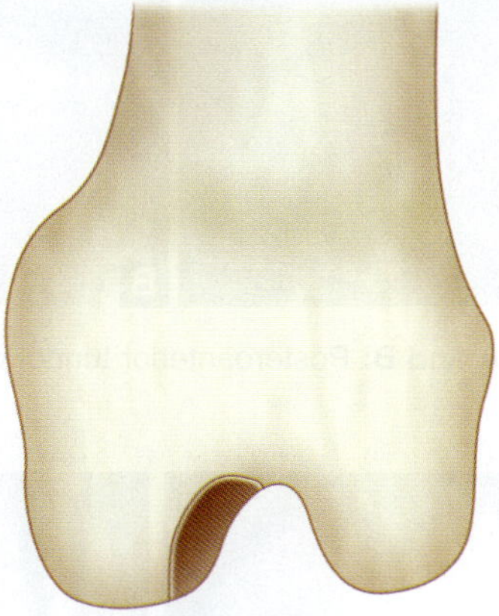

Fig. 25.314: Lesion over lateral surface of medial condyle (classical)

Stage IV (Fig. 25.313): Lesions consist of a completely detached fragment that is completely displaced from the crater bed. This is also termed a loose body.

Site of Lesion of Osteochondritis of Knee (Figs 25.314 to 25.318)

Clinical Features

- Pain is the most common symptom
- Clicking sound
- Locking, in variable positions

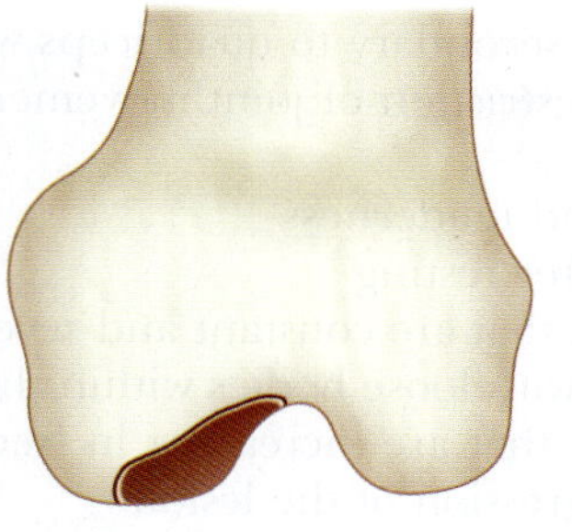

Fig. 25.315: Extended classical lesion

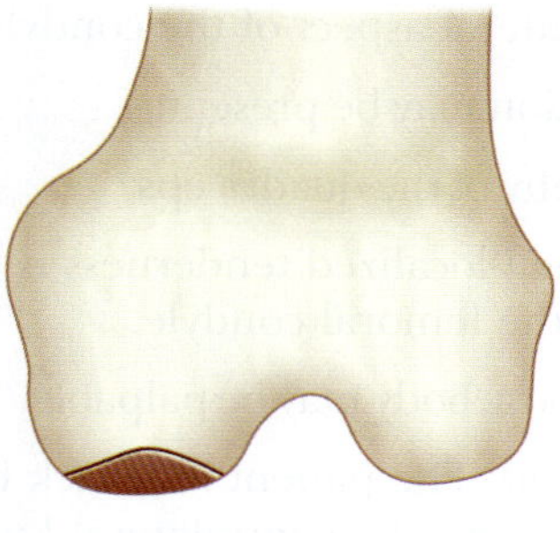

Fig. 25.316: Inferocentral region of medial condyle

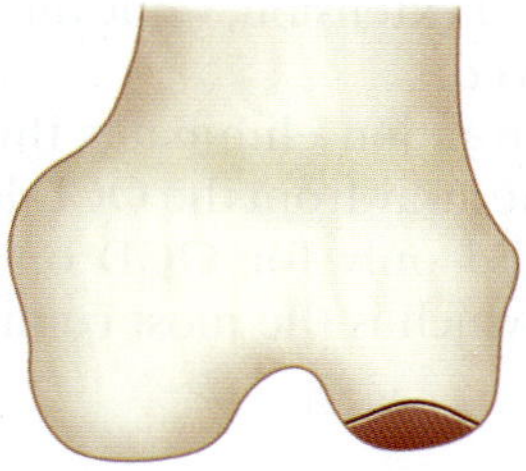

Fig. 25.317: Inferocentral region of lateral condyle

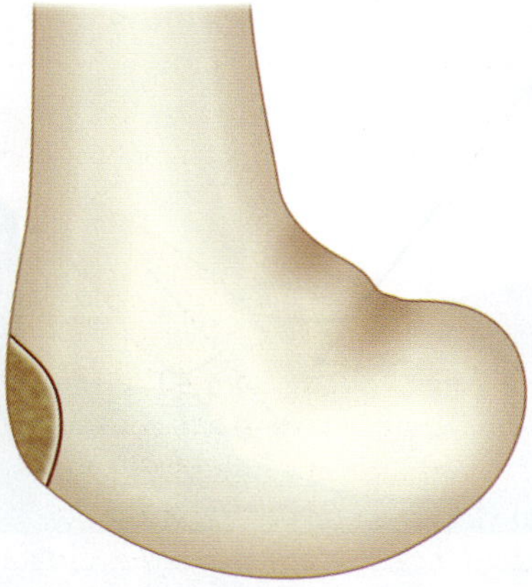

Fig. 25.318: Lesion on the anterior condylar surface

- Givingway, secondary to quadriceps weakness
- Terminal restriction of joint movement
- Limping
- Swelling and tenderness
- Stiffness after resting
- Symptoms, that are constant and severe are typically associated with loose bodies within the knee.
- Symptoms, that are increasing in frequency may indicate progression of the lesion.

On Examination

Gait: The affected leg may be externally rotated, during gait, in an attempt to avoid impingement of the tibial spine, on the lateral aspect of the condyle.

Effusion: Effusion may be present.

Atrophy: Atrophy of the quadriceps.

Tenderness: Well localized tenderness is found, by deep pressure over the femoral condyle.

Loose body: Loose body may be palpable.

Range of motion: The patient may lack full knee extension, compared with the contralateral knee.

Wilsons Sign

- Knee is flexed to 90° and internally rotated. On extension of knee, patient complains of pain at about 25° to 30° of extension, while on external rotation pain gets relieved.
- External rotation eliminates the pain, by taking the tibial spine away from the OCD lesion. Therefore, this test is valid only for OCD on the medial femoral condyle, which is the most common area in the knee for OCD.

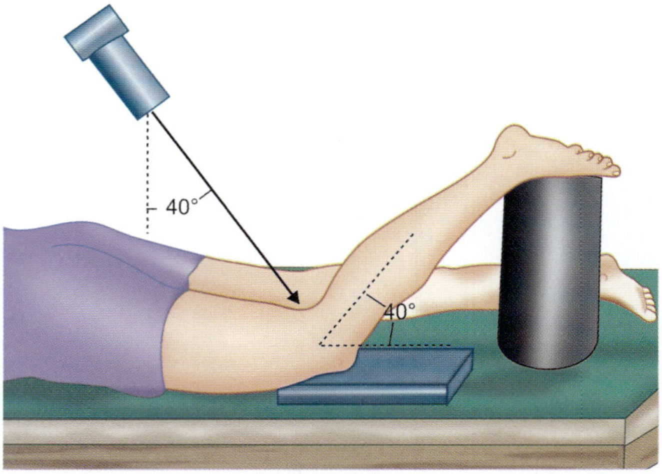

Fig. 25.319: Intercondylar notch view

Intercondylar Notch View and Tunnel View (Figs 25.319 and 25.320)

- Place the patient supine, flexing the knee to 45° over a casette and directing the rays perpendicular to the film.
- Posteroanterior tunnel view, as shown in Figures 25.320A and B, reveals the lesion best done, by placing the patient prone, flexing the knee to 60° and directing the tube in the caudle direction, so that the rays intercept the joint at an angle of 30°.

MRI Staging–Ninety-seven Percent Sensitivity (Figs 25.321A and B)

Stage I: Thickening of articular cartilage and low signal changes (stable), as shown in Figure 25.322.

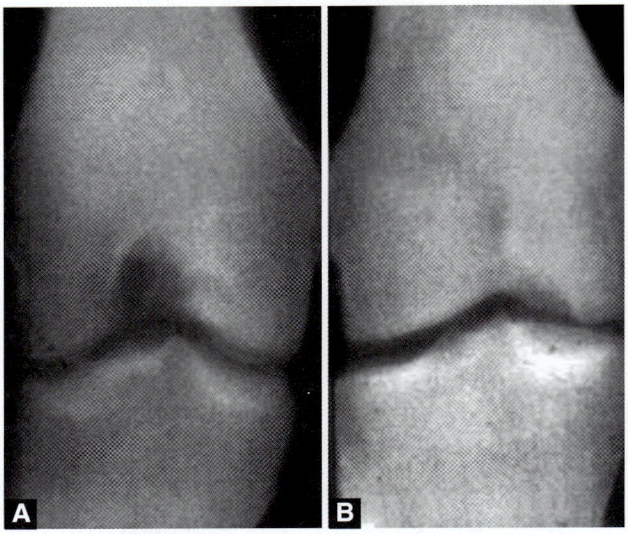

Figs 25.320A and B: Posteroanterior tunnel view

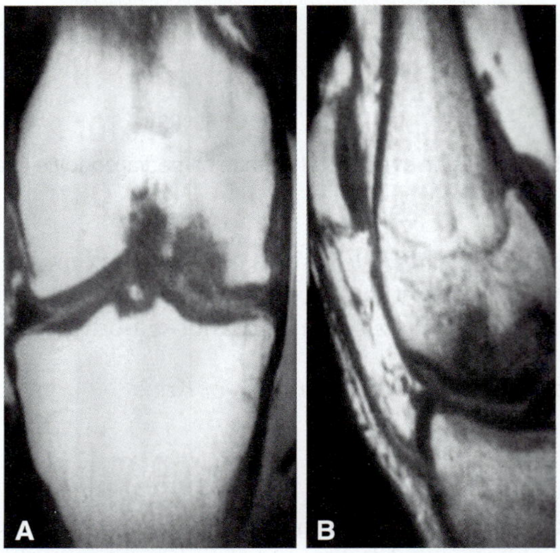

Figs 25.321A and B: MRI, showing OCD of knee joint

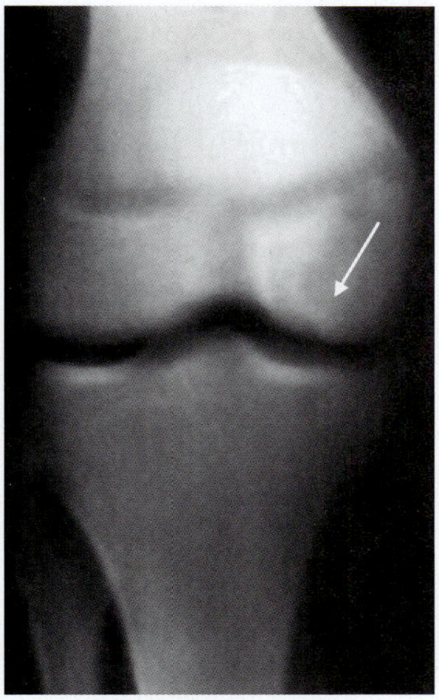

Fig. 25.322: X-ray showing stage I, OCD

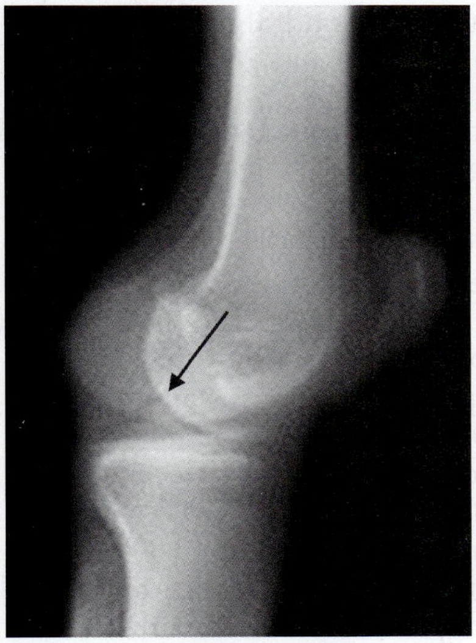

Fig. 25.323: X-ray showing stage II, OCD

Stage II (Fig. 25.323): Articular cartilage breached, low-signal rim behind fragment indicating fibrous attachment (stable).

Stage III (Fig. 25.324): Articular cartilage breached, high signal changes, behind fragment and underlying subchondral bone (unstable).

Stage IV: Loose body (unstable).

Diagnostic Procedures

Some authors advocate the use of arthroscopy as a diagnostic tool in addition to MRI prior to invasive procedures.

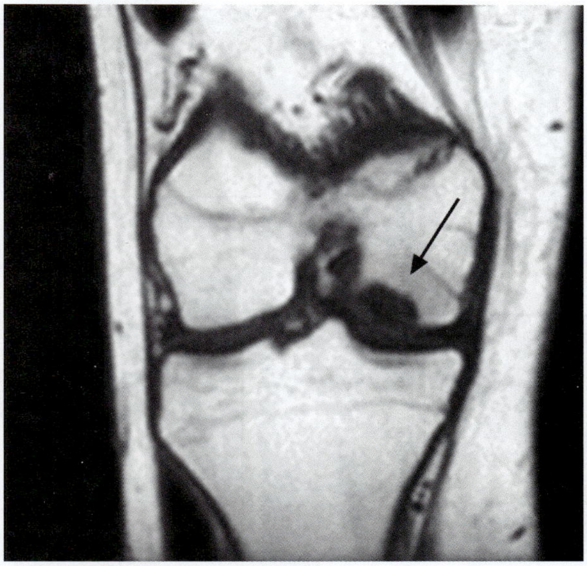

Fig. 25.324: X-ray showing stage III, OCD

Treatment Option

Certain important variables can affect the choice of treatment. The general rule is, younger the patient, the better the prognosis. Guidelines for treatment are outlined by the following categories:

Category I: Girls, younger than 11 years and boys younger than 13 years. These patients, usually do well with nonoperative treatment.

Category II: Girls, aged 11 to 15 years and boys aged 13 to 17 years. These patients are near skeletal maturity. Treatment depends on the looseness of the lesions.

Category III: Physeal closure and skeletal maturity have occurred. Treatment is based on the size and stability of the lesion.

■ Arthroscopic Stages (Fig. 25.325)

Stage I: Depressed osteochondral fracture

Stage II: Osteochondral fragment, attached by an osseous bridge

Stage III: Detached nondisplaced fragment

Stage IV: Displaced fragment.

■ Treatment

Conservative Treatment

Conservative treatment includes, limitation of activity and protected weight-bearing to allow healing and prevent further displacement. Children should be offered a knee immobilizer during this time, to limit the stress at the

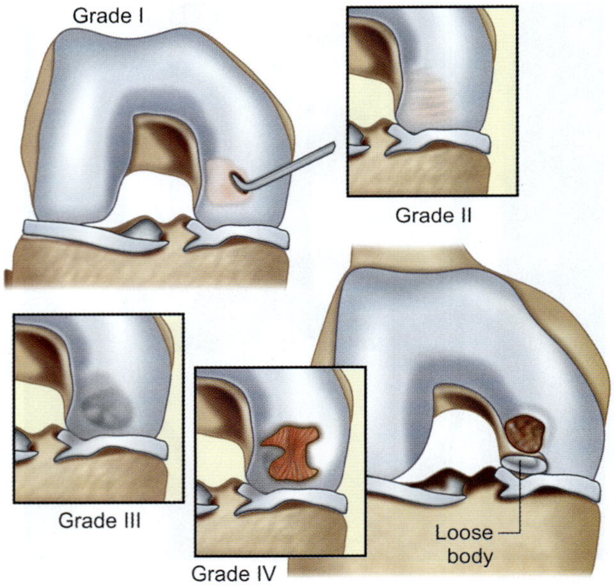

Fig. 25.325: Arthroscopic staging of OCD

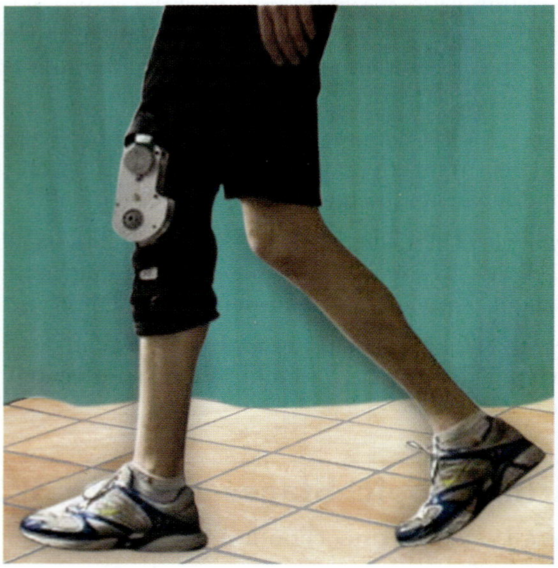

Fig. 25.326: Children should be offered a knee immobilizer, to limit the stress at the lesion

lesion, as shown in Figures 25.326 and 25.327. After 3 months patients, who are still symptomatic or whose repeat radiographs and do not show improvement should be offered surgery.

Surgical Treatment Options

- Arthroscopic drilling
- Arthroscopic fixation
- Microfracture chondroplasty

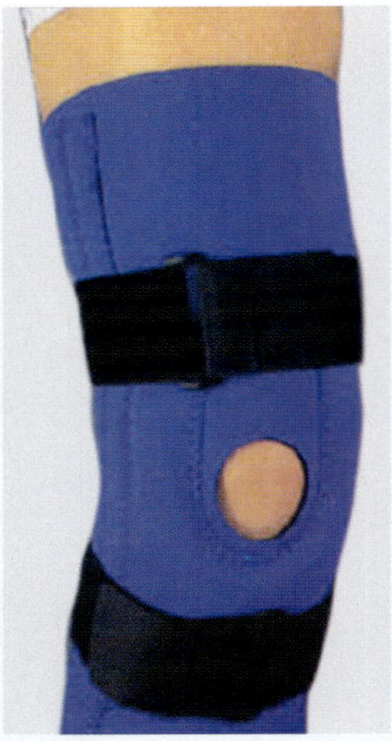

Fig. 25.327: A type of knee immobilizer

- Mosaicplasty (autologous osteochondral transfer)
- Autologous chondrocyte implantation (ACI)
- Allograft, osteochondral graft
- Articular cartilage and paste grafting.

Treatment Procedure Depending on the Type of Lesions

Stable Lesions (Types I and II)

- Adolescents (physis open)
- Brace or plaster of Paris (POP) cast for 6 to 8 weeks.
- Stop sports, strenuous activities
- Follow-up (F/U) bone scans and MRI
- Takes 10–18 months
- Less successful in adults
- Nonhealing surgery
- Debridement and drilling
- On failure of conservative treatment:
  - Decompression of the lesion
  - Opening of the vascular channels
  - Brace and nonweight-bearing (NWB) for 6 weeks
  - Regular follow-up
  - Fixation of fragment can be done.

Type III and Rarely Type IV

- Debridement of crater fixation of osteochondral fragment with either biodart, K-wire or headless screw.
- Knee ROM exercises should start from day 2.
- Brace and NWB for 6–8 weeks
- Regular follow-up, repeat MRI or arthroscopy.
- The base of the lesion is abraded to viable subchondral bone, as shown in Figures 25.328 and 25.329.

Debridement of the cartilage defect: The edges are brought back to a right angle and any detached cartilage is

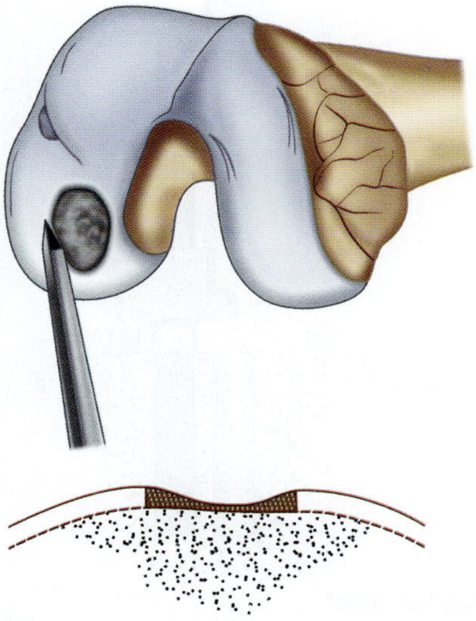

Fig. 25.328: The base of the lesion is abraded to viable subchondral bone

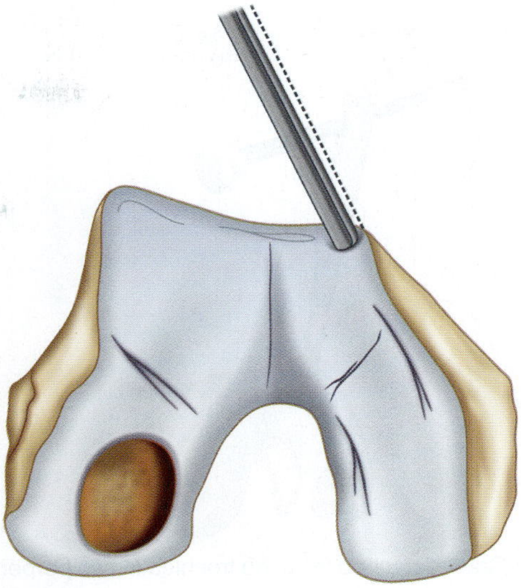

Fig. 25.330: The tubular chisel

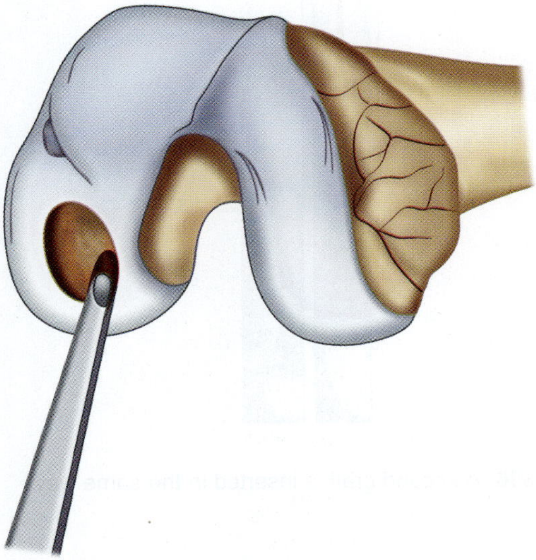

Fig. 25.329: The graft is harvested perpendicular to the surface of the donor site

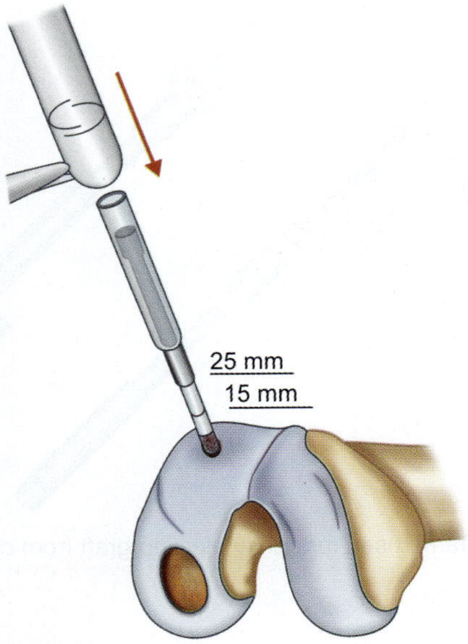

Fig. 25.331: The tubular chisel, driven by hammer

removed. The graft is harvested perpendicular to the surface of the donor site. The tubular chisel is driven by hammer to the desired depth, avoiding any overheating that could put the viability of the graft at risk (Figs 25.330 and 25.331). The graft is detached from the trochlea in two perpendicular toggling movements, without rotating the chisel. The degree of movement must be carefully judged, to avoid fracturing the rim of the trochlea, as illustrated in Figure 25.332. The graft is gently ejected from the chisel, as shown in Figure 25.333, using tamp and an appropriately sized guide. The graft is inserted, using a guide tube and a graduated tamp. This is illustrated in Figure 25.234. The level of the graft is adjusted, as shown in Figures 25.235 and 25.236. A second graft is inserted in the same way, about 1 mm from the preceding graft. Appearance on completion of the procedure, grafts in place and donor sites shown in Figure 25.237.

Type IV and Type V

- Arthoscopic debridement of crater
- Arthrotomy.

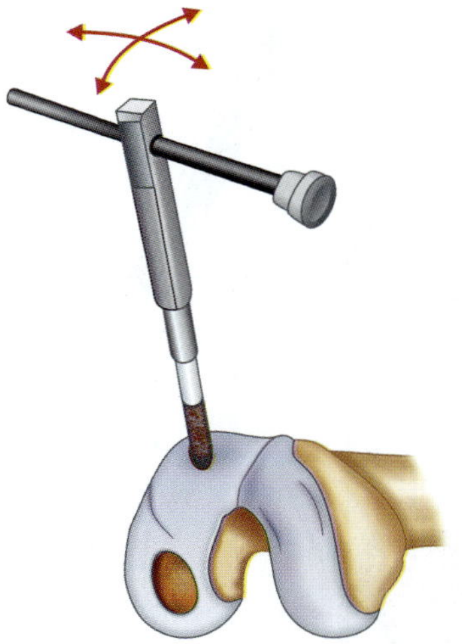

Fig. 25.332: Graft, detached from the trochlea in two perpendicular toggling movements

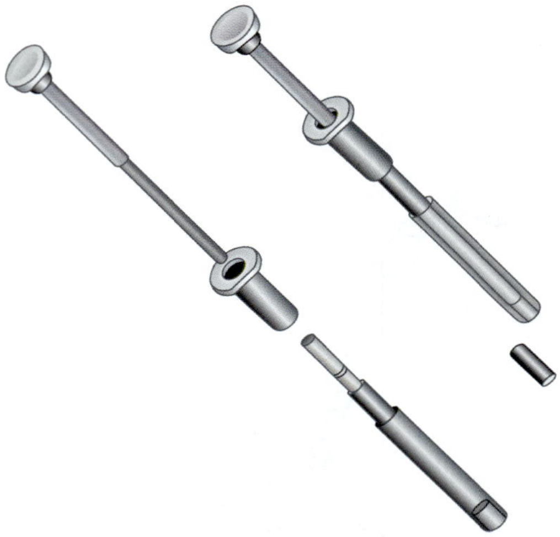

Fig. 25.333: Tamp used for gently ejecting graft from chisel

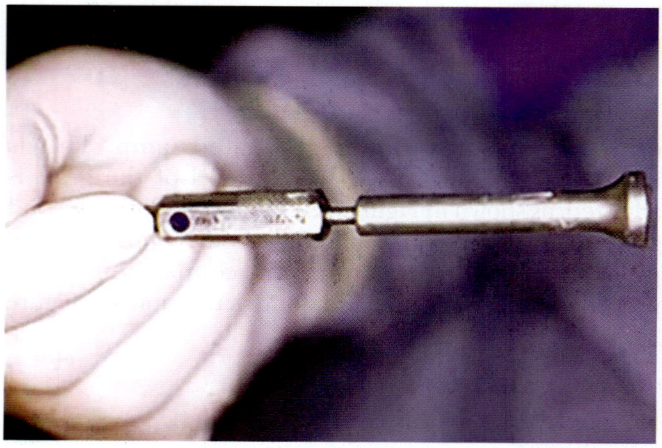

Fig. 25.334: A graduated tamp

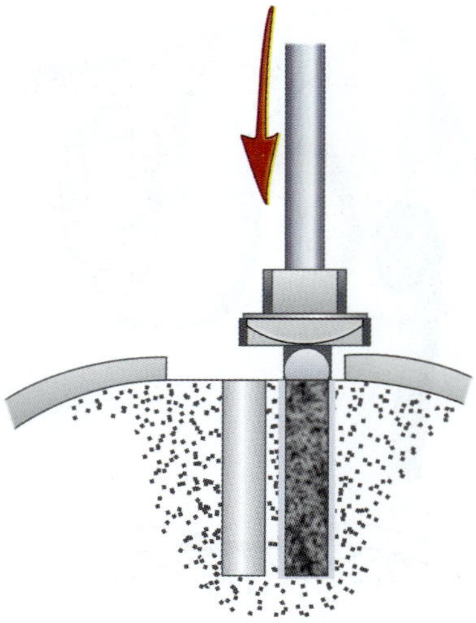

Fig. 25.335: A guide tube

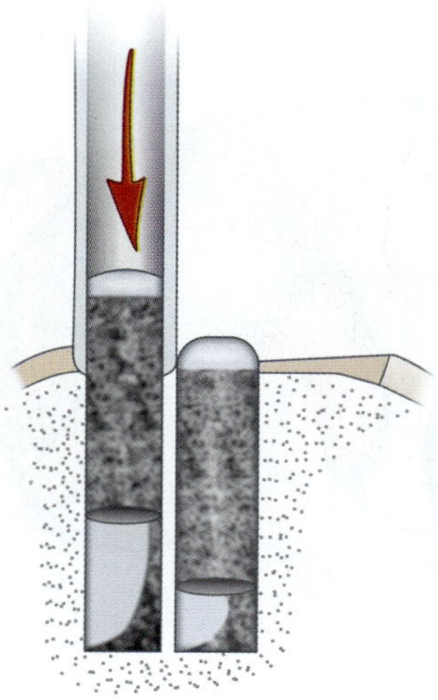

Fig. 25.336: A second graft is inserted in the same way

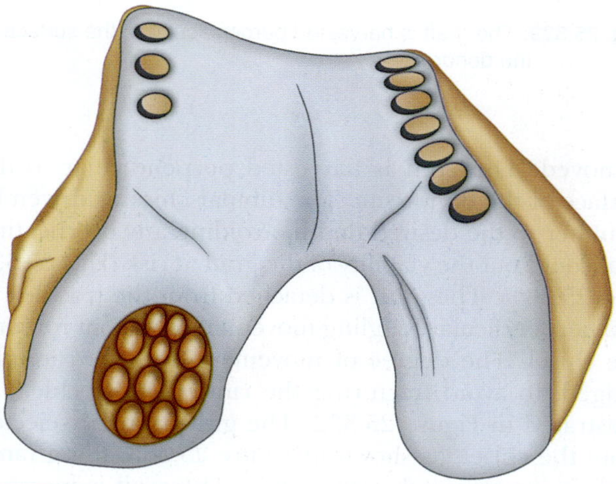

Fig. 25.337: Appearance on completion— grafts in place and donor sites

Osteochondral Autograft (Mosaicplasty)

- Arthroscopic procedure for loose body
- Debridement
- Mosaicplasty, e.g. miniarthrotomy
- 6.5 mm diameter grafts
- 3.5 mm diameter grafts
- *Postoperative:* 1.5 months, NWB 3 months PWB.
- Full weight-bearing (FWB) 6 months.

Autologus Cartilage Implantation

- Allograft transplant can be used
- Osteochondral grafts from a bone or tissue bank
- Risks include graft rejection and infection
- Autologous chondrocyte implantation shown in Figures 25.338 and 25.339

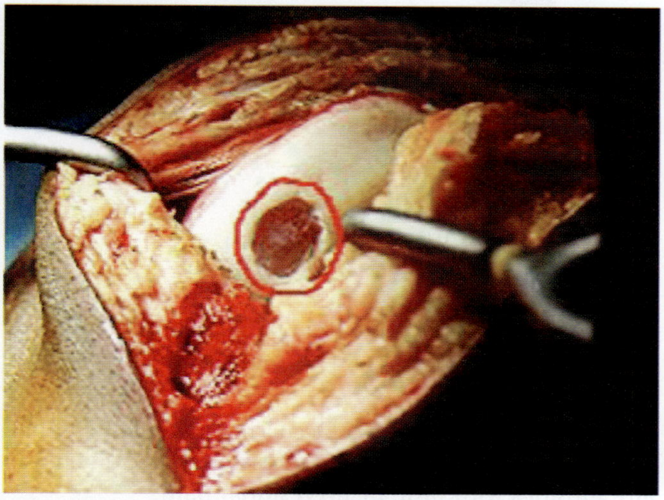

Fig. 25.338: Autologous cartilage implantation preparation

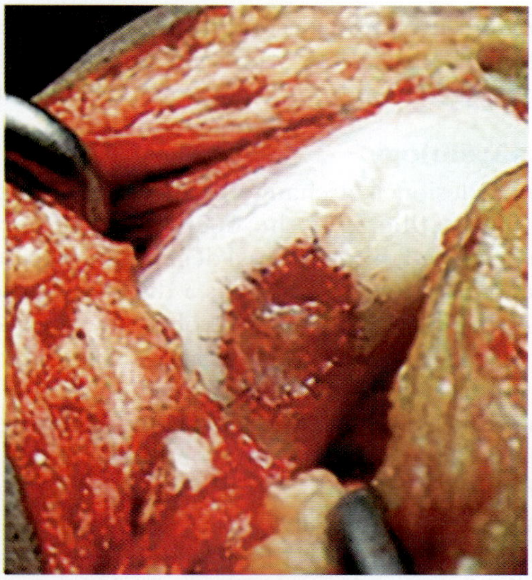

Fig. 25.339: Autologous chondrocyte implantation done

- Cartilage cells cultured from patient's biopsied cartilage
- Implanted into the defect, after suturing the defect with periosteal patch
- Costly, nonavailability in India and requires two procedures.

Articular Cartilage Paste Grafting

- The goal in treating arthritic lesions, traumatic lesions and failed OCD lesions with articular cartilage paste grafting is the same
- The intent is to stimulate a healing response, which covers the lesion with a protective layer of fibrocartilage and/or hyaline cartilage
- The regenerated cartilage protects the underlying bone and serves to reduce pain and swelling
- Articular cartilage paste grafting has been successfully applied to OCD lesions as both a primary treatment and as a salvage procedure for the defects, which fail other attempts at repair.

Treatment Options

- Take home message
- OCD knee is not very rare. Diagnosis is mainly radiological
- MRI must be done, for assessing stability
- Treatment depends upon size and stability of fragment
- *Closed lesions:* Articular cartilage is continous
- *Open lesion:* Disruption of cartilage
- *Stage I lesion:* Nonoperative treatment
- *Stage II lesion:* Conservative, if symptomatic then, scopy and drilling
- *Stage III lesion:* Fixation by biodarts or osteochondral pins, headless screws or K-wires
- *Stage IV lesion:* Mosaicplasty.

■ Chondromalacia Patellae (Fig. 25.340)

It is characterized by softening of the articular cartilage of patella of diverse origin. Also known as, patellofemoral pain syndrome or anterior knee pain. Chondromalacia literally means, softening of the cartilage and patellae means, the knee cap. Hence, chondromalacia patellae means, softening of the articular cartilage of the knee cap, as shown in Figure 25.341.

Historical Background

- Earliest described by Budigner, in 1906.
- First used by Aleman, in 1917.

Etiology

Jackson divided the etiological factors into two main types:

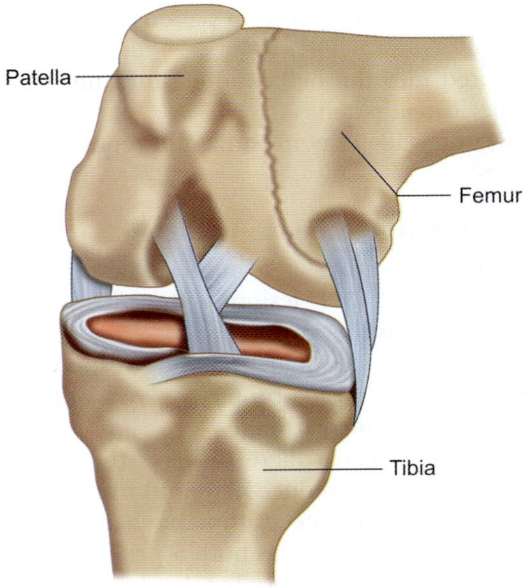

Fig. 25.340: Chondromalacia patellae and synovial chondromatosis

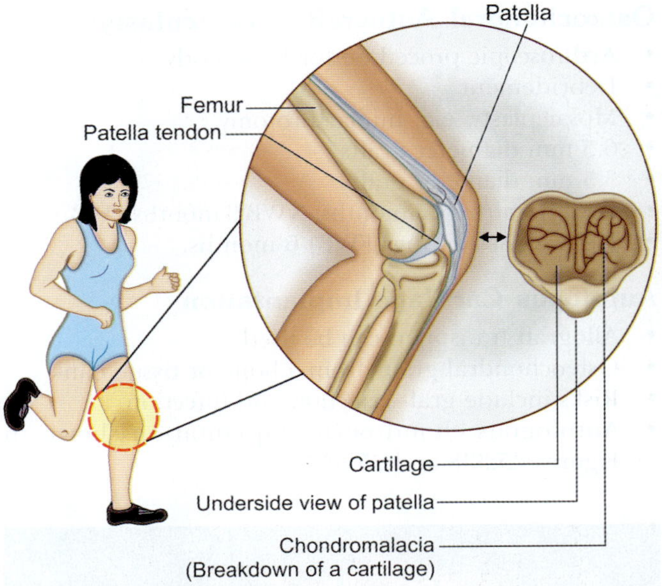

Fig. 25.341: Chondromalacia patellae

Biomechanical Causes

Acute: Dislocation of patella with a chondral or osteochondral fracture, direct trauma (fall or a blow to the patella) or fracture of patella resulting into an incongruous surface.

Chronic: Chronic causes include:

- Recurrent subluxation or dislocation of patella, secondary to femoral dysplasia, small patella, patella alta, femoral anteversion, external tibial torsion and anterior cruciate ligament (ACL) insuffiency
- Increased quadriceps angle
- Quadriceps muscle imbalance, either due to weakness or abnormal attachment of vatus medialis
- Patella alta
- Post-traumatic malalignment following femoral shaft fracture
- Excessive lateral pressure syndrome
- Meniscal injury
- Reflex sympathetic dystrophy
- Medial femoral condylar ridge.

Biochemical Causes

Disease

- Rheumatoid arthritis
- Recurrent hemarthrosis
- Alkaptonuria
- Peripheral synovitis
- Sepsis and adhesions.

Iatrogenic

- Repeated intra-articular steroid injections
- Prolonged immobilization.

Degenerative

Primary osteoarthritis.

Types

Three types of chondromalacia patellae are usually seen in girls, with female to male ratio is 3: 2. These types are described as follows:

Primary or idiopathic type: Occurring in adolescents and young adults, causing chronic persistent pain, which usually subsides with little or no residual pain.

Secondary adolescent type: Resulting from direct trauma to the patella or due to repeated trauma, e.g. patellar displacement. It leads to osteoarthritis with advancing age.

Adult type: Develops in second decade of life, when OA changes develop without symptoms and progress, with advancing age and become symptomatic at middle age.

Pathophysiology

The initial lesion is a change in the ground substance and collagen fibers, at the deep levels of cartilage. Goodfellow, used the term basal degeneration to describe this lesion. Basal degeneration is a disorder of the deep layers of the cartilage, which involves the surface layer late in its development. This change is tangible, but not visible and the surface is smooth and intact. It is attributed in sulfated mucopolysaccharides, in the ground substance. Changes occur most commonly at one of two sites, in the deep layer of cartilage.

- First site, is an area about 1 cm in diameter around the ridge, that separates the lateral facet from the medial facet, as shown in Figure 25.342.

- Second area is around the inferior part of the central ridge that separates the medial and the lateral facet.

Stages of Lesion of Basal Degeneration (Fig. 25.343)

Basic disorder is because of mechanical overload of the patellofemoral joint. More commonly due to repetitive overload. It can be due to either:

- *Malcongruence of patellofemoral surface:* Due to some abnormal shape of patella or interconylar groove.

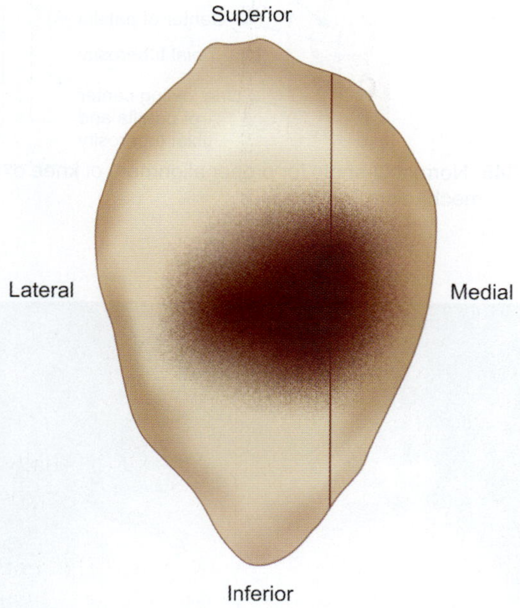

Fig. 25.342: Dark area represents most common area of patellar chondromalacia, most severe in cenral zone but extended equally onto medial and lateral facets

- Malalignment of the extensor mechanism or relative weakness of the vastus medialis, which causes the patella to tilt, subluxate or bear more heavily on one facet, than the other during flexion and extension.
- Overload means, either direct stress on a load bearing facet or sheer stress in the depth of the articular cartilage at the boundary between high contact and low contact areas.

Classification

Given by, Vigorita and Morgan. They divided the disease into four stages or grades, these are shown in Figure 25.344.

Stage I

- Changes include minimal articular cartilage changes.
- Cartilage may have localized softening, with minimal or no break in the surface.
- A blunt instrument pressed on the surface, may sink into the cartilage and cartilage may appear slightly discolored and soft.

Stage II

Changes include an area of fibrillation or fissuring an irregular surface.

Stage III

Changes have definite fibrillations, with fissuring extending down to the subchondral bone, which presents a classic arthroscopic picture described as crab meat appearance.

Stage IV

Changes are those in which the articular cartilage has disappeared, allowing exposure and erosion of the subchondral bone.

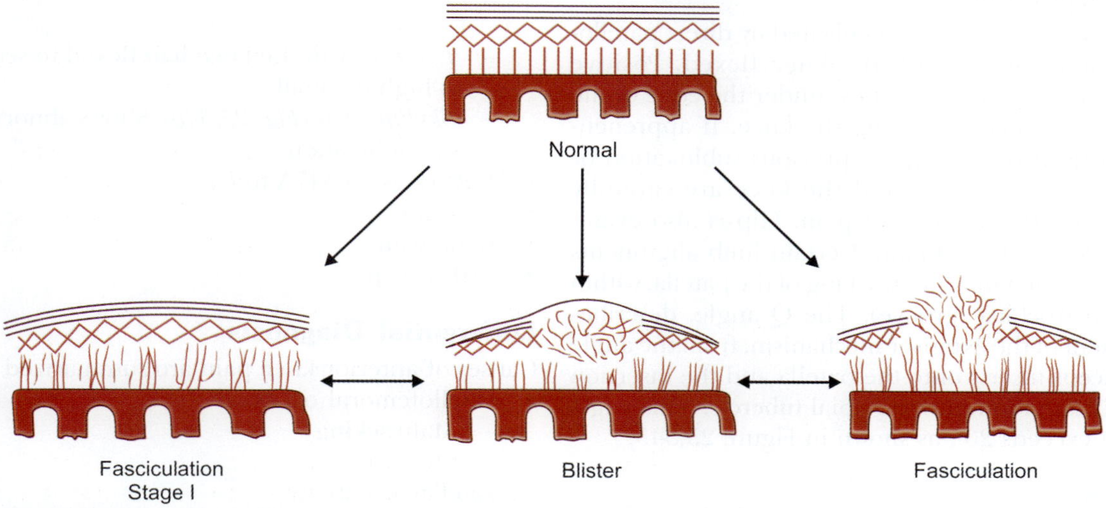

Fig. 25.343: Different stages of basal degeneration in chondromalacia patellae

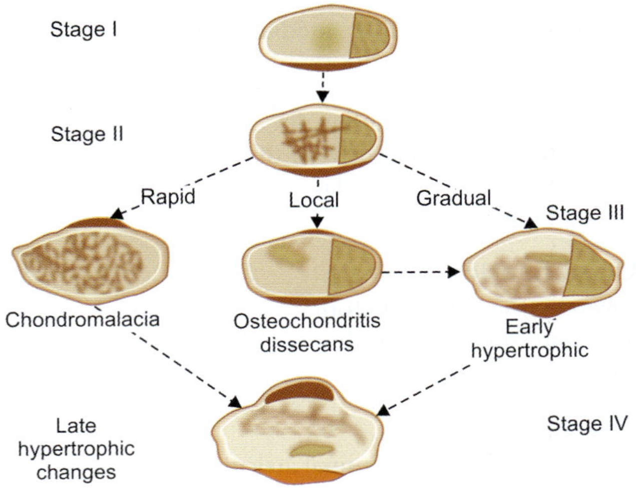

Fig. 25.344: Different stages of chondromalacia patellae, given by Vigorita and Morgan

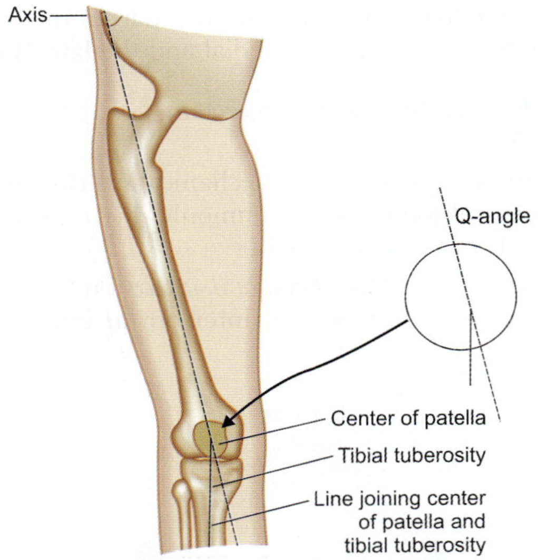

Fig. 25.345: Normal Q-angle for proper alignment of knee extensor mechanism

Clinical Features

- Diffuse aching pain, over the front or anteromedial aspect of the knee.
- Pain worsens when the knee functions under load in flexion, such as when going up or down stairs, squatting, kneeling and prolonged sitting.
- Prolonged sitting, with the knee in flexion, causes pain, which is relieved by extension. Also called cinema sign, movie sign or theater sign.
- History of catching or giving way may be present.

Physical Examination

Examination should begin with the patient standing, to observe overall limb alignment. Quadriceps muscle atrophy, may be present.

Genu Varum or Valgum

Retropatellar tenderness: It get elicited by direct patellofemoral compression, with the knee flexed. Positive patellar grinding test. Tenderness under the edge of the patella and crepitus on moving the knee. If apprehension test is positive, it suggests previous subluxation or dislocation. Structures around the knee are carefully examined for other sources of pain. Hip is also examined to exclude referred pain. Certain limb alignments may predispose to improper tracking of the patella, within the femoral trochlea (groove). The Q angle, describes the alignment of the extensor mechanism, from the angle the quadriceps inserts onto the patella and the insertion of the patella tendon into the tibial tubercle. This angle should not exceeds 20°, as shown in Figure 25.345.

Diagnosis

- X-ray
  - Anteroposterior (AP)
  - *Lateral:* With the knee half flexed to see if patella is high or small.
  - *Skyline view (Fig. 25.346):* Shows abnormal tilting or subluxation
- MRI (Figs 25.347A to C)
- CT scan
- Bone scan
- Arthroscopy.

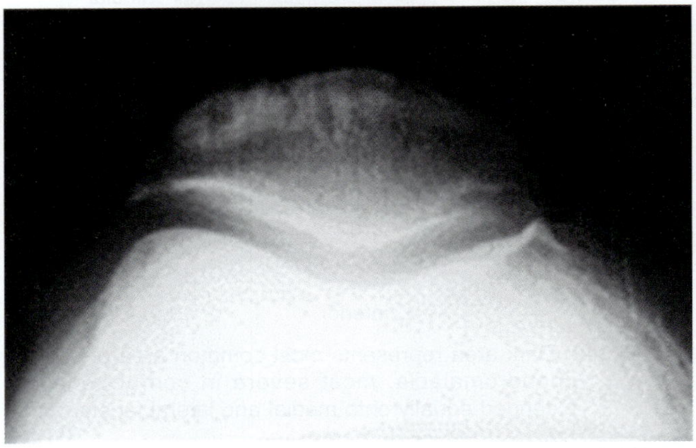

Fig. 25.346: X-ray skyline view, depicting alignment of patella

Differential Diagnosis

Causes of anterior knee pain are summarized as:

- Patellofemoral overload
  - Maltracking
  - Overuse
- Patellar instability
  - Patellar subluxation
  - Patellar tilt

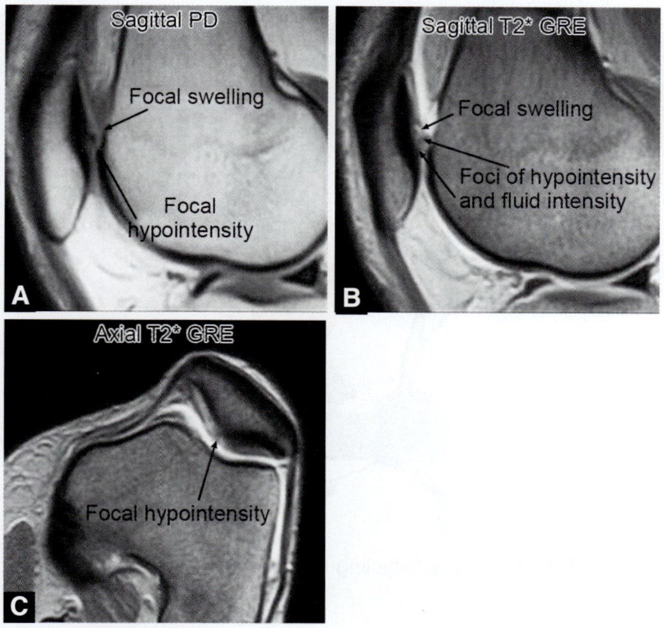

Figs 25.347A to C: MRI of knee

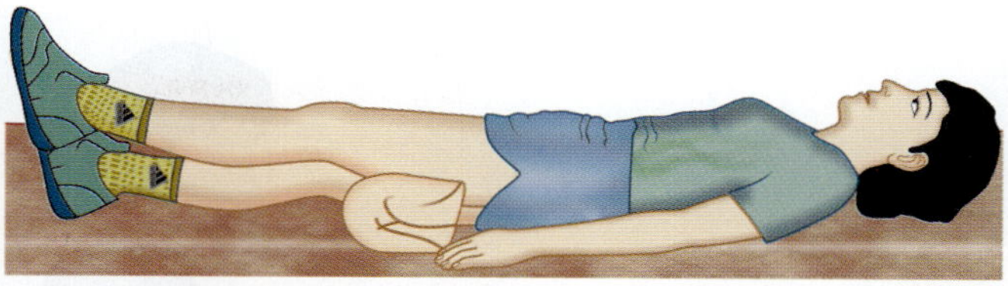

Fig. 25.348: Short arc knee extension exercises in lying down position

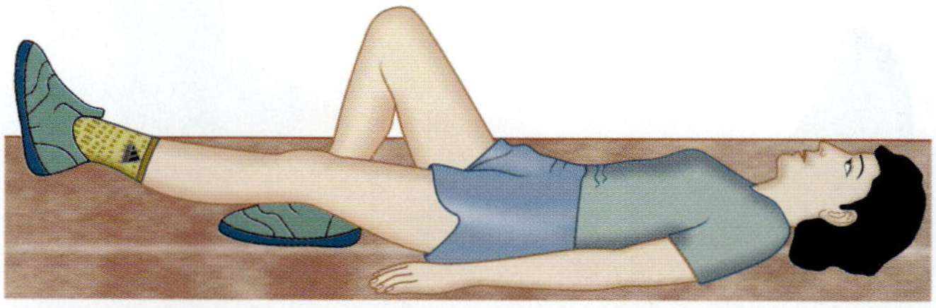

Fig. 25.349: SLR exercises performed in supine

- Intra-articular pathology
  - Plica syndrome
  - Meniscal disorders
  - OCD
  - Patellofemoral arthritis
- Peripatellar disorders
  - Bursitis
  - Tendinitis
  - Apophysitis
- Disorders of patella
  - Bipartite patella
  - Bone tumors
- Reffered pain
  - Hip disorders, e.g. slipped capital femoral epiphysis.

Treatment

Conservative Management

Anti-inflammatory drugs: Regardless of the above, the best way to minimize the chances of developing chondromalacia patellae is to warm up and stretch out before sports, especially quadriceps and hamstrings. If possible, varying between sports. For example, alternate, running swimming with bicycling. Avoid squatting, kneeling, stairs and hill running if possible. In addition, there are some exercises that are helpful in preventing and helping the symptoms of anterior knee pain. These exercises should be done regularly, twice a day. If symptoms are already present, it will take about 6 weeks before one get the benefit of the exercise. So the key is to be consistent and persistent. Short arc extensions are done, while sitting up or lying down. Use a rolledup towel, to support thigh, while keeping leg and foot in the air for 5 seconds. Lowering foot, as one bend the knee slowly. Repeat ten times for each leg, twice a day, as illustrated in Figure 25.348.

Straight leg raises (SLR) are done, while lying down. Lifting whole lower limb at the hip, with the knee extended and keep it up in the air for five seconds. Then lower down slowly. Repeat ten times for each leg, twice a day, this is illustrated in Figure 25.349. Quadriceps isometric exercises are performed in sitting up position, with both legs extended. Tighten quadriceps muscles, by pushing the knees down onto the floor. Hold for 5 seconds. Repeat ten times for each leg, as shown in Figure 25.350, twice a day. Stationary bicycling on low tension setting, improves exercise tolerance, without stressing the knees. Adjusting the seat high enough, so that the leg is straight on the down stroke. Start with 15 minutes a day and work up to 30 minutes a day. This is shown in Figure 25.351.

Operative Treatment

Surgery should be considered only in following cases:

- Demonstrable abnormality, which can be correctable by surgery only.
- Conservative treatment, has been tried for 6 months, but no relief.
- Patient is genuinely incapacitated.

Goal

- Goal of the treatment is to improve patellar alignment and patellofemoral congruence.
- To reduce patellofemoral pressure.

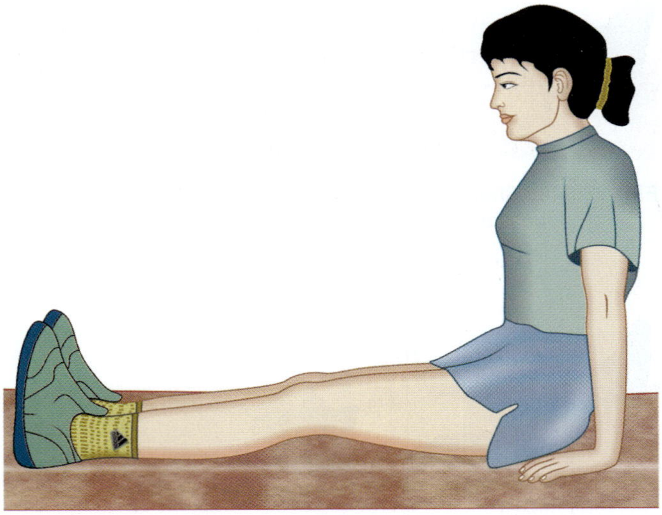

Fig. 25.350: Isometric quadriceps exercises

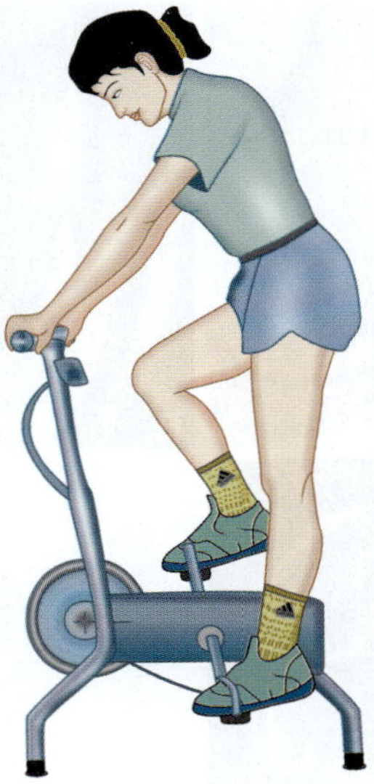

Fig. 25.351: Stationary bicycling on low tension setting

Surgical Procedures

Various surgical procedures are employed, which can be described as follows:

- *Chondroplasty:* Arthroscopic patellar shaving.
- *Excision:* Local excision of defects with drillng of subchondral bone, replace the defect by formation of fibrocartilage
- Facetectomy
- *Lateral release:* Lateral knee capsule and extensor retinaculum are divided longitudinally, either open or arthoscopically. Sometimes succeeds on its own, but more often patellofemoral realignment, either by proximal or distal realignment.
- *Proximal realignment:* Achieved by combined open release of the lateral retinaculum and reefing of the oblique part of the vatus medialis.
- Mechanical decompression, of the patellofemoral joint by elevating anteriorly the tibial tuberosity (Maquet procedure). Closed physis is prerequisite.
- *Patellectomy:* Last resort, but patient, with severe discomfort are grateful for the relief, it brings after other operations have failed.

■ Synovial Chondromatosis

Synonyms and related keywords:

- Synovial chondrometaplasia (Figs 25.352 to 25.354)
- Articular chondromatosis
- Osteochondromatosis
- Chondrocalcinosis articularis
- Tenosynovial chondrometaplasia
- Joint chondromata
- Diffuse endochondromatosis.

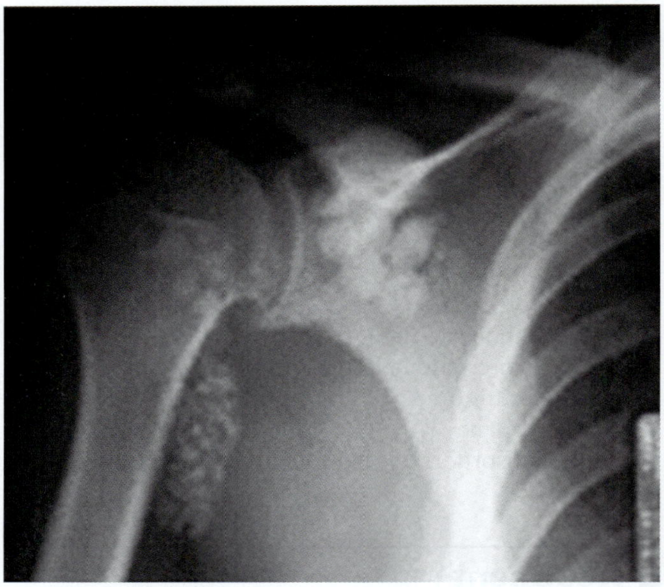

Fig. 25.352: Synovial chondrometaplasia of shoulder

Introduction

Defined as a benign condition, characterized by synovial membrane proliferation and metaplasia. The synovial lining of a joint, bursa, or tendon sheath, undergoes nodular proliferation and fragments may break off from the synovial surface into the joint. After nourished by synovial fluid, the fragments may grow, calcify or ossify. The intra-articular fragment, may vary in size from a few millimeters to a few centimeters.

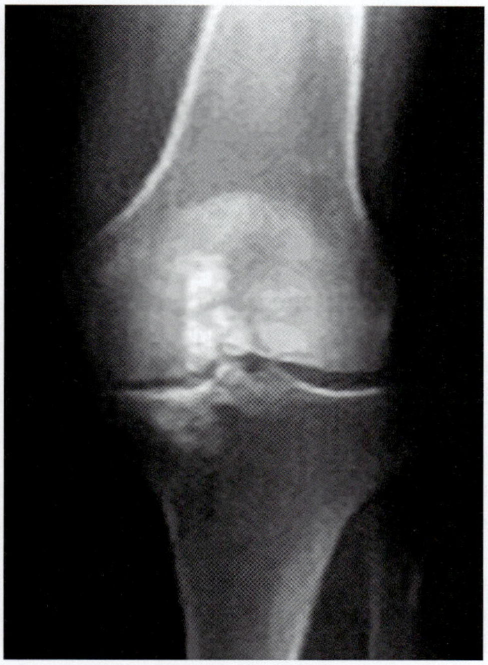

Fig. 25.353: Synovial chondrometaplasia of knee

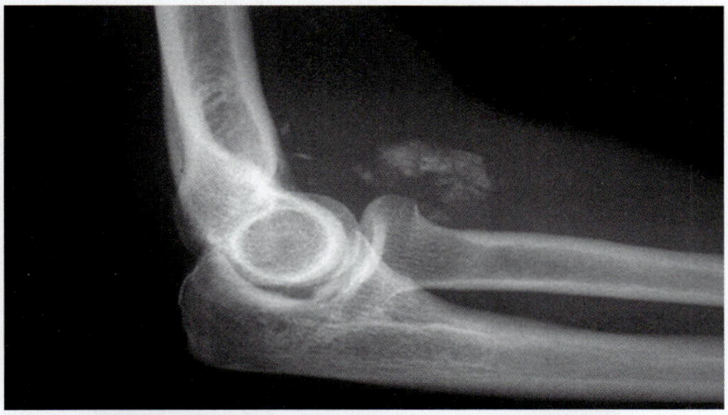

Fig. 25.354: Synovial chondrometaplasia of elbow

Incidence

Sex: Shows a predilection of two to four fold for males over females.

Age: Individuals of all ages can be affected, but the disease is often diagnosed in persons aged 20 to 50 years.

Etiology

Synovial chondromatosis (SOC) occurs, either as a primary or secondary form.

Primary Synovial Chondromatosis

Described as the presence of ectopic cartilage in synovial tissue and as loose bodies in the joint cavity, with or without calcification (osteochondromatosis) and without, an identifiable joint pathology. Whether this represents, synovial metaplasia or a true neoplasia is unclear. The true etiology remains unknown, but most authorities favor the metaplastic theory.

Secondary Synovial Chondromatosis

The secondary form is synovial chondromatosis, in the setting of pre-existent osteoarthritis, rheumatoid arthritis, osteonecrosis, osteochondritis dissecans, neuropathic osteoarthropathy, tuberculosis or osteochondral fractures. Free chondral or osteochondral fragments, formed by underlying disease, implant into the synovium and induce metaplastic cartilage around them.

Pathophysiology

Primary synovial chondromatosis appears to occur in three phases, as Milgram described in 1977:

Phase I

Active intrasynovial disease without loose bodies.

Phase II

Transitional lesions, with osteochondral nodules in the synovial membrane and osteochondral bodies, lying free in the joint cavity.

Phase III

Multiple free osteochondral bodies, with quiescent intrasynovial disease.

Involvement is typically monoarticular, with the large joints, being most frequently affected. The knee joint is involved in 60 to 70 percent of cases. The shoulder, elbow and hip are the next most frequently involved joints. Reports have described involvement of multiple other joints and locations, including the temporomandibular joint, spinal facet joints, the acromioclavicular joint, wrist joint, ankle joint, biceps tendon sheath and extra-articular locations.

Investigations

Lab Studies

- *Erythrocyte sedimentation rate:* Results are expected to be normal in persons, with primary synovial chondromatosis, but they may be elevated in persons, with secondary synovial chondromatos due to systemic inflammation from a condition, such as rheumatoid arthritis
- C-reactive protein
- Complete blood count (CBC), with differential count
- Rheumatoid (RA) factor.

Diagnostic Procedures

Arthrocentesis: It is used to obtain a sample of synovial fluid, if the physical findings suggest infection. Send the sample for a cell count, crystal examination, Gram staining and cultures. All findings, should be within normal limits in persons, with primary synovial chondromatosis.

Synovial biopsy: Done for histopathological evaluation.

Histologic Findings

Primary Synovial Chondromatosis

On hematoxylin and eosin staining, thick and villous formation to the synovial membrane, with islands of clustered chondrocytes is seen. The chondrocytes in the nodules are usually arranged in loose clusters, though a nonclustered uniform distribution may occur. In two thirds of cases, the chondrocytes show, mild-to-moderate nuclear atypia, with pleomorphism, enlarged, openfaced nuclei and frequent binucleation. Mitotic figures are rarely found. Osteoclast like giant cells and chondroblasts, with a dense eosinophilic cytoplasm may rim the nodules. If calcification occurs, it is distributed in a patchy and irregular pattern. In late stages, the nodules may undergo, true ossification via vascular invasion and endochondral bone formation.

Secondary Synovial Chondromatosis

Foci of implanted articular cartilage, with and without subchondral necrotic bone are found. The chondrocytes of implanted cartilage, usually lack significant atypia or binucleation and any calcification occurs in a zonal and ringlike fashion.

Imaging Studies

- Plain radiography, with orthogonal views of the affected joint.
- Findings are frequently normal.
- If loose bodies undergo ossification, they may be visible in the joint space. The pattern of mineralization varies with size. Large nodules have large, stippled or ringlike calcified areas. Small nodules have flecks of calcium.
- Pressure erosions (saucerization) and cyst formation, can be seen in adjacent bone, although this is more typical for joints with lax capsules (hip).
- In 30 percent of cases, no matrix mineralization is present and loose bodies appear as foci, with opacity similar to that of water.
- In secondary synovial chondromatosis, changes consistently, with the underlying disease process are evident.
- Frontal radiograph, of the shoulder shows multiple, rounded and calcified bodies in the axillary recess and in the subscapularis bursa, as shown in Figure 25.355.
- AP and lateral radiograph, of the knee shows multiple, calcified bodies in the proximal tibiofibular joint in a patient, with synovial osteochondromatosis. This is shown in Figure 25.356.
- Frontal and lateral radiograph of a patient, with synovial osteochondromatosis of the knee joint. The bodies are located in the popliteal space of the knee. Radiographs are shown in Figures 25.357 to 25.359.

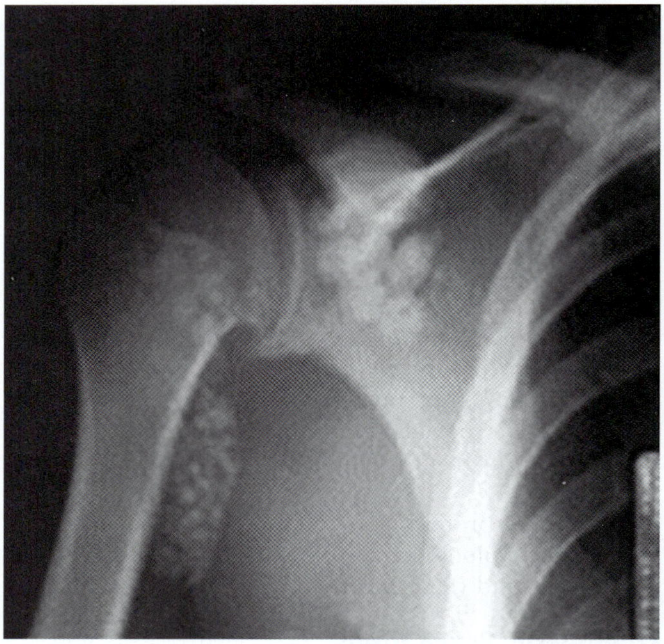

Fig. 25.355: Frontal shoulder radiograph shows multiple, rounded and calcified bodies in the axillary recess and in the subscapularis bursa

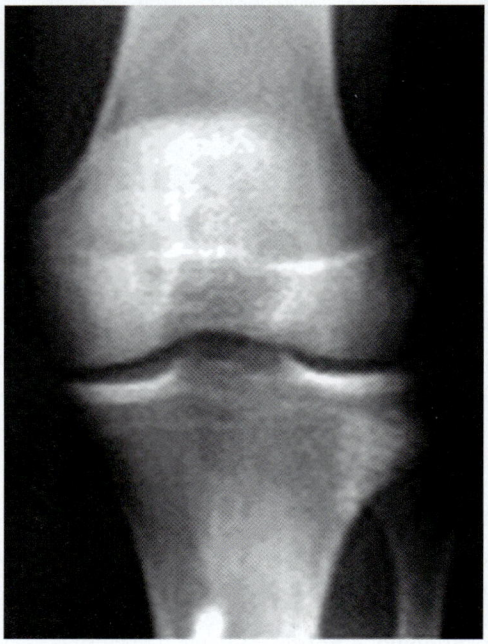

Fig. 25.356: AP view of knee joint, shows multiple, calcified bodies in the proximal tibiofibular joint

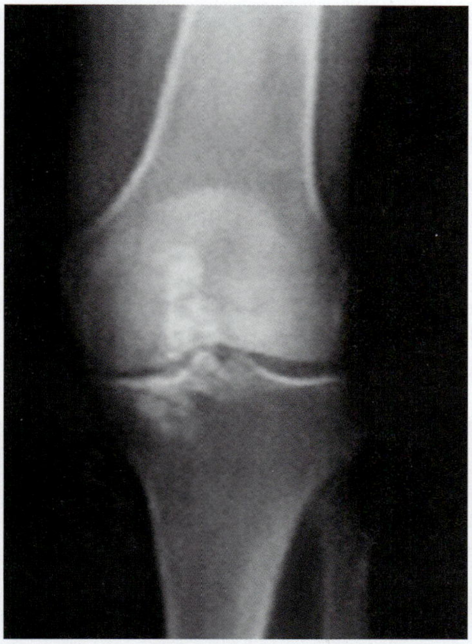

Fig. 25.357: Frontal radiograph of a patient with synovial osteochondromatosis of the knee joint

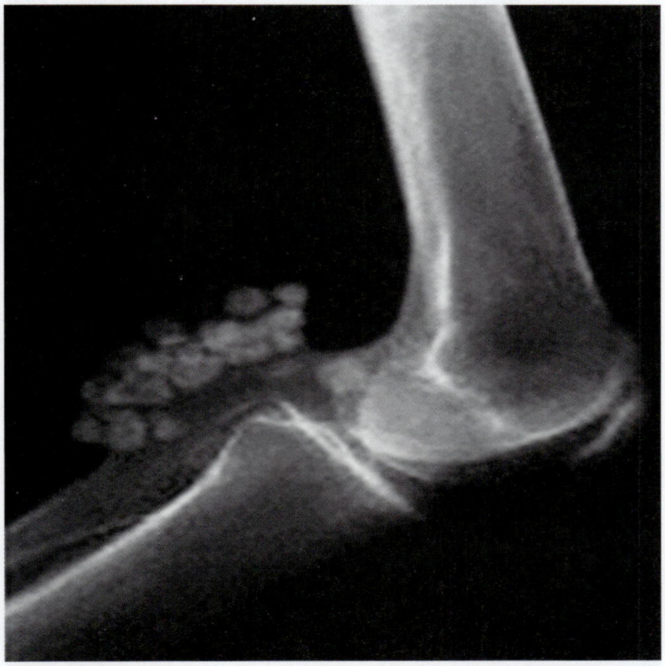

Fig. 25.358: Lateral radiograph of a patient, with synovial osteochondromatosis. The bodies are located in the popliteal space of the knee

Magnetic Resonance Imaging

Cartilaginous nodules have intermediate signal intensity on T1 weighted images and high signal intensity on T2 weighted images, with decreasing intensity, as the amount of calcium in the nodule decreases, this is illustrated in Figure 25.360. The addition of intra-articular gadolinium based contrast material, increases the sensitivity for detecting lesions.

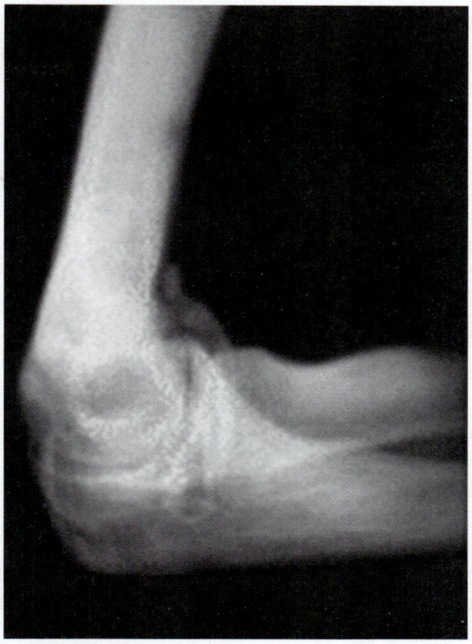

Fig. 25.359: Radiograph of a patient with synovial osteochondromatosis of the elbow joint. The bodies are located in the cubital space of the knee

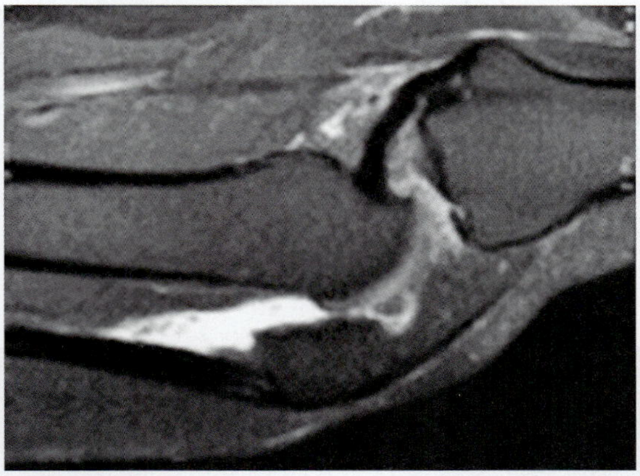

Fig. 25.360: MRI of knee

CT Scan

This is useful only for identifying calcified loose bodies. Unmineralized nodules, typically cannot be visualized. Sagittal T2 weighted MRI, through the knee in an adult, with synovial chondromatosis demonstrates, abnormal signal intensity in the suprapatellar pouch. Also note hypertrophic synovium, in the intercondylar notch region and a normal posterior region.

Nuclear Medicine

Radionuclide studies may be obtained, when the plain radiographic features are not clear. The affected areas, usually show increased radionuclide uptake on technetium –99m bone scan. Delayed bone scan shows, diffusely increased uptake, around the tibiotalar joint. This indicates, increased metabolic activity and is consistent with synovitis around the ankle.

Differentials

- Pigmented villonodular synovitis.
- *Other problems to be considered:* Rice bodies of tuberculosis and rheumatoid arthritis
- Synovial hemangioma.

Treatment

Medical Therapy

Nonsteroidal anti-inflammatory drugs can be used, along with transcutaneous therapies (e.g. ultrasound and thermal therapies), for reduction of inflammation. Patients with primarily mechanical symptoms, do not benefit significantly from nonoperative therapy.

Surgical Therapy

Treatment includes, arthroscopic examination and excision of loose bodies, with limited synovectomy of involved synovium only. The treatment of patients, with SOC involves surgical excision of the proliferating synovium. Because recurrence is frequent after surgery, total synovectomy has been suggested as the preferred treatment for the condition.

Arthroscopic (Figs 25.361 to 25.363)

Arthroscopic appearance of synovial chondromatosis, loose bodies in the shoulder.

Complications

The most common complications include, stiffness and recurrence of mechanical symptoms, due to loose body generation. In most series, rates of recurrent symptoms that required repeat arthroscopic surgery were less than 20 percent. With aggressive postoperative rehabilitation, use of the arthroscopic approach typically helps prevent stiffness.

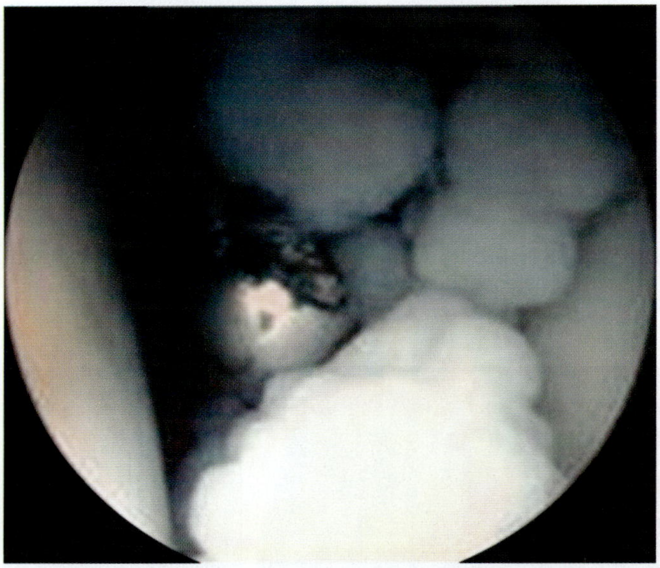

Fig. 25.362: Arthroscopic image of pedunculated SOC

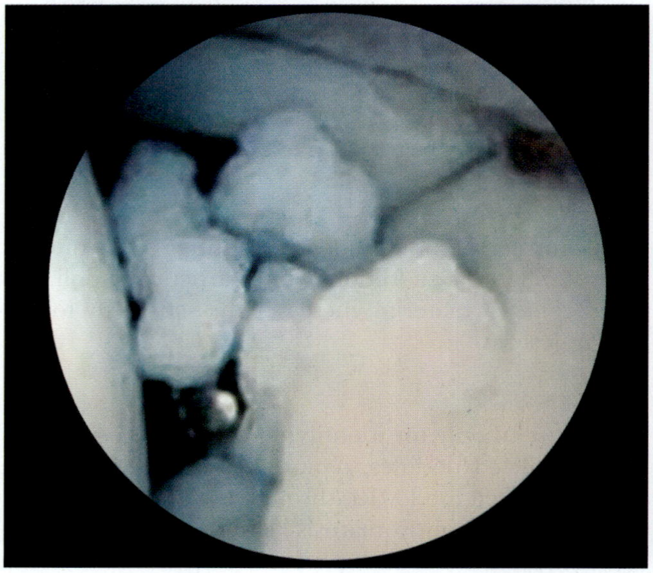

Fig. 25.361: Arthroscopic appearance of synovial chondromatosis, loose bodies in the shoulder

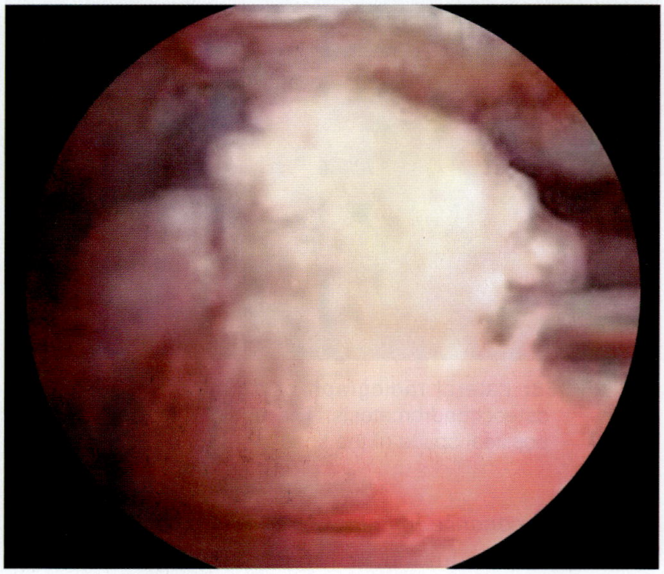

Fig. 25.363: Synovial chondromatosis of the knee

TUMORS AROUND KNEE

- Benign
- Malignant
- Benign tumors around knee
- Bone forming tumors
- Osteoid osteoma
- Chondroblastoma
- Cartilaginous tumors
- Osteochondroma
- Chondromyxoid fibroma
- Fibrous lesions
- Giant cell tumors
- Cystic lesions
- Unicameral cyst
- Aneurysmal bone cyst
- Malignant tumors around knee
- Chondrosarcoma
- Osteosarcoma
- Adamantinoma
- Fibrosarcoma
- Hystiocytic lymphoma
- Ewings sarcoma
- Metastatic tumors.

■ Osteoid Osteoma

Osteoid osteoma is a benign osteoblastic tumor.

Sex: Male : Female = 2:1

Age: Young adults between 10 and 25 years of age found in the first three decades of life, but an occasional lesion has been reported in older patients.

Location: The proximal femur is the most common location. Osteoid osteoma is found in the diaphysis or the metaphysis of the proximal end of the bone more often than the distal end.

Incidence: Approximately 10 percent of benign bone tumors are osteoid osteoma, 5 percent are subperiosteal and 5 percent of sciatica are due to osteoid osteoma.

Pathology

Vascular mesenchymal type of connective tissue stroma, with proliferating fibroblasts and osteoblasts, surrounds abundant pink staining osteoid tissue. Osteoid forms irregular branching network. Surrounding the poorly formed tissue at the center of lesion, there is marked bony proliferation. Marrow is fibrous, cartilage is never found.

Clinical Features

The typical patient has pain that gets worse at night and relieved by aspirin (aspirin tumor). The person may limp. When the lesion is near a joint, swelling, stiffness and contracture may occur. When in a vertebra, scoliosis may occur. Occasionally, osteoid osteoma occurs with minimal pain. In children, overgrowth and angular deformities may occur. Systemic symptoms are absent.

Radiographic Findings

Small rarefied lesions, less than 2 cm in diameter in cortex, subcortical or subperiosteal regions is seen, which is surrounded by thick sclerotic bone. Rarefied lesions have small dense center of ossification, called nidus. CT or MRI are useful to identify and localize the lesion. A bone scan is helpful in detecting small lesions, which may be overlooked on roentgenograms. The double density sign, which is a focal area of increased activity, with a second smaller area of increased uptake superimposed on it, is said to be diagnostic of osteoid osteoma.

Treatment

Conservative: Rest to the part and analgesics (aspirin).

Surgical: To affect a cure the entire nidus must be removed. Block resection of the nidus is done. However, if the lesion is in cortical bone, this method increases the risk of subsequent fracture. An alternative method suggested by Johnston, is to shave the reactive bone with a sharp osteotome, until the nidus is encountered then curette the exposed nidus. A CT guided percutaneous resection allows precise localization and removal of the nidus, through a small access without the need for removal of an excessive amount of bone. Percutaneous radiofrequency ablation of osteoid osteomas is also carried out. It is believed that their results are equivalent to operative excision. For rare intra-articular situations, arthroscopically assisted excision is performed. MRI guided cryotreatment may also be performed.

Recurrence and Malignancy

After complete removal of tumor along with nidus recurrence is very rare. No malignant change has ever been documented.

■ Chondroblastoma

It is a cellular, vascular and cartilaginous tumor of young adults. Occurs about the epiphyseal line. Destroys cancellous bone and contains calcium deposits.

Clinical Picture

Age: Before obliteration of epiphyseal line, i.e. 10–20 years of age.

Sex: Males predominate.

Location: Ends of long bones about the knee and humerus are mostly affected.

Position: About one side of epiphyseal line, chiefly in the metaphysic, it may extend to the epiphysis.

Symptoms and Findings

- History of trauma
- Pain, tenderness and swelling in most cases
- Occasionally limp and joint effusion.
- Course is rapid, from 1 month to 2 years.

Roentgenographic Findings

Well delineated area of rarefaction of cancellous bone, extending over and beyond epiphyseal line. Main mass of the tumor is either in metaphysis or the epiphysis. The position is often eccentric.

Pathology

Macroscopically: Tumor appears as a dark red, hemorrhagic and friable tissue, within which, small yellow zones of calcification, bluish white translucent nodules of cartilage and a few spicules of necrotic bone are scattered. The tumor extends, irregularly through the metaphysis, destroys the epiphyseal line at one side and occasionally invades subperiosteal space.

Microscopically: Large sheets of compact round or polyhedral cells, similar to mesenchymal tissue form the basic tumor tissue. Focal areas of calcification, distributed throughout the cellular tumor tissue are typical. A scattering of giant cells lies adjacent to areas of hemorrhage and necrosis. In some areas, tumor cells can be seen undergoing transformation to cartilage cells. About necrotic zones, a reparative process occurs by resorption of calcific detritus and organization of hemorrhage. Many blood spaces with or without a single layer of endothelium occur throughout the tumor.

Roentgenographic Findings

The cortex may be thinned or rarely penetrated. The tumor borders are irregular, fuzzy and vague. Mottled area of increased density, throughout the tumor represents calcium deposits.

Treatment

Curettage and obliteration of the cavity by bone grafts.

■ Osteochondroma

It is most common benign bone tumor. Accounts for 20–50 percent of benign bone tumors and 10 to 15 percent of all bone tumors. Approximately, 15 percent of patients with osteochondromas have multiple lesions. It is an offshoot from the spongy bone tissue, covered with a cartilaginous cap.

Age: Common during the growth period.

Sex: Male preponderance (male : female ratio is 1.5:1)

Area: Metaphysis of long tubular bones, especially around knee.

Location: Favors, site of tendinous attachments of strong muscles.

Theory of Histogenesis

- Exact cause is not known
- Cambium layer of periosteum retains throughout its life, ability to form cartilage and bone.
- Due to perverted activity of periosteum, it reverts to its role as perichodrium.
- At point of tendinous insertion, there is focal accumulation of embryonic connective tissue.

Clinical Features

Symptoms

- Usually symptom less
- Patient may complaint of pain, swelling, bursitis, malignant change, fracture, neuropathies, etc.

Signs

- Firm nontender swelling, fixed to bone around the joints.
- An inflamed bursa causes tenderness and local warmth.
- Decreased joint movements, tumor causing mechanical block.

Roentgenographic Findings

Plain radiographs are normally enough to diagnose osteochondromas. Pathognomonic radiographic findings associated with an osteochondroma include:

- The lesions protrude on host bone as pedunculated or sessile (broad based). Sessile lesions cover a broad area resulting in a widened metaphysic or a trumpet shaped deformity on X-ray. Lesions with stalks are found more distally.
- It occurs either in metaphysic or in diaphysis as the main epiphyseal line grows away from the lesion. It is never found in epiphysis.
- The cortes and cancellous bone of osteochondroma blend with cortex and cancellous bone of the host. This is the main radiographic finding.
- All osteochondromas, especially pedunculated ones are directed away from the growing ends of bones.
- Calcifications of cartilaginous cap can be seen as areas of opacities on X-ray.

Classification

Osteochondromas are of two types:

- *Stalked*
- *Broad based or sessile*: Sessile lesions cover a wide area and as a result cause metaphyseal widening or a "trumpet shaped deformity" on X-ray.

Treatment

Usually it requires no treatment. Surgical excision consists of an en bloc resection. It is indicated when:
- Joint interference
- Painful bursitis
- Fracture of the bony stalk
- Malignant changes
- Pressure on the neighboring vessels and nerves.

Prognosis

The risk of malignant transformation to chondrosarcoma in hereditary multiple osteochondromatosis is unknown, but can be 25 to 30 percent compared to approximately 1 percent for a solitary osteochondroma.

■ Chondromyxoid Fibroma

A rare tumor of bone, occurring mainly in adolescents and young adults. Least common benign cartilaginous tumor.

Etiology

Age: Second and third decades and less often in childhood.

Sex: No predominance.

Location: Most commonly, metaphyseal region of large tubular bone of lower limb.

Clinical Feature

- The tumor causes mild or no pain
- Slowly increasing local swelling
- Palpable and tender tumor mass fixed to the underlying bone
- When the tumor develops in people younger than 10 years, the symptoms are more pronounced and the course is rapid.

Roentgenographic Findings

The lesion is a translucent mass of variable size, located eccentrically in the metaphysis. On the medullary aspect of the lesion, the margin is scalloped and sclerosed. Over its outer aspect, the cortex is expanded and thinned and may appear interrupted. In a child, at the edge of the base of the tumor, triangular periosteal bone formation, unlike Codman's triangle, often forms. A faint trabecular pattern is apparent. Pseudoloculation represents ridges and corrugations of the inner sclerotic wall.

Pathology

Gross appearance: Tumor excised in toto. The outer surface is covered by a thin shell of newly formed periosteal bone or the periosteum itself. Its location in a large tubular bone is eccentric, but within a small tubular bone. It sometime occupies the entire width, producing a fusiform swelling.

On Cut Surface

A solid tumor mass is of grayish or bluish gray color, somewhat translucent and resembling cartilage. Sometimes containing small cavities with mucoid tissue. The consistency is usually firm. Calcified areas are unusual. The surface of the tumor mass toward the spongiosa is sharply demarcated, lobulated and surrounded by a thin, scalloped border of dense bone.

Pathology

Microscopic: The tumor is composed of lobulated or pseudolobulated areas of stellate cells with indistinct cytoplasmic borders, lying within the central portion of lobule and widely separated by intercellular mucin like material. The cells send out long, branching cytoplasmic processes.

Pathology

The nuclei are single, ovoid and of moderate size, although a few cells have large and multiple nuclei. Sparse collagen fibers form a widespread reticulum at the center of the lobule. At the periphery of the lobule, the appearance is more cellular and more collagenous. The hypercellularity, pleomorphism, bizarre shaped, hyperchromic and often multiple nuclei are characteristics that strongly suggest malignancy.

Differential Diagnosis

- Chondrosarcoma
- Myxosarcoma.

Treatment

Local excision and filling the cavity with autogenous bone. Wide en bloc excision can be performed. If tumor reoccurs, then additional studies should be done to determine whether malignant transformation has occurred and appropriate treatment like local excision or amputation should be done.

■ Giant Cell Tumor

Benign giant cell tumor is an osteolytic tumor, arising from the epiphysis and is common in young adults. Though it is benign, it can be locally malignant.

Sex: Male:Female ratio is 3:2.

Age: It is common between 15 and 35 years of age (80% occur in more than 20 years of age and the average age group is 35 years).

Sites: Giant cell tumor may occur in the sacrum and upper end of femur.

Pathology

Grossly, the tumor consists of ragged, friable and bleeding tissue, filled with old or fresh blood clot, with different sized cysts and cavities. Color varies from red and brown. Epiphyseal end of the bone is distorted. Tumor extension in the joint cavity is usually not seen and there is no evidence of periosteal reaction. Microscopically the tumor is encompassed by a fibrous capsule at the periphery. Presence of abundant tumor giant cells is quiet characteristic. These cells are characterized by their larger size and multiple nuclei more than 150 in number, which are distributed throughout the cell. Appearance of spindle cell, indicate malignant potential.

Histological Grading (Jaffe's Criterion)

Grade I

- Presence of characteristic stromal cell
- Little intercellular collagen
- Spindle cells are adjacent to the necrotic tissue.

Grade II

Random distribution of giant cells are seen among the stromal cell.

Grade III

Nuclei of giant cells are identical to those of the stromal cells.

Clinical Features

The course of the tumor is chronic. Unlike, osteogenic sarcoma, pain is not the presenting feature but trauma is present. The patient complains of swelling, which is situated on one side of the bone. Skin over the tumor is stretched, but there is no dilated vein. Tenderness is moderate or absent, egg shell crackling sensation may be present or absent. Invasion in the joint is rare and joint effusion is rare. Pathological fracture is a late feature.

Radiology

An osteolytic area is seen near the epiphysis. The cortex is thin and expanded. There is no periosteal new bone formation. Thin septa of bone transverse the interior of bone and gives it soap bubble appearance. The cortex may be disrupted in late stages. Joint extension is rare.

Companacci's Radiographic Grading

Grade I: Cystic lesion.
Grade II: Cortex is thin but not perforated.
Grade III: Cortex is perforated with extension in the soft tissue.

Ennekings Staging of Benign Giant Cell Tumor (GCT)

Stage I

- Latent, incidence is 10 to 15 percent
- Discovered accidentally, no symptoms
- Pathological fractures may be present.

Stage II

- Active, incidence is 70 percent
- Symptomatic, pathological fracture may be present
- Benign.

Stage III

- Aggressive, incidence is 10 to 15 percent
- Symptomatic rapidly growing
- Benign
- Cortex is perforated.

Treatment

- Intralesional excision by extended curettage is the treatment of choice.
- Curettage and bone grafting
- En bloc resection
- Curettage and acrylic bone cementation
- Curettage and cryosurgery
- Arthrodesis
- Arthroplasty
- Radiotherapy.

■ Unicameral Bone Cyst

Unicameral bone cyst (UBC) is a thin walled cavity in metaphysis of long bone, adjacent to the growth plate and migrate away from it as it matures. Pathological fracture is common but rarely affect epiphyseal growth plate.

Etiology

- Unknown
- Popular theory is local trauma
- Local venous congestion
- Increase in intraosseous pressure
- Reactive bone resorption
- Cyst fluid containing, prostaglandin IL and IB
- Bone resorption.

Types

Active Cyst

- Under 10 years
- Fill most of the metaphysis
- Thin bony wall
- Continue to enlarge
- Pathological fractures.

Passive Cyst

- Over 12 years
- Separated from growth plate
- Thick bony wall
- Cease to expand
- Less likely.

Pathology

Gross

- Area of fusiform expansion
- Periosteum lifts away
- *Underlying tissue:* Egg shell thin, semi translucent, bluish and easily penetrated
- *Cavity:* Single chamber containing yellow fluid following a healed fracture, cavity divided by fibro-osseous septae.

Microscopic

The connective tissue composed of fibroblasts lying on vascular collagenase tissue, containing multinucleated giant cells, foam cells containing hemosiderin, lipids and cholesterol crystals.

Clinical Features

Asymptomatic, until trivial trauma occurs. Local aching pain, due to fracture through the cyst wall. Local swelling and tenderness. Intermittent limp in weight-bearing bones. Pathological fractures in about 50 percent cases.

Infarction of the thinned cortex in about 25 percent cases. Displacement of the cyst down the shaft. Growth disturbances, e.g. coxa vara deformity in proximal femoral region, shortening and overgrowth.

Diagnosis

- X-ray shows, a large, well localized, radiolucent and expansile defect in metaphysis. Regional cortex attenuated. Pseudo-locuolated form, following a fracture healing. Fallen leaf sign (fragment of cortex in the cyst)
- CT scan, useful only if lesion is in pelvis
- MRI is not useful, as it demonstrates only fluid signals
- Bone scan shows, light peripheral uptake with cold center.
- Aspiration of fluid and injection of radio-opaque substance. Aspirated fluid shows, increased level of prostaglandin E2 (PG E2)
  - Open biopsy and cytology are also useful in diagnosis.

Treatment

Goal

Prevention of pathological fracture.

Modalities

- Curettage and bone grafting, this technique is having high recurrence rate
  - For active cyst, recurrence rate is 50 percent
  - For passive cyst, it is 10 percent
- *Steroids:* Methyl prednisolone, 80 to 200 mg is infused into the cavity
- Autologous bone marrow injection
- Multiple drill holes.

■ Aneurysmal Bone Cyst

Aneurysmal bone cysts (ABCs) is a benign cystic lesion of bone, composed of blood filled spaces, which are separated by connective tissue septa, containing fibroblast, osteoclast (type giant cells) and reactive woven bone. Aneurysmal bone cysts are benign, solitary, expansile and erosive lesion of bone.

Incidence: One percent of benign bone lesion.

Age: Most frequent in children (85% cases are less than 20 years old).

Sex: Female: Male is 2:1.

Radiological Classification of Juxta-physeal Aneurysmal Bone Cyst (Campanacci's Classification)

Type I: Cyst in middle with little or no expansion.

Type II: Lesion substitutes the whole bone segment.

Type III: Eccentric interosseous lesion with little or no expansion.

Type IV: Subperosteal cyst and superficial erosion of cortex.

Type V: Periosteum eroded and expands into soft tissue.

Aneurysmal Bone Cysts can be Tumors of Undefined Neoplastic Nature

Primary Lesion (De Novo)

Incidence: 70 percent of ABCs

Cause: Trauma or vascular disturbances.

Secondary with Precursor Lesion

Incidence: 30 percent.

Cause: Common precursor lesion is GCT 19 to 39 percent cases.

Other Precursor Lesion

Osteoblastoma, fibroma, chondroblastoma, osteosarcoma, UBC, etc.

Recommended Surgery

- Curettage with bone grafting
- Curettage with cementing
- Cryosurgery
- En bloc excision with or without reconstruction of skeletal defect.

■ Chondrosarcoma

It is a malignant, slow growing tumor. It arises from cartilage cell. It ranges from being locally aggressive to high grade malignancy.

Incidence: Second in frequency to osteosarcoma.

Site: Common in proximal femur.

Sex: Males commonly affected more than females (male to female ratio is 1.5:1).

Location: Long bone from diaphyseal metaphyseal region.

Age: 20 to 60 years, are most commonly affected.

Classification

Primary

- Central (medullary) type
- Juxtacortical (peri or parosteal)
- Clear cell chondrosarcoma
- Mesenchymal chondrosarcoma
- Dedifferentiated chondrosarcoma.

Secondary

Arising from pre-existing benign condition, like exostosis or multiple enchondroma.

Pathology

Macroscopically: Tumor is lobulated and appears as white or bluish mass. Firm in consistency. Areas of myxomatous degeneration and softening. Irregular patchy areas of calcification seen.

Microscopically: Masses of cartilage cell with more than one nucleus and are hyperchromatic.

Histologically: Histologically, tumor is graded as:
Grade I: Low grade
Grade II: Intermediate grade
Grade III: High grade.

Clinical Features

Pelvic tumors present with urinary frequency or obstruction or may masquerade as a groin muscle pulls. Patient complains of swelling with history of dull aching pain. Swelling is hard in consistency with lobulated surface. Grows very slowly and may causes mechanical restriction of joint movements.

Radiological Features

Central tumors: Central lytic lesion, with calcification gives fluffy, cotton wool, popcorn or breadcrumb appearance. It invades the soft tissue little or with no periosteal reaction.

Peripheral tumors: Very large tumors and central part is calcified.

Treatment

Surgery is the treatment of choice

- *Low and medium grade lesion*
  - Require wide excision.
- *High grade lesion*
  - Radical excision and chemotherapy.
- *Palliative radiotherapy*
  - It is done, when tumor is present in an inaccessible area.

Prognosis

Poor in axial skeleton and proximal bone tumors, childhood and young adults. Cytologically, suggesting high grade malignancy and secondary chondrosarcoma. Survival time after treatment is 10 years.

■ Osteosarcoma

It is a malignant primary bone tumor arising from multipotent mesenchymal tissues of bone. It is characterized by direct formation of bone or osteoid, by proliferating tumor cells.

Incidence: It is a common malignant tumor, commonly occurs in young, between 10 and 20 years of age.

Sites: Most commonly occur in distal femur followed by proximal tibia.

Exciting factors: The predisposing factors of the tumors are:

- *Virus*
  - Deoxyribonucleic acid (DNA) viruses, e.g. polyoma and sendai virus (SV40) and
  - Ribonucleic acid (RNA) viruses, e.g. Harvey and moloney sarcoma virus is known to produce tumors in animals but not in humans.
- *Radiation*: A dose of 2000 rads can set malignancy in the bone.
- *Chemicals*: Beryllium compounds, methyl cholanthrene, etc.

Distribution of Osteosarcoma in Body (Fig. 25.364)

Clinical Features

- Pain is the initial and dominating symptom.
- Bony swelling appears after some week.
- Swelling progressively increases in size.

Clinical Examination

General Examination

General health deteriorates, with anemia, loss of weight and cachexia. Patient develops pulmonary symptoms due to secondaries.

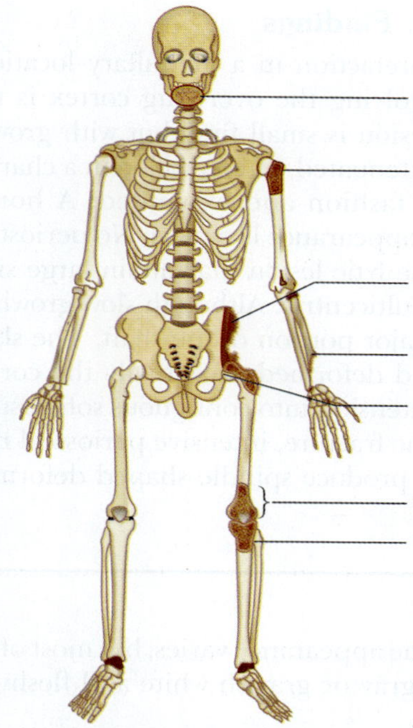

Fig. 25.364: Illustration showing distribution and incident rate of osteosarcoma in various parts of the body

On Examination

- Swelling is fusiform
- Skin is stretched, shiny and vascular, with prominent veins
- Swelling is warm to touch and shows pulsations if tumor is highly vascular
- It is firm to hard in consistency
- In late stages, the tumor fungates.

Classification of Osteosarcoma

Primary Osteosarcomas

- Conventional type
  - Osteoblastic
  - Chondroblastic
  - Fibroblastic
  - Small cell
  - Telangiectatic
- Surface (juxtacortical) osteosarcoma
  - Parosteal osteosarcoma.
  - Periosteal osteosarcoma.
  - High grade surface osteosarcoma.

Secondary Osteosarcoma

- Postirradiation.
- Pagets sarcoma
- Solitary or multiple osteochondromatosis
- Bone infarction
- Chronic osteomyelities.

Miscellaneous

- GCT
- Fibrous dysplasia
- Chondroblastoma
- Osteoblastoma
- Rare osteosarcoma
  - Li-Fraumeni syndrome
  - Osteosarcoma of the jaw
  - Multicentric osteosarcoma.

Pathology

Grossly: It is a large tumor, with areas of destruction, gives an appearance of a leg of mutton. Consistency range from hard to soft. Color of tumor could be white if fibroblastic, yellowish white if osteoblastic and bluish if cartilaginous. At the areas of rapid growth, there are areas of cavitations, necrotic foci and hemorrhages. Sun ray appearance, due to the bone deposition along the vessels. Codman's triangle is the reactive bone formation parallel to the bone.

Histology: Small spindle cells, with hyperchromatic nuclei. Shape may be round, cuboidal or columnar. Cells are pleomorphic in nature. Giant cells are often present. Matrix may be myxomatous, cartilaginous or osseous. Areas of hemorrhages may be present.

Radiological Features

Tumor arises from metaphyseal region of the bone either centrally or from cortex. Mottled area of rarefaction with areas of osteosclerosis. When it extends beyond the cortex, the periosteum is raised and there is new bone formation in lines at right angle to the cortex, this cause sun ray appearance on X-ray. Codman's triangle is seen at the junction of normal bone and tumor area. It is reactive new bone formation subperiosteally.

Ghost shadow: Chest X-ray (CXR) may show secondaries in chest.

Treatment

The aim of treatment is to confirm the diagnosis and to evaluate the spread and to execute adequate treatment. Confirmation of diagnosis is done clinicaly, histologically, radiologically and by laboratory findings. Evaluation of the spread of the tumors is done. Lungs are the common area of metastasis. CXR should be done. CT and MRI will detect the extent of tumor and soft tissue involvement. Bone scan will detect skip lesions.

Surgery

- *Early and radical ablation* is the surgery of choice
- *Limb salvage*: If no joint involved
- *En bloc resection* of proximal femur.
- *Reconstruction*: Bipolar with long stem

- Combined with allograft
- Total femoral replacement

- *Amputation*: Amputation remains the mainstay. Level of amputation, is upper end of femur (hind quarter amputation and hip disarticulation).
- Newer techniques
  - Limb salvage with tumor endoprosthesis
  - *In juxta-articular:* Intraepiphyseal resection and biological reconstruction.
- *Megavoltage radiotherapy:* Radiation is given preoperatively to decrease the viable cells that get disseminated into bloodstream. Useful adjuvant in the treatment of resectable tumors. Radiation destroys tumor cells with minimal effect on uninvolved parts. Total dose is 6000–8000 rads or 230 rads per day or 1000 rads per week.
- *Chemotherapy*: It is given pre-and postoperatively to control the micrometastasis. Drugs are methotrexate, citrovorum factor, endoxan and cisplatinum.
- *Immunotherapy*: Relatively, new concept. The sensitized lymphocytes from the survivors are infused into the patient. Follow-up is every 6 to 8 weeks for recurrence and metastasis.

Prognosis

Without therapy death occurs in 2 to 6 months. With surgery and chemotherapy, five years of disease-free life, seen in 70 percent of patients.

■ Adamantinoma

A rare, but distinctive primary bone tumor. The designation adamantinoma was originally given because of its histologic resemblance to the benign, but locally invasive tumor of proliferating odontogenic epithelium, embedded in a fibrous stroma, now is generally called ameloblastoma.

Age: Incidence seems to be between 10 and 35 years.

Incidence: Blacks are more predisposed.

Location: In appendicular skeleton, the tibia is the favored location.

Clinical Picture

The tumor develops, insidiously over the years. At first, it may be asymptomatic and discovered on X-rays, or the first indication may be a pathological fracture. The initial symptoms can be pain, swelling, tenderness and the acute development of symptoms associated with pathological fracture. The tumor is locally invasive, spreading slowly but progressively without metastasizing even after unsuccessful removal. Despite, a protracted local invasion, which suggests that the tumor is benign, metastasis have been recorded to regional lymph nodes, lungs, abdominal viscera ribs and tibia to humerus.

Roentgenographic Findings

A sharply defined rarefaction in a medullary location, that eccentrically involving the overlying cortex is the main finding. The lesion is small first, but with growth the cortex becomes attenuated, often eroded in a characteristic saw toothed fashion and expanded. A honey combed or loculated appearance is typical. No periosteal reaction is noted. The lytic lesion may attain large size. The lesion is often multicentric. Although slow growing, comes to occupy a major portion of the shaft. The shaft becomes widened and deformed. Eventually the cortex is penetrated, with extension into contiguous soft tissues. Following a pathologic fracture, intensive periosteal new bone formation may produce spindle shaped deformity of the bone.

■ Pathology

Gross appearance: The appearance varies, but most often the tumor is yellow, gray or grayish white and fleshy or firm in consistency.

Microscopically: Three basic patterns are observed. These are summarized as below:

- Elongated anastomosing masses of stellate epithelial cells are seen. The peripheral cells are columnar and arrange in a palisade fashion. The central cells of these masses are stellate and produce a reticulum appearance. A characteristic epithelial ameloblastic pattern is produced, with convoluted and infolded double layered structures and scanty intervening stroma.
- Discrete islands of basal cells with peripheral palisading and central cystic degeneration. This is a follicular ameloblastic pattern.
- Islands of squamous epithelium and pearl formation. The stroma is fibrous. Islands of spindle cells are characteristic feature.

Treatment

- Curettage and bone grafting
- Curettage with bone cementing
- If CT scan and X-rays suggest, that the tumor is limited in extent and confined to the bone, en bloc excision can be done. This is accompanied by removal of suspiciously enlarged lymph nodes.
- If recurrence is there, then amputation is indicated.

■ Fibrosarcoma

It is a malignant cytoplasm, the basic cell of which is the fibroblast in varying degree of anaplasia, as shown in Figure 25.365. Histologically, it is identical with a fibrosarcoma, which arises from soft tissue structures.

Clinical Picture

Age: Present in over 30 years of age.

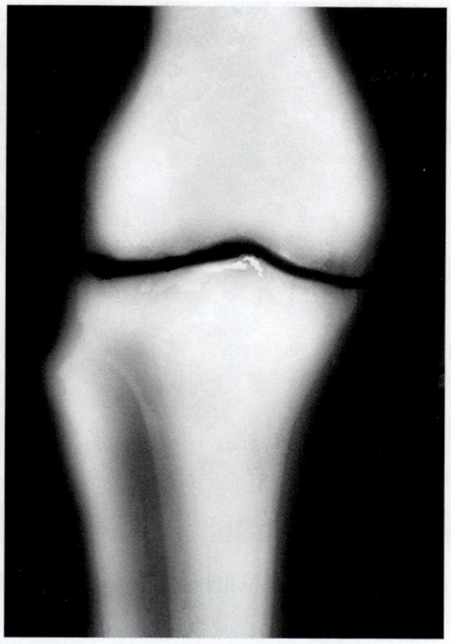

Fig. 25.365: Fibrosarcoma of proximal tibia

Site: Long bones especially the femur. Also in ribs, skull, vertebrae and mandible.

Position: Subperiosteal area of diaphysis, metaphysis or originates in medulla and then penetrates through to subperiosteal space. It is a solitary lesion.

Symptoms

- Gradual onset of continuous pain
- Worse at night
- Gradual appearance of swelling, which is smooth, firm, rubbery textured and firmly fixed to the underlying bone.
- Occasionally, tumor is infiltrative and fixes overlying soft tissues, thereby restricting joint motion.
- Pathological fracture is rare
- Metastases to lungs and other subperiosteal spaces can occur.

Roentgenographic Changes

A soft tissue shadow, slightly denser than muscle is seen. The shadow is usually a single lesion, extraosseous but immediately adjacent to the cortex of long bone. Directly beneath the tumor shadow, is a saucer shaped cortical erosion of varying depth. At the upper and lower corners of the periosteal shadow, slight triangles of reactive bone (Codman's triangles) may be seen. Slight calcific densities are sometimes seen within the shadow. If the tumor is very malignant and infiltrative, sharp borders of the shadow are lost. When the tumor has penetrated the cortex, the latter is riddled with small lytic areas. The medulla is then involved and shows vague areas of rarefaction. When tumor rarely originates within the medulla, a central irregular moth eaten area of rarefaction appears.

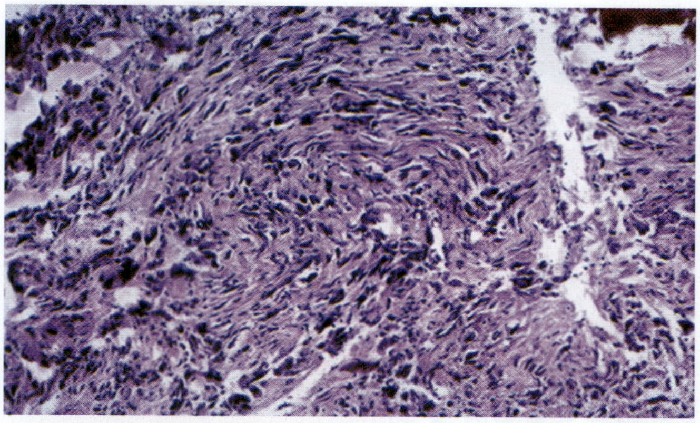

Fig. 25.366: High-grade fibrosarcoma with numerous mitotic figures seen in the spindle cells that are forming collagen fiber

Pathology

Gross appearance: The tumor is a well encapsulated, firm, white, fibrous and glistening mass beneath the elevated periosteum on one side of a long bone. On cut section, strands of fibrous tissue are arranged in striations, whorls or are criss crossed. The cortex may be uninvolved and the tumor may peel away easily from the bone. If the tumor has invaded cortex, the tumor is separated with difficulty and the underlying bone, presents a saucer shaped depression of varying depth. When the tumor is markedly invasive, the cortex is thoroughly destroyed, the medulla infiltrated and the bone markedly weakened so that pathological fracture occurs.

Microscopically: Fibrosarcoma consist mainly of a cellular tissue composed of small oat shaped cells resembling mesenchymal cells (most malignant), as shown in Figure 25.366. A less malignant fibrosarcoma, consist of cells which are more differentiated. The preponderant cell is the spindle cell. The least malignant tumor is composed chiefly of fibroblasts and more intercellular material of the eosinophilic collagenous type.

Treatment

Main line of treatment is amputation.

■ Hystiocytic Lymphoma

Lymphoma may involve bone primarily or secondarily.

Occurrence: Lymphoma can occur at any age but becomes more common in the sixth and seventh decades of life.

Sex: The male to female ratio is approximately 1.5:1.

Location: The femur is the most common bone involved, followed by the pelvis.

Signs and symptoms: Most patients complain of localized pain or swelling.

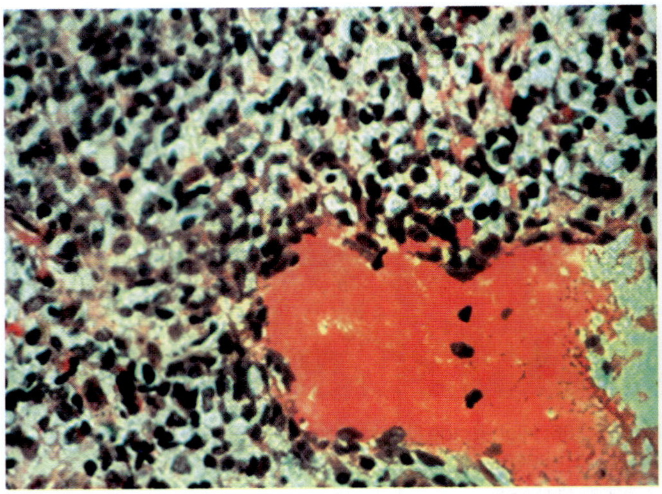

Fig. 25.367: An infiltrate of large lymphoid cells with prominent nucleoli is seen on histologic evaluation of this primary bone lymphoma

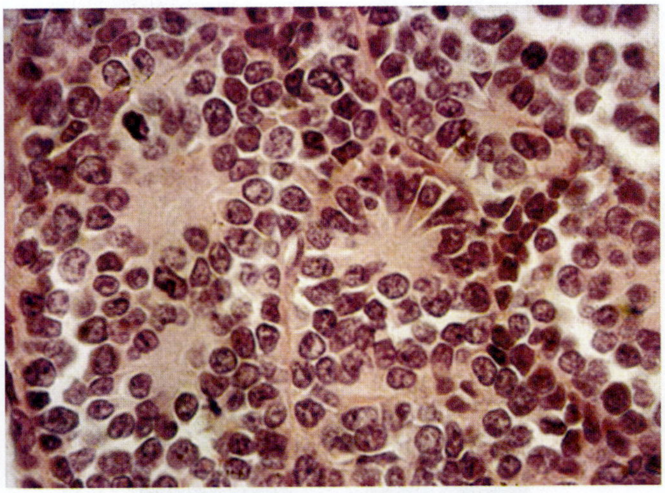

Fig. 25.368: Ewings sarcoma with uniform round cells

Roentgenographically: Lymphoma usually appears as an ill defined area of bone destruction, frequently diaphyseal and often has a permeative appearance. The cortex may be thickened, but a periosteal reaction is rarely seen.

Microscopically: Osseous lymphomas are composed of a mixture of both large and small lymphoid cells, with both cleaved and noncleaved nuclei, as shown in Figure 25.367.

Prognosis

Patients with primary lymphoma of bone have a better prognosis (approximately 55%, can have 5 years of survival) than those with systemic disease (less than 25% can survive till 5 years).

Treatment

The primary treatment of lymphoma is chemotherapy. Local control usually is attained, with radiation treatment. Surgical intervention is therefore, rarely needed but may be indicated for treatment of impending or actual pathological fractures.

■ Ewings Sarcoma

- Ewings sarcoma was first described by Ewing in 1928.
- It arises from primitive mesenchymal cells of the medullary cavity.
- This is a rare primary malignant bone tumor (10–14%), of all malignant bone tumors affecting children.
- It is lethal tumor, with poor survival rate of five years.

Incidence: Common between 4 and 25 years of age group (80%).

Sex: More common in males.

Site: Diaphysis of long bones, i.e. femur, tibia, fibula and humerus. About 20 percent of bone tumors are seen in flat bones.

Clinical Features

General Examination

- Moderate fever
- Anemia
- Pain and swelling.

Local Examination

- Visible or palpable tender swelling
- Rapidly increasing in size
- Local temperature elevation, with dilated vein.
- Location in rib may be associated with pleural effusion.
- Constitutional symptoms, like fever, sweating, chill, anemia and leukocytosis, creates confusion, as it mimics acute osteomyelitis.

Pathology

Macroscopically: Tumor is pale and soft mass, with minimal bone tissue. Areas of cystic degeneration and hemorrhages. There is simulation of osteomyelitis, by the presence of milky pus like fluid, due to degeneration. From the medulla, it reaches to the surface through the Haversian canal.

Microscopically: Tumor is very cellular with minimal stromal tissue, as shown in Figure 25.368. Characteristic cells are small, polyhedral with pale cytoplasm and large nucleus. Appearance is monotonously uniform. In some areas, there is pseudorosette formation, simulating rosette formation by neuroblastoma. Tumor can be differentiated

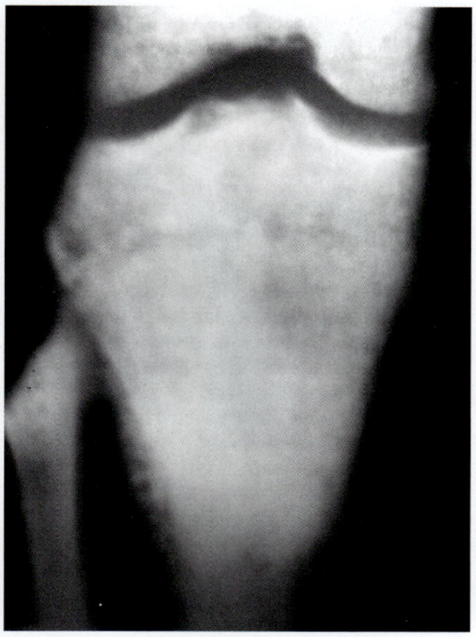

Fig. 25.369: X-ray of knee, with Ewings sarcoma

from reticulum cell sarcoma, as it stains for glycogen positively by positive cytoplasmic vesicles (PAS) in reticulum cell sarcoma silver stain is positive.

Radiographic Features (Fig. 25.369)

- Lesion can be lytic, sclerotic or mixed.
- Diaphyseal lesion, with irregular destruction (moth eaten appearance or cracked ice appearance)
- Periosteal new bone formation is in layer giving an onion peel appearance.
- Permeative margins.

Laboratory Test

- Increased erythrocyte sedimentation rate (ESR).
- Leukocytosis
- Anemia
- Urine for vanillylmandelic acid
- Immunohistochemical markers.
- Electron microscopy study
- Tissue for glycogen stain
- Special staining with HBA-71, which recognizes a product of MIC-2 gene has been suggested to be specific for Ewings sarcoma and neuroectodermal tumors.
- Ewing sarcoma is associated with chromosomal transformation (chromosomes 11 and 22). The tumor marker includes, neurone specific enclose myeloperoxidase.

Differential Diagnosis

- Osteomyelitis
- Osteosarcoma
- Malignant lymphoma.

Treatment

Tumor is highly sensitive to radiation, it melts like snow. Combination of radiotherapy and chemotherapy is used for the treatment. Recurrence rate is 20 to 30 percent because of radiation induced sarcomas. Therefore, surgical resection for the control of primary lesion is used.

Radiation: Highly sensitive to radiation and is mainstay of treatment. The dose is 4000 rads for entire limb and 1000 rads, as boost to tumor (which melts like a snow).

Surgery: Amputation, conservative surgery like debulking or limb saving surgery.

Prognosis

Unfavorable prognostic factor includes:

- Male patients
- Humerus, if involved
- Pelvic bone, if involved
- Distant metastasis.

Primary irradiation with amputation has two years of survival rate (15%). A combination of chemotherapy and radiotherapy with surgery, improves the survival rate of 50 to 75 percent for 3 to 5 years.

SYNOVIAL FLUID EXAMINATION

The analysis of synovial fluid should be a part of diagnostic evaluation of patients presenting with joint effusions, since the nature of underlying synovial tissue reaction is often reflected in synovial fluid findings. Evaluation of synovial fluid, aspirated from joints and the histopathological study of synovium, obtained by closed needle biopsy have been found to be a very useful investigative procedure in the diagnosis of joint diseases.

The procedure is quite simple and free from complications when compared to open methods. This diagnostic procedure is simple and safe. It has following advantages:

- Less surgical trauma to the patient
- Less time consuming
- Reliable procedure
- Does not require hospitalization of patient
- Does not require costly instruments and equipments.

■ Synovial Joint

Knee joint (a synovial joint) and constituent structures are shown in Figure 25.370.

■ Synovial Fluid

The word "synovia" was first coined by a Greek physician (Paracelsus). He noticed its superficial resemblance to egg white and described it as joint oil. Diarthrodial joints are lined at their margins by synovial membrane. Synovial

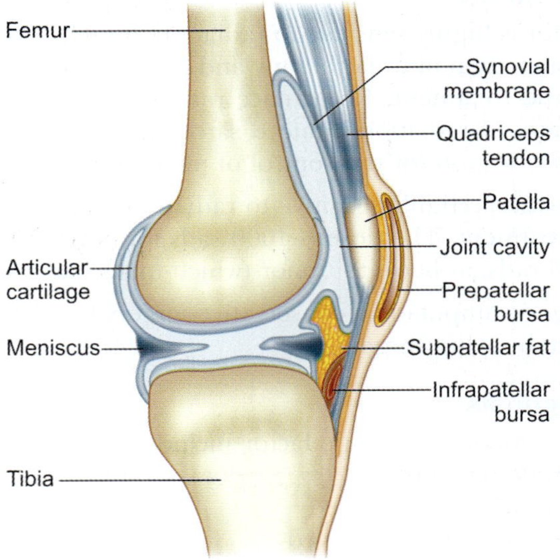

Fig. 25.370: Knee joint, a synovial joint, with constituent structures and their anatomical location

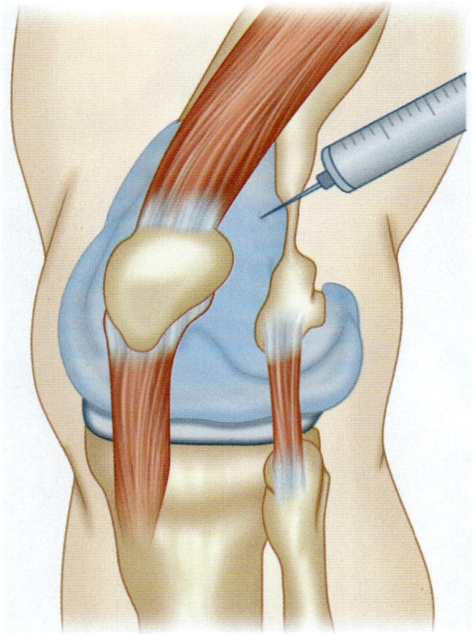

Fig. 25.371: Arthrocentesis of the knee joint

membrane is consists of lining cells facing the joint space, the underlying connective and adipose tissues are richly supplied by the vascular network. The lining or synovial flattened cells form a compact interlacing layer one to three cell in depth with thickness of 20 to 40 μ.

Synovial fluid has been described as being dialysate from plasma and is enriched with mucopolysaccharides, e.g. hyluronate, which is being synthesized by synovial cells (the presence of this gives characteristic viscosity to the fluid). Synovial fluid is a clear viscous yellow fluid which does not clot on standing, since it does not contain fibrinogen. Hence, synovial fluid is incoagulable. Synovial fluid contains 96 percent water and 4 percent solutes. The viscosity of synovial fluid depends on the concentration of hyaluronic acid and is lowered in ageing, osteoarthritis and following trauma.

Functions of Synovial Fluid

- Lubrication
- Nutrition (supply to articular cartilage)
- Defense mechanism (leukocytes and antibodies).

Indications for Joint Needle Aspiration

- Crystal induced arthropathy
- Hemarthrosis
- Limiting joint damage from an infectious process
- Symptomatic relief of a large effusion
- Unexplained joint effusion
- Unexplained monoarthritis.

Contraindications to Joint Needle Aspiration

- Bacteremia
- Inaccessible joints
- Joint prosthesis
- Overlying infection in the soft tissues
- Severe coagulopathy
- Severe overlying dermatitis
- Uncooperative patient.

Procedure of Arthrocentesis of Knee Joint (Fig. 25.371)

The usual site of aspiration is between patella and femoral condyles, either medially or laterally. Approach involves with aseptic precautions insertion of a needle 2 cm above and 2 cm lateral to the superior lateral aspect of the patella at an angle of 45° into the joint cavity. Synovial fluid is aspirated and collected in empty test tubes.

Arthrocentesis of other joints is shown in Figure 25.372.

Hip Joint Arthrocentesis

Lateral, anterior or posterior approaches are possible. In the anterior approach, the needle is inserted perpendicular to the skin at a point distal to and 2.5 cm lateral to the middle of the inguinal ligament, using the pulsation of femoral artery beneath the middle of ligament as a guide.

Wrist Joint Arthrocentesis

The needle is inserted into the joint from dorsal aspect just medial to anatomical snuff box.

Elbow Joint Arthrocentesis

Elbow is kept in acute flexion and the needle is inserted on the posterior aspect just lateral to olecranon.

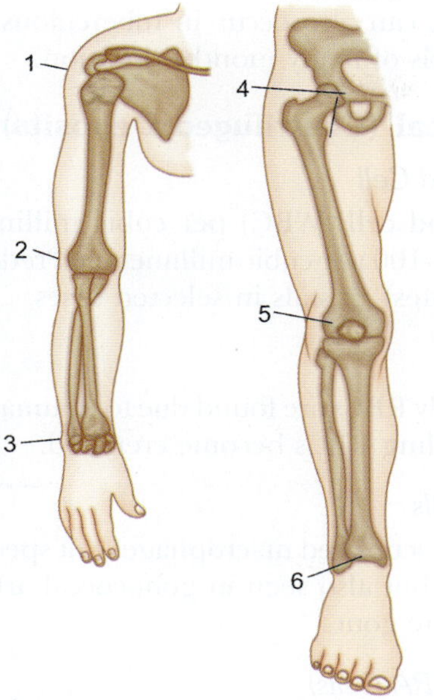

Fig. 25.372: Arthrocentesis of other joints—hip, knee and ankle (LL), wrist, elbow and shoulder (UL) joints —1. Shoulder joint; 2. Elbow joint; 3. Wrist joint; 4. Hip joint; 5. Knee joint; 6. Ankle joint

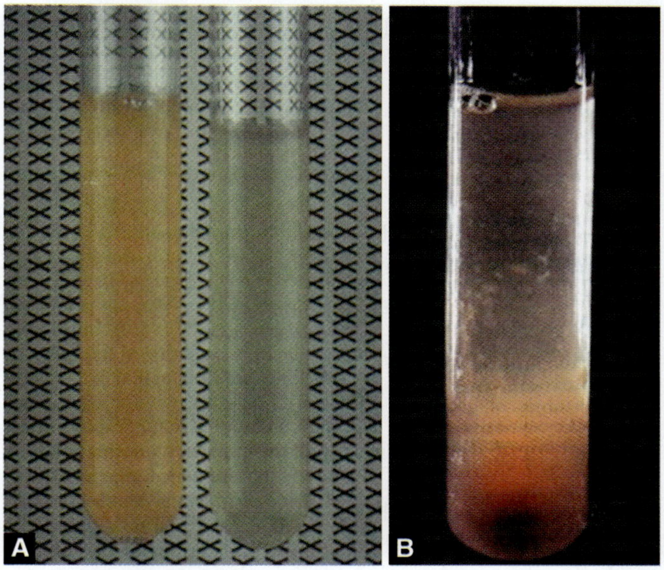

Figs 25.373A and B: Gross physical analysis of synovial fluid—(A) Color noted by holding against white background; (B) Color can vary from blood stained, straw to yellow colored

Ankle Joint Arthrocentesis

In the ankle, the needle is inserted at the lateral aspect of joint about 2.5 cm proximal and 1.3 cm medial to lateral malleolus.

■ Synovial Fluid Analysis

The gross appearance is often suggestive of particular type of effusion (Figs 25.373A and B). Aspirated fluid is analyzed under following headings.

Gross Analysis (Physical Analysis)

Color: Noted by holding the fluid against white background. The color can vary from blood stained, straw to yellow colored.

Clarity: It could be clear, cloudy or turbid.

Viscosity: This can be assessed by two methods:

- *String method:* A drop of fluid is held between the two fingers and the fingers are separated.
- *Drop method:* A drop of fluid is dropped from the needle and the time taken by drop is noted.

Mucin Clot Test (Rope's Test)

Glacial acetic acid is mixed with synovial fluid to check clot formation. Characteristics of various clots formed are:

Good clot formation: It is tight, ropy and suspended in clear solution. It does not break on tilting the tube.

Fair clot formation: A soft mass in a slightly cloudy solution.

Poor clot: Numerous soft friable masses.

Very poor clot: Few flakes of mucin suspended in turbid solution.

Fibrin clot test: It varies from 1 to 4 plus. When the fluid clots as soon as it is collected in the tube, it is 4 plus. Small soft clot at the end of one hour of aspiration is 1 plus. Other two grades fall in between. Wet mount preparation is done, to look for doubly refractile crystals of gout.

Specific Gravity

Based on the physical appearance the synovial fluid is grouped into the following groups:

Group I: Noninflammatory

Clear pale yellow to yellowish viscous fluid which usually does not clot is consistent with noninflammatory fluid, for example:

- Osteoarthritis, a degenerative joint disease
- Trauma
- Rheumatic fever
- Chronic gout or pseudogout
- Scleroderma
- Polymyositis
- Systemic lupus erythematosus
- Erythema nodosum

- Neuropathic arthropathy (with possible hemorrhage)
- Sickle-cell disease
- Hemochromatosis
- Acromegaly
- Amyloidosis.

Group II: Inflammatory

The inflammatory fluid is turbid yellow, tends to clot on standing and is of poor viscosity, for example:

- Reactive arthritis
- Psoriatic arthritis
- Acute rheumatic fever
- Acute gout or pseudogout
- Scleroderma
- Rheumatoid arthritis (RA)
- Polymyositis
- Systemic lupus erythematosus (SLE)
- Ankylosing spondylitis
- Inflammatory bowel disease arthritis
- Infection (viral, fungal or bacterial) including lyme disease
- Acute crystal synovitis.

Group III: Septic

The grossly purulent fluid of septic arthritis shows no mucin clot at all. Pyogenic bacterial infection or septic arthritis.

Group IV: Hemorrhagic

Consists of bloody or xanthochromic fluid due to recent or old trauma and other condition, for example:

- Trauma
- Tumors
- Hemophilia or coagulopathy
- Scurvy
- Ehlers-Danlos syndrome
- Neuropathic arthropathy
- Pigmented villonodular synovitis.

Biochemical Composition

Proteins in gram percentage (Normal 1.07–2.13%). Periam Ann et al. concluded that the level of synovial fluid protein, closely approaches to that of plasma in inflammatory disease.

Blood: Synovial fluid sugar level difference in milligram percentage. When glucose is being determined, the patient should be fasting for about 12 hours because equilibrium between blood and synovial fluid occurs slowly. Ropes and Bauer found that normal synovial fluid glucose is 10 mg/dl less than that of blood. A difference of 10 to 15 mg/dl is found in noninflammatory diseases and 20 mg/dl to more than 50 mg/dl is found in inflammatory group. Absolute synovial fluid sugar content of less than 30 mg/dl is observed only in septic arthritis, although it can also occur in tuberculous and rheumatoid arthritis of many months duration.

Cytological (Centrifuged Deposits)

White Blood Cell

White blood cell (WBC) per cubic millimeter (normal count is 13–100 per cubic millimeter). Predominant WBC (Lymphocytes) crystals in selected cases.

RBC

Occasionally RBCs are found due to trauma by the needle. Long standing RBCs become crenated.

Reiter's Cells

These are vacuolated macrophages not specific to Reiter's syndrome, but also seen in gonococcal arthritis, psoriasis and acute gout.

Ragocytes (RA Cells)

These are neutrophils containing inclusion bodies. These bodies contain fibrin, phagocytized extracellular material and rheumatoid factor. These cells are also found in gout and septic arthritis.

LE Cells

It is a polymorph engulfing the altered homogenous nucleus of another cell. These cells may be seen in SLE and RA.

Cartilage Cells

Seen in patients of osteoarthritis.

Physical Properties of Synovial Fluid in Normal and Diseased Joint

Polarized Microscopy for Crystals

The types of crystals that can be seen in synovial fluid are:

- *Monosodium urate crystals (Figs 25.374A and B)*: They are needle like, may be intracellular (acute gout) or extracellular. They are strongly negatively birefringent. Chalky deposits of monosodium urate crystals are seen in chronic gout.
- *Calcium pyrophosphate dihydrate (CPPD):* These are rod like crystals and weakly positive birefringent. They are commonly seen in degenerative arthritis, but also seen in pseudogout, hyperparathyroidism, diabetes mellitus and occasionally gout.
- *Cholesterol crystals*: Flat rectangular crystals with notched corners and maltese crosses. These are strongly negative birefringent. Sometimes seen in rheumatoid arthritis, chronic inflammatory arthritis and osteoarthritis.
- *Hydroxyapetite crystals*: Looks like shiny coins. Three major syndromes associated are:

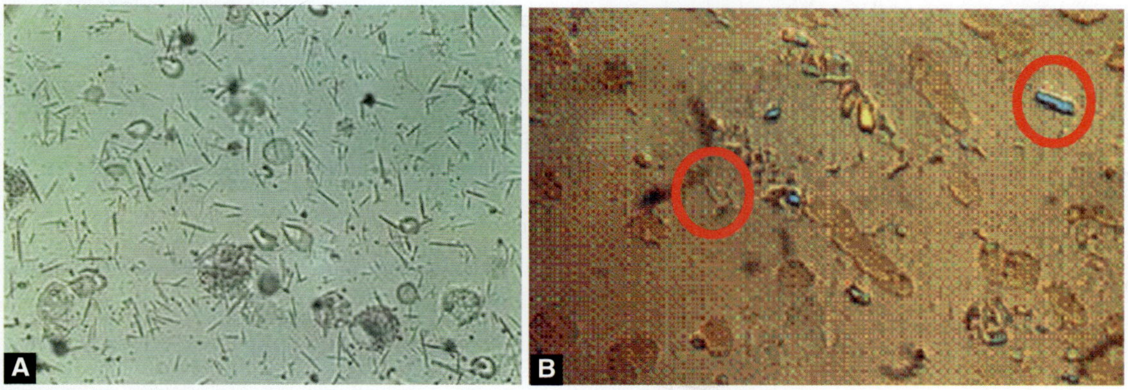

Figs 25.374A and B: Monosodium urate crystals found in synovial fluid

- Acute calcific periarthritis
- Acute calcific arthritis
- Chronic arthritis

- *Basic calcium phosphate (BCP):* Most commonly seen in calcific periarthritis seen as clumps and globules, are nonbirefringent. Associated conditions are:
  - Chronic BCP arthritis
  - Milwaukee shoulder knee syndrome
  - Mixed BCP-CPPD disease (see above)
  - Osteoarthritis
  - Metastatic calcinosis
- *Calcium oxalate*: Variable bipyramidal morphology. Strongly positively birefringent. Associated conditions are:
  - Chronic dialysis arthritis
  - Arthritis of primary oxalosis
- *Cryoglobulin crystals*: Most commonly seen in paraproteinemias. These are polygonal shaped, positively birefringent.
- Other crystals and associated anomalies
  - *Corticosteroid crystals:* Arthritis flares post-injection, birefringent crystals
  - *Cystine crystals:* Associated anomaly is called cystinosis
  - *Xanthine crystals:* Xanthinuria
  - *Charcot-Leyden crystals:* Hypereosinophilic syndromes
  - *Aluminum phosphate:* Hemodialysis
  - Talc from exam gloves (Artifact)
  - Apatite (Stained by Alizarin red S)

Cytological Properties of Synovial Fluid in Normal and Diseased Joint

I. *Bacteriological properties of various joint diseases are:*

Grams Staining

In septic arthritis the following organisms can be seen. This is demonstrated in Table 25.12:

Table 25.12: Shows various subgroups based on their age and disease causing bacterias in those subgroups

Subgroup	*Likely pathogens*
Neonates	*Staphylococcus aureus* *Enterobacteriaceae* Group B streptococci
Children under 5 years	*S. aureus* *Haemophilus influenzae* type B Streptococci
Children 5 years or older	*S. aureus* *Streptococcus* species
Adolescents and adults with possible STD	*Neisseria gonorrhoeae* *S. aureus*
Adults unlikely to have STD	*S. aureus* *Streptococcus* species *Enterobacteriaceae*
Adults with joint prosthesis or infection after procedure or surgery	*S. epidermidis* *S. aureus* *Streptococcus* species Gram-negative bacilli including *Pseudomonas* species

- Gram positive:
  - *Staphylococcus aureus*
  - Streptococci (*S. haemolyticus*)
  - *Enterobacter*
- Gram negative:
  - *Neisseria gonorrhoae*
  - Pneumococci
  - *Haemophilus influenzae*
  - *Salmonella*
  - *Pseudomonas*
  - *E.coli*
  - *Brucella spp. (melitensis, abortus, suis, canis)*
  - *Kingella kingae*

Acid Fast Staining

Acid fast staining of the centrifuged sample shows positive result, if there is an active infection by tubercle bacilli

Flow chart 25.3: Synovial fluid examination based upon different pathologies

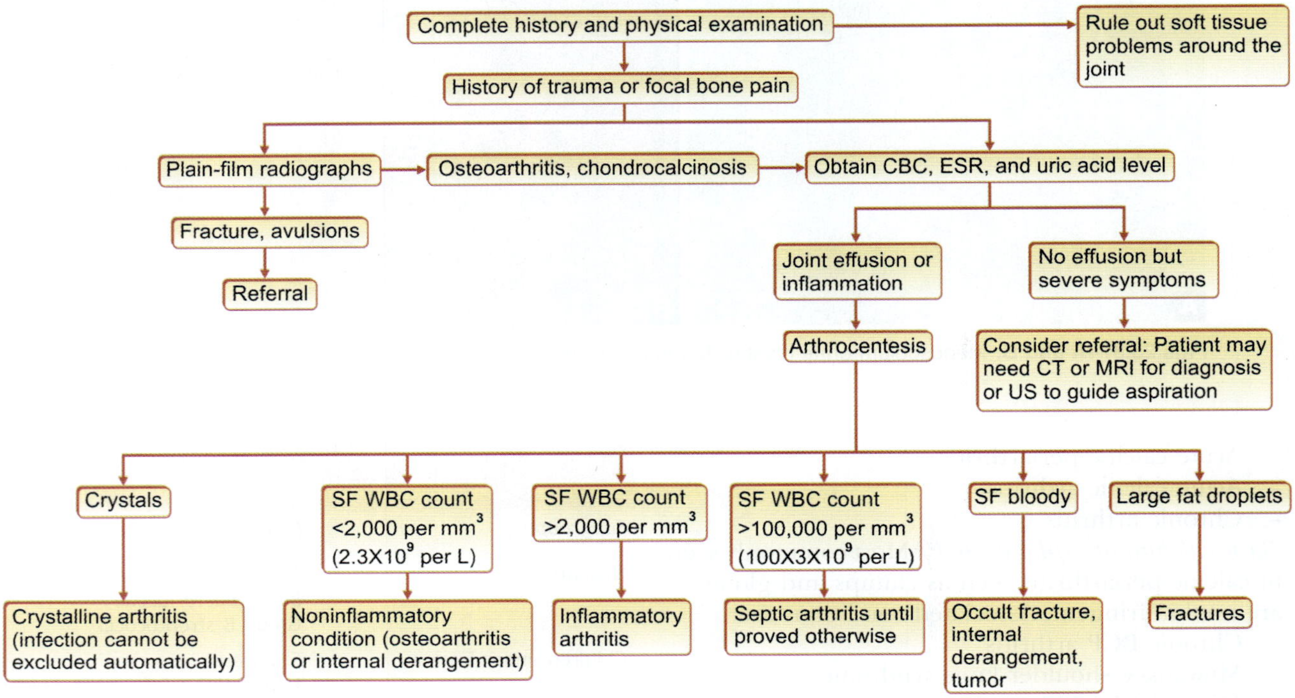

(*Mycobacterium tuberculosis, M. bovis*). Greater the number of the bacilli severe is the infection.

Wet Mount Preparation

Copper sulfate staining demonstrates fungus, like *Candida spp.*

II. *Immunological studies of synovial fluid*

Normal synovial fluid contains only ten percent of immunoglobulin levels of normal serum. These include following tests and studies:

- *Rheumatoid factor:* The cellular origin of rheumatoid factor is plasma cell. About 70 to 80 percent of patients with RA will have circulating rheumatoid factor.
- Rose-Waaler sheep cell agglutination test (SCAT)
- Hemerythrocyte agglutination test (HEAT)
- Latex fixation test
- Other diseases positive for RA factor include, SLE, liver cirrhosis, TB, syphilis, leprosy, filariasis and kala-azar, etc.

Various joint diseases, e.g. rheumatoid arthritis, tubercular arthritis, septic arthritis, gouty arthritis, osteoarthrosis can be diagnosed by synovial fluid study and biopsy. The physical, biochemical and cytological properties of synovial fluid are more or less specific to a particular group of diseases. The procedure is reliable, simple, safe and inexpensive. It may help in better understanding of the pathophysiology of various diseases. Synovial fluid examination based upon different pathologies has been elaborated in Flow chart 25.3.

26 Foot and Ankle

- Ankle Anatomy
- Examination of the Foot and Ankle
- Congenital Anomalies of Foot and Ankle
- Fractures of the Foot and Ankle Joint
- Epiphyseal Injuries Around Foot and Ankle
- Ligament Injuries Around Ankle
- Inflammation of Foot and Ankle and Neuropathic Foot
- Deformities of the Foot and Ankle
- Foot Pain and Osteochondritis Dissecans of Foot and Ankle
- Ankle Arthrodesis
- Ankle Arthroplasty
- Tumors Around Foot and Ankle
- Lower Limb Orthotics
- Lower Limb Prosthesis

ANKLE ANATOMY

The ankle joint is a complex and a three-bone joint. It consists of the tibial plafond (including the posterior malleolus, articulating with the body of the talus), the medial malleolus and the lateral malleolus. The joint is considered saddle-shaped, with a larger circumference of the talar dome laterally than medially, as shown in Figures 26.1A to C.

Tibia

The lower end of the tibia is formed by five surfaces: inferior, anterior, posterior, lateral and medial. The

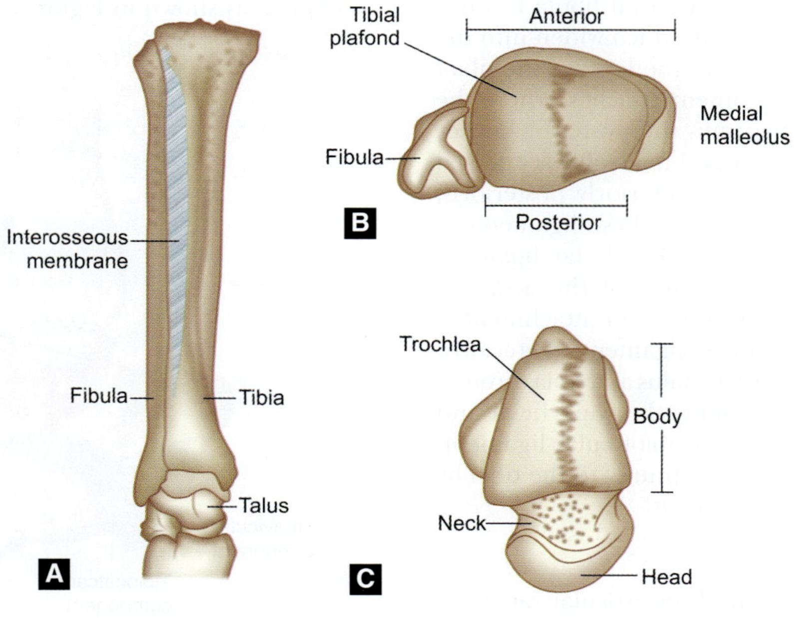

Figs 26.1A to C: Ankle joint anatomy

inferior surface is articular, concave anteroposteriorly and slightly convex transversely, dividing the surface into a wider lateral and narrower medial segment. The posterior border of the ankle joint is lower than the anterior border.

The posterior border is in continuity with the posterior surface of the medial malleolus. This segment has an oblique groove medially, which is directed downward and inward that corresponds to the tendon of the tibialis posterior muscle. The distal lateral border of the tibia is concave with anterior and posterior tubercles. The anterior tubercle is the site of origin of the anterior tibiofibular ligament. The posterior tubercle is the site of attachment of the deep component of the posterior tibiofibular ligament. The medial surface of the distal tibial articulation is directed obliquely downward and inward. It is prolonged distally by the medial malleolus.

The articular surface is comma shaped, with a larger surface anteriorly. The posterior border includes the groove for the tibialis posterior tendon. The medial malleolus is composed of two colliculi, separated by the intercollicular groove. The anterior colliculus is larger, extending approximately 0.5 cm distal to the posterior colliculus.

The deep talotibial component of the deltoid ligament inserts in the intercollicular groove and on the contiguous surfaces of the adjacent colliculi. The superficial deltoid ligament inserts on the medial surface and the anterior border of the anterior colliculus.

Fibula

The lower end of the fibula is a complex bony structure, giving rise to multiple ligaments and housing the lateral articular surface of the ankle. The distal fibula has two major surfaces, lateral and medial, which widen into the three-surfaced lateral malleolus at the level of the tibial plafond. The interosseous ligament attaches, where the lateral surface twists and becomes the posterior border of the lateral malleolus. The lateral malleolus is encased in strong ligamentous attachments anteriorly, posteriorly, inferiorly and superiorly. Anteriorly, these ligamentous attachments include the anterior tibiofibular ligament and the main and secondary bands of the anterior talofibular ligament. Inferiorly, the main attachment is through the stout calcaneofibular ligament. Posteriorly, the fibula is firmly connected to the talus and tibia through the posterior talofibular ligament, the superficial and deep components of the posterior tibiofibular ligament. Superiorly, the fibula is held in continuity to the tibia by the tibiofibular interosseous ligament.

Talus

The talus is almost covered entirely by articular cartilage, with no musculotendinous attachments. The superior surface is convex from front to back and it is slightly concave from side to side. The dome of the talus is trapezoidal, with its anterior surface wider than its posterior surface. This shape confers increased ankle stability with dorsiflexion. The medial and lateral articular facets of the talus are contiguous with the superior articular surface. On average, the talar dome bone is denser than tibial plafond bone and generally, it is not injured in ankle fractures. As the lateral border is larger than the medial border and the anterior border is longer than the posterior, Inman described this surface as a section of a frustrum of a cone with a medial apex. This is partially responsible for the ankle joint's variable axis of rotation.

Ligaments

Ankle stability is conferred by bony architecture and ligament capsular structures. There are three distinct groups of ligaments supporting the ankle joint:

1. The medial collateral ligament,
2. The lateral collateral ligaments, and
3. The syndesmotic ligaments.

1. *The medial collateral ligament:* It stabilizes the medial side of the ankle anteriorly and posteriorly. It is strong, flat, triangular consisting of five components. The deep portion of the deltoid ligament is probably the most important and provides the greatest restraint against lateral translation. The two components, the anterior and posterior deep tibiotalar ligaments, attach to the undersurface of the medial malleolus and the body of the talus. Both deep components are intra-articular but extrasynovial. The posterior deep tibiotalar ligament is the strongest of the entire deltoid complex, as shown in Figure 26.2.

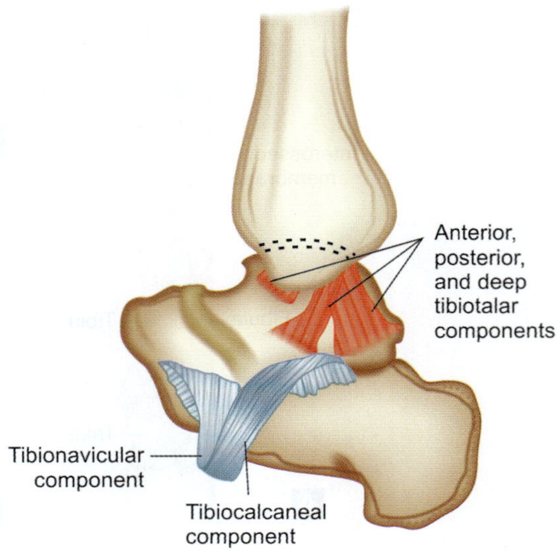

Fig. 26.2: Deltoid ligament

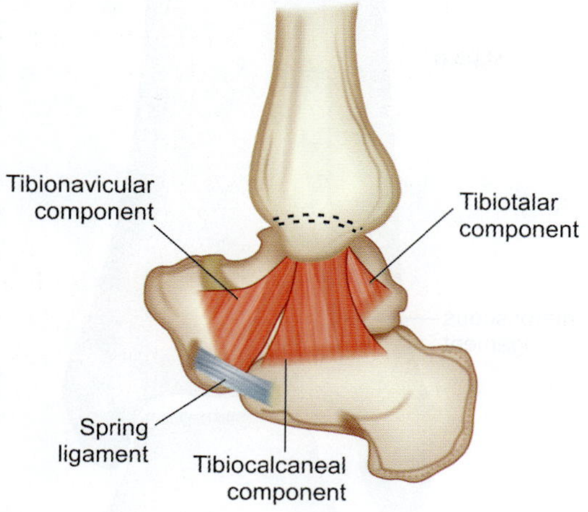

Fig. 26.3: Different components of deltoid ligament

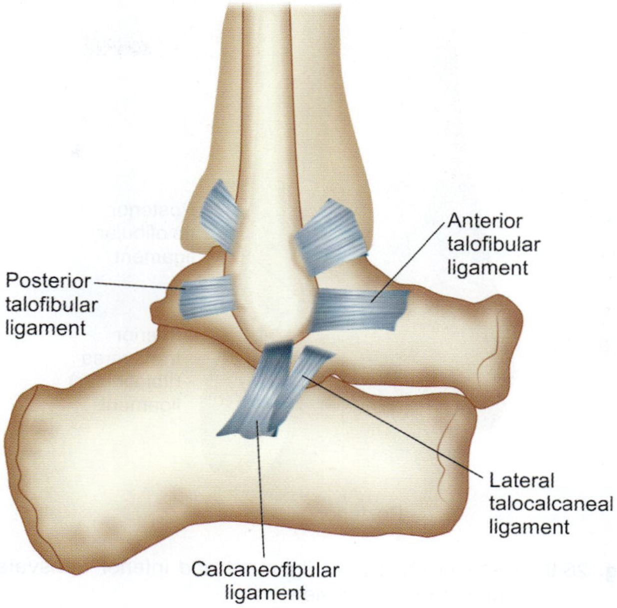

Fig. 26.4: Different components of lateral collateral ligaments

The superficial portion of the deltoid ligament consists of the other three components: the tibionavicular component anteriorly, the tibiocalcaneal component in the middle and the posterior tibiotalar component posteriorly. The superficial and deep components equally resist valgus tilting of the talus and are secondary restraints against anterior translation of the talus, as shown in Figure 26.3.

2. *The lateral collateral ligaments:* Three primary ligaments that stabilize the ankle vary in structure.
   - *The anterior talofibular ligament:* It is attached posteriorly to the anterior border of the lateral malleolus and anteriorly to the neck of the talus where it blends with the anterolateral joint capsule. It is the weakest and most often injured of the lateral ligaments. It primarily functions to resist anterior translation of the talus.
   - *The calcaneofibular ligament:* It is stronger than the anterior talofibular ligament. Attached superiorly to the tip of the lateral malleolus, extends deep to the peroneal tendons and inserts inferiorly on the lateral surface of the calcaneus (it is the only lateral ligament that is extracapsular).
   - *The posterior talofibular ligament:* It is the strongest of the lateral ligaments. It is attached anteriorly to the digital fossa of the fibula and posteriorly to the lateral tubercle on the posterior aspect of the talus, as shown in Figure 26.4.
3. *The syndesmotic ligaments:* Maintaining the relationship of the distal tibia and fibula is the syndesmosis, consisting of four components.
   - The anteroinferior tibiofibular ligament, attaches medially to the anterior tibial tubercle, extends inferior and lateral, and inserts on the anterior fibula. Occasionally, a slip of this ligament (Baxter ligament) inserts distal on the fibula and may cause impingement symptoms at the anterolateral aspect of the talus, as illustrated in Figure 26.5.
   - The posteroinferior tibiofibular ligament is the strongest component (the interosseous membrane is not part of the syndesmosis). It runs in a similar direction, as the anteroinferior tibiofibular ligament.

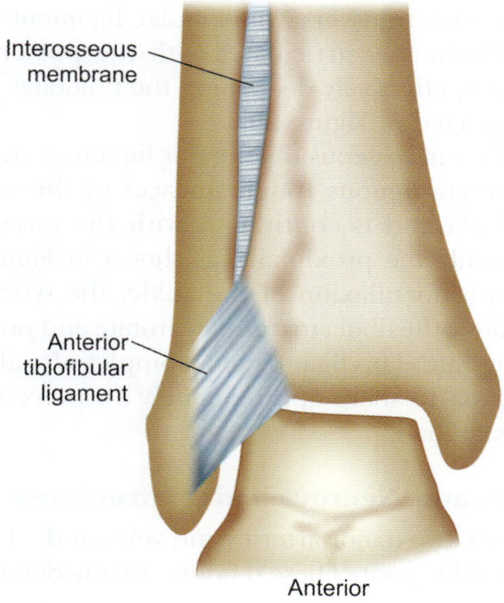

Fig. 26.5: Syndesmotic ligaments

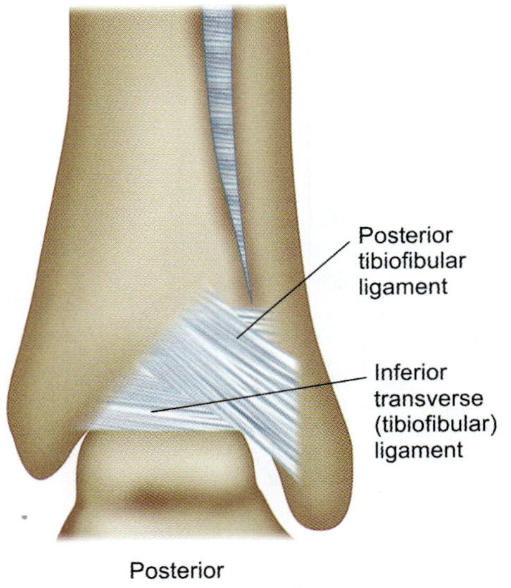

Fig. 26.6: Posterior tibiofibular ligament and inferior transverse ligament (posterior view)

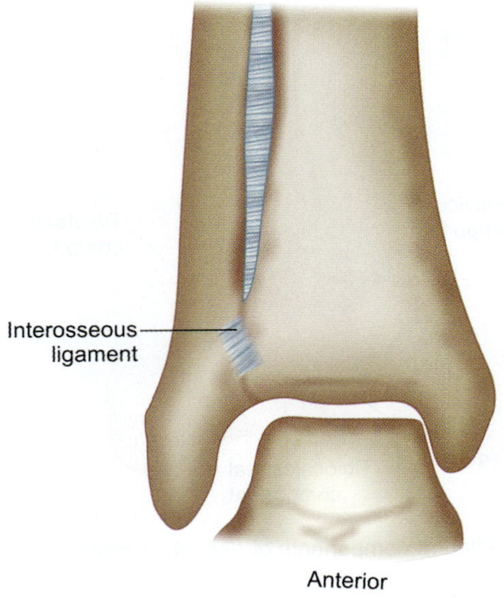

Fig. 26.7: Anterior view of foot showing attachment of interosseous ligament

- The inferior transverse tibiofibular ligament is deep and inferior to the posteroinferior tibiofibular ligament. On its anterior surface, the inferior transverse tibiofibular ligament forms a labrum that articulates with the posterolateral talus, effectively deepening the tibiotalar joint, as depicted in Figure 26.6.
- The interosseous tibiofibular ligament attaches to the contiguous rough surfaces of the tibia and fibula and is continuous with the interosseous membrane proximally, as shown in Figure 26.7. With dorsiflexion of the ankle, the syndesmosis allows the fibula to translate, rotate and proximally migrate. This ligamentous complex also allows the fibula to share approximately 16 percent of the axial load.

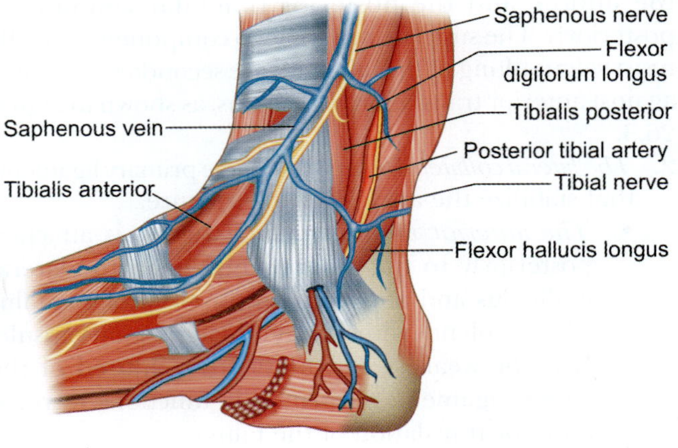

Fig. 26.8: Structures seen on medial side of the foot

Tendons and Neurovascular Structures

Five nerves, two major arteries and veins and 13 tendons cross the ankle joint. These tendons are divided into four groups:

1. *The posterior group:* It includes, the achilles and plantaris tendons. The achilles is the most power plantar flexor of the ankle, the plantaris is a small, perhaps vestigial and inconstant tendon that can be used to supplement tendon or ligament repairs in the ankle or elsewhere. Immediately lateral to the achilles tendon lies the sural nerve, which innervates the skin on the lateral heel and lateral border of the foot.
2. *The medial side of the ankle:* The flexor tendons are transmitted under cover of the laciniate ligament. This stout ligament courses from the calcaneus to the medial malleolus and has several septa separating its contents. Immediately posterior to the medial malleolus lies the posterior tibial tendon, which not infrequently is lacerated, incarcerated, or ruptured from medial malleolar fractures or osteotomies performed for visualization or reduction of talar fractures. Posterior and lateral to the tibialis posterior are in order, the flexor digitorum longus tendon, the posterior tibial artery and associated veins, the tibial nerve and the flexor hallucis longus tendon, as illustrated in Figure 26.8.
3. *Anterior group (Fig. 26.9):* Anterior to the medial malleolus courses the saphenous vein and accompanying nerves. These lie immediately medial to the tibialis anterior tendon. On the anterior aspect of the ankle, the extensor retinaculum restrains the extensor tendons, anterior tibial vessels and the deep

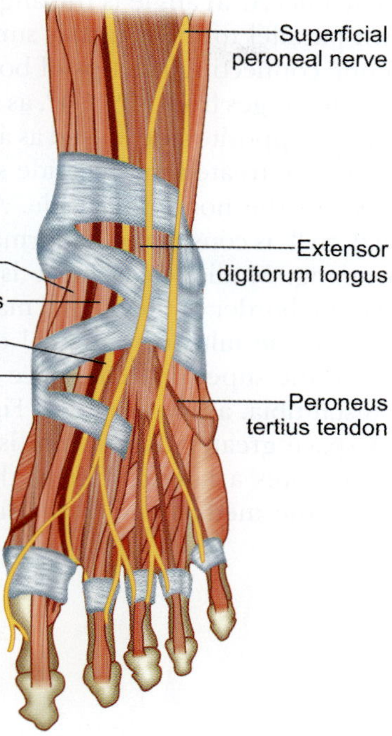

Fig. 26.9: Anterior view of foot

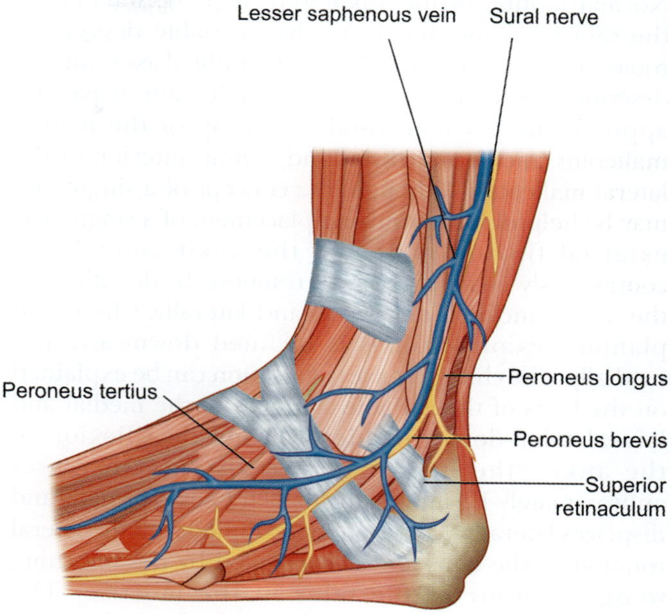

Fig. 26.10: Lateral aspects of foot and structures present on the lateral aspects of the foot

peroneal nerve. The extensor retinaculum proximal to the ankle runs from the anterior medial subcutaneous surface of the tibia to the anterolateral surface of the fibula. Distal to the ankle, the inferior extensor retinaculum is Y-shaped, with its base lateral on the calcaneus. Under the extensor retinaculum are transmitted from medial to lateral, the tibialis anterior tendon, the extensor hallucis longus tendon, the deep peroneal nerve and anterior tibial vessels, the extensor digitorum longus tendon and the peroneus tertius tendon. In approaches to the anterior aspect of the ankle, a relatively safe interval is between the tibialis anterior tendon and the extensor hallucis longus tendon. Superficial to the extensor retinaculum, lie the terminal branches of the superficial peroneal nerve. The superficial peroneal nerve fans into two or three major terminal branches that cross the ankle joint to innervate the dorsum of the foot.

4. *Lateral group (Fig. 26.10):* The peroneal tendons are transmitted under the superior peroneal retinaculum, posterior to the fibula. At the level of the ankle, the peroneus longus tendon is more external and the peroneus brevis lies up against the lateral malleolus. In cases of severe sprains and some fractures of the ankle and calcaneus, the peroneus longus and brevis tendons can become dislocated anterior to the fibula. Lateral approaches to the fibula can injure the superficial peroneal nerve proximally and the sural nerve distally. These nerves and their terminal branches sometimes are best exposed and protected during fixation of fibular fractures.

Tarsal Tunnel Syndrome

It is analogous to carpal tunnel syndrome, but instead of median nerve entrapment beneath the transverse carpal ligament, the tibial nerve is constricted beneath the flexor retinaculum (laciniate ligament). This unyielding fibrous roof extends from the medial malleolus posteriorly and inferiorly to the medial side of the tuberosity of the calcaneus and is 2.5 to 3 cm wide with indistinct borders.

Its proximal border is continuous with the investing deep fascia of the calf and distally its anterior margin is continuous with the deep fascia of the medial part of the sole. Projecting from this fibrous roof to the calcaneus are septa, which separate the posterior tibial, flexor digitorum longus and flexor hallucis longus tendons. Between the latter two tendons, the tibial nerve, posterior tibial artery and accompanying veins pass through the "tarsal tunnel." The tibial nerve may be constricted by pressure from without or within this tunnel. Sources of constriction beneath and adjacent to the tarsal tunnel include bone fragments from displaced distal tibial, talar or calcaneal fractures. Tenosynovitis or ganglia of an adjacent tendon sheath and bone, soft-tissue encroachment in rheumatoid arthritis or ankylosing spondylitis, varicosities, neural tumor (neurilemoma) or perineural fibrosis.

Biomechanics of the Ankle Joint

Normal motion of the ankle joint is predominantly in the sagittal plane, but it involves variable degrees of rotation around the vertical and longitudinal axes. Inman, described the empiric axis of the ankle joint as passing approximately 5 mm distal to the tip of the medial malleolus and 3 mm distal and 8 mm anterior to the lateral malleolus. Although, the concept of a single axis may be helpful for optimizing placement of a single-axis external fixator, in reality the ankle joint has a continuously changing axis of rotation. In dorsiflexion, the axis is inclined downward and laterally, whereas in plantar flexion the axis is inclined downward and medially. The changing axes of rotation can be explained on the basis of the variable contours of the medial and lateral talar dome trochlea. During dorsiflexion of the ankle, the intermalleolar distance increases approximately 1.5 mm as the fibula rotates externally and displaces laterally. This motion is coupled with the lateral rotation of the talus and is controlled by the matching wedge contour of the talus in the mortise. The syndesmosis firmly binds the tibia to the fibula. With the deltoid ligament, it contributes to the rotational stability of the talus in the ankle mortise and it allows the talus to assume a close-packed configuration with dorsiflexion during the stance phase of gait. Stability of the ankle joint in stance appears to be conferred mostly by articular congruity. The mortise view is taken with the patient's leg internally rotated approximately 15°, so the beam of the X-ray is perpendicular to the transmalleolar axis, as shown in Figure 26.11. The articular surface of the talus should be congruous with the distal tibia and the clear space between the talus and the medial malleolus, distal tibia and lateral malleolus should be equal.

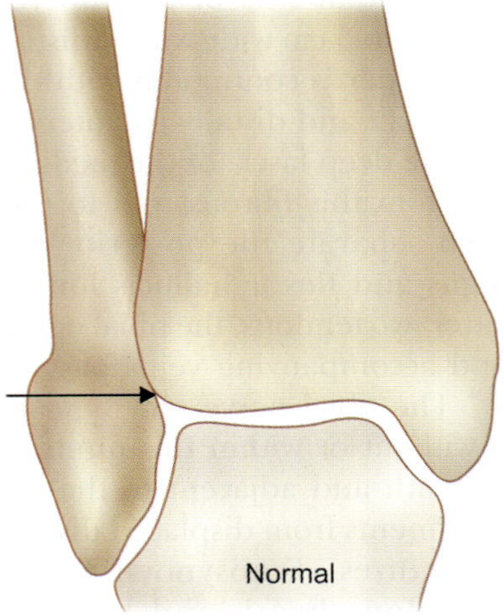

Fig. 26.11: The mortise view of ankle, taken with the patient's leg internally rotated approximately 15°, so the beam of the X-ray is perpendicular to the transmalleolar axis

The talocrural angle is the angle subtended by a line drawn parallel to the articular surface of the distal tibia and one connecting the tips of both malleoli. Normally, the angle ranges from 83° ± 4°, as shown in Figure 26.12. When the opposite side is used as a control, the talocrural angle of the treated injured side should be within a few degrees of the noninjured side. Any difference greater than 2° to 3° is considered abnormal and indicates fibular shortening. Medial clear space is the distance between the lateral border of the medial malleolus and the medial border of the talus (the medial clear space) should be equal to the superior clear space between the talus and the distal tibia, as illustrated in Figure 26.13.

A space greater than 4 mm is considered abnormal and indicates a lateral shift of the talus. The distance between the medial wall of the fibula and the incisural

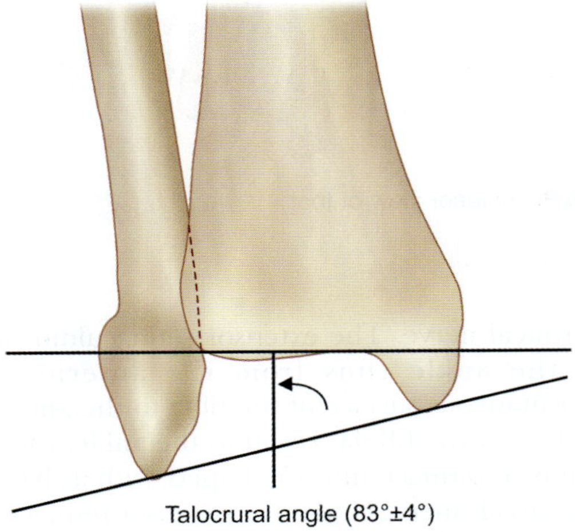

Fig. 26.12: The talocrural angle is the angle subtended by a line drawn parallel to the articular surface of the distal tibia and one connecting the tips of both malleoli

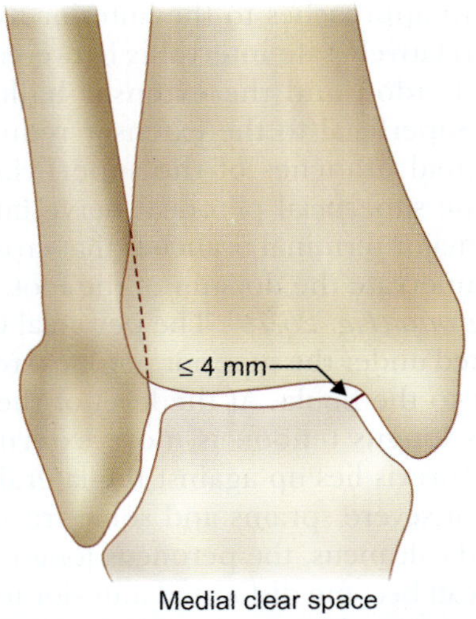

Fig. 26.13: Medial clear space is the distance between the lateral border of the medial malleolus and the medial border of the talus

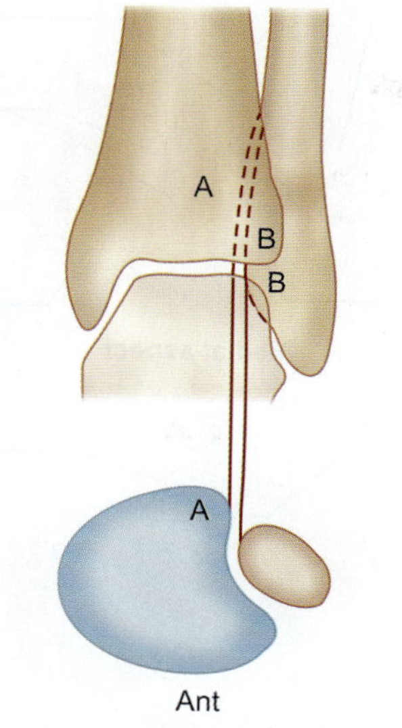

Fig. 26.14: The distance between the medial wall of the fibula and the incisural surface of the tibia, the tibiofibular clear space should be less than 6 mm

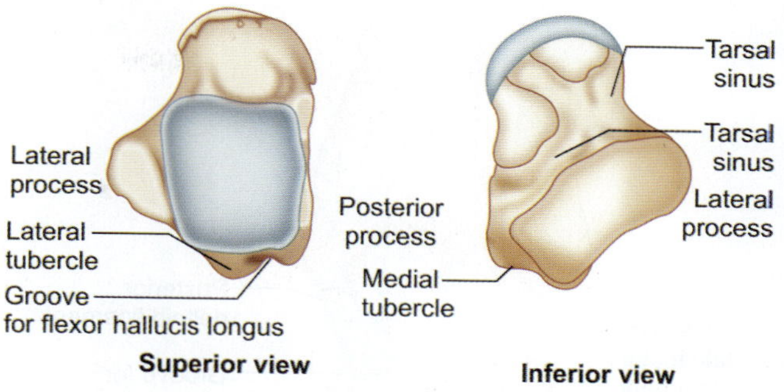

Fig. 26.15: Articular surfaces of the talus

surface of the tibia, the tibiofibular clear space should be less than 6 mm, as shown in Figure 26.14.

■ Foot

The foot supports the body weight and provides leverage for walking and running. It is unique in that it is constructed in the form of arches, which enable it to adapt its shape to uneven surfaces. It also serves as a resilient spring to absorb shocks, such as in jumping.

Bones of the Foot

The bones of the foot are:

- The tarsal bones
- The metatarsals
- The phalanges

The tarsal bones are the calcaneum, the talus, the navicular, the cuboid and the three cuneiform bones. Only the talus articulates with the tibia and the fibula at the ankle joint.

Hindfoot

Talus

Majority of its surface is covered in articular cartilage, as shown in Figure 26.15. There are multiple capsular and ligamentous sites of attachment and no muscles attach to the talus itself. Because of the lack of muscular soft tissue attachments and due to the limited space available for vascular foramina, the talus is particularly predisposed to difficulties with blood supply. Trauma associated with capsular or ligamentous disruption may be complicated by osteonecrosis of the body of the talus.

The trochlea, or superior surface, supports the body weight and transmits loads to the inferior aspect of the tibial plafond. Medially and laterally the articular cartilage extends plantarward to articulate with the medial and lateral malleoli. The neck of the talus has less cartilaginous coverage than the remainder of the talus and deviates medially by about 15 to 20°. This part of the bone is more susceptible to fracture compared to the body of the talus.

The head of the talus has rounded cartilaginous facets to articulate with the navicular anteriorly. The spring ligament wraps around the inferior aspect of the talar head. The deltoid ligament attaches to the medial aspect of the talar body.

There is a wide area of attachment for the deltoid ligament extending from the talar body onto the medial aspect of the neck. The inferior side of the talus is also predominantly covered by cartilage to form the articulation with the posterior facet of the calcaneus. The surface is wider anteriorly compared to posteriorly, such that the medial and lateral sides of the trochlea converge in a posterior direction. The lateral process of the talus is a large, broad-based, wedge-shaped prominence of the talar body. Includes two articular surfaces:

- Dorsolaterally, it articulates with the fibula
- Inferomedially, the lateral process articulates with the anterior portion of the posterior facet of the calcaneus.

The lateral talocalcaneal ligament originates from the tip of the lateral process. The posterior process of the talus is derived from two tubercles. The medial tubercle and the lateral tubercle are separated by a groove, within which courses the flexor hallus longus tendon. The posterior talofibular ligament is attached to the lateral tubercle. The posterior third of the deltoid ligament is attached to the medial tubercle, as shown in Figure 26.16.

The talus is 60 percent covered by articular cartilage, as a result a very limited surface area is available to provide adequate vascular perforation. Blood vessels enter the talus via capsular and ligamentous attachments and are

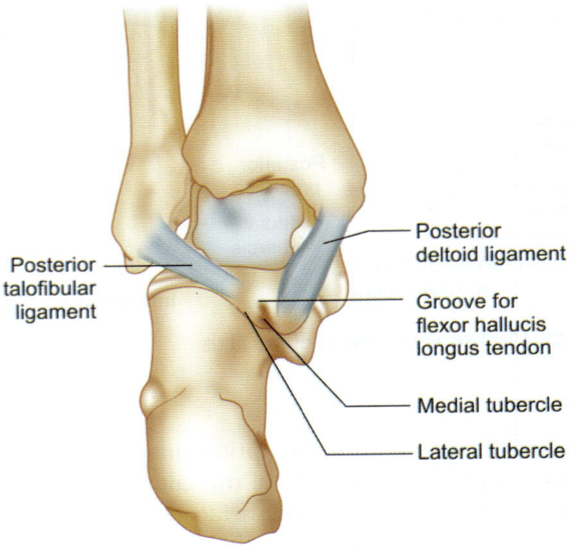

Fig. 26.16: Ligamentous attachments around talus

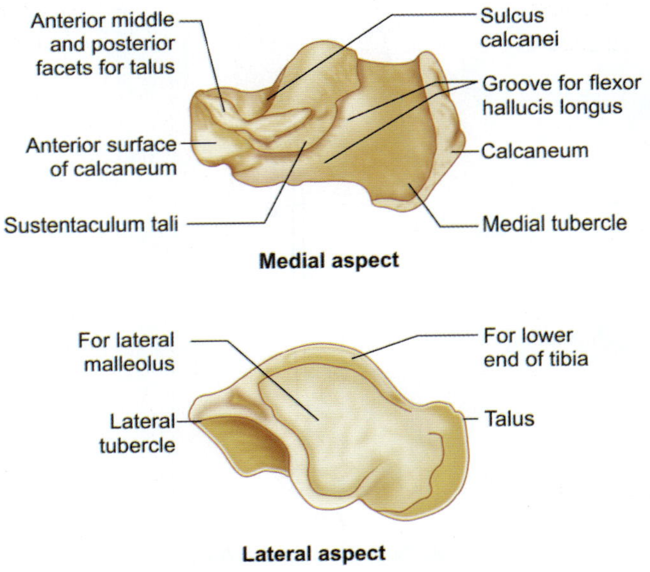

Fig. 26.17: Articular surfaces of calcaneus

therefore vulnerable to injury, such that osteonecrosis can be a complication of many fractures and dislocations of the talus. A critical anastomotic sling of vessels lie in the tarsal sinus and tarsal canal, lying inferior to the neck of the talus. Within the tarsal canal and the tarsal sinus, the critical anastomosis perforates the inferior neck, to form the primary source of blood supply to the body of the talus. The tarsal sinus is bounded by the calcaneus inferiorly, the body of the talus posteriorly and the talar head and neck anteriorly. The tarsal canal lies between the talus and calcaneus just behind and below the tip of the medial malleolus. The artery of the tarsal canal arises from the posterior tibial artery. The deltoid branches arise from the artery of the tarsal canal and supply the medial third of the talar body. From the anterior tibial or dorsalis pedis artery, come multiple branches to the dorsal aspect of the talar neck. From the peroneal artery come branches to the posterior process and a branch to form the artery of the sinus tarsi. The talar body therefore, receives most of its blood supply from the anastomotic sling in the tarsal canal and sinus. The talar head is nursed by branches of the dorsalis pedis, arising from the dorsal neck vessels and also from the artery of the tarsal sinus. Undisplaced fractures of the talar neck are associated with interosseous disruption of the branches of the arteries of the tarsal sinus and tarsal canal. However, the major vascular sling should remain intact. With increasing displacement, branches from the dorsalis pedis artery as well as the artery of the tarsal canal and artery of the tarsal sinus can be disrupted. These findings confirm the clinical observation that the rate of osteonecrosis depends upon the degree of fracture displacement.

Calcaneus (Fig. 26.17)

It is an odd-shaped bone. The superior surface consists of three articular facets (the anterior, middle and posterior) that articulate with the talus. The posterior facet is the major weight-bearing surface and the largest facet.

The middle facet is anterior and medial and is located on the sustentaculum. It is often contiguous with the anterior facet. The sustentaculum sits under the talar neck and is medial to the calcaneal body. It is attached to the talus by the interosseous talocalcaneal ligament and by the deltoid ligament medially. The flexor hallucis longus tendon runs below the sustentaculum. Laterally, the peroneal tendons run obliquely along the lateral wall of the calcaneus and sit in two shallow grooves, with a bony prominence between them known as the peroneal tubercle. The entire calcaneal surface behind the posterior facet is known as the posterior tuberosity. On its plantar surface, it has two processes, the lateral and medial. The lateral process is the origin of the abductor digiti quinti (minimi) muscle. The medial process is the origin of the abductor hallucis muscle and the major weight-bearing structure in the hindfoot. The Achilles tendon inserts on the posterior surface of the tuberosity.

Midfoot

Five bones comprise the midfoot the navicular, cuboid and medial, middle and lateral cuneiforms, as shown in Figure 26.18. This anatomic unit plays a distinct role in the normal mechanics of foot function. There is no bony weight-bearing contact with the ground in this area in the normal foot structure. Despite the presence of many large, broad, flat articular surfaces, this collection of bones

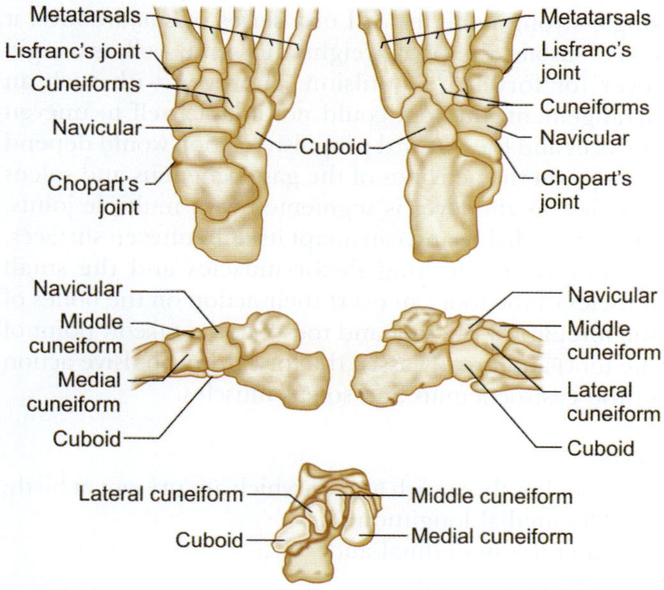

Fig. 26.18: Anatomy of midfoot

is also relatively immobile compared to the rotatory and accommodative functions of the hindfoot and forefoot.

The stability or resistance to movement in these articulations is due in large part to the numerous dense plantar ligaments, which tightly bind the osseous structures in the midfoot together. These ligaments also carry over to the hindfoot and medial forefoot, providing strong mechanical links between the three sections of the foot. The fact that the normal arch shape of the weight-bearing foot can be maintained without the need for muscle action, demonstrates the inherent stability supplied by these dense ligamentous structures. The strength and stability of the whole structure is dependent on the tensile strength of the plantar-based intersegmental ties between the osseous structures. The only motor unit to completely insert into the midfoot is the tibialis posterior. Its multiple insertions on the plantar surface of the midfoot bones are intertwined with the plantar ligamentous structures to provide dynamic support and mechanical overload protection. The medial arch provides a protective conduit and alcove for the neurovascular structures and intrinsic musculature of the plantar aspect of the foot. These muscles are extremely important to the function and stability of the weight-bearing surfaces of the forefoot. During weight-bearing, the midfoot acts as a mechanical actuator transmitting the rotational motion of the hindfoot complex to the forefoot. The midfoot, because of its axial rigidity, is also responsible for the weight-bearing relationship of the hindfoot to the forefoot. The midfoot motion is small compared to the motion of the subtalar complex and metatarsophalangeal joints, but it plays a role in shock absorption during weight-bearing. The structural integrity of the five bones and their positional relationship to each other are key to retaining midfoot function.

Maintenance of the normal relationship of the weight-bearing surfaces of the hindfoot to the maintenance of talonavicular, calcaneocuboid, and fifth tarsometatarsal joint motions.

Navicular

It is the keystone of the medial longitudinal arch of the foot. It is wider dorsally and medially than plantarly and laterally. The medial prominence, known as the navicular tuberosity, provides the interim attachment point for the tibialis posterior on its medial inferior surface. Proximally, the articular surface is concave and articulates with the talus. This joint enjoys a significant arc of motion and serves to transmit the motion of the subtalar joint to the forefoot. It is classically the point, from which forefoot inversion and eversion is initiated. The distal articular surfaces of the navicular have three separate, broad facets that articulate with each of the three cuneiforms. These joints provide little motion because they mainly play a role in the dissipation of loading stresses. Laterally, the navicular appears to rest on the dorsal medial aspect of the cuboid with a variable articular surface. The ligamentous support for this bone is dense. Thick ligaments plantarly and dorsally support the naviculocuneiform joints. The spring and superficial deltoid ligaments provide strong support to the plantar and medial aspects of the talonavicular joint. These are aided by the calcaneonavicular ligaments dorsally and laterally. There are also strong ligamentous connections between the cuboid and navicular laterally and posteriorly.

Cuboid

It is the sole osseous structure of the midfoot, considered part of the lateral support column of the foot. Its saddle-shaped articulation with the calcaneus acts as a stress valve for the imperfectly matched movements of the talonavicular and subtalar joints. The dorsal calcaneal tuberosity and medial cuboid tuberosity are fashioned to provide bony stability to the joint and prevent dorsal or lateral migration of the cuboid in a weight-bearing situation. Thick plantar and medial ligaments support those respective areas of the articulation. Distally, the cuboid provides separate articular facets for each of the fourth and fifth metatarsals. There are variable articular surfaces on the dorsomedial aspect of the cuboid, where the navicular and lateral cuneiform come into contact with the cuboid. The thick, broad, longitudinal plantar ligament provides support along the plantar and medial borders of the calcaneocuboid joint. A variable pattern of plantar and dorsal ligaments provides loose support at the tarsometatarsal joints. These tarsometatarsal joints provide for nearly all of the dorsal and plantar motion of the lateral column of the foot. The peroneus longus courses along the lateral and plantar surfaces of the cuboid on its way to the base of the first metatarsal. The importance of the cuboid in the overall function of the foot lies primarily in its structural position as a lateral column spacer, secondarily, in the function of the fourth and fifth tarsometatarsal joints and thirdly in calcaneocuboid joint motion.

Three Cuneiform Bones

Sit in the middle of the medial column of the foot and provide the rigid support for the medial longitudinal arch. They constitute the apex of the transverse arch that provides a stable conduit for the plantar musculotendinous and neurovascular structures. All are wedge shaped along the axial axis. The medial cuneiform has a plantar base and a dorsal crest. The middle and lateral cuneiforms are reversed, with dorsal bases and plantar crests. Proximally, each cuneiform articulates with approximately one-third of the distal navicular. Each cuneiform articulates with its respective metatarsal distally.

There are numerous ligamentous attachments between these three bones and the surrounding structures. Between each of the two cuneiform pairs, there are three distinct connecting ligaments. The weakest link structurally is the medial cuneiform, with its sloping proximal articulation with the navicular and relative paucity of ligamentous attachments to other structures.

Of importance also is the fact that there are no ligamentous connections between the first and second metatarsal, to stabilize the first ray and dissipate any rotatory forces. Isolated loading of the first metatarsal is resisted only by the strength of the medial cuneiform attachments.

Foot as a Weight-Bearer and a Lever (Figs 26.19A and B)

The foot has two important functions: (1) to support the body weight and (2) to serve as a lever to propel the body forward in walking and running. If the foot possessed a single strong bone instead of a series of small bones, it could sustain the body weight and serve well as a rigid lever for forward propulsion. However, with such an arrangement, the foot could not adapt itself to uneven surfaces and the forward propulsive action would depend entirely on the activities of the gastrocnemius and soleus muscles. As the lever is segmented with multiple joints, the foot is pliable and can adapt itself to uneven surfaces.

Moreover, the long flexor muscles and the small muscles of the foot can exert their action on the bones of the forepart of the foot and toes (i.e. the takeoff point of the foot) and greatly assist the forward propulsive action of the gastrocnemius and soleus muscles.

Arches of the Foot

The foot has three such arches, which are present at birth:
1. The medial longitudinal,
2. Lateral longitudinal and
3. Transverse arches.

In the young child, the foot appears to be flat because of the presence of a large amount of subcutaneous fat on the sole of the foot. The medial margin of the foot, from the heel to the first metatarsal head, is arched above the ground because of the important medial longitudinal arch. The pressure exerted on the ground by the lateral margin of the foot is greatest at the heel and the fifth metatarsal head and least between these areas because of the presence of the low-lying lateral longitudinal arch. The transverse arch involves the bases of the five metatarsals and the cuboid and cuneiform bones. This is, in fact only half an arch, with its base on the lateral border of the foot and its summit on the foot's medial border.

Bones of the Arches

Medial longitudinal arch: This consists of the calcaneum, the talus, the navicular bone, the three cuneiform bones and the first three metatarsal bones, as shown in Figure 26.20.

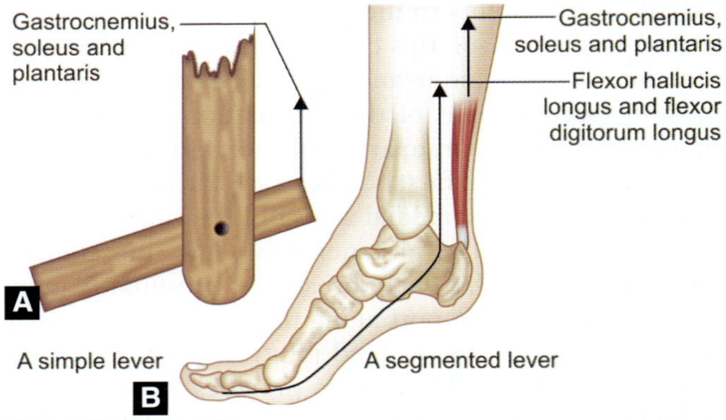

Figs 26.19A and B: (A) Wooden plank shown as a lever; (B) Foot function as a lever, with the forward propulsive action of the gastrocnemius and soleus muscles

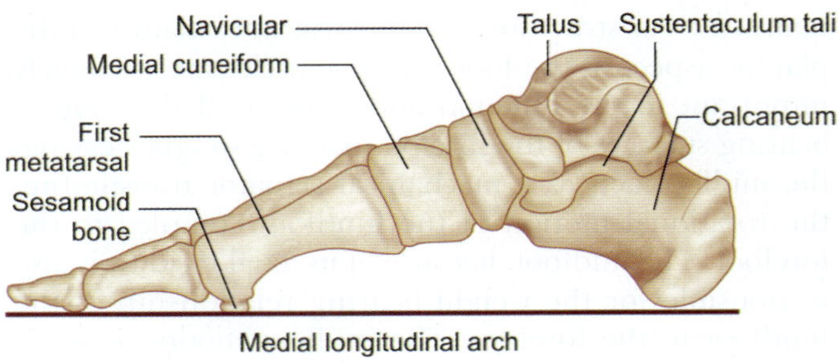

Fig. 26.20: Bony components forming medial longitudinal arch

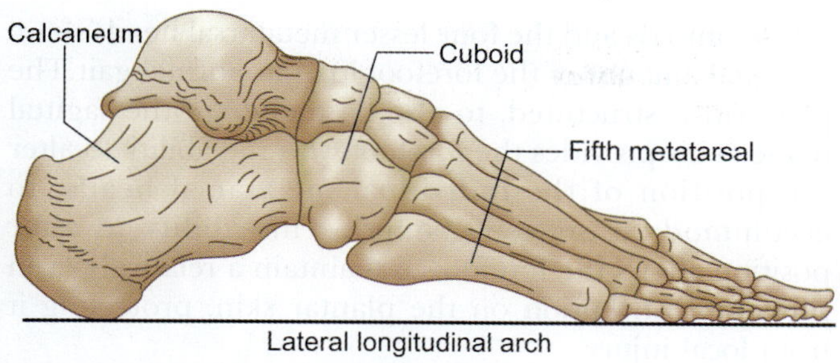

Fig. 26.21: Bony component forming lateral longitudinal arch

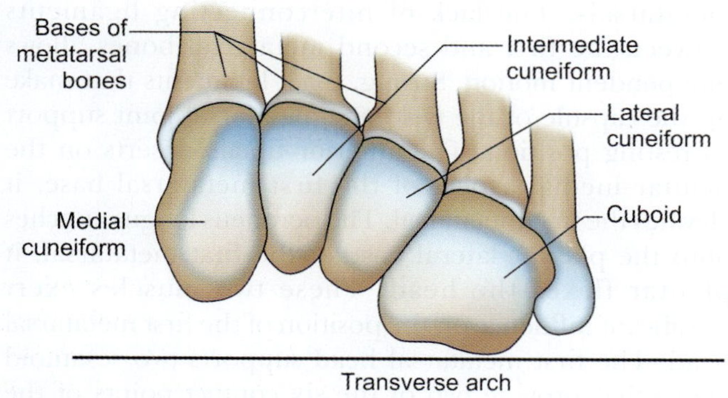

Fig. 26.22: Components of transverse arch

Lateral longitudinal arch: This consists of the calcaneum, the cuboid and the fourth and fifth metatarsal bones, as shown in Figure 26.21.

Transverse arch (Fig. 26.22): This consists of the bases of the metatarsal bones and the cuboid and the three cuneiform bones.

Mechanisms of Arch Support

Examination of the design of any stone bridge reveals the following engineering methods used for its support:

- *The shape of the stones:* The most effective way of supporting the arch is to make the stones wedge shaped, with the thin edge of the wedge lying inferiorly. This applies particularly to the important stone that occupies the center of the arch and is referred to as the "keystone", as shown in Figure 26.23.
- *The inferior edges of the stones are tied together:* This is accomplished by interlocking the stones or binding their lower edges together with metal staples. This method effectively counteracts the tendency of the lower edges of the stones to separate, when the arch is weight-bearing, as illustrated in Figure 26.24.
- *The use of the tie beams:* When the span of the bridge is large and the foundations at either end are insecure, a tie beam connecting the ends effectively prevents separation of the pillars and consequent sagging of the arch, as shown in Figure 26.25.

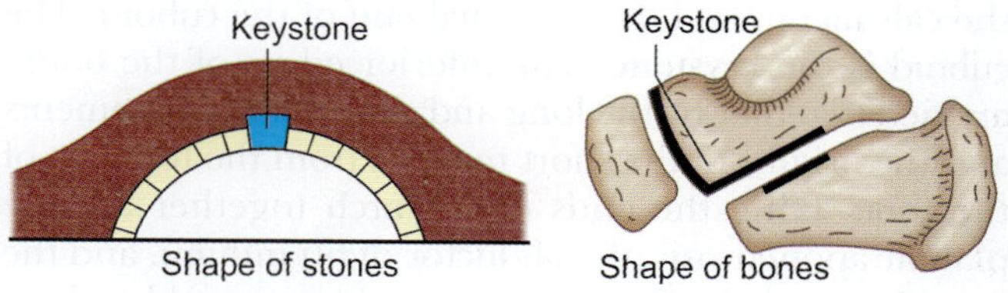

Fig. 26.23: Mechanism of supporting the arch is by making the stones wedge shaped, especially to "keystone"

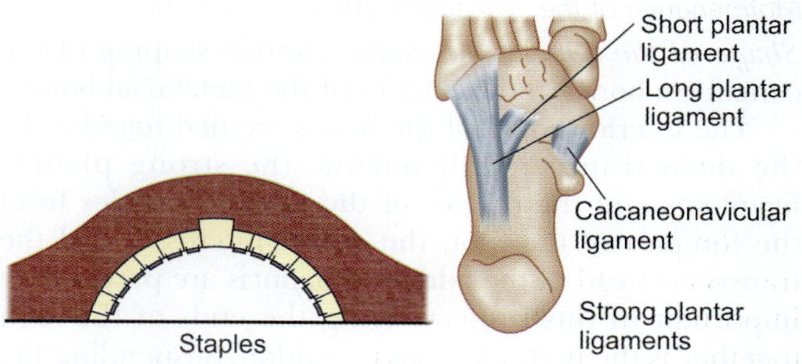

Fig. 26.24: Next step is tying the inferior edges of the stones

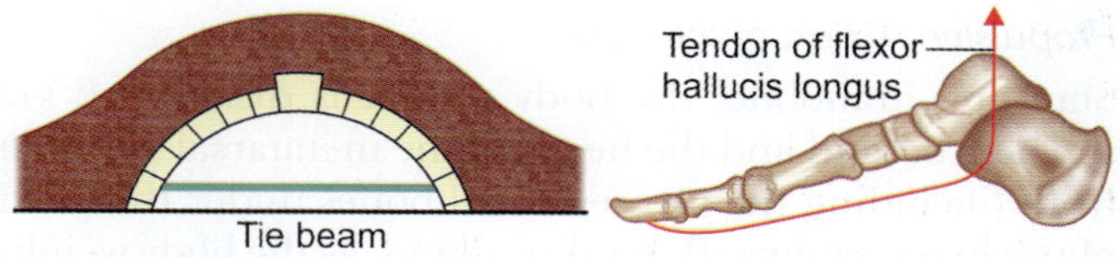

Fig. 26.25: A tie beam connecting the ends, effectively prevents separation of the pillars

Maintenance of the Medial Longitudinal Arch

Shape of the bones: The sustentaculum tali holds up the talus, the concave proximal surface of the navicular bone receives the rounded head of the talus and the slight concavity of the proximal surface of the medial cuneiform bone receives the navicular. The rounded head of the talus is the keystone in the center of the arch. The inferior edges of the bones are tied together by the plantar ligaments, which are larger and stronger than the dorsal ligaments. The most important ligament is the plantar calcaneonavicular ligament. The tendinous extensions of the insertion of the tibialis posterior muscle play an important role in this respect. Tying the ends of the arch together are the plantar aponeurosis, the medial part of the flexor digitorum brevis, the abductor hallucis, the flexor hallucis longus, the medial part of the flexor digitorum longus and the flexor hallucis brevis.

Suspending the arch from above are the tibialis anterior and posterior and the medial ligament of the ankle joint.

Maintenance of the Lateral Longitudinal Arch

Shape of the bones: Minimal shaping of the distal end of the calcaneum and the proximal end of the cuboid. The cuboid is the keystone. The inferior edges of the bones are tied together by the long and short plantar ligaments and the origins of the short muscles from the forepart of the foot. Tying the ends of the arch together are the plantar aponeurosis, the abductor digiti minimi, and the lateral part of the flexor digitorum longus and brevis.

Suspending the arch from above are the peroneus longus and the brevis.

Maintenance of the Transverse Arch

Shape of the bones: The marked wedge shaping of the cuneiform bones and the bases of the metatarsal bones.

The inferior edges of the bones are tied together by the deep transverse ligaments, the strong plantar ligaments and the origins of the plantar muscles from the forepart of the foot, the dorsal interossei and the transverse head of the adductor hallucis are particularly important in this respect. Tying the ends of the arch together is the peroneus longus tendon. Suspending the arch from above are the peroneus longus tendon and the peroneus brevis.

Propulsive Action of the Foot

Standing immobile, the body weight is distributed via the heel behind and the heads of the metatarsal bones in front (including the two sesamoid bones under the head of the first metatarsal). While walking, as the body weight is thrown forward, the weight is born successively on the lateral margin of the foot and the heads of the metatarsal bones. As the heel rises, the toes are extended at the metatarsophalangeal joints and the plantar aponeurosis is pulled on thus, shortening the tie beams and heightening the longitudinal arches. The slack in the long flexor tendons is taken up, thereby increasing their efficiency. The body is then thrown forward by the actions of the gastrocnemius and soleus (and plantaris) on the ankle joint, using the foot as a lever and by the toes being strongly flexed by the long and short flexors of the foot providing the final thrust forward. The lumbricals and interossei contract and keep the toes extended, so that they do not fold under because of the strong action of the flexor digitorum longus. In this action, the long flexor tendons also assist in plantar flexing the ankle joint. In running, the weight is borne on the forepart of the foot and the heel does not touch the ground. The forward thrust to the body is provided by the mechanisms described for walking (above).

Forefoot

The forefoot serves two purposes during gait. As a unit it provides a broad plantar surface for load sharing. The two sesamoids and the four lesser metatarsal heads share an equal amount of the forefoot load in normal gait.The platform is structured, to also be mobile in the sagittal plane. This provides the forefoot with the ability to alter the position of the individual metatarsal heads, to accommodate uneven ground. This ability to alter position allows the forefoot to maintain a relatively even pressure distribution on the plantar skin, protecting it from local injury.

First Metatarsal

It is shorter and wider than that of the lesser four metatarsals. The lack of interconnecting ligaments between the first and second metatarsal bones allows independent motion. Strong, thick ligaments that make up the capsule of the first tarsometatarsal joint support its resting position. The anterior tibialis inserts on the plantar medial aspect of the first metatarsal base, it elevates the first metatarsal. The peroneus longus attaches onto the plantar lateral base of the first metatarsal, it plantar flexes the head. These two muscles exert significant influence on the position of the first metatarsal head. The first metatarsal head supports two sesamoid bones that provide two of the six contact points of the forefoot. This translates to the first ray, essentially supporting one-third of the forefoot weight at any one time.

Central Metatarsals

The four lesser metatarsals each provide only one contact point on the plantar weight-bearing surface. At the base of each of these bones is a series of three ligaments (dorsal, central and plantar), which act to stabilize and support each with their neighbor. The central three have no extrinsic motor insertions. Their role is for structural support. They do provide for the origin of dorsal and plantar interossei muscles. There is the thick transverse metatarsal ligament distally, which connects the metatarsals indirectly by linking the plantar plates of the adjacent metatarsophalangeal joints. There is also a cascade of allowable increase in motion through the tarsometatarsal joints, beginning at the second metatarsal and going out to the fifth. It is this increase in motion in the sagittal plane that allows for significant adaptability to terrain by the metatarsal heads.

Fifth Metatarsal

It does have major motor insertions at its base. The peroneus brevis attaches on the dorsal aspect of the tubercle of the fifth metatarsal and acts as a balancing force to forefoot dorsiflexion, counteracting the natural inversion tendency of the tibialis anterior. The peroneus tertius attaches on the dorsal aspect at the proximal metaphyseal diaphyseal junction, acts as an antagonist to posterior tibialis function, to maintain the position of

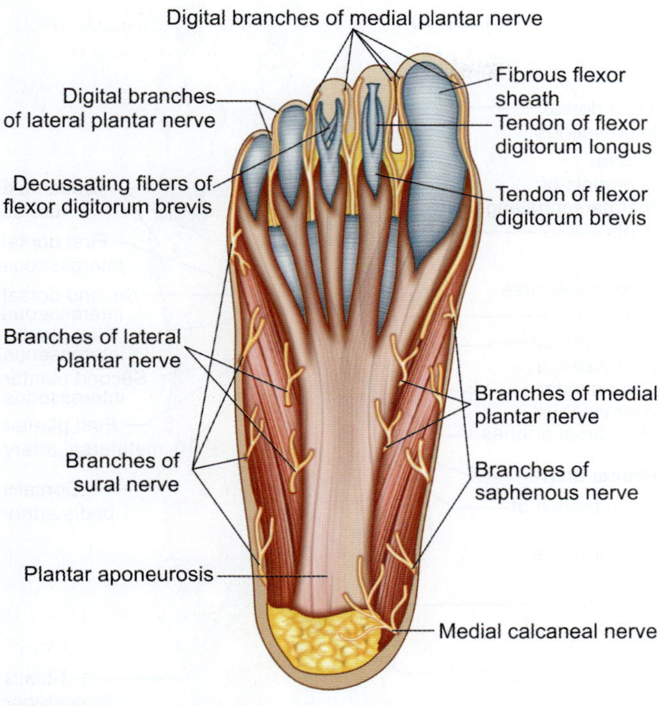

Fig. 26.26: Sole of the foot, with the base of the aponeurosis divides into five slips that pass into the toes

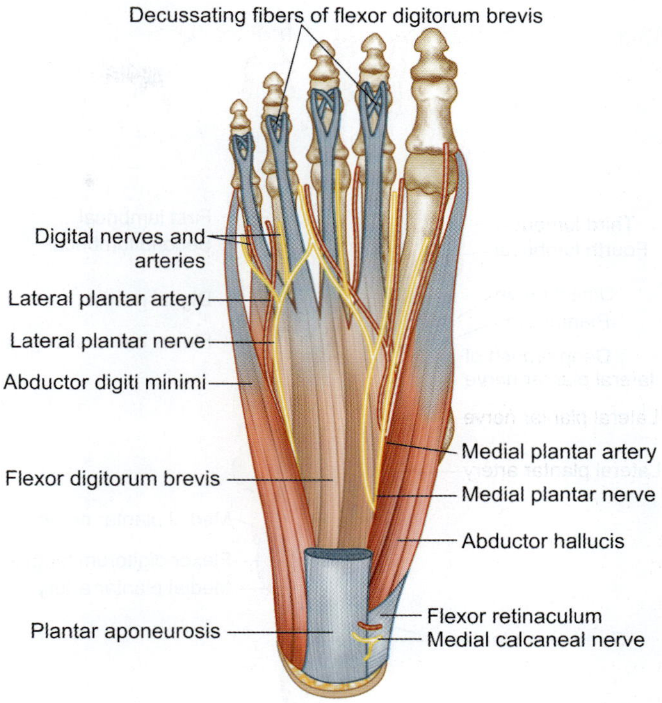

Fig. 26.27: Muscles in the first layer of the sole

the foot under the talus. There is also a strong attachment of the plantar fascia to the plantar aspect of the tubercle. In this area are two sesamoid bones, which should not be mistaken for a displaced fracture.

Sole of the Foot

Skin: The skin of the sole of the foot is thick and hairless. It is firmly bound down to the underlying deep fascia, by numerous fibrous bands. Shows a few flexure creases at the sites of skin movement. Sweat glands are present in large numbers. The sensory nerve supply to the skin of the sole of the foot is derived from the medial calcaneal branch of the tibial nerve, which innervates the medial side of the heel, branches from the medial plantar nerve, which innervate the medial two-thirds of the sole and branches from the lateral plantar nerve, which innervate the lateral third of the sole. The plantar aponeurosis is a triangular thickening of the deep fascia that protects the underlying nerves, blood vessels and muscles. Its apex is attached to the medial and lateral tubercles of the calcaneum. The base of the aponeurosis divides into five slips that pass into the toes, as shown in Figure 26.26.

Muscles of the Sole of the Foot

The muscles of the sole are conveniently described in four layers from the inferior layer superiorly. Unlike, the small muscles of the hand, the sole muscles have few delicate functions and are chiefly concerned with supporting the arches of the foot. Although, their names would suggest control of individual toes, this function is rarely used in most people.

First Layer (Fig. 26.27)

- Abductor hallucis
- Flexor digitorum brevis
- Abductor digiti minimi

Second Layer (Fig. 26.28)

- Quadratus plantae
- Lumbricals
- Flexor digitorum longus tendon
- Flexor hallucis longus tendon

Third Layer (Fig. 26.29)

- Flexor hallucis brevis
- Adductor hallucis
- Flexor digiti minimi brevis

Fourth Layer (Fig. 26.30)

- Interossei
- Peroneus longus tendon
- Tibialis posterior tendon

Arteries of the Sole of the Foot

- *Medial plantar artery:* The smaller of the terminal branches of the posterior tibial artery.
- *Lateral plantar artery:* The larger of the terminal branches of the posterior tibial artery. On reaching

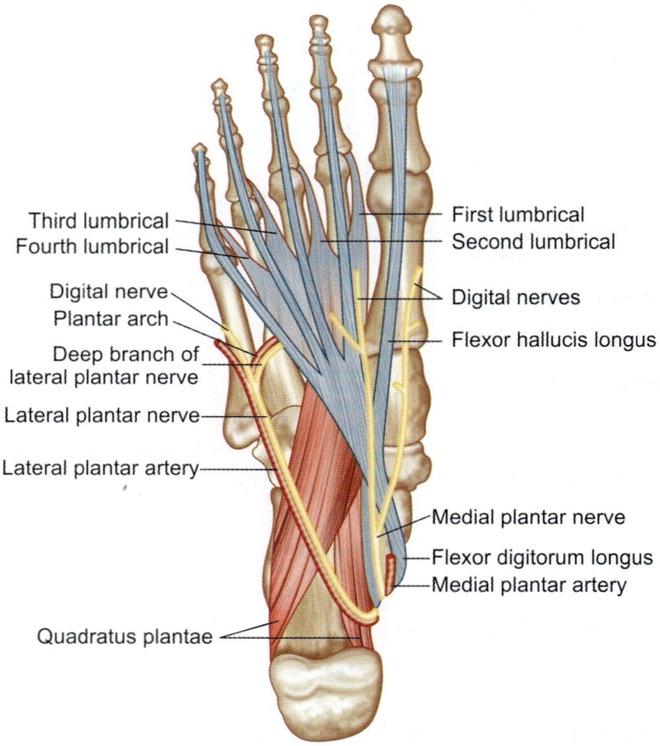

Fig. 26.28: Muscles in the second layer of the foot

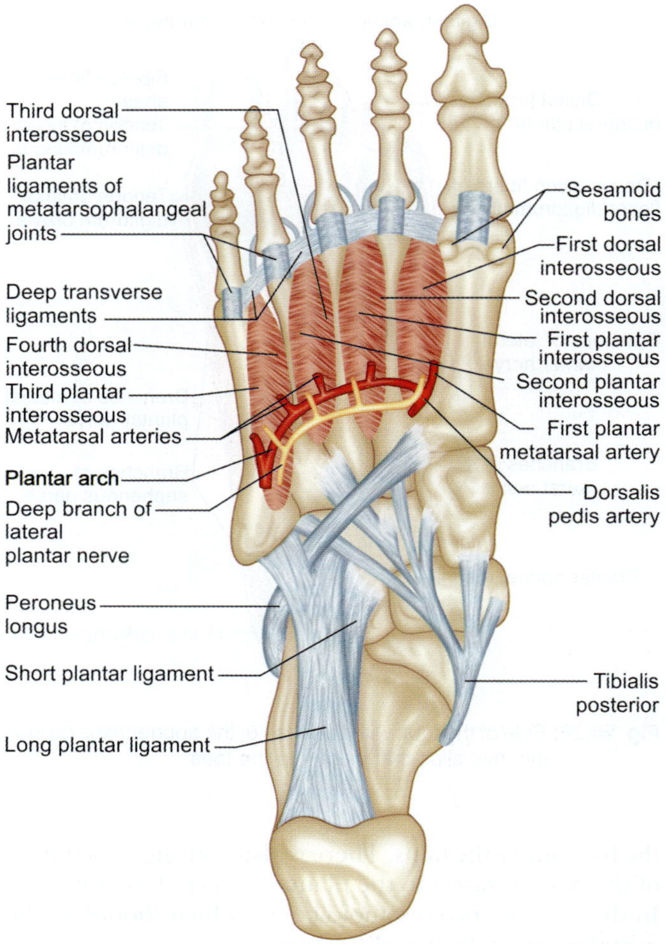

Fig. 26.30: Structures comprising fourth layer of the foot

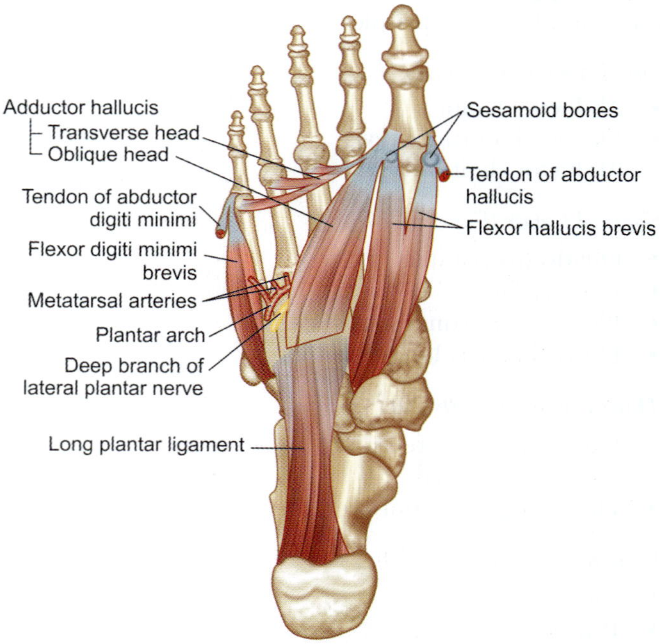

Fig. 26.29: Muscular attachments in the third layer of the foot

the base of the fifth metatarsal bone, the artery curves medially to form the plantar arch.

- *Dorsalis pedis artery (the dorsal artery of the foot):* On entering the sole between the two heads of the first dorsal interosseous muscle, the dorsalis pedis artery immediately joins the lateral plantar artery.

Veins of the Sole of the Foot

Medial and lateral plantar veins accompany the corresponding arteries and they unite behind the medial malleolus to form the posterior tibial venae comitantes.

Dorsum of the Foot

Skin is thin, hairy and freely mobile on the underlying tendons and bones. The sensory nerve supply to the skin on the dorsum of the foot is derived from the superficial peroneal nerve, assisted by the deep peroneal, saphenous and sural nerves. Dorsal venous arch (or network) lies in the subcutaneous tissue over the heads of the metatarsal bones and drains on the medial side into the great saphenous vein and on the lateral side into the small saphenous vein.

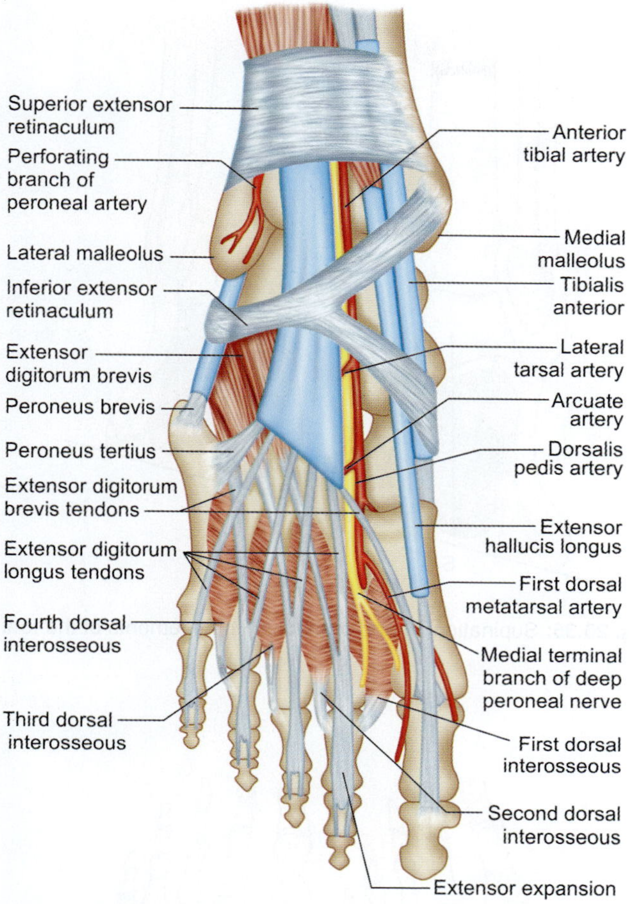

Fig. 26.31: Muscles of the dorsum of the foot

Muscles of the Dorsum of the Foot (Fig. 26.31)

- Extensor digitorum brevis
- The insertion of the long extensor tendons.

Artery of the Dorsum of the Foot

- *Dorsalis pedis artery:* It begins in front of the ankle joint, as a continuation of the anterior tibial artery. It terminates by passing downward into the sole between the two heads of the first dorsal interosseous muscle, where it joins the lateral plantar artery and completes the plantar arch
- Lateral tarsal artery, which crosses the dorsum of the foot just below the ankle joint
- Arcuate artery, which runs laterally under the extensor tendons, opposite the bases of the metatarsal bones. It gives off metatarsal branches to the toes
- First dorsal metatarsal artery, which supplies both sides of the big toe.

Compartment to the Foot

There are nine separate compartments to the foot (Fig. 26.32)

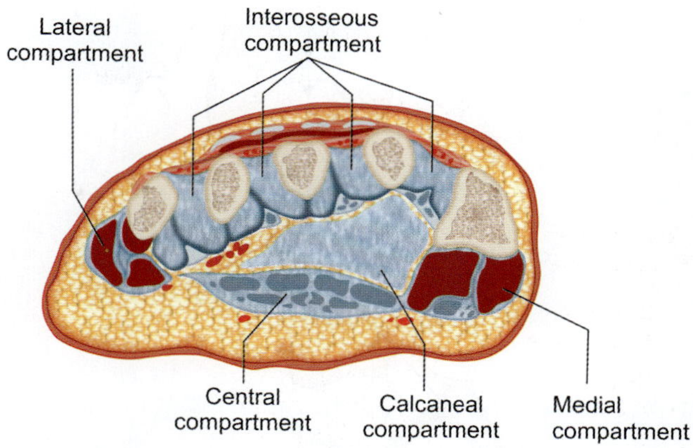

Fig. 26.32: Different compartments of the foot

- The medial compartment contains the abductor hallucis and flexor hallucis brevis muscles and is located plantar and medial to the first metatarsal.
- The lateral compartment contains the abductor digiti minimi and the flexor digiti minimi brevis and is found on the inferolateral surface of the fifth metatarsal.
- The central compartment is divided into superficial and deep portions.
  - The deep or calcaneal compartment contains the quadratus plantae muscle.
  - The superficial portion contains the flexor digitorum longus and brevis muscles.
- Dorsally, between each of the metatarsals lie the dorsal and plantar interosseous muscles, which appear to lie in a separate compartment defined by each intermetatarsal space.
- The calcaneal compartment, on the plantar aspect of the forefoot distal and deep to the quadratus plantae is the oblique head of the adductor hallucis, which also appears to have its own fascial compartment.

Tripod Action of the Foot

To maintain perfect ground contact each foot acts as a tripod, with the legs of the tripod represented by the calcaneus and the heads of the first and fifth metatarsals, as shown in Figure 26.33.

To maintain balance, the center of gravity must fall within the area covered by one or both feet and to facilitate this each foot must be capable of movement in two planes, as illustrated in Figure 26.34.

Planes of Movement

In the X-axis nearly all movement occurs in the ankle, and this allows balance to be maintained when going up and down slopes.

In the Z-axis supination (S) occurs when the soles of the feet are turned inwards to face one another. Pronation

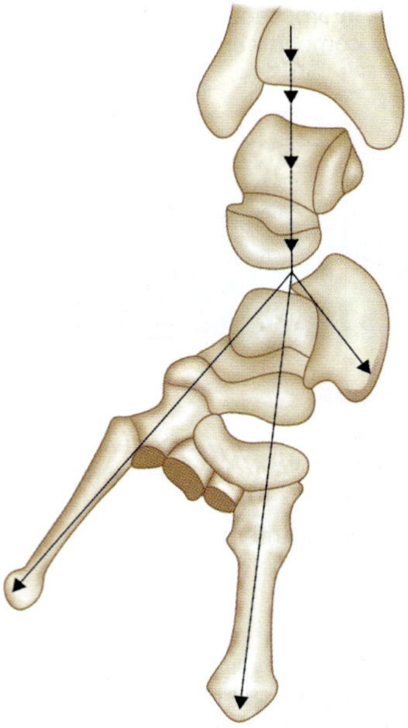

Fig. 26.33: Tripod action of the foot, formed by calcaneus and heads of the first and fifth metatarsals

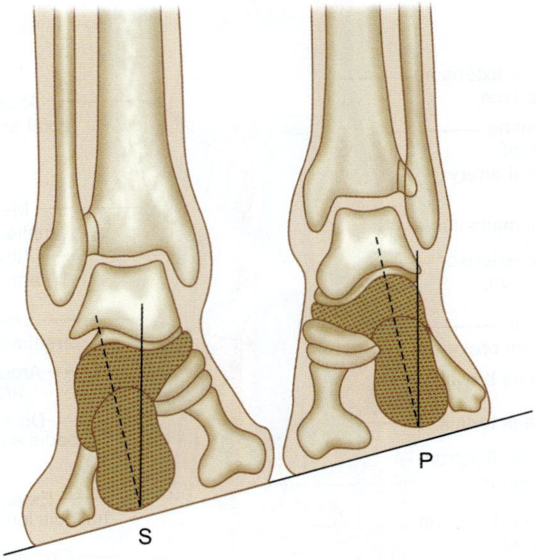

Fig. 26.35: Supination(S) and pronation(P) movements of the foot

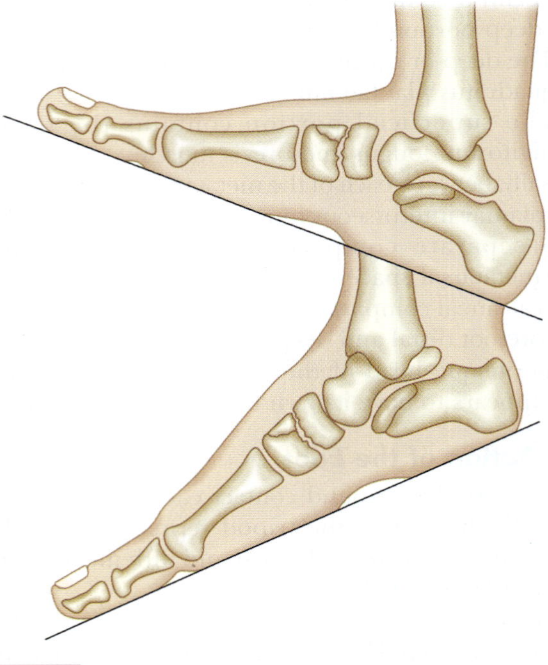

Fig. 26.34: Biplanar movement of the foot

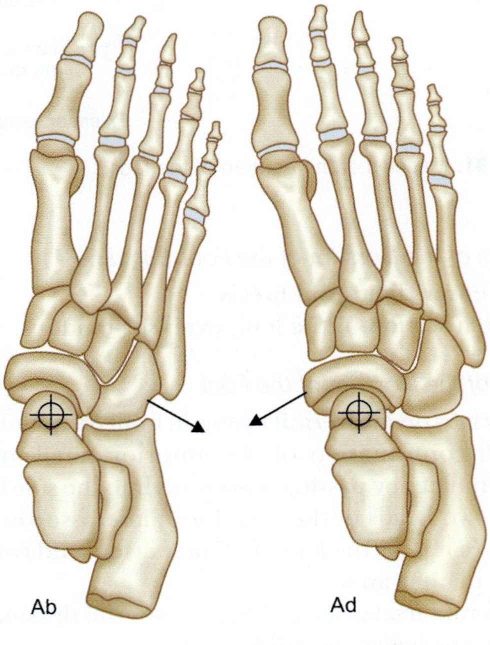

Fig. 26.36: Abduction (Ab) and adduction (Ad) movements of the foot

(P) involves movement in the opposite direction. This allows the feet to adapt to a surface sloping at right angles to the direction of travel. The major part of this movement involves the subtalar joint, as illustrated in Figure 26.35.

In the Y-axis, a very limited range of abduction and adduction of the forefoot may occur. Most of this occurs at the midtarsal joint but some takes place in the tarsometatarsal joints and the ankle, as shown in Figure 26.36.

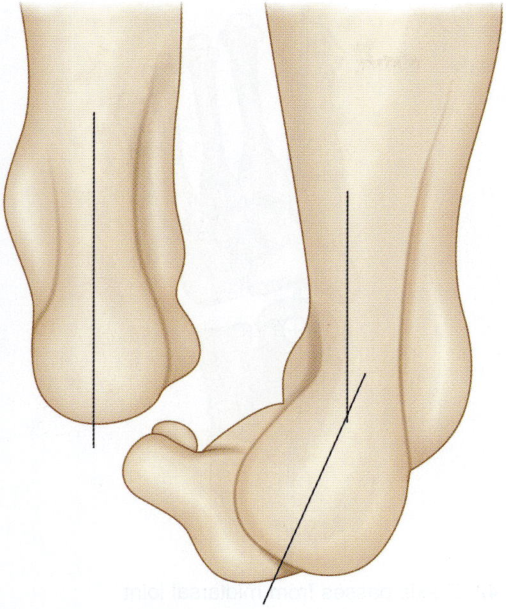

Fig. 26.37: Foot inversion (varus) movement, compared to position of the foot in neutral position

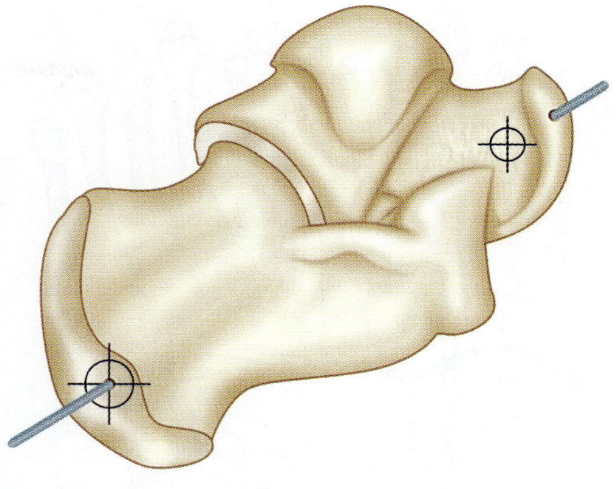

Fig. 26.38: Talus and axis of movements across talus

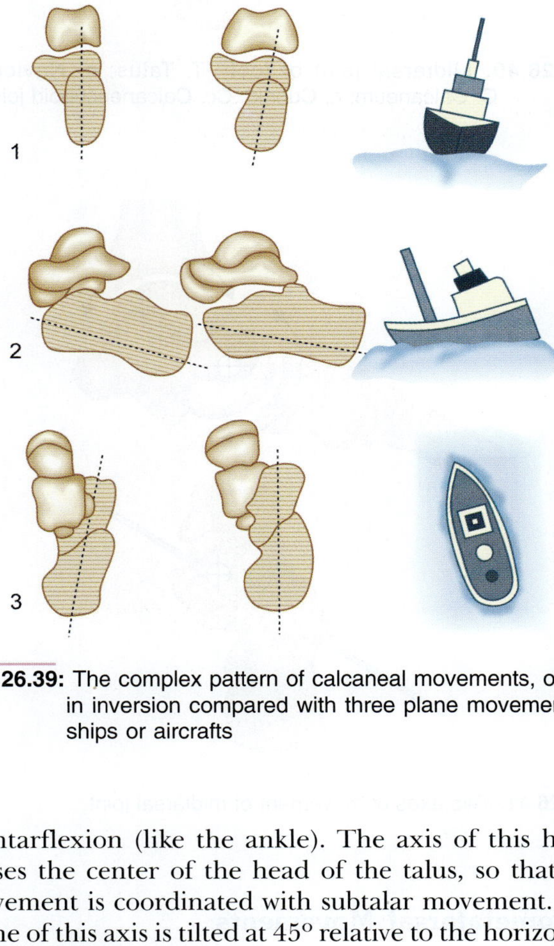

Fig. 26.39: The complex pattern of calcaneal movements, occurs in inversion compared with three plane movements of ships or aircrafts

Inversion

Inversion of the heel occurs when the calcaneus tilts into varus. This movement occurs in the subtalar joint. As the heel tilts, it carries the rest of the foot with it and this results in supination of the foot (varus tilting of the heel results in pronation of the foot), as shown in Figure 26.37.

Subtalar Movements (Fig. 26.38)

Movement at the subtalar joint, which involves two pairs of articular surfaces is highly complex, the only joint they resemble being those between the radius and ulna. There is, however a relatively fixed axis of movement, which passes through the center of the head of the talus in front and through the posterolateral tubercle of the calcaneus behind.

The complex pattern of calcaneal movements that occurs in inversion are sometimes compared with three plane movements of ships or aircrafts: the calcaneus (1), pitches (2) and yaws (turns) (3) under the talus, as shown in Figure 26.39.

Midtarsal Joint (Fig. 26.40)

This links the hindfoot with the midfoot. It is formed by the head of the Talus (T) and the navicular (n) on the medial side and on the lateral by the calcaneus (C) and the cuboid (c). The latter calcaneocuboid joint (Cc), which permits only a limited range of movements, ensures that when the heel moves the rest of the foot follows.

The joint has in effect two axes of movement. First, it acts as a hinge, allowing slight dorsiflexion and plantarflexion (like the ankle). The axis of this hinge passes the center of the head of the talus, so that this movement is coordinated with subtalar movement. The plane of this axis is tilted at 45° relative to the horizontal, as shown in Figure 26.41.

In addition to movements in (roughly) the X-axis, a limited amount of pronation and supination (Z-axis) is possible: the navicular slides and rotates round the head of the talus and the cuboid slides on the calcaneus. This axis of rotation also passes through the center of the head of the talus, this is illustrated in Figure 26.42.

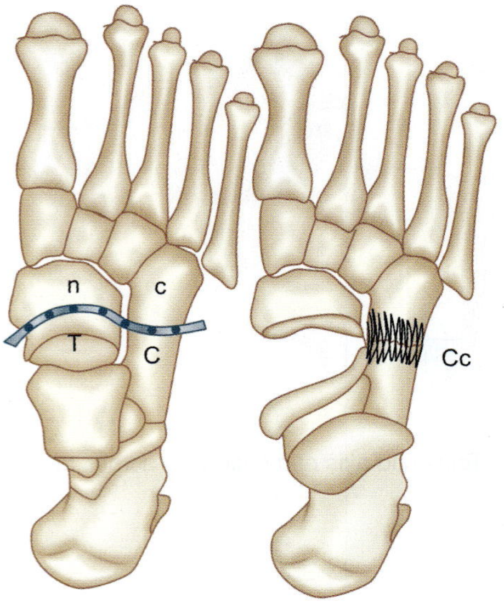

Fig. 26.40: Midtarsal joint of foot—T. Talus; n. Navicular; C. Calcaneum; c. Cuboid; Cc. Calcaneocuboid joint

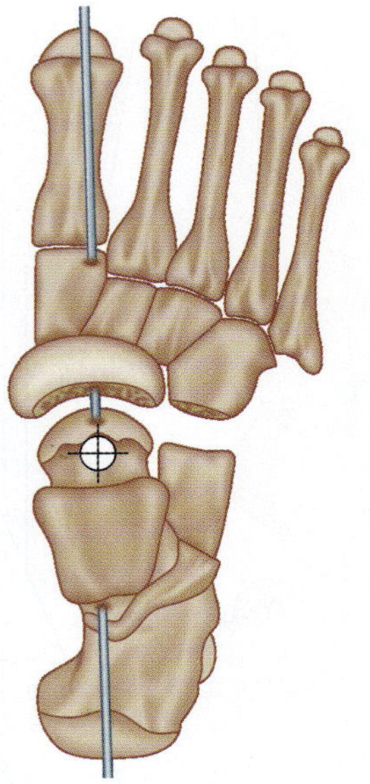

Fig. 26.42: Z-axis passes from midtarsal joint

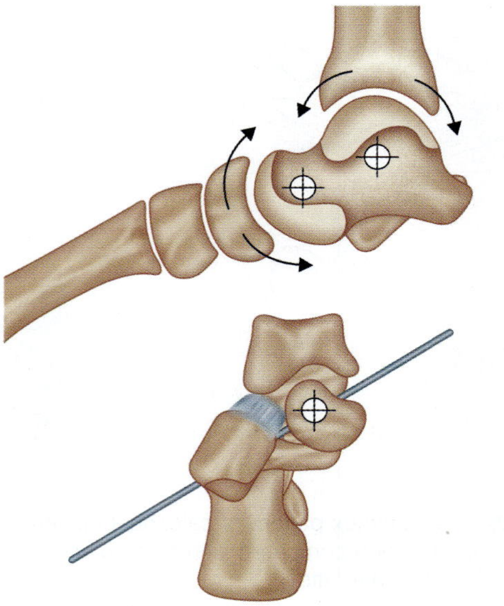

Fig. 26.41: Two axes of movement of midtarsal joint

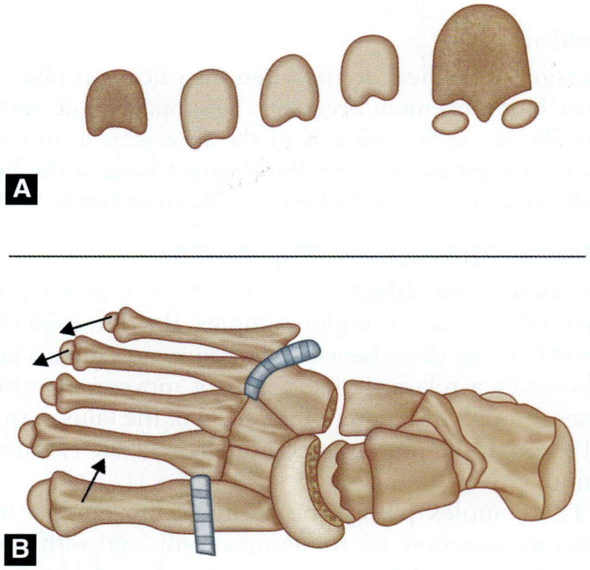

Fig. 26.43A and B: Tarsometatarsal joint of the foot

Tarsometatarsal Movements

Whereas the heads of the first and fifth metatarsals form the anterior limbs of each foot tripod, the other metatarsal heads can adopt to any irregularity in the surface of the ground. Elevation and depression of the first metatarsal head and of the other (particularly the fourth and fifth) can contribute an appreciable amount of overall supination of the foot, as shown in Figure 26.43.

Heel Posture

Figures 26.44A to E show heel posture.

The Arches

The Medial Longitudinal Arch (Fig. 26.45)

It is the most important and the one primarily affected in pes planus and pes cavus. It is formed by the talus (T), calcaneus (C), navicular (N), cuneiforms (Cn) and the

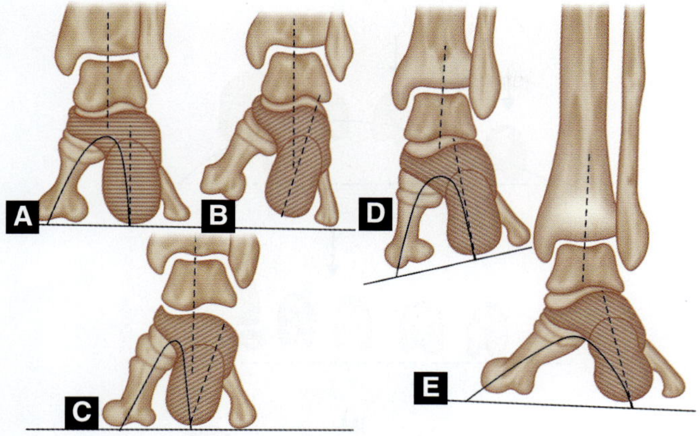

Figs 26.44A to E: (A) Normally the weight bearing foot the axis of the heel is in alignment with the tibia; (B) If the heel posture is abnormal and tilts into varus, the under normal circumstances the foot would supinate and the first metatarsal head would not contact the ground; (C) To correct this, the foot distal to the subtalar joint must pronate, and this leads to accentuation of the medial longitudinal arch; (D) If on the other hand, the heel posture is one of valgus; (E) Then to allow the metatarsal heads to contact level ground the foot distal to the subtalar joint must supinate, leading to flattening of the medial arch

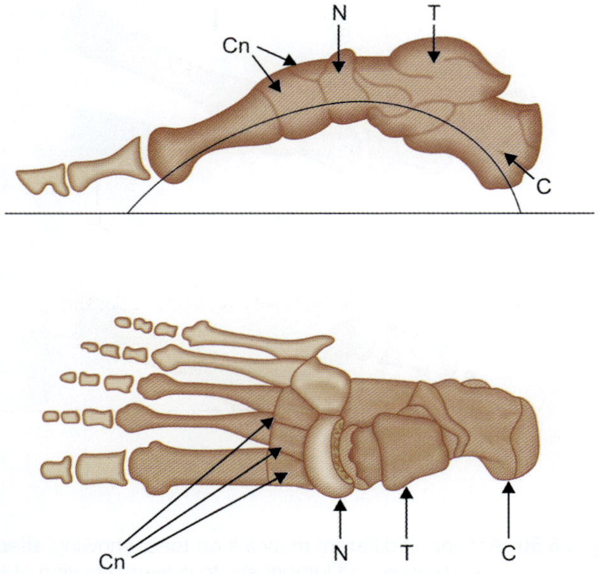

Fig. 26.45: The medial longitudinal arch—T. Talus; C. Calcaneus; N. Navicular; Cn. Cuneiforms

medial three metatarsals. The medial longitudinal arch is supported by the spring ligament (S), which shoulders the head of the talus, as shown in Figure 26.46. The plantar fascia (P), which acts as a tie. Abductor

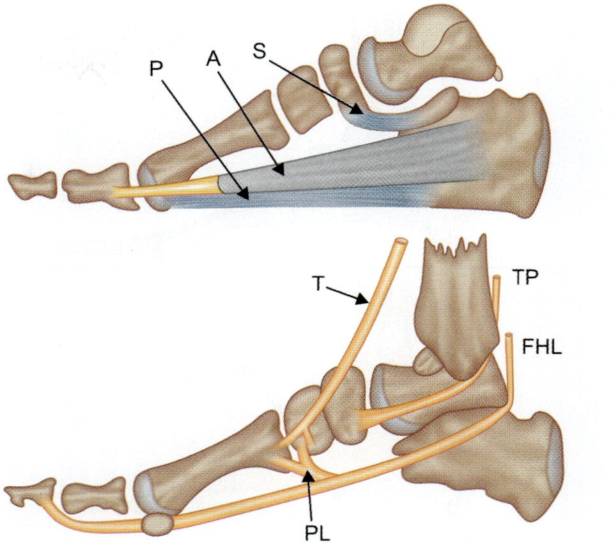

Fig. 26.46: Structures supporting medial longitudinal arch—S. Spring ligament; P. Plantar fascia; A. Abductor hallucis; T. Tibialis anterior; PL. Peroneus longus; TP. Tibialis posterior; FHL. Flexor hallucis longus

hallucis (A) and flexor digitorum brevis, which act as spring ties. Tibialis anterior (T), which lifts the center arch (and with peroneus longus (PL) forms a stirrup like support for it). Tibialis posterior (TP), which adducts the metatarsal joint and reinforces the action of the spring ligament. Flexor hallucis longus (FHL), which acts as a spring tie and helps support the head of the talus.

Lateral Longitudinal Arch (Fig. 26.47)

It is formed by the calcaneus, cuboid and fourth and fifth metatarsals. It is very shallow and generally flattens out on weight-bearing. It is supported by the long and short plantar ligaments (LS), the plantar fascia (P), flexor digitorum brevis, flexor and abductor digiti minimi, peroneus tertius (PT), peroneus brevis (PB) and peroneus longus (PL).

Transverse Arch (Fig. 26.48)

It is formed by the cuneiforms (C) and the cuboids (CU). It stretches across the sole in the coronal plane.

It is half an arch, the whole arch is completed by the other foot. It is of no clinical significance. The shape of the cuneiforms helps maintain the arch, the anterior arch lies in the coronal plane, its bony components comprise the metatarsal head. It is not a feature of the weight bearing foot. The metatarsal heads are prevented from spreading out (splaying) by the intermetatarsal ligaments (IM) and the intrinsic muscles, especially the transverse head of the adductor hallucis (AH), as shown in Figure 26.49.

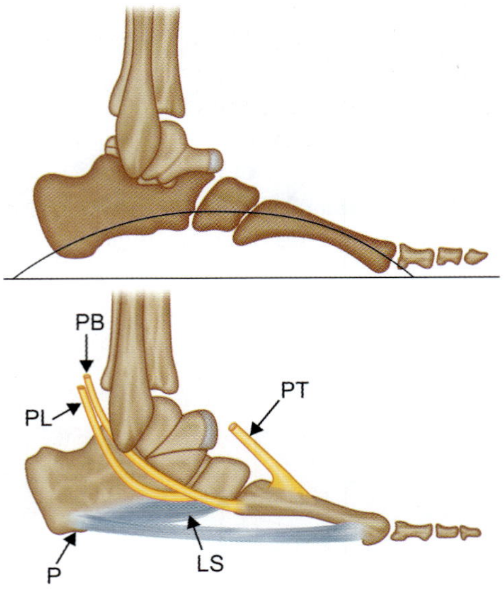

Fig. 26.47: Structures forming lateral longitudinal arch—LS. Long and short plantar ligaments; P. Plantar fascia; PT. Peroneus tertius; PB. Peroneus brevis; PL. Peroneus longus

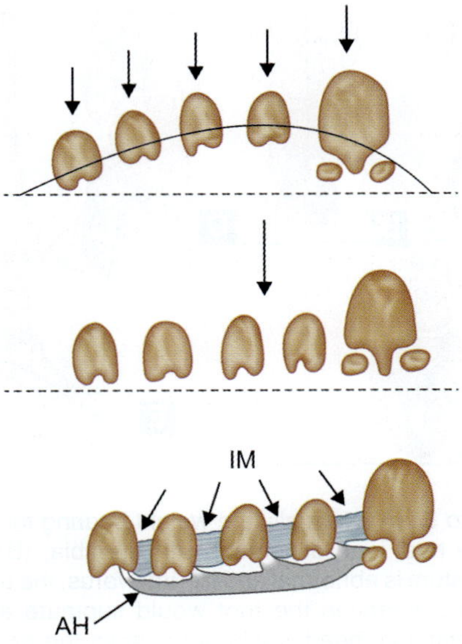

Fig. 26.49: Anterior arch of foot, comprising metatarsal heads—IM.Intermetatarsal ligaments; AH. Adductor hallucis

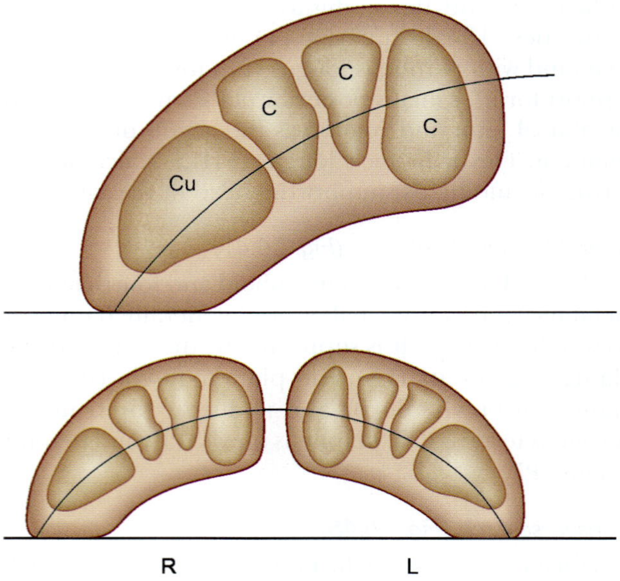

Fig. 26.48: The transverse arch of the foot—C. Cuneiforms; Cu. Cuboids; R. Right; L. Left

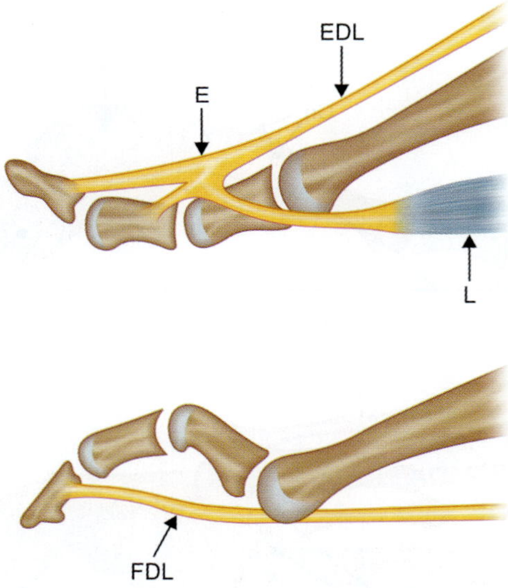

Fig. 26.50: Actions of different muscles on toes, showing affect of interosseous and lumbricals, to prevent clawing of toes by preventing excessive pull of flexor digitorum longus

Toes (Fig. 26.50)

Extensor digitorum longus (EDL) extends the MP and both IP joints of each toe. The interosseous and lumbricals muscles; R. Right; L. Left (L), through their attachments to the extensor expansions (E) extend the toes at the proximal and distal interphalangeal joints and flex the MP joints. If they become weak or fail, the unchecked pull of the flexor digitorum longus (FDL) results in clawing of the toes.

EXAMINATION OF THE FOOT AND ANKLE

■ Inspection

Look for any deformity of shape suggesting an old fracture (A), sinus scars, suggesting old infection (B), as shown in Figure 26.51.

Look for deformity of posture (e.g. plantar flexion owing to short tendocalcaneus, talipes deformity, drop foot), as illustrated in Figure 26.52.

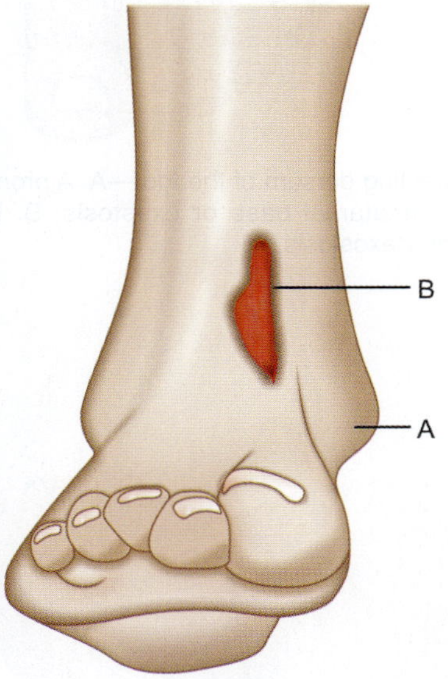

Fig. 26.51: Inspecting presence of deformity—A. Deformity of shape suggesting an old fracture; B. Sinus scars suggesting old infection

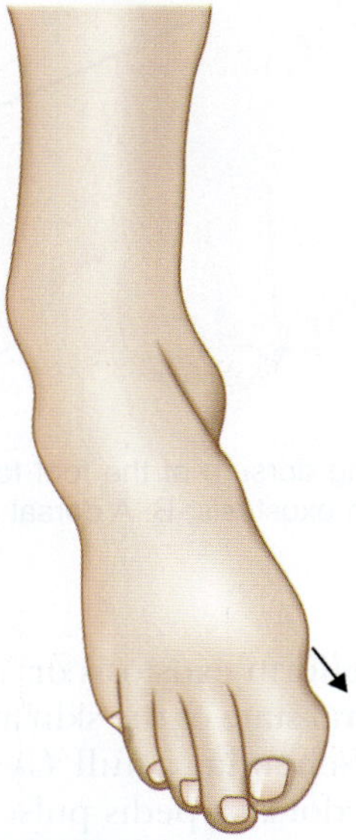

Fig. 26.52: Inspecting deformed posture

Look for bruising swelling or edema. If there is swelling, note whether it is diffuse or localized, unilateral or bilateral, as depicted in Figure 26.53.

Tenderness localized at the malleoli following injury, radiographic examination is necessary, as shown in Figure 26.54.

Note whether the foot is normally proportioned. If not look at the hands and asses the rest of the skeleton, as shown in Figure 26.55.

Heel (Fig. 26.56)

Is there a calcaneal prominence (calcaneal exostosis), with overlying callous or bursitis. Is there deformity of the heel, suggesting old fracture or talipes deformity.

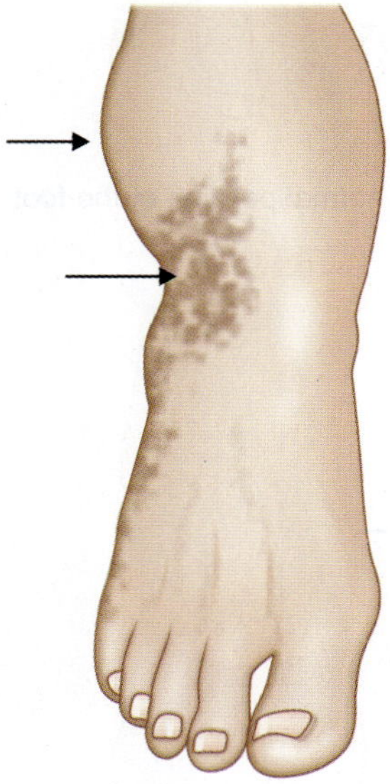

Fig. 26.53: Inspecting presence of swelling or edema

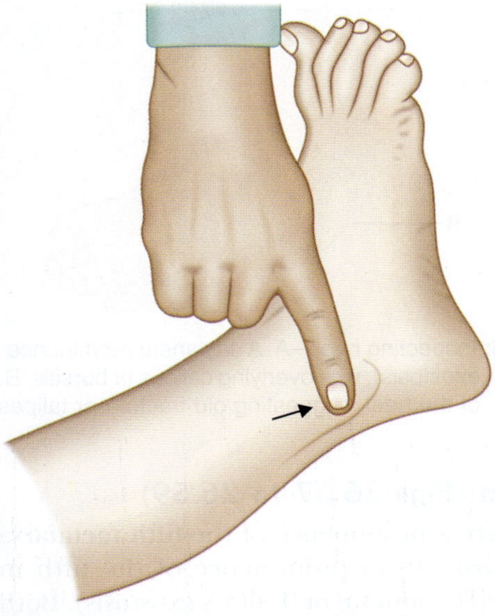

Fig. 26.54: Inspecting for localized tenderness at the malleoli

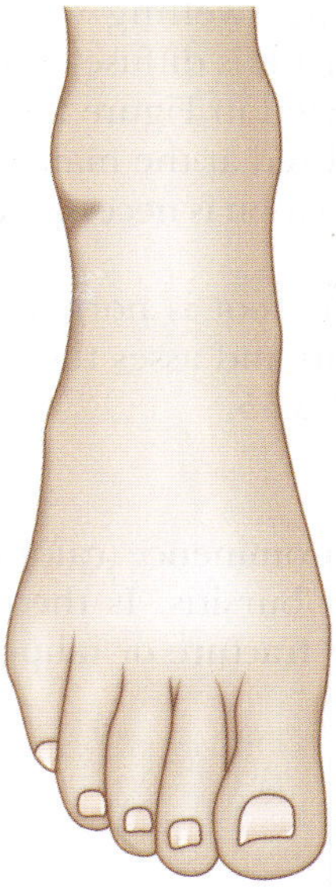

Fig. 26.55: Inspecting normal position of the foot

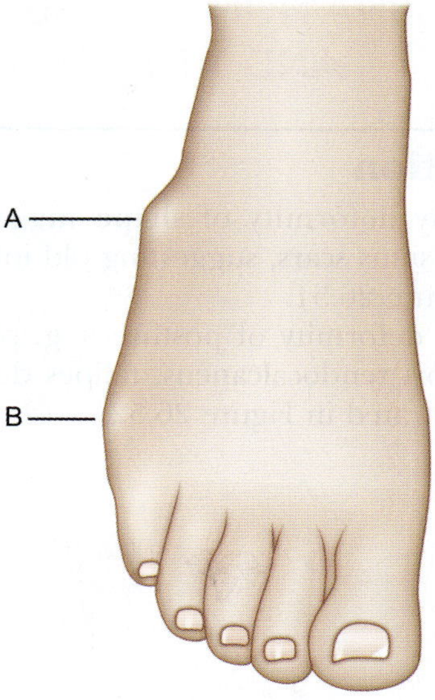

Fig. 26.57: Inspecting dorsum of the foot—A. A prominence of the fifth metatarsal base or exostosis; B. Bunionette or Tailor's exostosis

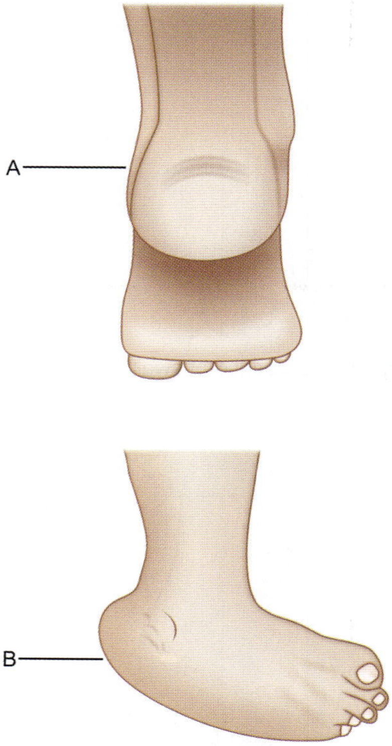

Fig. 26.56: Inspecting heel—A. A calcaneal prominence (calcaneal exostosis), with overlying callous or bursitis; B. Deformity of the heel, suggesting old fracture or talipes deformity

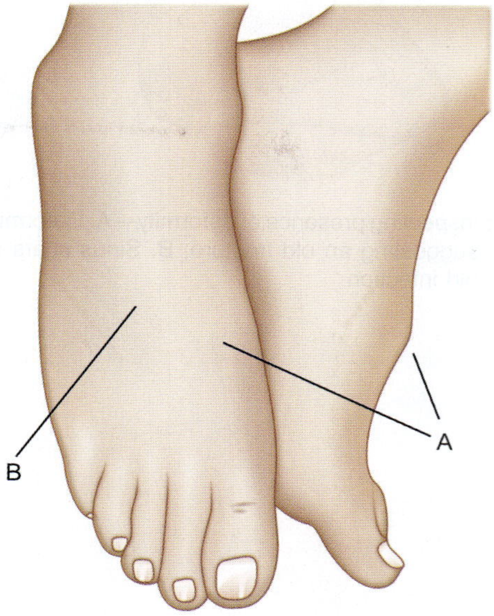

Fig. 26.58: Inspecting dorsum of the foot for any ganglion—A. A cuneiform exostosis; B. A dorsal ganglion

Dorsum (Figs 26.57 to 26.59)

- Is there a prominence of the fifth metatarsal base or exostosis, from prominence of the fifth metatarsal head (Bunionette or Tailor's exostosis). Both can be a source of local pressure symptoms.
- Is there a cuneiform exostosis or a dorsal ganglion.
- Note the general state of the skin and nails. If there is evidence of ischemia, a full CVS examination is required. The dorsalis pedis pulse should be sought routinely.

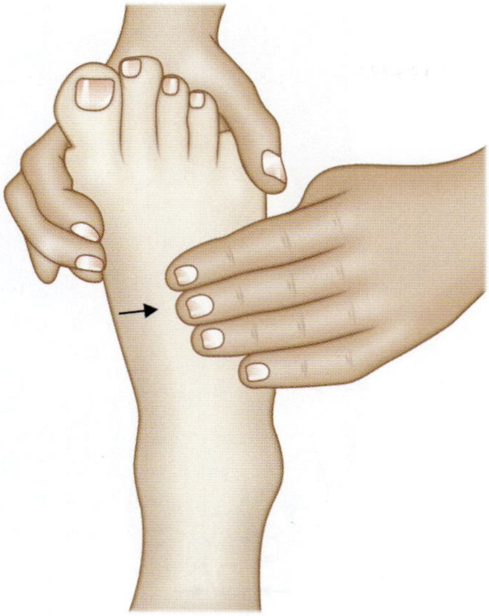

Fig. 26.59: Inspecting the dorsum of the foot for skin and nails or signs of ischemia arrow showing dorsalis pedis pulse palpation

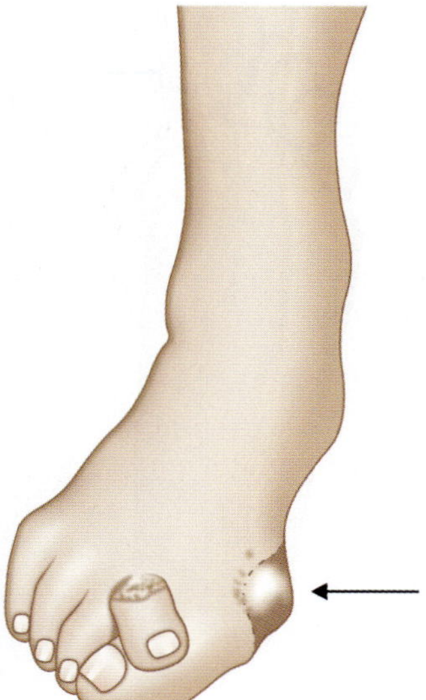

Fig. 26.61: Look for the presence of any bursa over the great toe

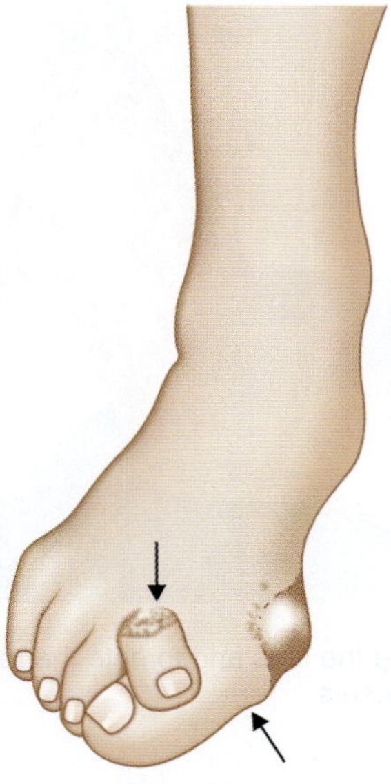

Fig. 26.60: Hallux valgus–deformed great toe

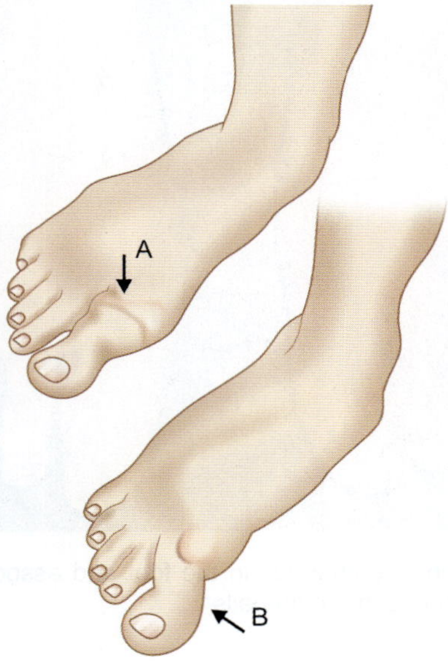

Fig. 26.62: Inspecting the great toe for any thickening or deformities—A. The toe is thickened at the MP joint, suggesting hallux rigidus (osteoarthritis); B. Hallux flexus

Great Toe (Figs 26.60 to 26.64)

- Note any hallux valgus deformity.
- Note the presence of any bursa over the MP joint (bunion) and whether active inflammatory changes are present. Discoloration of the joint with acute tenderness is suggestive of gout.
- Note whether the toe is thickened at the MP joint, suggesting hallux rigidus (osteoarthritis) or held in a flexed position, hallux flexus (osteoarthritis).
- Note the presence of excess callus under the great toe. This is highly suggestive of hallux rigidus.
- *Great toenail:* Note whether the great toenail is deformed (onychogryphosis), ingrowing (accompanied by inflammation), elevated (suggestive of subungual exostosis) or uneven in texture and growth (fungal infection or psoriasis).
- *Sign of ischemia:* Thinning of the skin, diminished hair growth, loss of subcutaneous fat, shininess and trophic changes in the nail, which become brittle and show transverse ridges, minor ulcerations in pressue areas such as heel, malleoli, ball of the foot and tip of the toes, as shown in Figure 26.64.

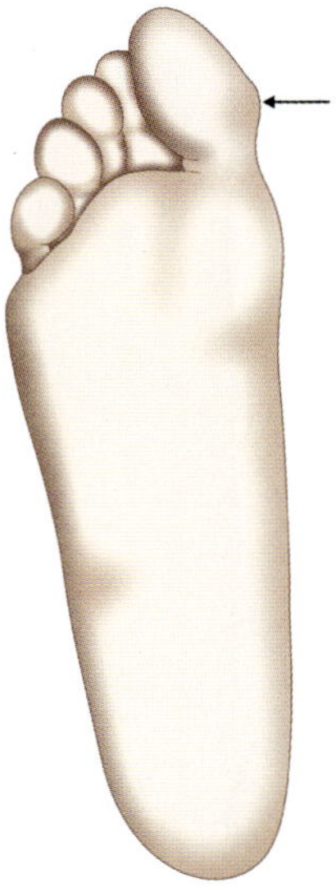

Fig. 26.63: Inspecting plantar aspect of great toe

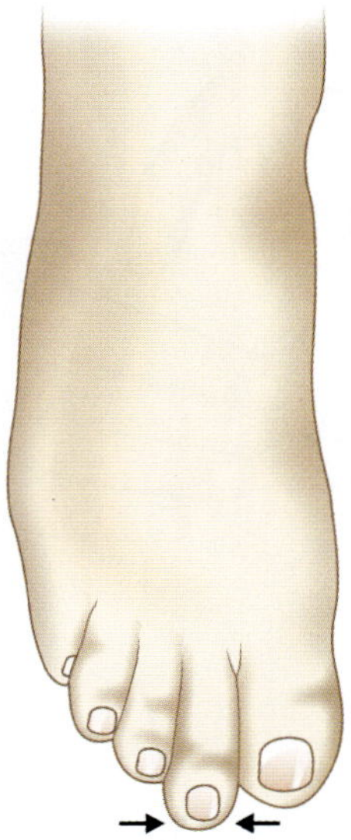

Fig. 26.65: Inspecting the relative lengths of the toes or any clawing

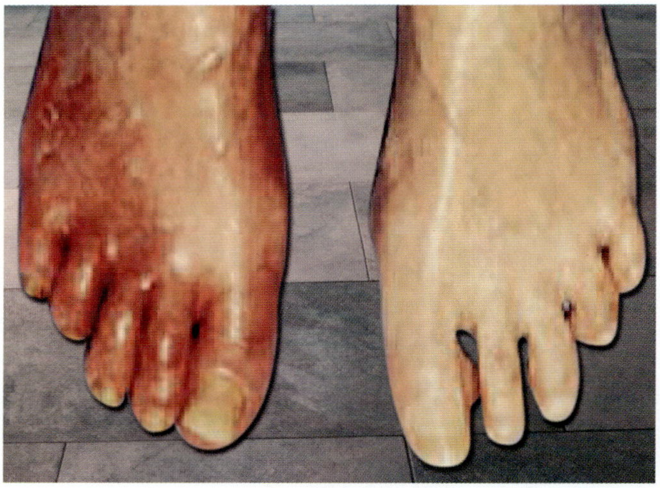

Fig. 26.64: Ischemic changes in the foot and associated trophic changes in the toenails

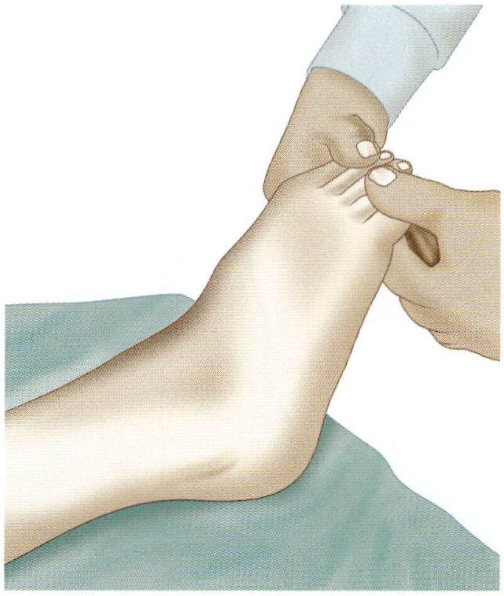

Fig. 26.66: Flexing the toes and to note the relative lengths of the metatarsals

Toes (Figs 26.65 to 26.71)

- Note the relative lengths. A second toe longer than the first, occasionally become clawed or throw additional stress on its MP joint. It may be associated with Freiberg's disease.
- Flex the toes and note the relative lengths of the metatarsals. Abnormally short first and fifth metatarsals are a potential cause of forefoot imbalance and pain.
- *Curly toes:* In this deformity a degree of fixed flexion develops in the IP joint and the MP joints. It is generally caused by interosseous muscle weakness. In grade A, the toe is mildly flexed, with or without some adduction. In grade B, there is some degree of under or overriding. Grade C the nail is not visible form the dorsum, as shown in Figures 26.67A to C.
- *Claw toes:* The toes are said to be clawed, when they are extended at the metatarsophalangeal joints and flexed at the interphalangeal joints. If all toes are involved, this suggests there may be an associated pes cavus or some cause of intrinsic muscle insufficiency, as shown in Figure 26.68.
- *Hammer toe deformity (Fig. 26.69):* The toe is flexed at the proximal IP joint and extended at the MP joint and distal IP joint. The second toe is most commonly affected, often owing to an associated hallux valgus deformity. There is usually a callus at the proximal IP joint, as a result of pressure against the shoe.

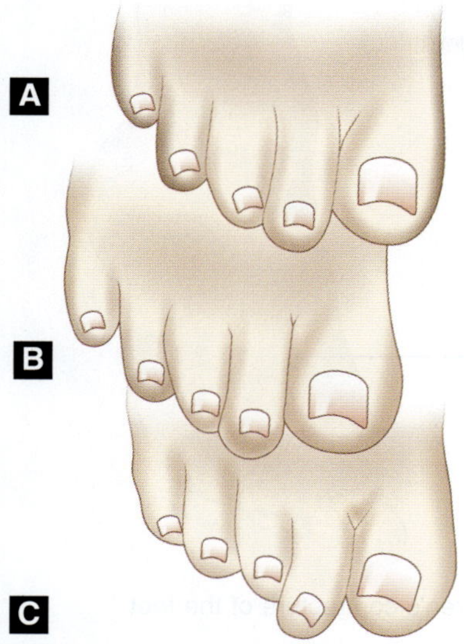

Figs 26.67A to C: Different grades of curling toes

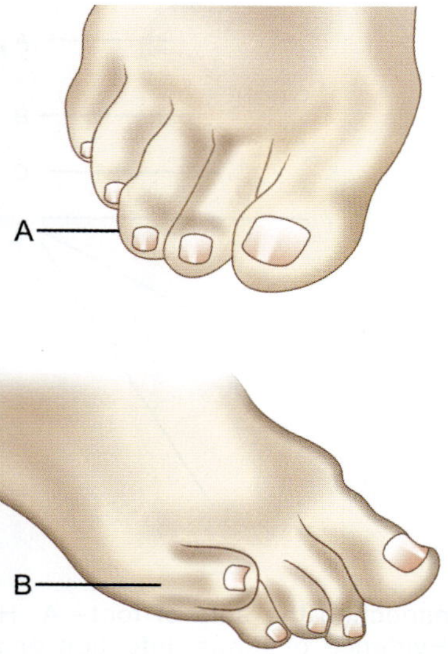

Fig. 26.70: Mallet toes and quinti varus deformity— A. A mallet toe deformity; B. An overlapping fifth toe or quinti varus

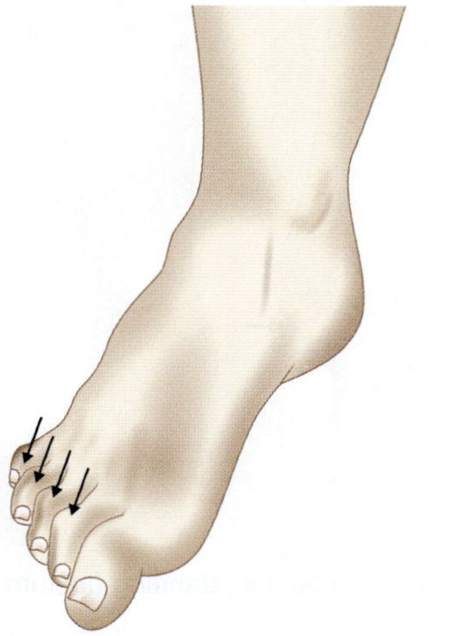

Fig. 26.68: Claw toes deformity

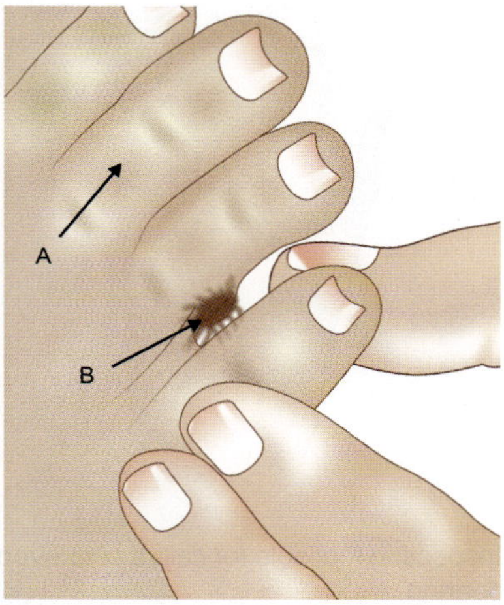

Fig. 26.71: Inspecting presence of corns–hard and soft—A. Hard corns; B. Soft corn

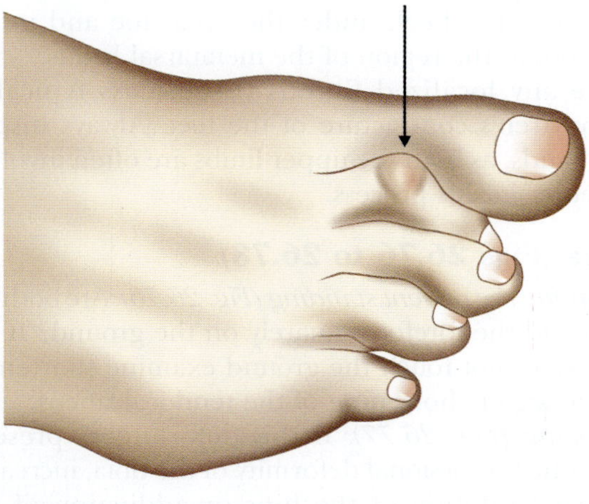

Fig. 26.69: Hammer toe deformity

- Note the presence of a mallet toe deformity (flexion deformity of the distal IP joint). There is usually a callus under the tip of the toe. Note an overlapping fifth toe or quinti varus (often congenital), as shown in Figure 26.70.
- Note the presence of hard corns. These are areas of hyperkeratosis that occur over bony prominences and are generally caused by pressure against the shoes. Soft corns are macerated hyperkeratotic lesions occurring between the toes and are not associated with friction or pressure, as illustrated in Figure 26.71.

Sole (Figs 26.72 to 26.75)

- Note hyperhidrosis, evidence of fungal infection or athletes foot and ulceration of sole, suggesting pes cavus or neurological disturbance.

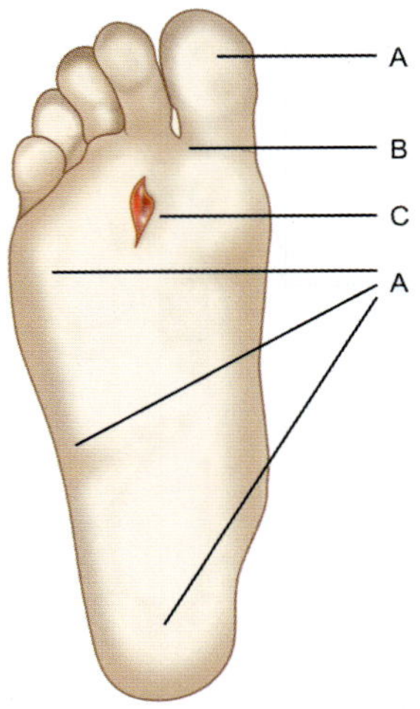

Fig. 26.72: Inspecting the sole of foot—A. Hyperhidrosis; B. Evidence of fungal infection or athletes foot; C. Ulceration of sole

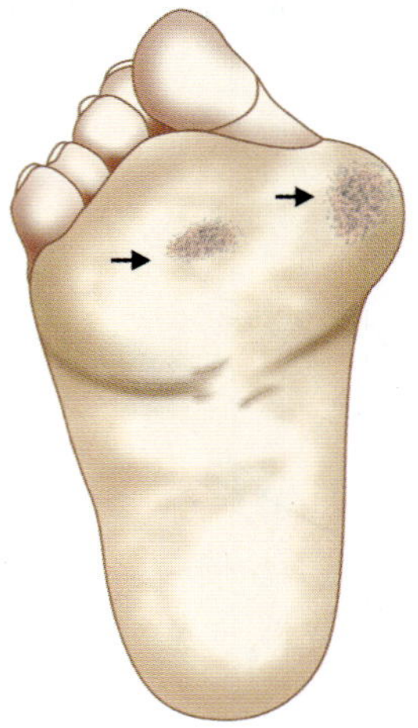

Fig. 26.73: Inspecting foot sole for callus or uneven areas of weight bearing

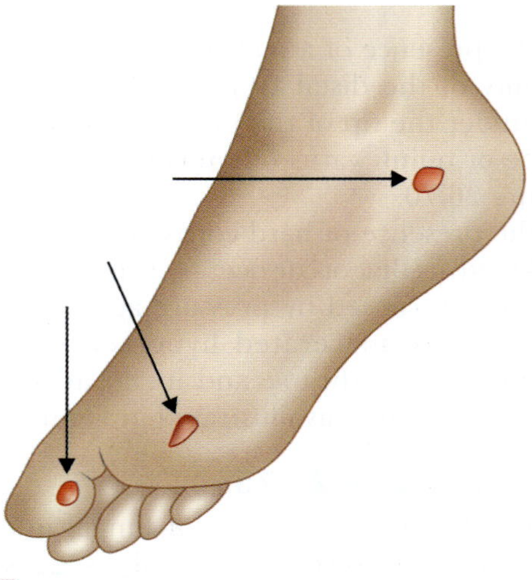

Fig. 26.74: Verruca (plantar wart)

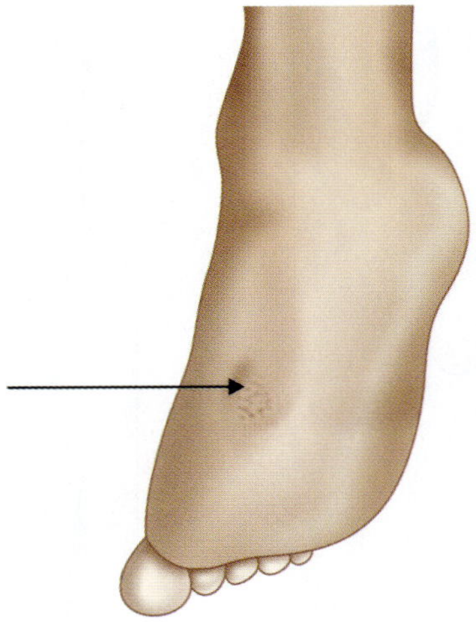

Fig. 26.75: Dupuytren's contracture of the feet

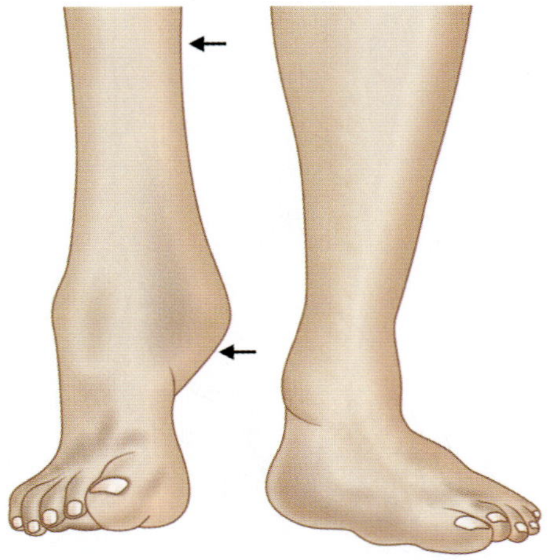

Fig. 26.76: Examining patient in standing posture

- Note the presence of callus, indicating uneven or restricted area of weight bearing.
- Note the presence of verruca (plantar wart). Classically occurs at the heel, under the great toe and in the forefoot in the region of the metatarsal heads.
- Note any localized fibrous tissue mass typical of Dupuytren's contracture of the feet. Always inspect the hands, as both the upper limbs are often involved together in this process.

Posture (Figs 26.76 to 26.78)

- *Examine the patient standing (Fig. 26.76):* Are both the heel and the forefoot squarely on the ground? If the heel does not touch the ground examine shortening of the leg or shortening of the tendocalcaneus.
- *Intoeing (Fig. 26.77):* If this deformity is present, examine for torsional deformity of the tibia, increased internal rotation of the hips or adduction of the forefoot.

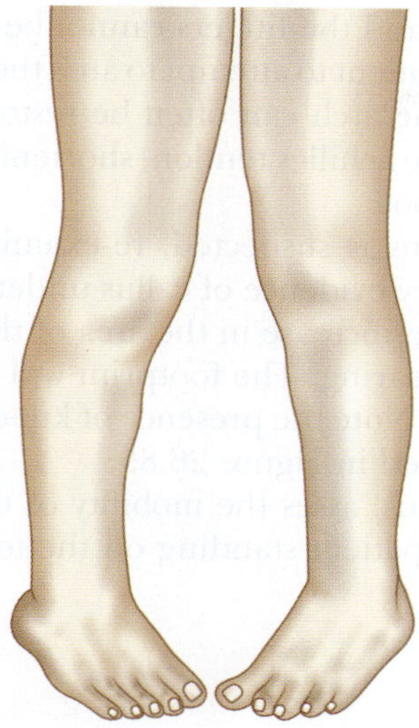

Fig. 26.77: Intoeing

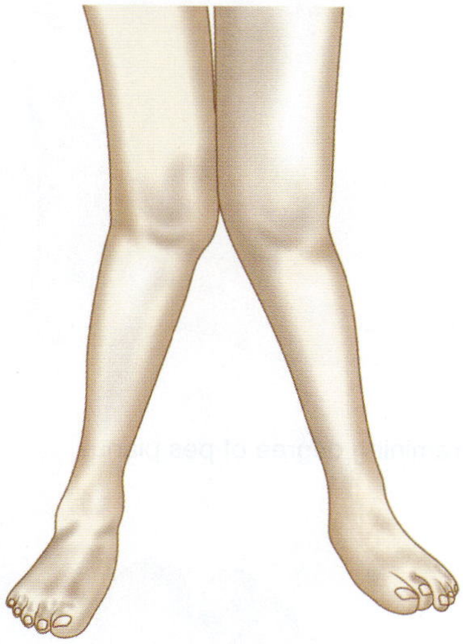

Fig. 26.78: Genu valgum

- *Genu valgum (Fig. 26.78):* It is frequently associated with flat foot. Most commonly seen as a growth disturbance of the knee or as a complication of osteoarthritis.
- *Eversion (Fig. 26.79):* If the foot is everted this suggests a peroneal spastic foot, a painful lesion on the lateral side of the foot or if less marked, pes planus.
- *Inversion (Fig. 26.80):* If the foot is inverted it suggests muscle imbalance from stroke or other neurological disorder, hallux flexus or rigidus, pes cavus, residual talipes deformity or painful condition of the forefoot.
- *Splaying (Fig. 26.81):* Note whether there is any broadening of the forefoot. This is often the result of intrinsic muscle weakness and may be associated with pes cavus, callus under the metatarsal heads, hallux valgus, anterior metatarsalgia and trouble with shoe fitting.

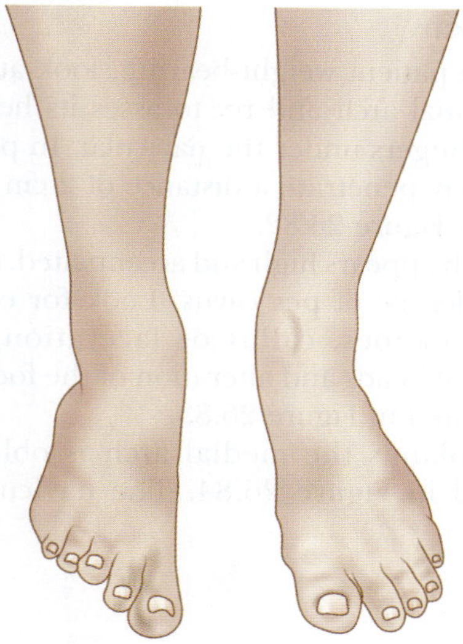

Fig. 26.79: Foot eversion deformity

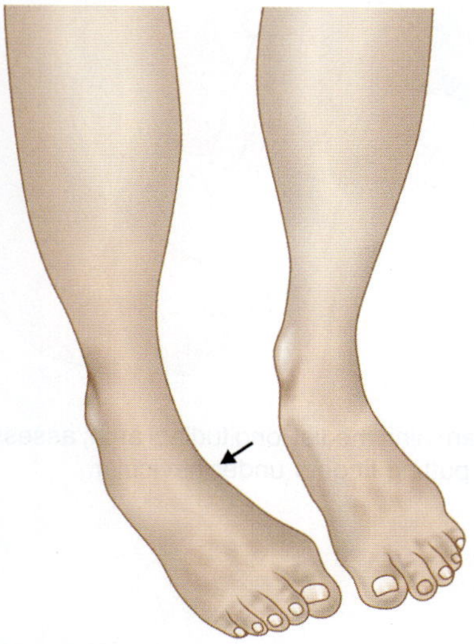

Fig. 26.80: Foot inversion

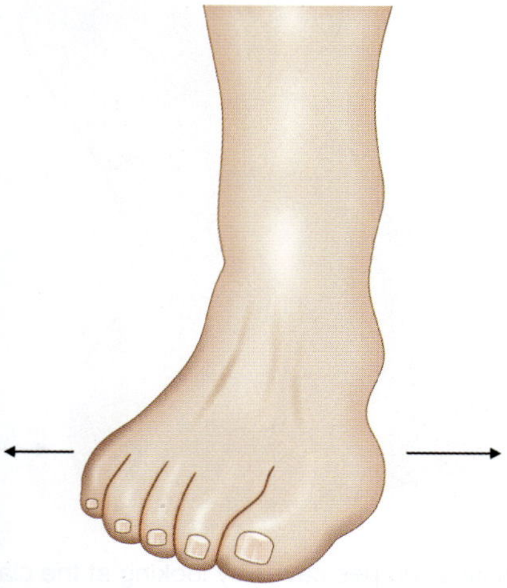

Fig. 26.81: Splaying of foot

Medial Arch

- With the patient weight-bearing, look at the medial longitudinal arch and try to asses its height. Try to slip the fingers under the navicular. In pes cavus the finger may penetrate a distance of 2 cm or more, as shown in Figure 26.82.
- If the arch appears high and accentuated, this suggests a high degree of pes cavus. Look for confirmatory clawing of toes, callus or laceration under the metatarsal heads and alteration of the footprints, this is illustrated in Figure 26.83.
- In pes planus the medial arch is obliterated, as depicted in Figure 26.84. The navicular is often prominent and the fingers cannot be inserted under it. Ask the patient to attempt to arch the foot. In mobile arch foot the arch can often be restored voluntarily. Examine the achilles tendon, shortening of which can cause flat foot.
- If pes planus is suspected, re-examine the sole for confirmatory evidence of callus under the metatarsal head and an increase in the area of the sole involved in weight-bearing. The footprint will be abnormal in these cases. Note the presence of knock knees. This is demonstrated in Figure 26.85.
- In pes planus, asses the mobility of the foot first, by asking the patient standing on the toes, while at the

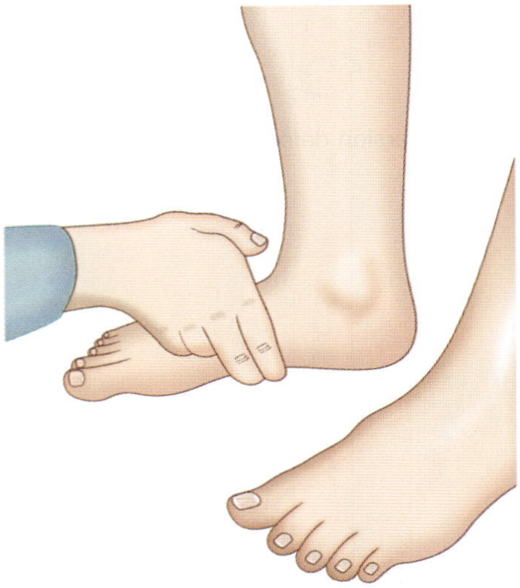

Fig. 26.82: Examining medial longitudinal arch, assessing its height, by putting fingers under navicular

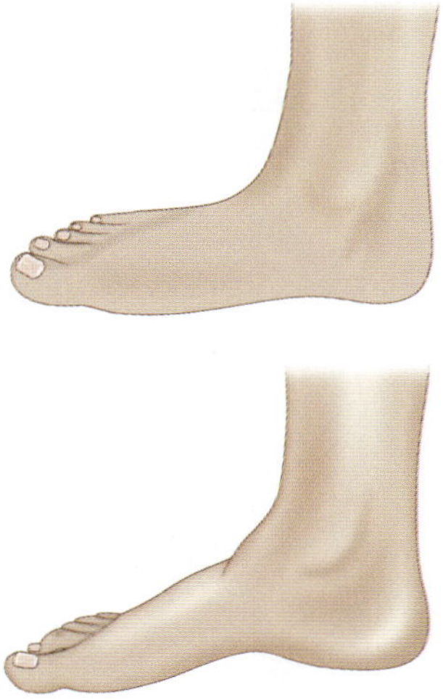

Fig. 26.84: Examining degree of pes planus

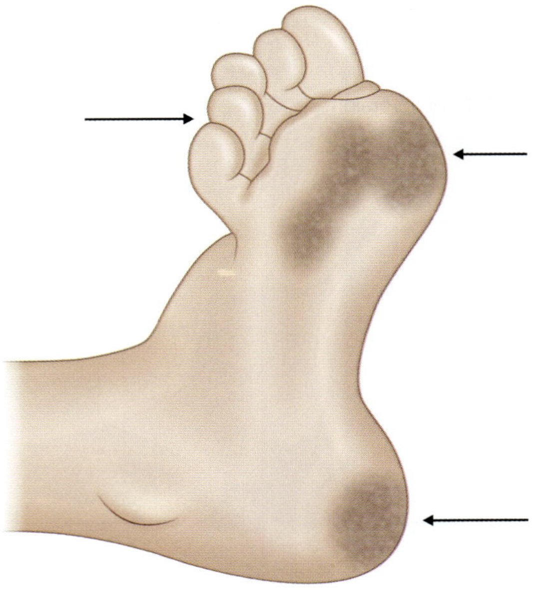

Fig. 26.83: Assessing pes cavus by looking at the clawing of toes, callus or laceration under metatarsal heads

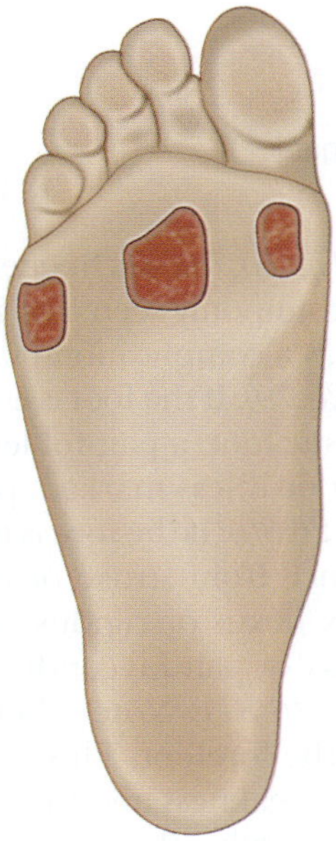

Fig. 26.85: Callus under the metatarsal head, confirmatory to pes planus

same time examining the alteration in shape of the foot. Later, carefully note the range of inversion and eversion, as demonstrated in Figure 26.86.

Heels

- Look at the foot from behind, paying particular attention to the slope of the heel, as shown in Figures 26.87A and B
- Again ask the patient to stand on his toes observing the heels. If the heel posture corrects, it indicates a mobile subtalar joint. Persisting deformity suggests loss of movement which may be due arthritic changes, tarsal coalition, loss of spring ligament or posterior tibialis function or shortening of the tendocalcaneus, as shown in Figure 26.88.

Gait (Fig. 26.89): Watch the patient walking first barefooted and then with shoes. Examine from all sides.

Skin temperature (Fig. 26.90): Grasp the foot and asses the skin temperature comparing with the other side. A warm foot is particularly indicative or rheumatoid arthritis or gout.

Footprint (Fig. 26.91)

- It is sometimes helpful to see the pattern of weight distribution in the foot.
- Typical patterns, shown in pes planus (Figs 26.92A to C)

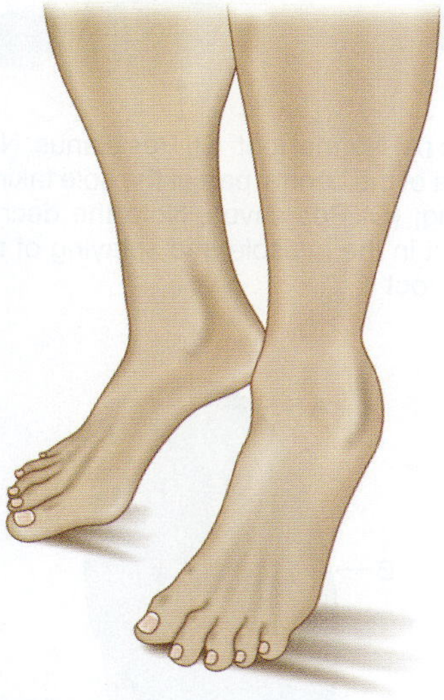

Fig. 26.86: Assessing the mobility of the foot, by asking the patient standing on toes

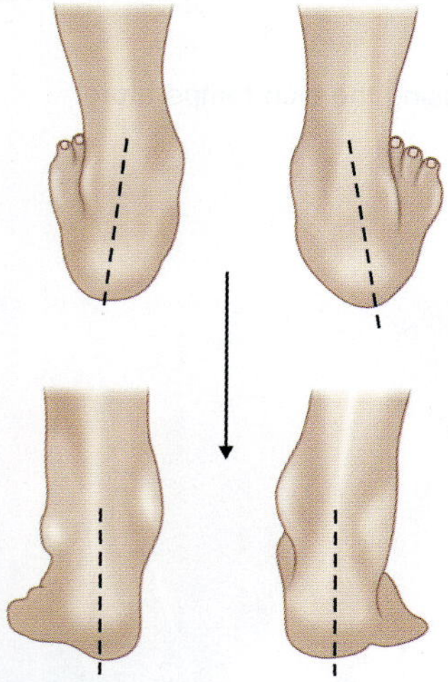

Fig. 26.88: Observing the heel by looking at its position on weight-bearing

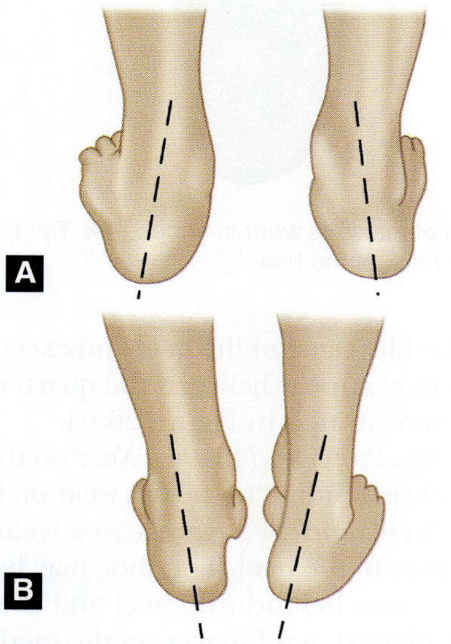

Figs 26.87A and B: (A) Valgus heels are associated with pes planus (B) Varus heels with pes cavus

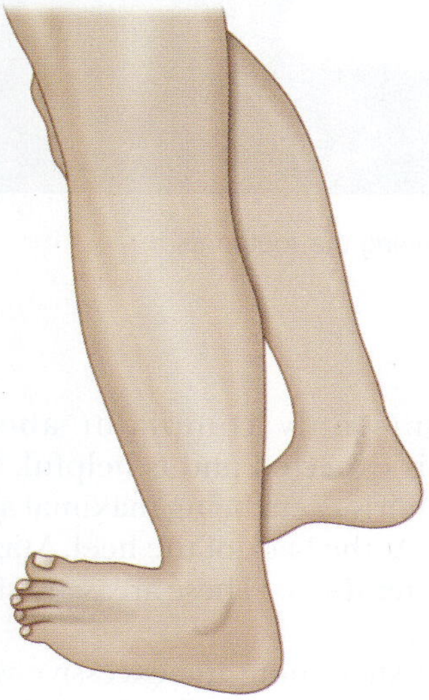

Fig. 26.89: Examining patient's gait

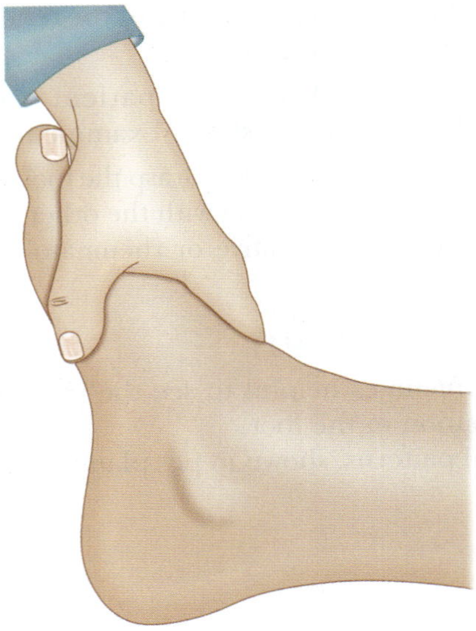

Fig. 26.90: Assessing the skin temperature

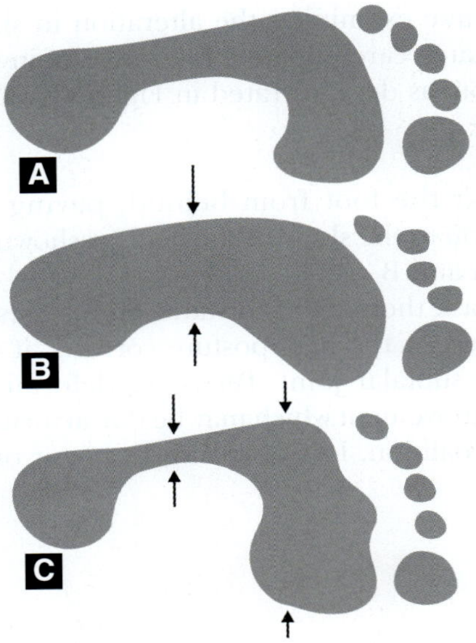

Figs 26.92A to C: (A) Normal foot; (B) Pes planus. Note the increase in area of the central part of the sole taking part in weight bearing; (C) Pes cavus. Note the decrease in area of contact in the midsole and splaying of the anterior part of the foot

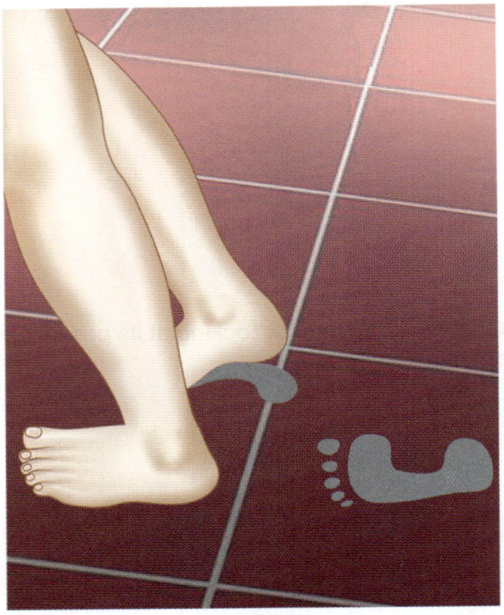

Fig. 26.91: Examining the footprints

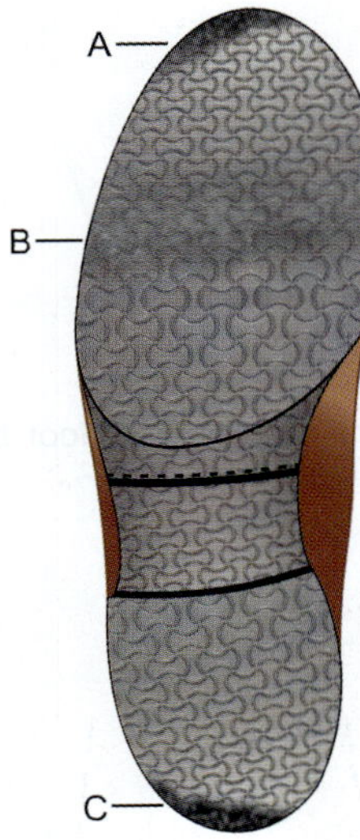

Fig. 26.93: Areas of maximal wear in shoes— A. Tip; B. Tread; C. At the back of the heel

Shoes

- The patients only complaint about footwear. Inspection is expected and is helpful. In the normal sole wear is fairly even, being maximal across the tread and the tip. At the back of the heel. Maximum wear is also to the lateral side. These areas are shown in Figure 26.93.
- In too short shoe, note the excessive wear at the toe and heel. A gap may appear above the sole. The toe cap may bulge and the inside of the shoe may be marked by the toes. The heel may give at the seam. There may be blistering of the heel and excessive sock wear. A gap may appear between the quarter and the ankle, as demonstrated in Figure 26.94.
- *Pes planus (Figs 26.95 and 26.96):* Wear on the medial side of the sole extending to the tip, wear on the outer side of the heel and in severe cases wear on the diagonal corner of the heel. The shoe may be twisted, when viewed from behind (the heel and the sole are on different planes), scuff marks on the medical side, the upper bulges over the sole on the medial side and the quarter bulges away from the foot.

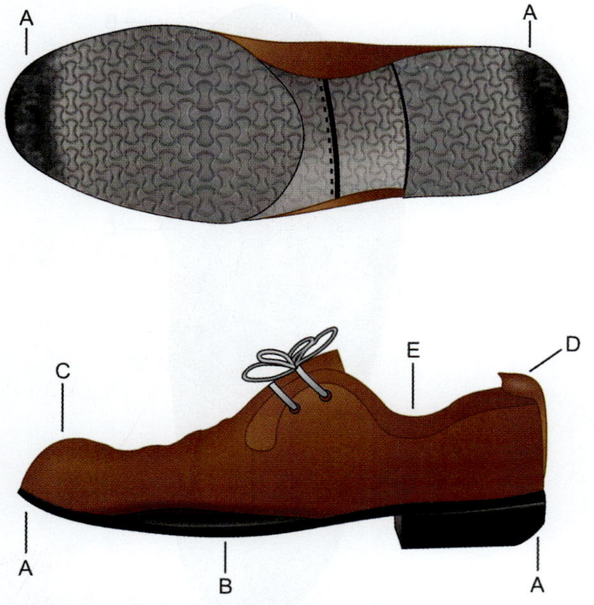

Fig. 26.94: Shoes areas which undergo wear—A. The excessive wear at the toe and heel; B. A gap may appear above the sole; C. The toe cap may bulge and the inside of the shoe may be marked by the toes; D. The heel may give at the seam. There may be blistering of the heel and excessive sock wear; E. A gap may appear between the quarter and the ankle

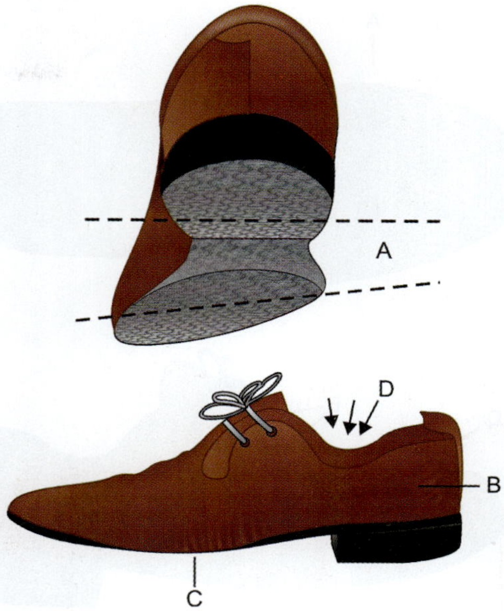

Fig. 26.96: Twisting and bulging of shoes in pes planus—A. The shoe may be twisted when viewed from behind (the heel and the sole are on different planes); B. Scuff marks on the medical side; C. The upper bulges over the sole on the medial side; D. The quarter bulges away from the foot

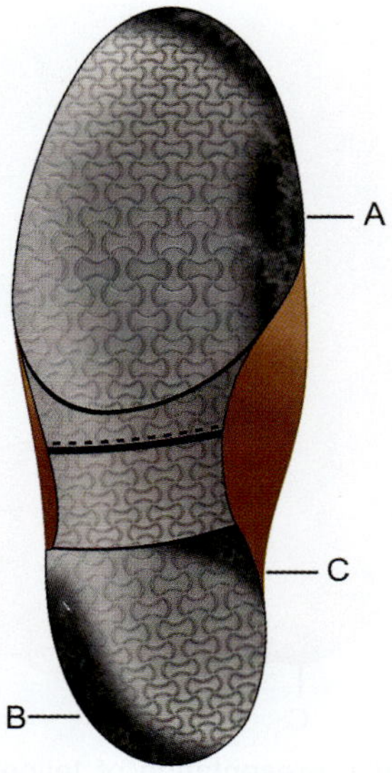

Fig. 26.95: Wearing pattern of shoes sole in pes planus—A. Wear on the medial side of the sole extending to the tip; B. Wear on the outer side of the heel; C. In severe cases wear on the diagonal corner of the heel

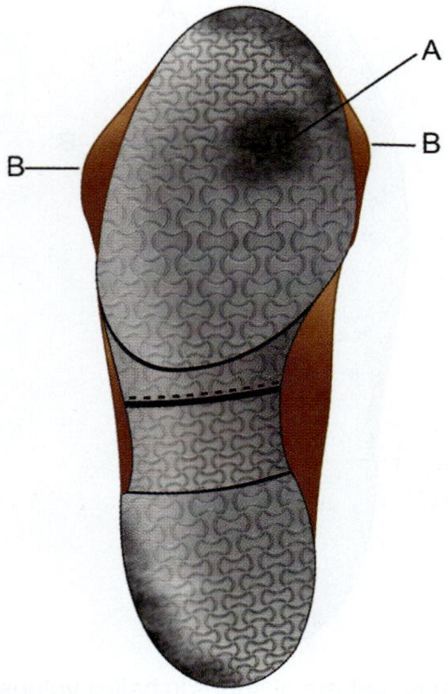

Fig. 26.97: Shoe wearing pattern in splay foot—A. Excess wear on region of the first and second metatarsal; B. The upper bulges over the sole anteriorly

- *Splay foot (Fig. 26.97):* Excess wear on region of the first and second metatarsal. There is an upper bulges over the sole anteriorly.
- *Pes cavus (Fig. 26.98):* Excessive wear under the metatarsal head region, excessive wear at the back of the heel, raising of toes, creases and giving way of lacings.
- *Hallux valgus (Fig. 26.99):* There is often excessive wear as in splay foot of the first and second metatarsal heads

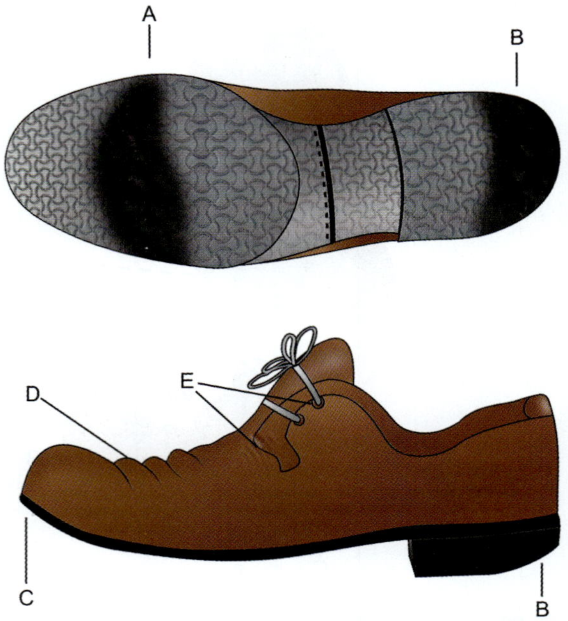

Fig. 26.98: Wearing shoe pattern in pes cavus— A. Excessive wear under the metatarsal head region; B. Excessive wear at the back of the heel; C. Raising of toes; D. Creases; E. Giving way of lacings

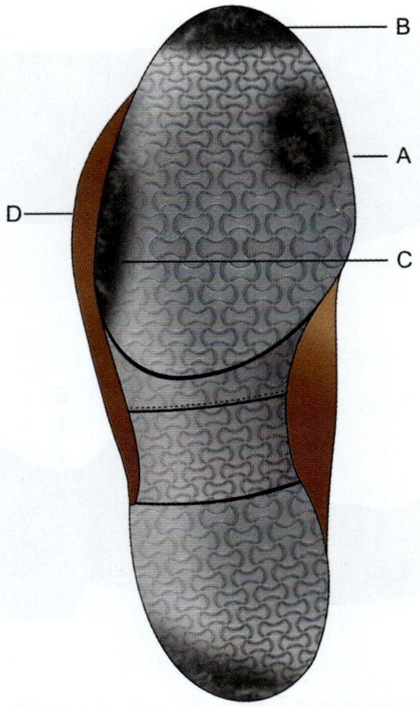

Fig. 26.100: Shoe wearing pattern in hallux rigidus—A. Excessive wear under the first metatarsal head; B. At the tip of the sole; C. Excessive wear on the lateral side (walking on the side of the foot); D. Lateral overhang and the toe of the shoe may be upturned

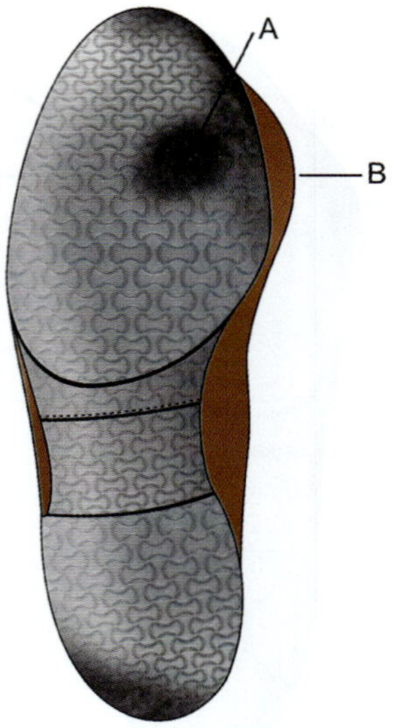

Fig. 26.99: Wearing pattern of shoes in hallux valgus—A. Excessive wear, as in splay foot of the first and second metatarsal heads; B. Bulging of the upper, to accommodate the prominent first metatarsal head

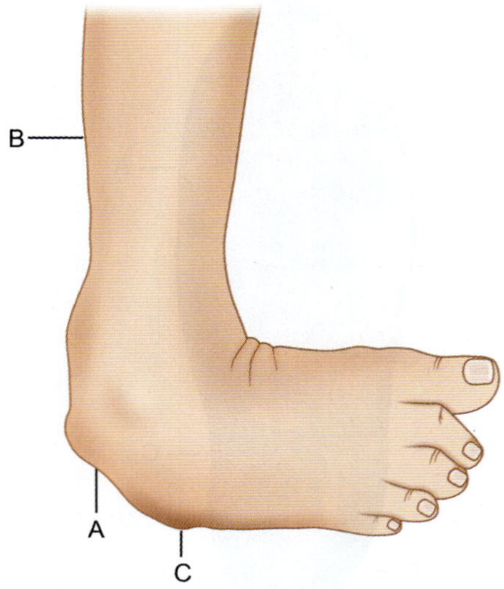

Fig. 26.101: Typical presentation of talipes equinovarus—A. Persisting varus of the heel; B. Atrophy of the calf muscles; C. Callus, where the child walks on the lateral border of the foot

and bulging of the upper to accommodate the prominent first metatarsal head.

Hallux rigidus (Fig. 26.100): Excessive wear under the first metatarsal head and at the tip of the sole, excessive wear on the lateral side (walking on the side of the foot), lateral overhang. The toe of the shoe may be upturned.

Club Foot

- *Talipes equinovarus (Fig. 26.101):* In the untreated case there is persisting varus of the heel atrophy of the calf muscles, callus where the child walks on the lateral border of the foot.

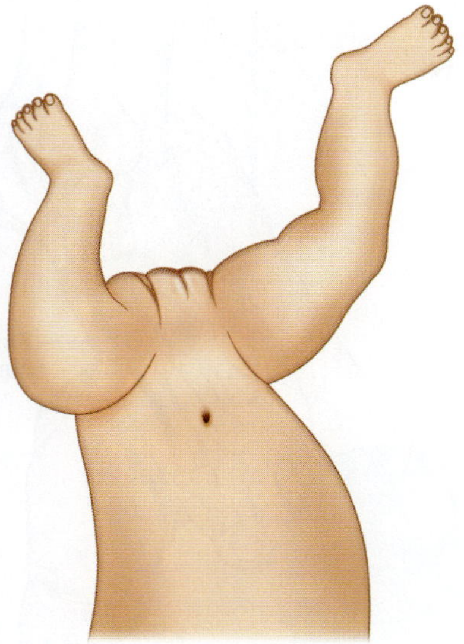

Fig. 26.102: Observing the deformity when child kicks confirm the equinovarus deformity

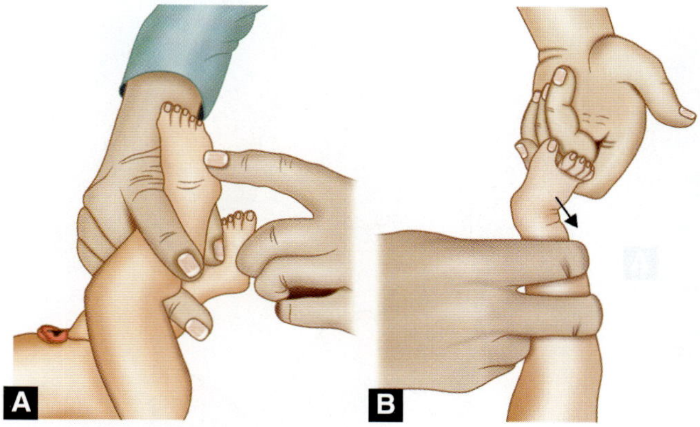

Figs 26.103A and B: (A) Examining the child with the foot in the inverted position, by lightly scratching the side of the foot; (B) The normal foot the child will respond by dorsiflexion of the foot, eversion and fanning of the toes, while such reactions are absent in case of deformity

- The newborn child often holds the foot in plantar flexion and inversion, giving a false impression of deformity. Observe the child as it kicks to see, if the deformity is maintained, as shown in Figure 26.102.
- If the child maintains the foot in the inverted position, support the leg and lightly scratch the side of the foot. In the normal foot the child will respond by dorsiflexion of the foot, eversion and fanning of the toes. This reaction does not take place in the presence of the deformity, as demonstrated in Figures 26.103A and B.
- If the child does not respond in a normal fashion, gently dorsiflex the foot. In the normal child, the foot can be brought either into contact with the tibia or very close to it. This is illustrated in Figure 26.104.
- In the less common talipes deformity, the foot is held in a position of dorsiflexion. In the normal infant the foot can be plantarflexed to such a degree that the foot and tibia are in line, as illustrated in Figures 26.105A and B.

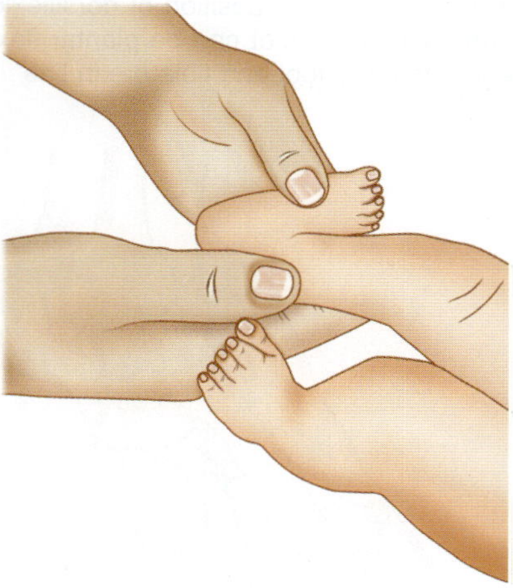

Fig. 26.104: Examining the foot equinovarus in a child by gently dorsiflex the foot. In the normal child, the foot can be brought either into contact with the tibia or very close to it, which is absent in child with the deformity

■ Palpation

Bony Palpation

Medial Aspect

Have the patient sit on the edge of the examining table with his feet dangling free. Stabilize the foot and lower leg with one hand holding the foot around the calcaneus. Head of the first metatarsal bone and the metatarsophalangeal joint, as shown in Figure 26.106. They are palpable at the ball of the foot. Note any bony excrescence. The joint is most frequently involved in gout and bunions. Probe proximally, along the medial shaft of the first metatarsal bone.

First metatarsocuneiform: The metatarsal flares light at the base and meets the first cuneiform bone. It articulates with the base of the first metatarsal in a simple joint providing gliding movement, as illustrated in Figure 26.107.

Navicular tubercle: Continue moving proximally along the medial border of the foot. The next bony prominence encountered is the tubercle. It articulates proximally with

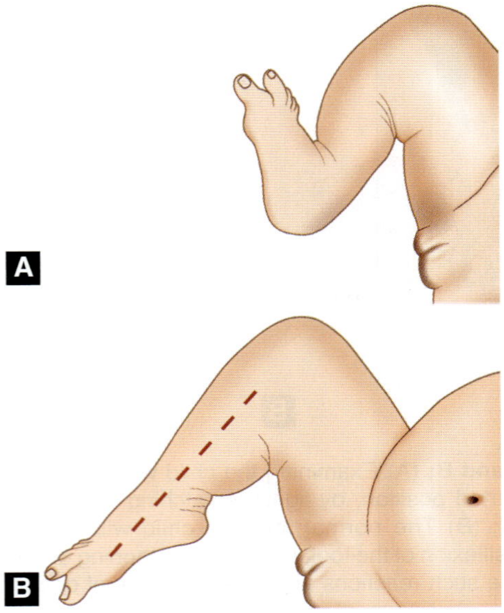

Figs 26.105A and B: Talipes equinovarus with the foot held in dorsiflexion— (A) In the less common talipes deformity, the foot is held in a position of dorsiflexion; (B) In the normal infant the foot can be plantar flexed to such a degree that the foot and tibia are in line

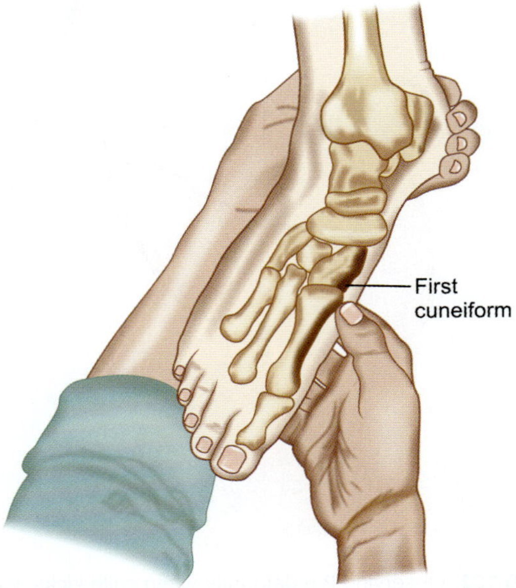

Fig. 26.107: Palpating metatarsocuneiform

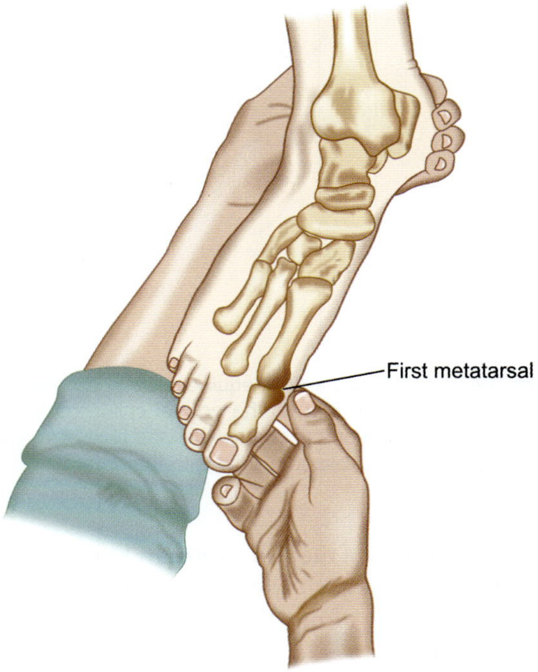

Fig. 26.106: Palpating medial aspect of the foot and first metatarsal joint

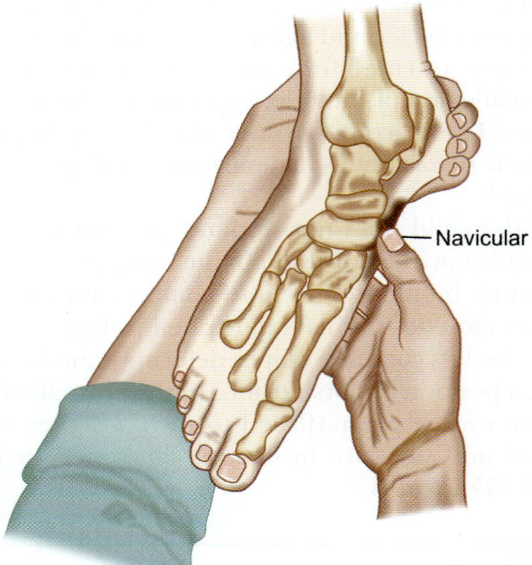

Fig. 26.108: Palpating navicular tubercle on medial side of the foot

the talar head, distally with the three cuneiforms and laterally with the cuboid, as shown in Figure 26.108.

Head of the talus: It is present immediately proximal to the the navicular and can be easily palpable during eversion and inversion of the foot. The resultant motion between the talus and navicular is palpable. Eversion causes the head of the talus to become more prominent. This is illustrated in Figure 26.109.

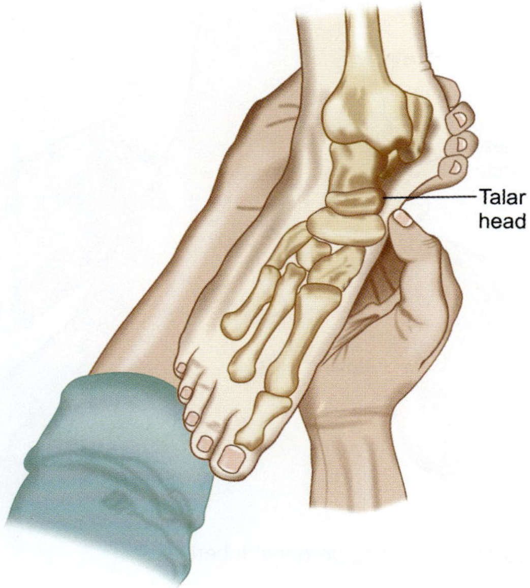

Fig. 26.109: Palpating head of talus

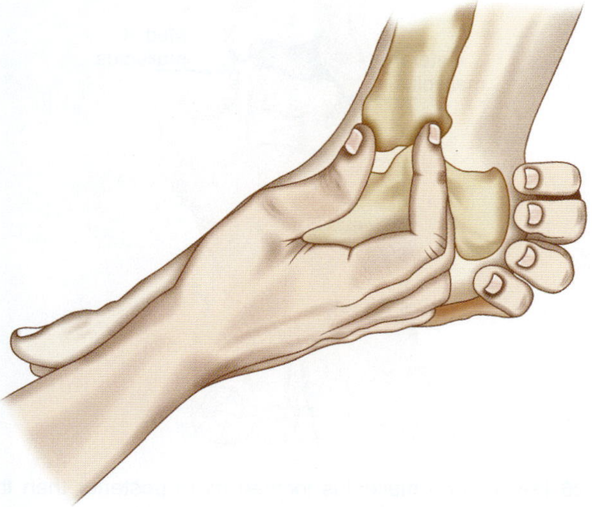

Fig. 26.110: Palpating medial malleolus

Medial malleolus: From the head of the talus, probe proximally. The malleolus embraces the medial talus adding bony stability, as shown in Figure 26.110.

Sustentaculum tali: Move plantarwards one finger breath from the distal end of the malleolus. It is small and may not be palpable at all. It helps in supporting the talus and server as an attachment of the spring ligaments, as illustrated in Figure 26.111.

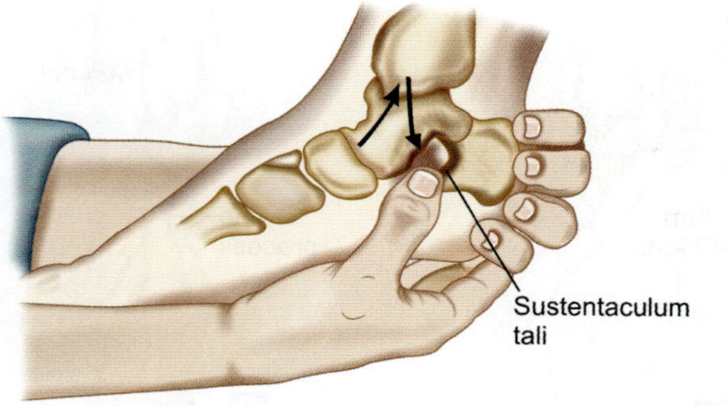

Fig. 26.111: Palpating sustentaculum tali

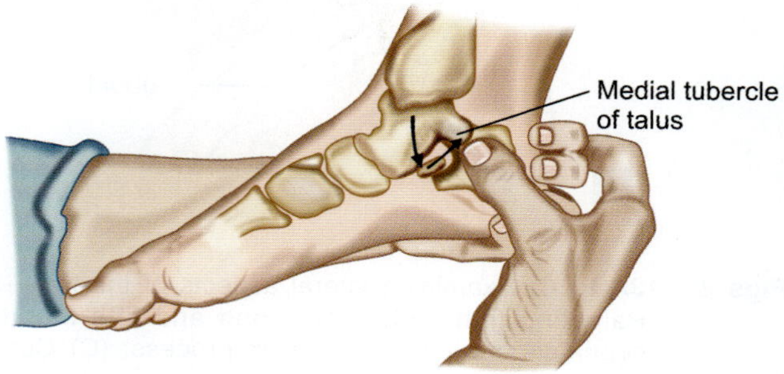

Fig. 26.112: Palpating the medial tubercle of the talus

Medial tubercle of the talus: It is small and is barely palpable. It lies immediately posterior to the distal end of the medial malleolus. It is the point of insertion of the medial collateral ligament, as depicted in Figure 26.112.

Lateral Aspect

Fifth metatarsal bone and fifth metatarsophalangeal joint, situated at the lateral side of the ball of the foot. Probe proximally, along the shaft to its flared base, the styloid process. Directly behind the flare is a depression, which is further, accentuated by the groove of the cuboid, created by the peroneus longus muscle tendon, as shown in Figures 26.113A to C.

Calcaneus: Move proximally along the foots lateral borde. It is subcutaneous and easily palpable, as shown in Figure 26.114.

Peroneal tubercle: It lies on the calcaneus, distal to the lateral malleolus. It is a significant landmark, as it separates the peroneus brevis and the longus tendons, as shown in Figure 26.115.

Lateral malleolus: Located at the distal end of the fibula, more posterior then the medial malleolus, as shown in Figure 26.116. If the thumb is placed on the most anterior portion of the lateral malleolus and the foot is plantar flexed, the anterolateral dome of the talus becomes

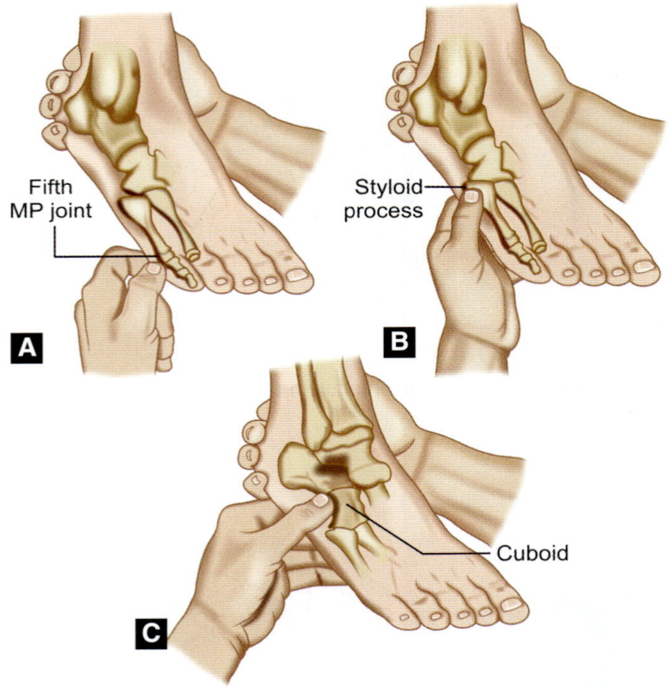

Figs 26.113A to C: Examining lateral aspects of the foot—(A) Palpating fifth metatarsal bone and fifth metatarsophalangeal joint; (B) Styloid process; (C) Cuboid groove

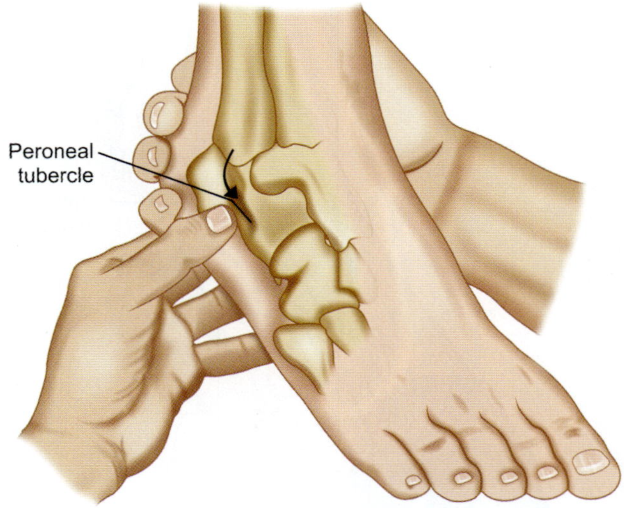

Fig. 26.115: Palpating peroneal tubercle

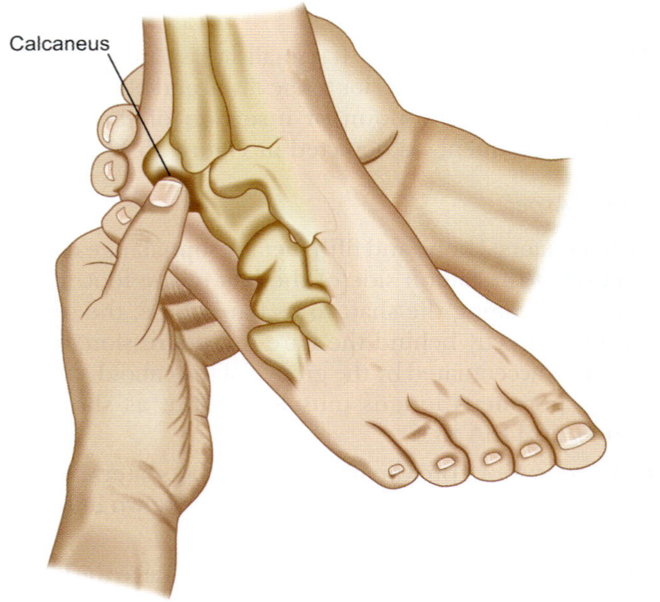

Fig. 26.114: Palpating calcaneus on lateral aspect of the foot

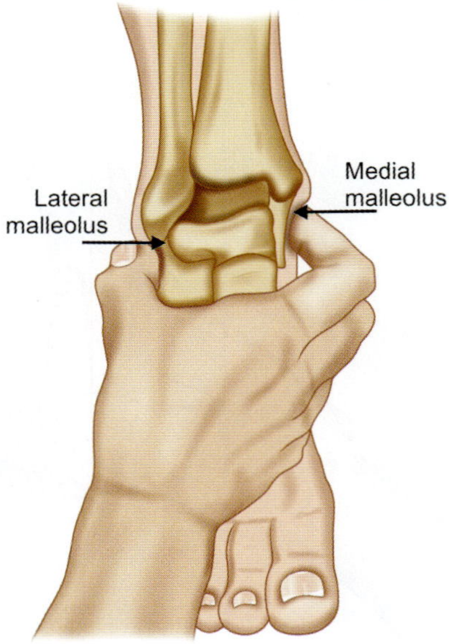

Fig. 26.116: Lateral malleolus located more posterior than the medial malleolus

palpable, as it rotates out from under the ankle mortise, as shown in Figure 26.117.

Dome of the talus (Fig. 26.118): The foot is kept in inversion and plantar flexion. A small portion of the dome becomes palpable. A greater portion is palpable on the lateral side than on the medial.

Inferior tibiofibular joint: It lies immediately proximal to the talus. Since, the anteroinferior tibiofibular ligament overlies this joint, clear palpation is impossible, the bones of the joint may be separate following ankle injury (diastasis), as depicted in Figure 26.119.

Sinus tarsi area: Stabilize the foot at the calcaneus with one hand and place the thumb of the free hand into the soft tissue depression just anterior to the lateral malleolus. This depression lies directly over the sinus tarsi, which is filled by the extensor digitorum brevis muscle and overlying pad of fat. If the foot is inverted, the lateral

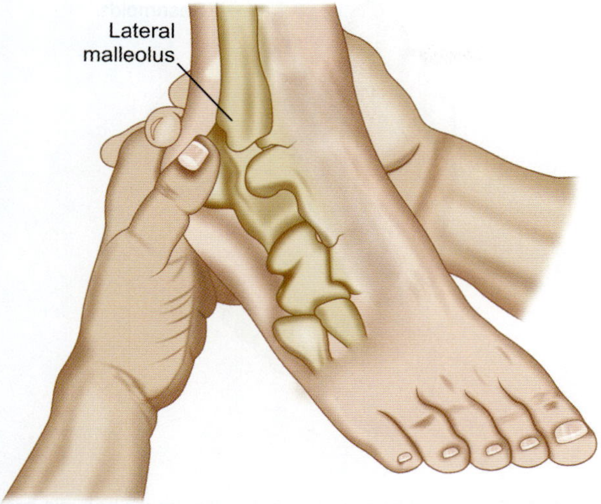

Fig. 26.117: Palpating lateral malleolus on lateral aspect of the foot

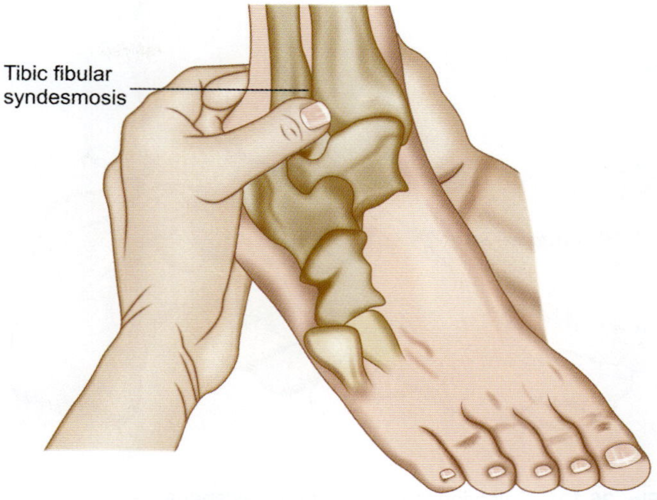

Fig. 26.119: Palpating the inferior tibiofibular joint

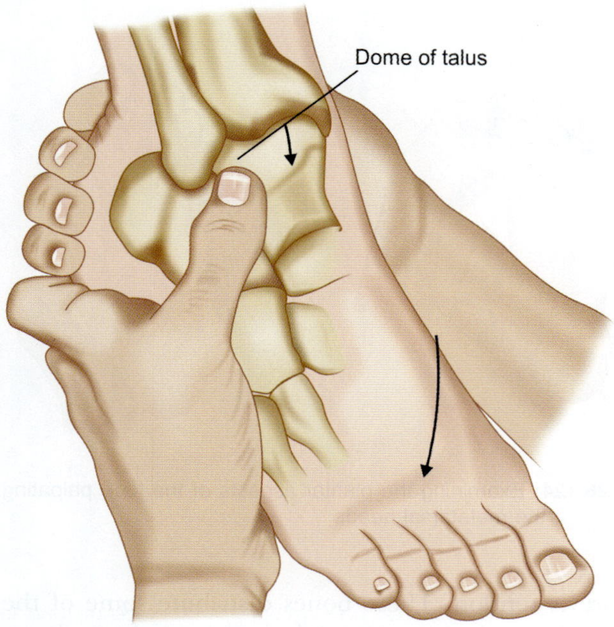

Fig. 26.118: Palpating the dome of talus

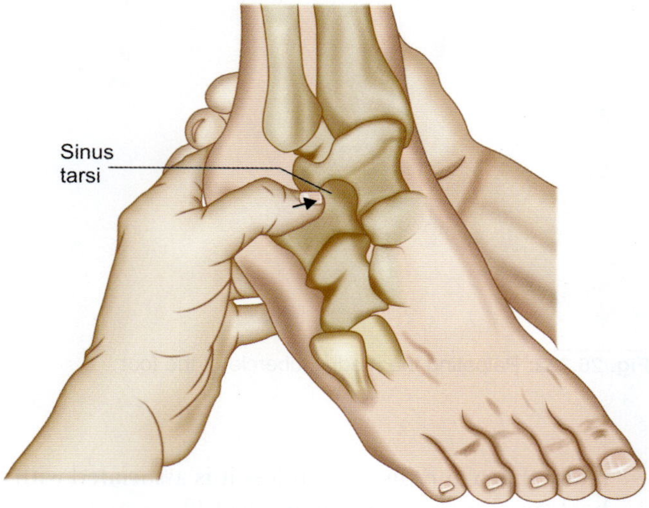

Fig. 26.120: Palpating sinus tarsi area

side of the talar neck may be palpable through the soft tissues. It is through this area that subtalar arthrodesis is performed, as illustrated in Figure 26.120.

Area of the Hindfoot

- Have the patient relax the foot. Place your thumb and finger in the soft tissue depression on either side, to the Achilles tendon.
- *Dome of the calcaneus:* The bare posterior third of the dome protrudes from behind the ankle joint. Plantarward the bone flares at it base. This flare may become excessive following a compression fracture of the posterior third of the osclacis, as shown in Figure 26.121.
- *Medial tubercle:* It lies in the medial planter surface of the calcaneus. It is broad and large and gives attachment to the abductor hallucis muscle medial and the flexor digitorum brevis muscle and the plantar aponeurosis anteriorly. The medial tubercle is weight bearing, whereas the lateral tubercle is not. It is not

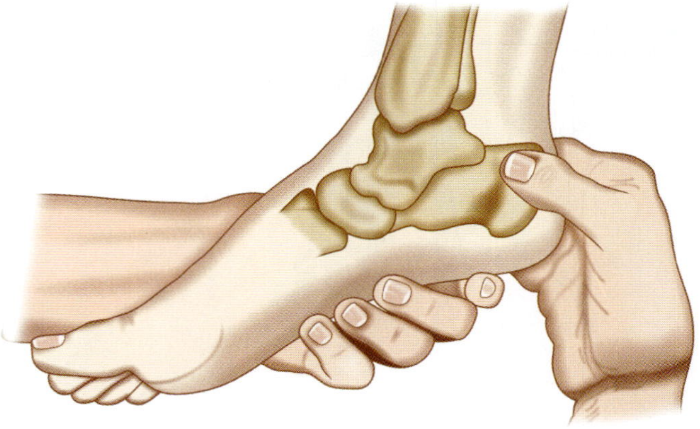

Fig. 26.121: Palpating the dome of the calcaneus

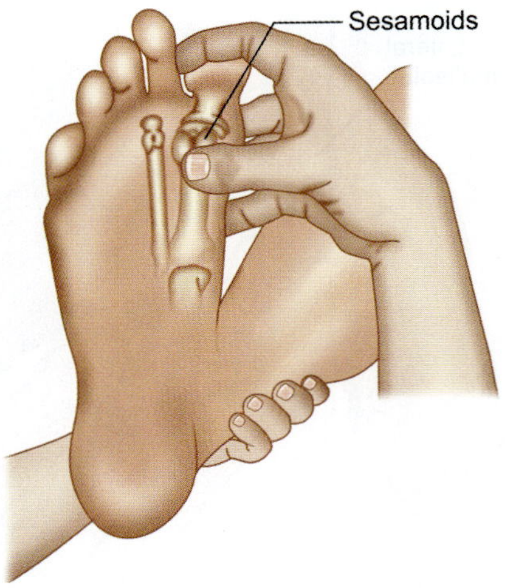

Fig. 26.123: Sesamoid bones, present in the flexor hallucis brevis tendon

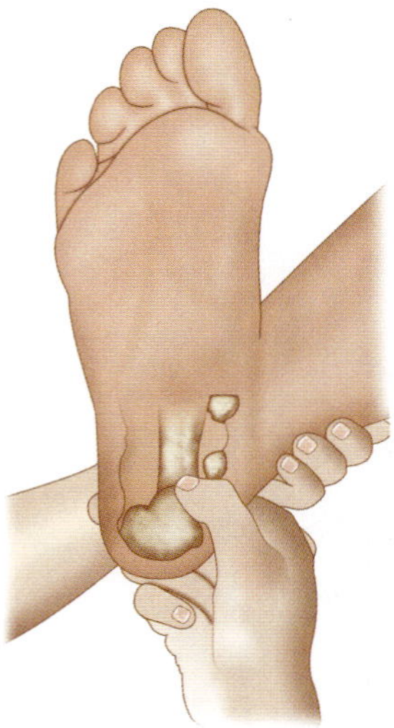

Fig. 26.122: Palpating the medial tubercle of the foot

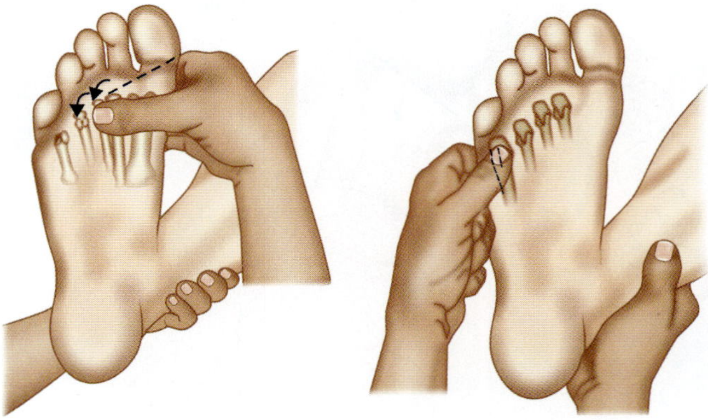

Fig. 26.124: Examining the plantar aspects of the foot, palpating the metatarsal heads

really sharp and distinct, unless it is associated with a heel spur, as shown in Figure 26.122.

Plantar Surface

- Examination is difficult due to the overlying fascial bands, the pad of fat and large callosities. Have the patient extend his leg with the sole of the foot facing you, stabilize the lower limb by holding the leg posterior to the ankle joint.
- *Sesamoid bone:* From the medial tubercle of the calcaneus, palpate distally along the medial longitudinal arch past the base of the first metatarsal bone to the first metatarsophalangeal joint. Pressing firmly on the first metatarsal, the two small sesamoid bones can be felt that lie within the flexor hallucis brevis tendon. These bones distribute some of the weight bearing pressure of the body's weight, as shown in Figure 26.123.
- *Metatarsal heads (Fig. 26.124):* Move laterally and palpate each metatarsal heads by placing the thumb over the plantar surface and the index finger over the dorsal aspect. Determine, if any one is disproportionately prominent. If one is, it must bear an unaccustomed weight amount of weight and is subject to a variety of problem.

Soft Tissue Palpation

Lateral Ligament

- *Complete tear:* Swelling is rapid and if seen within two hours of injury is egg shaped and placed over the

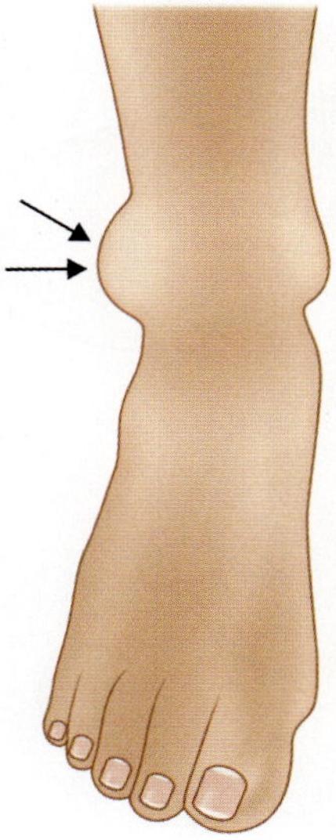

Fig. 26.125: Swelling due to tear of lateral ligament

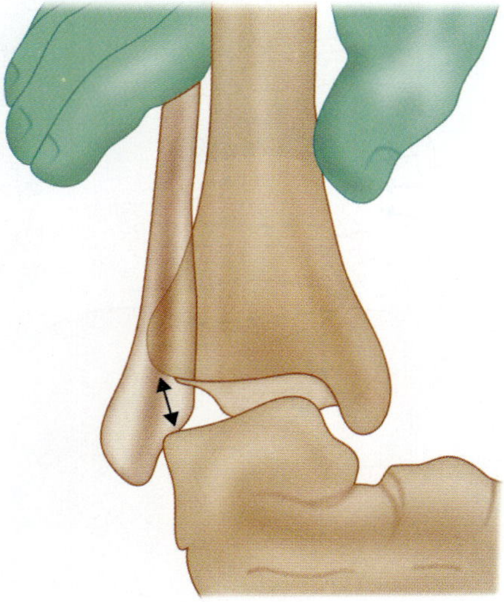

Fig. 26.127: On X-ray, if tilting of the talus in the ankle mortise is demonstrated, repeat the examination on the other side and compare

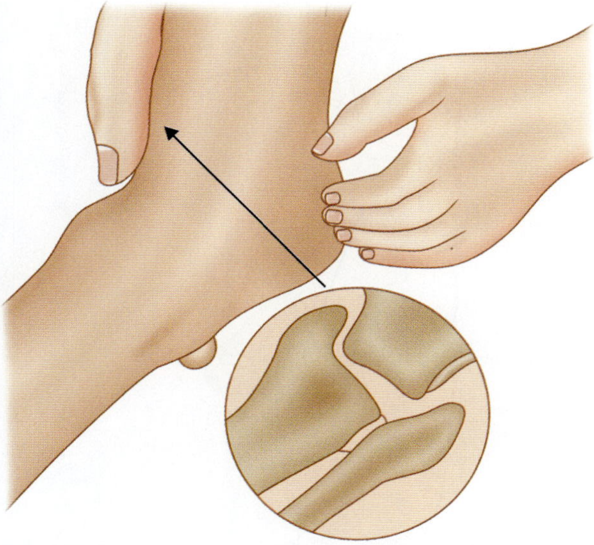

Fig. 26.126: Opening up of lateral side of the ankle between tibia and the talus on forcibly inverting the foot

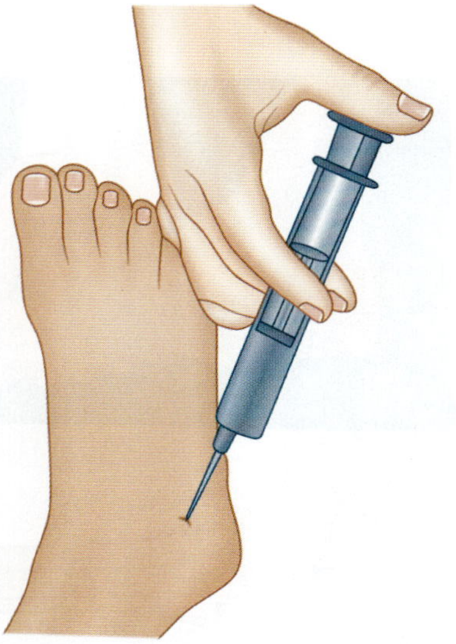

Fig. 26.128: Injection of a local anesthetic, widely in the region of the lateral ligament

lateral malleolus (McKenzie's sign), as shown in Figure 26.125.

- Stress testing:
  - Grasp the heel and forcibly invert the foot, feeling for any opening up of the lateral side of the ankle between the tibia and the talus, as shown in Figure 26.126.
  - On X-ray, if tilting of the talus in the ankle mortise is demonstrated, repeat the examination on the other side and compare, as demonstrated in Figure 26.127.
  - If the injury is fresh and painful, examination may be more readily permitted with the injection of a local anesthetic widely in the region of the lateral ligament, as shown in Figure 26.128.
  - Testing the anterior talofibular component, with the patient prone, press downwards on the heel, looking for anterior displacement of the talus, which is often accompanied by dimpling of the skin on either side. This is illustrated in Figure 26.129.
  - Stress testing for anterior tibiofibular ligament (Fig. 26.130).

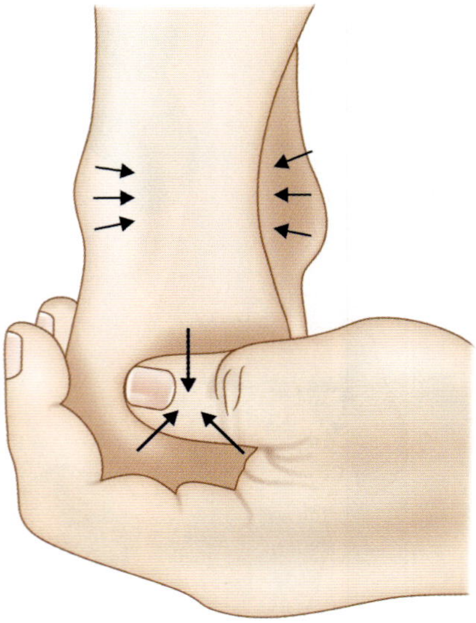

Fig. 26.129: Testing the anterior talofibular component, with the patient prone, press downwards on the heel, looking for anterior displacement of the talus, which is often accompanied by dimpling of the skin on either side

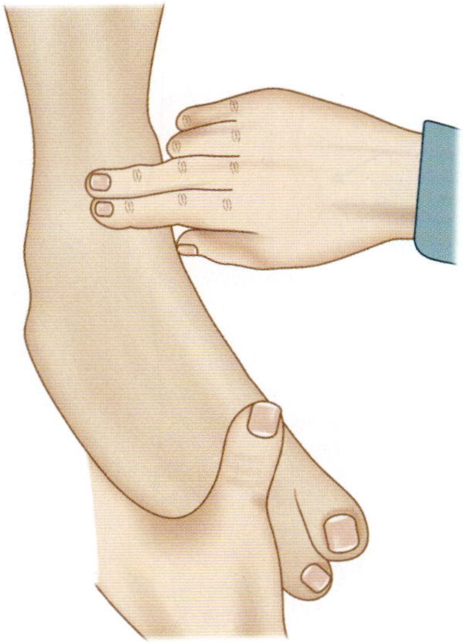

Fig. 26.131: Tenderness over the ankle joint line in case of inferior tibiofibular ligament

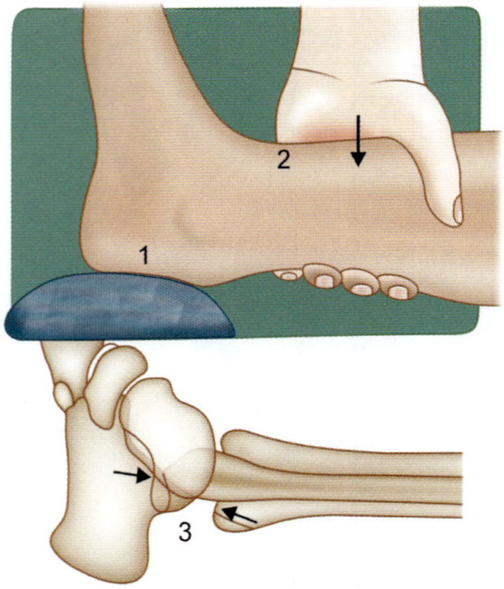

Fig. 26.130: Stress testing for anterior tibiofibular ligament and anterior displacement—1. Radiographs taken in the prone position, alternatively with the patient supine, support the heel on a sand bag; 2. Press firmly down on the tibia for 30° a gap on the X-ray between the talus; 3. The tibia of more than 6 mm is regarded pathological

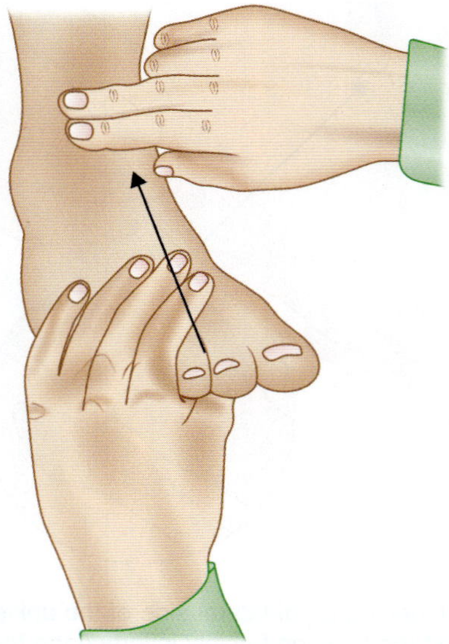

Fig. 26.132: Inferior tibiofibular ligament pain on dorsiflexion due to tear

Inferior Tibiofibular Ligament

- In tears of this component, tenderness is present over the ligament just above the line of the ankle joint, as shown in Figure 26.131.
- Ligament pain is produced by dorsiflexion of the foot, which displaces the fibula laterally, as shown in Figure 26.132.
- Grasp the heel and try to move the talus directly laterally in the ankle mortise. Lateral displacement indicates a tear in the ligament, as illustrated in Figure 26.133.

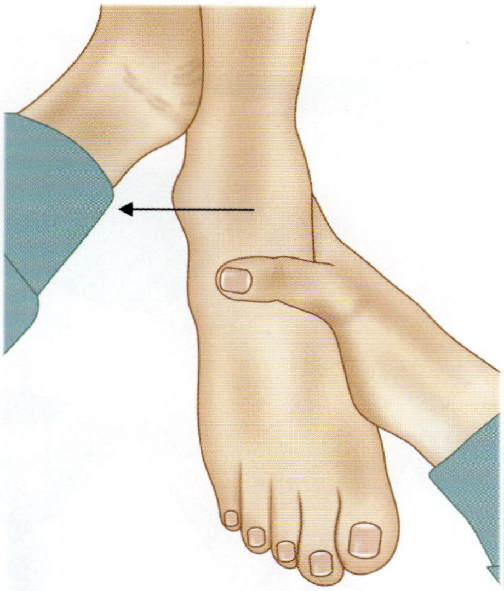

Fig. 26.133: On moving the talus directly laterally in the ankle mortise, if causes lateral displacement, indicates a tear in the ligament

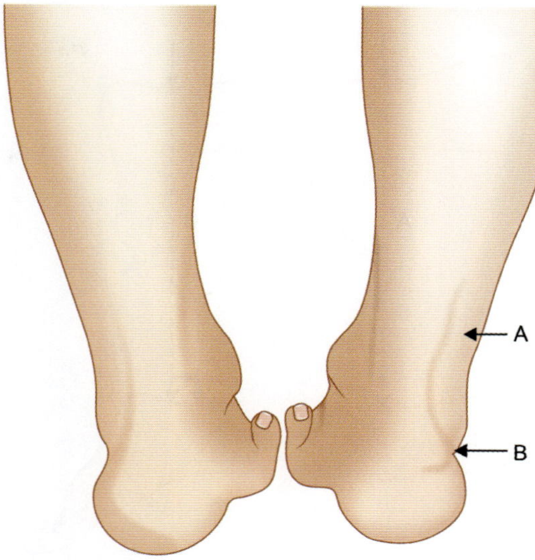

Fig. 26.135: Palpating achilles tendon—A. Diffuse swelling, redness of the skin or Hagland deformity; B. This is a bony exostosis, affecting the posterosuperior aspect of the heel on its lateral side

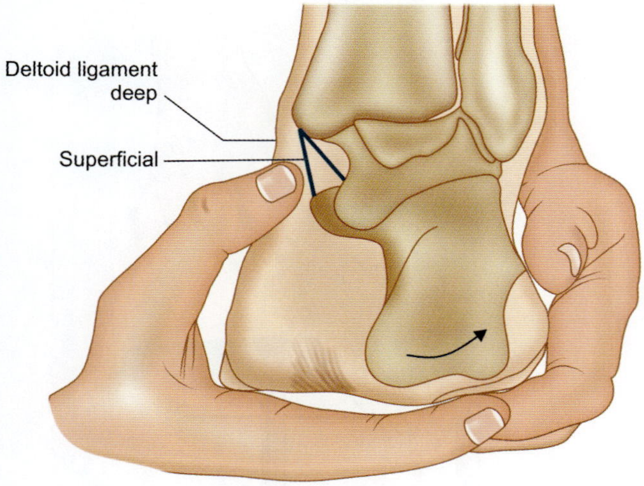

Fig. 26.134: Palpating deltoid ligament

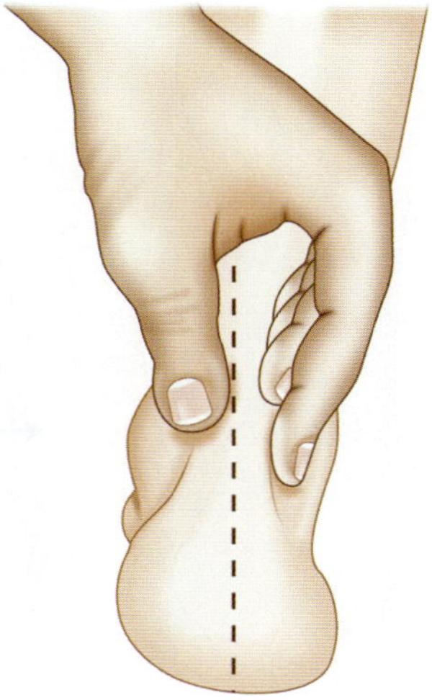

Fig. 26.136: Marked pain on squeezing the tendon indicates tendinosis

Deltoid Ligament (Fig. 26.134)

Is palpable just beneath the medial malleolus and is not easily palpable. Pain elicited during its palpation, may indicate a tear from an eversion ankle sprain.

Tendocalcaneus (Achilles Tendon)

- *Suspected tendinopathy:* The patient should be prone with the feet over the edge of the couch. Inspect and compare sides note any local diffuse swelling, redness of the skin or Hagland deformity, this is a bony exostosis, affecting the posterosuperior aspect of the heel on its lateral side, as shown in Figure 26.135.

Look for tenderness, normally situated 3 to 5 cm proximal to the tendon insertion. Check of any localized increase in temperature. Palpate the tendon, noticing any localized swelling and nodularity. Gently squeeze the tendon. Marked pain is a feature of tendinosis, as illustrated in Figure 26.136. If tenderness is found, note whether is changes with dorsiflexion and plantar flexion of the foot. Pain secondary to paratendinitis, the site of maximum pain will remain fixed. If due to tendinitis alone, it will move with the tendon (Fig. 26.137).

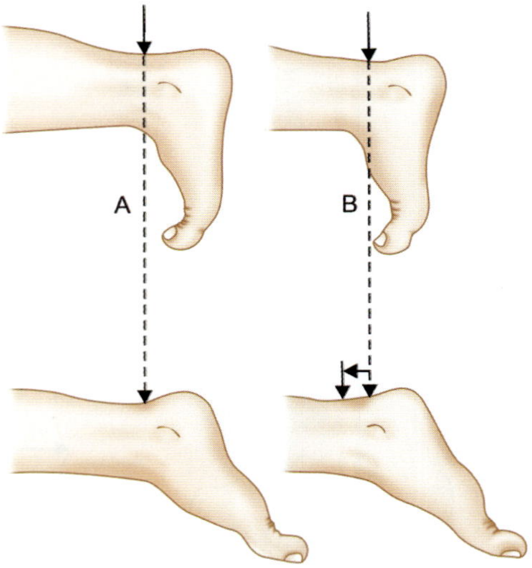

Fig. 26.137: Pain on foot movements, used to differentiate between pain due to paratendinitis and tendinitis—A. Pain secondary to paratendinitis the site of maximum pain will remain fixed; B. If due to tendinitis alone it will move with the tendon

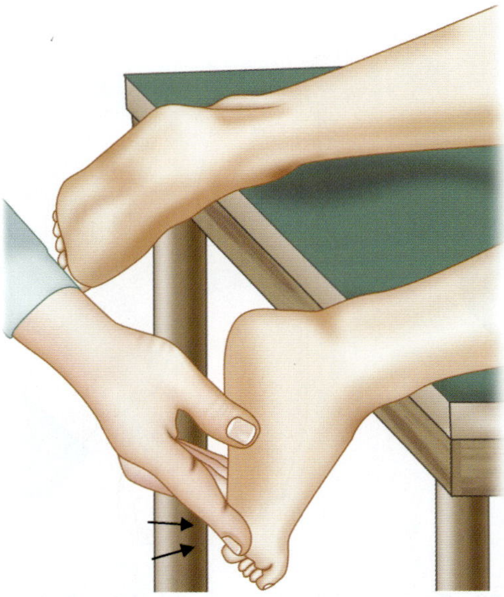

Fig. 26.139: Compairing plantar flexion of foot for both sides

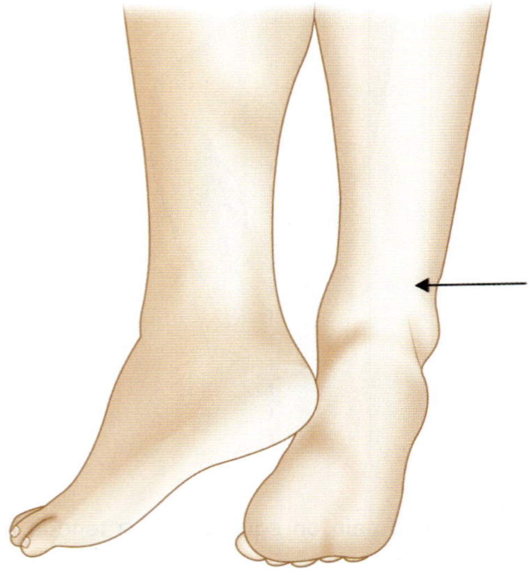

Fig. 26.138: Arrow showing deformed tendoachilles due to rupture

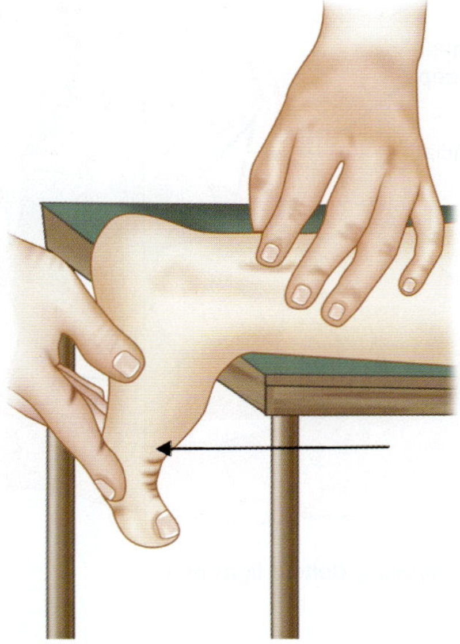

Fig. 26.140: Gap in the tendon on resisted plantar flexion due to tendon rupture

- *Suspected tendon rupture*
  - The patient should be examined with the feet over the end of the couch. Defects in the contour of the tendon may be obvious, as shown in Figure 26.138.
  - Test the power of plantar flexion, by asking the patient to press the foot against your hand, compare one side with the other and note the shape of each contracting calf and the shape of the tendon, as illustrated in Figure 26.139.
  - Palpate the tendon, while the patient continues resistance against plantar flexion. Any gap in the tendon should be obvious, as shown in Figure 26.140.
  - *Thompson test (Fig. 26.141):* Normally, when the calf is squeezed the foot moves as the ankle plantar-flexes. Loss of this movement is pathognomic of acute rupture.

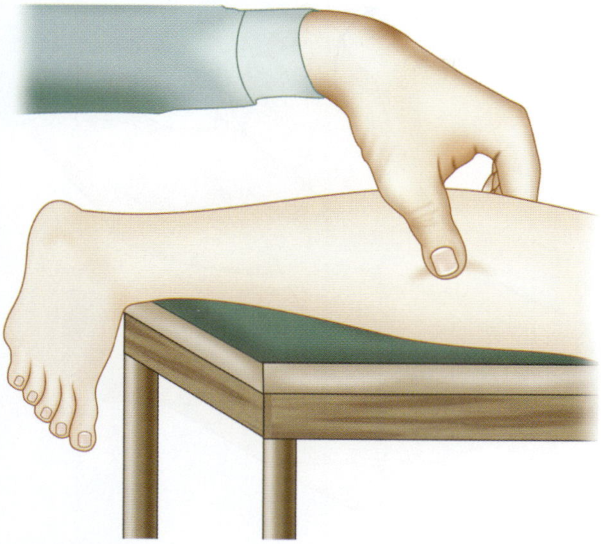

Fig. 26.141: Thompson test

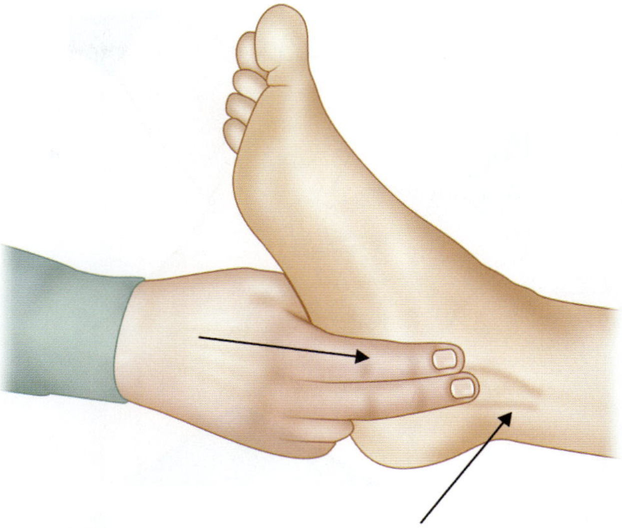

Fig. 26.143: Looking for presence of synovitis in relation to flexor tendons (arrow)

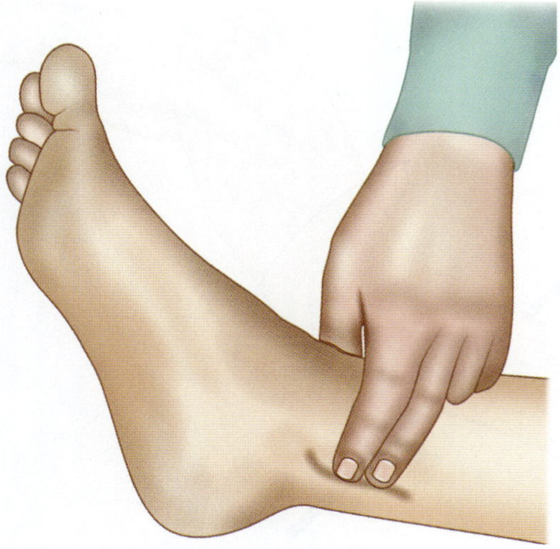

Fig. 26.142: Palpating long extensor tendons for pain

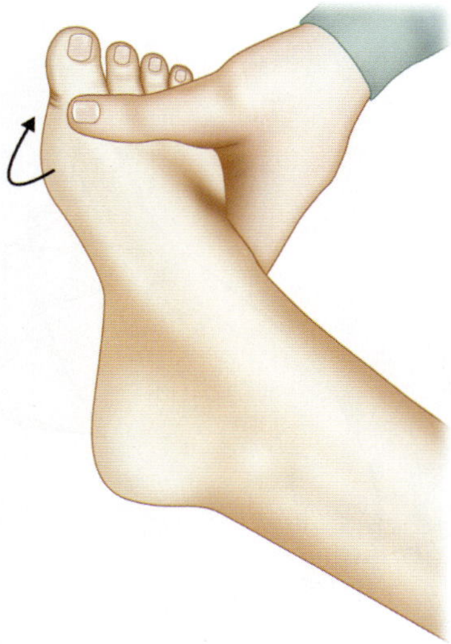

Fig. 26.144: Pain on plantar flexing and everting foot due to tenosynovitis of tibialis posterior tendon

Tenosynovitis

Medial

- Look for tenderness along the line of the long extensor tendons. Tenderness is usually diffuse and linear in pattern, as demonstrated in Figure 26.142.
- Look for synovitis in relation to the flexor tendons. Demonstrate the presence of any excess fluid, by milking the sheaths in a proximal direction, as shown in Figure 26.143.
- Plantar flex and evert the foot. This may produce pain, where tenosynovitis involves the tibialis posterior tendon, as illustrated in Figure 26.144.
- With the foot held in plantar flexion and eversion, look for tenderness or gaps in the line of the tibialis posterior tendon. Spontaneous rupture is seen most frequently in flat foot and rheumatoid arthritis, as demonstrated in Figure 26.145.

Lateral (Figs 26.146 to 26.148)

- Examine the peroneal tendons for tenderness and excess synovial fluid in their sheaths.
- Force the foot into plantar flexion and inversion. This will give rise to pain and increased tenderness along the line of the peroneal tendons, if tenosynovitis is present.

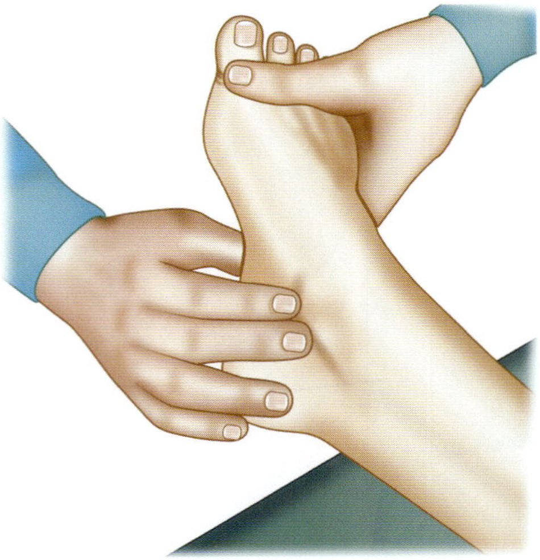

Fig. 26.145: Palpating tibialis posterior tendon on plantar flexing and everting the foot

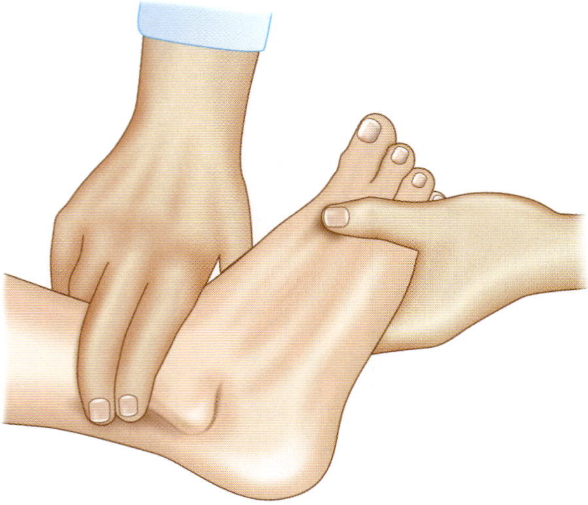

Fig. 26.146: Examining the peroneal tendons for tenderness and excess synovial fluid in their sheaths

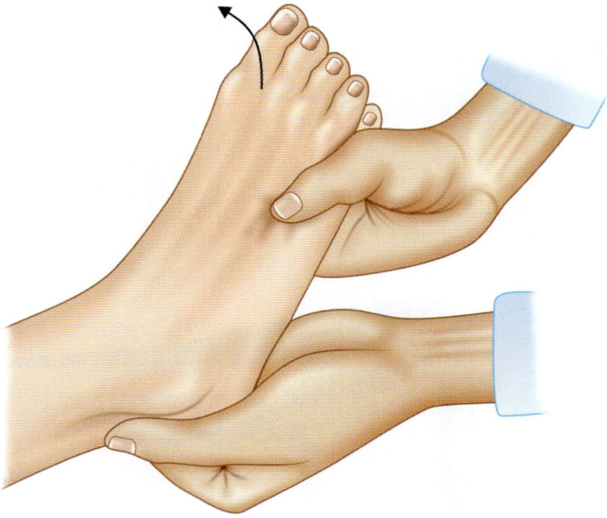

Fig. 26.147: Pain on plantar flexing and inverting the foot in case of tenosynovitis of peroneal tendons

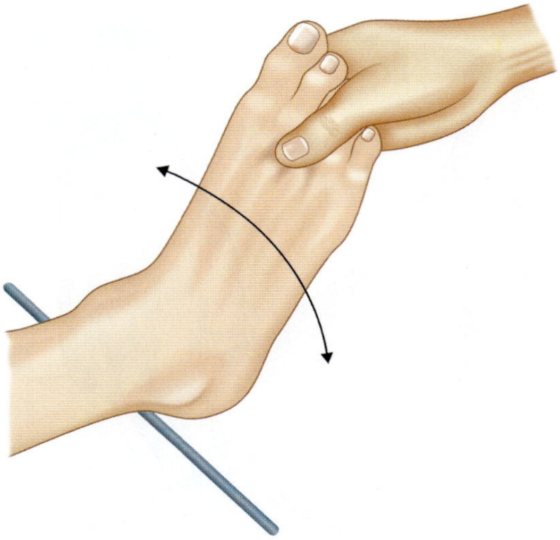

Fig. 26.148: Swinging foot backwards and forwards to feel any crepitation

- Feel for crepitus along the line of the tendon sheaths behind both the malleoli, as the foot is swung backwards and forwards between inversion and eversion. Confirm by auscultation.

Peroneal Tendons

Lightly palpate the peroneal tendons with the finger. Look and feel for displacement of the tendons, as the patient everts the foot against light resistance, displacement occurs in a condition known as snapping peroneal tendons, as illustrated in Figure 26.149.

Heel

Tenderness around the heel is present in Sever's disease, superior calcaneal exostosis and tendocalcaneus bursitis, planter fasciitis and inferior calcaneal exostosis and pes cavus, as shown in Figure 26.150.

Forefoot (Figs 26.151 to 26.154)

- Diffuse tenderness under the metatarsal heads is common in anterior metatarsalgia, pes cavus and pes planus, gout and rheumatoid arthritis.
- Tenderness under the second metatarsal head and over the second metatarsophalangeal joint is found

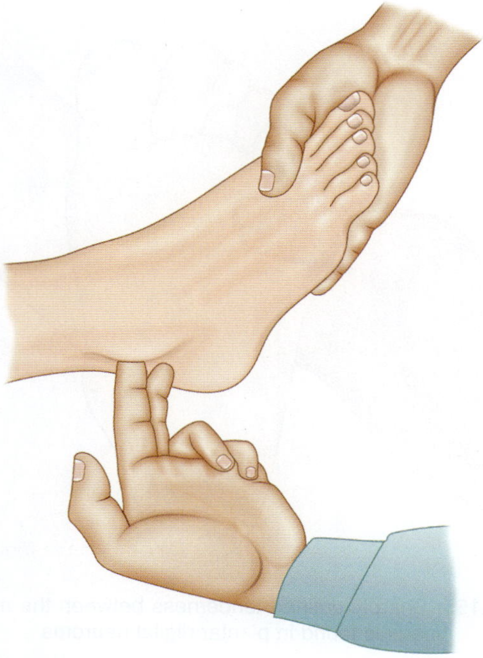

Fig. 26.149: Palpating peroneal tendon

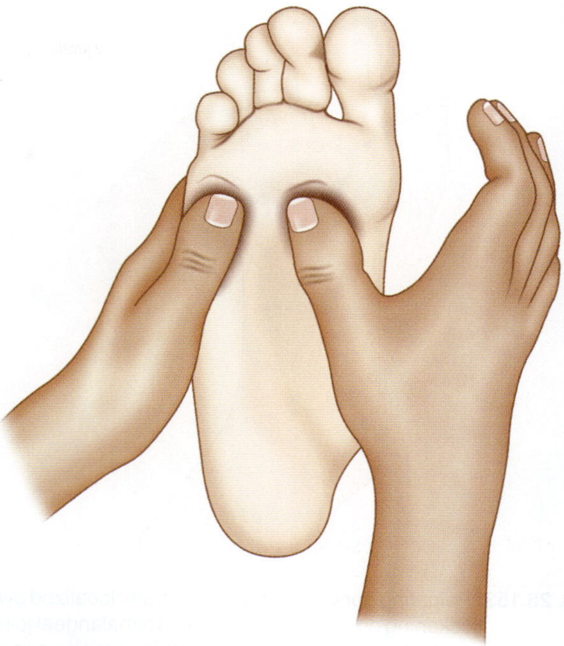

Fig. 26.151: Examining metatarsal head for tenderness or swelling

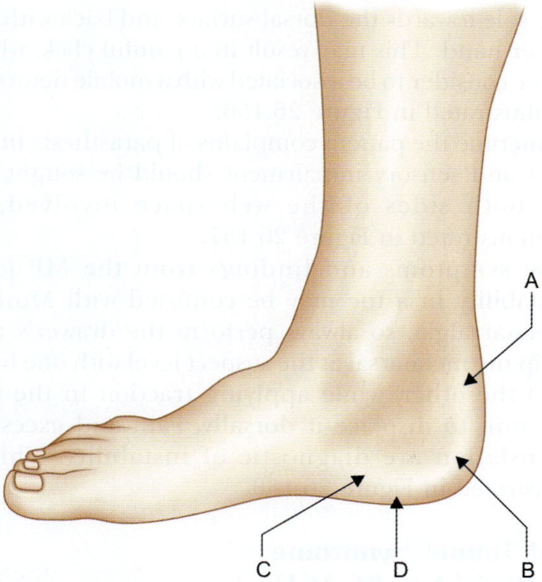

Fig. 26.150: Examining heel for the presence of different pathology— A. Sever's disease; B. Superior calcaneal exostosis and tendocalcaneus bursitis; C. Plantar fasciitis and inferior calcaneal exostosis; D. Pes cavus

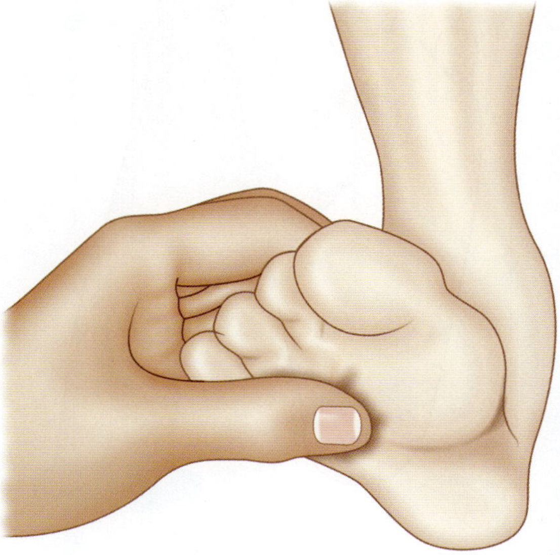

Fig. 26.152: Tenderness under the second metatarsal head and metatarsophalangeal joint in case of hallux valgus or rheumatoid arthritis

when the toe subluxes, as a sequel to hallux valgus or rheumatoid arthritis.

- Puffy localized swelling on the dorsum of the foot, palpable thickening on the second metatarsophalangeal joint, pain on plantar flexion of the toe and joint tenderness are diagnostic of Freiberg's disease.
- Tenderness on both plantar and dorsal surface of the second or third metatarsal necks or shafts occurs in march fracture.

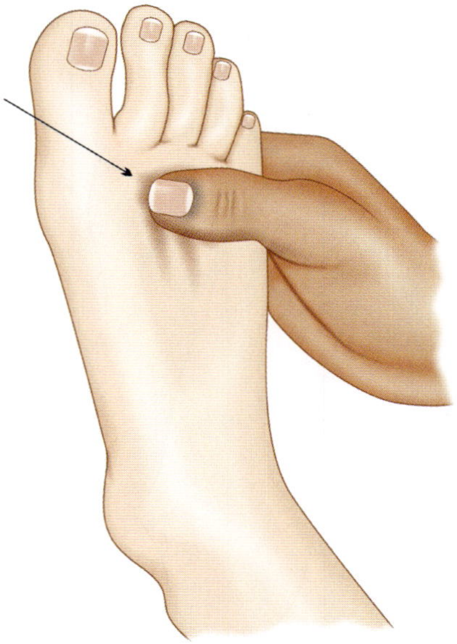

Fig. 26.153: Palpating dorsum of the foot for puffy localized swelling, thickening on the second metatarsophalangeal joint, pain on plantar flexion of the toe and joint tenderness

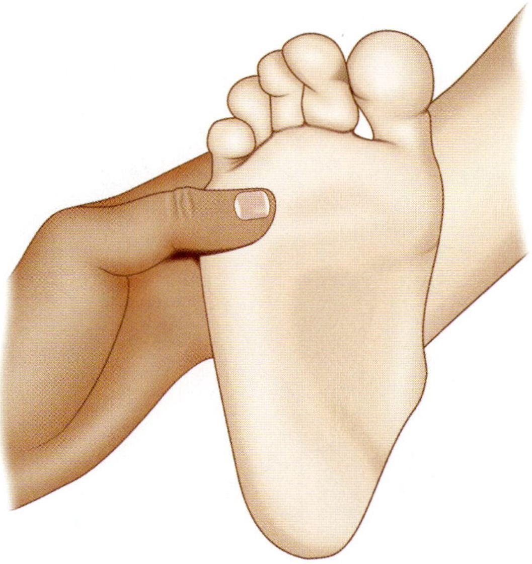

Fig. 26.155: Sharply defined tenderness between the metatarsal heads is found in plantar digital neuroma

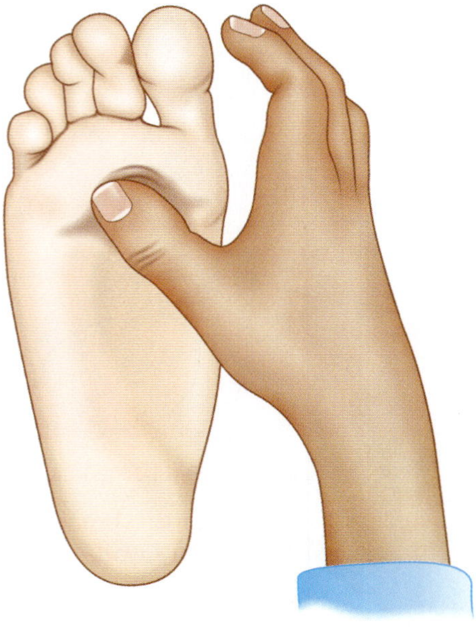

Fig. 26.154: Examining plantar and dorsal aspect of second and third metatarsal necks or shaft in march fracture

Suspected Plantar Neuroma (Morton's Metatarsalgia)

- Sharply defined tenderness between the metatarsal heads is found in plantar digital neuroma, as illustrated in Figure 26.155.
- Compress the metatarsal heads, note whether this produces the patients symptoms of pain a possible parasthesia (Mulder's sign). Repeat, while simultaneously pressing in a coordinated fashion from the sole towards the dorsal surface and back with the other hand. This may result in a painful click, which some consider to be associated with a mobile neuroma, as illustrated in Figure 26.156.
- Sometime the patient complains of parasthesia in the toes and sensory impairment should be sought out on both sides of the web space involved, as demonstrated in Figure 26.157.
- The symptoms and findings from the MP joint instability in a toe may be confused with Moron's metatarsalgia, so always perform the drawer's test. Grip the metatarsal at the suspect level with one hand and the other, while applying traction to the toe, attempt to displace it dorsally. Pain and excessive translation are diagnostic of instability. This is illustrated in Figure 26.158.

Tarsal Tunnel Syndrome (Figs 26.159 to 26.161)

Tenderness may occur over the posterior tibial nerve in this syndrome, where the presenting symptoms are usually of local pain and parasthesia in the foot. Tapping over the posterior tibial nerve may give rise to parasthesia in the sole of the foot (Tinel's sign). The sensation over the whole of the sole of the foot and the toes in the area of supply of the medial and lateral plantar nerves. Compare both sides. Sensory loss is uncommon in this syndrome. *The dorsiflexion-eversion test (Kinoshita et al.):* Maximally dorsiflex the ankle and the MP joints of all three toes,

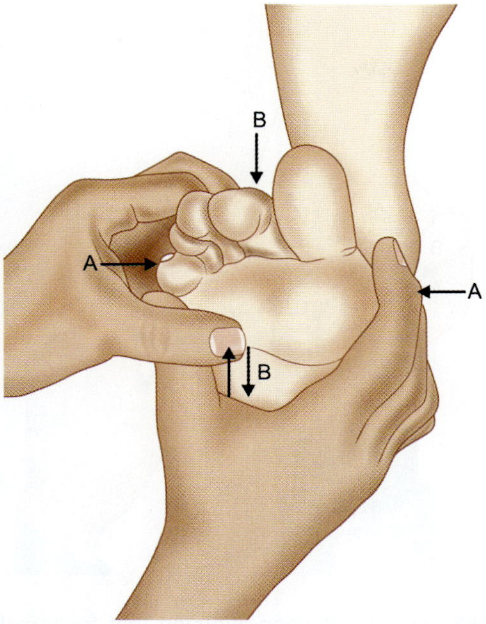

Fig. 26.156: Examining the presence of mobile neuroma—A. Compress the metatarsal heads and repeat, while simultaneously pressing in a coordinated fashion from the sole towards the dorsal surface; B. Back with the other hand

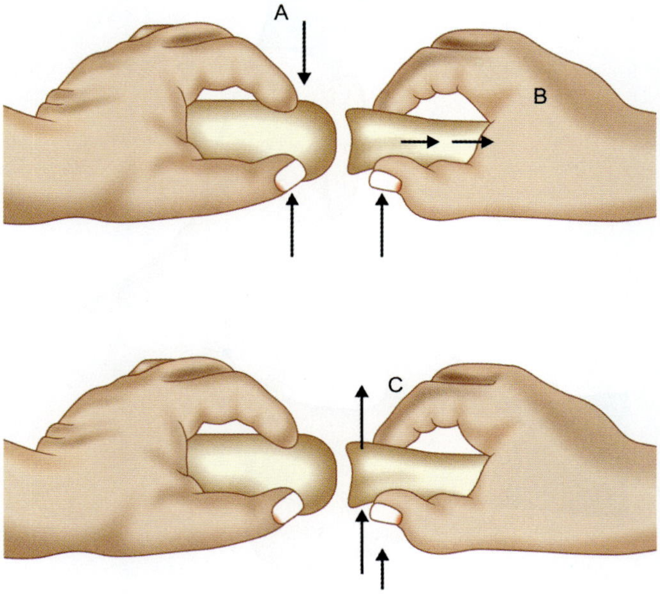

Fig. 26.158: Drawer test for finding MP joint instability—A. Grip the metatarsal at the suspect level with one hand; B. The other, while applying traction to the toe; C. Attempt to displace it dorsally

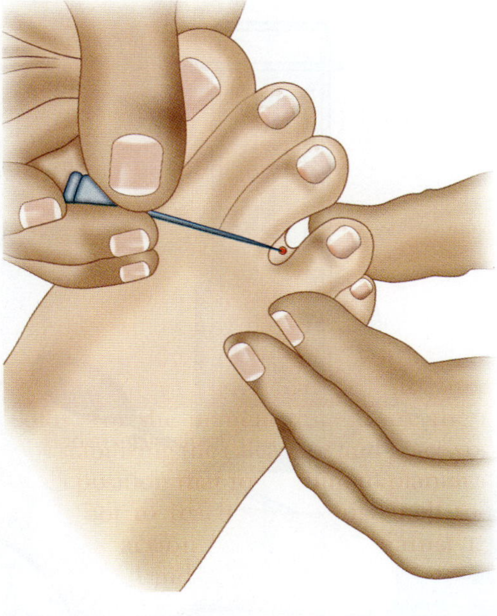

Fig. 26.157: Parasthesia in the toes and sensory impairment should be sought out on both sides of the web space involved

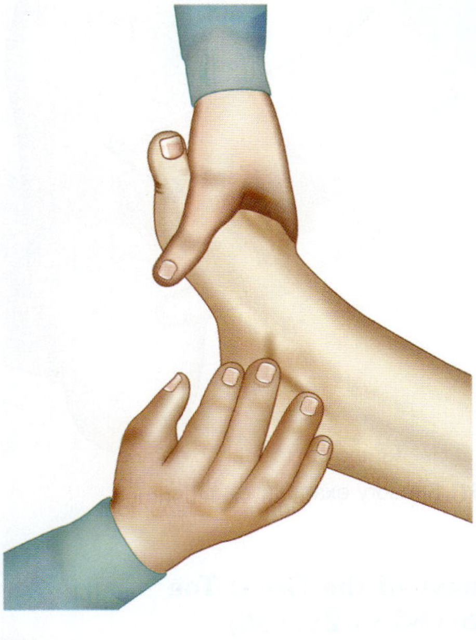

Fig. 26.159: Tenderness over the posterior tibial nerve in tarsal tunnel syndrome

firmly evert the foot and hold this position. In a positive case the patient's symptoms will be reproduced. Look also for increased local tenderness, accompanying the maneuver, as shown in Figure 26.162.

The tourniquet test (Fig. 26.163): In doubtful cases, apply a tourniquet to the calf and inflate to just above the systolic blood pressure. If this brings on the symptom the diagnosis is confirmed.

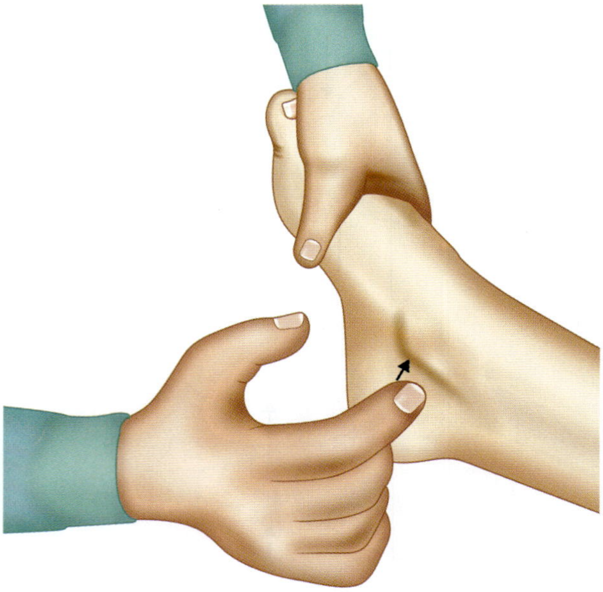

Fig. 26.160: Tinel's sign is positive in tarsal tunnel syndrome

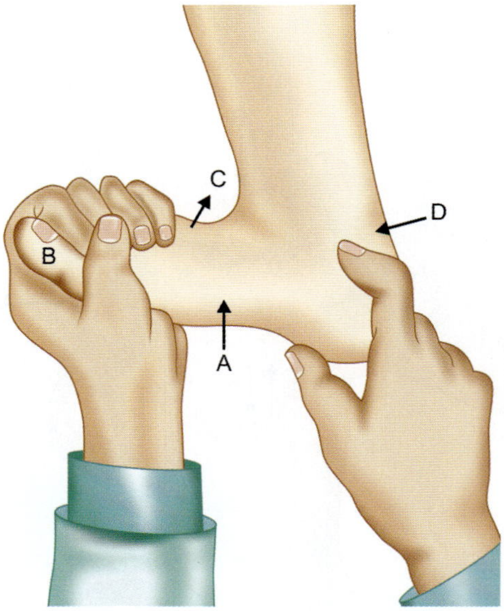

Fig. 26.162: The dorsiflexion-eversion test for tarsal tunnel syndrome— A. Maximally dorsiflex the ankle; B. Dors flex MP joints of all three toes; C. Firmly evert the foot and hold this position. In a positive case the patients symptoms will be reproduced; D. Look also for increased local tenderness accompanying the maneuver

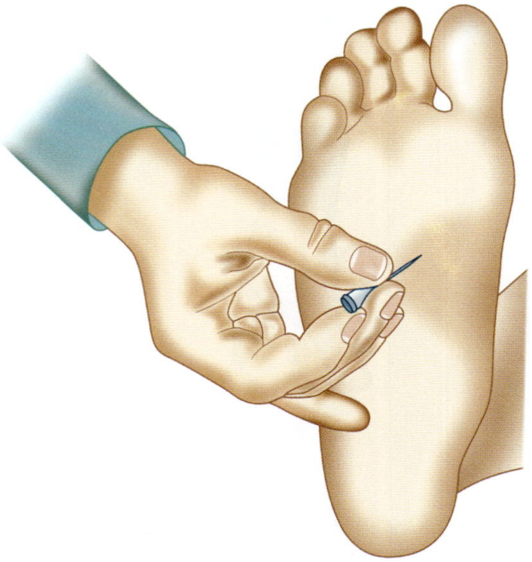

Fig. 26.161: Sensory examination of foot

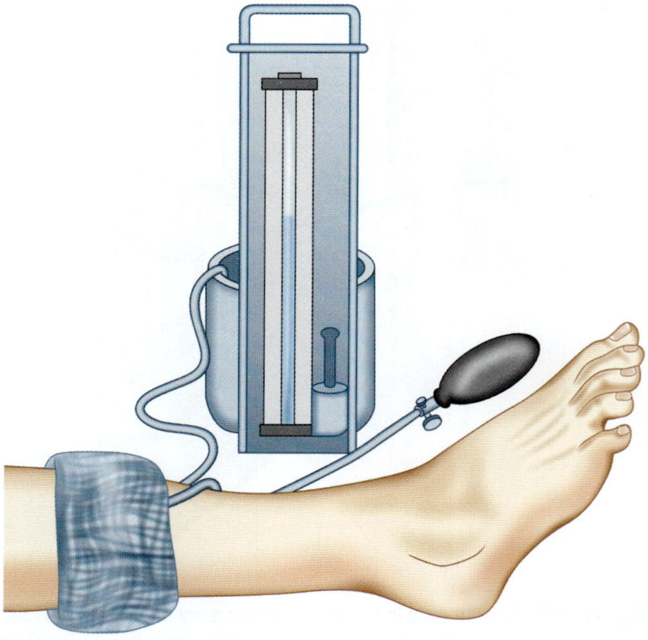

Fig. 26.163: The tourniquet test

Tenderness of the Great Toe (Figs 26.164 to 26.166)

In gout, tenderness is most often acute, but diffusely spread around the whole metatarsophalangeal joint and often the entire toe. There is often a reddish-blue discoloration of the skin. In hallux valgus tenderness is often absent or confined to bunion or painful corns on adjacent toes. In hallux rigidus there is usually tenderness over the exostosis, which arises on the metatarsal head and proximal phalanx.

Great toe nail (Fig. 26.166): In subungual exostosis, pain is produced by squeezing the toe in the vertical plane. In ingrowing nail, pain is produced by side to side pressure.

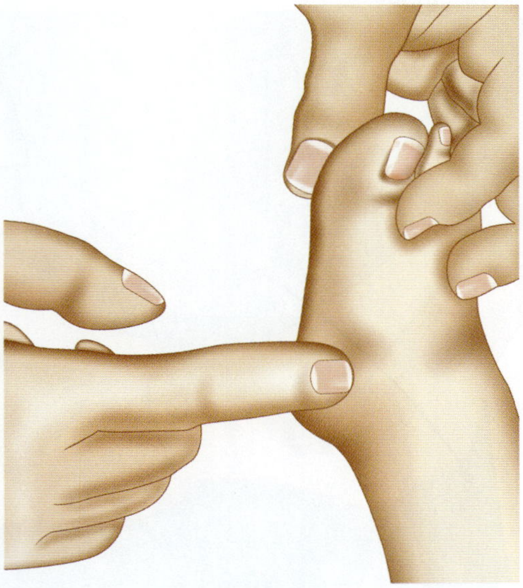

Fig. 26.164: Examining signs of diffuse tenderness and discoloration of the skin

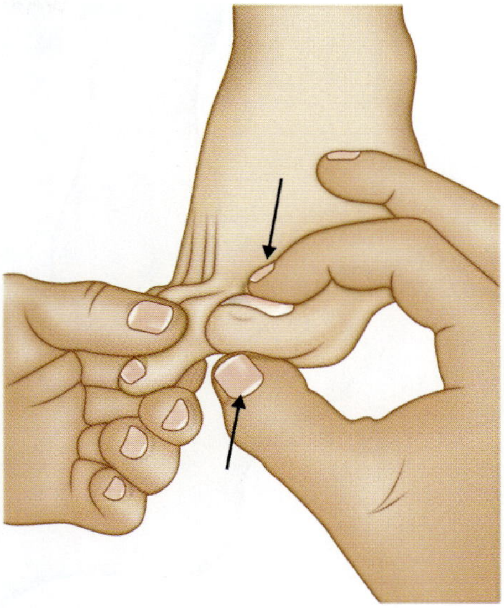

Fig. 26.166: Examining the great toe nail by squeezing or applying side-to-side pressure

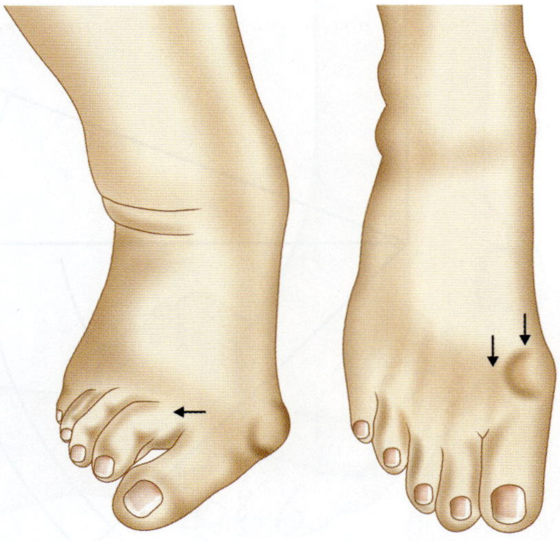

Fig. 26.165: In hallux valgus, tenderness is often absent or confined to bunion or painful corns on adjacent toes. In hallux rigidus, there is usually tenderness over the exostosis, which arises on the metatarsal head and proximal phalanx

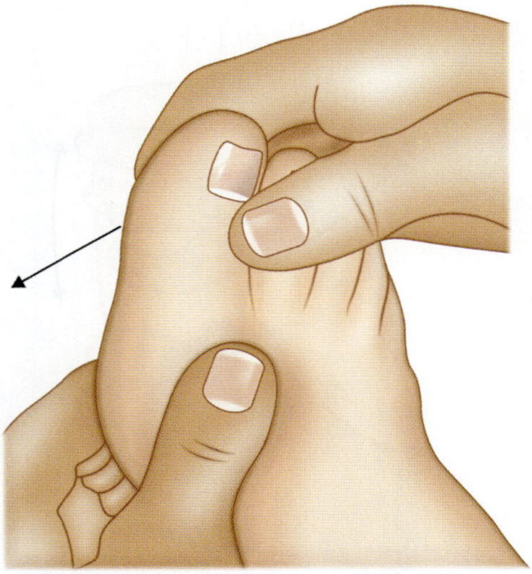

Fig. 26.167: Moving great toe to feel any crepitation in case of degenerative joint disease

Crepitus (Fig. 26.167)

Move the great toe in an up and down direction, while palpating the metatarsophalangeal joint. Repeat with the IP joint. Crepitus, indicating osteoarthritis change is constant in the MP joint in hallux rigidus. IP joint crepitus is considered a contraindication for MP joint fusion. Place a hand across the front of the ankle and passively dorsiflex and plantarflex the foot. Crepitus suggests articular surface damage.

■ Joint Movements

Articular Surfaces

Forcibly plantarflex the foot, to allow palpation of the anterior part of the superior articular surface of the talus. Tenderness occurs in arthritic conditions and in the osteochondritis of the talus. A tender exostosis may be present in cases of "footballer's ankle", as shown in Figures 26.168 and 26.169.

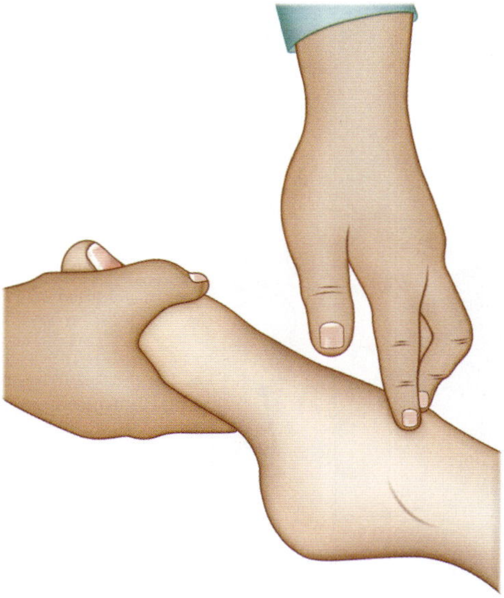

Fig. 26.168: Palpating anterior part of the superior articular surface of the talus by forcibly plantar flexing the foot

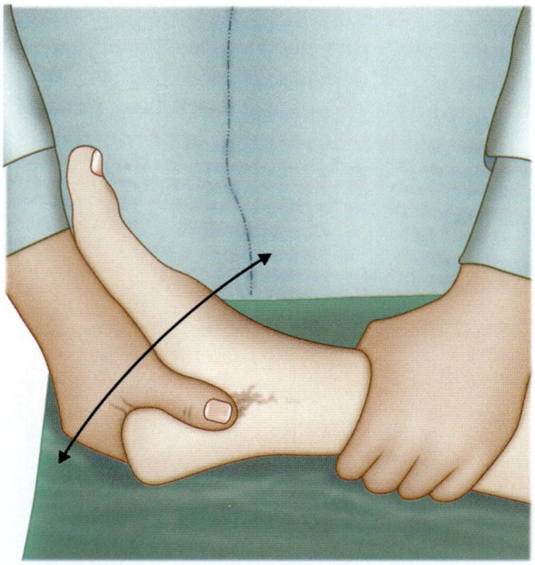

Fig. 26.170: Plantarflexing the ankle joint to measure ROM

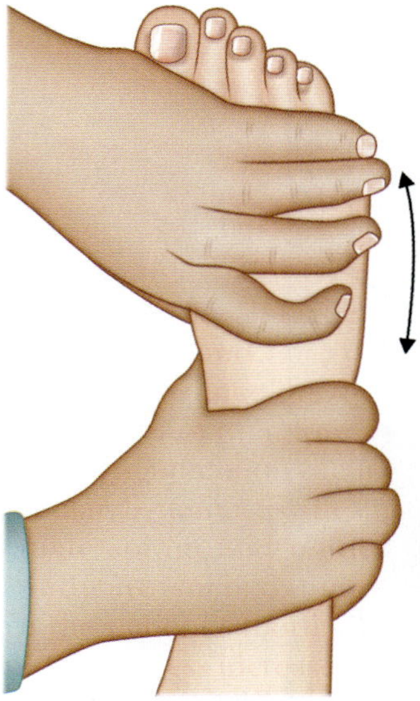

Fig. 26.169: Examining articular configuration by performing joint movement

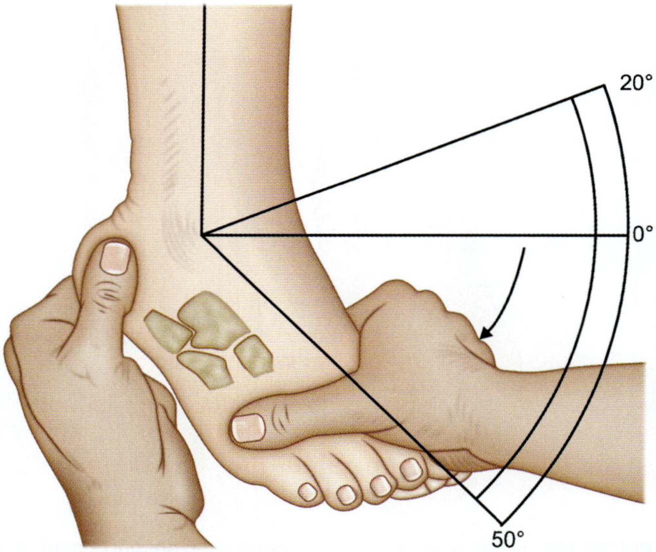

Fig. 26.171: Normal range of movement of ankle joint

Ankle Joint Movements (Figs 26.170 to 26.173)

First confirm that the ankle is mobile and that any apparent movement in not arising at the midtarsal or more distal joint. Firmly grasp the foot proximal to the midtarsal joint. Try to produce dorsiflexion and plantarflexion. Measure planter flexion from zero position. This lies at right angles to the line of the leg. Normal range 50° to 55°.

Dorsiflexion: always compare the sides. Normal range 15° to 20°. If dorsiflexion is restricted bend the knees. If this restores normal range, the achilles tendon is tight. If it makes no difference, joint pathology (osteoarthritis, rheumatoid arthritis or infection) is the likely cause.

Movements of Foot (Figs 26.174 to 26.176)

- *Supination:* Ask the patient to turn the soles of the feet towards one another. The patellae should be vertical. Normal range is approximately 35°.
- *Pronation:* Ask the patient to turn the feet outwards. Normal range is approximately 20°. If supination and pronation are restricted, fix the heel with one

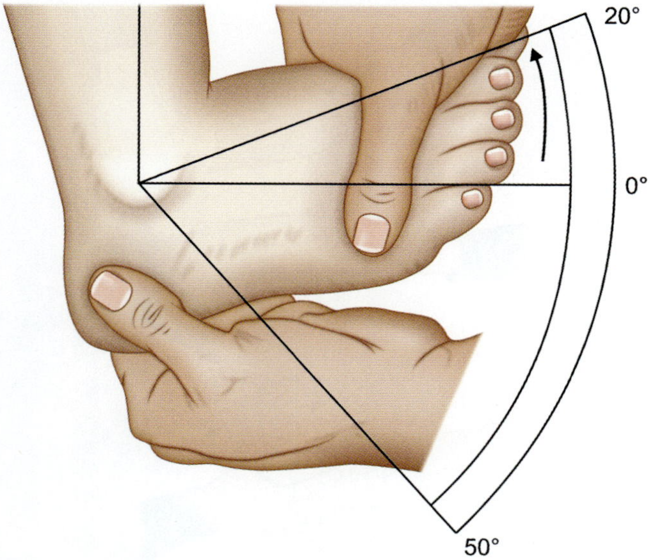

Fig. 26.172: Measuring ROM for ankle dorsiflexion

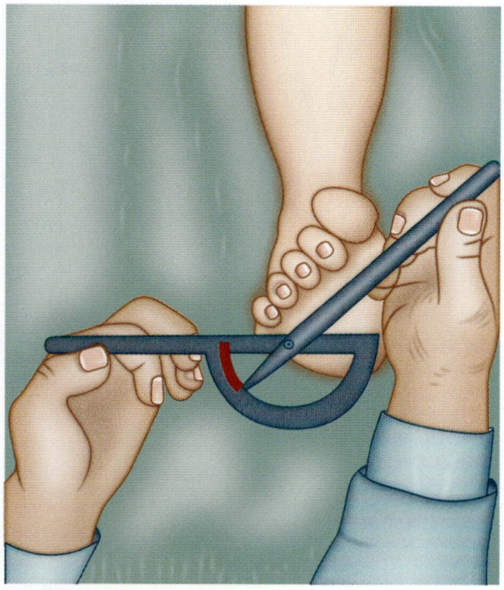

Fig. 26.174: Measuring the ROM of supination

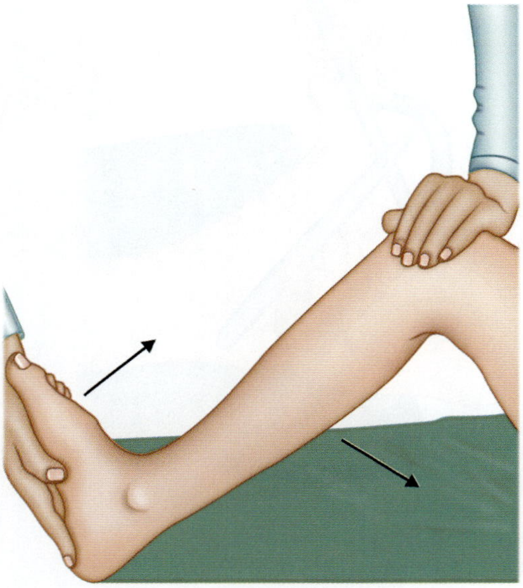

Fig. 26.173: Restoration of dorsiflexion by flexing the knee

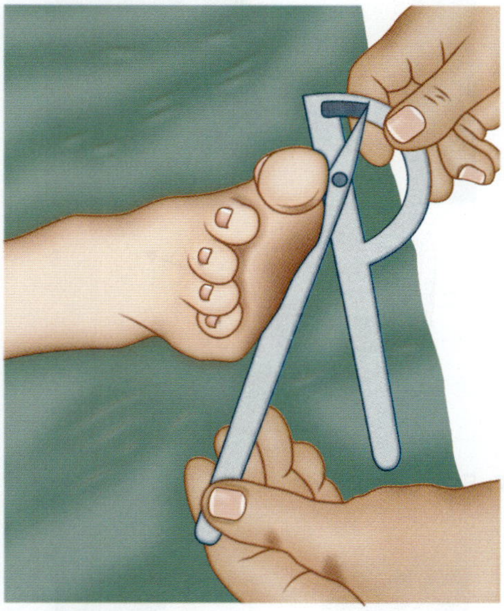

Fig. 26.175: Measuring foot pronation

hand and with the other, assist the patient to repeat the movements. No further reduction in the range indicates a stiff subtalar joint. The presence of some mobility, indicate that the midtarsal and tarsometatarsal joint preserve some mobility.

- *Eversion (Fig. 26.177):* Turn the patient face down with the feet over the edge of the couch. Evert the heel and note the presence of movement in the subtalar joint by position of the heel. Normal range is approximately 10°.
- *Inversion:* Repeat the above procedure, forcing the heel into inversion. Normal range is approximately 20°. Loss of movement indicates a stiff subtalar joint (e.g. old calcaneal fracture, rheumatoid or osteoarthritis and spastic flat foot), as shown in Figure 26.178.
- Test for mobility in the first, fourth and fifth metatarsal joints, by steadying the heel with one hand and attempting to move the metatarsal heads individually in a dorsal and plantar direction (Fig. 26.179).

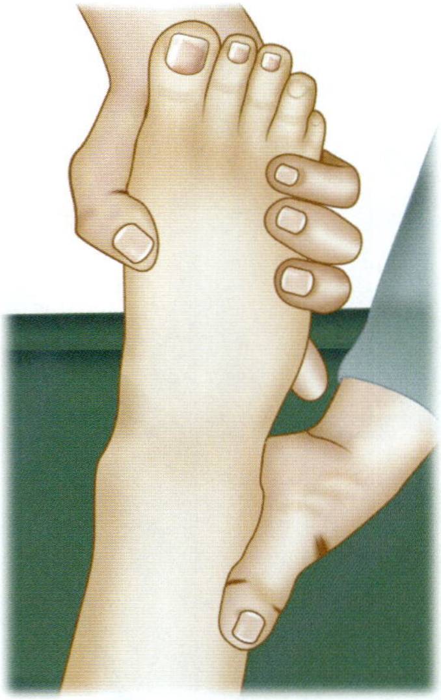

Fig. 26.176: Eliciting midtarsal joint movements

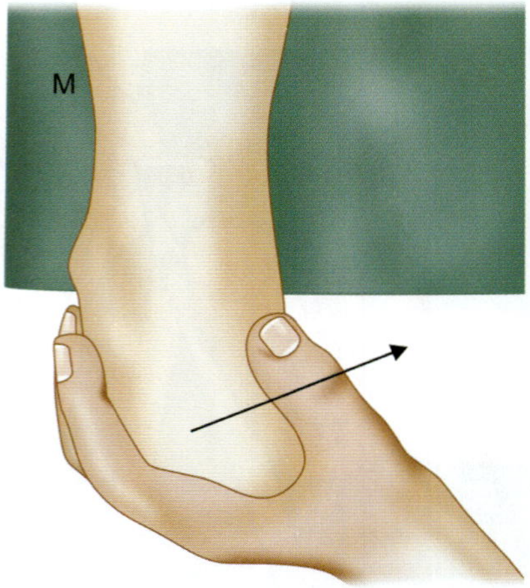

Fig. 26.177: Foot eversion movement

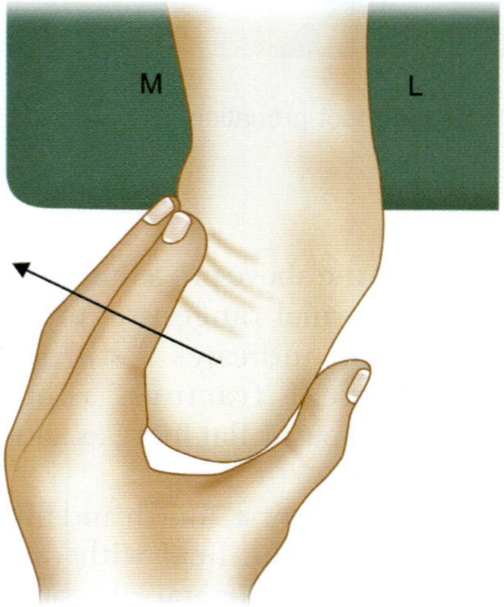

Fig. 26.178: Foot inversion (movement from neutral to medial side)

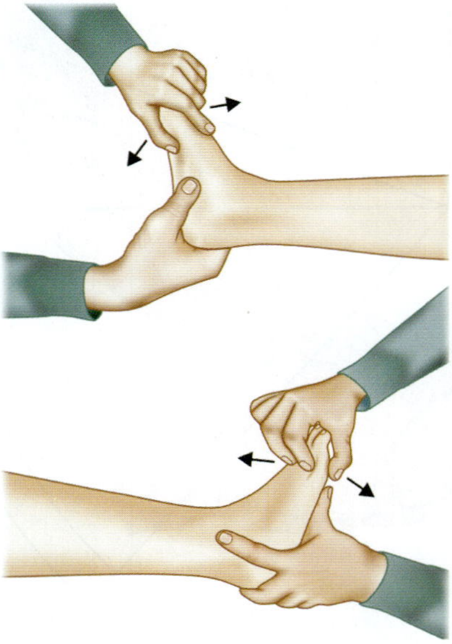

Fig. 26.179: Testing the mobility of metatarsal joints of the foot

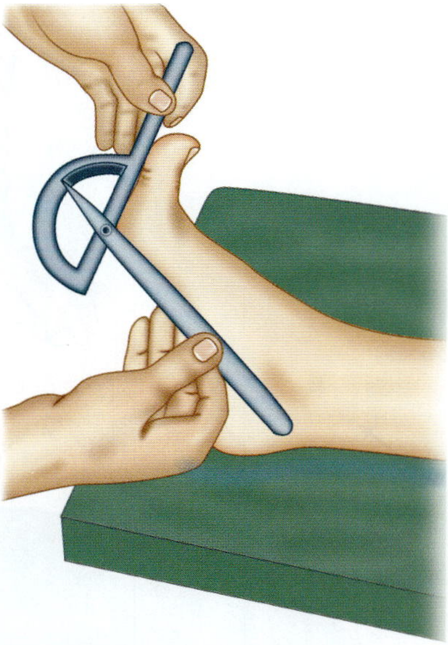

Fig. 26.180: Measuring ROM of MTP joints

Great Toe (Figs 26.180 to 26.182)

- Normal range in extension at the metatarsophalangeal joint is 65°.

Normal range in flexion at the metatarsophalangeal joint is 40°. Metatarsophalangeal joint movements are severely restricted in hallux rigidus. There is often little impairment in hallux valgus unless secondary arthritic changes are quite severe.

Range of motion in the IP joint. Normal flexion is 60°. Normal extension is 0°. Restriction is common after fractures of the terminal phalanx, and is generally regarded as a contraindication to metacarpophalangeal joint fusion.

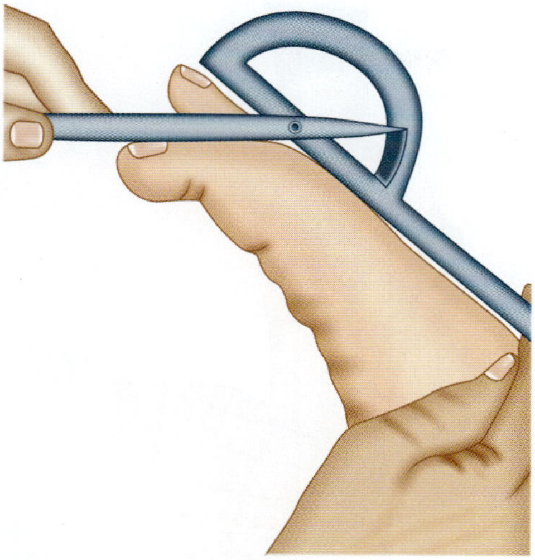

Fig. 26.181: Measuring MTP joint ROM

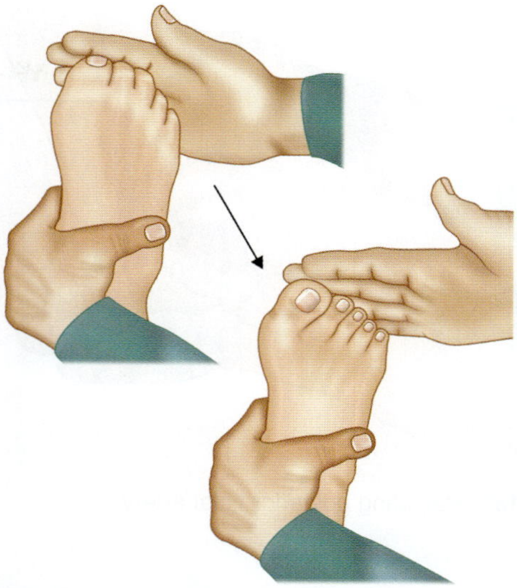

Fig. 26.183: Measuring overall mobility of toes by curling and straightening

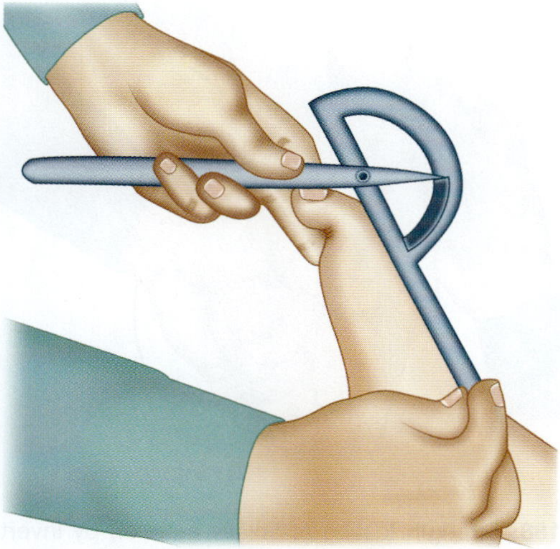

Fig. 26.182: ROM of IP joints

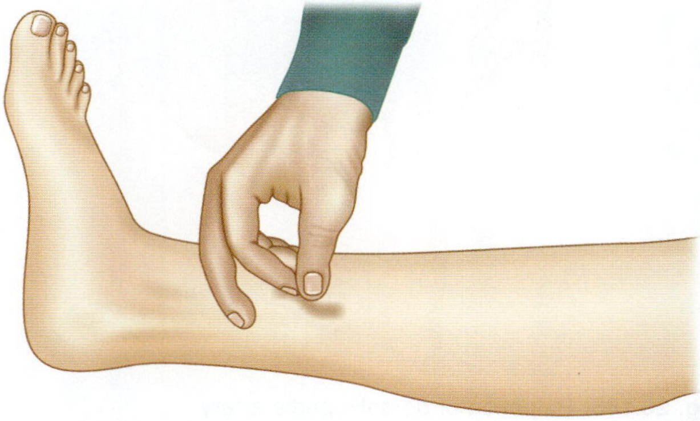

Fig. 26.184: Examining skin to get idea about the blood circulation in foot

Lesser toes: Overall mobility may be roughly assessed alternately curling and straightening the toes. Restriction is often seen in gout, rheumatoid arthritis, Sudeck's dystrophy and ischemic conditions of the foot and leg, as shown in Figure 26.183.

Blood Circulation

- If the skin is cold, note the skin temperature gradient along the limb. Observe any trophic changes or discoloration of the skin suggestive of ischemia, as shown in Figure 26.184.
- *Posterior tibial artery (Fig. 26.185):* It lies between the tendons of the flexor digitorum longus and flexor hallucis longus behind the medial malleolus. Easier to palpate, when the foot is in a relaxed nonweight-bearing position and the tendons are slack.
- *Dorsal pedis artery:* When attempting to palpate the dorsalis pedis artery, the vessel lies just lateral to the tendon of the extensor hallucis longus and its pulsations should be felt by compressing it against the middle cuneiform, as illustrated in Figure 26.186.
- *Anterior tibial artery:* Try to feel the anterior tibial artery near the midline of the ankle, just above the joint line, as demonstrated in Figure 26.187.
- The posterior tibial artery is often difficult to find and is helpful to invert the foot while palpating behind the medial malleolus.

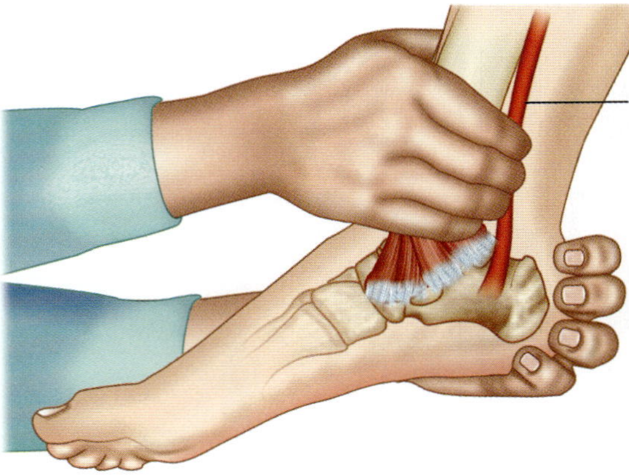

Fig. 26.185: Palpating posterior tibial artery

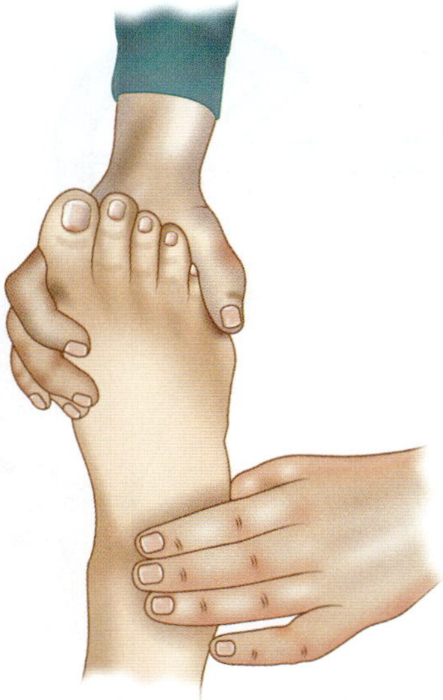

Fig. 26.187: Palpating anterior tibial artery

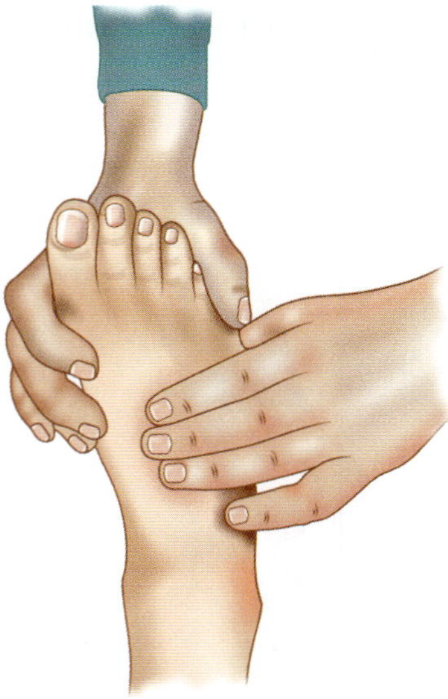

Fig. 26.186: Palpation of dorsalis pedis artery

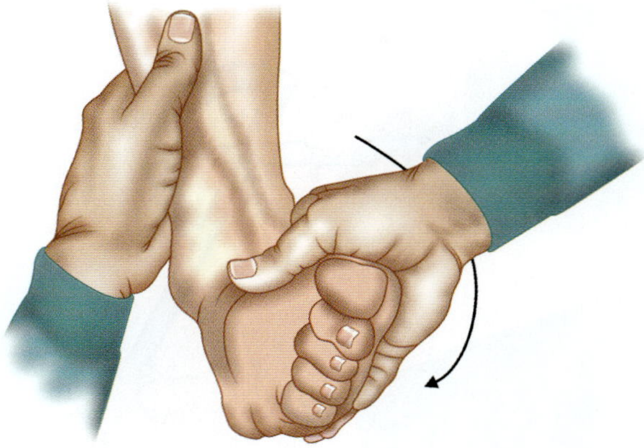

Fig. 26.188: Strength testing of tibialis anterior, by inverting the foot

- Note any cyanosis of the foot, when dependent and blanching on elevation.

Neurological Examination

Muscle Testing

Dorsiflexors

Majority lies in the anterior tibial compartment. They share a common innervation and any pathology, which prevent the nerve from functioning results in foot drop.

- *Tibialis anterior (deep peroneal nerve L4):* Ask the patient to walk on his heels with the foot inverted. The tendon can be seen, where it crosses the anteromedial portion of the ankle joint. Patients unable to perform may exhibit drop foot or steppage gait. For the manual test the patient should sit on the edge of the bed. Support his lower leg and place your thumb near the dorsum of the foot in such a position that he must dorsiflex and invert his foot to reach it. Then try to force his foot into plantar flexion and eversion by pushing against the first metatarsal head and shaft. Palpate the tendon as you perform the test, as shown in Figure 26.188.
- *Extensor hallucis longus (deep peroneal nerve, L5):* Ask the patient to walk on his heel with his foot inverted or everted. The tendon should stand out clearly on the way to it insertion at the proximal of the distal phalanx of the great toe. For the manual test, support the foot as above and place your thumb in such a way that he must dorsiflex his toe to reach it. Oppose his dorsiflexion by placing your thumb on the nail bed

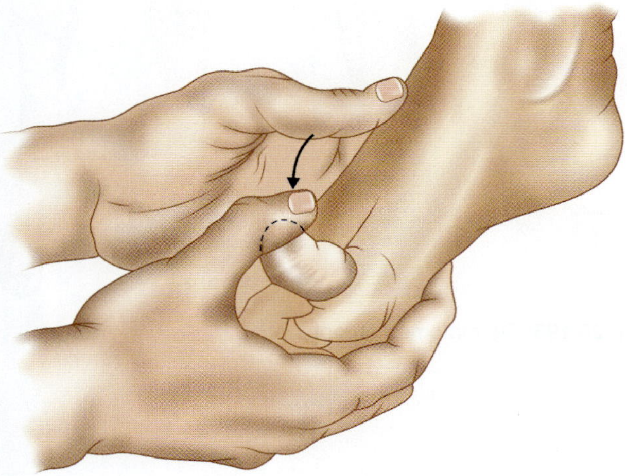

Fig. 26.189: Testing extensor halluces longus muscle by opposing dorsiflexion, by placing your thumb on the nail bed of the great toe

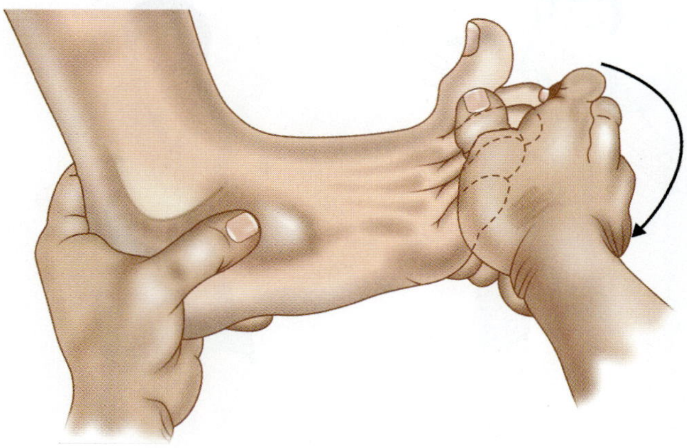

Fig. 26.190: Testing extensor digitorum longus

of the great toe. If the thumb is placed across the IP joint, the extensor hallucis brevis is also being tested. This is illustrated in Figure 26.189.

- *Extensor digitorum longus (deep peroneal nerve L5):* Instruct the patient on his heel. The tendon should stand out on the dorsum of the foot, fanning out to insert into slip on the dorsal surface of the middle and distal phalanges of the four lateral toes. For the manual test, secure his calcaneus and place the thumb of your free hand in such a position that he must extend his toes to reach it. Then oppose this motion by attempting to bend them plantarward, as shown in Figure 26.190.

Plantar Flexors

- *Peroneus longus and brevis (superficial peroneal nerve, S1):* Instruct the patient to walk on the medial borders of his feet. The tendons of the peronei should become prominent where they turn around the lateral malleolus. For the manual test, secure the patients ankle by stabilizing the calcaneus and place your other hand in a position that forces him to plantar flex and evert his foot to reach it with his small toe. Then oppose this action by pushing against the fifth metatarsal head and shaft with the palm of your hand, as shown in Figure 26.191.
- *Gastrocnemius and Soleus (tibial nerve S1, S2):* The common tendon of insertion for these muscles is the most prominent tendon behind the malleoli. As the gastrocnemius is stronger than all the other muscle combined, it is difficult to detect existing weakness by manual testing. Therefore, observe these muscles in function. First ask the patient to walk on his toes, an act he will be unable to perform, if there is muscle weakness. Then instruct him to jump up and down on the balls of his feet, one at a time to force the calf muscles to support almost two and a half time the body weight. If he lands flat footed or is otherwise incapable of performing this test, there is probably atleast minimal weakness of the calf muscle, as shown in Figures 26.192A and B.

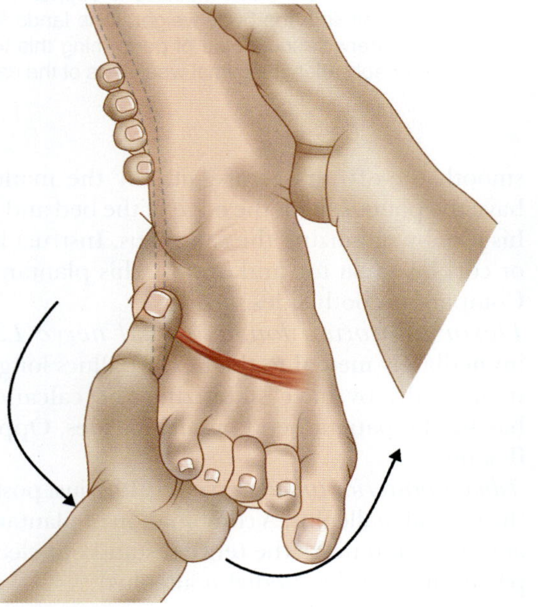

Fig. 26.191: Testing peroneus longus and brevis muscles

- *Flexor hallucis longus (tibial nerve, L5):* Lies medial to the achilles tendon. To evaluate this simply observe the patients gait. The muscle action is integral to the

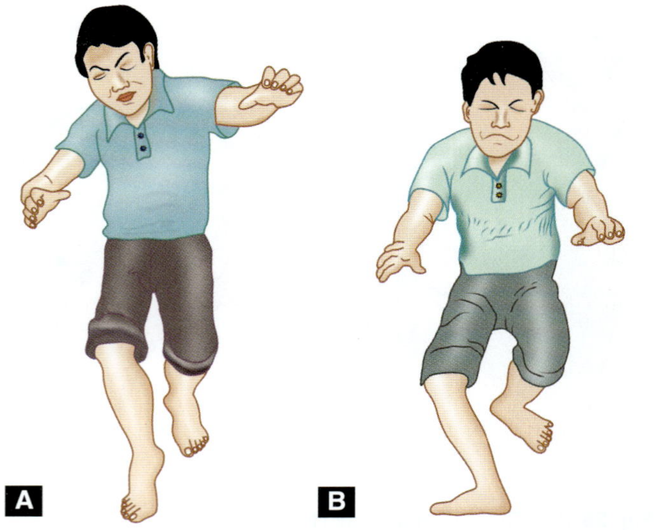

Figs 26.192A and B: Testing calf muscles strength—(A) First ask the patient to walk on his toes, an act he will be unable to perform, if there is muscle weakness; (B) Then instruct him to jump up and down on the balls of his feet, one at a time to force the calf muscles to support almost two and a half time the body weight. If he lands flat footed or is otherwise incapable of performing this test, there is probably atleast minimal weakness of the calf muscle

smooth toe-off phases of gait. For the manual test, have the patient sit on the edge of the bed and support his foot by stabilizing the calcaneus. Instruct him end or curl his great toe and oppose this plantar flexion. Compare on both sides.

- *Flexor digitorum longus (tibial nerve L5):* Lies immediately medial to the flexor hallucs longus. Test it manually by have stabilizing the calcaneus and having the patient bend or curl his toes. Oppose this flexion.
- *Tibialis posterior (tibial nerve L5):* Lies just posterior to the medial malleolus. A combination of plantar flexion and inversion make the tendon stand out clearly as it passes around the medial malleolus.

Sensation Testing

- Skin over the lower leg and foot is supplied by nerves emanating from the lumbar and sacral regions.
- L4 dermatome crosses the knee joint and over the medial side of the leg (medial to the crest of the tibia, the medial malleolus and the medial side of the foot).
- L5 dermatome covers the lateral side of the leg (lateral to the crest of the tibia) and dorsum of the foot.
- S1 dermatome covers the lateral side of the foot, as shown in Figure 26.193.
- The sensation of each peripheral nerve should be tested.
- The medial side of the foot is supplied by the saphenous nerve

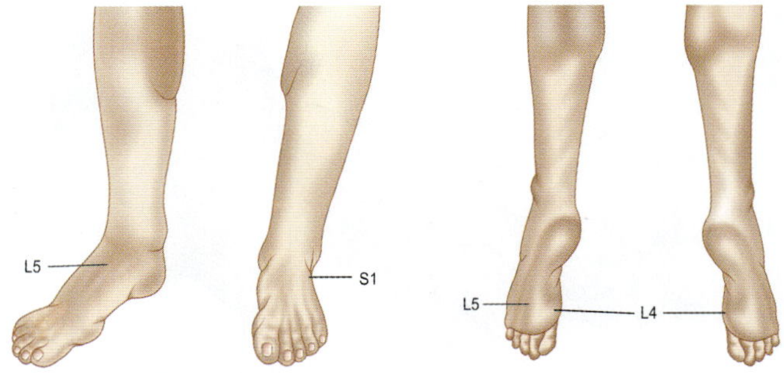

Fig. 26.193: Dermatomes of foot

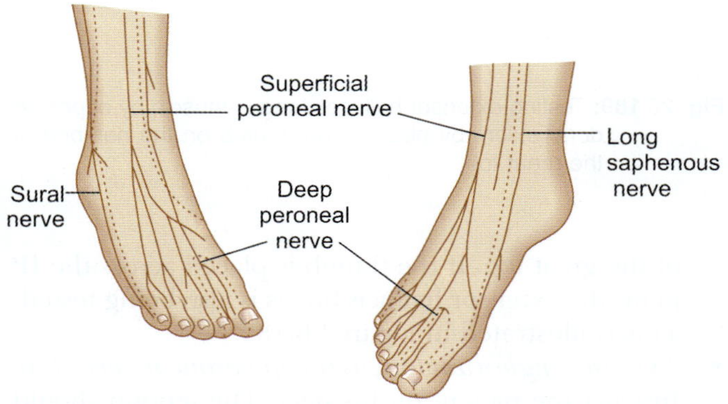

Fig. 26.194: Peripheral nerve supply of foot

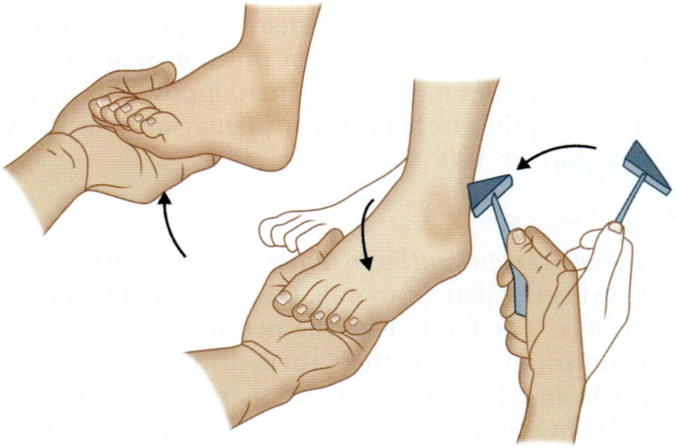

Fig. 26.195: Testing the achilles tendon reflex

- The dorsum by the peroneal nerve.
- The lateral side by the sural nerve, as shown in Figure 26.194.

Achilles Tendon Reflex (Fig. 26.195)

It is a deep tendon reflex mediated through the gastrocnemius-soleus muscles. Supplied predominantly by the S1 cord level. Ask the patient to sit on the edge of the examining table with his legs dangling and put the tendon into slight stretch by dorsiflexing the foot. Locate the tendon and tap it with flat end of a neurologic hammer

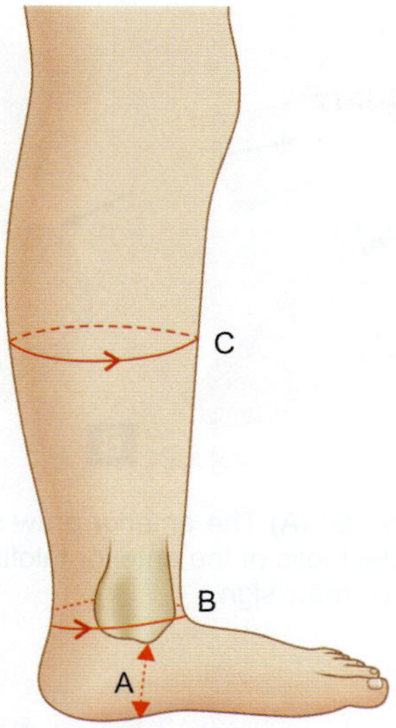

Fig. 26.196: Linear and circumferential measurement of the leg and foot—A. The distance between the tip of the medial malleolus to the sole (along a line dropped vertically from the medial malleolus) indicates roughly the height of the talus, calcaneum and heel pad; Measurements around the ankle; B. Indicates decrease or increase in the girth of the ankle; C. Indicates increase or decrease in muscle bulk

to induce a sudden involuntary plantar flexion of the foot. If the patient is bedridden, cross his leg over his opposite knee so that the ankle join is free. Prime the tendon by slightly dorsiflexing the foot. Then strike the tendon using the hammer.

Measurements

Ankle (Fig. 26.196)

Linear Measurements

The distance between the tip of the medial malleolus to the sole (along a line dropped vertically from the medial malleolus) indicates roughly the height of the talus, calcaneum and heel pad. Affections of any of these can cause disparity in this measurement.

Circumferential Measurement

- Measurements around the ankle–indicates decrease or increase in the girth of the ankle.
- Measurements around the ankle–indicates increase or decrease in muscle bulk.

Oblique Circumferential Measurements (Figs 26.197A to C)

It should be done across the point of the heel and front of the ankle. In calcaneus deformity this will increase. In equinus deformity, it will decrease.

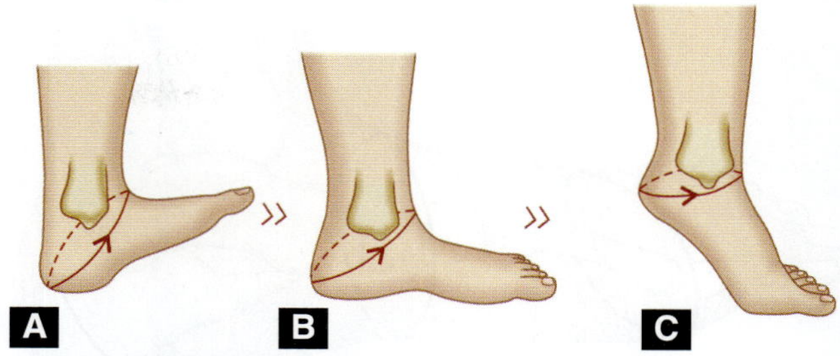

Figs 26.197A to C: Oblique circumferential measurements—(A) In calcaneus deformity; (B) In neutral position; (C) In equinus deformity

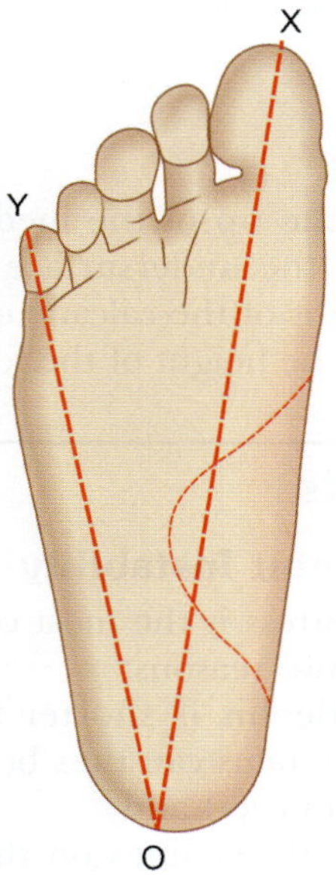

Fig. 26.198: Longitudinal measurement

Foot

Longitudinal Measurements

It is measured in two axes, from the most prominent point on the back of the heel (O) to the tip of the greater toe (X) and from the first point to the tip of the fifth toe (Y), as shown in Figure 26.198. The relationship between the long lever arm (tip of the medial malleolus to tip of the great toe and tip of the lateral malleolus to tip of the fifth toe on the outer side) and short level arm (tip of the medial malleolus to the most prominent heel point on the medial side and tip of the lateral malleolus to the tip of the most prominent heel point on the lateral side) of the foot should be symmetrical on both sides.

Circumferential Measurement (Fig. 26.199)

It is done at three levels: The metatarsal head level, maximum height of the medial arch just behind the ankle.

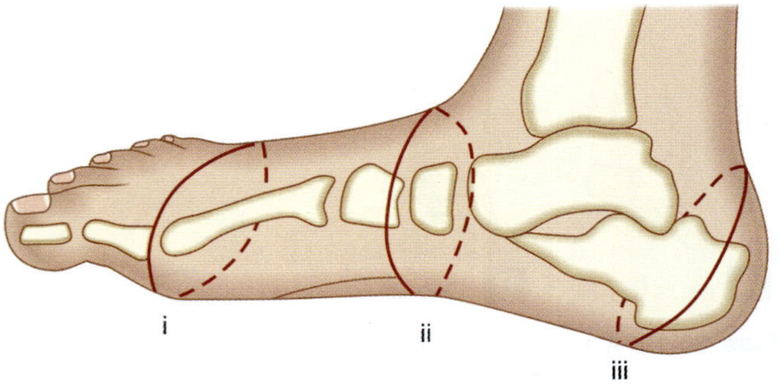

Fig. 26.199: Circumferential measurement— (i) At the metatarsal head level; (ii) Maximum height of the medial arch; (iii) Just behind the ankle

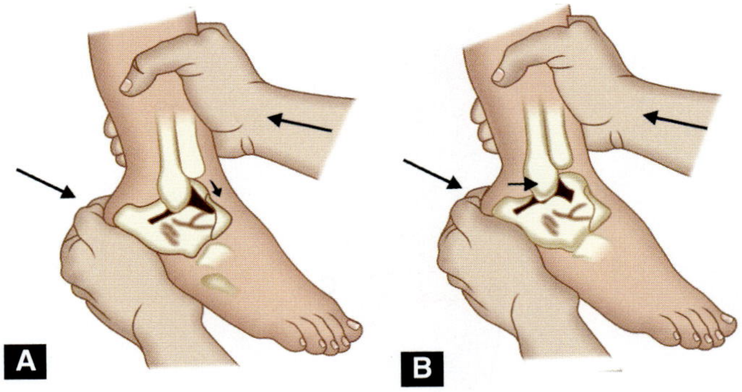

Figs 26.200A and B: (A) The anterior draw sign test to evaluate the intactness of the anterior talofibular ligament; (B) A positive draw sign

Vertical Measurement

The distance from the tip of the medial malleolus or lateral malleolus to the undersurface of the sole–any variation in the height of the calcaneum and heel-sole-cushion will disturb the height of the foot.

■ Special Tests

Tests for Ankle Joint Instability

Excessive inversion stress is the most common cause of the ankle injury for two reasons:

- The medial malleolus is shorter than the lateral malleolus and the talus can thus be forced to invert further, than it can evert and
- The ligamentous thickenings on the lateral side of the joint are separate and therefore, not as strong as the massive deltoid ligament on the medial side. The anterior talofibular ligament is the most commonly involved in ankle sprain and tenderness along its course may indicate such damage. To test this ligament, turn the patient's foot into plantar flexion and inversion. If the stress increases his pain, there is a distinct possibility that the ligament is sprained or torn. Such a tear would allow the talus to slide forward on the tibia, since the anterior talofibular ligament is the only structure preventing forward subluxation of the talus.

Anterior Draw Sign (Figs 26.200A and B)

The patient should sit on the edge of the examining table with his legs dangling and his feet in a few feet of plantar flexion. Place one hand on the anterior aspect of the lower tibia and grip the calcaneus in the palm of your other hand. Then draw the calcaneus anteriorly, while pushing the tibia posteriorly. Normally, the ligament is tight in all directions of the ankle joint and there should be no forward movement. Under abnormal condition, the talus slides anteriorly from under the cover of the ankle mortise; a clunk might be felt as it moves.

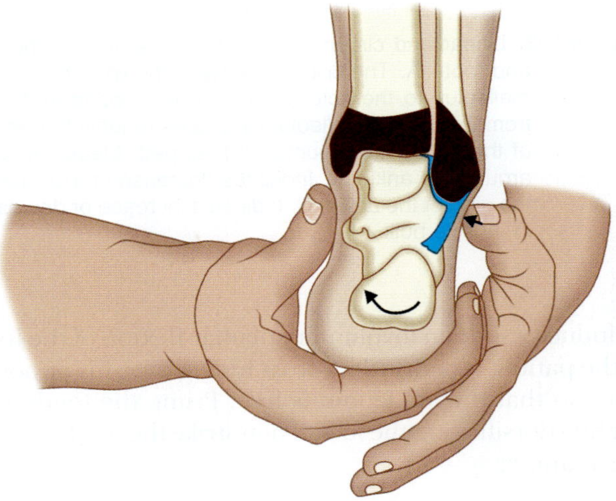

Fig. 26.201: Inverting calcaneus for checking integrity of anterior talofibular ligament and the calcaneofibular ligament

The anterior talofibular ligament and the calcaneofibular ligament must be torn, to produce gross lateral instability. To check the integrity of the ligament, invert the calcaneus, as demonstrated in Figure 26.201.

If the talus gaps and rocks in the ankle mortise, the ligaments are damaged with resultant lateral instability, as shown in Figure 26.202.

The posterior talofibular ligament can be torn only in conjunction with the other lateral ligaments, it takes a massive trauma to the ankle joint, such as dislocation to damage this joint. To test the stability of the deltoid ligament on the medial side, stabilize the patient's leg around the tibia and the calcaneus and evert his foot. If the ligament is torn, a gross gap might be felt at the ankle mortise. A stress X-ray is the best way to confirm these findings.

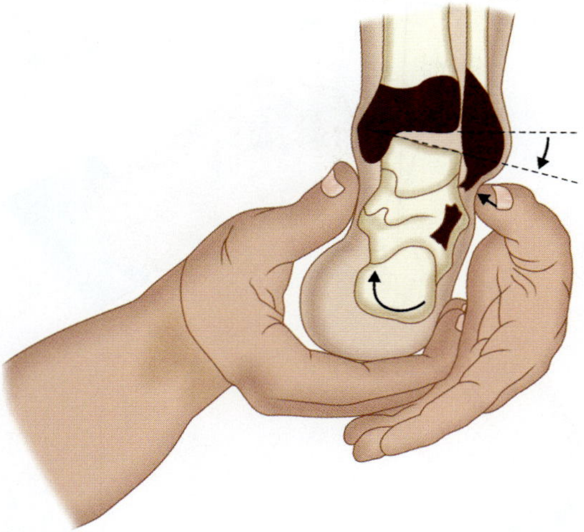

Fig. 26.202: Gap in the talus indicating ligamentous damage with lateral instability

Test for Rigid or Supple Flat Feet (Figs 26.203A and B)

Observe the patient, as he stands on his toes and while he is seated. If the medial longitudinal arch is absent in all positions, the patient has rigid flat feet. If the arch is present, while he is on his toes or sitting and absent, only when he stand, his flat feet are supple and correctable with longitudinal arch supports, as shown in Figures 26.204A and B.

Tibial Torsion Test (Figs 26.205A and B)

First locate the bony points at either end of the tibia: the tibial tubercle below the knee and the two malleoli at the ankle. Normally a line drawn between the malleoli is rotated 15°, from a perpendicular line drawn from the tibial tubercle to the ankle. If there is internal tibial torsion, the malleolar line may face directly anteriorly close to the perpendicular line.

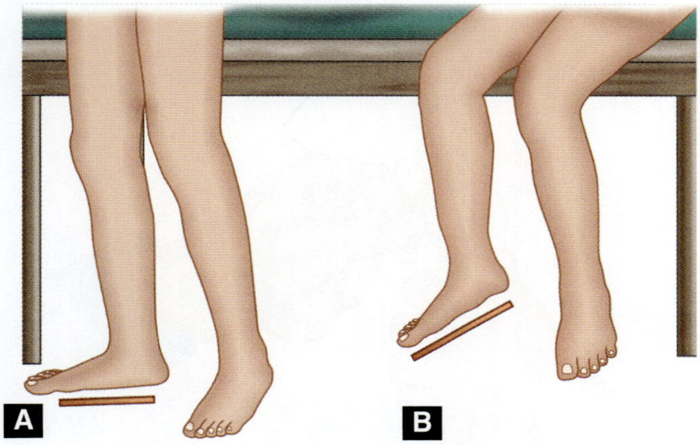

Figs 26.203A and B: Test for rigid or supple flat feet—(A) Testing in standing position; (B) Sitting position

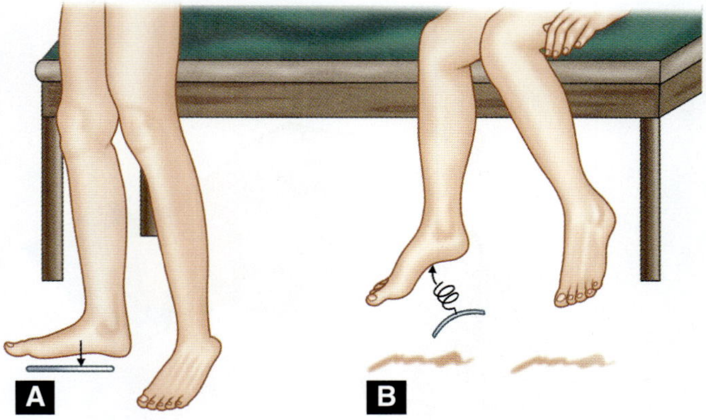

Figs 26.204A and B: (A) Obliteration of arch on standing; (B) Arch reappear in sitting

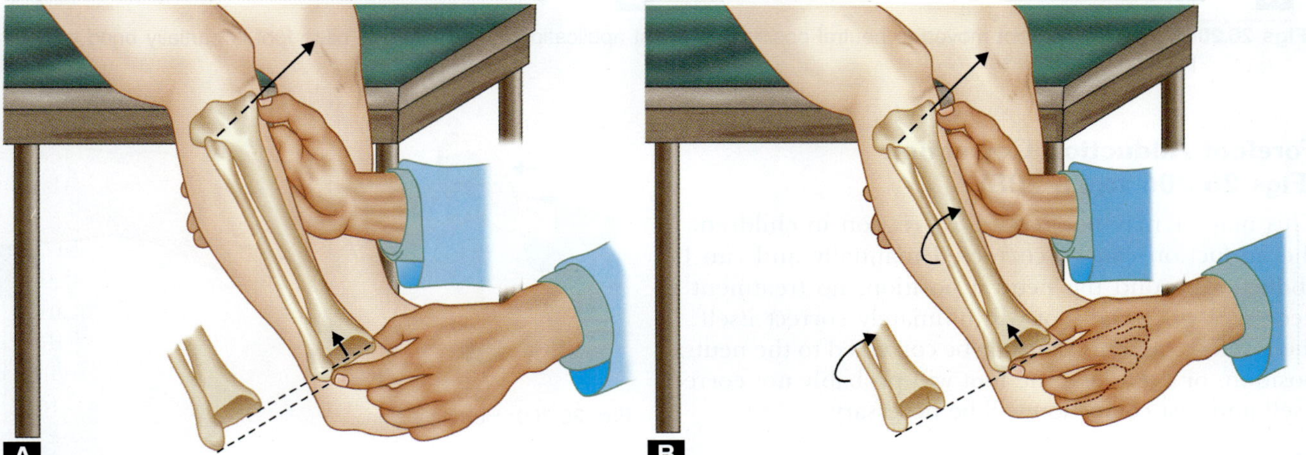

Figs 26.205A and B: Tibial torsion test—(A) Locating the bony points at either end of the tibia; (B) If there is internal tibial torsion, the malleolar line may face directly anteriorly close to the perpendicular line

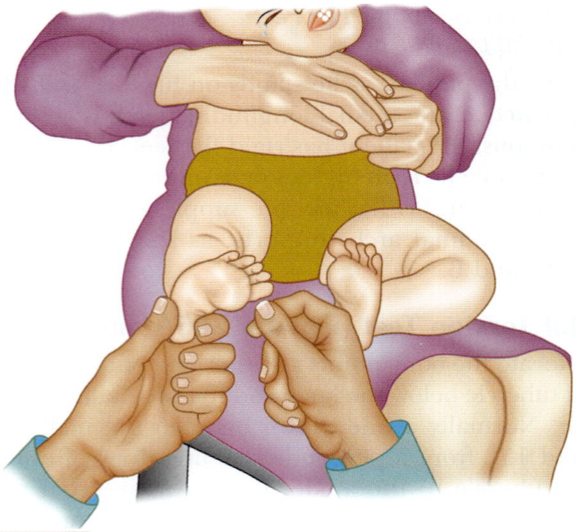

Fig. 26.206: Forefoot adduction deformity

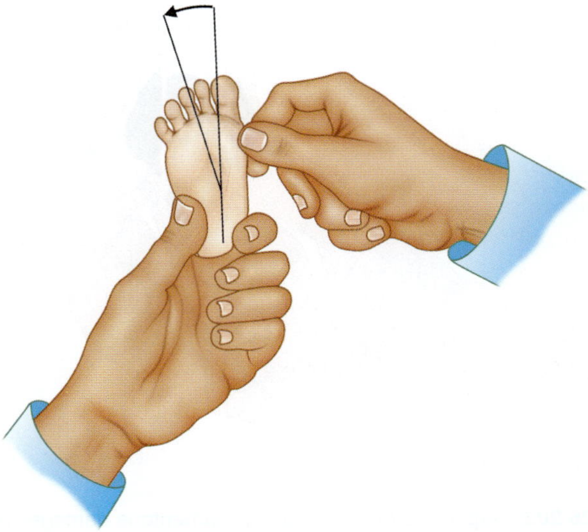

Fig. 26.207: Test, whether the adduction can be corrected manually or foot can move into abduction

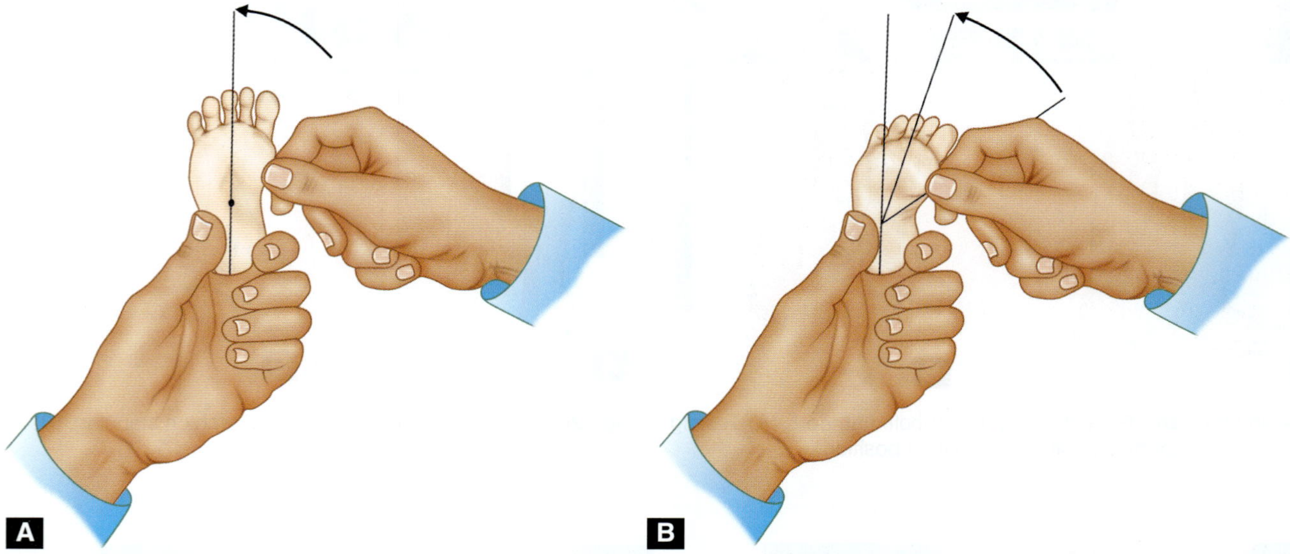

Figs 26.208A and B: (A) Foot moved to neutral position; (B) Cast application is necessary in case foot is partially bring to neutral position or even less

Forefoot Adduction Correction (Figs 26.206 to 26.208)

This may or may not require correction in children. If the adduction can be corrected manually and can be abducted beyond the neutral position, no treatment is necessary since the foot will ultimately correct itself. If the forefoot can only partially be corrected to the neutral position, or even less, the foot will probably not correct itself and cast correction will be necessary.

Homan's Sign (Fig. 26.209)

To test deep vein thrombophlebitis: Forcibly dorsiflex the patients ankle, when the leg is extended. Pain in the calf due to this maneuver, indicates a positive homan's sign. Tenderness elicited upon deep palpation of the calf muscle is further evidence of DVT.

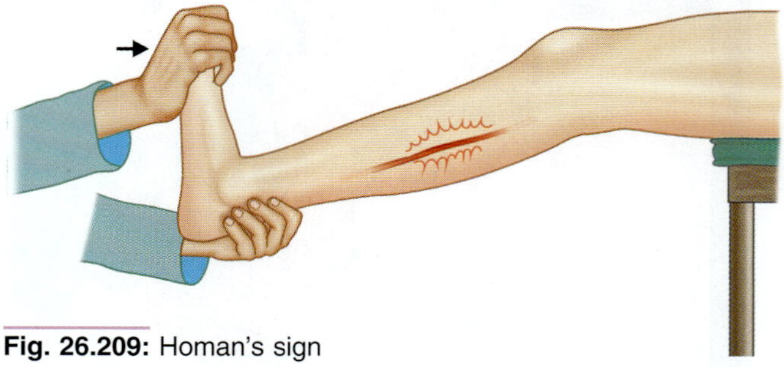

Fig. 26.209: Homan's sign

CONGENITAL ANOMALIES OF FOOT AND ANKLE

Common congenital anomalies of foot and ankle include:
- Polydactyly
- Syndactyly
- Macrodactyly
- Cleft foot (partial adactyly)
- Contracture or angulation of the toes
- Congenital hallux varus
- Congenital metatarsus adductus
- Congenital clubfoot (talipes equinovarus)
- Congenital vertical talus.

Polydactyly

The most common anomaly of the toes is polydactyly, characterized by the presence of supernumerary digits. Others are syndactyly (webbed toes), macrodactyly (enlarged toes) and congenital contracture or angulation. Any of these conditions may require surgery. When surgery is contemplated for anomalies of the toes, several factors must be considered, including cosmesis, pain and difficulty in fitting shoes. Polydactyly of the toes may occur in established genetic syndromes, but occurs most commonly as an isolated trait with an autosomal dominant inheritance pattern and variable expression. X-ray showing polydactyly is shown in Figure 26.210. The overall incidence of polydactyly is approximately two cases per 1000 live births. Surgical treatment of polydactyly is amputation of the accessory digit.

Preoperative radiographs should be obtained to detect any extra metatarsal articulating with the digit, which should be amputated with its associated digit. Occasionally, a combined polydactyly-syndactyly deformity requires more complex surgical correction, such as resection of the more peripheral digit, using residual skin for coverage. Polydactyly-syndactyly is shown in Figure 26.211. In preaxial polydactyly, the most medial great toe usually is excised. The remaining great toe should have a careful repair of the capsule, if necessary to prevent residual hallux varus, Kirschner wire fixation is used for 4 to 6 weeks.

Venn-Watson Classification (Figs 26.212A and B)

Macrodactyly

Macrodactyly occurs when one or more toes have hypertrophied and are significantly larger than the surrounding toes or fingers, as shown in Figure 26.213.

The most common associated conditions are neurofibromatosis and hemangiomatosis. Surgery is indicated to relieve functional symptoms, primarily pain or difficulty in fitting shoes. The cosmetic goal is to alter the grotesque appearance of the toes and foot and to achieve a foot similar in size to the opposite foot.

Surgical Option

Many operative procedures have been described for the treatment of macrodactyly including:
- Reduction syndactyly
- Soft-tissue debulking combined with stectomy or epiphysiodesis
- Toe amputation
- Ray amputation

Kotwal and Farooque described a staged procedure, in which defatting was done on one side of the digit,

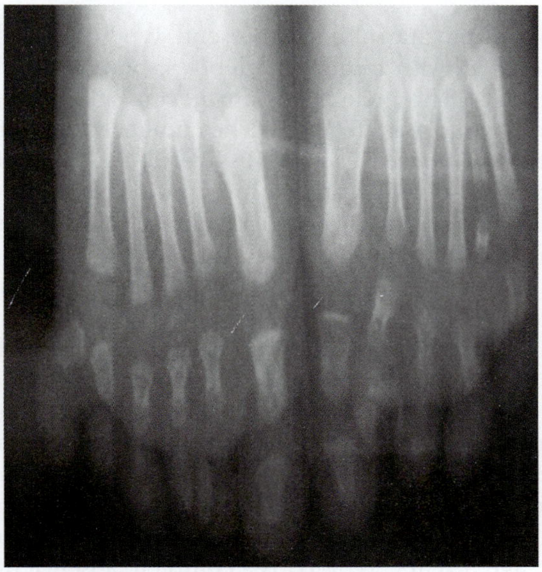

Fig. 26.210: X-ray showing polydactyly

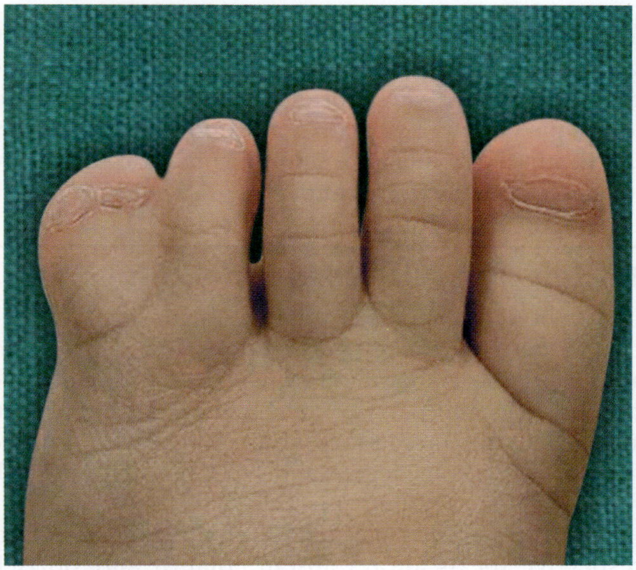

Fig. 26.211: Palpation of posterior tibial artery pulsations

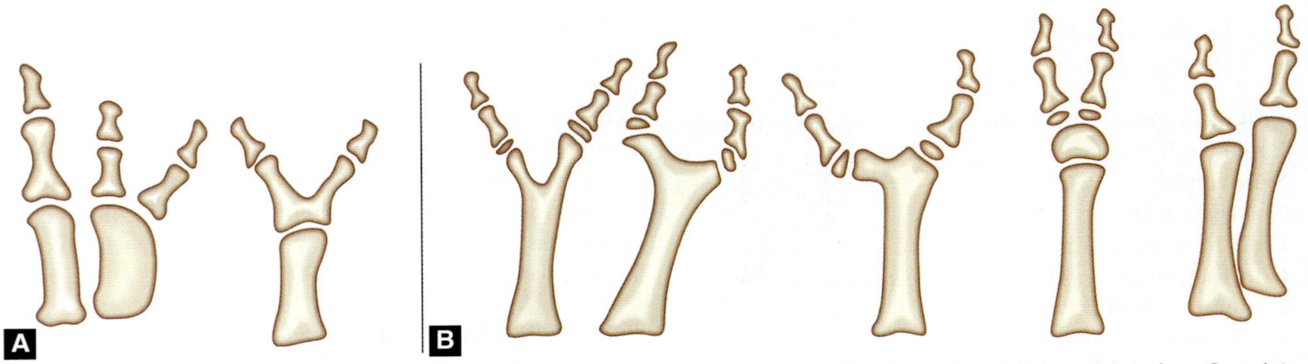

Figs 26.212A and B: Venn-Watson classification of polydactyly

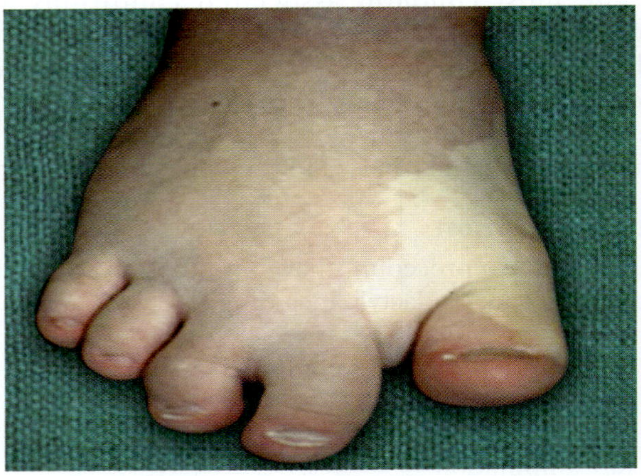

Fig. 26.213: Macrodactyly in foot

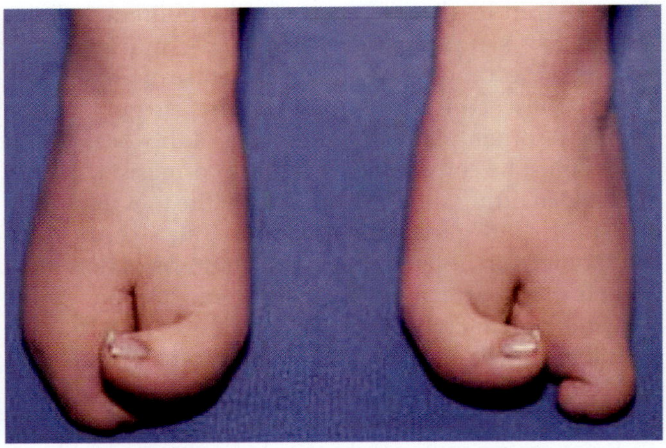

Fig. 26.214: Cleft foot

usually the convex to reduce the thickness by 10 to 20 percent. Three months later, deflating was done on the other side, along with shortening of the bone. In their technique an entire phalanx was removed, the capsules of the adjacent joints were sutured and a Kirschner wire was inserted for stabilization.

■ Cleft Foot (Partial Adactyly)

Cleft foot (lobster foot) is an anomaly in which a single cleft extends proximally into the foot, sometimes as far as the midfoot, as shown in Figure 26.214. Generally, one or more toes and parts of their metatarsals are absent, and often the tarsals are abnormal. Although the deformity varies in degree and type, the first and fifth rays usually are present.

If a metatarsal is partially or completely absent, its respective toe is always absent. Blauth and Borisch classified the deformities into six types based on the number of metatarsal bones present. Type I and type II are cleft feet with minor deficiencies, both having five metatarsals. The metatarsals are normal in type I and partially hypoplastic in type II. The number of identifiable metatarsals decreases progressively: Type III—four metatarsals; type IV—three metatarsals; type V—two metatarsals and type VI—one metatarsal. Abraham et al. described a simplified clinical classification, on which they based treatment recommendations. Type I has a central ray cleft or deficiency (usually second or third rays or both) extending up to the midmetatarsal level without splaying of medial or lateral rays. For this type of cleft foot, Abraham et al. recommended soft-tissue syndactylism with partial hallux valgus correction if needed. Type II has a deep cleft up to the tarsal bones with forefoot splaying, for which they recommended soft-tissue syndactylism, with first-ray osteotomy if needed, before age 5 years. Type III is a complete absence of the first through third or fourth rays, for which they did not

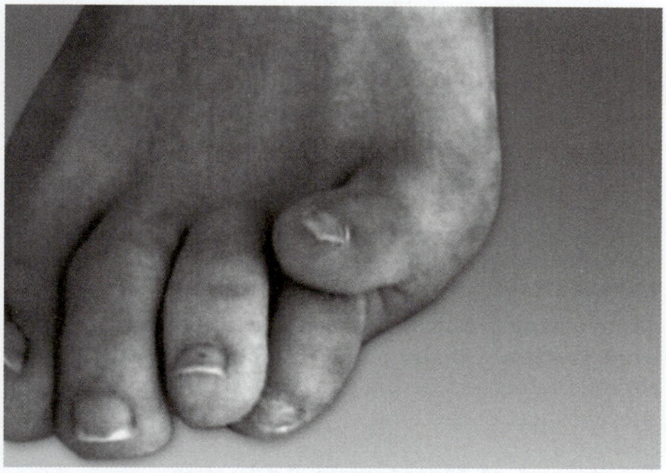

Fig. 26.215: Congenital contracture, angulation or subluxation of the fifth toe

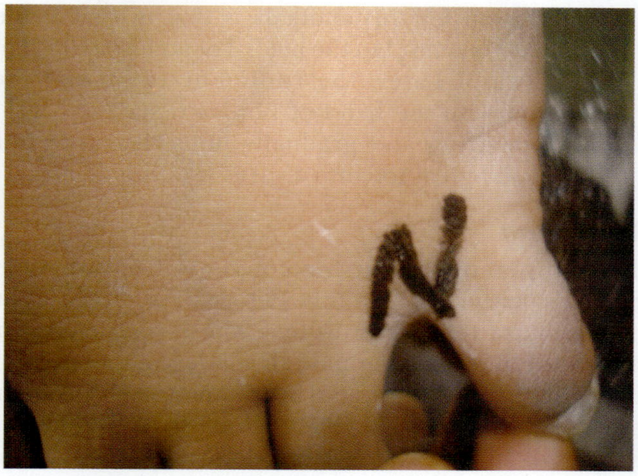

Fig. 26.216: Thordarson's, soft-tissue release and cutaneous Z-plasty used for correction of congenital over-riding fifth toe

recommend surgery. Abraham et al. recommended syndactylism for all type II cleft feet in the first 3 years of life while the forefoot is still supple. Any surgery for cleft foot should improve function and appearance. When the cleft extends proximally between the metatarsals, the skin of the apposing surfaces within the cleft is excised, but dorsal and plantar flaps are left that close the cleft when sutured together. If a metatarsal has no corresponding toe, it is resected, and the cleft is closed. Any bony or joint deformity of the first or fifth ray should be corrected at the time of surgery. This may require capsulotomies and osteotomies of any retained rays. If pin fixation is used, the pins and short leg cast are removed 6 weeks after surgery, and a short leg walking cast may be worn for an additional 4 to 6 weeks.

Contracture or Angulation of the Toes

Congenital contracture, angulation or subluxation of the fifth toe is a fairly common familial deformity, but rarely causes symptoms, as shown in Figure 26.215. The anomaly is rarely disabling, and surgery usually is indicated only to improve function of the foot. The direction of angulation of the fifth toe determines the operative procedure.

Surgical procedures for the correction of an angulated toe include:

- Soft-tissue correction alone
- Soft-tissue correction with proximal phalangectomy amputation
- Thordarson described a soft-tissue release and cutaneous Z-plasty used for correction of congenital overriding fifth toe, as shown in Figure 26.216.

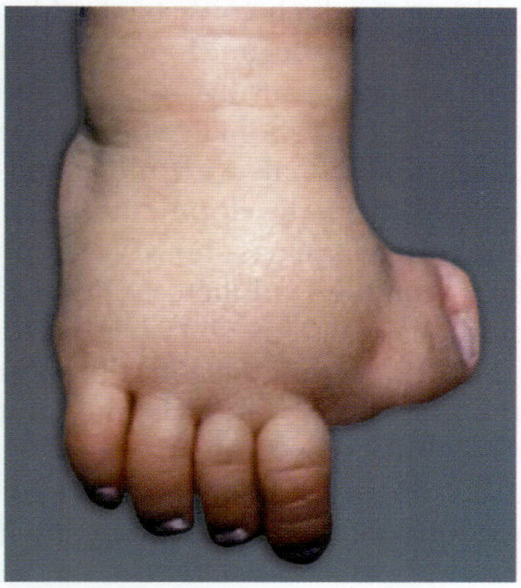

Fig. 26.217: Congenital hallux varus

Congenital Hallux Varus

Congenital hallux varus is a deformity in which the great toe is angled medially at the metatarsophalangeal joint. It should not be confused with varus deformity of the first metatarsal (metatarsus primus varus), in which the metatarsophalangeal joint is not deformed. The varus deformity of the toe varies in severity from only a few degrees to 90°, as shown in Figure 26.217. Congenital hallux varus usually is unilateral and is associated with one or more of the following:

- a short, thick first metatarsal,
- accessory bones or toes,
- varus deformity of one or more of the four lateral metatarsals and
- a firm fibrous band that extends from the medial side of the great toe to the base of the first metatarsal. The

explanation for this anomaly is that two great toes originate *in utero*, but the medial or accessory one fails to develop. Later, the rudimentary medial toe, together with the band of fibrous tissue, acts like a taut bowstring and gradually pulls the more fully developed great toe into a varus position.

Treatment

The proper treatment for congenital hallux varus depends on the severity of the deformity and the rigidity of the contracted soft structures. The Farmer technique is effective in correcting mild or moderate deformity. If the deformity is complicated by traumatic arthritis of the metatarsophalangeal joint, arthrodesis of this joint is indicated. In rare cases, if the deformity is too severe either to be corrected or to undergo arthrodesis, amputation is indicated.

■ Congenital Metatarsus Adductus

Metatarsus adductus, which consists of adduction of the forefoot in relation to the midfoot and hindfoot, is a common anomaly, often causing in-toeing in children. It can occur as an isolated anomaly or in association with clubfoot. Among individuals with metatarsus adductus, 1 to 5 percent also have developmental dysplasia of the hip or acetabular dysplasia as shown in Figure 26.218.

Clinically, metatarsus adductus can be classified as mild, moderate or severe, as described by Bleck. In the mild form, the forefoot can be clinically abducted to the midline of the foot and beyond. The moderate form has enough flexibility to allow abduction of the forefoot to the midline, but usually not beyond. In rigid metatarsus adductus, the forefoot cannot be abducted at all. There also may be a transverse crease on the medial border of the foot or an enlargement of the web space between the great and second toes. In general, mild metatarsus adductus resolves without treatment. Moderate or severe metatarsus adductus is best treated initially by serial stretching and casting for 6 to 12 weeks or until the foot is clinically flexible. Metatarsus adductus may be seen as a residual deformity in patients previously treated surgically or non-surgically for congenital clubfoot. This residual metatarsus adductus can be rigid, indicating fixed positioning of the forefoot on the midfoot and hindfoot or it can be dynamic, caused by imbalance of the anterior tibial tendon during gait. The rigidity or flexibility of the forefoot should be determined before undertaking any surgical correction in an older child. Late sequelae of metatarsus adductus may include an increased risk of stress fractures of the lateral metatarsal bones, due to altered biomechanics that placed greater loads across the lateral aspect of the foot.

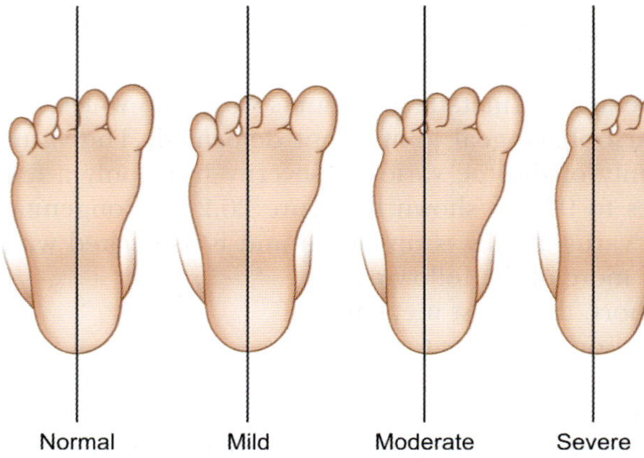

Fig. 26.218: Congenital metatarsus adductus

Treatment of Metatarsus Adductus

- Mild deformities resolve, hence require no treatment
- Serial stretching and casting, rarely indicated for moderate and severe deformities
- Surgery is indicated in severe deformity uncorrected by conservative treatment

Surgical indications include:

- Pain
- Objectionable appearance
- Difficulty in fitting shoes 2 to 4 years
- Tarsometatarsal capsulotomies (Heyman, Herndon and Strong)
- ≥4 year multiple metatarsal osteotomies (Berman and Gartland), medial cuneiform and lateral cuboid double osteotomy.

Berman and Gartland Metatarsal Osteotomy

Approach all five metatarsal bases dorsally. Make two longitudinal dorsal incisions, one between the first and second metatarsals and the other overlying the fourth. With a small power drill make a dome-shaped osteotomy in each with the apex of the dome proximally. Align the metatarsals and transfix the foot in the corrected position with small, smooth Steinmann pins inserted proximally through the shafts of the first and fifth metatarsals and across the osteotomies in these bones.

After Treatment

A short leg cast is applied with the foot in the corrected position. At 6 weeks, the cast and pins are removed and weight bearing is begun, commonly in a walking cast for 3 to 6 weeks.

■ Congenital Vertical Talus

Congenital vertical talus, rocker-bottom flatfoot, or congenital rigid flatfoot must be distinguished from flexible pes planus commonly seen in infants and children. Congenital vertical talus may be associated with numerous neuromuscular disorders, such as

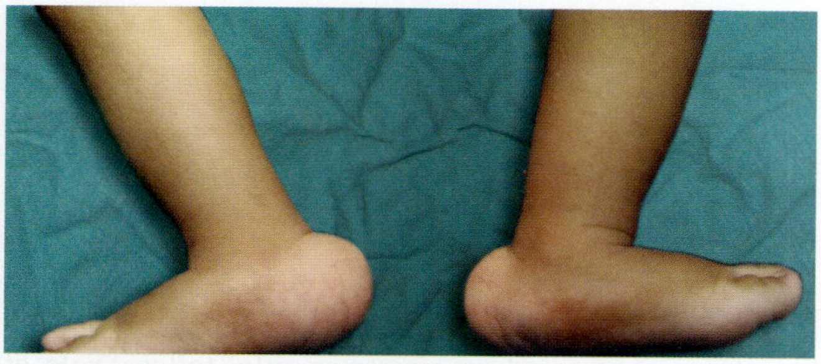

Fig. 26.219: Congenital vertical talus

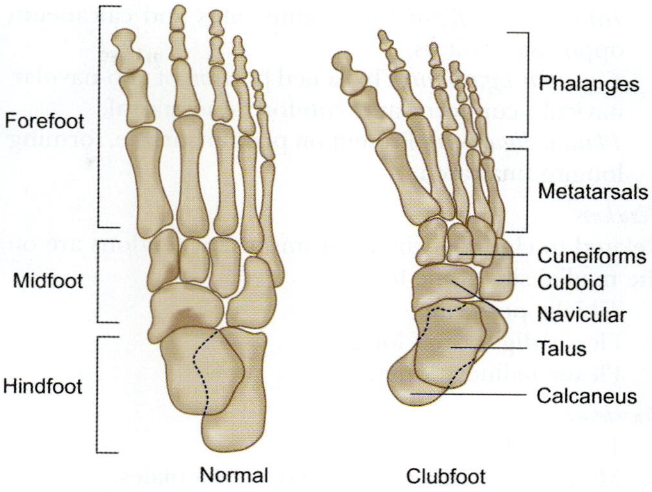

Fig. 26.220: Comparison of anatomy of normal foot and clubfoot

arthrogryposis and myelomeningocele, but it also may occur as an isolated congenital anomaly, as shown in Figure 26.219.

Congenital vertical talus usually can be detected at birth by the presence of a rounded prominence of the medial and plantar surfaces of the foot, produced by the abnormal location of the head of the talus. The talus is so distorted plantarward and medially as to be almost vertical. The calcaneus also is in an equinus position, but to a lesser degree. The forefoot is dorsiflexed at the midtarsal joints and the navicular lies on the dorsal aspect of the head of the talus. The sole is convex and there are deep creases on the dorsolateral aspect of the foot anterior and inferior to the lateral malleolus. As the foot develops and weight bearing is begun, adaptive changes occur in the tarsals. The talus becomes shaped like an hourglass, but remains in so marked an equinus position that its longitudinal axis is almost the same as that of the tibia and only the posterior third of its superior articular surface articulates with the tibia. The calcaneus remains in an equinus position also and becomes displaced posteriorly and the anterior part of its plantar surface becomes rounded. Callosities develop beneath the anterior end of the calcaneus and along the medial border of the foot superficial to the head of the talus. When full weight is borne, the forefoot becomes severely abducted and the heel does not touch the floor. Adaptive changes occur in the soft structures. All the capsules, ligaments and tendons on the dorsum of the foot become contracted. The posterior tibial and peroneus longus and brevis tendons may come to lie anterior to the malleoli and act as dorsiflexors rather than plantar flexors. Congenital vertical talus can be difficult to distinguish from severe pes planus, although the two can be differentiated by the use of appropriate radiographs. Routine radiographs should include anteroposterior and plantar flexion lateral views, the latter confirm the diagnosis of congenital vertical talus.

Treatment

Congenital vertical talus is difficult to correct and tends to recur. Gentle manipulations followed by immobilization in a cast are beneficial, however in that the skin, the fibrous tissue structures and the tendons on the anterior aspect of the foot and ankle are stretched. Reduction of the talonavicular joint rarely is possible by conservative means alone. Consequently, open reduction usually is necessary. The exact surgery indicated is determined by the age of the child and the severity of the deformity. In children, 1 to 4 years, open reduction and realignment of the talonavicular and subtalar joints is done. In children, 3-years-old or older, who have a severe deformity, navicular excision is required at the time of open reduction. In children, 4 to 8 years, open reduction and soft-tissue procedures combined with extra-articular subtalar arthrodesis and children of 12 years age or older are best treated by triple arthrodesis for permanent correction of the deformity.

Congenital Clubfoot (Talipes Equinovarus)

Relevant Anatomy (Fig. 26.220)

Joints

- Ankle joint between tibia and talus
- subtalar joint between talus and calcaneum
- Talo navicular joint
- Calcaneocuboid joint

Foot is divided into:

- Hindfoot
- Midfoot
- Forefoot

Ligaments

- *Deltoid ligaments:* This is the medial collateral ligament of ankle. It has superficial and deep component.
- *Spring ligament:* It joins anterior end of the calcaneum to the navicular.

- *Interosseous ligament:* It joins talus and calcaneum opposing surfaces.
- *Capsular ligament:* Thickened portion of talo-navular, naviculo-cuniform and cuniform-metatarsal.
- *Plantar ligament:* Present on plantar surface, forming longitudinal arch.

Tendons

Related to club foot the most important tendons are on the medial site of the foot:

- Tibialis posterior
- Flexor digitorium longus
- Flexor halluces longus

Incidence

- 1.2/1000 live births
- Males are commonly affected than females.

Types of CTEV (Etiology)

- *Osseous type:* Club-foot associated with absence of tibia and fibula and pseudoarthosis of tibia
- *Muscular type:* Arthrogryposis multiplex congenital
- *Neuropathic type:* Due to spina bifida
- *Idiopathic type:* Commonest variety.

Clinical Type

- *Mild:* All deformities are correctable
- *Moderate:* Two deformities are correctable
- *Severe:* All deformities are not correctable
- *Rigid severe:* CTEV of foot, relapsed recurrence of deformities after treatment
- Neglected CTEV.

Theories of CTEV

- Turco's medial displacement of navicular and calcaneum around talus
- Brockman's congenital atresia of talonavicular joint
- McKay's three-dimentional bony deformity of subtalar complex
- Intrauterine, due to compression of foetus *in utero*
- Genetic; general population 1:800 in sibling 1:3 and in twins 1:35
- *Germ plasm theory:* Germ plasm defect in talus and soft tissue changes
- *Soft tissue theory:* Soft tissue changes with bony defect
- *Prenatal muscle imbalance theory:* Weak pronators, overacting extensors and invertors.

Pathoanatomy

Soft tissue structures contracted on medial side follows rule of three:

Three muscles

- Flexor digitorum longus
- Tibialis posterior
- Flexor hallues longus

Three ligaments

- Deltoid
- Spring
- Plantar

Three capsules

- Subtalar
- Tarsal
- Tarsometatarsal joint

Structures contracted on posterior side, follows rule of two:

Two muscles

- Tibialis posterior
- Tendoachellis

Two ligaments:

- Talofibular
- Calcaneofibula

Two capsules

- Ankle joint
- Subtalar joint

Changes at bones and joints:

- *Calcaneus:* Varus position dorsiflexed
- *Talus:* Displaced medially and plantarwards
- *Navicular:* Medially displaced and rotated
- *Cuboid:* Displaced medially and articulated with non articular surface of calcaneum
- *Metatarsals:* Deviated medially
- *Tibia:* Medial torsion
- *Talocalcaneum articulation:* Dislocated in CTEV.

Clinical Features

In club-foot five classical primary deformities are present and in response secondary deformities are present, together they form Club foot complex.

Club Foot Complex

A. Primary deformities:
   - Equinus of ankle
   - Heel varus
   - Cavus of midfoot
   - Forefoot adduction
   - Internal tibial torsion

B. Secondary deformities:
   - Foot size is decreased in 50 percent
   - Medial border is concave and lateral border is convex
   - Forefoot is plantar flexed upon hindfoot
   - Skin is stretched upon dorsum of foot and deep skin creases on heel and medial side across the sole
   - Callosities are present over the lateral aspect of the dorsum of foot
   - Atrophy of muscles in posterior and anterior compartment of leg.
   - Bony prominence seen on lateral side of foot.

Severity assessment: Pirani score (given score from 0, 0.5 or 1 to each component). Maximum score is 10. Number of score usually correlates with number of casting needed. Other assessment–Dimeglio.

Examination of Foot

Dorsiflexion test: It is a screening test. In newborns it is possible to dorsiflex the foot till it is dorsum surface touches anterior part ot tibia. Not possible in CTEV.

Scratch test: It is performed to detect muscle imbalance.

Medial scratch test: Medial sole scratched, foot everts and test peroneals.

Lateral scratch test: Lateral sole scratch, foot inverts and test inverters.

Plumbline test: It detects tibial torsion. A line drawn from center of patella to tibial tubercle, when extended dow, cuts the foot at first and second intermetatarsal space normally. This is called plumbline. In CTEV due to medial rotation of tibia it cuts through third and fourth intermetatarsal space.

X-Ray (Fig. 26.221)

Radiograph is most important investigation. It helps to see the exact angle of deformity of CTEV. The most important angle is talocalcaneum on anterior and lateral view. The other angles are talometatarsal on anterior view and tibiocalcaneal on lateral view.

Normal range of radiographic angles for comparison to clubfoot (Figs 26.222A and B)

- *Talocalcaneal angle:*
  - Anteroposterior view: 30° to 55°
  - Dorsiflexion lateral view: 25° to 50°
- *Tibiocalcaneal angle:*
  - Stress lateral view: 10° to 40°
- *Talus–first metatarsal angle:*
  - Anteroposterior view: 5° to 15°

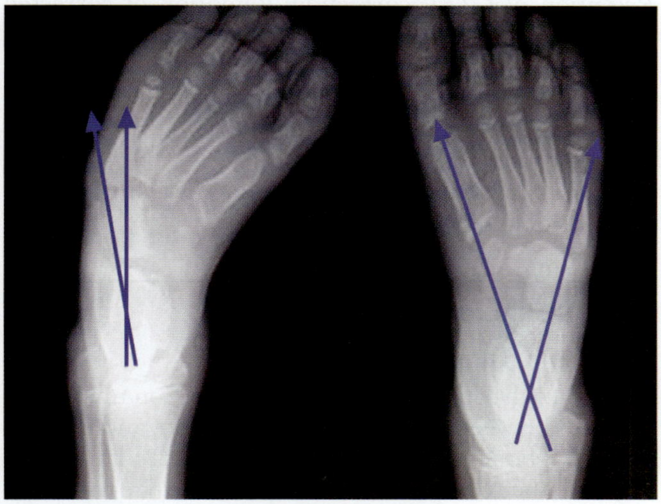

Fig. 26.221: X-ray angles in CTEV

Talocalcaneal-Index

The formula for talocalcaneal-index (TC-index) is given below:

TC-index = TC angle (AP view + lateral view of TC angle)

It should be at least 40°, which is less in CTEV. The study of talocalcaneal angle on the radiographs, indicates the extent of varus. Other angles are:

- Talometatarsal
- Tibiocalcaneal.

Management in CTEV

- Conservative management.
- Surgical management.
- External fixation (Jess).

Conservative Management

Manipulation alone: Birth to 30 days. In newborn manipulation is done by mother. She is taught to dorsiflex and evert the foot. Maintain it for 5s and to repeat it after every 5 minutes.

Manipulation with casting: Three months to one year by Ponseti or Kites method. At one month of age, deformities are corrected by subsequent casting in following order every 2 weeks for 6 to 8 weeks (Kite's method)

- Forefoot adduction (AD)
- Varus of heel (V)
- Equinus of hindfoot (E)

This order is followed to prevent Rocker Bottom foot (RB).

Ponseti technique: There is a specific technique of deformity correction, specific order of deformity correction and specific technique of serial casting. Success rate >90 percent with Ponseti technique.

- Specific order of deformity correction include:
  - *Correct the cavus:* By supinating the forefoot
  - *Correct the forefoot adduction:* By abducting the forefoot with other thumb pressing on the talar head. This also corrects the hindfoot varus, by letting the talus rotates on the calcaneum.
  - *Correct the equines:* By TA (heel cord) tenotomy

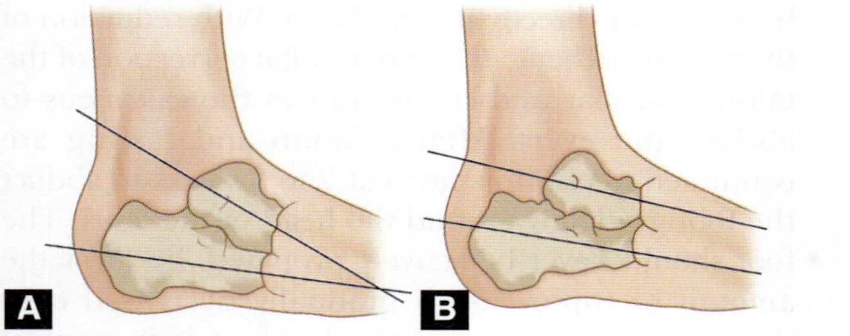

Figs 26.222A and B: (A) Normal angle of the calcaneous to talus axes, upon dorsiflexion of baby's normal foot; (B) Abnormal parallel calcaneus and talus axes, upon dorsiflexion of baby's clubfoot

- Specific technique of serial casting include:
  - Above knee casting with 90° flexion, to prevent dislodging
  - Proper moulding just above the heel and behind the knee, to prevent dislodging as well
  - Weekly serial casting to enhance manipulation and correction
  - Remove the cast just about to reapply the new one (to maximize time in cast)

The Ponseti method consists of two phases:
1. Treatment phase
2. Maintenance phase.

1. *Treatment phase:* The treatment phase should begin as early as possible, optimally within the first week of life. Gentle manipulation and casting are done weekly. Each cast holds the foot in the corrected position, allowing it to reshape gradually. Generally, five to six casts are required to correct the alignment of the foot and ankle fully. At the time of the final cast, most infants (≥ 70%) require percutaneous Achilles tenotomy to gain adequate lengthening of the Achilles tendon. The first cast application corrects the cavus deformity by aligning the forefoot with the hindfoot, supinating the forefoot to bring it in line with the heel and elevating (dorsiflexing) the first metatarsal. It may be easier to apply the cast in two stages: first, a short leg cast to just below the knee, then extension above the knee, when the plaster sets. Long leg casts are essential to maintain a strong external rotation force of the foot, beneath the talus and to allow adequate stretching of the medial structures, especially the posterior tibial tendon. One week after application, the first cast is removed and after about 1 minute of manipulation, the next toe-to-groin cast is applied. Manipulation and casting at this stage are focused on abducting the foot around the head of the talus, with care to maintain the supinated position of the forefoot and avoid any pronation. During these manipulations, the navicular can be felt reducing over the talar head, by a thumb placed on the head of the talus (left thumb for a right clubfoot and right thumb for a left clubfoot).

   A crucial point in the Ponseti technique is that the heel is never directly manipulated. With reduction of the talar head beneath the navicular, correction of the talus, navicular and cuboid causes the calcaneus to abduct and evert. Manipulation and casting are continued weekly for the next 2 to 3 weeks to abduct the foot gradually around the head of the talus. The foot should never be actively pronated, however the amount of supination is gradually decreased over these several casts, until the forefoot is in neutral position relative to the longitudinal axis of the foot. The final cast is applied with the foot in the same maximally abducted position and dorsiflexed 15°. In most children, a percutaneous Achilles tenotomy is done to prevent development of a rocker-bottom deformity. The foot is casted in the final position of approximately 70° of abduction and 15° of dorsiflexion for 3 weeks. Five or six casts usually are necessary to correct the clubfoot deformity.
2. *Maintenance phase*: When the final cast is removed, the infant is placed in a brace that maintains the foot in its corrected position (abducted and dorsiflexed). The brace (foot abduction orthosis) consists of shoes mounted to a bar in a position of 70° of external rotation and 15° of dorsiflexion. The distance between the shoes is set at about 1 inch wider than the width of the infant's shoulders. This brace is worn 23 hours each day for the first 3 months after casting and then while sleeping for 2 to 3 years. Bony surgeries are done from 4 to 11 years.

Dwyer's osteotomy: Open-wedge osteotomy of calcaneum to correct the varus of the heel. Minimum age is 4 years.

Dilwyn-Evan's procedure: It consists of soft tissue release with calcaneocuboid fusion. Neglected and recutorent CTEV between 4 and 8 years.

Wedge osteotomy: Wedge of bone from the midtarsal area is removed. Wedge is cut on dorsal lateral side. Neglected culbfeet between 8 and 11 years.

Triple arthrodesis: Fusion of three joints of foot subtalar, calcaneocuboid and talonavicular. Performed after 12 years of age. Jess is done after 2 years. Different components are corrected by gradual stretching using external fixator. Works on principle of differential distraction. Jess is gradual, controlled supervised deformity correction. Medial side is 1 mm is distracted and lateral side 0.5 mm is distracted. Till all the deformities are corrected, maintain the correction for the same period, it took to correct the deformity. Then remove the fixator and POP cast is given or CTEV shoes.

Retention of CTEV correction: Retention of corrected deformity is done by one of the following methods to prevent relaspe:
- Dennis Browne splint, used during night
- Phelps Brace, used during daytime
- Below knee walking calliper
- CTEV shoes, used when child starts walking up to 5 years of age.

■ Tarsal Coalition

What is a Tarsal Coalition?

A tarsal coalition is an abnormal connection/union that develops between two bones in the hindfoot and midfoot (the tarsal bones), as shown in Figure 26.223. This union may be either complete or incomplete and the condition may be congenital or acquired.

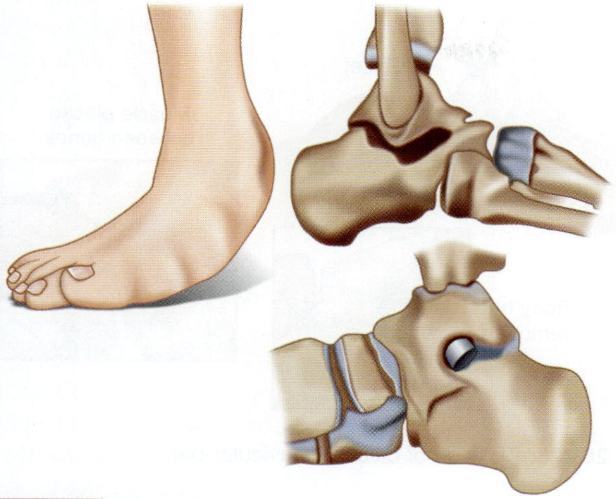

Fig. 26.223: Tarsal coalition

Coalitions can be:
- Bony (synostosis)
- Cartilaginous (synchondrosis)
- Fibrous (syndesmosis)

Classification

The classification of tarsal coalitions is based on the bones affected. The two most common types (comprise the majority):
- Calcaneonavicular
- Talocalcaneal

Although, calcaneocuboid, talonavicular and cubonavicular tarsal fusions also occur, they are less common. Sometimes the conditions are also called calcaneonavicular bar and talocalcaneal bar. The term "bar" refers to the abnormal "bar of bone" between the two bones. There is not a fully formed bar of bone between the two bones of the coalition in every case.

Pathophysiology

Congenital or developmental, coalition appears to represent a failure of primitive mesenchymal differentiation. It is possible for some coalitions to resolve during childhood, as a result of weight-bearing biomechanical activity. Inherited as an autosomal dominant trait with almost complete penetrance. Acquired secondary to trauma, infection, surgery or articular disorders. Tarsal fusions can be associated with other musculoskeletal conditions, such as hand-foot-uterus syndrome, carpal coalition, symphalangism, arthrogryposis, Apert syndrome (acrocephalosyndactyly) and Nievergelt-Pearlman syndrome.

Frequency

Most investigators report that tarsal coalition has an incidence of 1 percent or less. The rate may be higher because patients are commonly asymptomatic and tarsal coalition is incidentally discovered. Bilateral coalitions occur in approximately 50 percent of cases, and they are most often associated with calcaneonavicular coalition. Talocalcaneal and calcaneonavicular coalitions account for approximately 90 percent of the cases of tarsal coalitions.

Sex: Most investigators note a slight male predominance.
Age: Patients usually experience symptoms during their second decade of life. Once ossification of the coalition occurs, the patient may begin experiencing pain due to restrictions in motion.

Signs and Symptoms

While many people who have a tarsal coalition are born with this condition, the symptoms generally do not appear until the bones begin to mature, usually around ages 9 to 16 years. The signs and symptoms of tarsal coalition may include one or more of the following:
- Pain (mild to severe) when walking or standing. Pain is usually located on the outside of the foot just below the fibula
- Tired or fatigued legs
- Muscle spasms in the leg, causing the foot to turn outward when walking
- Flatfoot (in one or both feet)
- Walking with a limp
- Stiffness of the foot and ankle.

Diagnosis

- A tarsal coalition is difficult to identify until a child's bones begin to mature.
- In addition to examining the foot, the surgeon will order X-rays.
- AP, lateral and oblique projections are generally considered for the visualization of the coalitions.
- Calcaneonavicular coalition is viewed best on a 45° internal oblique radiograph, as shown in Figures 26.224A and B.
- Talocalcaneal coalitions, shown in Figure 26.225.

Harris-Beath (axial) views of the hindfoot are useful for visualizing the posterior and middle facets. With the ankle slightly dorsiflexed at 10°, the beam is directed through the hindfoot at a 45° angle. The angle is adjusted if the facets are still not well demonstrated. Obliteration or irregularity of the facets is indicative of a coalition. Additional diagnostic imaging tests, such as a CT scan or MRI may also be needed.

Treatment

Non-surgical Approaches

The goal of non-surgical treatment of tarsal coalition is to relieve the symptoms and reduce the motion at the affected joint. One or more of the following options may

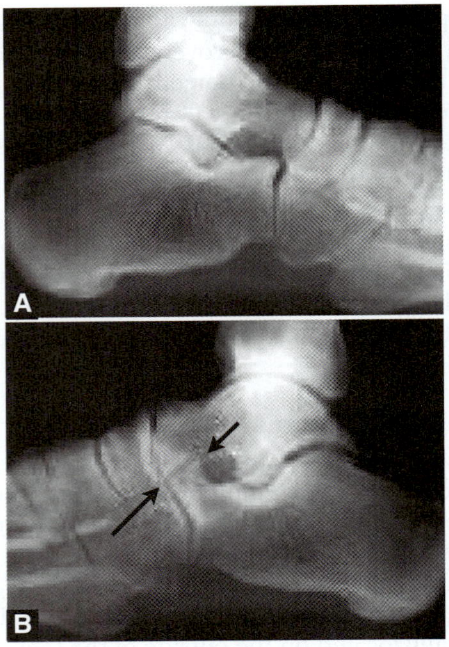

Figs 26.224A and B: Calcaneonavicular coalition is viewed best on a 45° internal oblique radiograph. Arrows showing coailation

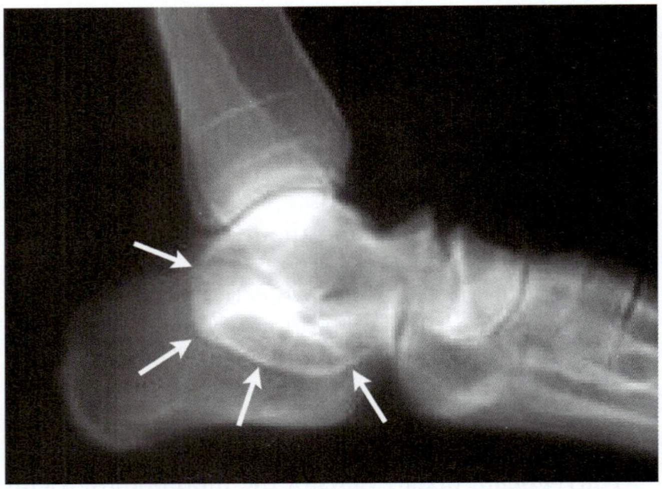

Fig. 26.225: Arrows showing talocalcaneal coalitions

be used, depending on the severity of the condition and the response to treatment:

Oral medications: Non-steroidal anti-inflammatory drugs (NSAIDs), such as ibuprofen, may be helpful in reducing the pain and inflammation.

Physical therapy: Physical therapy may include massage, range-of-motion exercises, and ultrasound therapy.

Orthotic devices: Custom orthotic devices can be beneficial in distributing weight away from the joint, limiting motion at the joint and relieving pain.

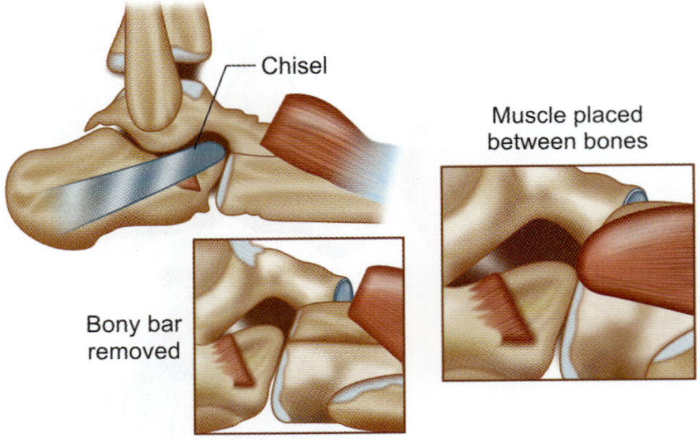

Fig. 26.226: Excision of calcaneonavicular bar

Steroid injections: An injection of cortisone into the affected joint reduces the inflammation and pain. Sometimes more than one injection is necessary.

Immobilization: Sometimes the foot is immobilized to give the affected area a rest. The foot is placed in a cast or cast boot and crutches are used to avoid placing weight on the foot.

Injection of an anesthetic agent: Injection of an anesthetic into the leg may be used to relax spasms and is often performed prior to immobilization.

Surgical Approaches

If the patient's symptoms are not adequately relieved with non-surgical treatment, surgery is an option. Surgery for tarsal coalition falls into two categories:

- To remove or excise the bar and attempt to restore normal motion between the two bones
- To fuse the affected joints together solidly
  - Excision of calcaneonavicular bar (Fig. 26.226)
  - Excision of talocalcaneal bar (Fig. 26.227)
  - Subtalar arthrodesis (Fig. 26.228)
  - Triple arthrodesis (Fig. 26.229).

Tibial Hemimelia

First described by Otto in 1941. Tibial hemimelia is a rare anomaly, characterized by deficiency of the tibia with relatively intact fibula. Also known as congenital longitudinal deficiency of the tibia, congenital dysplasia of the tibia, paraxial tibial hemimelia, tibial dysplasia and congenital deficiency or absence of the tibia, as shown in Figure 26.230. It may present as an isolated anomaly or be associated with a variety of skeletal and extraskeletal malformations, as illustrated in Figure 26.231.

Associated syndromes (Fig. 26.232): At least four distinct syndromes have tibial hemimelia as a component:

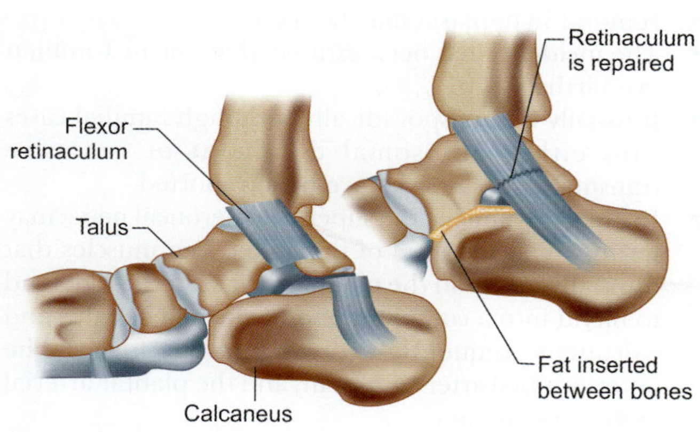

Fig. 26.227: Excision of talocalcaneal bar

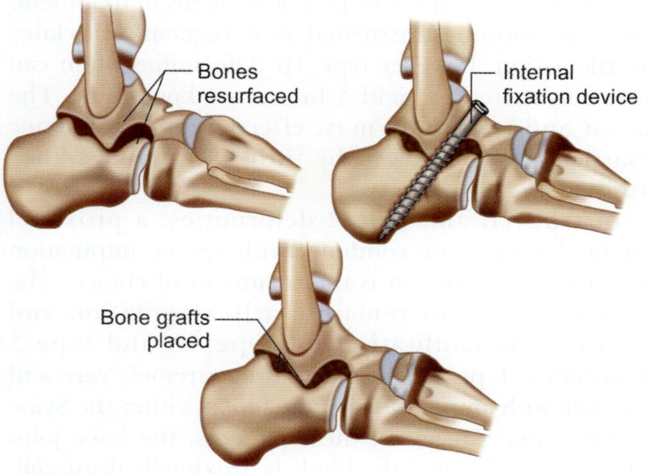

Fig. 26.228: Subtalar arthrodesis

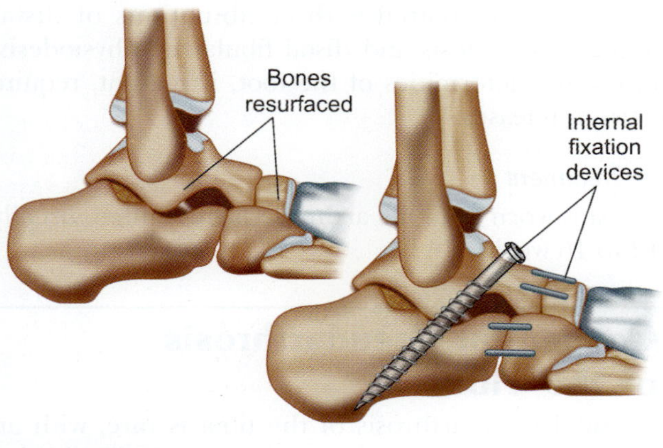

Fig. 26.229: Triple arthrodesis

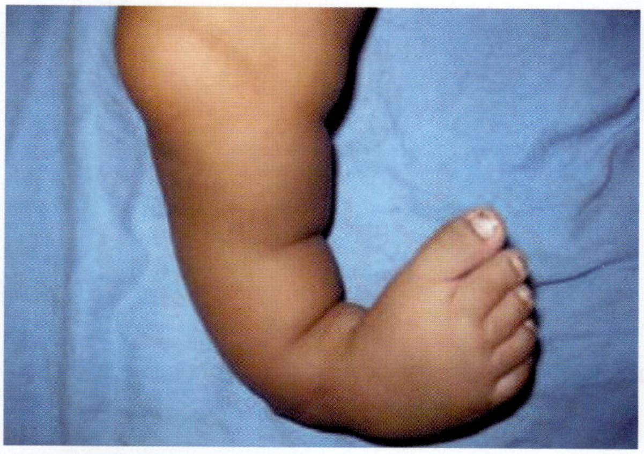

Fig. 26.230: Tibial hemimelia

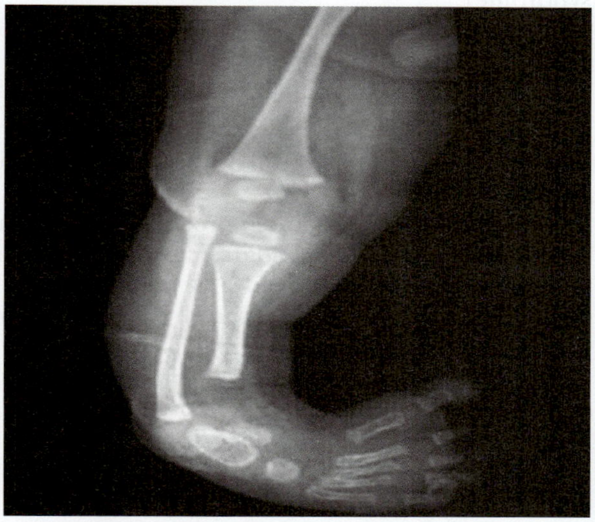

Fig. 26.231: Tibial hemimelia, may present as an isolated anomaly or be associated with a variety of skeletal and extraskeletal malformations

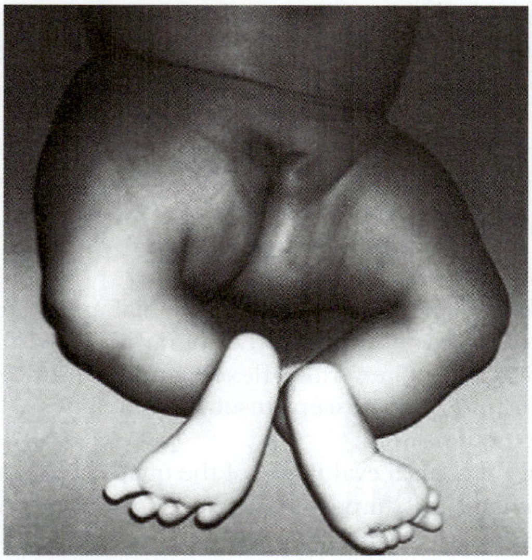

Fig. 26.232: Tibial hemimelia with associated syndromes

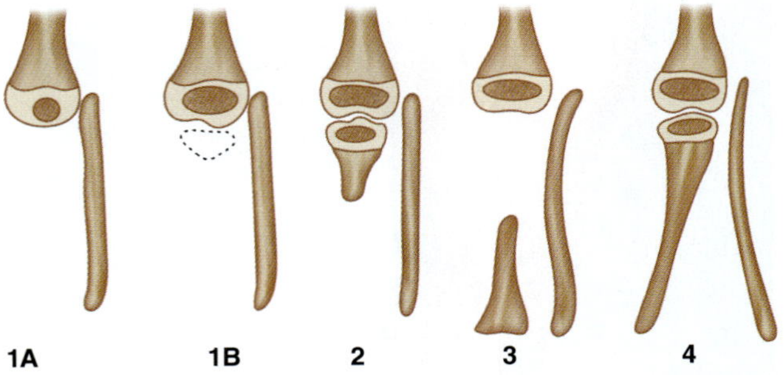

Fig. 26.233: Jones classification of tibial hemimelia (based on radiological criteria)

- Polydactyly triphalangeal thumb syndrome (Werner syndrome)
- Tibial hemimelia diplopodia
- Tibial hemimelia–split hand/foot syndrome
- Tibial hemimelia–micromelia–trigonal brachycephaly syndrome.

Jones classification (Based on radiological criteria) (Fig. 26.233)

- In type 1A, fibula is dislocated proximally, tibia is not radiographically evident and distal femoral epiphysis is smaller than on normal side
- In type 1B, fibula is dislocated proximally and proximal tibial cartilaginous anlage may be visible at birth on ultrasound or MRI, but not on plain radiographs
- Type 2 deformity has proximal dislocation of fibula and radiographically visible proximal tibia with normal-appearing knee joint
- In type 3 deformity, fibula is dislocated proximally, distal tibia is radiographically visible, but proximal tibia is not seen
- In rare type 4 deformity, fibula has migrated proximally, with diastasis of distal tibiofibular joint (congenital diastasis of the ankle joint and congenital tibiofibular diastasis).

Presentation

- The involved leg is short, and the fibular head is palpable, if it is proximally displaced
- The foot is held in severe equinovarus and the hindfoot is stiff
- In older children, the proximal tibial anlage may be palpable, even if it is not radiographically visible.
- The knee is generally flexed and in more severe deformities, quadriceps insufficiency causes a lack of knee extension
- Careful clinical evaluation of the quadriceps extensor mechanism is important because this has significant prognostic value regarding the potential for reconstruction of the knee
- Femoral hypoplasia may be seen
- The incidence has been estimated at one in 1 million live births
- It usually occurs sporadically, although familial cases with either autosomal dominant or recessive transmission patterns have been reported
- In tibial hemimelia, the superficial peroneal nerve may terminate at the level of the ankle. Leg muscles that normally insert on the plantar surface of the foot tend to blend into a common tendon sheet. The talus and calcaneus frequently are congenitally fused. The anterior tibial artery is absent, and the plantar arterial arch is incomplete.

Treatment

The type of surgical treatment depends on the radiographic classification and clinical appearance. For severe deficiencies, amputation and prosthetic rehabilitation are the most practical means of treatment. Type 1A deformities are treated most frequently with knee disarticulation, however type 1B deformities often can be reconstructed to yield a functional knee joint. The easiest and frequently most effective option is knee disarticulation, followed by fitting with above-knee prosthesis.

In type 1B and type 2 deformities, a proximal tibiofibular synostosis combined with a Syme amputation or distal reconstruction is the treatment of choice. The primary treatment remains early amputation and prosthetic rehabilitation for type 1A and type 3 deformities. Type 3 deficiencies are extremely rare and is treated with amputations of the foot at either the Syme or the Chopart level. In these patients, the knee joint generally is stable and the fibula is proximally displaced. These patients function well as below-knee amputees. In some patients, tibiofibular synostosis may be possible.

For patients with type 4 deficiencies, treatment must be individualized. Syme amputation provides excellent function. Customized reconstruction of the ankle joint, to retain the foot and ankle also has been described. Most patients can be treated with combinations of distal tibiofibular synostosis and distal fibular epiphysiodesis. Equinovarus deformities of the foot, if present, require soft-tissue releases.

After Treatment

The cast is worn until the arthrodesis has united, usually at 12 to 16 weeks.

■ Congenital Pseudarthrosis of the Tibia

Congenital pseudarthrosis of the tibia is rare, with an incidence of approximately one in 250,000 live births.

Most large series report 50 to 90 percent association of this disorder with the stigmata of neurofibromatosis, including skin and osseous lesions.

Classification (Boyd)

Boyd classified congenital pseudarthrosis of the tibia into the following six types:

Type I: Pseudarthrosis occurs with anterior bowing and a defect in the tibia present at birth. Other congenital deformities also may be present and these may affect the management of the pseudarthrosis.

Type II: Pseudarthrosis occurs with anterior bowing and an hourglass constriction of the tibia present at birth. Spontaneous fracture or fracture after minor trauma, commonly occurs before 2 years of age. This is the so-called high-risk tibia. The tibia is tapered, rounded and sclerotic and the medullary canal is obliterated. This type is the most common, is often associated with neurofibromatosis, and has the poorest prognosis. Recurrence of the fracture is common during the growth period, but decreases in frequency with age and generally ceases to occur after skeletal maturation.

Type III: Pseudarthrosis develops in a congenital cyst, usually near the junction of the middle and distal thirds of the tibia. Anterior bowing may precede or follow the development of a fracture. Recurrence of the fracture after treatment is less common than in type II and excellent results after only one operation have been reported to last well into adulthood.

Type IV: Pseudarthrosis originates in a sclerotic segment of bone in the classic location without narrowing of the tibia. The medullary canal is partially or completely obliterated. An "insufficiency" or "stress" fracture develops in the cortex of the tibia and gradually extends through the sclerotic bone. With completion of the fracture, healing fails to occur and the fracture widens and becomes a pseudarthrosis. The prognosis for this type generally is good, especially when it is treated before the insufficiency fracture becomes complete.

Type V: Pseudarthrosis of the tibia occurs with a dysplastic fibula. A pseudarthrosis of the fibula or tibia or both may develop. The prognosis is good, if the lesion is confined to the fibula. If the lesion progresses to a tibial pseudarthrosis, the natural history usually resembles that of type II pseudarthrosis.

Type VI: Pseudarthrosis occurs as an intraosseous neurofibroma or schwannoma that results in a pseudarthrosis. This is extremely rare. The prognosis depends on the aggressiveness and treatment of the intraosseous lesion.

Treatment

Treatment of congenital pseudarthrosis of the tibia depends on the age of the patient and the type of pseudarthrosis. A true congenital pseudarthrosis of the tibia does not heal when treated by casting alone. The decision must be made, whether to attempt to secure union or if amputation is the treatment of choice. Factors favoring amputation include, anticipated shortening of more than 2 or 3 inches (5–7.5 cm), a history of multiple failed surgical procedures and stiffness and decreased function of a limb that would be more useful after an amputation and fitting with a prosthesis. For the tibia with a cyst in the medullary canal (type III), prophylactic curettage and autogenous iliac bone grafting are recommended. The limb is immobilized in plaster, until the graft has united and then a patellar tendon-bearing brace is worn, until skeletal maturity is reached. A tibia with anterior bowing and a narrow, sclerotic canal (type II or the high-risk tibia) often fractures during the first 2 years of life. Initially, bracing may be beneficial for an anterolaterally bowed tibia with a narrow canal, in which a fracture has not developed. Well-adjusted knee-ankle-foot orthosis, with an anterior shield in the prepseudarthrotic stage delayed fracture and pseudarthrosis and allowed patients to reach an older age before undergoing surgical treatment. When a fracture does occur, the treatment is surgery.

In an infant or young child, bone grafting is indicated as early as feasible. Although, the likelihood of obtaining union increases with increasing age, especially after puberty, the longer grafting is delayed, the shorter and more poorly developed the leg will be. When union is obtained in a young child, weight bearing in a brace results in more normal development of the limb. Bone grafting procedures remain the mainstay of treatment for congenital pseudarthrosis of the tibia. The most commonly used technique in recent years is the intramedullary rodding technique described by Anderson. A more recent technique is the free vascularized bone graft with either fibular or iliac crest grafts. The procedure requires experience with microvascular techniques. For most established pseudarthrosis, initial treatment should be intramedullary rodding and bone grafting. Vascularized fibular grafts may be indicated for pseudarthroses, with gaps of more than 3 cm and for pseudarthroses, in which multiple surgical procedures have failed.

FRACTURES OF THE FOOT AND ANKLE JOINT

Ankle Fractures

Ankle fractures are among the most common fractures treated by surgeons. Incidence of various fracture patterns:

- *Isolated malleolar fractures:* Two-thirds of ankle fracture
- *Bimalleolar fractures:* One-fourth of ankle fracture
- *Trimalleolar fractures:* 7 percent.

Classification

- A number of methods are available to classify the ankle fractures. Simple way is to describe the fracture in terms of:
  - Open or closed
  - Status of the overlying soft tissues (blister, swelling)
  - Bony structure involved (bimalleolar or trimalleolar)
- Another method is to classify in terms of:
  - *Stable fractures:* No displacement and are able to withstand physiologic forces.
  - *Unstable fractures:* Medial or posterior malleolar fractures, medial clear space widening or tibio-fibular disruption. This guides the method of treatment.
- Systematic classifications are:
  - Lauge-Hansen classification
  - Danis-Weber classification
  - OTA classification

Lauge-Hansen Classification

It is based on the fracture patterns observed from a series of experiments by Lauge-Hansen, in which cadaveric ankles were placed in either supination or pronation and loaded to failure by either a translational or rotational force. In the Lauge-Hansen system, the injury starts at the tension side of the ankle and proceeds in the direction of the applied force.

Supination-External-Rotation Pattern

Four designations of this fracture are numbered from 1 to 4, as follows:

1. Supination external rotation 1 describes failure of the anterior talofibular ligament (essentially an ankle sprain).
2. Supination external rotation 2 describes a fracture of the fibula tipically a posterolateral distal fragment with the anteromedial fracture line at the level of the plafond.
3. Supination external rotation 3 is failure of the posterior inferior tibiofibular ligament or a posterior malleolar fracture (Volkman's fracture).
4. Supination external rotation 4 describes a medial malleolus fracture or deltoid ligament rupture.

Supination-Adduction (SAD) Pattern

- Supination-adduction 1 injuries involve a fracture of the lateral malleolus, at the level of the joint line or more distal (typically transverse).
- Supination-adduction 2 injuries have an additional vertical fracture of the medial malleolus.

Pronation-External Rotation Injuries

- Pronation-external rotation 1 injuries begin with a fracture of the medial malleolus.
- Pronation-external rotation 2 injuries involve a failure of the anterior tibiofibular ligament.
- Pronation-external rotation 3 injuries demonstrate a high oblique or spiral fibula fracture beginning above the level of the joint.
- Pronation-external rotation 4 fractures add an injury to the posterior tibiofibular ligament or posterior malleolus fracture.

Pronation-Abduction Injuries

Fracture of the medial malleolus or rupture of the deltoid ligament. This is followed by a failure of the anterior tibiofibular ligament. Progressive force leads to a high (above the joint line) comminuted fracture of the fibula, as shown in Figure 26.234.

Danis-Weber Classification

Danis-Weber classification is based on location and appearance of fibula fracture, as shown in Figure 26.235.

- *Type A below syndesmosis:* Internal rotation and adduction
- *Type B at level of syndesmosis:* External rotation leads to oblique fracture
- *Type C above syndesmosis:*
  - C1: Abduction injuries with oblique fracture of the fibula proximal to the disrupted tibiofibular ligaments.
  - C2: Abduction-external rotation injuries, with a more proximal fracture of the fibula and more extensive disruption of the interosseous membrane.

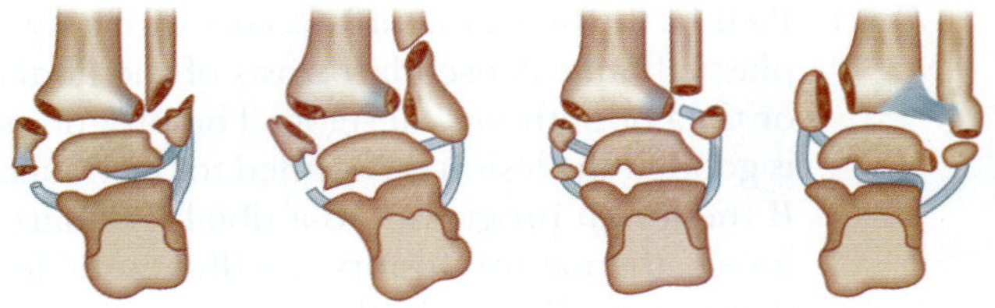

Fig. 26.234: Pronation-abduction injuries

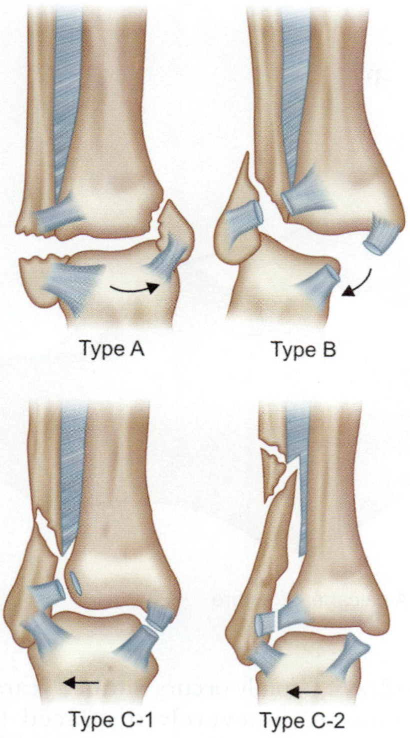

Fig. 26.235: Danis-Weber classification of ankle fractures

It was felt that Weber A fractures could be treated non-operatively, Weber B fractures required stabilization of the fibula and Weber C fractures required syndesmotic stabilization, in addition to fixation of the fibula.

AO/OTA Classification

Type A: Fibula fracture below syndesmosis (infra-syndesmotic)
- A1—isolated
- A2—with fracture of medial malleolus
- A3—with a posteromedial fracture

Type B: Fibula fracture at level of syndesmosis (trans-syndesmotic)
- B1—isolated
- B2—with medial lesion (malleolus or ligament)
- B3—with a medial lesion and fracture of posterolateral tibia.

Type C: Fibula fracture above syndesmosis (suprasyndesmotic)
- C1—diaphyseal fracture of the fibula, simple
- C2—diaphyseal fracture of the fibula, complex
- C3—proximal fracture of the fibula.

Clinical Presentation

These fractures result from low energy torsional forces and present with swelling, deformity and inability to bear weight.

Examine the following:
- Condition of the skin
- Neurovascular status
- Tenderness over tibia, fibula and midfoot
- Squeeze to rule out syndesmotic injury

Radiology

Three views (AP, lataral and mortise) should be obtained and evaluated for fracture and talar subluxation or dislocation. Evaluation of the talocrural angle, medial clear space and tibiofibular clear space will aid in determining proper alignment. The talocrural angle is the angle subtended by a line drawn parallel to the articular surface of the plafond and one connecting the tips of the malleoli. The angle is normally 4° to 11°. Medial clear space distance greater than 4 mm or greater than the superior clear space is a sign of lateral talar subluxation. Syndesmotic clear space greater than 6 mm on either view, indicates injury to the syndesmosis.

Treatment

Primary Management

Dislocation, if present should be reduced on emergency basis. Goal is to reduce the talus under the tibial plafond, to minimize the amount of abnormal soft tissue pressure, which can lead to pressure ischemia. Any open injuries should be cleared of gross debris and covered with a sterile dressing and appropriate prophylactic antibiotics should be administered. The ankle should be immobilized in a well padded splint and the extremity elevated to minimize soft tissue swelling. In undisplaced and radiographically stable fractures, definitive treatment is ankle support (short leg cast, CAM walker, air cast) with a brief period of protected weight bearing. For fractures that are displaced, but an anatomic reduction is achieved, these fractures may be treated in a long leg cast with frequent radiographic assessment. For displaced or unstable fractures, operative fixation is often indicated. It has been shown that even a 1 mm lateral talar shift, results in a 42 percent increase in contact loading of the tibiotalar joint, which may lead to early post-traumatic arthritis.

Methods of Fibular Fixation

Traditional fixation consists of a lateral approach, followed by direct manual reduction, placement of a lag screw and lateral neutralization plating. Recent locking plate technology may provide stronger fixation and allow for bridge plating in severely comminuted fractures. In SER injuries, posterolateral plating has the advantage of counteracting the fracture deformation forces and posterior to anterior distal screw placement (taking advantage of the longer AP diameter and the stronger bone on the posterior surface). Posterior antiglide plating (using the plate to assist in fracture reduction), may be employed for oblique fractures that displace posteriorly.

Long oblique fractures in a stable ankle may be amenable to lag screw fixation only. Intramedullary rods and K-wires have also been used as primary or supplemental fixation for more proximal injuries.

Methods of Fixation of Medial Malleolus

Transverse medial malleolus fractures are often stabilized with one or two screws in a lag fashion. Tension banding with Kirschner wires can be employed for small fracture fragments. For vertical fractures of the supination-adduction type, a medial antiglide plate or transverse lag screw placement is effective.

Posterior Malleolus

The posterior malleolus often is effectively reduced when the fibula is stabilized. Indications for operative fixation include:

- Greater than 25 to 30 percent involvement of the plafond
- Greater than 2 mm step off
- The posterior malleolus may be stabilized with lag screws from an anterior or posterior direction or with a posteriorly placed buttress plate.

Syndesmotic Injuries

There has to be anatomic reduction, restoration of fibular length and rotation. The syndesmosis may be stabilized via a number of methods and techniques. Two screws are more stable than one screw and 3.5 mm and 4.5 mm screws perform similarly. A fully threaded screw placed from the fibula to the tibia engaging either 3 or 4 cortices can stabilize the syndesmosis. Some authors prefer three cortices, as this theoretically allows some motion at the syndesmosis, which is thought to be more physiologic. Larger screws placed over four cortices are easier to remove, especially when broken. Additionally, the screw breakage rate is lower when three cortices are engaged. However, some authors prefer the increased rigidity of four cortices. The timing of weight bearing and whether to remove the screw prior to allowing weight bearing is controversial. Newer methods of syndesmotic fixation, include suture fixation that may allow physiologic motion. Dorsiflexion of the ankle, during syndesmotic fixation has not been shown to be important in determining ankle function.

Complications

- *Malunion:* Typically occurs with fibula in shortened and externally rotated position.
- *Nonunion:* Uncommon. Medial malleolar fractures are more likely to result in nonunion.
- *Infection and wound complications:* Increased in older patients, alcoholics, and diabetics.
- Stiffness

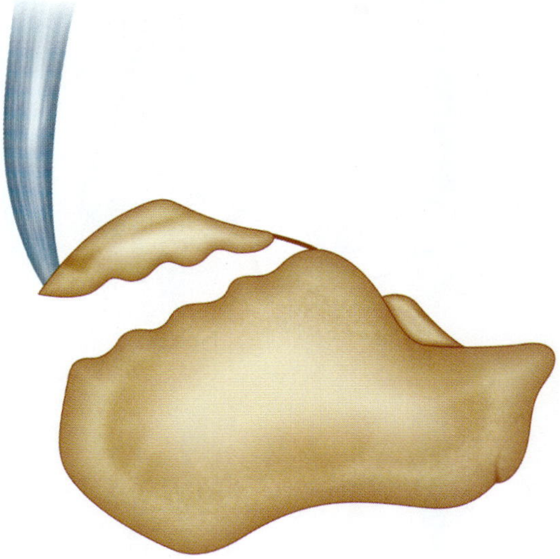

Fig. 26.236: A calcaneal fracture

- *Ankle arthritis:* Usually occurs within 2 years of injury. More common in severely displaced fractures, bimalleolar fractures and those involving the posterior malleolus.
- Broken hardware

■ Fracture of Calcaneus

Calcaneal fractures can be extra-articular (not involving the subtalar joint) or intra-articular (involving the subtalar joint). Extra-articular fractures include fractures of body, anterior process or tuberosity.

Generally extra-articular fractures should be treated with cast or brace immobilization and nonweight-bearing for the first 6 weeks. An exception is the displaced tuberosity avulsion fracture, which serves as the attachment of the Achilles tendon. Open reduction and internal fixation of this fragment with a large, partially threaded cancellous screw is advised. A calcaneal fracture is shown in Figure 26.236.

Intra-articular Fractures

Intra-articular fractures account for approximately 75 percent of calcaneal fractures. Mechanism of injury include, as an axial load force is applied to the posterior facet of the calcaneus through the talus, shear forces are directed through the posterior facet toward the medial wall of the calcaneus. The ensuing primary fracture line is almost always present and extends from the proximal, medial aspect of the calcaneal tuberosity, through the anterolateral wall, usually in the vicinity of the crucial angle of Gissane. As the axial force continues, two things happen: (1) the medial spike attached to the

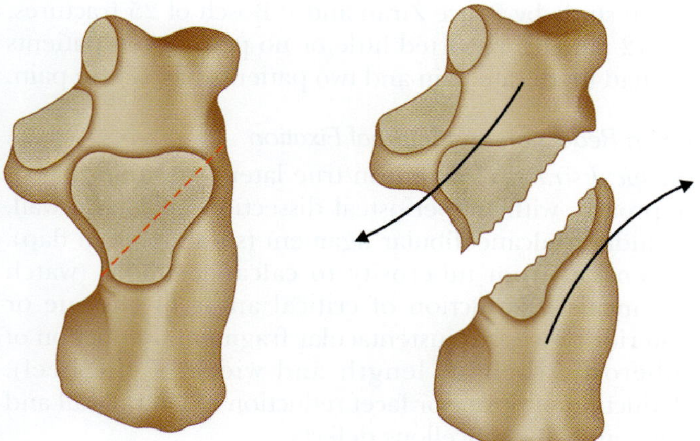

Fig. 26.237: Intra-articular fracture due to axial force

sustentaculum is pushed farther toward the medial heel skin and (2) various secondary fracture lines occur in the region of the posterior facet. This is illustrated in Figure 26.237. Sometimes anterior fracture extends toward the anterior process and may exit into the calcaneocuboid joint.

Classification

- Sander's classification
- Rowe types 1 to 5 (types 4 and 5 intra-articular)
- *Essex Lopresti:* Extra-articular, intra-articular, tongue fracture and joint depression calcaneal fracture.

Sander's Classification

Choose the coronal CT image that shows the posterior facet in widest profile and mark two vertical lines to divide the posterior facet into three equal sections, hence (A-lateral, B-central, C-medial) and the final line marks the vertical border of the sustentaculum:

Type I: Undisplaced fractures
Type II: Fractures: Two part
Type III: Fractures: Three part fracture with depression of posterior facet
Type IV: Severely comminuted.

Essex-Lopresti Classification

- Extra-articular fractures
- *Intra-articular:* Joint depression calcaneal fractures, here the fracture line producing the posterior facet fragment, exits behind the posterior facet and anterior to the attachment of the Achilles tendon
- *Tongue fractures:* If fracture exits distal to the Achilles tendon insertion, it is called a tongue type. This is shown in Figure 26.238.

Radiographic Evaluation

A lateral radiograph is used to assess height loss (loss of Böhler angle) and rotation of the posterior facet, as shown

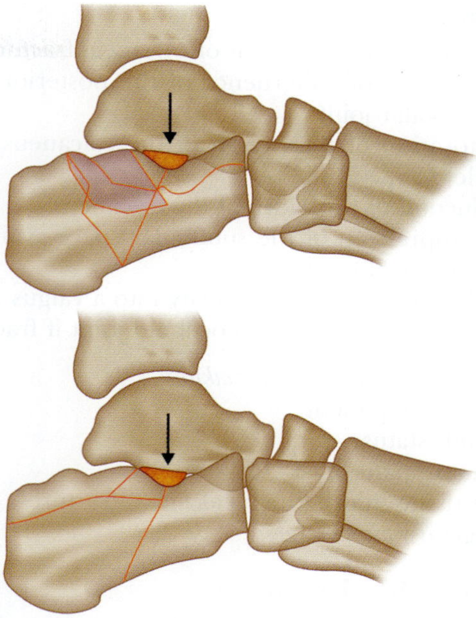

Fig. 26.238: Tongue fracture exiting distal to achilles tendon

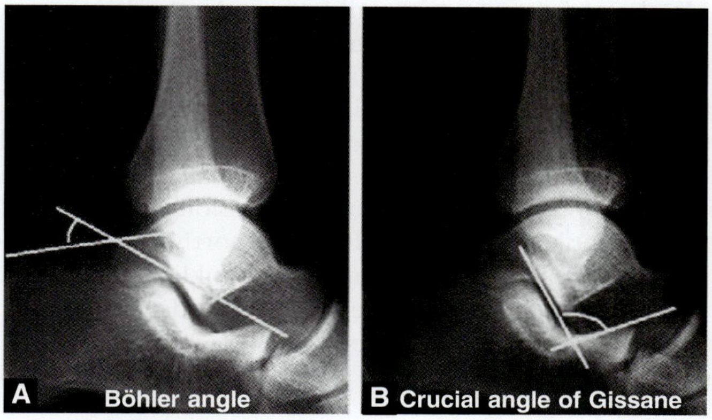

Figs 26.239A and B: Lateral radiographs, to assess height loss (loss of Böhler angle) and rotation of the posterior facet

in Figures 26.239A and B. The axial (or Harris) view is made to assess varus position of the tuberosity and width of the heel. Anteroposterior and oblique views of the foot are made to assess the anterior process and calcaneocuboid involvement. Single Brodén view, obtained by internally rotating the leg 40°, with the ankle in neutral, then angling the beam 10° to 15° cephalad, is made to evaluate congruency of the posterior facet.

CT scans are obtained to evaluate the injury completely. The scans should be ordered in two planes—the semicoronal plane, oriented perpendicular to the normal position of the posterior facet of the calcaneus and the axial plane, oriented parallel to the sole of the foot.

Treatment

Goals common to treatment of calcaneal fractures:

- Restoration of congruence of the posterior facet of the subtalar joint
- Restoration of the height of the calcaneus (Böhler angle)
- Reduction of the width of the calcaneus
- Decompression of the subfibular space available for the peroneal tendons
- Realignment of the tuberosity into a valgus position
- Reduction of the calcaneocuboid joint if fractured.

Factors affecting the decision making:

- Age of the patient
- Health status
- Fracture pattern
- Soft-tissue injury (open calcaneal fractures)
- Surgeon's experience.

Nonoperative Treatment

Most crucial measurement is degree of continuity of posterior facet, which is best determined by CT scan. All fractures are initially treated by strict bed rest and elevation, until acute swelling has subsided. Non-displaced fractures, with mild or moderate decrease in Böhler's angle are initially treated by early mobilization, avoidance of weight bearing for 6 weeks. Early mobilization with protection from weight bearing is maintained until fracture union occurs. Historical treatment has included closed reduction (Böhler), with distraction and medial lateral compression that may need to be supplemented by orthotic support with a custom-molded insole, rocker-bottom shoe or ankle-foot orthosis. When nonoperative treatment fails, considering subtalar arthrodesis is often indicated.

Percutaneous Fixation

Indication: Patients with inadequate soft tissues, i.e. diabetics with fracture blisters, where risk of dehiscence is high. Goal is to regain calcaneal height and width and to take the calcaneus out of varus alignment and no attempt is made to reconstruction the articular surface.

Technique

- Manual position across the calcaneal body.
- Large threaded Steinman pin is placed through the posterosuperior portion of the calcaneal tuberosity.
- Longitudinal traction is applied across the Steinman pin with a valgus vector applied as well.
- Threaded Steinman pin is inserted through the posteroinferior corner of the calcaneus, across posterior facet and into the talar body.
- This stabilizes the valgus reduction.
- Threaded Steinman pin is inserted through the posterior calcaneus into the cuboid.
- In study by Bruce Ziran and P Bosch of 25 fractures, 12 patients reported little or no pain, seven patients had moderate pain and two patients had severe pain.

Open Reduction and Internal Fixation

Surgical strategy: Patient in true lateral position. J or L approach, with subperiosteal dissection off lateral wall, including calcaneofibular ligament (sural nerve in flap). Extension from tuberosity to calcaneocuboid (watch peroneals). Reduction of critical angle of Gissane or anterior process to sustentacular fragment. Reduction of tuberostiy (height, length and width of the heel). Reduction of posterior facet reduction of lateral wall and bone graft for cancellous defects.

Plate fixation: Early ROM, nonweight-bearing 10 to 12 weeks. Hardware out equal to 1 year.

Primary Subtalar Fusion

It is indicated for fractures with more than three parts. Restores length of gastrocnemius-soleus complex, corrects flat foot and relieves the narrow peroneal space. Many surgeons point out that primary fusion is easier than delayed fusion because the soft tissues around the fracture site are scarred and shortened and the normal anatomy must be restored and they advise against the wait and see attitude, since this often causes the patient up to 6 months of pain and lost wages, whereas with fusion, the patient may move on their life.

Anterior Process Fracture of Calcaneus

Two types: (1) Avulsion and (2) compression fractures:

- *Avulsion fractures is the more common mechanism:* Adduction, plantar flexion and tension placed on bifurcate ligament, bifurcate ligament connects the anterior process of the calcaneus to both the cuboid and navicular bones
- *Compression fracture:* Mechanism of injury is forceful abduction of forefoot with compression of the calcaneocuboid joint, anterior articular surface of calcaneus is fractured and fragment can be displaced superiorly and posteriorly, resulting in joint incongruity.

Examination: Pain and tenderness may be located in region of sinus tarsi, point of maximal tenderness will be 2 cm anterior and 1cm inferior to anterior talofibular ligament, which should help distinguish this injury from a lateral ankle sprain.

X-ray: Lateral X-ray of hindfoot will best demonstrate compression type of fracture, lateral oblique views most frequently will show avulsion fracture, small inconsistent ossicle and calcaneus seconndatrium, lies just adjacent to anterior process and must not be confused with fresh fracture.

Treatment: When diagnosed early, immobilized in short leg cast for 4 weeks and full recovery may take 6 to 9 months.

■ Talar Fractures

Talar Head Fractures

Constitute 5 to 10 percent of talar injuries.

Mechanism of Injury

- Axially directed loading
- Compression of the talar head and a dorsal compression fracture of the anterior tibial plafond. The head of the talus with loss of support of the talonavicular joint may be associated with clinical instability of the triple joint complex. Injuries to the calcaneocuboid and subtalar joints are common with this injury.

Treatment

Open reduction and internal fixation, using an anteromedial approach, medial to the anterior tibial tendon. Stable fixation is accomplished with partially threaded cancellous lag screws or with headless, fully threaded compression screws. Osteonecrosis of this segment of the head has been reported to be 10 percent and if degenerative arthrosis occurs, talonavicular arthrodesis may be indicated.

Talar Neck Fractures

Hawkins Classification

Type I talar fractures: Non-displaced fractures of the talar neck without dislocation.

AVN: Ten percent important challenge is ensuring that anatomic reduction is obtained with no varus rotation. Treatment is closed, usually with short leg cast with foot in slight equinus. Nonweight-bearing for 4 weeks then weight bearing is allowed in cast for another 8 weeks or until healing is evident by X-ray (evidenced by trabeculations across fracture site).

Type II talar fractures: Displaced fracture of the talar neck with subluxation or dislocation of the subtalar joint (subtalar joint subluxation is usually dorsal) and the ankle remains aligned; type II injuries are caused by the destruction of the talocalcaneal ligament. Closed reduction is difficult of the dorsal and supination deformity, if possible then 8 to 12 weeks is necessary for healing (trabeculation across the fracture site) ORIF is needed if there is more than 3 to 5 mm of dorsal displacement and any rotational deformity and AVN (30%).

Type III talar fractures: Displaced fractures of talar neck with dislocation of body of talus from both subtalar joint and the ankle joint; when body dislocates, it is usually found on posterior medial aspect adjacent to the Achilles tendon; in this location, there can be compression of neurovascular structures and care must be taken, when approaching by open means the dislocated body of the talus; talocalcaneal ligament is ruptured, when there is dorsal displacement of the distal fragment, after rupture of this ligament, it is difficult to control distal talar neck fracture by closed means; requires ORIF: retrograde K wires can be placed through fractures and out postero-lateral aspect cannulated screws can be used through the posterolateral aspect, using the wires. AVN occurs in 90 percent cases.

Type IV subtalar, tibiotalar, and talonavicular joint subluxation or dislocation: Talar neck fracture with dislocation of the head fragment, open type IV fractures are associated with high rate of infection (30%), despite aggressive debridement and infection. Salvage treatment, consider placement of methyl methacrylate spacer shaped, like a talus, there are documented cases of patients being pain free for several years with this method of treatment.

Complications

Complications are related to the degree of displacement. One of the most common complications of talus fractures is avascular necrosis due to injury to the artery of the tarsal canal, which supplies the body and branches of the dorsalis pedis and peroneal arteries, which supply the head and neck.

Risk of avascular necrosis is stratified according to the Hawkins classification:

Hawkins type I: 0–15 percent
Hawkins type II: 20–50 percent
Hawkins type III: 20–100 percent
Hawkins type IV: 100 percent

Open fractures can occur in up to 15 to 25 percent of injuries, reflecting the high-energy mechanism of injury. There is an infection rate of up to 40 percent in open talus fractures. Post-traumatic arthritis occurs in 40 to 90 percent of cases. Delayed union or nonunion occurs in approximately 15 percent of cases and malunion is also a concern. Other complications include skin slough secondary to prolonged dislocation, interposition of the long flexor tendons and foot compartment syndrome.

Fractures of Posterior Process of Talus (Fig. 26.240)

Anatomy: It comprises of two tubercles—Medial and lateral undersurface of tubercles comprise posterior 25 percent of posterior facet of the subtalar joint. FHL runs between these tubercles and can have synovitis in this area (ballet dancers). Lateral tubercle serves as attachment of posterior talofibular ligament. Lateral tubercle has an articular surface and a fracture through this tubercle is

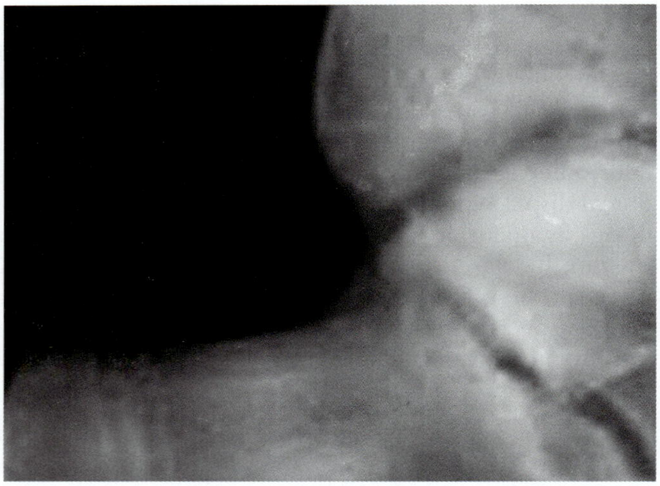

Fig. 26.240: Fractures of posterior process of talus

often associated with arthrosis. Medial tubercle, serves as attachment for posterior 1/3 of deltoid ligament and serves as the medial limb of the bifurcate talocalcaneal ligament inferiorly.

Fracture of Lateral Tubercle of Posterior Process (Shepherd's Fracture)

Mechanism

- Inversion of ankle may avulse tubercle leaving posterior talofibular ligament (PTFL) intact
- Fracture may also occur when ankle is forced into extreme equinus.

Clinical Findings

Patients will present with ankle sprain symptoms: Posterolateral ankle tenderness may be elicited; decreased and painful motion of ankle and subtalar joints, active flexion of great toe may also produce pain as FHL moves over fracture site (between medial and lateral tubercles).

Fracture of Medial Tubercle

Look for tenderness and perhaps a mass just posterior to medial malleolus and pain with motion of great toe (due to motion of FHL), treatment may involve excision of the fragment. Minimally displaced fractures are treated with short leg cast for 4 to 6 weeks some suggest casting in 15° of plantar flexion.

Complications

- Nonunions are uncommon
- Patient will note persistent pain with extreme plantar flexion and limitation of subtalar motion
- Surgical excision of the ununited fragment through a posterolateral ankle arthrotomy may relieve the pain.

Fractures of Lateral Process of Talus

Anatomy: Broad based, wedge shaped prominence of lateral talar body with an articular surface dorsolaterally for fibula and inferomedially for anterior aspect of posterior facet. Lateral talocalcaneal, cervical, bifurcate and anterior talofibular ligaments originate from tip of this process.

Mechanism of injury: Occur when the foot is dorsiflexed and inverted. Shearing stress is transmitted from calcaneus to lateral process, causing fracture of variable size, which may enter into posterior facet.

Classification (Hawkins)

- Non-articular chip fracture
- Single large fragment involving both talofibular articulation and subtalar joint.
- Comminuted fracture involving both articulations.

Clinical findings: Point tenderness over lateral process just anterior and inferior to the tip of lateral malleolus. Resemble an ankle sprain, patient may note persistent pain and loss of motion, if fracture extends into posterior facet of subtalar joint.

Radiographs: Fracture may involve up to one-third of posterior facet of subtalar or ankle joint. Note that radiographs will frequently underestimate the size of the fracture fragment.

- Broden's medial and lateral oblique axial views will help evaluate posterior facet
- Mortise view help define size of fragment and amount of articular involvement, taking the mortise view in plantar flexion along with 20° to 25° of internal rotation will place the lateral process in profile and will flex the forefoot out of the way.

CT scan: Allows accurate sizing and assessment of articular displacement of posterior facet.

Nonoperative Treatment

Undisplaced fractures are treated with nonweight-bearing cast immobilization for approximately 4 to 6 weeks. Nonunion is frequent complication of displaced lateral process fracture that are treated nonoperatively.

Operative Treatment

Unreduced, displaced fractures may lead to nonunion, with residual malalignment of the subtalar joint and persistent pain. Large fragments are treated with ORIF, fractures larger than 1 cm and fracture with more than 2 mm displacement probably should be treated surgically. Small comminuted fragments, treated with excision of fragments.

Complications: Nonunion is frequent complication of displaced lateral process fracture that are treated non-operatively, subtalar arthrosis, whether treated operatively

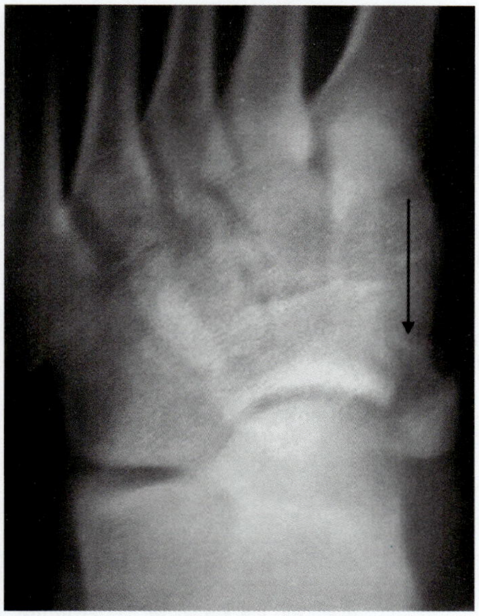

Fig. 26.241: Navicular tuberosity fractures (arrow)

or nonoperatively, many patients will develop subtalar arthrosis and may require late subtalar arthrodesis.

Navicular Fractures

- Avulsion fractures
- Tuberosity fractures
- Body fractures

Avulsion Fractures

- Usually dorsal lip (essentially severe sprain)
- *Treatment*
  - Immobilization and progressive weight-bearing
  - Excision of fragment if painful.

Tuberosity Fractures

- Avulsion by posterior tibial tendon and spring ligament, as shown in Figure 26.241. Usually minimally displaced.
- May have associated calcaneocuboid impaction.
- ORIF is done, depending on degree of displacement (>5 mm).

Body Fractures

- High energy trauma with axial foot loading
- Frequently associated with talonavicular subluxation
- CT scans helpful for preoperative planning
- Anatomic reduction is essential
- *Body fractures classification*
  Sangeorzan type 1: Coronal fracture plane
  Sangeorzan type 2: Primary fracture dorsolateral to plantar medial with medial displacement of major fragment and forefoot.
  Sangeorzan type 3: Comminution of the body in the sagittal plane with forefoot laterally displaced.
- *Treatment*
  - ORIF if any displacement
  - Anteromedial incision along medial aspect tibialis anterior
  - Second anterolateral incision to help reduce lateral fragment
  - May require stabilization or fusion to cuneiforms
  - Avoid fusion of essential talonavicular joint if at all possible
- *Prognosis:* With adequate reduction most have good result, but few are normal. Type 3 worst prognosis:
  - Only half are adequately reduced in Sangeorzan series (60% of joint surface).
  - 6 out of 21 developed osteonecrosis with one collapse.

Navicular Stress Fractures

- *Incidence:* Uncommon
- *Etiology:* Repetitive stress and poor blood supply
- Running most common, but can occur in all patients active in sports
- *Diagnosis:* Vague arch pain with midfoot tenderness
- Delay in diagnosis common
- *X-rays:* AP, lateral and oblique
- CT and bone scans if uncertain
- Treatment
  - *Incomplete fracture:* Nonweight-bearing cast until healed (variable time)
  - *Complete fracture or nonunion:* ORIF with screws perpendicular to fracture plane with or without bone graft
- *Complications:* Nonunion or persistent pain.

Fracture of Cuboid

Cuboid fractures are rare as isolated injuries. These bones frequently are injured as part of a wider injury pattern, involving the Lisfranc (most common) or Chopart joint. Cuboid fractures can be classified into avulsion or compression types. Small avulsions may occur with inversion-type ankle sprains and generally respond to conservative treatment. Compression fractures's mechanism of injury is "nutcracker" axial loading with plantar flexion and forefoot abduction.

Treatment: Most are minimally displaced and can be treated in a nonweight-bearing cast for 4 weeks, followed by weight bearing casts for 4 weeks. A well-molded arch support often is used afterward. For severe displacement with shortening of the lateral column, consideration should be given to open reduction and internal fixation with bone grafting.

Cuneiform Fractures

- Isolated fractures quite rare
- Displacement of these fractures is unusual
- Healing with few complications is likely
- Mechanisms of injury:
  - *Direct trauma:* Most common and heal rapidly with non-operative treatment
  - Indirect trauma (Lisfranc variants)

Lisfranc's Joint Injuries

It includes any bony or ligamentous injury, involving the tarsometatarsal joint complex. It is named after the Napoleonic-era surgeon, who described amputations at this level without ever defining a specific injury.

Anatomy

Lisfranc's joint articulation is between the three cuneifoms and cuboid (tarsus) and the bases of the five metatarsals.

Osseous stability is provided by the Roman arch of the metatarsals and the recessed keystone of the second metatarsal base. Lisfranc's ligament is large oblique ligament that extends from the plantar aspect of the medial cuneiform to the base of the second metatarsal (there is no transverse metatarsal ligament from 1 to 2), as shown in Figures 26.242A and B. Interosseous ligaments connect the two through five metatarsal bases, both dorsal and plantar (stronger and larger). Secondary stabilizers, plantar fascia, peroneus longus and intrinsincs.

Incidence

Generally considered rare (1 per 55,000 people per year or 15/5500 fractures). As index of suspicion increases, so does incidence. Approximately, 20 percent of Lisfranc's injuries may be overlooked (especially in polytraumatized patients).

Mechanisms of Injury

- *Trauma:* Motor vehicle accidents account for one-third to two-thirds of all cases (incidence of lower extremity foot trauma has increased with the use of air bags).
- Crush injuries
- *Sports injuries:* Sports-related injuries are also occurring with increasing frequency. Mechanisms of injuries can be direct or indirect. Typical of athletic injury include, axial loading to plantar flexed foot results in hyperplantar flexion and ligament rupture. Rarely associated with open injury or vascular compromise. Indirect injury can be due to twisting injuries leading to forceful abduction of the forefoot, often resulting in a second metatarsal base fracture and/or compression fracture of the cuboid ('nutcracker').

Associated Fractures

- Base of second metatarsal
- Avulsion of navicular

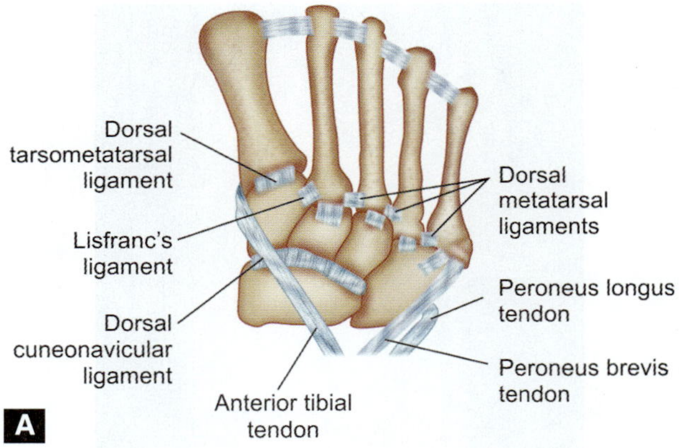

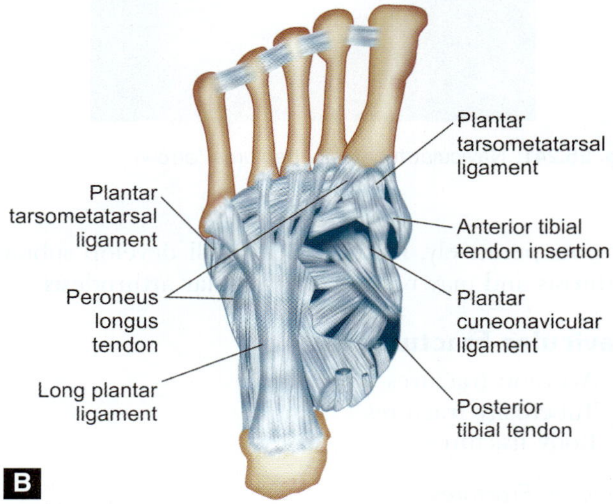

Figs 26.242A and B: Lisfranc's joint articulation between the three cuneifoms and cuboid (tarsus) and the bases of the five metatarsals—(A) Dorsal view; (B) Plantar view

- Isolated medial cuneiform
- Cuboid

Classification

- *Classification by Quenu and Kuss (1909):* Can be classified as homolateral, isolated and divergent, as shown in Figures 26.243A to C. Modified by Hardcastle in 1982 and further modified by Myerson in 1986. It fail to encompass all injury patterns especially crush injuries. Guide treatment, but do not establish prognosis.
- *Classification by Hardcastle (1982):* This is shown in Figures 26.244A and B.
- Classification Myerson (1986).

Diagnosis

Requires a high degree of clinical suspicion

- Twenty percent misdiagnosed
- Forty percent no treatment in the first week. Be wary of the diagnosis of "midfoot sprain"

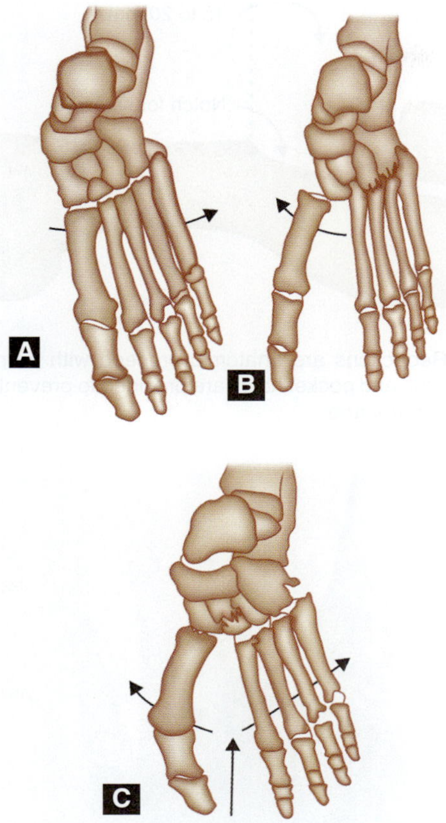

Figs 26.243A to C: Quenu and Kuss classification of Lisfranc's joint injury—(A) Homolateral; (B) Isolated; (C) Divergent

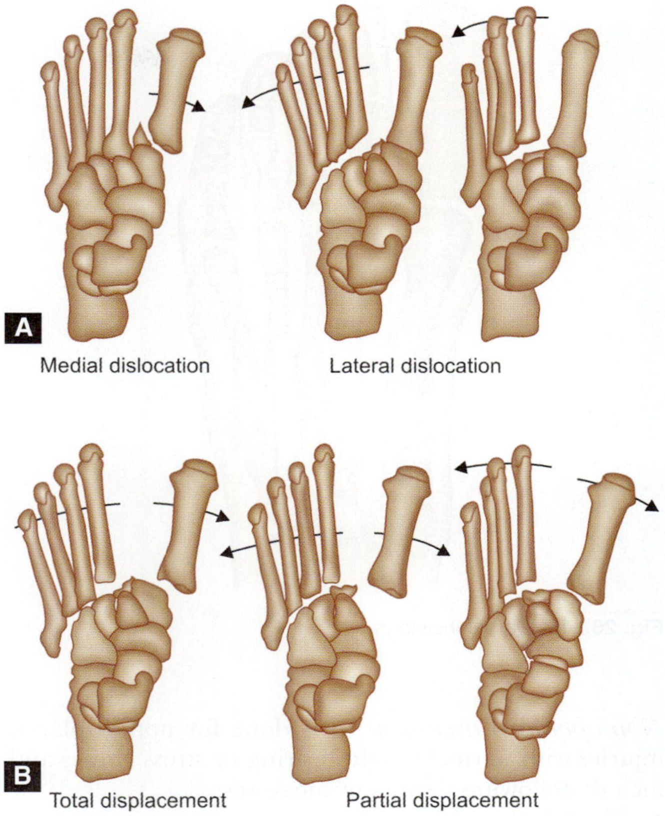

Figs 26.244A and B: Classification of Lisfranc's fracture by Hardcastle, showing—(A) Type B, with partial incongruity; (B) Type C, with divergent incongruity

Clinical Findings

- Midfoot pain with difficulty in weight bearing.
- Swelling across the dorsum of the foot.
- Deformity variable due to possible spontaneous reduction.
- Ecchymosis may appear late.
- Local tenderness at tarsometatarsal joints.
- Gentle stressing plantar/dorsiflexion and rotation will reveal instability.
- Check neurovascular status for compromise of dorsalis pedis artery and/or deep peroneal nerve injury.
- Assessing for possible compartment syndrome.

Radiographic Evaluation

- AP, lateral and 30° oblique X-rays are mandatory.
- *AP:* The medial margin of the second metatarsal base and medial margin of the middle cuneiform should be aligned.
- *Oblique:* Medial base of the fourth metatarsal and medial margin of the cuboid should be aligned.
- *Lateral:* The dorsal surface of the first and second metatarsals should be level to the corresponding cuneiforms.
- Standing views provide "stress" and may demonstrate subtle diastasis.
- Comparison views are very helpful.

Associated Fractures

- Base of second metatarsal
- Avulsion navicular
- Isolated medial cuneiform
- Cuboid

Additional Imaging

- True stress views or fluroscopy
- CT Scans
- Bone scan for persistent pain, with no radiographic findings
- *If suspicious:* Repeat X-rays and keep looking.

Treatment

- Early recognition is the key to preventing long-term disability.
- *Anatomic reduction is necessary for best results:* Displacement of > 1 mm or gross instability of tarsometatarsal, intercuneiform or navicular cuneiform joints is unacceptable.
- Goal is to obtain or maintain anatomic reduction.

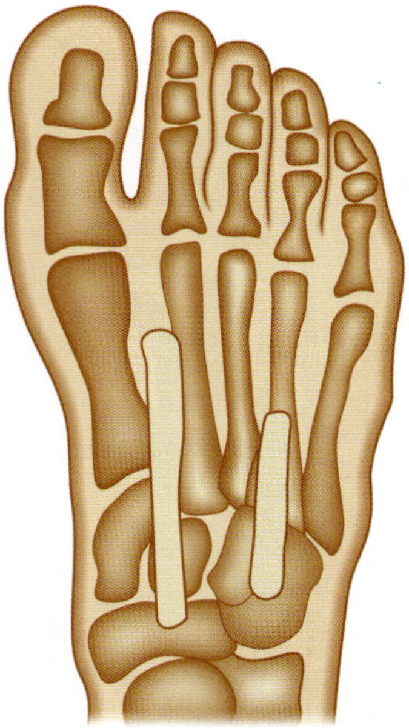

Fig. 26.245: Dorsal incisions

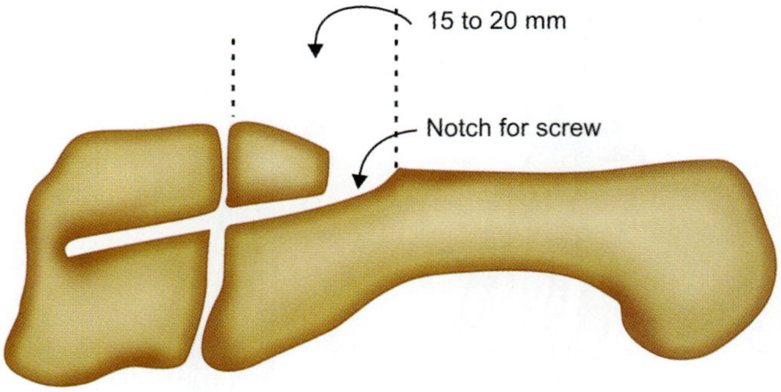

Fig. 26.246: Reductions are anatomic proceed with permanent fixation and pocket holes are provided to prevent dorsal cortex fracture

Non-operative treatment: It is done for non-displaced injuries with normal weight bearing or stress X-rays and include following treatment measures:

- Short leg cast
- 4 to 6 weeks nonweight-bearing
- Repeat X-rays to rule out displacement as swelling decreases
- Total treatment 2 to 3 months.

Operative treatment: Surgical emergencies.

- Open fractures
- Vascular compromise (dorsalis pedis)
- Compartment syndrome

Techniques: One to three dorsal incisions, as shown in Figure 26.245

- First incision centered at TMT joint and along axis of second ray, lateral to EHL tendon.
- Identify and protect NV bundle
  - Reduce and provisionally stabilize second TMT joint
  - Reduce and provisionally stabilize first TMT joint
  - If lateral TMT joints remain displaced use second or third incision(s)
- If reductions are anatomic proceed with permanent fixation:
  - Screw fixation is preferable for the medial column.
  - "Pocket hole" to prevent dorsal cortex fracture, as shown in the Figure 26.246.
  - Screws are positional not lag
  - To aid reduction or if still unstable use a screw from medial cuneiform to base of second metatarsal.

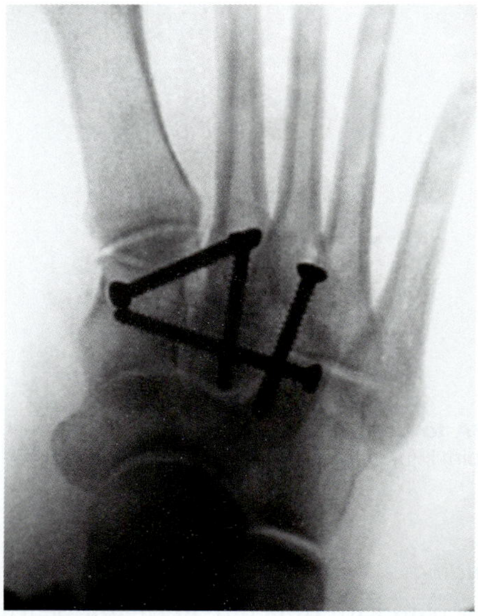

Fig. 26.247: Using an intercuneiform screw in case of intercuneiform instability

  - If intercuneiform instability exists use an intercuneiform screw, as shown in Figure 26.247.
  - The lateral metatarsals frequently reduce with the medial column and pin fixation for mobility is acceptable.
  - Postoperative management include:
    - Splint 10 to 14 days, nonweight-bearing
    - Short leg cast, nonweight-bearing 4 to 6 weeks
    - Short leg weight bearing cast or brace for an additional 4 to 6 weeks
    - Arch support for 3 to 6 months
  - Hardware removal:
    - Lateral column stabilization can be removed at 6 to 12 weeks
    - Medial fixation should not be removed for 4 to 6 months
    - Some advocate leaving screws indefinitely unless symptomatic

Complications

- Post-traumatic arthritis
  - Present in most, but may not be symptomatic
  - Related to initial injury and adequacy of reduction
  - Treated with arthrodesis for medial column
  - Interpositional arthroplasty may be considered for lateral column
- Compartment syndrome
- Infection
- Complex mediated pain syndrome
- Neurovascular injury
- Hardware failure

Prognosis

- Long rehabilitation (>1 year)
- Incomplete reduction leads to increased incidence of deformity and chronic foot pain
- Incidence of traumatic arthritis (0 – 58%) and related to intra-articular surface damage and comminution.

Fractures of the Metatarsals

Fifth metatarsal is the most common metatarsal to fracture. It include fractures of the proximal and distal portions of fifth metatarsal.

Classification of fractures of the base of the fifth metatarsal:

Type I: Acute fractures at the metaphyseal-diaphyseal junction
- IA nondisplaced
- IB displaced or comminuted or both

Type II: Fractures at the metaphyseal-diaphyseal junction with clinical or radiographic evidence of previous injury (i.e. pain, sclerosis).

Type III: Fractures of the styloid process of the fifth metatarsal
- IIIA Without involvement of the fifth metatarsocuboid joint
- IIIB With involvement of the fifth metatarsocuboid joint.

Treatment

Treatment depends on the type of fracture and physical demands of the patient.

Type IA: Nonweight-bearing cast for 6 to 8 weeks followed by weight bearing cast till union

Type IB: Conservative treatment is enough, but for athletes open reduction and internal fixation is recommended. Nonunion rate is 7 to 28 percent

Type II: Nonweight-bearing casting for 8 weeks, may yield satisfactory results. Refracture is common in this category

Type III: These are treated satisfactorily in a short leg cast for 3 weeks followed by a well-molded arch support. Although nonunions of type III fractures may occur, they rarely are painful and can be treated with excision of the fragment.

For type I and type II fractures that require surgical intervention, two operative treatments have proved successful:

- Fixation with a medullary 4.5 mm malleolar screw.
- Corticocancellous inlay bone grafting with clearing of the medullary canal of all sclerotic bone.
  - Spiral fractures of the distal fifth metatarsal are common and occur frequently in dancers and professional athletes.
  - The mechanism of injury has been reported to be rotational, with rolling over on the outer border of the foot, while standing on the ball of the foot with the ankle fully plantar flexed (demipointe position).
- Other methods include:
  - Cast immobilization
  - Symptomatic treatment with bandaging and full weight bearing
  - Closed reduction with percutaneous pinning
  - Open reduction and internal fixation.

Stress Fractures of Metatarsals

Who is at Risk?

- They occur most commonly in women, especially during the early years of menopause in the phase of rapid bone resorption.
- Stress fractures also have been noted to occur in athletes, especially ballet dancers and athletes engaged in cutting and jumping sports.
- Military recruits in their first few weeks of training also are vulnerable to so called march fractures.
- Individuals with diabetes and sensory and motor neuropathy, rheumatoid arthritis, Charcot-Marie-tooth disease or stroke may be at risk as well.

Clinical Findings

- Gradual onset of pain directly over the second metatarsal neck region 2 to 4 weeks after beginning a running or aerobics program.
- Swelling over the area usually is noted.
- The diagnosis is suspected on history and physical examination.
- Initial radiographs made within 2 weeks after the onset of symptoms may be negative and bone scan or MRI may assist in the diagnosis in questionable cases. Generally, repeat radiographs at 4 to 6 weeks after injury reveal periosteal new bone formation.

- Differential diagnoses include entrapment neuritis of the superficial peroneal nerve, radiating pain from a more proximal tarsometatarsal joint arthrosis and idiopathic or overuse synovitis of the adjacent metatarsophalangeal joint.

Treatment

- Generally, conservative management with rest or cast immobilization results in resolution of symptoms.
- Subsets of fractures that may be especially difficult to manage, include stress fractures of the proximal second metatarsal.
- It is important to inform the patient that a stress fracture at the second metatarsal, occasionally it may result in a slight dorsiflexion malunion and transfer of weight to the third metatarsal, which is at risk for the development of a stress fracture.
- Surgical intervention rarely is required for stress fractures, however open reduction and plating may be required, if significant bony healing has occurred in a malunion.

Acute Fractures of Metatarsals

The mechanism of injury usually is direct, such as a motor vehicle accident, which is reported to be the most common. Factors cited as contributing to the poor outcome included sagittal plane displacement, open fracture and severe soft-tissue injury. Mild lateral plane displacement may be tolerated, however sagittal plane displacement of a metatarsal head either in extension or plantar flexion or excessive shortening of a metatarsal leads to metatarsalgia and chronic forefoot pain. For this reason, closed reduction and percutaneous pinning from a dorsal approach is recommended. Occasionally, the displacement is severe enough to require open reduction and internal fixation.

Phalangeal Fractures

Most of the phalangeal fractures are treated successfully with conservative measures. Occasionally, an intra-articular fracture severely displaced into the interphalangeal joint of the great toe may require open reduction and internal fixation to prevent deformity and arthritic changes. The fracture and the joint are exposed, the fracture is reduced anatomically and with a power drill small 0.045 inch Kirschner wires are inserted for internal fixation. These pins are bent and left outside the skin and generally removed 3 to 4 weeks after surgery, when the fracture has stabilized.

Sesamoid Fractures

It is most commonly seen in association with metatar sophalangeal joint dislocation. Chronic stress fractures of the sesamoids, most commonly seen in long-distance runners and ballet dancers. Medial or tibial sesamoid is the more commonly injured sesamoid because it generally is larger than the fibular sesamoid and is seated more directly beneath the metatarsal head.

Differentiating fracture from a bipartite sesamoid:

- Fractured sesamoid bones tend to be roughly divided into equally sized sections, bipartite sesamoids tend to have one larger fragment and one smaller fragment.
- Bipartite sesamoids tend to have smooth, rounded edges and fractured sesamoids tend to have irregular, jagged edges.

Physical examination usually shows tenderness and swelling in the region of the sesamoid. Limited extension of the great toe and pain, with passive extension of the great toe are usually present. The patient may have a shortened stance phase of gait and usually descends stairs with the injured foot leading. Radiographic evaluation should include standard anteroposterior and lateral views.

Treatment

If the sesamoid fragments are of roughly equal size and the displacement is significant (>5 mm), open reduction with internal fixation. Internal fixation generally involves use of an 18-gauge wire looped around the proximal and distal poles and placed in a figure-of-eight over the sesamoid. Bone grafting from the calcaneus or the supramalleolar area of the distal tibia may be helpful in achieving union. Minimally displaced or non-displaced fractures of the sesamoid and stress fractures can be treated initially with cast immobilization, incorporating a toe plate for 3 to 4 weeks. Repeat casting for another 3 to 4 weeks may be necessary, if symptoms have not resolved. After this, the toe is protected by placing a lightweight steel shank and a toe rocker in an athletic shoe.

Operative Treatment

The following options are available for surgical treatment:

- Complete excision of the sesamoid
- Partial excision of a painful bipartite sesamoid or nonunion of a sesamoid fracture
- Cancellous bone grafting to promote union.

The tibial sesamoid has a significant function in increasing the lever arm and action of the flexor hallucis brevis muscle and in protecting the flexor hallucis longus tendon, so complete excision should be avoided. If a partial sesamoid excision is done, the patient should be informed preoperatively that the remaining sesamoid fragment may need to be excised as well. Repairing the flexor hallucis brevis mechanism is crucial regardless of which treatment method is chosen. Indications for complete sesamoidectomy are comminuted fractures with no large fragments and the loss of articulating cartilage, either on the articular side of the sesamoid or on the overlying surface of the metatarsal head.

EPIPHYSEAL INJURIES AROUND FOOT AND ANKLE

■ Introduction

All long bones of a growing child consist of an epiphysis, physis and metaphysic, at each end separated by the diaphysis, as shown in Figure 26.248. Physis is a Greek word (phyein), which means nature or to generate.

Diaphysis

Dia means between (the physes). The diaphysis is the initial and Primary Center of Ossification (PCO). It becomes the central shaft of a long bone and is composed of mature, lamellar bone with a strong cortical exterior. It enlarges circumferentially by periosteal, membranous osseous tissue apposition on the original enchondral model, but does not grow longitudinally. All long bones (humerus, radius, ulna, femur, tibia, fibula, clavicle, metacarpals, metatarsals, phalanges, and ribs) have one PCO, located in the diaphysis. Flat bones (scapula and innominate) and vertebrae have multiple primary centers of ossification.

Metaphysis

Meta means adjacent to (the physis). The metaphyses denote the flaring ends of the central shaft of along bone and are composed of endosteal, spongy, trabecular bone surrounded by the exterior thin cortical bone.

Epiphysis

Epi means upon (the physis). The chondro-osseous epiphysis rests upon the physis and articulates with the adjacent bone. Most, but not all, epiphyses contain at least one secondary center of ossification (SCO).

Physis (Fig. 26.249): The physis is the reference point of a growing bone and differentiates immature bone from mature bone. The physis is a complex structure, discoidal in form and often referred to as a "plate", i.e. the epiphyseal growth plate. Its cellular anatomy is defined in terms of layers:

- Germinal
- Proliferative
- Columnar
- Hypertrophic

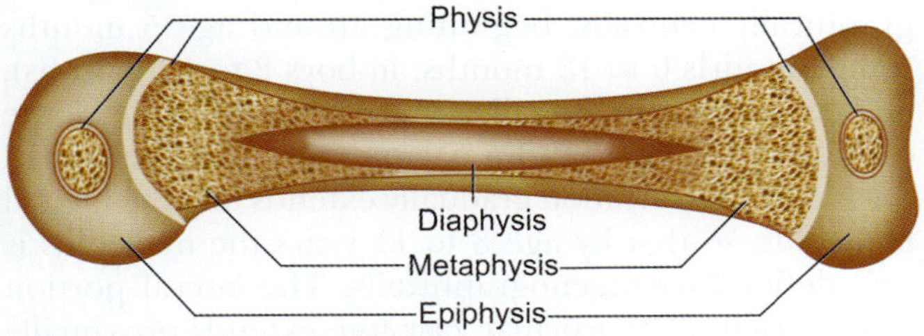

Fig. 26.248: Long bone of a growing child

- Provisional calcification, each with a designated function.

The germinal zone is also called the resting or reserve zone. Its functions include storage of nutrients and accumulation of stem cells. The proliferative and columnar zones provide for cell division, differentiation of chondrocytes oriented in columns and matrix production. In the hypertrophic zone the cells enlarge in size and show enhanced metabolic activity with an established program of apoptosis. At the zone of provisional calcification vascular channels invade the dead columnar cells and mineralization of the intercellular matrix occurs, later to be replaced by osteoblasts and bone. The physis is avascular. Its supply of oxygen and nutrients is provided by epiphyseal vessels small arterial branches arise at right angles to the main epiphyseal artery (arteries) in the SCO and pass through small cartilage canals in the resting zone to terminate at the top of the cell columns in the proliferative zone.

Zone of Ranvier: The periphery of the growth plate, the periphysis, surrounds the physis of tubular bones. It contains fibrovascular tissue, undifferentiated mesenchymal tissue, differentiated epiphyseal and physeal-cartilage (the zone of Ranvier) and the osseous ring of lacroix, as shown in Figure 26.250. The zone of Ranvier is responsible for latitudinal growth and Lacroix's perichondral ring provides mechanical support for the physis.

Blood Supply of the Physis

The blood supply of the physis derives from three independent sources:

- Epiphyseal arteries
- Intramedullary metaphyseal arteries
- The periosteal arteries of the circumferential zone of Ranvier.

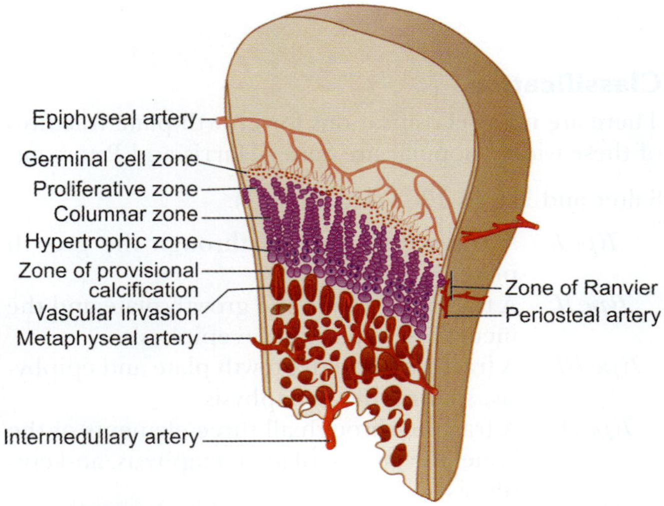

Fig. 26.249: Cellular anatomy of physis

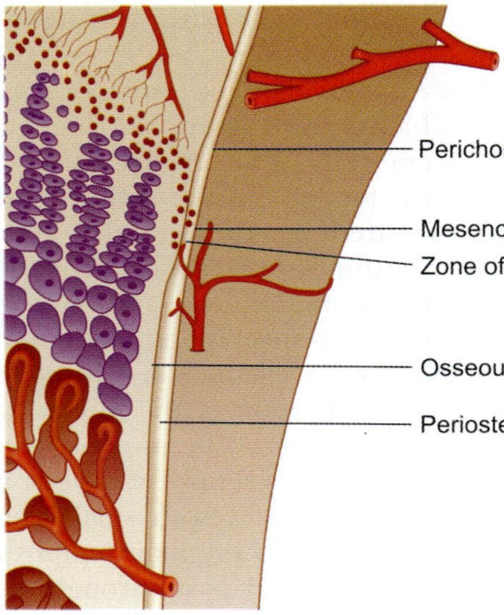

Fig. 26.250: Showing the zone of Ranvier and the osseous ring of lacroix

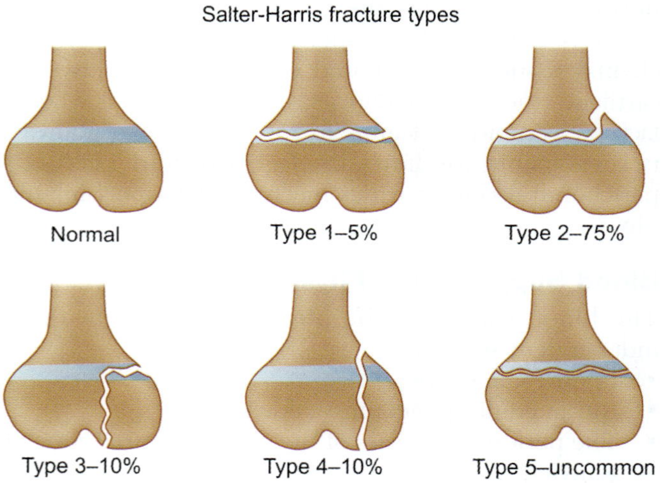

Fig. 26.251: Salter and Harris classification of growth plate fractures

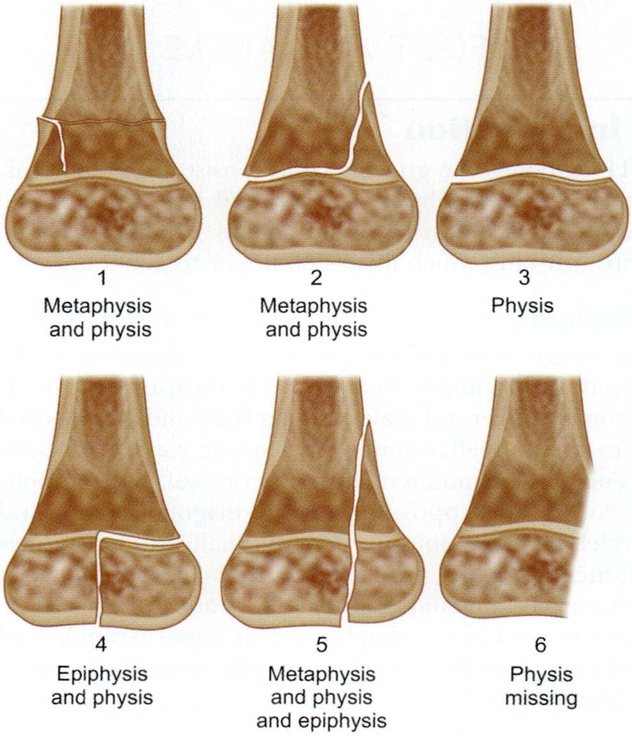

Fig. 26.252: Peterson's classification of growth plate fractures

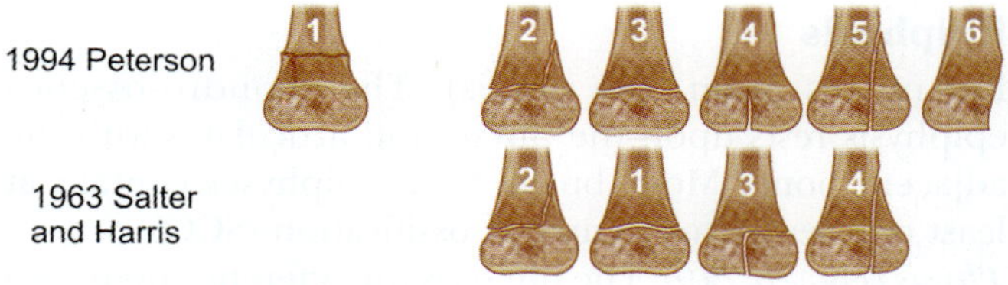

Fig. 26.253: Comparison between Salter-Harris and Peterson's classifications

Classification

There are many classifications for growth plate fractures of these widely popular are Salter-Harris and Peterson.

Salter and Harris 1963 (Fig. 26.251):

- *Type I:* A transverse fracture through the growth plate
- *Type II:* A fracture through the growth plate and the metaphysis, sparing the epiphysis
- *Type III:* A fracture through growth plate and epiphysis, sparing the metaphysis
- *Type IV:* A fracture through all three elements of the bone, the growth plate, metaphysis, and epiphysis
- *Type V:* A compression fracture of the growth plate.

- Peterson's classification (Fig. 26.252)
- Comparison (Fig. 26.253)

Distal Tibia

At birth the distal tibial epiphysis is entirely cartilaginous. The secondary center of ossification appears roentgenographically centrally, beginning around age 5 months (range in girls 0 to 12 months, in boys 2 to 12 months), and expands centrifugally. The lateral portion of the ossification center is more narrow (wedge shaped) than the medial. Ossification gradually extends into the medial malleolus, so that by age 8 to 11 years the malleolus is well defined roentgenographically. The lateral portion of the distal tibial articular cartilage extends proximally nearly the entire longitudinal length of the epiphysis to

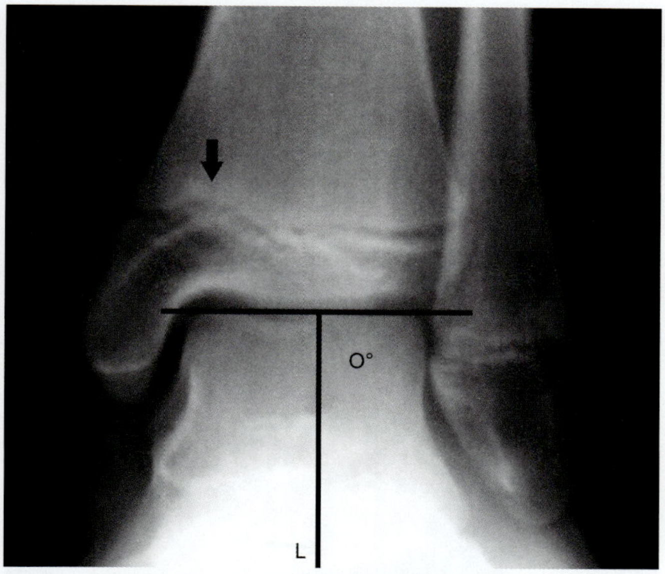

Fig. 26.254: Poland's hump or Kump's bump (arrow) seen in the distal tibia

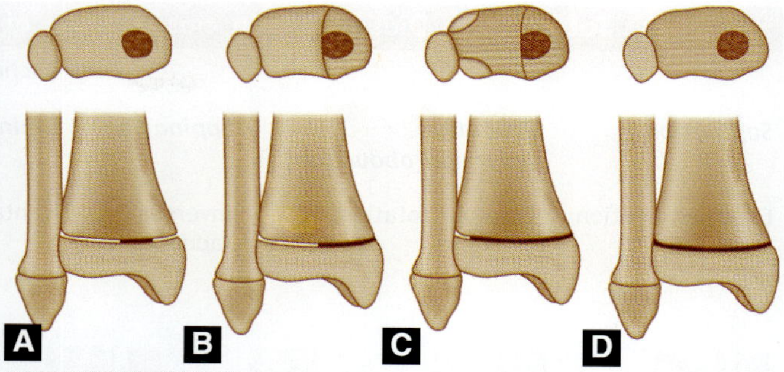

Figs 26.255A to D: Order of epiphyseal closure of distal tibia

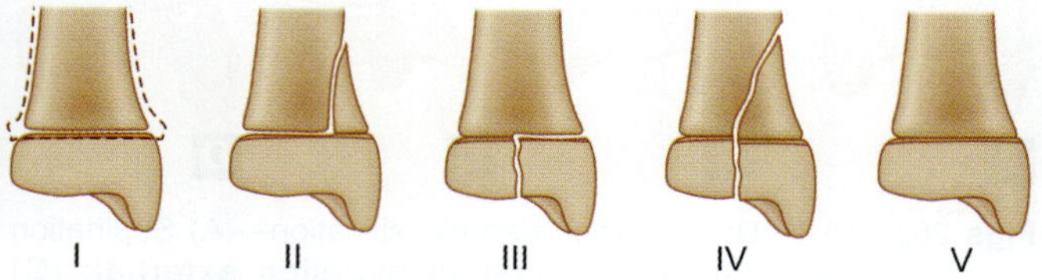

Fig. 26.256: Salter-Harris anatomic classification

form an articulation with the distal fibula. In the neonate the physis is flat, and the epiphyseal cartilage has many vascular canals. By age 2 to 3 years, the physis develops undulations, most prominently anteromedially. By age 8 to 11 years these multiple undulations, sometimes called papillae or mammary processes, are evident roentgenographically. By age 12 years or so the growth of this anteromedial area lags slightly behind the remaining physis producing a mild curve, apex proximally. This has been called Poland's hump or Kump's bump, as shown in Figure 26.254.

This dome shape of this portion of the physise makes it roentgenographically indistinct. This should not be misinterpreted as an injury or premature physeal arrest secondary to trauma. The physis in this "hump" area is the first to close. Physeal closure begins centromedially in the area of Poland's hump and progresses first anteromedially then posterolaterally and occurs progressively over a period of 18 months, as shown in Figures 26.255A to D.

Complete closure of the distal tibial physis varies widely, from age 12 to 17 years (median, 14 years 10 months) in girls and from age 15 to 20 years (median 16 years 10 months) in boys. Distal tibial and fibular physeal closure occur at approximately the same time in both girls and boys.

Fractures of Distal Tibia

Tibial physeal fractures most commonly occur between the ages of 8 and 15 years. As the distal tibial physis closes in an asymmetric pattern over a period of about 18 months, injuries sustained during this period can produce fracture patterns that are not seen in younger children with completely open physes. This group of fractures has been labeled transitional fractures because they occur during the transition from a skeletally immature ankle to a skeletally mature ankle. The fractures included in this group are juvenile Tillaux and triplane fractures, recently, two new types of transitional fractures have been identified. The adolescent pilon fracture and the incisural fracture.

Classification

Classifications of ankle fractures are of two broad types: anatomic and mechanism of injury. Anatomic classifications divide fractures into groups based on the parts of the epiphyses or metaphyses that make up the fracture fragments.

Salter-Harris Anatomic Classification (Fig. 26.256)

Mechanism-of-injury classifications are based on the nature of the force that creates the fractures and often include the position of the foot at the time the force is applied. An important benefit of mechanism-of-injury classifications is that they provide clues that may be helpful in planning closed reduction: the mechanism of injury is simply reversed to reduce the fracture.

Dias: Tachdjian classification of physeal injuries of the distal tibia and fibula, as illustrated in Table 26.1 and Figures 26.257A to D.

Dias-Tachdjian Classification of Physeal Injuries (Figs 26.257A to D)

Axial compression: Axial compression is a Salter-Harris type V injury of the distal tibial physis.

Table 26.1: Dias-Tachdjian classification of physeal injuries of the distal tibia and fibula

Dias-Tachdjian (child)						
Supination	*Pronation (eversion abduction)*	*Supination*	*Supination*	*Axial compression*	*Juvenile tillaux*	*Triplane*
External rotation	External rotation	Inversion (adduction)	Plantar flexion			

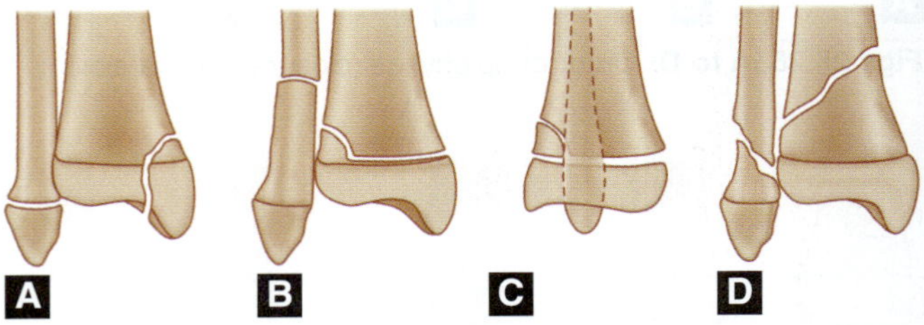

Figs 26.257A to D: Dias-Tachdjian classification—(A) Supination inversion; (B) Pronation eversion external; (C) Supination plantar flexion; (D) Supination external rotation

Juvenile Tillaux fracture: The juvenile Tillaux fracture is a Salter-Harris type III fracture involving the anterolateral distal tibia, as shown in Figure 26.258.

The triplane fracture has the appearance of a Salter-Harris type III fracture on an anteroposterior X-ray and of a Salter-Harris type II fracture on a lateral X-ray, as illustrated in Figures 26.259A and B.

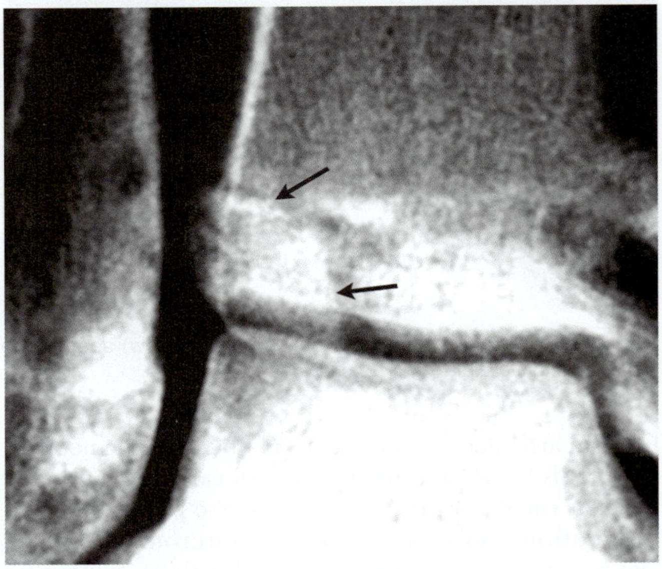

Fig. 26.258: Juvenile Tillaux fracture (arrows)

Pediatric Pilon Fractures

The pediatric pilon fracture is defined as any fracture of the tibial plafond with articular and physeal involvement, variable talar and fibular involvement.

Letts et al. classification:

- *Type I:* Fractures have minimal comminution and no physeal displacement
- *Type II:* Fractures have marked comminution and less than 5 mm of physeal displacement
- *Type III:* Fractures have marked comminution and more than 5 mm of physeal displacement.

Incisural fractures: Fractures that on anteroposterior and mortise views appear to be Tillaux fractures, with the fractured piece appearing smaller than usual and essentially non-displaced. On CT scan the fracture line does not extend through the anterior cortex, as is seen in a typical Tillaux fracture, as shown in Figures 26.260A and B.

It appears, therefore, that the fragment is not the result of avulsion by the anterior tibiofibular ligament, the accepted mechanism of injury for a Tillaux fracture, but rather that the fragment is avulsed by the intraosseous ligament and represents the pediatric equivalent of an adult diastasis injury.

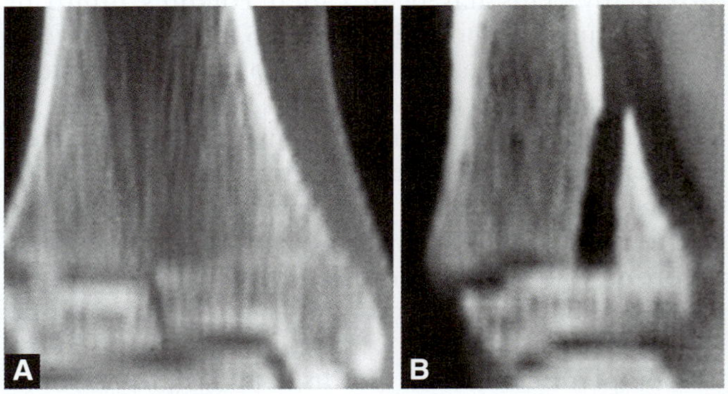

Figs 26.259A and B: Triplane fracture

Signs and Symptoms

- Patients with significantly displaced fractures have severe pain and obvious deformity.
  - The position of the foot relative to the leg may provide important information about the mechanism of injury and should be considered in planning reduction

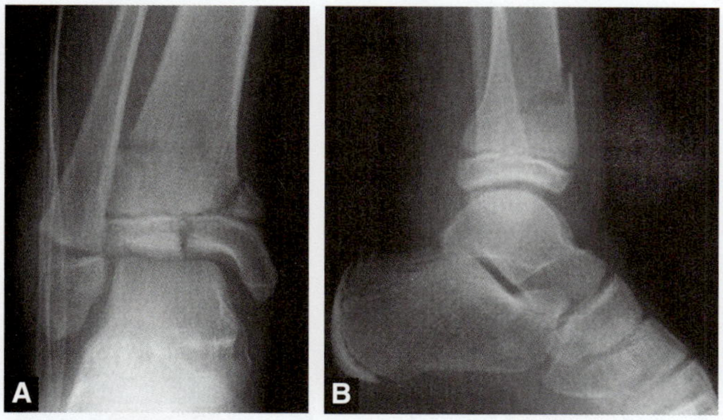

Figs 26.260A and B: Incisural fractures

- The status of the skin, pulses, sensory and motor function should be determined and recorded. Tenderness, swelling, and deformity in the leg and foot should be noted
- It is important in patients with tibial epiphyseal fractures to carefully evaluate the contralateral ankle clinically and by X-ray.

Diagnosis

- By clinical evaluation
- *X-rays:* AP, lateral and mortice views should be taken
- *Stress views:* The anterior tibiofibular ligament view is made by positioning the foot in 45° of plantar flexion and elevating the medial border of the foot 15°. The calcaneofibular ligament view is obtained by rotating the leg 45° inward
- CT scan
- MRI for any ligamenous laxity and osteochondral injuries associated with fractures.

Treatment

- Salter-Harris types I, II fractures of the distal tibia can be caused by any of four mechanisms:
  1. Supination-inversion
  2. Supination-plantar flexion
  3. Supination-external rotation
  4. Pronation-eversion-external rotation
- The treatment depends upon:
  - Mechanism of injury
  - Associated fibula fracture
  - Displacement of the fractures.

Cast immobilization is generally sufficient treatment for nondisplaced Salter-Harris type I and II fractures of the distal tibia. Recommended treatment ranges from a below-knee cast worn for 4 weeks to a long nonweight-bearing cast worn for 3 weeks, followed by 3 weeks of immobilization in a short-leg walking cast. Closed reduction of significantly displaced Salter-Harris type I and II fractures should be attempted. Due to fears of

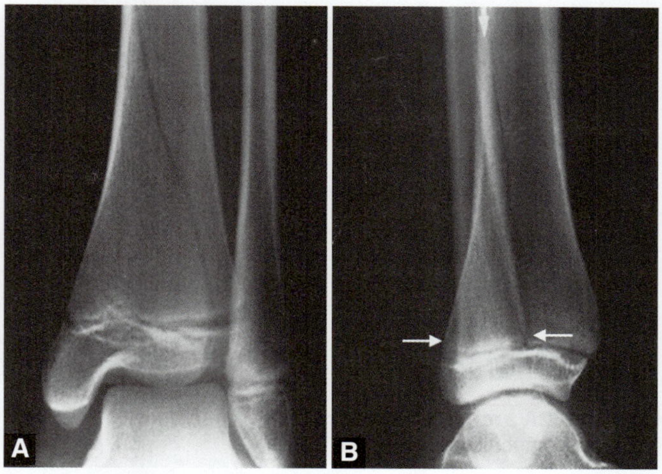

Figs 26.261A and B: X-ray shows Salter-Harris type two fractures in a 12-year-old child. Arrows shows posterior displacement

iatrogenic damage to the distal tibial physis during closed reduction, many researchers recommend the use of general anesthesia with adequate muscle relaxation for all patients with Salter-Harris type I and II distal tibial fractures.

Indications for ORIF include:

- Grossly displaced fractures
- Interposition of soft tissue between the fracture fragments (neuro vascular bundle)
- Interposition of periosteum between the fragments.

Distal tibia type II fracture. Twelve years 2 month old girl injured her left ankle. The ankle was swollen. an AP and lateral roentgenograms show type II fracture with large posterior metaphyseal fragment attached to the epiphysis (arrows) with 2 mm or less posterior displacement, as shown in Figures 26.261 and 26.262.

A Robert Jones compression bandage was applied with the foot in neutral dorsiflexion. Five days later a short leg nonweight-bearing cast was applied. Three weeks later the cast was removed and the patient started active motion and progressive weight bearing.

Salter-Harris Types III and IV Fractures

Salter-Harris type III and IV fractures share the same mechanism of injury (supination-inversion), and their treatment and prognosis are similar. These injuries usually are produced by the medial corner of the talus being driven into the junction of the distal tibial articular surface and the medial malleolus. As the talus shears off the medial malleolus, the physis also may be damaged. Nondisplaced Salter-Harris types III and IV fractures can be treated with above-knee cast immobilization, but care must be taken to be sure no displacement is present, which may require CT evaluation, and that no displacement

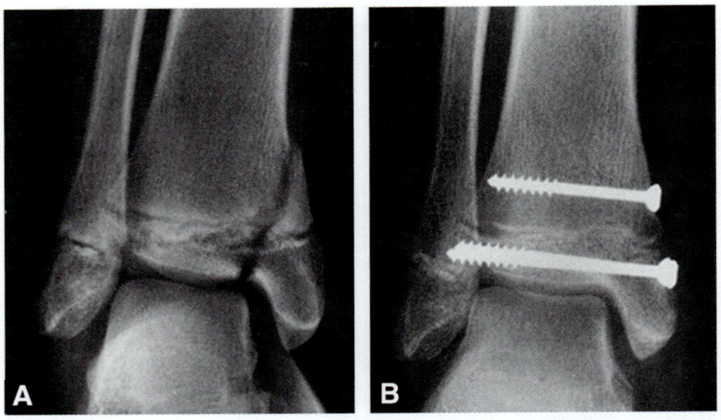

Figs 26.262A and B: Salter-Harris type IV treated with ORIF with cancellous screw

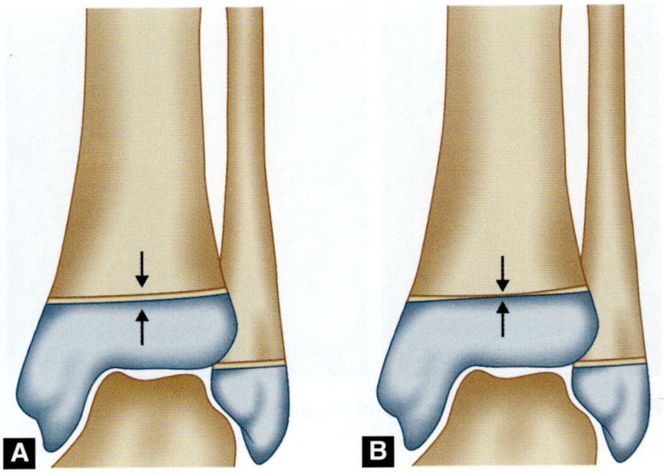

Figs 26.263A and B: Salter-Harris type V fractures of the ankle. Arrows showing axial compression

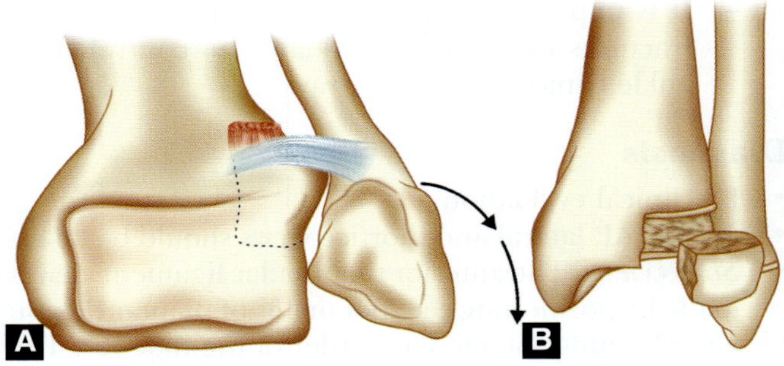

Figs 26.264A and B: (A) The anteroinferior tibiofibular ligament avulses a fragment of the lateral epiphysis; (B) Corresponding to the portion of the physis that is still open

occurs after casting. If anatomic reduction cannot be obtained by closed methods, open reduction with internal fixation should be performed. Options for internal fixation include smooth Kirschner wires (K-wires), small fragment cortical and cancellous screws and 4 mm cannulated screws. Several reports have advocated the use of absorbable pins for internal fixation of ankle fractures. The main advantage of absorbable pins and screws is that hardware removal is avoided. These fractures also require open reduction for inspection of the joint and replacement or removal of loose osteochondral fragments. Internal fixation devices should be inserted within the epiphysis, parallel to the physis, and should avoid the physis and ankle joint.

Salter-Harris type IV treated with ORIF with cancellous screw (Figs 26.262A and B).

Salter-Harris Type V Fractures

Salter-Harris type V fractures of the ankle are believed to be caused by severe axial compression and crushing of the physis, as shown in Figures 26.263A and B.

These injuries are not associated with displacement of the epiphysis relative to the metaphysis, which makes diagnosis of acute injury impossible from plain X-rays. The diagnosis can be made only on follow-up X-rays when premature physeal closure is evident. As of the uncertain nature of this injury, no specific treatment recommendations have been formulated. Treatment usually is directed primarily toward the sequelae of growth arrest that invariably follow Salter-Harris type V fractures. Compression-type injury of the tibial physis. Early physeal arrest can cause leg length discrepancy.

Juvenile Tillaux Fractures

It occurs when, with external rotation of the foot, the anteroinferior tibiofibular ligament through its attachments to the anterolateral tibia avulses a fragment of bone corresponding to the portion of the distal tibial physis that is still open. The fracture described in adults by the French surgeon Tillaux. The fibula usually prevents marked displacement of the fracture and clinical deformity generally is absent. Swelling usually is slight, and local tenderness is at the anterior lateral joint line, in contrast to ankle sprains, in which the tenderness tends to be below the level of the ankle joint. Juvenile Tillaux fracture. Mechanism of injury, the anteroinferior tibiofibular ligament avulses a fragment of the lateral epiphysis (A) corresponding to the portion of the physis that is still open (B) (Figs 26.264A and B).

Both below-knee and above-knee casts have been used for immobilization of non-displaced juvenile Tillaux and triplane fractures. Fractures with more than 2 mm of displacement require closed or open reduction. Closed reduction is attempted by internally rotating the foot and applying direct pressure over the anterolateral tibia. If necessary, percutaneous pins can be used for stabilization

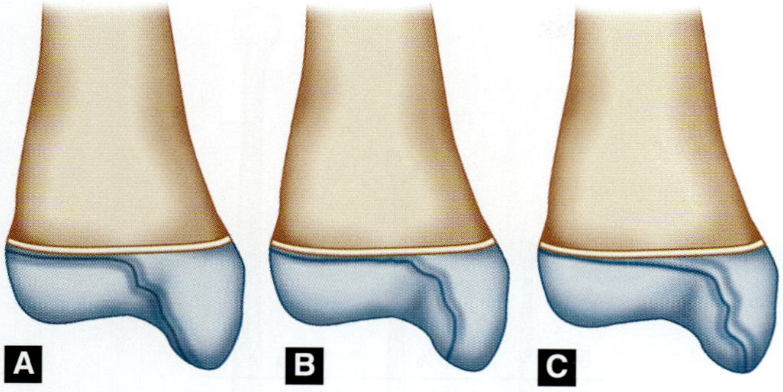

Figs 26.265A to C: Types of triplane fractures

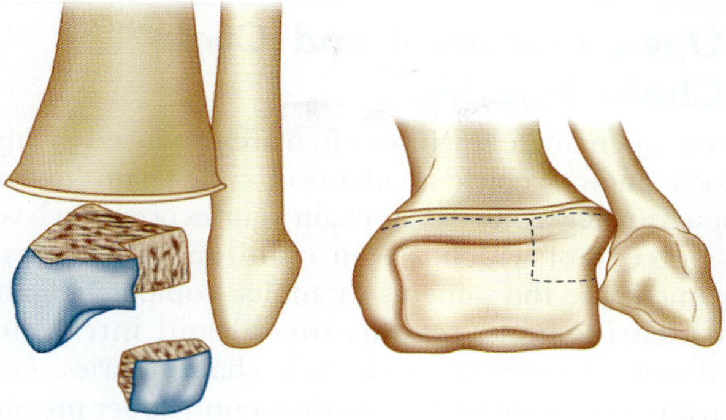

Fig. 26.267: Anatomy of a three-part lateral triplane fracture (left ankle)

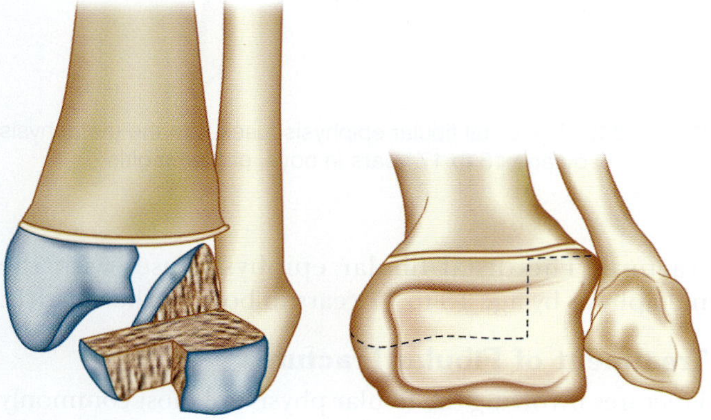

Fig. 26.266: Anatomy of a two-part lateral triplane fracture (left ankle)

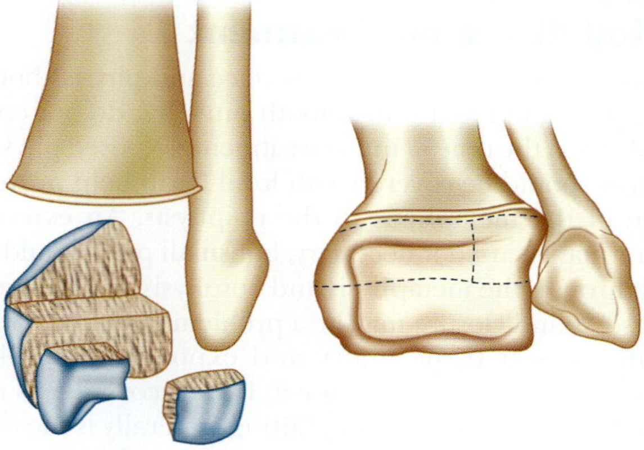

Fig. 26.268: Anatomy of a four-part lateral triplane fracture (left ankle)

of the reduction. If closed reduction is not successful, open reduction is required. Occasionally, percutaneously inserted pins can be used to manipulate the displaced fragment into anatomic position and then advanced to fix the fragment in place.

Triplane Fractures (Figs 26.265A to C)

Triplane fractures are divided into—• Two-part; • Three-part; • Four-part. Two-part and three-part triplane fractures are divided into three types:

Type I: Intramalleolar intra-articular fracture

Type II: Intramalleolar, intra-articular fracture outside the weight-bearing surface

Type III: Intramalleolar, extra-articular fracture.

Anatomy of a two-part lateral triplane fracture (left ankle). Note the large posterolateral epiphyseal fragment with its posterior metaphyseal fragment. The anterior portion of the medial malleolus remains intact, as illustrated in Figure 26.266.

Anatomy of a three-part lateral triplane fracture (left ankle). Note the large epiphyseal fragment with its metaphyseal component and the smaller anterolateral epiphyseal fragment. This is shown in Figure 26.267.

Anatomy of a four-part lateral triplane fracture (left ankle). The anterior epiphysis has split into two fragments, and the posterior epiphysis is the larger fragment with its metaphyseal component, as depicted in Figure 26.268.

Non-displaced triplane fractures (those with less than 2 mm of displacement) and extra-articular triplane fractures can be treated with long-leg cast immobilization with the foot in internal rotation for lateral fractures and in eversion for medial fractures. Fractures with more than 2 mm of displacement (65% of the injuries in Karrholm's series) require reduction. Closed reduction of lateral triplane fractures is attempted by internally rotating the foot. Based on the mechanism of injury, the most logical maneuver for reduction of medial triplane fractures is abduction. If closed reduction is shown to be adequate by fluoroscopic examination a long-leg cast is applied or percutaneous screws are inserted for fixation if necessary. If closed reduction is unsuccessful, open reduction is required. This can be accomplished through an anterolateral approach for lateral triplane fractures or through an anteromedial approach for medial triplane fractures. Fractures of the incisura-casting with immobilization is the treatment of choice.

■ Open Fractures and Cycle Chain Injuries

Severe open ankle fractures often are produced by high-velocity motor vehicle accidents or cycle chain injuries. Approximately 25,000 cycle chain injuries occur each year, 20 percent of which are in children. Principles of treatment are the same as in adults: copious irrigation and debridement, tetanus toxoid and intravenous antibiotics. In children with cycle chain injuries, grass, dirt, and debris are blown into the wound under pressure, and removal of these embedded foreign objects requires meticulous mechanical debridement.

■ Modalities of Treatment

In most patients, the articular surface and physis should be aligned and fixed with smooth pins that do not cross the physis at the time of initial treatment. Exposed physeal surfaces should be covered with local fat to help prevent union of the metaphysis to the epiphysis. An external fixator may be used if necessary, but small pins should be used through the metaphysis and epiphysis, avoiding the physis. Wound closure may be a problem in patients with significant soft tissue injury and exposed bone. Skin coverage with local tissue is ideal. If local coverage is not possible, split-thickness skin grafting generally is the next choice. Free vascular flaps and rotational flaps may be required for adequate coverage.

Distal Fibula (Fig. 26.269)

The distal fibular physis is transverse at birth. With growth it becomes convoluted and contains peripheral lappet formations. These convolutions reduce the likelihood of separation and displacement. The distal fibular secondary center of ossification (SCO) may be present at one year of life and is usually present by the third year. The distal fibular epiphysis may have an accessory SCO, referred to as the os subfibulae. When present it may become roentgenographically apparent by age 6 or 7 years and might easily be confused with a fracture of the tip of the lateral malleolus. At birth the fibula has 20 percent of its final length. The distal fibular physis provides more growth than the proximal fibular physis until the fibula has reached 30 percent of its length. Then the proximal fibular physis becomes the dominant growth center. By age 7 years the proximal fibular physis has become themore dominant growth center, so that by maturity the distal physis has contributed only 40 percent of the length of the fibula. The level of the fibular physis relative to the distal tibia also changes with growth. In the neonate it is located at the level of the mid tibial epiphysis. By age three (and thereafter) it is level with the tibiotalar joint. This knowledge is valuable when assessing any ankle fracture. The distal fibular epiphysis fuses with the metaphysis by age 15 to 17 years in boys, earlier in girls.

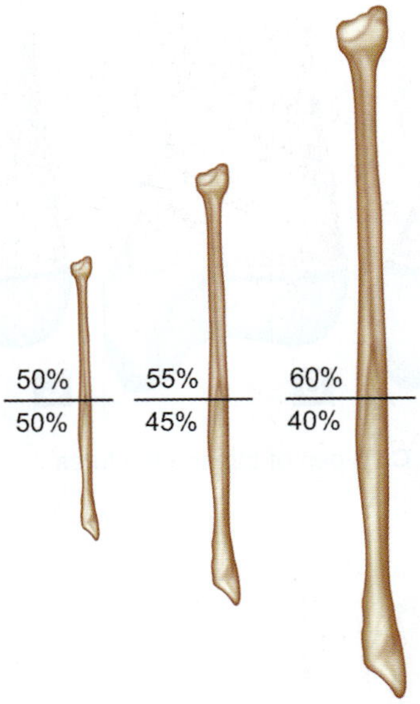

Fig. 26.269: The distal fibular epiphysis fuses with the metaphysis by age 15 to 17 years in boys, earlier in girls

Treatment of Fibular Fractures

Fractures involving the fibular physis are most commonly Salter-Harris type I or II fractures that are caused by a supination inversion injury. Isolated fibular fractures usually are minimally displaced and can be treated with immobilization in a below-knee cast for 4 to 6 weeks. Significantly displaced fibular fractures accompany Salter-Harris types III and IV tibial fractures and usually reduce when the tibial fracture is reduced. Internal fixation of the tibial fracture generally results in stability of the fibular fracture such that cast immobilization is sufficient. If the fibular fracture is unstable after reduction and fixation of the tibial fracture, fixation with a smooth intramedullary or obliquely inserted K-wire is recommended. In older adolescents in whom growth is not a consideration, an intramedullary rod or plate-and-screw device can be used as in adults. Avulsion fractures from the lateral malleolus occur in children with inversion sprain-type injuries to the ankle. These may fail to unite with cast immobilization. Patients with such nonunions may have pain without associated instability. In such patients, simple excision of the ununited fragment usually relieves their pain. When the nonunions are associated with instability, reconstruction of one or more of the lateral ankle ligaments is required.

Complications

- *Physeal arrest:* Premature complete closure of the distal tibial physis following fracture of the medial malleolus is unlikely. Premature partial closure, however, is common. The incidence is much higher when the initial treatment is non-operative. This may be due to the incompleteness of reduction. Non-anatomic reduction of the physis by closed or open reduction markedly increases the probability of partial arrest. Frequent and prolonged follow-up, with a standing radiograph at 3 to 6 months intervals up to 18 months, even when preceding ones are normal, may detect an early bar. As the bar forms in the healing fracture site, growth ceases locally. The lateral tibial and distal fibular physes continue to grow resulting in an increasing ankle varus deformity. The developing bar is usually relatively small (20% or less) and excellent results have been noted following bar excision. Ankle varus deformity of 10° or more accompanying a physeal bar is unlikely to correct spontaneously and may be treated by osteotomy. The site of deformity is at the metaphyseal-physeal junction so an osteotomy in the distal metaphysis just proximal to the epiphysis affords the best correction. A medial open wedge osteotomy with bone grafting has the advantage of adding a little length. Illiac creast bone graft or the graft from the ipsilateral fibula can be used.

- *Irreducible:* Interposition of soft tissue, usually periosteum between the fracture fragments of the medial malleolus is not uncommon. The interposed tissue must be surgically extricated to avoid nonunion or physeal arrest.
- *Nonunion:* Nonunion is an under-reported complication and when it occurs it is a major problem. As the talus fits snugly between the two malleoli, it is impossible to excise the tibial pseudarthrotic scar tissue and still have the medial malleolus in contact with the remaining distal tibia. Insertion of a bone graft to accomplish ankle congruity and motion ensures a physeal bar. In some instances it may be better to leave the nonunion untreated until the physis is closed or nearly closed before attempting osteosynthesis.
- Malunion
- Overgrowth
- Degenerative arthrosis
- Osteomyelitis

Metatarsals

The metatarsals have epiphyses and physis at both ends, but develop secondary center of ossification (SCO) at only one end. The mechanism of bone elongation by physeal growth is similar whether a SCO develops or not. The first metatarsal distal epiphysis and the lateral four metatarsal proximal epiphyses do not usually develop secondary center of ossification, yet their physes provide 20 to 30 percent of metatarsal longitudinal growth. Metatarsal epiphysis begin to ossify in the third year of life, as shown in Figure 26.270.

Multiple ossification centers within the epiphyses of metatarsals are not unusual and gradually coalesce into a single SCO. In general, the foot matures early. It grows relatively slowly after 5 years of age. Completion of foot growth occurs earlier than growth of other bones. By age 12 years the average foot in boys has achieved 96 percent of total length and in girls 88 percent of total length. Thus, physeal injuries of the metatarsals are less likely to cause significant length disturbance or functional impairment after age 12 years. First and fourth metatarsals, showing multiple ossification centers, as shown in Figure 26.271.

Fractures of the metatarsals are the most common fractures of the foot in children, accounting for up to 60

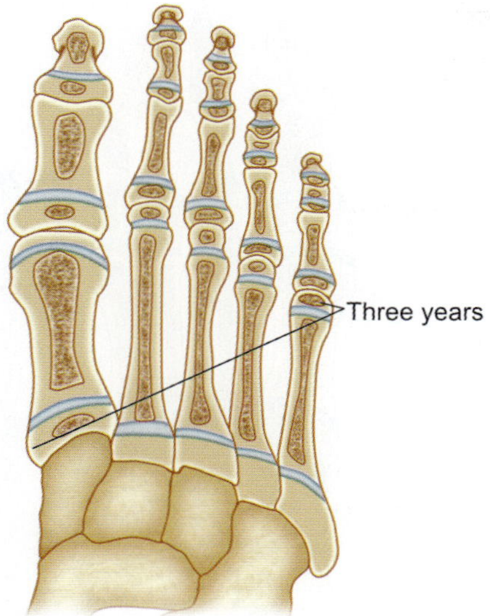

Fig. 26.270: Metatarsal epiphyses begin to ossify in the third year of life

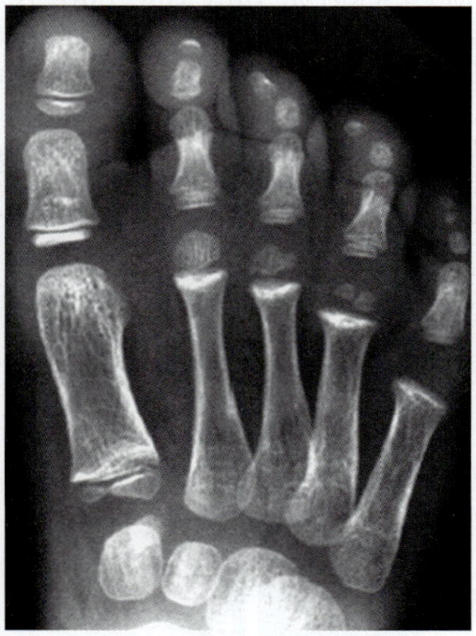
Fig. 26.271: Multiple ossification centers of metatarsal

percent of all pediatric foot fractures. In children younger than 5 years of age, 75 percent of metatarsal fractures involve the first metatarsal, whereas in children older than 10 years the most commonly fractured foot bone is the fifth metatarsal.

Mechanism of injury: The mechanism of metatarsal fractures may be either direct or indirect. Direct injuries result from the impact of falling objects or crush injuries typically involving bicycles or motor vehicles. Indirect injuries are caused by axial loading, inversion, rotation, or a combination of these.

Classification

Salter-Harris classification holds good for metatarsal fractures. Swelling and tenderness are often the only signs present. Deformity is uncommon. AP and oblique roentgenographs are the most useful since on lateral films the metatarsals obscure each other, as shown in Figures 26.272A and B.

Management: Most metatarsal fractures in children can be treated non-operatively. Initial management depends on the severity of the injury. With marked swelling and soft tissue injury, posterior below knee splint is applied once swelling is reduced below knee cast is given. Partial weight-bearing is allowed, and immobilization is continued for 3 to 6 weeks depending on the age of the child and the amount of fracture displacement. Displaced physeal fractures may require reduction under general anesthesia. Closed reduction is usually successful, but if the fracture is unstable, percutaneous pinning can be performed using image intensification.

Phalanges of the Foot

Foot phalanges, like metatarsals, have epiphyses and physes at each end, but typically have a secondary center of ossification (SCO) at only one end. SCO appear roentgenographically at different times in each phalanx in each toe. In the great toe the distal phalanx SCO appears first between 8 and 21 months, and the proximal phalanx later, between 15 and 36 months. In the lateral four toes the opposite is true; the SCO of the proximal phalanges appear first, between 9 and 36 months, and of the distal phalanges between 24 and 36 months. The order of appearance of proximal phalangeal SCO is third toe, fourth toe, second toe, and fifth toe. The order of appearance of the SCO of the distal phalanges is the fourth toe, third toe, second toe, and fifth toe. The SCO of all phalanges appear a few months earlier in girls, as shown in Figure 26.273.

The physes are typically flat and transverse. However, those of the proximal phalanges vary considerably in shape, from flat to cone shaped with the apex projecting distally into an accommodating crater of the metaphysic. They should not be confused with injury or sequelae of injury. Another variant is bracket, as shown in Figure 26.274.

Epiphyses in Early Life

In girls physis closes between 11 and 14 years of age and in boys it is between 13 and 15. Swelling, deformity, and tenderness will vary greatly with the severity of fracture. Nailbed injuries are common with fractures of the distal phalanx, particularly the great toe.

Management: Closed fractures rarely require reduction type 1 fractures of the lesser toe and great toe are common. Taping the toe to one or both adjacent toes almost universally results in a well-aligned and well-healed fracture in 3 to 4 weeks. A hard-soled shoe with the dorsum of the toe portion removed is sufficient for weight bearing.

Fractures that would benefit from reduction are those with intra-articular displacement involving more than 25 percent of the articular surface, those with more than

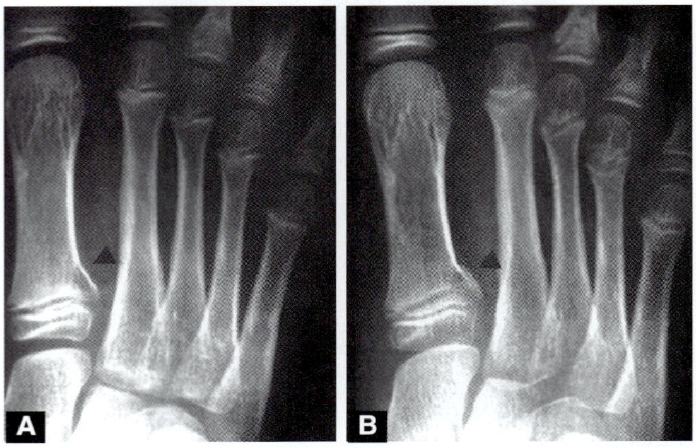

Figs 26.272A and B: X-ray showing metatarsal fractures

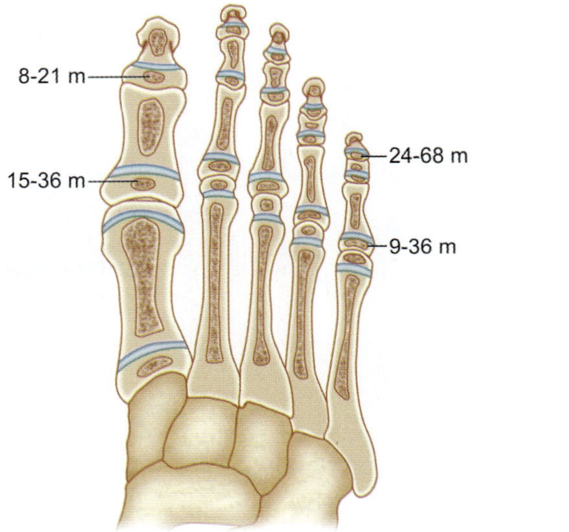

Fig. 26.273: Appearance of secondary ossification centers of phalanges of foot

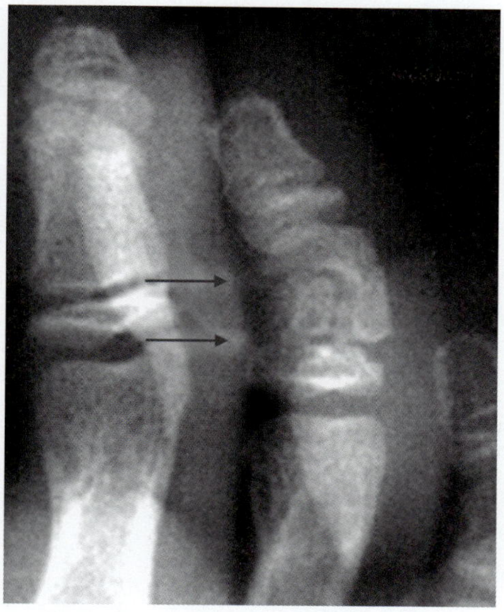

Fig. 26.274: The physes are typically flat and transverse. However, those of the proximal phalanges vary considerably in shape, from flat to cone shaped with the apex projecting distally into an accommodating crater of the metaphysic, arrow showing bracket physis

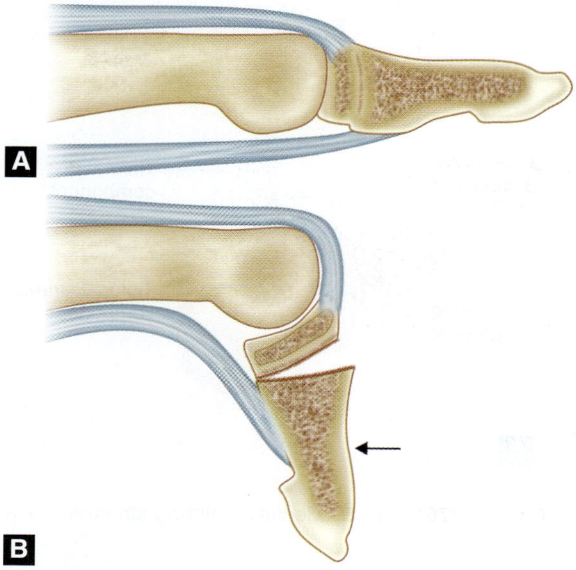

Figs 26.275A and B: Stubbed toe due to plantar flexion injuries

2 mm displacement, and markedly angulated fractures of any type. If reduction is unstable it may be maintained by percutaneous pinning. Open fractures require irrigation, debridement and antibiotics. Nailbed injuries involving the germinal matrix should be repaired. The injured toe should be soaked in a warm water and anti-infection solution until the skin of the foot wrinkles, three times a day for one week to extract any pus.

Stubbed toe: The extensor digitorum longus inserts primarily into the dorsum of the epiphysis of the distal phalanx, while the flexor digitorum inserts primarily into the metaphysis of volar aspect thus plantar flexion injuries produce stubbed toe, as shown in Figures 26.275A and B. The "stubbed great toe", particularly if compound is best protected by a short leg walking cast with a toe plate extension.

LIGAMENT INJURIES AROUND ANKLE

Anatomy

Medially

Stabilizing the medial side of the ankle, anteriorly and posteriorly is the strong, flat and triangular deltoid ligament consisting of five components, as shown in Figures 26.276 and 26.277. Deltoid ligament is divided into superficial and deep components.

- Deep components are:
  - Anterior deep tibiotalar ligament
  - Posterior deep tibiotalar ligament
- Superficial components are:
  - Anteriorly tibionavicular component
  - Middle tibiocalcaneal component
  - Posteriorly tibiotalar component

Both deep components are intra-articular, but extrasynovial. The posterior deep tibiotalar ligament is the strongest of the entire deltoid complex. Superficial and deep components equally resist valgus tilting of the talus and are secondary restraints against anterior translation of the talus.

Laterally (Fig. 26.278)

Three primary ligaments that stabilize the ankle vary in structure. The anterior talofibular ligament is 2 to 2.5 mm thick, 15 to 20 mm long and 6 to 8 mm wide and is attached posteriorly to the anterior border of the lateral malleolus and anteriorly to the neck of the talus, where it blends with the anterolateral joint capsule. It is the weakest and most often injured of the lateral ligaments. It primarily functions to resist anterior translation of the talus. The calcaneofibular ligament is 20 to 25 mm long, 6 to 8 mm thick and is stronger than the anterior talofibular ligament. It is attached superiorly to the tip of the lateral malleolus, extends deep to the peroneal tendons and inserts inferiorly on the lateral surface of the calcaneus (it is the only lateral ligament that is extracapsular). The posterior talofibular ligament is

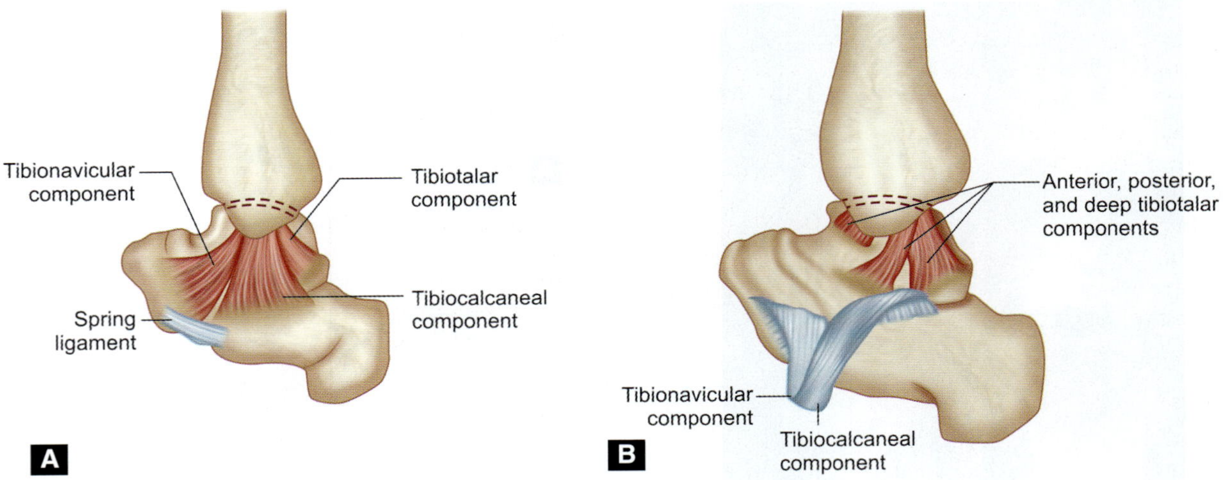

Figs 26.276A and B: Medial stabilizing structures of ankle and foot

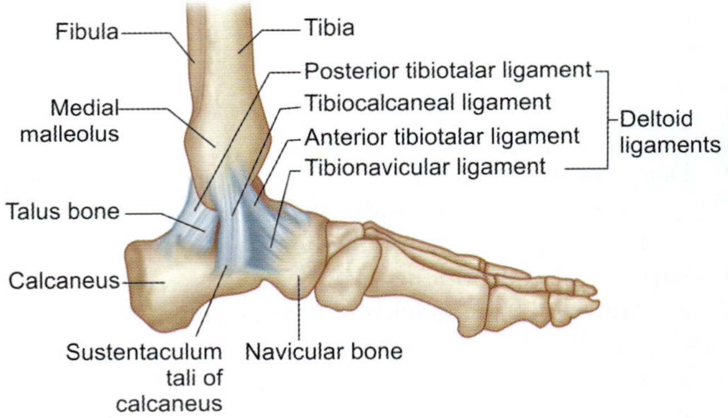

Fig. 26.277: Ankle and foot (medial view)

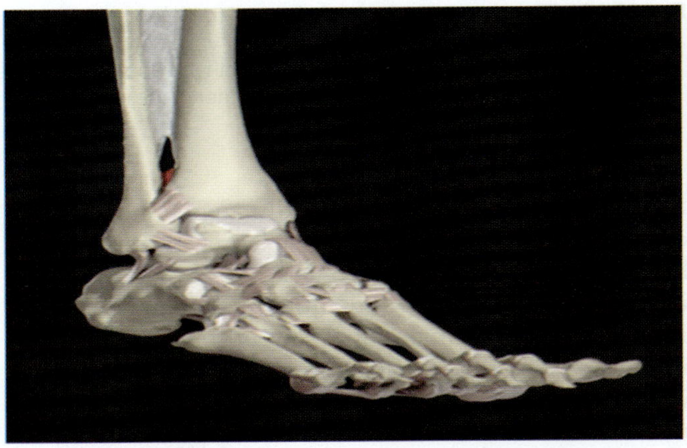

Fig. 26.279: Components of syndesmosis

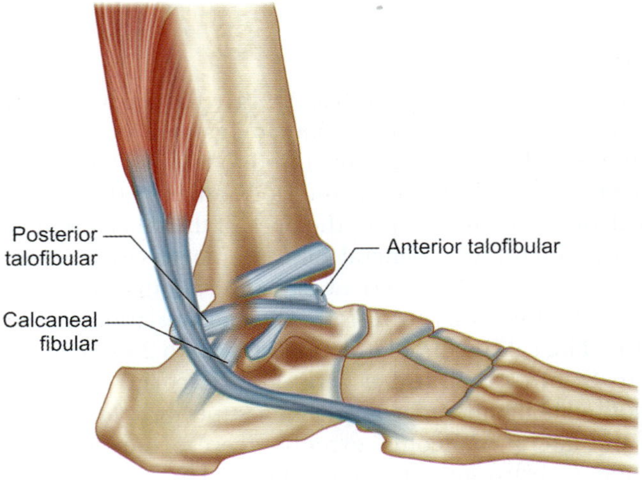

Fig. 26.278: Ankle and foot (lateral view)

30 mm long, 5 mm wide and 5 to 8 mm thick and is the strongest of the lateral ligaments. It is attached anteriorly to the digital fossa of the fibula and posteriorly to the lateral tubercle on the posterior aspect of the talus.

Syndesmosis (Fig. 26.279)

Maintaining the relationship of distal tibia/fibula is the syndesmosis, consisting of four components:

1. Anterior tibiofibular ligament
2. Posterior tibiofibular ligaments
3. Inferior transverse tibiofibular ligament
4. Intraosseous ligament

Major Functions of Ligaments

- Provide proprioceptive information for joint function
- Provide static stability to the joint and prevent excessive motion
- Act as guides to direct motion.

Acute Ligament Injuries

- Most common acute sports injury
- Commonly seen in sports like basketball and jumping sports
- Mechanism of injury is inversion and plantar flexion of the foot, when landing off balance or clipping another player's foot
- Eighty-five percent of all ankle sprains involve some plantar flexion of the ankle and inversion of the foot
- The remaining 15 percent consist of eversion mechanisms, which are often the result of an outside force, such as being fallen on from the outside.

Diagnosis

A careful physical examination is essential to avoid misdiagnosis. The following structures must be palpated because they may be associated with a complaint of ankle pain. The anterior tibiofibular, calcaneofibular, bifurcate, syndesmotic and deltoid ligaments. The medial and lateral malleoli, the fifth metatarsal base and the insertion of the peroneus tertius onto the dorsal fifth metatarsal base, the anterior process of the calcaneus and lateral process of the talus and the Achilles, peroneal, posterior tibial, flexor hallucis longus and flexor digitorum longus tendons.

Clinical Examination (Fig. 26.280)

- Swelling
- Echymosis
- Tenderness
- Decreased range of motion

Examine Ligaments (Fig. 26.281)

– *Medial:* Deltoid/anterior, medial and posterior portions
– *Lateral:* Anterior talofibular ligaments
– Syndesmotic ligaments

Provocative Tests

Injection of local anesthetic into the peroneal sheath and lateral gutter of the ankle before provocative maneuvers of the ankle, often improves the examination of the lateral ligaments by decreasing guarding and muscle spasm.

Eversion Stress Test

Knee is bent 90° and gastrocnemius is relaxed. The heel is held from below by one hand, while the other hand holds the lower leg. The hand on the heel is placed somewhat inferior, medial and is used to push the calcaneus and talus into eversion, while the other hand grips the lower leg laterally and pushes medially. It is to test deltoid ligament, the talus often shifts laterally with eversion stress on radiograph.

Inversion Stress Test (Fig. 26.282)

Knee is flexed 90° and gastrocnemius is relaxed. The heel is held from below by one hand, while the other hand holds the lower leg. The hand on the heel is placed somewhat inferior lateral and is used to push the calcaneus and talus into inversion, while the other hand grips the lower leg medially and pushes laterally. Note an end point. It is to test calcaneofibular ligament, posterior talofibular ligament and anterior talofibular ligament. Tilting of the talus 15° indicated rupture of the anterior talofibular ligament alone, that tilting 15° to 30°

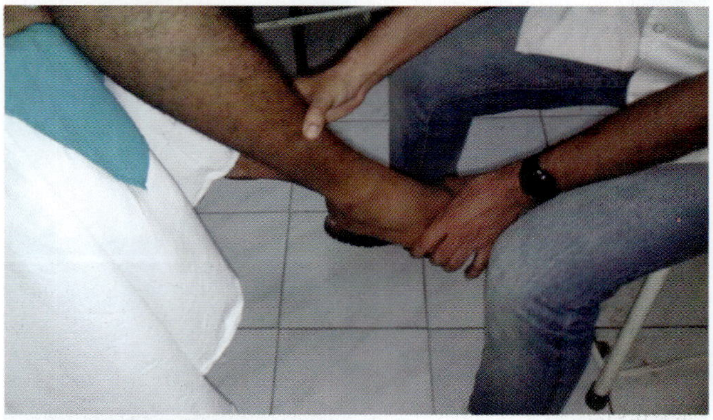

Fig. 26.281: Foot ligaments examination

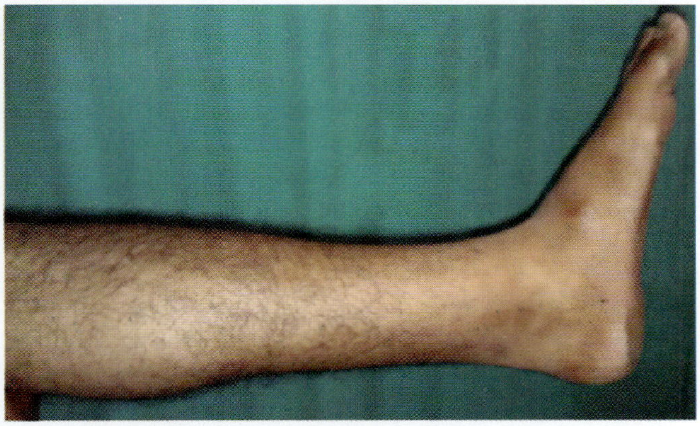

Fig. 26.280: Clinical findings in acute ligament injuries

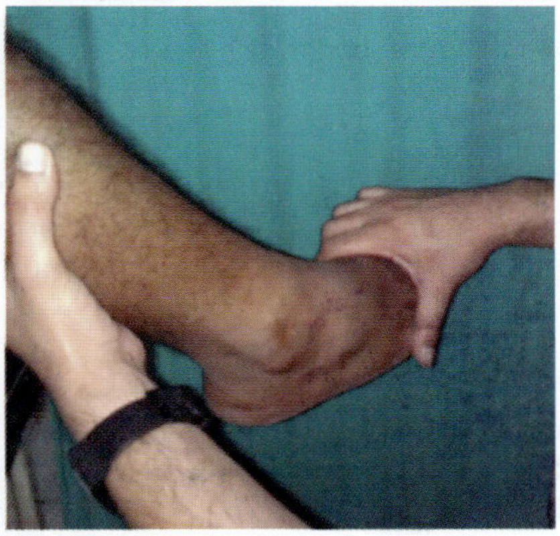

Fig. 26.282: Inversion stress test

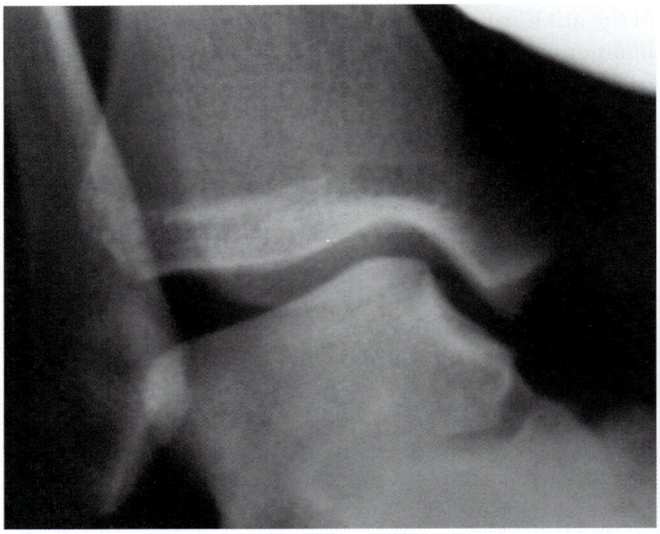

Fig. 26.283: Tilting of the talus determine ligament rupture

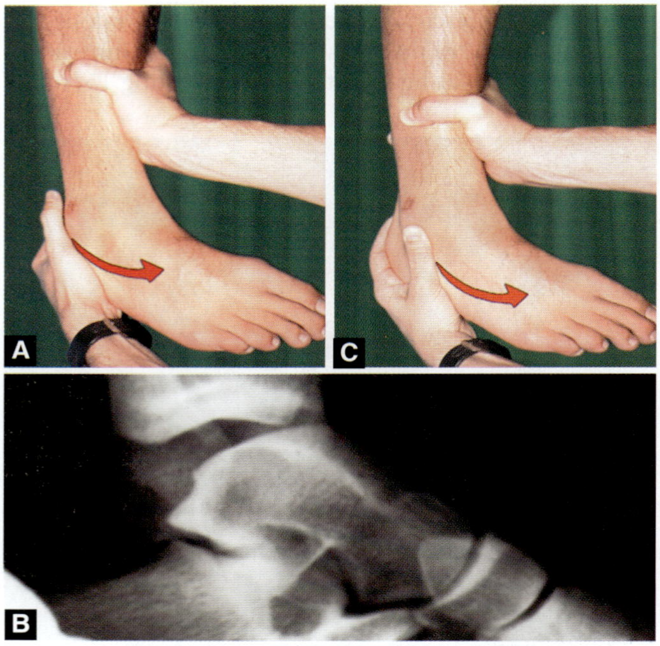

Figs 26.284A to C: Anterior drawer's test

indicated rupture of the anterior talofibular and calcaneofibular ligaments and that tilting more than 30° indicated that all three of the lateral ligaments were ruptured (Fig. 26.283).

Anterior Drawer's Test (Figs 26.284A to C)

Knee is flexed 90° and gastrocnemius is relaxed. One hand holds the lower tibia and exerts a slight posterior force and the other hand is around the posterior aspect of the calcaneus and attempts to bring the calcaneus and talus

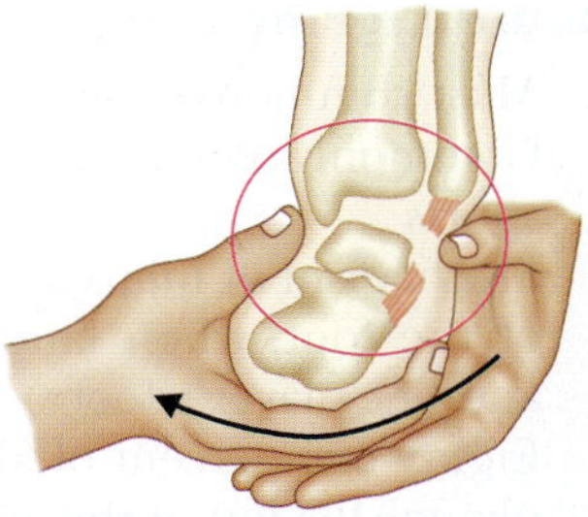

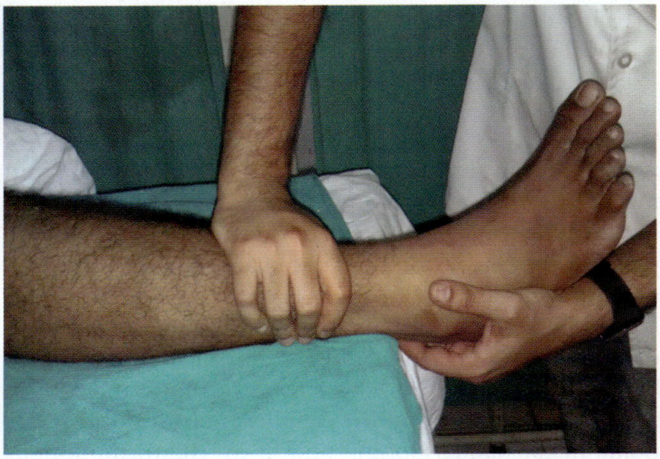

Fig. 26.285: Talar tilt test

forward on the tibia. Also done by stabilization of foot and talus on table and pushing tibia and fibula posteriorly. It is to test anterior talofibular ligament/anteromedial capsule. Anterior displacement of the talus relative to the tibia.

Talar Tilt Test (Fig. 26.285)

It is performed to determine extent of inversion or eversion injuries. With foot at 90°, calcaneus is inverted and excessive motion indicates injury to calcaneofibular ligament and possibly the anterior and posterior talofibular ligaments. If the calcaneus is everted, the deltoid ligament is tested, as shown in Figures 26.286A and B.

Kleiger's Test (Fig. 26.287)

Used primarily to determine extent of damage to the deltoid ligament and may be used to evaluate distal ankle syndesmosis, anterior/posterior tibiofibular ligaments and the interosseus membrane. With lower leg stabilized, foot is rotated laterally to stress the deltoid.

Medial Subtalar Glide Test (Fig. 26.288)

It is performed to determine presence of excessive medial translation of the calcaneus on the talus. Talus is stabilized in subtalar neutral, while other hand glides the calcaneus medially. A positive test presents with excessive movement, indicating injury to the lateral ligaments.

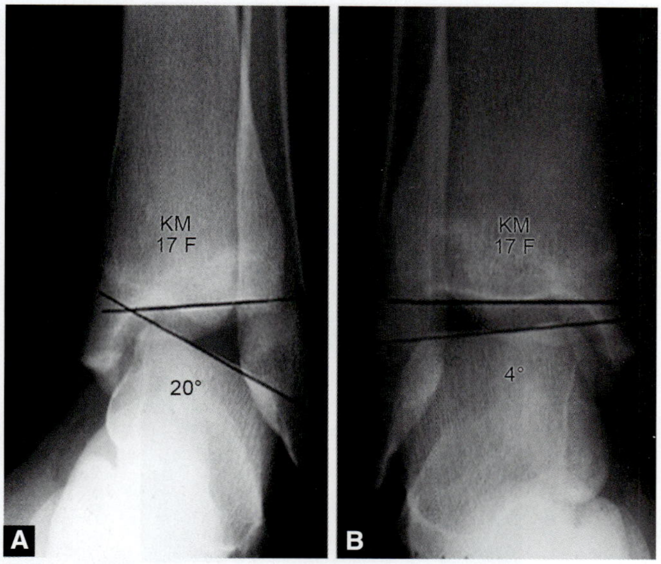

Figs 26.286A and B: X-rays, showing various talar tilts

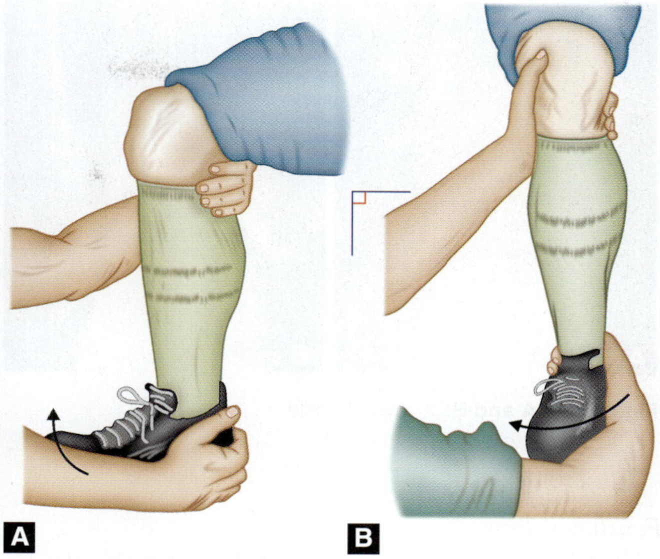

Figs 26.289A and B: External rotation test

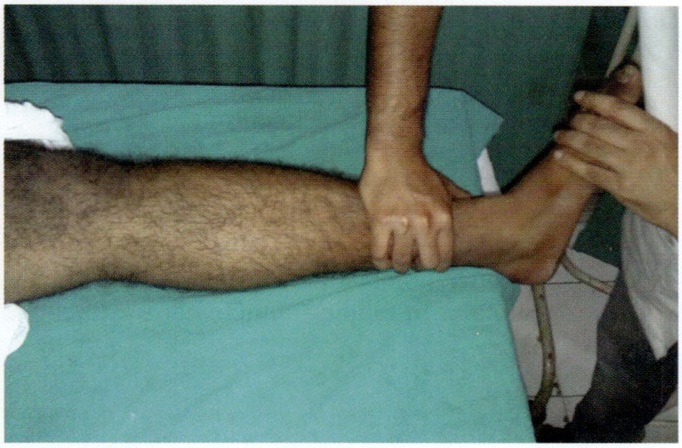

Fig. 26.287: Kleiger's test

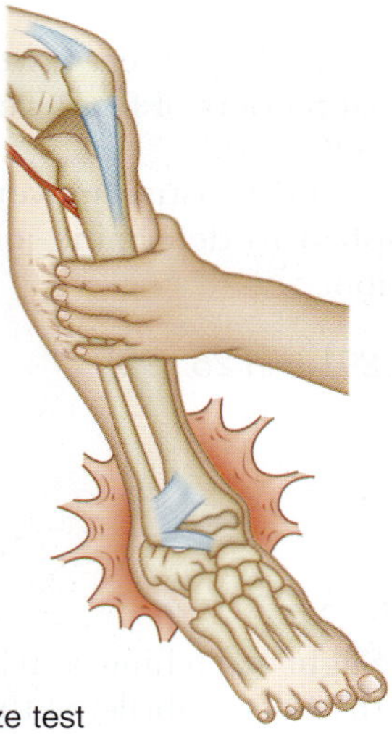

Fig. 26.290: Squeeze test

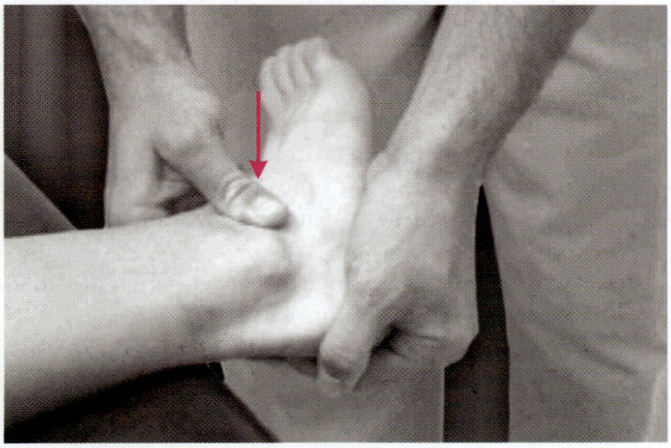

Fig. 26.288: Medial subtalar glide test

External Rotation Test (Figs 26.289A and B)

Foot should be in neutral position with the lower leg stabilized. Examiner should then externally rotate the foot. If this causes pain then must consider a tear of the anterior tibiofibular ligament. Depending on severity the interosseous membrane may be involved. Pain will be at site of the anterior tibiofibular ligament.

Squeeze Test (Fig. 26.290)

Perform the squeeze test just above the anterior tibiofibular ligament. Squeeze the bones together firmly and slowly, hold and then quickly release. If there is pain upon release at the area of the anterior tibiofibular ligament, then a sprain of that ligament is highly suspected.

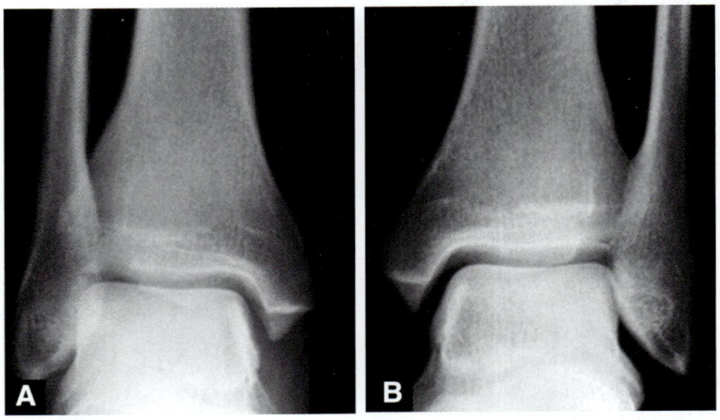

Figs 26.291A and B: X-rays of ankle

Functional Tests

- While weight bearing the following should be performed
- Walk on toes (plantar flexion)
- Walk on heels (dorsiflexion)
- Walk on lateral borders of feet (inversion)
- Walk on medial borders of feet (eversion)
- Hops on injured ankle
- Passive, active and resistive movements should be manually applied to determine joint integrity and muscle function.

Imaging (Figs 26.291 and 26.292)

- X-rays
- MRI
- USG

Classification

Grade 1 sprain: Slight stretching and some damage to the fibers (fibrils) of the ligament.

Grade 2 sprain: Partial tearing of the ligament. If the ankle joint is examined and moved in certain ways, abnormal looseness (laxity) of the ankle joint occurs.

Grade 3 sprain: Complete tear of the ligament. If the examiner pulls or pushes on the ankle joint in certain movements, gross instability occurs.

Classification of Ankle Ligament Injury and Treatment Recommendations (Clanton)

On the Basis of Stability

- Type I, stable ankle to clinical testing (with anesthesia, if necessary).
- Type II, unstable ankle with positive anterior drawer test or positive talar tilt test or both.

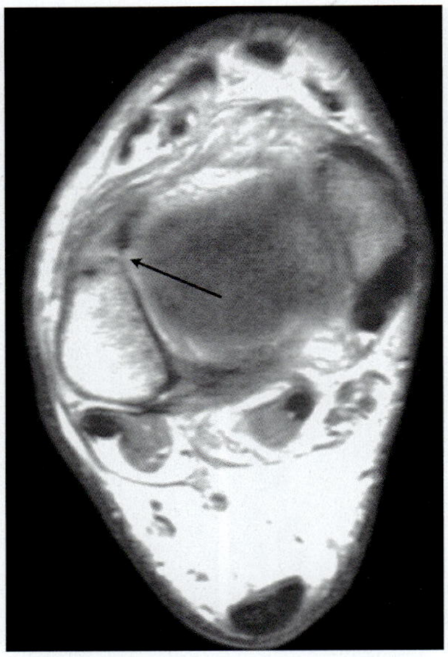

Fig. 26.292: MRI of foot and ankle

On the Basis of the Type of Patient

- Grade 1, non-athlete or older patient—functional treatment
- Grade 2, athlete or high-demand patient.

On the Basis of the Radiographic Stress Testing

- Type A, negative radiograph stress test—functional treatment
- Type B, positive tibiotalar stress test—surgical repair
- Type C, subtalar instability—functional treatment.

Treatment

Conservative Management

Indicated for type 1, type 2 and type 3 sprains, using selective functional treatment, which consists of a short "select" period of protection with taping or bracing that allows early weight bearing, followed by functional range-of-motion exercises and neuromuscular training of the ankle).

RICE (Fig. 26.293)

— *Rest:* Stay off the ankle, crutches may be needed.
— *ICE:* 15 minutes a 4 to 5 times a day.
— *Compression:* Ice wrap with horse shoe keeps the swelling down.
— *Elevation:* Keep ankle above heart level when possible, allows gravity to pump out swelling.

Goals of RICE: (Fig. 26.294)

— Limit swelling reduction
— Reduce pain
— Return to sport/activity quicker

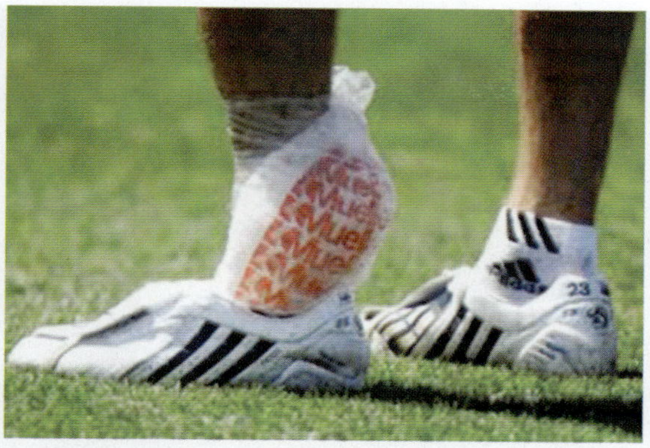

Fig. 26.293: Conservative treatment for ankle ligament injuries include ice application on the injured part

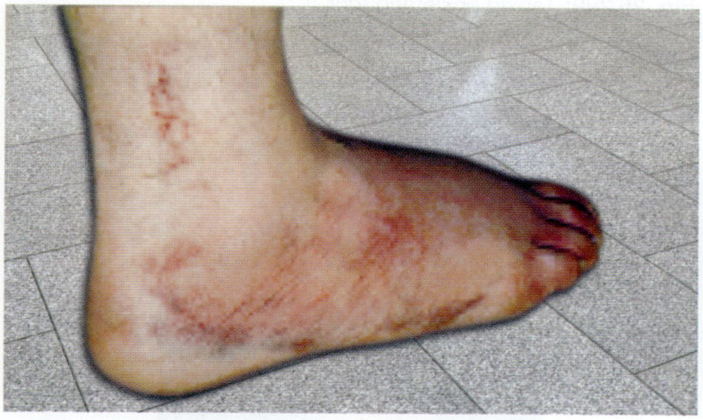

Fig. 26.294: Swelling and ecchymosis of the foot

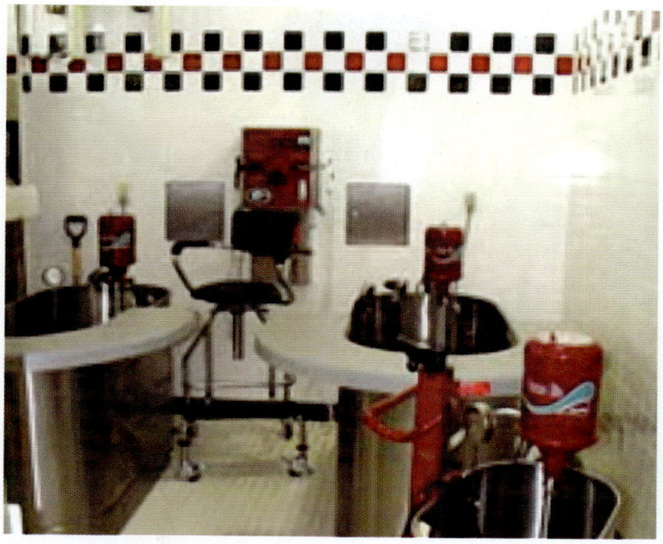

Fig. 26.295: Whirlpool treatment for foot and ankle injuries

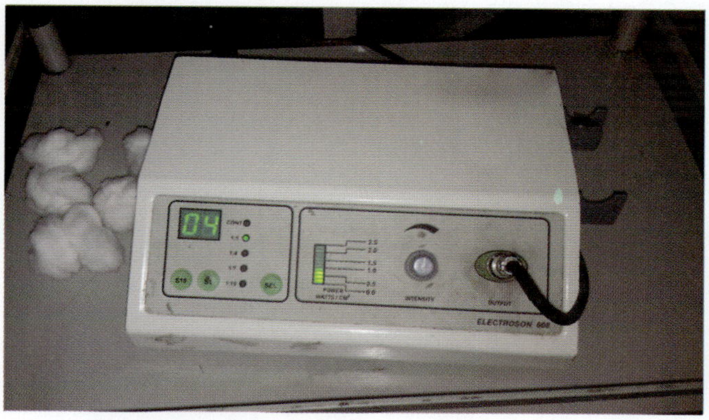

Fig. 26.296: Ultrasonic treatment

Modalities used: These are enumerated below:

- *Cold whirlpool (Fig. 26.295):*
  - 15 minutes a couple times a day
  - Vasoconstricts vessels around ankle
  - Stimulates pain killing receptors
  - Slows cell metabolism
  - Aids in reducing swelling
- *High voltage:*
  - Assists in activating pain killing receptors
  - Assists in muscle stimulation around ankle joint to aid in edema removal.
- *Ultrasound (Fig. 26.296):*
  - Assists in edema removal.
  - Assists in bringing digestive enzymes to clean debris cells of the injured ankle.
- *Rehabilitation exercises (Fig. 26.297):*
  - Range of motion exercises
  - One leg stands
  - Biomechanical ankle platform system (BAPS) board
  - Towel curls
  - Toe pick-ups
  - Toe rises (Fig. 26.298)
  - Theraband
- *Taping (Fig. 26.299):*
  - Psychologically better feeling to the athlete
  - Tight fitting at first
  - Tape looses a large percentage of its support within the first 15 to 20 minutes of competition.
- *Wrapping (Fig. 26.300):*
  - Purpose of wrapping is injury prevention.
  - Wrapping will not eliminate sprained ankle, but it does minimize the severity of the sprain.
- *Ankle braces:*
  - Many varieties and types
  - Lace up (Fig. 26.301)
  - Hinged
  - Air casts (Fig. 26.302)
  - All offer different levels of support.

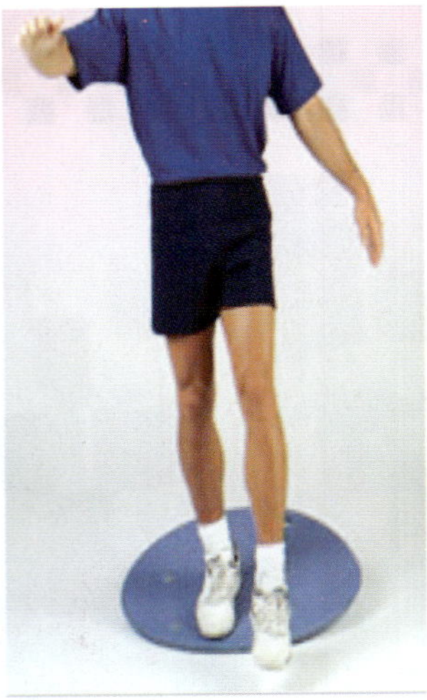

Fig. 26.297: BAPS board exercises

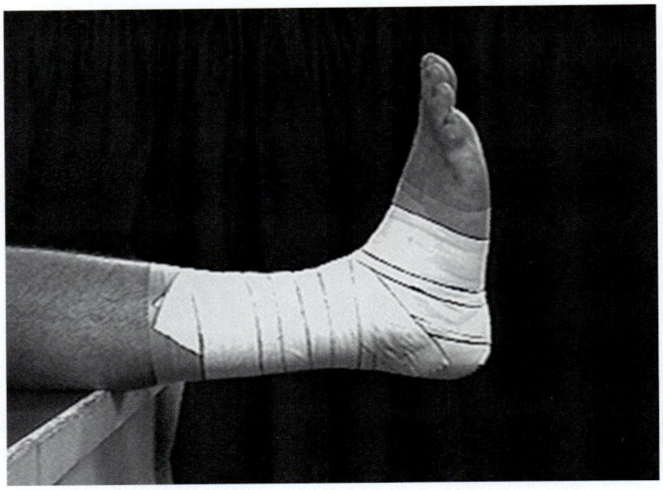

Fig. 26.299: Taping ankle and foot

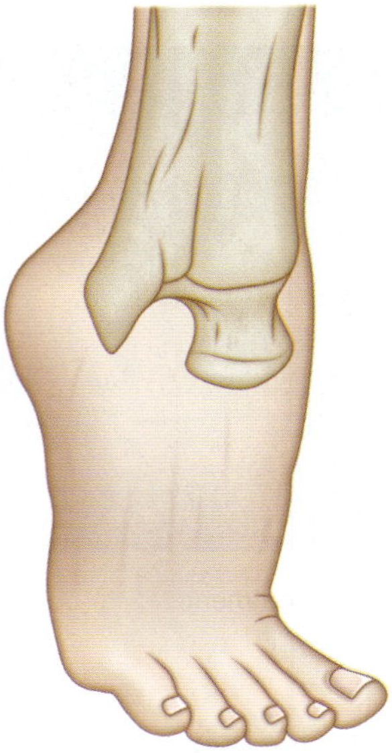

Fig. 26.298: Toe raising exercises

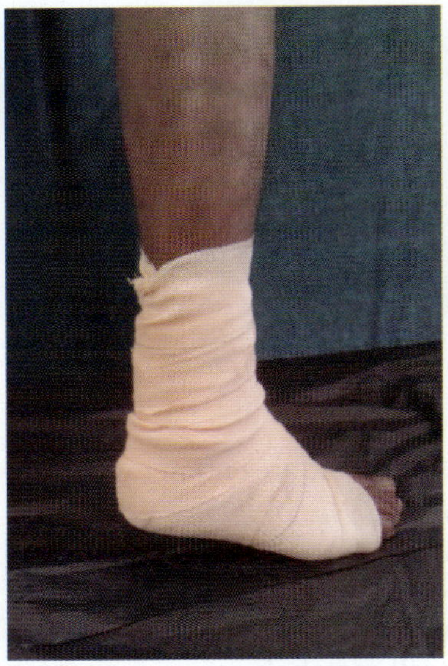

Fig. 26.300: Wrapping ankle and foot

- Large and competitive business market for ankle braces.

Surgical Treatment

Indications

- Large bony avulsions
- Severe ligamentous damage on the medial and the lateral sides of the ankle
- Indicating a major joint injury
- Severe recurrent injuries

Goal of the Treatment is to Prevent Chronic Instability

- *Repair of acute rupture of the deltoid ligament* (Figs 26.303 and 26.304): Anteromedial incision is done, as shown in Figure 26.303. Suture the ligament with non absorbale sutures after the fixation of lateral malleolus fracture, if any, as shown in Figures 26.304A and B.
- *Repair of acute rupture of the ligaments of the distal tibiofibular joint (Fig. 26.305):* Make an incision 5 cm long parallel to the anterior border of the distal fibula and expose the distal tibiofibular joint. Press the fibula

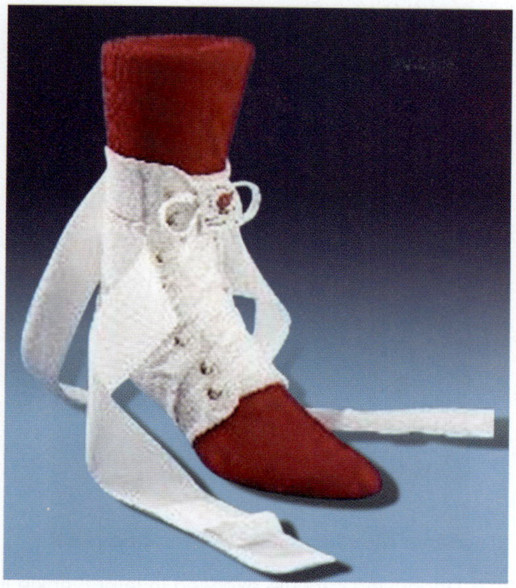

Fig. 26.301: Lace up ankle braces

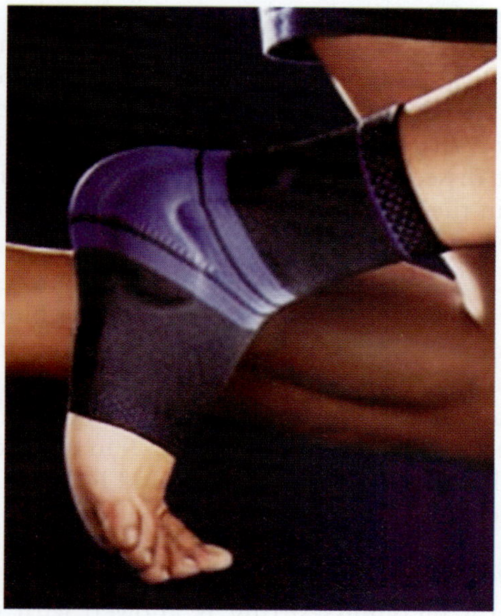

Fig. 26.302: Air casts

into the groove in the tibia to shift the fibula and the talus medially into normal position. Suturing or reattaching the ligaments is unnecessary. With the ankle dorsiflexed 30°, insert a screw transversely through the fibula into the tibia approximately 1 to 1.5 cm proximal to the ankle joint. If the foot is held in equinus during screw fixation, the narrowest part of the talus is engaged in the ankle mortise, and for later dorsiflexion the widest part of the talus must be forced into this narrowed space between the malleoli.

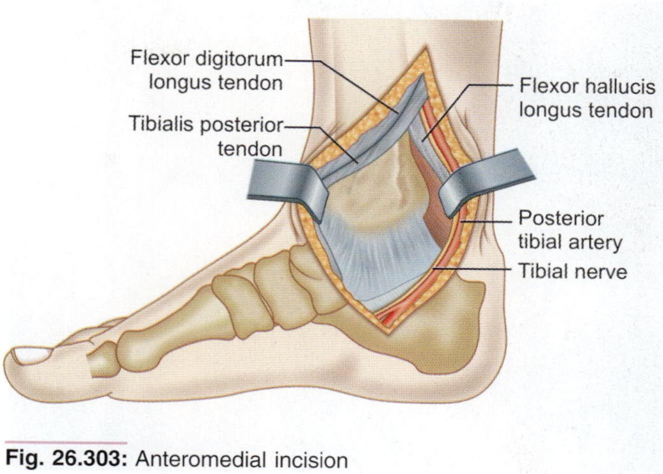

Fig. 26.303: Anteromedial incision

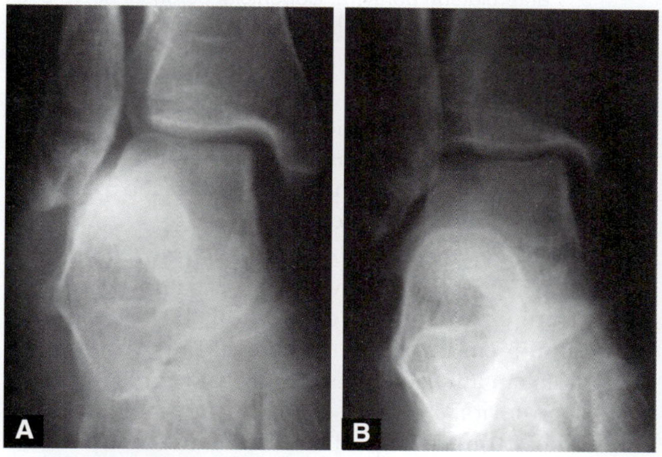

Figs 26.304A and B: (A) Preoperative X-ray; (B) Postoperative X-ray

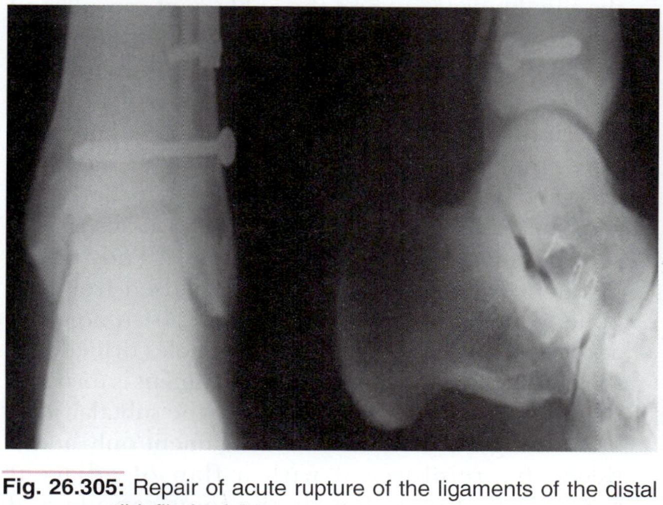

Fig. 26.305: Repair of acute rupture of the ligaments of the distal tibiofibular joint

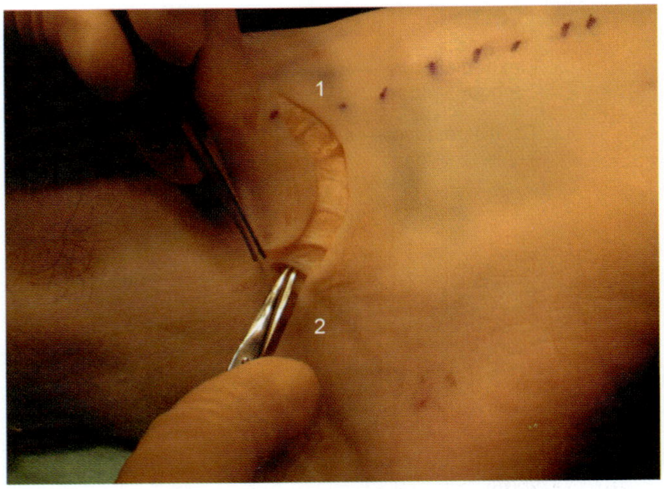

Fig. 26.306: Repair of acute rupture of the lateral ligaments—1. The skin incision, runs from just lateral to the anterolateral portal; 2. Superficial peroneal nerve back towards the peroneal tendons

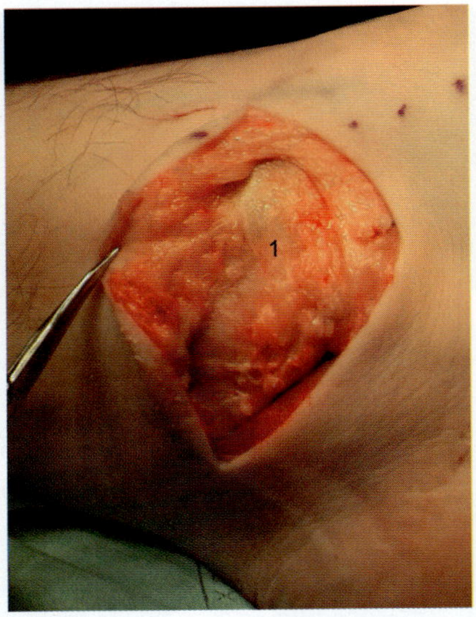

Fig. 26.307: Underlying capsule exposed in lateral ankle ligament repair

Check the position of the screw and the reduction of the talus by radiographs in the operating room, to ensure that the talus has been replaced precisely against the medial malleolus.

- *Repair of acute rupture of the lateral ligaments (Fig. 26.306):* To avoid venous stasis and necrosis of skin edges and nerve disruption, begin a curved incision 5 cm proximal to the distal tip of the fibula and 1.5 cm anterior to its margin and curve it distally and posteriorly to end distal to the fibula half the distance from the tip of the fibula to the tip of the heel. Identify and preserve the branches of the superficial peroneal nerve anteriorly and the sural nerve distally and preserve as many superficial veins as possible. Section the aponeurotic tissue overlying the tibiofibular joint and the ankle joint capsule and expose tears in these areas by blunt dissection. Incise the peroneal sheath and retract the peroneal tendons to expose the calcaneofibular ligament and the anterior portion of the posterior talofibular ligament. Stress the lateral ligaments for stability at the ankle and subtalar joints by forcibly inverting the foot, while they are exposed. With appropriate non-absorbable suture material, approximate the torn ends of the ligaments or when ligaments are avulsed from the bone, suture the ends of the ligaments to adjacent aponeurotic tissue or through small holes drilled into the bone. When the talocalcaneal ligament is torn and there is subtalar instability, stabilize the subtalar joint by suturing the calcaneofibular ligament only and if necessary reinforce it with a flap of adjacent aponeurotic tissue. Repair the joint capsule and peroneal sheath, close the wound and apply a plaster cast from the toes to the tibial tuberosity with the ankle in neutral position. The skin incision, runs from just lateral to the anterolateral portal (1) and *superficial peroneal* nerve back towards the *peroneal tendons* (2) A blunt dissection at right angles to the skin incision and in the line of the sural and superficial nerves is undertaken to isolate these.

Lateral ankle ligament repair (Figs 26.307 to 26.311): Underlying capsule is exposed following a blunt swab dissection of the fat layer. The avulsed anterior talofibular ligament (2) is in good condition and can be reattached to the lateral talus (1). A good demonstration of the uninjured, calcaneofibular ligament (2) in the bed of the peroneal tendons (1). The capsule and ligaments being tightened with multiple sutures.

After Treatment

For lateral ligaments sitting is allowed with the leg dependent for 30 to 60 seconds each half hour and when dependency is tolerated well, crutch walking is instituted. The initial cast should be changed after 2 weeks and the sutures should be removed. After 2 more weeks, weight bearing with crutches is allowed. At 6 weeks, the cast is discarded and range-of-motion exercises and manual resistive exercises, to gain inversion and eversion strength are begun. Dorsiflexion and plantar flexion exercises are prescribed as soon as practical. For distal tibiofibular ligaments, a cast is applied from the base of the toes to the tibial tuberosity. At 3 weeks, the cast is removed and a walking boot cast is applied and worn for 4 weeks. At 8 weeks, the screw across the joint should be removed and

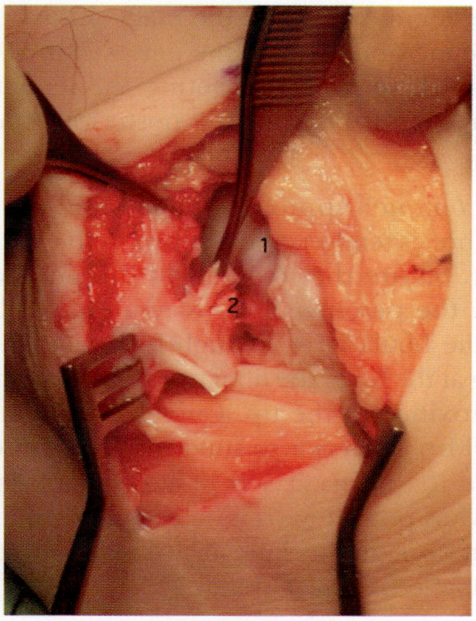

Fig. 26.308: Lateral ankle ligament repair, showing underlying structures—1. Lateral talus; 2. The avulsed anterior talofibular ligament

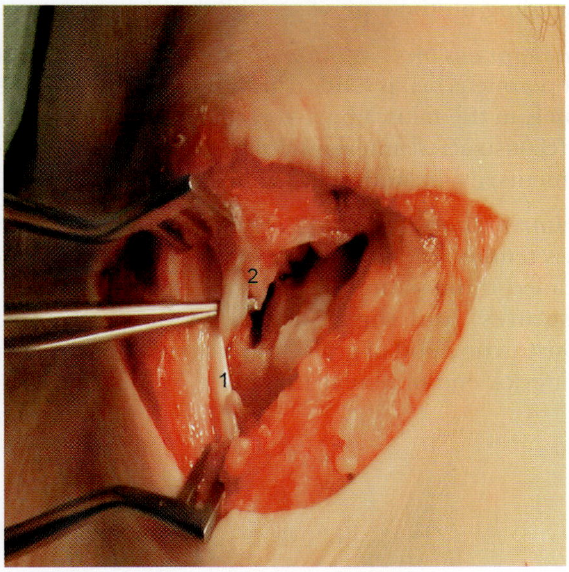

Fig. 26.309: Lateral ankle repair, showing calcaneofibular ligaments—1. Peroneal tendons; 2. Calcaneofibular ligament

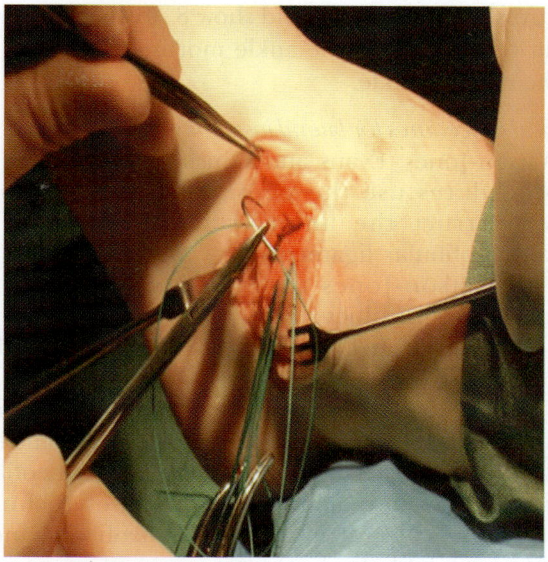

Fig. 26.310: Capsules and ligaments being tightened with multiple sutures

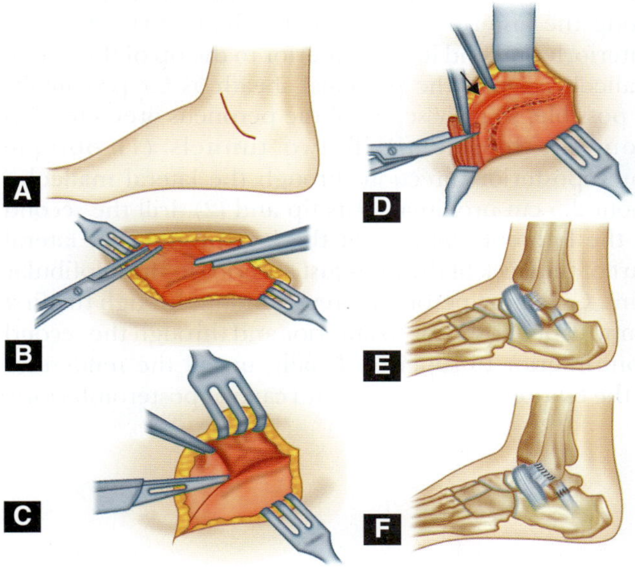

Figs 26.311A to F: Steps of lateral ankle repair

because its head is just beneath the skin, its removal is usually fairly easy. Prompt removal is necessary because the screw becomes loose and sometimes breaks within the tibiofibular joint.

Chronic instability after injury

- It is common complication of acute ligament injury
- At first it should be treated conservatively with braces
- Findings would be:
  - Disabling pain
  - Persistent instability
  - Stress radiographs showing 8° to 10° of talar tilt
- Should first be treated conservatively, if it is symptomatic:
  - Stirrup brace
  - Ankles tape
  - A muscle-strengthening program
- When disabling pain and instability persist, however reconstruction of the lateral ligaments should be considered.

- Stress radiographs should show 8° to 10° of increased tilt of the talus in the ankle mortise, compared with the normal ankle.

Surgical procedures for lateral instability

- Watson-Jones, Evans and Elmslie operations. These procedures use the peroneus brevis tendon to reconstruct the anterior talofibular and the calcaneofibular ligaments.
- The Watson-Jones technique may present two technical difficulties
  - The tunnel in the neck of the talus may be difficult to drill
  - The peroneus brevis tendon may be too short
- The Evans technique was designed to overcome these difficulties, but it reconstructs only the calcaneofibular ligament, whereas the Watson-Jones technique attempts reconstruction of the calcaneofibular and the anterior talofibular ligaments.

Watson-Jones procedure: Make a lateral incision over the ankle beginning proximally at the junction of the middle and distal thirds of the fibular shaft, continue it distally along the anterior border of the shaft, curve it gently anteriorly and end it 5 cm anterior to the tip of the lateral malleolus. Open the peroneal sheath as far proximally as possible, sharply separate the peroneus brevis tendon from the muscle. Drill two tunnels (1) oblique anteroposterior direction through the lateral malleolus about 2.5 cm proximal to its tip and (2) drill the second in the longitudinal axis of the leg through the lateral part of the neck of the talus just anterior to the talofibular joint. Guide the peroneus brevis tendon through the first tunnel from posterior to anterior and through the second from inferior to superior. Finally, unroll the remainder of the tendon to make it flat and carry it posteroinferiorly across the lateral surface of the malleolus, after making an oblique incision through the periosteum at this level, as shown in Figure 26.312. Suture the tendon to itself and to the periosteum on the posterior aspect of the malleolus.

Evans technique: Approach, divide and mobilize the peroneus brevis tendon, as described in the Watson-Jones technique. Suture the free end of the peroneus brevis muscle to the peroneus longus tendon. Drill a tunnel through the fibula large enough to receive the tendon, beginning at the tip of the fibula and emerging posteriorly 3.2 cm proximal to the tip. Guide the tendon through the tunnel from inferior to superior and suture it under tension, to the adjacent soft tissue at both ends of the tunnel. Evans procedure can be used, only if anatomical reconstruction of the lateral ankle ligaments is not feasible, as shown in Figure 26.313.

Larsen technique (Figs 26.314A and B): The tendon was pulled through two canals in the lateral malleolus and fixed in a hole in the calcaneus. The direction of the tendon in relationship to the calcaneus and talus varied depending on the type of instability.

Split peroneus brevis tendon graft: Sammarco described a split peroneus brevis tendon graft routed through osseous tunnels in the talus, fibula and calcaneus and sutured to the reconstructed anterior talofibular and calcaneofibular ligaments, as illustrated in Figures 26.315A to E.

Chrisman-Snook (*Figs 26.316A to D):* Split of peroneus brevis tendon. Mobilized half of peroneus brevis tendon threaded through anterior talocalcaneal ligament (held by sutures) and through hole in fibula. Complete reconstruction end of graft sutured to its anterior portion at anterior end of fibular tunnel.

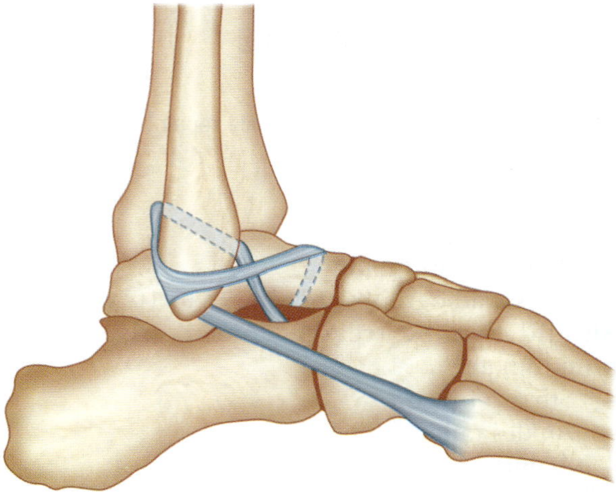

Fig. 26.312: Watson-Jones procedure

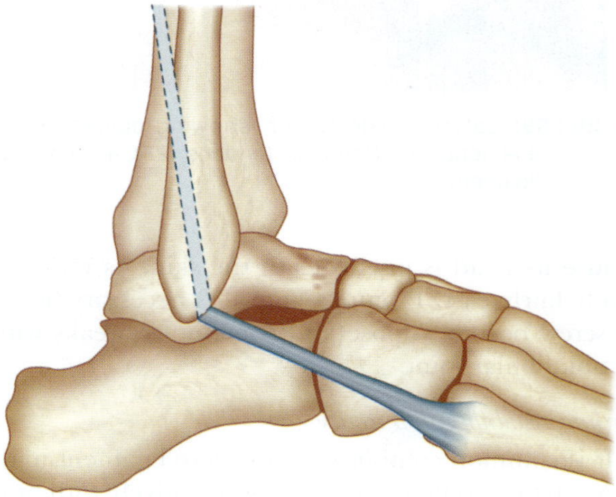

Fig. 26.313: Evans procedure of correcting lateral instability

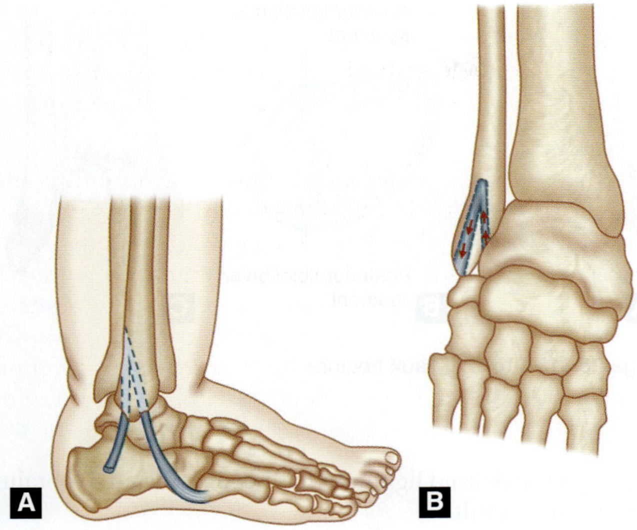

Figs 26.314A and B: Larsen's technique

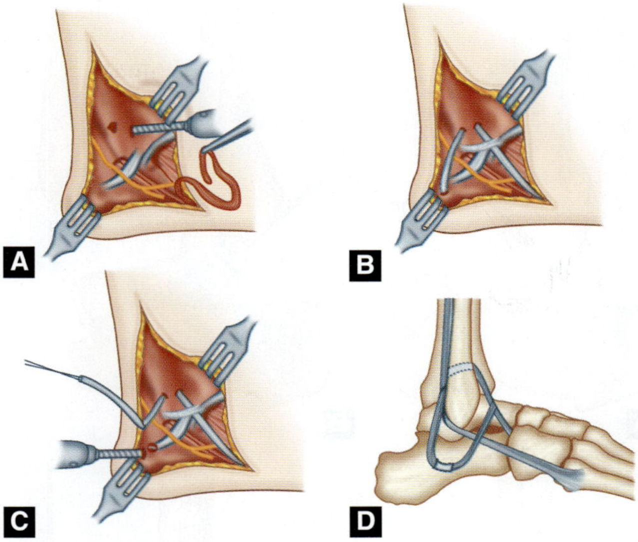

Figs 26.316A to D: Chrisman-Snook procedure

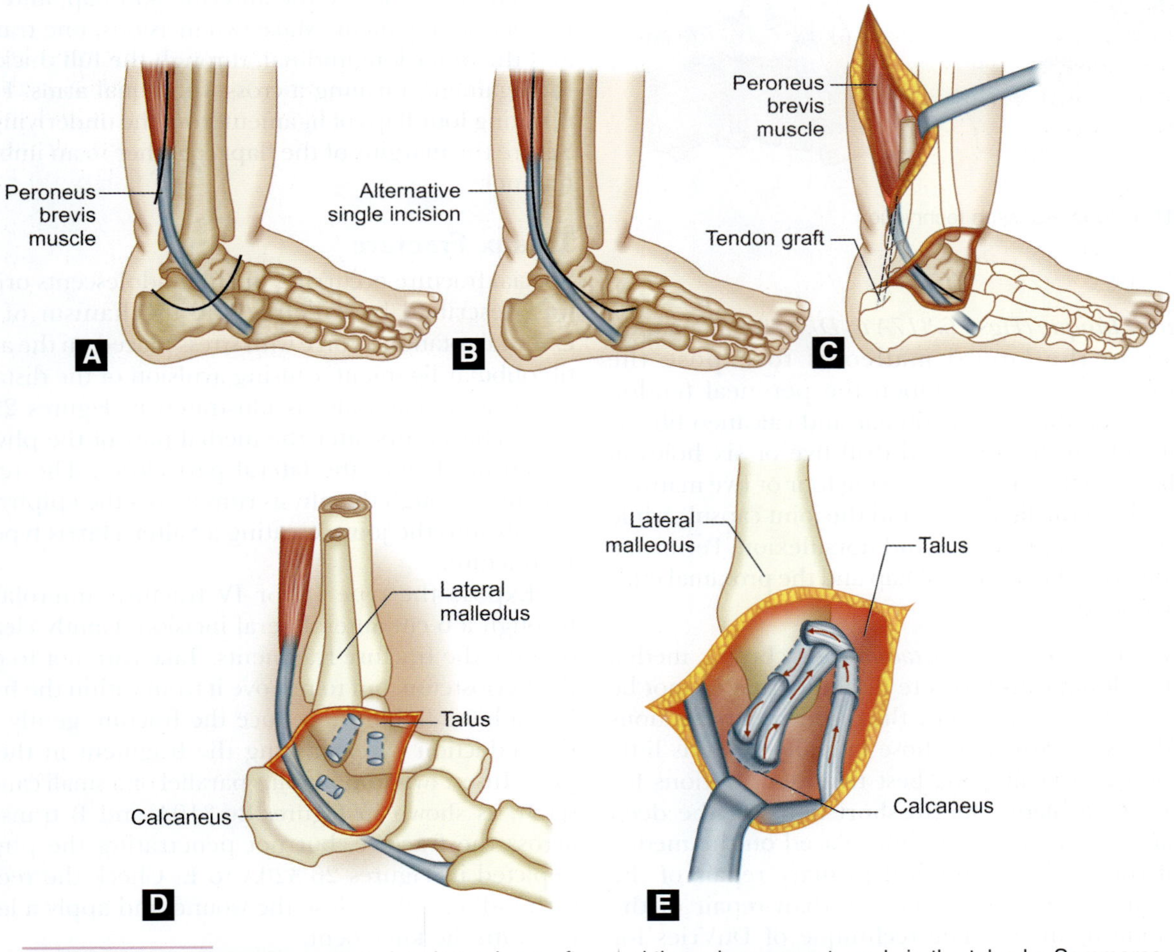

Figs 26.315A to E: A split peroneus brevis tendon graft routed through osseous tunnels in the talus by Sammarco

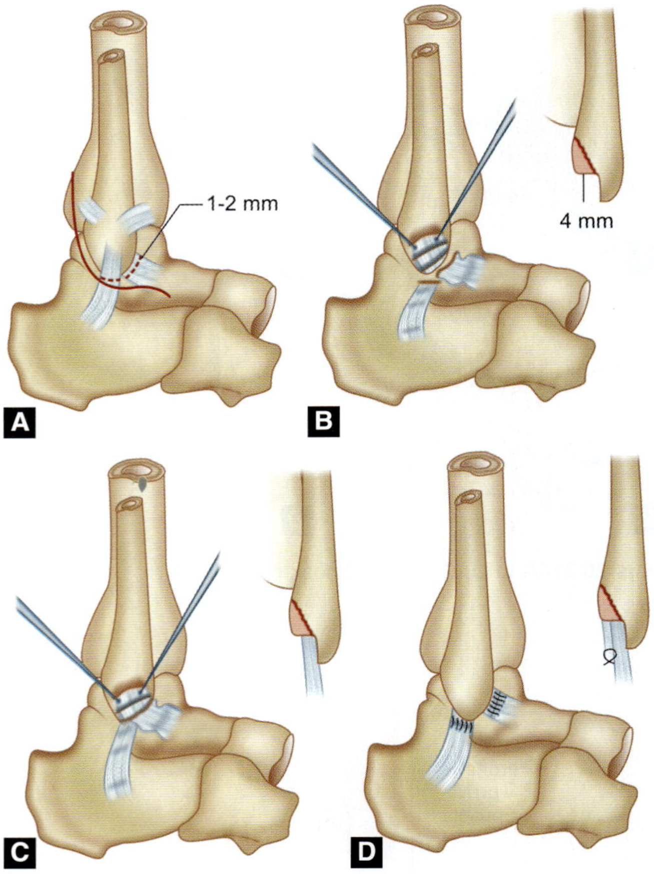

Figs 26.317A to D: Karlsson technique

Karlsson technique (Figs 26.317A to D): Make an incision posterior to the lateral malleolus to expose the calcaneofibular ligament. Open the peroneal tendon sheath, and identify the talofibular and calcaneo fibular ligaments. Open the joint and drill five or six holes in the fibula with a 2 mm drill bit. Using four or five mattress sutures, tighten the ligaments and the joint capsule while the foot is held in pronation and dorsiflexion. Perform a duplication with the periosteal flap and the proximal ends of the ligaments.

Medial repair of chronic instability: As chronic medial instability seldom causes severe disability that cannot be treated conservatively, because the reconstructive options have had less success than those laterally, there is little information concerning the best treatment options for this difficult problem. Due to short fibers of the deep deltoid and the increased tension placed on the medial aspect of the ankle, anatomical primary repair of the deltoid ligament is less satisfactory than repair of the lateral ankle ligament. The technique of DuVries for

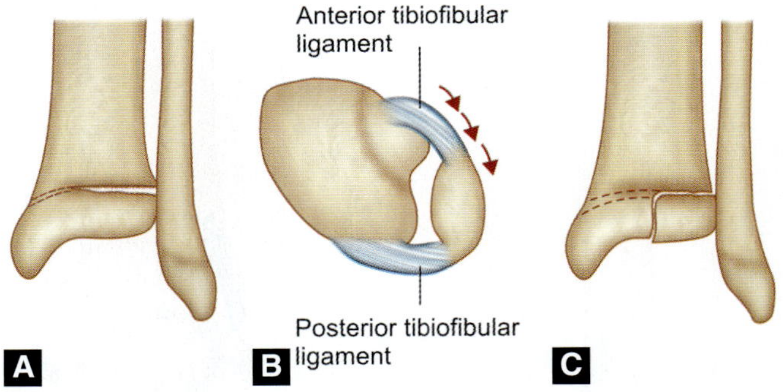

Figs 26.318A to C: Tillaux fracture

repair of the deltoid ligament has been reported to obtain satisfactory results.

DuVries technique: Make a curved incision over the medial aspect of the ankle beginning posterior to the medial malleolus, coursing distally and anteriorly about 2 cm distal to the malleolus, and ending over the tuberosity of the navicular. Elevate the anterior skin flap, and expose the deltoid ligament. Make two incisions, one transverse and the other longitudinal, through the full thickness of the ligament, forming a cross with equal arms. Free the resulting four flaps of ligament from the underlying bone. Suture the margins of the flaps together in an imbricated manner.

Tillaux Fracture

Special fracture occurring in older adolescents originally was described by Tillaux. The mechanism of injury external rotational force with stress placed on the anterior tibiofibular ligament, causing avulsion of the distal tibial physis anterolaterally, as illustrated in Figures 26.318A to C. This occurs after the medial part of the physis has closed but before the lateral part closes. The resultant fracture through the physis runs across the epiphysis and distally into the joint, creating a Salter-Harris type III or IV fracture.

Expose the type III or IV fracture anterolaterally, through a 6 cm anterolateral incision. Gently clean and observe the fracture fragments. Take care not to disrupt the periosteum, but to remove it from within the fracture. Use a bone holder to reduce the fracture gently. Check the reduction by examining the fragment in the ankle joint. Insert two smooth pins parallel or a small cancellous screw, as shown in Figures 26.319A and B transversely across the fracture, but not penetrating the physis, as depicted in Figures 26.320A to E. Check the reduction with radiographs. Close the wound and apply a long leg cast with the knee bent.

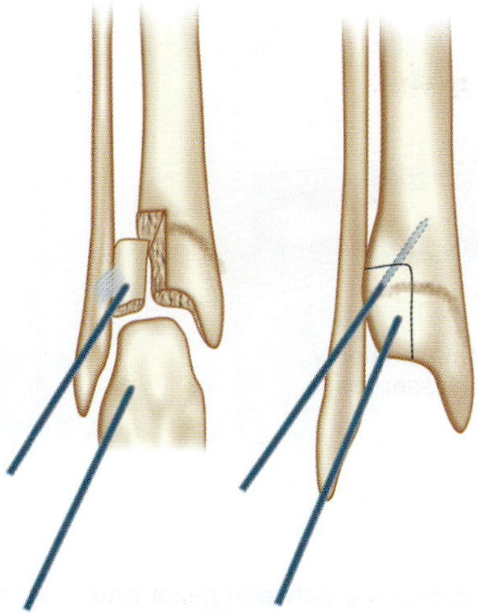

Figs 26.319A and B: Inserting two smooth pins parallel or a small cancellous screw transversely across the fracture, but not penetrating the physis

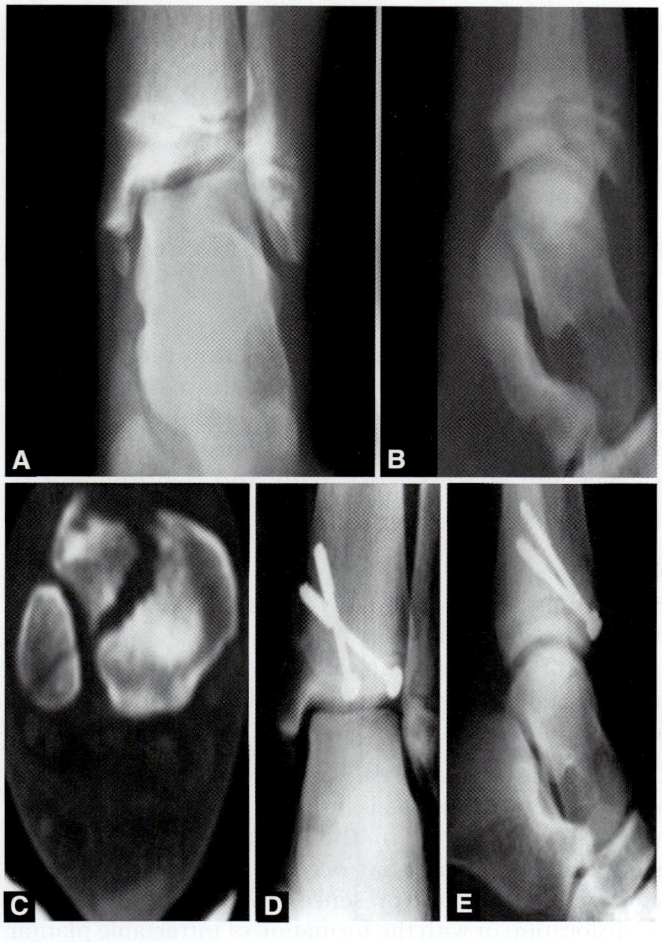

Figs 26.320A to E: X-ray showing Tillaux fracture reduction procedure

INFLAMMATION OF FOOT AND ANKLE AND NEUROPATHIC FOOT

I. Autoimmune:
- Rheumatoid arthritis
- Sero negative inflammatory arthritis
  - Ankylosing spondylitis
  - Psoriatic arthritis
  - Inflammatory bowel disease
  - Reactive arthritis (Reiter's syndrome)
  - Crystalline arthropathies (Metabolic)– Gout, pseudogout, calcium hydroxy-apatite crystal arthritis

II. Infective (septic, tubercular, fungal).

■ Rheumatoid Arthritis (Forefoot, Midfoot, Hindfoot)

Eighty-nine percent of rheumatoid arthritis (RA) patients are with arthritis of foot and ankle. About 17 percent of patients with RA present initially with symptoms affecting the joints of the feet. Different stages of RA are elaborated in the Table 26.2.

RA Forefoot

Of patients with RA, 89 percent have forefoot involvement and patients often present with this involvement within 1 year of diagnosis. The earliest manifestation of rheumatoid arthritis of the forefoot is synovitis of the metatarsophalangeal joints. Enzymes like proteases and collagenases are released from the diseased synovium.

These enzymes destroy articular cartilage and disrupt ligament-bone interphases. Fluid distention of the joint capsule and weakening of the capsular ligaments allow the toes to sublux dorsally at the MP joint. Normal alignment of MP joints and toes is due to the balance between flexor and extensor mechanisms and joint capsules, as shown in Figure 26.321. In RA, imbalance occurs with progressive dorsal subluxation of MP joints. Progression of deformities leads to pressure atrophy of fat pad, over protruding metatarsal heads, callus formation and ulceration, as shown in Figure 26.322.

Table 26.2: Stages of rheumatoid arthritis

Stage 1:	Discomfort, synovitis without significant joint space narrowing; no bony deformity
Stage 2:	Minimal erosive articular changes; early involvement without fixed deformity
Stage 3:	No significant joint erosion; soft-tissue deformity present
Stage 4:	Severe hallux valgus, lesser MTP-joint dislocation with fixed hammer-toe or claw-toe deformities, articular destruction, pes planovalgus, hindfoot arthritis

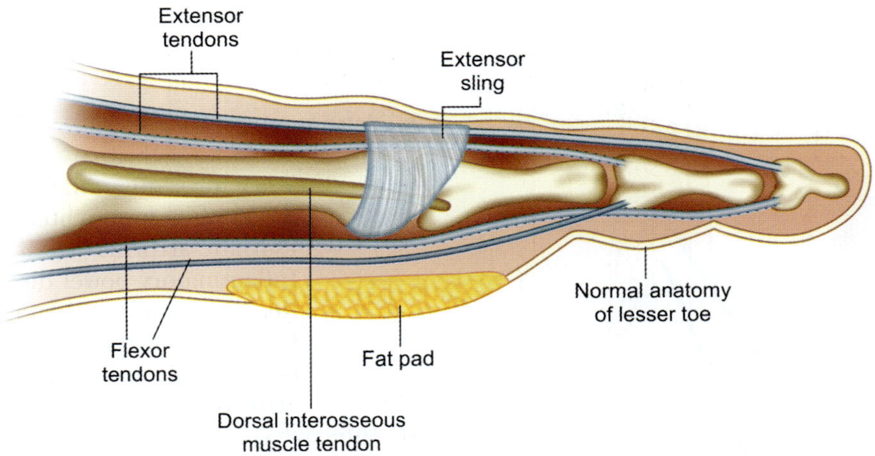

Fig. 26.321: Normal alignment of MP joints and toes due to the balance between flexor and extensor mechanisms and joint capsules

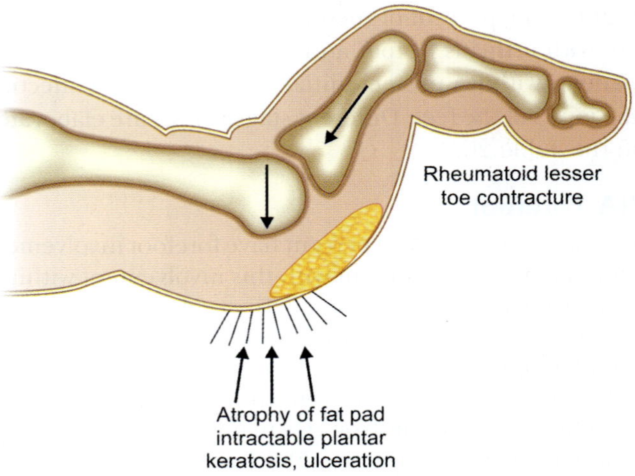

Fig. 26.322: Progression of deformity

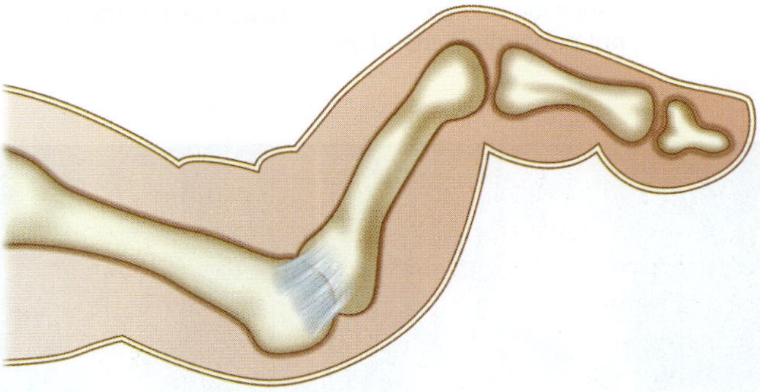

Fig. 26.323: Progression of deformity into flexion contracture

Flexion contracture of the middle and distal digital joints of the lesser toes and interphalangeal joint of the great toe. Painful corns over the dorsum of the middle joints and end corns at the nail-pulp junction. Finally, dislocation of MP joint occurs and the proximal phalanx is ankylozed to dorsal aspect of metatarsal head, as shown in Figure 26.323.

Treatment

The principles of non-operative treatment involve: (1) maintaining a good gait pattern and (2) independent ambulation or restoring adequate gait by minimizing inflammation, reducing pain, and supporting inflamed joints. Initially, patients are advised extra deep shoes with a wide, high toe box and a molded insert that allows for bony prominences. Semirigid orthosis is more effective than a soft orthosis. Rocker soles and steel shanks may help relieve midfoot pain and counteract stiffness. Orthotic devices help to redistribute plantar weight-bearing forces, which may decrease discomfort associated with pressure areas and support unstable joints. Toe sleeves and spacers, corn pads and debridement of plantar callosities also may help.

Surgery

Surgery usually is required because of continued pain increasing deformity.

Patient dis-satisfaction with unattractive footwear that needs frequent modifications, as old deformities progress or new deformities develop.

Lesser metatarsophalangeal joint synovectomy: Synovectomy of the lesser MTP joints is indicated for the treatment of painful joints early in the disease process, before significant deformity has occurred. This procedure is contraindicated in the presence of MTP joint subluxation or dislocation or with the formation of intractable plantar keratoses. Excision of hypertrophic synovial tissue may slow or arrest the degenerative process, decrease distention of MTP joints and reduce the soft-tissue deformation that would lead in time to subluxation and dislocation. Center a dorsal longitudinal incision over the involved MTP joint. With multiple joint synovectomies, use a second and/or fourth interspace incision to expose adjacent joints. Using the extensor tendon as a guide, carry the dissection down through the extensor hood and incise the capsule, exposing the MTP joint. Resect proliferative synovial tissue on the medial and dorsolateral aspects, taking care to remove any synovium beneath the collateral ligaments. Carry the resection as far in the plantar direction, as possible. Forefoot arthroplasty is directed primarily at the metatarsophalangeal joint deformity. Adequate bony resection to allow the phalanges to realign loosely with the metatarsals is mandatory. The goals of forefoot arthroplasty are to relieve pain, correct deformity with concomitant cosmetic improvement, improve ambulatory function and ideally, allow a reasonable variety of footwear.

Techniques of forefoot arthroplasty

Hoffmann's procedure: Removal of metatarsal heads through transverse plantar incision.

Fowler's procedure (Fig. 26.324): Through a dorsal transverse incision, removal of the base or up to one half of the proximal phalanges, shortening and contouring of the metatarsal heads to provide a uniform weight bearing surface and removal of an ellipse of plantar skin, to allow repositioning of the forefoot pad.

Thompson and Mann technique (Fig. 26.325): Metatarsophalangeal joint is exposed through dorsal approach. Distal 3 to 5 mm of metatarsal head is removed with sagittal saw. Base of proximal phalanx is removed. Lesser metatarsophalangeal joints are approached through dorsal incisions in second and fourth web spaces. Followed by, resection of metatarsal heads.

After fusion, site has been stabilized with Kirschner wires, interfragmentary screw is inserted, if bone stock is strong enough. Followed by fixation of arthrodesis site with six-hole, one-quarter tubular AO plate or pinning of arthrodesis site with one-eighth inch threaded Steinmann pins and 0.045 inch Kirschner wires in lesser toes, as shown in Figures 26.326A to D.

RA Midfoot

Deformity resulting from articular destruction in the intercuneiform, naviculocuneiform, metatarsalcuneiform and metatarsalcuboid joints is uncommon in patients with rheumatoid arthritis. Involvement of the first metatarsocuneiform joint is most common and may lead to instability with collapse of the medial longitudinal arch, with or without hallux valgus.

Management

An arthrodesis of the first metatarsocuneiform joint and possibly the medial cuneiform navicular articulation would correct part of this deformity, but seldom completely restores the arch. A percutaneous lengthening of the Achilles tendon should be added, if the tendon is tight after the collapsed arch has been restored and dorsiflexion of the ankle to at least 10° is impossible.

RA Hindfoot

Involvement of the hindfoot in chronic rheumatoid arthritis is not uncommon. Seventy-two percent of women and 59 percent of men with chronic rheumatoid arthritis had involvement of the subtalar and midtarsal joints. Isolated talonavicular arthritis may be one of the earliest findings with rheumatoid arthritis. Cystic changes of the inferior aspect of the talus associated with hindfoot rheumatoid arthritis.

The typical findings with chronic rheumatoid arthritis are midfoot and hindfoot pain, swelling, flattening of the longitudinal arch, forefoot rotation in axial plane and progressive valgus of the hindfoot, as shown in Figures 26.327A and B.

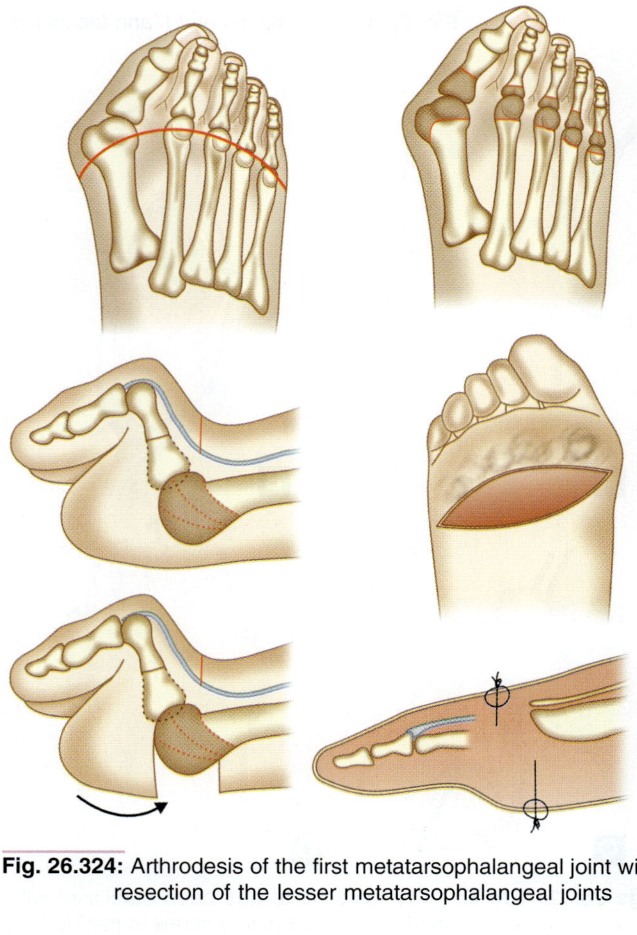

Fig. 26.324: Arthrodesis of the first metatarsophalangeal joint with resection of the lesser metatarsophalangeal joints

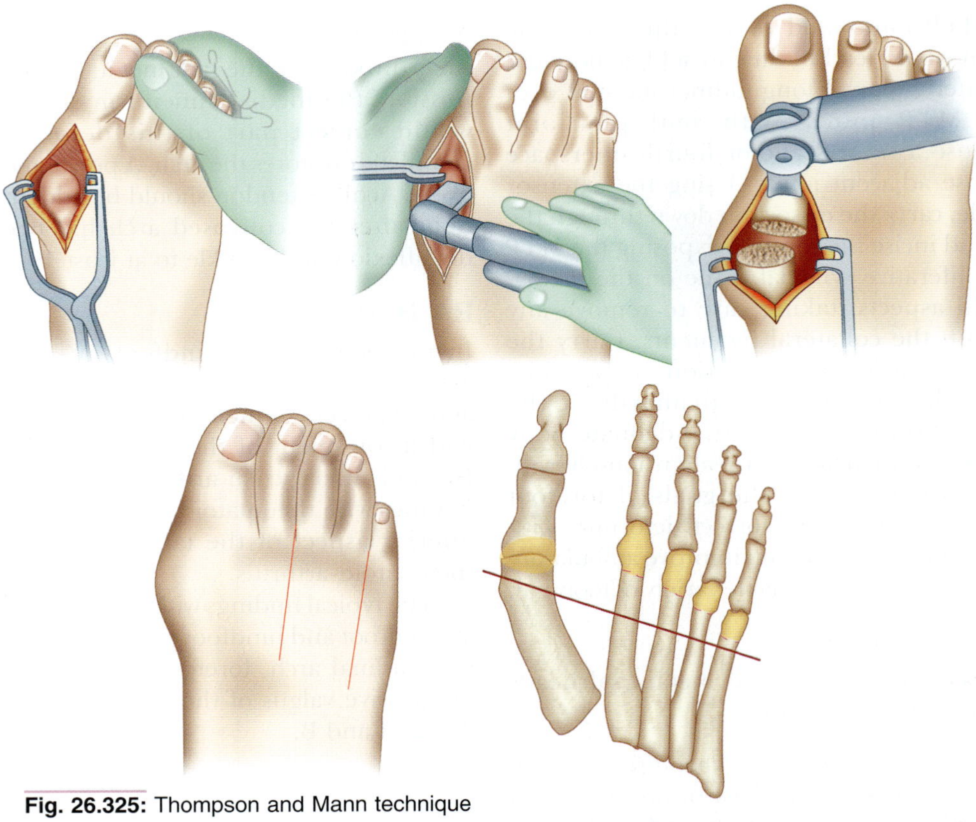

Fig. 26.325: Thompson and Mann technique

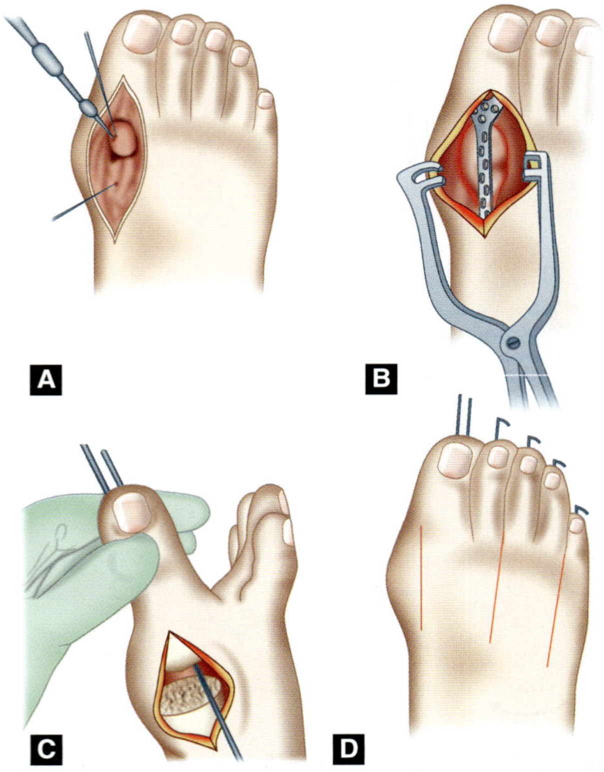

Figs 26.326A to D: After fusion, site has been stabilized with Kirschner wires, interfragmentary screw is inserted

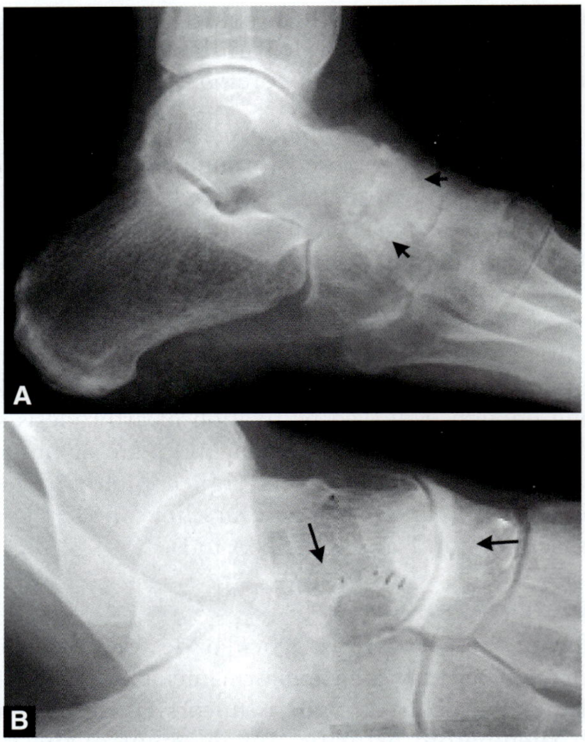

Figs 26.327A and B: X-rays showing, typical findings with chronic rheumatoid arthritis, midfoot and hindfoot pain, swelling, flattening of the longitudinal arch, forefoot rotation in axial plane and progressive valgus of the hindfoot. Arrows showing cysts and exosions

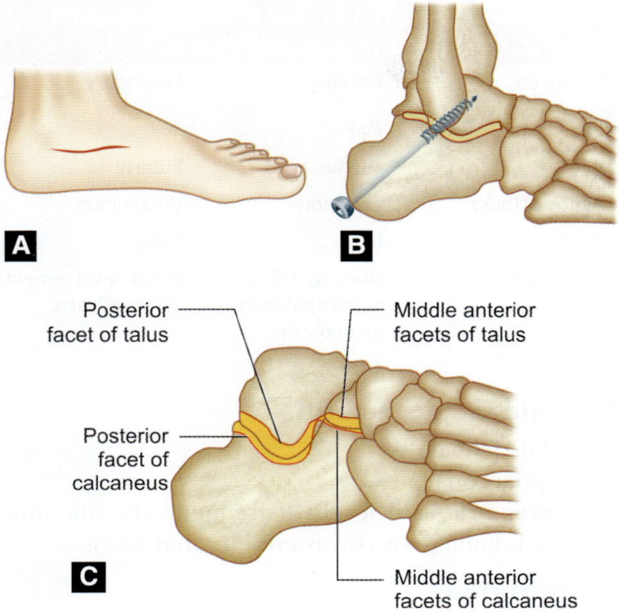

Figs 26.328A to C: Procedures of arthrodesis

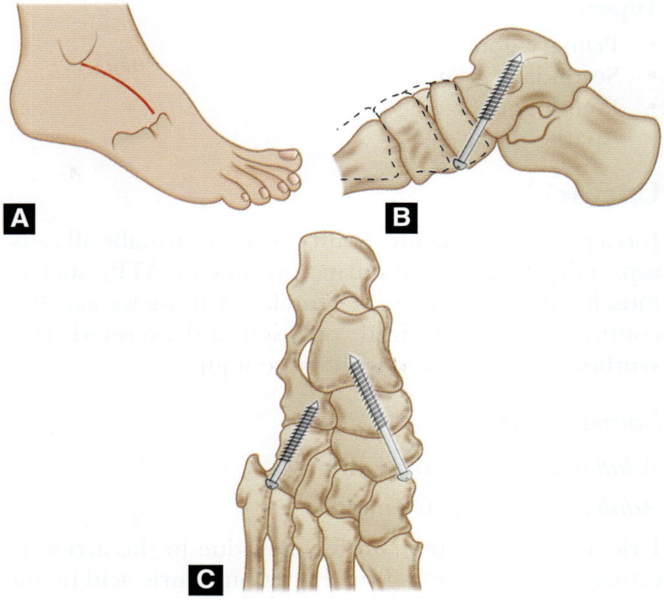

Figs 26.329A to C: Triple arthrodesis

Management

- Conservative care includes proper footwear, rest to relieve swollen and inflamed joints from the stresses of weight-bearing, padding and longitudinal arch supports. When progressive deformity occurs or unrelenting pain is refractory to conservative treatment, surgery of the hindfoot may be necessary.
- *Synovectomy:* Persistent synovitis and synovial hypertrophy of the tibiotalar joint that is unrelieved after 6 months of medical therapy is an indication for synovectomy, provided that major articular damage has not already occurred.
- *Subtalar arthrodesis (Figs 26.328A to C):* A subtalar joint arthrodesis is indicated to correct heel valgus, if the midtarsal joint and tibiotalar have been spared by the rheumatoid destructive process, if not, a triple arthrodesis is indicated. The goal of surgical treatment is to restore hindfoot stability in the appropriate position, 5° to 10° of hindfoot valgus should remain. Two incisions are used, one anterolateral and one medial, combined with internal fixation of the talonavicular and calcaneocuboid joints with two large smooth Steinmann pins, staples or screws.
- *Triple arthrodesis (Figs 26.329A to C):* With progressive involvement of the transverse tarsal joint or with more severe and irreducible valgus of the hindfoot, perform a triple arthrodesis, not only to stabilize the hindfoot but also to correct the deformity. In the patient with hindfoot involvement and a rigid forefoot, the objective is to obtain a plantigrade foot. Therefore, a triple arthrodesis is usually necessary. Straight lateral incision 1 cm, inferior to the tip of the fibular malleolus. Extend it distally over the anterolateral border of the calcaneus and cuboid. All eburnated or subchondral bone is removed from talonavicular joint to expose bleeding, cancellous bony surfaces. If correction is desired, bone grafting may be necessary. Talonavicular fixation, calcaneocuboid and talonavicular cannulated screw fixation.

Gouty Arthritis

History

- The term "gout" commonly is used to refer to the painful arthritis attacks.
- It derives from an ancient term "*gutta*", which referred to arthritis at the base of the big toe over 2000 years ago.
- The uric acid crystals were first noted with a microscope by Anton van Leeuwenhoek in 1684.
- Alfred Garrod first described the uric acid crystals in the tissues of the skin and joints of patients with gout.

Definition

Gout is a hereditary condition of disturbed uric acid metabolism, in which urate salts are deposited in articular, periarticular and subcutaneous tissues. Gouty arthritis is defined as peripheral arthritis (joint inflammation) and pain resulting from the deposition of sodium urate crystals in one or more joints.

Types

- Primary gout
- Secondary gout
- Pseudogout
- Apatite disease

Uric Acid

It is a purine metabolite. Source include virtually all cells, especially those rich in purine precursors (ATP), such as muscle, whether it is "our" muscles or those we eat. It is continuously synthesized, released and excreted. It is synthesis is accelerated with tissue injury.

Normal Range

Adult male: 3.5 to 7.0 mg/dl

Adult female: 2.5 to 6.0 mg/dl

Uric acid level is lower in females, due to the action of estrogen, on promoting the excretion of uric acid by the kidney.

Biochemistry (Flow chart 26.1)

Primary vs Secondary Gout (Table 26.3)

■ Primary Gout

Asymptomatic Hyperuricemia

- Uric acid levels >8 mg/dl in men; >7 mg/dl in women
- Not actively treated.

Acute Gouty Arthritis

- Intermittent painful attacks in single joint
- Uric acid levels normal in 30 percent of patients
- If elevated uric acid, do not initially manipulate

Flow chart 26.1: Uric acid metabolism

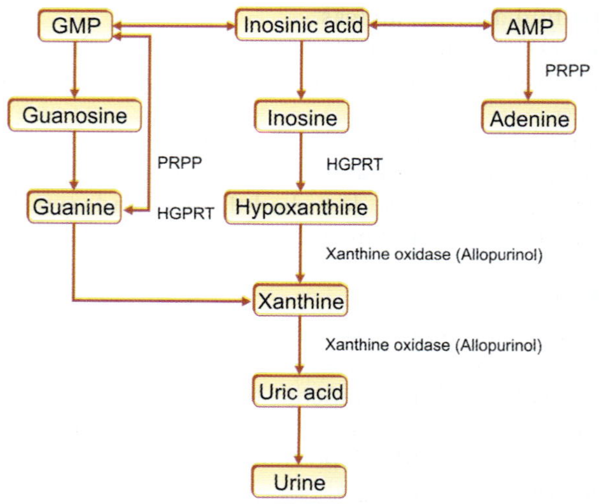

Table 26.3: Criterion for determining primary and secondary gout

Criterion	*Primary*	*Secondary*
Sex	M>F	M=F
Age	Middle aged	Elderly
Acute attacks	Common	Uncommon
Tophi	Late	Early
Association	Obesity, HTN, hyperlipidemia, alcoholism	Renal involvements, osteoarthritis

Chronic Gouty Arthritis

- Joint deformity
- Tophaceous
- Lower uric acid levels, if frequent arthritic attacks, renal damage or consistent elevated levels.

Distribution

Gender

- Most common in middle age men
- Seen in up to 10 percent of males
- Common in postmenopausal women.

Geographic

- New Zealanders
- Pacific islanders.

Age

- Second to fourth decade
- In children, it is rare, but is severe and crippling.

Genetic

Runs in families and is not sex linked.

Epidemiology

Incidence rate of 1.5 to 2.6/1000 individuals.

Predisposition

- Genetic predisposition
- Cancers and blood disorders
- Alcohol abuse
- Obesity
- Hypothyroidism
- High intake of purine containing food
- Lead poisoning (moonshine whisky)
- Radiation treatment
- Age
- Duration of hyperuricemia
- Starvation
- Renal failure
- Pharmacologic agents (thiazides, cyclosporine, pyrazinamide, ethambutol, nicotinic acid, warfarin, low dose salicylates).

Triggering Factors

- Injury
- Surgery
- Withdrawal of steroids
- Vascular disturbance
- Consumption of large quantities of alcohol
- Disturbed electrolyte imbalance
- Decreased urinary 17-ketosteroid
- Consumption of large quantities of purine rich foods
- Fatigue
- Emotional stress
- Illness
- Foods that are rich in purines are enumerated in Table 26.4.

Drugs that can Decrease Uric Acid

- Allopurinol
- High-dose aspirin
- Azathioprine
- Clofibrate
- Corticosteroids
- Estrogens
- Glucose infusion
- Guaifenesin
- Mannitol
- Probenecid, warfarin

Hyperuricemia

Hyperuricemia may indicate:
- Acidosis
- Alcoholism
- Diabetes
- Gout
- Hypoparathyroidism
- Lead poisoning
- Leukemia
- Nephrolithiasis
- Polycythemia vera
- Renal failure
- Toxemia of pregnancy
- Purine-rich diet
- Severe exercise

Table 26.4: Foods rich in purines

Anchovies	Asparagus
Beans	Broths
Consommé	Fish roe
Herring	Lentils
Meat gravies	Mushrooms
Mussels	Peas
Sardines	Scallops
Shellfish	Sweetbreads
Brewer's yeast	Baker's yeast
Organ meats (liver, kidney, tongue, Tripe)	

Hypouricemia

Hypouricemia may indicate:
- Fanconi's syndrome
- Wilson's disease
- SIADH
- Low purine diet

Signs and Symptoms (Fig. 26.330)

Acute:
- Suddenly appears in 12 to 24 hours
- Usually occurs overnight (metabolic changes)
- *Skin:* Red-purplish, tight and shiny
- Joints are painful, swelling, warmth
- Recurrent attacks develop
- Fever, chills, malaise
- Tachycardia
- Frequently at night
- 1 to 2 joints affected at a time
- Cooler joints affect more commonly because urate crystals form at cool temperatures
- Podagra or pain in the first metatarsophalangeal joint is the classic presentation.

Intracritical periods: Joints are virtually free of symptoms, although crystal may be found.

Chronic

- Progressive joint damage
- More frequent attacks
- Crippling deformity
- Disability
- Restricted joint motion

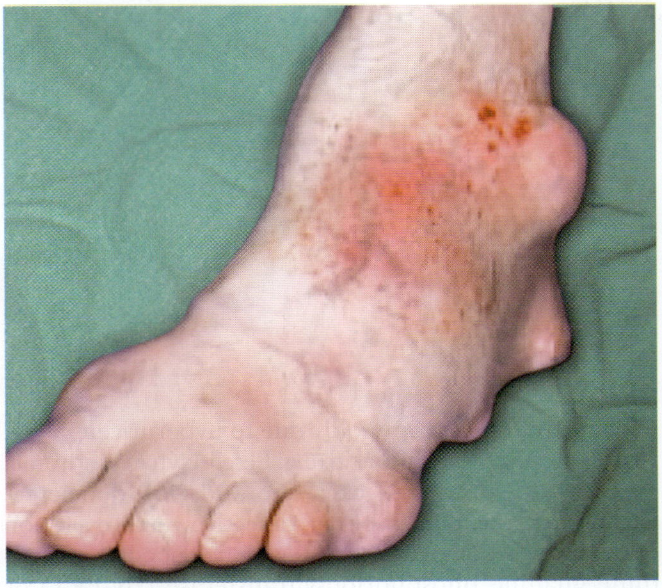

Fig. 26.330: Typical representation of foot in primary gout

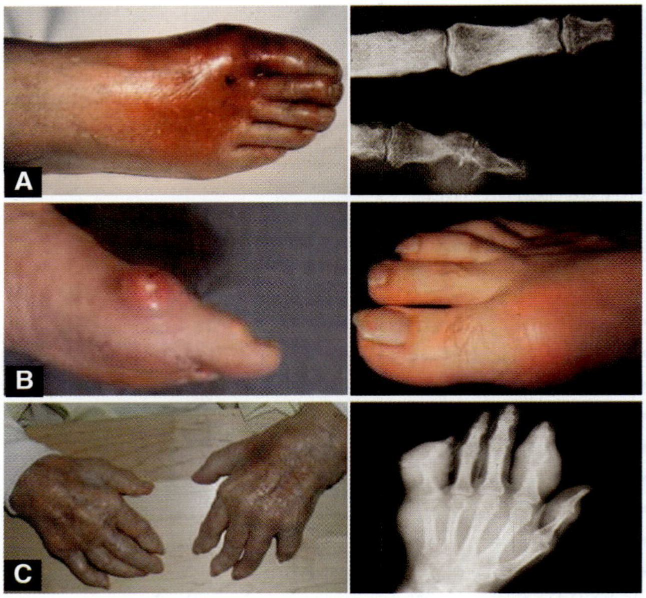

Figs 26.331A to C: Joint involvements in gouty arthritis—(A and B) Foot involvement; (C) Hand involvement

Flow chart 26.2: Pathogenesis of the primary gout

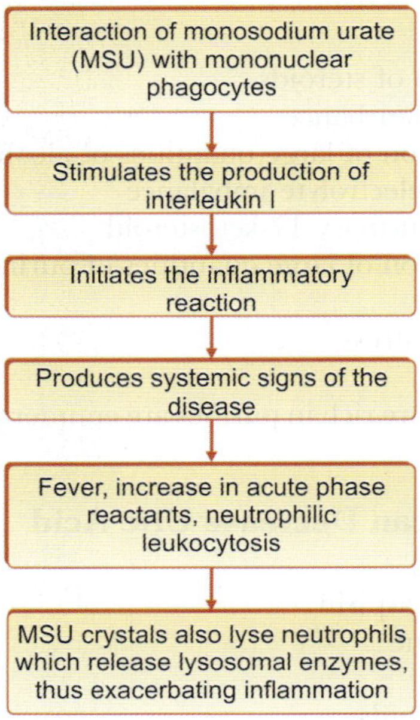

- Hard lumps of urate crystals (tophi) in
  - Synovium
  - Bone
  - Skin around joint
  - Kidney
  - Achilles tendon
  - Elbows

Common Joints Affected (Figs 26.331A to C)

- First metatarsophalangeal joint
- Feet
- Tarsal joints
- Ankles
- Fingers
- Wrist
- Elbow

Rare Joints

- Spine
- Hips
- Shoulders

Etiology

Primary gout most commonly due to hyperuricemia due to *under-excretion* of uric acid, e.g. Lesch-Nyhan syndrome, excess PRPP, decreased excretion and G6P deficiency. Secondary gout due to either defective renal excretion or overproduction of uric acid, e.g. deficiency of hypoxanthine guanine phosphoribosyltransferase (HGPRT) or defective regulation of purine biosynthesis.

Pathogenesis (Flow chart 26.2)

Flow chart 26.2 shows pathogenesis of the primary gout.

Associated Conditions

- Blood (hematopoietic) diseases
- Psoriasis
- Thyroid (myxoedema)
- Parathyroid (hypo and hyperparathyroidism)
- Hypertension
- Myocardial infarction
- Advanced renal diseases
- Obesity
- Down's syndrome
- Glycogen storage disease, type I
- Sex-linked uricaciduria, with a deficiency of HGPRT is associated with excessive uric acid production, uric acid kidney stones and severe gouty arthritis nephropathy at an early age.

Diagnosis

- Distinctive symptoms
- Examination of the joint
- Laboratory results:
  - High serum uric acid levels (may be normal in acute attack)
  - Increased serum white blood cells
  - High 24 hour urinary uric acid
- Joint aspiration (tophus or fluid): Negatively birefringent needle-shaped urate crystals.
- *X-ray:*
  - Joint destruction

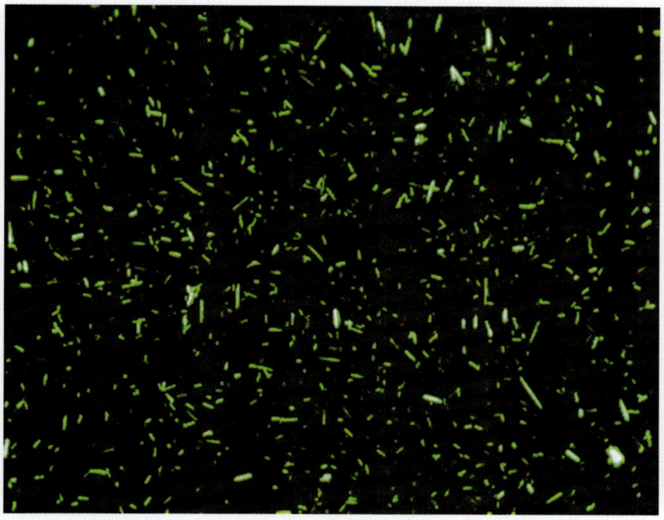

Fig. 26.332: Crystals of sodium urate that can be visualized under polarized light

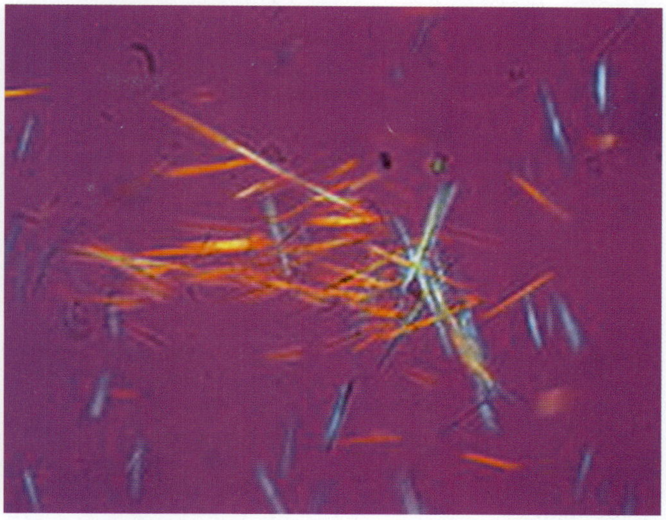

Fig. 26.333: Intensely birefringent needle-like crystals intra and extracellularly

- Tophi that displaces the bone and produces cysts.
- Crystals of sodium urate that can be visualized under polarized light (Fig. 26.332).
- Intensely birefringent needle-like crystals intra and extracellularly (Fig. 26.333).

The American College of Rheumatology has 11 criteria and the presence of six or more suggests that gout is present.

1. More than one attack of active arthritis
2. Maximum inflammation develops within one day
3. Oligoarthritis attack
4. Redness observed over joint
5. First metatarsalophalangeal joint painful or swollen
6. Unilateral first metatarsalophalangeal joint attack
7. Unilateral tarsal joint attack
8. Tophus (proven or suspect)
9. Hyperuricemia
10. Asymmetrical swelling within a joint on radiography
11. Complete termination of an attack

Differential Diagnosis (Table 26.5)

Table 26.5: Differential Diagnosis

Acute gout	*Chronic gout*
• Septic arthritis	• RA
• Cellulitis	• Multiple myeloma
• Pseudogout	• Chronic lead intoxication

Treatment

I. *Acute*
- Relieve pain, inflammation, etc.
- Anti-inflammatory drugs

II. *Long-term*
- Prevent recurrences
- Prevent progression, organ damage, death
- Control serum urate
  - Anti-inflammatories
  - Uricosurics
  - Inhibitors of uric acid synthesis
- *Diet:* Reduce foods high in purines
- Decrease alcohol intake
  - Increase water consumption
- Weight loss
- Adjust current medications (e.g. HTN medicines)
- Add gout medications (take them even if feeling worse)
- Medicines for acute stage:
  - NSAIDs (e.g. indomethacin, celecoxib)
  - Glucocorticoids (e.g. prednisone)
  - Colchicine
- Medicines for chronic stages:
  - Allopurinol
  - Uricosuric drugs (e.g. probenecid, sulfinpyrazone)

III. *Naturopathic treatment*
1. *Drink water:* Percentage of body weight (e.g.150 lb pt =75 oz H_2O/day; 96 oz during attack; 64 oz regularly daily; 30% more than expel)
2. *Supplements:*
   - Quercetin — Inhibits uric acid production
   - Bromelain — Anti-inflammatory
   - Vitamin E
   - Flaxseed oil
   - Avoid vitamin C and niacin (vitamin B_3) (increases uric acid levels)

Table 26.6: Etiology of secondary gout, as defective renal excretion or overproduction

Etiology: Defective renal excretion or overproduction		
Excretion	Intrinsic renal disease Low dose aspirin Cyclosporine	Diuretic therapy Nicotinic acid Ethanol abuse
Hyperuricemia	Starvation Dehydration Diabetic ketoacidosis	Lactic acidosis Pre-eclampsia
Overproduction	Lymphoprolif disease Myeloprolif disease Cyanotic CHD	Hemolytic anemia Polycythemia
Treatment	Underlying cause and Allopurinol	

3. *Eat:*
   - Unsweetened cherries lowers uric acid levels
   - Blueberries, blackberries and dark pigmented berries

Secondary Gout

Etiology

- Defective renal excretion or overproduction, this is explained in Table 26.6.
- Infections, e.g. Madura foot

Madura Foot

Synonyms

- Mucormycosis
- Maduromycosis
- Eumycetoma
- Actinomycetoma

Introduction

It is a chronic, progressive, local infection caused by fungi or bacteria, involving the feet, upper extremities or back and characterized by formation of multiple sinuses. First documented in Madras, India, in 1842 and acquired its name Madura foot because of its prevalence in the Indian province of Madura. Men aged 20 to 40 are most often affected, presumably because of trauma incurred during work outdoors.

Epidemiology

The disease is endemic in the tropics and subtropics and is named after the region of India where it was first described in 1842. Although, currently uncommon in temperate regions, it does occur in the southern USA and cases are found in the homeless, and AIDS sufferers. The incidence of mycetoma is likely to rise in temperate regions due to increases in worldwide travel and since mycoses are not notifiable, the incidence in the UK is unknown.

Risk Factors

Mycetoma typically presents in agricultural workers (hands, shoulders and back from carrying contaminated vegetation and other burdens. In individuals who walk barefoot in dry, dusty conditions. Minor trauma allows pathogens from the soil to enter the skin.

Etiology

Fungi: *Mycetomatis. M.grisea, Fusarium spp* 20 other fungal species.

Bacteria: *Actinomycetes, Nocardia, Streptomyces.* Actinomycetes is a gram-positive filamentous bacteria as per microbiologists (it is commonly referred as a fungus in many orthopedic textbooks). *Actinomyces* are anaerobic, while *Nocardia* and *Streptomyces* are aerobic. *Nocardia* stain partially acid-fast, *Actinomyces* and *Streptomyces* are not acid-fast.

Pathophysiology

Nocardia and other *Actinomycetes, Mycetoma* occurs mainly in tropical or subtropical areas. Spread through contiguous subcutaneous areas, multiple draining sinuses exude characteristic "grains" of clumped organisms. Tissue reactions may be suppurative or granulomatous depending on the specific causative agent. All genera may produce granules, *Actinomyces* almost always produce granules.

Clinical Features (Figs 26.334 and 26.335)

First lesion may be a papule, a fixed subcutaneous nodule, a vesicle with an indurated base or a subcutaneous abscess that ruptures to form a fistula to the skin surface. Gradual and progressive extension and destruction of contiguous muscles, tendons, fascia and bones. There is neither systemic dissemination nor signs and symptoms suggesting generalized infection.

Three Stages

1. Formation of soft tissue granuloma and sinuses
2. Loss of definition of cortex followed by erosion of bone
3. Periosteal reaction and cavitations of bones

Advanced Stage

Muscle wasting, deformity and tissue destruction prevent use of limbs. In advanced infections, extremities appear swollen, a club-shaped mass of cystic areas with multiple draining and intercommunicating sinus tracts and fistulase that discharge thick or serosanguinous exudates containing characteristic grains. Fistulae do not occur before 3 months. Secondary infections present in untreated cases, as shown in Figure 26.336.

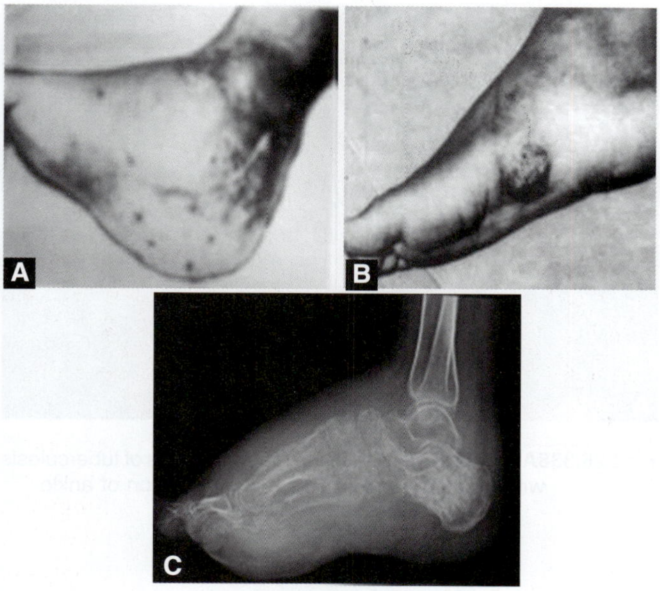

Figs 26.334A to C: Clinical presentation of Madura foot

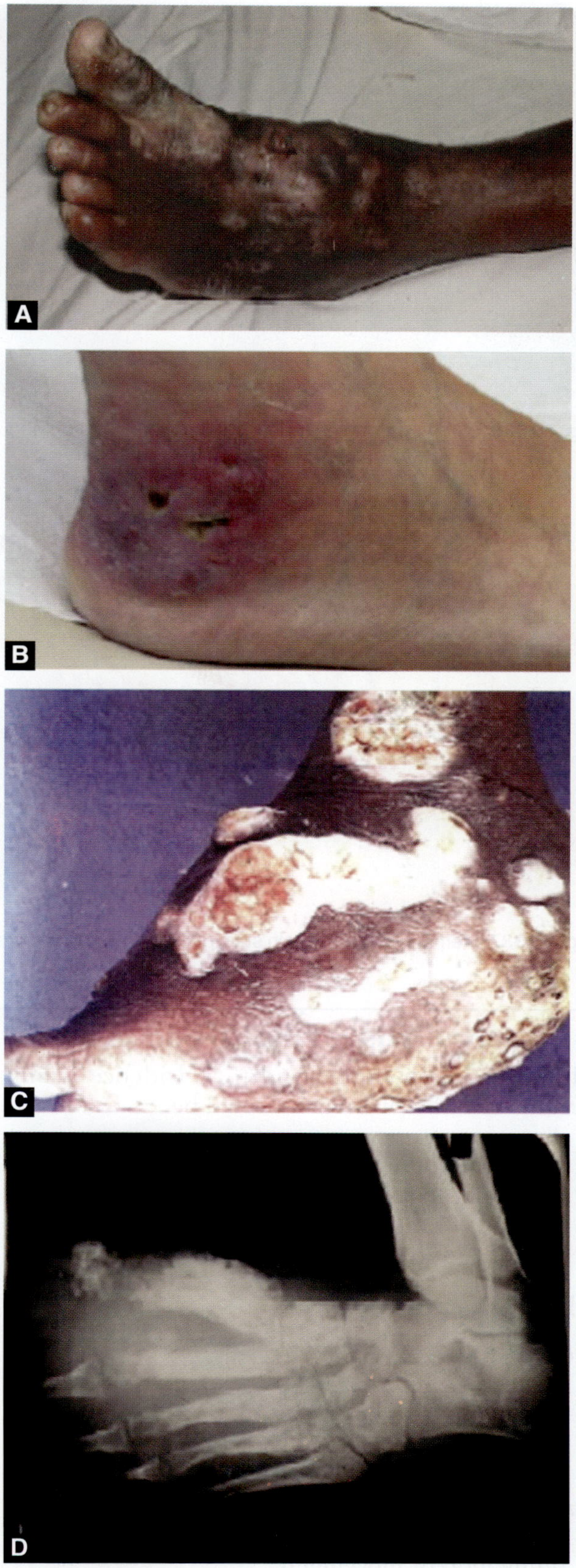

Figs 26.335A to D: Clinical presentation of Madura foot in different stages of disease progression

Diagnosis

- Culture from discharge, microscopy is diagnostic.
- Sulphur granules seen on microscopy, as illustrated in Figure 26.337.
- Polymorphonuclear infiltrate and may be accompanied by a granulomatous reaction, with varying proportions of epithelioid cells, plasma cells and giant cells.
- Resolution of eosinophilia is prognostic.

Differential Diagnosis

The main differential diagnoses are chronic bacterial osteomyelitis, tuberculosis or the early phase of Buruli ulcer. Other deep fungal infections such as blastomycosis or coccidomycosis and also leishmaniasis, yaws and syphilis should be considered.

Management

Due to the slow, relatively pain-free progression of the disease, *mycetoma* is often at an advanced stage when diagnosed. Surgical debridement, followed by prolonged appropriate antibiotic therapy for several months is required for *Actinomycetoma*. *Eumycetomas* are only partially responsive to antifungal therapy, but can be treated by surgery due to their normally well circumscribed nature. More recently, successful treatment with itraconazole has been reported. Excision of affected tissue is the treatment of choice. Some healthy tissue to be removed and functionally important tissue may be preserved. Amputation of completely involved foot and reconstructive skin grafting/plastic procedures.

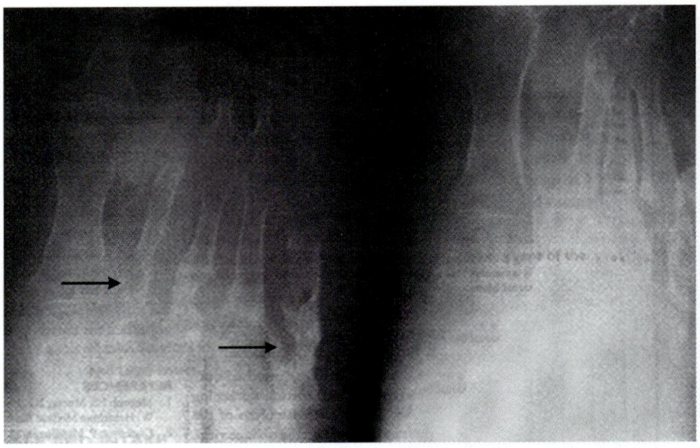

Fig. 26.336: X-ray showing changes in advanced stage of Madura foot. Arrows showing destruction of the bone

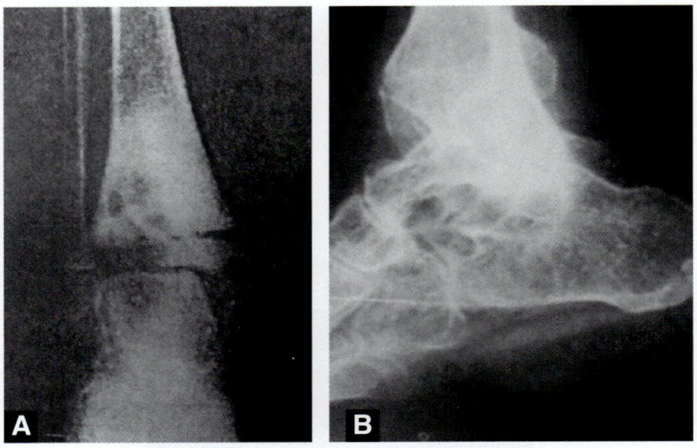

Figs 26.338A and B: X-rays showing manifestations of tuberculosis with marked osteoporosis and destruction of ankle

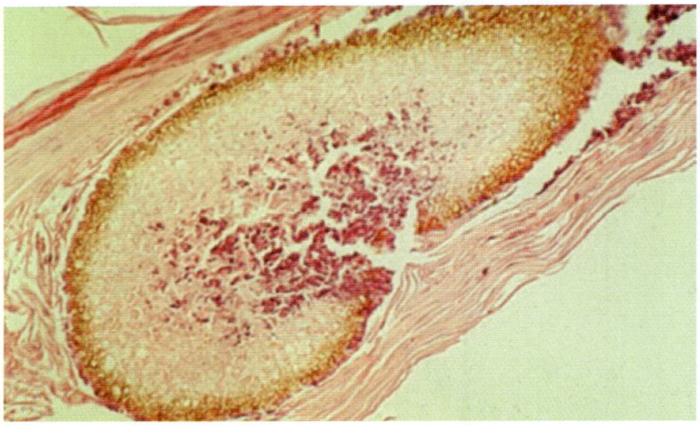

Fig. 26.337: Hematoxylin and eosin stain of *Mycetoma* of Madurella

Tuberculosis of Foot and Ankle

This is very uncommon and the incidence is only 5 percent. Sites of involvement could be:
- Synovium
- Distal end of tibia
- Malleoli
- Talus
- Calcaneum (rarely)

Clinical Features

Early stage
- Pain
- Limp
- Swelling
- Ankle is held in plantar flexion

Late stage
- Pathological anterior dislocation of the ankle
- Limitation of movements
- Wasting of calf muscles
- Sinus formation

Radiology (Figs 26.338A and B)

- Marked osteoporosis
- Destruction of ankle

Treatment

- Chemotherapy is the mainstay of the treatment.
- Below knee plaster cast for 8 to 12 weeks.
- Synovectomy and joint debridement during earlier stage.
- Arthrodesis for advanced and persistence disease.

Neuropathic Foot

Neuropathic arthropathy may be defined as a relatively painless, progressive and degenerative arthropathy of single or multiple joints caused by an underlying neurological deficit.

Background

- M > F
- Age > 40 years
- Originally described in 1868 by Jean Martin Charcot
- Patients with tabes dorsalis
- Massive joint destruction, subluxation and dislocation was seen
- Today, most common in diabetics, commonly in the lower extremity

Etiology (Table 26.7)

Pathogenesis

- Has yet to be fully known

Table 26.7: Etiology of neuropathic foot

• Diabetic neuropathy
• Syphilis (tabes dorsalis)
• Syringomyelia
• Meningomyelocele/spina bifida
• Nerve injury—spinal cord or peripheral nerves
• Congenital insensitivity to pain
• Leprosy
• Charcot-Marie-Tooth syndrome

- Sensory and autonomic neuropathy nearly universally present
- Arteriovenous shunting thought to play a role
- Normal blood supply and hyperglycemia also seen
- Repetitive microtrauma may be inciting factor
- *Two theories:*
  - Neurotraumatic (German)
  - Neurovascular (French)

Neurotraumatic Theory

This theory proposes that Charcot arthropathy results from repetitive mechanical trauma from weight bearing on insensate extremity. This trauma can lead to intracapsular effusions, ligamentous laxity and joint instability. Absence of protective sensation allows continued loading of fractured extremity. Heightened healing response are seen.

Neurovascular Theory

This theory proposes that Charcot is a sequel of increased peripheral blood flow, resulting from autonomic sympathectomy. Autonomic sympathectomy produces a failure of the normal regulatory mechanisms that control blood flow. Autonomic dysfunction causes arteriovenous shunting and vasodilatation. Increases rate of blood flow to extremity. It is correlated with increased osteoclastic activity, marked demineralization of bone, increases susceptibility to subluxation, fracture and collapse.

Pathogenesis

Today, most agree that both theories play a role in Charcot. Combination of osteopenia, bone hyperemia, joint instability and sensory motor deficits predisposes to changes seen with Charcot.

Investigations

- Full blood count (helps distinguish from osteomyelitis), urine examination, creatinine, LFT's, calcium, vitamin B_{12}, folate, VDRL, glucose and increased or decreased glycosylated hemoglobin.
- Joint aspiration may be necessary to exclude septic arthritis.
- MRI can help distinguish between soft tissue infection and osteomyelitis.

Table 26.8: Radiographic findings in neuropathic foot

Radiographic hallmarks
6 D'S
• Dense subcondral bone—sclerosis
• Degeneration—marginal osteophytes
• Destruction of articular cartilage
• Deformity
• Debris
• Dislocation

Radiographic Findings (Table 26.8)

Charcot Foot

Radiographic Hallmarks (Fig. 26.339)

- Bony destruction, fragmentation
- Bony remodeling
- Joint destruction, subluxation and dislocation

Radiographic Staging

Stage I: Developmental (acute) stage

Stage II: Coalescence (quiescent) stage

Stage III: Consolidation (resolution) stage

Stage I: Developmental or acute (Fig. 26.340)

- Hyperemia due to autonomic neuropathy weakens bone and ligaments.
- Diffuse swelling, joint laxity, subluxation, frank dislocation, fine periarticular fragmentation and debris formation.

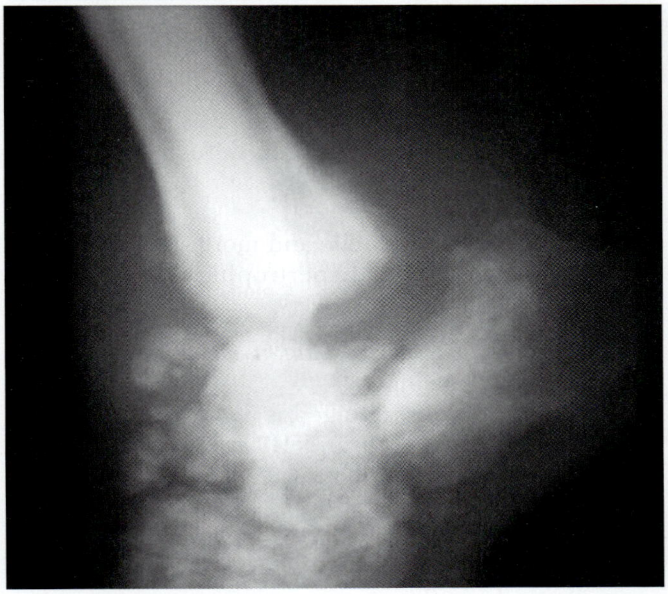

Fig. 26.339: Radiographic findings in Charcot foot

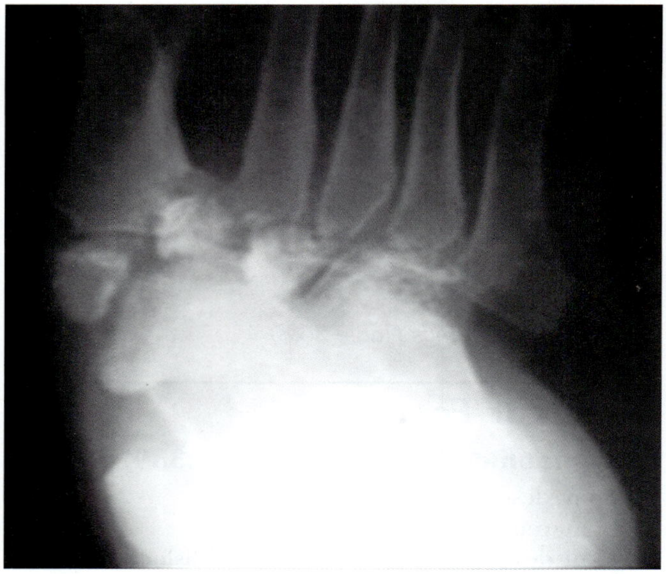

Fig. 26.340: X-ray findings in stage I of Charcot's foot

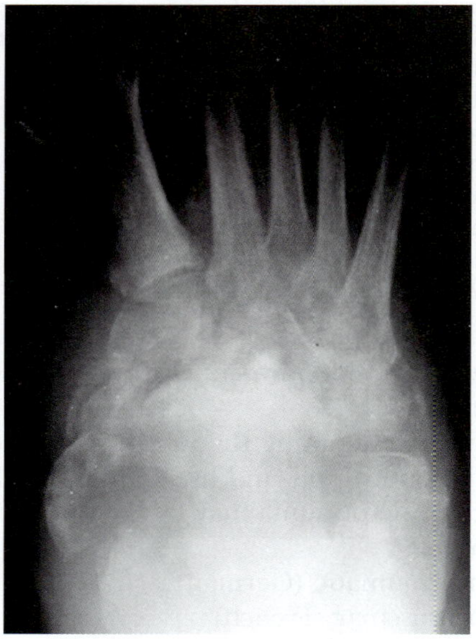

Fig. 26.342: X-ray findings in stage III of Charcot's foot

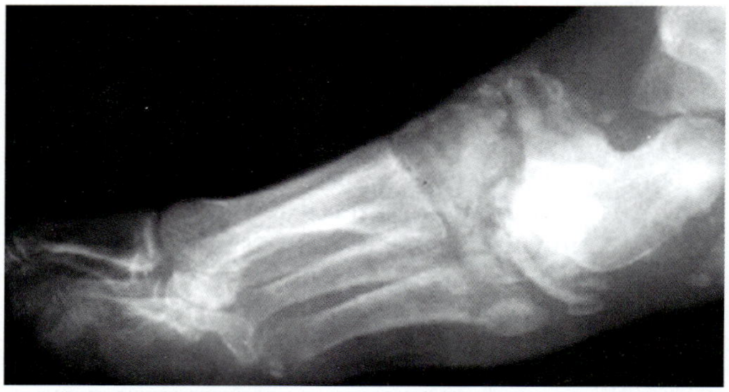

Fig. 26.341: X-ray findings in stage II of Charcot's foot

Stage II: Coalescence or Quiescent (Fig. 26.341)

- Absorption of osseous debris, fusion of larger fragments
- Dramatic sclerosis
- Joints become less mobile and more stable
- Aptly known as the "hypertrophic" or "subacute" phase of Charcot

Stage III: Consolidation or resolution (Fig. 26.342)

- Osseous remodeling
- For clinical purposes, stage I is regarded as the acute phase, while stages II and III are regarded as the chronic or quiescent phase.

Charcot and diabetes mellitus

- Average disease history of 10 to 12 years or more.
- Generally poor glycemic control.
- Reported incidence varies widely in literature, from 0.08 to 0.5 percent up to 16 percent of diabetics.

Syphilitic lesions of joints

Children with congenital syphilis sometimes develop bilateral serous symmetrical synovitis in the knee joints. They present with painless swelling of both knees with marked effusion. These are called Clutton's joints. In the secondary stage of syphilis, patients complain of fleeting joint pains. This is called syphilitic arthralgia and is worse at nights. Diagnosis is by the concomitant presence of other secondary syphilitic arthralgia and is worse at nights. Diagnosis is by the concomitant presence of other secondary syphilitic manifestations. In the tertiary stage of syphilis, patients with tabes dorsalis may manifest a neuropathic joint lesion called Charcot's joint. This is characterized by painless swelling in the knee with gross disorganization and instability. This is one of the neuropathic joints.

Charcot-Marie disease

A hereditary motor and sensory neuropathy transmitted most often as an autosomal dominant trait and characterized by progressive distal wasting and loss of reflexes in the muscles of the legs (and occasionally involving the arms). Onset is usually in the second to fourth decade of life. This condition has been divided into two subtypes, hereditary motor and sensory neuropathy (HMSN) types I and II. HMSN I is also associated with abnormal nerve conduction velocities and nerve hypertrophy, features not seen in HMSN II.

Clinical Presentation (Fig. 26.343)

- Charcot joints are usually painless but large effusions.
- Soft tissue swelling, deformity, instability, crepitus, etc.

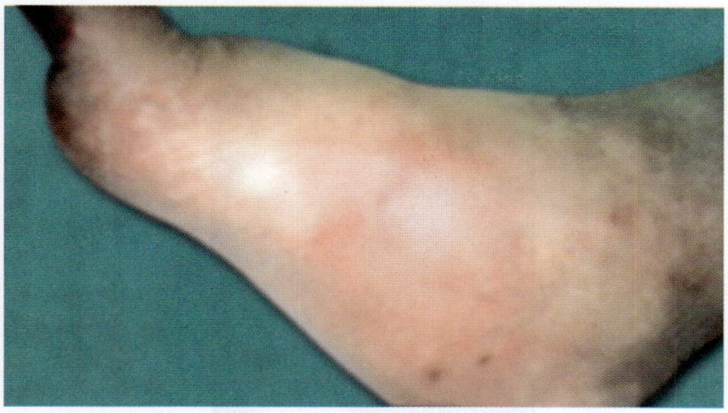

Fig. 26.343: Charcot's foot in acute stage

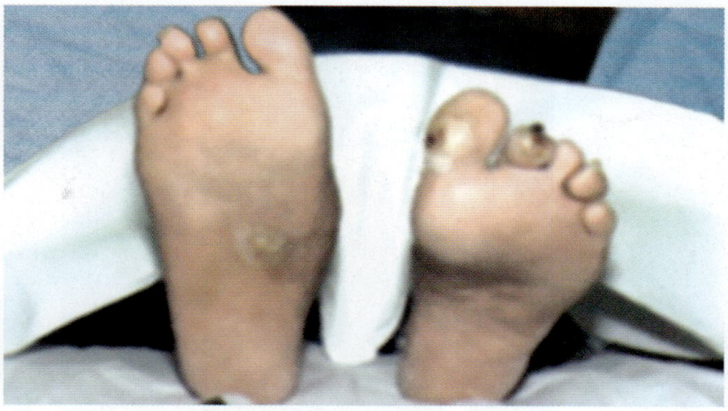

Fig. 26.344: A rocker bottom foot deformity

- Subluxation and fracture are characteristic features during the course of the disease.
- Usually, there is a large effusion that can be very inflamed, mimicking septic or inflammatory arthritis. It mainly affects ankle and joint in mid and forefoot. Joint degenerates into "bag of bones" in advanced disease, can produce massive destruction of joint surfaces with resorption of adjacent bone. Generally painless, but flare up may be painful.
- Red, hot and swollen foot.
- Typically painless or only mildly painful unilateral swelling of extremity.
- Can mimic cellulitis, gout, osteomyelitis and even DVT.
- Plain films may appear normal initially.
- Orthopedic examination may reveal joint hyper mobility with crepitus with or without cutaneous ulceration.
- As disease progresses, longitudinal and transverse arches of foot may collapse, creating a rocker bottom foot, as shown in Figure 26.344.
- Some degree of sensory deficit always present.
- Deep tendon reflexes, vibratory sensation, and proprioception may be diminished or absent.
- Due to autonomic sympathectomy, may see bounding pulses, calor, rubor, tumor and anhidrosis positive or negative.

Management

- Primarily non-surgical
- In acute phase, may need hospital admission, intravenous antibiotics and immobilization.
- *Chronic phase:* Plaster-cast boot to immobilize joint. May be needed for several months until joint is quiescent—with frequent assessments and serial radiographs.
- Reduction of stresses through joint—minimize weight bearing.
- Life-long protection of the involved joint e.g. individualized footwear, analgesia as necessary (NSAID's).
- Bisphosphonates inhibit bone reabsorption and may hasten healing.
- Surgery to the joint is necessary in the minority of cases.

Treatment

Primary goals is stability, plantigrade foot and to keep the foot free of ulceration. Selection of treatment plan is phase dependent, location, severity, and the positive and negative ulceration.

Conservative versus surgical: Initially, consists of immobilization during acute phase to prevent disease progression, generally via total contact casting. Some disagreement in the literature, as to whether or not to permit any weight bearing during this time. Others modalities are: pneumatic walker brace, etc.

Total contact cast permits ambulation, while uniformly distributing weight bearing pressures over the entire foot surface. After acute phase has passed, long-term or permanent bracing is often needed. Gradual return to protected weight bearing. Examples: Charcot Restraint Orthotic Walker (CROW), patellar tendon-bearing braces, custom-molded shoes (Fig. 26.345), AFO, etc. Patellar tendon-bearing brace is used to transfer weight bearing forces from the orthosis through the patellar tendon, thereby decreasing weight bearing forces through the foot and ankle, as shown in Figure 26.346.

Surgical Treatment

Only considered after all conservative measures exhausted. Surgical intervention is necessary in some cases of continued ulceration, gross instability, presence of infection, limb shortening and difficulty in shoe gear. Guidelines of surgery include correct timing, adequate

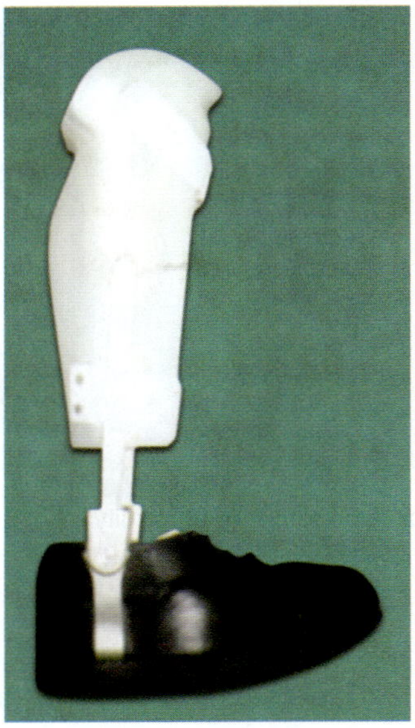

Fig. 26.345: Custom-molded shoes

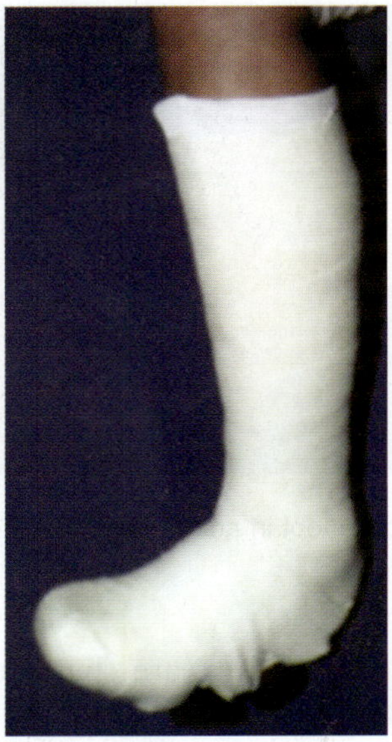

Fig. 26.346: Total contact cast

fixation and a long postoperation nonweight-bearing period. Ideally, the prompt identification of patients in the early stages of neuroarthropathy would enhance treatment outcomes and reduce patient morbidity. Treatment is very patient dependent. Ostectomy, arthrodesis, midtarsus closing wedge osteotomy and external fixation. Bone mineral density alterations have been documented in Charcot patients. For example, localized osteopenic changes. There's increasing interest in the use of bisphosphonates.

Bisphosphonates

Pyrophosphate analogs that inhibit osteoclastic bone resorption, used commonly in diseases characterized by abnormal bone turnover. For example, Paget's disease, osteoporosis, osteolytic bone metastasis and others.

Pamidronate

Most commonly used bisphosphonate is pamidronate (Aredia), a second generation bisphosphonate. It acts by adsorbing onto hydroxyapatite crystals in newly synthesized bone matrix, blocking access of osteoclast precursors to this matrix and inhibiting bone resorption.

Conclusion

- Charcot a potentially devastating sequel of diabetes mellitus.
- Treatment requires careful initial management and long-term follow-up.
- Conservative, surgical treatment options can be augmented with the pharmacologic use of bisphosphonates.

DEFORMITIES OF THE FOOT AND ANKLE

Deformities of the hallux

- Bunion
- Hallux rigidus
- Hallux flexus

Deformities of the lesser toe

- Hammer toe and claw toe
- Mallet toe
- Combined hammer toe and mallet toe deformity
- Bunionette (Tailor's bunion)
- Ingrowing toe nail (Onychocryptosis)
- Acquired pes planus
  - Flexible pes planus
  - Rigid pes planus
  - Accesory navicular
- Neurogenic disorders
- Cavus foot
- Drop foot

Disorders of the Hallux

- Bunion
- Hallux rigidus
- Hallux flexus

Bunion (Fig. 26.347)

Bunion is often described as a bump on the side of the big toe and is often seen in hallux valgus deformity. The

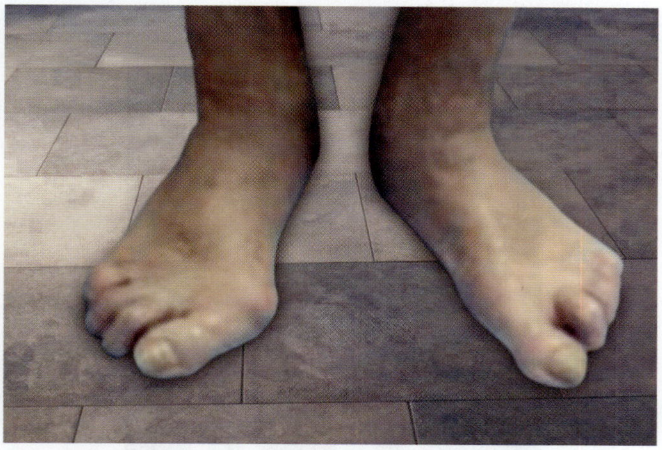

Fig. 26.347: Bunion formation a hallux disorder

hallux valgus deformity is characterized by lateral deviation of the proximal phalanx on the metatarsal head.

Etiology

Biomechanical Instability

The most common yet most difficult to understand etiology is biomechanical instability. Contributing factors, if present include gastrocnemius or gastroc soleus equinus, flexible or rigid pes plano valgus, rigid or flexible forefoot varus, dorsiflexed first ray, hypermobility or short first metatarsal.

A. *Arthritic/metabolic conditions*
   - Gouty arthritis
   - Rheumatoid arthritis
   - Psoriatic arthritis
   - Connective tissue disorders, such as Ehlers-Danlos syndrome, Marfan syndrome, Down syndrome and ligamentous laxity

B. *Neuromuscular disease*
   - Multiple sclerosis
   - Charcot-Marie tooth disease
   - Cerebral palsy

C. *Traumatic compromise*
   - Malunions
   - Intra-articular damage
   - Soft-tissue sprains
   - Dislocations

D. *Structural deformity*
   - Malalignment of articular surface or metatarsal shaft
   - Abnormal metatarsal length
   - Metatarsus primus elevatus
   - External tibial torsion
   - Genu varum or valgum
   - Femoral retrotorsion

Pathophysiology

As a result of this lateral subluxation of the proximal phalanx on the metatarsal head, several secondary changes occur. These include following:

- Contracture of the lateral joint capsule
- Attenuation of the medial joint capsule
- A medial eminence of varying size
- Pronation of the hallux, as the deformity becomes more severe
- Medial deviation of the first metatarsal, giving rise to an increase in the intermetatarsal angle. This leads to an uncovering of the sesamoids, which are anchored in their lateralward position by the adductor halluces.

As the hallux valgus deformity becomes more severe, the impingement of the hallux against the second toe can lead to destabilization of the second metatarso-phalangeal joint. As the deformity increases, the weight bearing of the hallux and first metatarsal is diminished, resulting in increased weight bearing by the second metatarsal head, which results in metatarsalgia.

Diagnosis

Physical Examination

Observe the alignment of the foot and lower extremity. Note the deformity of the great toe and lesser toes. Note any pain about the metatarsophalangeal joint, synovial thickening or crepitation. If pain is persistent, it is important to localize this pain to the dorsal or plantar aspect of the joint because a sesamoid problem may be present. Neurovascular status of the foot.

Radiographic Examination (Figs 26.348 and 26.349)

Obtain anteroposterior (AP) and lateral radiographs of the foot weight bearing. Measure the first metatarsophalangeal joint angle, which should be less than 15°. The intermetatarsal angle should be less than 8°. Look for arthrosis in the first metatarsophalangeal joint and assess whether the joint is congruent or incongruent. Measure the distal metatarsal articular angle (DMAA), which is the relationship of the articular surface to the long axis of the metatarsal. Normally, this should be less than 10° of lateral deviation.

Treatment

Conservative Management

Using broad, soft-soled shoes, preferably with a low heel, that provide adequate room for the great toe and the medial eminence

Protocol for Surgery (Flow chart 26.3)

One of the most important factors in the outcome of bunion surgery is the correct selection of the operative procedure. The first consideration is whether the deformity is in a congruent or an incongruent joint. If

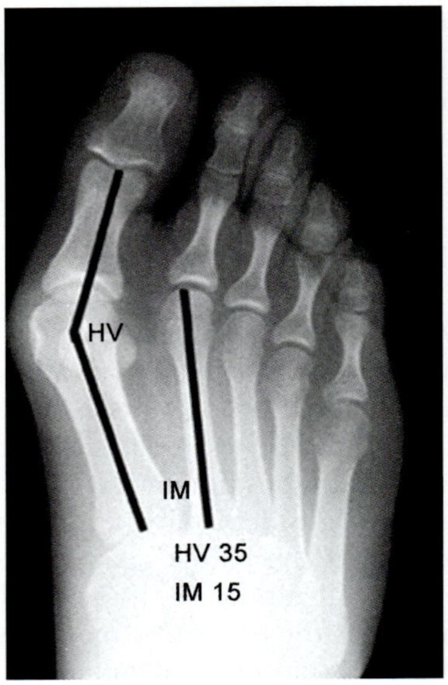

Fig. 26.348: Hallux valgus of foot, degree of deformation is given HV. Hallux valgus; IM. Intermetatarsal angle

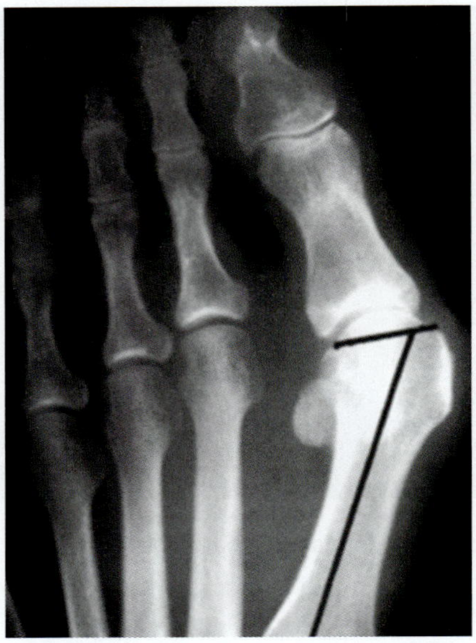

Fig. 26.349: Lateral radiograph for measuring the distal metatarsal articular angle, which is the relationship of the articular surface to the long axis of the metatarsal

Flow chart 26.3: Protocal for surgery

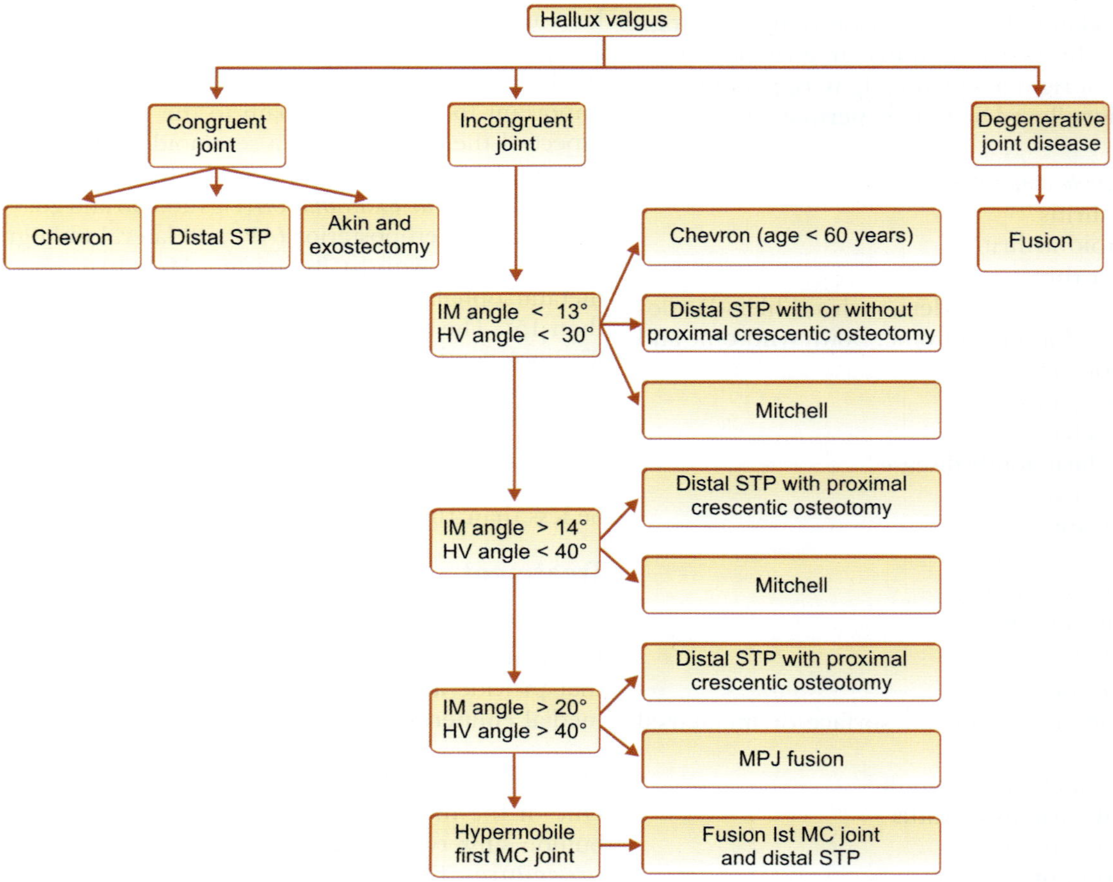

Key: STP. Soft-tissue procedure; IM. Intermetatarsal; HV. Hallux valgus; MC. Metatarsocuneiform; MPJ. Metatarsophalangeal joint

the joint is congruent, the proximal phalanx cannot be rotated on the metatarsal head, to correct the deformity and if the deformity is incongruent, however, the proximal phalanx can be rotated on the metatarsal head to correct the deformity. In a congruent joint, use a chevron procedure to correct the deformity. If the DMAA is increased, use a medial closing wedge with a chevron osteotomy, rotating the metatarsal head medially and thereby correcting the DMAA. Other procedures include a distal soft-tissue procedure or an Akin procedure (osteotomy of the proximal phalanx) along with excision of the medial eminence. If the hallux valgus deformity is associated with an incongruent joint, the operative procedure depends on the severity of the deformity. If the hallux valgus is mild with a hallux valgus angle of less than 30° and the intermetatarsal angle is less than 13°, use a chevron osteotomy or distal soft tissue procedure to correct the deformity. If the deformity is moderate with a hallux valgus of 40° or less, and the intermetatarsal angle is 20° or less, use a distal soft-tissue procedure and a proximal metatarsal osteotomy to correct the deformity. Note that a chevron osteotomy cannot correct a deformity of this magnitude. If the deformity is severe with a hallux valgus angle of more than 40° and the intermetatarsal is greater than 20°, use a distal soft-tissue procedure with proximal osteotomy, if there is minimal arthrosis. If arthrosis is present or the deformity is too severe, then consider an arthrodesis. If there is significant arthrosis of the metatarsophalangeal joint, an arthrodesis is probably the procedure of choice. Place the hallux at about 15° of valgus and 10° to 15° of dorsiflexion in relation to the ground.

Any procedure chosen must take into account the following structural components:

- Valgus deviation of the great toe (hallux valgus)
- Varus deviation of the first metatarsal
- Pronation of the hallux, first metatarsal or both
- Hallux valgus interphalangeus
- Arthritis and limitation of motion of the first metatarsophalangeal joint
- Length of the first metatarsal relative to lesser metatarsals
- Excessive mobility or obliquity of the first metatarsomedial cuneiform joint
- The medial eminence (bunion)
- The location of the sesamoid apparatus
- Intrinsic and extrinsic muscle-tendon balance and synchrony.

McBride Operation

In this surgery the lateral deforming forces of the conjoined tendons of adductor halluces and the lateral head of flexor halluces brevis are transferred from the proximal phalanx into the lateral side of head of first metatarsal. The tendon is passed through a hole in the metatarsal and this releases the deforming force on the proximal phalanx.

Metatarsal Osteotomy

It is indicated in hallux valgus, when no arthritis is present in metatarsophalangeal joint. It corrects deformity, by shifting the axis of the metatarsal laterally towards the second metatarsal and is supplemented by soft tissue procedures, which involve tightening of the medial capsule of metatarsophalangeal joint to realign the toe in correct position.

Operation by Mitchell

Metatarsophalangeal joint is exposed by dorsal incision and small exostosis is removed from the medial aspect of metatarsal head. Osteotomy is made at the junction of head with the neck, using parallel saw cuts, distal being incomplete. The head is pushed laterally and locked in position.

Other Types

- Metatarsal neck wedge osteotomy (reverdin)
- Basal osteotomy
- Hohmann neck osteotomy
- Oblique neck osteotomy
- *Kellers operation:* When osteoarthritis is established in an old patient then arthroplasty is indicated. It involves the removal of bunion and excision of the proximal half of the proximal phalanx of great toe and shortening of the toe.
- *Arthrodesis of first metatarsophalangeal joint:* The base of the phalanx and the head of the metatarsal are denuded of the articular cartilage and the osteophytes are trimmed. The joint is fixed in 5° of dorsiflexion and held by a transfixation screw.
- *Bunionectomy:* Consists of removing the exostosis with a careful reefing and repair of medial joint capsule. It is indicated in elderly patient with slight valgus deformity.

  Akin procedure (Figs 26.350A and B): An Akin procedure is a medial closing-wedge osteotomy of proximal phalanx.
- Can be utilized as an isolated procedure or in conjunction with excision of the medial eminence.
- Do not perform this procedure if the metatarsophalangeal joint is incongruent.
- It is a useful salvage procedure for a mild recurrent hallux valgus deformity with a stable metatarsophalangeal joint.
- Perform the Akin procedure through a medial incision.
- Make a dorsomedial capsular incision to expose the medial eminence.
- Expose the medial eminence by sharp dissection and excise it with a sharp thin osteotome.

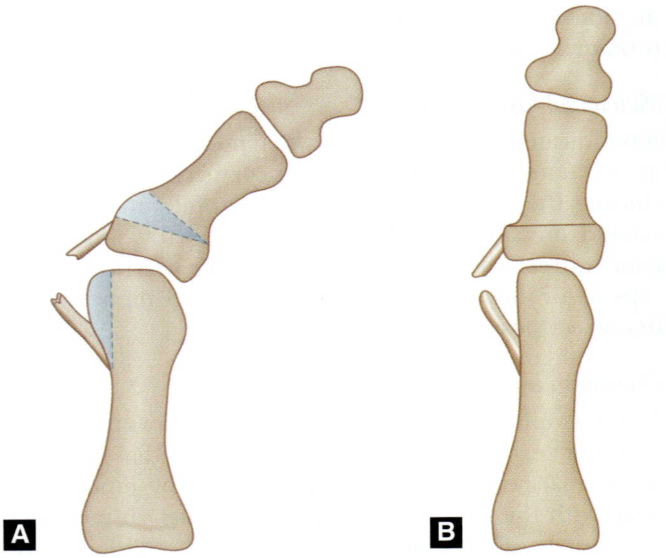

Figs 26.350A and B: Akin procedure

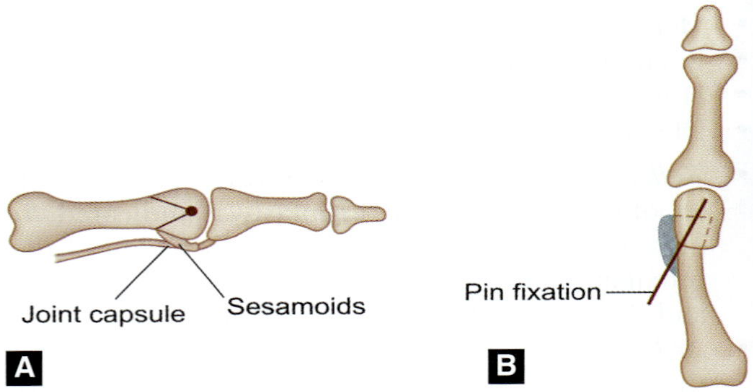

Figs 26.351A and B: Chevron procedure

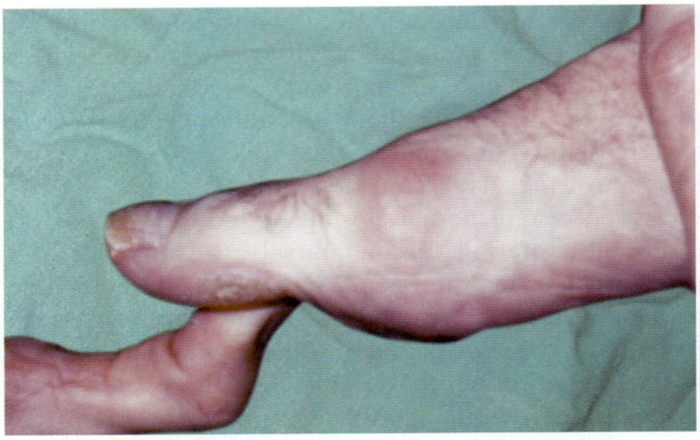

Fig. 26.352: Distal soft tissue procedures in front of hallux rigidus

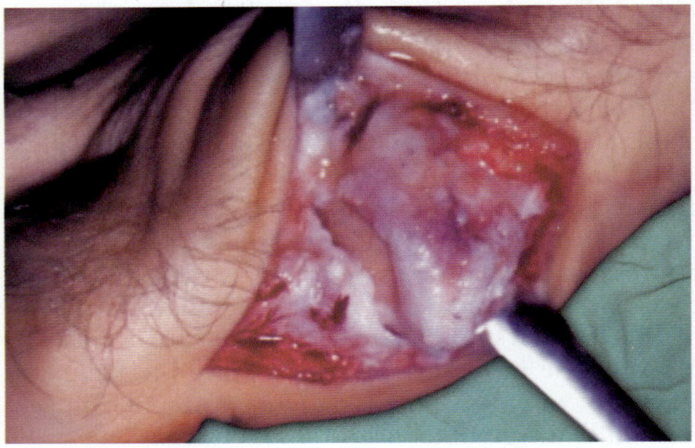

Fig. 26.353: Distal soft tissue procedure for Hallux rigidus

Chevron Procedure (Figs 26.351A and B)

This procedure is done for mild to low-moderate hallux valgus deformity. Involves a V-shaped cut in the metatarsal head that allows it to be displaced up to 5 mm laterally. Avascular necrosis of the metatarsal head is an unusual complication.

Distal Soft Tissue Procedure

The distal soft tissue procedure with and without a proximal crescentic metatarsal osteotomy is indicated for a wide range of deformity from mild to severe.

■ Hallux Rigidus (Figs 26.352 and 26.353)

It refers to limitation of motion of the metatarsophalangeal joint of the great toe. Pathogenesis of hallux rigidus is still not clearly defined. Cartilage damage is believed to initiate the synovitis, which leads to further cartilage destruction, osteophyte proliferation and subchondral bone destruction. The process may begin in adolescence, when a single traumatic event at the metatarsophalangeal joint damages the dorsal articular surface of the metatarsal head. Repeated microtrauma also may cause articular cartilage damage.

Other suggested causes include:

- Osteochondritis dissecans of the first metatarsal head secondary to an osteochondral fracture over the dorsal convexity of the joint surface.
- Hyperextension of the first metatarsal, an abnormally long first metatarsal.
- Severe pronation of the foot.

Adult hallux rigidus most often is caused by degenerative arthritis of the first metatarsophalangeal joint, whereas in adolescents, hallux rigidus usually results from localized cartilage damage to the first metatarsal head.

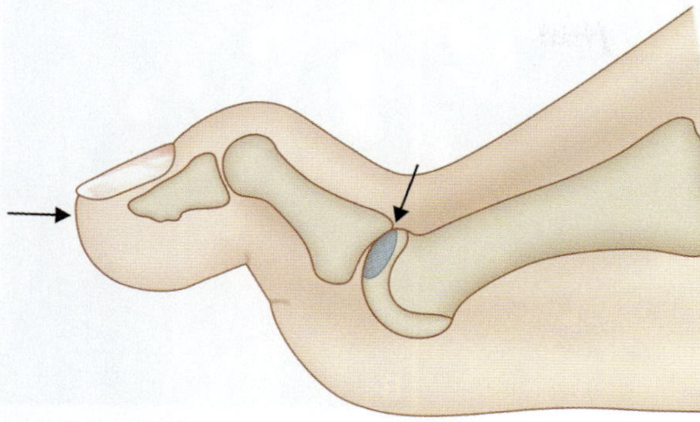

Fig. 26.354: Radiographic finding is a small depression in the dome of metatarsal head (arrows)

Most common microscopic finding in patients with hallux rigidus, include a cleavage lesion in the articular cartilage of the first metatarsal head without any detached subchondral bone and the earliest radiographic finding is a small depression in the dome of the metatarsal head, as shown in Figure 26.354.

The cleavage lesion on the metatarsal head is always between the apex of the dome and the dorsal margin of the articular surface. When the hallux is extended, abutment of the proximal phalanx against the cleavage lesion in the articular cartilage produces pain and instinctive flexion of the joint, limiting extension. As the disease worsens, an osteophyte at the dorsal articular margin of the metatarsal head presents a mechanical abutment to extension. This is the usual condition of the patient at the initial presentation.

Grading of Severity of Hallux Rigidus (Coughlin and Shurnas) (Table 26.9)

Table 26.9: Grading of severity of hallux rigidus by Coughlin and Shurnas

Grade radiograph	*Pain*	*MTP joint motion*
0. Normal	None	Stiffness or slight loss
1. Minor narrowing of MTP joint space	Intermittent	Mild restriction
2. Moderate joint space narrowing, osteophyte formation	More constant	Moderate restriction
3. Severe joint space narrowing, extensive osteophyte formation	Constant (no pain at midrange of MTP joint motion)	Moderately severe restriction (<20 degree total motion)
4. Same as grade 3	Pain at midrange of passive MTP joint motion	Same as grade 3

Treatment

- In most patients, operative correction is required to relieve pain and improve function.
- The most common type of self-care was use of a shoe with an ample toe box.

Operative Treatment

- Cheilectomy (chiseling away bony irregularities at osteochondral margin of a joint cavity that interfere with movements of joint).
- Dorsal wedge osteotomy at the base of the proximal phalanx or distal first metatarsal, especially for adolescent patients.
- Arthrodesis of the first metatarsophalangeal joint only if loss of joint space is evident not only on the anteroposterior and lateral views, but also on the oblique view of the first metatarsophalangeal joint, as shown in Figures 26.355A to C. Arthrodesis for patients with grade 4 hallux rigidus or grade 3 hallux rigidus, with more than half of the metatarsal head cartilage remaining.

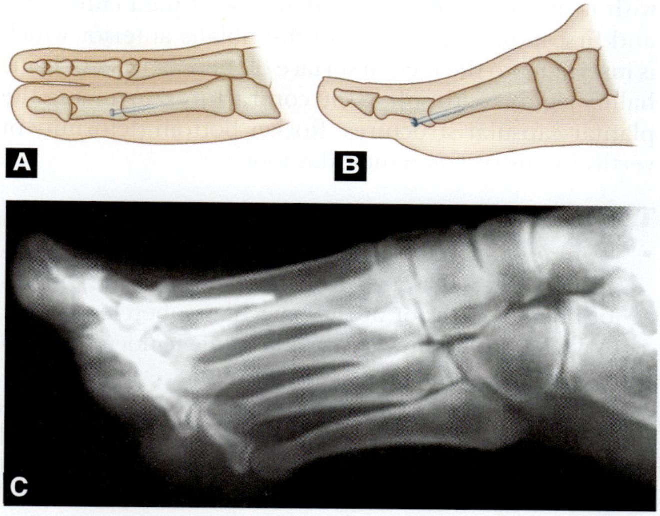

Figs 26.355A to C: Arthrodesis of the first metatarsophalangeal joint

- Modern fixation techniques with interfragmentary compression screws or dorsal plates have produced high rates of fusion.
- Resection arthroplasty (Keller procedure), in which the extensor halluces brevis and capsular tissue were used as interposition materials. Hemiarthroplasty of the proximal phalanx, with a metallic resurfacing component. Silicone-rubber and single-stem replacement arthroplasty.

Hallux Flexus

Static deformity, which occurs initially during walking, but may become fixed and rigid. Marked plantar flexion of the proximal phalanx of the big toe, with some degree of dorsiflexion of the first metatarsal, resulting in dorsal bunion formation. Normal longitudinal arch is lost and the talonavicular break is often present, with abnormality of the cuneiform which is tilted upwards. Soft tissue contractures occur, particularly of the capsule, flexor halluces longus and brevis tendons, so that there is loss of mobility of the first metatarsophalangeal joint.

Etiology

Poliomyelitis: Paralysis of all the foot muscles except for a normal gastrocnemius-soleus group posteriorly and normal flexors of the toes, as well as flexor hallucis brevis. Certain tendon transfer operations in which there is failure to achieve balance between the peroneus longus with its insertion into the lateral side of med cuneiform and first metatarsal base and the tibialis anterior which is inserted into the medial surface of these bones. Arthritic hallux rigidus with soft tissue contractures, involving the plantar capsular structures. Rocker bottom deformity of vertical talus or congenital flat foot.

Treatment

- *Lapidus technique:* The insertion of tibialis anterior is transferred backwards to be attached on the tendon of tibialis posterior at the navicular tubercle
- A wedge osteotomy is carried out naviculocuneiform-metatarsal joints
- The flexor halluces longus tendon is divided at its insertion and transferred proximally to be inserted through an oblique hole drilled in the neck of first metatarsal
- Plantar capsulotomies may be necessary.

Deformities of the Lesser Toe

Anatomy and Physiology

Each of the lesser toes consists of three phalanges, the proximal, middle and distal phalanx. Barriers to deformities include the medial and lateral collateral ligaments of the metatarsophalangeal (MP) joints, as well as of the proximal and distal interphalangeal joints.

Hammer Toe

- Rigid hammer toe
- Flexible hammer toe

Rigid Hammer Toe (Figs 26.356A and B)

It cannot be passively correctable to the neutral position. A rigid hammer toe is defined as a fixed flexion deformity of the PIP joint.

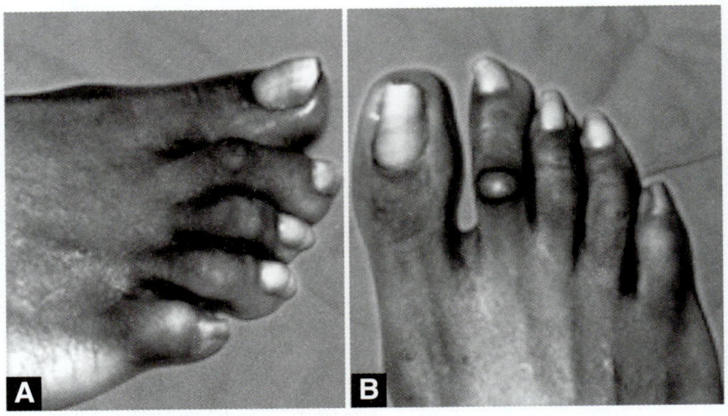

Figs 26.356A and B: Rigid hammer toe

Etiology

- Flexible hammer toe is often a tight Flexor Digitorum Longus (FDL) tendon.
- A disproportionately long lesser toe or a shoe with a tight toe box can also cause a fixed hammer toe deformity.
- Hammer toe deformity can also be due to poor shoe wear or the formation of a hallux valgus deformity, which can push the second toe into a hammered or overlapped position.

Symptoms

- This deformity can cause symptoms over the dorsum of the PIP joint, where the toe rubs against the top of the toe box or at the tip of the toe, where the toe hits the sole of the shoe
- If the hammer toe produces sufficient distal migration of the plantar fatty cushion, pain under the metatarsal head can result.

Treatment

- Shoe modifications, including extra depth shoes, soft insoles and metatarsal pads, can help to alleviate symptoms
- Surgical correction
- Evaluation of the entire foot for related deformities, such as a tight FDL tendon or a hallux valgus deformity is important prior to any surgical treatment.
- A hallux valgus deformity can reduce the space lateral to the hallux, which prevents reduction of a second toe into a reduced position. If this condition exists, a hallux valgus repair should be strongly considered.
- A PIP joint arthroplasty, such as described by DuVries consists of the resection of the distal condyle of the proximal phalanx. It results in a fibrous ankylosis that allows approximately 15° or 20° of motion.
- An alternative is bony arthrodesis of the PIP joint.

Complications of Surgery

- Swelling is the most common complication
- Recurrence of a hammer toe deformity

- Floppy toe can result, if too much of the shaft of the proximal phalanx is removed along with the distal condyle
- Migration of the intermedullary pin used to fix PIP joint.

Flexible Hammer Toe

- A flexible hammer toe deformity can decrease or be completely eliminated with plantar flexion of the MP joint or of the ankle
- This can be passively corrected
- These deformities are usually caused by tightness of the FDL tendon.

Treatment

A flexible hammer toe is treated with a Girdlestone-Taylor flexor tendon transfer, if surgery is indicated. This transfer, often combined with the release of deforming forces at the MP joint can produce satisfactory results. An arthroplasty of the PIP joint is sometimes combined with the tendon transfer if there is some element of a fixed component.

Surgery

Distal condyle of the proximal phalanx is excised as in a fixed hammer toe repair, if there is noncorrectable deformity. Each half of the FDL tendon is brought from plantar to dorsal along both sides of the shaft of the proximal phalanx, and is sutured into the extensor hood. This is done with PIP joint of the toe extended and with the MP joint in slight flexion. Close all wounds and hold the toe in neutral position with a postoperative dressing. Fix the toe with a K-wire, if a fixed PIP joint deformity was treated.

Complications

Possible neurovascular injury from pressure or swelling around the area of the tendon transfer, producing vascular or neurologic compromise. Other difficulties, such as swelling and recurrence of deformity can occur. Different deformities, their characteristics and treatment plan are described in Table 26.10.

■ Deformities of the Metatarsophalangeal Joint

- Mild dorsiflexion deformities
- Fixed dorsiflexion deformity
- Subluxation or dislocation of the joint

Treatment

Mild dorsiflexion deformities often can be treated with extensor tenotomy. If the deformity is of such a magnitude that this treatment is not sufficient, an open release of the joint capsule may be necessary. An open extensor tenotomy and capsulotomy will correct many subluxation deformities, although it is important to ensure release of the medial and lateral collateral ligaments. After correcting the soft-tissue deforming forces, toe is held in a neutral position and an intermedullary K-wire is inserted. Wooden postoperative shoe is given until the pin is removed. When a severe deformity is present, a soft-tissue procedure is often not adequate and an arthroplasty of the MP joint is necessary.

Complications

- Redislocation of the MP joint is the most common complication of this procedure
- Neurologic or vascular compromise can occur

Table 26.10: Different deformities, their characteristics and treatment

Deformity	*Characteristics*	*Treatment*
Flexible hammer toe	No fixed contracture at MTP of PIP joint	Usually nonoperative rarely; flexor-to-extensor transfer using FDL
Rigid hammer toe with MTP subluxation	Fixed flexion contracture at PIP; MTP subluxation in extension	Resection of condyles of proximal phalanx, dermodesis; lengthening of EDL, tenotomy of EDB; MTP capsulotomy, collateral ligament sectioning
Rigid hammer toe with MTP subluxation claw toe	Fixed flexion contracture at PIP; MTP subluxation in extension	Resection of condyles of proximal phalanx, dermodesis; lengthening of EDL, tenotomy of EDB; MTP capsulotomy collateral ligament sectioning.
Rigid hammer toe with MTP dislocation	Fixed flexion contracture at PIP; complete MTP dislocation	Resection of condyles of proximal phalanx dermodesis; lengthening of EDL, tenotomy of EDB; MTP capsulotomy, collateral ligament sectioning MTP arthroplasty or Well osteotomy.
Crossover toe	Fixed flexion contracture at PIP; MTP subluxation in varus or valgus	Resection of condyles of proximal phalanx dermodesis collateral ligament/capsular repair, EDB transfer
Mallet toe	Fixed flexion contracture at DIP	Resection of condyles of middle phalanx, dermodesis; FDL tenotomy

Abbreviations: DIP. Distal interphalangeal joint; EDB. Extensor digitorum brevis; EDL. Extensor digitorum longus; FDL. Flexor digitorum longus; MTP. Metatarsophalangeal joint; PIP. Proximal interphalangeal joint.

Crossover Second Toe

A significant hallux valgus deformity can cause pressure on the second toe and lead to dorsal subluxation or dislocation of the second toe, placing the great toe adjacent to the third toe. This results in attenuation of the second MP joint's fibular collateral ligament and possibly even the formation of a rent in it. The tibial collateral ligament can sometimes contract. As the deformity progresses, dorsal subluxation and possibly dislocation of the second MP joint can occur. Evaluate instability of the joint using the anterior drawer sign of the lesser MP joint, as described by Thompson and Hamilton.

Thompson and Hamilton's anterior drawer sign: Grasp the proximal phalanx of the lesser toe between the thumb and index finger and stabilize the metatarsal with the other hand. Then manipulate the toe in a vertical fashion. If instability exists, there is subluxation at the MP joint and pain may exist.

Treatment

- Nonsurgical treatment includes taping the second toe in a reduced position or using open-toed or extra-depth shoes.
- Surgical repair includes extensor tenotomy, dorsal capsulotomy and collateral ligament release, with intramedullary K-wire fixation of the toe.
- For severe deformity, MP joint arthroplasty to both decompress the joint and allow reduction of the proximal phalanx is done.
- Reefing of the lateral capsule may also be used to strengthen the reconstruction and decrease the chances of recurrence of the deformity.
- Perform correction of the hallux valgus deformity at the same time, to prevent the hallux from again displacing the second toe.

Complications

- Swelling
- Recurrence
- Loss of motion at the MP joint from postsurgical scarring and fibrous arthrodesis is a common complication.
- Neurovascular compromise (occasionally).

Claw Toe

- A claw toe is a deformity of the MP joint that occurs together with a flexion deformity of either the proximal or distal interphalangeal joints.
- When evaluating a claw toe, examine both the MP and the involved interphalangeal joint to determine whether the involved deformity is fixed or flexible at each joint.
- Carefully evaluate the hallux for a valgus deformity, which could prevent reduction of the second toe into its normal position. If there is a hallux valgus deformity, it might interfere with the second toe.

Treatment

- Fibrous arthroplasty as described for the surgical treatment of hammer toe.
- Extensor tenotomy and capsulotomy, with release of the medial and lateral collateral ligaments as necessary.
- This is often enough to correct all deformities.
- However, a flexor tendon transfer, as described in the treatment of flexible hammer toe is sometimes also required.
- If severe subluxation or dislocation of the MP joint is present, a resection arthroplasty of the MP joint might be necessary.

Complications

- Redislocation of the MP joint:
  - It can result from inadequate shortening of the MP head or stiffness from inadequate rehabilitation after pin removal.
  - Incomplete soft-tissue release may also be a factor contributing to recurrence.
- Compromise of the vascular supply at the toe can occur from tension or spasm of the interdigital vessels.

Mallet Toe (Fig. 26.357)

Mallet toe is a flexion deformity of the distal interphalangeal joint. It often causes pain because the tip of the toe rubs on the inner sole of the shoe. Mallet toe is usually a fixed deformity and is less common than hammer toe.

Surgical Correction of Mallet Toe

Mallet toes that are flexible can occasionally be treated with percutaneous tenotomy of the FDL tendon. With a fixed deformity, it is necessary to decompress the distal interphalangeal joint. Excise an ellipse of skin from the dorsal aspect of the distal interphalangeal joint and after release of the extensor apparatus and the collateral ligaments, excise the distal condyle of the middle phalanx with a bone cutter. This technique is similar to that described for correction of rigid hammer toe.

Complications

- Possible neurovascular injury
- Swelling
- Recurrence of deformity

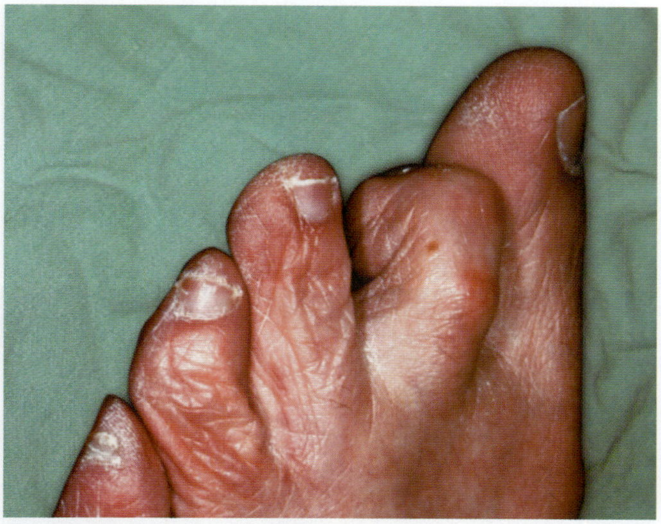

Fig. 26.357: Mallet toe

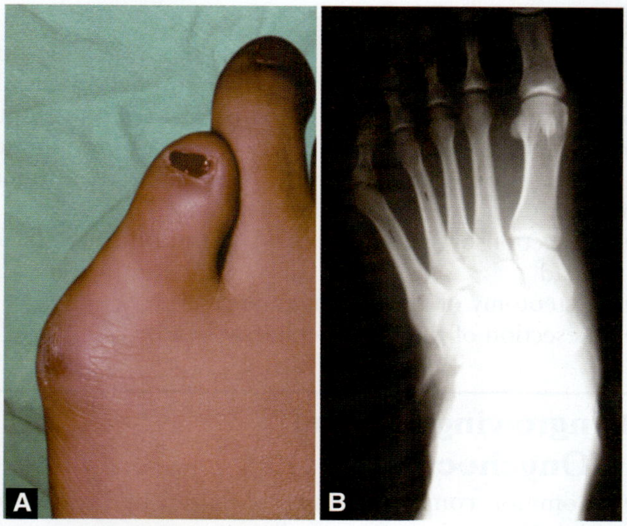

Figs 26.358A and B: (A) Tailor's bunion or bunionette; (B) X-ray showing enlargement of the lateral aspect of fifth metatarsal

■ Tailor's Bunion or Bunionette (Figs 26.358A and B)

Tailor's bunion or bunionette is a term applied to an enlargement of the lateral aspect of the fifth metatarsal head that produces various degrees of pain, swelling and tenderness. This enlargement of the lateral aspect of the fifth metatarsal head may present as either hypertrophy of soft tissue overlying the fifth metatarsal, a congenitally enlarged or dumbbell-shaped fifth metatarsal head, an abnormal lateral angulation of the fifth metatarsal shaft, or a combination of these conditions.

Etiology

Structural etiology: Persistent embryonic splaying of the fifth metatarsal, caused by incomplete or imperfect development of the transverse intermetatarsal ligament. Development of a Tailor's bunion deformity is attributed to one of following mechanisms:

- A supernumerary bone that attaches to the lateral aspect of the fourth metatarsal head, forcing the fifth metatarsal head laterally
- Spreading of the metatarsals resulting in a wide intermetatarsal angle.

Pressure on the lateral side of the fifth metatarsal head caused by sitting with crossed legs. The functional etiologies of a Tailor's bunion deformity are attributed to abnormal biomechanics. The functional etiology of a Tailor's bunion deformity consists of following factors:

- Excessive subtalar joint pronation
- Uncompensated varus position of the forefoot
- Rearfoot in a fully pronated subtalar joint
- A congenitally plantar-flexed fifth metatarsal
- Idiopathically, an absence of the transverse pedis muscle or an enlarged fifth metatarsal head.

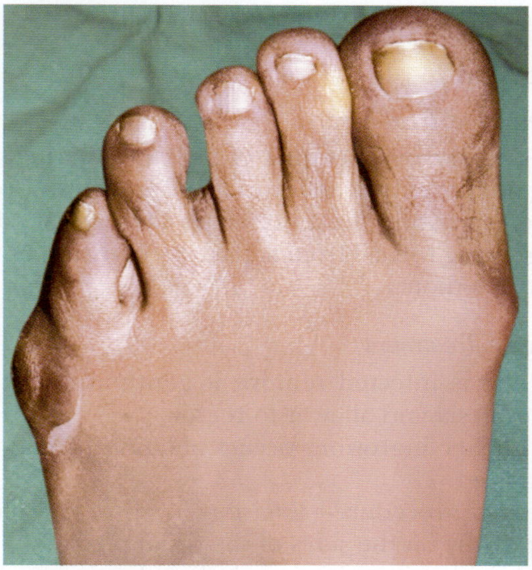

Fig. 26.359: Tailor's bunion or bunionette

Clinical Features

- With continuous pressure over this bony prominence, a bursa develops and enlarges because of chronic irritation, as shown in Figure 26.359
- Ulceration may ensue
- An intractable keratosis may develop over a prominent bunionette because of shoe pressure
- In diabetes, advanced Charcot-Marie-Tooth disease or certain types of spinal dysraphism with poor sensibility, this complication can result in loss of the entire fifth ray or even the foot
- A diffuse callus or localized intractable keratosis can develop beneath the plantar aspect of the fifth metatarsal head.

Treatment

Treatment with metatarsal pads or bars, wide toe box shoes and semirigid shoe inserts with a relief (or "well") beneath the plantar aspect of the condyle or one-eighth to one-fourth inch foam rubber between the prominence and the shoe may relieve the symptoms. If surgical treatment becomes necessary, the choices are:
- Resection of the lateral third of the fifth metatarsal head
- Osteotomy of the fifth metatarsal and
- Resection of the fifth metatarsal head.

■ Ingrowing Toenail (Onychocryptosis)

- Common complaint which is caused by pressing of the shoe against the toenail.
- The nail is driven into the soft part of the toe and results in pain.
- Prophylaxis—nail should be cut square at right angles to its long axis and not in a lunar shape.

Treatment

Conservative Treatment

It consists of correct cutting of nail and wearing of easy fitting stockings and shoes to avoid pressure. It can be treated separating the anterior tip and lateral edges of an ingrowing toenail from adjacent soft tissues by cotton with a collodion.

Operative Treatment

- If nail is infected remove it gently under general anesthesia and allow it to regrow
- If further ingrowing occurs ablation of nail bed is required
- Zadik's procedure—Excision of all of the nail bed especially on the sides of the distal phalanx
- Marginal nail avulsion and phenolization
  Acquired Flat Foot (Pes Planus) (Figs 26.360A and B)
- Refers to loss of the normal medial longitudinal arch
- May be osseous, ligamentous, muscular-paralytic, spastic postural or static
- Osseous–trauma to bones (run over fracture, fracture of navicular or calcaneus) or from disease of bones
- Ligamentous variety may follow rupture or avulsion of plantar ligaments from their attachments
- Paralytic and spastic muscular types the flattening of the arch is secondary to weight bearing on foot whose position has been altered by muscle imbalance.

Etiology

- Flat foot arises when the postural muscles of the longitudinal arch becomes unable to fulfill their function.

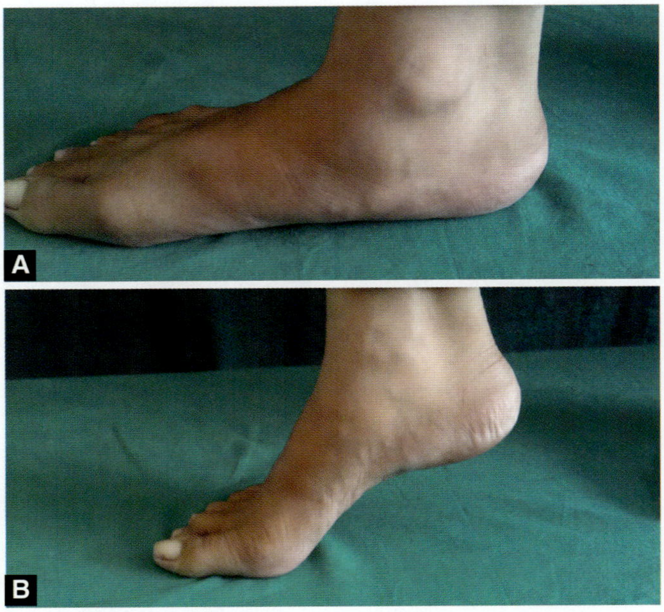

Figs 26.360A and B: Acquired flat foot, as the arch appears again on raising the toe

- Normally, the arch transmits the weight through subtalar mid tarsal region into the ground, when the stress passes normally through the bones, but a little further forward then plantar and interosseous ligaments take the strain. This ligament strain calls into play the muscles, which shift the strain back into normal area. This is the balancing act of the foot.
- *Two reasons for pes planus or loss of longitudinal arch:*
  - Calcaneus may be at fault and heel is drawn up in equinus deformity.
  - The medial anterior pillar may be at fault and the big toe is off the ground as a result of the varus deformity.
- Certain predisposing factors
  - General muscle hypotonus
    Convalsence after ill
    Rapid growth
    Severe trauma
- Excessive fatigue of normal muscles
  - Occupations which require standing or working for long hours
  - Rapid gain in weight (e.g. menopause)
- Shoe wear

Pathology

- In the earliest stages there may be few or no appreciable changes.
- As the calcaneonavicular ligament yields, the head of the talus is pressed forwards, downwards and medially. The calcaneum may deviate medially and its anterior end depressed, resulting in the sustentaculam tali and

head of the talus and tuberosity of navicular forming prominences on the medial side of foot.
- The long and short plantar ligaments yield, followed by yielding of deltoid.

Symptoms

- Feet feel tired after use, later feet become stiff after sitting or resting and are most uncomfortable in the morning
- Inelastic and clumsy gait
- Tendency to walk with feet everted and not to rise on toes
- Pain—more severe on standing than on walking
- Tenderness—navicular, inferior calcaneonavicular ligament, sole of the foot and below the first meta tarsal head
- Gait—raising of the heel is avoided, to prevent strain on tarsal and metatarsal ligaments. Patient carefully lifts ball and heel of the foot together. The toes are turned outwards
- Pressure symptoms—medial part of shoe wear out more quickly. Skin along the medial border of the heel and foot is thickened and painful. Callosities may form in weight bearing areas, and over little toe.

Types

- Foot strain or incipient flat foot. It is the earliest stage and corresponds to the period, when pressure is being first exerted on the ligaments. There is no evident deformity
- Mobile or flexible flat foot
- Rigid flat foot.

Flexible Pes Planus

Pes planus in children and adults usually is flexible and on nonweight bearing, a normal-appearing arch is present. If an acceptable medial longitudinal arch does not appear with non weight bearing, pes planus is termed fixed or rigid. The arch may not develop fully until the child is 7 to 10 years old.

Etiology

- Due to faulty postural activity of the muscles
- Due to short tendo achillis
- Due to varus deformity of fore foot
- Due to spinal dysraphism (e.g. spina bifida, diastematomyelia, lumbosacral lipomata)
- Other anatomical abnormalities are present, including:
  - Valgus posture of the heel.
  - Mild subluxation of the subtalar joint, in which the head of the talus tilts medially and plantarward, appearing foreshortened on the standing dorsoplantar radiograph.
  - Eversion of the calcaneus at the subtalar joint.
  - Lateral angulation (abduction) at the midtarsal joint (talonavicular and calcaneocuboid joints).
  - Supination of the forefoot relative to the hindfoot, which places the first ray plantigrade.
  - Achilles tendon frequently is shortened, accentuating the valgus of the hindfoot.

Clinical Examination

- When the child stands there is a flattening of the longitudinal arches, which disappears on standing on toes.
- Due to short tendo achillis the malalignment of the body weight disappears on tip-toeing, but when the foot is correctly aligned it is in equinus.
- Valgus deformities of the knees.

Radiography

- Standing radiographs in the anteroposterior and the lateral planes and nonstanding lateral oblique views are necessary to evaluate the severity of the deformity, by showing the talocalcaneal divergence on the dorsoplantar view and plantar flexion of the talus on the lateral view
- Lateur et al. in 1994, described the "C" sign on lateral radiographs of the ankle, as being suggestive of evidence of talocalcaneal subtalar coalition. However, more recently Brown et al. found it to be more specific for pes planus than subtalar coalition
- A "sag" at the talonavicular and naviculocuneiform joint or tarsometatarsal joint or both can be assessed. The oblique view in a 9 to 14 year-old-child, may show a calcaneonavicular bony bar or suggest a synchondrosis.

Treatment

An arch support is placed in a leather shoe with a firm heel counter, an extended medial counter, a steel shank, a Thomas heel and a medial heel wedge. Continuous use of a molded orthosis over an extended period can result in an improved arch radiographically and clinically. The issue of whether the use of orthoses results in permanent correction of a flexible pes planus deformity has not been settled. In a symptomatic child with severe flexible pes planus (3–9 years old), with marked heel valgus, forefoot abduction and a prominent talar head protruding medially, a custom orthosis is recommended.

I. *Surgical management*: Crego and Ford conclusions for surgical correction of pes planus. Any procedure for the correction of flexible pes planus should be done for disabling pain and then only after exhausting every means of conservative management. It should not be performed for cosmetic reasons only. The surgeon, the patient and the parents must be willing to exchange a loss of inversion and eversion of the foot for the relief of pain and disability. Arthrodesis for relieving painful pes planus have been most successful, when the subtalar joint is included, although midtarsal arthrodesis without inclusion of the subtalar joint has gained in popularity. The techniques described here are as follows:

- Durham pes planus plasty (Caldwell; Coleman)
- Plantar flexion osteotomy of medial cuneiform (Hirose and Johnson)
- Triple arthrodesis (triplane)
- Posterior calcaneal displacement osteotomy (Koutsogiannis)
- Anterior calcaneal lengthening-distraction wedge osteotomy (Mosca)
- Evans Procedure

The Durham plasty combines advancement of the posterior tibial tendon and osteoperiosteal flap with arthrodesis of the navicular—first cuneiform joint. In triple arthrodesis of all three joints (subtalar, talonavicular and calcaneocuboid), if an arthrodesis is indicated. The patient's bone age should be 12 years or older. In a symptomatic patient with flexible pes planus and excessive heel valgus, a calcaneal osteotomy is intended to displace the posterior part of the calcaneus medially to restore normal weight bearing alignment. The Evans procedure involves lengthening the lateral column, by placing a bone graft from the tibia into the anterior process of the calcaneus. Medial and lateral columns are equalized in length. This procedure preserves the calcaneocuboid joint and pushes the navicular bone medially in relation to the talus.

Accessory Navicular

The accessory navicular is an accessory bone that is also called the accessory scaphoid, prehallux, os tibial, os tibial externum, naviculare secundarium and navicular secundum. The accessory navicular sits posteromedial to the navicular and it ossifies between 9 and 11 years of age. There are three types of accessory navicular, as determined by radiographic appearance.

- Type I is an ossicle that lies within the posterior tibial tendon
- Type II is connected to the navicular by a cartilaginous bridge
- Type III is a cornuate-shaped navicular from fusion of the accessory bone to the navicular

There is some controversy as to whether the accessory navicular can cause pes planus. Generally, the patient has a flatfoot deformity and the accessory bone interferes with the normal mechanics of the posterior tibial tendon and the removal of the accessory navicular would allow a straighter pull of the tendon and thus improvement of the flatfoot deformity.

Diagnosis

Physical examination will reveal a bony prominence of the proximal medial border of the navicular with tenderness over the accessory bone. There can be associated local edema and erythema. The accessory bone is usually visible on plain radiographs of the foot. A bone scan may help to localize and differentiate the pathologic cause of medial arch pain, but it is rarely necessary.

Treatment

Nonoperative: Most cases of accessory navicular are asymptomatic and less than 1 percent require surgical treatment. Nonoperative treatment is generally effective and consists of rest from activity, nonsteroidal anti-inflammatory medication and shoewear modification. A wider shoe will relieve the pressure over the bony prominence. With a flatfoot deformity, a medial arch in a custom orthotic device may reduce the stress on the medial longitudinal arch. Acute symptoms associated with an injury, even a minor sprain, can be treated with a short course of cast immobilization for 3 to 6 weeks.

Surgical: Excision of the accessory bone with advancement of the posterior tibial tendon is known as the Kidner procedure. However, there is little advantage to advancing the tendon.

Rigid Pes Planus

The etiology of rigid pes planus is different from that of a flexible deformity. Usually, there is a bony abnormality, such as tarsal coalition, congenital vertical talus or arthritis. Of these, tarsal coalition is the most common cause and can present as peroneal spastic flatfoot. Other causes include, secondary degenerative changes in subtaloid and mid tarsal joints due to clubfoot, old trauma rheumatoid arthritis os osteoarthritis. The cause of tarsal coalition is a failure of mesenchymal segmentation and the resulting connection of two tarsal bones may be fibrous (syndesmosis), cartilaginous (synchondrosis) or bony(synostosis). The tarsal coalition is an inherited disease that is autosomal dominant. Tarsal coalition should be suspected in adolescents with painful and stiff pes planus. The most common age of presentation is the teen years, but patients can develop initial symptoms in their twenties. Most patients complain of pain about the tarsal area and stiffness and tightness of the peroneal and toe extensor muscles. They complain of difficulty with sports activities or even with standing and walking. Physical examination shows a rigid hindfoot, loss of the medial longitudinal arch and fixed forefoot abduction. Spasm of the peroneal tendons, can be seen by placing the foot into inversion. The result is contraction of the peroneus brevis or longus or both.

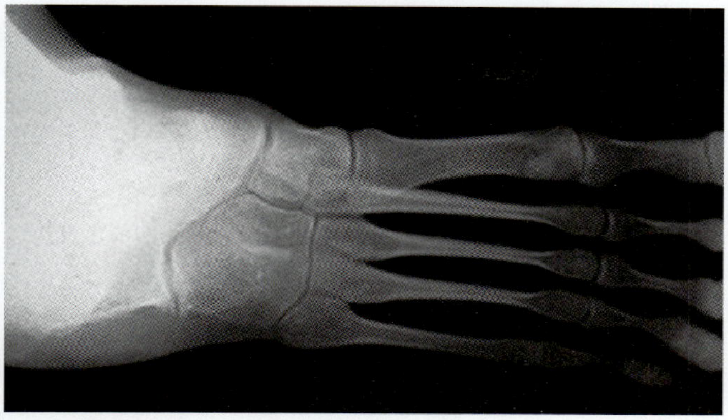

Fig. 26.361: Radiograph showing rigid pes planus with naviculocalcaneal coalition

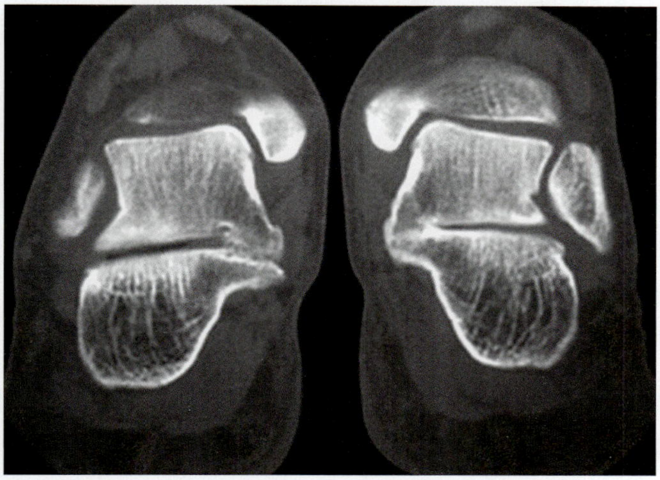

Fig. 26.362: CT scans demonstrating the rigid pes planus

Radiographs (Figs 26.361 and 26.362)

Radiographs may show a naviculocalcaneal coalition on the oblique view of the foot. The Harris view (posterior axial) can show a talocalcaneal coalition, but CT scans are more helpful in demonstrating this.

Nonoperative Treatment

Rest, nonsteroidal anti-inflammatory medication and cast immobilization will be helpful to some patients. Use a cast for at least 3 weeks; usually 6 to 8 weeks are required for relief of symptoms. Later, a shoe modification, such as a heel cup, a medial arch support or a medial heel wedge, may allow patients to return to weight-bearing activities.

Surgical Treatment

Resection of tarsal coalition is the treatment of choice in a child with a middle facet coalition or a posterior facet coalition that comprises less than 25 percent of the joint surface and that is symptomatic and unresponsive to nonoperative treatment. Contraindications to coalition resection, include degenerative arthritis, associated deformity and involvement of greater than 50 percent of the posterior facet.

■ Peroneal or Spasmodic Pes Planus

- Acute condition
- Commonly seen in young adolescents with pain, tightness or spasm of the peroneal muscles and an eversion deformity of the foot
- Onset is usually after starting work or changing to an occupation involving much standing.

Etiology

- *Congenital:* Tarsal anamolies and inter tarsal bridges, e.g. calcaneonavicular, talocalcaneal bars, calcaneocuboid bars and anamolies of navicular.
- *Acquired*
  - Tuberculous lesions
  - Rheumatoid arthritis
  - Osteoarthritis
  - Nonspecific tarsal joint synovitis
  - Trauma
  - Occupational strains

Pathology

The pathology of the peroneal spasm is probably that of a reflex muscle reaction, but there is no established relationship between the sensory innervation to talonavicular joint and that supplying peroneal muscles.

■ Cavus Foot (Figs 26.363A to D)

Cavus foot is a deformity of the foot, characterized by an excessively high longitudinal plantar arch that results from an equinus position of forefoot in relation to hind foot.

Etiology

Three main groups have been identified. In majority the origin is obscure. In second group the deformity arises as a result of paralytic disease in three ways:

- Contracture during acute stage, e.g. poliomyelitis
- Postural deformity
- Muscle imbalance during growth period

Third group occurs in association with certain neurological diseases or developmental deformity of spine.

Classification

Idiopathic

- Most common
- Develops after three years of age
- Males and females are equally affected
- Often associated with spina bifida occulta

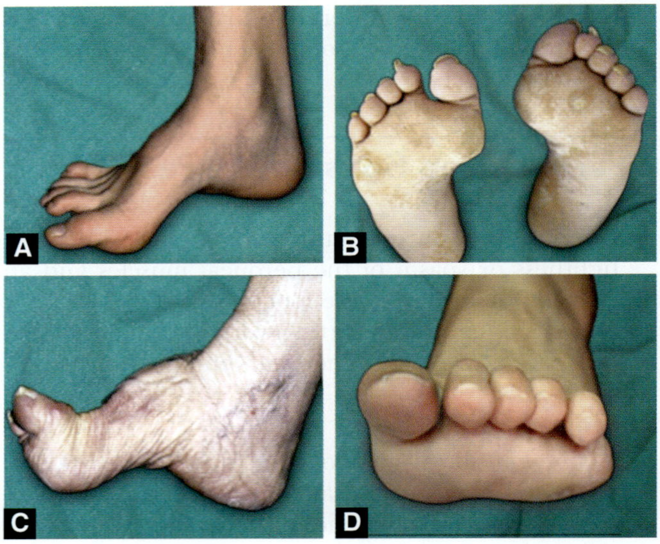

Figs 26.363A to D: Cavus foot deformity

Secondary

- Neurologic disease
  a. Spinocerebellar heriditory degeneration of molaret
  b. Friedreich's ataxia
  c. Poliomyelitis
  d. Diseases of conus medullaris or cauda equina
     – Diastematomyelia
     – Cauda equina tumor
  e. Pyramidal or extrapyramidal syndromes
     – Cerebral palsy
  f. Progressive peroneal palsy
     – Charcot-Marie-Tooth disease
- Direct trauma to foot
- Myopathies, e.g. muscular dystrophy
- Plantar fibromatosis
- Congenital talipus equinovarus

Theories of Pathogenesis

Mechanism of idiopathic pes cavus is unknown. The two main theories related to muscle imbalance are:

- *Weakness of intrinsics (Duchenne)*
  – The intrinsics fail to flex the metatarsophalangeal joints and extend the interphalangeal joints
  – Theory is untenable because paralysis of intrinsics produces a planovalgus foot.
- *Over activity of intrinsics*
  – Persistant function of short toe flexors and intrinsics in an otherwise flat foot results in the development of cavovarus foot.
  – Sharrad principles of paralytic deformity for secondary pes cavus:
    - Acute contacture—develops rapidly in acute stage of paralytic disease (poliomyelitis).
    - Postural contracture—immobility and edema encourage deposition of collagen.
    - Muscle imbalance—in the growing child, progresses in spite of stretching and splinting.

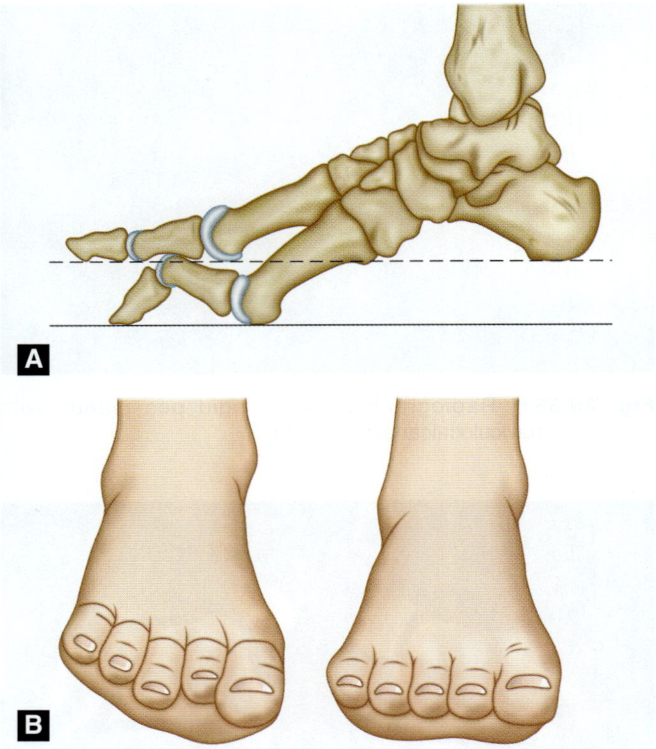

Figs 26.364A and B: Pathologic anatomy of cavus of foot

Pathologic Anatomy (Figs 26.364A and B)

Following description relates to idiopathic or primary pes cavus.

- *Dropping of forefoot*
  – Deformity initially develops in first ray, which gradually drops down.
  – The naviculocuneiform and cuneiform metatarsal joints become rigid.
  – The first metatarsal gardually loses its passive range of dorsiflexion, while other metatarsals remail mobile until late.
  – Entire foot becomes everted, which becomes rigid and resists passive correction.
- *Contracture of plantar fascia*
  – Increases the height of longitudinal arch
  – Cavus is increased, by pronation of the forefoot and inversion of heel.
- *Varus of heel*
  – As the forefoot becomes fixed in eversion, in order that all metatarsals can be placed evenly on the floor, the outer forefoot must invert
  – This movement carries the hindfoot inward at midtarsal joint

- Gradually, the varus becomes fixed and pronounced.
- *Clawing of toes*
  - Proximal phalanges are hyperextended and middle and distal phalanges are flexed.

Examination

- A through search for underlying disease.
- Examine the parents and siblings because of high incidence in idiopathic pes cavus, degenerative disease of spino cerebellar tracts and spina bifida.
- Include examination of feet, aneurologic evaluation including examination of muscles and X-ray studies of feet and entire spine.

Types of Deformity

a. *Simple Pes Cavus*
- Forefoot equinus evenly distributed
- All metatarsals bear weight equally
- Heel in neutral position or slight valgus

b. *Pes Cavovarus*
- Medial column alone in plantar flexion and resists passive dorsiflexion.
- Fifth metatarsal is easily dorsiflexed.
- Forefoot pronated 20° to 30° hindfoot in neutral position.
- Initially, hindfoot inversion is flexible and reducible and spontaneously subsides, when the fixed equinus and pronation of first metatarsal are corrected. Later varus of hindfoot becomes fixed and requires separate correction.

c. *Calcaneocavus*
- Results from paralysis of triceps surae
- Heel assumes vertical position
- Forefoot in equinus in relation to hindfoot

d. *Equino Cavovarus*
- Typical deformity of uncorrected clubfoot.

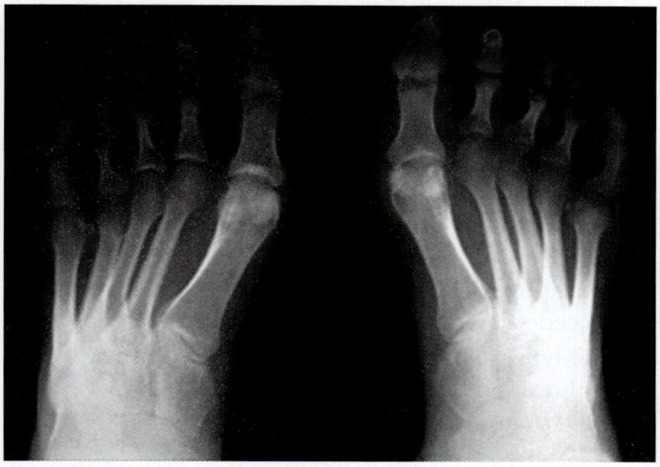

Fig. 26.365: Foot cavus in standing weight bearing position, depicting apex of the deformity

Roentgenographic Findings (Fig. 26.365)

Standing weight bearing films demonstrate the apex of the deformity. Normally, the proximal and distal articular surfaces of the innercuneiform are parallel. In pes cavus, forefoot downward inclination is maximal at innercuneiform and proximal and distal articular surfaces of the cuneiform converge outward to the plantar aspect of foot. In anteroposterior standing view, the talocalcaneal angle is decreased when heel inversion is fixed help corroborate any metatarsus adductus component suspected clinically. In lateral weight bearing view, the angle of the cavus can be demonstrated by the intersection of two lines corresponding to the axis of first metatarsal and the other through the axis of either talus or calcaneus. A standing lateral view allows assessment of ankle joint position, calcaneal pitch and midfoot and forefoot position, especially the degree of plantar flexion of the first ray, as shown in Figure 26.366. The standing lateral radiograph also allows estimation of the contribution of the hindfoot (talus and calcaneus), midfoot (navicular and cuboid-cuneiform) and forefoot (Lisfranc) to the cavus deformity.

Other radiographic findings that may be helpful include:

- Degenerative changes, even slight, in the tibiotalar, subtalar or midtarsal Lisfranc joints.
- Rotation of the talus in the ankle mortise, which probably is caused by talar dorsiflexion and varus at the subtalar joint.
- Dystrophic ossification in soft tissue, suggesting tendon or ligament injury on the oblique view.

Clinical Presentation

- Hyperextension of the toes at the metatarsophalangeal joints
- Hyperflexion at the interphalangeal joints
- Pronation and adduction of the forefoot (forefoot valgus)
- A "bony" dorsum of the midfoot with wrinkled skin folds on the medial plantar aspect

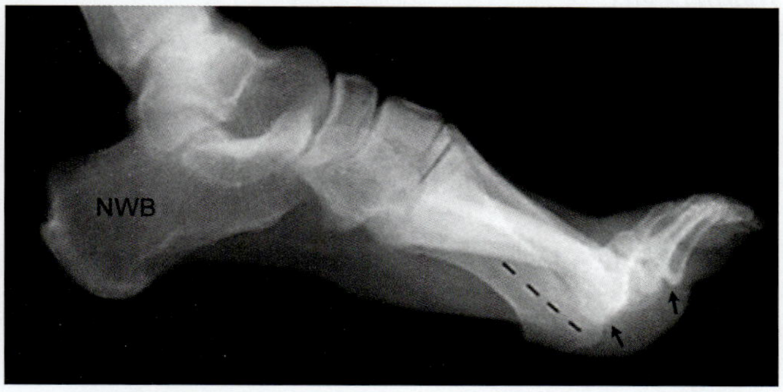

Fig. 26.366: X-ray showing foot cavus deformity and other radiographic findings (NWB: Nonweight bearing)

- Lengthened lateral border of the foot and shortened medial border
- Calluses beneath the metatarsal heads
- Varied stiffness of the subtalar joint, fixed or flexible varus deformity of the heel
- Tightness of the Achilles tendon with or without an equinus contracture

Clinical Features

Can be divided into a series of stages

First Degree

- Foot appears normal, deformity appearing when foot is relaxed
- Child is clumsy with history of repeated falls and the child catches his toes against low objects such as edge of the carpet
- Corrects easily by pushing up on the first metatarsal bone
- Only physical sign positive at this stage is slight extensor weakness, which can be demonstrated by difference in circumference of two calves.

Second Degree

- In addition of flexion of forefoot, there is dorsiflexion of great toe at the MP joint and flexion at IP joint
- Plantar fascia is felt to be tense and contracted
- Characteristic deformity, include clawing can be made to disappear by upward pressure on the ball of great toe.

Third Degree

- In addition to dropping of first ray, the other metatarsals participate in equinus deformity
- The calcaneus begins to invert and resists passive reduction
- The arch of the foot is markedly raised, while all the toes are clawed and tendocalcaneus may begin to appear contracted
- The plantar structures are further shortened and all the toes are now dorsiflexed at MP joint and flexed at IP joints
- Painful corns are seen
- Foot tires easily.

Fourth Degree

- In addition to cavus and the hammer toes, there is adduction at tarsometatarsal joints, resulting in varus deformity
- Rigid and painful foot
- Walking becomes increasingly painful.

Fifth Degree

- Seen only in some paralytic conditions, like polio
- Toes are blue and cold
- Whole foot is contracted into rigid equinovarus with high arch
- Tender callosities

  – Patients with cavus deformity, as a residual of poliomyelitis usually have different physical findings.

A weak gastrocnemius-soleus opposite a strong anterior tibial, may cause a calcaneus deformity of the hindfoot with or without hindfoot varus or valgus, depending on which muscle groups around the ankle are strong. The post poliomyelitis cavus foot has anterior and posterior (or forefoot and hindfoot) components to the deformity unlike Charcot-Marie-Tooth disease. Due to intact sensation and the nonprogressive nature of the deformities, patients with post poliomyelitis cavus feet have a better or at least more predictable, prognosis than patients with Charcot-Marie-Tooth disease.

Treatment Principles

- Directed towards correcting the primary deformity, equinus and pronation of forefoot
- Correction that is limited to secondary deformities, like contracted plantar fascia clawed toes and varus heel is sufficient and affects partial improvement
- The neurologic disturbance should be clearly defined and muscle imbalance analyzed before surgical measures can be taken
- Precautions should be taken in the care of immature foot to avoid compromising joint motion and growth.
  - Gentle manipulative stretching
  - Surgery is limited, if possible to soft tissues
  - Surgical trauma to bone structures should avoid growth areas and midtarsal joints
- When the deformity is recognized early, it should be treated conservatively
  - Forefoot is forced into inversion and dorsiflexion
  - Heel is manipulated into eversion
  - Toes are plantarflexed at metatarsophalangeal joint
- Following this, a transverse lift is placed behind metatarsal heads
- A lateral three-eighth inch sole wedge counteracts inversion of forefoot on weight bearing
- Progressive, increasingly resistant cavus deformity requires surgical correction
- In immature foot, the operative procedure is mainly directed to soft tissues, to avoid compromising growth of foot
- When late structural changes have occurred, the forefoot is fixed in marked equinus and bony procedures are necessary, which should always be preceded by plantar release
- The type of surgical procedure is determined by:
  - Location of apex of cavus
  - Type of pes cavus
  - Nature of hindfoot deformity
  - Stability of heel

- Toe deformities and
- Degree of muscle weakness

Treatment

First Degree

- Daily manipulations—flatten arch by supinating forefoot and everting heel
- Exercise dorsiflexors without allowing cocking of toes.
- Anterior arch bar in shoe
- Night splint–dorsiflexion pressure applied behind metatarsal heads
- Progress may be arrested by re-educating the small muscle function by intrinsic exercises
- If not Girdlestone flexor to extensor transfer is performed.

Second Degree

Equinus and pronation of first ray become irreducible and associated with early contractures of plantar fascia and clawing of large toe. Shoe fitted with metatarsal bar gives relief. Adequate treatment is by operation—the plantar fascia is divided (if the plantar structures are barely contracted they can be released by subcutaneous fasciotomy. If the contracture is greater, the aponeurosis and the underlying muscles are stripped from the calcaneus–Steindler stripping) and the tendon of extensor halluces longus is divided at its insertion and passed through the neck of first metatarsal—Jones tenosuspension. Arthrodesis of IP joint with tenodesis of extensor halluces brevis to improve take off.

Third Degree

It is same as second degree. In immature foot, dynamic correction is accomplished by transferring the long extensors to metatarsals. This is particularly effective in reinforcing weak anterior tibial. Muscle slide operation–all the structure on the sole of the foot, which arise from undersurface of calcaneum are seperated from bone. Structures are erased right forward to the calcaneocuboid joint laterally and talonavicular medially. Extensors of the toe are divided.

- *Extensor shift procedure:* Objective is to remove the deforming force that hyper extends the metacarpophalangeal joint and use it to elevate the metatarsals. The extensor hallusces longus tendon is divided 1 inch proximal to interphalangeal joint. The toe is tightened and the tendon stump is fixed to a drill hole in the proximal phalynx.
- *Dwyer procedure:* Osteotomy of the posterior portion of calcaneus restores the valgus position of the heel. The weight bearing stresses on the fore part of the foot, improve the equinus deformity. This operation is effective only in growing foot.

Fourth and Fifth Degrees

Various components of the deformity become pronounced and resist passive correction. More radical measures directed towards bone resection are necessary. It can be corrected by dividing the bones across at the level of midtarsal joint by wedge tarsectomy/osteotomy.

Tarsal osteotomy of Japas: Anterior tarsal wedge osteotomy and fusion of first metatarsocuneiform navicular joints.

Various Surgical Techniques

The operative treatment of cavus deformity requires correction of the separate components within the foot and ankle. The recommended techniques are described for each component.

- *Claw toes:* In patients with traumatic pes cavus, only the claw toe deformities and possibly tight plantar fascia may require surgical treatment, leaving the bony midfoot deformity to appropriate shoe and orthotic management. For fixed contractures at the metatarsophalangeal and interphalangeal joints, the following are recommended:
  - Lengthening of the extensor halluces longus and extensor digitorum longus
  - Tenotomy of the extensor digitorum brevis and the extensor halluces brevis
  - Dorsal capsulotomy of the metatarsophalangeal joints
  - Resection of the head and neck of the proximal phalanges
  - Release of the plantar fascia
  - Arthrodesis of the interphalangeal joint of the hallux or plantar plate release and sectioning of the collateral ligaments, at the interphalangeal joint of the hallux with temporary Kirschner wire fixation.
- *Forefoot equinus:* Occasionally, in an adolescent foot, soft-tissue procedures alone correct the forefoot equinus sufficiently to avoid osteotomy or arthrodesis. Gould technique, as shown in Figures 26.367 and 26.368 includes:
  a. Double plantar fasciotomies
  b. Closing wedge greenstick dorsal proximal metatarsal osteotomies
     - Jones technique includes, tendon suspension (extensor halluces tendon) of the first metatarsal and interphalangeal joint arthrodesis.
     - Equinus of the forefoot also may require the Hibbs procedure, which involves transfer of the extensor digitorum longus to the middle cuneiform.
     - Another procedure for forefoot equinus advocated by Jahss is arthrodesis of all

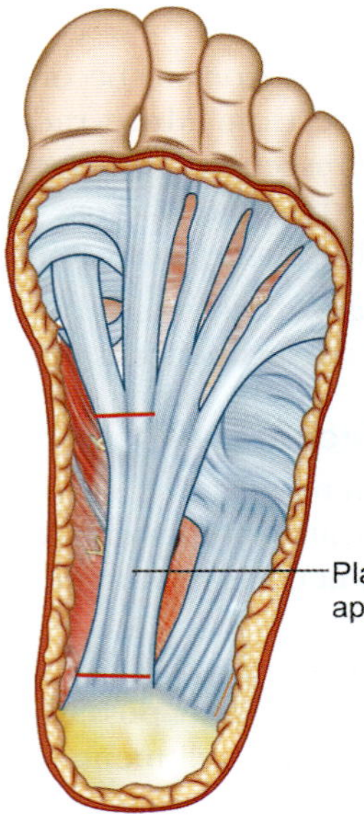

Fig. 26.367: Plantar aspect of the foot

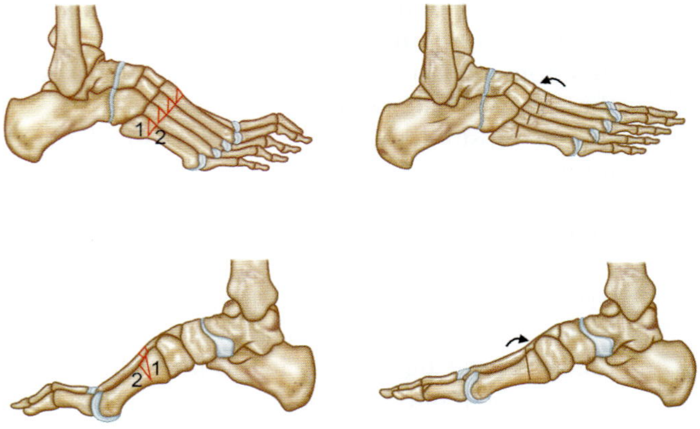

Fig. 26.368: Correction of cavus deformity of foot

tarsometatarsal joints with out plantar fascial release.

- *Midfoot cavus:* Cavus deformity can occur at the midtarsal joints (talonavicular-calcaneocuboid) or naviculocuneiform joints, but is most common at the former. Depending on the rigidity of the deformity, plantar fascial release combined with calcaneal or metatarsal osteotomy, may correct the deformity sufficiently to achieve a plantigrade foot. For mild-to-moderate fixed cavus deformity at the midfoot, the following osteotomies have been described.
  1. *Anterior tarsal wedge osteotomy by Cole* (Fig. 26.369)
  2. *Jahss technique for tarsometatarsal truncated wedge arthrodesis* (Figs 26.370A to F)
  3. *V-osteotomy of the tarsus by Japas* (Figs 26.371A and B): It consists of a V-osteotomy, in which the apex of the V is proximal and at the highest point of the cavus, usually within the navicular. One limb of the V extends laterally and the other medially through the first cuneiform to the medial border. No bone is excised, instead the proximal border of the distal fragment of the osteotomy is depressed plantarward, while the metatarsal heads are elevated, correcting the deformity and lengthening the plantar surface of the foot. The technique is recommended for moderate deformity in children 6 years old or older. Deformities of the hindfoot or midtarsal joint are not corrected by this osteotomy and may require later correction by triple arthrodesis or the Dwyer osteotomy.
  4. *Combined cavus (calcaneocavus deformity):* Although a hindfoot crescentic calcaneal osteotomy, with or without midtarsal osteotomy has been recommended for calcaneocavus deformity. If appropriate bony wedges are removed, however, the Dwyer procedure can correct the varus and calcaneus posture of the hindfoot. Only a certain amount of midfoot-forefoot cavus can be corrected by any calcaneal osteotomy and a triple arthrodesis usually is a better choice for severe and fixed equinocavovarus deformity.
  5. *Dwyer calcaneus osteotomy* (Figs 26.372A to C): Remove a wedge of bone from the calcaneus just inferior and posterior to the peroneus longus tendon and parallel with it. Make the base of the wedge 8 to 12 mm wide and taper the wedge to, but not through the medial cortex. Break the medial cortex, and close the gap.
  6. *Crescentic calcaneal osteotomy of Samilson* (Figs 26.373A and B): For ambulatory patients with symptomatic calcaneocavus feet. On a lateral radiograph, the calcaneus must be relatively vertical, and the apex of the cavus must be posterior to the midtarsus. The operation does not correct midtarsal or forefoot cavus, but does correct hindfoot cavus (calcaneocavus).
  7. *Calcaneocavovarus and cavovarus deformity:* Most often seen in patients with Charcot-Marie-Tooth disease, but occasionally this deformity occurs after

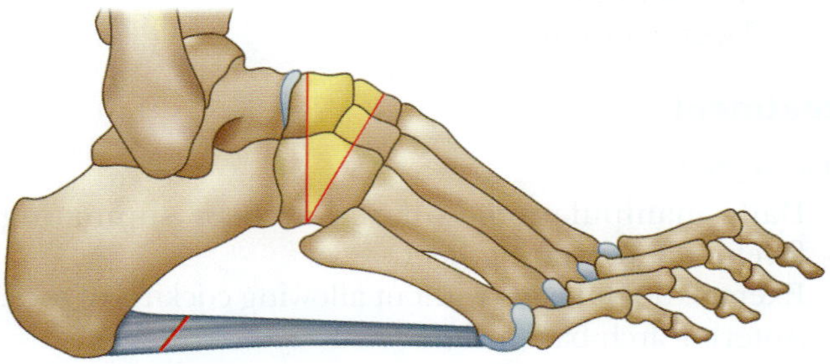

Fig. 26.369: Anterior tarsal wedge osteotomy by Cole

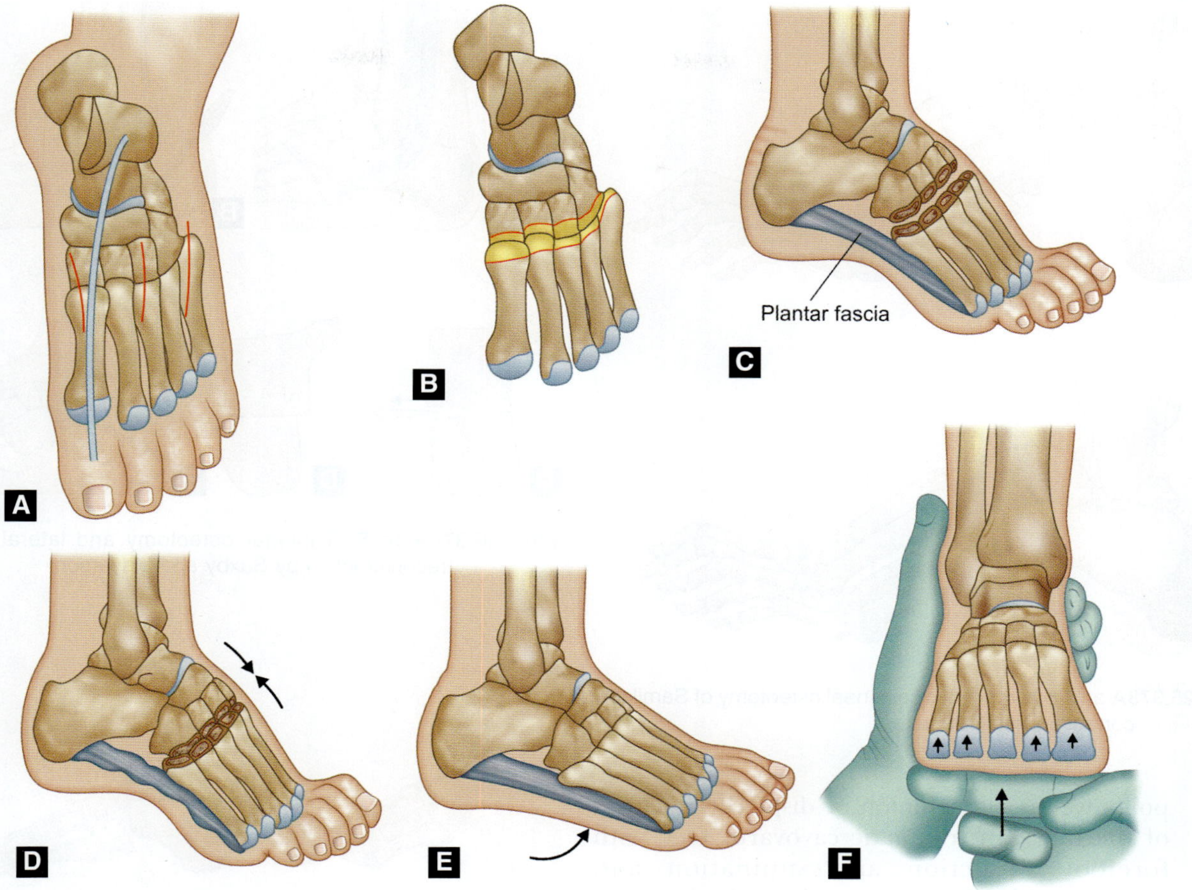

Figs 26.370A to F: Jahss technique for tarsometatarsal truncated, a wedge arthrodesis—(A) Skin incision; (B) Amount of bone resected; (C to E) Truncated-wedge principle permitting ready closure. Plantar fascia tightens up when wedge is closed, adding stability and eliminating need for internal fixation; (F) Checking level of metatarsal heads

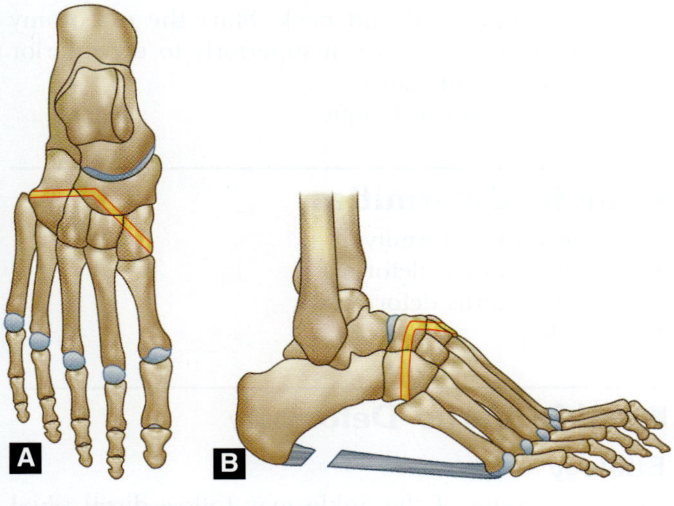

Figs 26.371A and B: V-osteotomy of the tarsus by Japas

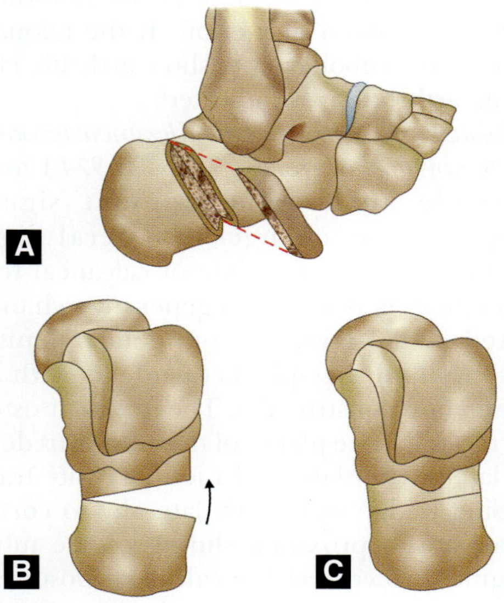

Figs 26.372A to C: Dwyer calcaneus osteotomy

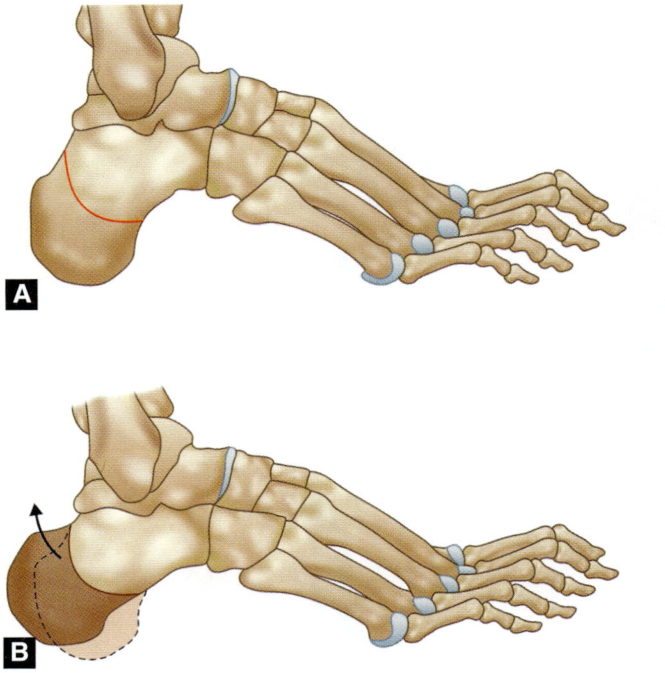

Figs 26.373A and B: Crescentic calcaneal osteotomy of Samilson, correcting hindfoot cavus

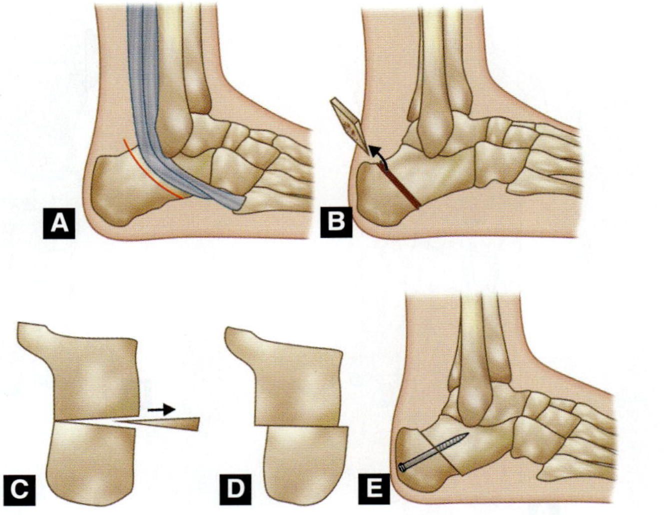

Figs 26.374A to E: Triplanar osteotomy and lateral ligament reconstruction by Saxby and Mayerson

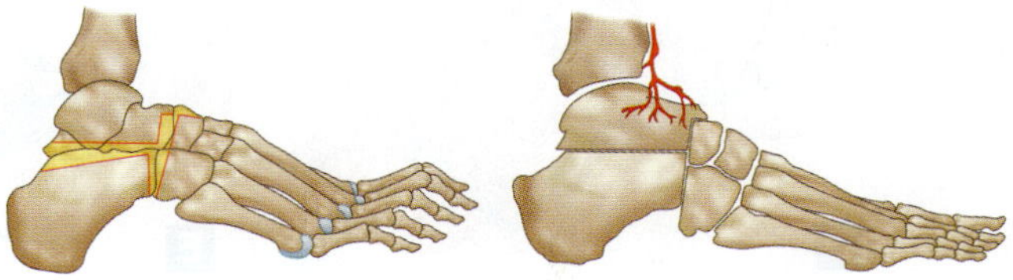

Fig. 26.375: Triple arthrodesis

poliomyelitis or malunion of displaced fractures of the talus. In traumatic cavovarus feet, with forefoot adduction and supination and radiographically intact talonavicular and calcaneocuboid joints, subtalar arthrodesis (removing more bone laterally) combined with lateral closing wedge (7–10 mm) osteotomy of the anterior aspect of the calcaneus 1 cm proximal to the calcaneocuboid joint (reverse Evans osteotomy) may correct the deformities, while allowing some degree of midtarsal motion. If the talonavicular or calcaneocuboid joints show arthritic changes, triple arthrodesis is indicated.

8. *Triplanar osteotomy and lateral ligament reconstruction by Saxby and Mayerson (Figs 26.374A to E):* For unstable ankle joints without significant degenerative changes a lateral ligament reconstruction at the time of calcaneal triplanar osteotomy is done. If degenerative changes are noted in the midtarsal or subtalar joints, they recommend a triple arthrodesis with lateral ligament reconstruction. The triplanar osteotomy corrects all three planes of the cavovarus deformity by lateral translation of the tuberosity fragment, closing wedge osteotomy laterally to correct the varus and a proximal sliding of the tuberosity fragment to correct the calcaneal posture of the hindfoot.
9. *Triple arthrodesis (Fig. 26.375):* Calcaneocavovarus and cavovarus deformity associated with arthritic changes of the subtalar and midtarsal joints. Wedge of bone is removed by osteotomy of the anterior aspect of the calcaneus, the posterior aspect of the navicular and the inferior aspect of the talar head and neck. Start the osteotomy inferiorly and carry it superiorly to the inferior surface of the talus.
10. Lambrinudi technique.

■ Ankle Deformities

- Ankle varus deformity
- Hindfoot valgus deformity
- Hindfoot varus deformity
- Foot drop

■ Ankle Varus Deformity

Etiology

Varus deformity of the ankle may follow distal tibial fracture or distal tibial epiphyseal fractures; deformities due to distal tibial epiphyeal injuries are often progressive;

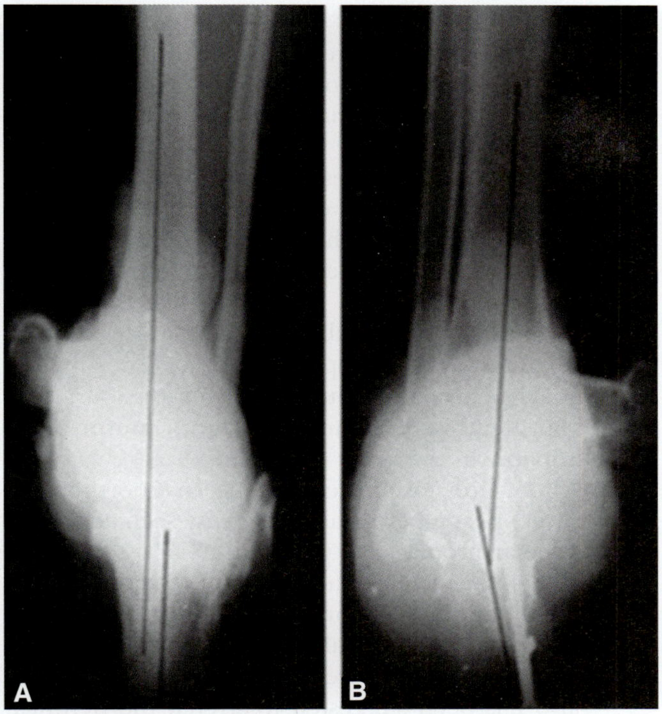

Figs 26.376A and B: Weight bearing X-rays of ankle and foot

deformities due to tibial plafond injuries are usually static (from malreduction at the time of the original procedure).

Sequelae: If left untreated, the varus deformity may lead to DJD of the ankle.

Diagnosis

- History of epiphyseal injuries or trauma earlier
- Weight bearing X-rays (Figs 26.376A and B)

Treatment

It involves a one stage opening wedge valgus osteotomy, since the affected leg is most often short, an opening wedge rather than a closing wedge osteotomy is indicated. Fibular osteotomy performed through a small lateral incision, tibial osteotomy site use a longitudinal medial incision, make the osteotomy parallel to the joint line, but leave a small posterolateral portion of the distal tibia intact (for stability). In adults, attempt to place the osteotomy site at the level of the initial fracture, if this is not possible then make the osteotomy cut 5 cm above the distal end of the medial malleolus. In children, consider making the osteotomy cut about 2 to 3 cm proximal to the physis, make the opening wedge correction and then use calipers to determine the necessary width of the bone graft. K-wires can be used to stabilize the graft controversies, physeal bone-bridge resection ipsilateral and contralateral growth plate arrest in situations in which bone bridge resection is not advisable, growth plate excision is indicated. Be sure to arrest the fibular growth plate as well (which contributes to varus deformity).

Complications

- Some patients will note a decrease in ROM.

■ Hindfoot Valgus Deformity

Spastic pes valgus foot is a flexible deformity until adolescence; spastic peroneal muscles pull the forefoot laterally and with it supporting plantar ligaments for the talar head, resulting in plantar flexed talus; left untreated, the natural history may result in midfoot sag and lateral near complete break down in the midfoot.

Anatomical Relationships

- Plantar flexion of the talus and calcaneus.
- Excessive valgus, external rotation and dorsiflexion of the calcaneus in relationship to the talus.
- Navicular dorsiflexed and abducted on the head of the talus.
- Forefoot is supinated in relationship to the hindfoot.

Examination

- Note correctability of the hindfoot in relation to the forefoot
- Look for equinus contracture (with the hindfoot placed in varus)
- Skin changes may occur over the medial aspect of the talar head

Treatment

Nonoperative treatment: Patient's with spastic deplegia will often not tolerate orthotic management.

Treatment methods:

1. *Grice arthrodesis:* Subtalar extra-articular arthrodesis that was originally devised by Grice for the management of pes valgus due to flaccid paralysis muscle imbalance (Polio). Modifications of the Grice procedure have also been widely used for treating hindfoot valgus deformity in CP.
2. Subtalar arthrodesis.
3. Triple arthrodesis
4. *Calcaneal lengthening:* Modified Evan's calcaneal lengthening technique; indicated for chronic pain, brace intolerance, and skin changes.

■ Hindfoot Varus Deformity

It is usually accompanied by equinus deformity.

Etiology

- An uncorrected or relapsed club foot
- As part of pes cavus deformity

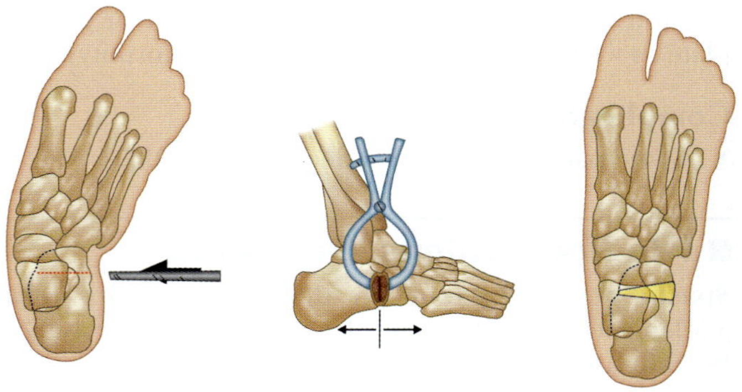

Fig. 26.377: Dilwyn Evans operation for varus correction

- As a result of neurological disorders, like spina bifida or cerebral palsy or poliomyelitis
- As part of arthrogryphosis multiplex congenita
- Spastic hemiplegia
- Presents as an inverted and small heel, a tight tendo calcaneus forefoot abduction and inversion rotation at the mid tarsal joints. There may also be some cavus deformity as well as clawing of the toes and lateral rotation of tibia.

Treatment

- *Jones operation*: Extensor halluces longus is placed through the neck of the first metatarsal bone, with the fusion of interphalangeal joint of great toe.
- *Dilwyn Evans operation (Fig. 26.377):* Extensive medial soft tissue release with lengthening of tight tendons together with calcaneo cuboid arthrodesis. Lengthens the calcaneus by a transverse osteotomy of the calcaneus and the insertion of a bone graft to open a wedge and lengthen the lateral border of the foot.
- *Dwyer operation*: Aimed at correcting varus by increasing the medial height of calcaneus and placing it directly under the line of weight bearing.

Foot Drop

- Foot drop is a deceptively simple name for a potentially complex problem.
- Can be defined as a significant weakness of ankle and toe dorsiflexion.
- Foot drop can be associated with a variety of conditions, such as dorsiflexor injuries, peripheral nerve injuries, stroke, neuropathies, drug toxicities or diabetes.
- The causes of foot drop may be divided into three general categories:
  - Neurologic
  - Muscular
  - Anatomic

Etiology

- Foot drop may follow direct injury to the dorsiflexors. This subcutaneous tendon (tibialis anterior) rupture usually occurs after a minor trauma with the foot in plantar flexion.
- Compartment syndromes also may lead to foot drop.
- Neurologic causes of foot drop include mononeuropathies of the deep peroneal, common peroneal or sciatic nerves. Lumbosacral plexopathy, lumbar radiculopathy, motor neuron disease or parasagittal cortical or subcortical cerebral lesions also can manifest as foot drop.
- Peroneal neuropathy caused by compression at the fibular head is the most common compressive neuropathy in the lower extremity.
  - A foot drop of particular concern to orthopedic surgeons is a peroneal nerve palsy seen after total knee arthroplasty or proximal tibial osteotomy.
  - Ischemia, mechanical irritation, traction, crush injury and laceration can cause intraoperative injury to the peroneal nerve.
  - Correction of a severe valgus or flexion deformity also has been suggested to stretch the peroneal nerve and lead to palsy.
  - Postoperative causes of peroneal nerve palsy include hematoma or constrictive dressings.
- A common behavioral cause of foot drop is habitual crossing of the legs. These cases typically resolve with discontinuation of the habit.
- Foot drop also may be seen as a combination of neurologic, muscular, and anatomic dysfunction, e.g. Charcot foot.

Pathophysiology

The pathophysiology of nerve damage commonly causing foot drop is as follows:

The functional integrity of an axon and its target depend on the continued supply of trophic substances synthesized in the neuronal perikaryon and transported down the axon, known as axoplasmic flow. A laceration interrupts this flow. A crush injury may compromise it as well. A double-crush phenomenon occurs when a proximal insult in a nerve root diminishes axoplasmic flow, making it more susceptible to injury. A distal lesion further compromises the flow and clinical palsy results. This is the phenomenon thought to be responsible for the increased risk of foot drop after hip replacement in a patient with pre-existing spinal stenosis. The spinal stenosis causes the proximal compromise and intraoperative stretch of the sciatic nerve provides the distal insult.

Clinical Presentation

Direct injury to the dorsiflexors with acute dorsiflexor injury due to laceration or contusion, both cause and effect are readily apparent on clinical examination. If the patient develops a degenerative rupture of the tibialis anterior muscle, foot drop may be observed, but the cause may not be immediately apparent. Patient stands with the foot everted and has some loss of dorsiflexion, when attempting to heel-walk. The degree of foot drop varies depending on time elapsed since the rupture.

- *Compartment syndromes:* Increased pain with passive stretch of the involved muscles is a consistent diagnostic indicator of a compartment syndrome. Pain out of proportion to the injury usually is the initial presenting symptom. The time of presentation of foot drop varies with the compartment involved.
  - *Anterior compartment syndrome:* Clinical presentation of an acute anterior compartment syndrome includes pain with passive toe flexion, some weakness of toe extension and diminished sensation in the first web space because of deep peroneal nerve compression. The extensor halluces longus usually is the first muscle to show weakness. Anterior compartment syndrome may follow trauma to the extremity, but also can be observed in March gangrene. Local erythema, heat and brawny edema over the anterior compartment are present. Regardless of the cause, wide fasciotomy of the anterior compartment must be performed to salvage the ischemic muscles.
  - *Deep posterior compartment syndrome:* An acute deep posterior compartment syndrome presents as pain and some weakness of toe flexion and ankle inversion. Pain on passive toe extension is referred to the calf. Diminished sensation over the sole of the foot, especially on the medial side is noted, resulting from posterior tibial nerve compression. Foot drop develops because of ischemic contracture of the posterior compartment and is seen if the acute syndrome is not treated. Once again, wide fasciotomy of the involved compartment is mandatory at the time of acute presentation.
  - *Chronic compartment syndrome:* This occurs in athletes in their third or fourth decade, who have exercise-induced pain in the lower leg or foot within 20 to 30 minutes of beginning to exercise. Often, this occurs after a recent increase in intensity or duration of training or after a change in the training routine. The symptoms resolve after 15 to 30 minutes of rest. The anterior compartment is the most commonly involved, may have diminished sensation in the first dorsal web space. Recording of intracompartmental pressures before, during and after exercise can provide useful diagnostic information, as to which compartments may be involved. Nonsurgical treatment of a chronic compartment syndrome is only successful, if the patient is willing to discontinue the inciting activity. The surgical treatment of choice is fasciotomy of the involved compartment.
- *Neurologic defects:* Equinovarus deformity associated with toe contracture is the most common lower extremity manifestation of stroke. This can be differentiated from a peripheral neuropathy on examination, by eliciting hyperactive deep tendon reflexes and a positive Babinski sign.
- *Gait:* Patients with a paretic foot drop bear weight on the heel during initial foot strike, whereas those with a spastic deformity strike with the forefoot.
- *L5 compression:* In addition to weakness in the peroneal nerve distribution, the tibialis posterior is weak. back pain, sciatica and limitation of straight leg raising also are seen. Motor conduction velocity may remain normal.
- *Peroneal neuropathy:* It may be spontaneous, traumatic or less frequently progressive and is characterized by weakness in dorsiflexion without back pain, sciatica or other symptoms. Foot drop from neuropathy may develop in patients, who have undergone bariatric surgery, especially those who experience rapid postoperative weight loss. Micronutrient deficiencies (e.g. vitamin B_{12}) may be a factor in these cases. There is combination of neurologic, muscular and anatomic dysfunction. Patients typically are diabetic and develop loss of protective sensation and proprioception, leading to unperceived trauma. This is coupled with an autonomic neuropathy that results in loss of sympathetic vasoconstriction and enhanced pedal blood flow, causing demineralization and subsequent bone weakness. Unperceived trauma, demineralization and bone weakness culminate in destruction of the tarsal bones. This, in turn forms a bony block at the ankle joint and foot drop.

Diagnosis

- *Laboratory studies:* Work-up of foot drop proceeds according to the suspected cause a spontaneous unilateral foot drop in a previously healthy patient requires further investigation into metabolic causes, including diabetes, alcohol abuse and exposure to toxins. The following tests would be helpful:
  - Fasting blood sugar
  - Hemoglobin A_{1c}
  - Erythrocyte sedimentation rate
  - C-reactive protein
  - Serum protein electrophoresis
  - Blood Urea Nitrogen (BUN)
  - Creatinine
  - Vitamin B_{12} levels
- *Imaging studies*
- *Plain films*: To uncover any bony injury, when anatomic dysfunction (e.g. Charcot joint) is suspected.

- *Ultrasonography:* If bleeding is suspected in a patient with a hip or knee prosthesis.
- *Magnetic resonance neurography:* It is used in case of a tumor or a compressive mass lesion to the peroneal nerve is being investigated.

Diagnostic Procedures

Electromyogram: In addition to the metabolic disorders, the differential diagnosis of spontaneous foot drop includes spasticity, dystonia, motor neuron disease, L5 radiculopathy, lumbosacral plexopathy, sciatic nerve palsy, compressive peroneal neuropathy, peripheral neuropathy and some myopathies. An electromyogram (EMG) is useful in differentiating among these diagnoses.

Treatment

- *Medical therapy:* If painful paresthesias develop, they can sometimes be effectively managed with sympathetic blocks or synovectomy. Alternative treatments are antidepressants, optimizing glucose control in diabetic patients and managing vitamin deficiencies with supplements of B_1, B_6 or B_{12} can also be useful. If foot drop is not amenable to surgery, an ankle-foot orthosis (AFO) often is used. The specific purpose of an AFO is to provide toe dorsiflexion, during the swing phase, medial and/or lateral stability at the ankle during stance and if necessary, pushoff stimulation during the late stance phase. In patients, in whom foot drop is due to hemiplegia, peroneal nerve stimulation can be considered.
- *Surgical repair:* If foot drop is secondary to lumbar disc herniation, consider discectomy. Foot drop following hip replacement can also be treated with sciatic nerve decompression, particularly if there is any concern about bleeding at the operative site. Surgical management of peroneal nerve lesions demonstrated that neural repair is the first priority in selected patients with peroneal nerve palsy. For foot drop from deep peroneal nerve injuries of less than 1 year duration, transfer of functional fascicles to deep peroneal innervated muscle groups, using either the superficial peroneal or tibial nerve, as a donor can be done. If a foot drop is chronic and accompanied by contracture, Achilles tendon lengthening may be necessary to achieve adequate dorsiflexion. In patients, in whom foot drop is due to neurologic and anatomic factors (e.g. polio, Charcot joint), arthrodesis may be the preferred option. The goal is to achieve a stable, well-aligned foot and ankle. This may be accomplished via ankle arthrodesis, Lisfranc arthrodesis and triple or pantalar arthrodesis with or without Achilles tendon lengthening.

Surgical Techniques

a. *Tendon transfers:* A common method of tendon transfer moves the posterior tibial tendon, with or without complementary Achilles tendon lengthening.
b. *Bridle procedure:* This procedure involves insertion of the posterior tibial tendon into the second cuneiform bone, combined with anastomosis of the posterior tibial tendon transfer to the anterior tibial tendon and a rerouted peroneus longus tendon in front of the lateral malleolus to balance the foot in dorsiflexion. In a neurotendinous transposition, the lateral head of the gastrocnemius is transposed to the tendons of the anterior muscle group with simultaneous transposition of the proximal end of the deep peroneal nerve. The nerve is sutured to the motor nerve of the lateral head of the gastrocnemius. This restores active voluntary dorsiflexion of the foot and automatic walking. This transfer avoids use of an antagonist muscle to the paralytic group of muscles, avoiding retraining to achieve dorsiflexion.

Complications

- As with any surgical procedure, wound infection may occur.
- Nerve graft failure also can occur.
- In tendon transfer procedures, recurrent deformity is reported.
- In arthrodeses or fusion procedures, there may be pseudoarthrosis, delayed union or nonunion.

FOOT PAIN AND OSTEOCHONDRITIS DISSECANS OF FOOT AND ANKLE

■ Foot

What do we know about foot?

- The foot is a complex structure of 26 bones and 33 joints, layered with an intertwining web of more than 120 muscles, ligaments, and nerves.
- It serves the following functions:
  - Supports weight
  - Acts as a shock absorber
  - Serves as a lever to propel the leg forward
  - Helps maintain balance by adjusting the body to uneven surfaces

Divisions of Foot

A foot can be divided into following parts (Fig. 26.378):

- Forefoot
- Midfoot
- Hindfoot

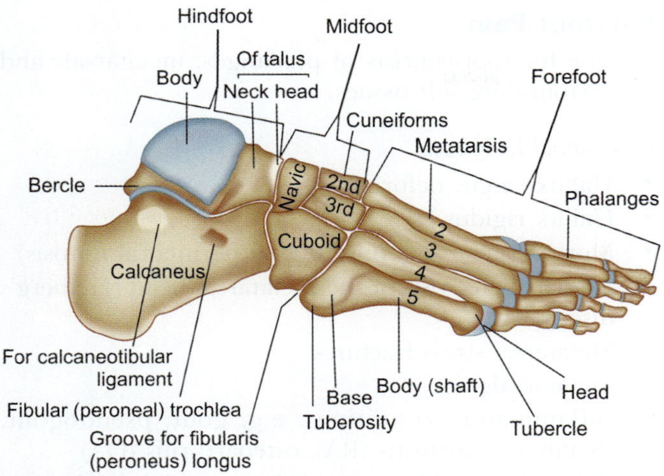

Fig. 26.378: Division of a foot into forefoot, midfoot and hindfoot

Hindfoot Pain (Heel Pain)

The hindfoot consists of talus, calcaneum and surrounding soft tissues.

Causes of Pain in the Posterior Heel

- Achilles tendonitis
- Retroachilles bursitis
- Retrocalcaneal bursitis

Causes of Pain in the Plantar Aspect of Heel

- Plantar fasciitis
- Plantar fascia rupture
- Heel pad atrophy
- Tarsal tunnel syndrome
- Neuroma
- Bone cyst
- Osteomyelitis
- Fracture
- Tumor

Various Foot Conditions and Associated Pathological Characteristics (Table 26.11)

Depending on the structures and associated symptoms, various pathological foot conditions can be divided into:

- Neurological
- Soft tissue related
- Skeletal origin
- Miscellaneous origin

Table 26.11: Different structures involved in various foot conditions and their characteristics

Condition	Characteristics
Neurologic:	
Abductor digiti quinti nerve entrapment	Burning in heel pad
Lumbar spine disorders	Pain radiating down the leg to the heel, weakness, abnormal reflexes
Problems with the medial calcaneal branch of the posterior tibial nerve	Medial and plantar heel pain
Neuropathies	Common in patients who abuse alcohol and in patients with diabetes Diffuse foot pain, night pain
Tarsal tunnel syndrome	Pain, burning sensation, and tingling on the sole of the foot
Soft tissue:	
Achilles tendonitis	Pain is retrocalcaneal
Fat pad atrophy	Pain in area of atrophic heel pad
Heel contusion	History of trauma
Plantar fascia rupture	Intense tearing sensation on bottom of foot
Posterior tibial tendonitis	Pain on the inside of the foot and ankle
Retrocalcaneal bursitis	Pain is retrocalcaneal
Skeletal:	
Calcaneal epiphysitis (Sever's disease)	Heel pain in adolescents
Calcaneal stress fracture	Calcaneal swelling, warmth, and tenderness
Infections	Osteomyelitis Systemic symptoms (e.g. fever, night pain)
Inflammatory arthropathies	More likely with bilateral plantar fasciitis Multiple joints affected
Subtalar arthritis	Heel pain is supracalcaneal
Miscellaneous:	
Metabolic disorders	
Osteomalacia	Diffuse skeletal pain, muscle weakness
Paget's disease	Bowed tibias, kyphosis, headaches
Sickle cell disease	Acute episodes of pain involving long bones, pelvis, sternum, ribs Dactylitis in young children
Tumors (rare)	Deep bone pain, night pain, constitutional symptoms
Vascular insufficiency	Pain in muscle groups that is reproducible with exertion, abnormal vascular examination

Midfoot Pain

- The midfoot is composed of three cuneiform bones, the cuboid, the navicular and the surrounding soft tissues.

Differential Diagnosis

Common conditions: These include

- Navicular stress fracture
- Midtarsal joint sprain
- Extensor tendinopathy
- Flexor tendinopathy
- Tibialis posterior tendinopathy
- Plantar fascia strain

Less Common

- Cuneiform stress fractures
- Cuboid stress fractures
- Stress fracture at base of second metatarsal
- Peroneal tendinopathy
- Abductor hallucis strain
- Cuboid syndrome
- Tarsal coalition
- Kohler's disease (in young children)

Not to be missed

- Lisfranc's injury (fracture or dislocation)
- Osteoid osteoma
- Complex regional pain syndrome (after knee or ankle injury)

Forefoot Pain

- The forefoot consists of phalanges, metatarsals and surrounding soft tissues.

Differential Diagnosis

- Hallux valgus deformity
- Hallux rigidus
- Morton's neuroma (interdigital perineural fibrosis)
- Avascular necrosis of the metatarsal head (Freiberg's disease)
- Metatarsal stress fractures
- Metatarsalgia
- Inflammatory conditions, e.g. gout, pseudogout, rheumatoid arthritis (RA), osteoarthritis (OA)
- Ill fitted shoes like pointed shoes or high heels
- Various foot abnormalities, associated pathology and region affected is illustrated in Table 26.12.

■ Osteochondritis Dissecans of the Talus

The earliest report of osteochondritis dissecans (OCD) was published in 1888 by Konig, who characterized a loose body formation associated with articular cartilage and subchondral bone fracture. In 1922 Kappis, described this process in the ankle joint.

Table 26.12: Different causes and affected regions of various types of foot abnormalities

	Malformation (M)	*Inflammation (I)*	*Neoplasm (N)*	*Trauma (T)*	*Systemic disease (S)*
Skin	Ingrown toe nail	Herpes zoster	-	Callus	-
	-	Cellulitis	-	Bunion	-
Subcutaneous tissue and fascia	-	Cellulitis	-	-	-
	-	Plantar fascitis	-	-	-
Arteries	-	Vasculitis	-	Hemorrhage	Diabetes
	-	-	-	Contusion	Periarteritis nodosa
	-	-	-	Aneurysm	Buerger disease
Veins	Varicose vein	Thrombophlebitis	-	Hemorrhage	Buerger disease
Nerves	Hypertrophic polyneuritis	Tuberculosis of spine	Neuroma	Contusion	Diabetic neuropathy
	Peroneal muscular atrophy	-	Cauda equina tumor	Compression	-
	Plantar entrapment syndrome	-	-	Laceration	-
Bones	Pes planus	Osteomyelitis	Primary and metastatic neoplasms	Fracture	Hyperparathyroidism
	Pes cavus	Kohler disease	-	-	Sickle cell anemia
	Talipes equinovarus	-	-	-	-
Joints	-	Rheumatoid arthritis	-	Traumatic synovitis	Gout
	-	Gout	-	-	Rheumatic fever
	-	Osteoarthritis	-	-	Reiter syndrome
	-	Pseudogout	-	-	-

Definition

- Osteochondritis dissecans is a localized injury or condition affecting an articular surface, that involves separation of a segment of cartilage and subchondral bone.

Frequency

- Most often, they affect the knee, followed by the elbow and the talus
- Lesions of the talus account for 4 percent of all osteochondral lesions in the body.

Relevant Anatomy

- The dome of the talus is covered by the trochlear articular surface, which supports the weight of the body
- The talar dome is trapezoidal in shape, and its anterior surface is on average 2.5 mm wider than the posterior surface
- The medial and lateral articular facets of the talus articulate, with the medial and lateral malleoli
- The articular surface of these facets is contiguous with the superior articular surface of the talar dome
- Approximately 60 percent of the talar surface is covered by articular cartilage
- The talus has no muscular or tendinous attachments
- Most of the blood supply of the talus enters through the neck via the sinus tarsi
- The artery of the sinus tarsi is formed from branches of the peroneal and dorsalis pedis arteries
- The dorsalis pedis artery, supplies the head and neck of the talus
- The artery of the tarsal canal, branches from the posterior tibial artery
- The sinus tarsi artery and the tarsal canal artery, join to form an anastomotic sling inferior to the talus, from which branches enter the talar neck.

Etiology (Figs 26.379A and B)

- Once thought to be nontraumatic/avascural necrosis (AVN)
- Most agree now of its traumatic origin
- Osteochondral fragment is disrupted
- If stable, new capillaries may cross fracture and revascularize fragment
- If not stable or displaced, AVN and fragmentation occurs and becomes separated and behave like a loose body
- Lesions are located, either posteromedial or anterolateral on the talus (Figs 26.379A and B)
- *Posteromedial lesions:* Often asymptomatic, with no history of trauma. There is less risk of osteoarthritis
- *Anterolateral lesions:* Usually symptomatic, associated with trauma

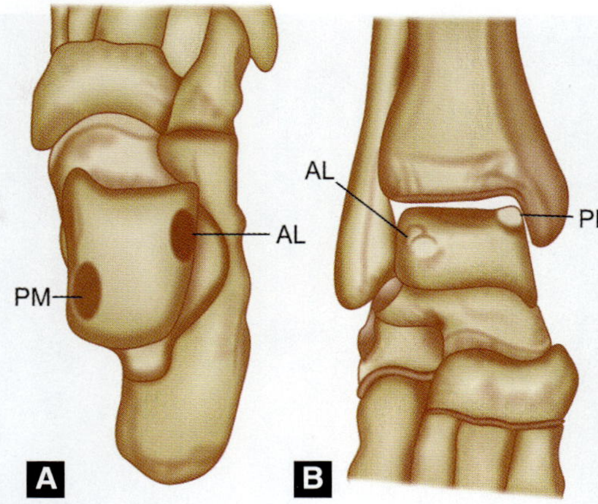

Figs 26.379A and B: Osteochondritis dissecans of the talus, showing various talar lesions—AL. Anterior lesion; PM. Posterior medial

- Ninety-eight percent of lateral lesions and 70 percent of medial lesions are associated with trauma.

Mechanism of Injury

Mainly caused by inversion injuries of the foot. Mechanism of injuries for various commonly occuring lesions are illustrated below:

Anterolateral Lesions

Associated mechanism of injury for anterior lesion is as follow:

- Result from inversion and dorsiflexion forces, which cause the anterolateral aspect of the talar dome to impact the fibula.
- These lesions are usually shallower and more wafer shaped than medial lesions, possibly because of a more tangential force vector, that results in shearing type forces.

Posteromedial Lesions

- Result from a combination of inversion, plantarflexion and external rotation forces, which cause the posteromedial talar dome to impact the tibial articular surface with a relatively more perpendicular force vector.
- Are deeper and cup shaped.

Clinical Features

- Ankle pain usually localized to the side of the talar lesion
- Intermittent swelling
- Patient may complaint of catching or grinding, instability and frequent giving way
- History of ankle sprain is common
- May have crepitus with movements
- Joint effusion is common

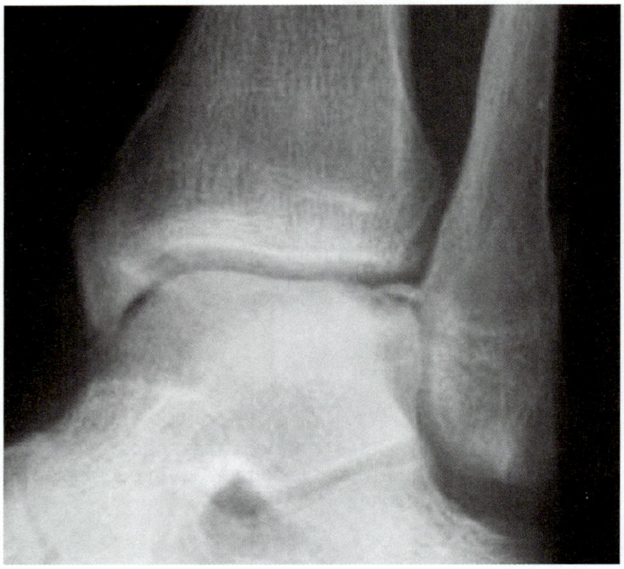

Fig. 26.380: X-ray of ankle (AP view)

- Tender along tibiotalar joint line either anterolaterally or posteromedially depending on lesion location.

Investigations

X-rays *(Fig. 26.380)*

- Anteroposterior (AP), lateral and mortise views of the ankle. Lesions appear as a well circumscribed area of sclerotic subchondral bone separated from the remainder of the epiphysis by a radiolucent line.
- If not traumatic history, consider X-ray of contralateral ankle. Contralateral lesions found in 10 to 25 percent of the time
- Stress radiographs indicated if instability detected, on examination.

MRI (Figs 26.381A and B)

- MRI should be performed on patients, suspected of having talar OCD.
- MRI allows determination of location of lesion as well as integrity of articular cartilage.

CT Scan (Fig. 26.382)

CT provides best definition of bone fragments seen on plain X-ray, but not as helpful at detecting subtle lesions.

Bone Scan

Bone scan can identify lesions, but is not helpful in determining integrity of articular cartilage.

Classification or Staging

Several staging systems have been developed on the basis of the first system, which Berndt and Harty proposed in 1959.

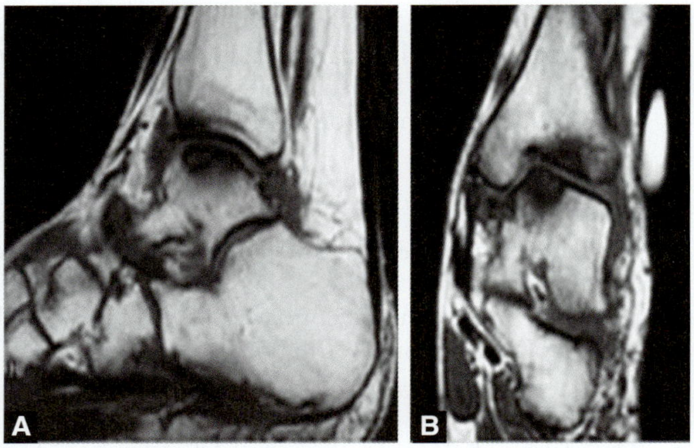

Figs 26.381A and B: MRI of ankle

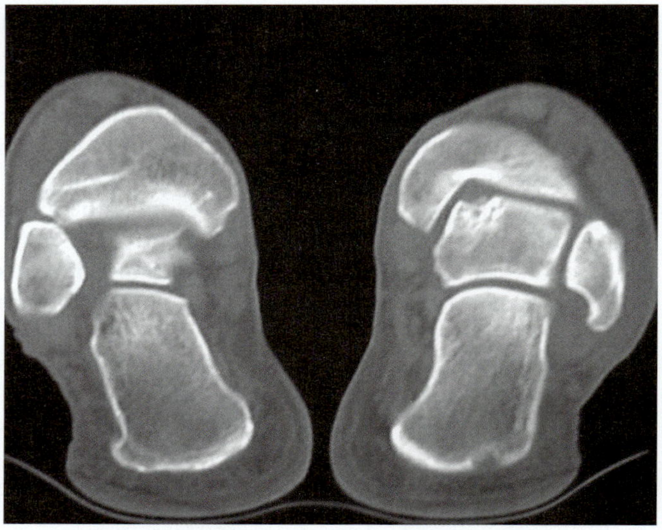

Fig. 26.382: CT scan of foot and ankle

Berndt and Harty Staging (Figs 26.383A to D)

- *Stage 1:* As the foot is inverted on the leg, the lateral border of the dome is compressed against the face of the fibula, while the collateral ligament remains intact.
- *Stage 2*: Further inversion ruptures the lateral ligament and begins avulsion of the chip.
- *Stage 3:* Chip may be completely detached, but remain in place.
- *Stage 4*: Chip may be displaced by inversion.

Hepple et al MRI Staging (Figs 26.384A to F)

- *Stage 1*: Only articular cartilage is damaged
- *Stage 2*: Cartilage injury with underlying fracture. This stage can further be divided into following substages as follows:
  - Stage 2A: Cartilage injury with underlying fracture and edema.

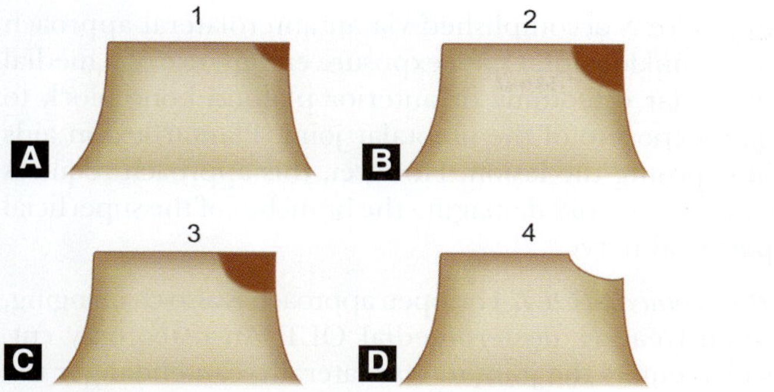

Figs 26.383A to D: Different stages of talus OCD by Berndt and Harty—(A) Stage 1, a small compression fracture; (B) Stage 2, incomplete avulsion of a fragment; (C) Stage 3, complete avulsion without displacement; (D) Stage 4, complete avulsion with displacement

- Stage 2B: Cartilage injury with underlying fracture but no edema.
- *Stage 3*: Detached (rim signal) but not displaced fragment.
- *Stage 4*: Displaced fragment.
- *Stage 5*: Subchondral cyst formation.

Cheng et al Arthroscopic Staging System

- *Stage A*: Smooth, intact, but soft or ballotable; stable
- *Stage B*: Rough surface and stable.
- *Stage C*: Fibrillation/fissuring, but is stable.
- *Stage D*: Flap present or bone exposed and is unstable.
- *Stage E*: Loose, undisplaced fragment and is unstable.
- *Stage F*: Displaced fragment and is unstable.

Staging Systems for Osteochondritis Dissecans

- Various stages of OCD and their characteristics features, seen in different investigation techniques are illustrated in Table 26.13.

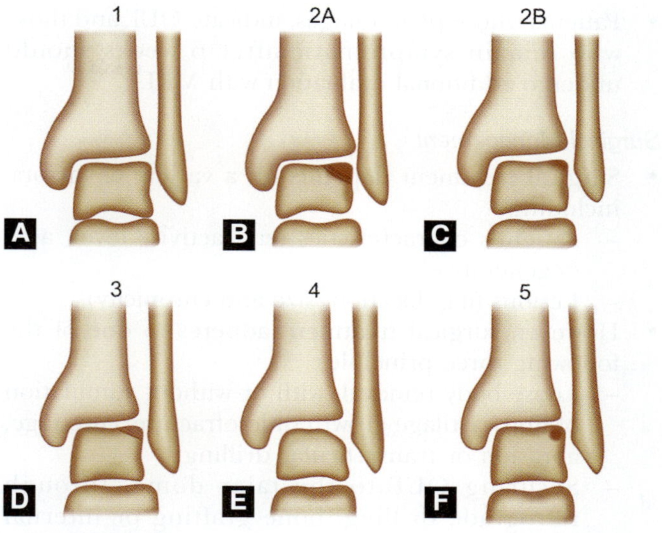

Figs 26.384A to F: Hepple et al MRI staging of talus OCD—(A) Stage 1. Cartilage damage; (B) Stage 2A. Cartilage damage with edema and fracture; (C) Stage 2B. Fracture without edema; (D) Stage 3. Detached, undisplaced fracture; (E) Stage 4. Displaced fragment; (F) Stage 5. Subchondral cyst formation

Treatment

- Conservative treatment
- Surgical treatment

Conservative Management

- Conservative management of osteochondral lesions of the talus (OLT) should be attempted first.
- Symptomatic patients with negative findings on plain radiographs should undergo an initial period of immobilization, followed by physical therapy.
- Studies have shown that a trial of conservative therapy does not adversely affect surgery, which is performed after conservative therapy has failed.

Table 26.13: Characteristic features of stages of OCD, seen in different investigative techniques

Stage	*Arthroscopy*	*MRI*	*Radiographs*
1.	Irregularity and softening of articular cartilage; no definable fragment	Thickening of articular cartilage; low signal changes	Compression lesion; no visible fragment
2.	Articular cartilage breached; definable fragment, not displaceable	Articular cartilage breached; low signal rim behind fragment indicating fibrous attachment	Fragment attached
3.	Articular cartilage breached; definable fragment, displaceable, but attached by some overlying cartilage	Articular cartilage breached; high signal changes behind fragment indicating synovial fluid between fragment and underlying subchondral bone	Nondisplaced fragment without attachment
4.	Loose body	Loose body	Displaced fragment

- Patients whose plain images, indicate OLT and those who remain symptomatic after 6 weeks should undergo additional evaluation with MRI.

Surgical Management

- Surgical treatment depends on a variety of factors, including:
  - Patient's characteristics (e.g. activity level, age, degenerative changes)
  - Lesions (e.g. location, size and chronicity)
- However, surgical treatment adheres to one of the following three principles:
  - Loose body removal, with or without stimulation of fibrocartilage growth (microfracture, curettage, abrasion or transarticular drilling)
  - Securing OLT to the talar dome, through retrograde drilling, bone grafting or internal fixation
  - Stimulating the development of hyaline cartilage through osteochondral autografts [(osteochondral autograft transfer system (OATS), mosaicplasty)] allografts or cell culture (Carticel, Genzyme Biosurgery, Cambridge, Mass).

Treatment for Different Stages of OLT

Stage I

There are small areas of compression of subchondral bone. Treatment include, an initial period of no weight bearing with cast immobilization, followed by progressive weight bearing and mobilization to full ambulation by 12 to 16 weeks.

Stage II

Partially detached osteochondral fragment (a flap). Treatment include, an initial period of no weight bearing with cast immobilization, followed by progressive weight bearing and mobilization to full ambulation by 12 to 16 weeks.

Stage III

The most commonly seen stage. There is a completely detached fragment, which remains in the underlying crater bed.

Treatment: Posteromedial lesions treated with immobilization and nonweight bearing for 3 to 6 months. Lateral lesions are treated with arthroscopy.

Stage IV

Completely detached fragment with complete displacement from the crater (a loose body). Treatment include arthroscopy.

Surgical Exposures

Anterolateral OLT: When anterolateral osteochondral lesions of the talus (OLT) are treated, open surgical exposure is accomplished via an anterolateral approach to the ankle joint. Open exposure entails, use of a medial malleolar osteotomy or anterior plafond bone block to gain exposure of the tibiotalar joint. Plantarflexion aids in exposing the lesion. However, this approach requires caution, to avoid damaging the branches of the superficial peroneal nerve.

Posteromedial OLT: The open approach is also challenging, when treating posteromedial OLT. An osteotomy cut, which enters the joint too far laterally, can endanger the weight bearing plafond and a cut, which enters the joint too far distally on the medial malleolus, limits exposure. Screw holes must be predrilled before osteotomy. In addition, care must be taken to avoid injury to the allograft, nerve, vein, anterior tibial tendon, posterior tibial tendon, flexor digitorum longus (FDL), posterior tibial artery and tibial nerve. An apex proximal chevron bone cut, provides excellent visualization in chevron medial malleolar osteotomy. Posteromedial OLT have also been treated, by using a combined anterior and posterior arthrotomy exposure. This approach allows access to 80 percent of the talar dome, while it avoids the medial malleolar osteotomy in most cases. Arthroscopic treatment of OLT can be accomplished, using wide angle 2.7 mm arthroscopes, which provide more maneuverability than traditional 4 and 5 mm arthroscopes. Noninvasive joint distraction techniques, enable easier visualization of the entire talar dome.

Treatment of a Completely Detached Lesion

Removal of the loose body and debridement of the bony bed are indicated. The base of the bed should be debrided back to bleeding bone and the edges should be trimmed back to viable cartilage. Studies have shown that excision, curettage and drilling provide the best outcome.

Treatment of Intact Lesions

Transmalleolar drilling (Fig. 26.385): Drilling of the subchondral bone creates channels, to enable revascularization of the fragment. Drilling can be accomplished, using existing arthroscopic portals, a curved meniscus repair needle guide and transmalleolar drill holes.

Retrograde drilling (Fig. 26.386): Sinus tarsi approaches to posteromedial lesions, also known as retrograde drilling or transtalar drilling, do not disrupt the articular surface. Retrograde drilling can facilitate bone grafting, which is ideal for large subchondral cystic lesions, with intact articular cartilage. The COLT (Interpore Cross, Irvine, Calif), provides for accurate positioning of the drill hole and a cannula for bone graft delivery. Studies have shown good clinical and radiographic results, using transarticular or transmalleolar drilling and retrograde or transtalar drilling.

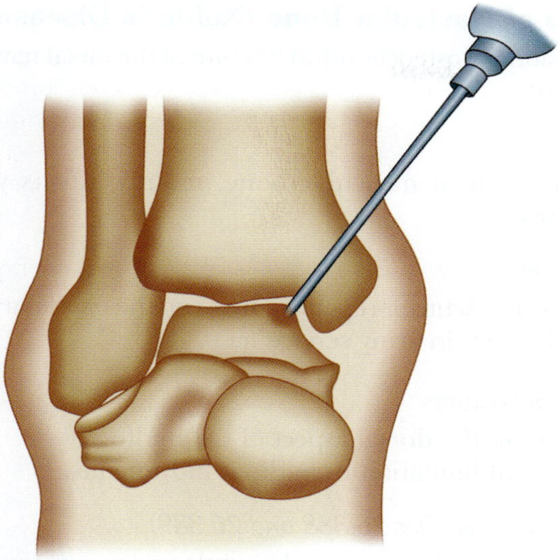

Fig. 26.385: Transmalleolar drilling procedure for treatment of intact lesions

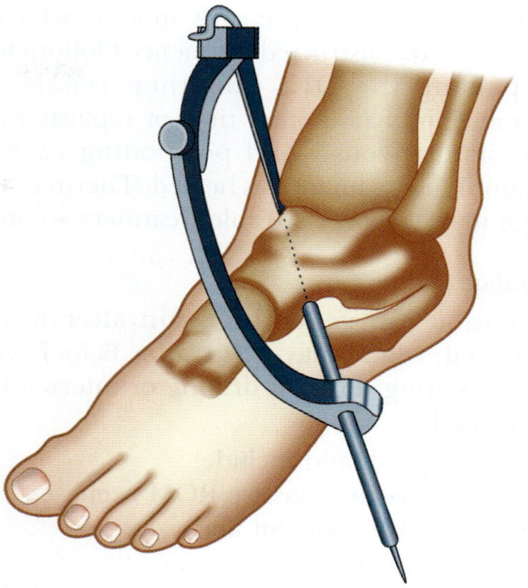

Fig. 26.386: Retrograde drilling procedure for treatment of intact lesions

Internal Fixation

The use of traditional bone screws, passed in an antegrade fashion is discouraged because of irreparable damage to the intact articular cartilage. Screw fixation typically is used only for anterolateral lesions because of the difficulty in gaining good exposure for posteromedial lesions. Kirschner wires can be inserted in retrograde way through a nonarticular portion of the talus. Bioabsorbable pins can be advanced immediately below the articular surface and then cut off at the skin.

Bone Grafting

Autologous Osteochondral Grafting (OATS) Mosaicplasty (Fig. 26.387)

These techniques involve, grafting a plug from the femoral trochlea or condyle into the OLT on the talar dome. The OATS procedure transplants a single plug into the OLT and mosaicplasty is used to harvest and transplant multiple plugs. Single plug grafts, result in reduced ingrowth of the fibrocartilage, although donor site morbidity may be greater, because of harvesting a single larger plug. The mosaicplasty procedure is said to provide a better match to the talar dome contour and surface area of the defect, although 20 to 40 percent of the defect is filled with fibrocartilage. In some studies, plugs were harvested from the ipsilateral medial or lateral articular facet of the talus. Those studies reported that no structural failures occurred in the graft or donor site.

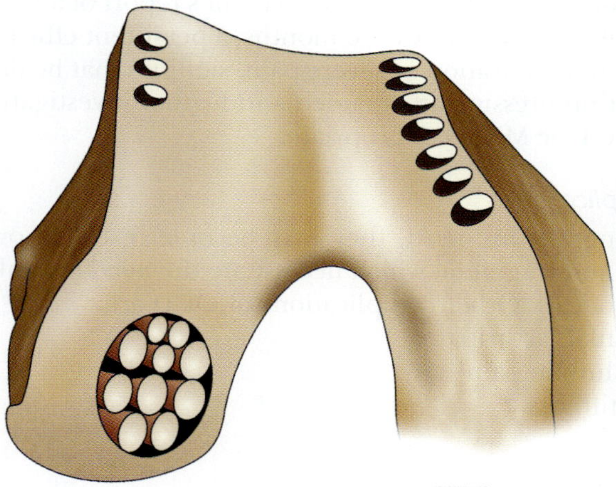

Fig. 26.387: Autologous osteochondral grafting mosaic plasty

Autologous Chondrocyte Transplantation (ACT)

Patients first should undergo diagnostic arthroscopy, cartilage biopsy, chondrocyte extraction and culture. An average of 2.5 weeks later, arthrotomy, malleolar osteotomy, bone debridement and chondrocyte transplantation should be performed. Patients should be kept on nonweight bearing status for 6 to 7 weeks. Routine arthroscopic examination, performed 6 months after the transplant, shows cartilage like tissue, completely covering the OLT. Many studies, described good early results with autologous chondrocyte transplantation, with better functional outcomes.

Coexisting OLT and Ligamentous Instability

Acute ankle ligament injuries with a large unstable fragment, typically first undergo surgical repair of the talar lesion. The ligament is allowed to heal postoperatively. Treatment decisions for treating chronic OLT, with chronic ankle instability are less clear.

Postoperatively, OLT require early motion, which is not appropriate for reconstructed ligaments. Options include, first repairing the OLT and then repairing the ligamentous injury at another time or repairing the two injuries simultaneously and postponing early ankle motion, until the ligament has healed. Thermal capsular shrinkage may also be a possible treatment solution.

Postoperative Care

Rehabilitation can generally begin after healing is demonstrated, which may occur after 6 to 7 weeks of nonweight bearing status, if drilling or internal fixation was performed.

- Physiotherapy should include:
  - Ankle active and passive ROM exercises
  - Strength development and
  - Proprioceptive training

Treatment Follow-up

Pain following operative treatment of OLT is common for up to a year. MRI changes, including edema are slow to resolve and often match the patient's report of an achy feeling in the joint. After 6 months, a persistent effusion, a catching sensation or severe pain, signifies that healing is not progressing as intended and further investigation with CT or MRI is appropriate.

Complications

If allografts are used, they may become resorbed over time and fragment, which necessitate the need for ankle arthrodesis. Other complications of OCD are:

- Ankle arthritis
- Chronic pain
- Stiffness

OCD of Navicular Bone (Kohler's Disease)

Occasionally osteochondral fracture of the tarsal navicular is seen.

Age

OCD of tarsal navicular bone, mainly affects young patients.

Etiology

Traumatic: Acute or repetitive stress on the navicular bone. Usually seen in army service men.

Clinical Features

- Pain in the dorsal aspect of the midfoot
- Painful limitation in midfoot movements.

Investigations (Figs 26.388 and 26.389)

Radiographic findings can be subtle and in some patients may mimic Mueller-Weiss syndrome or stress fracture of the tarsal and navicular. CT or MRI helps confirm the diagnosis. OCD of the tarsal navicular is limited to the proximal articular surface

Treatment

Conservative treatment: Below knee walking cast for 6 to 8 weeks. The cast is better in moderate varus (10–15°), that is associated with moderate equinus (10–20°). In this position, the navicular is relaxed from posterior tibialis strain. Arch supports can be prescribed following the cast period and used for an average of 6 months. In mild cases, soft arch supports may be the only treatment necessary.

Surgical treatment: It includes:

- Excision
- Curettage

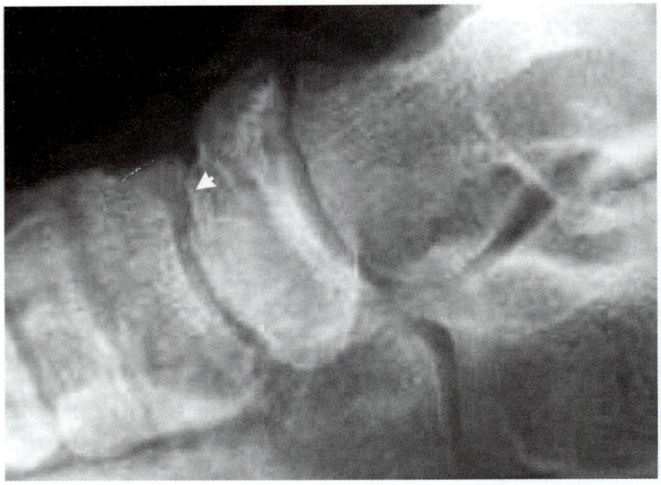

Fig. 26.388: X-ray of foot showing tarsal bones (navicular)

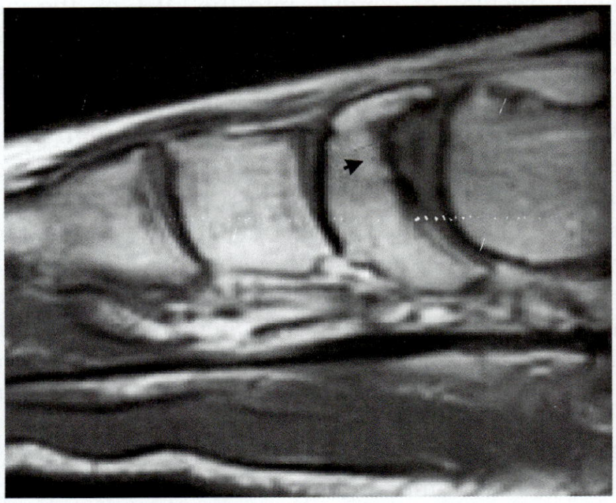

Fig. 26.389: MRI of foot showing tarsal bones (navicular)

- Drilling
- Fusion

OCD of Cuneiforms

Osteochondritis of tarsal cuneiforms is a rare entity, barely reported in the medical literature.

OCD of Cuboid

Osteochondritis of the cuboid is uncommon.

Avascular Necrosis of the Metatarsal Head (Freiberg's Disease)

Anterior metatarsalgia, which involves head of second metatarsal. In 1914 Alfred H. Freiberg, first described the painful collapse of the articular surface of the second metatarsal head.

Site

The second metatarsal is most commonly affected, although the third and fourth can occasionally be involved.

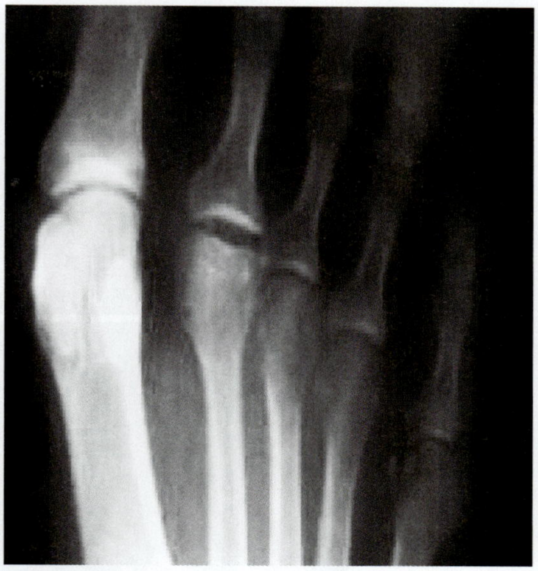

Fig. 26.390: X-ray showing Freiberg's disease

Age

Most common in adolescents.

Sex

Female are more vulnerable to male, female to male ratio is 4:1.

Etiology

Avascular necrosis of the metatarsal head. Traumatic insult or repetitive stress with microfractures, at the junction of the metaphysis and the growth plate. These fractures deprive the epiphysis of adequate circulation. Disease is more common in patients whose first metatarsal is shorter than second metatarsal, which increases weight on second metatarsal head.

Clinical Features

- Pain in the forefoot, usually localized to the head of the second metatarsal
- Wearing of high heeled shoes makes condition worse
- Localized swelling and limitation of motion in metatarsophalangeal (MP) joint.

Investigations

Radiography (Fig. 26.390): Radiographic changes are characteristic, initially the epiphysis becomes sclerotic early in disease, joint space is widened and lateron it narrowed down. Irregular bony surfaces, sclerosis and bone spurs at margins, give the appearance of osteoarthritis, epiphysis becomes fragmented, followed by osteolysis and reconstitution of bony architecture. Metatarsal head becomes irregular, widened and flattened at articular surface.

Bone scan: It shows photopenia, decreased uptake in early stages and increased uptake as the metatarsal head is reconstituted.

MRI: It is helpful for the preoperative evaluation, to show the full extent of the lesion.

Staging by Smillie (Figs 26.391A to D)

Stage I: The earliest sign is fissuring of the epiphysis. Radiographic changes at this stage may be so subtle, that they are generally missed with routine radiographs.

Stage II: Later central depression of the articular surface, becomes evident as subchondral cancellous bone is resorbed. The articular cartilage hinges on an intact plantar bridge.

Stage III: The central depression is seen to be resulting in medial and lateral projections at the margins. The plantar hinge remains intact at its plantar isthmus.

Stage IV: This stage, demonstrates that the central portion has sunk below the surface and is free of the plantar hinge, thus becoming a loose body. Fractures of the medial and lateral projections are present, with folding of the projections over the central loose body.

Stage V: The final stage shows marked flattening and deformity of the metatarsal head with secondary degenerative changes. The central loose body may have been resorbed at this stage. The shaft of the metatarsal becomes thickened and dense.

Treatment

Conservative treatment: Initial management, includes proper foot wear with metatarsal bar or pad placed

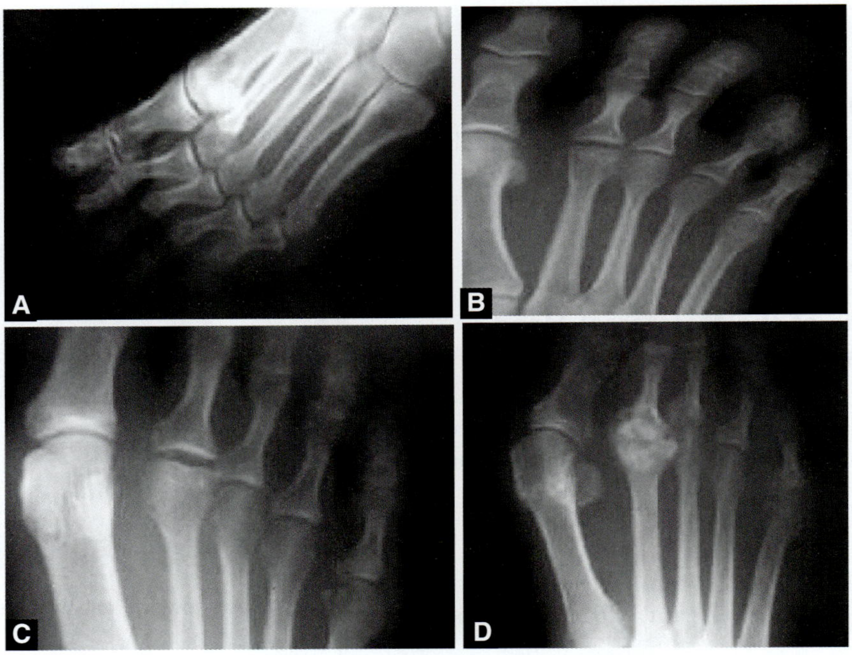

Figs 26.391:A to D: Different stages of avascular necrosis of the metatarsal head (Freiberg's disease), (see text)

beneath the involved bone. Limit activity for four to six weeks. With severe symptoms, consider immobilizing foot in short leg walking cast, until symptoms subside, usually in 3 to 4 weeks.

Surgical treatment: The progression of Freiberg disease is variable in time course and severity. While some stage I, stage II and stage III, lesions may resolve spontaneously. Patients, who do not respond to conservative measures and patients with stage IV and stage V lesions, may require surgery. Several surgical options have been advocated. Simple debridement and loose body removal were originally described by Freiberg. Other procedures described include:

- Various osteotomies
- Elevation of the depressed metatarsal head with bone grafting
- Core decompression
- Metatarsal head excision
- Shortening of the metatarsal
- Proximal phalanx hemiphalangectomy
- Total joint arthroplasty

Simple Debridement Procedure

Freiberg's original monograph, reported that two of his six patients had good results with debridement. The report only infers that these two patients presented with advanced stage disease based on the presence of loose bodies. Simple debridement can be combined with other procedures, such as excision of the metatarsal head, hemiphalangectomy and loose body excision.

Bone Grafting

Originally described by Smillie. In an attempt to restore joint congruity, a cancellous bone graft is used to elevate the depressed metatarsal articular surface. The technique, involves creating a slot in the metatarsal shaft, through which the sclerotic bone can be drilled. The metatarsal articular surface is then elevated and supported by a bone graft. This procedure is recommended for stage I, II or III lesions, in which an intact cartilage flap is present.

Osteotomies

Several different osteotomies, have been described. The common goal of all osteotomies is to redirect the loading of the MTP joint, away from the damaged area of the articular surface.

The two basic procedures are:

- Dorsal closing wedge osteotomies
- Shortening osteotomies.

Dorsal Closing Wedge Osteotomies

Gauthier and Elbaz, were the first to describe a dorsal closing wedge osteotomy, for the treatment of Freiberg disease. They performed dorsiflexion osteotomy of the neck of the metatarsal. The dorsal closing wedge osteotomy, reorients the intact cartilage on the plantar surface to articulate with the base of the proximal phalanx. Some authors modified this procedure, e.g. dorsal closing wedge osteotomy combined with synovectomy and debridement and temporary fixation with Kirschner wires (K-wires).

Shortening Osteotomies

The use of a shortening osteotomy is based on the observation that, when involved, the second metatarsal usually is the longest of the metatarsals. Several authors believe that this subjects the involved metatarsal to repetitive injury and abnormal loading. With shortening, overloading of the metatarsal is reduced and thus the relief of symptoms.

Procedure: The metatarsal is shortened, approximately 4 mm through a dorsal incision and is fixed with a small T-plate.

Complications: Stiffness of the involved ray.

Resection Arthroplasty

Resection arthroplasty, although advocated in the past, has fallen out of favor for the initial treatment of Freiberg disease. Various methods have been described, including resection of the base of the proximal phalanx or of the metatarsal head. Resection can be combined with soft tissue interposition arthroplasty or even syndactylization of the toes or it can be performed without these other procedures. Resection arthroplasty is an inherently destructive procedure. Development of transfer lesions, occurs as a result of rendering the affected metatarsal incompetent. Additionally, potential complications from any of the resection techniques, include progressive hallux valgus and excessive shortening.

Total Small Joint Arthroplasty

Total small joint arthroplasty, utilizing silicone prosthesis, also has been described for the treatment of Freiberg disease.

Advantages over resection arthroplasty include:

- Maintenance of length
- Improved joint motion
- Better weight distribution, if condyles are preserved.

Complications are similar to those for resection arthroplasty, other potential problems, inherent in the implants themselves, include:

- Synovitis
- Infection
- Dislocation

Other Procedures

Core decompression: Done for the treatment of early stage lesions, include multiple drilling of metatarsal head with K-wire (0.45 inch).

Osteochondral plug transplantation: Done for late stage lesions. The osteochondral plug, is harvested from a nonweight bearing site of the upper lateral femoral condyle of the ipsilateral knee.

Treatment Algorithm

Common to all of these procedures, is the goal of diminishing pain and restoring joint function. Different authors have suggested treatment algorithms, based on the stage of the disease and the presenting symptoms.

Daniels Algorithm

- Grafting and joint elevation as per Smillie, for patients with stage II disease.
- Grafting or dorsiflexion osteotomy as per Gauthier and Elbaz, for patients with stage III disease.
- Metatarsal shortening, for patients with stage IV or stage V disease.
- Daniels cautioned, against the use of resection or joint arthroplasty, to avoid potential problems with transfer lesions.

Helal and Gibb Algorithm

- Grafting and elevation of the collapsed articular surface, for patients with stage I or stage II disease.
- For later stage lesions, i.e. stages III to V, these authors, suggested tailoring the treatment to the patient's symptoms.
- They recommended, using an osteotomy, to treat patients with pressure metatarsalgia and using replacement arthroplasty, to treat patients suffering from arthritic symptoms of pain with joint motion.
- However, it is important to recognize, that currently, no consensus exists, as to which procedure works best for all patients.
- In general, if conservative treatment fails, the least destructive and invasive procedures should be considered first, for patients with early stage disease, the more invasive joint altering procedures, reserved for advanced cases or for patients, in whom other forms of treatment have failed.

Differential Diagnosis

- Ewing's sarcoma
- Stress fracture
- Osteosarcoma

ANKLE ARTHRODESIS

■ Introduction

Ankle arthrodesis eliminates pain and improves function even in the most severely disabled patient. Ankle fusion previously lost popularity and ankle replacements were designed, but they could not demonstrate the same success rate as THR or TKR in terms of long-term survivorship. So ankle arthrodesis currently is the most successful treatment of ankle pain, arthritis and instability. Arthrodesis of ankle is performed more frequently than arthrodesis of the hip or knee. It can be intra-articular, extra-articular or combined. Extra-articular techniques are useful in children, where joint surfaces are cartilage and in treating patients with active infection like TB.

Historical Perspective

First reported by, E Albert. Later in 1906 Lexer described, intramedullary fixation for hindfoot and ankle fusion. Plantar fusion for flail ankles and other sequelae of poliomyelitis, paralysis or TB. Sir John Charnley (1951), two parallel steinmann pins inserted into distal tibia and talus respectively and tightened with screw clamps, to prevent shear and gapping between the cut bone surfaces. Schneider/Morgan devised arthroscopic technique for ankle fusion (1983).

Anatomic and Physiologic Considerations

Composite joint formed by the syndesmosis of distal tibia and fibula and the diarthrosis of the tibia, fibula and talus. A linkage of axial structures to plantar structures. All together eleven ligaments bind the ankle and four major retinaculae can be found. Thirteen tendons traverse the joint, but no muscles cross the hinge or originate from or insert into the talus. Five major nerves and two arteries as well as a network of veins surround the ankle.

Biomechanics

A hinge joint with some additional motion due to the truncated conical structure of talus. An "incomplete mortise" being 0 to 6 mm broader anteriorly than posteriorly, but it is an extremely congruent joint, which makes it quite prone to fractures. The syndesmosis accommodates the geometry of the talus, by allowing for minor splaying of the tibia and fibula, as well as rotation and distal-proximal migration of the fibula. In full plantar flexion to dorsiflexion, there is a 1.5 mm lateral motion and 2° to 5° external rotation of the fibula and 4° of external rotation of the talus. Fibula downward motion, during the weight bearing phase of gait and 0.9 mm dorsal translation of fibula. ROM 30° dorsiflexion to 45° plantar flexion. In dorsiflexion there is additional abduction and pronation, while in plantar flexion we find slight adduction and supination. The actual joint axis changes with motion: in dorsiflexion the axis runs just below the malleoli, in plantar flexion the axis runs from a proximal lateral point to a distal medial point.

Indications

- Degenerative OA of tibiotalar joint
- Post-traumatic tibiotalar OA
- Severe RA of ankle
- AVN of talus
- Unstable, infected, painful or deformed ankles (Salvage procedure).
- Chronic instability with non-reconstructable muscle weakness.
- Chronic instability that is not reconstructable.
- Septic ankles
- Salvage of failed TAR
- Extreme equinus deformity
- Deformity as a complication of compartment syndrome.
- Marked varus or valgus deformity, unable to be corrected by osteotomy.

Optimal Position

- 0° to 5° of valgus
- 5° to 10° of external rotation

Slight posterior displacement of talus. Attempt should be made to create broad and flat, cancellous surfaces that are placed into apposition such that hindfoot is aligned to leg and forefoot to hindfoot to create a plantigrade foot. Some advocate talus being positioned posterior to tibia, as it improves the lever arm of the calcaneus and reduces the anterior lever arm and makes easier for the foot to clear the ground, while walking and decreases the stress at the knee, but also decreases the contact area for fusion.

Aim

- To provide a solid, pain free fusion of the ankle in the optimum position.
- Minimize risk of complications.

Clinical Diagnosis

- ROM and joint contracture of the hip/knee assessed.
- Gait analysis
- ROM of ankle, alignment referable to the lower extremity (tibia, patella, hip), its function during gait as well as proprioception qualities, muscle control and the ligamentous stability.
- Adjacent joints are examined for ROM alignment and arthritis.
- OA in adjacent joints
- After arthrodesis of the ankle dorsi/plantar flexion will be compensated for by subtalar, transverse tarsal and tarsometatarsal joints.
- Warmth, swelling, synovial proliferation, rheumatoid nodules, joint effusion, skin affections and open wounds.
- The main indication: pain, resulting from a severely damaged or/and malaligned joint.
- It is generally accepted, not to perform arthrodesis in active infection, in poor blood supply and poor compliance.

Radiographic Diagnosis

AP and Lateral View

- To assess the distal tibiofibular joint Mortise view (Wruhs, 1987).
- Whole leg or at least the knee joints X-rays, to appreciate the lower extremity axis and different effects of loading forces.
- In certain cases CT or MRI is helpful, e.g. AVN talus.

- *Bone scan preoperatively:* In assessing ankle arthritis or concurrent subtalar arthritis.

Relative Contraindications

Conditions that produce diminished sensations and sensory neuropathies: Charcot arthropathy, previous spinal cord injury, myelomeningocele, diabetes, infection, open ulcers (incidence of non-union may be higher). Severe peripheral vascular disease, that is unreconstructable.

Alternatives

Orthotics

- A double-upright brace with a patellar tendon bearing support
- A locked ankle with solid ankle cushion heel (SACH)
- A rocker bottom sole with ankle foot orthosis (AFO)

Nonsteroidal Anti-inflammatory Drugs

- Intra-articular corticosteroids
- Intra-articular hyaluronic acid
- An open or arthroscopic ankle debridement of impinging bone spurs and synovitis.
- *Preoperative:* A short leg cast or a walkerboot, to simulate fusion and assess pain relief with the semirigid external splinting.

Preoperative Considerations

- Sensory deficits disease may make ankle arthrodesis difficult
- Consent with a thorough explanation (after surgery the foot allows dorsiflexion/plantar flexion of foot of 10°–25°)
- Cessation of smoking, as it increases non union 16 times
- Sensorymotor status/posterior tibial and dorsalis pedis
- External rotation of ipsilateral hip
- Heel cord contracture should be noted by maximally inverting and dorsiflexing the foot to lock the subtalar joint
- Soft tissue envelope for a possible compromise after previous surgeries or trauma and to plan the exact surgical approach, so that there is minimal tension on the wound edges.

Approaches of Ankle Arthrodesis

- *Anterior approach:* Through the anterior tibial tendon sheath supplemented with anteromedial/anteriolateral approach.
- *Transmalleolar or transfibular approach:* Gives slightly better access to posterior aspect of ankle.
- *Posterior approach:* For isolated tibiotalar fusion in patients with compromised anterior skin and for tibiotalar calcaneal arthrodesis.

Technique

Principles of Surgery

- Create broad, congruent cancellous bone surfaces
- Stabilize with rigid internal fixation
- Align hindfoot to the lower extremity and the forefoot to the hindfoot to create a plantigrade foot. Preserving the malleoli has significant advantages: defining the correct position of the ankle, avoids rotational malalignment.

  Higher incidence of union can be ascertained by following factors:
  - Safer positioning of the screws
  - Allows for better vascular perfusion
  - If fusion is needed to be done at young age, conversion to a total ankle replacement still possible at an older age, if the malleoli are still present.

Arthroscopic (Myerson 1991): Used if there is little or no malalignment of the ankle joint. Invasive or non-invasive joint distraction is required to distract the joint prior to insufflating the joint with Ringer's Lactate. The anteromedial, anterolateral and posterolateral portals. Anteromedial means just medial of the anterior tibial tendon at the level of the joint. The anterolateral portal be made lateral to the peroneus tertius avoiding the nerve. The posterolateral access is gained between fibula and Achilles tendon under direct vision from the interior of the ankle joint.

Anterior synovectomy and debridement: Denuding the articular surfaces of remaining cartilage, also denude in medial and lateral gutter to expose bleeding subchondral bone, but maintain the contour of bony surfaces, internal or external fixation *in situ* in the position described above. Two to three percutaneous, cannulated or non-cannulated cancellous screws, parallel or converging.

Advantages: Less blood loss, a shorter time to union and a higher union rate because of the minimal interruption of the surrounding soft tissue with subsequent better blood supply. Fewer complications in patients with compromized healing potential (vascular disease, diabetes, RA, history of corticosteroid use, prior skin or soft tissue flaps).

Disadvantages: Deformities cannot be corrected, if they are more than a few degrees and severe bone deficiencies cannot be addressed well.

Miniopen: Similar to the arthroscopic technique, but the portals are extended to an anterolateral and anteromedial 1.5 to 2 cm incision. The advantages and disadvantages correspond with arthroscopic technique.

- *Anteromedial incision:* Medial to tibialis anterior tendon at the level of ankle joint.
- *Anterolateral incision:* Lateral to peroneus tertius tendon avoiding the branches of the superficial peroneal nerve.
- Debridement, denuding of articular surfaces
- Removal of cartilage in posterior one-fourth of joint with a small retrograde currette
- *In situ* fixation in the position described above
- 2 or 3 screw
- Possible iliac crest grafting
- Meticulous closing of anterior capsule
- This technique is usually quicker than the arthroscopic technique and yields similar results.

Other techniques

a. *Blair*: This method uses an anterior distal tibial sliding graft, allows nearly normal appearance of the foot with little shortening of the extremity
b. *Morris*: Morris modified Blair's technique by placing a screw in the tibial inlay and using a longitudinal Steinmann pin
c. *Lionberger*: Using a pediatric hip compression screw for fixation
d. *Anterior sliding graft technique (Patterson, 1997):* Described a technique with an anterior sliding graft to provide fixation and fusion
e. *Technique proposed by R Mann:* Transfibular approach with resection of distal fibula allows good joint visualization, as illustrated in Figures 26.392A to D. Two matched parallel osteotomy cuts on distal tibia and talar dome. Two parallel interfragmentary compression screws from sinus tarsi into tibia with screw tip engaging into medial tibial cortex. Screw heads buried in sinus tarsi. Partial or total resection of medial malleolus, in cases of total resection additional screw or other fixation device should be considered. Sometimes augment with medial staples. Slight limb shortening of about 4 to 9 mm, but without problems with the peroneal tendons. The deltoid arterial blood supply to the medial talus is preserved. The arthrodesis usually does not require bone grafting.

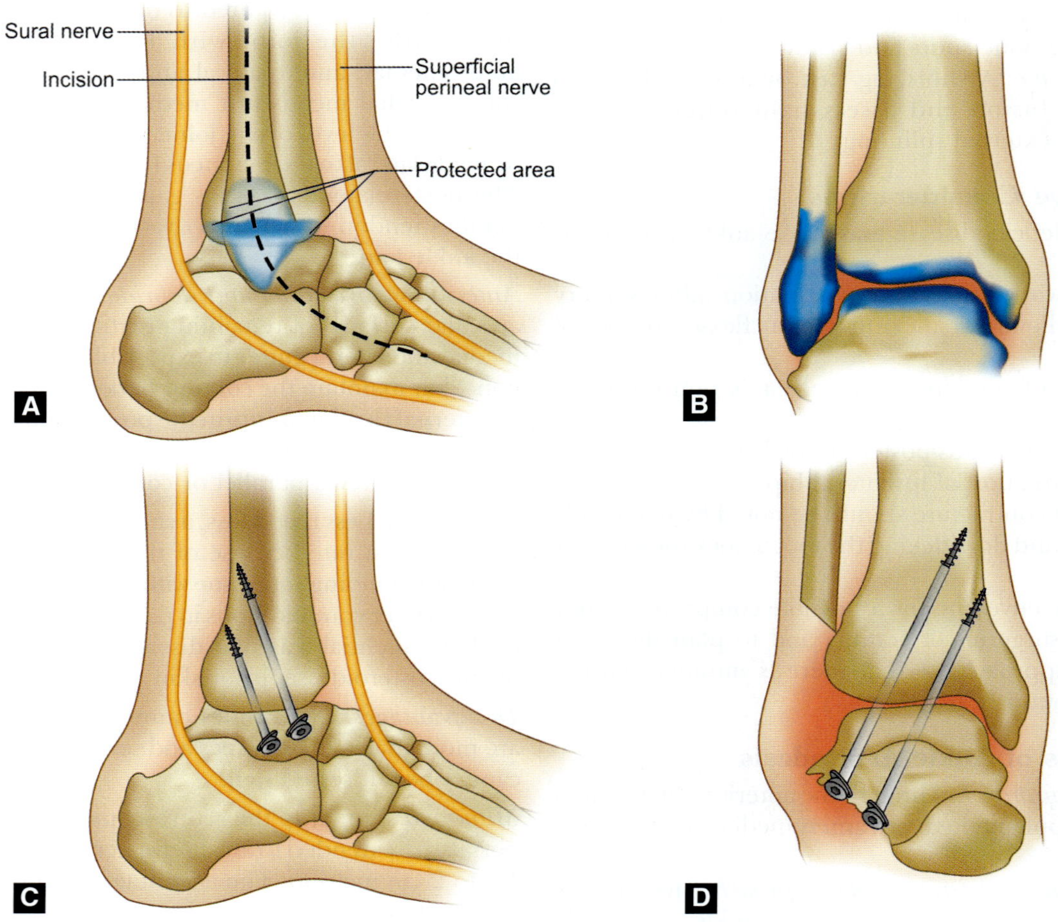

Figs 26.392A to D: Transfibular approach with resection of distal fibula

Disadvantages

- Disruption of the sinus tarsi and difficult placement of the screws with two parallel screws having less stability than crossed screws
- With flat surfaces it can sometimes be very difficult to align the joint properly
- Resection of the fibula supposedly interferes with proper blood supply and subluxation of the peroneal tendons
- Usually this technique results in greater shortening and the lack of the medial and lateral malleolus provides less stability than with other techniques, but allows for the greatest correction of angular deformities.

Open Method

- Lateral approach with subperiosteal dissection of the tibia and talus from the lateral side
- Possible correction of deformity with subsequent wedge resection at the tibial plafond or talus
- Insert lamina spreader over K-wires, that have been placed percutaneously into talus and tibia medially and laterally and distract joint
- Remove cartilage from all surfaces of tibia and talus and curette
- Drill all surfaces with 2.5 mm drill, to enhance penetration of subchondral bone and to increase surface area
- Position ankle in correct position and transfix with guide wires for 6.5 or 7.3 mm screws under manual compression, so that the surfaces are flush
- Check under fluoroscope
- Insert 7.3 mm screw beginning with the posterolateral one first
- Insert 6.5 or 7.3 mm screws medially and laterally.
- Insert autologous bone graft from excised medial one half of fibula to front and back of joint
- Fix lateral part of fibula onto fusion site with one or two 4.0 cancellous screws
- Check peroneals that they do not sublux.

Bone Grafting

- The usual ankle arthrodesis does not require bone grafting, if flush surfaces are accomplished
- Partial fibula onlay (lateral) with the medial one half of the fibula used as cancellous bone
- With greater deformity an iliac crest bone graft to bridge a large defect in failed TAR or consider the use of bank bonegraft
- Some prefer to use graft every time, by creating a trough 2.5 cm wide and 2.5 cm deep into the tibia and talus
- A tricortical block of iliac crest wedged into trough, with cancellous bone graft facing the tibial bed, as shown in Figures 26.393A and B

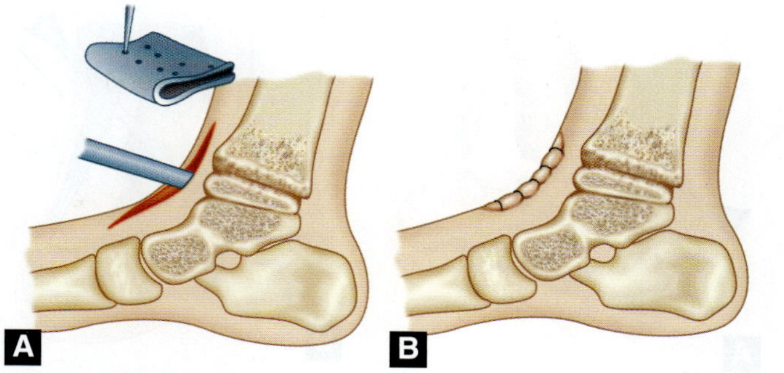

Figs 26.393A and B: A tricortical block of iliac crest wedged into trough, with cancellous bone graft facing the tibial bed

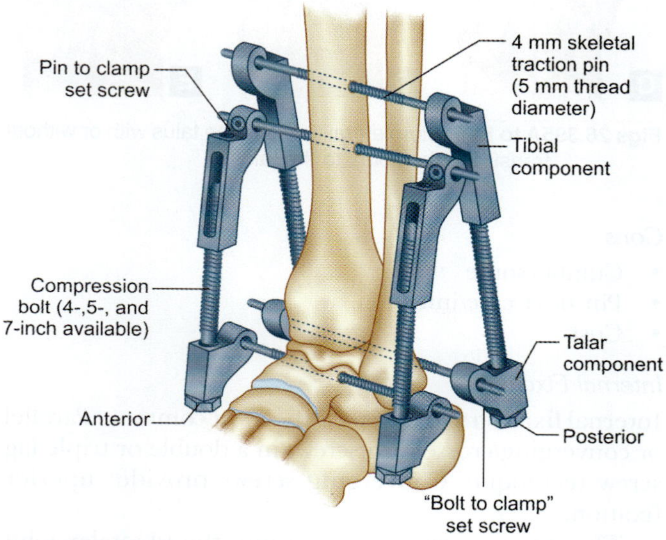

Fig. 26.394: Monoplanar with 2–3 pins in the tibia and 2 pins in talus

- Rarely do surgeons use free transfer vascularized bone grafts.

Fixation Techniques (Fig. 26.394)

External fixator exists in varying designs:

- Monoplanar, such as the AO fixator (2–3 pins in the tibia, 2 pins in talus).
- Orthofix two pins in the tibia, one pin in the talus and one pin in the calcaneus.
- Multiplanar, such as the Ilizarov and the tripod Calandruccio apparatus.

Pros

- Useful for difficult cases
- Active infection
- Nonunion
- Salvage—failed arthroplasty
- Poor bone quality
- Poor soft tissues

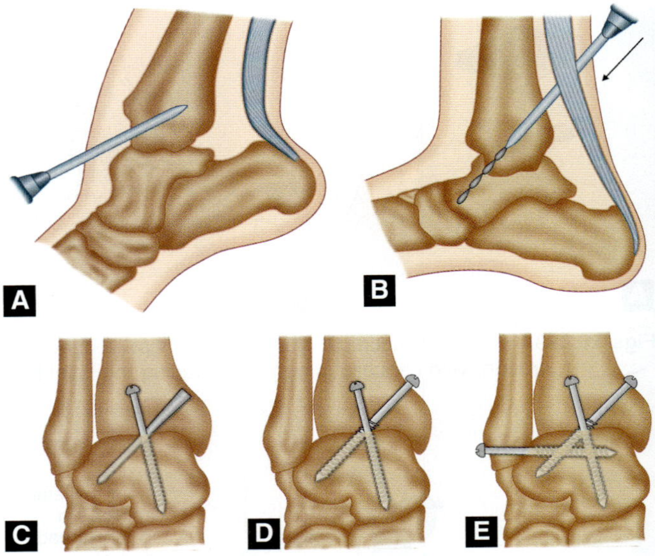

Figs 26.395A to E: Posterolateral tibia into the talus with or without transfixing the fibula to the talus

Cons

- Cumbersome
- Pin tract care/infection
- Cost

Internal Fixation

Internal fixation with screws is the most common. Parallel or converging/crossed lag screws in a double or triple lag screw technique. Converging screws provide superior fixation.

The three screws are placed into the tibiotalar joint from the:

1. Anterolateral,
2. Anteromedial and
3. Posterolateral tibia into the talus with or without transfixing the fibula to the talus, as shown in Figures 26.395 to 26.397.

Plate Fixation

- Lateral plate
  - A large or small fragment T-plate to lateral side (compression type).
  - A pediatric 90° osteotomy, with compression plate can be applied.
  - Double T-plate fixation is stronger than the fibular strut fixation (lateral fibular strut fixed is with 2 × 4.5 mm screws in tibia) with the crossed screw fixation (6.5 mm).
- Anterior plate is bent to hold the joint in the desired position:
  - Severe osteoarthritis
  - Joint destruction
  - Salvage procedures

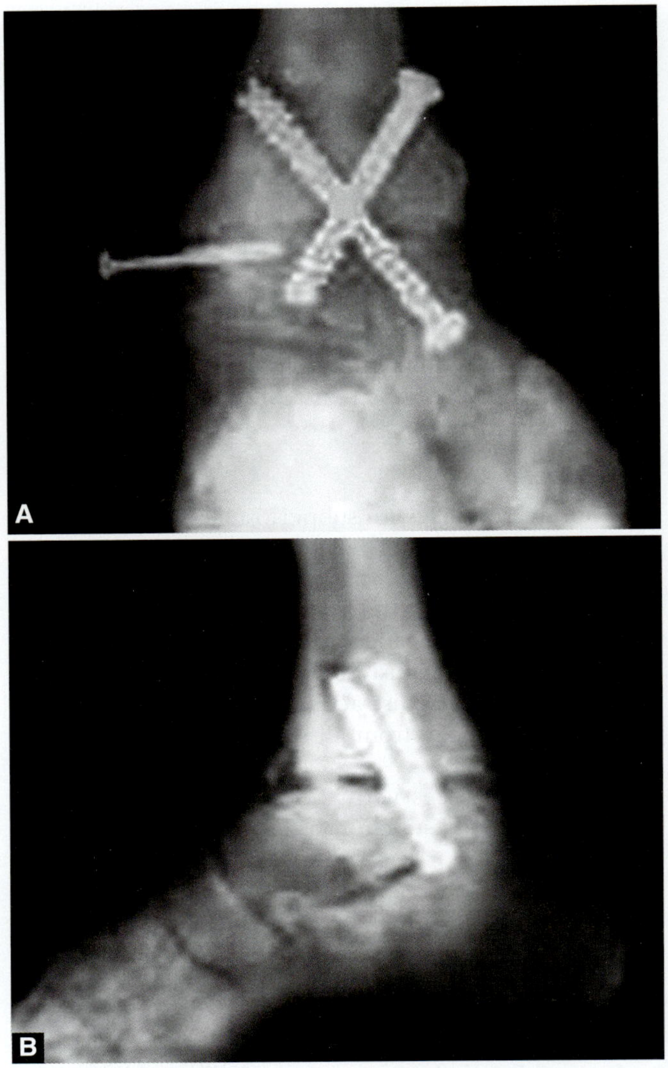

Figs 26.396A and B: X-rays showing fixation of fracture by screws

- Posterior plate requires a posterior approach, where the arthrodesis is fixed with a 90° osteotomy plate, where the blade is in the talus, as shown in Figures 26.397 and 26.398.

Postoperative

- Routine closure
- POP slabs initially
- Below knee plaster of paris (BKPOP) and nonweight bearing (NWB) 6–8 weeks
- Then weight bearing (WB) in cast for further 6 to 8 weeks.

Pros

- Patient convenience
- Ease of insertion
- Good to excellent results

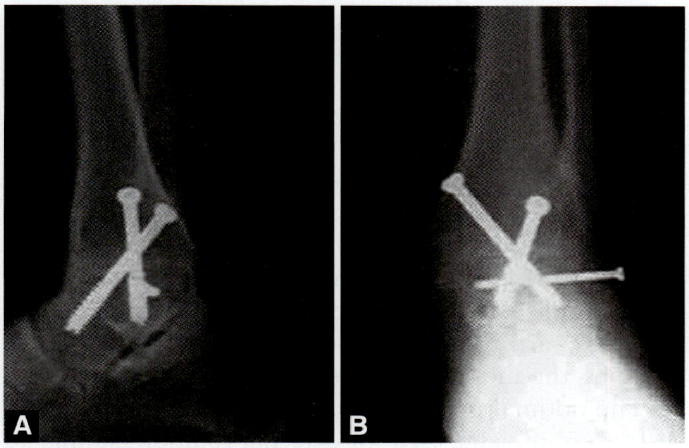

Figs 26.397A and B: Posterior plate fixation

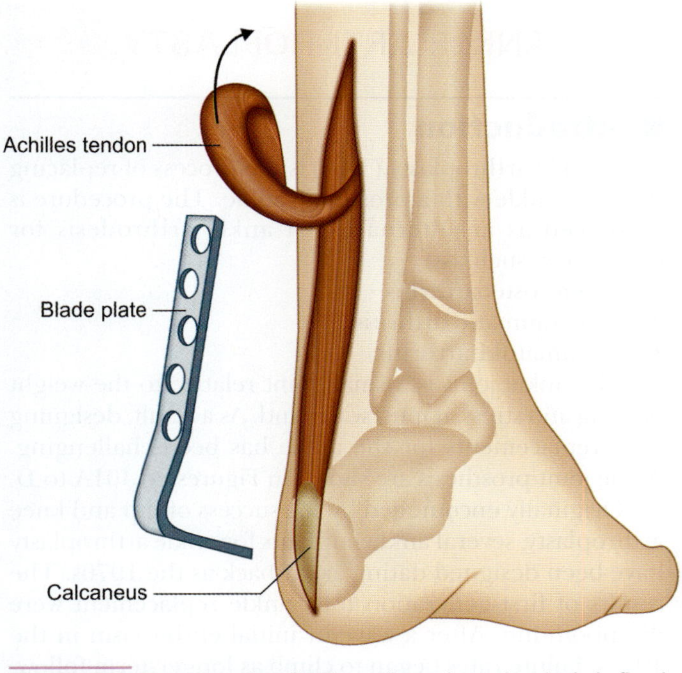

Fig. 26.398: Posterior plate fixation, where the arthrodesis is fixed with a 90° osteotomy plate

Complications

- Nonunion (pseudarthrosis)
- Malunion
- Infection
- Neurovascular injury, neuroma
- Skin necrosis

Results

- Eighty to ninety percent fusion rates
- Most patients satisfied with pain relief
- Hindfoot motion limited—uneven ground difficult
- Difficult to run
- Most can wear normal shoes

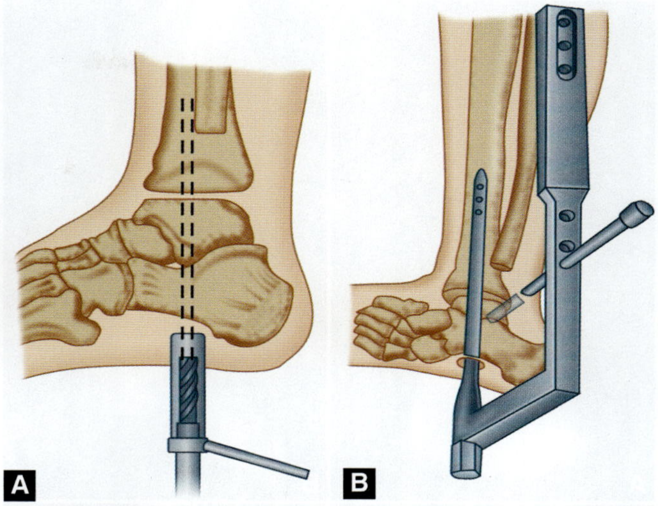

Figs 26.399A and B: Salvage technique—(A) Intramedullary nail; (B) External fixator

- Rocker bottom shoe may help gait
- Gait velocity slowed 16 percent
- Three percent increase oxygen consumption
- Shortened stride length
- Increase external rotation at hip

Salvage Techniques

If the posterior half of the talus shows AVN, an anterior tibial sliding graft is recommended. If the posterior two-thirds of the talus is affected by AVN, the talar body may even be removed and a tibiocalcaneal fusion is advisable. Large slabs of iliac crest graft are needed for this type of reconstruction. After a failure far anterior approach is recommended, with preservation of the malleoli, if possible. The results suggest that electrical implantable stimulation may be a useful adjunct to rigid internal fixation and bone grafting for ankle and hindfoot fusions in high-risk patients. Nonunions might cause subtalar involvement, so in revision surgery that joint has to be addressed additionally and also be fused using screws, intramedullary nail or external fixator or even a plate, as shown in Figures 26.399A and B.

The revision retrograde intramedullary nailing (Figs 26.400A to D): Post-traumatic arthrosis and bone loss following distal tibial plafond fractures, concomitant subtalar arthrosis and/or severe osteopenia, such as in patients with rheumatoid arthritis. In sagittal plane to counteract muscular forces generated in gait. A medial malleolar osteotomy, combined with a medial translation of the talus will reduce risk of neurovascular and FHL injury and will increase the strength of fixation. The ideal position for pantalar arthrodesis is approximately 5° of valgus. A double plate fixation or anterior plate in cases with bone loss with fibular bone graft or iliac crest is possible.

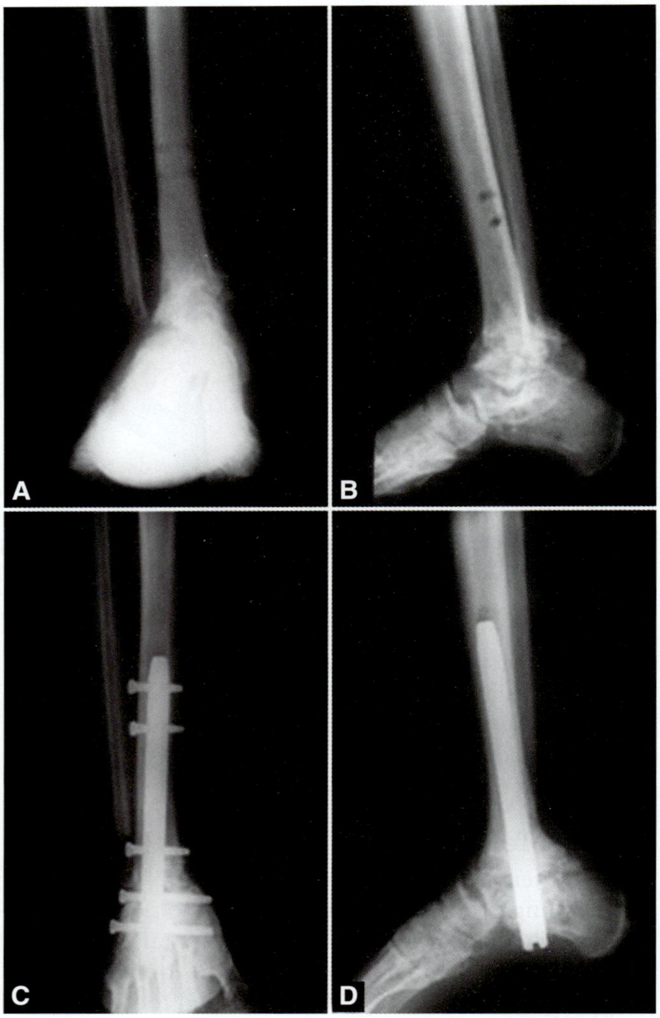

Figs 26.400A to D: X-rays showing intramedullary technique as a salvage procedure

■ Summary

- Evaluation and examination of the patients, who are not suitable for that procedure.
- Vascular and neurological status and to obtain weight bearing X-rays of the ankle, in some cases a CT, to judge the deformity.
- Careful preoperative planning.
- *A possible correction of the deformity and the proper fixation technique:* 2 to 3 internal screws (posterolateral, anterolateral and anteromedial) are widely used. Internal plate and external fixator are alternatives and best choices in certain situations, e.g. large bony defects.
- The arthroscopic or mini open technique, as they allow large bony services to oppose and they least compromise the surrounding soft tissue.
- Great care to meticulously denude the articular surfaces, without burning the bone and to create fresh bleeding surfaces.
- Intraoperative autologous bone grafting can be performed, either using the medial part of the fibula or iliac crest cancellous bone graft in larger defects, with the remaining lateral fibula, as an onlay to further reinforce the fusion.
- Different bone configurations are demonstrated to accomplish a solid arthrodesis, with the insitution and flat top arthrodesis, after correction of the deformity, being the most popular ones.
- The optimal position of the ankle is neutral flexion, 0° to 5° of valgus, 10° of external rotation, similar to the contralateral foot and posterior translation of talus under tibia (5 mm).

ANKLE ARTHROPLASTY

■ Introduction

Total ankle arthroplasty (TAA) is the process of replacing diseased ankle with a prosthetic ankle. The procedure is employed as an alternative of ankle arthrodesis for conditions, such as:

- Severe osteoarthritis
- Post-traumatic arthritis
- Rheumatoid arthritis

The ankle joint is a small joint relative to the weight bearing and stress, it must withstand. As a result, designing joint replacements for the ankle has been challenging. Ankle joint prosthesis are shown in Figures 26.401A to D.

Originally encouraged by the success of hip and knee arthroplasty, several ankle implants for ankle arthroplasty have been designed dating as far back as the 1970s. The results of first-generation total ankle replacement were disappointing. After a wave of initial enthusiasm in the 1970s, failure rates began to climb as longer-term follow-up was reported.

Causes of Failure

The soft tissues about the ankle are thin and frequently compromised by previous trauma, surgery, systemic disease

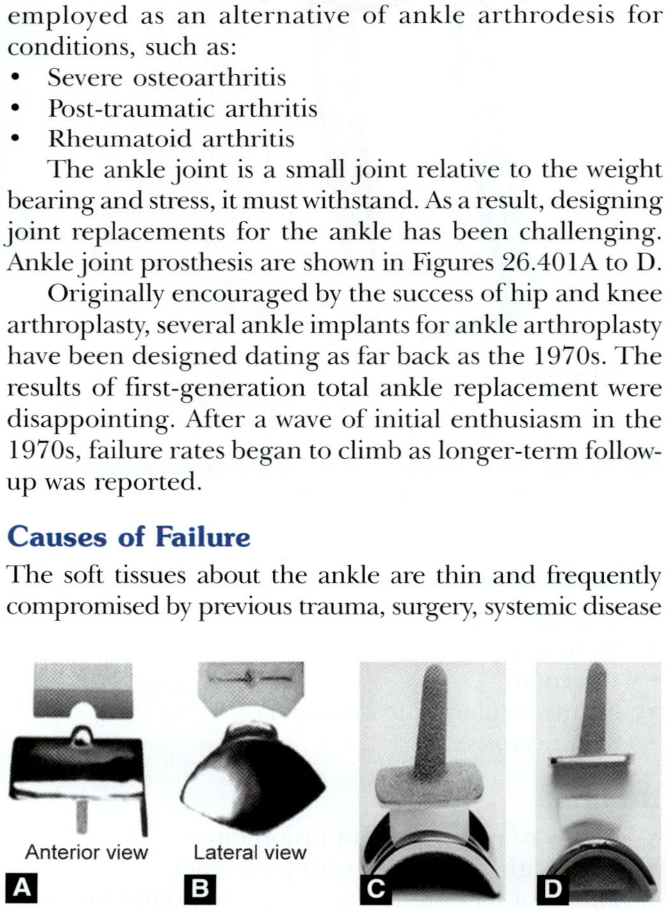

Figs 26.401A to D: Ankle joint prosthesis

and steroid use. The vascularity of these thin soft tissue flaps can be easily impaired with hematoma formation. Delayed wound healing has been reported to occur in as many as 40 percent of patients and most long-term series cite rates of deep infection of 3 to 5 percent. With most early prostheses meeting failure from subsidence, wear and loosening within a few years following implantation. Rates of loosening with these cemented designs ranged from 25 to 75 percent within 3 years. Poor results lead most surgeons to abandon implant arthroplasty and return to ankle arthrodesis, as their treatment of choice for the severely arthritic ankle. The forces at the ankle are large and the surface area for bone support. The size and shape of the talus make expansion of the surface area for fixation very difficult and greatly minimize options for prosthetic revision. The quality of bone in the distal tibia frequently may be questionable and the bone strength is not uniform across the distal tibia. The proximity of the medial and anterior neurovascular structures also increases the likelihood of serious complication. Due to poor implant survival, as well as wound difficulties, ankle arthroplasty was largely abandoned for the last two decades of the twentieth century, with ankle arthrodesis being the primary treatment for the arthritic ankle. Improved prosthesis designs have sparked renewed interest in ankle joint replacement procedures for the treatment of trauma, osteoarthritis and rheumatoid arthritis.

Contraindications

Absolute

- Active infection
- Peripheral vascular disease
- Charcot arthropathy

Relative

- Severe osteoporosis
- Osteonecrosis of talus
- Severe malalignment or instability

Design

Two basic different designs exist:

1. A two component fixed-bearing design:
   - Constrained
   - Semiconstrained
   - Unconstrained
2. A three component mobile-bearing design.

These designs differ not only in the bearing surface, but also in the portion of the ankle joint that they replace. Constraint of the implant is defined as the ability to limit rotational, anteroposterior and medial-lateral displacements to within normal ranges. One such design incorporates a fusion of the syndesmosis, to share the load between the distal tibia and fibula. The second design principle is a three-component, mobile-bearing implant. Both have shown survivorship rates of 93 percent, rejuvenating interest in this treatment modality.

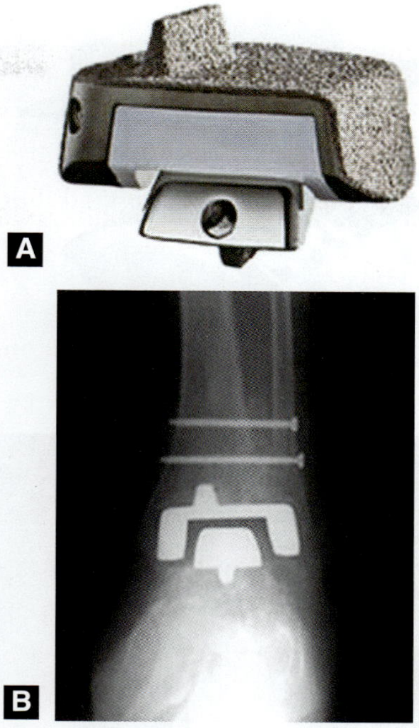

Figs 26.402A and B: Agility ankle prosthesis

Agility Ankle (Figs 26.402A and B)

Is a prototypical two-component design that allows limited medial-lateral shift as well as axial rotation. In contrast to the mobile-bearing designs, it replaces both medial and lateral malleolar surfaces and requires that an arthrodesis of the distal tibiofibular syndesmosis be performed at the time of implantation, which eliminates fibular motion as a source of loosening for the implant. This type of implant requires a greater segment of bone resection in both longitudinal and transverse dimensions than the mobile-bearing designs. This allows a larger surface area for bone ingrowth, although the risk of tendon injury, particularly posteromedially, may be higher.

After Treatment

Postoperatively, the involved limb is immobilized in a well-padded splint, until the incisions have healed adequately. A removable controlled ankle motion (CAM) walker boot may be substituted to allow initiation of early range-of-motion activities. Patients are kept nonweight-bearing, however for approximately 8 to 10 weeks until sufficient early bone ingrowth has occurred at the prosthetic-bone interface and the distal syndesmosis arthrodesis has adequately solidified, as necessary. Aggressive ankle motion is continued. Ideally, ankle range of motion should be adequately restored during this interval to allow a near-normal heel-to-toe gait. Weight-bearing is advanced initially in the CAM boot, which supports and stabilizes the ankle and limits shear and rotational forces on the

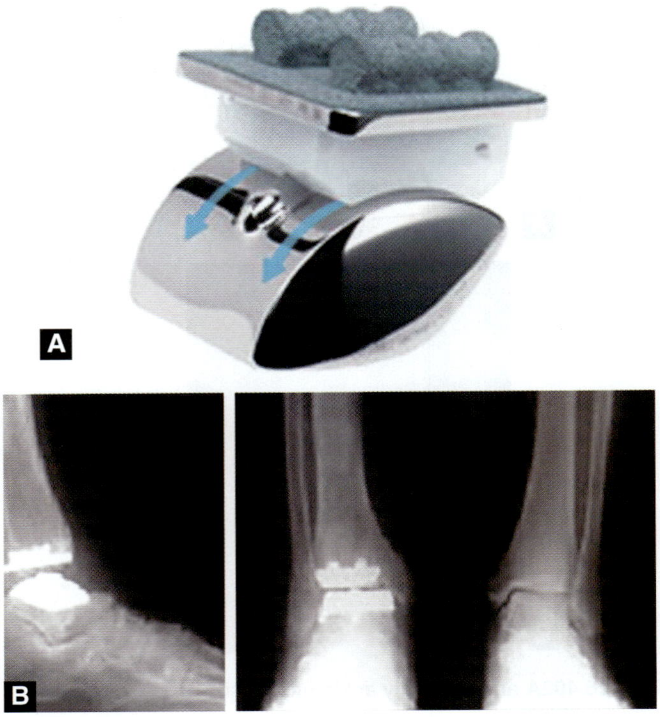

Figs 26.403A and B: STAR a mobile-bearing design

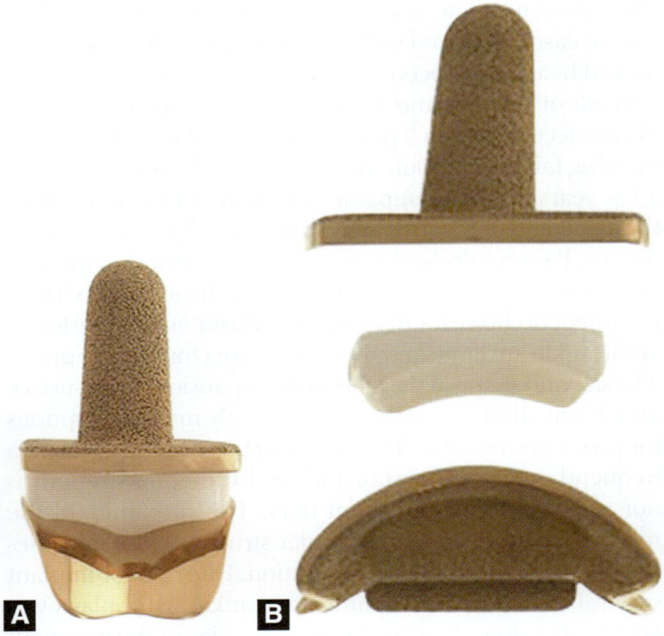

Figs 26.404A and B: Buechel-Pappas ultra total ankle

prosthesis. The patient is gradually weaned from the CAM boot over the ensuing weeks, as activity levels are gradually increased.

Three Component Mobile-Bearing Design

The Scandinavian total ankle replacement (STAR), as shown in Figures 26.403A and B and the Buechel-Pappas Ultra total ankle shown in Figures 26.404A and B are prototype examples of the three-component mobile-bearing design. Instead of totally replacing the ankle mortise, a flat plate with porous backing serves as the distal tibial articular surface that articulates with a metal talar dome component through a mobile-bearing that is flat on its tibial surface and conforms on the talar surface.

Design Background

1974–BP cylindrical fixed bearing design (Fig. 26.405): The first design was a two piece component, consisting of a metal tibial and a plastic talar component. Failure of this design occurred from three major reasons:

1. Lack of axial rotation resulting in tibial loosening due to torque.
2. Talar component subsidence secondary to talar dome resection.
3. Wear of polyethylene due to a metal edge of the tibial component wiping over the bearing surface.

These problems were common to all fixed bearing ankle devices of the period, such as the Mayo and Oregon Ankles.

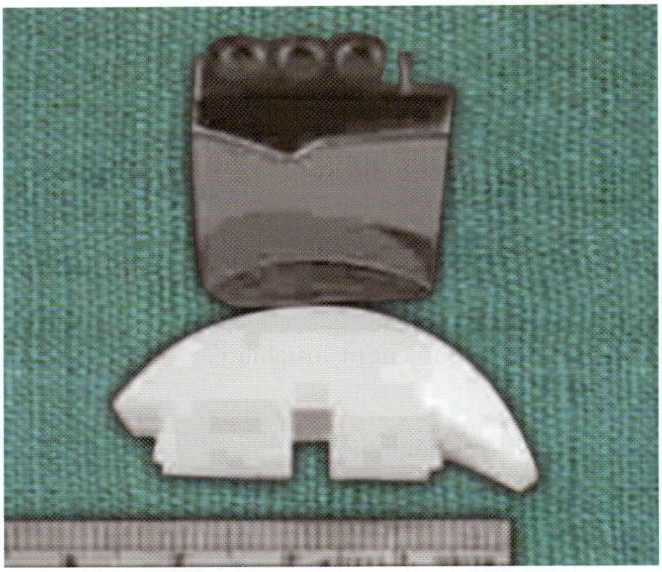

Fig. 26.405: Cylindrical fixed bearing design

1976—Trunnion cylindrical design (Fig. 26.406): Due to the problems identified after review of devices similar to the 1974 design, the need to have congruent articulating contact, without restriction to axial rotation was apparent. This lead to the adaptation of the mobile bearing concept, which was first used in the shoulder in 1974, to the ankle. The rotating trunnion device allowed axial rotation with congruity.

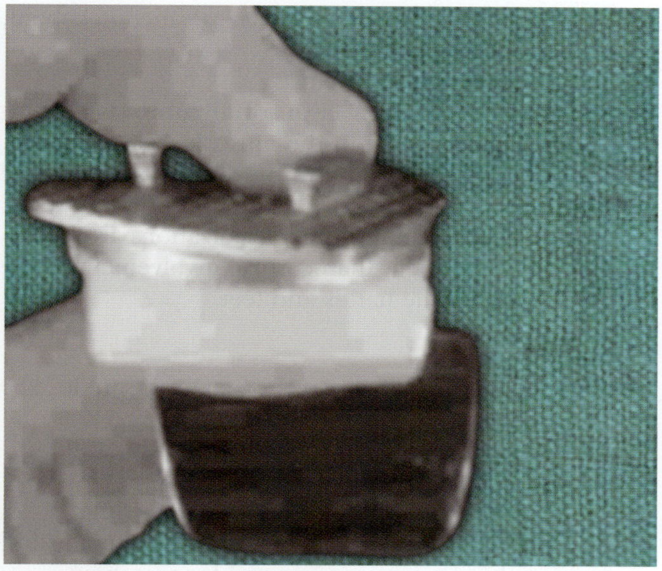

Fig. 26.406: Trunnion cylindrical design

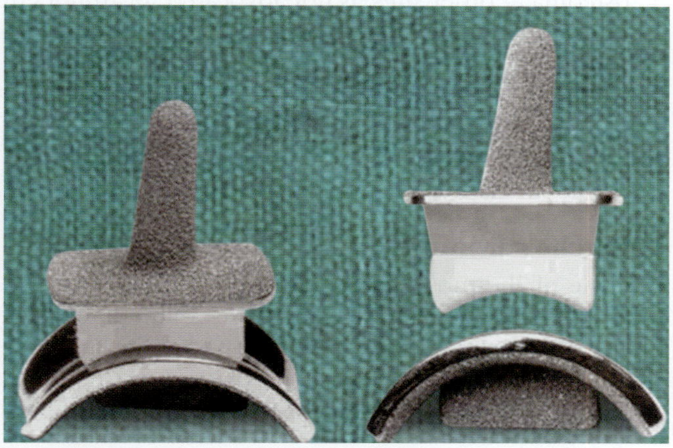

Fig. 26.407: Original meniscal bearing design

1978—Original meniscal bearing design (Fig. 26.407): Although, the trunion ankle performed as expected initially, the New Jersey Meniscal Bearing knee replacement was developed in 1977 and the benefits of lack of constraint were apparent. These benefits included congruent articular surfaces and the reduction of constraint forces. This design worked except for three infrequent problems:

1. Mechanical bearing subluxation due to talar necrosis with component subsidence and tilting (15%).
2. Fracture of the tibial plate (5%).
3. Fracture of the meniscal bearing.

1989—current meniscal bearing design (BP low contact stress total ankle replacement): In response to the infrequent problems discovered with the original meniscal bearing design, and discoveries made in wear reduction resulting from thin ceramic films, the current design encompassing the following changes was developed:

- Titanium alloy is used instead of CoCr due to its superior biocompatibility, resulting from less toxic and fewer corrosion products.
- Improved ingrowth into porous coating.
- Avoidance of nickel sensitivity condition (metal allergy).
- Strength
- Material properties (elastic modulus) closer to bone for better elastic compatibility.
- Reduced cost

Devices currently available for ankle replacement are:

- Agility™ total ankle system, a two-component design.
- Scandinavian total ankle replacement (STAR), a three-component design.
- Buechel-Pappas (BP) ultra total ankle replacement, a three-component design.
- TNK ankle, a two-component
- Salto Talaris total ankle prosthesis and Eclipse total ankle implant.

■ Complications

Intraoperative

Malalignment: Varus malpositioning can lead to medial impingement, stiffness, excessive lateral foot pressure and edge wear. Valgus malalignment may result in lateral impingement, arch pain from overstretching and edge wear. Medial translation of the tibial component causes a higher risk of medial malleolar fracture. Lateral translation places excessive tension on the deltoid, which tips the talus into varus.

Fracture: Medial and lateral malleolar fractures can occur intraoperatively from overzealous cuts or malpositioning of the cutting jig. They should be fixed, if recognized intraoperatively, or malposition of the component or poor implant fixation and subsequent loosening may occur.

Tendon injury: The posterior tibial tendon and the peroneal tendons are at risk if saw blades penetrate too far posteriorly.

Postoperative

Syndesmotic nonunion: Nonunion of the syndesmosis is a complication unique to the agility prosthesis because this is the only prosthesis that requires a syndesmosis fusion to provide support to the tibial component. Nonunion may lead to loosening of the tibial component, with angular change or subsidence. With the use of one screw, there is a longer time to union as opposed to the use of two screws.

Wound problems: Wound healing problems are common because there is a thin soft-tissue envelope around the ankle as opposed to the hip and knee. These complications can be minimized with proper soft-tissue handling technique, including making the incision long enough to minimize excessive retraction and avoiding overdistraction with the external fixator.

Infection: Infection should be treated as with other joint arthroplasties. Deep infection should be treated with aggressive debridement, an antibiotic cement spacer and delayed fusion.

Component instability and lysis: Migration of 5 mm or more or angular change of 5° or more may lead to a poor clinical outcome. The talar component subsides more often than the tibial component and progressive lysis or circumferential lucency may lead to a poor outcome.

TUMORS AROUND FOOT AND ANKLE

■ Introduction

Foot and ankle tumors are rare entity, but must be kept in differential diagnosis of musculoskeletal complaints. Meticulous work-up of all lesions must be undertaken. Majority of tumors in foot and ankle are benign, but occassionally primary sarcoma can be present. This chapter will outline the common bone and soft tissue tumors of bone and ankle, their classic characteristics and typical presentation as well as management protocols.

Osteoid Osteoma (Figs 26.408 and 26.409)

- Common benign tumor
- *Site:* prediliction for lower extrimity
- Five to ten percent cases seen around foot and ankle
- Most commonly, it involves talus, calcaneum, cuboid, cunieform, first metatarsal.
- *Sex:* 2:1, male predominence
- According to Edeiken et al. of all sites of osteoid-osteoma involvement in the musculoskeletal system, cortical bone is by far the most common and the subperiosteal region is the least common. However, cancellous and subperiosteal localizations are known to be more frequent than cortical involvement in the small bones of the hands and feet.

Clinical Presentation

- Aching discomfort in either the foot or the ankle. The pain occurs predominantly at night
- Pain is exacerbated by weight-bearing and walking
- Aspirin can provide relief
- Some patients may present with local swelling.
- *Treatment:* Surgical managemet involves removal of entire nidus, by curretage or en bloc resection.
- Radiofrequency ablation treatment so widely recommended with excellent results for osteoid-osteoma at other sites, is not advocated for tumors in the small bones of feet and spine.

Enchondroma (Fig. 26.410)

It is a common benign lesion of hyaline cartilage. Most commonly seen in small bones of hands and feet. It is discussed in chapter for tumors around shoulder.

Osteochondroma (Figs 26.411 and 26.412)

It is one of the most common tumors around foot and ankle. In cases of (multiple osteochondroma) diaphyseal aclasis, foot and ankle is a common site for multiple exostoses. Subungual exostosis is common in the distal phalanx of great toe. There is history of definite trauma.

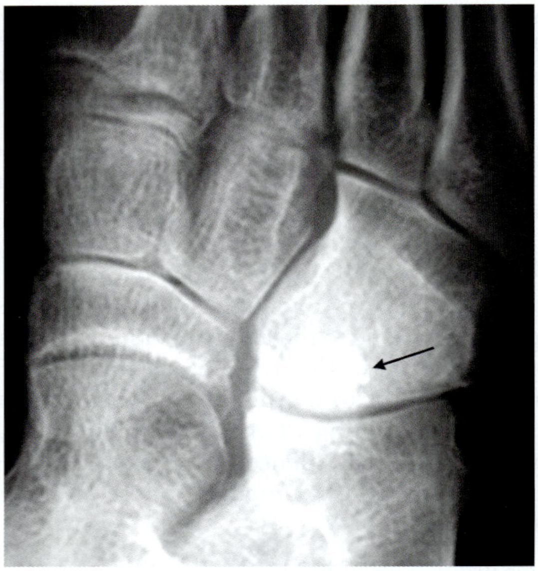

Fig. 26.408: Osteoid osteoma in cuboid (arrow)

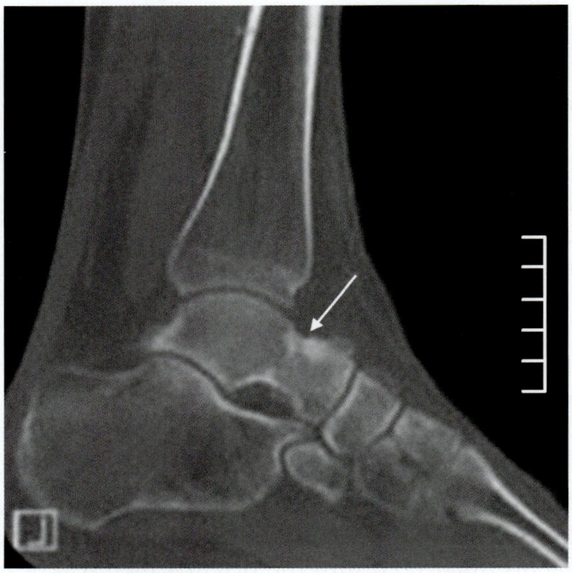

Fig. 26.409: Osteoid osteoma in talus (arrow)

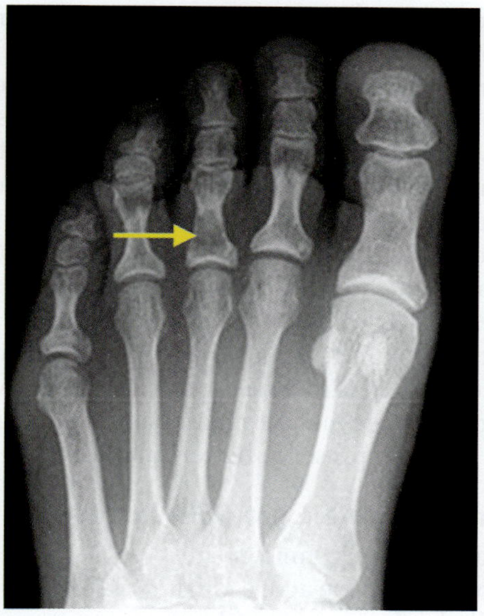

Fig. 26.410: Enchondroma in small bones of feet

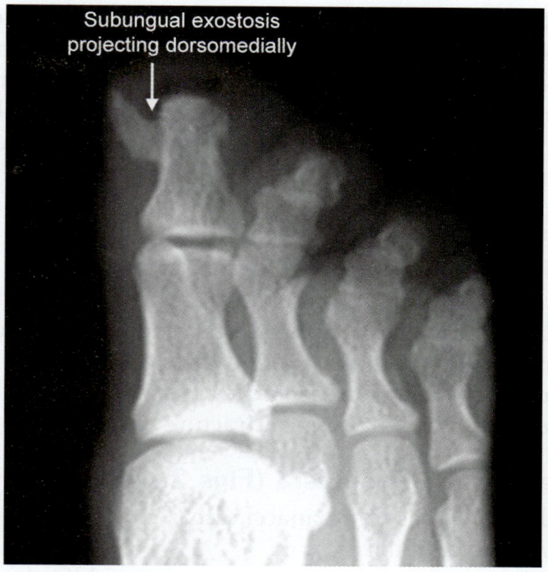

Fig. 26.412: Subungual exostosis is common in the distal phalanx of great toe

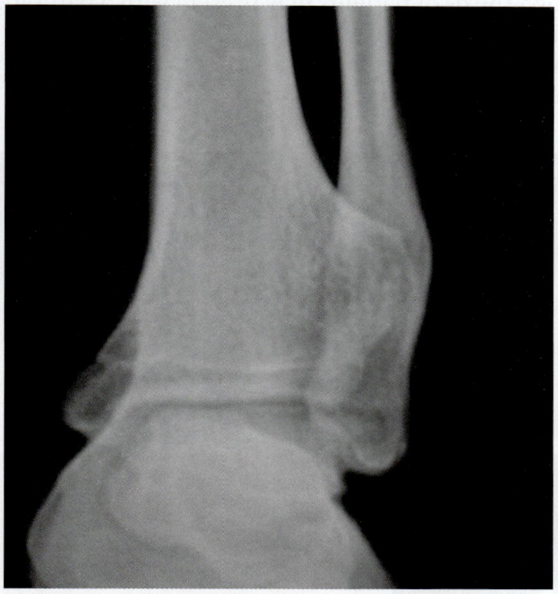

Fig. 26.411: Osteochondroma around foot and ankle

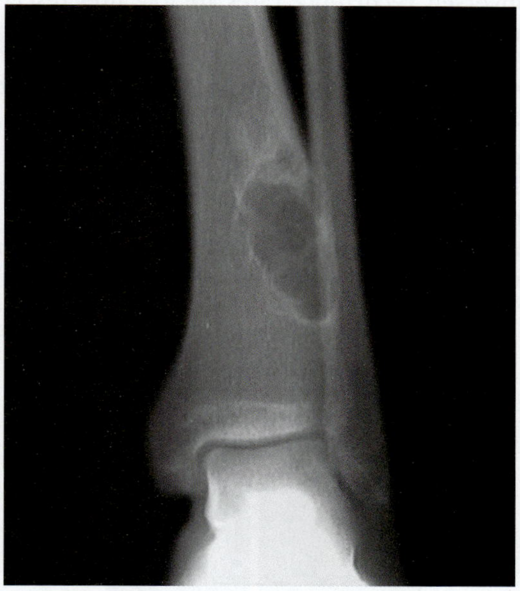

Fig. 26.413: Nonossifying fibroma in the metaphysic of tibia

Excision is indicated, when elevation of nail produces pain. History and location distinguishes this entity from true osteochondroma.

Nonossifying Fibroma (Fig. 26.413)

- Also known as metaphysesal fibrous defects, fibrous cortical defects, fibroxanthomas
- Most common complication is pathological fracture
- Incidence around foot and ankle: 40 percent in tibia and 10 percent in fibula
- Treatment is curettage, only done for larger lesions to prevent pathological fracture.
- Recurrence is rare.
- Distinction between fibrous cortical defect and fibroxanthoma is based on size and natural history.

- FCD are asymptomatic, small, < 3 cm, eccentrically located. Most of these spontaneously disappear. Conversely, fibroxanthoma are > 3 cm, eccentric intramedullary lesion that about the cortex. They have a typical superficial scalloping pattern in adjacent cortex.

Fibrous Dysplasia

- Most commonly fibrous dysplasia around foot and ankle is seen in polyostotic type.
- Radiographic appearance is characteristic with lucent area having granular ground glass appearance.
- Surgical treatment is indicated when significant deformity or pathological fracture occurs.

Osteofibrous Dysplasia (Figs 26.414A and B)

- Also known as Campanacci disease
- *Site:* Tibia, fibula
- Although, lesion is usually seen in middle third of tibia, it may encroach on metaphysis
- Tibia is enlarged and often bowed anterolaterally
- Recurrence rates are high after curretage or marginal resection in children
- Conversely recurrence rates are low after resection in adult patients.

Desmoplastic Fibroma (Figs 26.415A to E)

- Desmoplastic fibroma is an extremely rare, locally aggressive benign bone tumor
- It has been reported in all age groups, but is more common in the second and third decades
- The long tubular bones are involved most often
- Pain typically is the chief complaint.

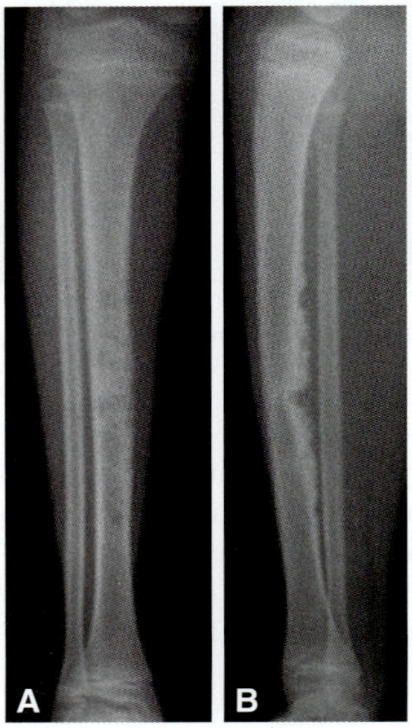

Figs 26.414A and B: Osteofibrous dysplasia

- Radiographs typically reveal a well-circumscribed lytic lesion, with a narrow zone of transition and frequently a thin rim of reactive bone. Cortical destruction may be present. The lesion sometimes appears septate
- On MRI, desmoplastic fibroma, may show low signal intensity on T1 and T2-weighted images. The lesional tissue is dense and tough
- Microscopically, it is hypocellular and fibroblastic and contains much collagen and few mitoses.

Treatment: This tumor does not metastasize, but local recurrence is common after simple curettage. Most recommended treatment is wide resection. Aggressive extended curettage may be a reasonable option in selected patients to try to preserve better function.

Unicameral Bone Cyst (UBC) (Fig. 26.416)

- Calcaneum is a common site
- Lesions are most active during skeletal growth and usually heal spontaneously.

Clinical Features

- Usually asymptomatic unless a pathological fracture has occurred.
- Two-thirds of patients may present with a pathological fracture.
- X-ray reveal a centrally located, purely lytic lesion with a well-marginated outline.

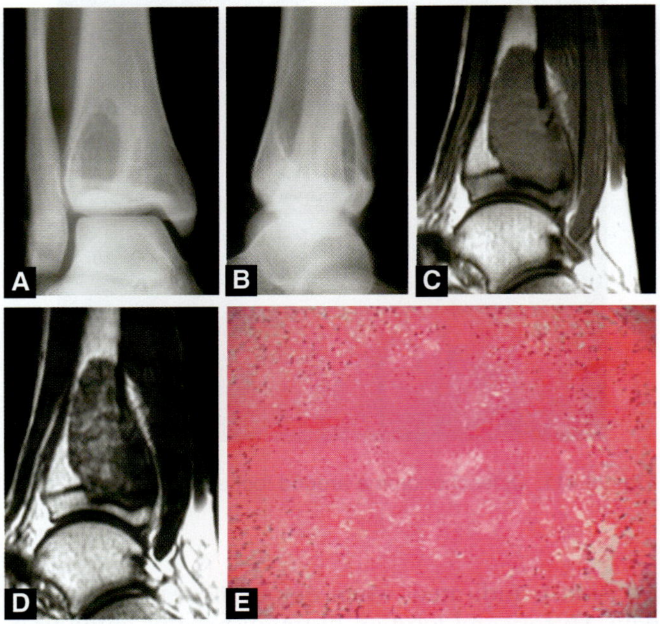

Figs 26.415A to E: Desmoplastic fibroma—(A and B) X-rays reveal a well-circumscribed lytic lesion, with a narrow zone of transition and frequently a thin rim of reactive bone; (C and D) On MRI, desmoplastic fibroma, may show low signal intensity on T1 and T2-weighted images. The lesional tissue is dense and tough; (E) Microscopically, it is hypocellular and fibroblastic and contains much collagen and few mitoses

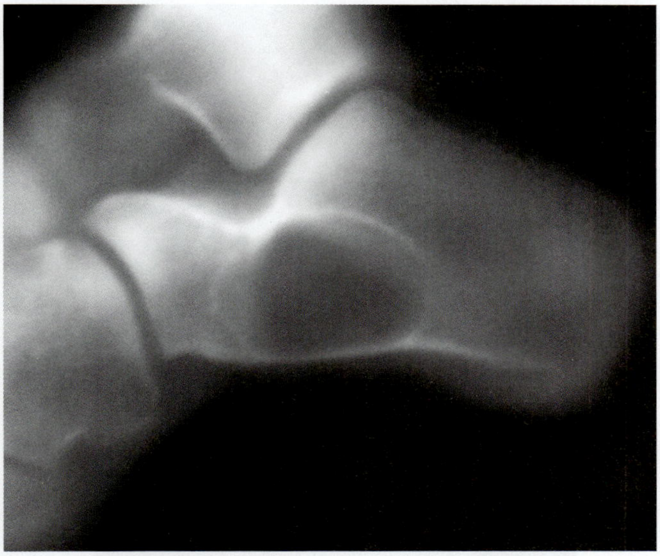

Fig. 26.416: Unicameral bone cyst

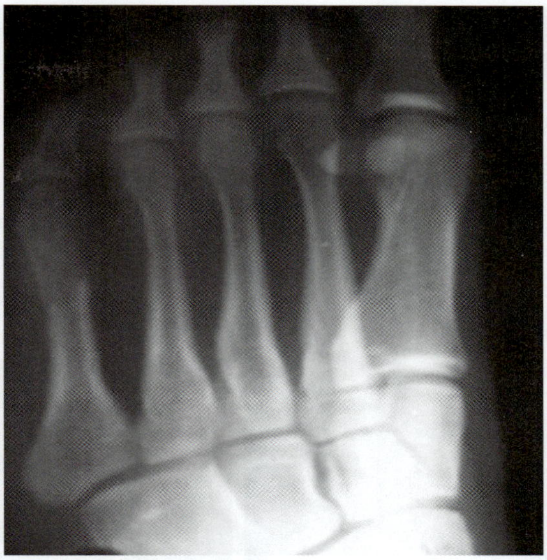

Fig. 26.417: Aneurysmal bone cysts in foot

- The cyst may expand concentrically, but never penetrates the cortex.
- Prominent osseous ridges on the inner cortical wall may give it a multiloculated appearance.
- No periosteal reaction is present, unless there has been a fracture.
- Lesions in the lower extremities usually are treated with curettage with or without bone grafting or internal fixation
- Other methods of treatment are: Aspiration, injection using, steroids, bone marrow aspirate and demineralized bone matrix.

Aneurysmal Bone Cyst (Figs 26.417 and 26.418)

- Aneurysmal bone cysts (ABC) are locally destructive, blood-filled reactive lesions of bone and are not considered to be true neoplasms
- *Site:* In foot and ankle it can occur in tibia, fibula and metatarsals
- *Age-sex:* Before second decade of life with slight female predominance.

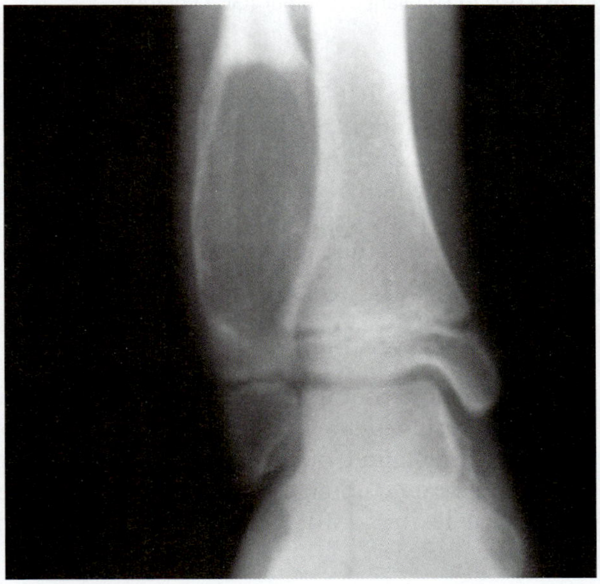

Fig. 26.418: Aneurysmal bone cysts in fibula

Clinical Features

- Mild to moderate pain present for several weeks to months
- X-ray shows expansile lytic lesion that elevates periosteum, but remained contained by thin shell of cortical bone
- MRI, shows multiloculated cavities and fluid levels, when differentiating between a UBC and ABC presence of a double density fluid level and intralesional septations indicates ABC.

Treatment

Extended curettage with a bone graft substitute is usually advised.

The recurrence rate after curettage is 10 to 20 percent.

Recurrence can be treated with the same approach as the primary lesions.

Giant Cell Tumor (Figs 26.419A to C)

- Giant cell tumor (GCT) around foot and ankle is rare.
- Incidence is 4 percent of all GCT

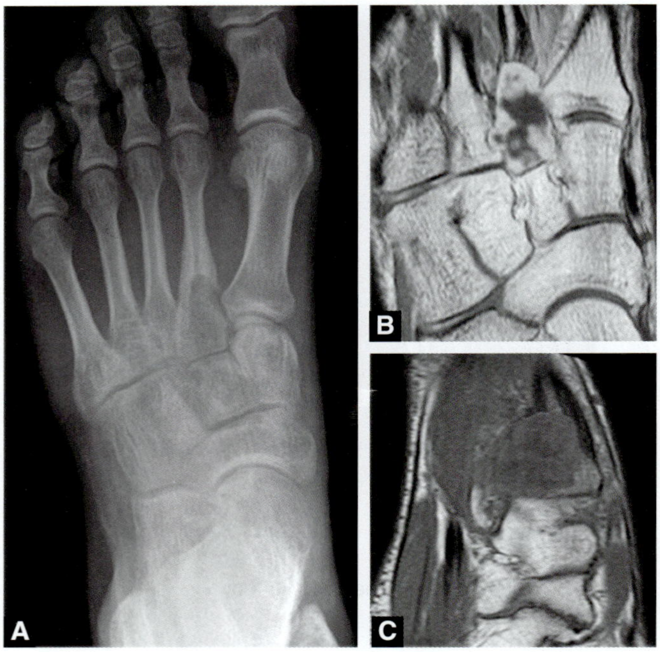

Figs 26.419A to C: Giant cell tumor (GCT) of foot

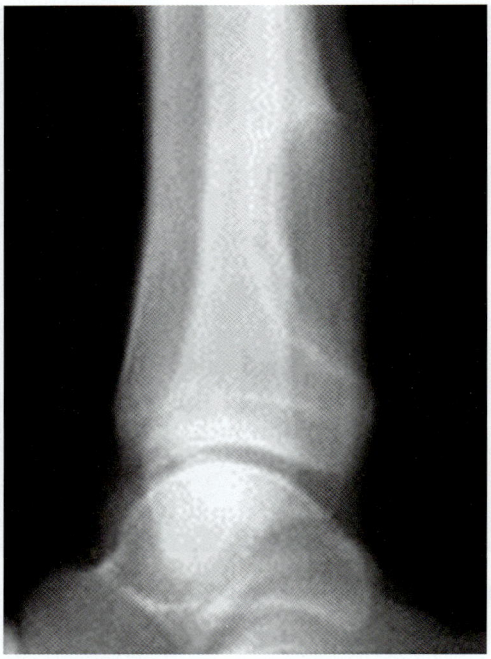

Fig. 26.420: Chondromyxoid fibroma

- Giant cell tumor (GCT) is a radiolucent, epiphyso-metaphyseal tumor that most commonly has a distinct bony margin and is associated with extensive subchondral bone erosion.
- There can be bony expansion, cortical destruction or frank extension of the tumor mass into the soft tissues.

Treatment alternatives for GCT include:
- Curettage, with or without local adjuvant treatment
- Marginal resection
- Local adjuvant therapy used in conjunction with curettage includes, the application of phenol, bone cement (cementation) or liquid nitrogen (cryotherapy)
- Recurrence rate curettage alone is 20 to 30 percent for active lesions and 5 percent after marginal resection.

Chondromyxoid Fibroma (Fig. 26.420)

- Chondromyxoid fibroma is a rare lesion of cartilaginous origin, representing less than 0.5 percent of all bone tumors.
- *Age:* 10 to 30 years. Any bone may be involved, but the tibia is the most common location.
- *Symptoms:* Patients typically complain of pain, if the tumor is located in the hands or feet, a painless mass or swelling may be the chief complaint.
- *X-ray:* It usually is a well-circumscribed lesion with a rim of sclerosis in the metaphysis of a long bone and have a bubbly appearance.
- Treatment consists of resection or extended curettage with bone grafting.

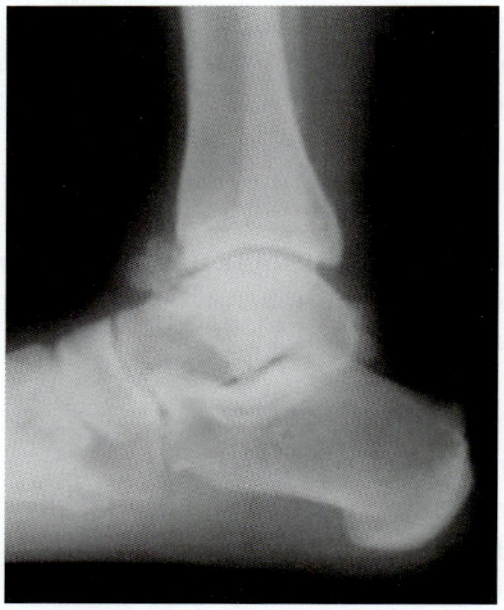

Fig. 26.421: Synovial chondromatosis

- Local recurrence occurs in about 20 percent of patients and is treated with repeat surgery.
- Sarcomatous change is rare.

Synovial Chondromatosis (Fig. 26.421)

- It is a monoarticular synovial proliferative disease, in which cartilaginous or osteocartilaginous metaplasia occurs within the synovial membrane of joints, bursae or tendon sheaths.
- Synovial chondromatosis is most common in the knee and hip, but almost any joint, bursa or tendon sheath may be affected.

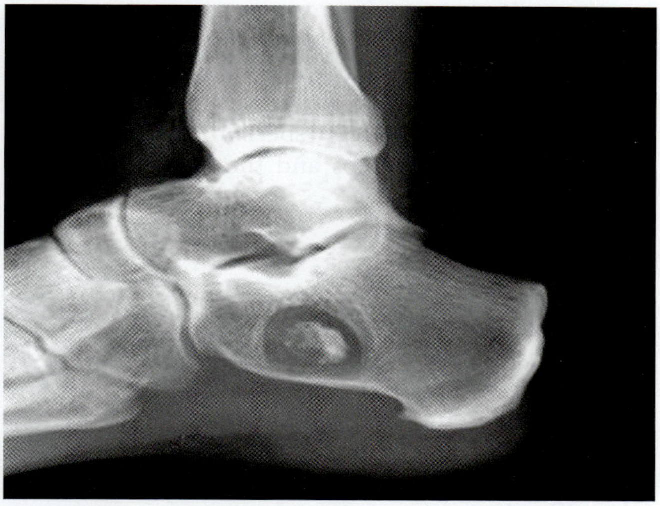

Fig. 26.422: Intraosseous lipoma

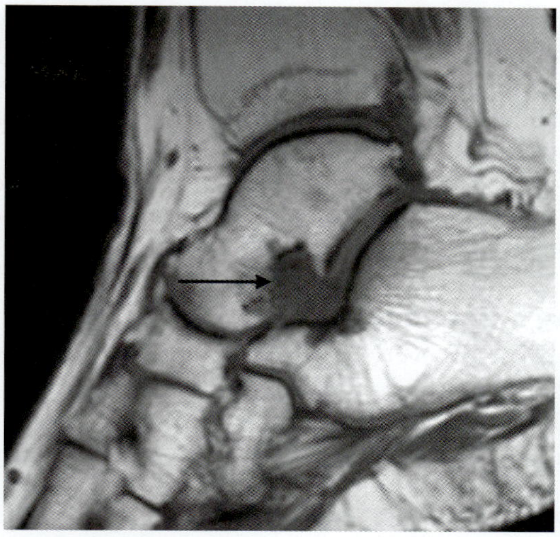

Fig. 26.423: Intraosseous ganglion cyst in talus (arrow)

- It has been classified into three phases:
  - Early, with synovial chondrometaplasia but no loose bodies
  - Transitional, with active synovial disease and loose bodies
  - Late, with loose bodies but no synovial disease.
  - X-ray, shows loose bodies, but often MRI is needed to establish the diagnosis
  - Treatment consists of synovectomy and removal of the loose bodies, either by arthroscopy or by open operation
  - Recurrence after surgery is common and there are rare reports of malignant transformation to chondrosarcoma.

Intraosseous Lipoma (Fig. 26.422)

- Rare lesion, true incidence is unknown
- Most common sites calcaneum
- Asymptomatic lesions and are discovered incidentally
- Biopsy is rarely necessary because imaging usually is diagnostic
- Surgery is indicated only for rare symptomatic lesion. In these cases, simple curettage ususally is curative.

Intraosseous Ganglion Cyst (Fig. 26.423)

- Typically occurs in the ends of the long bones of middle aged men
- Most common site being distal end of tibia
- X-rays and MRI, show uniloculated/multiloculated well demarcated lytic defects with a thin rim of sclerotic bone
- Treatment involves local excision of soft tissue and curetteage of involved bones.

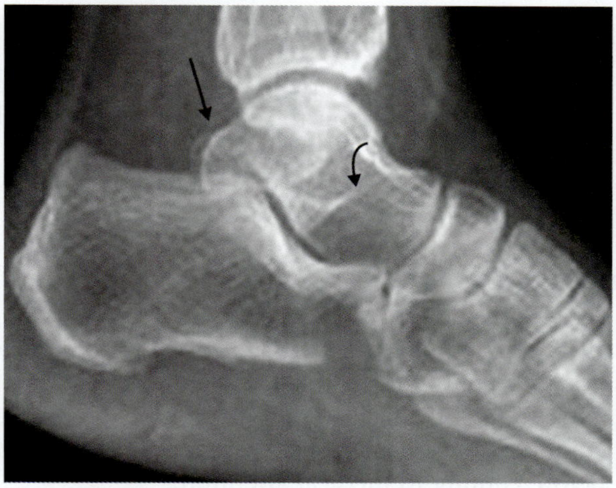

Fig. 26.424: Intraosseous Schwannoma of foot

Intraosseous Schwannoma (Fig. 26.424)

- Intraosseous Schwannoma is a very rare tumor accounting for only 0.1 percent of all primary bone
- It occurs most often in the head, neck, and flexor surfaces of upper and lower extremities
- Schwannomas are found at all ages but most commonly between age 20 and 50
- Symptoms commonly presents with swelling. It may be symptomless in 25 percent
- *X-ray:* It is unilocular or multilocular, lytic, sharply demarcated defects that often expand the involved bone.
- Perilesional sclerosis may surround the area of central lucency and associated with bone resorption and may be rarely associated with pathological fracture.

- There are three mechanisms, by which schwannoma may involve a bone are:
  - The tumor may arise centrally within a bone
  - The tumor may arise within a nutrient canal and produce canal enlargement.
  - Soft tissue or periosteal tumor may cause secondary erosion and penetration into a bone.
- *Treatment:* Curettage and bone grafting.

Ewing's Sarcoma

- It occurs in every bone of the foot.
- About one-third are located in hindfoot among them 20 percent occur in calcaneum
- *Age:* 10 to 20 years.

Symptoms

- Pain and diffuse swelling
- *X-ray:* Small lytic lesion with no matrix or soft tissue calcification
- MRI is essential for surgical planning and demonstrates soft tissue extent
- CT scan to see bony extent.
- *Treatment:* Chemotherapy, radiation therapy, surgical resection depending on the stage and extent of the disease.
- Patients with the tumor in the fore foot had survival of 70 percent and of hindfoot was 33 percent.

Synovial Sarcoma

- *Age:* Young adults
- It is most common soft tissue sarcoma in the foot accounting around 18 to 22 percent
- They frequently have an indolent course initially. It is common for a mass to be present for several years before coming to medical attention.
- Finally, synovial sarcomas frequently are relatively small (<5 cm) at presentation.
- This may be attributed to the fact that many patients complain of pain, rather than an enlarging mass.
- The term originates from the histological appearance of the cells, which can resemble synovial cells. The tumors do not arise from synovial tissue.
- Plain radiographs frequently show amorphic calcification within the tumor.
- Microscopically, the tumors frequently show a biphasic growth pattern with nests of epithelioid cells surrounded by spindle cells.
- Treatment is wide resection. Radiation can be used as adjuvant treatment for large tumors or for any case, in which the margins are close. Radiation can be administered preoperatively or postoperatively.
- Lymph node metastasis is common and should be evaluated carefully on physical examination.

LOWER LIMB ORTHOTICS

Orthotic is a mechanical aid to improve the function of the extremity and to maintain it in the maximum possible anatomic position. Caliper is a specialized type of orthosis prescribed for lower limbs and the main component/ material is metal.

Functions

- Stabilizes a flail joints
- Prevents deformities
- Corrects deformities
- Prevents unwanted movements
- Facilitates useful movements
- Provides rest to a part.

Classification

According to joint it supports, these can be classified as:

Example	H	K	A	F	O
Will support	Hip	Knee	Ankle	Foot	Orthosis

(O=Orthosis)

- Foot orthosis (FO)
- Ankle orthosis (AO)
- Ankle-foot orthosis (AFO)
- Knee orthosis (KO)
- Knee-ankle foot orthosis (KAFO)
- Hip orthosis (HO)
- Hip knee-ankle foot orthosis (HKAFO)

Compound Orthosis

Orthosis that cross more than five body segments, composed of two or more less complex devices, e.g. thoracolumbosacral orthosis (TLSO) and HKAFO.

Materials

- Stainless steel-durable
- Aluminum-lighter
- *Plastics: Accuracy of fit, cosmetic, permit a closer fit* (polypropylene, polyethylene)

Hybrid orthosis: Orthotic made of both metals and plastics.

■ Below Knee Orthosis (Fig. 26.425)

Function: Control of the ankle and foot joints.
Components: Two uprights, calf band, mechanical ankle joint.
Prerequisite: Lower limb orthoses must be appropriately attached to shoes.

Shoes (Fig. 26.426)

- Serves variety of functional and cosmetic purposes
- Minimizes pressure on sensitive, deformed structure

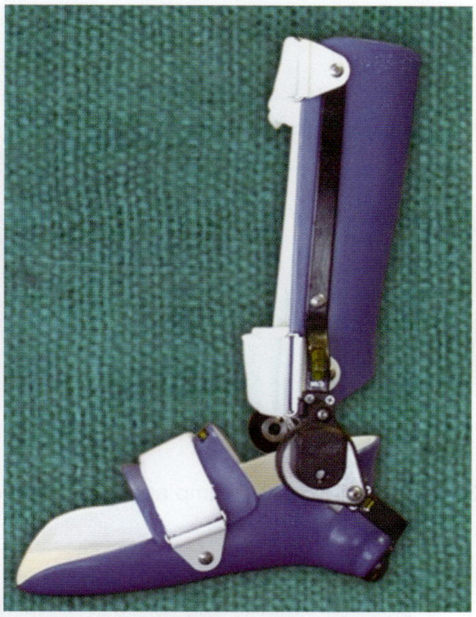

Fig. 26.425: Below knee orthosis

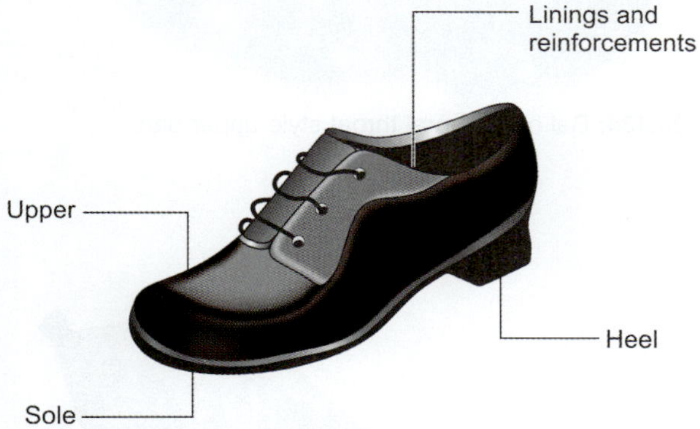

Fig. 26.426: Shoe and its components

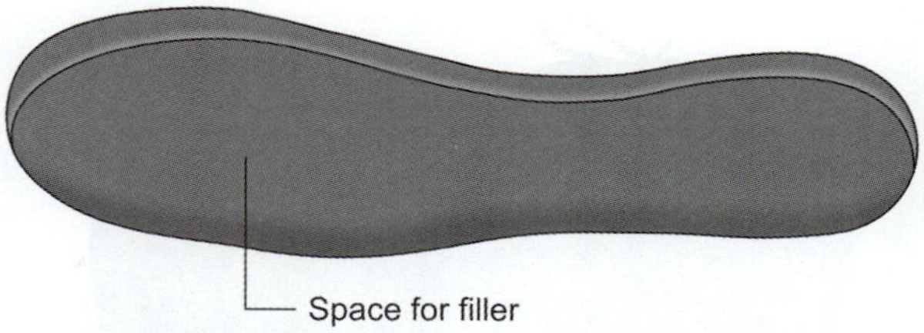

Fig. 26.427: Inner sole and space occupied by the space below it

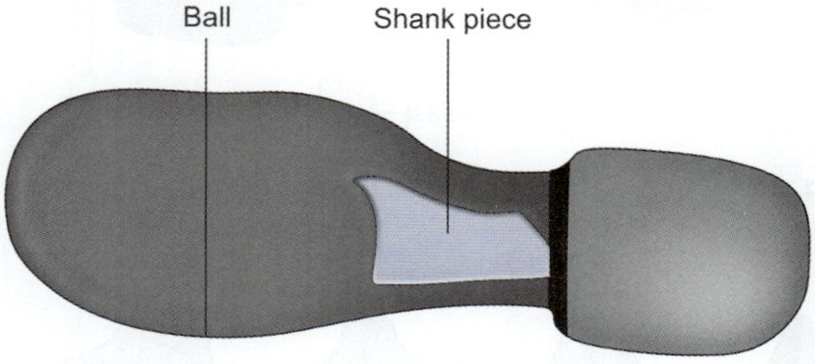

Fig. 26.428: Sole with ball area

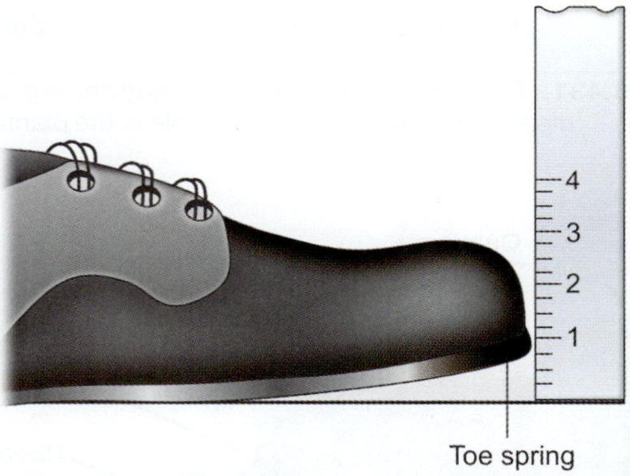

Fig. 26.429: Toe spring, a space between the floor and anterior portion of the sole

- Can be modified to redistribute weight towards pain free areas, to improve the comforts
- Forms foundation for orthosis.

Parts

Bottom: Insole, outsole, waist and heel

Upper: Vamp, quarters and toe cover.

Sole (Fig. 26.427)

- Outer sole, contacts the floor and is made of leather
- Inner sole, lies under the foot preferably made of leather. Below the inner sole, a space occupied by a compressible filler, which separates the inner from outer sole. Above the inner sole is stitched a welt, a narrow strip of leather, which is attached to the upper portion of the shoe.
- Ball is a widest part of the sole, should corresponds to the metatarsal heads, as shown in Figure 26.428.

Shank area: It is an area between the ball and anterior border of the heel, which is reinforced by a shank piece (preferably a corrugated metal).

Toe spring (Fig. 26.429): It is a space between the floor and anterior portion of the sole allows rocker effect to facilitate toe off reduces wrinkling of the upper part of the shoe.

Heel: Proximal section (firm leather), distal section or plantar section (medium or firm rubber in men, hard rubber in women and children), which contacts the ground. Anterior surface of the heel is the breast, as shown in Figure 26.430.

Pitch of the heel: Inclination of the posterior surface of the heel from the vertical.

Heel is measured from the outer sole to the plantar surface of the heel.

- *Spring heel:* 3 to 5 mm high
- *Oxford heel:* 19 to 25 mm

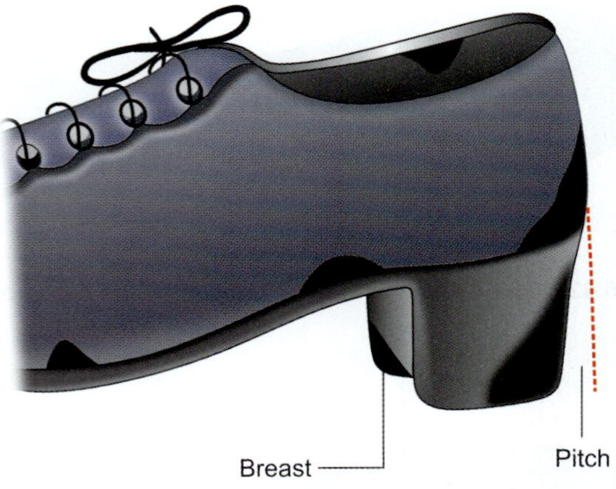

Fig. 26.430: Heel of shoes with its breast and pitch

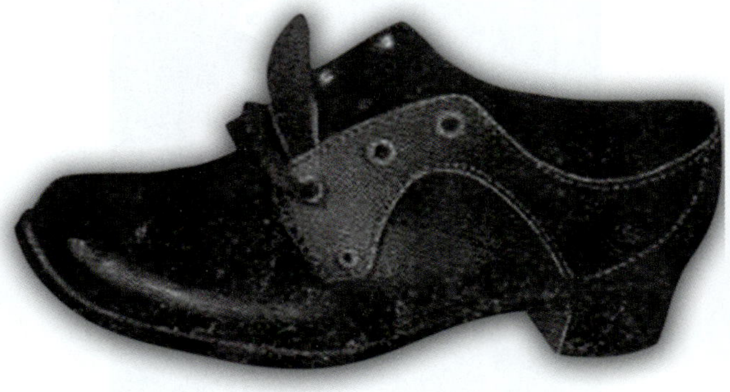

Fig. 26.433: Blucher throat style vamp and upper part of shoe

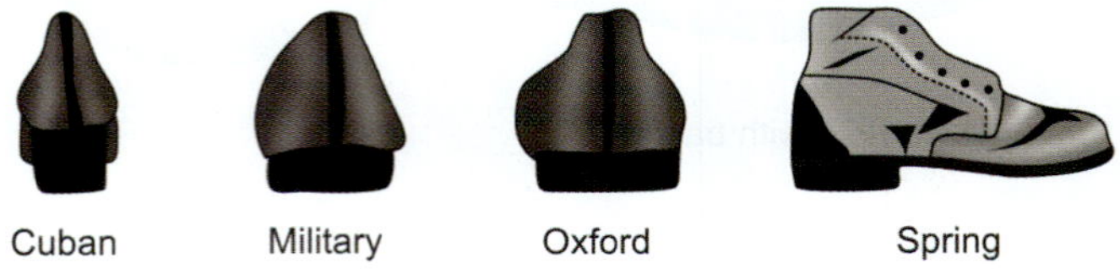

Fig. 26.431: Different types of heels depending upon the measurements from the outer sole to the plantar surface

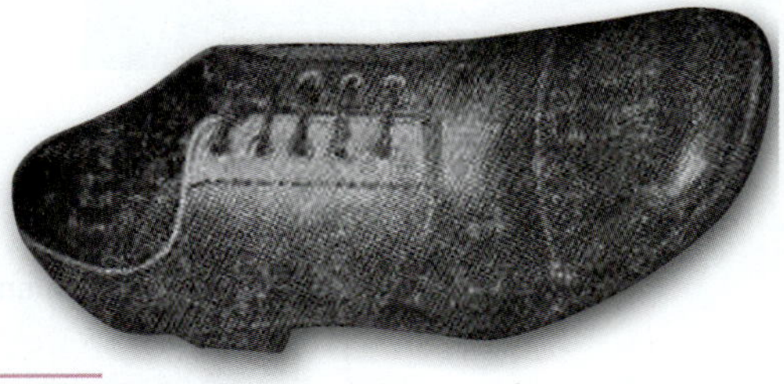

Fig. 26.434: Bal or Balmoral throat style upper part

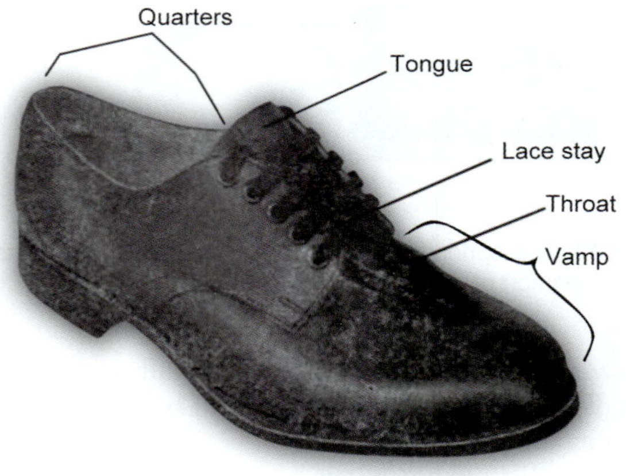

Fig. 26.432: Upper part of shoe, showing vamp and quarter

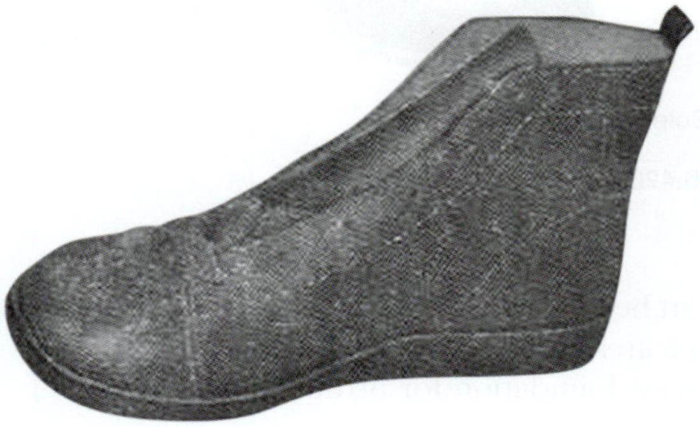

Fig. 26.435: Lace to toe throat style (surgical boot)

- *Military heel:* 31 mm
- *Cuban:* 38 mm (used for most orthopedic purposes), as illustrated in Figure 26.431.

Higher the heel, greater the pitch, more narrow the bearing surface on the floor.

Upper (Fig. 26.432)

Part above the sole, consisting vamp (anterior section), quarters (posterior section).

Tongue: Strip of the leather lying under the laces. Base of the tongue is throat.

- *Blucher throat style (Fig. 26.433):* Anterior margin of the lace stays are loose quarters lie over the vamp and contain the lace stays permits reflecting the tongue completely back, which facilitates donning.
- *Bal or Balmoral throat style (Fig. 26.434):* Vamp covers the forward edges of the quarters not possible to completely open the shoe completely over the forefoot.
- *Lace to toe throat style (surgical boot),* lace stays extend to the toe, as shown in Figure 26.435.

Lace stay: Part containing the eyelets (minimum 4 or preferably 5 pairs) for the lace.

Lining: A cotton vamp lining absorbs perspiration.

Low shoe or Oxford shoe (Fig. 26.436): Quarters extend to a level just below the malleoli.

High shoe or boot (Fig. 26.437): It covers the malleoli, reduces the piston action, and grips the foot better (resists back and forth sliding of the foot). Restricts ankle and subtalar joint movements.

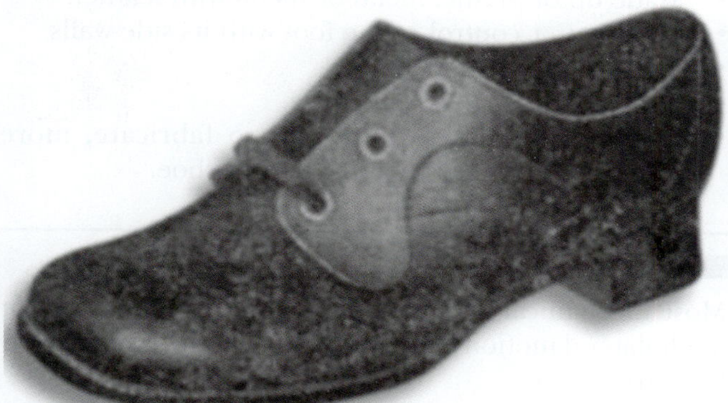

Fig. 26.436: Low shoe or Oxford shoe

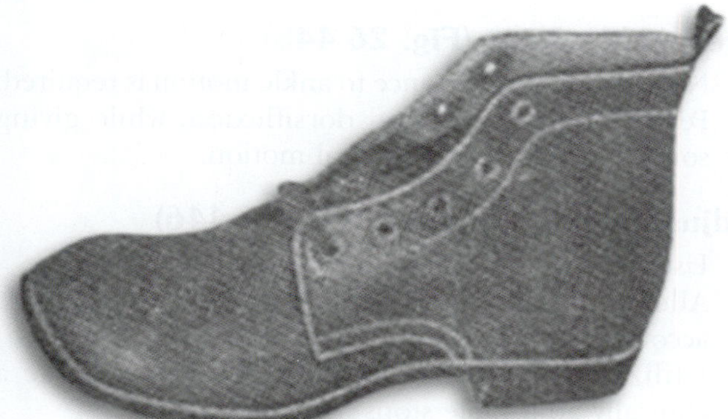

Fig. 26.437: High shoe

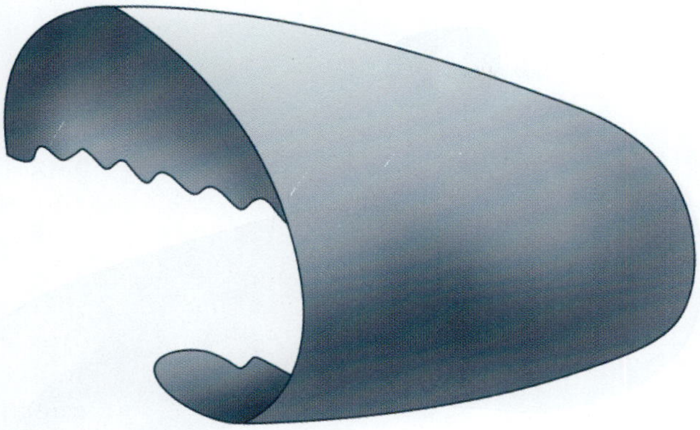

Fig. 26.438: Toe box

Toe box (Fig. 26.438): Reinforcement of the toe box, which guards the dorsum of the toes and preserves the contour of the vamp.

Counter (Fig. 26.439): Reinforcement at the anatomical heel.

Closures (Figs 26.440A and B): Adjustable-cotton lacing, elastic laces and nonadjustable-Velcro flaps, zippers.

Last-model of the weight bearing foot, on which the shoe is built.

Construction: Goodyear welt construction is recommended for orthopedic purposes. This method produces a shoe, which is absolutely smooth inside and is easiest to alter with external modifications, easier to repair and retains its shape best.

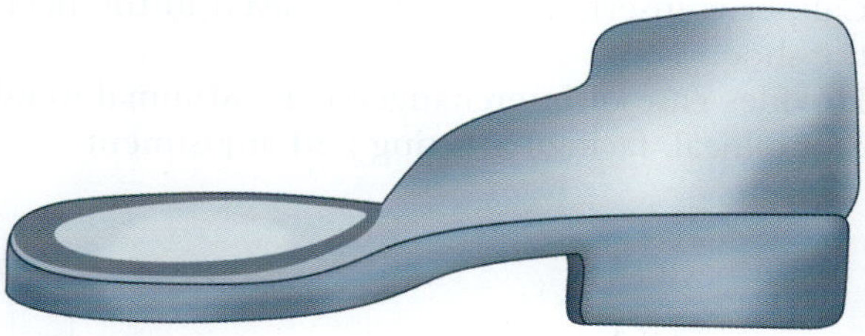

Fig. 26.439: Counter, reinforces the anatomical heel

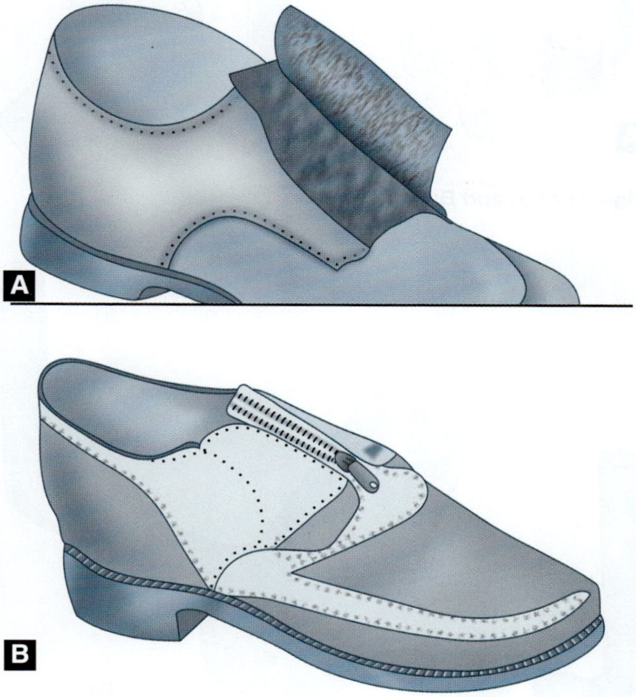

Figs 26.440A and B: Closures, with adjustable-cotton lacing, elastic laces and nonadjustable-Velcro flaps, zippers

Shoe Attachments

- Directly connecting attachments are: stirrup, caliper
- Incorporating shoe insert.

Stirrup (Figs 26.441A and B)

- Riveted to the sole of the shoe directly underneath the malleoli (anterior section of the heel)
- A permanent attachment between uprights and the shoe
- Can be employed with any type of ankle joint
- Allows fairly accurate correspondence of the mechanical and anatomical ankle joints
- Disadvantages are it may needs to split at the bottom to permit shoe changes
- Heavier, thicker and less durable than the solid stirrup.

Caliper (Fig. 26.442)

- Caliper is inserted into a tube placed in the heel of the shoe.
- Provides ease of interchangeability. Minimal weight, economical, facilitates fitting and adjustment

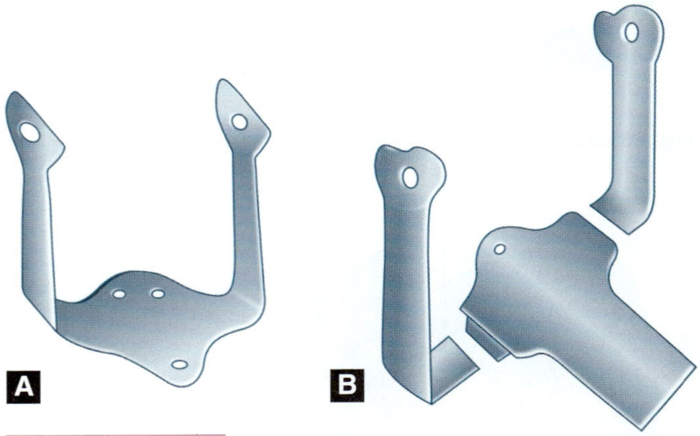

Figs 26.441A and B: Stirrups

- *Disadvantages:* Mechanical ankle joint is at the level of shoe heel, considerably distal to the anatomical joint will cause relative motion between the orthosis and the patient's limb.

Shoe Insert (Fig. 26.443)

- Stirrup can be incorporated in a shoe insert, which in turn fits into the shoe.
- Made up of plastic, metal or metal with leather.
- Gives better control of the foot with its side walls.
- Joints are well matched.
- Interchange of shoes is simple.
- Requires more skill and time to fabricate, more expensive and may require a larger shoe.

■ Ankle Joints

Most mechanical ankles are single axis joints (prevent mediolateral motion but control dorsiflexion and plantar flexion).

Little or no Motion Ankle (Fig. 26.444)

Not allowing any clearance between the apposing surfaces of the mechanical joint.

Free Ankle Joint (Fig. 26.445)

- No restraint or assistance to ankle motion is required.
- Permits full plantar and dorsiflexion, while giving some control of mediolateral motion.

Adjustable Ankle Joint (Fig. 26.446)

- Used, if the ankle condition is expected to change
- Allows the ankle to be set at different angles, to accommodate the altered patterns
- Utilizes serrated interlocking disks to provide a clinically adjustable stops
- Used as a positioning devise to be worn at night rather for daytime ambulance.

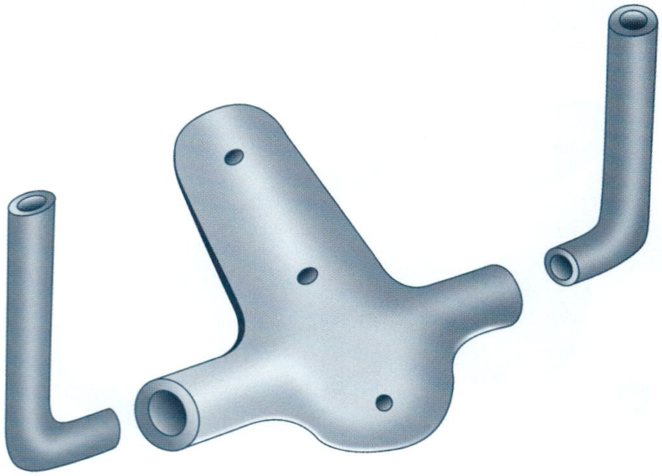

Fig. 26.442: A caliper

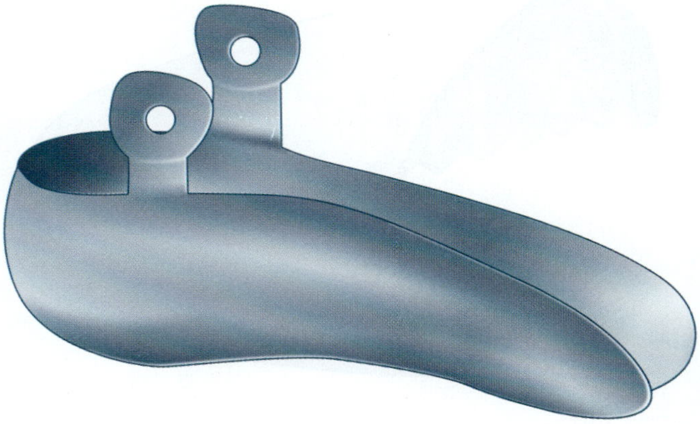

Fig. 26.443: A shoe insert

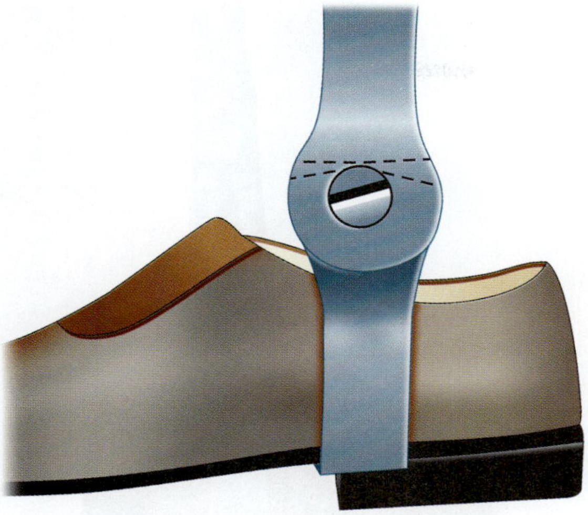

Fig. 26.444: Little or no motion ankle

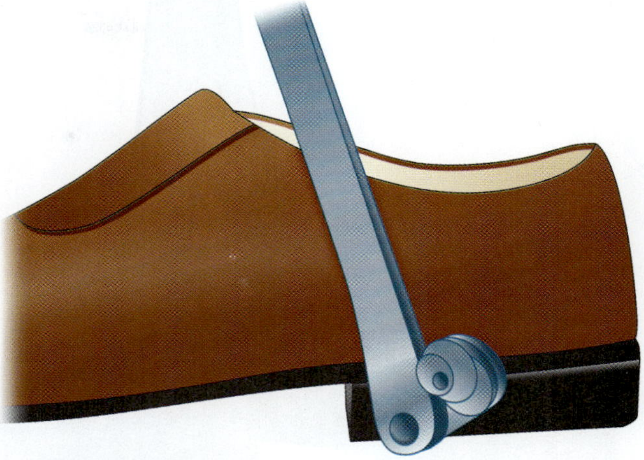

Fig. 26.446: Adjustable ankle joint

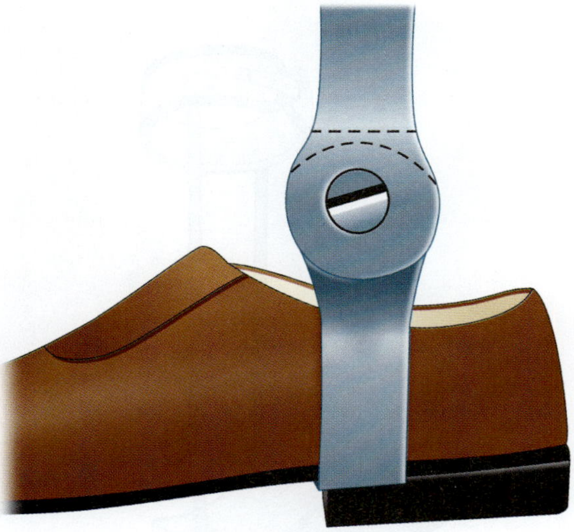

Fig. 26.445: Free ankle joint

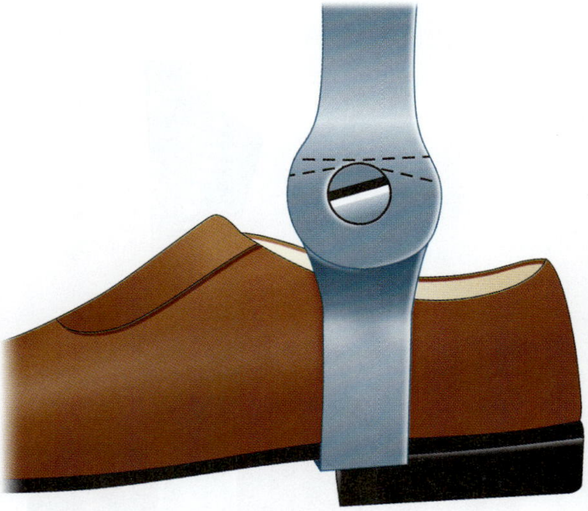

Fig. 26.447: Limited motion stops

Ankle Controls

- Stops
- Solid ankle
- Assists

Ankle Joint Stops

Allows any predetermined range of motion.

- *Plantar flexion (posterior) stop*: Used in foot drop. Allows unlimited dorsiflexion, but restricts plantar flexion.
- *Dorsiflexion (anterior) stop:* Allows plantar flexion but restricts dorsiflexion.
- *Limited motion stop (Fig. 26.447):* Restricts motion in both directions. Indicated when there is involvement of a number of muscles around ankle. The front and back of the top of the stirrup are cut at angles to the horizontal, leaving a predetermined clearance in relation to the proximal part of the joint. As the patient dorsiflexes, the anterior gap closes to prevent further motion, conversely plantar flexion closes the posterior gap.

Solid Ankle (Fig. 26.448)

- For rigid control of the ankle.
- Quite strong, but not adjustable.

Ankle Joint Assists

- Utilized as an aid to weakened muscles.
- Provided by the action of a spring, elastic strap, springiness of the material (Plastic or wire).
- Assists in simulating normal functions to some extent.

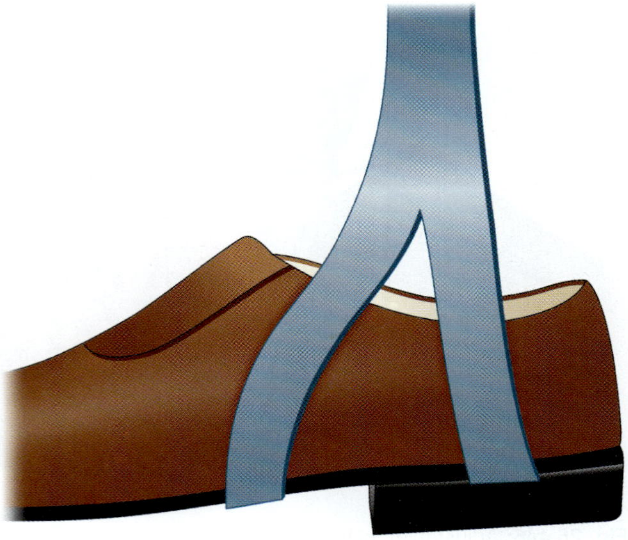

Fig. 26.448: Solid ankle

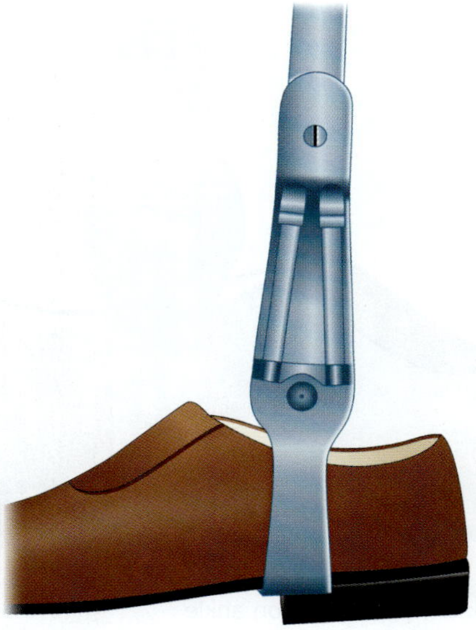

Fig. 26.450: Double action ankle assist

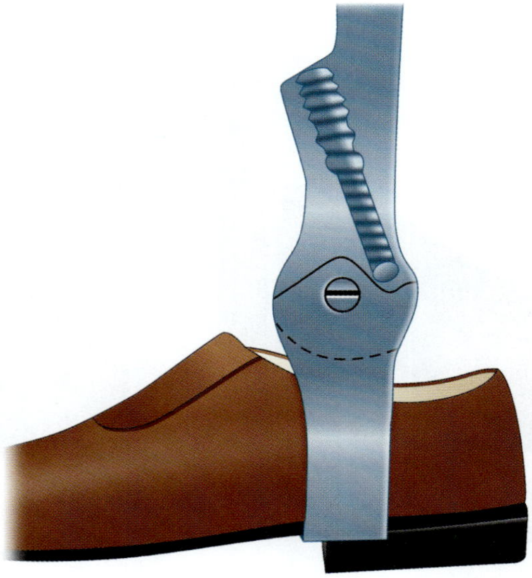

Fig. 26.449: Spring loaded dorsiflexion assist

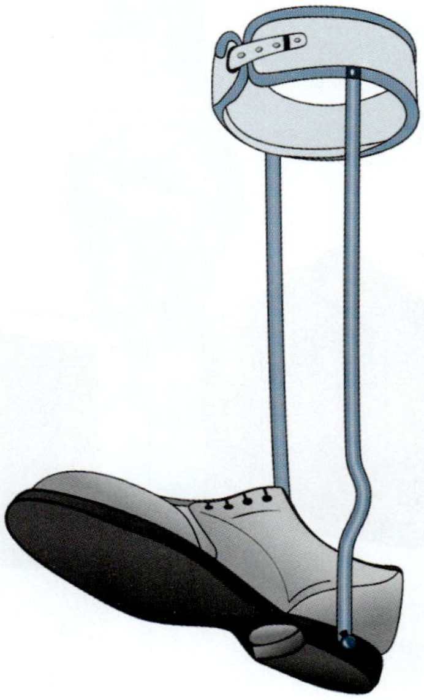

Fig. 26.451: Wire spring dorsiflexion assist

- Contraindicated in severe spasticity, where maximum control is required.
- *Spring loaded dorsiflexion assist (Fig. 26.449):* Helps to dorsiflex the foot during swing phase (recoiling of the spring), but allows controlled plantar flexion at heel strike (spring is compressed).
- *Double action ankle assist (Fig. 26.450):* Assists in both plantarflexion and dorsiflexion and adds more bulk to the joint.
- *Wire spring dorsiflexion assist (Fig. 26.451):* Accomplishes the motion by the recoil action of the springy material, of which the uprights and shoe attachment are light weight, cosmetically accepted easily adjustable. Does not offer ankle stability under great stress.

Bichannel Adjustable Ankle Lock (BiCAAL) Joint

Steel dowel replaces the springs and convert the joint to fully adjustable stops.

Double Axis Joints (Fig. 26.452)

- Provides necessary amounts of dorsiflexion and inversion or eversion
- Increases the bulk of the orthoses

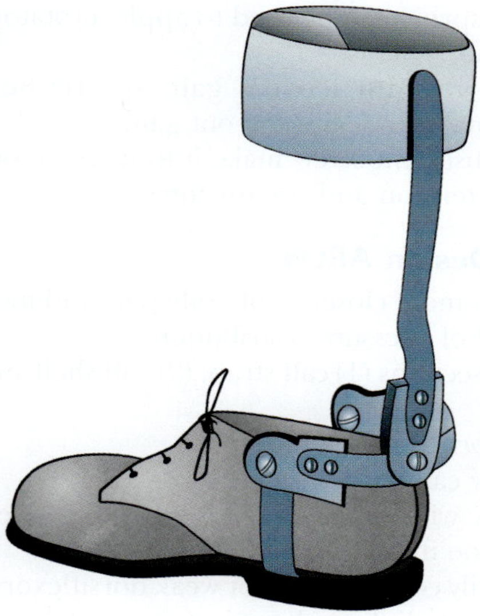

Fig. 26.452: Double axis joints

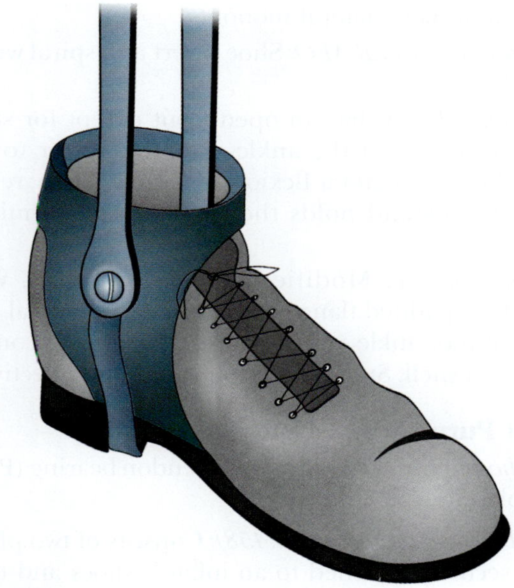

Fig. 26.453: Corrective straps and pads

Corrective Straps and Pads (Fig. 26.453)
- Provides additional control at the ankle
- *Valgus or varus correction straps:* Attached to the shoe and buckle around the opposite bar. The side of the shoe, to which the strap is attached on the deviation that is being corrected. The valgus correction strap attaches to the shoe medially, encompasses the medial malleolus and buckles around the lateral upright. The varus correction strap is attached in the opposite manner.

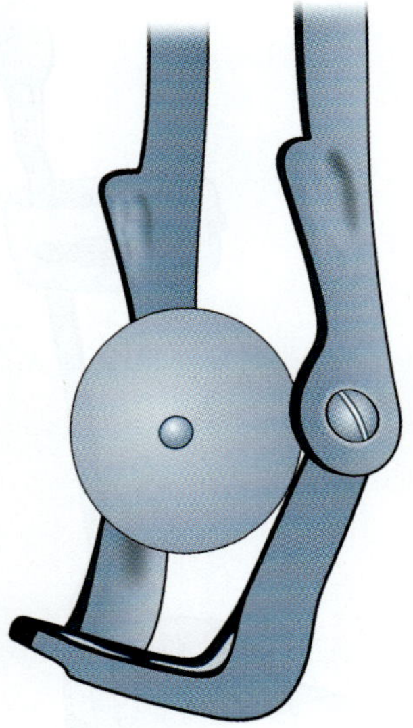

Fig. 26.454: Pads attached to the medial or lateral side of the joint

Buckled Inserter
- Greater mediolateral correction can be afforded
- Primarily for valgus correction
- A plastic shoe inserter with a rigid medial extension, incorporating a protective polyethylene foam relief pad over the malleolus. A nonstretchable leather/fabric strap, reverted to the top of the extension, buckles around the lateral upright.

Pad (Fig. 26.454)

Attached to the medial or lateral side of joint and are required to prevent deviations.

Uprights and Calf Band

Single bar orthoses (Fig. 26.455):
- More cosmetic (medial, lateral or posterior bar)
- Easily adjustable to accommodate deformities.
- Do not provide as much stability as bilateral upright.
- Medial upright, if extended to the epicondyle and provides better three point pressure systems.
- *Posteriorly placed single upright:* Motion at the ankle joint may cause the orthoses to displace up and down on the limb (calf band should be permitted to slide on the upright, to prevent motion of the calf band on the leg).

Calf band: The metal calf band with its leather cuff.
- Adds rigidity to the orthoses
- Maintains proper alignment of the uprights
- Secure the orthoses to the limb
- Provides a reaction point for the application of force to the limb
- Should be one inch below the neck of fibula

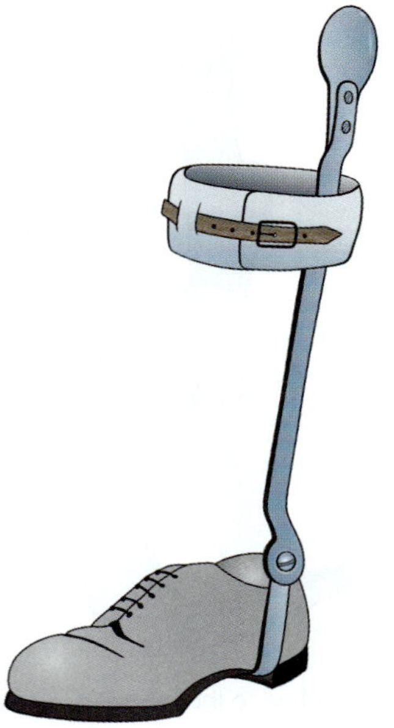

Fig. 26.455: Single bar orthoses

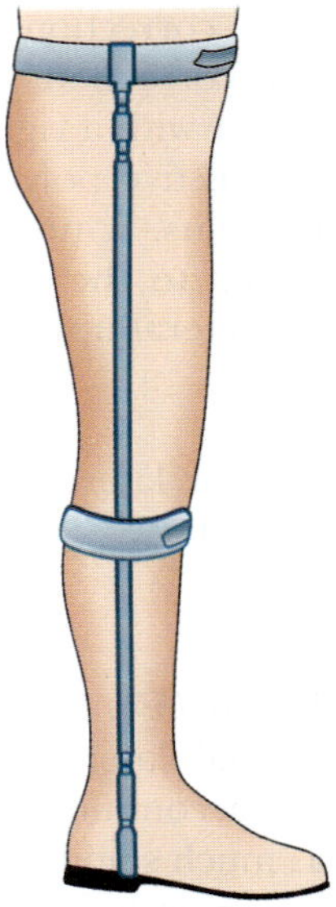

Fig. 26.456: Torsion shaft

- If a dorsiflexion stop is to be employed, the calf cuff will exert pressure anteriorly, therefore reversing of the calf band may be desirable. Anterior band is ease for donning.

Torsion Shaft (Fig. 26.456)

- Consists of a tightly coiled spring within a flexible housing.
- Upper end of the shaft attached to a well-fitted pelvic belt, lower end attached to the side of the shoe or to the lateral aspect of the calf band, the force developed by the spring can be used to apply a rotatory force to the limb.
- Useful in mild scissors gait, spastic hemiplegia, abnormal toe-in and toe-out gait.
- An adjustment screw make it to increase or decrease spring tension and rotator force.

Plastic Design AFOs

- Permits more closer fit of body part and more precise control of pressure distribution.
- Three sections (1) calf strap, (2) calf shell and (3) shoe insert.
- *Posterior leaf-spring AFO*
- Narrow calf shell.
- Narrow width at the junction between the calf shell and shoe insert-simulates ankle motion.
- Primarily compensates for weak dorsiflexors, does not control mediolateral motion.
- Similar disadvantages as single upright orthoses.
- *Modification:* More anterior calf shell linings. More resistance to plantar and dorsiflexion. Increased control of mediolateral motion.

Spiral and hemispiral AFO: Shoe insert and spiral with a calf band proximally.

Solid ankle AFO: It has an open front except for strap closure, trim lines at the ankle extend anterior to the malleoli. Prevents plantar flexion and dorsiflexion, resists varus or valgus and holds the foot in predetermined position.

AFO with flange: Modified solid ankle AFO, with polyethylene padded flange projecting from medial side (to control foot-ankle valgus) or lateral side (to control varus) of calf shell. Stabilizes the subtalar joint effectively.

Special Purpose BK Orthoses

PTB orthoses (Fig. 26.457): Patellar tendon bearing (PTB) brim replaces a calf cuff.

Dennis Brown splint (Fig. 26.458): Consists of two plates that are securely attached to an infant's shoes and then connected to a cross bar. Worn 24 hours a day in an attempt to correct rotation problems in the feet, tibia or hips. Used to hold the feet in varying degrees of dorsiflexion and hips in abduction. The footplates can be rotated on the cross bar to obtain a degree of rotation desired. Dorsiflexion of the ankles may be accomplished by appropriate bending of the cross bar.

Knee-ankle-foot Orthosis (KAFO) (Fig. 26.459)

- AFO with proximal extension, to encompass the knee joint
- Controls knee motion and alignment
- Support the body weight
- Uprights extend upwards to the knee joint

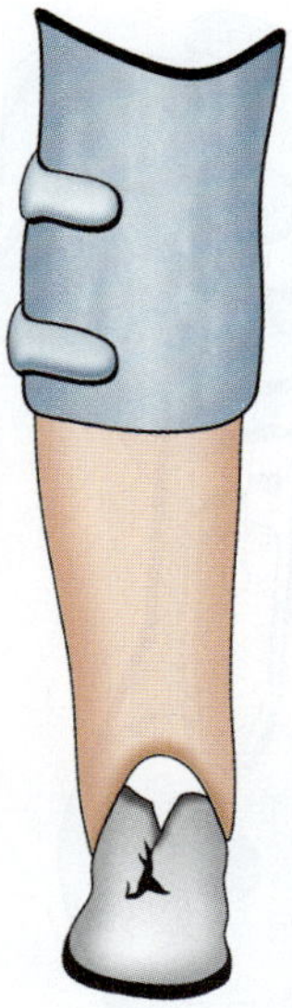

Fig. 26.457: PTB orthosis

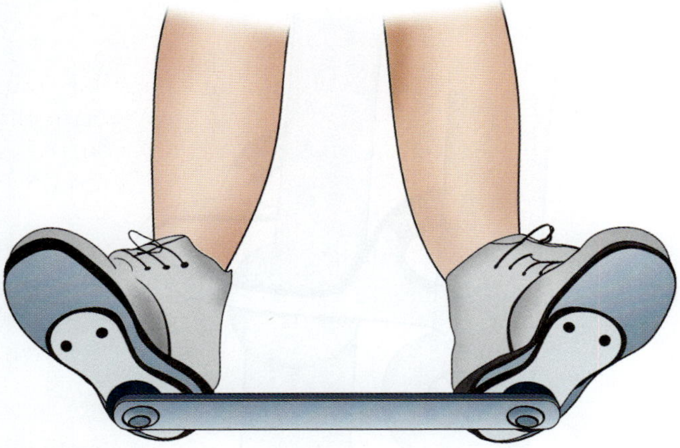

Fig. 26.458: Denis Brown splint

- Knee pads employed to assist in knee control
- Thigh upright are shaped to the contour of the thigh and held together by one or two high bands
- Distal components are same as AFO
- If control is needed at the hip a pelvic band and hip joint may be added.

Knee Joints

Mechanical knee joints have a fixed axis of rotation. Therefore, some shifting of the orthoses with respect to the limb occurs during flexion and extension of the knee, which can be minimized by proper placement of the mechanical joint or by using polycentric joints, meshing gears and a plate with two pivots (genucentric).

Types: Free motion, offset, locked and adjustable.

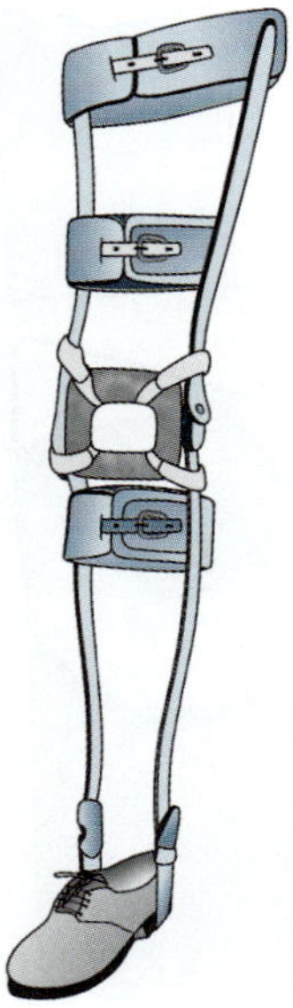

Fig. 26.459: KAFO splint

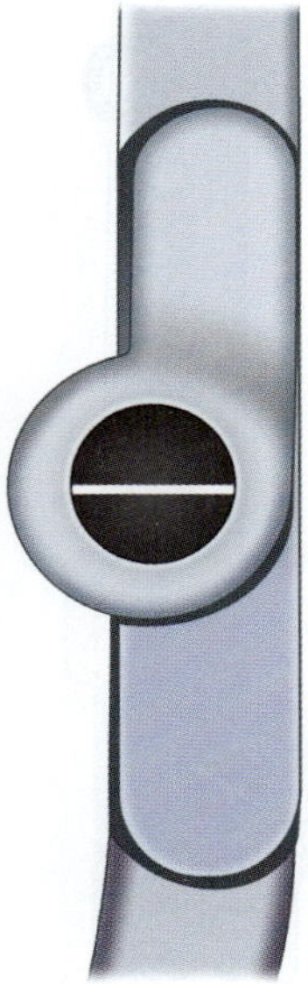

Fig. 26.460: Free motion knee joint

Free Motion Knee Joints (Fig. 26.460)

If an individual can control his knee against flexion (sufficient muscle power), but has a tendency towards mediolateral instability or recurvatum, a free knee joint can be used. The free knee prevents recurvatum, but since it permits the knee to flex during swing phase, it allows for a more natural gait than the locked knee.

Knee Locks

Drop-ring lock (Figs 26.461 and 26.462): To control flexion, the lock is usually located on the lateral bar. May be placed

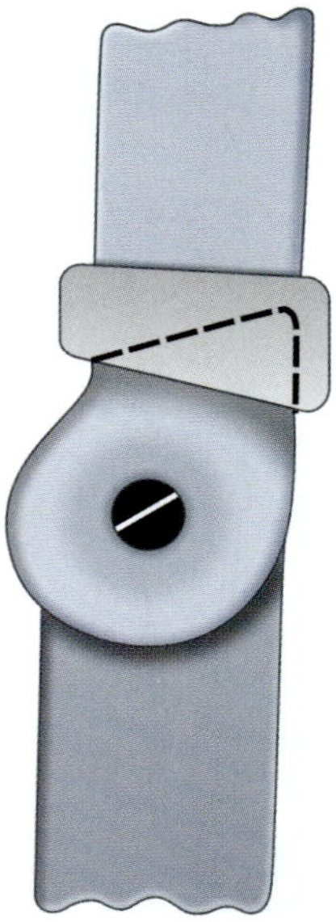

Fig. 26.461: Drop-ring knee lock

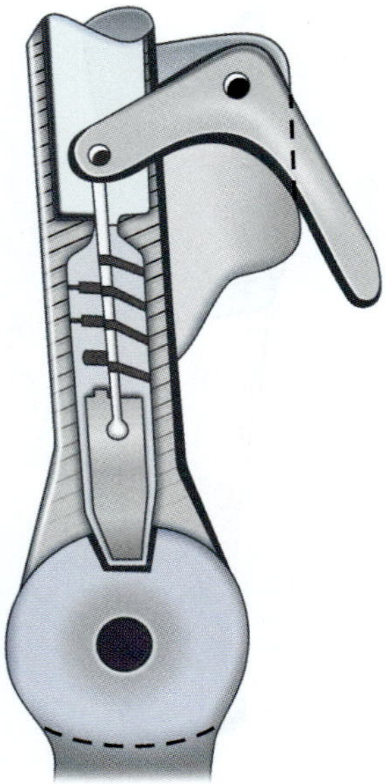

Fig. 26.463: The plunger or internal lock

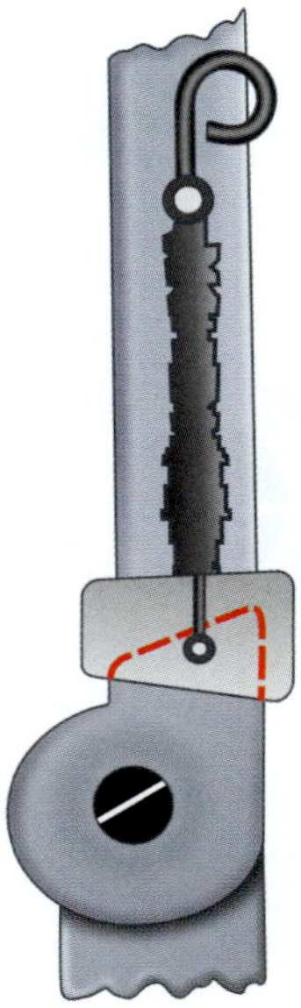

Fig. 26.462: Locking and unlocking the drop ring knee joint

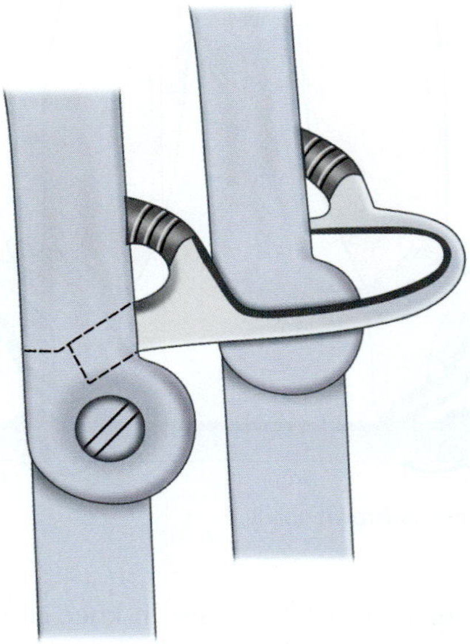

Fig. 26.464: Cam lock-pawl knee lock

medially, if upper limb on the same side of orthoses is involved. When the mechanical knee joint is in full extension, the ring drops over the joint manually or by gravity. The lock is simple and sturdy, but has a tendency to bend in presence of spasticity. A spring loaded pull rod located at thigh level added to the ring drives the drop lock down automatically, so that the person need not bend to lock or unlock the joint. Used only for a unilateral upright.

The plunger or internal lock (Fig. 26.463): Spring loaded pull rod with a cable attached to its lower end. When knee is fully extended, the plunger snaps into a notch on the proximal end of the lower uprights and the knee joint is automatically locked.

Cam Lock-pawl Knee Lock (Fig. 26.464)

- In case of severe spasticity
- Easy to release
- A spring loaded, cam shaped part which fits into a similarly shaped recess, when the knee joint is fully extended. In the extended position of the knee, the spring maintains the cam in the recess, locking the knee.

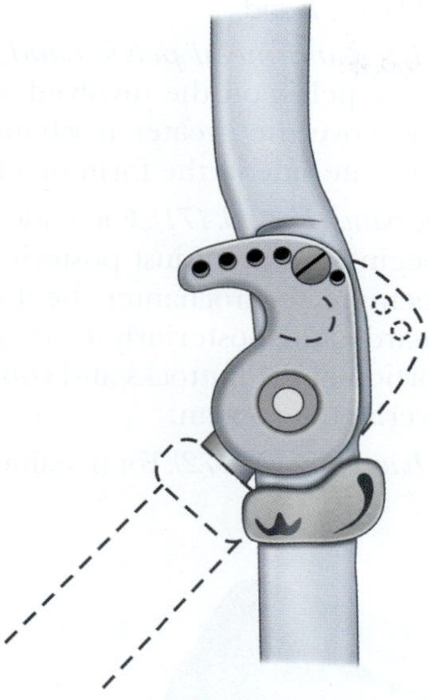

Fig. 26.465: Adjustable knee lock

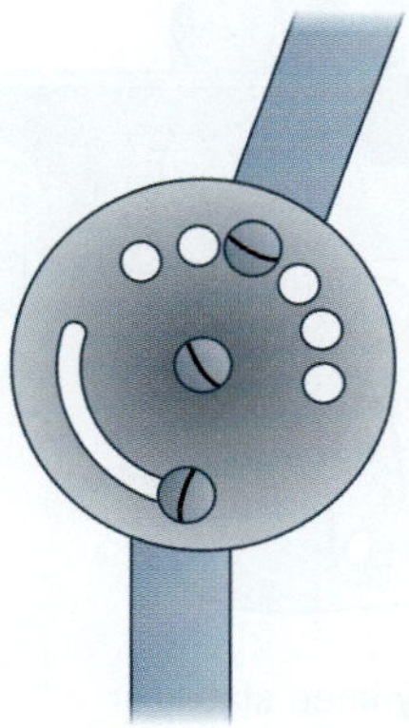

Fig. 26.466: Dial locking system

- A bail, which is a type of lever, used to unlock both sides simultaneously.

Swiss lock: In the absence of springs, elastic webbing from the bail to the calf band are used.

Adjustable Knee Lock (Fig. 26.465)

Useful, when change in the condition of the patient is anticipated or desired, such as in the gradual stretching of a knee flexion contracture. Example, fan lock incorporate a drop ring lock that maintains the desired knee position in standing and walking, but which can be unlocked to permit knee flexion when sitting.

Dial lock (Fig. 26.466): To restrict flexion or extension, but it permits free motion in the opposite direction.

Offset knee joint (Fig. 26.467): Mechanical knee joint is placed posterior to the uprights. Knee will extend, when the weight is transmitted through the bars. Knee is stable without a lock during stance phase and is free to bend during swing phase, allowing a more natural gait. Cannot be used, where there is knee flexion spasticity, hip or knee flexion contracture or with a plantar flexion stop. It is necessary for weight to be transmitted through the uprights, which is difficult without the addition of a thigh corset or quadrilateral cuff.

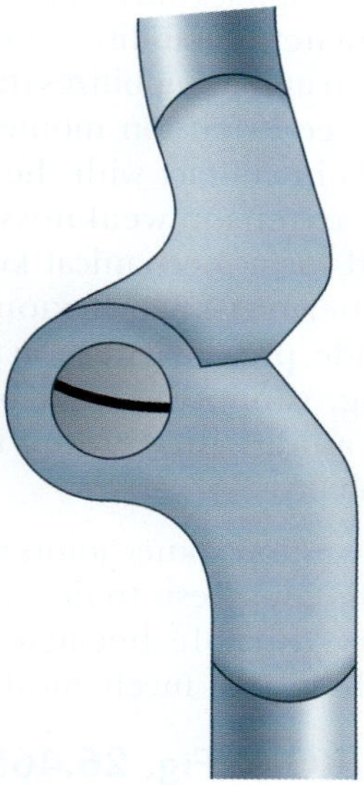

Fig. 26.467: Offset knee joint

Knee Cap

- Prevents knee flexion within the orthosis during stance phase.
- With medial/lateral strap, provides corrective force in genu varum or valgum.

Modifications of KAFO

Scott-Craig orthosis: Variation of metal KAFO. In spinal cord injured patients to stand and walk. Provides orthotic stabilization of knee, ankle and foot, passive or ligamentous stabilization to hip without additional components.

Consists of double uprights, one posterior thigh band, a hinged pretibial band, ankle joint with anterior and posterior adjustable pin stops, a cushion heel, a T-shaped footplate (embedded in the sole from heel to metatarsal heads).

Ankle joint in 10° of dorsiflexion is the key factor. The orthosis and the patients limbs, thus lean forward slightly. Balance is achieved by compensatory hyperextension of the hip joints, so that the center of gravity comes to a position posterior to the hip joints and anterior to the locked knee and ankle joints. Hinged pretibial band facilitates donning and doffing.

Floor reaction orthosis: Applies forces that resists recurvatum and provide mediolateral stability. The distal portion limits subtalar motion and immobilizes the ankle in slight equines so that a knee extension moment is produced, when the forefoot is in contact with the ground. In the presence of knee extensor weakness, this orthosis eliminates the need for a mechanical knee lock during stance phase and permits knee flexion during swing. Disadvantages include, proximal portion protrudes above the knee on sitting, cannot be used bilaterally, since positioning both ankles in equinus interferes with anteroposterior stability.

Modifications: Conventional knee joints and uprights are included to allow the prosthesis to flex at the knee joint, while sitting. Very durable because of its unitary construction and absence of mechanical parts.

Knee Orthoses (KOs) (Fig. 26.468)

Used, when only knee (mediolateral) control is required (not the foot and ankle). It consists of two lateral bars with thigh and calf cuffs. Bilateral or single knee pads may be used to control knee alignment. Example include Swedish knee cage, prevents recurvatum but permits flexion. Due to short lever arm, knee orthoses are not effective, when strong forces are required. Some tendency for theses orthoses to slip.

Three way knee stabilizer (Fig. 26.469): Pivotable attachments of straps, makes more cosmetic. No problem of prominence on sitting.

Hip Orthosis (HO)

- Controls selected motion of the hip
- Resists hip adduction.

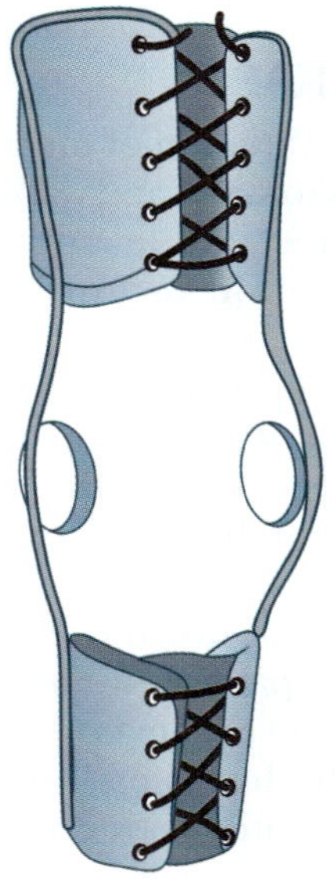

Fig. 26.468: A knee orthosis

Hip Joints and Pelvic Band

Unilateral pelvic band metal pelvic band (Fig. 26.470): Encompasses the pelvis on the involved side below the iliac crest and above the greater trochanter, continues around the opposite side in the form of a flexible belt.

Bilateral pelvic band (Fig. 26.471): Each side of the bilateral pelvic band begins at a point just posterior to the ASIS, midway between greater trochanter the iliac crests, then curves downwards and posteriorly to contact the most prominent portion of the buttocks and continues slightly upwards to overlie the sacrum.

Double pelvic band (Fig. 26.472): For maximum hip control.

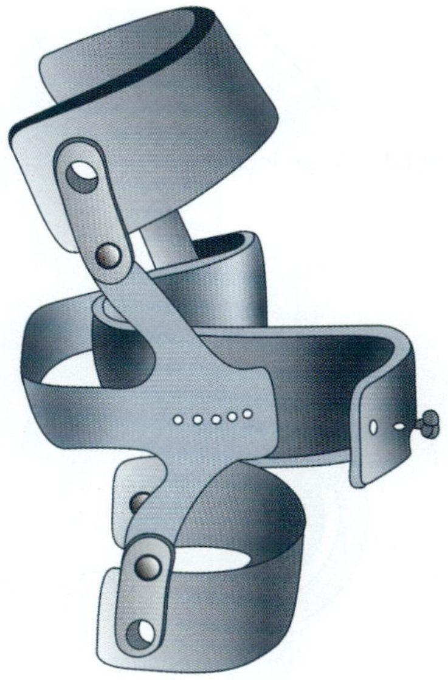

Fig. 26.469: Three way knee stabilizer

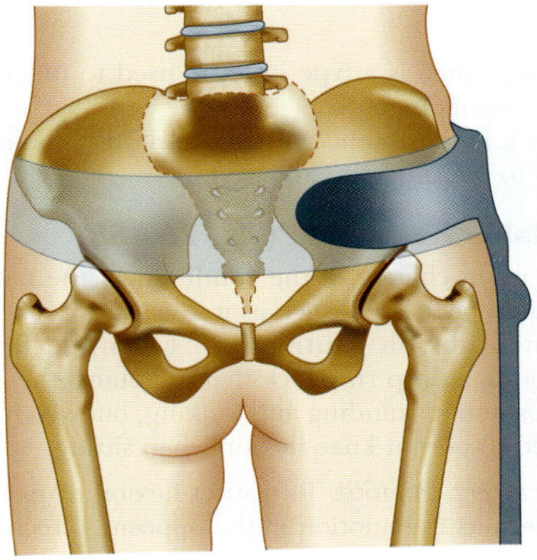

Fig. 26.470: Unilateral pelvic band metal pelvic band

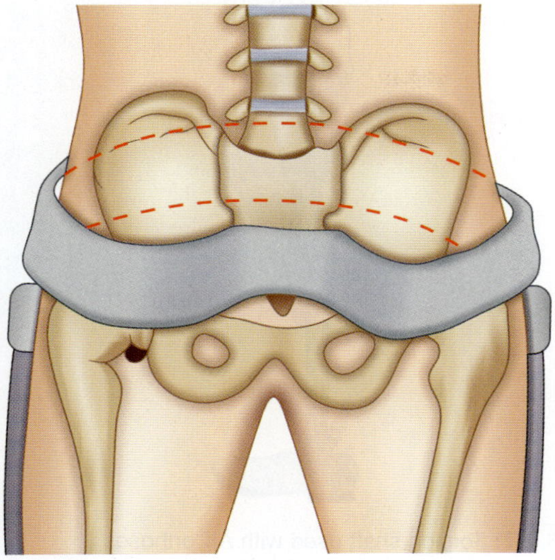

Fig. 26.471: Bilateral pelvic band

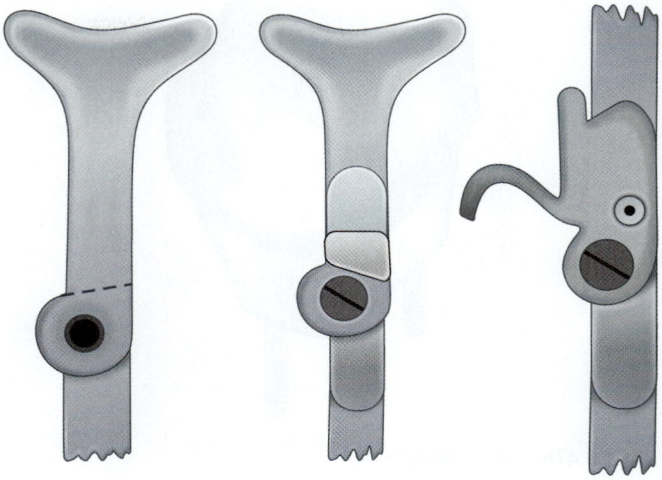

Fig. 26.473: Single-axis hip joints

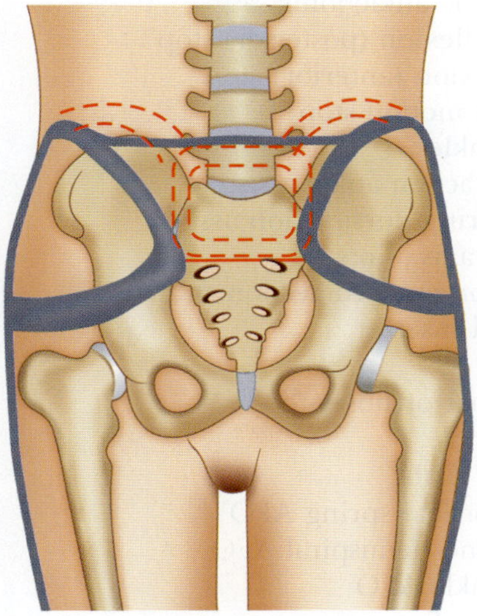

Fig. 26.472: Double pelvic band

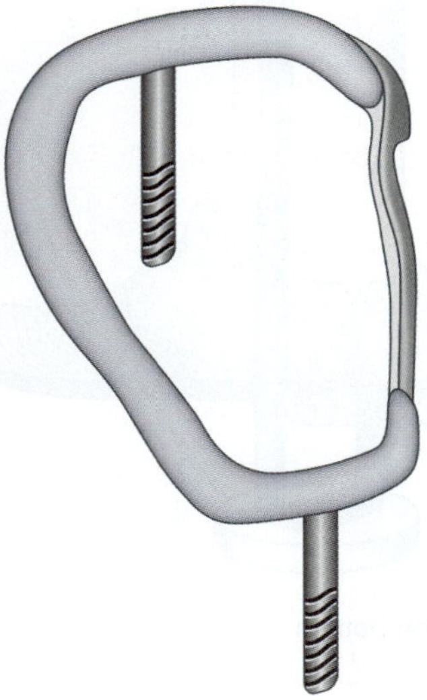

Fig. 26.474: Ischial ring

Hip-knee-ankle-foot Orthosis (HKAFO)

- To control the hip motion
- Attaching a hip joint and a pelvic band to the lateral upright of the KAFO.

Single axis hip joints (Fig. 26.473): It allows flexion and extension, but limited hyperextension. May include a lock to prevent flexion, while standing, whether locked or unlocked it controls mediolateral (abd-add) motion.

Double axis hip joints: It allows lateral motion in addition to flexion and extension used, where adduction and rotation control is desired.

Double position hip locks: Locking at both full extension and 90° of hip flexion. Useful for individuals with difficulty in maintaining the sitting position because of the spasticity of hip muscles.

Weight-bearing Devices

Ischial ring (Fig. 26.474): Simpler to fabricate. Weight-bearing surface is small. Little counterforce to maintain the ischial tuberosity on the ring.

Quadrilateral brim (Fig. 26.475): Gives good weight relief.

Patten bottom (Fig. 26.476): For complete weight relieving with quadrilateral brim. Weight is transmitted directly by the orthoses from the ischial tuberosity to the patten bottom. Ankle joint is eliminated, lateral uprights extend distal to the shoe. Requires contralateral shoe lift.

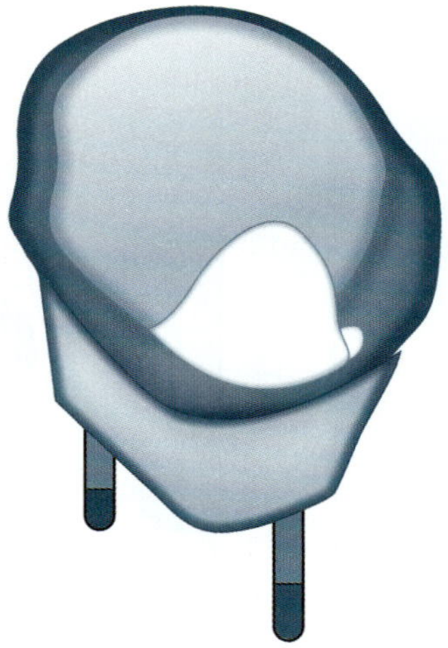

Fig. 26.475: Quadrilateral brim

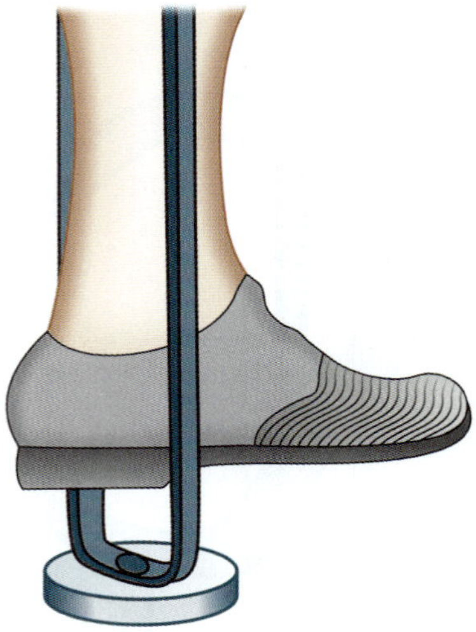

Fig. 26.476: Patten bottom

Torsion shaft used with AK orthoses (Fig. 26.477): Controls rotation at the hip, allows freedom of motion in all other directions. Used with a well-fitted pelvic band.

Special Purpose AK Orthoses

UCLA functional AK orthoses: It consists of a plastic quadrilateral thigh brim, offset knee joints, a plastic pretibial shell and hydraulic ankle joints. Provides stability at knee during stance phase, offers no resistance to flexion during the swing phase.

Below Knee Orthosis

- Shoes
- Stirrup
- Caliper
- Shoe insert

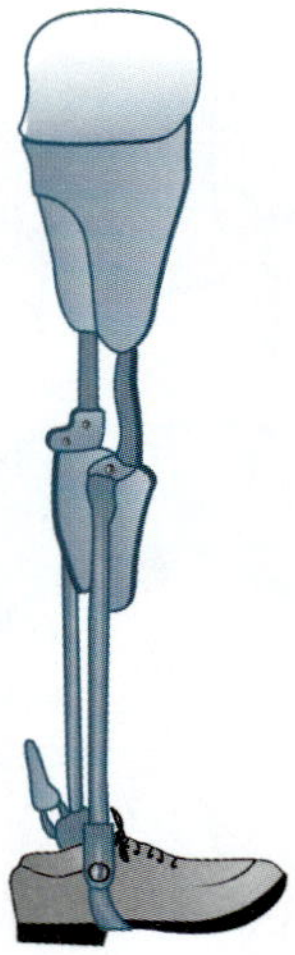

Fig. 26.477: Torsion shaft used with AK orthoses

- Little or no motion ankle
- Free ankle joint
- Adjustable ankle joint
- Plantar flexion (posterior) stop
- Dorsiflexion (anterior) stop
- Limited motion stop
- Solid ankle
- Double action ankle assist
- Wire spring dorsiflexion assist
- Double axis joints
- Valgus or varus correction straps
- Buckled inserter
- Pad
- Single bar orthoses
- Calf band
- Torsion shaft
- Posterior leaf-spring AFO
- Spiral and hemispiral AFO
- Solid ankle AFO
- AFO with flange
- PTB orthoses
- DB splint
- Knee-ankle-foot orthosis (KAFO)
- Free motion knee joints
- Drop-ring lock
- The plunger or internal lock
- Cam lock-pawl lock
- Swiss lock
- Adjustable knee lock
- Dial lock
- Offset knee joint
- Knee cap
- Scott-Craig orthosis
- Floor reaction orthosis
- Spring loaded dorsiflexion assist
- Knee orthoses (KOs)

- Swedish knee cage
- Unilateral pelvic band
- Bilateral pelvic band
- Double pelvic band
- Single axis hip joints
- Double axis hip joints
- Ischial ring
- Quadrilateral brim
- Patten bottom
- Torsion shaft used with AK orthoses
- UCLA functional AK orthoses

LOWER LIMB PROSTHESIS

■ Below-knee Prostheses

Basic components (Fig. 26.478): Foot-ankle assembly, shank, socket and suspension element.

Foot-ankle Assembly

All prostheses terminate in a foot-ankle assembly, which substitutes for the anatomic foot and ankle and satisfy several basic requirements. The assembly should:
- Provide a base for weight bearing
- Absorb shock at heal contact and rapidly reach foot-flat position
- Provide for metatasophalangeal hyperextension late in stance phase
- Resemble the general contour of the missing foot

In addition, many components offer additional functions, such as mediolateral motion or energy storage and return.

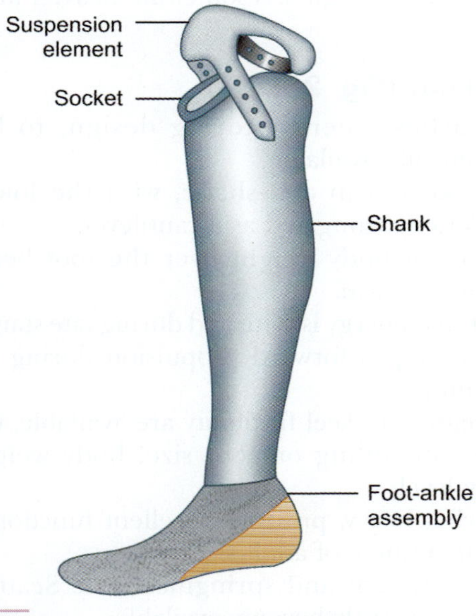

Fig. 26.478: Basic components of a prosthesis

Nonarticulated Components

Most below-knee prostheses incorporate a nonarticulated assembly. The foot is attached directly to the shank with neither a joint. No movement in the region corresponding to the natural ankle or natural appearance at the ankle. Durable, quieter and lighter than articulated components. The weight supporting structure inside the foot-designated as the keel. Keel is surrounded by resilient material in particular the heel area. Consequently, at heel contact, when the wearer first applies weight to the foot, the posterior material compresses, simulating plantar flexion and absorbing shock. As the individual moves forward, the keel provides a firm base of support. When weight has been transferred to the end of the keel, which is at a point corresponding to the metatarsophalangeal joints, the foot bends into to hyperextension, allowing the heel to lift from the ground. During swing phase, the unloaded foot reverts to a neutral position.

Solid Ankle Cushion Heel (SACH) Foot

The most frequently prescribed assembly. The cushion heel compresses when weight is applied, permitting the forefoot to approach the floor. The amount of this simulated plantar flexion depends on the resilience of the heel material and the weight and activity level of the wearer. Active or obese users require a firmer heel than feeble or slender individuals. As the keel is rigid, the SACH foot does not provide dorsiflexion.

SACH Foot with an Internal Keel (Fig. 26.479)

It consists of a wooden keel, covered by relatively incompressible foam and a synthetic rubber heel wedge. Belting, a strip of tough fabric, underlies the keel preventing it from puncturing the sole. A bolt through the keel attaches the foot to the shank. The material surrounding the keel does yield slightly upon application of weight, affording the patient a small amount of mediolateral and transverse motion to accommodate to irregular terrain.

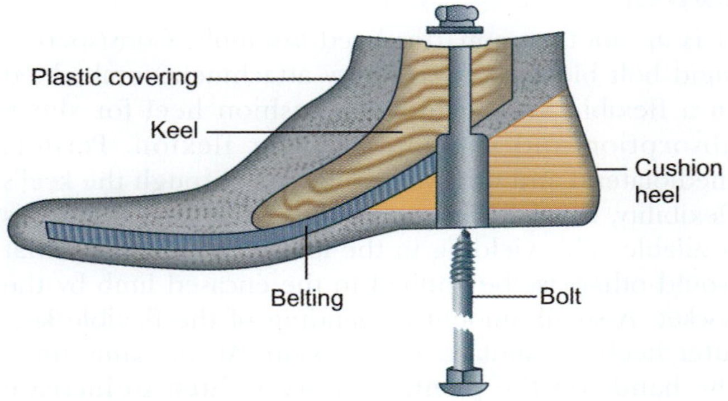

Fig. 26.479: SACH foot with internal keel

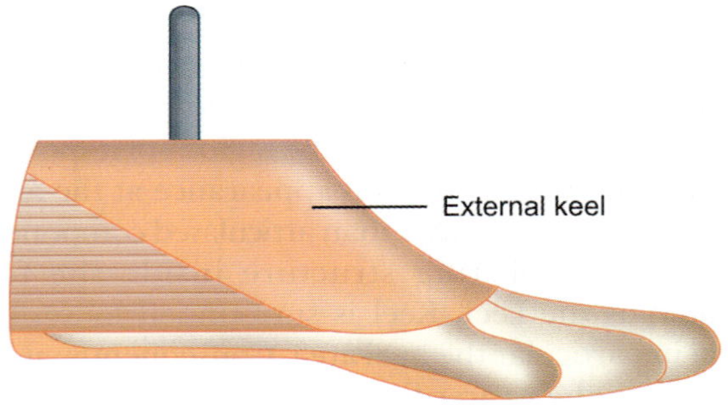

Fig. 26.480: SACH foot with external keel

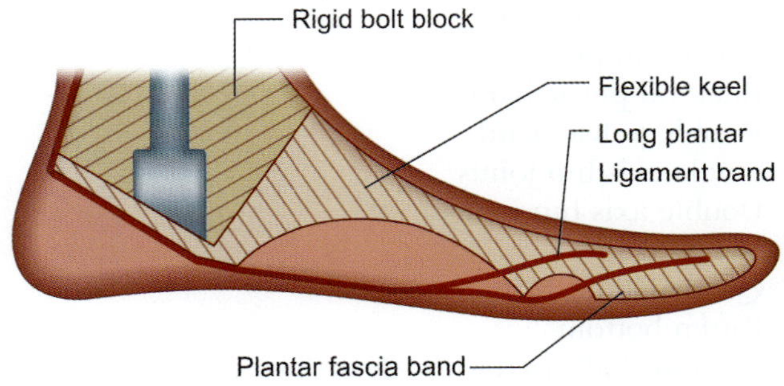

Fig. 26.481: SAFE foot

SACH Foot with an External Keel (Fig. 26.480)

The keel is wider than in the basic SACH foot. It has a greater mediolateral stability. Dorsum of the keel is exposed and can be covered with the same plastic laminate finishing, as on the shank, improving the appearance of the prosthesis. Mediolateral and transverse motion, however, are minimized.

SACH feet are relatively inexpensive and are manufactured in a wide range of sizes, suitable for young children's to large adult's feet. Models are available to accommodate flat-soled and high-heeled shoes as well as all amputation levels from Syme's upward. Versions with the forepart molded to suggest toes and toenails can be ordered, sometimes with a separation between the first and second toes to enable to wearing of thronged sandals.

Disadvantages

- The risk of delay in reaching the foot-flat position in early stance.
- If the patient does not transfer substantial weight to the prosthesis, the heel cushion will not compress adequately, the forefoot will fail to reach the floor quickly and the prosthesis will rotate forward on the heel as a pivot, thus tending to cause the knee to flex excessively.

Stationary Attachment/Flexible Endoskeleton (SAFE) Foot (Fig. 26.481)

It is an another nonarticulated assembly. Consists of a rigid bolt block (the stationary attachment) embedded in a flexible keel includes, a cushion heel for shock absorption and simulates plantar flexion. Permits mediolateral and transverse motion. Through the keel's flexibility, more frontal and transverse plane motion is available. This yielding in the foot reduces stresses that would otherwise be applied to the encased limb by the socket. A small amount of bending of the flexible keel after heel-off simulates dorsiflexion. At this same time, the bands on the plantar surface tighten to increase structural stability, similar to the plantar aponeurosis in the anatomic foot. Available in adult sizes, is heavier and more expensive. Can be used for all amputation levels, including Syme's.

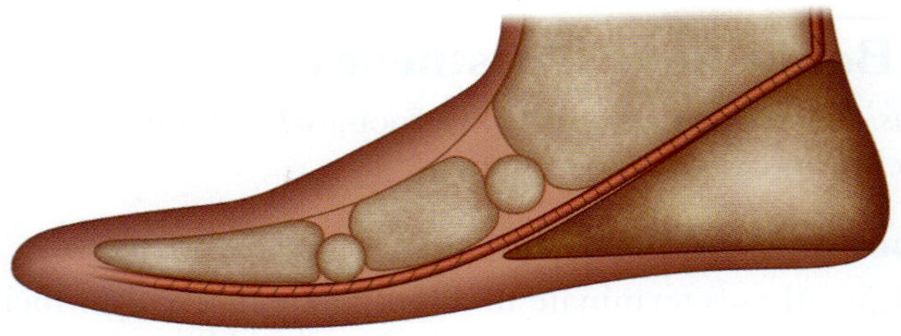

Fig. 26.482: STEN foot

Stored Energy (STEN) Foot (Fig. 26.482)

It includes a wood keel, which is in three pieces joined by two rubber plugs. Transfer of body weight over the foot first compresses the plugs, then permits them to recoil. With this design, the amount of energy return is quite modest. In all other respects, the STEN foot duplicates the SACH foot, though it is somewhat heavier and more expensive.

Seattle Foot (Fig. 26.483)

- The earliest energy storing design, to become commercially available.
- Delrin keel is in a C-shape, with the lower arm considerably elongated as a cantilever.
- Transfer of body weight over the foot bends the cantilevered arm.
- This stored energy is returned during late stance, thus contributing to forward propulsion during walking and running.
- Five degrees of keel flexibility are available, with the choice depending on foot size, body weight and activity level.
- Somewhat heavy, provides excellent function and is made in a range of adult sizes.
- Reduced weight and springiness (the Seattle Litte Foot) has recently become available.

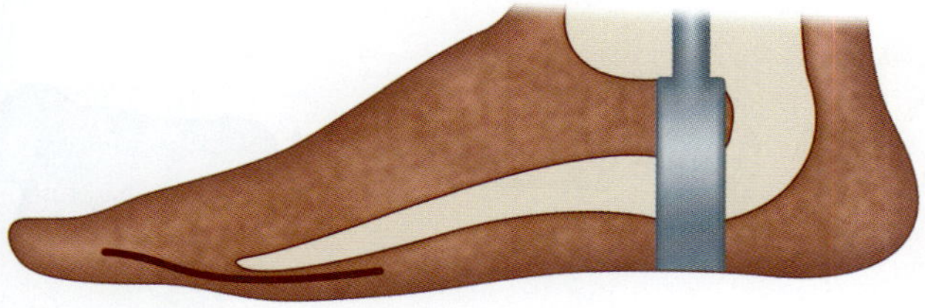

Fig. 26.483: Seattle foot

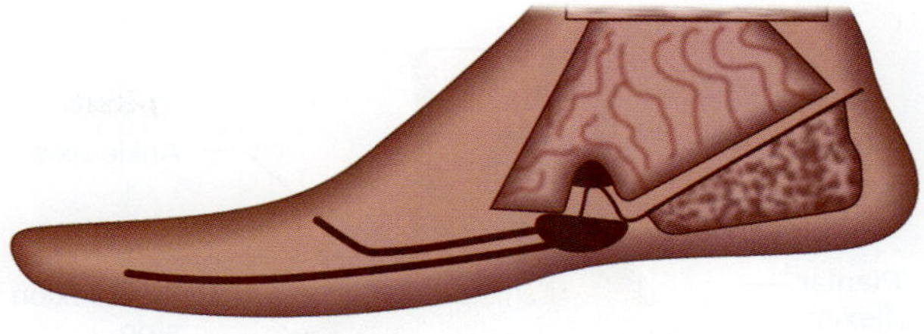

Fig. 26.484: Carbon copy II foot

Carbon Copy II (Fig. 26.484)

- Considerable energy is stored and returned.
- Keel is composed of two strong, but light plates constructed of carbon composites.
- The longer deflection plate, which terminates at the level of the distal interphalangeal joints, returns energy during walking.
- The shorter, upper plate is activated under very high loads (jumping or running).
- Relatively, lightweight and durable, but provides little mediolateral motion.
- It is manufactured in adult sizes to suit shoes of two low-heel heights.

Quantum

- Lightweight nonarticulated foot.
- Heel is in the form of a spring module, consisting of a lower and upper deflection plate attached to the ankle base.
- From the base, the plates project forward to the metatarsophalangeal joints and backward into the heel.
- No cushion heel.
- Simulated plantar flexion and impact absorption are provided by the heel deflection plates.
- The lower of the two plates that project forward is the primary spring that stores and returns energy during the last half of stance phase, while the secondary upper plate acts as an overload spring in case of unusually high forces.
- The spring module or keel, which is available in several degrees of firmness is encased in a semiflexible cosmetic shell, which yields to medial and lateral loads, affording the wearer inversion and eversion to accommodate ground irregularities.
- Manufactured in adult sizes to fit low-heeled shoes.

Flex-Walk

- Energy storing, nonarticulated foot-ankle assembly.
- Heel is made of lightweight carbon graphite composite.
- As in the Quantum foot, the keel extends forward to the metatarsophalangeal joint line and includes a heel section, which substitutes for a compressible cushion heel.
- Heel section comes in two versions suitable for either a high or a low-heeled shoe.
- Relatively broad keel provides little inversion-eversion; rather it is stable mediolaterally and resists torsion.
- Nine Flex-Walk modules of different resistance's are available with the choice based on the body weight and activity level of the user.
- The module is encased in a plastic foam cosmetic cover, to create a pleasing appearance and is sized for both adults and children.

Flex-Foot

The above description of the Flex-Walk applies equally to the distal portion of the Flex-Foot. Flex-Foot keel extends from the metatarsophalangeal joint line to the bottom of the below-knee socket or for above-knee wearers to the knee unit.

Heel forms the shank of the prosthesis. This shank portion acts as a long leaf spring. Stores and returns more energy than any other foot-ankle assembly. Lighter than one with other foot-ankle components. Requires sufficient space between the floor and the residuum end and is more expensive than other feet.

Articulated Components

Motion between the foot and shank can occur around an articulation in the region corresponding to the anatomical ankle.

More adjustable than nonarticulated alternatives and at early stance, plantar flex more readily. Heavier and more likely to develop looseness in the mechanism which causes unwanted noise.

Single Axis Assembly (Fig. 26.485)

- The base of the foot is connected to the ankle block by a bolt.
- The transverse ankle axis permits the foot to go into plantar flexion and dorsiflexion.
- All motion is around one axis.
- As the foot plantar flexes, a posterior bumper (a small cylinder of rubber behind the ankle axis) is

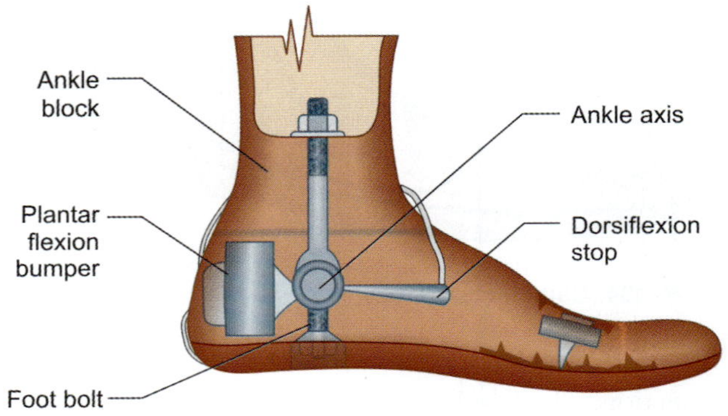

Fig. 26.485: Single axis assembly

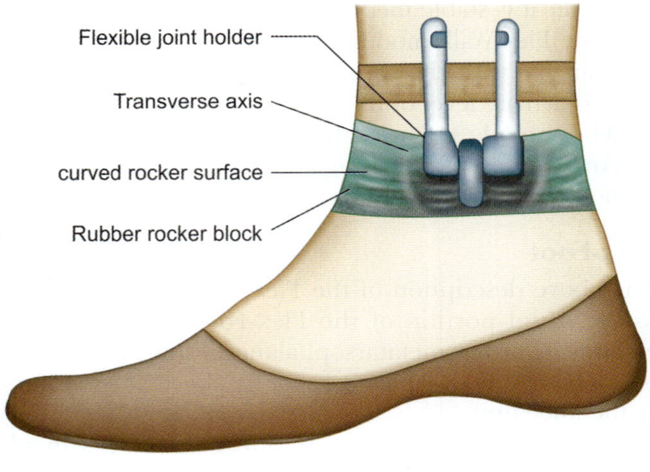

Fig. 26.486: Multiple-axis foot-ankle assembly

compressed, resisting the motion. The action of the bumper corresponds to the action of the dorsiflexors of the foot in the intact limb.

- The bumper permits about 15° of plantar flexion. In the opposite direction, motion is resisted by the dorsiflexion stop, which is positioned in front of the ankle axis.
- The dorsiflexion stop is made of firm rubber, felt or resilient plastic, and premits less than 5° of dorsiflexion.
- The toe section of the foot bends during the push-off phase of walking and returns to a neutral position in swing phase. This action is achieved by means of a flexible toe section or a toe break with a rubber bumper.

Multiple-axis Foot-ankle Assembly (Fig. 26.486)

- Permits movement in any direction: plantar flexion, dorsiflexion, inversion, eversion and a slight amount of rotation around a vertical axis.

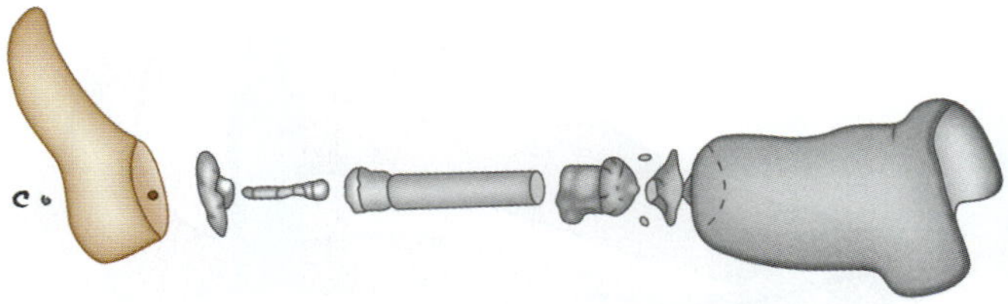

Fig. 26.487: Shank maintains the spatial relationship between the socket and foot

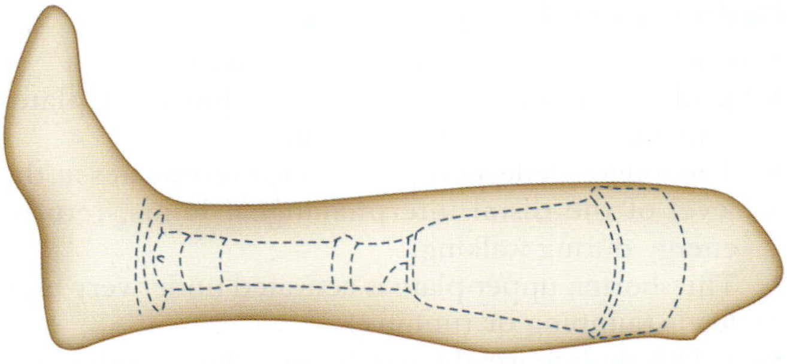

Fig. 26.488: A soft cosmetic cover surrounds the endoskeleton to provide a lifelike appearance.

- The lower end of the ankle block has a curved surface that rests on a rubber rocker block.
- Curved surface permits the foot to rotate around the transverse axis of the ankle joint, so that it can go into moderate plantar flexion and slight dorsiflexion. This transverse axis is positioned in a flexible joint holder, thus permitting mediolateral motion and slight rotation in the horizontal plane.
- Accommodates to uneven walking surfaces and absorbs some of the torsional forces created in walking, thus reducing torque to the limb by the socket.
- Relatively bulky, heavy, expensive and may require more maintenance.
- Greater latitude of movement may create instability in patients, who have marginal coordination.

Shank (Figs 26.487 and 26.488)

It may be of exoskeletal (crustacean) or of endoskeletal (central support or pylon) construction. Shank maintains the spatial relationship between the socket and foot, and transmits the load from the socket above to the foot below.

Exoskeletal shank is commonly made from light but strong and rigid plastic foam. Alternatively, wood may be used, in which case the space between the bottom of the socket and the ankle block should be hollowed to reduce weight. Whether foam or wood, a light and strong, waterproof finish is provided by an external lamination around the shank.

In the *endoskeletal type*, a metal or plastic tube connects the socket and foot-ankle assembly.

Advantages of a modest reduction in weight (more significant weight savings are provided for above-knee and hip-disarticulation prostheses) and incorporation of the means of adjusting the alignment of the prosthesis. A disadvantage is that the cosmetic cover is much less durable than the laminate finish.

Socket

Serves two essential purposes, containment of the tissues of the stump and transmission of body weight to the floor.

PTB Socket

Introduced in 1958, is by far the most frequently used design throughout the world. Made of laminated or molded plastic and provides an intimate fit over the entire area of the stump. The socket is shaped so that a substantial amount of weight is borne on the patellar tendon, the flares of the tibia and anteriorly on either sides of the tibial crest. The intimately fitted socket should be totally in contact with the entire residuum, including the distal end. This feature helps to prevent edema, provides some additional support area (although the end of the stump cannot usually tolerate much pressure) and probably provides better sensory feedback because of the greater area of contact. To enhance comfort, the basic PTB socket also incorporates a compressible liner or soft insert, commonly formed of Pe-Lite, a closed cell and polyethylene foam.

Hard Socket

A variant of the basic PTB socket, in which the soft insert is eliminated. Used for those with mature residua with good tissue covering and for those with severe perspiration problems. Less likely to be used for elderly amputees with poor tissue covering of the stump and for patients with continuing vascular problems, sensitive tissue or fluctuating stump size.

ISNY PTB Socket (Fig. 26.489)

In 1982, Ossur Kristinsson of Iceland proposed a socket design for the above-knee amputee, consisting of two separate structures, each of which provides one function. Further development of this idea took place at the Een-Holmgren company in Sweden, while an extension of this concept to the below-knee amputee has been undertaken, primarily at prosthetics and Orthotics, New York University, hence the designation "INSY" (Icelandic-Swedish-New York University). The ISNY Socket System for the below-knee amputee consists of a thin, flexible, vacuum-formed, thermoplastic PTB socket for tissue containment; and a rigid, carbon-fiber-reinforced and laminated frame for weight transmission. The frame consists of three struts (one posterior and two anterior), which connect the distal end-cup to the proximal segments covering the patellar-tendon medial flare, and popliteal areas.

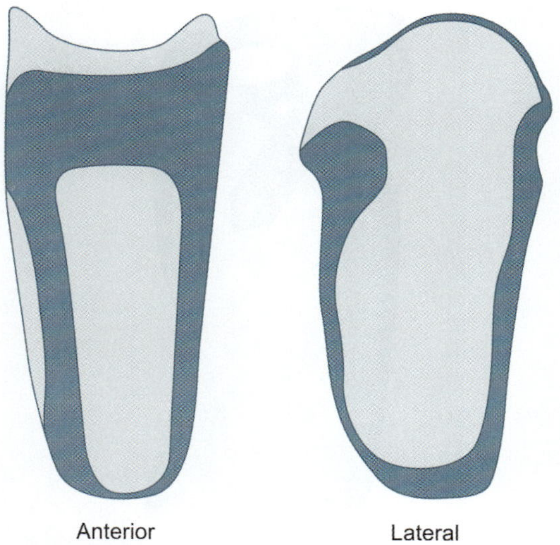

Fig. 26.489: The ISNY PTB socket

Advantages

- Enhanced comfort, because the socket's flexibility allows it to change shape to correspond with stump changes due to muscle contraction or motion.
- Thinness (1/16–3/32 inches) permits improved heat dissipation so that sockets feel cooler.
- Translucency of the thermoplastic, enables it to serve as both a check or trial socket as well as definitive or permanent socket.
- Ease and speed of socket modification and replacement are significantly increased.

Disadvantages: Thin thermoplastic socket is not as durable as the rigid laminated version and the appearance of the socket-frame combination may be displeasing.

Suspension Systems

Cuff Suspension (Fig. 26.490)

PTB prosthesis is suspended by means of a cuff, which is attached to the medial and lateral socket walls, passes over the superior edge of the patella and encircles the thigh above the femoral condyles. The cuff serves primarily to retain the prosthesis on the limb. Provides only slight assistance for mediolateral stability but resists forces that tend to move the knee into hyperextension. Most amputees, with the possible exception of those with short or painful residua, find the stump-socket pressures well within their tolerance with this type of suspension.

Supracondylar (SC) System

Employs medial and lateral walls higher than those of the original PTB design. The higher walls encompass the femoral epicondyles duly and terminates proximally with a smaller mediolateral diameter than that at the

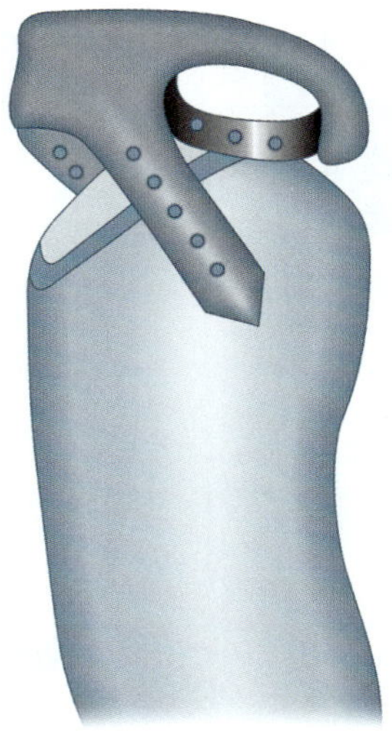

Fig. 26.490: A cuff suspension

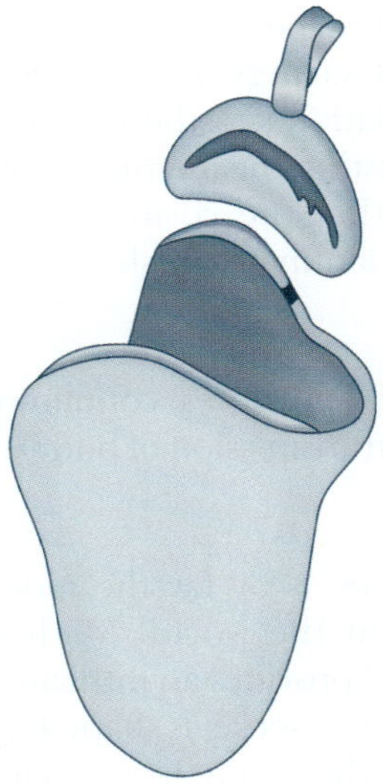

Fig. 26.491: A wedge suspension system

apices of the epicondyles. Therefore, once donned the prosthesis cannot slip down over the epicondyles.

Two Methods Facilitate Donning

1. The first involves forming the medial and lateral walls of the socket with sufficient width to permit the relatively protuberant epicondyles to enter the socket. Once the amputee has inserted the limb into the socket, the space is filled with a removable plastic wedge inserted between the socket wall and the medial epicondyle, as shown in Figure 26.491.
2. An alternate method, probably more commonly used, is to incorporate into the soft insert a contoured proximomedial buildup which serves the same function as the removable wedge. The compressible, but resilient buildup allows the epicondyles to enter the socket and yet retains firm suspension. Occasionally, if donning is difficult, a proximolateral soft insert buildup may be added.

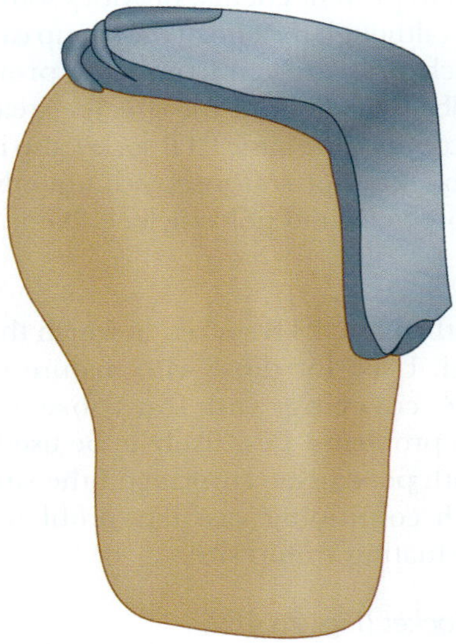

Fig. 26.492: Supracondylar/Suprapatellar (SC/SP) system

Supracondylar/Suprapatellar (SC/SP) System (Fig. 26.492)

It has similarly high medial and lateral socket walls, and in addition, has a high anterior wall which covers the entire patella.

The high molded anterior wall of the SC/SP not only helps retain the prosthesis on the limb, but effectively resists any tendency toward recurvatum. The proximal brims of both the SC and the SC/SP are somewhat more bulky and the high anterior brim of the SC/SP may protrude uncosmetically when the wearer sits.

Thigh Corset (Fig. 26.493)

Attached to the socket and shank, by the side bars and knee-joint assembly. In addition to suspending the prosthesis, it supports part of the body weight, provides mediolateral stability and increases sensory feedback. In some cases, a flexible waist belt and fork-strap assembly are used to aid in suspension. The fork strap is attached to the shank of the prosthesis and by an elastic strap to the waist belt. The elastic strap exerts an upward pull on the prosthesis to aid in suspension.

When the knee is flexed, the elastic strap is stretched further and the increased tension acts to extend the knee. A check strap, if used extends from the posterior aspect of the thigh corset to the shank and checks the motion of the shank, as the knee approaches full extension, preventing the metal stops of the knee joint from coming into abrupt and noisy contact.

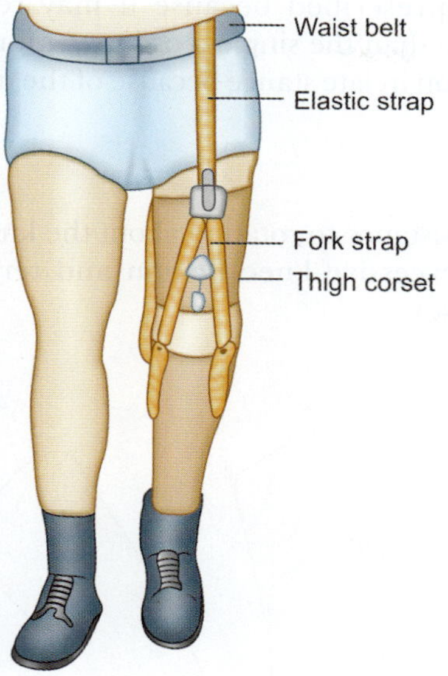

Fig. 26.493: A thigh corset

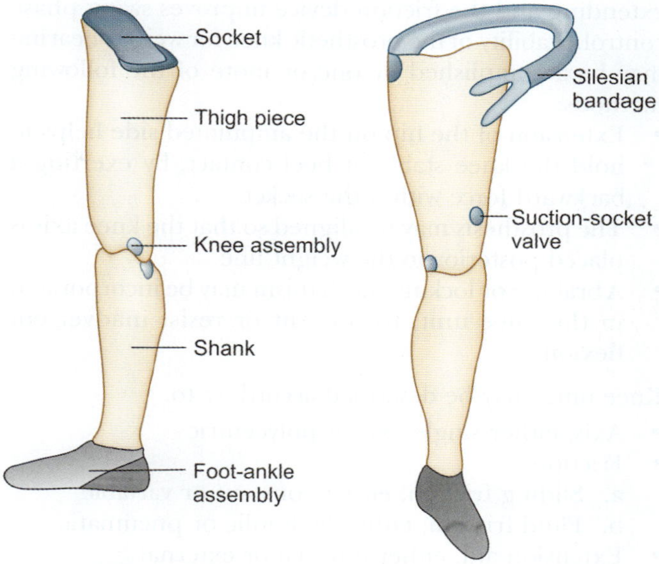

Fig. 26.494: Above-knee prosthesis with its components

Disadvantages: Thigh corset are bulky, adds to the weight of the prosthesis, its constricting effect may cause atrophy of the thigh and it may aggravate any edema in the amputated limb.

Rotator Unit

When an amputee walks, the socket tends to twist on the amputated limb, causing a shearing effect at the stump-socket interface. Some of the torsional forces are absorbed in the foot-ankle assembly, so that the residual torque is not troublesome. In other cases, particularly with active amputees, the torque applied to the stump is a source of discomfort.

To cope with this problem, a torque-absorber rotator mechanism may be used. It is not indicated for most below-knee amputees, but may be useful for those, who have thigh corsets or are active athletes encountering discomfort. The rotator unit is interposed between the lower end of the shank and the foot-ankle assembly. A resilient element that is incorporated between the upper and lower attachments of the unit permits the rotation of the shank to take place, while the foot is in contact with the floor. Different models are available for use with exoskeletal and endoskeletal shank construction.

■ Above-knee Prosthesis

Components (Fig. 26.494): The foot-ankle assembly, shank, knee assembly, socket and suspension device.

Foot-ankle Assembly

Any of the foot-ankle assemblies, described on below-knee prostheses and components, may be incorporated in the above-knee prosthesis. Knee stability may be a problem for the above-knee amputee and the anticipated activity level may be comparatively low. Consequently, fewer energy-storing feet and more single-axis feet are indicated. Also, the heel cushion of SACH-type feet usually will be more compressible.

Shank

It is a structure that connects the foot-ankle assembly to the knee unit. The exoskeletal shank is usually made of rigid foam or wood, covered with plastic laminate and differs from the shank of the below-knee prosthesis in that it does not contain a socket. In an endoskeletal system a shank tube, with adaptors at both ends, connects the foot-ankle assembly to the knee unit. A thigh tube with adaptors at both ends connects the knee unit to the socket. Desired alignment relationships are achieved by means of the adjustable adaptors, as shown in the Figure 26.495. After the endoskeleton and socket have been assembled and aligned, a foam rubber outer cover is applied and shaped to provide an acceptable appearance. As compared with the exoskeletal prosthesis, the endoskeletal system is appreciably lighter in weight and more attractive, however the covering deteriorates rather rapidly with repeated bending of the knee.

Knee Assembly

It consists of a wooden or plastic knee block, an axis within the block, a friction device, and an extension stop. The upper part of the knee block is attached either to the lower end of the socket, or to the thigh tube of an endoskeletal system. The axis permits the knee to bend, the extension stop prevents the knee from hyper extending and the friction device improves swing phase control. Stability of the prosthetic knee for weight-bearing may be accomplished by one or more of the following methods:

- Extension of the hip on the amputated side helps to hold the knee stable at heel contact, by exerting a backward force within the socket.
- The prosthesis may be aligned so that the knee axis is placed posterior to the weight line.
- A braking or locking mechanism may be incorporated in the knee unit, to prevent or resist inadvertent flexion.

Knee units may be described according to:

- Axis, either single axis or polycentric
- Friction
  a. Sliding friction, either constant or variable
  b. Fluid friction, either hydraulic or pneumatic
- Extension aid, either internal or external
- Braking or locking mechanism

Many combinations of these features are incorporated in various knee assemblies.

Knee Axis

Single axis (Fig. 26.496): In this common type of knee, flexion and extension occur around a single axis. Advantages are its simplicity (few moving parts) and minimal noise, maintenance and cost.

Polycentric axis (Fig. 26.497): The knee block and the shank are attached to each other, by means of multiple linkage, so that rotation occurs around a constantly shifting axis. Advantage is its inherent stability and it is, therefore, useful for patients with short above-knee amputations. Less often prescribed because it may require more maintenance than the single-axis knee. More difficult to initiate flexion in late stance because of the unit's marked stability.

Friction

Applying resistance to rotation about the knee axis helps to control excessive knee flexion and terminal-swing impact (noise).

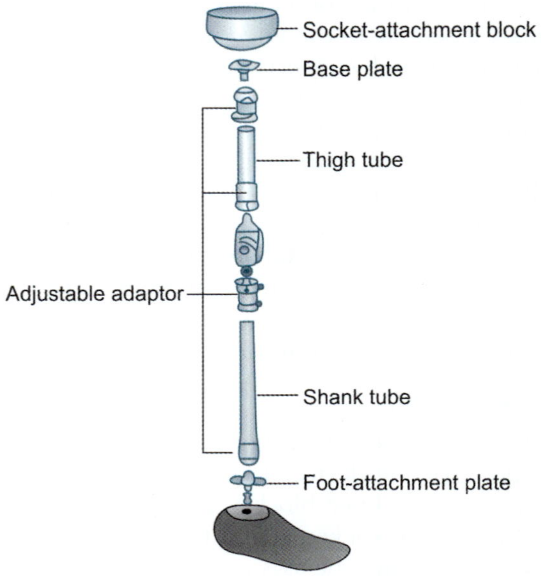

Fig. 26.495: Components of above-knee endoskeletal prosthesis

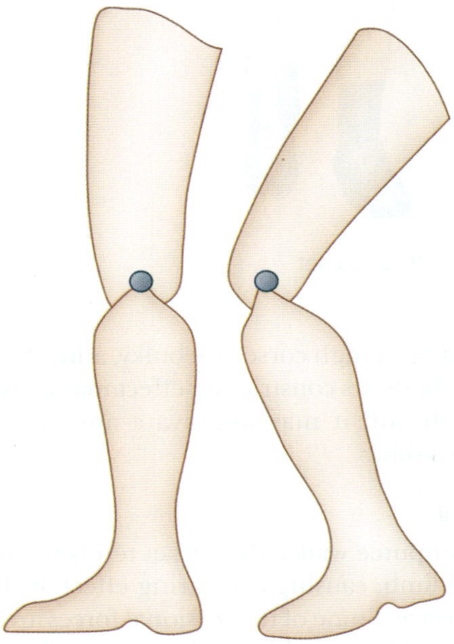

Fig. 26.496: Single-axis knee prosthesis

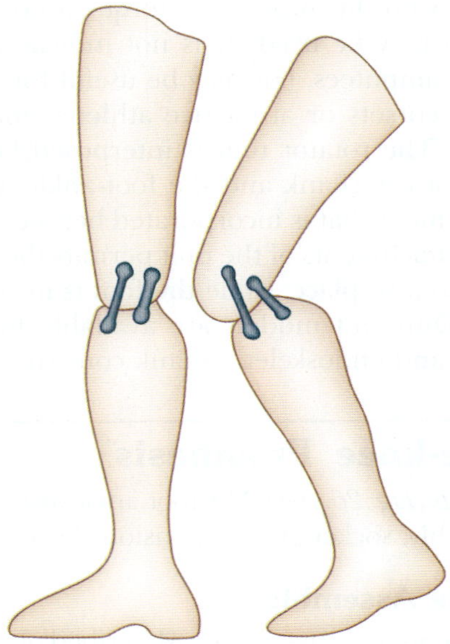

Fig. 26.497: Polycentric knee axis

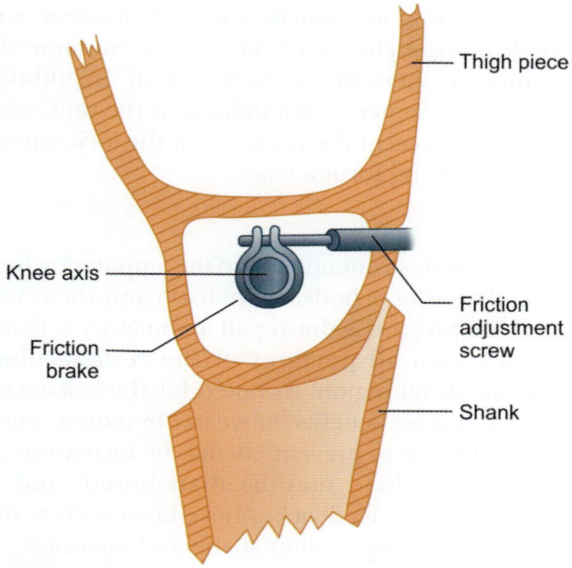

Fig. 26.498: Constant friction knee unit

Constant friction (Fig. 26.498): Most commonly used. Same amount of resistance is applied throughout swing phase. Resistance is usually achieved by a sleeve or split bushing and clamp, which slide around the knee bolt. The amount of friction is increased or decreased, by rotating the friction-adjustment screw, which tightens or loosens the sleeve or bushing. Simple, low in cost, light in weight, quiet, easy to adjust and requires relatively little maintenance. It does not, however produce normal swing phase kinematics, in which early and late swing are damped. On the other hand, if a swing phase of reasonably normal appearance does result, it will occur at only one cadence. Faster or slower walking will produce asymmetrical swing.

Variable friction (Fig. 26.499): Has provision to vary the degree of friction during each subphase of the swing of the shank. Provides relatively greater resistance at the beginning and at the end of swing phase and less friction during midswing. In one device of this type, variation of resistance is achieved by the action of several segmented friction elements, which rotate with the knee axis. As knee motion takes place, the individual segments contact the plate successively, providing increased resistance at the beginning and at the end of swing phase. A friction-adjustment wheel is rotated clockwise or counterclockwise to increase or decrease the friction. Variable friction device tend to have increased noise and higher maintenance is sometimes required because of the larger number of moving parts.

Fluid Control

Most fluid-controlled prosthesis are hydraulic (oil), but several pneumatic (air) systems are also available. Fluid-controlled units are designed to provide cadence-dependent motion. The adjustments initially made are retained more adequately, because these units are sealed to exclude outside material. In the typical hydraulic mechanism, oil is forced through a series of passages by a piston. The resistance encountered depends on the type of oil, the rate of flow (governed by the speed of shank swing) and the characteristics of the channels, which are usually patterned so that the resistance varies through the swing.

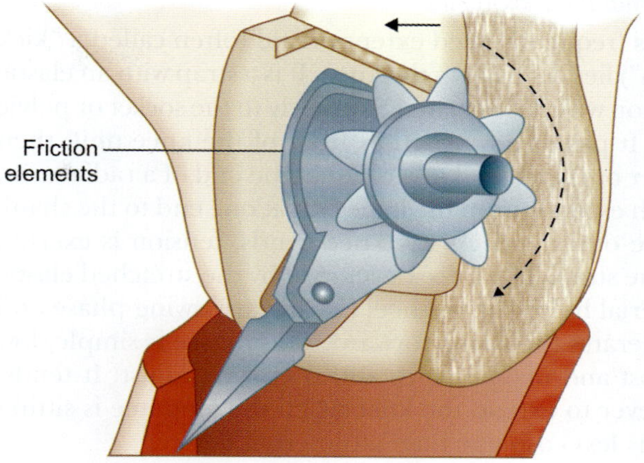

Fig. 26.499: Variable friction unit

Extension Aids

Some patients find that additional mechanical assistance is needed to control heel rise or to accelerate the shank during its forward swing. This may be accomplished by an extension aid. This assistive device is also useful, when the wearer takes short steps, as when working in a confined area.

Internal Extension Aid

The lever is a type of internal extension aid. The upper end of the lever is attached to the knee block at a point posterior to the knee center, while the lower end is attached to an extension bias spring, which is fastened at its other end to the upper part of the shank. As the knee bends, the spring is stretched, thus providing the force to restrain heel rise and to accelerate the shank forward during the initial part of the swing phase. In some instances, a compression spring is used instead of a tension spring, but the action is essentially the same. The internal extension aid is inconspicuous because it is contained within the prosthesis and it does not tend to cause the prosthetic knee to extend, when the wearer is seated. Occasionally, it can be noisy and it is difficulty to adjust on some knee models. All fluid-controlled units have extension bias quite similar in function to an internal extension aid.

External Extension Aid

A less frequently used extension aid (often called a "kick strap") lies external to the knee. It is a strap with an elastic portion which is fastened anteriorly to the socket or pelvic belt. It passes downward in front of the knee unit, then under or is attached to a roller at the end of a radial arm, which extends from the knee bolt at one end to the shank at the other end. As the knee bends, tension is exerted on the strap. The force developed by the stretched elastic material helps control heel rise in early swing phase and accelerates the shank forward. This device is simple, low in cost and maintenance and is easy to adjust. It tends, however to extend the knee when the amputee is sitting and is less cosmetic than an internal device.

Braking and Locking Mechanisms

Weight-activated friction brake: Stability may be attained by the use of a weight-activated friction brake. When weight is borne on the prosthesis, even if the knee is inadvertently flexed 20° to 25°, the friction brake automatically resists further knee motion, thus preventing buckling. During swing phase, the brake does not impede motion. Several models are available. In the design, the mechanism includes mating, wedge-shaped brake surfaces on the lower section of the knee block and upper section of the shank which are in very light contact during swing phase. When the amputee places weight on the prosthesis, the two brake surfaces are forced into firm contact, thus resisting inadvertent flexion. The primary advantage of a friction brake is the stability, which is inherent in the mechanism and only incidentally depends upon the amputee's strength and coordination. Accordingly, it is usually reserved for weak, elderly patients or for those whose vocational or avocational activities pose stability problems, which cannot be addressed by alignment or other means. Units with friction brakes have more moving parts, are slightly heavier are likely to be noisier, require more frequent adjustment and are more expensive. In addition, should the wearer wish to attempt them, activities such as step-over-step stair descent, which require knee motion under weight bearing are prevented by the brake.

Manual Lock

Maximum stability is achieved with a manual lock. When the knee is fully extended (as in rising from the seated to the standing position), the locking lever drops automatically to immobilize the knee. The amputee unlocks the unit by manipulating the locking lever. The manual lock is indicated for the amputee, who needs the utmost stability because of poor coordination or muscular weakness. Occasionally, it may be used for a more active person whose occupation requires a great deal of standing. When engaged, the manual lock forces the amputee to walk without flexing the prosthetic knee, which usually produces a halting, uncosmetic gait and problems with ground clearance. The latter difficulty is minimized if the prosthesis is shortened 1 cm (1/2 inch). In addition, the wearer must contend with unlocking the unit, when sitting and must accept the noisiness of the lock, when it engages upon rising form a chair.

Socket

Provide comfortable containment to the amputation limb, support and transfer of body weight to the prosthetic foot, control of the prosthesis during all ambulatory activities and contact with all portions of the residual limb, including the distal region. As noted for the below-knee socket, distal contact benefits the wearer by aiding venous return and helping to prevent edema, by increasing the area over which load may be distributed, and by augmenting sensory feedback. Above-knee sockets may be classified according to their shape and materials.

Quadrilateral Shape

The posterior socket wall, intended for substantial weight-bearing has a proximal brim lying directly under the ischial tuberosity and buttock. As the anterior wall must apply posteriorly directed forces, to maintain the position of the ischial tuberosity on the posterior brim, it is relatively close to and higher than the posterior wall. Thus, the quadrilateral socket proximally is narrow from anterior to posterior and relatively wide mediolaterally.

Ischial Containment Shape

Shaped, so that the tuberosity lies within the socket. The posterior wall extends higher than in the quadrilateral shape, as does the posterior half of the medial wall, which covers the pubic ramus rather than lying beneath it. Relatively, narrow in the mediolateral dimension, and relatively wide anteroposteriorly. Both sockets are intended to contact the amputation limb totally. Ischial containment sockets, with their higher trimlines, appear to be especially suitable for patients with very short amputation limbs and seem to satisfy younger individuals, who are active sports participants. For bilateral above-knee amputees, the narrow mediolateral dimension may improve perineal clearance during walking.

Materials

Both quadrilateral and ischial containment sockets may be fabricated of flexible or rigid materials. A flexible socket is molded of thin polyethylene or other thermoplastic and nests in a rigid frame. These sockets enhance comfort, adapt their shape, especially to chair seats, increase sensory input and are cooler because body heat dissipates through the thin walls. The customary thermoplastics used in prosthetics are transparent or translucent, thus one may view the amputation limb as the patient stands and walks. Flexibility improves suction suspension and wearers perceive the prosthesis, as being lighter in weight. Socket adjustments can often be accomplished easily, by spot heating the thermoplastic material and reshaping. The frame can be made of carbon-fiber reinforced polyester laminate or of other rigid materials. Due to its strength and rigidity, the frame need cover a small part of the socket, leaving most of the amputation limb encased in flexible material only. The frame can be attached to any appropriate knee unit, and any mode of suspension may be used with the flexible socket and rigid frame combination. In lieu of a flexible socket, the patient may be fitted with a rigid one, usually made of polyester laminate. Fabrication is somewhat simpler, thus the cost may be slightly less than for a flexible socket. In addition, the rigid socket may prove more durable for the exceptionally active user. A client habituated to a rigid socket may resist changing to a flexible one, though patient acceptance of flexible designs has been remarkably positive.

Suspension Device

The above-knee prosthesis may be suspended by:

- Suction alone or suction with auxiliary suspension.
- Partial suction with auxiliary suspension.
- No suction with complete reliance on a pelvic belt.

Suction suspension: The suction socket is ideal for an amputee, who has a well-shaped, fairly strong residuum. More preferred for younger and active patients. Has a one-way valve that allows air to be expelled from the socket in stance phase. During swing phase, when gravity tends to make the prosthesis drop from the thigh, suction created within the socket holds the prosthesis in place. When suction suspension is used, a very close fit of the brim is required to make the socket airtight. No sock is worn, since it would interfere with the airtight seal produced by the close proximal fit. The socket is donned with the aid of a donning sock or elastic bandage, which is applied to the residuum and used to pull the limb into the socket. The sock or bandage is removed, by pulling it through the valve hole in the distal aspect of the socket. Alternatively, the wearer may lubricate the thigh and socket with lotion and then slide into the socket. Suction suspension offered the wearer greater freedom of motion, increased use of the remaining musculature, decreased piston action between limb and socket and more comfort and improved appearance because all torso straps and belts are eliminated.

Due to mandatory close fit, suction may be unsuitable for elderly amputees because of relative difficulty of donning. In addition, residuum volume fluctuations may preclude maintenance of a snug suction socket fit. In some cases additional suspension may be needed to retain the suction socket or control its motion, particularly rotation or abduction. A Silesian bandage is often used for this purpose.

Partial Suction with Auxiliary Suspension

If the total suction socket cannot be utilized because of difficulty in donning the prosthesis, inability to tolerate the prosthesis without a sock or volume fluctuation, a partial suction socket and auxiliary suspension may be beneficial.

In this arrangement, a suction valve is used, but the amputee wears a sock, the socket is not as intimately fitted and the thickness of sock can be varied to accommodate changes in limb volume. The slightly looser fit enables the prosthesis to be donned without recourse to a sock or bandage for pulling in. During swing phase, the tendency of the prosthesis to drop from the limb is resisted by the partial suction developed in the socket for a brief period of time. This occurs because the fit of the socket impedes free airflow into the socket through the sock. Partial suction, however is not sufficient to secure the prosthesis without assistance, so auxiliary suspension must be used, usually in the form of a Silesian bandage, although a pelvic belt may be utilized if needed.

Silesian Bandage (Fig. 26.500)

A webbing band, which encircles the torso.

One end is attached to the lateral proximal aspect of the socket in the region of the greater trochanter. The other end is attached to the anterior wall of the socket on the vertical midline at ischial level. The Silesian bandage is used with total suction or partial suction suspension, to help control rotation of the prosthesis and lateral instability for amputees with weak musculature or with short or flabby residua. It provides a safety factor for active individuals with suction sockets, who engage in climbing or similar pursuits and has been used successfully as a psychological aid with amputees, who feel insecure with suction suspension alone.

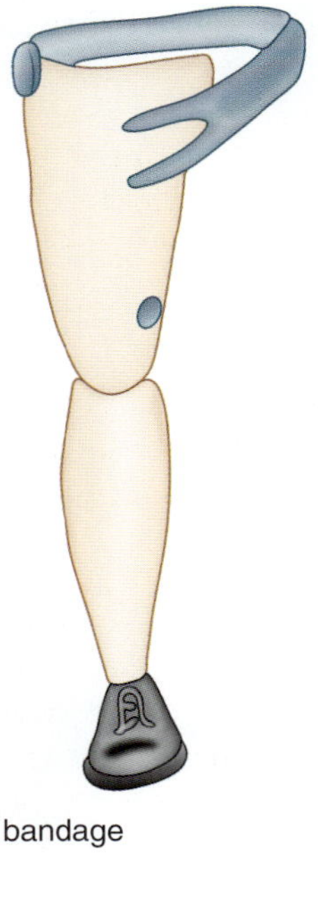

Fig. 26.500: Silesian bandage

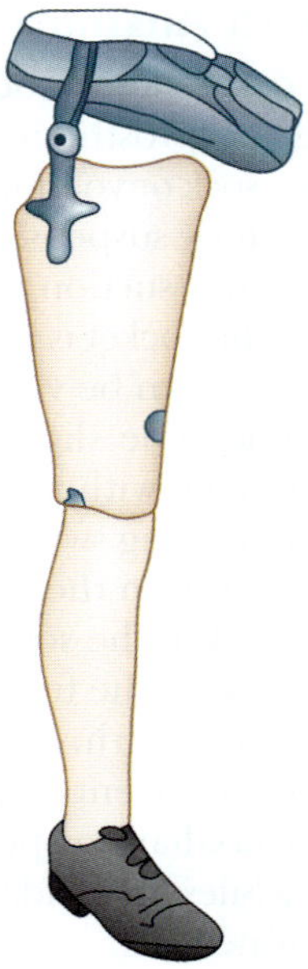

Fig. 26.501: A prosthesis with pelvic belt

Pelvic Belt (Fig. 26.501)

A pelvic belt may be used with partial-suction suspension or as the sole means of suspension, when suction or partial suction is not feasible. The pelvic belt is a wide leather or fabric strap, which encircles the torso and incorporates a band of rigid metal or semirigid plastic. A hip joint connects the band to the prosthesis at the lateral superior aspect of the socket.

The pelvic belt holds the prosthesis on the limb, controls rotation and promotes mediolateral stability. To minimize undesirable motion and pressure of the band, the hip joint must be placed slightly above and ahead of the greater trochanter to correspond as closely as possible with the normal hip joint. Amputees with short, weak or poorly shaped amputation limbs. Individuals, who are timid, feeble or poorly coordinated and those who are habituated to this mode of suspension may require a pelvic belt. This suspension restricts hip motions and tends to interfere with sitting comfort. Hip joints can be noisy, tear clothing, present maintenance problems and contribute to excessive piston action of the thigh in the socket. A leather belt absorbs perspiration and may cause skin problems. Also, the pelvic belt increases the weight of the prosthesis. Although, plastic bands and joints are somewhat lighter, their relative lack of rigidity may make them inappropriate for obese or very active clients or for those with very short amputation limbs.

Special Devices

In a few instances, none of the suspension devices described above can be used because of conditions, such as excessive obesity, pregnancy, scar tissue, skin disorders or deformity. In these circumstances, the prosthesis may be suspended by a shoulder harness, by attachment to a lumbosacral girdle or by a combination of methods individually devised to meet unusual requirements.

Rotator Unit

The shank torque absorber rotator unit, described in below-knee prostheses, is more apt to be used with above-knee prostheses, particularly if the wearer is very active. The unit is usually placed between the socket and the knee axis.

27 Spine

- Embryology and Anatomy of Vertebral Column
- Examination of Spine
- Congenital Deformities of Spine
- Imaging of the Spine
- Prolapsed Intervertebral Disk
- Degenerative Diseases of Spine
- Ankylosing Spondylitis
- Scoliosis
- Kyphosis
- Spina Bifida
- Tuberculosis of the Spine
- Nontubercular Infections of Spine
- Traumatic Quadriplegia and Paraplegia
- Spinal Orthosis

EMBRYOLOGY AND ANATOMY OF VERTEBRAL COLUMN

Embryology

- Vertebral column is derived from sclerotomes of somites. Somites are paraxial mesoderm which becomes segmented to form 42 to 44 somites that lie on either side of the neural tube (Figs 27.1A to C)
- Somites have three parts:

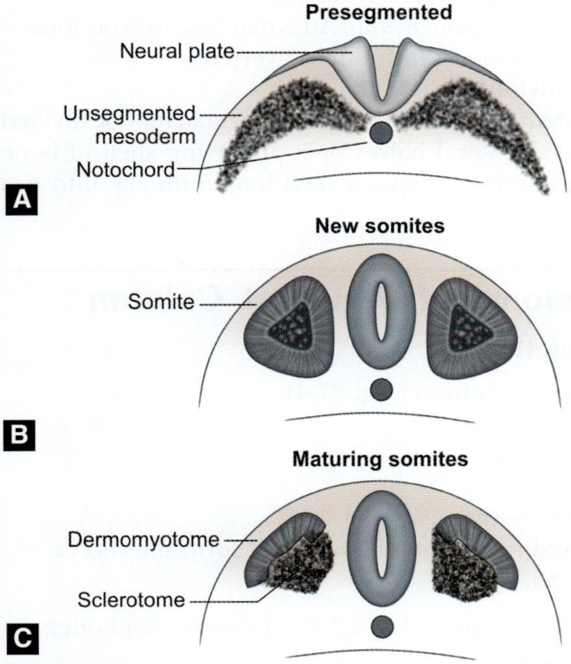

Figs 27.1A to C: Somites lying on either side of neural tube

  - *Ventromedial:* Sclerotome
  - *Lateral:* Dermatome
  - *Intermediate:* Myotome
- Sclerotome has three parts:
  - Cranial
  - Middle
  - Caudal
- A vertebrae is formed by fusion of caudal part of one sclerotome and cranial part of next sclerotome.
- The middle part forms intervertebral disk (Figs 27.2A to C).

Formation

- The cells of each sclerotome get converted into loose mesenchyme. This mesenchyme migrates medially and surrounds the notochord.

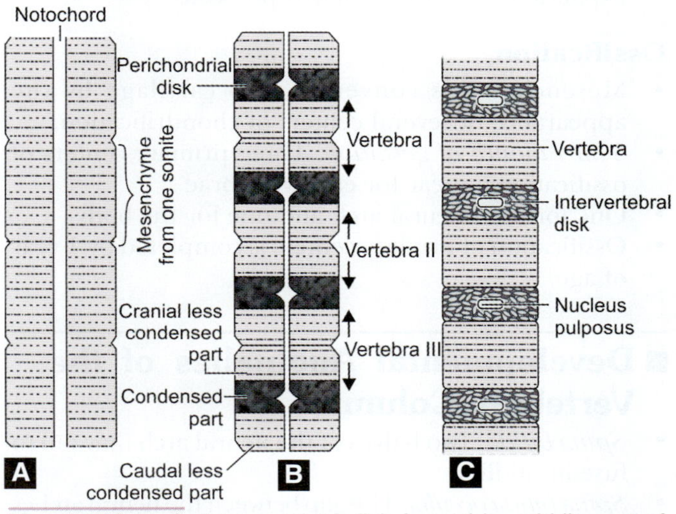

Figs 27.2A to C: Intervertebral disk formed by middle part of sclerotome

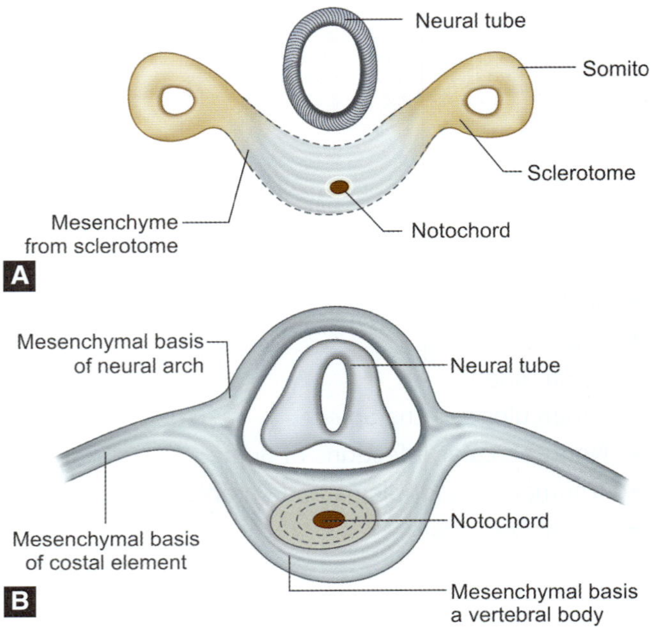

Figs 27.3A and B: (A) Formation of mesenchyme basis of the body of a vertebra from a sclerotome; (B) Extension of mesenchyme taking place laterally to be subsequently occupied by transverse processes and ventrally in body wall to be occupied by ribs

- The mesenchyme then extends backwards and surrounds neural tube
- Extension of mesenchyme also take place laterally to be subsequently occupied by transverse processes and ventrally in body wall to be occupied by ribs (Figs 27.3A and B).
- The neural arch, the transverse process and the costal elements are formed in the same way as the body
- The interspinous and intertransverse ligaments-formed in the same manner as the disk
- In the region of disk, the notochord becomes expanded and forms nucleus pulposus.

Ossification

- Mesenchyme is converted into cartilage by the appearance of several centers of chondrification.
- *Third month of gestation:* Three primary centers of ossification appear for each vertebrae
- One for each neural arch and one for the body
- Ossification of primary centers is completed by 1 year of age.

Developmental Anomalies of the Vertebral Column

- *Spina bifida:* Two halves of the neural arch may fail to fuse in midline
- *Spina bifida occulta:* The gap between the neural arches may not be obvious

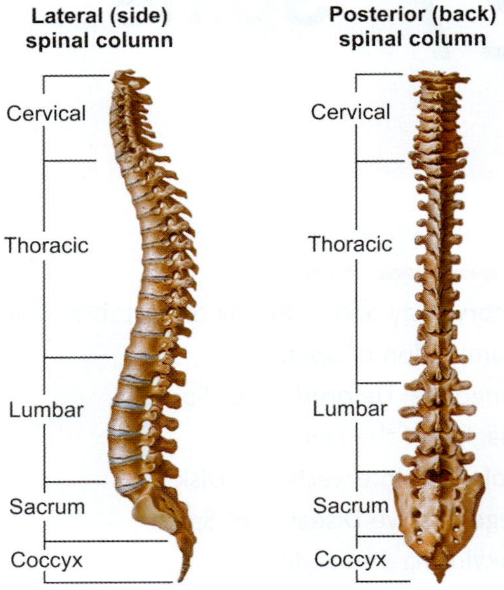

Fig. 27.4: Components of spine

- *Spina bifida manifesta:* When gap is large meninges and neural elements may bulge out leads to meningocele or meningomyelocele.
- *Hemivertebrae:* Vertebral body may ossify from two primary centers which soon fuse. One of these parts may fail to develop resulting in only half of the body being present.
- *Klippel-Feil syndrome:* Two or more vertebrae that are normally separate may be fused to each other in cervical region (Block vertebrae)
- *Occipitalization of atlas:* Atlas may fuse with occiput
- Sacralization of fifth lumbar vertebrae
- Spondylolisthesis
- *Diastematomyelia:* The vertebral canal may be divided into two lateral halves by a projecting shelf of bone which splits the spinal cord longitudinally into two halves.

Anatomy of Vertebral Column

Introduction

Spine made up from (Fig. 27.4):

- 7 cervical
- 12 thoracic
- 5 lumbar
- 5 fused sacral
- 4 fused rudimentary bones that form the coccyx.

Total = 33.

Curves of the spine (Fig. 27.5)—Primary (Kyphotic):

- Thoracic
- Sacrococcygeal

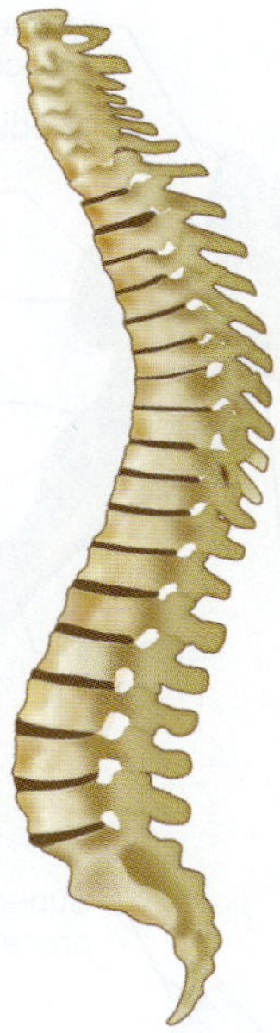

Fig. 27.5: Curves of spine

Secondary (Lordotic):
- Cervical
- Lumbar

■ Components of Typical Vertebrae (Figs 27.6A and B)

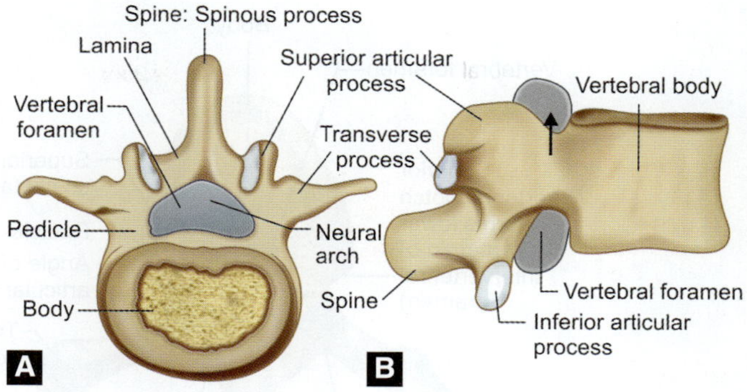

Figs 27.6A and B: Components of vertebrae

Structure of a Typical Cervical Vertebrae (Figs 27.7A and B)

- *Body:* Transverse diameter > AP diameter
- Smaller transverse processes
- Different orientation of joints
- Foramen transversarium for vertebral artery
- Smaller and thinner disks.

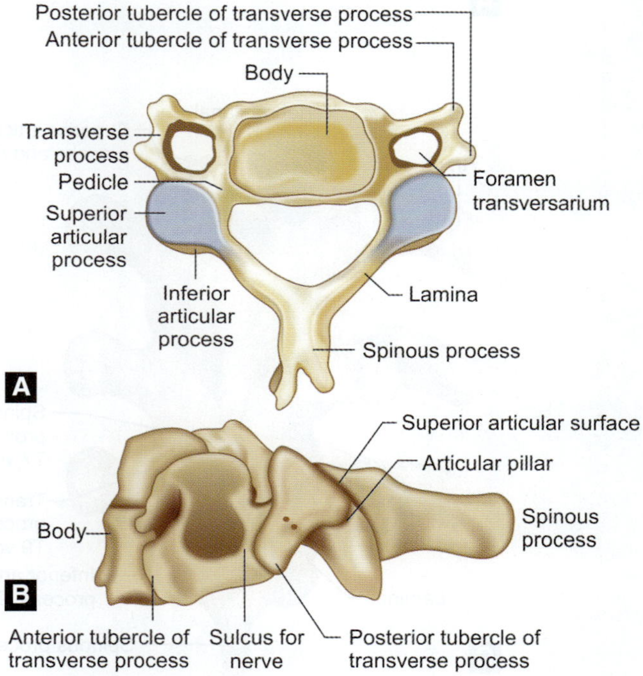

Figs 27.7A and B: Structure of cervical vertebrae

Atlas and Axis (C1 and C2) no Disk (Fig. 27.8)

- Pivot joint
- Mainly rotation about odontoid process
- Integrity of joint maintained by strong ligaments.

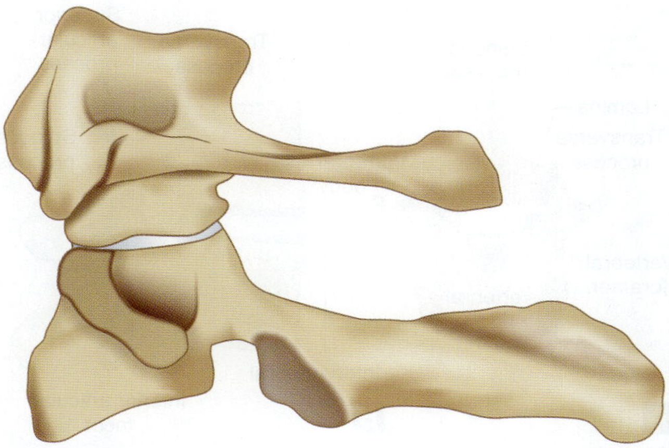

Fig. 27.8: Atlas and axis

Structure of a Typical Thoracic Vertebrae (Figs 27.9A to D)

- Heart shaped body
- Longer and more vertical spinous processes
- Small and circular vertebral foramen
- Thinner disks
- Facets for rib articulations.

Structure of a Typical Lumbar Vertebrae (Figs 27.10A and B)

- Large disks for weight-bearing and shock absorbing

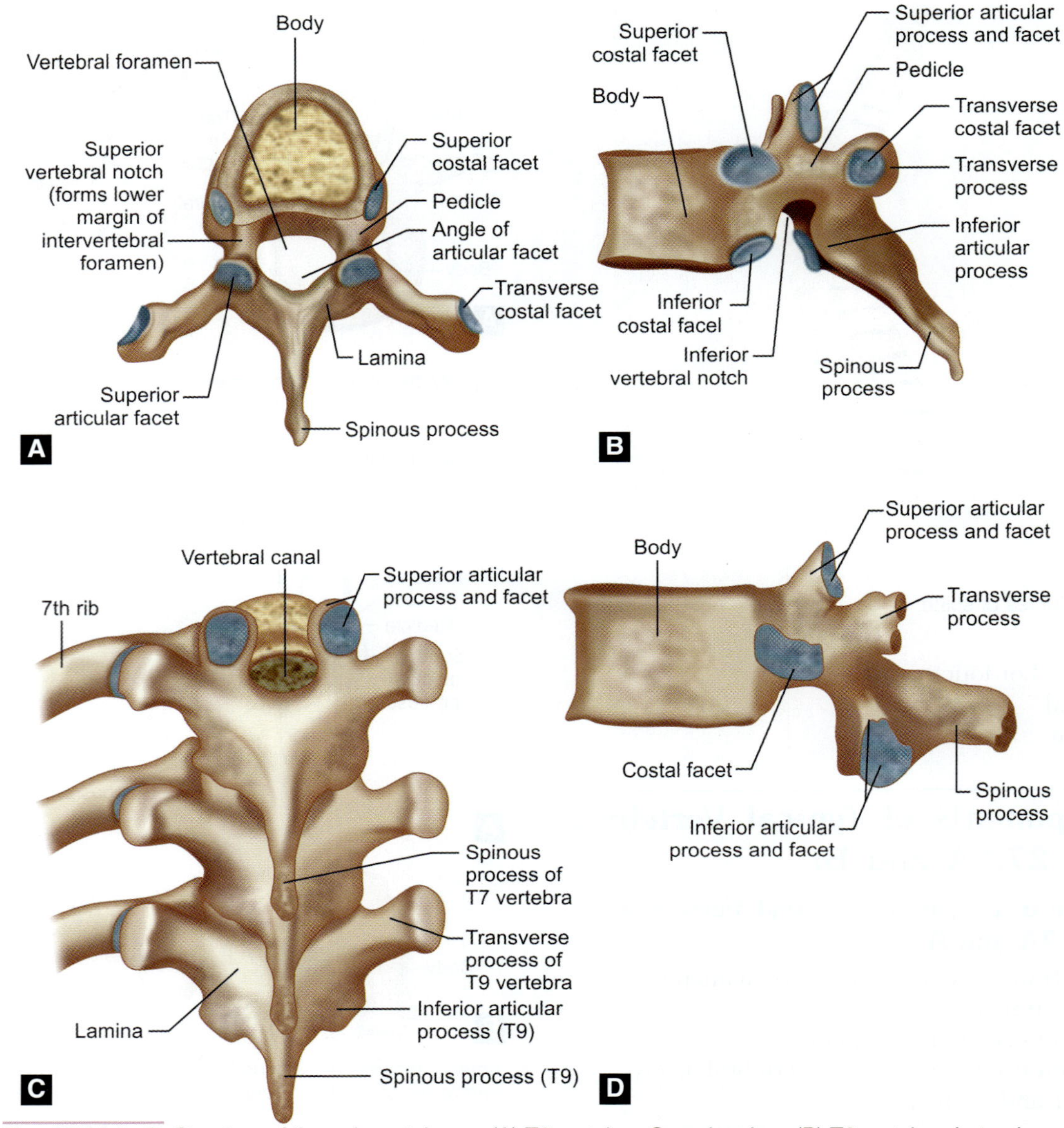

Figs 27.9A to D: Structure of thoracic vertebrae—(A) T6 vertebra: Superior view; (B) T6 vertebra: Lateral view; (C) T7, T8 and T9 vertebrae: Posterior view; (D) T12 vertebra: Lateral view

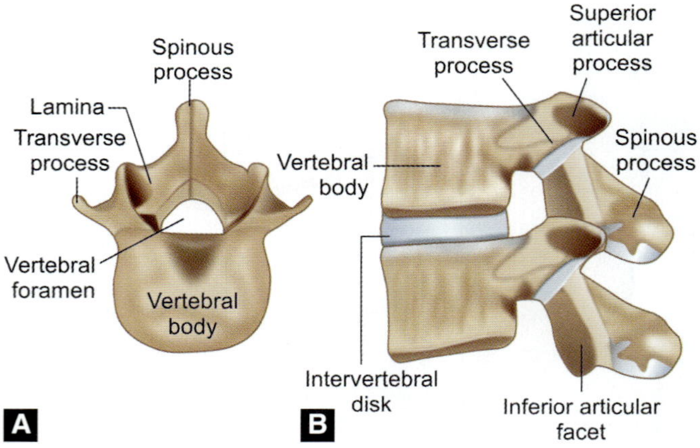

Figs 27.10A and B: Structure of lumbar vertebrae

- Large joints that limit movement
- Small range of overall movement

Structure of a Typical Sacral Vertebrae (Fig. 27.11)

- Fused vertebrae
- Sacral foramen for sacral nerve roots
- Form part of sacroiliac joint

Intervertebral Foramen (Figs 27.12 and 27.13)

- Formed between the pedicles above and below
- The vertebral body and disks in front
- The joint behind

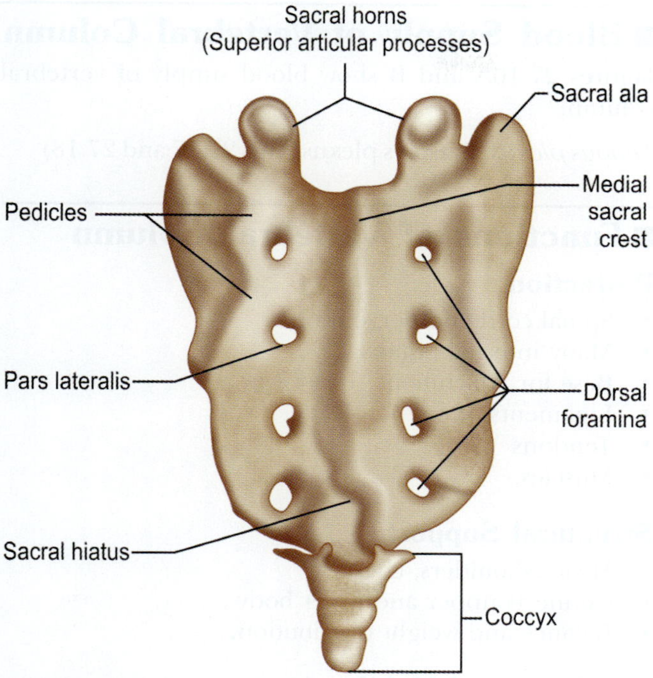

Fig. 27.11: Structure of sacral vertebrae

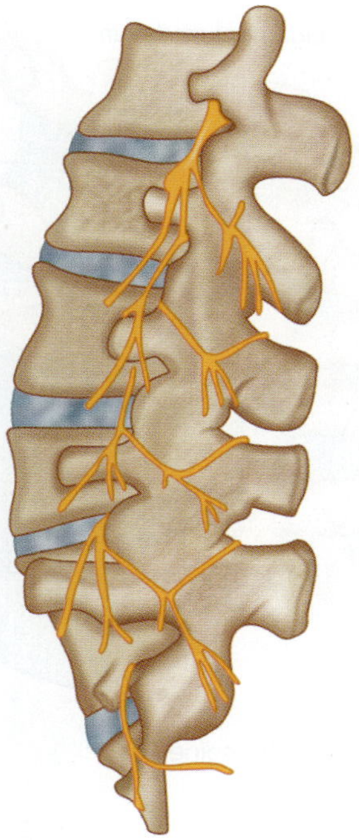

Fig. 27.13: Intervertebral foramen—lateral view

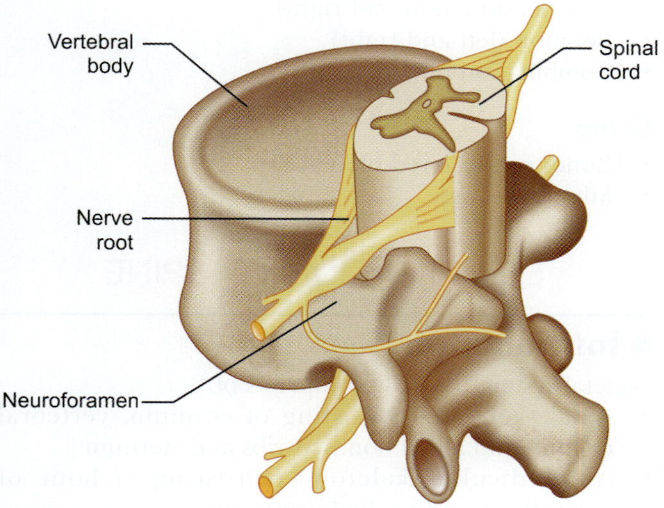

Fig. 27.12: Vertebra showing intervertebral foramen with nerve root

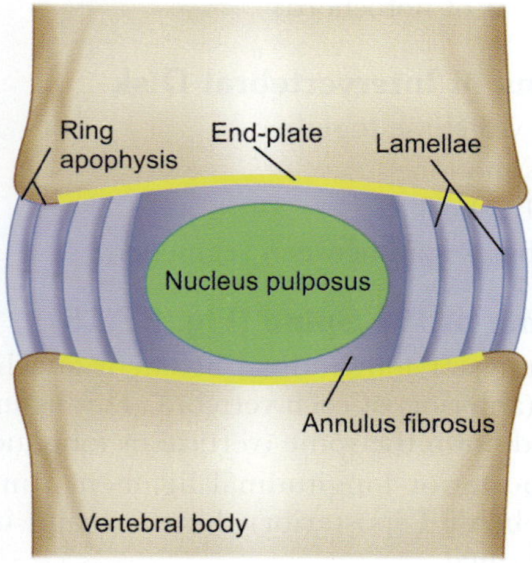

Fig. 27.14: Intervertebral disk

It contains

- Nerve root and sinuvertebral nerve
- Blood vessels
- Lymphatic vessels
- Fat
- Nerve root occupies 1/3rd of the space in the intervertebral foramen (Fig. 27.13)
- Contains the dorsal root ganglion

Intervertebral Disk (Fig. 27.14)

- The intervertebral disks are fibrocartilaginous cushions serving as the spine's shock absorbing system, which protect the vertebrae, brain and other structures (i.e. nerves)
  - Annulus fibrosus
  - Nucleus pulposus
  - Vertebral end-plate

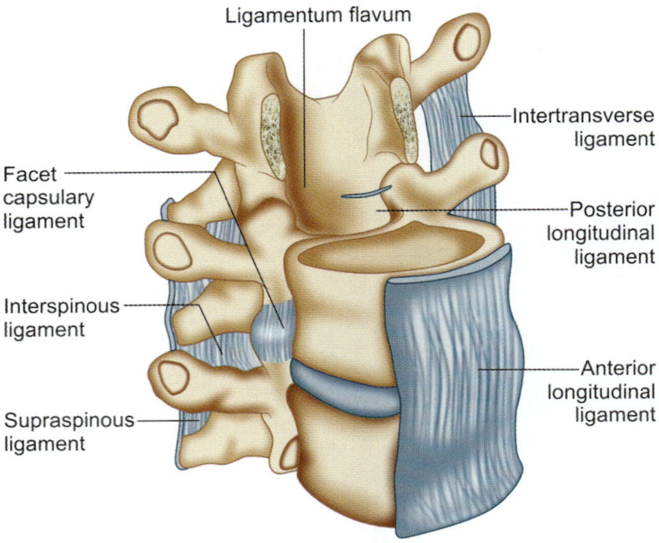

Fig. 27.15: Ligaments of the spine

- The annulus fibrosus is a strong radial tyre-like structure made up of lamellae (concentric sheets of collagen fibers connected to the vertebral end-plates)
- *Nucleus pulposus:* Gelatinous mass found in the center (remnant of notochord).

Functions of Intervertebral Disk

- Binds vertebrae together
- Allows motion
- Absorbs shock
- Distributes load between segments

Ligaments of the Spine (Fig. 27.15)

- The anterior longitudinal ligament attaches to the front (anterior) of each vertebra. This ligament runs up and down the spine (vertical or longitudinal)
- The posterior longitudinal ligament runs up and down behind (posterior) the spine and inside the spinal canal
- The ligamentum flavum forms a cover over the dura mater—a layer of tissue that protects the spinal cord. This ligament connects under the facet joints to create a small curtain over the posterior openings between the vertebrae
- Supraspinous ligament present only in thoracic and lumbar vertebrae. It connects the tips of 2 adjacent spinous process
- Ligamentum nuchae present only in cervical region. It connects the tips of the spine of cervical vertebrae.
- Capsular ligament at the margins of the articular facets of the superior and inferior articular processes of each vertebrae.

■ Blood Supply of Vertebral Column

Figures 27.16A and B show blood supply of vertebral column.

Venous plexus: Batson's plexus (Figs 27.17 and 27.18)

■ Functions of Vertebral Column

Protection

- Spinal cord and nerve roots
- Many internal organs
- Base for attachment
- Ligaments
- Tendons
- Muscles.

Structural Support

- Head, shoulders, chest
- Connects upper and lower body
- Balance and weight distribution.

Flexibility and Mobility

- Flexion (forward bending)
- Extension (backward bending)
- Side bending (left and right)
- Rotation (left and right)
- Combination of above.

Other

- Bones produce red blood cells
- Mineral storage.

EXAMINATION OF SPINE

■ Introduction

Skeletal system basically comprises of:
- Axial skeleton—consisting of cranium, vertebral column and allied bones as ribs and sternum
- Appendicular skeleton—consisting of bone of appendages in fins, limbs or wings.

■ Development of Spine (See Fig. 27.1)

The spine develops in concurrently overlapping stages which overlap each other
- *First stage:* Notochord—15 days of intrauterine life
- *Second stage:* Membrane stage—21 days of IUL
- *Third stage:* Cartilage stage—5 to 6 weeks and continues throughout the fetal stage
- *Fourth stage:* Bony stage—second month of IUL
  - Congenital anomalies can occur in any stage but usually occur due to defects in the membrane

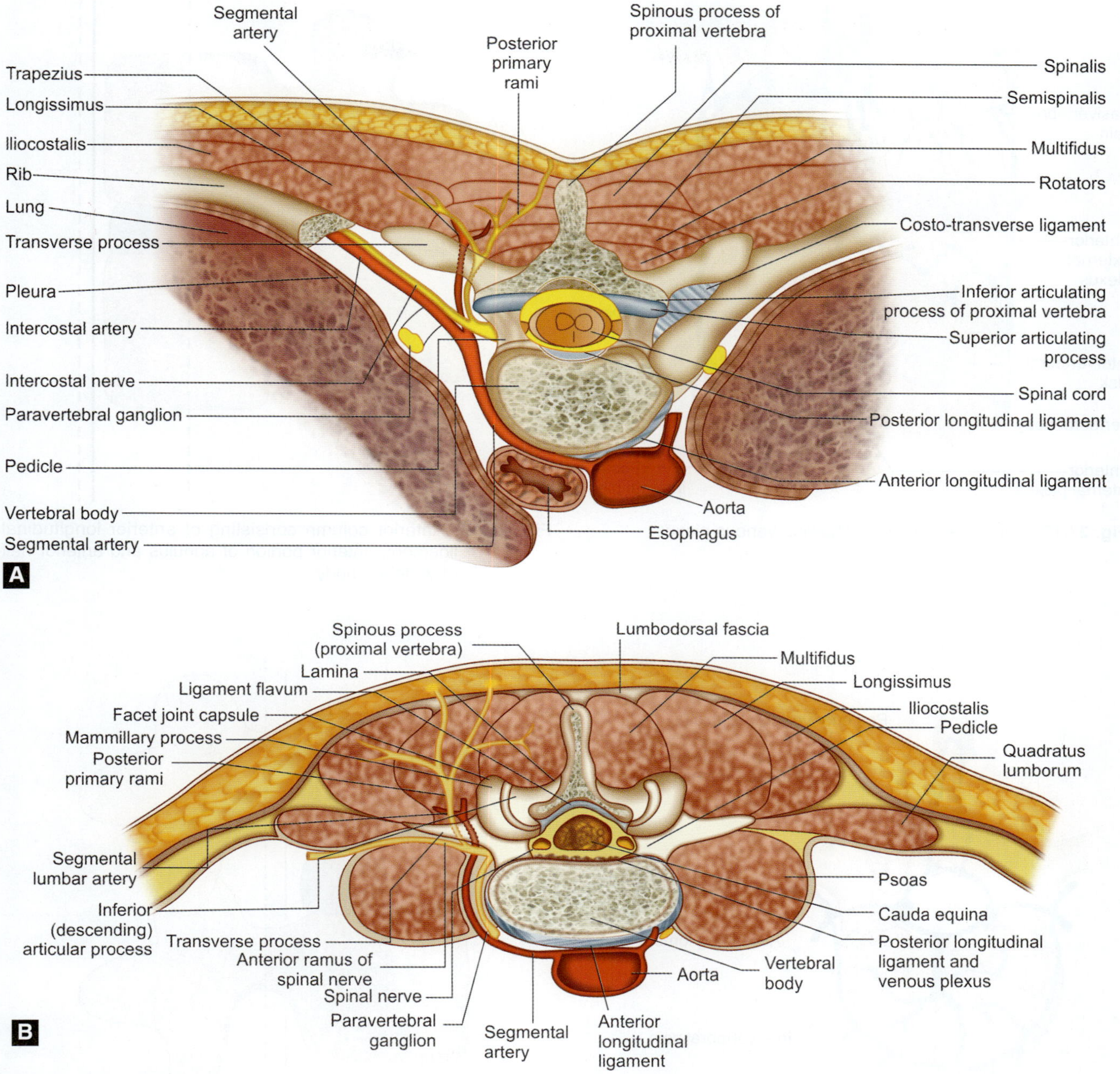

Figs 27.16A and B: Blood supply of vertebral column—(A) Thoracic region; (B) Lumbar region

stage, when mesenchyme first starts forming around the notochord.

Function of Spine

In bipeds, the spinal column assumes the following important structures:

- Encasement of spinal cord
- Transmit ion of weight of head, neck and trunk to lower limbs through the pelvis
- Maintenance of posture
- Forming a stout back support for the vital organs of the chest and abdomen
- Providing attachment to certain group of muscles responsible for maintenance of posture.

Stability of Spine

It depends on three column support (Denis, 1983):

- Anterior column consists of anterior longitudinal ligament, anterior portion of annulus and anterior half of vertebral body (Fig. 27.19)

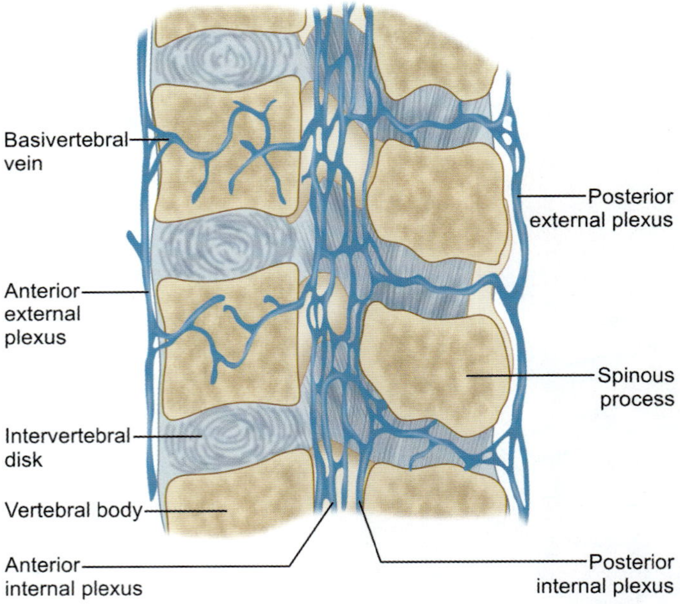

Fig. 27.17: Lateral view of spine showing venous plexus

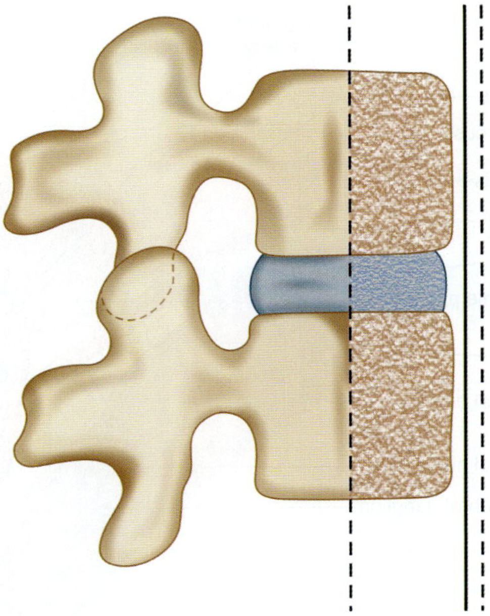

Fig. 27.19: Anterior column consisting of anterior longitudinal ligament, anterior portion of annulus and anterior half of vertebral body

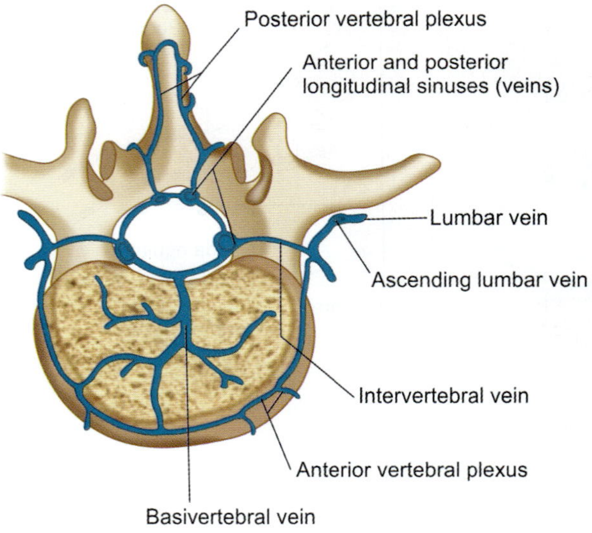

Fig. 27.18: Venous plexus

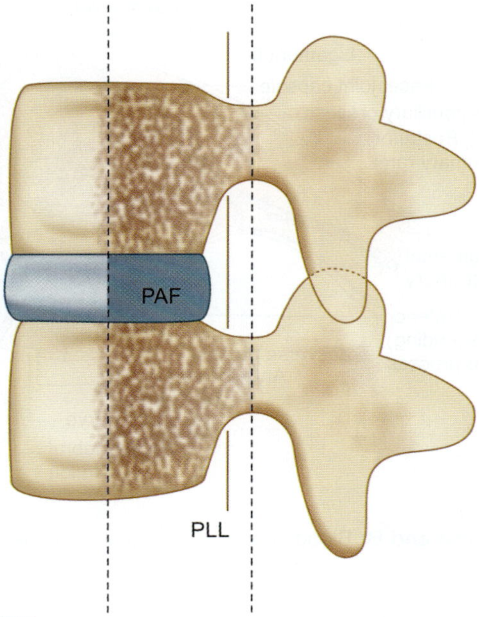

Fig. 27.20: Middle column

- Middle column consists of posterior longitudinal ligament, posterior portion of annulus and posterior half of vertebral body (Fig. 27.20)
- Posterior column consists of posterior bony arch and posterior ligamentous complex (Fig. 27.21).

Examination of Spine

- History taking
- General and systemic examination
- Gait analysis if patient can walk

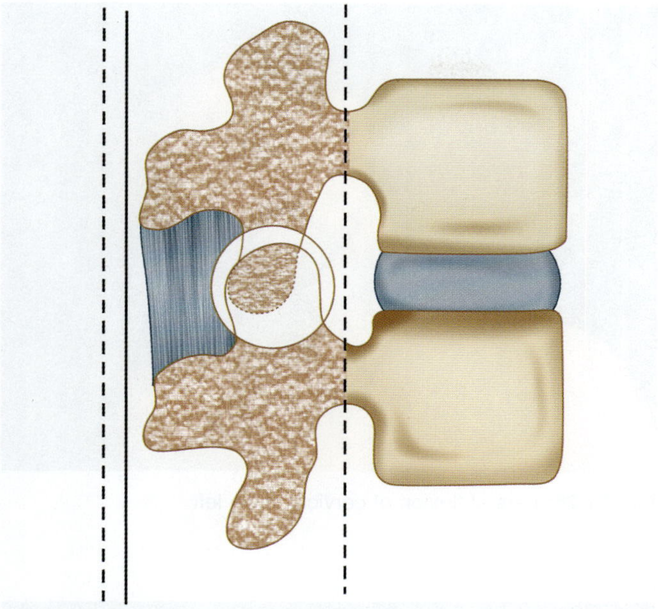

Fig. 27.21: Posterior column

- Local examination
  - Inspection
  - Palpation
    a. Bony palpation
    b. Soft tissue palpation
  - Range of motion
  - Neurological examination
  - Special test

Inspection

- Inspection begins as the patient arrives. Look at his gait, attitude and posture of his head
- Note the position of the head, the hairline, length of the neck and the levels of the shoulders, scapulae and the iliac crests
- From the sides and back, note the curvatures of the spine, the central furrow, paraspinal muscles and renal angle
- Look for any bulge in the loin region, fullness over or below the iliac crest and fullness of the dimple of venus.
- Look for any scars, sinuses or discoloration, lypomas, hairy patch (Fauns beard), dimple, puckering or café-au-lait spots.

Palpation

- General palpation is done by passing the palm from the occipital protuberance to the tip of the coccyx
- *Superficial palpation:* Look for hyperesthesia, abnormal prominence or depression, pulsation or increase in temperature
- Palpate the side of the chest, abdomen, iliac region, renal angle for abnormal swellings like cold abscesses.
- *Tenderness:* It is elicited by three methods (Fig. 27.22)

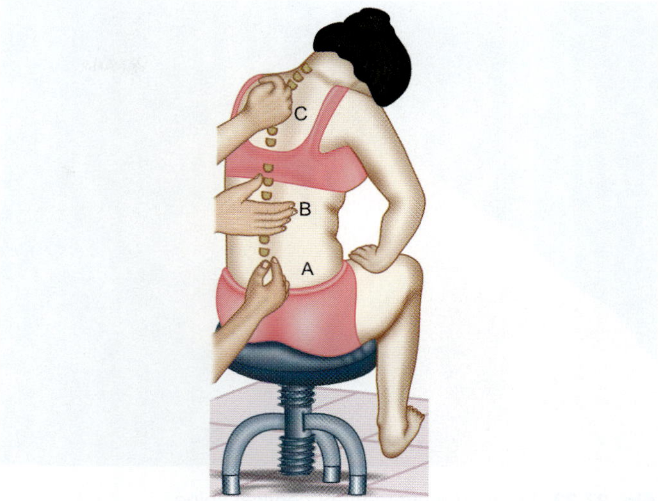

Fig. 27.22: Methods of elicitation of tenderness

Table 27.1: Range of movements of prime movers and nerve supply

Movements	Range of motion	Prime movers	Nerve supply
Flexion	With mouth closed, chin just touching the manubrium sterni	Sternocleido-mastoid muscle	Spinal accessory C2-C3
Extension	Till head comes in contact with posterior part of the upper trunk	Trapezius, semispinalis capitis, spenius capitis, splenius cervicis	Spinal accessory and C3-C4 posterior rami of spinal nerve
Side bending	0° to 45° on each side	Sternomastoid muscle	Spinal accessory C2-C3
Flexion	0°to 90°	Rectus abdominis	Lower intercostal nerves
Extension	0° to 30°	Sacrospinalis quadratus lumborum	D 11, 12, 13
Trunk rotators	0° to 30°	External oblique internal oblique	Iliohypogastric and ilioinguinal nerve
Side bending	0° to 30°	Quadratus lumborum	D12, 11, l2

- *Direct pressure tenderness:* Apply firm direct pressure on the spinous process
- *Twist tenderness:* Twisting pressure by thumb is applied on spinous process
- *Deep thrust tenderness:* A thrust is applied by fist over the spinous process.

Range of Movements

Prime movers and nerve supply (Table 27.1)
Cervical spine (Figs 27.23 to 27.28)

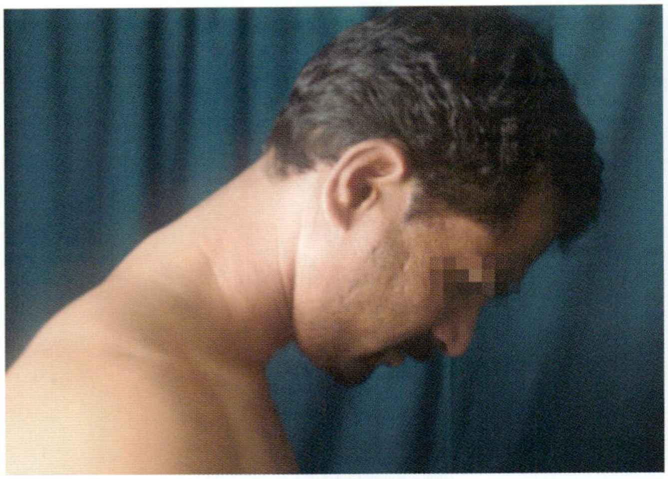

Fig. 27.23: Forward movement of cervical spine

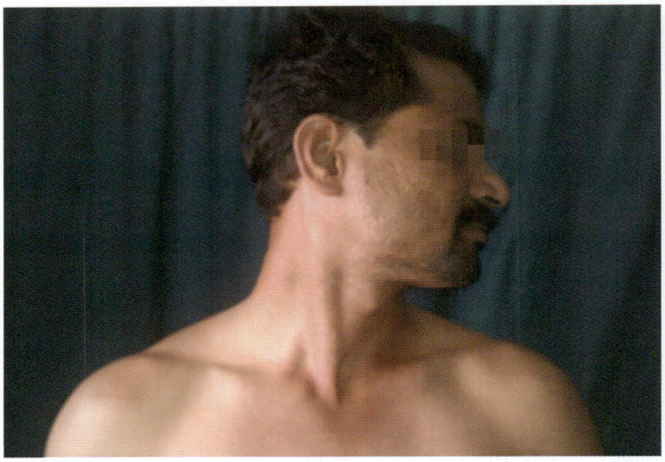

Fig. 27.24: Lateral rotation of cervical spine left

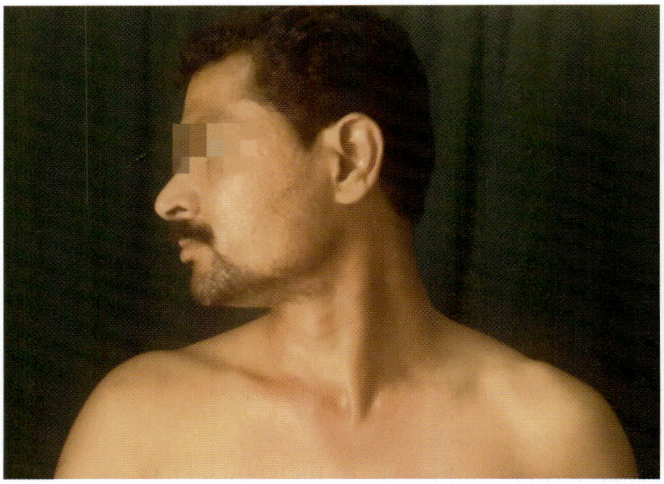

Fig. 27.25: Lateral rotation of cervical spine right

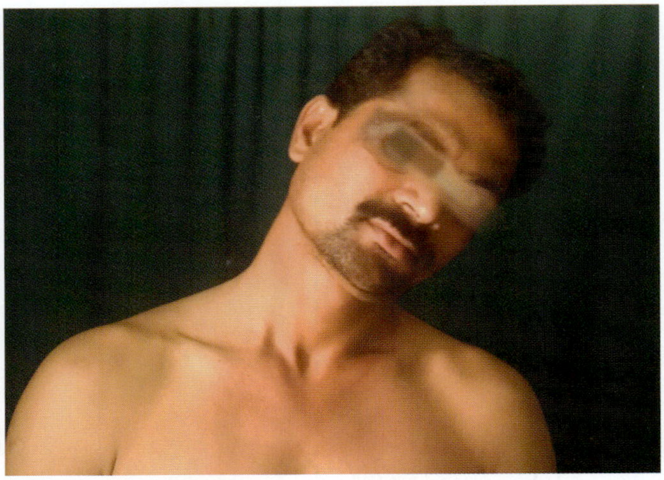

Fig. 27.26: Lateral flexion of cervical spine left

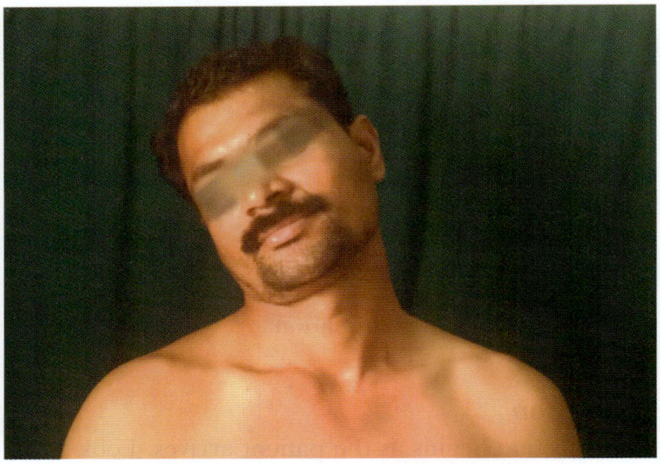

Fig. 27.27: Lateral flexion of cervical spine right

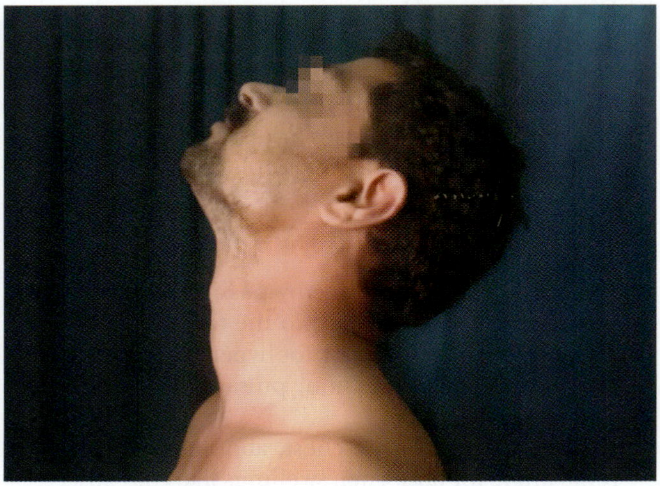

Fig. 27.28: Backward movement of cervical spine

Trunk (Figs 27.29 to 27.32)

Measurements

- Measurements are helpful in spinal deformities like kyphosis and scoliosis, to assess the degree of spinal curvature. (Fig. 27.33)
- Total length of spinal column can be measured from occipital prominence to coccyx
- *Iliocostal distance:* Measure from tip of last rib to highest point on iliac crest
- *Ilio-occipital distance:* It is distance from occipital protuberance to highest point on iliac crest.
- *Occipital acromial distance:* From occipital prominence to tip of acromion
- *Schober's test:* (Figs 27.34A and B)
  - Mark the T1/L1 and S1 vertebrae and measuring tape with patient in normal extension, i.e. upright posture
  - Ask patient to flex forward and note the distance between T1 and S1. Normal is 6 to 7 cm excursion.

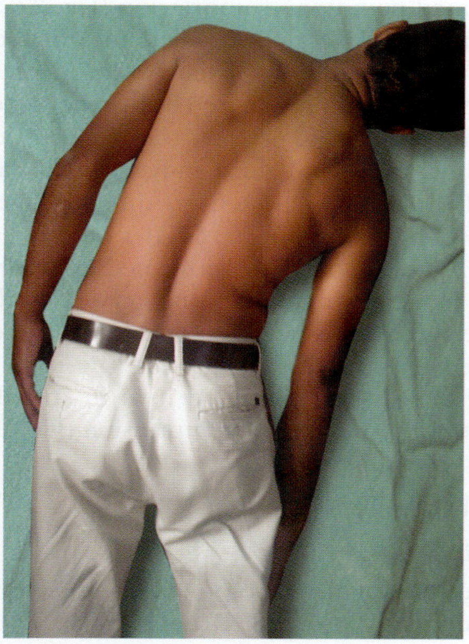

Fig. 27.29: Lateral flexion to right

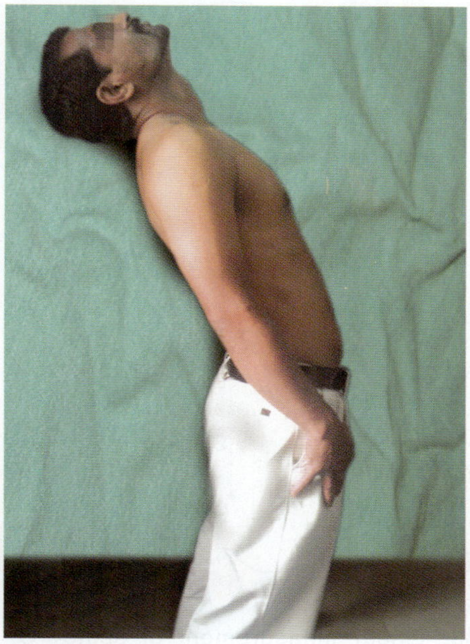

Fig. 27.31: Backward movement of trunk

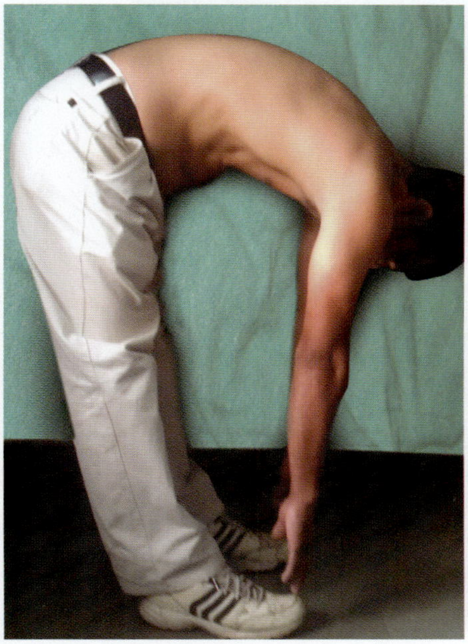

Fig. 27.30: Forward movement of trunk

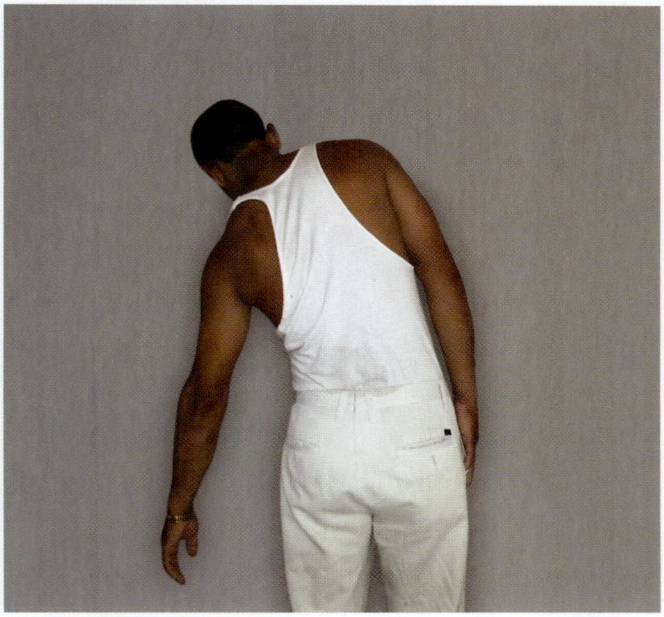

Fig. 27.32: Lateral flexion to left

- Modified Schober's test (Figs 27.35A and B):
  - Mark the S2 vertebrae and select a point 10 cm above and 5 cm below and ask patient to flex
  - Normal is 6 to 7 cm
  - Less than 5 cm is significant
- Flexion of thoracic spine can be measured with upper point 30 cm from S2 and normally is 3 cm
- Chest expansion measurement (Figs 27.36 and 27.37)

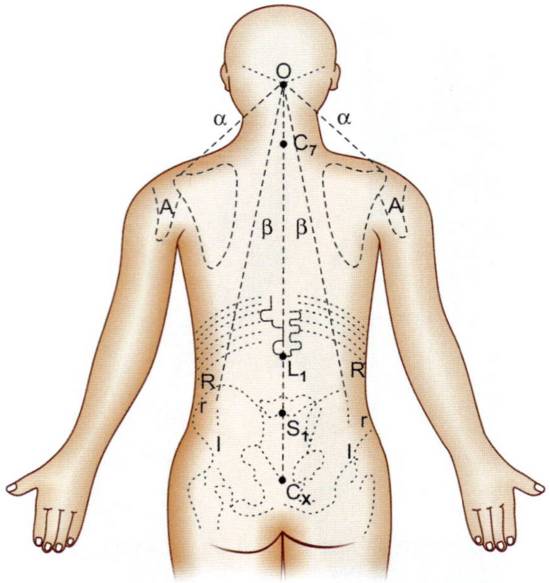

Fig. 27.33: Linear measurement of spine—O. Occipital protuberance; A. Acromion angle; I. Iliac crest; R. Tip of the last rib

Special Test

Cervical Spine

- *Distraction test:* Distraction test relives pain due to narrowing of foramen causing nerve root compression, it also relives pain by decreasing pressure on facet joint, in addition it may help to alleviate muscle spasm by relaxing contracted muscle (Fig. 27.38).
- *Compression test:* Narrowing of neural foramen, pressure on facet joint or muscle spasm can cause increased pain upon compression (Fig. 27.39)
- *Spurling test:* Neck is extended and rotated towards the involved side and axial compression is given. Pseudoradicular pain caused by degenerative diseases in spine radiates to occiput, scapula or sometimes to arm but not beyond elbow radicular pain caused due to PIVD, foramenal stenosis due to degeneration radiates below elbow (Fig. 27.40).
- *Lhermitte's maneuver:* Performed by asking seated patient to maximally flex the cervical and thoracic spine. Lhermittes sign is considered present when maneuver produces distal paresthesia in multiple extremity or the trunk. Positive in spinal stenosis resulting in spinal cord compression (Fig. 27.41).

Upper Limb Tension Test

Upper Limb Tension Test-1

- Is a series of maneuvers applied to upper limb to place tension on C5, C6 and C7 nerve root
- As median nerve is most stressed here it is described as median nerve dominant test

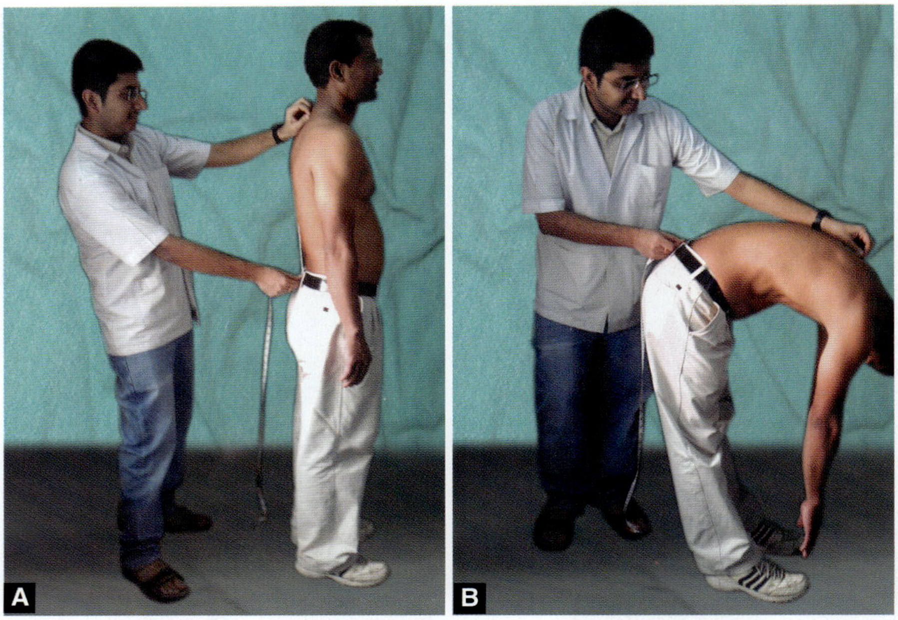

Figs 27.34A and B: Schober's test

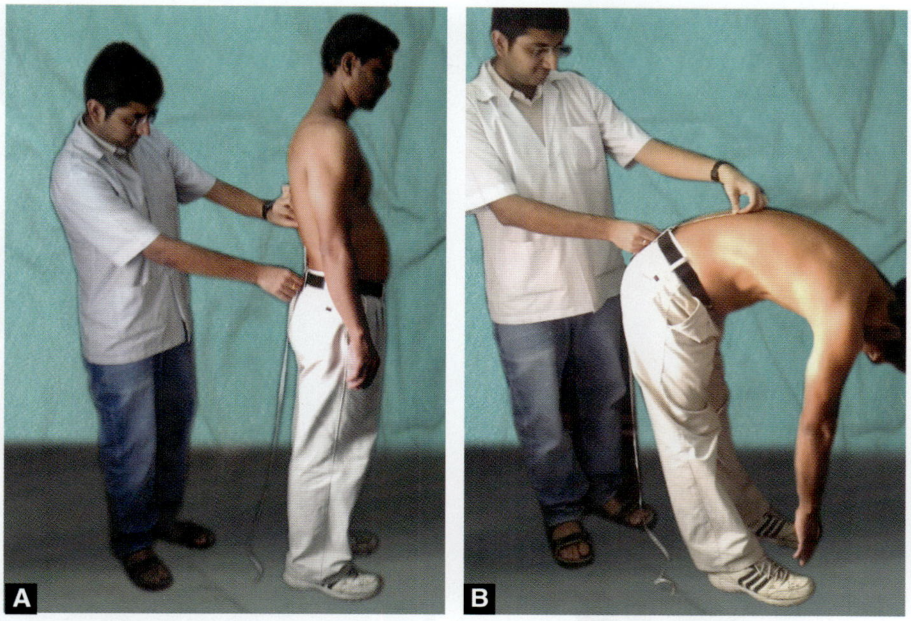

Figs 27.35A and B: Modified Schober's test

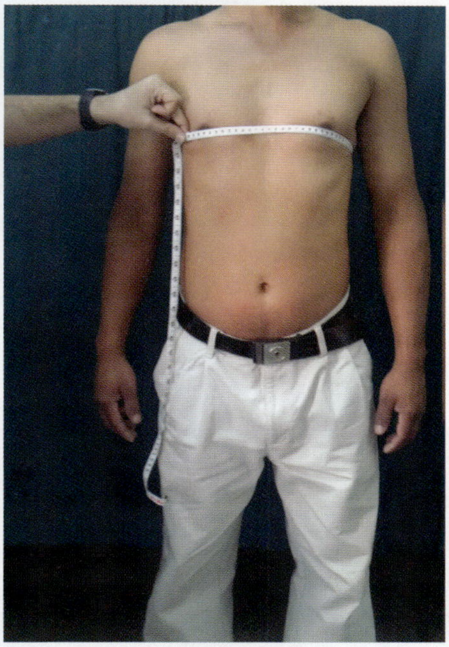

Fig. 27.36: Chest expansion measurement (during expiration)

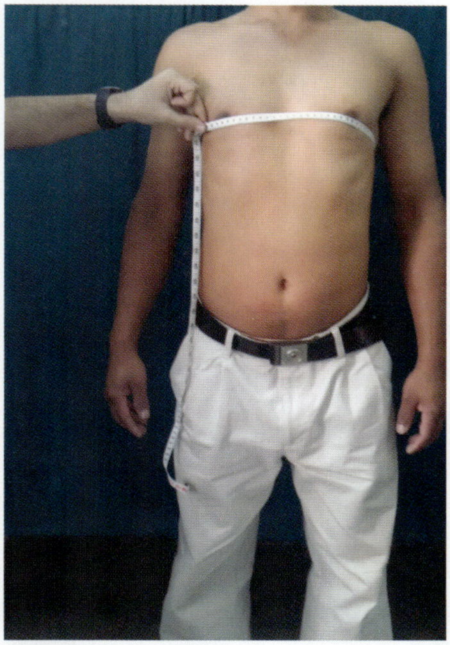

Fig. 27.37: Chest expansion measurement after full inspiration

- Procedure must be done carefully and gently and the examiner should maintain communication with patient to know the point at which radicular pain starts
- Upper limb tension test-1 (ULTT-1) produces pain in antecubital fossa in all subjects and should not be considered as abnormal response.

Maneuver of ULTT-1

- Position patient in relaxed supine position along the edge of the table.
  - With one hand gently hold the patient hand and with other hand stabilizes patients shoulder against

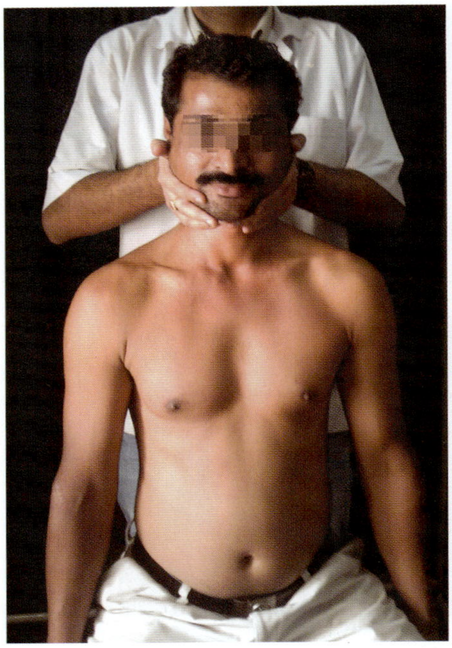

Fig. 27.38: Distraction test

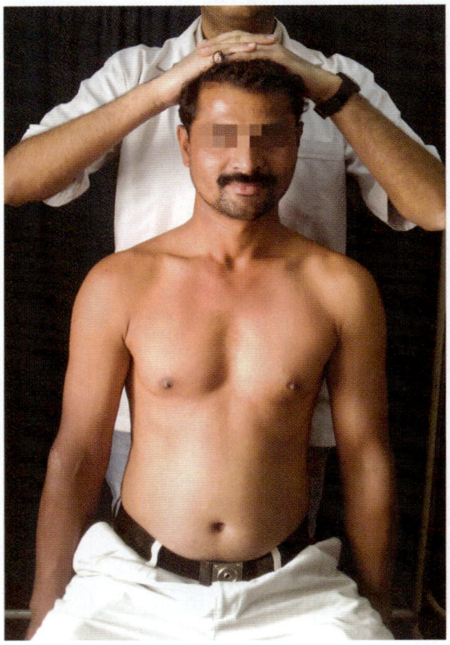

Fig. 27.39: Compression test

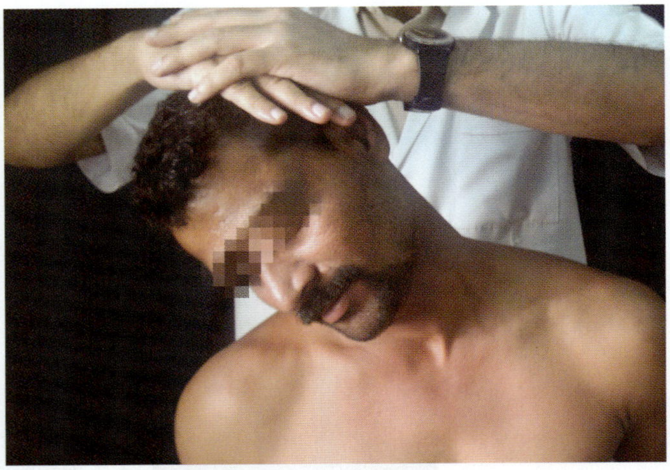

Fig. 27.40: Spurling test

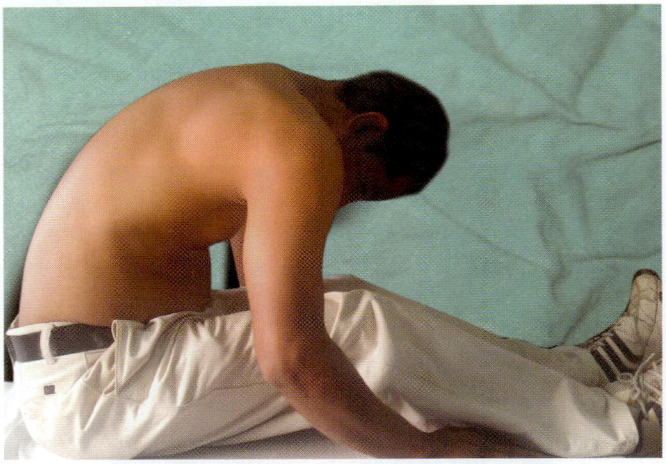

Fig. 27.41: Lhermitte's maneuver

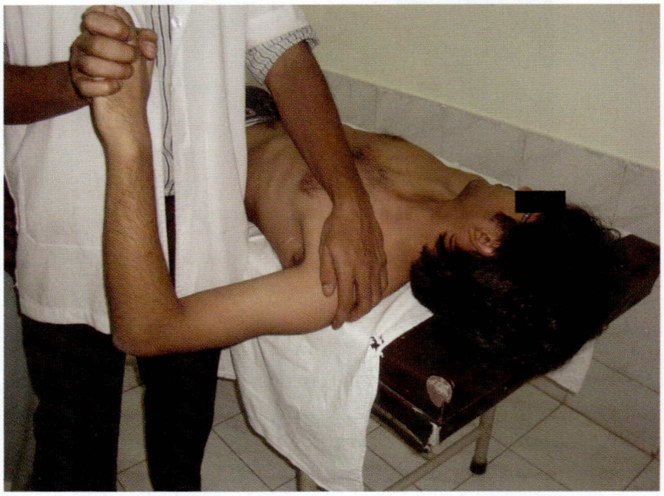

Fig. 27.42: Maneuver of ULTT-1

the examination table to prevent further elevation of shoulder abduct the arm to 90° (Fig. 27.42)

- Further abduct the arm to 110° (Fig. 27.43)
- While maintaining the position supinate the forearm and extend the wrist along with fingers (Fig. 27.44)

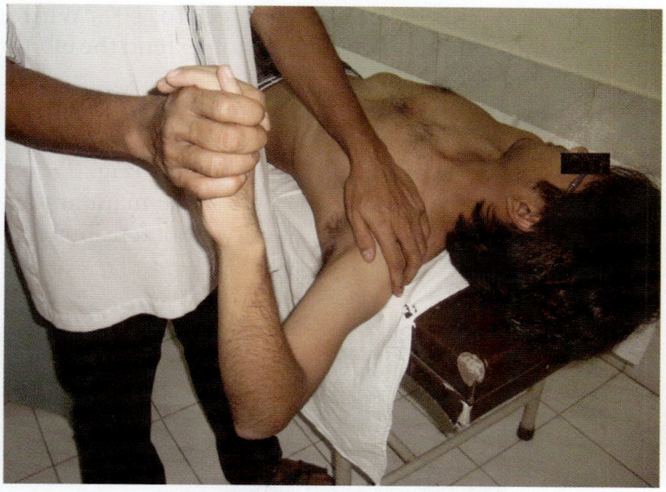

Fig. 27.43: Arm is abducted at 110°

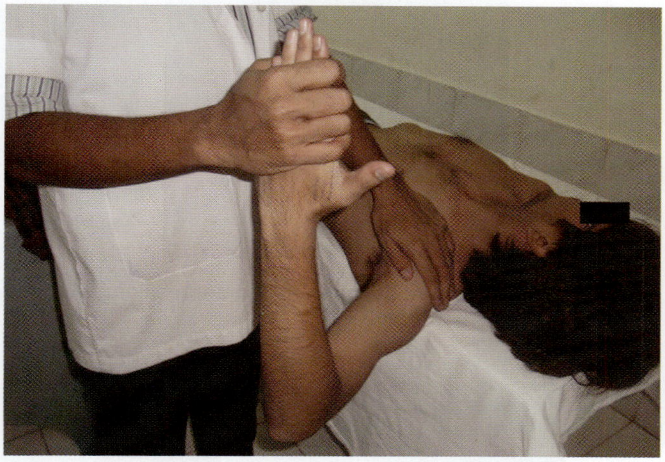

Fig. 27.44: Maintain the position and supinated the forearm and extend the wrist along with fingers

- Then rotate the patients shoulder to 90° (Fig. 27.45)
- Slowly extend the elbow (Fig. 27.46)
- Ask the patient to laterally bend the neck (Fig. 27.47).

- Pain is relived when neck is bent on same side and increases when neck is bent on opposite side
- Radicular pain radiating on lateral deltoid and mid-forearm nerve root is C5. Dorsoradial aspect of forearm involving index and thumb nerve root is C6, centrally down the forearm involving middle finger nerve root is C7.

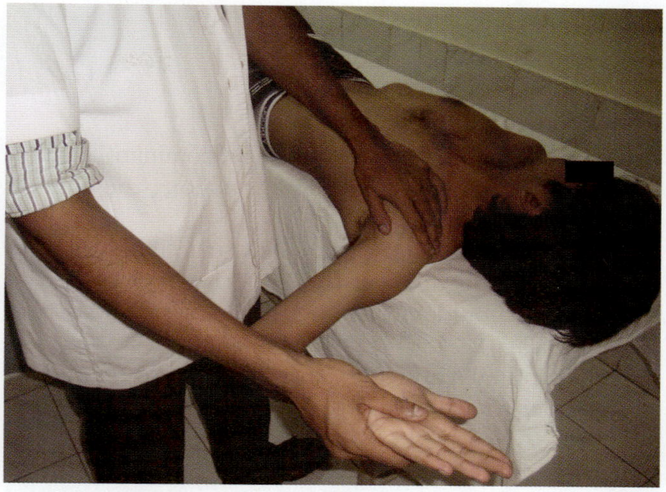

Fig. 27.45: Rotate the patient's shoulder at 90°

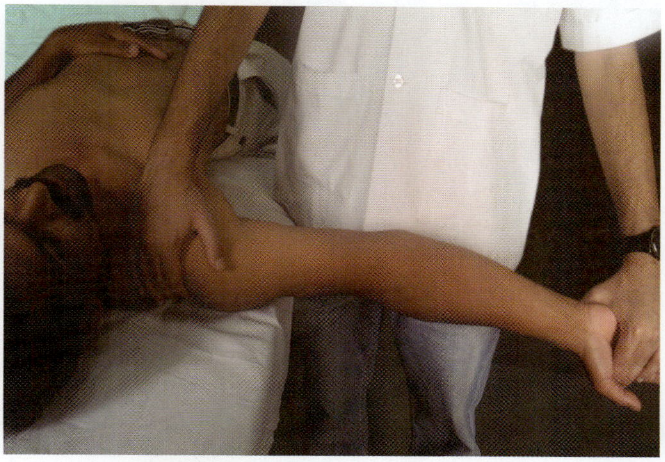

Fig. 27.46: Extend the elbow

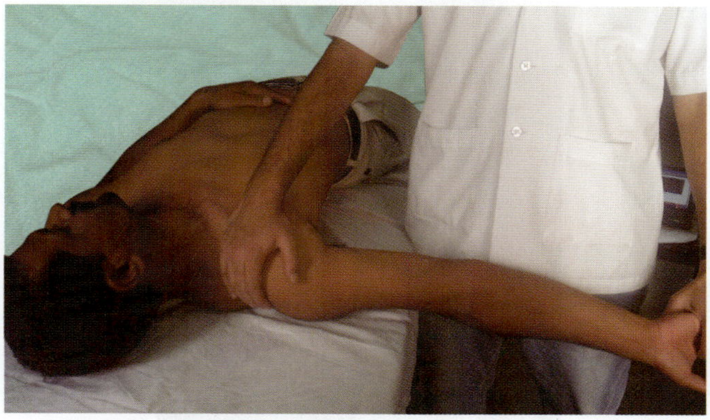

Fig. 27.47: Patient is asked to bend the neck laterally

Upper Limb Tension Test-2

- ULTT-2 has two variants:
  - Median nerve dominant
  - Radial nerve dominant

  Maneuver of ULTT-2: Median nerve dominant. Position patient in relaxed supine position along the edge of the table.
- Examiner stands on head side of the table with his thigh resting against the superior aspect of the patient's shoulder. Examiner hold patient's wrist and elbow (Fig. 27.48)
- In controlled manner, the examiner depresses patient shoulder with his thigh (Fig. 27.49)
  - Patient shoulder is abducted to 10°. While maintaining shoulder depression extend the elbow (Fig. 27.50)
- Then externally rotate the patients shoulder (Fig. 27.51)
- Dorsi-flex wrist with extension of fingers (Fig. 27.52)
- Abducting patient shoulder to 90° while maintaining shoulder depression increases nerve root tension (Fig. 27.53)

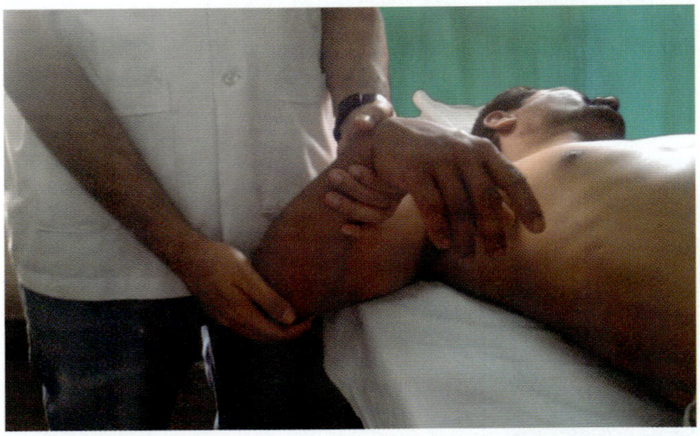

Fig. 27.48: Examiner holding patient's wrist and elbow

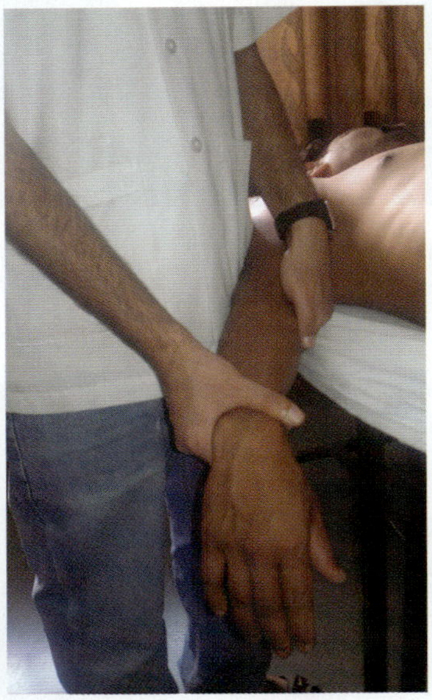

Fig. 27.50: While maintaining shoulder depression, elbow is extended

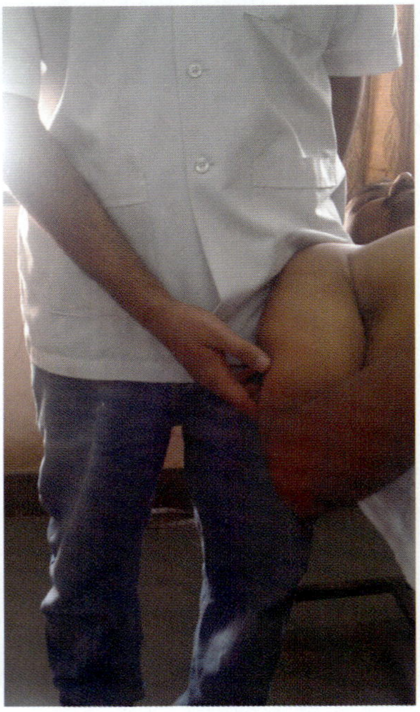

Fig. 27.49: Examiner depressing patient's shoulder with his thigh

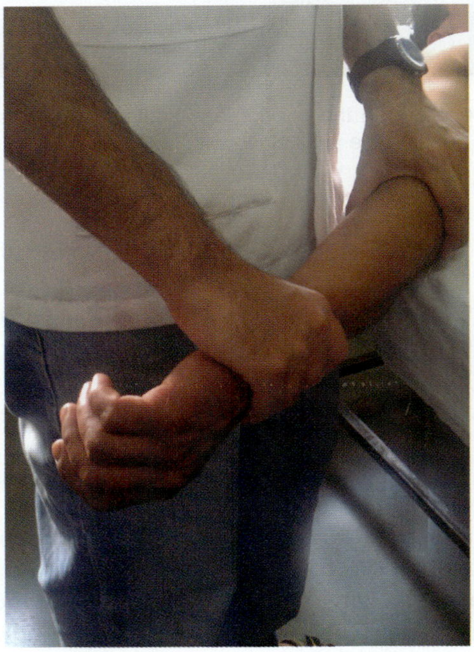

Fig. 27.51: Patient's shoulder is externally rotated

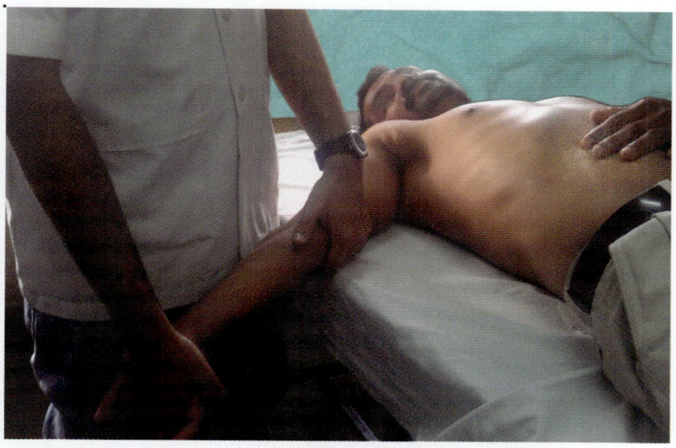

Fig. 27.52: Wrist is dorsi-flexed with extension of fingers

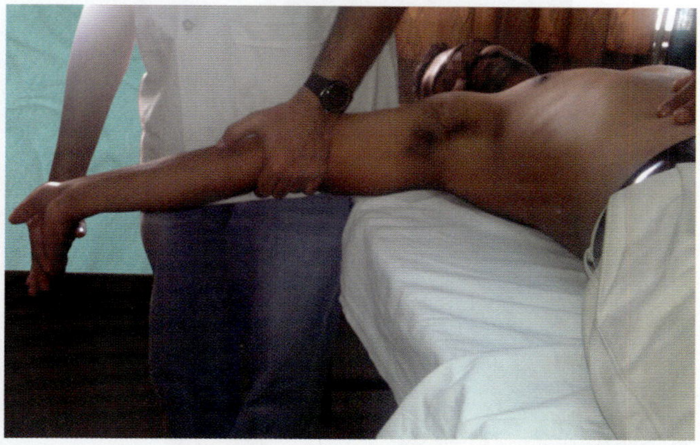

Fig. 27.53: Abducting patient shoulder to 90° while maintaining shoulder depression increases nerve root tension

- Maneuver of ULTT-2 radial nerve dominant. Position patient in relaxed supine position along the edge of the table
- Examiner stands on head side of the table with his thigh resting against the superior aspect of the patient's shoulder. Examiner holds patient's wrist and elbow (Fig. 27.54).
  - In controlled manner, examiner depresses patient shoulder with his thigh (Fig. 27.55)
  - Patient shoulder is abducted to 10°
  - Maintaining shoulder's depression extend the elbow (Fig. 27.56)
  - Then internally rotate the patient's shoulder (Fig. 27.57)
  - Palmar flexion of wrist with extension of fingers (Fig. 27.58).

Upper Limb Tension Test-3

- ULTT-3 is used to access possible irritation of C8 and T1 nerve root. It is designed for ulnar nerve dominance

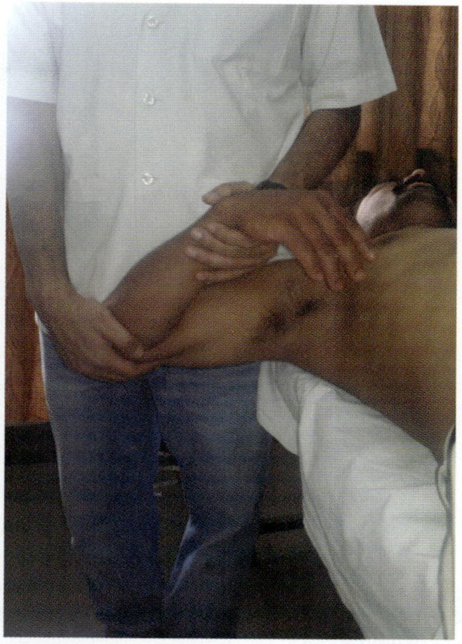

Fig. 27.54: Examiner holding patient's wrist and elbow, while standing on headside of table with his thigh resting against the superior aspect of the patient's shoulder

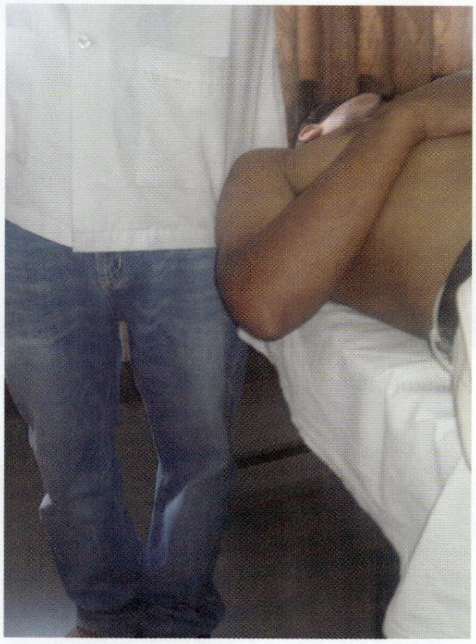

Fig. 27.55: In controlled manner, examiner depresses patient's shoulder with his thigh

- Maneuver of ULTT-3. Position patient in relaxed supine position along the edge of the table
- With one hand gently holding the patient's hand and with other hand stabilizes patients shoulder against the examination table to prevent further elevation of shoulder (Fig. 27.59)

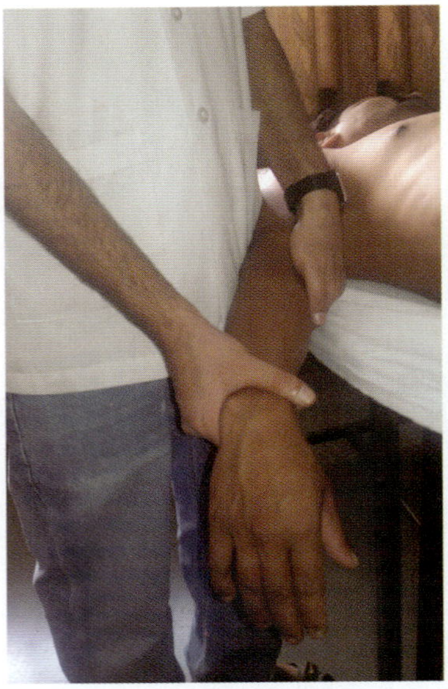

Fig. 27.56: While maintaining shoulder's abduction to 10°, elbow is extended

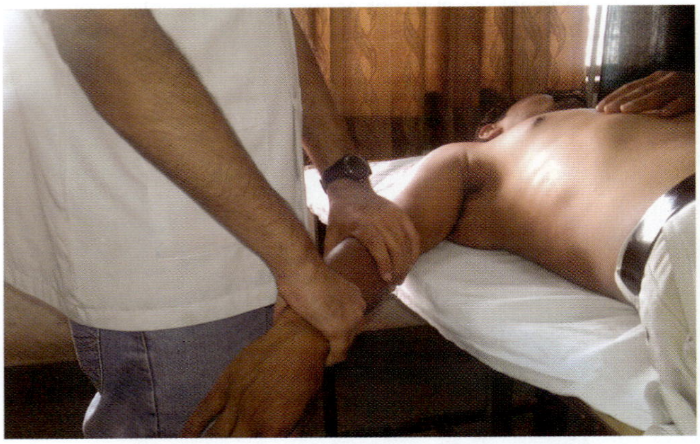

Fig. 27.57: Internal rotation of patient's shoulder is done

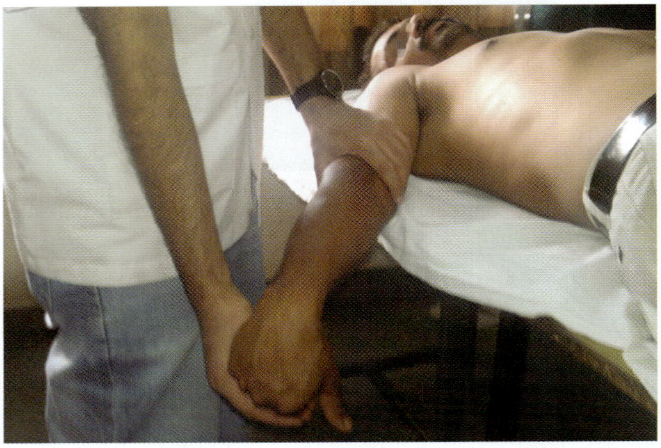

Fig. 27.58: Palmar flexion of wrist is done with extension of fingers

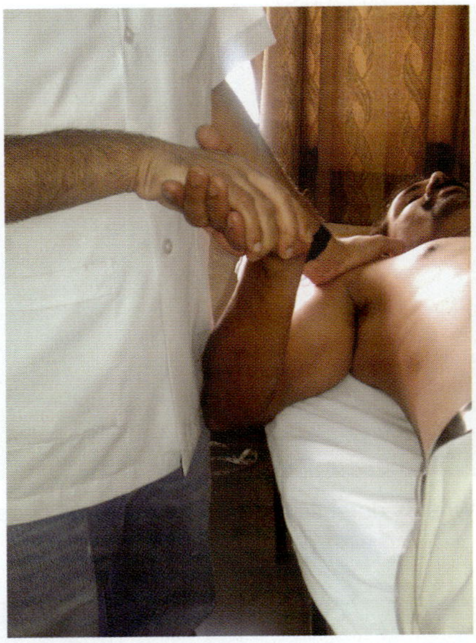

Fig. 27.59: With one hand gently hold the patient hand and with other hand stabilize patient's shoulder against the examination table to prevent further elevation of shoulder

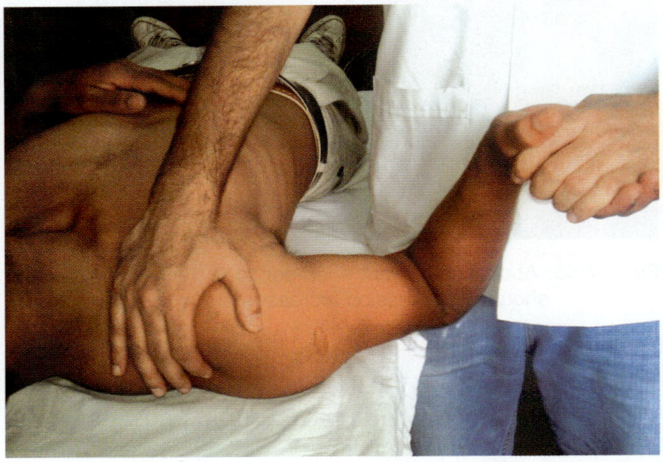

Fig. 27.60: With dorsi-flexed wrist, forearm is supinated

- The patient wrist is dorsi-flexed and forearm supinated (Fig. 27.60)
- Maintaining shoulder depression, flex the elbow (Fig. 27.61)
- Maximum flexion of elbow is done (Fig. 27.62)
- Patients arm is externally rotated and abducted to meet his or her ear (Fig. 27.63)
- Ask the patient to laterally bend the neck (Fig. 27.64)
- Pain is relived when neck is bend on same side and increases when neck is bend on opposite side.

Tension tests in lumbar disk prolapse are:

- Straight leg raising test
- Bowstring test

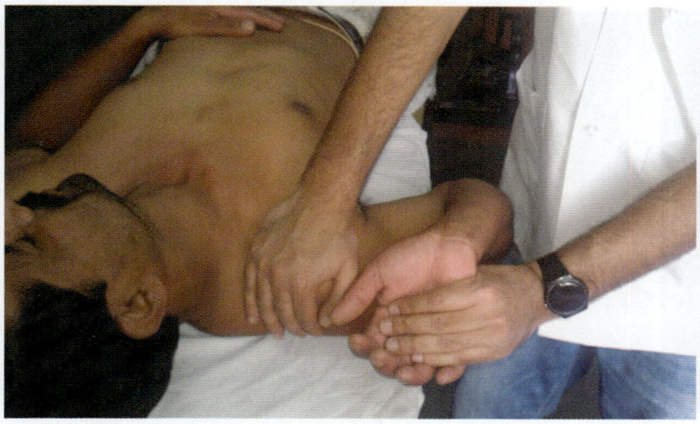

Fig. 27.61: While maintaining shoulder's depression, flex the elbow

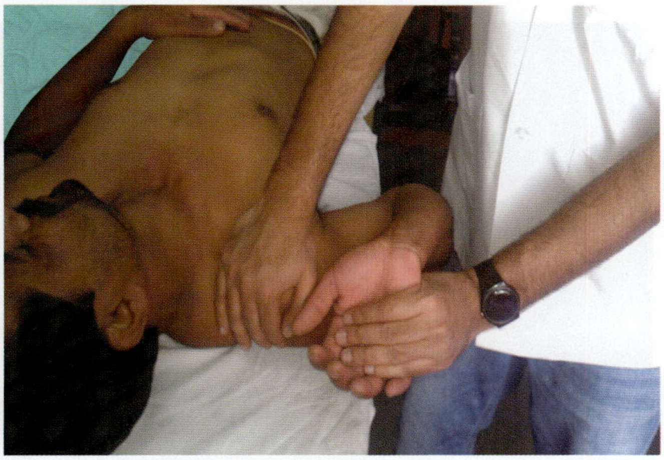

Fig. 27.62: Maximum flexion of elbow is done

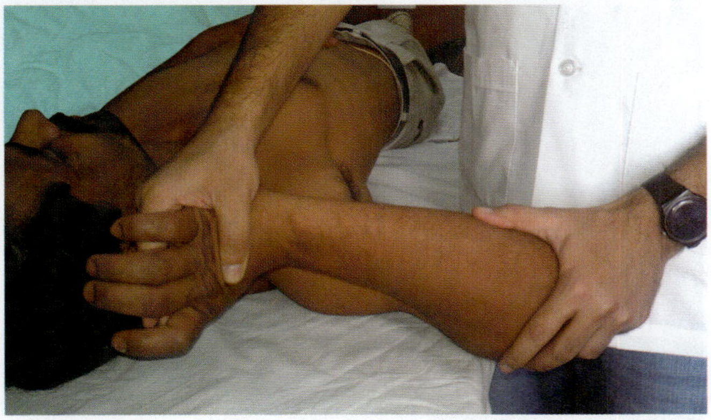

Fig. 27.63: Patient's arm is externally rotated and abducted to meet his or her own ear

- Well-leg raising test
- Lasegue's test
- Lateral flexion test of spine
- Sciatic stretch test
- Figure of 4 test

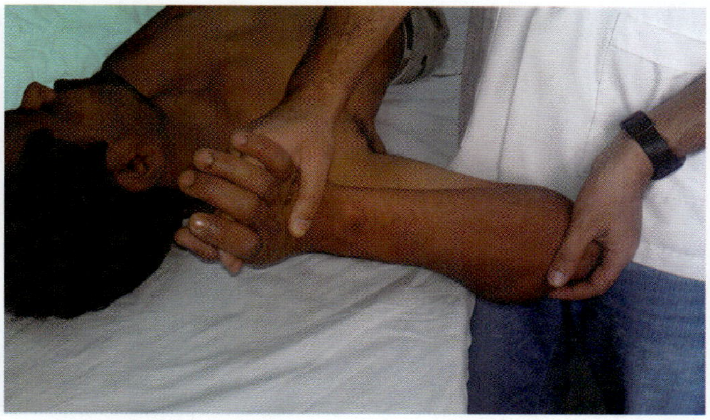

Fig. 27.64: Patient is asked to bend the neck laterally

- Sitting root test
- Femoral nerve stretch.

Straight Leg Raising Test (Fig. 27.65A)

- Straight leg raising (SLR) test is used to demonstrate a lumbosacral nerve root irritation due to a herniated disk
- It is a part of tension tests which are based upon the maneuvers which tighten the sciatic nerve and thus compress the inflamed nerve root against the herniated disk leading to pain
- Interpretation of SLR:
  - Pain or parasthesia up to 70° is suggestive of prolapsed disk
  - Pain above 70° is equivocal
  - Back pain suggests central disk prolapse—not indicative of root tension
  - Leg pain (buttock, thigh, leg) suggests lateral protrusion—indicative of root tension
- False positive SLR
  - Hamstring tightness might cloud the assessment of SLR

  Can be differentiated by following characteristics:
  - Discomfort is bilateral
  - Discomfort is distal in the thigh, in the region of the hamstring tendons
  - Does not radiate below the knee
- False negative SLR:
  - Generally seen in a loose jointed individual
  - Can be appreciated on examining the other limb (the person's ability to straight leg raise will be beyond 90°)
  - So to avoid both false positives and false negatives it is mandatory to examine both the lower limbs

Bowstring's Sign (Fig. 27.65B)

- It is probably single most important sign in diagnosis of tension and irritation of a nerve root caused by a ruptured intervertebral disk

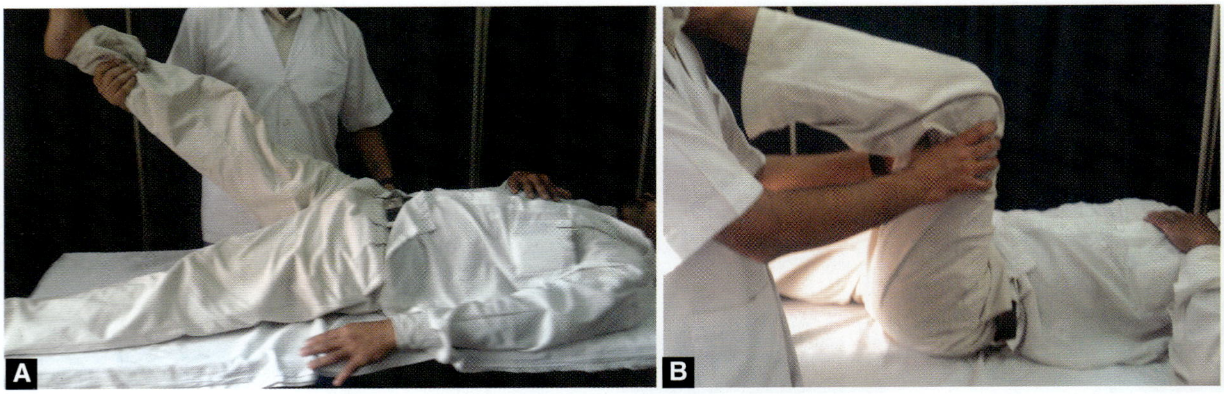

Figs 27.65A and B: (A) Straight leg raising test; (B) Bowstring's sign

- Carry out the SLR up to the point the patient experiences discomfort in the distribution of sciatic nerve, allow the knee to flex and the patient's foot is allowed to rest on the examiner's shoulder
- A sudden pressure is applied on the popliteal nerve in the popliteal fossa
- Positive test is a reproduction of radiating leg discomfort
- P.S: Pain in the popliteal fossa is not significant.

Well-Leg Raising Sign (Crossover Pain)

- This is considered positive when the a symptomatic leg is lifted and the symptomatic side becomes more painful
- Indicative of a disk herniation lying medial to the nerve root, either in the axilla of the nerve root or in the midline position.

Nonorganic Pain

- Patients with functional overlay or malingerers can be diagnosed by following maneuvers
- *Positive flip test:* Patient sits with knees dangling by the end of a table, knee and hip at 90° flexion. Knee is now extended fully; the position assumed by the leg will be equivalent to 90° SLR (Fig. 27.66)
- Patient with a root compression will throw his trunk backwards to avoid tension on the nerve, but a patient with a nonorganic pain will allow the examiner to fully extend the leg (Fig. 27.67)
- If the patient complains of increase of pain on flexion of knee and hip at the end of SLR, the patient is emotionally compromised or is a malingerer.

Fajersztajn Test

- SLRT is done until pain is produced then gentle dorsiflexion of the foot
- It is done to ascertain whether symptoms are increased. These are also known as Bragards sign (Fig. 27.68).

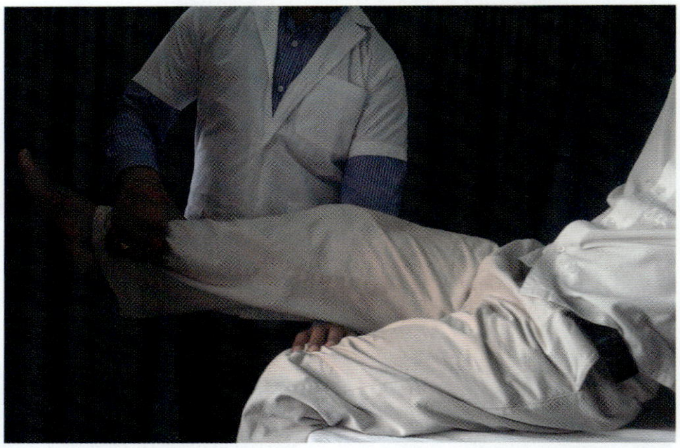

Fig. 27.66: Positive flip test

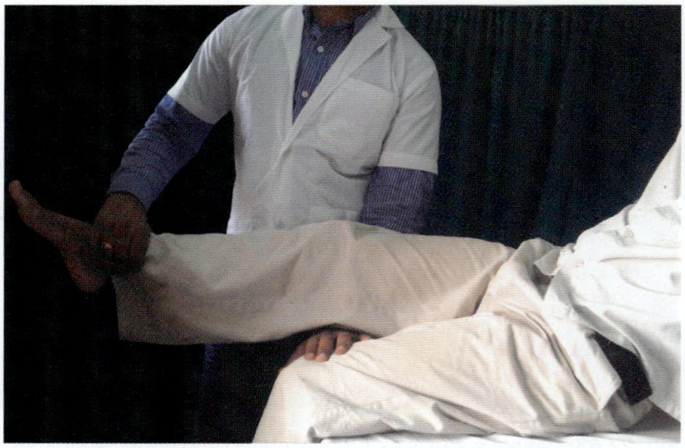

Fig. 27.67: Patient throwing his trunk backwards to avoid tension on the nerve

Lasegue's Test

Hip and knee gently flexed to 90°. The leg is then extended which reproduce the symptoms of sciatica.

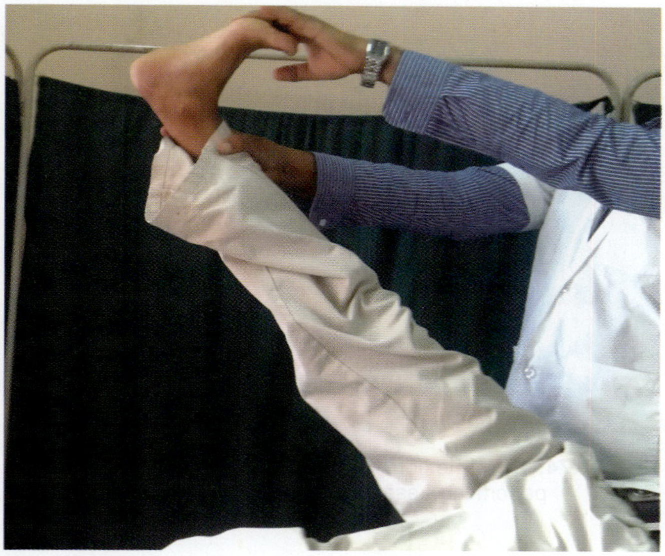

Fig. 27.68: Fajersztajn test

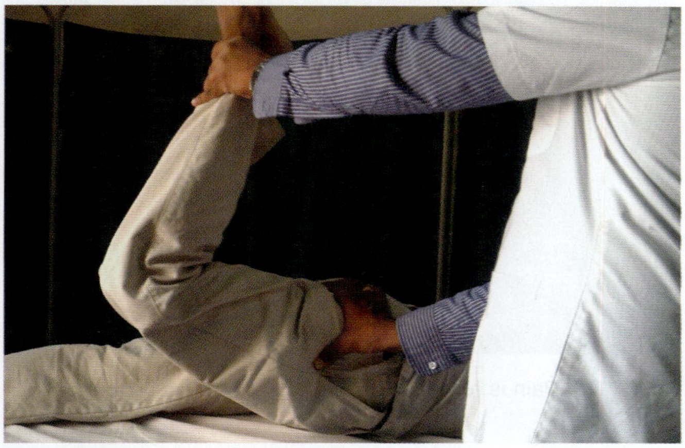

Fig. 27.69: Femoral stretch test

Femoral Stretch Test

Patient is in prone position. Knee is gradually flexed and then the hip extended this causes excursion in L2, L3 and L4 roots (Fig. 27.69).

Slump Test

- Patient sits on the side of table (Fig. 27.70)
- Patient is encouraged to flex thoracic and lumbar spine while still looking ahead (Fig. 27.71)
- Full flexion of cervical spine is done (Fig. 27.72)
- Extension of one knee is done thus performing SLRT (Fig. 27.73)
- Dorsi-flexion of foot on same side is done thus performing lasegue's test (Fig. 27.74)
- Test is positive if patient complains of radicular pain
- Pain get relived on extension of cervical spine (Fig. 27.75).

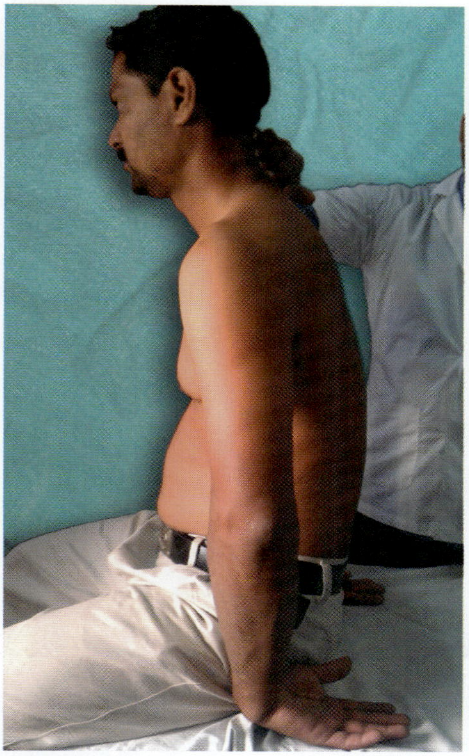

Fig. 27.70: Slump test

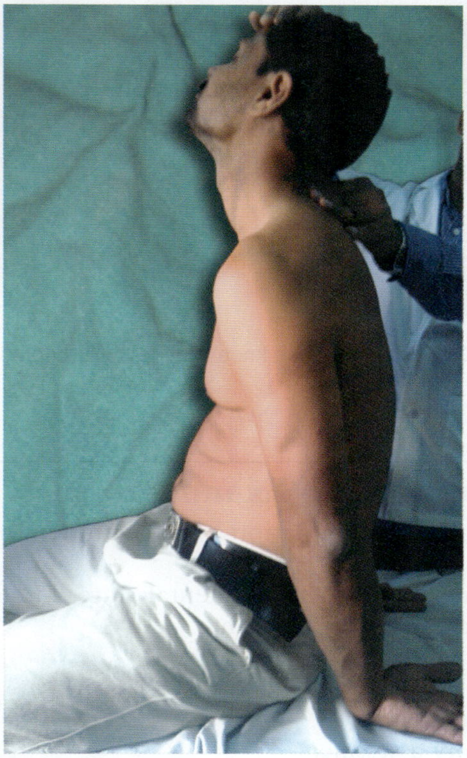

Fig. 27.71: Thoracic and lumbar spine is flexed while still looking ahead

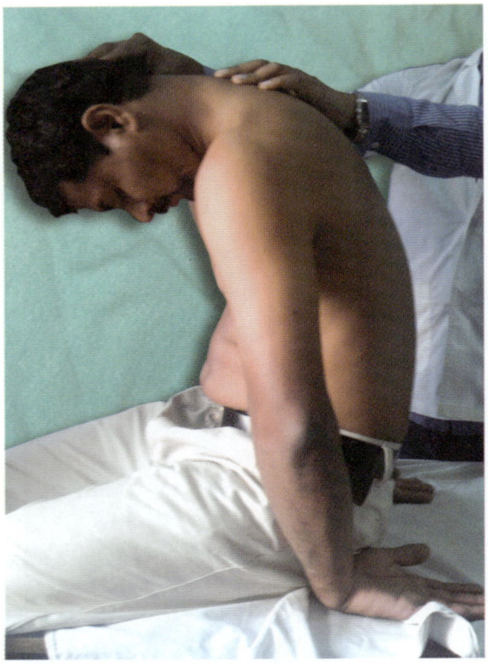

Fig. 27.72: Full flexion of cervical spine is done

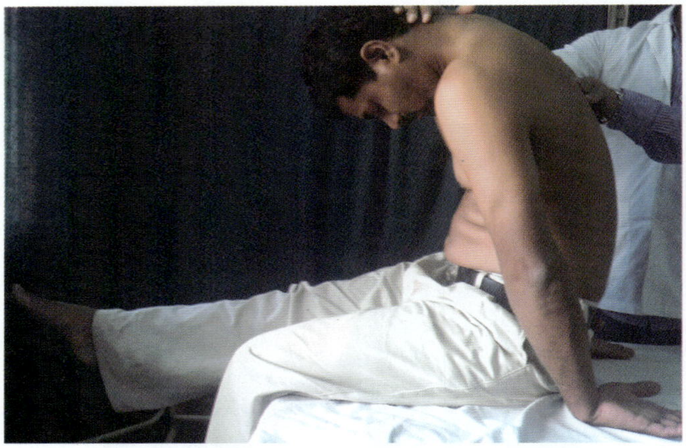

Fig. 27.73: Extension of one knee is done thus performing SLRT

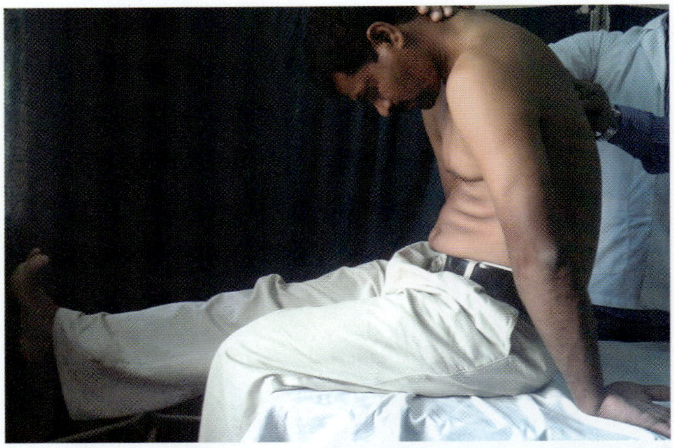

Fig. 27.74: Dorsi-flexion of foot on same side is done thus performing Lasegue's test

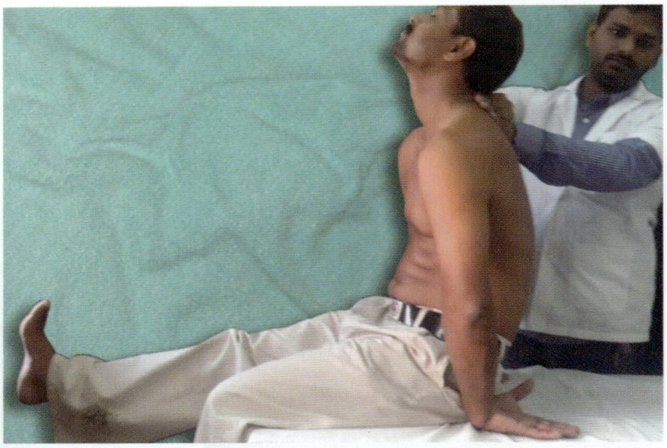

Fig. 27.75: Pain is relieved on extension of cervical spine

Neurological Examination

Neurological examination is done under following headings:

- A quick assessment of mental state, intelligence, speech, general appearance
- Cranial nerves
- Gait
- Posture
- Sensory assessment
- Vasomotor functions
- Reflexes
- Visceral assessment: Assessment, specially of bladder and bowel.

Gait Cycle (Table 27.2)

Continuous rhythmic alternative movements of lower limbs in order to propulse the body forward by moving center of gravity in forward direction with minimal expenditure of energy.

Two phases of gait are:

1. Cycle stance phase (Figs 27.76 to 27.79)
2. Swing phase 40 percent (Figs 27.80 to 27.83).

Motor Functions

- *Bulk of the muscle:* Look for atrophy, hypertrophy, flabbiness, pliability. Confirm by circumferential measurement.
- *Tone of muscle:* Look for hypotonia, hypertonia, clasp knife rigidity, lead pipe rigidity
- Powers of the muscle

Table 27.2: Different terminologies of gait cycle

Phase	*Traditional terminologies*	*Rancho Los Amigos Medical Center*
Stance phase	Heel strike	Initial contact
	Foot flat Mid-stance	Loading response Mid-stance
	Heel off	Terminal stance
	Toe off	Preswing
Swing phase	Acceleration	Initial swing
	Midswing	Midswing
	Deceleration	Terminal swing

Abnormal gait	*Diseases in which they are seen*
Scissors gait	Cerebral diplegia
High stepping gait (Steppage gait, equine gait)	Foot drop
Spastic gait	Hemiplegia
Lathyriatic gait	Lathyriasis
Waddling gait or duck gait	Congenital dislocation of hip, myopathies, pregnancy
Trendelenberg's gait	CDH, fracture neck femur, polioparalysis
Drunkards gait or reeling gait	Cerebellar in-coordination or in drunken state
Festinant gait or short shuffling gait	Parkinsonism
Antalgic or painful gait	Pain anywhere from foot to hip
Stamping gait	Tabes dorsalis
Quadriceps gait, hand to knee gait or five fingers quadriceps	Weak quadriceps
Calcaneus gait	Weakness of triceps surae
Gluteus maximus gait	Weak gluteus maximus muscle

Assessed on MRC scale	
Grade 0	Not even flicker of contraction
Grade 1	Flicker of contraction
Grade 2	Contraction of muscle with no assistance and gravity eliminated but moving the joint to full range of motion
Grade 3	Contraction of muscle against gravity
Grade 4	Contraction of muscle against gravity and moderate resistance
Grade 5	Normal

- Motor function assessment
  - C5 nerve root by testing deltoid muscle (Fig. 27.84)
  - C6 nerve root assessment by wrist extensors and biceps (Figs 27.85 and 27.86)
  - C7 nerve root assessment by wrist flexor, finger extensor and triceps brachii (Figs 27.87 to 27.91)
  - C8 muscle assessment is done by long finger extensors (Fig. 27.92)
  - T1 nerve root assessment done with finger abduction, first dorsal interossei and finger adduction (Figs 27.93 and 27.94)

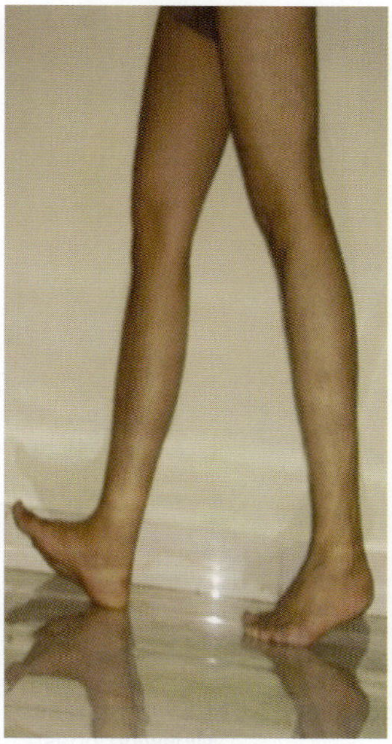

Fig. 27.76: Stance phase—Heel strike

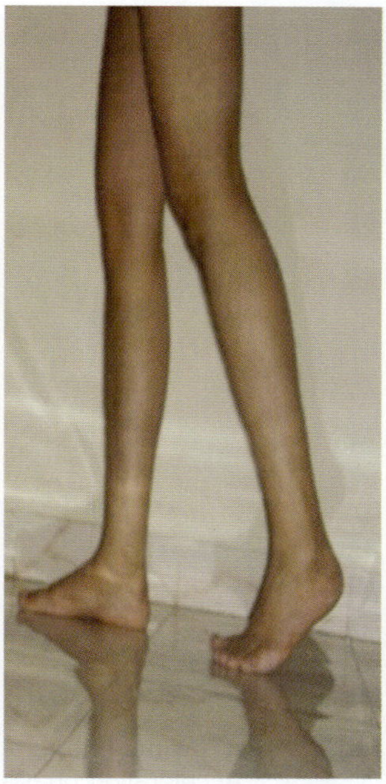

Fig. 27.77: Stance phase—Flat foot

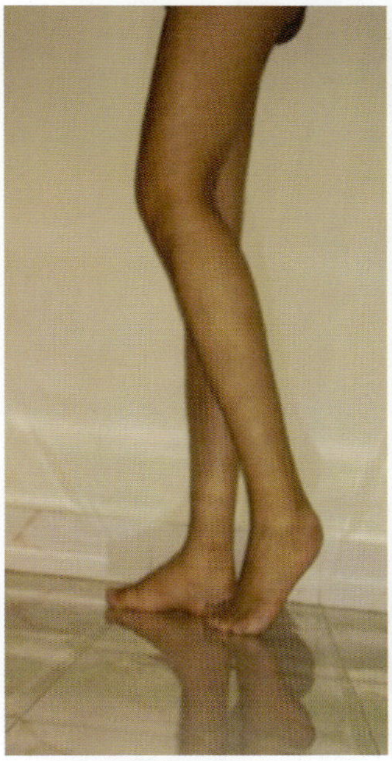

Fig. 27.78: Stance phase—Heal off

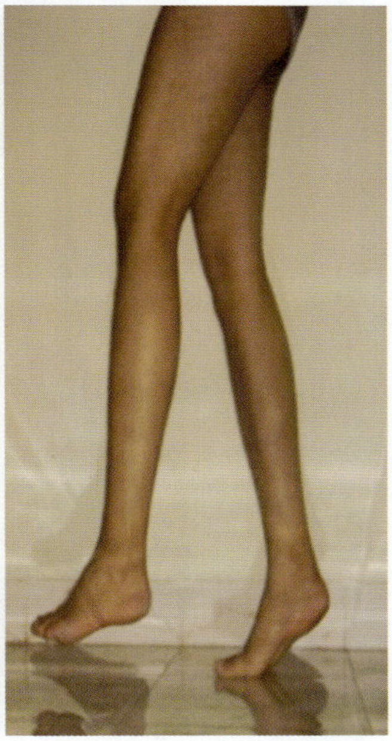

Fig. 27.79: Stance phase—Toe off

Beevor's Sign (Fig. 27.95)

Lower Limb Motor Assessment

- L1 and L2 motor function by assessing iliopsoas muscle
- Assessing L3 motor function of quadriceps muscle (Fig. 27.96)

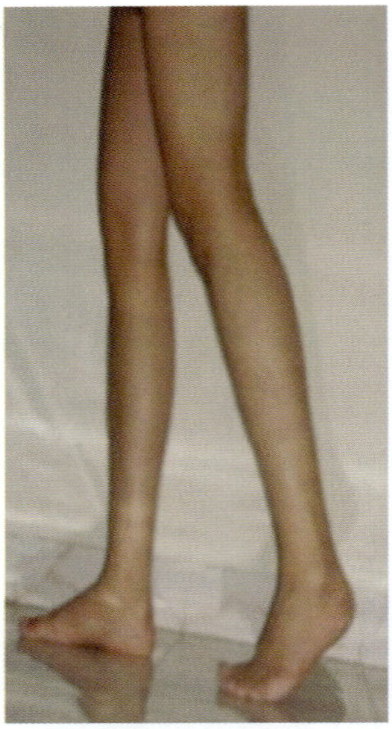

Fig. 27.80: Swing phase—Acceleration phase

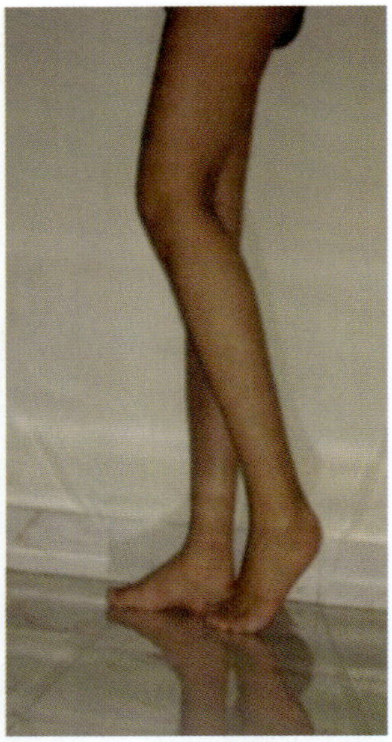

Fig. 27.81: Swing phase—Midswing phase

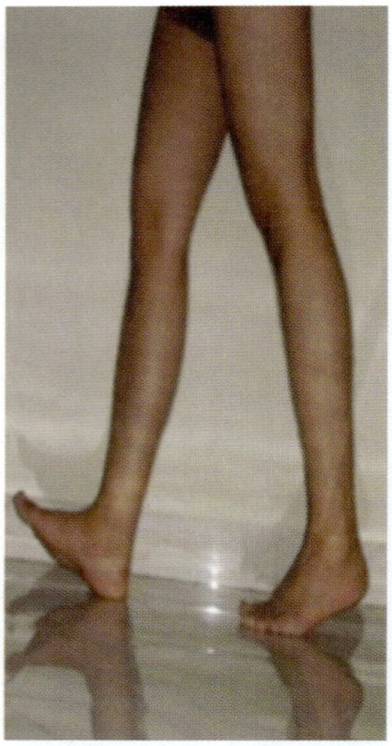

Fig. 27.82: Swing phase—Deceleration phase

- *Assessing L4 motor function:* Tibialis anterior strength (Fig. 27.97)
- Assessing L5 motor function extensor hallucis longus, extensor digitorum longus, gluteus medius (Figs 27.98 to 27.100)
- Assessing S1 motor function of gastroesoleus, peroneus longus and brevis, gluteus maximus (Figs 27.101 to 27.103)

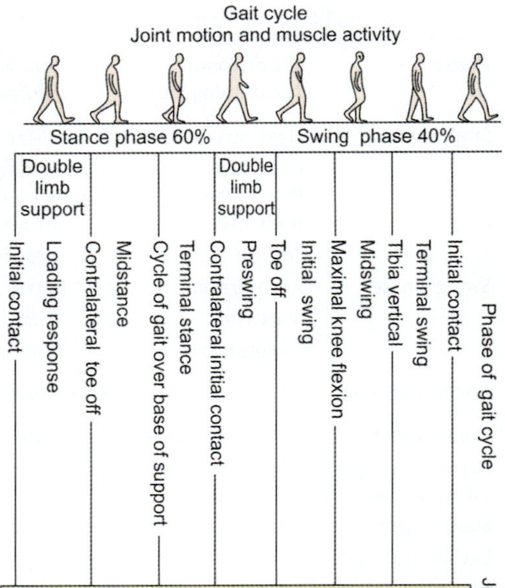

	Initial contact	Contralateral toe off	Cycle of gait over base of support	Contralateral initial contact	Toe off	Maximal knee flexion	Tibia vertical	Initial contact
Pelvic fwd rotation	5		0	–5			0	5
Hip flexion	30	30	5	–10	0	20	30	30
Knee flexion	0	15	5	0	40	60	30	0
Ankle plantar flexion	0	15	–5	–10	20	10	0	0
Subtalar supination	5	–10	–5	5	10			5

Fig. 27.83: Gait cycle: Joint motion and muscle activity

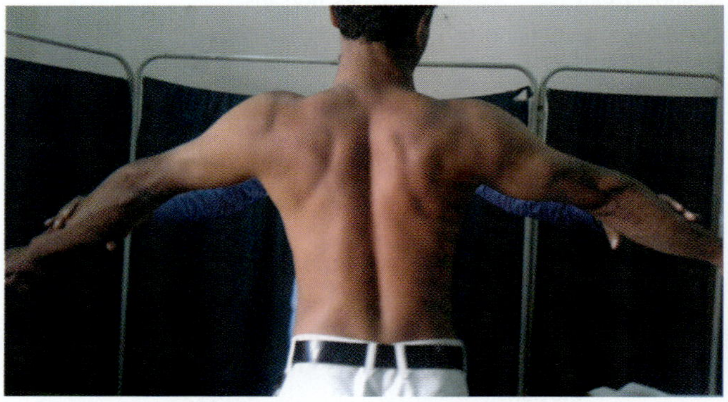

Fig. 27.84: C5 nerve root by testing deltoid muscle

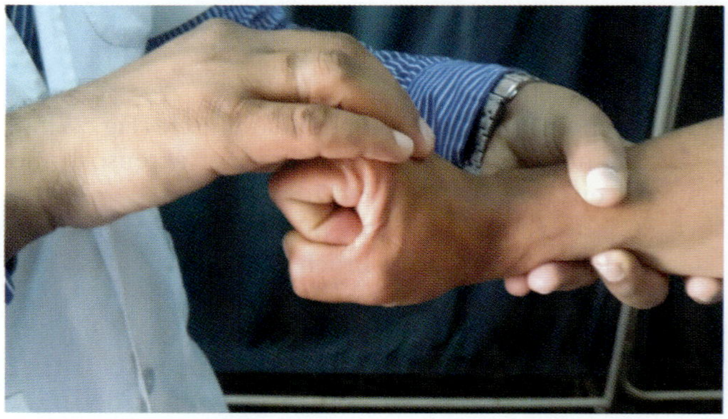

Fig. 27.85: C6 nerve root assessment by wrist extensors

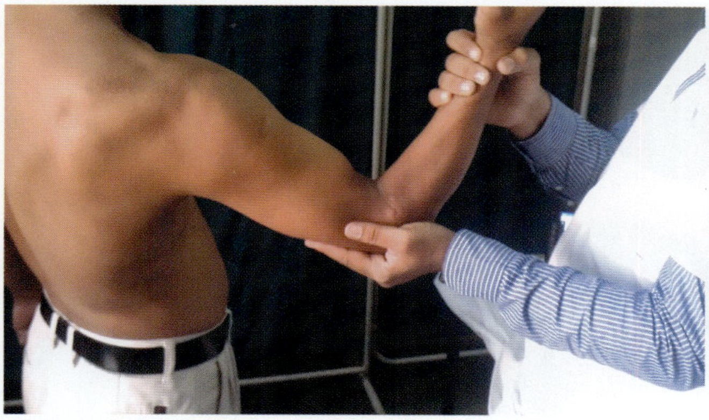

Fig. 27.86: C6 nerve root assessment by biceps

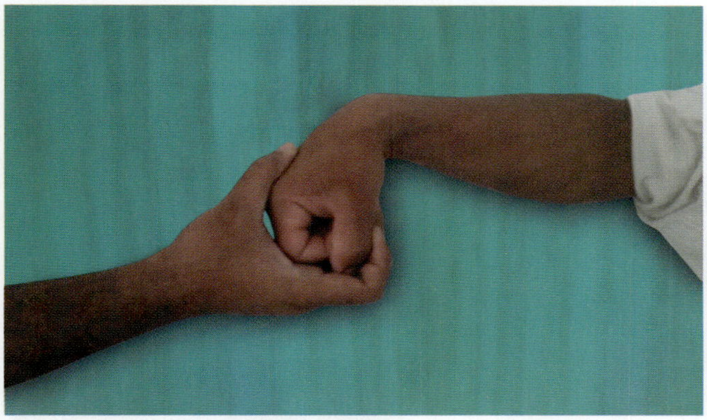

Fig. 27.87: C7 nerve root assessment—Finger extensors

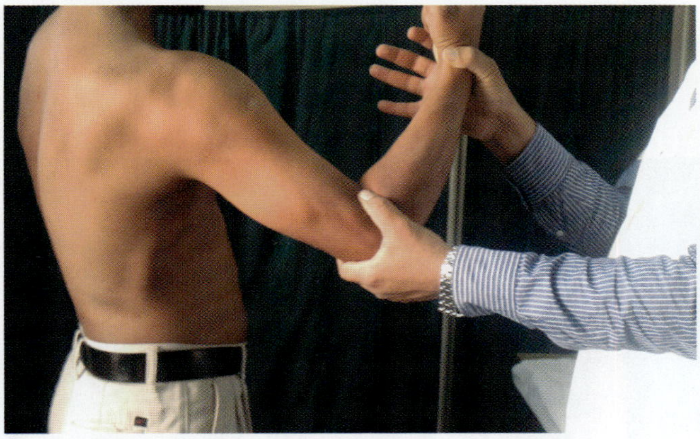

Fig. 27.88: C7 nerve root assessment—Elbow extension

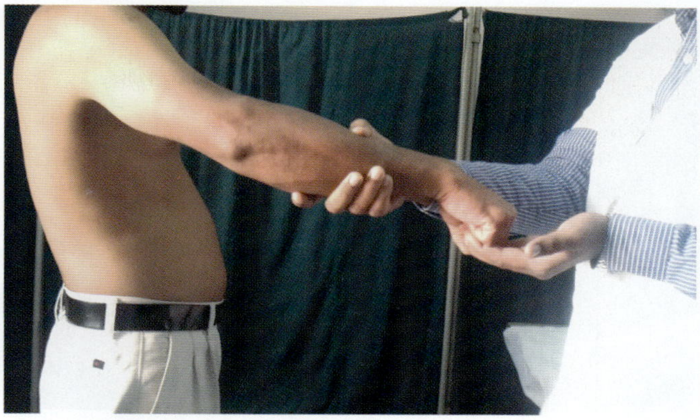

Fig. 27.89: C7 nerve root assessment by wrist flexion

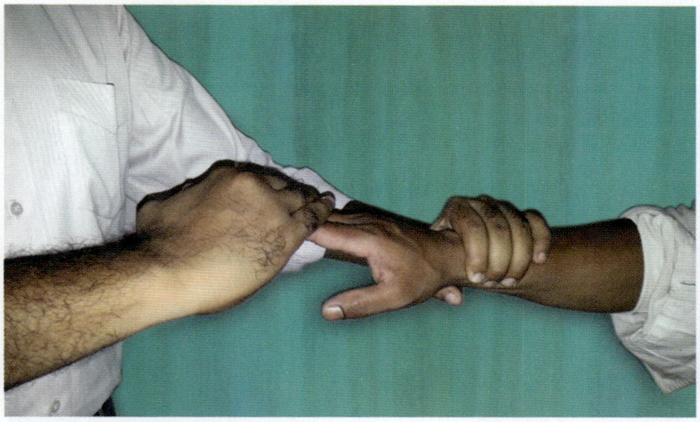

Fig. 27.90: Finger extension

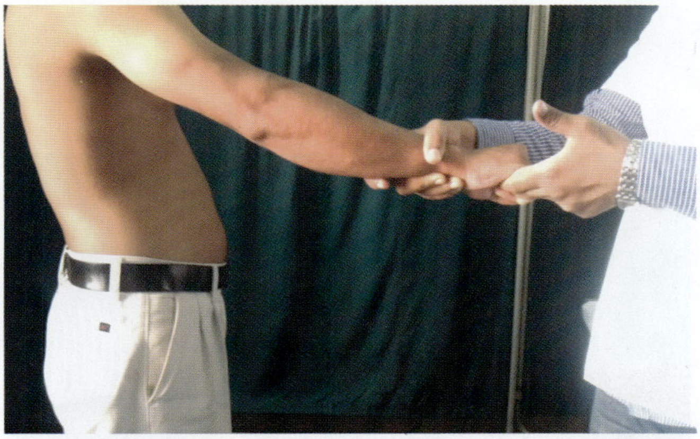

Fig. 27.91: C7 nerve root assessment

- *Co-ordination of movements:* Finger to nose test and Romberg's test
- *Involuntory movement:* Athetosis, chorea, dystonia, dyskinesia, tetany, tics.

Reflexes

Superficial reflexes (Figs 27.104 and 27.105).

For other reflexes (Table 27.3) for manifestations of nerve root compression at different levels (Table 27.4).

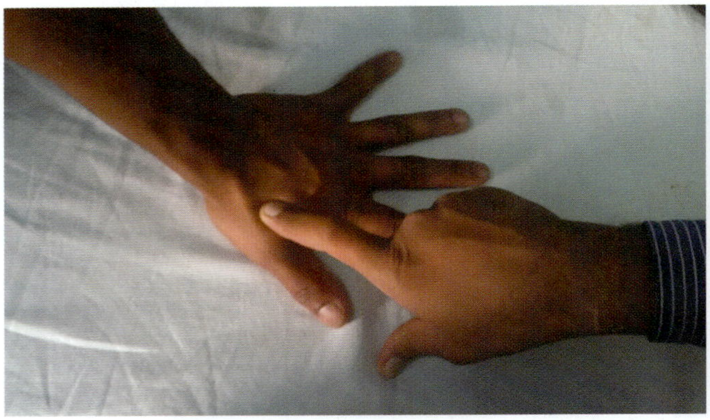

Fig. 27.92: C8 nerve root assessment by long finger extensors

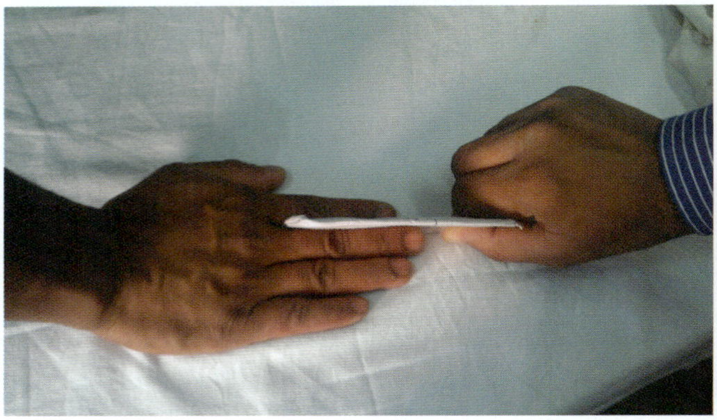

Fig. 27.93: T1 nerve root assessment by palmar interossei

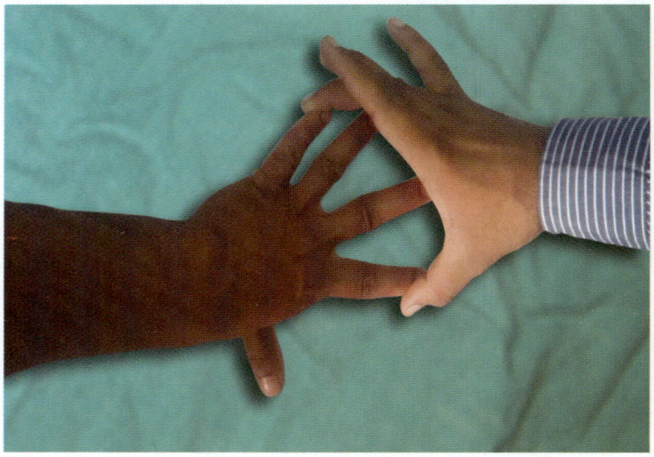

Fig. 27.94: T1 nerve root assessment by dorsal interossei

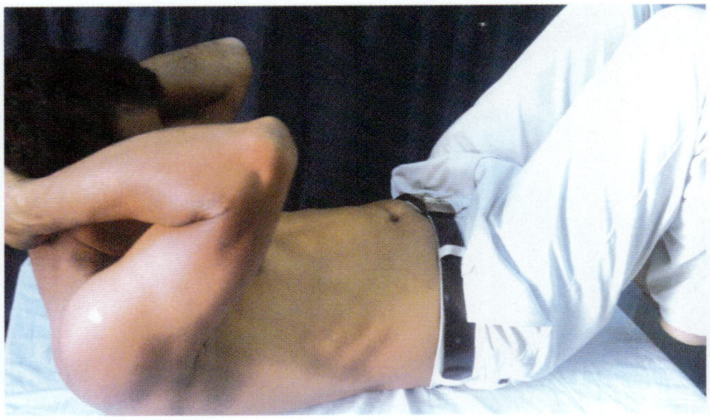

Fig. 27.95: Beevor's sign

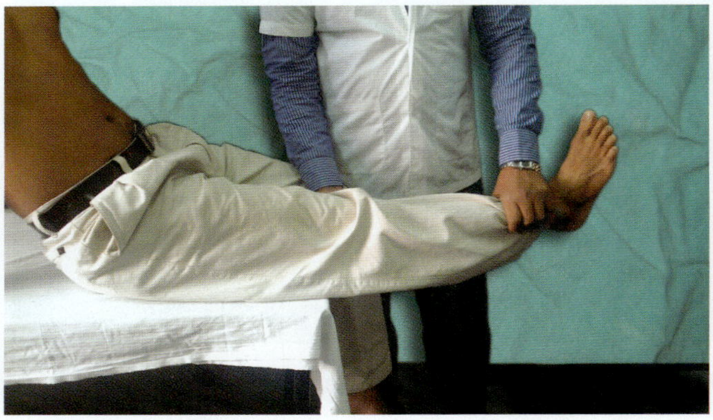

Fig. 27.96: Assessing L3 motor function of quadriceps

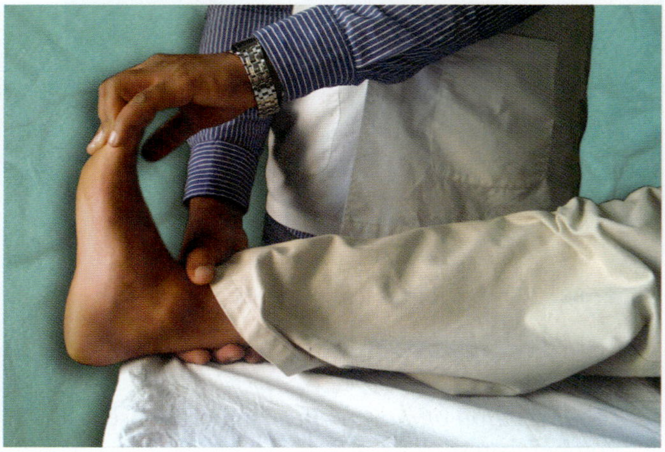

Fig. 27.97: L4 nerve root assessment by tibialis anterior

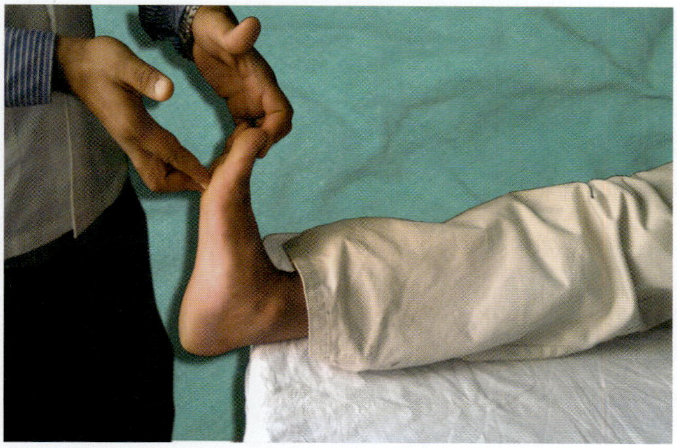

Fig. 27.98: L5 root assessment by extensor digitorum longus

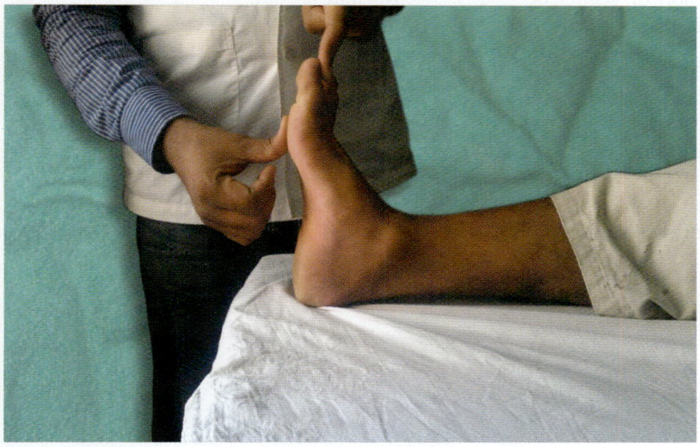

Fig. 27.99: L5 root assessment by extensor hallucis longus

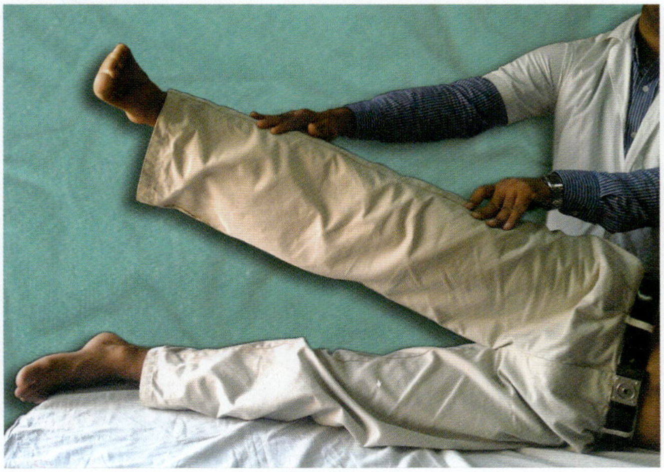

Fig. 27.100: L5 root assessment by gluteus medius

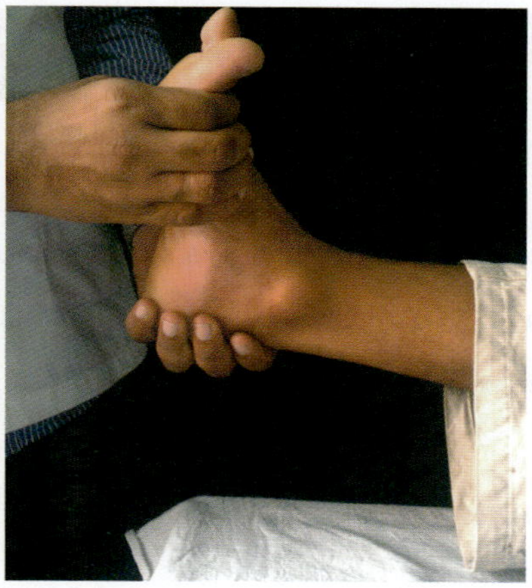

Fig. 27.101: S1 root assessment by gastrosoleus

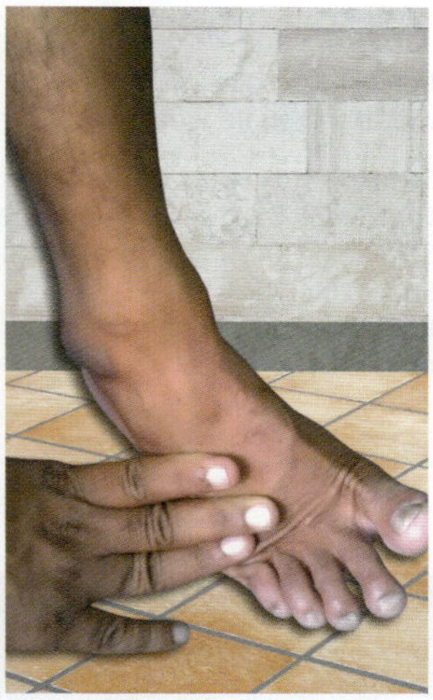

Fig. 27.102: S1 root assessment by peronei

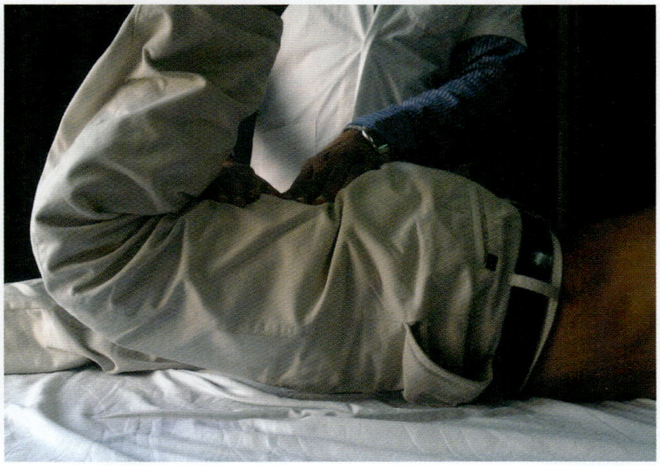

Fig 27.103: S1 root assessment by gluteus maximus

Table 27.3: Interpretation of reflexes

Reflex	*How to initiate*	*What to initiate*	*Inference*	*Cord level*
Trapezius reflex	Proximal to acromion tap the stretched muscle	Contraction of trapezius	Normal	C3-C4
Deltoid reflex	Tap on deltoid mass distal to acromion	Contraction of deltoid	Normal	C5-C6
Scapular reflex	Scratching of skin at interscapular region	Scapular muscle contraction	Normal	C5-T1
Abdominal reflex	Scratching of abdominal wall in oblique direction from all four quadrants from outer aspect towards midline	Contraction of abdominal muscle in testing quadrants	Normal, absent in UML lesion above their spinal lesion	T7-T12
Cremasteric reflex	With blunt pointed gently scratch upper medial side of thigh	Involuntary contraction of dartos muscle of scrotum	Normal	L1
Anal reflex	Scratch perianal skin or insert one lubricated gloved finger in anus	Contraction of anal sphincter no contraction	Normal cauda equina syndrome	S3-S4
Bulbocavernosus reflex	Pinching the dorsum of glans penis	Contraction of bulbocavernosus muscle	Normal	S3-S4
Throckmorton's reflex	Percuss the dorsum of foot at metatarsophalangeal joint	Extension of great toe and flexion of other toes	Normal	
Plantar reflex	Stroking the outer part of the sole from heel to base of outer toes Squeezing the heel cord (Gordon's sign) Squeezing the calf Pressing firmly along the medial surface of tibia (Oppenheim's sign)	Flexion of toe, dorsiflexion of foot, inversion of foot Extension of great toe spreading out and extension of other toes dorsiflexion of ankle Flexion of hip and knee (withdrawal reflex)	Flexor plantar response Extensor plantar response UMN lesion	L5-S1

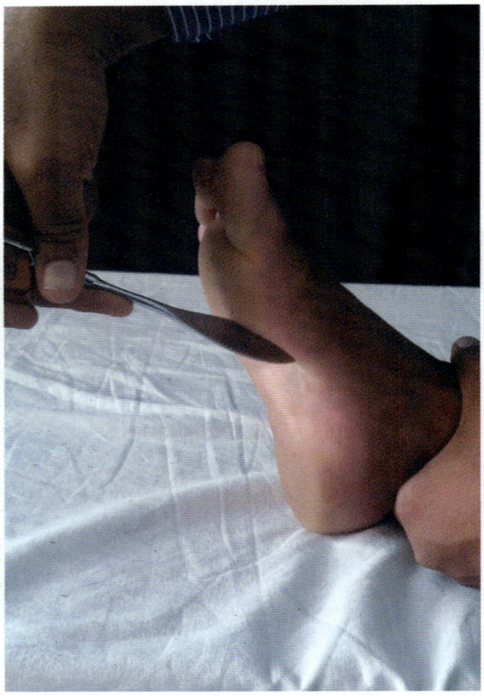

Fig. 27.104: Superficial reflexes

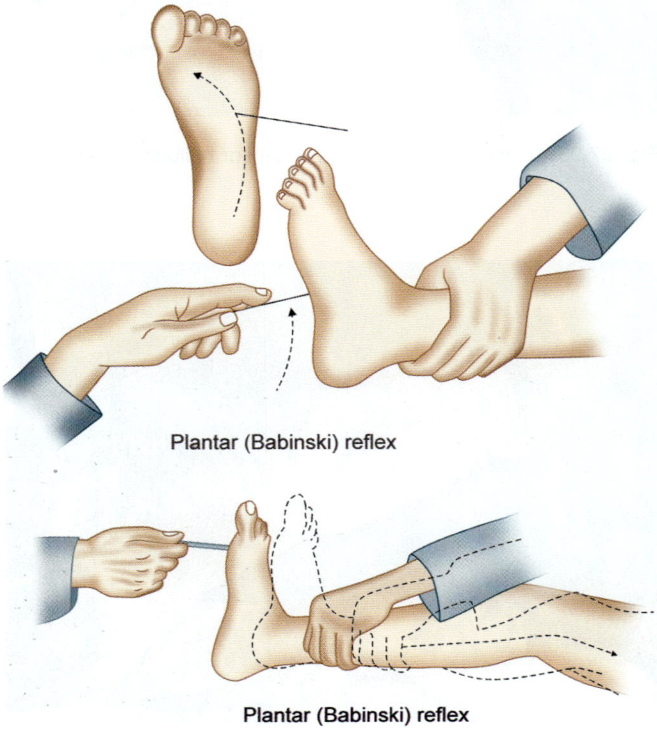

Fig. 27.105: Babinski reflex

Deep Tendon Reflexes

Knee jerk: L2, 3, 4 (Fig. 27.106).

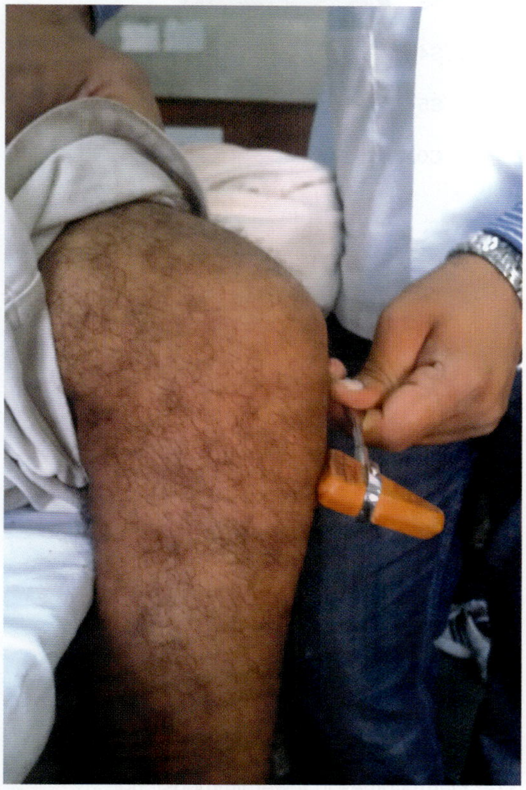

Fig. 27.106: Knee jerk

Patellar clonus: L2, 3, 4 (Fig. 27.107).

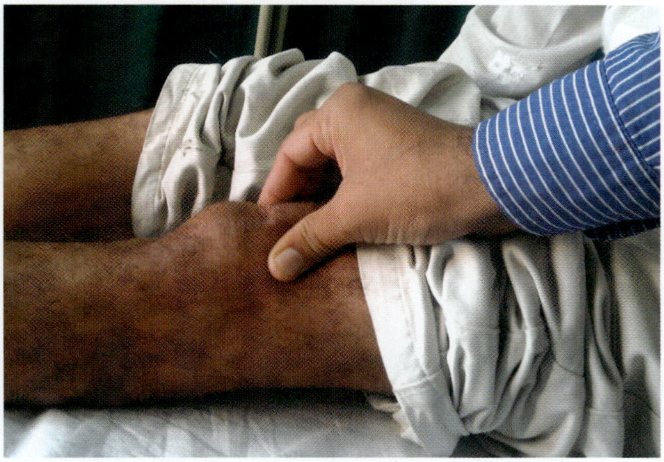

Fig. 27.107: Patellar clonus

Ankle jerk: S1, 2 (Fig. 27.108).

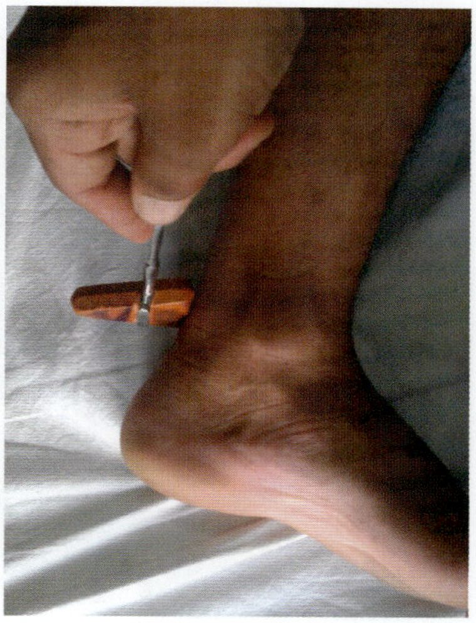

Fig. 27.108: Ankle jerk

Ankle clonus: S1, 2 (Fig. 27.109).

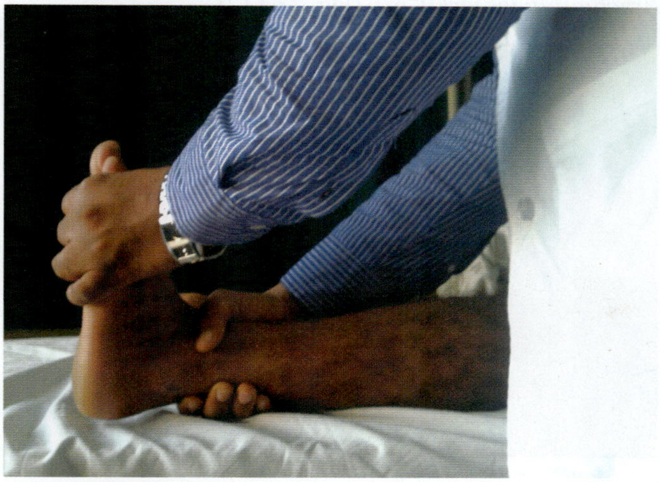

Fig. 27.109: Ankle clonus

Triceps jerk: C6, 7 (Fig. 27.110).

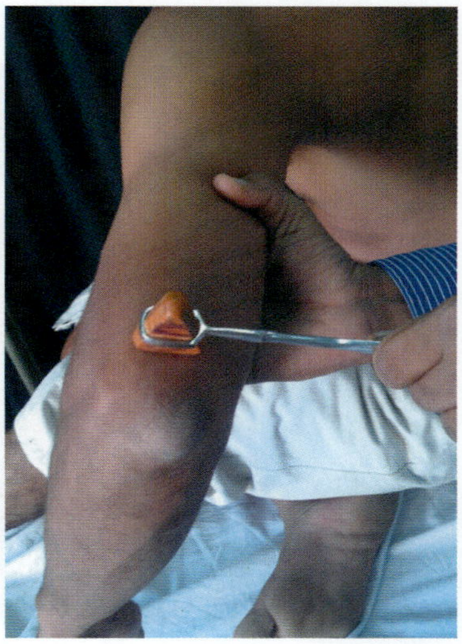

Fig. 27.110: Triceps jerk

Biceps jerk: C 5, 6 (Fig. 27.111).

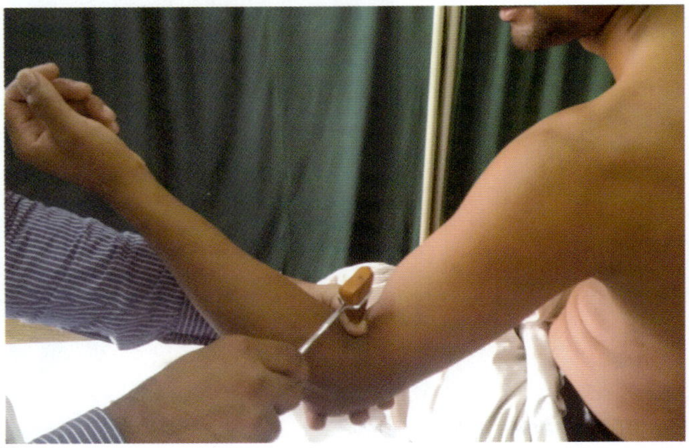

Fig. 27.111: Biceps jerk

Brachioradialis jerk: C5, 6 (Fig. 27.112).

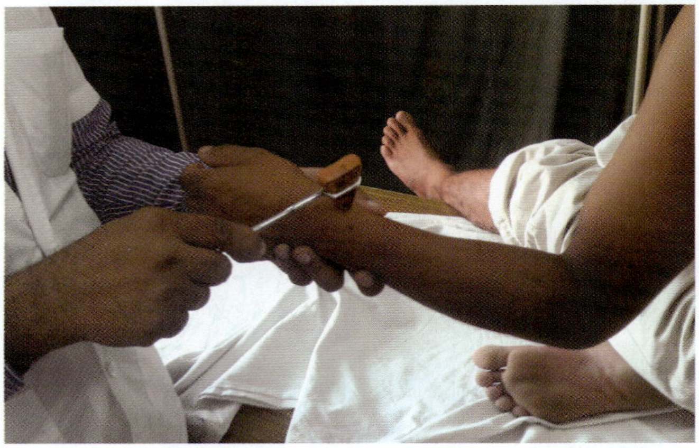

Fig. 27.112: Brachioradialis jerk

Jaw jerk: Increased contraction in UMN lesion above fifth cranial nerve (Fig. 27.113).

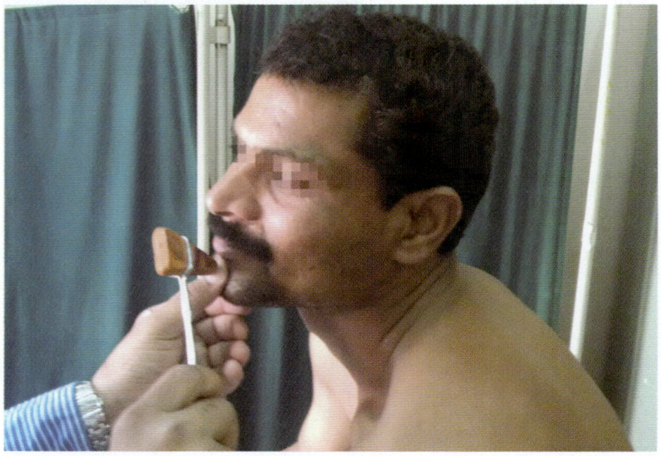

Fig. 27.113: Jaw jerk

■ Dermatomes

Figures 27.114 to 27.116 show dermatomes.

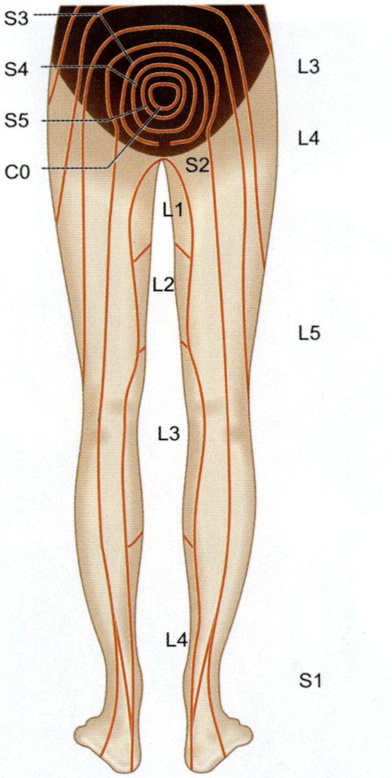

Fig. 27.114: Dermatomes in lower limb posterior

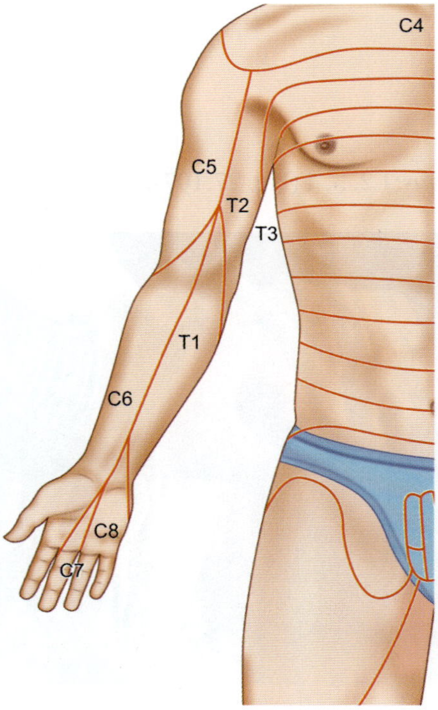

Fig. 27.115: Dermatomes in upper limb

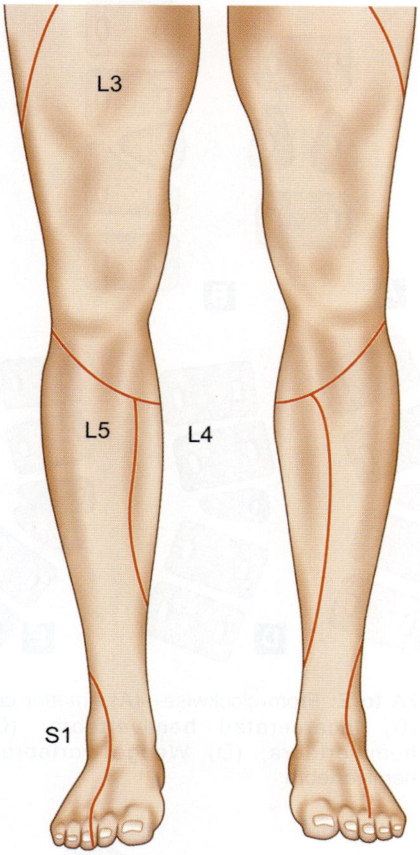

Fig. 27.116: Dermatomes in lower limb—Anterior

Vasomotor Changes

- Pallor, cynosis, redness, atrophy of skin, nailbed and subcutaneous tissues
- History of anhydrosis, oligohydrosis and hyperhydrosis should be inquired
- Determine by starch iodine test and Guttmans test
- *Visceral assessment:* Ask for bladder and bowel control.

Table 27.4: Finding of nerve root compression eight different levels

Nerve root compression	*Neurological findings*
C5 C4-C5 disk	*Motor weakness:* Deltoid, biceps (variable) *Sensory deficit:* Upper lateral arm and elbow *Reflex:* Biceps (variable)
C6 C5-C6 disk	*Motor weakness:* Biceps, extensor radialis longus and brevis *Sensory deficit:* Lateral forearm, thumb and index finger *Reflex:* Biceps, brachioradialis
C7 C6-C7 disk	*Motor weakness:* Triceps, wrist flexors *Sensory deficit:* Middle finger *Reflex:* Triceps
C8 C7-T1 disk	*Motor weakness:* Interossei, finger flexors, flexor carpi ulnaris *Sensory deficit:* Ring finger, little finger and ulnar border of palm *Reflex:* None
T1 T1-T2 disk	*Motor weakness:* Interossei *Sensory deficit:* Medial aspect of elbow *Reflex:* None
T12, L1, L2, L3, L4	*Motor deficit:* Iliopsoas weakness *Sensory:* Anterior part of the thigh *Reflexes:* None, patellar tendon variable
L4	*Motor deficit:* Quadriceps, hip adductors *Sensory:* Anterolateral thigh, anterior knee and medial leg *Reflexes:* Patellar tendon
L5	*Motor deficit:* Extensor hallucis longus, gluteus medius, extensor digitorum longus and brevis *Sensory:* Anterolateral leg, dorsum of foot and great toe *Reflexes:* None, tibialis posterior variable
S1	*Motor deficit:* Peroneus longus and brevis, tendoachillis, gluteus maximus *Sensory:* Lateral malleolus, lateral foot, heel and web of fourth and fifth toe *Reflexes:* Ankle reflex

CONGENITAL DEFORMITIES OF SPINE

Introduction

- Caused by anomalous vertebral development in the embryo.
- It can be simple and benign, with no spinal deformity or it can be complex with severe spinal deformity, e.g. cor pulmonale or even paraplegia.

Three major patterns of congenital spinal deformities

1. Hyperlordosis
2. Kyphosis
3. Scoliosis

Development of the Spine

- Molecular and cellular tissue interaction and increasing organ complexity are fundamental features of development during axial embryogenesis
- Alteration in the molecular and macromolecular process may lead to structural defects prenatally, postnatally or both.

Developmental Defects of Spine

These defects can further be classified into following heads:

Malformation

Failure of embryological differentiation, development or both, causing it to be absent or improperly formed, before the fetal period commences. The defect may continue to adversely affect spinal development, e.g. formation of hemivertebra.

Disruption

Structural defect resulting from destruction of a part, which normally formed during the embryonic period. Involves the limbs more frequently than the spine, e.g. amniotic band syndrome.

Deformation

- Alteration in the shape or structure of an individual vertebra or of entire spine during the fetal or postnatal periods. It can further be classified as:
- *Intrinsic deformation*: Reduced ability of the fetus or child to move away from normally imposed forces, which depends on the integrity of the neuromuscular system to respond effectively
- *Extrinsic deformation:* Result of reduction in the amount of space in which a developing fetus may move. These may be physiologic or pathologic
- Late gestational deformations have an excellent prognosis
- The earlier a deformation is recognized, the greater the likelihood of correcting it or at least preventing further deformation, e.g. with early bracing for idiopathic scoliosis.

Classification (Macewen's)

Failure of Formation (Figs 27.117A to E)

- Partial failure of formation (wedge vertebra)
- Complete failure of formation (hemivertebra).

Failure of Segmentation (Figs 27.118A and B)

- Unilateral failure of segmentation (unilateral unsegmented bar)
- Bilateral failure of segmentation (Block vertebra).

Mixed (Fig. 27.119)

Elements of both failure of formation and failure of segmentation.

Defects of Formation

These can be classified as:

- Anterior formation failure resulting in sharply angulated kyphosis (Fig. 27.120)
- Posterior formation failure is rare and can produce a lordotic curve
- Lateral formation failure is common and produces the classic hemivertebrae of congenital scoliosis.

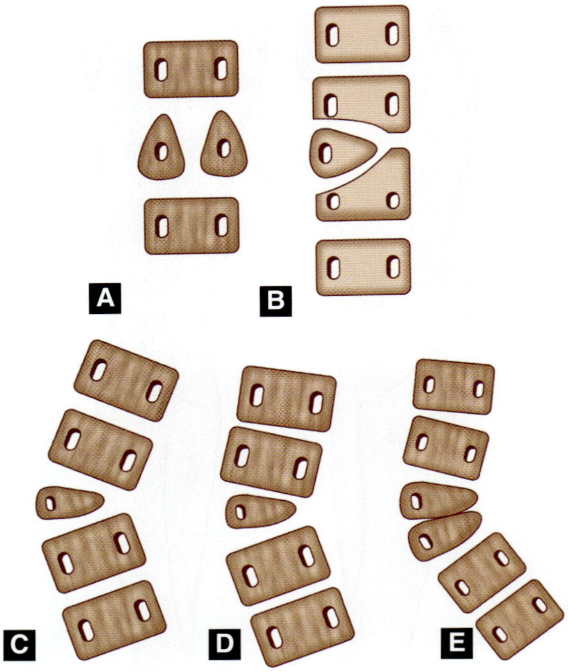

Figs 27.117A to E: From clockwise—(A) Anterior central defect; (B) Incarcerated hemivertebra; (C) Multiple hemivertebra; (D) Wedge vertebra; (E) Free hemivertebra

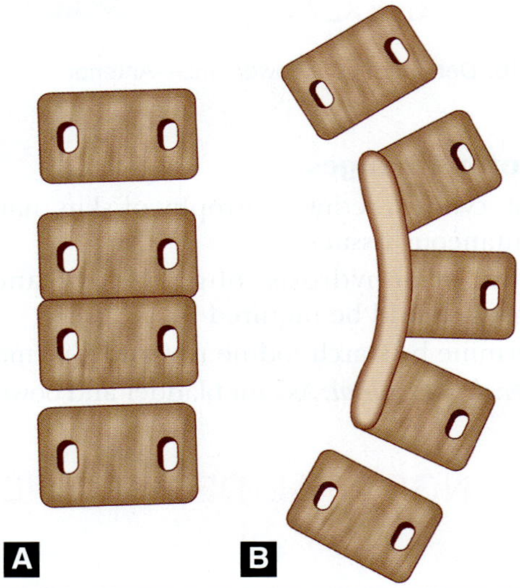

Figs 27.118A and B: Failure of segmentation of vertebra—(A) Block vertebra; (B) Unilateral unsegmented bar

Defect of Segmentation

Specific defects of segmentation may be classified as:

- Anterior segmentation failure (anterior unsegmented bar), leads to progressive kyphosis owing to the absence of anterior vertebral growth
- Posterior segmentation failure, if asymmetrical, results in lordotic deformities (Fig. 27.121)

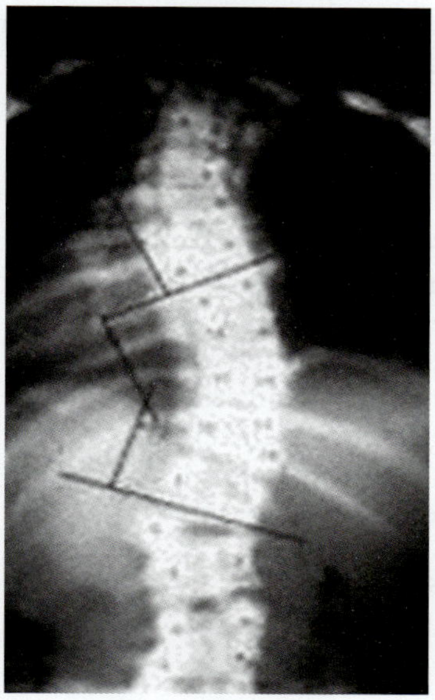

Fig. 27.119: Mixed elements of both failure of formation and failure of segmentation

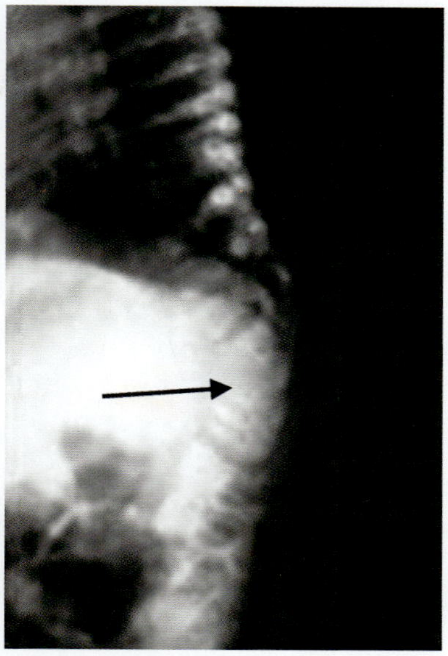

Fig. 27.121: X-ray of lateral view lumbar spine. Arrow showing posterior segmentation failure with lordosis

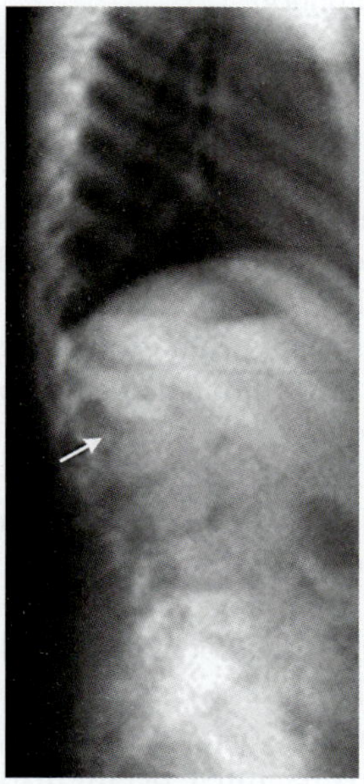

Fig. 27.120: Anterior formation failure resulting in sharply angulated kyphosis

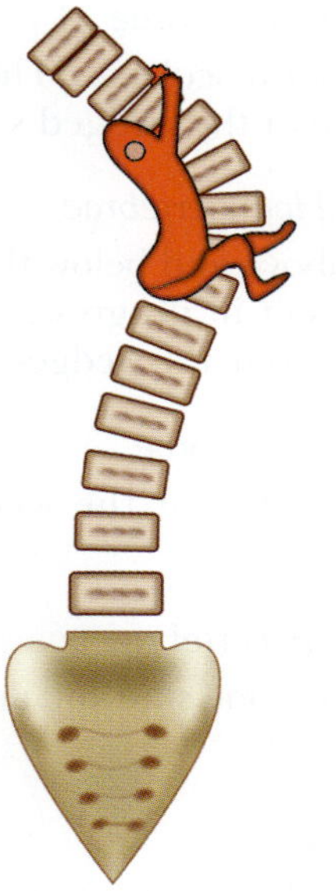

Fig. 27.122: Scoliosis with unilateral unsegmented bar

- Lateral segmentation failure (unilateral unsegmented bar), produces the worst and the most unrelenting scoliotic curves (Fig. 27.122)
- Total segmentation failure, produces block vertebrae, hence shortening of the spine
- Posterolateral and anterolateral segmentation failure is rare, but produces lordoscoliosis and kyphoscoliosis respectively.

Variations of Hemivertebrae (Fig. 27.123)

Incarcerated Hemivertebrae

It usually do not produce any abnormal alignment because the vertebral bodies above and below the abnormal segment are shaped so as to accommodate the hemivertebra.

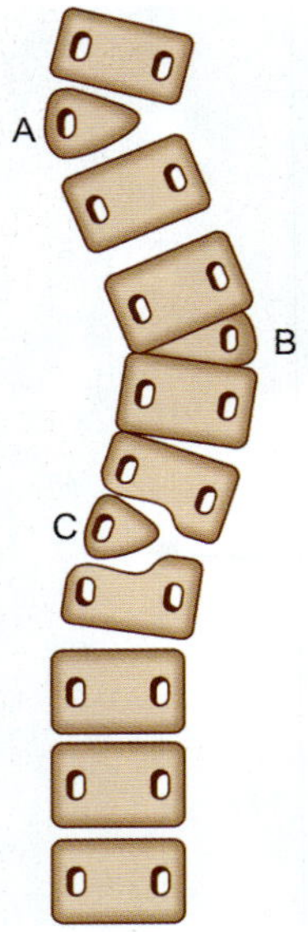

Fig. 27.123: (A) Fully segmented hemivertebrae; (B) Unsegmented hemivertebra; (C) Incarcerated hemivertebra

Nonincarcerated Hemivertebrae

It lies at the apex of a scoliosis. The curve magnitude depends on the size of the wedged segment.

Segmented or Free Hemivertebrae

Normal disks lies above and below the defective body. It is more likely to result in progressive curvatures due to unbalanced growth from, the wedge-oriented end-plates.

Nonsegmented Hemivertebrae

Lack disk spaces between the wedged and normal adjacent vertebral bodies.

Semi-segmented Hemivertebrae

Normal disk space on one side and are nonsegmented at the opposite end.

Prognostic Factors

- Type of anomaly that causes the most severe deformity is a unilateral unsegmented bar with contralateral hemivertebrae at the same level
- The least severe deformity is caused by a block vertebra
- Congenital scoliosis caused by unclassifiable anomalies, can be difficult to predict and requires careful monitoring. The poor prognosis is associated with a unilateral unsegmented bar with or without contralateral hemivertebrae. This should be treated immediately without waiting for a period of observation
- The rate of deterioration of the resulting scoliosis is most severe in the thoracic and thoracolumbar regions. It is usually less severe in the cervicothoracic and lumbar regions

Vertebral Anomalies Leading to Congenital Scoliosis

Risk of Progression (Highest to Lowest)

- Unilateral unsegmented bar with contralateral hemivertebra
- Unilateral unsegmented bar
- Fully segmented hemivertebra
- Partial segmented hemivertebra
- Incarcerated hemivertebra
- Nonsegmented hemivertebra.

Curve Progression

- Rapid and relentless
- Rapid
- Steady
- Less rapid
- May progress slowly
- Little progression.

Radiographic Evaluation

- Standard posteroanterior and lateral views of the entire spine
- Standing films are customary, as they show the characteristics of the curve under gravity, with its compensation and torsopelvic relationships
- Supine coned down views, are helpful to visualize defects and their patterns
- Bending films allow evaluation of rigidity or flexibility of the curves and their adjacent motion segments
- Tomography is a useful technique for evaluating congenital spinal deformities, especially for documenting the presence and extent of unsegmented bars and incarceration of hemivertebra
- CT and MRI are particularly useful in detailing bony canal anatomy and associated spinal cord dysraphism
- CT and MRI are also mandatory prior to surgical intervention because spinal cord tethering and diastematomyelia must be identified and released prior to correction of the curve.

Key Factors in Achieving Optimum Result in Patients with Deformities

- *Early diagnosis*: An opportunity exists for prophylactic surgery to balance the growth of the spine
- *Anticipation*
- *Prevention of deterioration:* It is easier to prevent a severe spinal deformity than to correct one. All patients require radiological assessment in every 4 to 6 months interval and once progression is established, immediate treatment is necessary to prevent further deterioration.

Nonoperative Treatment

Observation

Most common nonoperative management is mere observation and monitoring the curves for progression.

Orthotic Treatment

Very few cases of congenital scoliosis respond to brace treatment because the primary deformity is in the vertebrae and the curves tend to be rigid. Cases in which the natural history indicates a poor prognosis, orthotic treatment is contraindicated, viz. short stiff curves, an unsegmented bar, congenital lordosis and congenital kyphosis. The only congenital deformity in which bracing is useful is that of long curves with good flexibility and unbalanced scoliosis, secondary to an unbalanced hemivertebrae at the T12 or Tl5 levels. The brace of choice for high thoracic curves (apex T6 or above) is Milwaukee brace.

Operative Treatment

- Method of surgery selected, depends on the age of patient, site and type of vertebral anomaly, the size of curvature and the presence of other congenital anomalies. Successful surgical treatment depends on selecting the right procedure and applying it at the right time
- Progressive curves should be treated surgically, especially if they do not respond to orthotic treatment.

Basic Procedures for Surgical Treatment

Convex Growth Arrest

Designed to arrest the excessive convex growth, allow the concave growth to occur and correct the deformity. It is best applied to patient younger than five years.

Posterior Fusion

The aim of posterior fusion is not curve correction, but rather curve stabilization with the prevention of further increase in curve. It is the usual surgical procedure for an older child with a moderately severe curve that still is relatively flexible.

Combined Anterior and Posterior Fusion

It is used for thoracic, thoracolumbar or lumbar curves with a poor prognosis. The multiple discectomies provide an anterior growth arrest, which reduces or eliminates any bending of the fusion (crankshaft effect).

Hemivertebrae Excision

First performed in 1921 in Australia by Royale. Indicated for patients younger than five years and who have development of a secondary structural curve, with a fixed decompensation in which adequate alignment cannot be achieved with other procedures. It usually at the L4-L5 level.

Vertebrectomy

Most radical of all procedures. Performed in order to create mobility, but at the price of instability. A highly skilled surgeon or a very severe deformity is the strictly prerequisite.

■ Klippel-Feil Syndrome

- Klippel-Feil syndrome is a congenital fusion of the cervical vertebrae that may involve two segments, a congenital block vertebra, or the entire cervical spine (Fig. 27.124)
- Initially reported in 1912 independently, by *Maurice Klippel* and *André Feil* from France
- Characterized by patients with:
  - Short neck
  - Low hairline
  - Decreased cervical motion
- Fewer than 50 percent with congenital defects of cervical spine, have all three signs.

Etiology

- The true etiology and incidence of Klippel-Feil syndrome are unknown
- It involves congenital failure of segmentation of cervical vertebrae
- It results from failure of normal segmentation of cervical *somites* at 3 to 8 weeks gestation:

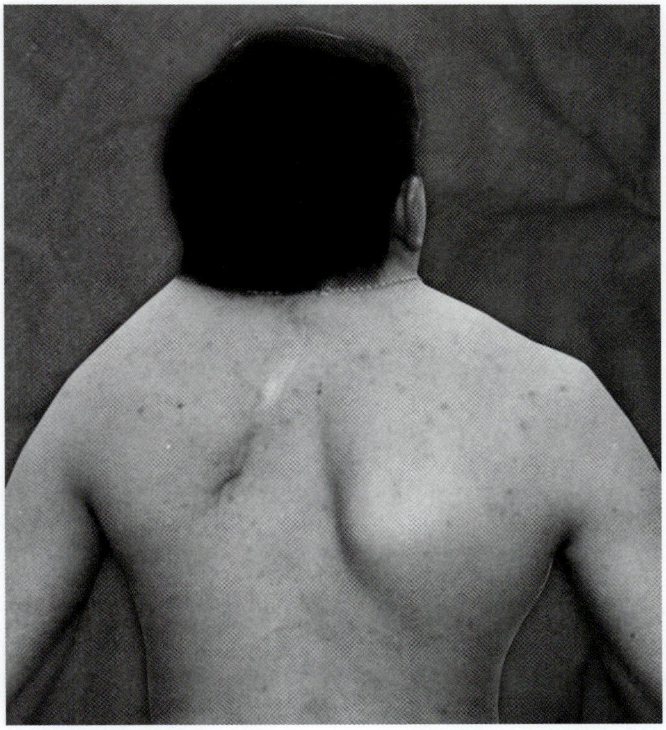

Fig. 27.124: A patient in the figure is having Klippel-Feil syndrome, with congenitally fused cervical vertebrae

- Result is multiple fused cervical segments
- Spectrum of deformity from fusion of two vertebrae to involvement of entire cervical spine
- Fusion of C2 and C3 is most common
- Familial Klippel-Feil syndrome gene locus, on the long arm of the eighth chromosome.

Associated Conditions

Consistently associated with congenital anomalies of other systems. Most common are:

- *Congenital scoliosis (Fig. 27.125)*
  - Seen in 60 percent cases
  - Majority of cases require treatment
- *Sprengel's deformity* (33%)
  - Failure of scapula decent
  - Attached to cervical spine by omovertebral bone or fibrous band
  - Synkinesis (mirror motions) (Fig. 27.126)
- *Renal disease*
  - Occurs in 33 percent cases
  - Aplasia is common and renal ultrasound in indicated
- *Congenital heart disease*
- *Brain stem abnormalities*
- Congenital cervical stenosis
- *Syndactyly* and *hypoplastic thumb* (Fig. 27.127)
- *Hearing loss*
  - It may occur in 30 percent of patients.

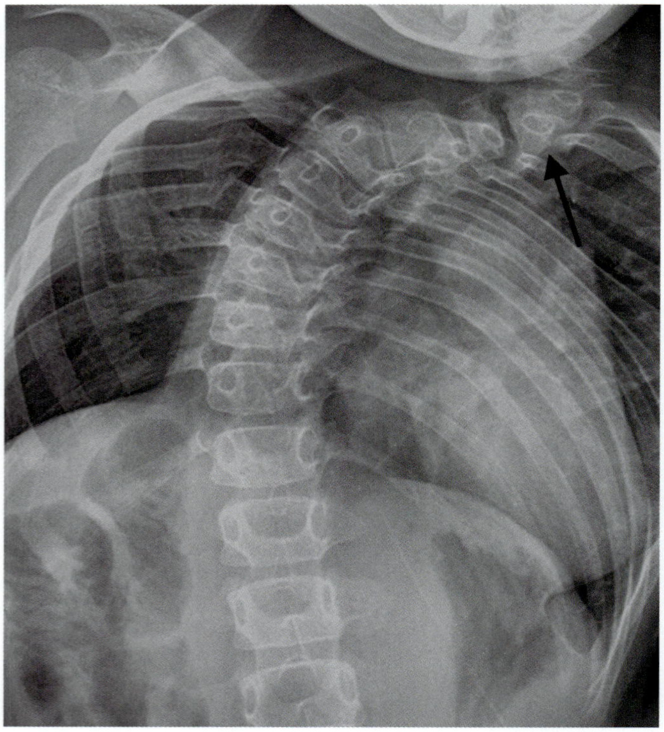

Fig. 27.125: X-ray showing congenital scoliosis, associated with Klippel-Feil syndrome arrow showing fused segments

Differential Diagnosis

- Juvenile rheumatoid arthritis
- Rheumatoid spondylitis.

Clinical Presentation

- Low posterior hairline
- Short neck
- Limited neck range of motion (especially lateral side bending)
- Torticollis
- Patients with extensive fusions present earlier
- Instability or hypermobility at unfused levels
- Cord compression in congenitally anomolous and narrow canal in young adults
- Scoliosis, 60 percent with curve greater than 15°. It can be congenital or compensatory
- Arnold Chiari malformation, with ataxia, dizziness and nystagmus
- Central nervous system (CNS) involvement:
  - Difficulty swallowing
  - Disturbed phonation

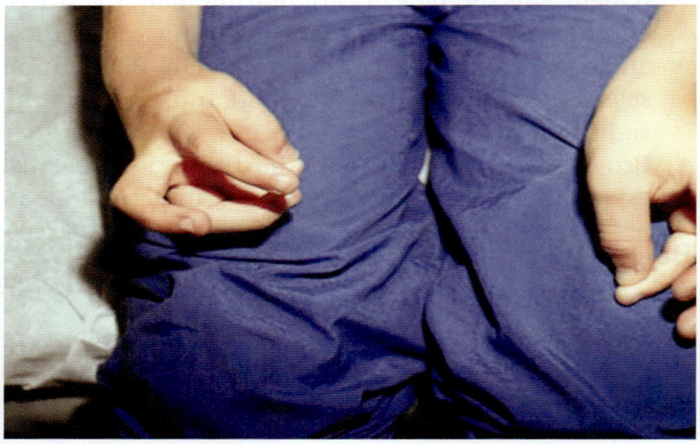

Fig. 27.126: Synkinesis (mirror motions of extremities)

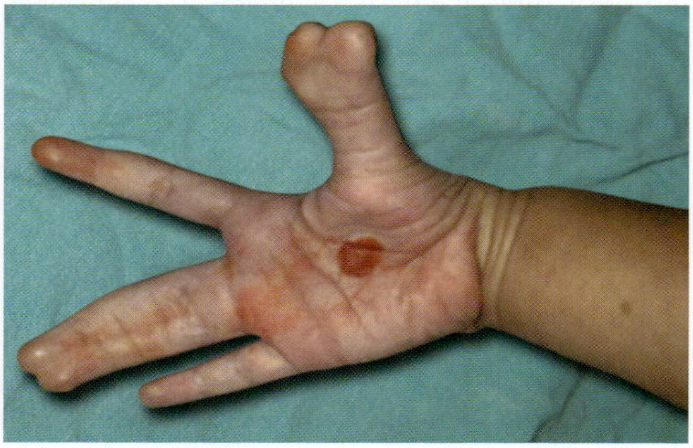

Fig. 27.127: Syndactyly and hypoplastic thumb

- Hydrocephalus
- Blurred vision
- Headache

- Vertebral artery involvement, although rare, may associated with syncope, seizures and ataxia.

Classification

Originally done by Feil

- *Type I*: Massive fusion of cervical spine
- *Type II*: Fusion of one or two cervical interspaces
- *Type III*: Thoracic or lumbar vertebrae involved

Samartzis and colleagues also suggested a new classification system, useful in predicting which patients may develop symptoms

- *Type I*: Patients have a single level fusion
- *Type II*: Patients have multiple, noncontiguous fused segments
- *Type III*: Patients have multiple, contiguous fused segments.

Investigations

X-ray

- Plain radiography is the basis for the diagnosis of Klippel-Feil syndrome
- Initial studies include anteroposterior (AP) and lateral views of the cervical spine
- Flexion-extension radiographs are indicated, if instability is suspected at the craniocervical junction or if two fused segments are separated by an open segment (Figs 27.128 and 27.129)
- Plain radiographs of the entire spine must be obtained to detect other spinal anomalies
- Examination of the chest wall for possible rib anomalies, such as multiple rib fusions is necessary. Rib fusions can be revealed with plain radiography
- Pizzutillo in 1994, evaluated flexion-extension radiographs to determine:
  - Alterations from normal motion
  - Potential neurologic risk.

Conclusion

- If hypermobility of upper cervical segment is present, there is a greatest risk of neurologic sequelae
- If hypermobility of lower cervical segment is present, then there is greatest risk of degenerative changes.

CT Scan

- Valuable tool to assess the bony anatomy
- Helpful in preoperative planning
- Obtain reconstructions.

MRI

- Identifies spinal cord abnormalities
- Flexion and extension MRI to identify cord compression or stenosis:
  - Ultrasonography of the kidneys is indicated to screen for renal anomalies
  - Intravenous pyelography should be performed, if further definition of a kidney abnormality is required (Fig. 27.130)

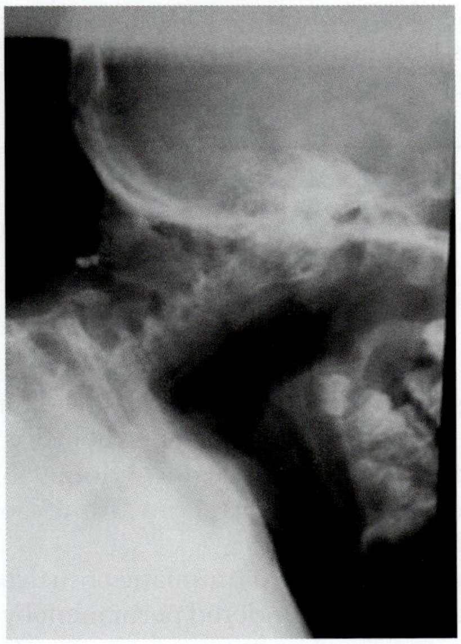

Fig. 27.128: Neck is flexed, while taking X-ray, if instability is suspected at the craniocervical junction or if two fused segments are separated by an open segment

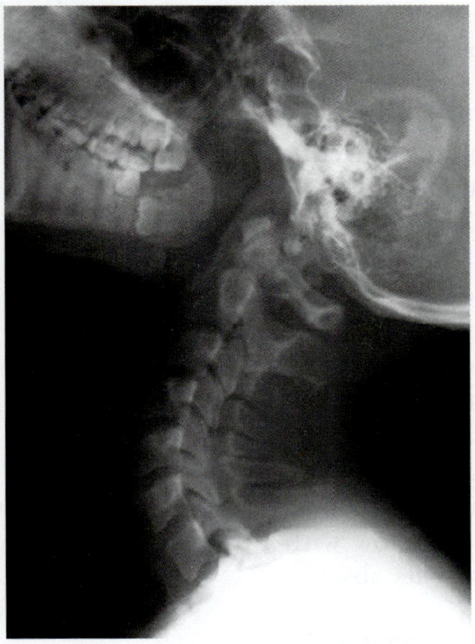

Fig. 27.129: X-ray taken, with neck in extension

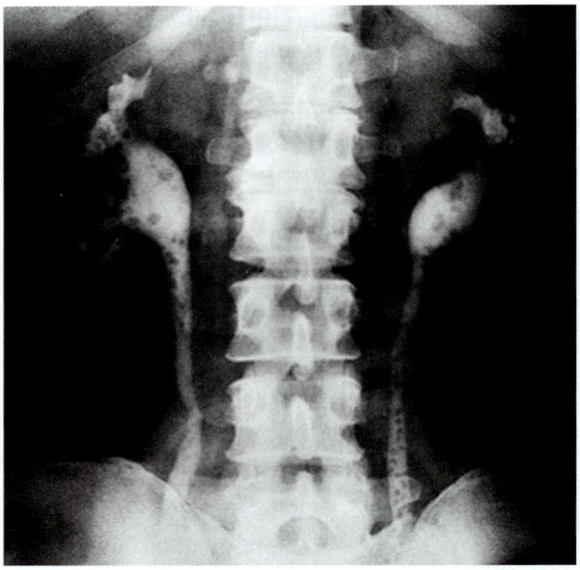

Fig. 27.130: Intravenous pyelography, for evaluating kidney abnormalities

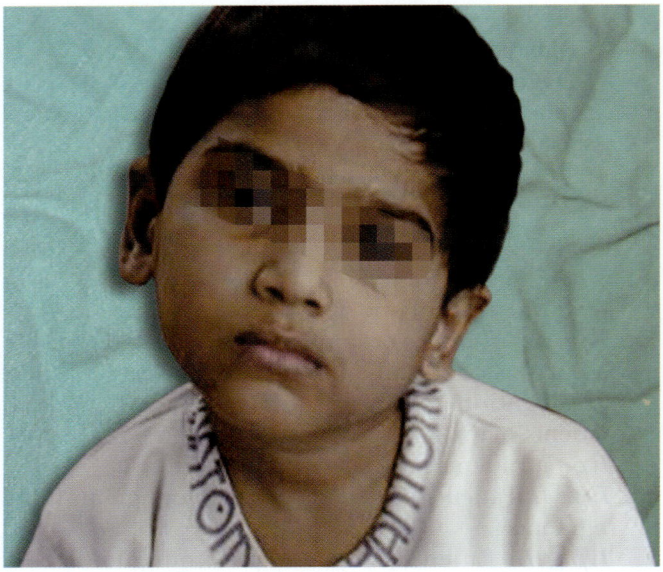

Fig. 27.131: A child with torticollis, having neck turned and tilted to the left side

- As there is high incidence of hearing loss with Klippel-Feil syndrome, an audiologist or otologist should evaluate all children.

Treatment

If patient is asymptomatic and no evidence of instability is present, then treatment include:
- Periodic flexion-exion radiographs
- Avoidance of contact sports
- Avoidance of occupations and recreational activities, with risk of head trauma.

Sports Participation
- *Type I*: Absolute contraindication for participation in contact sports
- *Type II*: Absolutely contraindicated in fusion of one or two interspaces, with:
  - Associated limited motion
  - Occipitocervical anomalies
  - Involvement of C2
  - Instability
  - Disk disease
  - Degenerative changes
- No contraindication in fusion of one or two interspaces at C3 or below with full cervical range of motion (ROM) or its absence.

Symptomatic Treatment
- Modification of activities
- Bracing
- Traction.

Surgical Intervention

Indication
- Progressive symptomatic segmental instability
- Neurologic compromise.

Surgical Techniques
- Occipitocervical arthrodesis
- Halo immobilization
- Atlantoaxial arthrodesis (Gallie, Brooks and Mageryl)
- Rib resection (Bonola's method)
- Soft tissue resection, Z-plasty and muscle resection for cosmetic improvement.

■ Torticollis

- Torticollis (Wryneck) is defined as rotational deformity of the cervical spine that causes turning and tilting deformity of the head and neck (Fig. 27.131).

Etiology

- Etiology is unknown, but may be due to birth trauma, like breech, forceps or improper delivery
- Ischemic changes of sternocleidomastoid, as it is supplied by an end artery, a branch of superior thyroid.
- It can also occur due to traumatic obstruction of veins of muscle, which is rendered permanent by obstructed venous tree and is evident by development of sternocleidomastoid tumor (Fig. 27.132). The tumor eventually disappear, its place being taken by fibrous tissue, which later contract.

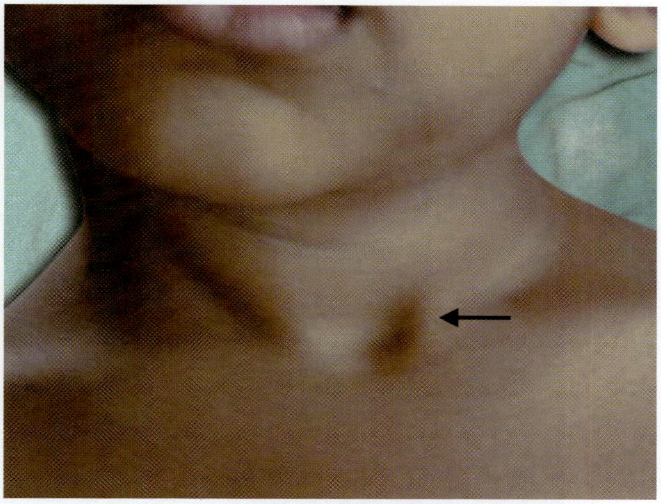

Fig. 27.132: A child develops sternocleidomastoid tumor

Causes

Congenital: It is due to contracture pulling of the sternocleidomastoid to same side, turning the face to opposite side.

Acquired

- Infective, e.g. tuberculosis of cervical spine
- Spasmodic due to neurological or psychological disorder cause marked spasm of the sternocleidomastoid
- Traumatic, e.g. sprain, dislocation and fracture of cervical spine
- Myositis or fibromyositis of sternocleidomastoid, exposure to cold causes myositis
- Unilateral muscle paralysis, e.g. polio
- Neuritis of spinal accessory nerve
- Ocular disturbances child turns head to one side to compensate for defective vision.

Clinical Features

Congenital

Primary changes: These include following:

- Head tilted to same side
- Face rotated to same side
- Taut sternocleidomastoid
- Macular changes.

Secondary changes

- Asymmetry of face
- Flattened frontal eminence, with marked protrusion of occipital region of the affected side
- Scoliosis capitis, where skull projected backwards on the affected side and projects forwards on opposite side
- Compensatory cervical scoliosis
- Prominence of mastoid process, with exostosis develop on it.

Acquired: Spasmodic sternocleidomastoid contraction.

Treatment

- *Conservative*
  - Nonsteroidal anti-inflammatory drugs (NSAIDs)
  - Physiotherapy
- *Surgery*
  - Surgery is delayed till fibroma is well formed
  - Open tenotomy till one year. Subcutaneous tenotomy can be done, but not advised, as there is risk of injuring great vessels at the root of the neck
  - After one year secondary deformity are less corrected
  - Unipolar release of muscle is advised in milder cases
  - For older children (3 to 5 years) or failed operation, bipolar release of muscle from both sides (Ferkel's procedure) or Z-plasty are tried.

IMAGING OF THE SPINE

Imaging of the spine is a very important step along with clinical examination to come to a specific diagnosis in most of the cases with spinal complaints. Radiography is the basic investigation to be carried out.

Further investigations which can be done, if required are:

- Computed tomography (CT) scan
- Myelography
- Magnetic resonance imaging (MRI)
- Bone scanning (Scintigraphy).

■ Radiography

- Radiography was discovered by Roentgen in 1896
- The simplest and most readily available diagnostic test for spinal complaints is radiography
- The routine views to be taken primarily include the anteroposterior and the lateral views. Additional special views can be taken whenever required.
- For the study of the X-rays the spine can be divided into:
  - Cervical spine
  - Thoracic spine
  - Lumbosacral spine.

Cervical Spine (Figs 27.133 and 27.134)

The various views that can be done are:

- Lateral view
- Anteroposterior view
- Open mouth view—for C1 to C3
- Oblique view
- Flexion-extension view.

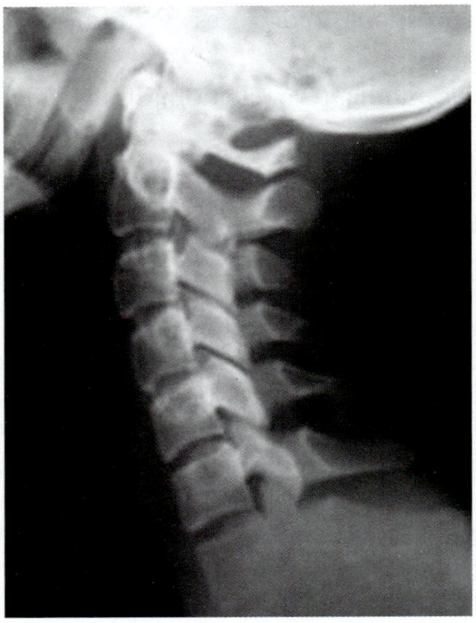

Fig. 27.133: Cervical spine

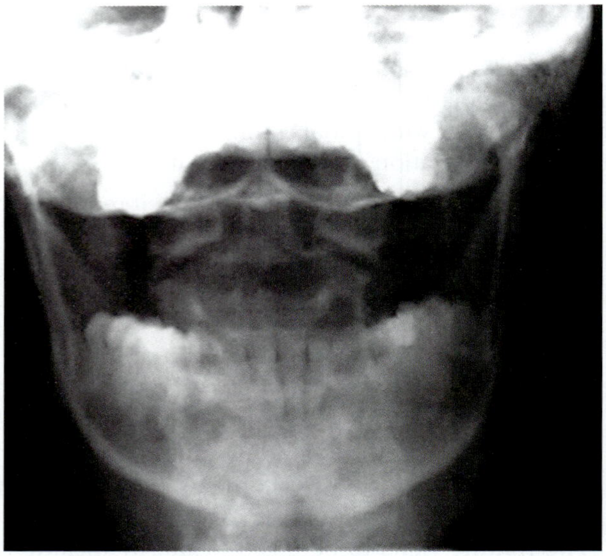

Fig. 27.134: Transoral view

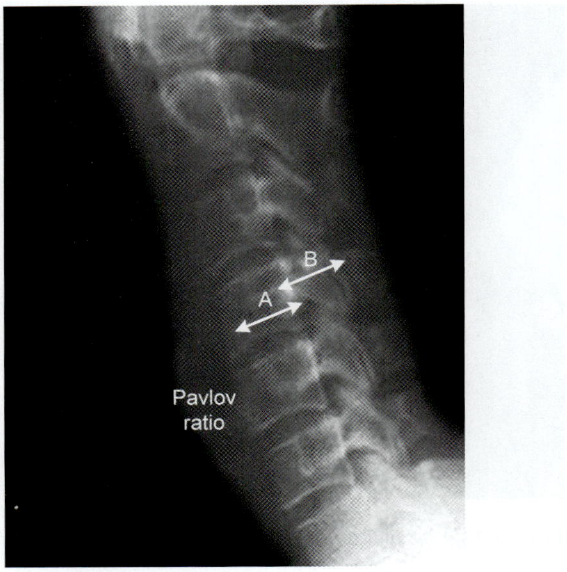

Fig. 27.135: Pavlov ratio

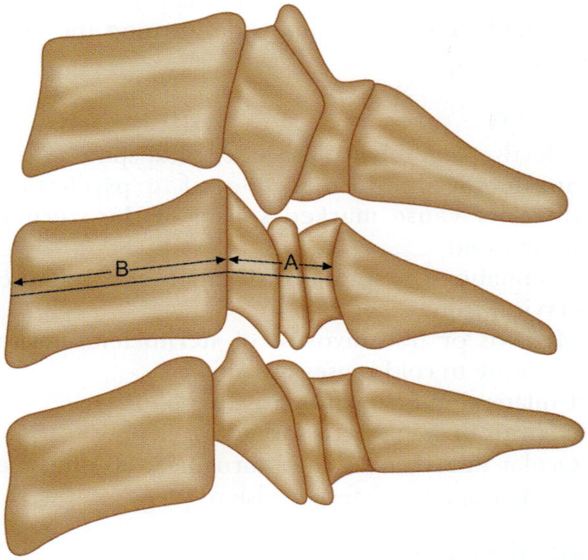

Fig. 27.136: Pavlov ratio—cervical canal with to vertebral body width ration (vide text)

Lateral View

- The cervical curve, which is normally slightly convex anteriorly, should be noted. Loss of curvature may be a positional error or due to muscular spasm.
- The shape of the vertebrae should be compared with each other. Vertebral collapse (TB, tumor, fracture) or fusion, wedging, etc. should be noted.
- The relationship of each vertebra to the one above and below is seen. Displacement is seen in subluxations or dislocations.
- *Disk space:* Narrowing if any
- Anterior lipping
- Posterior lipping
- Vertebral fusion
- Pharyngeal shadow should be seen
- *Pavlov ratio (Figs 27.135 and 27.136)*
  - Normally, the depth of the cervical canal is equal to that of the related vertebral body, i.e. ratio is 1.0
  - A ratio of 0.8 or less indicates narrow cervical canal and risk of cord compression.

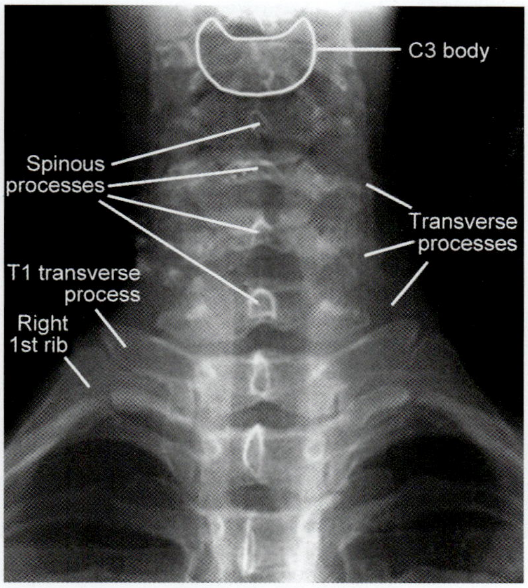

Fig. 27.137: Anteroposterior view of cervical spine

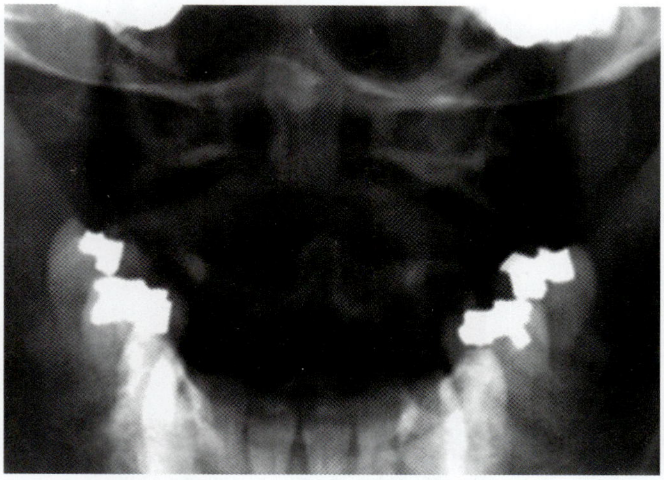

Fig. 27.139: Open mouth view of cervical spine

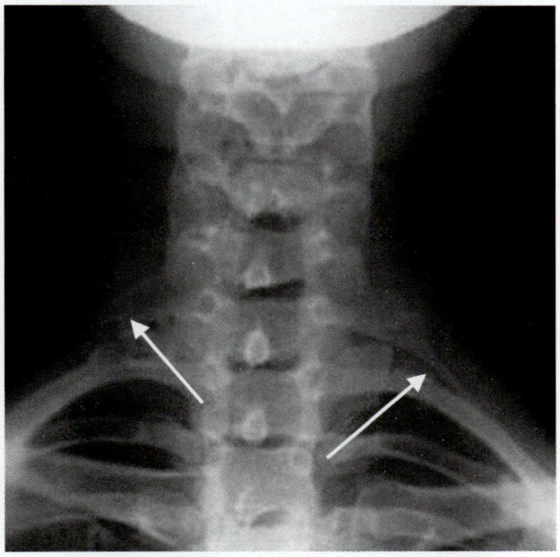

Fig. 27.138: Anteroposterior view of cervical spine, arrows showing cervical rib

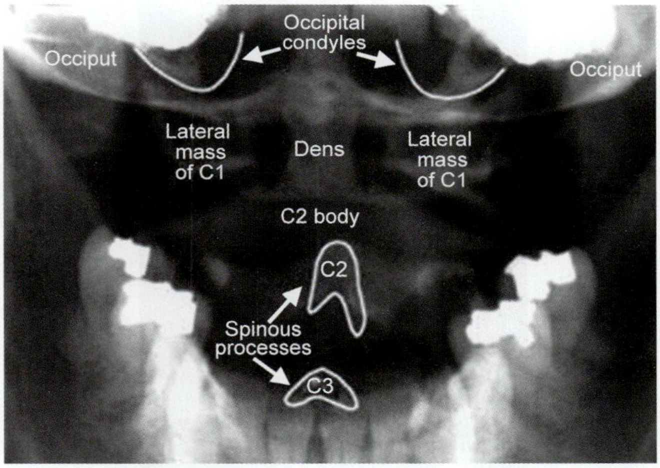

Fig. 27.140: Open mouth view of cervical spine showing various structures

Anteroposterior View (Figs 27.137 and 27.138)

Interpretation is difficult owing to superimposed structures, look for:

- Shape of the vertebra
- Any lateral wedging from fracture, tumor or infection
- Presence of any cervical rib.

Open Mouth View (Figs 27.139 to 27.140)

- It is done to look for pathology from C1 to C3
- Look for
  - Atlanto-occipital joint
  - Atlantoaxial joints
  - Lateral mass of atlas
  - Alignment of the odontoid
  - Fracture of the odontoid.

Oblique View (Figs 27.141 to 27.143)

- The oblique view in the cervical spine are done to see:
  - Localized lipping of the uncovertebral joints (Joints of Luschka)
  - The neural foramina
  - Overlapping (locked) facet joints
- A lateral view in flexion and extension helps in determining any instability of the spine.

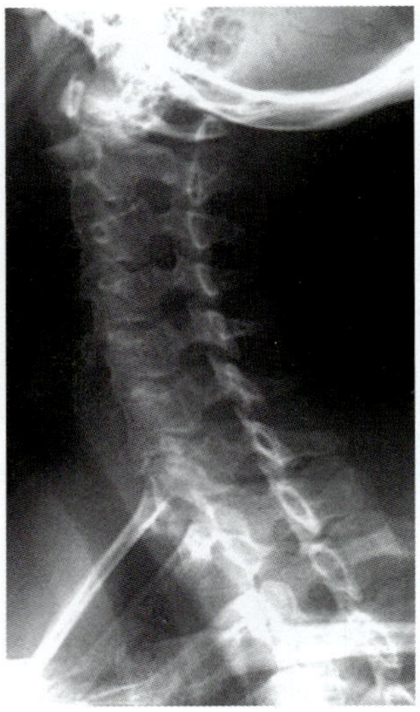

Fig. 27.141: Normal oblique view of cervical spine

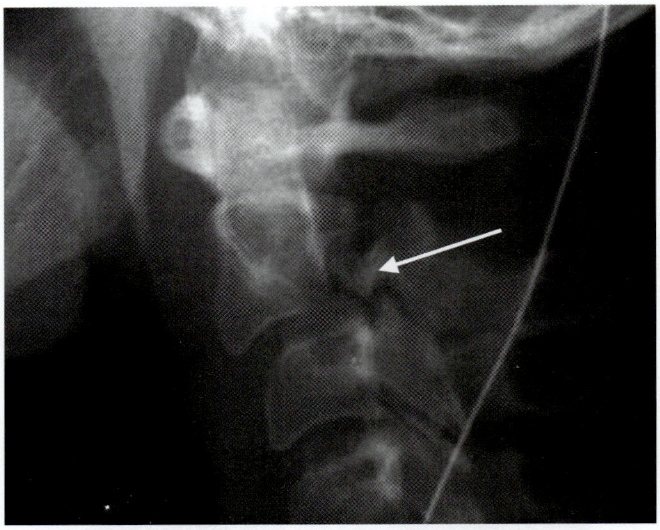

Fig. 27.143: Oblique view of cervical spine arrow showing break in pars interarticularis

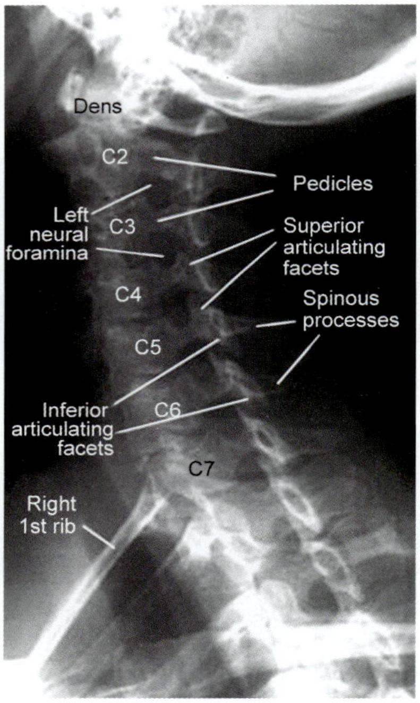

Fig. 27.142: Oblique view of cervical spine showing various structures

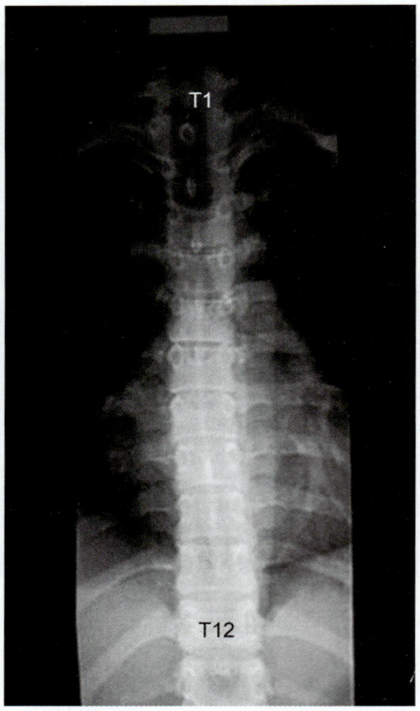

Fig. 27.144: Anteroposterior view of thoracic spine

■ Thoracic Spine

The routine views taken are:

- Anteroposterior view
- Lateral view.

Anteroposterior View (Figs 27.144 to 27.146)

- The shape, relationship of the vertebra, the intervertebral disk space are looked
- Any congenital abnormality of the vertebral development
- The presence of any structural scoliosis with rotation of the vertebra
- The soft tissue shadows at the sides of the vertebra, e.g. in TB there will be a fusiform swelling
- The presence of any localized lateral angulation of the spine due to lateral vertebral collapse from fracture, infection, tumor or osteoporosis.

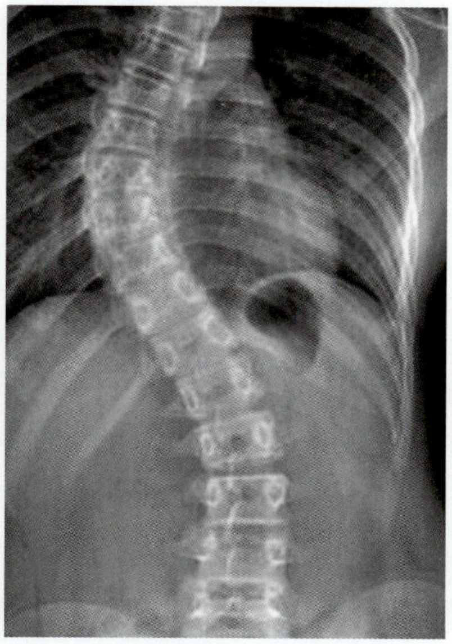

Fig. 27.145: Anteroposterior view of thoracic spine showing scoliosis

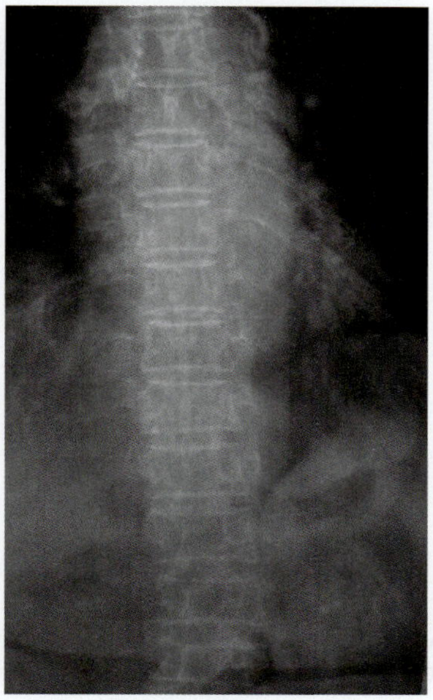

Fig. 27.146: Anteroposterior view of thoracic spine showing fusiform swelling

Lateral View (Figs 27.147 and 27.148)

- The normal kyphotic curve is noted. Increased curve is seen in senile kyphosis or Scheuermann's disease
- Any sharp alteration in the curve (angular kyphosis) which is found typically where there is pathology of one or two vertebra, e.g. fractures, TB or other infections, tumors and osteoporosis
- The intervertebral disk spaces are noted.

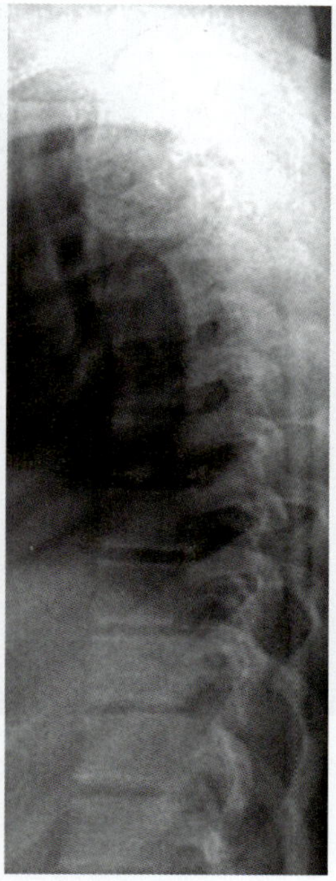

Fig. 27.147: Lateral view of thoracic spine

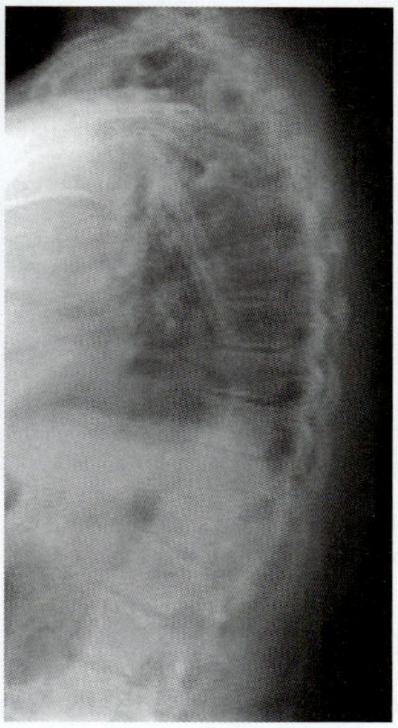

Fig. 27.148: Lateral view of thoracic spine showing angular kyphosis

Lumbosacral Spine

The commonly taken views are:

- Anteroposterior view
- Lateral view
- Oblique view

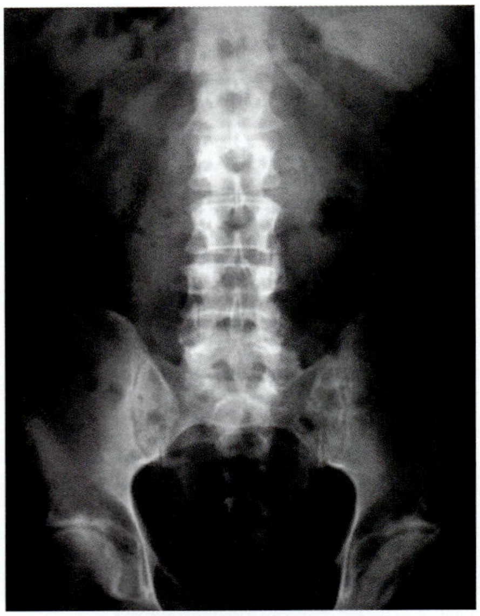

Fig. 27.149: Anteroposterior view of lumbosacral spine showing scoliosis

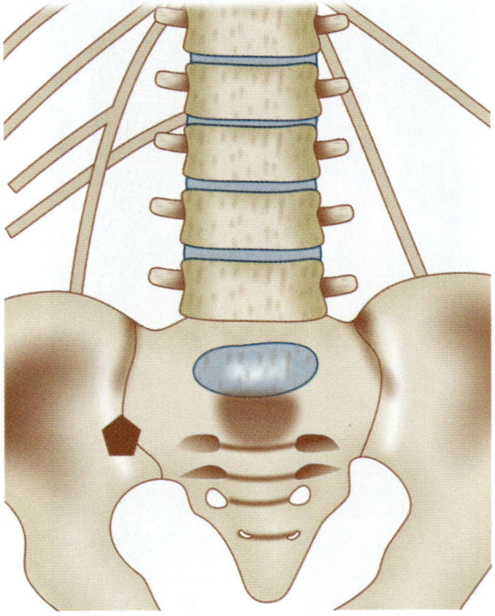

Fig. 27.151: Anteroposterior view of lumbosacral spine showing lateralization of psoas shadow due to abscess

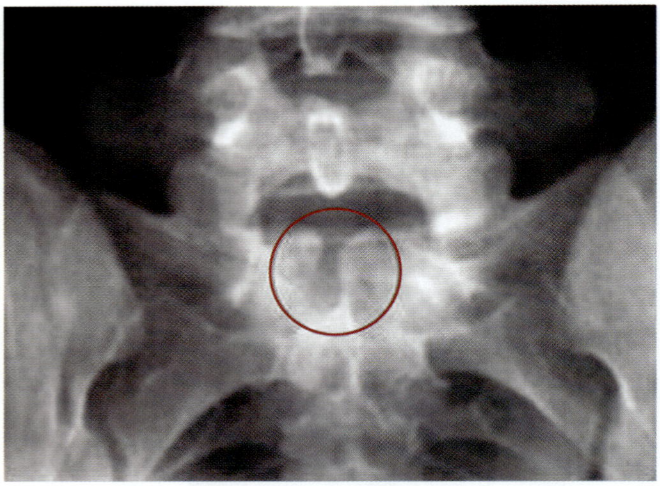

Fig. 27.150: Anteroposterior view of lumbosacral spine showing spina bifida of L5 vertebra

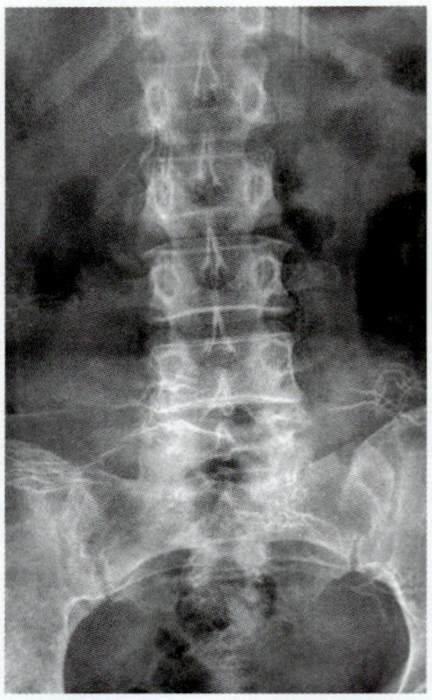

Fig. 27.152: Anteroposterior view of lumbosacral spine showing partial and complete sacralization of L5 vertebra

Anteroposterior View (Figs 27.149 to 27.152)

- The presence of any congenital abnormalities like congenital fusion is looked for
- Note anomalies of lumbosacral articulation like partial sacralization of L5
- Look for the presence of spina bifida
- Examine the psoas shadow for symmetry. Lateral displacement of the edge of the shadow and increased density suggests psoas abscess
- Look at the sacroiliac joints. Unilateral involvement (sclerosis, cystic changes or obliteration) occurs in TB and bilateral involvement is seen in ankylosing spondylitis.

Lateral View (Figs 27.153 and 27.154)

- The intervertebral disk spaces are seen
- Anterior or posterior lipping can be seen in chronic disk lesions or osteoarthritis
- Lipping is commonly seen at L5-S1 but can be seen at other sites also
- Note the relationship of each vertebra to its neighbor. Look for spondylolisthesis or retrolisthesis (usually associated in disk degeneration).
- The height of the vertebral bodies and its density is compared. Loss of height is seen in trauma, infection, tumor or osteoporosis.

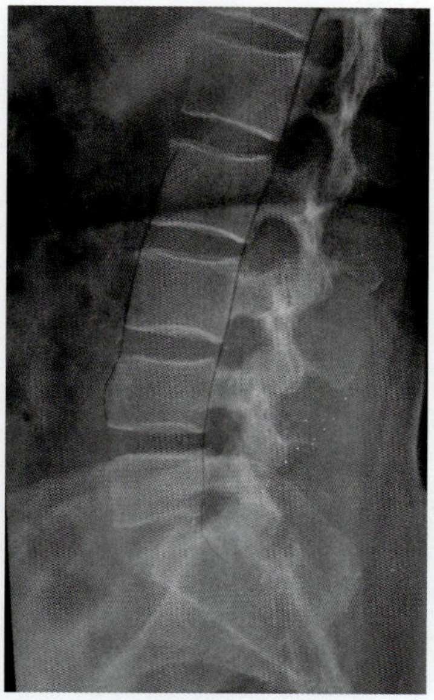

Fig. 27.153: Lateral view of lumbosacral spine showing lipping of vertebra note both anterior and posterior lipping of L4–L5

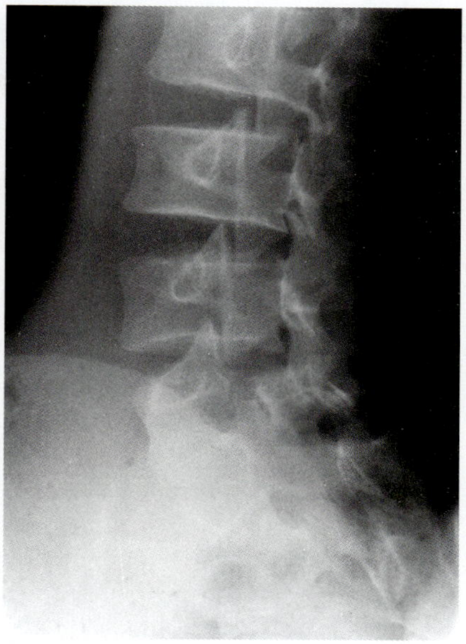

Fig. 27.155: Oblique view of lumbosacral spine

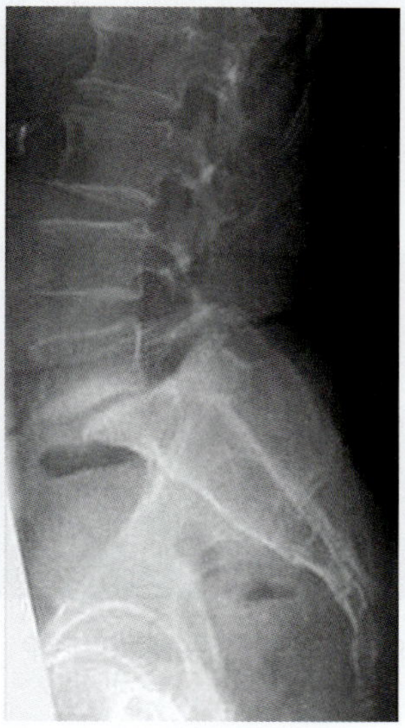

Fig. 27.154: Lateral view of lumbosacral spine

Oblique View (Figs 27.155 and 27.156)

- In the oblique view identify the "Scotty dog" shadow
- In spondylolisthesis, the dog becomes decapitated due to the forward slipping and the inferior articular process of the above vertebra encroaches on the neck
- In spondylolysis the neck is elongated or the neck develops a collar

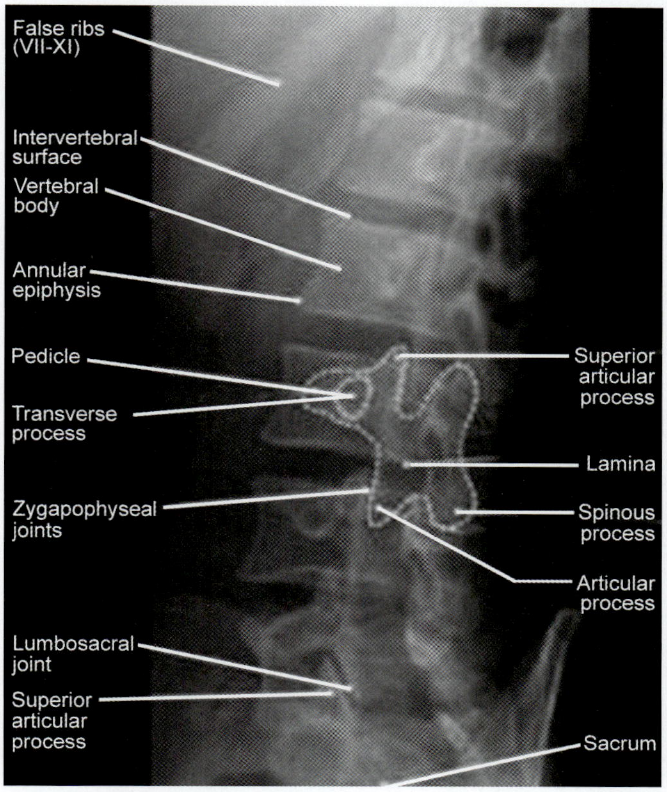

Fig. 27.156: Oblique view of lumbosacral spine showing scatty dog sign

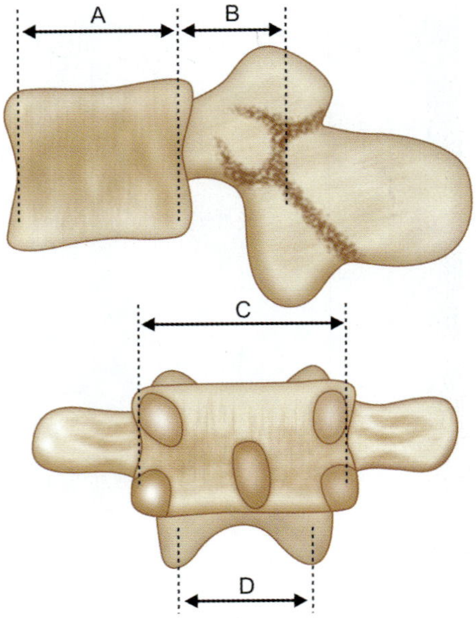

Fig. 27.157: Spinal stenosis—A. Body front to back; B. Spinal canal front to back; C. Width of vertebral body; D. Interpedicular distance

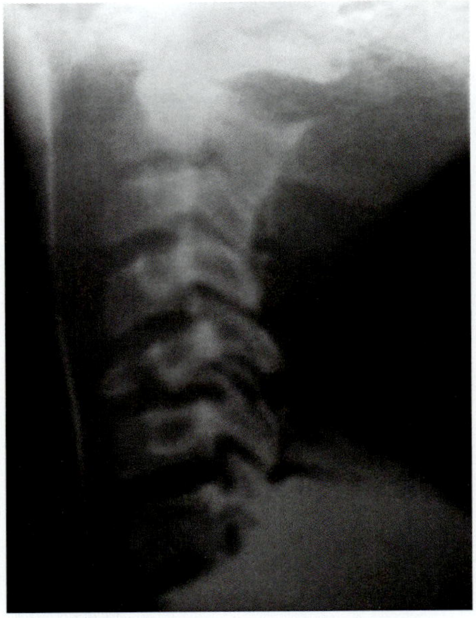

Fig. 27.158: Lateral view showing burst fracture C5

Calculation of Spinal Canal Stenosis

- In spinal canal stenosis the canal to body ratio is calculated
- It is A × B: C × D, where:
  - A = interpedicular distance
  - B = spinal canal front to back
  - C = width of vertebral body
  - D = body, front to back
- The normal range is 1:2 to 1:4.5
- Values greater than 4.5 suggest spinal stenosis (Fig. 27.157).

■ Computed Tomography

- Computed tomography (CT) was discovered by Godfrey Hounsfield in 1972
- CT is based on the principal that different tissues of the body absorb X-rays in different proportions depending on their molecular weight
- The scattering of the rays is eliminated by use of a very narrow X-ray beam and only a single slice of the body is radiographed
- The effects of superimposition are eliminated by viewing any point up to 360°
- The absorption coefficient of tissues is calculated in Hounsfield (H) units. Water is 0, air –1000 and bone +1000 units.
- The coefficient is also related to the amount of protein. A greater percentage of protein increases the H number. Similarly calcium has a higher H number.

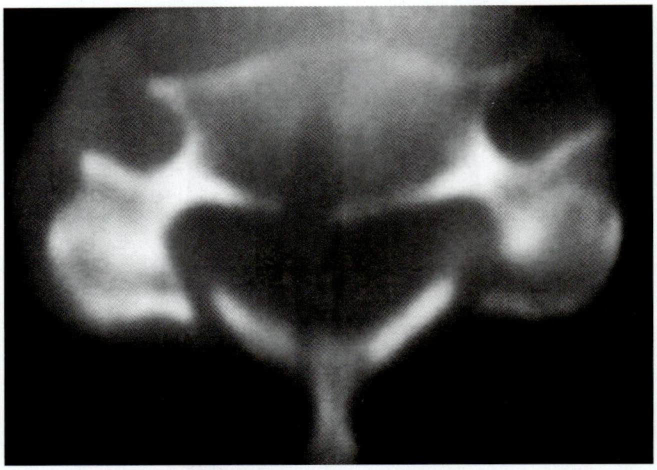

Fig. 27.159: CT scan showing traumatic spine

- CT of the spine is helpful in:
  - Traumatic spine
  - Spinal canal stenosis
  - Disk disease.

Traumatic Spine (Figs 27.158 to 27.160)

- In traumatic conditions, CT will show fractures that may not be well seen on plain radiography
- CT is useful to study the fracture area and to evaluate injury to the spinal cord, if any
- Fractures may be missed on X-ray and multiple injuries should be looked for, especially in the cervical spine

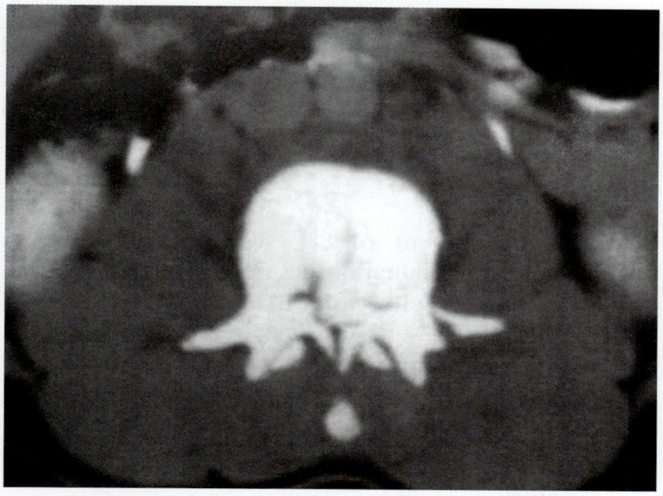

Fig. 27.160: Traumatic spine

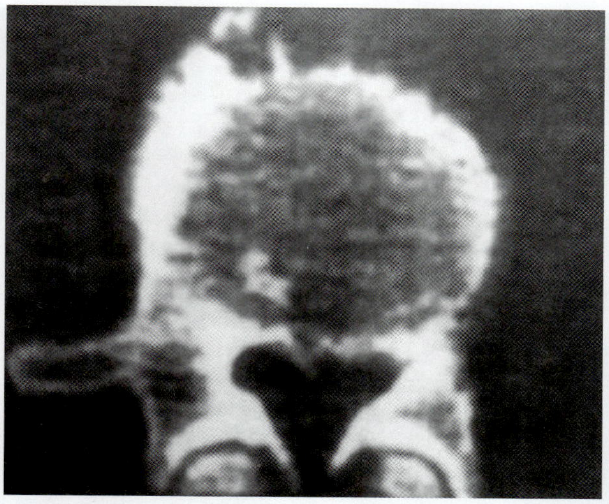

Fig. 27.162: CT showing spinal canal stenosis

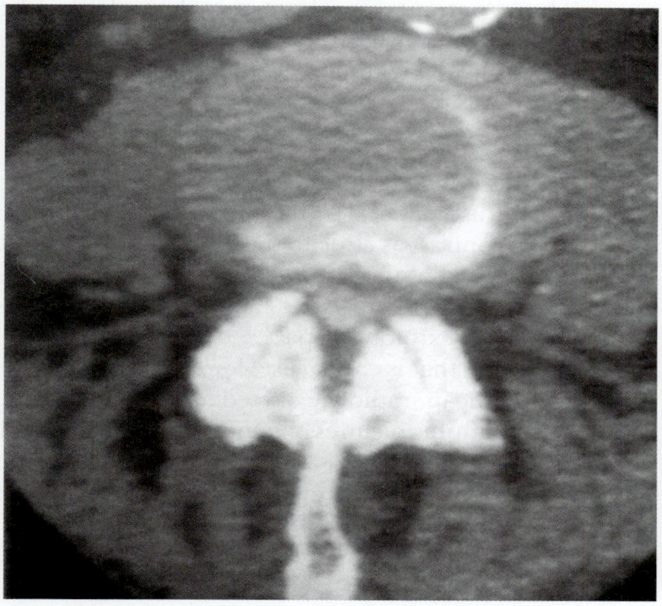

Fig. 27.161: Axial view showing spinal canal stenosis

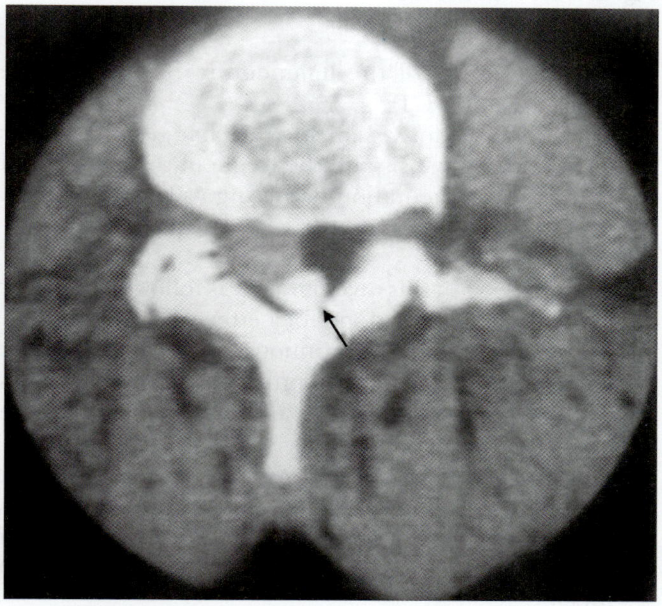

Fig. 27.163: Axial view showing disk calcification

- CT examination is important in burst fractures, as they may produce fragments protruding in the spinal canal and compress the cord or the nerve roots.

Spinal Canal Stenosis (Figs 27.161 and 27.162)

- CT is preferable to evaluate the bony canal
- There are two types of stenosis:
  - The canal has a narrow posterior angle, with hypertrophic articular processes and facet joints with osteophytes. There is narrowing of the medial aspect (lateral recess) of the neural canal on each side (trefoil configuration).
  - The canal is normal but there is thickening of the ligamentum flavum with bulging of the intervertebral disk.

Disk Disease (Figs 27.163 and 27.164)

- CT yields more information than MRI on the bones and joints in relation to osteoarthritic changes. It also shows the disks satisfactorily but does not demonstrate the spinal contents well.
- CT scan shows disk herniation and also demonstrates calcification in the disk. It also shows osteoarthritic changes and osteophyte formation.
- CT also shows disease of the apophyseal joints

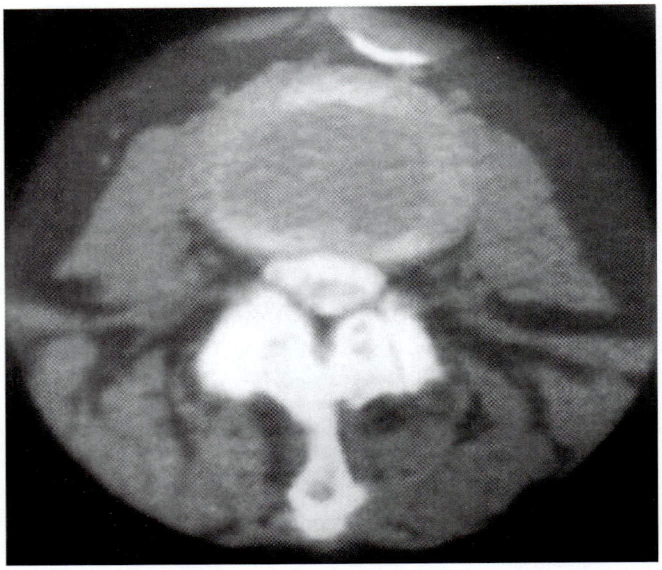

Fig. 27.164: Disk disease

- The thickening of the ligamentum flavum is more clearly seen on CT
- CT is superior for visualizing the changes in articular facets, osteophytosis and the frequent disruption and marginal fragmentation occurring at L3 to L5 to S1.

Recent Advances

- *Contrast CT:* In this myelography is followed by CT or CT with contrast is done for better visualization
- *Spiral CT:* It allows continuous rotation of the tube that can spiral down for an unlimited number of slices This gives continuous slices and reconstruction of the images in three dimensions
- *Single photon emission computed tomography (SPECT):* It is done with bone scanning. The gamma camera is rotated 360° and images obtained. Superimposition is minimized and the image can be obtained as a 3D image
- *Positron emission tomography (PET):* This is similar to SPECT. It is more sensitive for detection of tumors. In the spine, it is commonly employed for detection of tumor activity after chemotherapy.

Myelography

- Myelography with gases was first introduced by Dandy in 1919
- Positive contrast myelography using iodized oil was introduced by Sicard in 1922
- Steinhausen then introduced iophendylate (Pantopaque) in 1940. But it needed large needles to introduce the viscous fluid, post study removal of the contrast, late arachnoiditis and other complications.
- This led to the use of water soluble contrast agents
- Agents used today are iohexol (Omnipaque) and iopamidol (Isovue) as they are water soluble, cheap, relatively nontoxic, are premixed and do not have to be removed after the procedure.

Indications

- With the advent of CT scan and MRI scan, myelographic evaluation has decreased presently
- Almost all myelograms are followed by a CT examination
- The indications of myelogram are:
  - An equivocal CT or MRI in a patient who is suspected of having a surgical lesion
  - An obese patient who cannot fit in the CT or MRI gantry
  - Multilevel spinal stenosis, especially with scoliosis as scoliosis interferes with proper slicing in CT or MRI
  - Those patients in whom metal implants like pedicle screws will distort CT or MRI images
  - If CT or MRI scanning is not available.

Objective

The objective of doing myelography is:

- Place contrast material in the subarachnoid space
- Place the contrast as close to the lesion as possible yet not at the level of the lesion
- Assure that the contrast is not injected in extra-arachnoid or extradural space
- Use an agent that is easy to use, low viscosity, miscible with CSF, cheap, rapidly excreted and less toxic
- The radiographic pictures obtained should be of good quality
- The dose of the contrast medium is 180 to 240 mg/cc in 10 to 14 cc of fluid.

Technique

- The contrast can be introduced through a lumbar (L2 to L3), cisternal or a cervical (C1 to C2) puncture
- Lumbar puncture is routinely done
- The indications of a cervical puncture are: fusion of L2 to S1, severe arthritis of the lumbar spine, spinal instability, complete blocks at multiple levels, lumbar infection or for cervical myelography
- The patient is placed prone and a 22-guage spinal needle is inserted. Cerebrospinal fluid (CSF) backflow confirms subarachnoid placement of the needle.
- A small amount of contrast is injected. Diffuse image verifies that the contrast is mixing with CSF and a sharp image indicates subdural or extradural injection
- Films are obtained in AP, lateral and oblique views (Figs 27.165A to C).

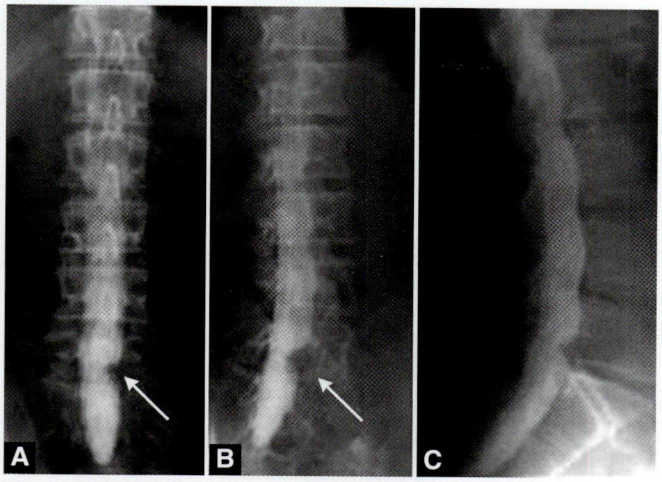

Figs 27.165A to C: Films are obtained in AP, lateral and oblique views (sites for cisternal puncture)

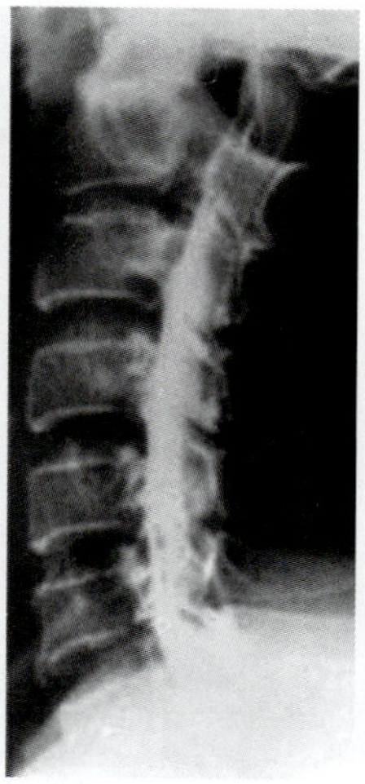

Fig. 27.167: Lateral view of cervical spine with contrast

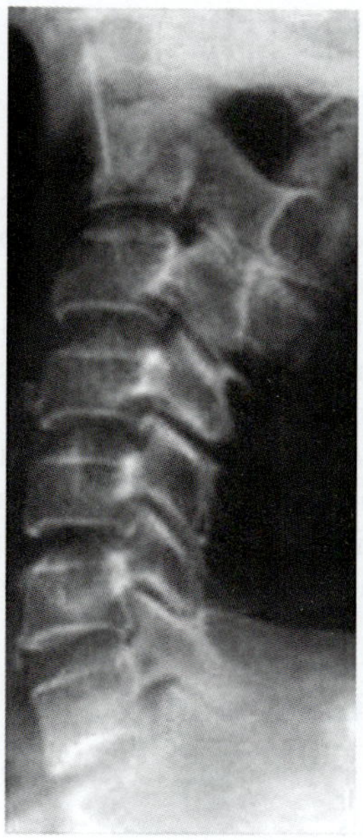

Fig. 27.166: Lateral view of cervical spine without contrast

Adverse Reactions

- Severe adverse reactions occur in 1:35000 procedures
- They are divided into anaphylactic, neurological and renal toxicity
- *Anaphylactic reaction:* They are rare with the newer agents. Screening of the patients should be done. Also corticosteroid and antihistamine treatment is given when indicated.
- *Neurological reactions:* Most frequent are headache, nausea and vomiting. Less frequent are increased pain, seizures, myoclonic spasms, psychomotor disturbances and vertigo.
- *Renal toxicity:* These are rare as the doses of the contrast is less. There is a possibility that a patient with pre-existing renal disease can have a toxic reaction.

Normal Myelogram

- The spinal canal will be visualized from L2 below
- The axillary pouch is the point of exit of the root that will run parallel to the thecal sac to emerge from the canal below the pedicle of the vertebra below
- A little contrast runs with the root for a variable distance, parallel to the thecal sac and sometimes may be seen curving under the pedicle (Figs 27.166 and 27.167).

Prolapsed Intervertebral Disk

Figures 27.168 to 27.170 show prolapsed intervertebral disk.

■ Magnetic Resonance Imaging

- Magnetic resonance imaging (MRI) is the major medical imaging development of the century
- MRI was developed by Purcell and Bloch, independently in 1946. But its use for image production was by Paul Lauterber in 1973.
- It provides a digital representation of tissue characteristics related to spatial location and can be obtained in any tissue plane
- The appearance of an MR image is a function of the chemical composition of the tissue
- Soft tissues are composed of around 70 percent water and 10 to 15 percent adipose which generate the signal.

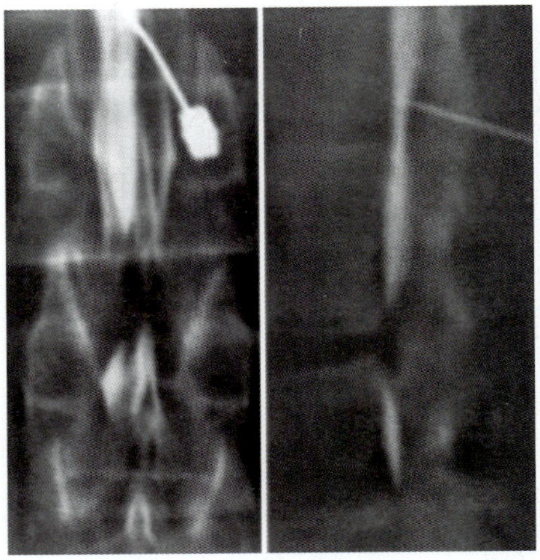

Fig. 27.168: Myelogram showing a prolapsed intervertebral disk

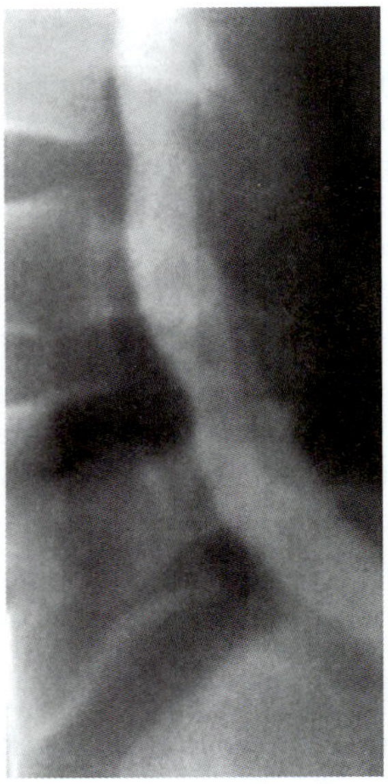

Fig. 27.169: Prolapsed intervertebral disk on myelogram

Fundamentals of MRI

Magnetic

There are two magnets essential to MRI:

- *External magnet:* It is part of the imaging machine and its strength is described in Tesla (T) units, like 0.5, 1.0, 1.5 T
- *Internal magnet:* These are the zillions of hydrogen atoms in the body.

Resonance

It is the matching of the frequency of the radiowaves used for excitation with the frequency of the spinning hydrogen atoms in the magnetic field. The hydrogen atoms have to be resonated with the correct frequency which changes their magnetic vector.

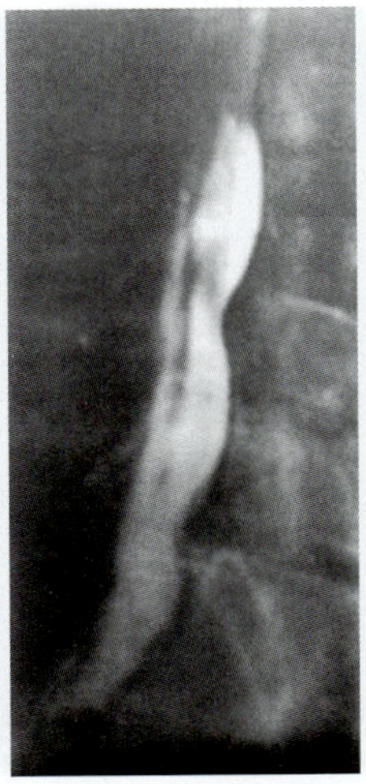

Fig. 27.170: Lumbar disk herniation on myelography

Why Hydrogen Atom?

- Hydrogen is a simple element with 1 proton in its nucleus
- It is everywhere in the body; water, lipids, proteins and nucleic acids
- The hydrogen ion in water contributes to the signal, lipids to a lesser extent and proteins and nucleic acid offers nothing to the signal
- The atom is positively charged and has a spinning or angular movement, which produces an internal magnetic field around the atom
- When these randomly oriented atoms are placed in an external magnetic field, some will align itself parallel to the magnetic field, producing a net magnetic vector
- Other atoms like sodium or potassium can also be used.

Common Terms Used in MRI

Pulse Sequence

There are three types:

1. *Spin-echo pulse sequence:* A combination of 90° and 180° radiofrequency (RF) waves result in hydrogen ion magnet deflecting out of its position and it spins like a top. The resulting signal is called the spin-echo.
2. *Gradient-echo pulse sequence:* These use less RF power, resulting in less angle deflection of H^+ ion and these sequences require less time for recovery. This results in less time for the image gathering.
3. *Fast spin-echo:* This delivers a faster image. Routine images take around 30 to 45 minutes for an image. FSE can get T2 SE images in less than five minutes.

Echo Time

It is the time between the initial RF pulse and the middle of the spin echo production when the antenna detects the signal.

Repetition Time

It is the time between one RF pulse and the next. By varying echo time (TE) and (TR) repetition time, various tissue relaxation times are produced and different tissue contrasts can be produced.

Relaxation Time

This is determined by the behavior of atoms in a magnetic field and can be used to produce images of varying tissue contrast. There are two types of relaxation:

T1 Relaxation time (T1-weighted images): It is the time required to restore 63 percent of the equilibrium population of atoms to align with the magnetic field following the excitation pulse. It is also known as spin lattice or longitudinal relaxation time.

T2 Relaxation time (T2-weighted images): It is the time required for 63 percent of the signal given to disappear irreversibly, caused by interaction of adjacent nuclei. It is also known as spin-spin or transverse relaxation time.

Each tissue has a characteristic T1 and T2 relaxation times which determine the signal intensity and thus the image produced.

The set up of the machine is:
- T1 to TR: 600 ms and TE: 30 ms. Slice thickness: 4-5 mm
- T2 to TR: 2000 ms and TE: 60/90 ms. Slice thickness: 4-5 mm.

Technique

- Place the patient in the magnetic coil
- Broadcast a predetermined radiofrequency into the body and the series of the RF pulse is repeated in cycles
- The hydrogen atoms absorb the energy from the RF and there is change in the net magnetic vector. During a gap in the pulse the atoms try to reorient, releasing energy they have absorbed
- This energy is picked up by an antenna
- It is recorded as digital data by the computer
- Computer converts digital data into varying shades of grey to produce an image.

MRI Gray Scale

The varying shades of gray produced are based upon:
- *Proton density:* The more number of free, mobile protons, brighter is the image and vice versa. Materials with high proton density are fat, CSF, blood and other fluids and these produce bright images. Materials with low proton density are calcium, air, cortical bone and fibrous tissue and these produce gray images.
- *T1 and T2 relaxation times:* Substances with the shortest T1 give off the brightest signal fat, lipid containing molecules or proteinaceous fluid. Substances with the longest T1 give low signal and appear gray (edema, CSF, pure fluid and tumors). In T2 images, longer the T2 relaxation time, brighter the signal and vice versa.
- Motion or flow of materials, e.g. blood.

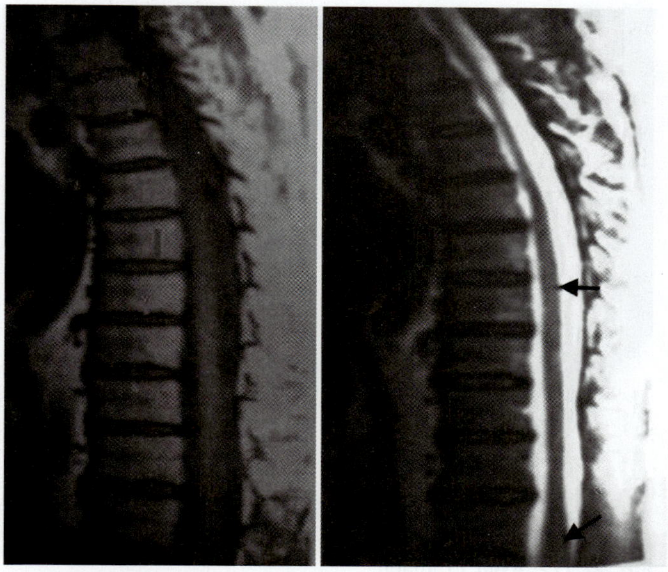

Fig. 27.171: Left sagittal T1 and right sagittal T2 image

Normal Anatomy of Thoracic and Lumbar Spine

Sagittal T1 Images (Fig. 27.171)

- Spinal cord—intermediate signal
- CSF—low (gray)
- Epidural fat—high
- Marrow—intermediate to high
- Dorsal root ganglion—intermediate.

Sagittal T2 Images

- Spinal cord—low
- CSF—high (white)
- Epidural fat—intermediate
- Marrow—intermediate to low
- Dorsal root ganglion—intermediate.

Axial T1 Images (Fig. 27.172)

- Spinal cord—intermediate
- CSF—low
- Marrow—high
- Interforaminal vein—low
- Dorsal root ganglion—low but well defined and surrounded by bright fat.
- Ligamentum flavum—intermediate.

Axial T2 Images (Fig. 27.173)

- Spinal cord—low
- CSF—high
- Marrow—low

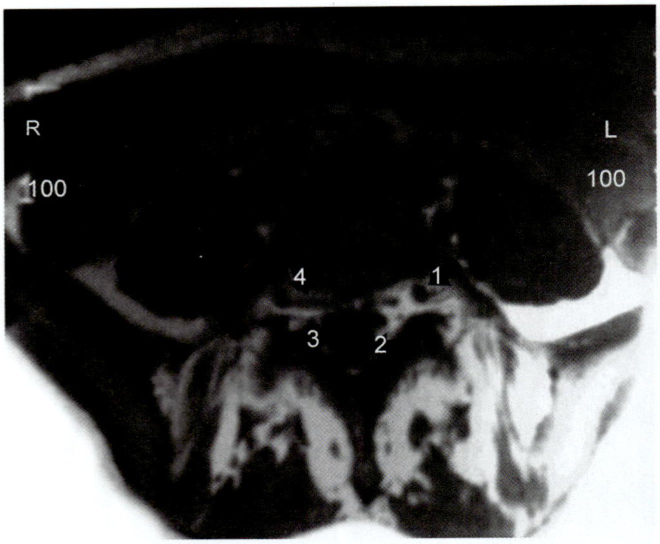

Fig. 27.172: Axial T1 image

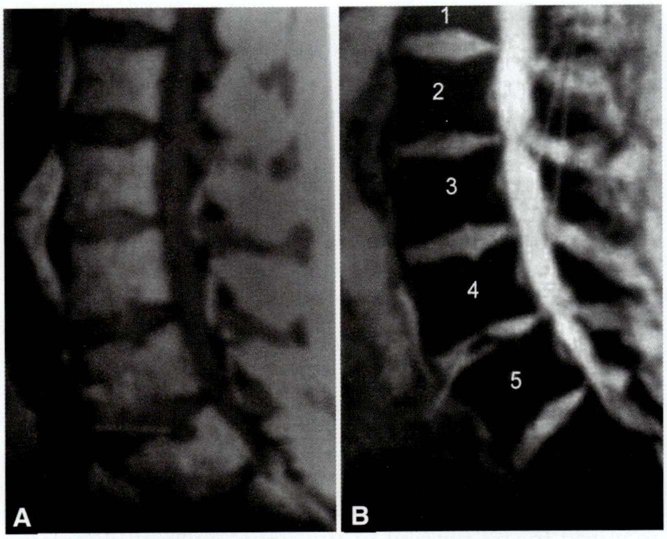

Figs 27.174A and B: Degenerative disk disease

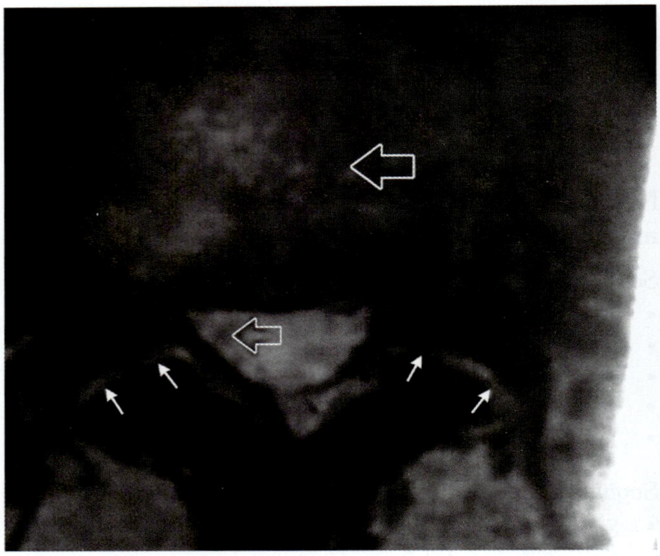

Fig. 27.173: Axial T2 image

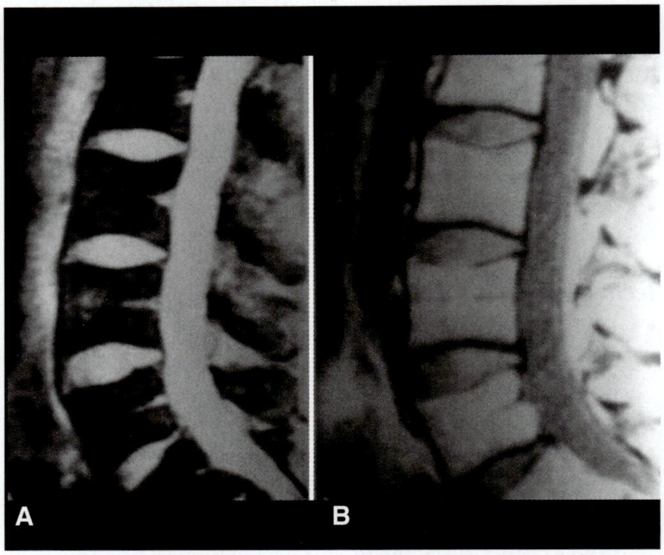

Figs 27.175A and B: T1 and T2 sagittal images showing degenerative disk disease (vide text)

- Facet hyaline cartilage—intermediate
- Ligamentum flavum—high
- Intervertebral disk—high.

Indications

- Degenerative disk disease
- Postoperative spine
- Infection
- Trauma
- Neoplasms—bone, soft tissue and cord
- Spondylolisthesis
- Marrow replacement disorders—leukemia, multiple myeloma, metastasis
- Abnormalities of the pediatric spine.

Degenerative Disk Disease

- Disk herniation is better seen in the T2 images as there is white CSF as the background
- Lateral or posterolateral disks are best seen in the axial images
- Schmorls nodes and vacuum phenomenon can also be seen (Figs 27.174 to 27.176).

End-Plate Changes (Modic)

- *Type I:* There is decreased signal intensity in T1 and increased on T2 and it represent subchondral vascularized fibrous tissue associated with end-plate fissuring and disruption

- *Type II:* There is increased signal intensity on T1 and iso or hypotense signal on T2. It represents fatty marrow endplate conversion
- *Type III:* There is low signal intensity on both T1 and T2 images. It represents sclerosis (Figs 27.177 to 27.179).

Fractures and Cord Trauma

- MRI has been used for traumatic and nontraumatic body fractures
- In 28 percent of cases supraspinous ligament disruptions associated with thoracolumbar burst fractures are identified on MRI
- In post traumatic myelopathy, there is low intensity on T1 and hyperintensity on T2
- Syringomyelia shows hyperintensity on T2 images
- Myelomalacia, i.e. gliosis induced microcystic degeneration of cord parenchyma is isointense or hyperintense to cord on T1 images
- Sacral fractures may mimic metastasis and show low intensity on T1 and high intensity on fat suppression images.

Infection

- MRI is more sensitive than X-ray or CT for detection of vertebral osteomyelitis
- Infection of vertebral body and the adjacent disk space is seen as low intensity on T1 images and high on T2 images
- TB spondylitis is characterized by intraosseous and paraspinal abscess formation, subligamentous extension of infection, destruction and collapse of the vertebral body and epidural space extension

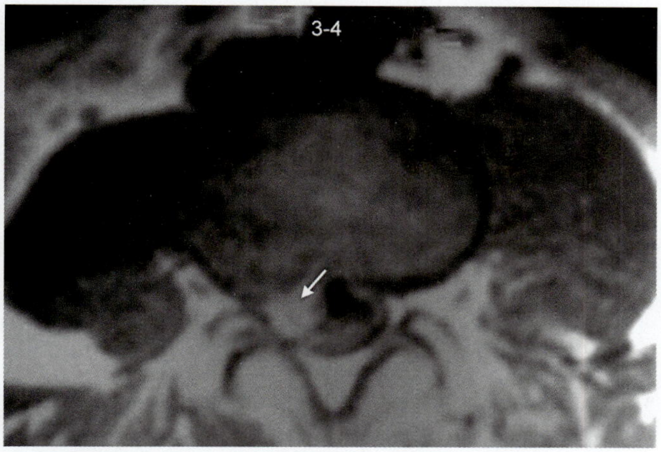

Fig. 27.176: Axial images showing disk herniation

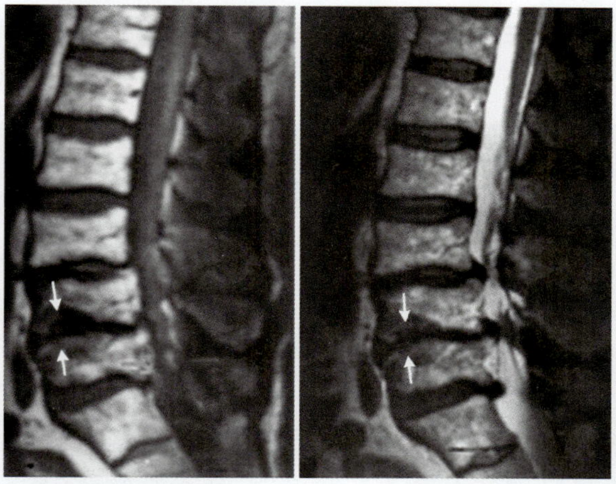

Fig. 27.178: MR images showing degenerative disk disease

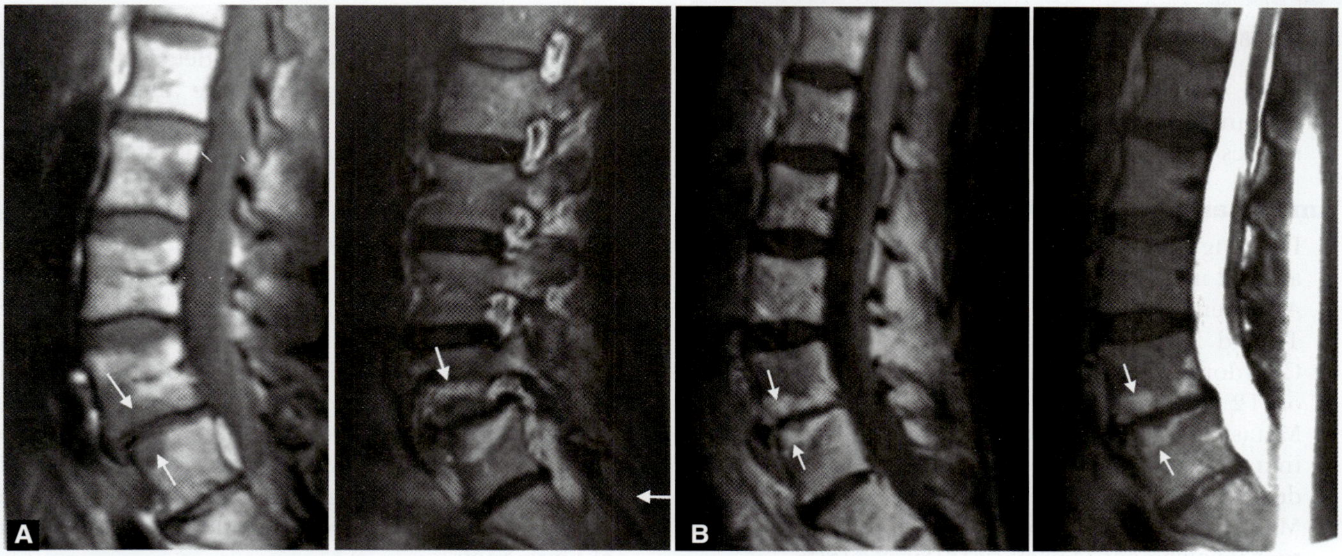

Figs 27.177A and B: (A) T1 and T2 sagittal images showing L4–L5 degenerative disk disease with spondylolisthesis; (B) Sagittal T1 and T2 images showing end-plate changes

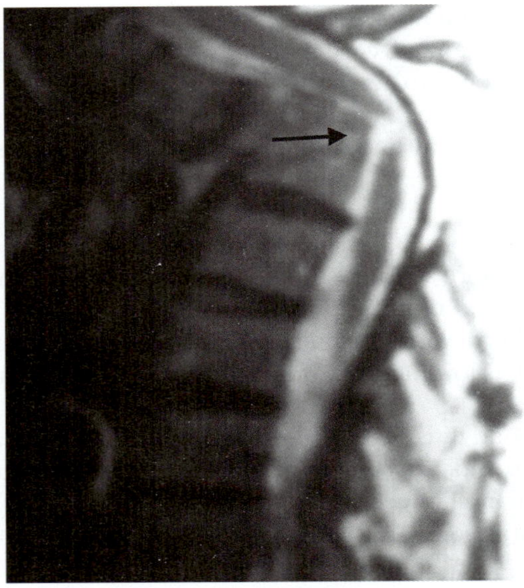

Fig. 27.179: Epidural abscesses demonstrated on T2 image

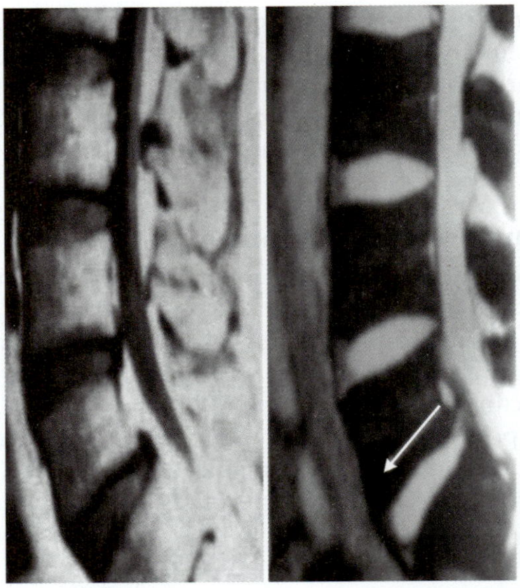

Fig. 27.181: The contors of the thecal sac having an hourglass or constricted outline

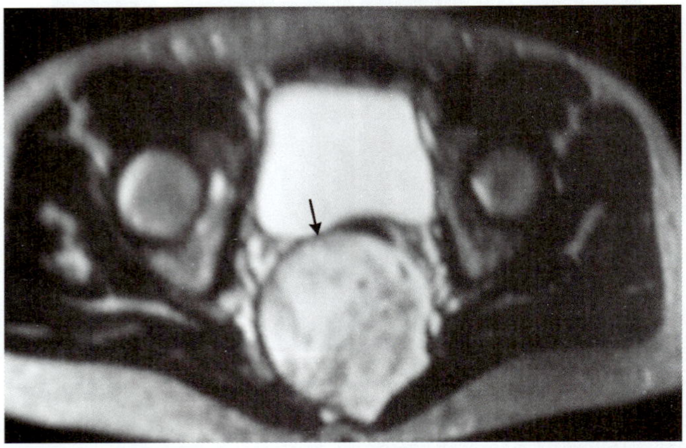

Fig. 27.180: Tarlov cyst

- Epidural abscesses are best demonstrated on T2 images (Fig. 27.179).

Tumors and Marrow Disorders

- Hemangiomas have increased signal intensity on T1 and T2 images
- ABC demonstrate inhomogenous signal intensity on T1 and T2 images
- Chordomas are hypointense on T1 and hyperintense on T2 images
- Metastatic tumors having osteoclastic activity have increased activity on T2 and osteoblastic have decreased activity on T2 images
- Meningeal cysts may present without or with nerve root involvement (Tarlov cyst) (Fig 27.180).

Spondylolisthesis

- MR images are less sensitive than CT
- The AP diameter is increased in spondylolytic listhesis and narrowed in degenerative listhesis
- Axial images demonstrate low signal intensity sclerosis, fragmentation or discontinuity in the region of the pars interarticularis
- Reactive changes in the end plates can be seen (Modic Type II)
- The contors of the thecal sac may have an hourglass or constricted outline (Fig. 27.181).

Postoperative Spine

- CT is important in assessing bony details, but MRI is useful in characterizing end-plate and associated marrow changes
- Stable fusions show modic type II changes and increased intensity on T1 and isointense on T2 images
- On T1, posterior scar has heterogenous intermediate intensity and iso to hyperintense on T2 compared to the discectomy scar
- Postoperative discitis shows decreased intensity in the marrow on T1 images, hyperintensity on T2 images
- Arachnoditis is classified as group I—central conglomeration of nerve roots within the thecal sac, group II—nerve roots are clumped peripherally to the meninges, producing an apparent empty thecal sac and group III—images show increased soft tissue signal, occupying the thecal sac with no discrimination of nerve roots.

Disadvantages

- The gantry is smaller and longer than CT and patient may have claustrophobia
- The scan time is longer and the patient may find it difficult to be still for the time required
- Patients with ferromagnetic materials in the body cannot be scanned:
  - Cerebral aneurysmal clips
  - Pacemakers
  - TENS units
  - Metallic cardiac valves
  - Life support devices
- Most orthopedic implants are not ferromagnetic and do not affect image quality, unless are directly in the field, e.g. pedicle instrumentation.

Recent Advances

- *Kinematic MRI:* It refers to the assessment of joint function with respect to various interactions of soft tissue and bony structures, and relative alignment of these structures through a specific range of motion. It is used in evaluation of the cervical spine, temporomandibular joint, patellofemoral joint, knee, wrist, ankle and the shoulder.
- *STIR and GRASS:* Short T1 inversion recovery (STIR) improves visualization of joint fluid. 3D gradient recalled acquisitions in steady state (GRASS) and spoiled GRASS (SPGR) images optimize trabecular bone detail and the anatomy.
- *3D MR rendering technique:* Here the 2D images obtained are converted into 3D by the computer. Finer structures can be visualized.
- *Fat suppression images:* The adipose tissue gives a strong signal on the normal view and may hinder detection of pathology. Here, fat suppression offers improved visibility and sensitivity.
- *Contrast enhanced MRI:* Contrasts used are compounds known as gadolinium chelates. They are deposited in tissues with high water content and increase their signal intensity.

Bone Scanning (Scintigraphy)

- Bone scanning is done by injecting radionuclide element in the body
- The radionuclide combines with specific cells. From there it emits gamma rays that are detected by a gamma camera
- The images are then interpreted
- Strontium was the first element used but recently the mostly used element is ^{99m}Tc
- Gallium 67 citrate (^{67}Ga) and indium-111-labeled leukocytes are also used.

Indications

- Location of metastatic bone tumors
- Early detection of bone infection, days before regular radiographic changes occur
- Detection of osteonecrosis (AVN)
- Unexplained bone pain (? Stress fractures)
- Dating of fracture age.

Technitium-99m-labeled Phosphorus

- ^{99m}Tc is the most frequently used radionuclide as it is readily available, cheap, easily incorporates in the bone; timing is convenient and has a low radiation dose
- The dose is 10 to 20 mCi
- Technitium is used in a linkage to diphosphonates (organic phosphates) for examination of bone
- The ^{99m}Tc in phosphorus quickly incorporates in bone within 15 minutes of IV injection. The exchange occurs at the interface of bone and extracellular fluid where active mineralization is taking place.
- The faster the bone turnover, the greater the ^{99m}Tc in deposit and more gamma rays are emitted by the site. This is the basis of the "hot spot".

Phases of the Scan

- The phosphorus labeled compound is injected intravenously and three phases of the scan are completed.
- *Phase I:* Flow phase:
  - The scan is done within 1 to 2 minutes to show whether the area of interest has a vascular supply. It is also known as the nuclear angiogram.
- *Phase II:* Immediate/equilibrium phase:
  - The scan is done 5 to 10 minutes after phase I scan and shows the vascular status of the lesion.
- *Phase III:* Delayed phase:
  - The scan is done 2 to 4 hours after the injection. At this time incorporation of the isotope onto the bone hydroxyapatite crystal is maximum and background tracer is been excreted by the kidneys.
- ^{99m}Tc is deposited where bone turnover is greatest, i.e. the hydroxyapatite crystals that are the most immature
- These sites are in growing bones at the epiphysis, metaphysis of long bones and the sacroiliac joints
- Abnormal or faster turnover occurs in tumors, infections, fractures and bone-soft tissue junctions where increased metabolic activity is occurring
- These sites show a "hot spot"
- Sites with decreased bone activity, like osteonecrosis or highly destructive tumors (multiple myeloma) will show no activity change or a "cold spot", i.e. decreased tracer activity compared with surrounding normal bone (Figs 27.182).

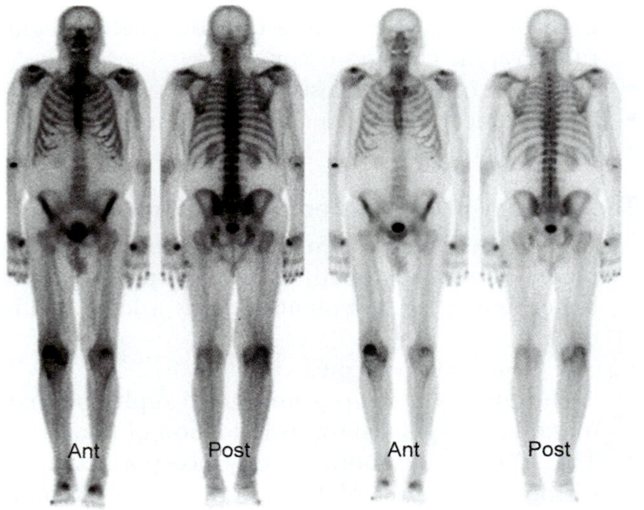

Fig. 27.182: Sites with decreased bone activity showing cold spot

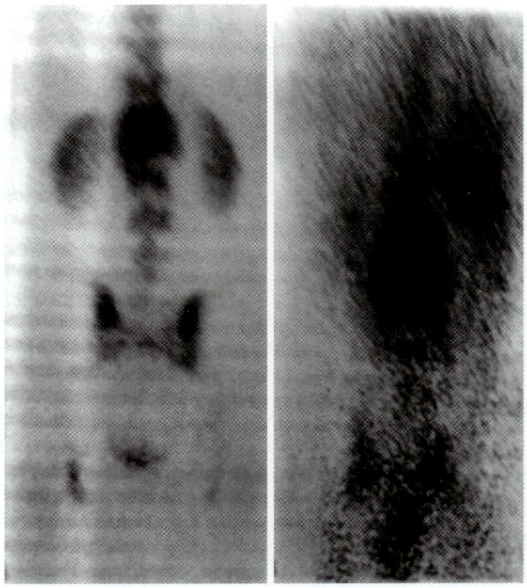

Fig. 27.183: A hot ^{99m}Tc scan with increased ^{67}Ga activity suggesting of bone infection

Gallium 67 Citrate

- ^{99m}Tc scanning identifies areas of increased turnover and is nonspecific for infection
- ^{67}Ga binds to transferrin and other proteins associated with inflammation and infection
- But, it emits four gamma rays which cause more exposure and the scan is less clear
- Also it is slowly excreted and the scan timing is 48 hours
- The value of gallium scanning is enhanced by doing ^{99m}Tc and ^{67}Ga scanning sequentially and comparing them
- A hot ^{99m}Tc scan with increased ^{67}Ga activity is suggestive of a bone infection (Fig. 27.183).

Indium-111-Labeled Leukocytes

- It has a greater specificity for musculoskeletal and other infective foci
- After harvesting the patient's own blood, the WBC are separated and labeled with indium-111
- These leukocytes are resuspended in the patient's plasma and reinjected
- 24 hours later gamma activity is measured
- It has accuracy in low-grade infection also
- ^{99m}Tc/indium-111 scanning is the method of choice for a patient suspected of having increased bone turnover from tumor or infection
- At best, an X-ray provides a limited interpretation of nonosseous events
- Myelography, an invasive procedure, provides an indirect evaluation of the disk by displaying the contor of the thecal sac and proximal nerve root sleeves
- CT is useful in delineating bone detail and direct axial scans of the spine provide soft tissue discrimination of the disk, nerve roots and thecal sac. However sagittal, coronal or oblique views cannot be directly acquired and fibrosis and scarring may be difficult to differentiate from disk material
- MRI supersedes CT and myelography in routine evaluation of spine for degenerative disk disease, trauma, infection, neoplasm, and intrinsic cord disease. It also provides the unique advantage of direct marrow imaging.

PROLAPSED INTERVERTEBRAL DISK

■ Intervertebral Disk and Relevant Anatomy

Development of spine starts from third week of intrauterine life and continues till third decade of life. There are 23 disks throughout the spine, absent only at atlantoaxial articulation. Disk is thinnest in thoracic spine and thickest in the lumbar spine. Disk lies interposed between the vertebrae, which are covered by thin cartilage plates, anterior longitudinal ligament and posterior longitudinal ligament, bound vertebral bodies and disk Disk is avascular, receives its nutrition by diffusion.

Structure of Intervertebral Disk

A disk consists of two parts:

1. *Central:* Centrally, lies nucleus pulposus made up of collagen fibrils, fibrocytes, chondrocytes, gelatinous material, water and salt

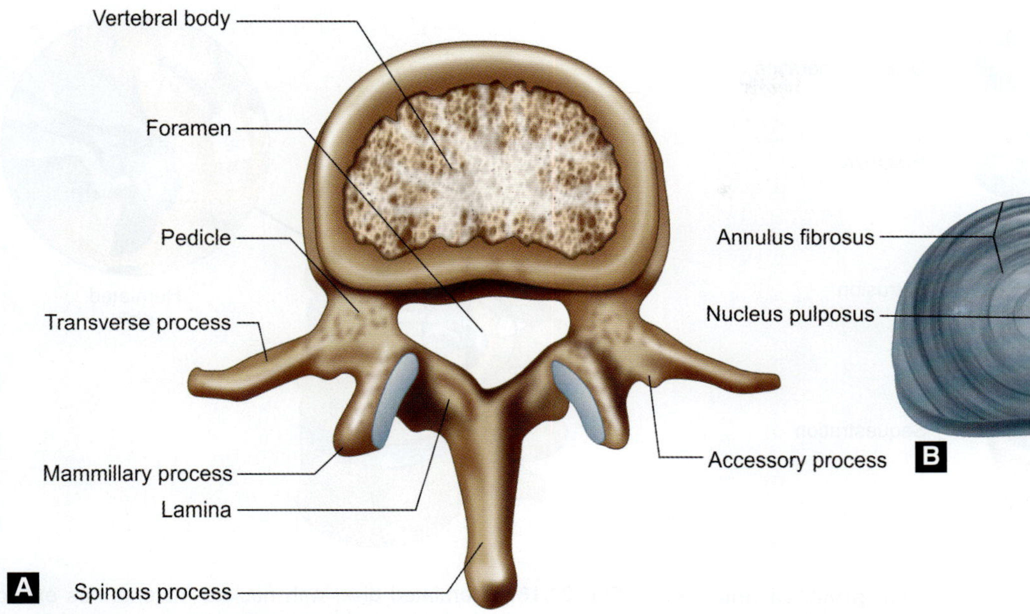

Figs 27.184A and B: (A) A thoracic vertebrae and its constituent structures; (B) An intervertebral disk

2. *Peripheral:* Peripherally, lies annulus fibrosus, a fibrocartilaginous substance. Thick anteriorly and thin posteriorly on posterolateral aspect. Hence, posterolateral disk prolapse is more common (Figs 27.184A and B).

Functions of Intervertebral Disk

- It gives mobility to spine
- Acts as shock absorber
- Increases the height of spine by 25 percent
- Distributes the load equally along the surface of the vertebral body
- Maintain the size of the vertebral foramen (Fig. 27.185).

Types of Disk Prolapse

There are four degrees of disk prolapse:

Intraspongi Nuclear Herniation

Nuclear material migrates from central region into the annular fibers, without any change in the configuration of outermost annular fibers.

Protrusion

Nuclear fibers causing bulging of annular fibers.

Extrusion

Nuclear material escapes through all the fibers, but still remains connected to nuclear material within the disk.

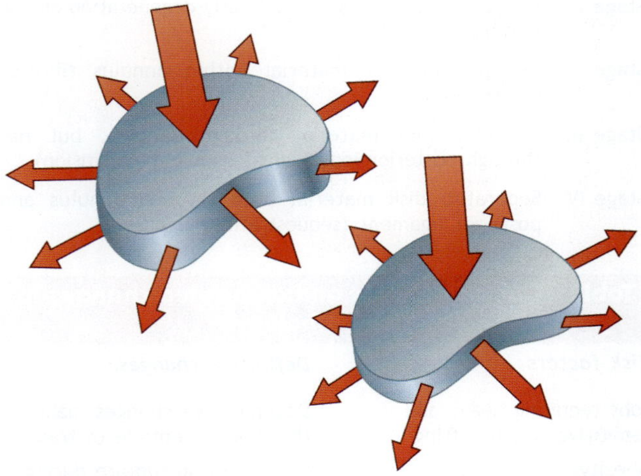

Fig. 27.185: Various forces acting on an intervertebral disk, shown by the directions of arrows

Sequestered Disk

Nuclear material has extruded through fibers of annulus fibrosus and lies in spinal canal, as free fragment (Fig. 27.186).

Pathological Staging (Eismont and Currier, 1989)

Different pathological stages are shown in the Table 27.5.

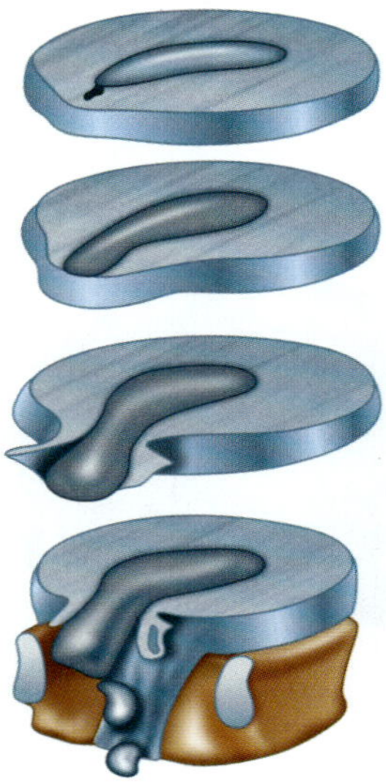

Fig. 27.186: Different degrees of disk prolapse and their physiological presentation

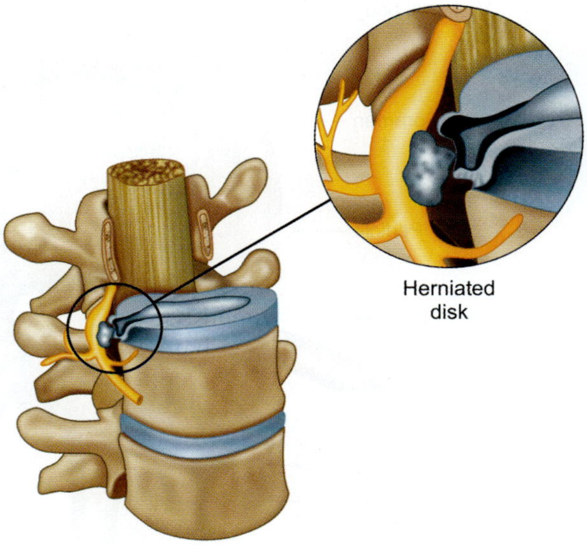

Fig. 27.187: Herniated disk, with nuclear material has extruded through fibers of annulus fibrosus

Table 27.5: Different pathological stages of disk herniation	
Stage I	Dehydration, desiccation and early degeneration of disk material
Stage II	Prolapse of disk material within annulus fibrosus (protrusion)
Stage III	Extruded disk material through annulus, but not through posterior longitudinal ligament (extrusion)
Stage IV	Separated disk material both through annulus and posterior ligament (sequestration)

Table 27.6: Risk factors and associated changes in disk pathology

Risk factors	*Definitive changes*
Jobs requiring heavy and repetitive weight lifting	Degenerative changes makes the disk susceptible to trauma
Obesity	Disk may also rupture during pregnancy and labor
Stressful occupation as in doctors, police, etc.	Disk may also rupture after prolonged bed rest due to disk softening
Women with great number of pregnancies	Disk rupture without any cause is definitely due to degenerative cause
Improper postural habits	
Operation of motor vehicles	
Rarely anxiety and depression, etc.	

Etiology of Disk Herniation (Table 27.6)

Etiology consist of risk factors and definitive causes, jobs requiring heavy and repetitive weight lifting and other factors (Figs 27.187 to 27.189).

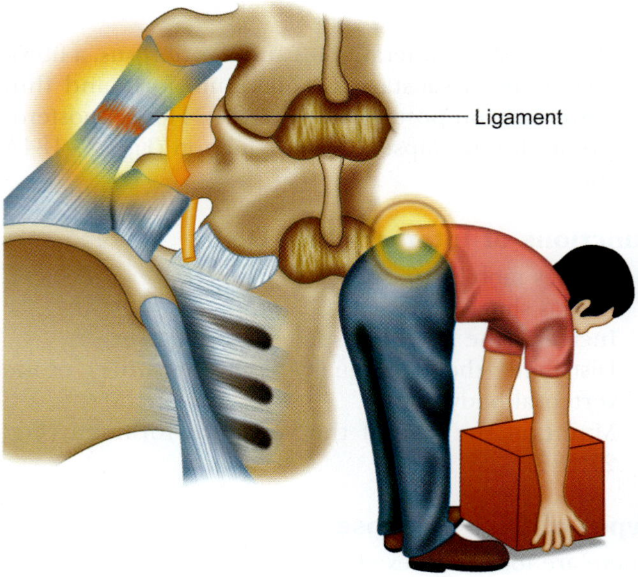

Fig. 27.188: Activities, like heavy weight lifting cause stress on surrounded ligaments and degenerative changes, make the disk susceptible to trauma

Cervical Disk Prolapse (Figs 27.190 and 27.191)

Clinical Features

More common in men, ratio of 1.4 to 1.

Symptoms

- Neck pain, medial scapular pain and shoulder pain

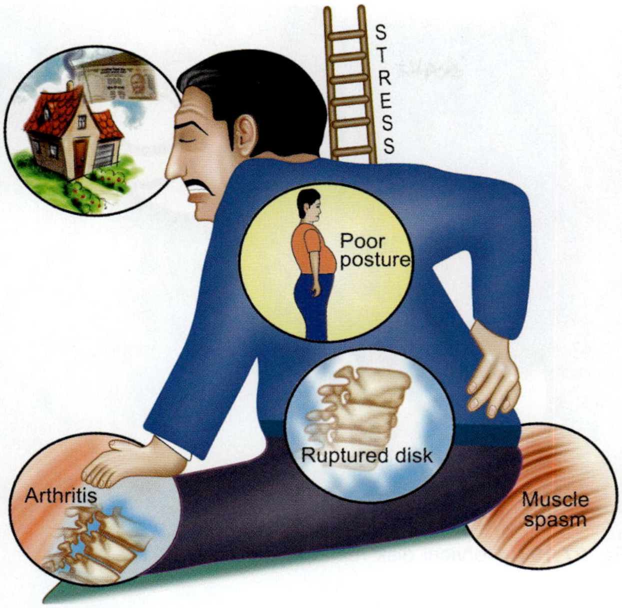

Fig. 27.189: Bad posture, occupational stress, unaccustomed activity and emotional stress

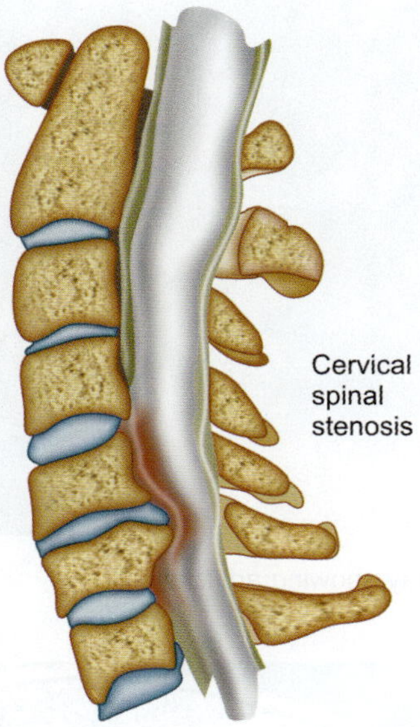

Fig. 27.190: Herniated cervical disk

- Some complains of headache, vertigo, tinnitus and ocular problems
- Radiating pain to arm with numbness and weakness in fingers
- Sometimes with generalized weakness of lower extremities and feeling of instability.

Signs

- Cervical paraspinal muscle spasm and limitation of neck motion

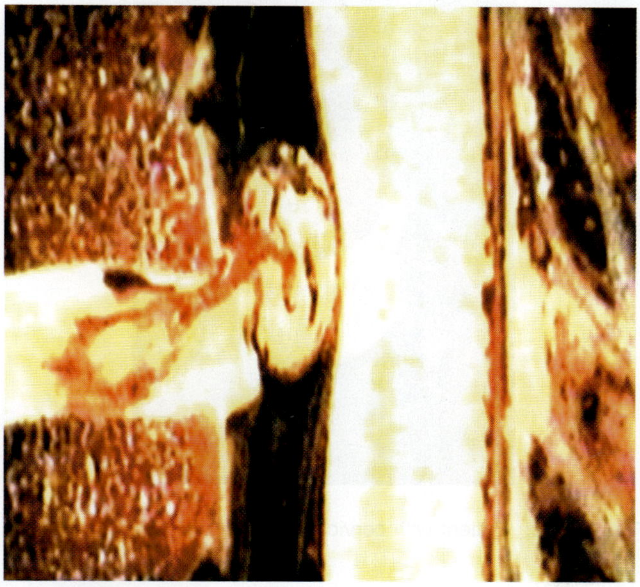

Fig. 27.191: Extrusion of prolapsed disk

- Loss of cervical lordosis, i.e. straight and stiff neck
- In case of midline herniation, signs of spinal cord compression like clonus, hyperactive reflexes and babinski reflex and less frequently spasticity and impairment of proprioception.

Examination of Cervical Spine

- Palpate for tender spot on spine
- Movement of the spine.

Special Tests

- Distraction test
- Compression test
- Upper limb tension test
- Spurling test.

Investigation

- *Routine investigation:* Complete hemogram with ESR, urine examination
- *Radiographs:* AP, lateral view is done. It shows straightening of spine, decreased height of disk, sclerosis and condensation of bone above and below the affected disk, calcification in nucleus pulposus or annulus fibrosus
- Myelography
- CT scan
- MRI.

Treatment

Nonoperative treatment: Analgesic, cervical braces, orthosis, cervical traction. Isometric neck and shoulder exercises as the acute pain subsides (Fig. 27.192).

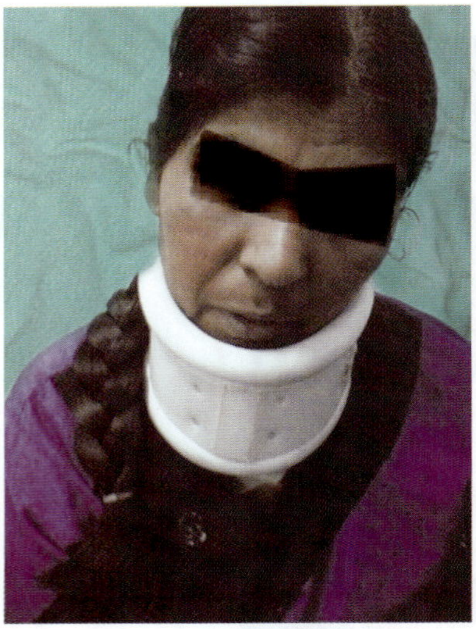

Fig. 27.192: Patient with cervical brace

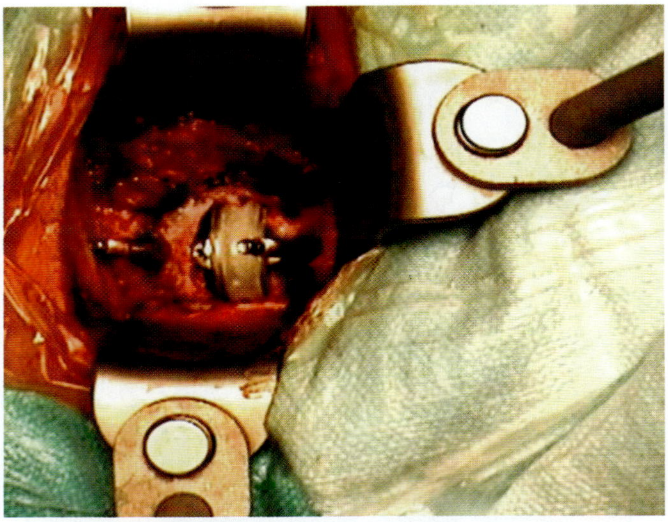

Fig. 27.193: Cervical disk replacement

Operative Treatment: Indications

- Failure of conservative therapy
- Increasing neurological deficit
- Cervical myelopathy, i.e. progressive
- Anterior or posterior approach is taken
- Anterior discectomy and interbody fusion is done by Coward and Smith Robbinson technique
- *Coward technique involves:* Making a round hole centered at disk space with large round iliac crest plug inserted
- *Smith robbinson technique:* Involves inserting a tricortical plug of iliac graft with cancellous side facing the cord and the cortical surface is fashioned to fill the intervertebral disk
- Patient are advised a semirigid collar for 8 to 12 weeks.

Cervical Disk Replacement (Figs 27.193 to 27.195)

■ Thoracic Disk Prolapse

- Extremely rare, incidence is 0.25 to 0.5 percent of all IVA ruptures
- Major reason is less motion of spine in thoracic region
- Most of the disk protrusion occurs in lower region of thoracic spine T9–T12.

Clinical Features

Symptoms

- Backache usually not well localized, describing it as aching, radiating to low back
- Band of tenderness due to involvement of thoracic nerve root irritation
- Spinal cord compression such as weakness of lower limb, bladder bowel dysfunction or ataxia

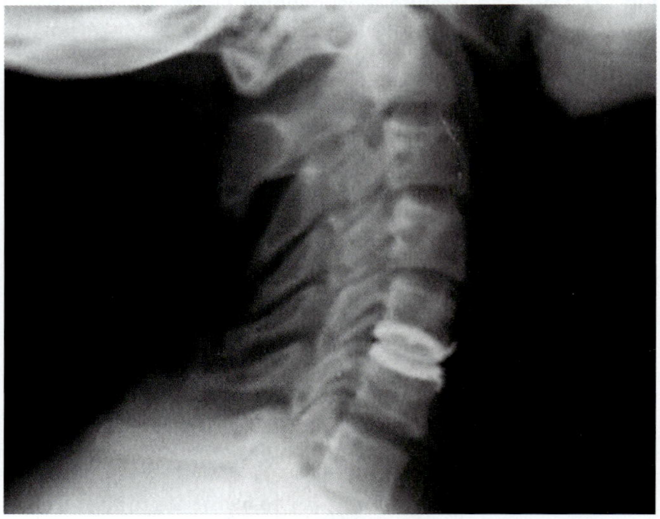

Fig. 27.194: X-ray showing artificial disk

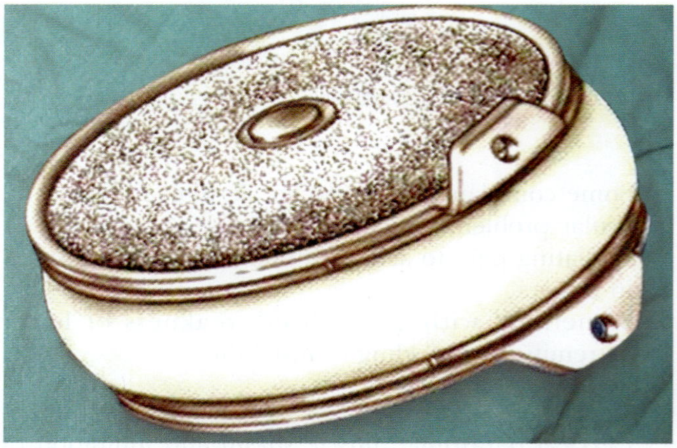

Fig. 27.195: Artificial disk

- Occasionally the initial presentation may be complete or incomplete paraplegia or sudden onset of Brown-Sequard syndrome.

Signs

- Weakness of lower abdominal muscle in addition to leg weakness which is bilateral
- Sensory loss is present
- Hyper-reflexia
- Plantars are extensor response
- Clonus present
- The disk protrusion may be lateral contralateral or central.

Treatment

- There is no evidence to indicate the value of conservative therapy.

Surgical Treatment

- Thoracic laminectomy
- Costo transversectomy.

Lumbar Disk Prolapse

- Most common in males
- The prolapse occurs mostly
  - just above or below the 5th lumbar vertebra, i.e. between L4-L5 and L5-S1 (Fig. 27.196).

Clinical Features

Symptoms

- Back pain increases with activity, prolonged sitting
- Pain relived by rest in semi-Fowlers position

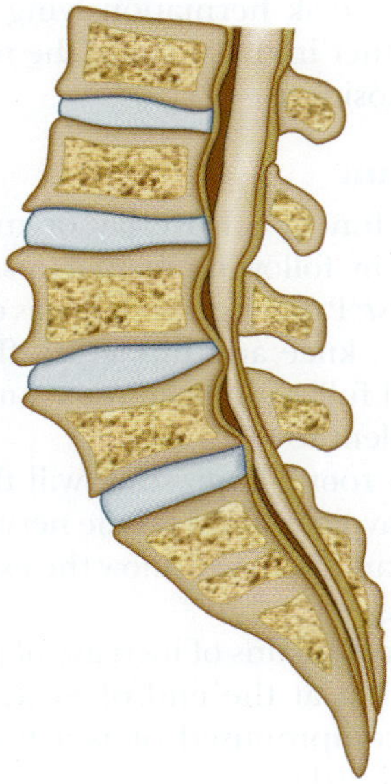

Fig. 27.196: L4-L5 disk prolapsed

- Pain exacerbated by straining, sneezing and coughing
- Radicular pain
- Weakness, numbness and parasthesia according to the nerve involved.

Signs

- In acute cases paraspinal muscle spasm
- Loss of lumbar lordosis
- Scoliotic deformity
- Point tenderness over the spinous process
- Decreased forward flexion of the spine (Fig. 27.197).

Tension tests in lumbar disk prolapse are:

- Straight leg raising test
- Well leg raising test
- Lasegue's test
- Lateral flexion test of spine
- Sciatic stretch test
- Figure of 4 test
- Bowstring test
- Sitting root test
- Femoral nerve stretch test.

Test for Nerve Root Tension

- *Straight leg raising test:* Straight leg raising test is used to demonstrate a lumbosacral nerve root irritation due to a herniated disk
- It is a part of tension tests which are based upon the maneuvers which tighten the sciatic nerve and thus compress the inflamed nerve root against the herniated disk leading to pain.

Straight Leg Raising Test (Fig. 27.198)

- Interpretation of SLR
- Pain or parasthesia up to 70° is suggestive of prolapsed disk
- Pain above 70° is equivocal
- Back pain suggests central disk prolapse—not indicative of root tension

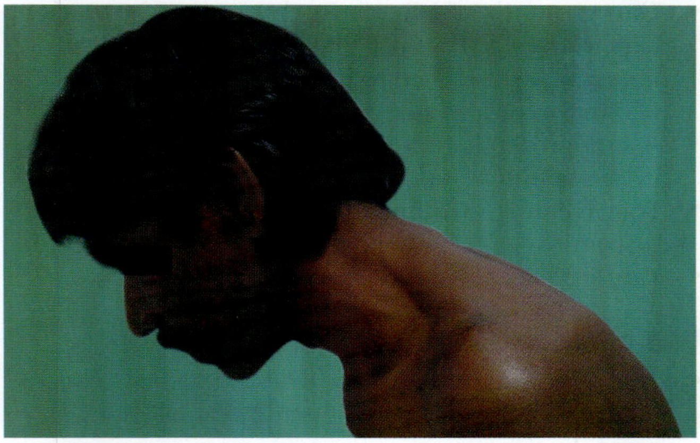

Fig. 27.197: Decreased forward flexion of the spine

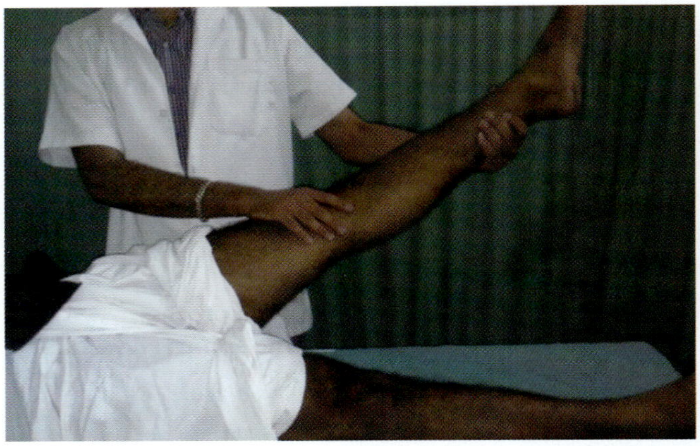

Fig. 27.198: Straight leg raising test

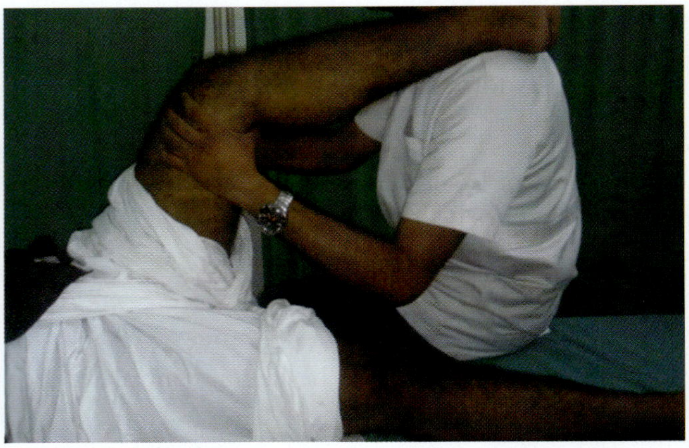

Fig. 27.199: Bowstring's sign

- Leg pain (buttock, thigh, leg) suggests lateral protrusion—indicative of root tension.

False positive SLR: Hamstring tightness might cloud the assessment of SLR.

Can be differentiated by following characteristics:
- Discomfort is bilateral
- Discomfort is distal in the thigh, in the region of the hamstring tendons
- Does not radiate below the knee
- False negative SLR
- Generally seen in a loose jointed individual
- Can be appreciated on examining the other limb (the person's ability to straight leg raise will be beyond 90°)
- So to avoid both false positives and false negatives it is mandatory to examine both the lower limbs.

Bowstring's Sign (Fig. 27.199)

- It is probably single most important sign in diagnosis of tension and irritation of a nerve root caused by a ruptured intervertebral disk
- Carry out the SLR up to the point the patient experiences discomfort in the distribution of sciatic nerve, allow the knee to flex and the patient's foot is allowed to rest on the examiner's shoulder
- A sudden pressure is applied on the popliteal nerve in the popliteal fossa
- Positive test is a reproduction of radiating leg discomfort
- Pain in the popliteal fossa is not significant.

Well-Leg Raising Sign (Crossover Pain)

- This is considered positive when the a symptomatic leg is lifted and the symptomatic side becomes more painful

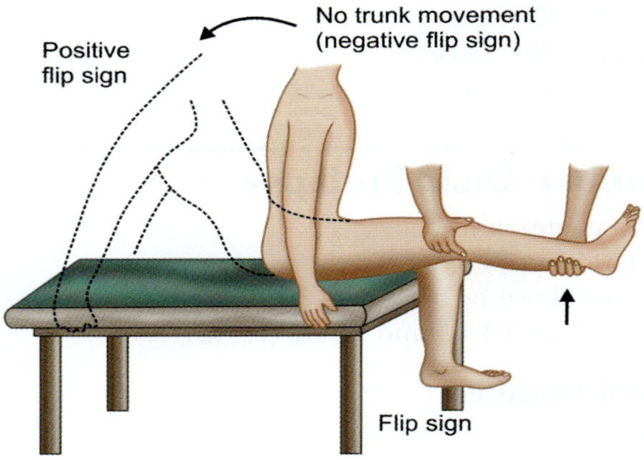

Fig. 27.200: Flip test

- Indicative of a disk herniation lying medial to the nerve root, either in the axilla of the nerve root or in the midline position.

Nonorganic Pain

- Patients with functional overlay or malingerers can be diagnosed by following maneuvers
- *Positive flip test:* Patient sits with knees dangling by the end of a table, knee and hip at 90° flexion. Knee is now extended fully; the position assumed by the leg will be equivalent to 90° SLR
- Patient with a root compression will throw his trunk backwards to avoid tension on the nerve, but a patient with a nonorganic pain will allow the examiner to fully extend the leg
- If the patient complains of increase of pain on flexion of knee and hip at the end of SLR, the patient is emotionally compromised or is a malingerer (Figs 27.200 and 27.201).

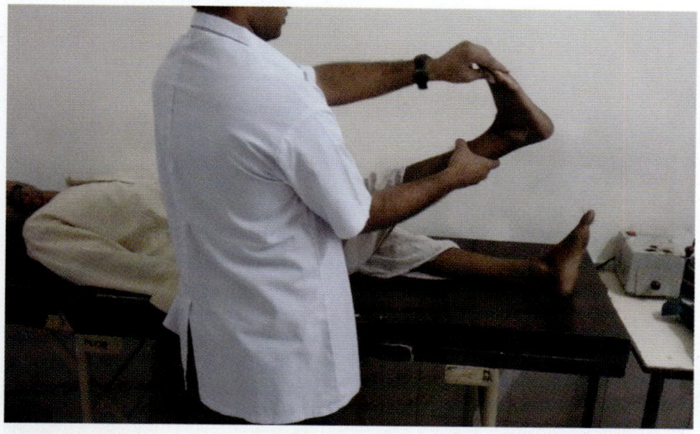

Fig. 27.201: Patient throwing his trunk backward to avoid pressure on the nerve

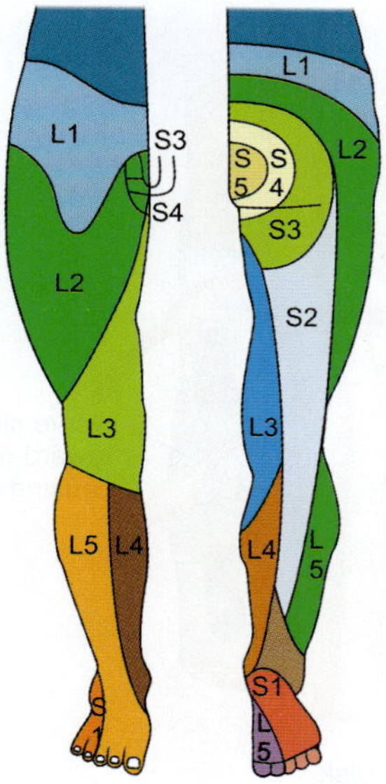

Fig. 27.202: The cutaneous and motor distribution of the nerve roots supplying the skin and muscles of the lower limbs

Fajersztajn Test

Straight leg raising test (SLRT) is done until pain is produced then gentle dorsiflexion of the foot is done to ascertain whether symptoms are increased. These is also known as Bragards sign.

Lasegue Test

Hip and knee gently flexed to 90°. The leg is then extended which reproduce the symptoms of sciatica.

Femoral Nerve Stretch Test

Patient is in prone position. Knee is gradually flexed and then the hip extended this causes excursion in L2, L3 and L4 roots. (Table 27.7 and Figs 27.202 and 27.203).

Table 27.7: Finding of nerve root compression

Nerve root compression	*Neurological findings*
T12, L1, L2, L3, L4	*Motor deficit:* Iliopsoas weakness *Sensory:* Anterior part of the thigh *Reflexes:* None, patellar tendon variable
L4	*Motor deficit:* Quadriceps, hip adductors *Sensory:* Posterolateral thigh, anterior knee and medial leg *Reflexes:* Patellar tendon
L5	*Motor deficit:* Extensor hallucis longus, gluteus medius, extensor digitorum longus and brevis *Sensory:* Anterolateral leg, dorsum of foot and great toe *Reflexes:* None, tibialis posterior variable
S1	*Motor deficit:* Peroneous longus and brevis, tendon achilles, gluteus maximus *Sensory:* Lateral malleolus, lateral foot, heel and web of fourth and fifth toe *Reflexes:* Ankle reflex

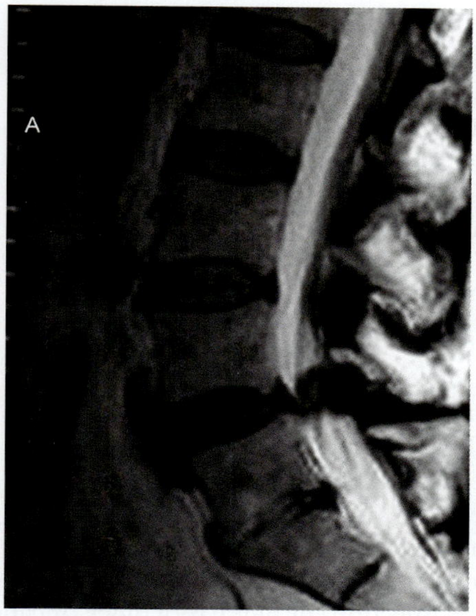

Fig. 27.203: L4-L5 disk prolapse

Cauda Equina Syndrome

- Large midline disk prolapse (Fig. 27.204)
- Compresses several nerve roots
- Sphincter disturbance
- Saddle anesthesia
- Prompt surgical intervention
- Common diseases that mimic disk disease
- Ankylosing spondylitis
- Multiple myeloma
- Vascular insufficiency

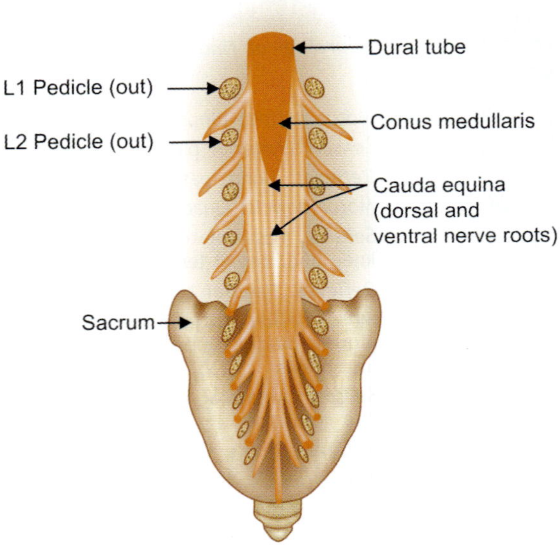

Fig. 27.204: Large midline disk prolapse

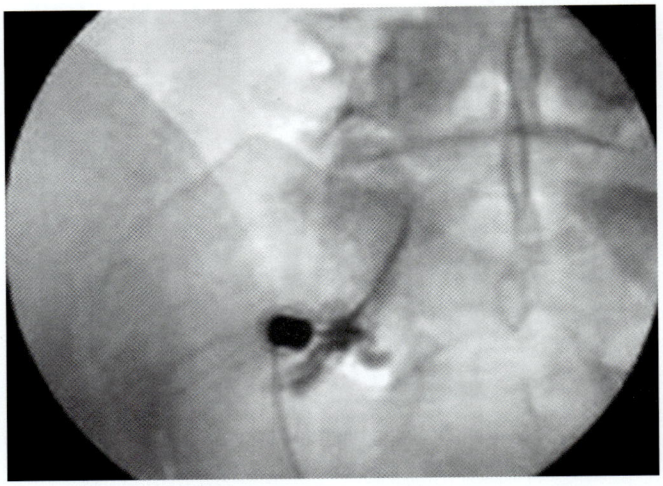

Fig. 27.205: Nerve root block under C-arm

- Arthritis of hip
- Osteoporosis with stress fracture
- Extradural tumors
- Peripheral neuropathy
- Herpes zoster
- SI joint dysfunction.

Treatment

Conservative

- Analgesic
- Lumbar traction
- Heat therapy
- Back exercises
- Bed rest
- Epidural injections
- Chemonucleolysis
- Epidural injections or nerve root block or caudal block
- Combination of long acting steroid with anesthetic agent
- Methyl-prednisolone is usually used.

Indications

- Painful SLRT or femoral stress test
- Patient with appropriate neurological deficit
- Patient with acute or chronic symptoms with different level of disk pathology nerve root block (Figs 27.205 to 27.207).

Contraindication

- Infection
- Hemorrhagic conditions
- Cauda equina syndrome.

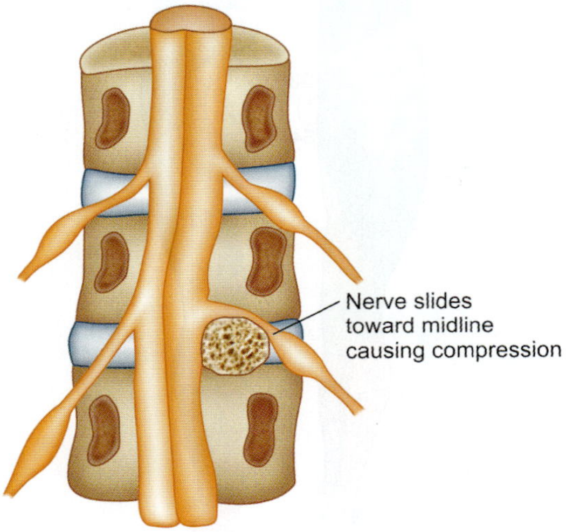

Fig. 27.206: Axillary disk

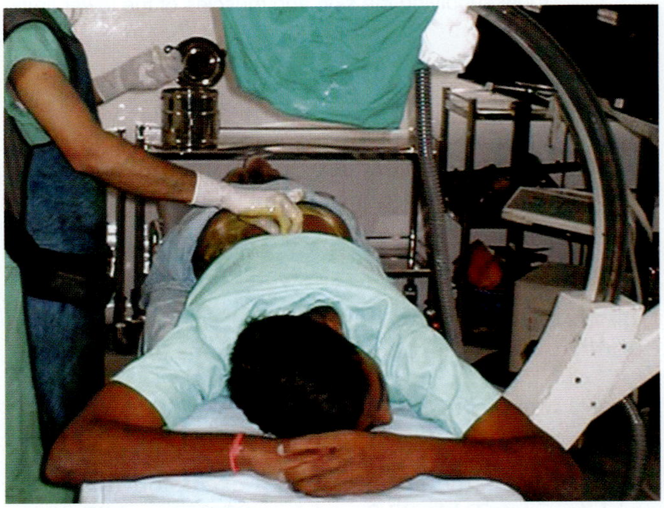

Fig. 27.207: Preparation for nerve root block

Complications

- Twenty-five percent rate of failure to place the drug in epidural space
- Bacterial meningitis
- Transient hypotension
- Severe paresthesia
- Headache, cardiac angina
- Chemonucleolysis
- Various substance are used to shrink or dissolve the disk such as chymopapain, collagenase, aprotienin, chondroitinase and cathepsins.

Indications

- Pain less than six months
- Leg pain greater than back pain
- Positive nerve root compression test
- Nerve root dysfunction.

Operative Treatment

Indications

- Advancing neurological deficit
- Paraplegia
- Acute bladder paralysis
- Severe persistent pain
- Failure of conservative management
- Hemi or partial laminectomy
- Total laminectomy
- Microdiscectomy
- Fenestration operation
- Microdiscectomy (Figs 27.208 to 27.210)
- Causes of failed back surgery
- Recurrent or persistent disk herniation
- Epidural fibrosis
- Facetal fractures
- Lateral recess stenosis
- Rarely adhesive arachnoiditis
- Recent surgical advances
- Automated percutaneous lumbar discectomy
- Arthoscopic microsurgical discectomy
- Percutaneous laser discectomy
- Percutaneous anterior arthoscopic microdiscectomy.

■ Discitis

- Discitis describes conditions in which the intervertebral disk is infected. These infections can develop through blood born bacteria being delivered to the disk space. Infections can spread from adjacent infections. Diagnostic testing can inadvertently introduce bacteria into the disk space.

Signs and Symptoms

- Fever and chills occurs early in the course of disk space infections
- Local pain occurs and increases as the infection progresses
- Muscle spasms develop in the areas adjacent to the infection
- If the infection spreads into the adjacent spinal canal, either compression or inflammation of the spinal cord and nerve roots can occur
- This can lead to varying degrees of weakness, numbness, tingling, urinary and bowel dysfunction.

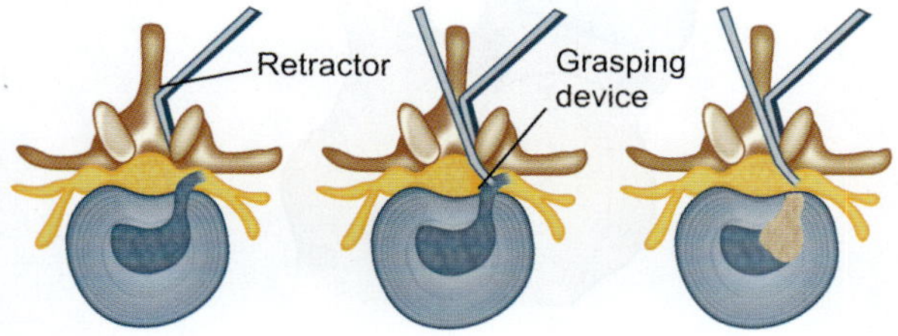

Fig. 27.208: Microdiscectomy

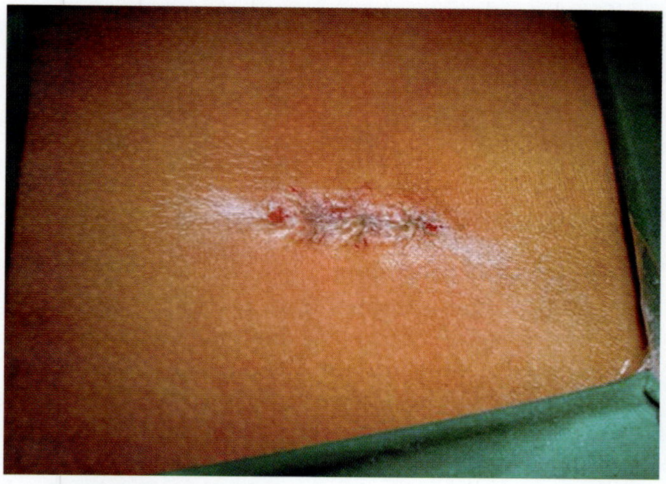

Fig. 27.209: Microdiscectomy scan

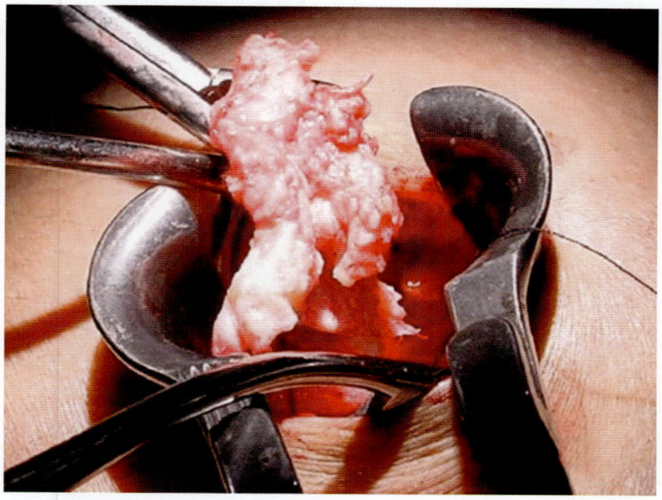

Fig. 27.210: Removal of disk material

Investigation

- Routine hemogram, ESR
- C-reactive protein
- CT scan
- MRI.

Treatment

Antibiotics

- Immobilization of spine
- Surgical treatment is reserved for the more advanced cases where there is an abscess, spinal instability or weakness, tumor involvement or in cases where bowel or bladder function are involved
- Debridement can be performed through an open or minimally invasive technique. Once the infected disk material is removed, your surgeon may wish to perform a fusion, a procedure in which the vertebrae on each side of the infected disk are joined together (fused) to eliminate movement between them.

DEGENERATIVE DISEASES OF SPINE

■ Spondylolisthesis (Fig. 27.211)

Lumbar Canal Stenosis

- Spondylolisthesis derives from two parts: Spondylos meaning "spine" and olisthanein meaning "to slip"
- Is defined as slow anterior displacement (luxation) of a vertebra at the lower lumbar spine, generally accepted as involving the lower most vertebrae slipping forward on the first sacral segment
- The essential lesion that permits the superimposed body weight to encourage forward displacement is an interruption in continuity of the pars interarticularis, that portion of the posterior arch that extends between superior and inferior articular process, usually the defect lies within the pars as it extends toward the inferior articular process.

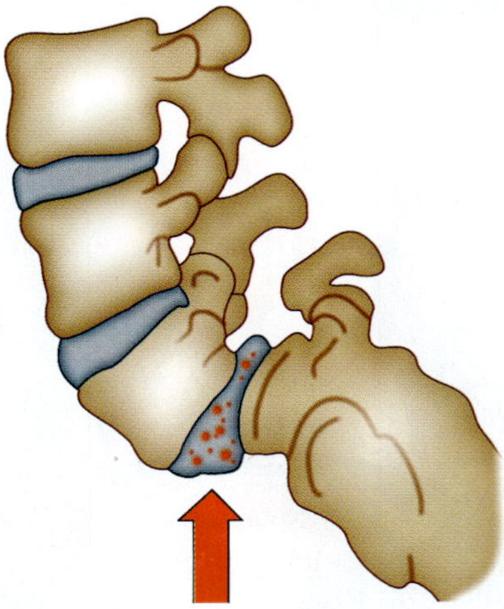

Fig. 27.211: Spondylolisthesis

Spondylolysis (Fig. 27.212)

- In spondylolysis, there is a defect in the *pars interarticularis* (which literally means "piece between the articulations")
- When the defect exists without forward slipping, the term spondylolysis (spondylos, "spine"; lysis, "to disintegrate") is used and could be unilateral (involving one side) or bilateral (involving both sides)
- Although the defect can be found at any level, the commonest vertebra involved is the 5th lumbar vertebra (or L5)
- Lateral lumbar spinal radiograph in a pediatric patient showing spondylolysis with grade 1 spondylolisthesis (Figs 27.213 and 27.214).

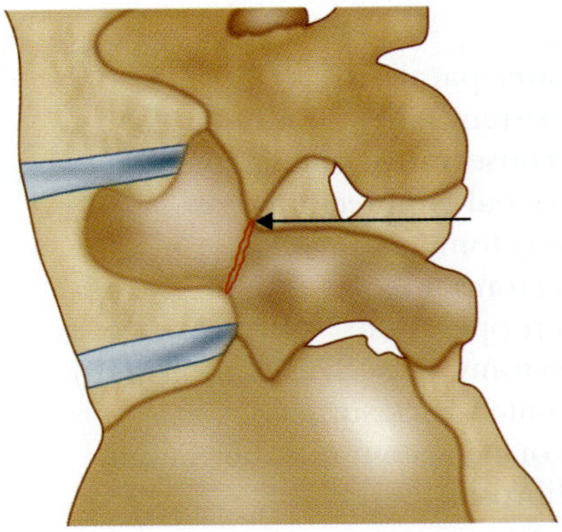

Fig. 27.212: Arrow shown spondylolysis

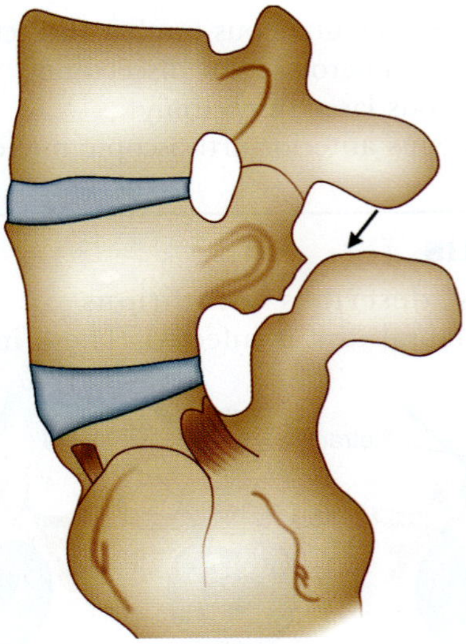

Fig. 27.213: Break in pars interarticularis

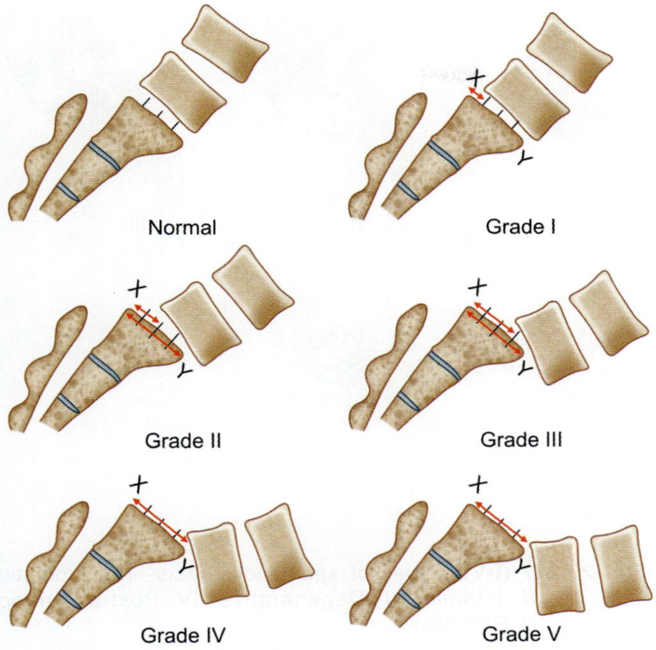

Fig. 27.214: Lateral lumbar spinal radiograph in a pediatric patient showing spondylolysis with grade 1 spondylolisthesis

Introduction

- The spine or vertebral column consists of a series of vertebrae held together to give support for the spinal cord and nerves arising from it
- Each vertebra consists of an anterior vertebral body and a posterior bony ring with two superior facets and two inferior facets that articulate with the neighboring vertebrae
- These articulations form the posterior facet joints that provide stability to the spine
- Spondylolysis is the most common cause of spondylolisthesis and is sometimes referred as isthmic spondylolisthesis, since the defect is in the isthmus.

Incidence

Sex

- Females are more prone to progressive displacement than males
- Congenital spondylolisthesis (dysplastic type) occurs with a 2:1 female-to-male ratio with symptoms beginning around the adolescent growth spurt
- Degenerative spondylolisthesis occurs more commonly in females with a 5:1 female-to-male ratio. The incidence increases after age of 40 years.

Age

- Acute isthmic spondylolysis occurs during the first and second decades of life
- Congenital spondylolisthesis usually manifests later in life

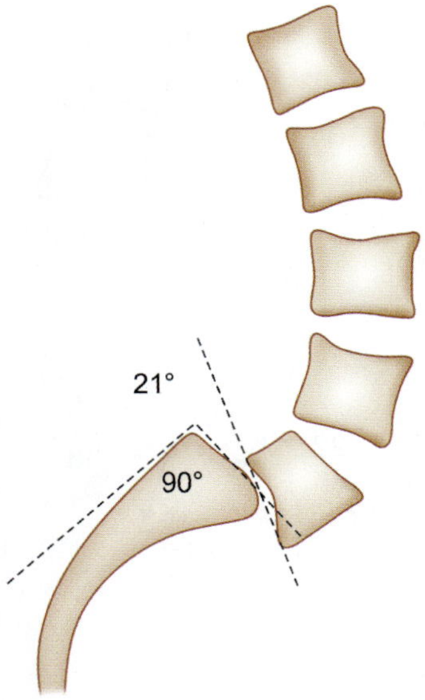

Fig. 27.215: Slip angle

- Degenerative spondylolisthesis occurs most commonly after the age of 40 years.

X-ray Classification (Fig. 27.215)

Severity of slip is estimated on the lateral view on X-ray and depends on the amount of contact left between the LF5 and S1 vertebral bodies:

- Grade 1 indicates more than 75 percent of contact
- Grade 2 indicates 50 to 75 percent of contact
- Grade 3 indicates 25 to 50 percent of contact
- Grade 4 indicates less than 25 percent of contact

Angular relationships are the best predictors of instability or progression of the deformity. Angle of slipping is formed by insertion of line drawn parallel to inferior aspect of L5 body and line drawn perpendicular to posterior aspect of body of S1 (Fig. 27.216).

Pathophysiology

- Facet joint in the lumbar spine is in the coronal plane
- Inferior articular process of the superior vertebra is located posteriorly
- Superior articular process of the inferior vertebra located anteriorly
- This configuration prevents forward movement of the vertebrae relative to each other.
- It locks in the superior vertebra relative to the inferior vertebra.

Importance of this anatomy is:

- The center of gravity of the human body is located anterior to the spine and exerts a forward slipping force on the spine, especially at the L5-S1 level

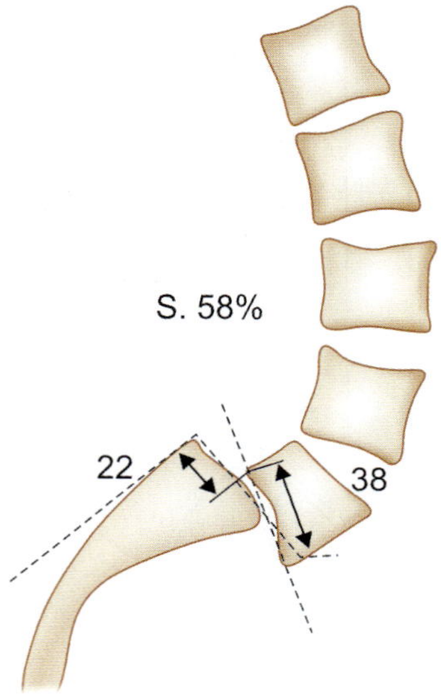

Fig. 27.216: Percentage of slip

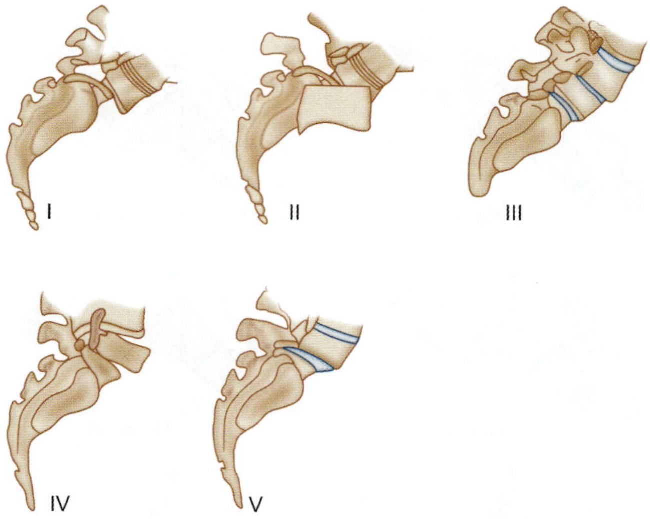

Fig. 27.217 (I-V): Types of spondylolisthesis—I. Dysplastic; II. Isthmic; III. Degenerative; IV. Post-traumatic; V. Pathological

- The anteriorly located center of gravity causes a rotating movement, with the axis of rotation oriented transversely at the L5-S1 level.

General Classification

- Congenital
- Isthmic
- Degenerative
- Traumatic
- Pathological
- Iatrogenic

Types of spondylolisthesis (Fig. 27.217)

Type I: Dysplastic

Type II: Isthmic

Type III: Degenerative

Type IV: Post-traumatic

Type V: Pathological

Type I: Dysplastic

- Congenital abnormalities of the upper sacral facets or inferior facets of the fifth lumbar vertebra that allow slipping of L5 or S1. There is no pars interarticularis defect in this type
- It refers to hypoplasia or indeed aplasia, of L5/S1 posterior facet joint, which does not allow slippage beyond 25 percent of the sagittal width of the spine
- A complete anterior dislocation (spondyloptosis) occurs when there is a period of attenuation of the pars intearticularis followed by the development of a frank secondary spondylosis.

Congenital

- Because it starts at birth or soon afterwards, there are a number of features which allow clear distinction of this category based upon plain radiographs or now with CT or MRI
- On the anteroposterior projection there is always a spina bifida occulta of L5 and a wide open sacrum
- In lateral projection, the upper border of the sacrum is rounded, indicating that the body of L5 has rolled round the top of the sacrum rather than simply having moved forward
- Accordingly, the inferior margin of L5 is reciprocally rounded and the L5 body is lordotically wedged
- It is the only true developmental type of spondylolisthesis, all others being acquired
- Congenital dysplastic spondylolisthesis (Fig. 27.218). On the right, the right pars has cracked through and the left has elongated but has remained intact. Note the spina bifida of lowermost lumbar vertebrae
- Lateral view (Fig. 27.219) is showing anterior displacement. The pars may stretch for years and then crack and come apart (Stress fracture).

Type II: Isthmic

- There is a defect in the pars interarticularis that allows forward slipping of L5 on S1. Three types of isthmic spondylolistheses are recognized:
  1. *Lytic:* A stress fracture of the pars interarticularis
  2. An elongated but intact pars interarticularis. Same as lytic type, except that fatigue microfracture presumably take place repeatedly, each healing and

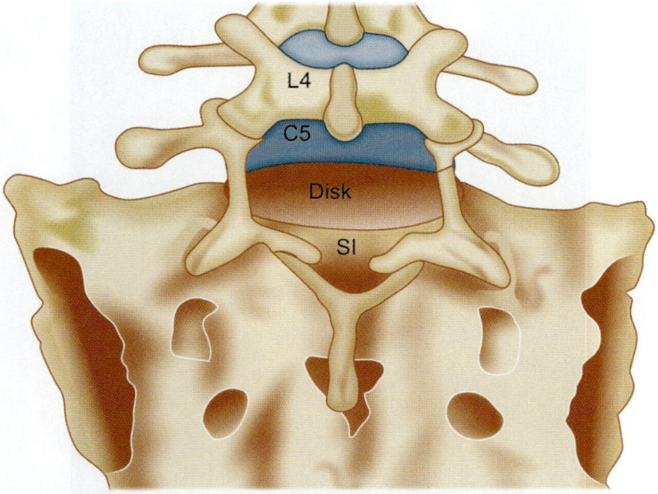

Fig. 27.218: AP view of developmental spondylolisthesis

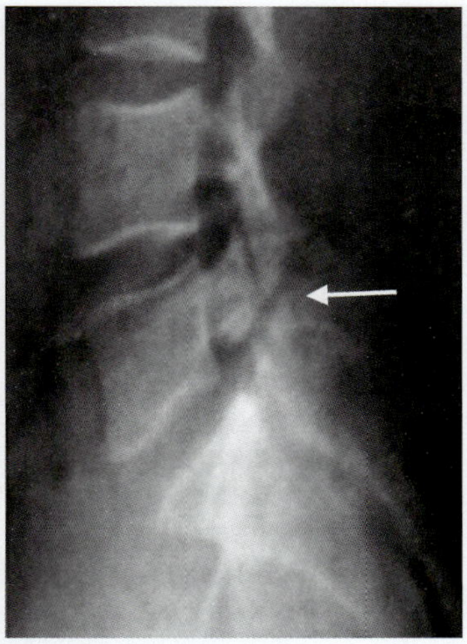

Fig. 27.220: Lateral view of isthmic

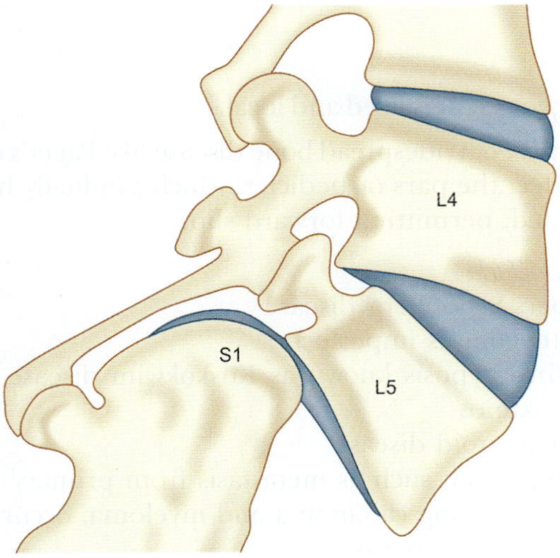

Fig. 27.219: Lateral view of developmental spondylolisthesis

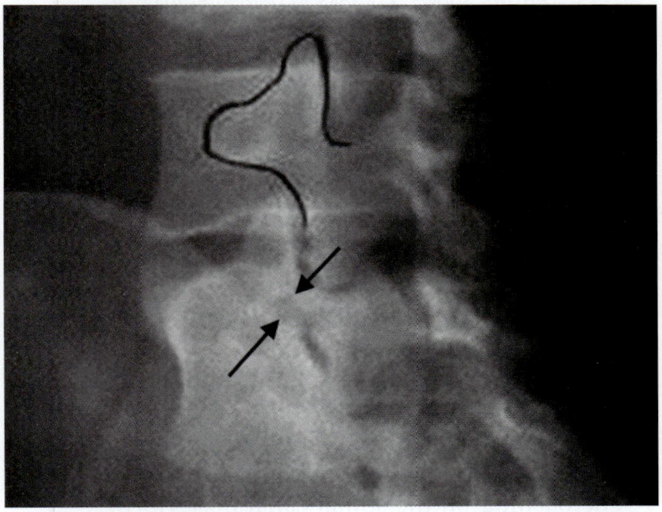

Fig. 27.221: X-ray showing isthmic type of spondylolisthesis with arrows showing decapitate sign (break in pars interarticularis)

contributing to progressive elongation of the pars as the vertebral body gradually displaces forward. There is strong hereditary component. The pars progressively thins out as it elongates and may remain in continuity or it may ultimately separate, leaving stumps of the pars and then recalcified as the lytic type

3. An acute fracture of the pars interarticularis always secondary to trauma. Most often the defect is not associated with slip and is termed spondylolysis. Infrequently, listhesis may develop heredity plays no part.

- The appearance of a Scottic dog with a collar will be outlined in the normal vertebra, with the pars defect (the collar) (Figs 27.220 to 27.222).

Type III: Degenerative

- This is a specific entity characterized by instability of paired zygapophyseal joints, which undergo progressive degeneration, permitting forward slipping of the cephalad vertebra
- It occurs most often at the L4-L5 level, infrequently at L3-L4 level and rarely at the lumbosacral level
- The degree of slip is limited and never exceeds 30 percent

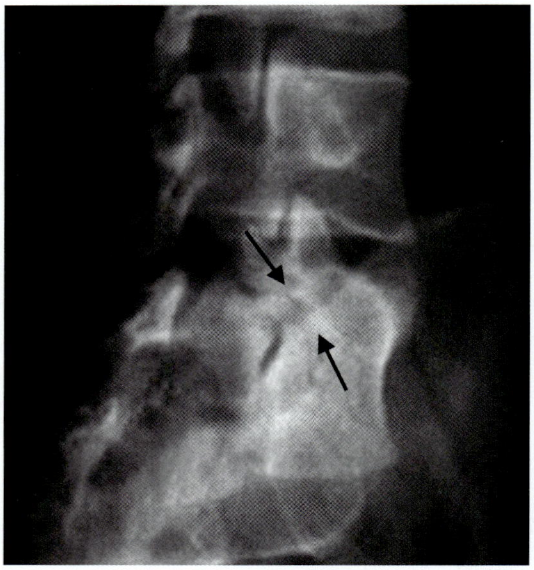

Fig. 27.222 X-ray showing isthmic type of spondylolisthesis with arrows showing breaks in pars interarticular

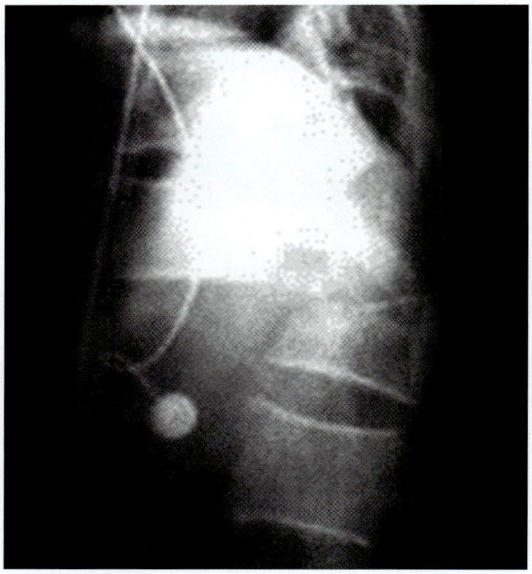

Fig. 27.223: Traumatic spondylolisthesis

- Women past the fifth decade are predisposed
- The superior articular process of subjacent vertebrae are progressively eroded over their posterior aspects but concomitantly develop hypertrophic bone anteriorly where they encroach on the lateral recesses of spinal canal
- The thick bone may compress a nerve root, which passes through lateral recess enroute to the neural foramen at the next level below
- As the articular process of the caudal vertebra are remolded and gradually come to lie in a forward position, the inferior articular processes of the cephalad vertebra are carried forward, its lamina encroaching on the spinal canal posteriorly
- The intervertebral foramina remain patent.

Type IV: Traumatic (Fig. 27.223)

This type results from fractures in the area of the bony hook other than the pars interarticularis, such as the pedicle, lamina or facet.

A gradual type of slippage can occur below a longstanding fusion of the spine.

This is referred to as 'spondylolisthesis acquisita' and belongs to the traumatic category.

Type V: Pathological

Because of local or generalized bone disease, the bone hook, which consists of the pars, pedicle and superior and, inferior articular processes, fails to withstand the forward thrust imposed by the superimposed by the superincumbent body weight and the vertebra slips forward.

Two types: Generalized and local.

Generalized: Widespread bone disease like Paget's disease may affect the pars or pedicles, which gradually become elongated, permitting forward slip.

Others include

- Albers-Schönberg disease
- Osteogenesis imperfecta
- Arthrogryposis known as Kuskokwim disease occurs in eskimos
- Rheumatoid disease
- Malignancy, such as metastasis from primary breast, prostate, lung carcinoma and myeloma, occur in the posterior elements
- Infections, such as blood-borne staphylococcal osteomyelitis, occurring in the posterior elements and may cause pathologic spondylolisthesis.

Local: This is an acquired form of spondylolysis or spodylolisthesis:

- Following an apparently successful lumbar spine fusion, the uppermost vertebra incorporated in the fusion mass may develop a defect through its pars
- This is considered a fatigue fracture, resulting from the stresses of movements (flexion and rotation) being transmitted to the end vertebra.

Clinical Features (Figs 27.224 to 27.226)

- Marked lordosis
- Lower back pain
- Localized tenderness over the spine just above the pelvis

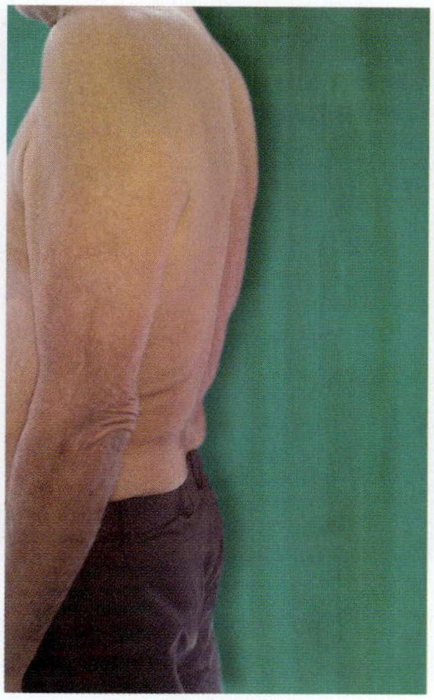

Fig. 27.224: Abdominal fold and marked lumbar lordosis

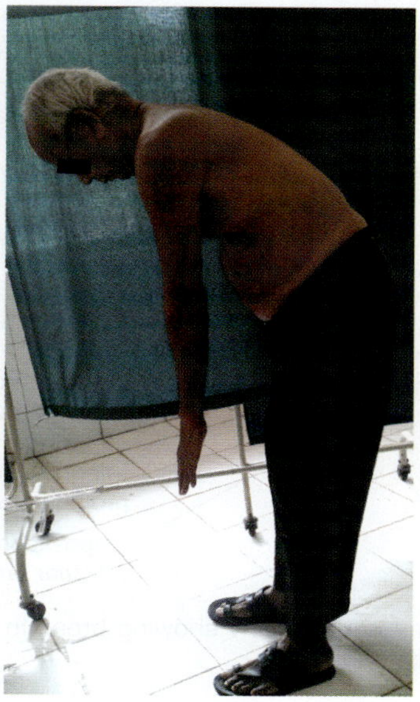

Fig. 27.225: Restriction of spine movements

- Pain in thighs
- Pain in buttocks
- Tight hamstrings
- Stiffness in back
- In advanced spondylolisthesis there is development of a waddling style of gait
- Because lumbosacral kyphosis the skin crease necessarily is anterior. Sideways view forward bending to show the very obvious lumbosacral kyphosis (Fig. 27.225)
- Note the flattening of the buttock, anterior protrusion of the pelvis, the visible lumbar slip off, and apparent shortening of the trunk. Displaying characteristic hamstring tightness, limiting his ability to touch his toes without flexing the knees (Fig. 27.226).

Mechanism of Pain

- Pain is the most common symptom of spondylolysis and spondylolisthesis
- Originates in area of lysis facet joint arthropathy
- Ligament sprain or strain
- Neural involvement
- Spinal canal narrowing and compressing cauda equina
- Radiculopathy due to inferior articular process of slipping vertebra impinging on nerve roots.

Investigations

- Lateral spine X-ray
- Anteroposterior spine X-ray
- Left and right oblique views
  - Plain radiographs may demonstrate congenital types and the changes of spondylosis
- In the trauma setting, fractures may be apparent

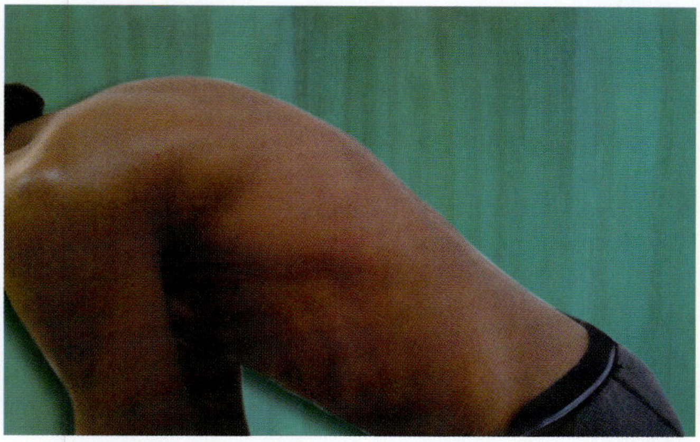

Fig. 27.226: Straightening of lumbar spine

- Other causes of the patient's symptoms may be demonstrated, such as an osteoid osteoma, Paget's disease and osteolytic lesions.

Importance of Lateral X-ray

- Classification based on lateral view
- Shows elongated pars
- Oblique views bilateral oblique view demonstrate "Scottie dog with collar" (Fig. 27.227).

Other Investigations

Role of CT Scan

- Demonstrate a horizontally oriented defect in the pars, which interrupts the normally complete bony ring of the posterior elements

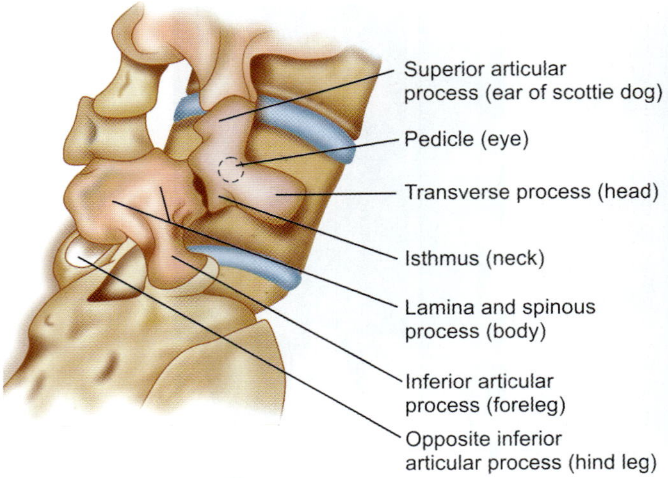

Fig. 27.227: X-ray oblique view showing break in the pars intra-articularis

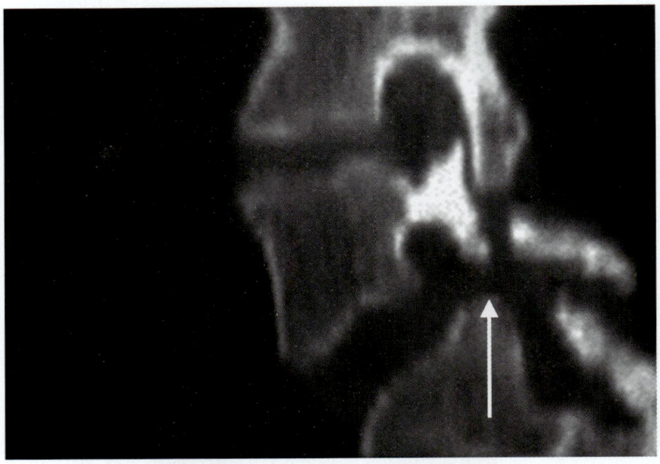

Fig. 27.228: CT scan showing acute spondylolisthesis

- Demonstrate findings of congenital/dysplastic and degenerative types of spondylolisthesis.

Other conditions such as:

- Disk disease
- Disk herniations
- Spondylosis and spinal canal stenosis
- Spina bifida
- Patients with radiculopathy, CT myelography can yield information regarding nerve-root impingement and its etiology, such as disk herniation, abscess or neoplasm
- A bone scan or SPECT scan is helpful in determining whether the process is acute or chronic (Figs 27.228 and 27.229).

Risk Factors for Progression of Spondylolisthesis

Clinical Risk Factors

- Growth years (9–15 years of age)
- Girls > boys
  - Episodes of back pain
  - Postural deformity or gait abnormality caused by hamstring spasm.

Roentgenographic Risk Factors

- Dysplastic (Type I) spondylolisthesis
- Dome-shaped, vertical sacrum
- Trapezoid-shaped L5 vertebral body
- 50 percent slip (Grades III and IV)
- Increasing slip angle
- Instability or excessive motion on flexion-extension views.

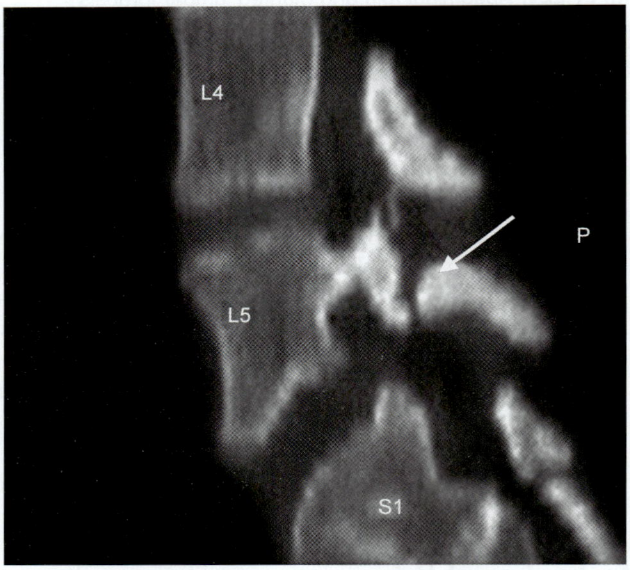

Fig. 27.229: CT scan showing chronic spondylolisthesis

Treatment

Aim of treatment is pain relief and increasing the patient's ability to function.

Nonoperative

- Bed rest
- No contact sports
- Restriction of vigorous activities
- Brace
- *Physiotherapy:* Back and abdominal muscle strengthening exercises
- Local heat and traction
- Injections of corticosteroids.

Operative Treatment

- For the repair of the defect
- Severe unremitting symptoms
- Neurological deficit develops
- Symptoms of instability
- Slip > 50 percent and progression of slippage.

Surgeries

- Decompression procedure (gill operation)
- Posterolateral fusion (Watkins). This is probably the best method that preserves much if supporting soft tissues, there is a high rate of fusion
- Posterolateral fusion (Wiltse)
- *Posterior fusion:* Postoperative additional slip is frequent until fusion is solid. There is high rate of pseudarthrosis. When posterior fusion must be done, intertransverse fusion must be added
- Laminectomy (removal of loose posterior element). Indicated only to relieve neurological deficit, laminectomy must be followed by an intertransverse fusion
- Anterior interbody fusion for subtotal olisthesis, the procedure is fraught with risk and of doubtful efficacy.

■ Spinal Canal Stenosis (Fig. 27.230)

Introduction

Spinal stenosis refers to narrowing of the spinal canal, nerve root canals or intervertebral foramina due to spondylosis and degenerative disk disease. There is decrease in sagittal diameter of the spinal canal. This process usually occurs in the cervical and lumbar spine; it seldom occurs in the thoracic spine (Figs 27.231 and 27.232).

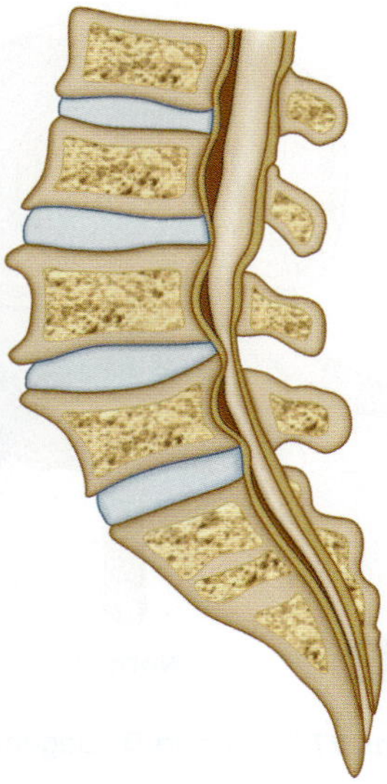

Fig. 27.230: Spinal canal stenosis

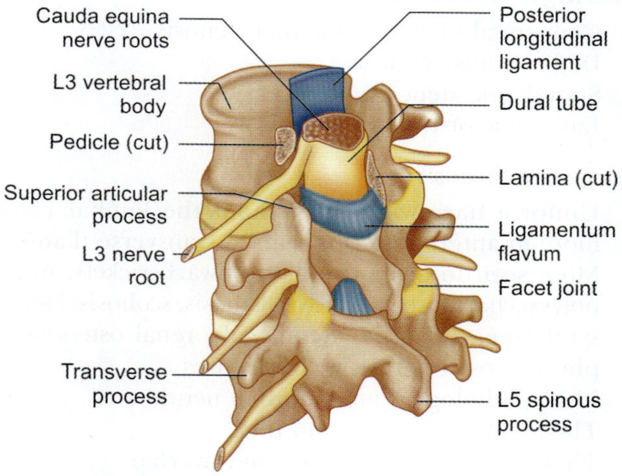

Fig. 27.231: Anatomy of lumbar spine

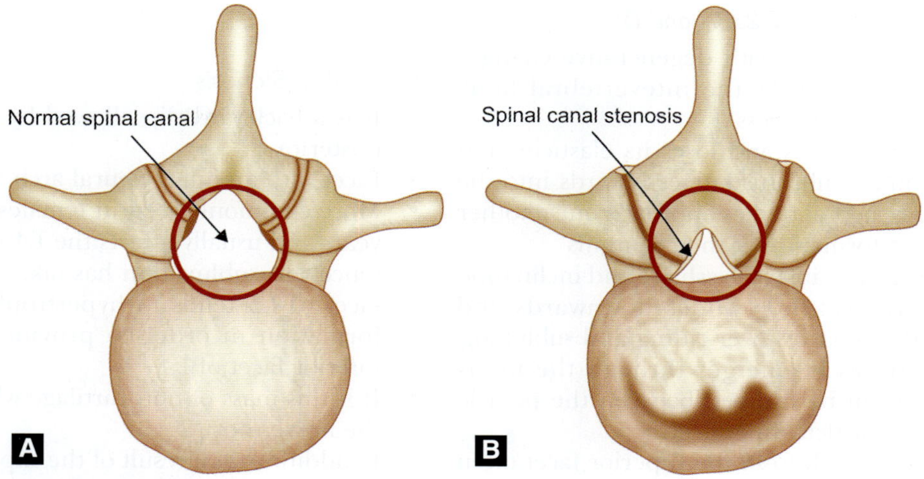

Figs 27.232A and B: Normal spinal canal

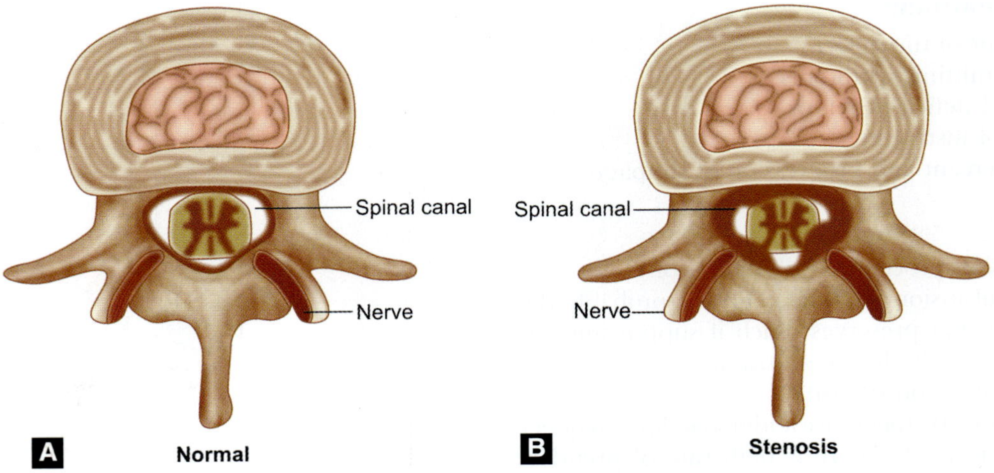

Figs 27.233A and B: Degenerative stenosis

Etiological Classification

- Congenital or developmental stenosis
- Degenerative stenosis
- Spondylitic stenosis
- Iatrogenic or traumatic stenosis

Congenital Stenosis

- Uniform narrowing throughout the lumbar canal, more in anteroposterior than in transverse diameter
- More seen in achondroplastic dwarf, rickets, mucopolysaccharidoses, spondylolisthesis, scoliosis, Down's syndrome, dysplasia, acromegaly, renal osteodystrophy and osteoporosis with fractures
- Main pathology is an abnormal neural arch
- The lamina are heavy and thick
- They may be for shortened and overlap
- In addition, they end in enlarged articulation at the facet.

Degenerative Stenosis (Figs 27.233A and B)

- Basically an arthropathy with degenerative changes which impinge on either the intevertebral bony foramen or the lateral recess
- As the disk degenerates and loses its elasticity and height, the annulus fibrosus bulges inwards into the canal and the vertebral bodies approach one another with osteophyte formation at their margins
- Because of the articular surface shape and inclination the upper vertebral body slides downwards and backwards with the facets over-riding and subluxing
- The nerve root, as it emerges through the intervertebral canal can be trapped between the pedicle and the superior articulating facet.
- Osteophytic outgrowth from the superior facet often adds to the compression.

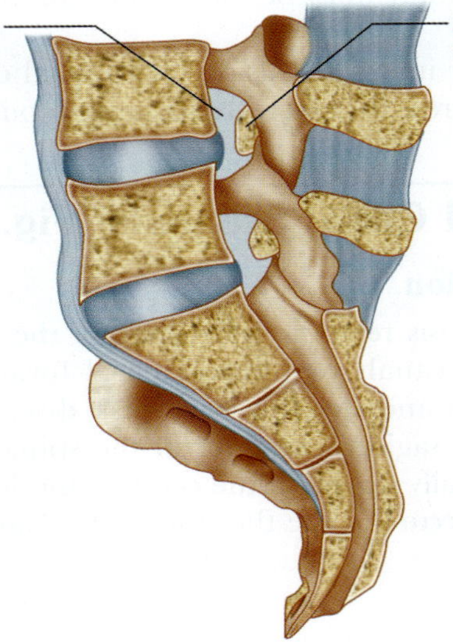

Fig. 27.234: Facet with an intact neural arch

Spondylitic Stenosis

- It is a backward slip allowed by a poorly developed posterior
- Facet with an intact neural arch (Fig. 27.234)
- More commonly seen in females after the age of 40 years and usually affects the L4-L5 level.
- Once this subluxation has taken place, the superior facet of L5 tends to hypertrophy with osteophytic formation in order to provide a support for the inferior facet of L4
- It is this mass of fibrocartilage which usually entraps the nerve root
- In addition, as a result of the slip there is a large step in the canal often resulting in marked stenosis.

Iatrogenic Stenosis

- Controversial whether results as a complication of spinal surgery
- It is unclear if this condition is due to say, hypertrophy of a posterior bone graft or to incomplete treatment of the stenotic condition with a recurrence of the original symptoms
- Most common stenosis is due to an infolding of the ligamentum flavum just superior to the fusion mass in association with a disk herniation.

Anatomical Classification

There are two types: Central and lateral recess.

1. Central canal stenosis, commonly occurring at an intervertebral disk level, defines midline sagittal spinal canal diameter narrowing that may elicit neurogenic claudication (NC) or pain in the buttock, thigh or leg. Such stenosis results from ligamentum flavum hypertrophy, inferior articulating process (IAP), facet hypertrophy of the cephalad vertebra, vertebral body osteophytosis and herniated nucleus pulposus (HNP)
2. Lateral recess stenosis (i.e. lateral gutter stenosis, subarticular stenosis, subpedicular stenosis, foraminal canal stenosis, intervertebral foramen stenosis) is defined as narrowing (less than 3 to 4 mm) between the facet superior articulating process (SAP) and posterior vertebral margin. Such narrowing may impinge the nerve root and subsequently elicit radicular pain. This lateral region is compartmentalized into entrance zone, midzone, exit zone and far-out stenosis.

Lateral Recess Stenosis

- The entrance zone lies medial to the pedicle and sap, and, consequently, arises from facet joint sap hypertrophy. Other causes include developmentally short pedicle and facet joint morphology, as well as osteophytosis and HNP anterior to the nerve root. The lumbar nerve root compressed below SAP retains the same segmental number as the involved vertebral level (e.g. L5 nerve root is impinged by L5 SAP).
- The mid zone extends from the medial to the lateral pedicle edge. Mid-zone stenosis arises from osteophytosis under the pars interarticularis and bursal or fibrocartilaginous hypertrophy at a spondylolytic defect
- Exit-zone stenosis involves an area surrounding the foramen and arises from facet joint hypertrophy and subluxation, as well as superior disk margin osteophytosis
- Far-out (extracanalicular) stenosis entails compression lateral to the exit zone. Such compression occurs with far lateral vertebral body end-plate osteophytosis and when the sacral ala and L5 transverse process impinge on the L5 spinal nerve.

Pathophysiology

- Intervertebral disks lose hydration and elasticity with age, and these losses lead to cracks and fissures. The surrounding ligaments also lose their elastic properties and develop traction spurs the disk subsequently collapses as a result of biomechanical incompetence, causing the annulus to bulge outward. As the disk space narrows, the annulus bulges and the facets override. This change, in turn, increases motion at that spinal segment and further hastens the damage to the disk. This process can cause tilting, slippage or rotation of vertebral bodies.
- Disk desiccation and degenerative disk disease (DDD) with resulting loss of disk height may induce segmental instability such instability incites vertebral body and facet joint hypertrophy. Inferior articular process (IAP) hypertrophy and promotes central spinal canal stenosis (Fig. 27.235).
- The ligamentum flavum also ossifies and becomes hypertrophic. The compressed disks result in shortening of the spinal column, which causes the ligamentum flavum to buckle inward and compress the spinal sac and nerve roots
- The spine responds to physiological stresses with bone growth at the superior and inferior margins of the vertebral body (osteophytes)
- Osteophytes can form anteriorly or posteriorly. Posterior osteophytes narrow the intraspinal diameter and also cause lateral recess stenosis. This results in spinal cord or nerve root impingement. Furthermore, arthritic degeneration causes formation of synovial cysts and hypertrophy of the facet joints, which further compromise the patency of the spinal canal and the neural foramina.

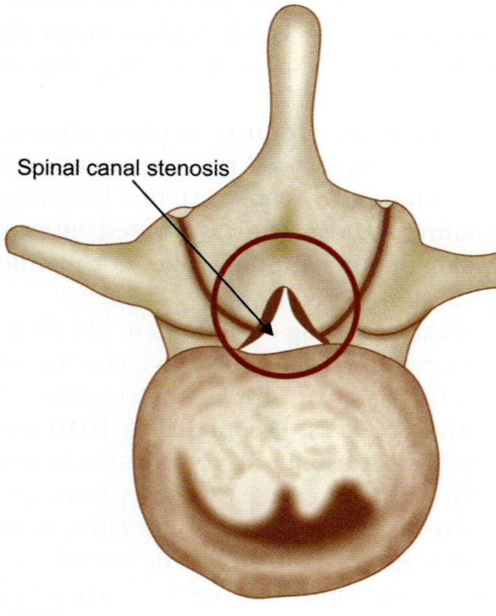

Fig. 27.235: Central spinal canal stenosis

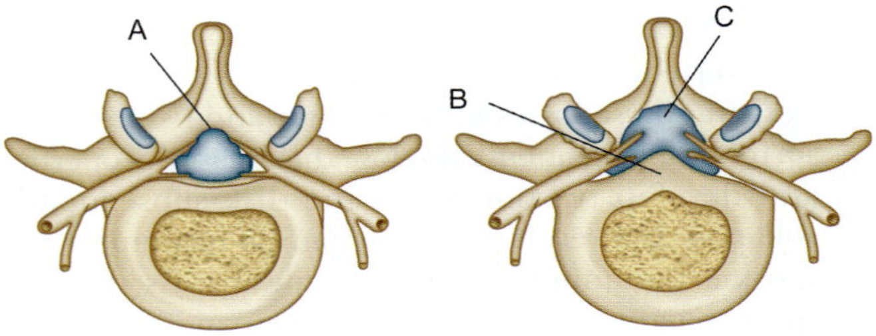

Fig. 27.236: A. Canal volume loss; B. Herniated nucleosus pulposus; C. Hypertrophied ligamentum flavum

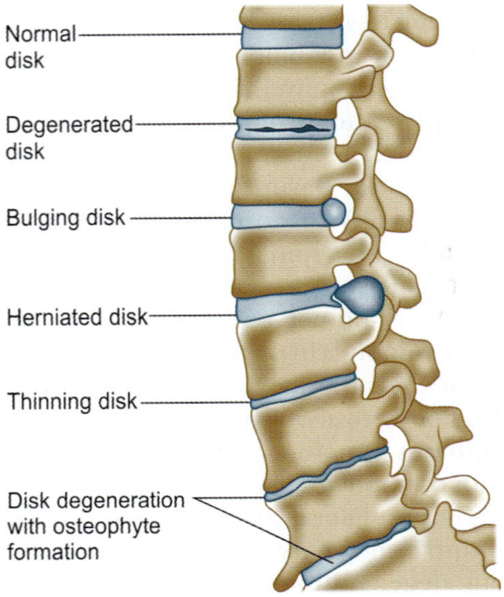

Fig. 27.237: Examples of disk problem

- Further canal volume loss results from herniated nucleosus pulposus. HNP, ligamentum flavum hypertrophy and disk space narrowing (Figs 27.236 to 27.239)
- Dynamic foraminal stenosis implies intermittent lumbar extension-provoked nerve root impingement from HNP, osteophytosis and vertebral body slippage. Such dynamic stenosis with associated intermittent position-dependent symptoms may not manifest on imaging studies.
- Other factors promoting development of LSS include shortened gestational age and synovial facet joint cysts with resulting radicular compression. Adult degenerative scoliosis, secondary to DDD-induced instability with subsequent vertebral rotation and asymmetric disk space narrowing, promotes facet hypertrophy and subluxation in the curve concavity. Degenerative spondylolisthesis, when combined with facet hypertrophy, causes both central canal and lateral recess stenosis.

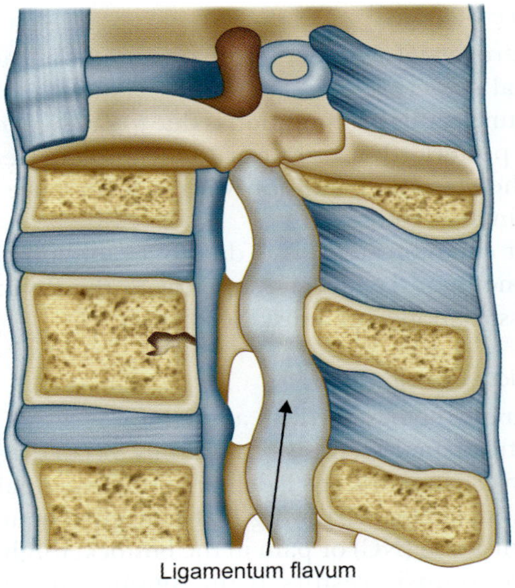

Fig. 27.238: Ligamentum flavum hypertrophy

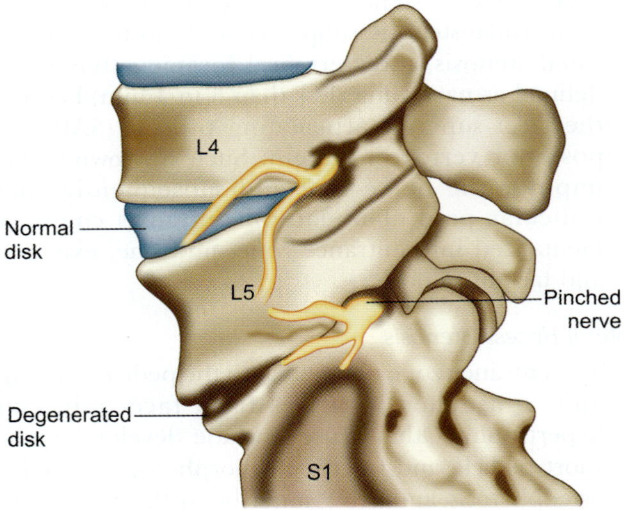

Fig. 27.239: Collapse of intervertebral space causing pinching of the nerve

■ Lumbar Canal Stenosis (See Figs 27.230 and Fig. 27.240)

History

- Lumbar canal stenosis (LCS) classically presents as bilateral neurogenic claudication (NC) (pain, weakness, numbness in the legs while walking or a combination thereof)
- Unilateral radicular symptoms may result from severe foraminal or lateral recess stenosis. Patients, typically aged more than 50 years, report insidious-onset with

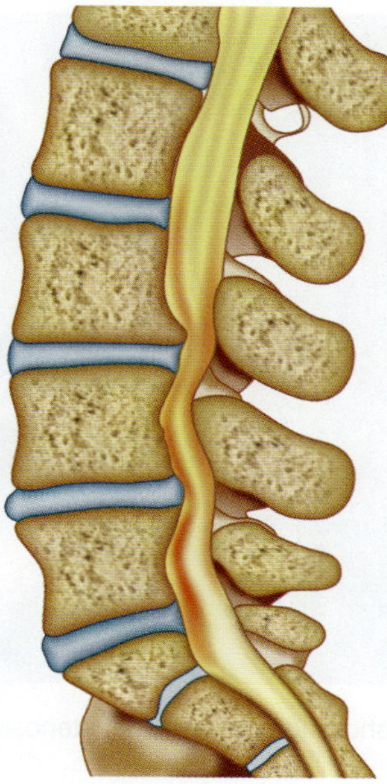

Fig. 27.240: Lumbar stenosis

NC manifesting as intermittent, crampy, diffuse radiating thigh or leg pain with associated paresthesis. Indeed, leg pain affects 90 percent of patients with LSS

- NC pain is exacerbated by standing erect and downhill ambulation and is alleviated with lying supine more than prone, sitting, squatting and lumbar flexion. Eighty percent pain diminution with sitting and 75 percent with forward bending
- Lumbar spinal canal and lateral recess cross-sectional area increases with spinal flexion and decreases with extension
- Furthermore, cross-sectional area is reduced 9 percent with extension in the normal spine and 67 percent with severe stenosis. The penning rule of progressive narrowing implies that the more narrowed the canal by stenosis, the more it narrows with spinal extension.

Neurogenic Claudication

- NC, unlike vascular claudication, is not exacerbated with biking, uphill ambulation and lumbar flexion and is not alleviated with standing
- LSS patients compensate for symptoms by flexing forward, slowing their gait, leaning onto objects and limiting distance of ambulation. Unfortunately, such compensatory measures, particularly in elderly osteoporotic females, promote disease progression and vertebral fracture.
- Pain radiates downward in NC and in contrast, upward in vascular claudication
- Proposed mechanisms for development of NC include cauda equina microvascular ischemia, venous congestion, axonal injury and intraneural fibrosis
- Ambulation-provoked cauda equina blood vessel dilation with subsequent circulatory stagnation in LCS patients with NC. They propose that ambulation dilates the epidural venous plexus, which, amidst narrow spinal canal diameter, increases epidural and intrathecal pressure. Such elevation of pressure ultimately compresses the cauda equina, compromises its microcirculation, and causes pain.
- Another pain generator may be the dorsal root ganglion (DRG), which contains pain-mediating neuropeptides, such as substance p, that possibly increase with mechanical compression
- Lastly, severe radiologic stenosis in otherwise asymptomatic individuals suggests inflammation, not just mechanical nerve root compression. Specific inflammation generators may include HNP, ligamentum flavum and facet joint capsule.

Physical Examination

- Physical examination findings frequently are normal in patients with LCS. Nevertheless, review of the literature suggests diminished lumbar extension appears most consistently, varies less and constitutes the most significant finding in LCS.
- Other positive findings include loss of lumbar lordosis and forward-flexed gait
- Radiculopathy may be noted with motor, sensory and/or reflex abnormalities. Asymmetric muscle stretch reflexes and focal myotomal weakness with atrophy occur more with lateral recess than central canal stenosis.
- Some report objective neurologic deficits in approximately 50 percent of LCS cases. Provocative maneuvers include pain reproduction with ambulation and prone lumbar hyperextension. Pain alleviation occurs with stationary biking and lumbar flexion.
- Katz and colleagues report physical examination findings most strongly associated with LCS include wide-based gait, abnormal Romberg Test, thigh pain following 30 seconds of lumbar extension and neuromuscular abnormalities; however, Fritz and colleagues state physical examination findings do not seem helpful in determining the presence or absence of LCS.
- Negative findings in the physical examination include skin color, turgor and temperature; normal distal lower extremity pulses; absence of arterial bruits and unremarkable dural tension signs. Lumbar segment mobilization often fails to reproduce pain and palpation locates no trigger points.

Differentials

- Chronic pain syndrome, diabetic lumbosacral plexopathy
- Radiation-induced lumbosacral plexopathy
- Diabetic neuropathy
- Fibromyalgia lumbar compression fracture lumbar spondylolysis and spondylolisthesis mechanical low back pain osteoarthritis, osteoporosis, rheumatoid arthritis, trochanteric bursitis

Other Problems

- Rheumatologic ankylosing spondylitis/spondyloarthropathy diffuse idiopathic skeletal hyperostosis (DISH). Infectious epidural, subdural, intradural abscess discitis metabolic osteomalacia parathyroid disease vitamin B_{12} or folic acid deficiency
- Developmental/congenital scoliosis vascular peripheral vascular disease (with vascular claudication) abdominal aortic dissection
- Psycogenic conversion disorder malingering
- Imaging studies.

Plain Radiograph (X-ray)

- Disk space narrowing
- Facet hypertrophy and arthrosis
- Spondylosis
- Degenerative scoliosis and spondylolisthesis
- Osteochondrosis
- Transitional segmentation
- Spinous process settling
- Shortened interpedicular distance
  - Interpedicular distance is considered subnormal if distance is less than 18 mm, commonly increases from upper to lower lumbar segments
  - Some sources define pure absolute central canal stenosis as a midsagittal canal diameter of less than or equal to 10 mm, pure relative at 10 to 12 mm. Midsagittal canal diameter less than 15 mm and transverse diameter less than 20 mm usually are considered abnormal
  - Posterior disk height of 4 mm or less and foraminal height of 15 mm or less may suggest foraminal stenosis; nevertheless, clinical correlation is required. No convincing correlation has been found between clinical symptoms and radiologic findings.

CT Scan

- CT scan provides excellent central canal, lateral recess and neuroforaminal visualization. Additionally, CT scan offers contrasts between intervertebral disk, ligamentum flavum and thecal sac. Unfortunately, CT scan, like MRI, yields a high false-positive rate [35.4% when correlated with surgically proven lumbar spinal stenesis (LSS)].

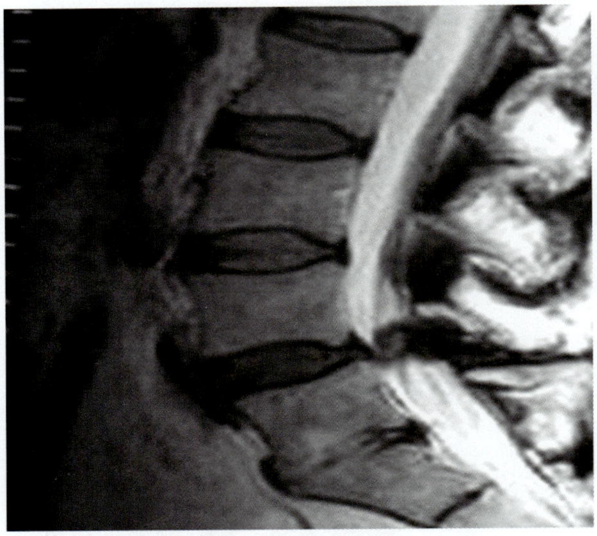

Fig. 27.241: MRI showing lumbar spinal stenosis

- Parasagittal reconstructed CT scan findings suggesting stenosis include posterolateral vertebral body or facet osteophytosis extending into the foramen.

Imaging Studies

1. *MRI* remains the imaging modality of choice for LSS.
   - Advantages include nonionizing radiation and superior multiplanar soft tissue visualization without osseous artifact. (Fig. 27.241)
   - Sagittal T1-imaged adipose tissue outlines neuroforaminal nerve root segments and dorsal root ganglia. Therefore, parasagittal MRI findings suggesting foraminal stenosis include paucity of T1-weighted perineural adipose tissue surrounding the nerve root and diminished foraminal size. Unfortunately, MRI abnormalities have been documented in 20 percent of asymptomatic subjects (Fig. 27.242).
2. *Myelography*: This test effectively documents central canal stenosis and remains superior in evaluating lumbar disk herniation. Predictive value of myelography versus CT scan has been reported as 83 percent versus 72 percent, respectively, for lumbar disk herniation and 93 percent versus 89 percent for LCS. Furthermore, myelography images the entire lumbar spinal canal and enhances stenotic segments due to hyperextension during imaging; however, it may miss lateral stenosis and HNP because the dural sac terminates at the lateral mid zone, preventing contrast spread to the distal nerve root sheath.
   - Myelography is less sensitive and specific than CT scan or MRI
   - Procedural complications include spinal headache, seizure, allergic reaction and nausea.

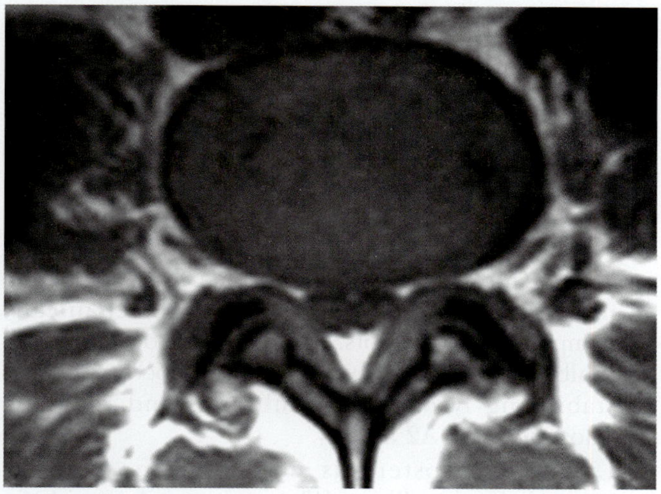

Fig. 27.242: MRI showing abnormality in 20% of asymptomatic subjects

3. *Electrodiagnosis (EDX)*
   Needle electromyography (EMG)
   Nerve conduction studies (NCS)
   Somatosensory evoked potentials (SSEP), evaluates nerve root and peripheral nerve function
4. *Needle electromyography* (EMG)
   - Needle EMG diagnoses lumbosacral radiculopathy by detecting increased insertional activity, spontaneous potentials (e.g. positive waves, fibrillations, fasciculations, chronic repetitive discharges), and decreased motor unit recruitment in paraspinal and lower extremity muscles innervated by the same nerve root
   - Limitations include inability to evaluate sensory and upper motor neurons
   - Multisegmental muscle innervation may cause false negative results by preserving motor unit function despite nerve root compromise. Such innervation may elicit multilevel abnormalities in severe lumbar spinal stenosis (LSS).
5. *EMG and NCS*
   - Nerve conduction studies (NCS) differentiates LCS from other confounding neuropathic conditions such as lumbosacral plexopathy, generalized peripheral neuropathy, and mononeuropathy (e.g. peroneal neuropathy at the fibular head, tarsal tunnel syndrome).
   - Canal stenosis may compress the cauda equina with resulting polyradicular insults. Such multiple lumbosacral radiculopathies, involving lower lumbosacral (especially S1) nerve roots, are often bilateral and asymmetric, and frequently may manifest NCS abnormalities. Such abnormalities include decreased or unelicitable posterior tibial and peroneal compound motor action potentials (CMAPs) reflecting axon loss, and unobtainable reflexes signifying bilateral S1 compression. Sensory nerve action potentials (SNAPs) remain unaffected (unless impingement occurs distal to the dorsal root ganglion), but may not be detectable in older persons.
   - Diagnostically, EMG complements MRI in assessing radiculopathy. Specifically, EMG rarely presents false-positive results and carries high specificity (85%). Conversely, MRI carries high sensitivity and poor specificity (50%) and consequently, demonstrates many false-positive asymptomatic abnormalities. Some advocate using highly specific EMG to determine whether structural abnormalities imaged on MRI carry functional and pathologic significance. Indeed, Robinson proposes that such use of needle EMG ultimately might prove helpful in avoiding costly and high-risk invasive interventions.

Histological Findings

- Thinning and fragmentation of the articular cartilage may be observed. The normal, smooth, white articular surface becomes irregular and yellow
- Continued loss of articular cartilage leads to exposure of areas of subchondral bone, which appears as shiny foci on the articular surface (eburnation). Fibrosis, increased bone formation and cystic changes frequently occur in the underlying bone.
- Loss of articular cartilage stimulates new bone formation, usually in the form of nodules (osteophytes) at the bone edges.

Treatment

- *Physical therapy:* Patients with LCS often benefit from conservative treatment and participation in a physical therapy (PT) program
- Lumbar extension exercises should be avoided in this population, as spinal extension and increased lumbar lordosis are known to worsen LSS
- Flexion exercises for the lumbar spine should be emphasized, as they reduce lumbar lordosis and decrease stress on the spine. Spinal flexion exercises increase the spinal canal dimension, thus reducing NC. William's flexion-biased exercises target increased lumbar lordosis, paraspinal and hamstring inflexibility and, abdominal muscle weakness. These exercises incorporate knee-to-chest maneuvers, pelvic tilts, wall-standing lumbar flexion and avoidance of lumbar extension.
- Others advocate stationary cycling and abdominal muscle strengthening. Passive modalities such as heat, cold, transcutaneous electrical nerve stimulation (TENS) and ultrasound may provide transient analgesia and increased soft tissue flexibility in LSS patients.

Medical Complications

In rare cases, central canal stenosis may provoke cauda equina syndrome with associated saddle anesthesia, bladder and/or bowel dysfunction and altered muscle reflexes. Additionally, patients with lateral recess stenosis-induced radiculopathy may manifest significant lower limb weakness or numbness. Lastly, intractable axial, radicular or neurogenic claudication pain may result.

Surgical Intervention

- LCS remains one of the most common conditions leading to lumbar spine surgery in adults aged 65 years and older
- Increasing rates of LCS surgery among the medicare population has been shown to be due possibly to imaging techniques that enable physicians to diagnose LCS more frequently
- Other contributing factors may include improved surgical techniques that might allow patients previously managed conservatively to undergo surgery, as well as a philosophy that LSS surgery prevents future morbidity
- Widely agreed upon indications for LCS surgery do not exist. Typically, patients undergo elective surgery to improve walking tolerance and disabling leg and back pain. Preoperatively, such disability infrequently is measured in objective quantitative terms. Surgical emergencies (e.g. cauda equina syndrome, rapid neurologic deterioration) rarely arise
- Surgical techniques include standard wide laminectomy and decompression, which first removes lamina and ligamentum flavum from the lateral borders of one lateral recess to the other and then decompresses entrapped nerve roots
- Foraminal enlargement surgery is used to address refractory foraminal stenosis-induced radicular pain. Other surgical decompressions include the following:
  - Laminotomy
  - Medial facetectomy
  - Medial or lateral foraminotomy.
- The Wiltse approach with foraminotomy is used for isolated foraminal stenosis by providing:
  - Widening the longissimus-multifidus muscle interval
  - Removing the lateral pars interarticularis and facet joint
  - Exposing the nerve root with subsequent decompression
- In addition to decompression and foraminal enlargement, some patients with segmental instability from facet joint removal and pain secondary to DDD may require fusion.
  - Fusion stabilizes the intervertebral segment while maintaining lordosis and foraminal size
  - Additional options include arthrodesis and instrumentation

Other Treatment

- Epidural steroid injection (ESI) provides aggressive-conservative treatment for LCS patients who demonstrate limited response to oral medication, physical therapy and other noninvasive measures
- Corticosteroids may inhibit edema formation from microvascular injury sustained by mechanically compressed nerve roots. Furthermore, corticosteroids inhibit inflammation by impairing leukocyte function, stabilizing lysosomal membranes and reducing phospholipase A2 activity.
- Lastly, corticosteroids may block nociceptive transmission in c fibers. When using oral steroids (in rapid tapering fashion), possible side effects may include fluid retention, skin flushing and shakiness.
- Local anesthetic may be combined with corticosteroids to provide immediate pain relief and diagnostic feedback on the proximity of the injectate to the putative pain generator.

Complications

- Serious complications, although rare, include infection (e.g. epidural or subdural abscess) and epidural hematoma
- Dural puncture (in 5% of lumbar interlaminar esis and 0.6% of caudal injections) with possible subsequent subarachnoid anesthetic/corticosteroid deposition may provoke neurotoxicity, sympathetic blockade with hypotension, and/or spinal headache; however, contrast-enhanced fluoroscopic guidance minimizes the possibility of dural puncture and intravascular injection
- Transient corticosteroid dose-related side effects include facial flushing, low-grade fever, insomnia, anxiety, agitation, hyperglycemia and fluid retention. Steroids may suppress the hypothalamic-pituitary axis for 3 months following the injection. Lastly, vasovagal reaction, nerve root injury, injectate allergy and temporary pain exacerbation can occur as well.

Precautions

- Anticoagulation therapy (e.g. warfarin, heparin) should be stopped a few days prior to injection. (Alternative methods of DVT prophylaxis, such as serial compression hose, should be instituted in the interim).
- Aspirin and other nonsteroidal anti-inflammatory drugs (NSAIDs) should be discontinued before the procedure in accordance with their half-life and hematologic profile.

■ Cervical Canal Stenosis (Figs 27.243 and 27.244)

Causes

Age

- Cervical spondylosis is a disease observed most commonly in elderly individuals
- Among those younger than 40 years, 25 percent have degenerative disk disease (DDD) and 4 percent have foraminal stenosis, as confirmed with MRI
- In those older than 40 years, almost 60 percent have DDD and 20 percent have foraminal stenosis, as confirmed with MRI.

Trauma

- The role of trauma in spondylosis is controversial
- Repetitive subclinical trauma probably influences the onset and rate of progression of spondylosis.

Work Activity

Cervical spondylosis is significantly higher in patients who carry loads on their head than in those who do not.

Genetics

- The role of genetics is unclear
- Patients older than 50 years who had normal cervical spine radiographic findings are significantly more likely to have a sibling with normal or mildly abnormal radiographic results

Incidence

Race: No apparent correlation between race and cervical spondylosis exists.

Sex: Both sexes are affected equally. Cervical spondylosis usually starts earlier in men than in women.

Age: Symptoms of cervical spondylosis may appear in those as young as 30 years and are most commonly in those aged 40 to 60 years. Radiological spondylotic changes increase with patient age, as 70 percent of asymptomatic persons older than 70 years have degenerative cervical spine changes in one form or another. Cervical spondylosis usually starts earlier in men than in women.

When cervical spondylosis develops in a young individual, it is almost always secondary to a predisposing abnormality in one of the joints between the cervical vertebrae, probably as the result of previous mild trauma.

Clinical History

Common clinical syndromes associated with cervical spondylosis include the following:

Cervical Pain

Intermittent neck and shoulder pain (cervicalgia) is the most common syndrome in clinical practice. This is a frustrating problem for physicians and patients, as often no associated neurologic signs are present.

Neck pain experienced with cervical spondylosis often is accompanied by stiffness, with radiation into the shoulders or occiput. It may be chronic or episodic, with long periods of remission.

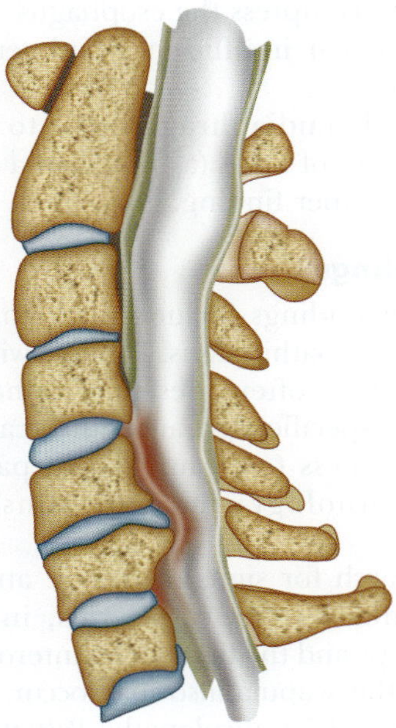

Fig. 27.243: Cervical spinal stenosis

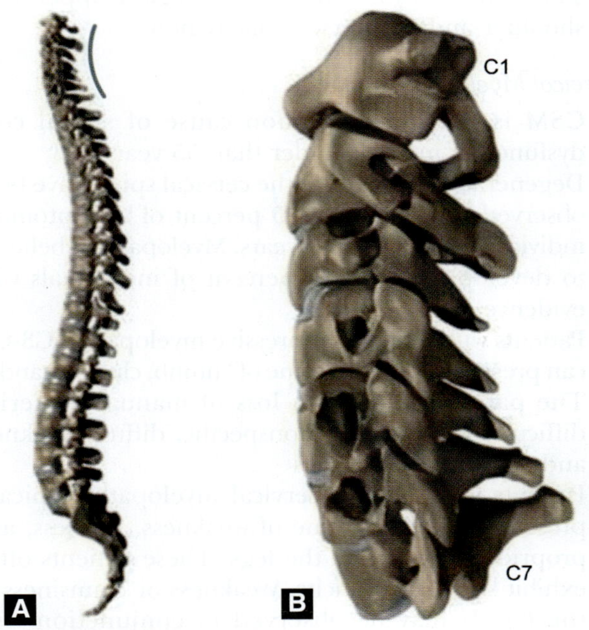

Figs 27.244A and B: Cervical spine

One-third of patients with cervicalgia from cervical spondylosis present with headache and over two-thirds present with unilateral or bilateral shoulder pain. A significant amount of these patients also present with arm, forearm and/or hand pain.

Cervical Radiculopathy

- Compression of the cervical nerve roots leads to ischemic changes that cause sensory dysfunction (e.g. radicular pain) and/or motor dysfunction (e.g. weakness). Radiculopathy most commonly occurs in those aged 40 to 50 years.
- An acute herniated disk or chronic spondylotic changes can cause cervical radiculopathy and/or myelopathy
- The most commonly involved nerve roots are the sixth and seventh cervical nerve roots, caused by C5-6 or C6-7 spondylosis, respectively. Patients usually present with pain, paresthesias, weakness or a combination of these symptoms
- The most commonly disk degeneration and collapses, leading to spur formation occurs at C5-6 and C6-7. A relative decrease in spinal motion occurs at these levels with a concomitant increase in spinal motion at C3-4 and C4-5.
- The resultant degeneration and abnormal motion lead to instability with anterolisthesis or retrolisthesis (subluxation of vertebral bodies out of the normal cervical alignment). Therefore, the cord tends to be compressed from spur formation at C5-6 and C6-7 and compressed from listhesis at C3-4 and C4-5. Often, this is accompanied by posterior canal compromise from ligamentum flavum hypertrophy.
- The pain usually is in the cervical region, upper limb, shoulder and/or interscapular region.

Cervical Myelopathy

- CSM is the most common cause of spinal cord dysfunction in adults older than 55 years
- Degenerative changes of the cervical spine have been observed in as many as 95 percent of asymptomatic individuals older than 65 years. Myelopathy is believed to develop in up to 20 percent of individuals with evidence of spondylosis
- Patients with a high compressive myelopathy (C3-C5) can present with a syndrome of "numb, clumsy hands." The patient describes a loss of manual dexterity; difficulty with writing; nonspecific, diffuse weakness and abnormal sensations
- Patients with a lower cervical myelopathy typically present with a syndrome of weakness, stiffness, and proprioceptive loss in the legs. These patients often exhibit signs of spasticity. Weakness or clumsiness of the hands may be observed in conjunction with weakness in the legs. Motor loss in the hands with relative sparing of the legs is a relatively rare syndrome.

Central Cord Syndrome

- An important cause of acute myelopathy that may be related to cervical spondylosis is central cord syndrome
- This syndrome typically occurs when an elderly patient experiences an acute hyperextension injury with pre-existing, acquired stenosis due to ventral osteophytes and infolding of redundant ligamentum flavum, resulting in acute cord compression.
- Patients usually present with a history of a blow to the forehead
- The syndrome consists of upper extremity weakness greater than lower extremity weakness, varying degrees of sensory disturbances below the lesion and myelopathic findings (e.g, spasticity, urinary retention).

Clinical Examination

- In CSM, the most typical examination findings are suggestive of upper motor dysfunction, including hyperactive deep tendon reflexes, ankle and/or patellar clonus, spasticity (especially of the lower extremities), Babinski sign and Hoffman sign.
- Less common manifestations:
  - Primary sensory loss may be present in a glove-like distribution
  - Tandem spinal stenosis is a simultaneous cervical and lumbar stenosis due to spondylosis. It is a triad of findings; neurogenic claudication, complex gait abnormality and a mixed pattern of upper and lower motor neuron signs
  - Dysphagia may be present if the spurs are large enough to compress the esophagus
  - Vertebrobasilar insufficiency and vertigo may be observed
  - Elevated hemidiaphragm, due to spondylotic compression of C3-4 (as noted in a case report), may be another finding.

Physical Findings

- Examination findings include neck pain, radicular signs and myelopathic signs. Patients with neck pain from spondylosis often present with neck stiffness. This is a nonspecific sign and other causes of neck pain and stiffness (e.g., myofascial pain, intrinsic shoulder pathology) must be considered and excluded.
- Carefully search for signs of muscle atrophy in the following muscles; supraspinatus, infraspinatus, deltoid, triceps and the first dorsal interosseus muscle
- Winging of the scapula also may occur, since it may occur with C6 or C7 radiculopathy. Palpate all muscles, since this may allow earlier detection of wasting than

visualization. Detecting weakness in either one myotomal distribution or 2 to 3 peripheral nerves likely excludes peripheral nerve injury as the cause. Muscle testing is important because muscle findings have more specificity than sensory or reflex findings.

- Perform a detailed sensory and reflex examination. Note that radicular findings often do not adhere strictly to textbook's dermatomal charts. Patients often experience more pain proximally in their limbs, while paresthesias dominate distally.

Spurling Test or Sign

The neck compression test (Spurling test or sign), if positive, is useful when assessing a patient for cervical radiculopathy.

This test is best performed by having the patient actively extend his or her neck, laterally flex and rotate to the side of the pain while sitting. Next, use careful compression by slight axial loading. This maneuver works by narrowing the ipsilateral neural foramina during flexion and rotation, while the initial extension causes posterior disk bulging.

While this maneuver has a low sensitivity for cervical radiculopathy, it has a specificity of nearly 100 percent. Other useful tests are the axial manual traction test and the shoulder abduction test.

Hoffman Sign

Hoffman sign is a reflex contraction of the thumb and index finger after nipping the middle finger. Although this sign usually is present with corticospinal tract dysfunction, unlike the Babinski sign, it also can be present in generalized hyper-reflexic states and in neurosis.

Thus, this sign is only valuable if it is associated with other upper motor neuron-related findings. The Hoffman sign is best elicited by positioning the patient's hand at rest, then stabilizing the proximal phalanx between the examiner's index and middle finger; with the examiner's thumb, the patient's distal middle finger is flicked downward. The sensitivity of this examination maneuver may be increased by examining the patient during multiple full flexion or extension of the neck (Dynamic Hoffman sign).

Hoffman sign may be insignificant if present bilaterally.

Special Test

Pectoralis Muscle Reflex

This is elicited by tapping the pectoralis tendon in the deltopectoral groove, which causes adduction and internal rotation of the shoulder if hyperactivity is present. It suggests compression in the upper cervical spine (C2-C4).

If the patient exhibits diffuse hyper-reflexia, then the jaw jerk may distinguish an upper cervical cord compression from lesions that are above the foramen magnum.

Lhermitte Sign

This consists of electric shock-like sensations that run down the center of the patient's back and shoot into the limbs during flexion of the neck.

This sign is not specific for CSM and classically is attributed to the posterior column's dysfunction. Other causes of Lhermitte sign include multiple sclerosis, tumors and other compressive pathology.

Muscle weakness in patients with CSM, weakness is most commonly seen in the triceps and/or hand intrinsic muscles, where upper extremity symptoms typically begin. Wasting of the intrinsic hand musculature is also a typical finding.

A thorough examination of patient's hands should also be performed. By having the patient make a fist and release it 20 times in 10 seconds, impairment or clumsiness may be observed that may suggest CSM.

The finger escape sign may also be present. To assess this, the patient holds his or her fingers extended and adducted. If the ulnar digits drift into abduction and flexion within 30 to 60 seconds, CSM may be present.

■ Lower Limb

Examination of the lower extremities classically reveals proximal motor weakness, most commonly in the iliopsoas followed by the quadriceps femoris; distal weakness is a less common finding.

The finding of lower extremity weakness and lower extremity upper motor neuron signs but absent upper extremity symptoms and signs should trigger a work-up for thoracic cord pathology.

Examine gait in any neurologic examination whenever possible. Patients with CSM typically exhibit a stiff or spastic gait, especially later in the course of their disease.

Differential Diagnosis

- Adhesive capsulitis Brown-Sequard syndrome
- Carpal tunnel syndrome
- Central cord syndrome cervical disk disease
- Cervical sprain and strain diabetic neuropathy
- Multiple sclerosis
- Neoplastic brachial plexopathy
- Osteoporosis and spinal cord injury
- Radiation-induced brachial plexopathy
- Rheumatoid arthritis
- Traumatic brachial plexopathy.

Imaging Studies

- Plain cervical radiography
- CT, with myelography
- MRI

Complications

Cervical spondylosis may result in complications including the following:

- Cervical myelopathy
- Paraplegia
- Tetraplegia
- Recurrent chest infection
- Pressure sores
- Recurrent urinary tract infection.

Treatment

Physical Therapy

Immobilization of the cervical spine is the mainstay of conservative treatment for patients with cervical spondylosis. Immobilization limits the motion of the neck, thereby reducing nerve irritation.

Soft cervical collars are recommended for daytime use only, but they are unable to appreciably limit the motion of the cervical spine. More rigid orthoses (e.g. philadelphia collar, minerva body jacket) can significantly immobilize the cervical spine. With the use of any of the braces, the patient's tolerance and compliance are considerations.

A program of isometric cervical exercises may help to limit the loss of muscle tone that results from the use of more restrictive orthoses. Molded cervical pillows can better align the spine during sleep and provide symptomatic relief for some patients.

Mechanical traction is a widely used technique. This form of treatment may be useful because it promotes immobilization of the cervical region and widens the foraminal openings.

The use of cervical exercises has been advocated in patients with cervical spondylosis. Isometric exercises often are beneficial to maintain strength of the neck muscles. Neck and upper back stretching exercises, as well as light aerobic activities, also are recommended. The exercise programs are best initiated and monitored by a physical therapist.

Passive modalities generally involve the application of heat to the tissues in the cervical region, either by means of superficial devices (e.g. moist-heat packs) or mechanisms for deep-heat transfer (e.g. ultrasound, diathermy).

Manual therapy (e.g. massage, mobilization, manipulation may provide further relief for patients with cervical spondylosis. Mobilization is performed by the application of a gentle pressure within or at the limits of normal motion, with the goal of increasing the rom. Manual traction may be better tolerated than mechanical traction in some patients.

Surgical Intervention

Indications for surgery include the following:

- Progressive neurologic deficits
- Documented compression of the cervical nerve root, spinal cord or both
- Intractable pain

The aims of surgery are to relieve pain and neuronal structured compression and to achieve stabilization in selected cases.

Approaches for surgery are anterior or posterior.

- *Anterior approaches include the following:* Diskectomy without bone graft, diskectomy with bone graft and cervical instrumentation
- *Posterior approaches include the following:* Decompressive laminectomy and foraminotomy, hemilaminectomy, and laminoplasty.

Approaches

Indications for surgery include intractable pain, progressive neurologic deficits and documented compression of nerve roots or of the spinal cord that leads to progressive symptoms. Surgery has not been proven to help neck pain and/or suboccipital pain.

Several approaches to the cervical spine have been proposed. The approach selected is determined by the type and location of pathology and by the surgeon's preference.

Cervical radiculopathy traditionally has been approached either via the anterior approach, which was first described by Robinson and Smith in 1955 or by the posterolateral approach, where a "keyhole" foraminotomy is performed.

The anterior approach allows excellent access to midline disease and visualization of pathology without manipulation of neural elements. Robinson and Smith proposed that the anterior approach coupled with fusion using iliac crest bone graft arrests progressive spondylotic spurring, causes existing osteophytes to eventually regress due to spinal stability promoted by fusion, decompresses and enlarges the neural foramen and spinal canal by the distraction of the disk space and minimizes surgical manipulation of the contents of the spinal canal, thereby minimizing complications.

The posterolateral approach to cervical radiculopathy has similar results as the anterior approach when used for the proper indications.

This approach is associated with greater initial postoperative discomfort but avoids the possibility of graft dislodgement and damage to neck structures. It is best used for nerve root decompression, when the pathologic entity is a lateral spondylotic spur or soft disk.

In this approach, a keyhole foraminotomy is made by removing the medial third of the facet joint and the most lateral aspects of the lamina at the involved level and side. The underlying lateral aspect of the ligamentum flavum then is removed to visualize the nerve root.

The impact of facetectomies on the stability of the cervical spine has been questioned. Bilateral 50 percent facetectomies have been demonstrated to expose the nerve by 3 to 5 mm without notable effect on stability. Bilateral facetectomies of 70 percent reduced the spine's ability to withstand stresses while increasing the exposure of the nerve root. In all likelihood, maintenance of the interspinous and most of the interlaminar ligaments is important in preserving stability in patients undergoing foraminotomy.

Traditionally, for cervical laminectomy, a posterior approach has been the treatment of choice.

During the previous 20 years, laminectomy increasingly has been recognized as not appropriate for all patients. Neurological deterioration, which has been reported after laminectomy are spinal instability and kyphotic deformities.

Laminectomy also is unable to address ventral osteophytic overgrowth via a posterior approach. Through an anterior cervical approach, one can directly remove osteophytes, disk material and even vertebral bodies if necessary to decompress the cord. With interposition of bone grafts and in some instances, cervical plates, (i.e. instrumentation), neck instability can be prevented.

In severe situations, extensive decompression is accomplished using multiple level vertebrectomies (corpectomy) and reconstruction with bone graft and instrumentation. Recent series by MacDonald, et al. have demonstrated good-to-excellent results with both the anterior and posterior approaches in as many as 70 percent of patients. Neither approach is proven superior, provided that the appropriate procedure is performed for the clinical indication. The number of elderly patients who seek surgical treatment for CSM is increasing steadily.

ANKYLOSING SPONDYLITIS

- Most common of spondyloarthropathies
  - Prevalence 0.2 to 0.86 percent
  - Male > female
  - 96 percent are HLA-b27 +ve.

Diagnosis

- Inflammatory back pain
- Limitation of spinal movement in all planes
- Early morning stiffness
- Radiological evidence of sacroiliitis

Etiology and Predisposing Factors

- Unknown etiology
- Strongly associated with HLA-b27 genetic marker (85%)
- Gram-negative organisms *(Klebsiella)*
- Young adults below 40 years
- Male/Female 10:1
- Lower frequency in black
- Pathology

Microscopic Appearance

- Abundant lymphocytes, moderate polymorphs and many plasma cells; much eosinophilic fibrin and fibrin like material and early feature; synovial cell hypertrophy and hyperplasia, many layers deep; edema and increased ground substance formation
- Superficial focal synovial tissue necrosis; vascular congestion. The persistence of fibrin is of critical importance to the formation of marginal granulation tissue pannus leading to joint destruction. Along with there is increased bone production adjacent to joint.

Gross Appearance

The cartilage and the articular cortices are destroyed and fibrous and bony bridging is frequent. The para-articular tissue are degenerated and calcified and frequently ossified.

Pathology

- The anterior longitudinal ligaments are specially affected by those processes with the bony bridging between vertebral segments producing a rigid bamboo spine. However, the anterior sporty structures are friable and easily ruptured by the forceful extension of spine (Figs 27.245A and B)
- The aorta and the inferior vena cava which lie in close proximity to spine anteriorly may be compressed and even ruptured by this sudden change of position. The apophyseal joints of the spine and the hip joint frequently are enclosed by bone. Knee less and rarely the shoulder affected.
- Clinical signs in as
- Axial disease
  - Decreased lumbar spine mobility
  - Reduced chest expansion
  - Poor mobility of cervical spine
  - Increasing stoop
- Peripheral arthritis
  - Hips, shoulders, knees
- Achilles tendonitis, dactylitis
- Uveitis.

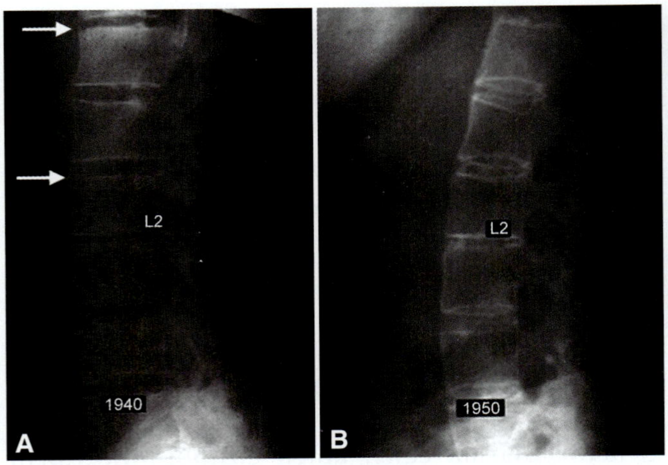

Figs 27.245A and B: Lumbar vertebrae in ankylosing spondylitis—Radiographs of lumbar vertebrae showing progressive disease in ankylosing spondylitis. Radiograph from 1940 (left panel) reveals "shiny coiners" (arrows) at anterior T11 and L2 vertebral bodies, an early sign of ankylosing spondylitis. A comparison of radiographs from 1940 and 1950 (right panel) also reveals progressive squaring of lumbar vertebrae. The 1950 radiographs demonstrate early development of a "bamboo" spine. *Courtesy of Mark Robinson, MD*

Clinical Features

Early Disease

- Pain in buttocks
- Lumbar back ache
- Early morning stiffness
- Restriction of chest movements.

Enthesopathies

- Peripheral joints involvement
- Dorsal and cervical spine pain.

Advanced Disease

- As time passes stiffness increases and extends to fresh areas so that in advanced stage the head, neck, entire spine, hips and shoulder are all stiff
- Some patients are stiff but many patients have a rounded shouldered back with spine so flexed that in some cases vision is confined to a point just ahead of them on walking.
- Mobility is diminished.

Physical Findings in Spine

The movements in spine are less free. Movements in spine are documented by forward flexion (Fig. 27.246).

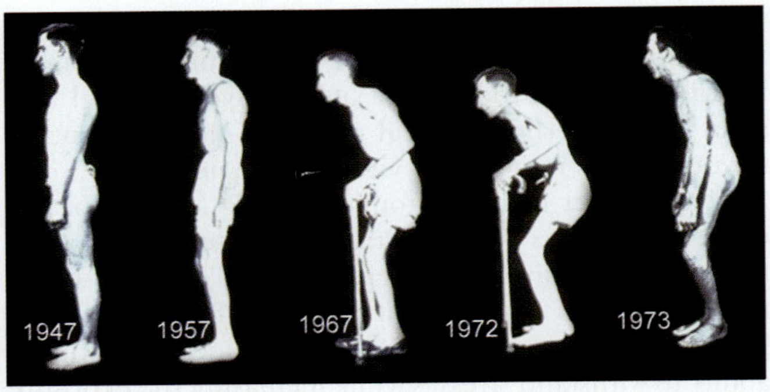

Fig. 27.246: Progression of postural changes with ankylosing spondylitis—this series of photographs shows the progressive postural changes of ankylosing spondylitis

Schober's Test

- Mark the T1/l1 and S1 vertebrae and measuring tape with patient in normal extension, i.e. upright posture
- Ask patient to flex forward and note the distance between T1 and S1. More than 10 cm excursion is normal.

Modified Schober's Test

- Mark the S2 vertebrae and select a point 10 cm above and 5 cm below, and ask patient to flex
- Normal is 6 to 7 cm
- Less than 5 cm is significant
- Examination of sacroiliac joints
- Direct tenderness over SI joints.
- Active SLRT
- Pump handle test
- Ganslen's test
- Active abduction against resistance

Investigations in as:

- Pelvic X-ray (Fig. 27.247)
  - Sacroiliitis
  - Juxta-articular sclerosis and erosions
- Lumbar spine
  - Squaring of vertebrae
  - Syndesmophytes
  - Bamboo spine
- Laboratory tests
  - Raised acute phase response
  - Anemia of chronic disease
- Symmetrical sacroilitis ankylosing spondylitis

Grading of Sacroiliitis

- Grade 0 : Normal
- Grade 1 : Probably abnormal
- Grade 2 : Definite marginal sclerosis
- Grade 3 : Definite erosion and sclerosis
- Grade 4 : Complete obliteration.

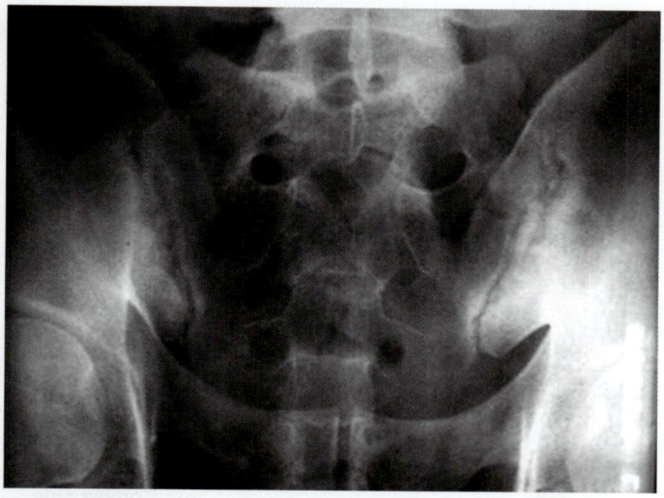

Fig. 27.247: X-ray showing sacroiliitis with juxta/articular sclerosis and erosion

■ Diagnostic Criteria 1961 (Bone Criteria)

Clinical Criteria

- Low back pain and stiffness for more than three months with patient not relieved by rest
- Pain and stiffness in thoracic region
- Limited motion of lumbar spine
- Limited chest expansion
- History of iritis
- Radiological criteria X-ray showing bilateral sacroiliac changes.

Diagnosis

Radiological criteria + one clinical criterion
Four clinical criteria.

■ New York Criteria 1969 (Bennett and Wood)

Diagnosis

- Limitation of motion of the lumbar spine in all plain of motion that is forward flexion, later flexion and extension.
- History of presence of pain at dorsolumbar joint or lumbar spine.
- Limitation of chest expansion to <1" measured at the level of fourth intercostals space.

Grading

Definite ankylosing spondylitis:

- Bilateral sacroiliitis with at least one clinical criteria
- Unilateral sacroiliitis with clinical criteria that is limited lumbar motion in all three plains
- Grade two bilateral sacroiliitis with clinical criteria. Two and 3 (i.e. pain in dl or l spine and limitation of chest expansion).

Treatment

- General measures
  - Patient education
  - Genetic counseling
  - Avoid smoking
  - Regular exercise especially swimming is of tremendous help
- Physiotherapy and joint exercise
- Occupational therapy
  - Exercise is most important, with attention to posture
  - Hydrotherapy and physiotherapy with lifelong exercise program
- NSAIDs
  - Indomethacin 75 mgbd
- DMARDs in those with peripheral arthritis
  - Sulphasalazine/methotrexate
- *Surgical management*
  - Flexion deformity can be measured by chin brow to vertical angle which can be corrected by various osteotomies as follows
  - Smith-Peterson osteotomy
  - Pedicle subtraction osteotomy
  - Three egg shell osteotomy
- *Complications in as*
  - *Hip disease:* Twenty percent of patients who develop as in their teens will need 1 or 2 hip replacements within 15 years of disease onset
  - *Knee disease:* Occasionally results in need for total knee replacement
  - *Spinal fracture:* Increased risk with rigid spine and secondary osteoporosis
  - Apical fibrosis and aortic regurgitation rarely
- *Human leukocyte antigen:* Though, it is not a component of immune system, HLA system is considered important in the regulation of the immune system. HLA stands for human leukocyte antigens because these antigens were first described on leukocytes. The major importance of human histocompatibility antigens of HLA system lies in matching donor and recipient for organ transplantation.

HLA

Out of the various genes for histocompatibility antigens, most of the transplantation antigens are located on the portion of chromosome 6 of all nucleated cells of the body and platelets. This is called major histocompatibility complex (MHC). These genes occupy four loci A, B, C, D on the short arm of chromosome 6 and exhibit marked variations in allelic genes at each locus. So, product of HLA antigens is highly polymorphic.

Three Classes

- *Class 1:* Have loci as HLA-A, HLA-B and HLA-C. CD8 lymphocytes carry receptors for class 1 MHC and are used to identify the cells having them.
- *Class 2:* Have single locus as HLA-D. These antigens have further three loci, dr, dq and dp. Class 2 MHC is identified by B cells and CD4 or T helper cells
- *Class 3:* They are some components of the complement system coded on HLA complex but not associated with HLA expression and are not used in antigen identification.
- Role of HLA complex
- Organ transplantation
- Regulation of immune system
- Association of diseases with HLA:
  - Inflammatory
  - Autoimmune disorders
  - Inherited disorders of metabolism.

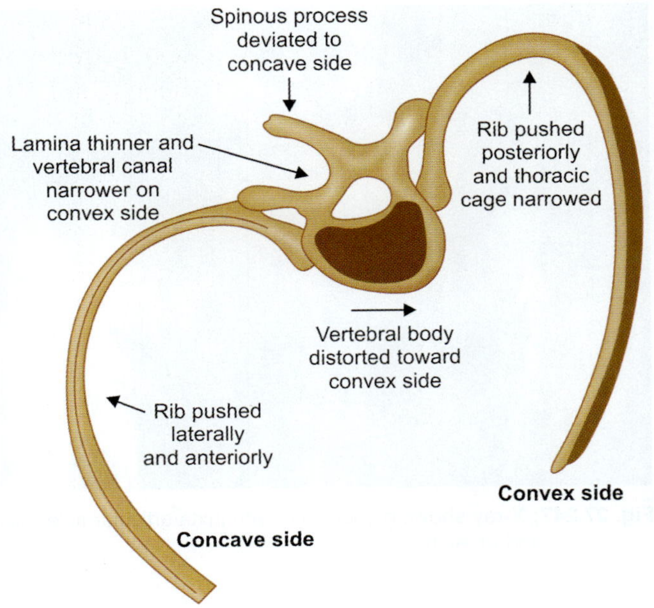

Fig. 27.248: Lateral curvature and vertebral rotation in scoliosis with associated anatomical changes

SCOLIOSIS

Scoliosis is lateral deviation of the normal vertical line of the spine, which when measured by X-ray, is greater than 10°. Scoliosis consists of lateral curvature of the spine with rotation of the vertebrae within the curve.

■ Anatomy

The normal thoracolumbar spine is relatively straight in the sagittal plane and has a double curve in the coronal plane. Normally there should be no lateral curvature of the spine.

Pathoanatomy (Fig. 27.248)

Scoliosis is a complicated deformity that is characterized by both lateral curvature and vertebral rotation. As the disease progresses, the vertebrae and spinous processes in the area of the major curve rotate toward the concavity of the curve. On the concave side of the curve, the ribs are close together. On the convex side, they are widely separated. As the vertebral bodies rotate, the spinous processes deviate more and more to the concave side and the ribs follow the rotation of the vertebrae. The posterior ribs on the convex side are pushed posteriorly, causing the characteristic rib hump seen in thoracic scoliosis. The anterior ribs on the concave side are pushed anteriorly.

■ Classification of Scoliosis

Nonstructural Scoliosis

- Postural scoliosis
- Compensatory scoliosis.

Transient Structural Scoliosis

- Sciatic scoliosis
- Hysterical scoliosis
- Inflammatory scoliosis.

Structural Scoliosis

- Idiopathic (70-80% of all cases)
- Congenital
- Neuromuscular
  - Poliomyelitis
  - Cerebral palsy
  - Syringomyelia
  - Muscular dystrophy
  - Amyotonia congenita
  - Friedreich's ataxia
- Neurofibromatosis
- Mesenchymal disorders
  - Marfan's syndrome
  - Morquio's syndrome
  - Rheumatoid arthritis
  - Osteogenesis imperfecta
  - Certain dwarves
- Trauma
  - Fractures
  - Irradiation
  - Surgery

■ Congenital Scoliosis

Congenital scoliosis is caused by the presence of vertebral anomalies that result in an imbalance of the longitudinal growth of the spine. Critical time in the development of the spine embryologically is in the fifth to sixth week, at the time of segmentation processes. Some type of anomaly must be visible on the X-ray of the spine before a diagnosis of congenital scoliosis can be made. It is often rigid and correction can be difficult: thus it is important to detect these curves early and to institute appropriate treatment while the curve is small.

Patient Evaluation

Some specific physical findings should be sought in patients with congenital scoliosis.

- *The skin of the back:* Hair patches, lipomata, dimples, and scars, which may indicate an underlying anomalous vertebra
- Evidence of neurological involvement, such as a clubfoot, calf atrophy, absent reflexes, and atrophy of one lower extremity
- Urological anomalies are present in 18 percent of the cases
- Congenital heart disease in 7 percent of the cases
- Diastematomyelia occurs in approximately 5 percent of patients, as shown in Figure 26.249
- The deformity produced by a failure of formation is much more difficult to predict than that caused by failure of segmentation
- Analysis of the growth status is the most important factor in predicting the possibility of progression of these congenital deformities, as illustrated in Figures 27.250A and B.

Treatment

There are three types of curves responded to brace management:

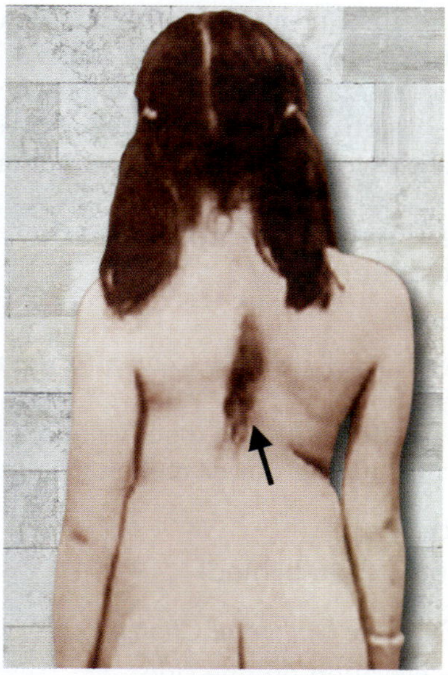

Fig. 27.249: Hair patch associated with diastematomyelia and congenital scoliosis

- Longer and flexible curves
- Curves that could be corrected either in traction or on side bending
- Curves with a mixture of anomalous and non-anomalous vertebrae. Short, sharp and rigid curves do not respond to brace treatment.

Congenital Scoliosis Treatment (Figs 27.251A to D)

As 75 percent of congenital curves are progressive and only 5 to 10 percent can be treated with bracing, surgery remains the fundamental treatment.

■ Neuromuscular Scoliosis

It can be associated with many neuromuscular diseases. These are enumerated in Table 27.8.

■ Adolescent Idiopathic Scoliosis

- What is the prevalence of idiopathic scoliosis in the general population?
- What is the likelihood of curve progression necessitating treatment in a child with scoliosis?
- What problems may occur in adult life if scoliosis is left untreated and the curve progresses?

Factors related to progression of adolescent idiopathic scoliosis are given as follows:

- Girls tend to show a greater tendency towards scoliosis than boys
- Premenarchal
- Risser sign of 0 (no iliac apophyses ossified)
- Double curves greater than single curves
- Thoracic curves more than lumbar curves

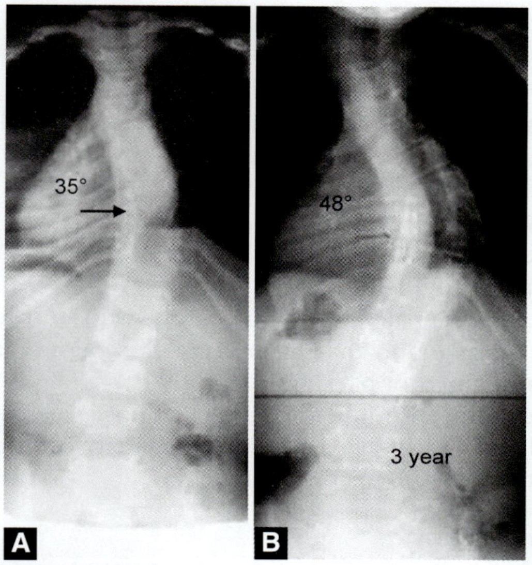

Figs 27.250A and B: Progression of curve with normal convex growth and deficient concave growth due to unsegmented bar—(A) Initial curve of 35°; (B) Three years later, curve is 48°

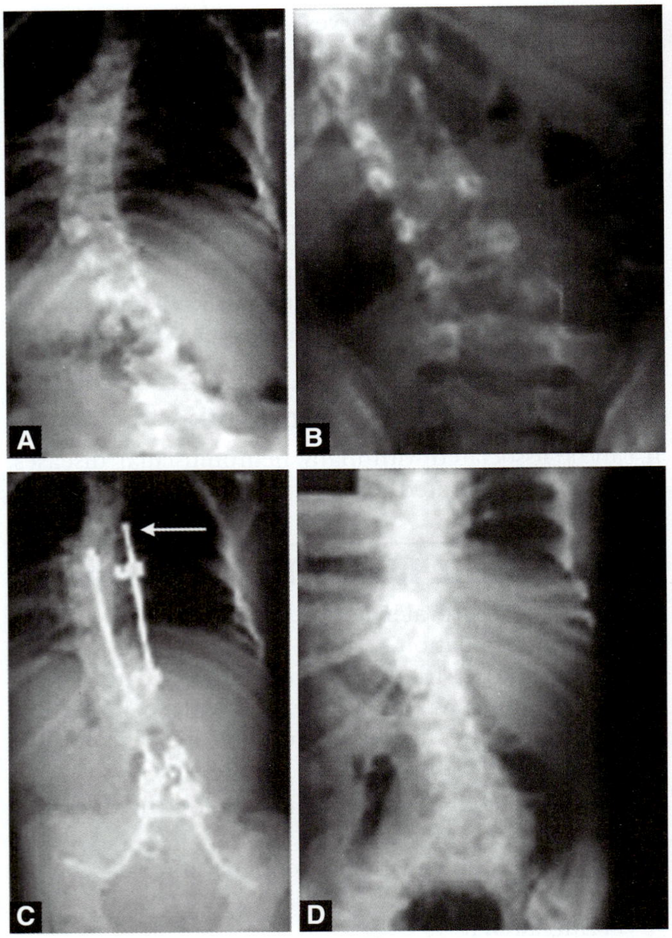

Figs 27.251A to D: (A) and (B) Hemivertebra; (C) After hemivertebral excision and fusion with short segmented rods and cross links; (D) After rod removal

- More severe curves
- Untreated idiopathic scoliosis.

Major considerations in the natural history of untreated adolescent idiopathic scoliosis in adults are as follows:

- Back pain
- Pulmonary function
- Psychosocial effects
- Mortality
- Curve progression
- Weinstein et al. in a long-term follow-up study of over 40 years found that 80 percent of scoliotic patients complained of backache
- Mortality in adult idiopathic scoliosis seems to be related to thoracic curves greater than 100 degrees, with resultant cor pulmonale.

Examination

- Characteristics of the deformity should be recorded.
- The height of the patient while standing and while sitting should be measured and recorded

Table 27.8: Neuropathic conditions associated with neuromuscular scoliosis

Neuropathic
Upper motor neuron
• Cerebral palsy
• Spinocerebellar degeneration
• Friedreich ataxia
• Charcot-Marie-tooth
• Roussy-Levy
• Syringomyelia
• Spinal cord tumor
• Spinal cord trauma
Lower motor neuron
• Poliomyelitis
• Other viral myelitides
• Traumatic
• Spinal muscle atrophy
• Werdnig-Hoffmann
• Kugelberg-Welander
• Dysautonomia
• (Riley-Day syndrome)
• Arthrogryposis
• Muscular dystrophy
• Duchenne
• Limb-girdel
• Facioscapulohumeral
• Fiber-type disproportion
• Congenital hypotonia
• Myotonia dystrophica

- A thorough neurological examination should be performed to determine if an intraspinal neoplasm or a neurological disorder is the cause of scoliosis.
- Particular attention should be given to the abdominal reflexes, as often they are the only neurological abnormalities found with some intraspinal disorders.

Technique: Forward Bending Test (Most Accurate)

Patient Position

- Patient with a fully visible spine after he removes his shirt
- Forward bending with feet together and knees straight
- Allow arms to hang down freely (or palms opposed).

Examiner Position

Observe patient from behind.

Abnormal Findings: Unilateral Changes

- Rib cage elevation on one side
- Prominent unilateral lumbar paravertebral muscle.

Technique: Scoliometer (Measures Trunk Rotation)

Patient positioned as in the case of forward bending mentioned above.

Scoliometer Position

- Place scoliometer on midline, i.e. perpendicular to the spine
- Position at vertebral level of maximum rib prominence.

Interpretation

- Inclination exceeding 5 to 7 degrees requires workup
- Seven degrees correlates with 20 degrees Cobb angle.

Technique: Adam's Test (Used for School Screening)

Patient is positioned as in the case of forward bending mentioned above.

Examiner Position

Examiner sits towards the head of the patient.

Abnormal Findings

Same as for the forward bending exam mentioned above.

X-rays

- PA and lateral X-rays of the spine, including the iliac crest distally and most of the cervical spine proximally.
- Right and left bending films usually are obtained only when the patient is being evaluated for surgery or bracing.
- An AP X-ray of the hand and wrist should be made to determine skeletal age, which is considered in addition to other signs of maturation, including ossification of the vertebral ring apophysis, iliac apophysis excursion (Risser sign), as shown in Figures 27.252A to C and physical signs of maturity, such as breast development and pubic hair.

Lateral Bending Film

Figures 27.253 and 27.254 show lateral bending films.

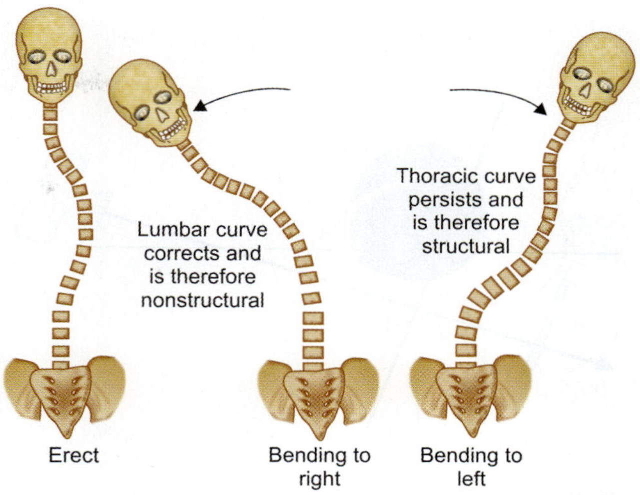

Fig. 27.253: Different lateral bending positions

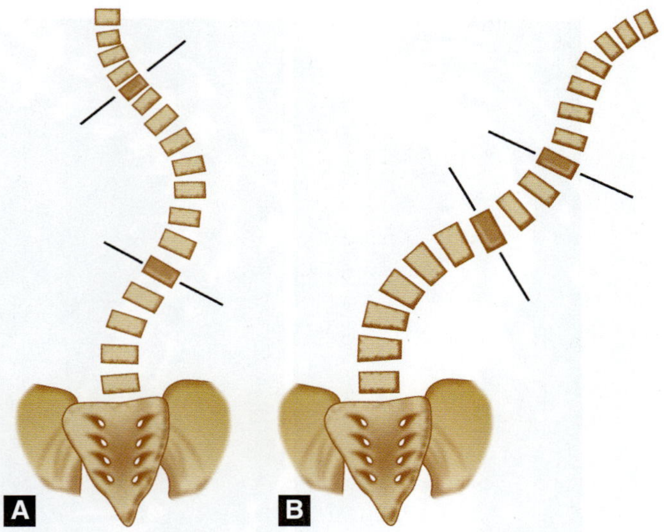

Figs 27.254A and B: (A) Anteroposterior diagrams of uppermost and lowermost instrumented vertebrae; (B) Upper and lower rigid vertebral bodies are shown on bending films

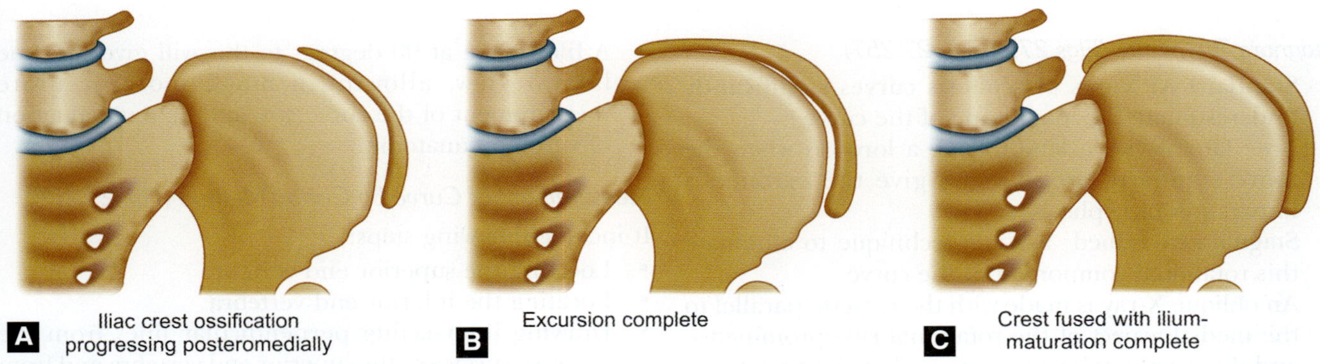

Figs 27.252A to C: Iliac apophysis excursion (Risser sign)

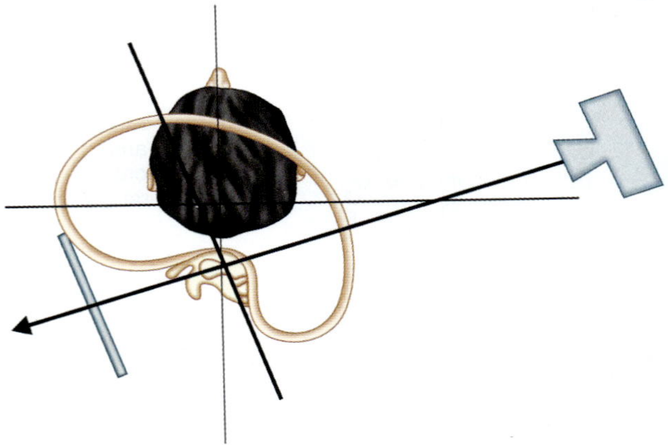

Fig. 27.255: Stagnara derotation view

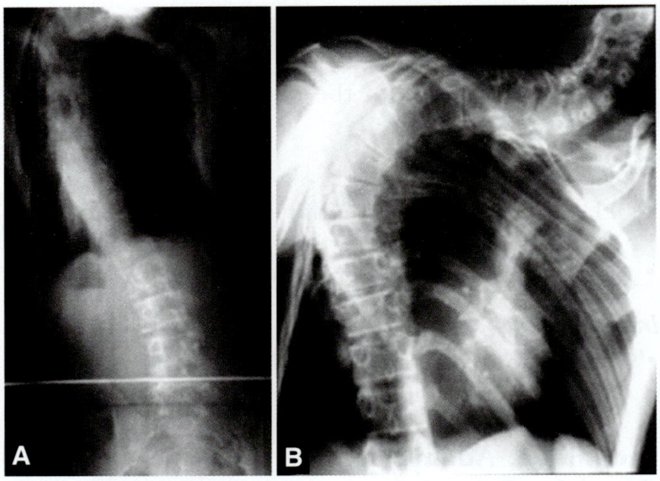

Figs 27.257A and B: (A) Standard posteroanterior roentgenogram of large scoliosis; (B) Stagnara view showing better detail of curve, size, and vertebral anatomy

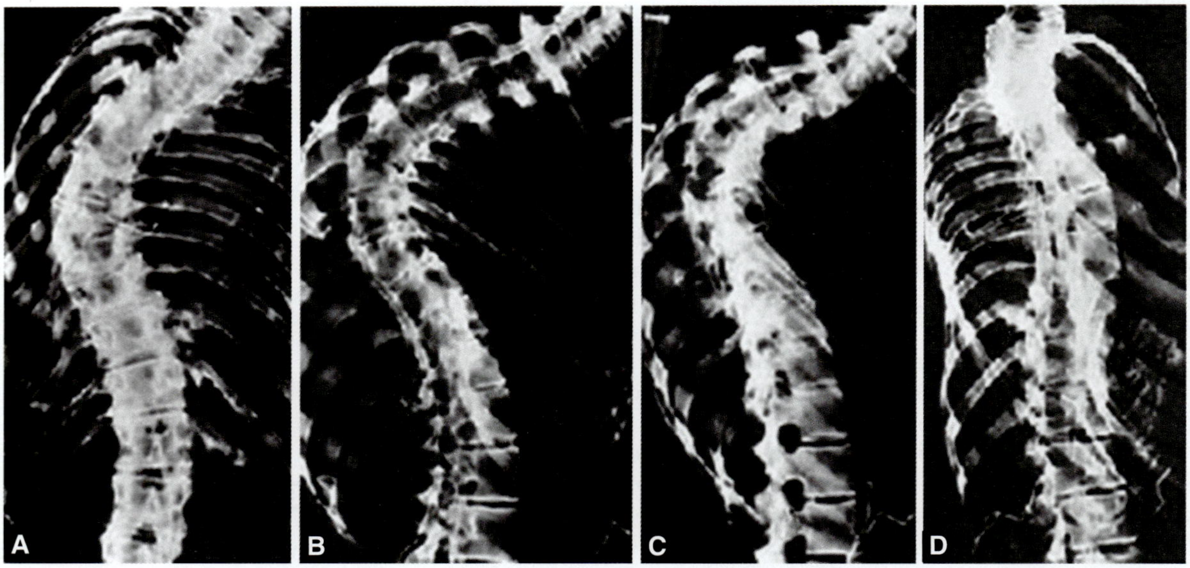

Figs 27.256A to D: Roentgenograms at four points during rotational cycle of articulated scoliotic spine show changes in Cobb angle with rotation—(A) On anteroposterior view, apparent Cobb angle of 87 degrees; (B) True Cobb angle of 128 degees; (C) On lateral view, apparent kyphosis of 61 degrees; (D) True apical lordosis of 14 degrees

Stagnara Technique (Figs 27.255 to 27.257)

- Standard AP views of scoliosis curves significantly underestimate the magnitude of the curve
- True lateral views demonstrate a lordosis when the more standard lateral views give the erroneous impression of kyphosis
- Stagnara described a X-ray technique to eliminate this rotational component of the curve
- An oblique X-ray is made with the cassette parallel to the medial aspect of the rotational ribe prominence and the roentgen beam positioned at right angles to the cassette
- A film made at 90 degrees to this will give the true lateral view, allowing a much more accurate measurement of the curve size and better evaluation of vertebral anatomy.

Measurement of Curve by Cobb's Method (Fig. 27.258)

It include following steps:

- Locating the superior end vertebra
- Locating the inferior end vertebra
- Drawing intersecting perpendicular lines from the superior surface of the superior end vertebra and from the inferior surface of the inferior end vertebra

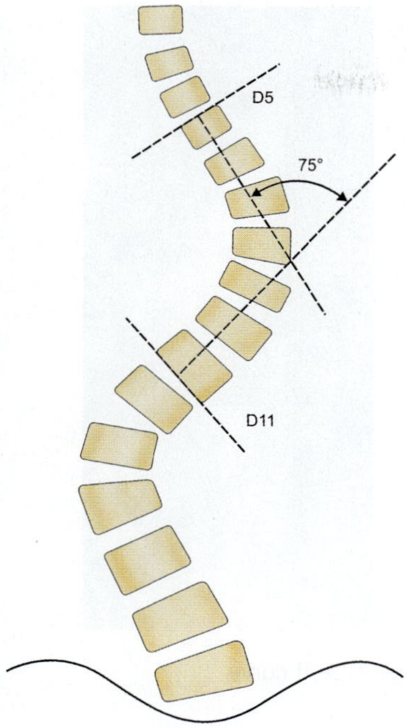

Fig. 27.258: Diagram of Cobb's method

- The angle of deviation of these perpendiculars from a straight line is the angle of the curve
- If the end plates are obscured, the pedicles can be used instead
- The end vertebra of the curve is the one that tilts the most into the concavity of the curve being measured.
- When moving away from the apex of the curve, the next intervertebral space below the inferior end vertebra or above the superior end vertebra is wider on the concave side of the curve.
- Within the curve the intervertebral spaces usually are wider on the convex side and narrower on the concave side.
- When significantly wedged, the vertebrae themselves, rather than the intervertebral disk spaces, may be wider on the convex side of the curve and narrower on the concave side.

Vertebral Rotation Method of Nash and Moe (Fig. 27.259)

- If the pedicles are equidistant from the sides of the vertebral bodies, no vertebral rotation is present (zero rotation).
- The grades progress up to grade IV rotation, in which the pedicle is past the center of the vertebral body.

Perdriolle Torsion Meter (Fig. 27.260)

- The vertebra's pedicle shadow-offset and the edges of the vertebral body are marked and then measured with the torsion meter

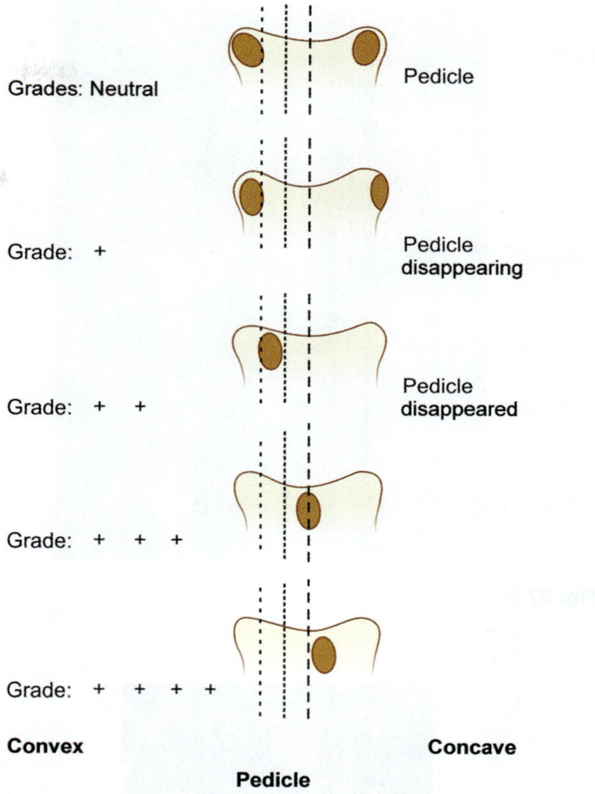

	Convex	Concave
Grade: Neutral	No asymmetry	No asymmetry
Grade: +	Migrates within first segment Early distortion	May start disappearing Early distortion
Grade: ++	Migrates to second segment	Gradually disappears
Grade: +++	Migrates to middle segment	Not visible

Fig. 27.259: Pedicle method of determining vertebral rotation. Vertebral body is divided into six segments and grades from 0 to 4+ are assigned, depending on location of pedicle within segments. Because pedicle on concave side disappears early in rotation, pedicle on convex side, easily visible through wide range of rotation, is used as standard

- Theoretically a CT scan is much more accurate in evaluation of vertebral rotation, but CT scanning is inappropriate in routine scoliosis evaluation.

King's Classification (Figs 27.261 to 27.265)

- The classification system of King et al. is used to describe thoracic curves
- Identification of curve types using the King's classification begins with a careful physical examination.
- The location and magnitude of the thoracic rib hump and lumbar rotational prominence should be noted, as well as any elevation of the shoulder.
- Roentgenographic evaluation should include standing posteroanterior, lateral, and side-bending roentgenograms. The side-bending films are used to determine flexibility of the individual curves.

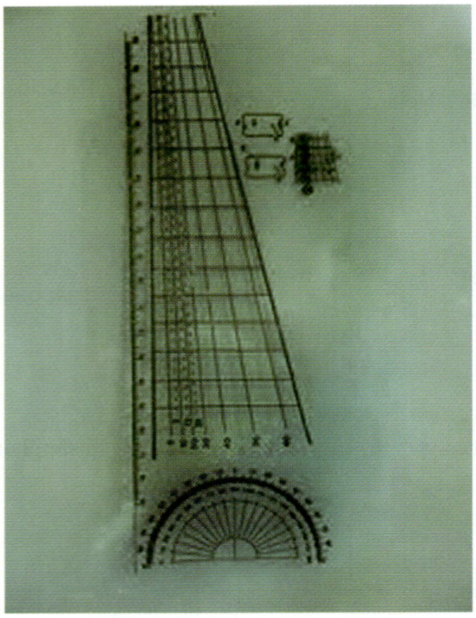

Fig. 27.260: Perdriolle torsion meter

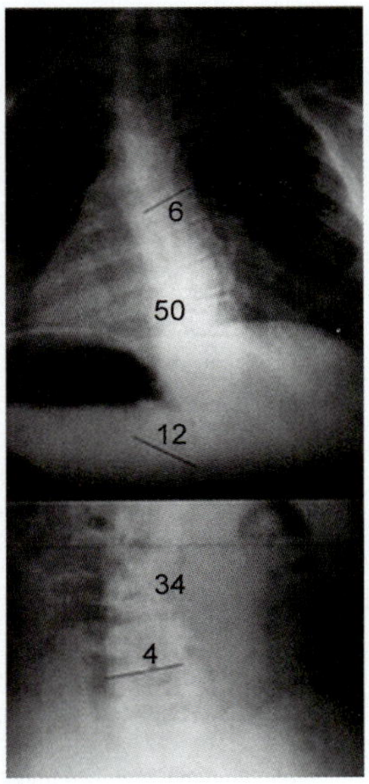

Fig. 27.262: King's type II curve

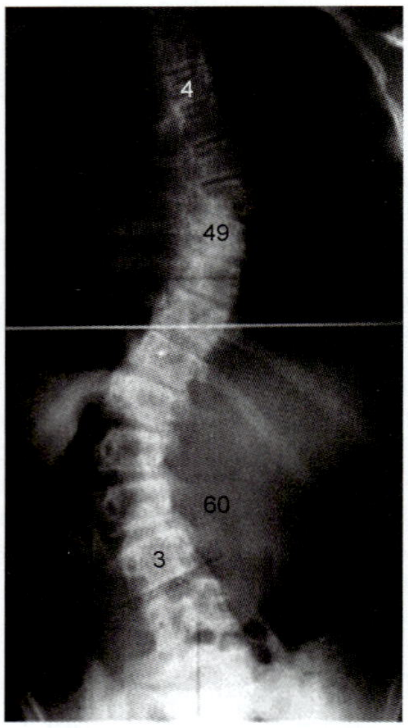

Fig. 27.261: King's type I curve

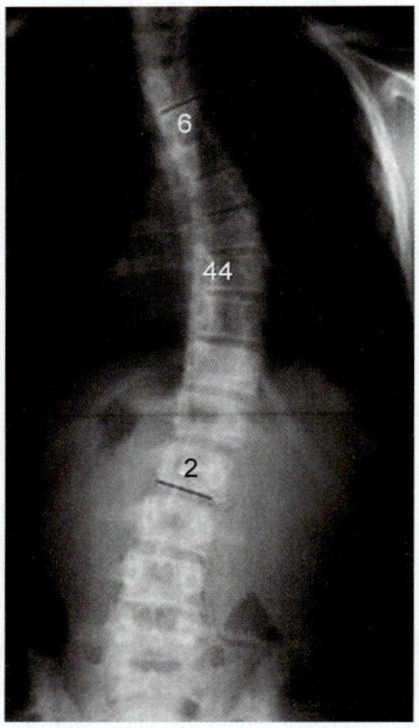

Fig. 27.263: King's type III curve

- A King type I curve is recognized easily because the lumbar curve is larger than the thoracic curve. Occasionally, the thoracic and lumbar curves are nearly equal, but the lumbar curve is less flexible on side bending. Clinically, the lumbar rotational prominence is larger than the rib hump.
- A type II curves have created more confusion than any other curve pattern. As defined by King, type II thoracic scoliosis is a combined thoracic and lumbar curve pattern. On roentgenograms the thoracic curve is larger than or equal to the lumbar curve. The lumbar curve must cross the center sacral line. On supine side-bending roentgenograms the lumbar curve is more flexible than the thoracic curve. On clinical examination the thoracic rib hump is larger than the lumbar rotational prominence.
- A type III curve is a thoracic scoliosis with the lumbar curve not crossing the midline. The lumbar curve is very flexible on side-bending roentgenograms. On clinical examination the thoracic rib hump is quite apparent, and the lumbar prominence may be quite small or nonexistent.
- A type IV curve is a single long thoracic curve, with L4 tilted into the curve and L5 balanced over the pelvis.

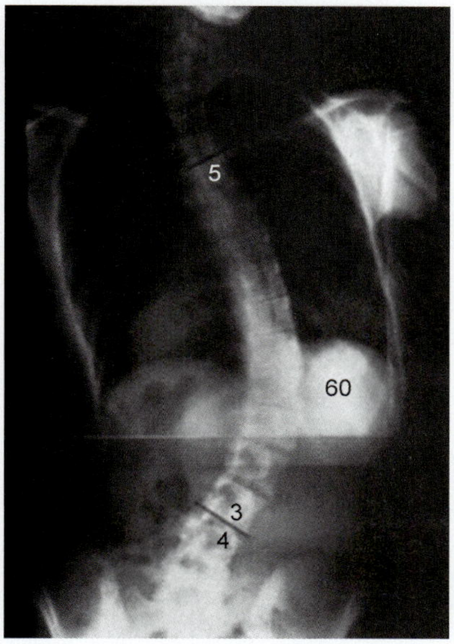

Fig. 27.264: King's type IV curve

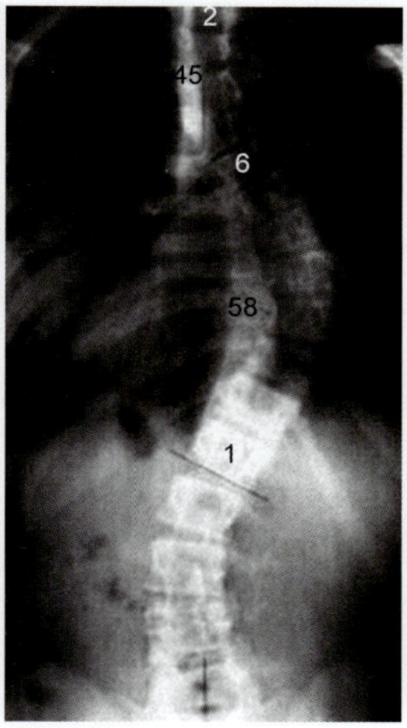

Fig. 27.265: King's type V curve

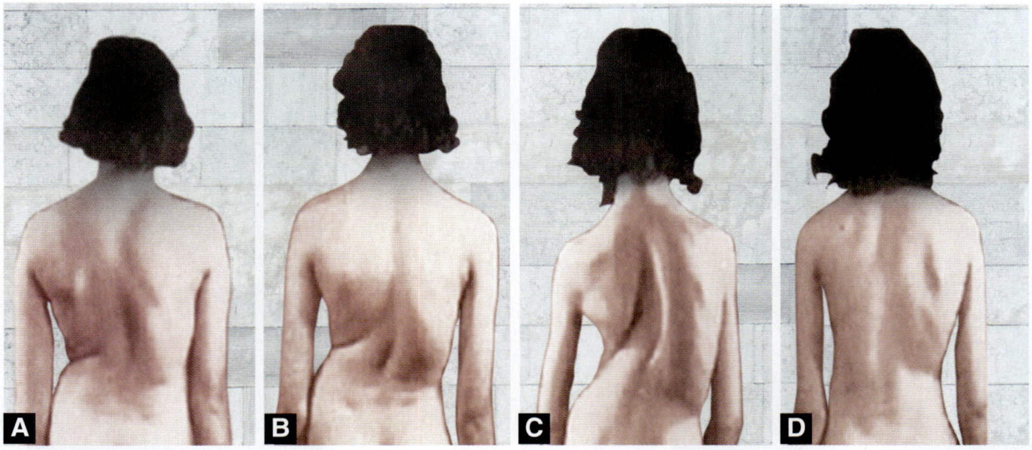

Figs 27.266A to D: Scoliosis deformity varies with pattern of curve. In each patient shown, angle of primary curve or curves is 70 degrees, but pattern of curve is different. Left to right, lumbar, thoracolumbar, thoracic, and combined thoracic and lumbar curves

- A type V curve is a double structural thoracic curve. On roentgenograms the first thoracic vertebra is tilted into the concavity of the upper curve, which is structural on side-bending films. Clinical examination frequently demonstrates an elevation of the left shoulder. On forward bending there is an upper left thoracic rib hump and a lower right thoracic rib prominence.

King's Classification

Pattern of the Curve (Figs 27.266A to D)

- *Single major lumbar curve (Fig. 27.267):* The lumbar curve has its apex between the L1-L2 disk and L4. These curves produce an asymmetry of the waistline with prominence of the contralateral hip that parents often assume is caused by a short leg on the side of the curve.
- *Single major thoracolumbar curve (Fig. 27.268):* The thoracolumbar curve apex is at T12 or L1. This curve tends to produce more truncal imbalance than the other curves. This decompensation from the midline often produces a severe cosmetic deformity.
- *Combined thoracic and lumbar curves (double major curves) (Fig. 27.269):* Symmetrical double major curves generally cause less visible deformities because the curves are nearly the same degree in size and the trunk usually is well balanced.

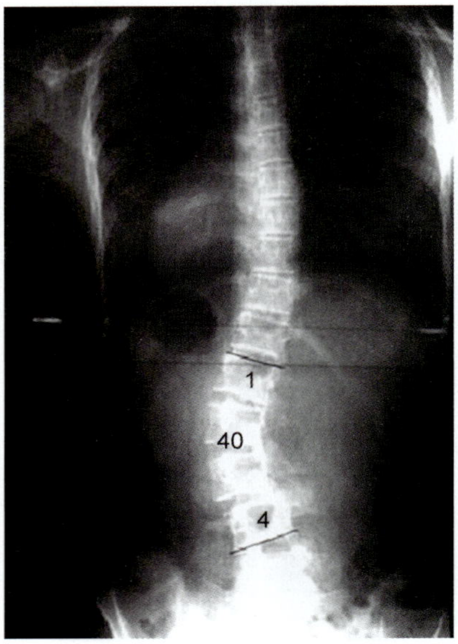

Fig. 27.267: Asymmetry of the waistline

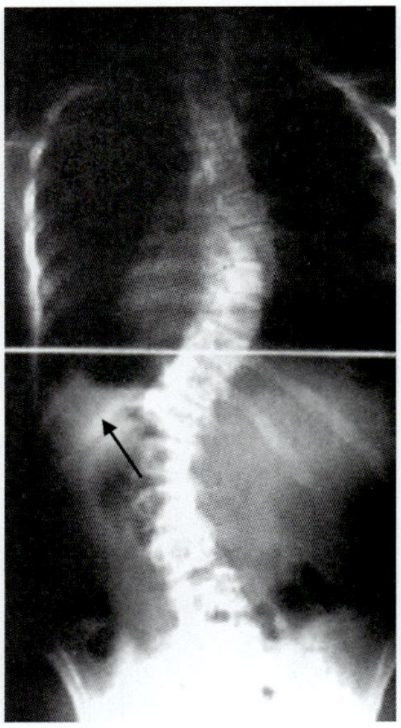

Fig. 27.269: X-ray showing two major curves, arrow showing rib lumb

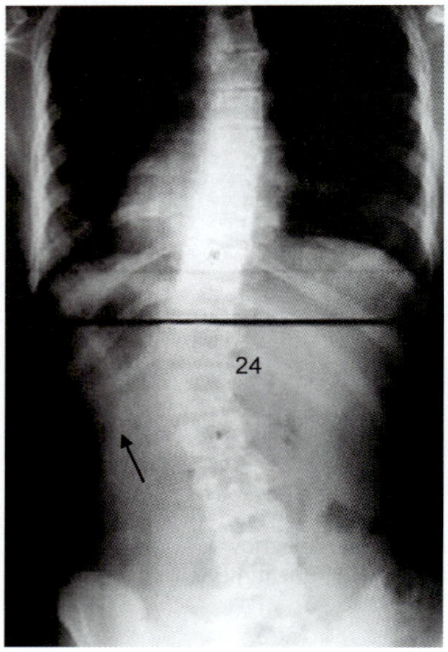

Fig. 27.268: Arrow showing severe cosmetic deformity due to single major thoracolumbar curve at T12-L1

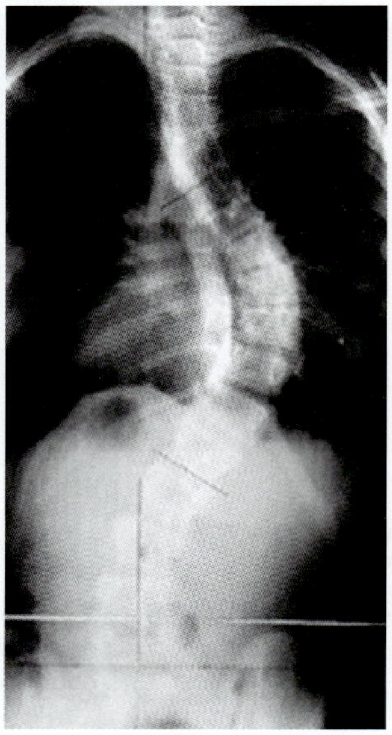

Fig. 27.270: Single major thoracic curve

- *Single major thoracic curve (Fig. 27.270):* This curve pattern is generally a convex right pattern. The rotation of the involved vertebrae may be obvious because of the thoracic location of the curve. The curve produces prominence of the ribs on the convex side, depression of the ribs on the concave side, and elevation of one shoulder, resulting in an unsightly deformity. Included in these single major thoracic curve categories are the King and Moe types II, III, and IV curves.
- *Double major thoracic curve (Fig 27.271):* Short upper thoracic curve, often extending from T1 to T5 or T6, with rotation of the vertebrae and other structural changes in combination with the lower thoracic curve extending from T6 to T12 or L1. Upper curve usually is convex to the left, and the lower usually is convex to the right. Deformities not as severe as in those with a single thoracic curve, but because of asymmetry of the neckline produced by the upper curve, this pattern is more deforming than combined thoracic and

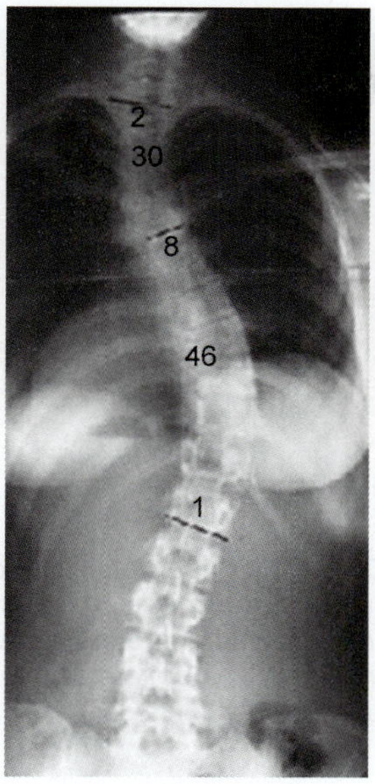

Fig. 27.271: Double major thoracic curve

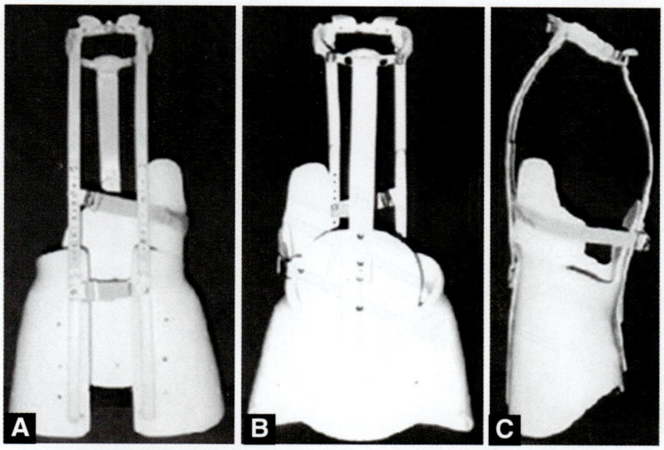

Figs 27.272A to C: Full Milwaukee brace for right thoracic curve

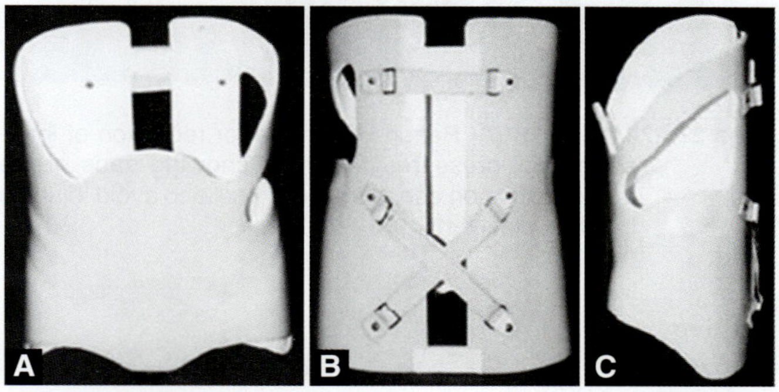

Figs 27.273A to C: Boston brace for right thoracic, left lumbar curve

lumbar curves. If only the lower thoracic curve is corrected by fusion and instrumentation, the upper curve may not be flexible enough to allow correct posture and may lead to a cosmetically unacceptable result.

Nonoperative Treatment

- For curves of 30 to 40° in a skeletally immature patient, orthotic treatment at the initial evaluation is necessary.
- Curves of 30 to 40° in skeletally mature patients, generally do not require treatment; follow-up with yearly standing PA X-rays for 2 to 3 years after skeletal maturity, then every 5 years throughout life.

Orthotic Treatment

In adolescent idiopathic scoliosis—for a flexible curve of 20 to 30° in a growing child with documented progression of 5° or more. Curves in the 30 to 40° range in growing children are treated at initial evaluation. Although, surgery usually is indicated for curves in the 40 to 50° range in growing children, orthotic treatment may be considered for some curves, such as a cosmetically acceptable double major curve of 40 to 45°. Orthotic treatment is not used in patients with curves of more than 50°.

Braces

A. Cervical-thoracic-lumbar-sacral orthoses (CTLSOs): Milwaukee brace
B. Thoracic-lumbar-sacral orthoses (TLSOs): Boston brace and the Wilmington plastic jacket.

The basic principle of both types is control of lumbar lordosis by producing a forward pelvic tilt of the pelvic girdle. If the apex of the thoracic curve is at the seventh thoracic vertebra or below, a TLSO is appropriate. A CTLSO is used for high thoracic curves with an apex above the seventh thoracic vertebra, as shown in Figures 27.272 and 27.273.

Results: Approximately 50 percent improvement in the curve is obtained after about six months in the brace, after which improvement gradually lessens. When the brace is discontinued, the average curve is slightly better than before bracing, but at 5 years follow-up, the average curve is about the same as at the start of the treatment. Therefore, the brace should be presented to the family and the patient as a holding device. Boston brace controlled idiopathic scoliosis in 80 percent of the patients in whom the apex of the curve was at T7 or below.

Traction

It is not commonly used nowadays. Halo—a device that provides stable fixation and comfort for the patient. The halo device may still be useful in few selected patients. It may be used for added external immobilization in post-surgery case, to maintain correction until fusion occurs. Also used in patients with cervical spine fractures.

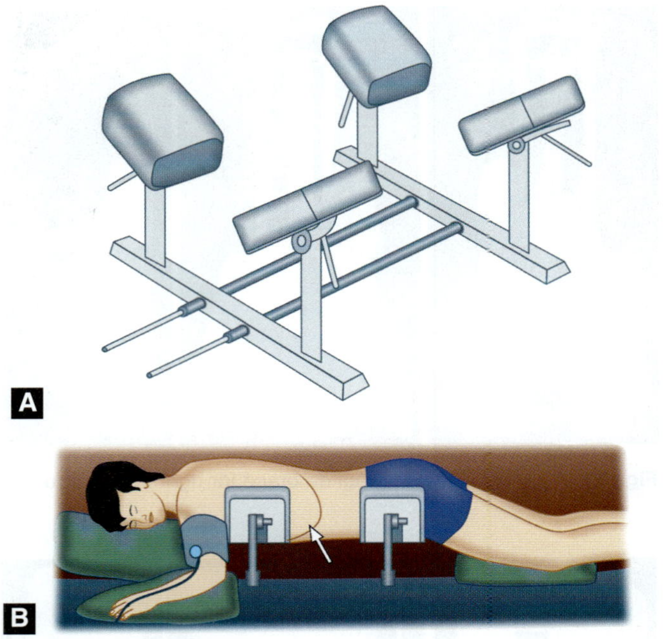

Figs 27.274A and B: (A) Relton-Hall frame for reduction of intra-abdominal pressure; (B) Arrow showing pads of the frame resting on chest and not in axilla to avoid injury to brachial plexus

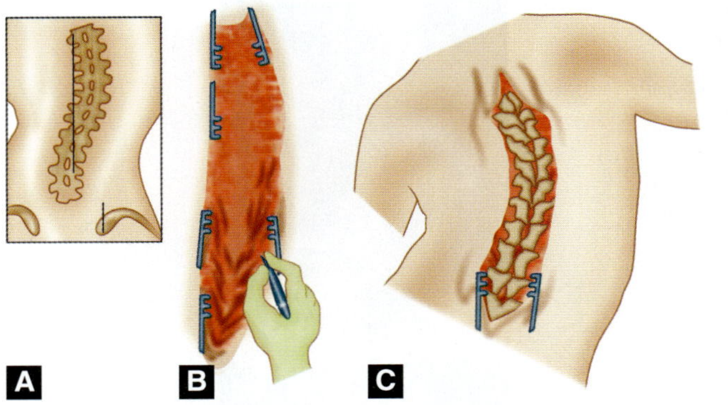

Figs 27.275A to C: (A) Skin incisions for posterior fusion and autogenous bone graft; (B) Incisions over spinous processes and interspinous ligaments; (C) Weitlaner retractors used to maintain tension and exposure of spine during dissection

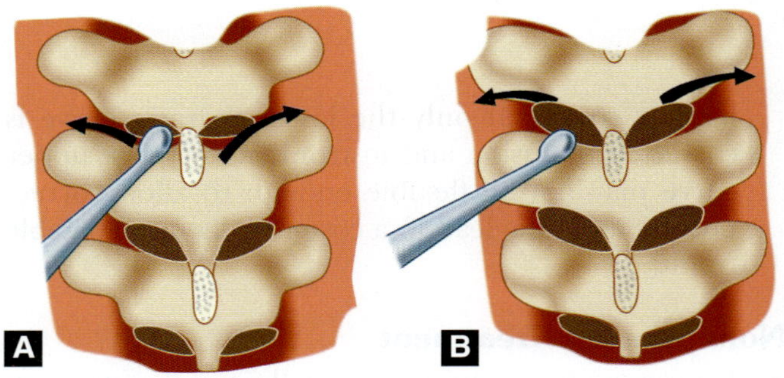

Figs 27.276A and B: Cobb curettes used to clean facets of ligament attachments

Casting

Underarm casts are seldom used. If postoperative immobilization is needed, TLSO is a better modality.

Operative Treatment

Position (Figs 27.274A and B)

Shoulders should not be abducted greater than 90° to prevent pressure or stretch on the brachial plexus. The pressure points should be carefully padded. The upper pads of the frame rest on the chest and not in the axilla, again to relieve pressure on any nerves from the brachial plexus.

Stagnara Wakeup Test

- Gold-standard
- The anesthesia is decreased or reversed after correction of the spinal deformity. The patient is brought to a conscious level and asked to move both the lower extremities.
- Once voluntary movement is noted, anesthesia is returned to the appropriate level and the surgical procedure is completed.

Posterior Approach (Figs 27.275 and 27.276)

Posterior fusion—principles

Extra-articular or intra-articular fusion. Intra-articular fusion techniques include the facet joints. Avascular tissue should be removed from the graft bed surface of the bone and the facets should be decorticated to provide a large maximally exposed surface area for vascular ingrowth and allow delivery of more osteoprogenitor cells. Smoking has been found to significantly inhibit fusion. Iliac crest remains the single best source of graft material, combining osteogenic, osteoconductive and osteoinductive properties. Autogenous bone from rib, obtained from a thoracoplasty can also be used.

Allografts: Paralytic scoliosis, in which large amounts of bone graft are needed and the iliac crests often are small or are used for instrumentation.

Alternatives: Tricalcium phosphate/hydroxyapatite.The farther the fusion is from the instantaneous axis of rotation, the better the fusion will prevent or minimize movement of that axis of rotation. If the fusion is performed for scoliosis and the amount of bone available is limited, concentrate the bone graft on the concave side of the curve because this bone will be subjected to compressive forces as opposed to tension forces on the convex side. Thoracolumbar and lumbar areas are the areas associated with the highest incidence of pseudarthrosis.

Spinal instrumentation

It is main role is to correct the deformity as much as possible and to stabilize the spine in the corrected position while the fusion mass becomes solid. The fusion mass in a well-corrected spine is subjected to much lower bending moments and tensile forces than the fusion mass in an uncorrected spine. Patients with a solid spinal fusion rarely have progression of their scoliosis. The purpose of instrumentation, therefore, is to lower the rate of pseudarthrosis and to improve the amount of correction obtained at the surgery. Harrington distraction rod combined with posterior arthrodesis and immobilization in a cast or brace for 6 to 9 months—standard surgical treatment for adolescent idiopathic scoliosis. Incidence of neurological injury with this technique is less than 1 percent. The rate of pseudarthrosis less than 10 percent. The major correcting force with the Harrington instrumentation is a distraction force.

Disadvantage of Harrington's (Figs 27.277A and B)

Multihook Segmental Instrumentation

Cotrel-Dubousset (CD) and Texas Scottish Rite Hospital (TSRH) systems—these systems provide multiple points of fixation to the spine and allow both compression and distraction on the same rod. Improved correction of the thoracic hypokyphosis. Preservation of lumbar lordosis when instrumentation extends into the lower lumbar spine. Improvement in the rib prominence deformity because of a derotation effect. No postoperative immobilization is required.

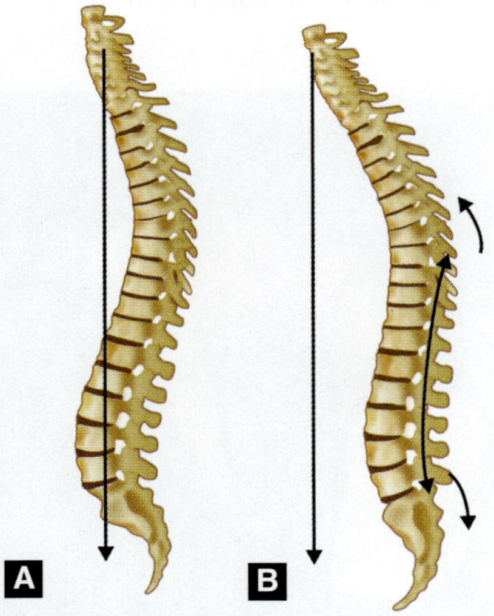

Figs 27.277A and B: Effects of distraction rod in lumbar spine. If contouring for lordosis is inadequate, lumbar spine can be flattened by distracting force. Also note kyphotic deformity just superior to distraction rod.

The basic principles are as follows:

- Distraction forces (forces directed away from the apex of the curve) decrease lordosis or contribute to kyphosis.
- Compression forces (towards the apex of the curve) decrease kyphosis or create lordosis.
- To create kyphosis, the concave side must be approached first.
- To create lordosis the convex side must be approached first, and the forces must be directed toward the apex of the curve.
- At the thoracolumbar junction, distractive forces should not be applied, and in rod bending, the lordotic bend of the rod should be initiated at the T12-L1 interspace, as shown in Figure 27.278.

Surgical Technique

Multihook Segmental Instrumentation Systems

- Exposure
- Level identification
- Hook site preparation
- Facetectomy on the side of rod insertion
- Rod contouring
- Hook insertion and placement of the first rod
- Seating of the hooks without attempting to correct the curve
- Rotation of the rod to correct the curve
- Distraction or compression of the hooks on the first rod
- Contouring of the second rod
- Facetectomy on the second side
- Insertion of the second rod

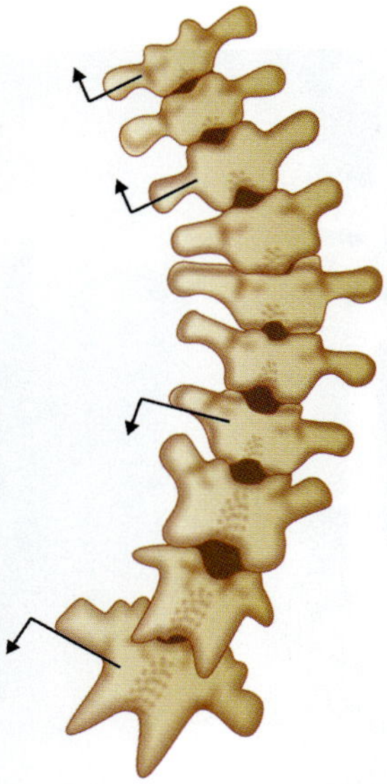

Fig. 27.278: Four-hook construct for insertion of concave rod for correction of King's type III curve without junctional kyphosis

- Distraction or compression of the hooks on the second rod
- Cross linking of the rods
- Decortication
- Placement of autogenous iliac bone graft
- Closure

Types of Hooks

There are two types of hooks: Pedicle and laminar. The pedicle hooks are designed for secure fixation in the thoracic spine by insertion into the facet and impingement on the thoracic pedicle. Pedicle hooks are used in an upgoing direction at T10 or higher vertebrae. The laminar hooks are for most other areas of the spine. These can be placed around either the superior or inferior edge of the lamina, according to the desired direction of forces.

Complications (Fig. 27.279)

- In contouring the rod, it should be remembered that the goal of the surgery is to restore normal sagittal contours.
- Excessive bending of the rod should be avoided, if possible.
- If between the rod and hook is too large, the lamina can break as the rod is being inserted into the hook. In this case it may be necessary to contour the rod further.

Pedicle Fixation

- Instrumentation that uses the pedicle as a source of purchase for bone screws from the posterior approach into the vertebral body.
- Popular form of spinal fixation.

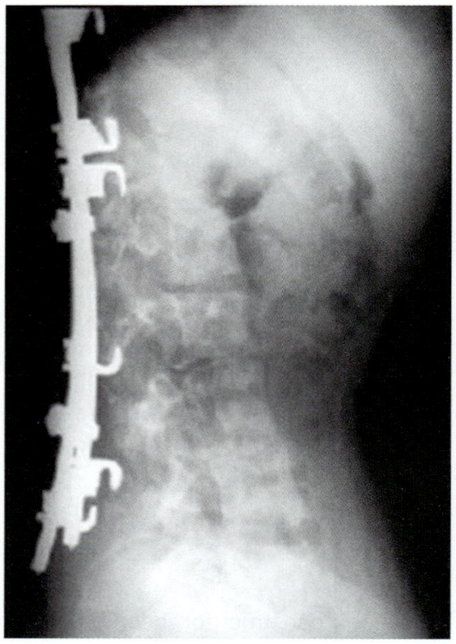

Fig. 27.279: Cut-out of lower hooks caused by improper contouring of rods

- Its role in the treatment of adolescent idiopathic scoliosis is still being debated.

Complications of Scoliosis Surgery

Early Complications

- Neurological injury
- Infection
- Ileus
- Atelectasis
- Pneumothorax
- Dural tear
- Wrong levels
- Urinary complications.

Late Complications

- Pseudarthrosis
- Loss of lumbar lordosis
- Superior mesenteric artery syndrome
- Thoracoplasty
- Of all the deformities caused by idiopathic scoliosis, the posterior rib prominence is generally the patient's main concern
- With rigid curves, the trunk does not always derotate despite current advanced multihook segmental spinal instrumentation systems
- If necessary for cosmetic or psychological reasons, resection of the convex ribs can improve the postoperative cosmetic result of the surgery, as shown in Figures 27.280 and 27.281.

Anterior Instrumentation for Idiopathic Scoliosis

Two basic types: flexible and rigid.

- *Flexible:* Zielke and Harms systems.
- *Rigid systems:* Anterior TSRH system.

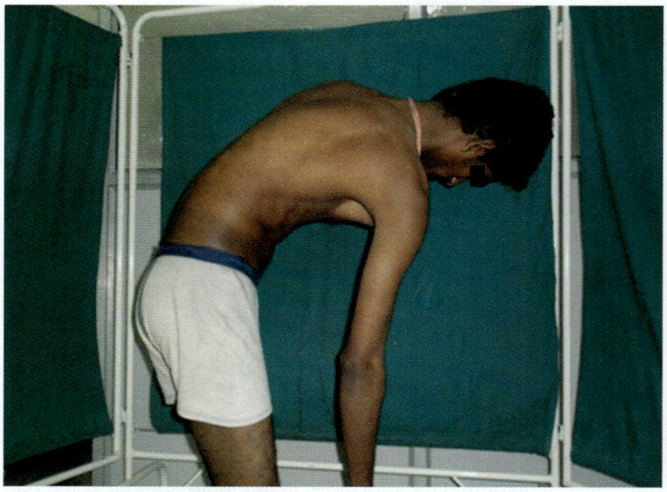

Fig. 27.280: Posterior rib prominence in adolescent patient with idiopathic scoliosis

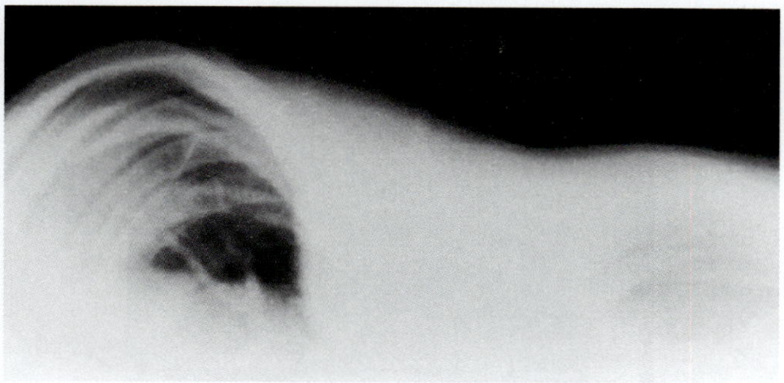

Fig. 27.281: Rib prominence on roentgenogram

In certain thoracolumbar and lumbar curves, anterior instrumentation provides better derotation and better correction of the curve in the coronal plane. Often the deformity can be corrected by fusing fewer motion segments than in the case, if the same curve was approached posteriorly. In lumbar curves, translational correction of the apical vertebra is better than that obtained with posterior multihook segmental instrumentation systems.

Criteria for Anterior Instrumentation

- Patient should not be obese.
- The curves should be flexible and should correct more than 50 percent on bending films.
- The compensatory thoracic curve above should be less than 30° and also should correct more than 50 percent on bending films.
- The fractional curve below also must be carefully evaluated and must be flexible enough to correct on bending films, as illustrated in Figures 27.282A to E.

Thoracoabdominal Approach

Figures 27.283A to D show thoracoabdominal approach.

Conclusion

- It is important to consider the etiology of the scoliosis.
- Treatment modality depends on age, degree of curve and its possibility of progression.
- Observation/orthotics/surgery.
- Posterior fusion/Harrington instrumentation/multihook segmental instrumentation/anterior instrumentation/pedicle screws.

KYPHOSIS

It is defined as the backward convexity of the spine. Kyphosis of 50° or more in the thoracic spine region is usually considered to be abnormal.

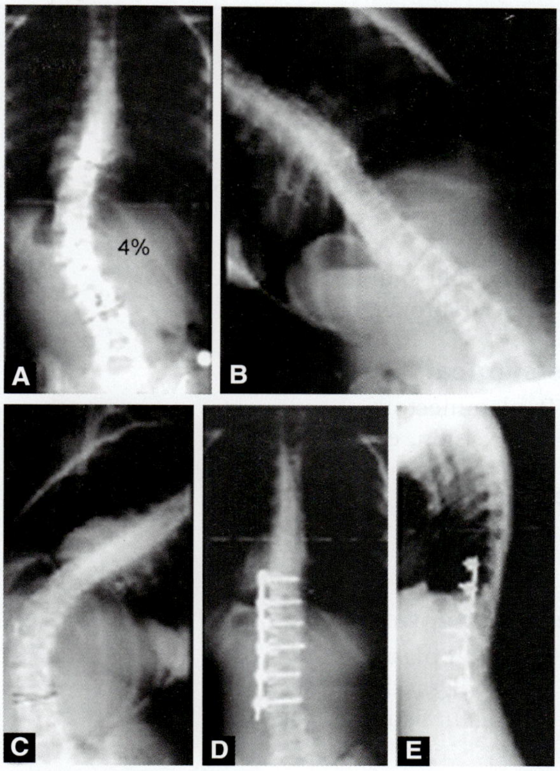

Figs 27.282A to E: (A) Flexible 43 degrees thoracic curve; (B) Correction on bending film; (C) Correction of fractional curve on bending film; (D) and (E) After anterior fusion with TSRH instrumentation

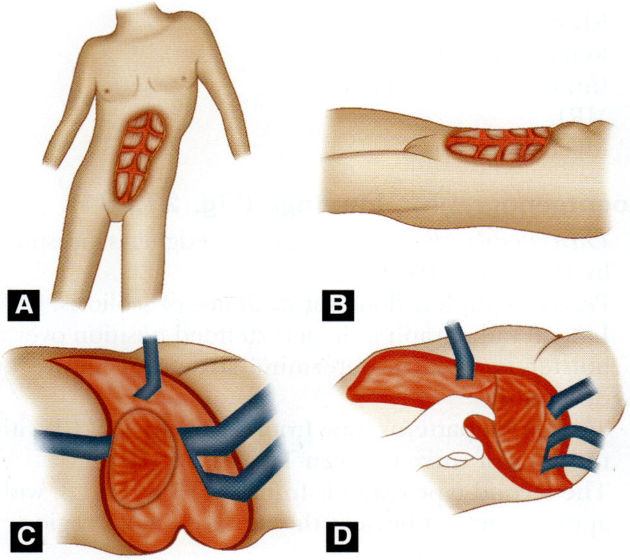

Figs 27.283A to D: (A) and (B) Skin incision for thoracolumbar approach; (C) Transthoracic detachment of diaphragm; (D) Retroperitoneal detachment of diaphragm

Causes

Congenital

- Defect of segmentation
- Defect of formation
- Mixed, e.g. Scheuermann disease
  - Postural
  - Paralytic
- Poliomyelitis (anterior horn cell)
- Upper motor neuron

Postsurgical

- Postlaminectomy
- Postexcision, e.g. tumor.

Metabolic

- Osteoporosis
- Senile.

Developmental

- Achondroplasia
- Mucopolysaccharidoses
- Osteogenesis imperfecta
- Others.

Clinical and Roentgenographic Evaluation

- Neurological evaluation
- Genitourinary abnormalities
- Cardiac anomalies
- Klippel-Feil syndrome
- Renal ultrasonography
- Intraspinal abnormalities
- MRI
- Myelogram.

Roentgenographic Findings (Fig. 27.284)

- *On a lateral radiograph:* Degree of wedging is measured by Dickson method.
- PA radiograph is done for evidence of scoliosis.
- Lateral radiograph in hyperextended position over a bolster is done to determine structural nature of deformity.
- Two curves patterns, one from T1/T2 to T12/L1 with the apex of curve between T6 and T8
- The second type extends from T4/T5 to L2/L3, with apex of curve at or near the thoracolumbar region.

Measurement of Angles

Dickson's Method

Figures 27.285A to C show Dickson's method.

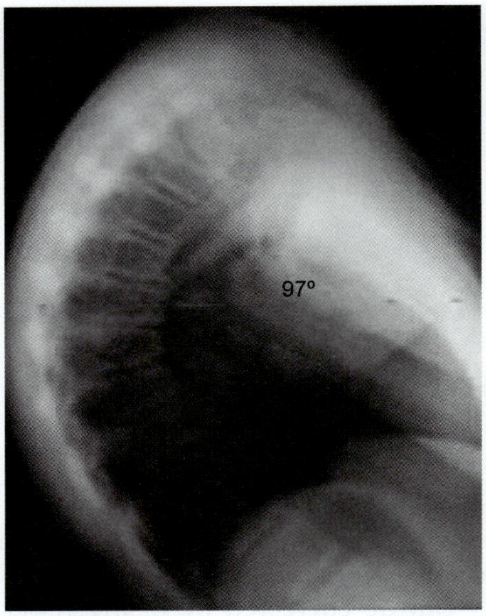

Fig. 27.284: Wedging as seen in lateral X-ray of spine

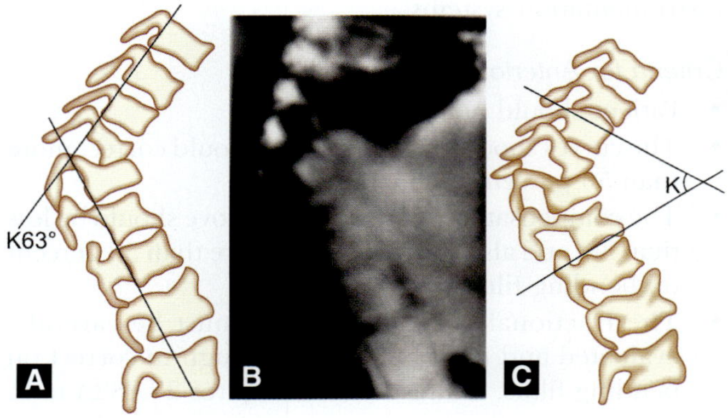

Figs 27.285A to C: A line is drawn along posterior margins of bodies of healthy vertebra, both above and below. Alternatively, lines are drawn along superior and inferior end-plates of each vertebral body and the angle of intersection is measured

Treatment

Nonoperative Treatment

Observation for four to six months with repeat lateral radiograph until the growth is complete. Exercises are not effective, but can help to maintain flexibility, correct lumber lordosis and strengthen extensors muscles of spine. Thoracic type with more than 50° is managed by Milwaukee brace. Boston lumbar kyphosis orthosis is used for correction of curves less than 70°.

Operative Treatment

Operative treatment is necessary as treatment of congenital kyphosis with an orthosis is ineffective. Operative mainly depend upon severity of deformity, age and presence or absence of neurological symptoms. Anterior release with posterior instrumentation and fusion is generally done. Currently posterior double rod, multihook segmental instrumentation systems are most commonly used.

SPINA BIFIDA

Introduction

Spina bifida is a congenital defect, which affects the spinal column. It is the most common amongst the group of birth defects, known as neural tube defects, which affect the central nervous system (brain and spinal cord), as shown in Figures 27.286 and 27.287.

Development of Spinal Cord (Fig. 27.288)

- Neural grooves start appearing on third-fourth weeks of intrauterine life (IUL)
- Deepens into furrow and closes off to form the neural canal, which later develops entire CNS
- The lumen persists, as central spinal canal. Canal separated from the ectodermal covering of the body, by an ingrowth of mesoderm
- Meninges arises from loose mesenchymal tissues
- Anterior to the neural canal is a solid rod of cells called notochord
- Around the notochord the vertebral bodies develop, as depicted in Figure 27.289.
- Two projections from each body, extending backwards to form vertebral arch.

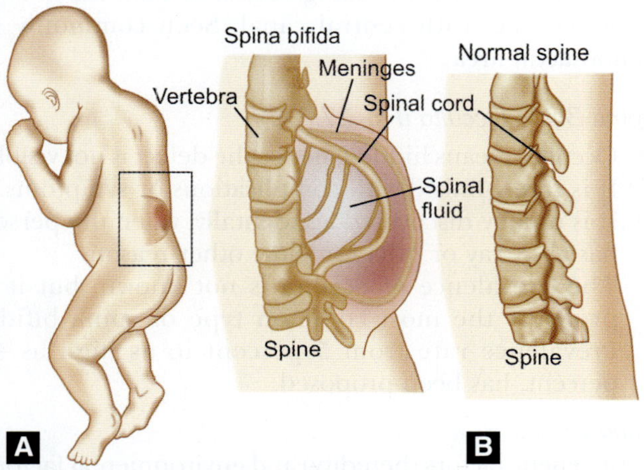

Figs 27.286A and B: (A) Spina bifida with its external and internal presentation; (B) Normal spine

- Two-halves of the arch fuse behind in the thoracic region and extend up and down the spine.
- When this fusion fails, there is a gap in vertebral neural arch, which is called "spina bifida"
- Most commonly in lumbosacral region.

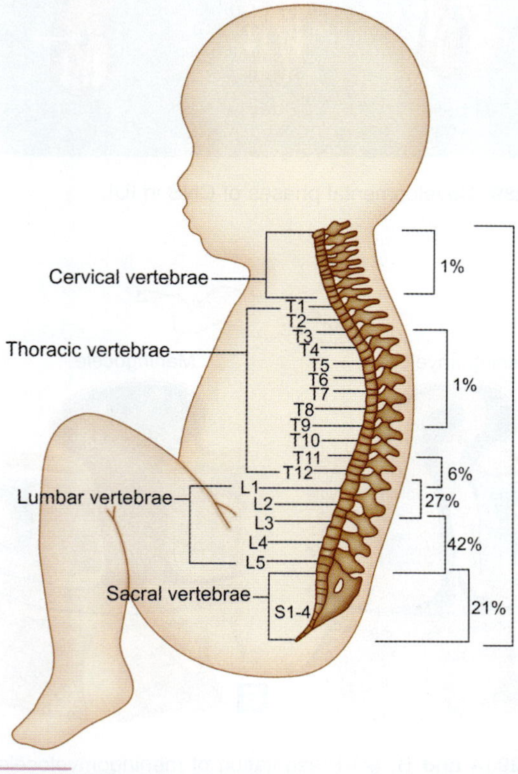

Fig. 27.287: The levels of lesion and frequency of spina bifida at various levels

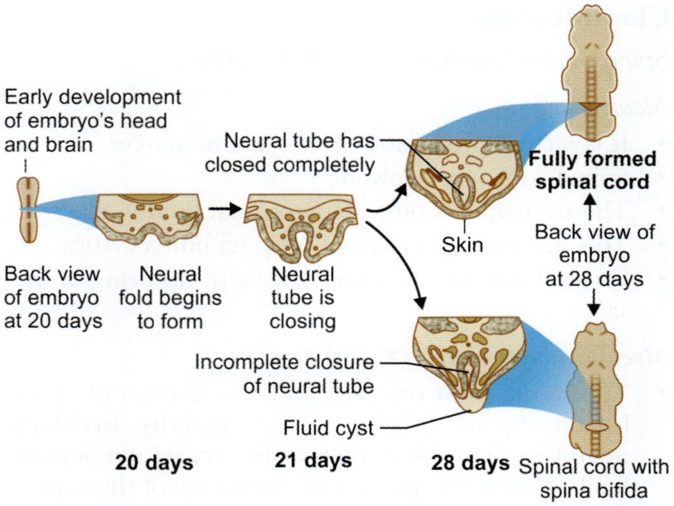

Fig. 27.288: Comparison of the development of a fully formed spinal cord, which shows spina bifida. Note the fluid cyst and open skin overlying the open neural tube in the case of spina bifida

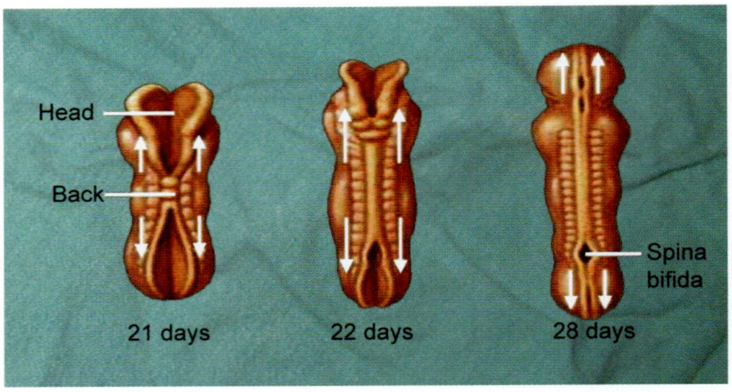

Fig. 27.289: Developmental phases of CNS in IUL

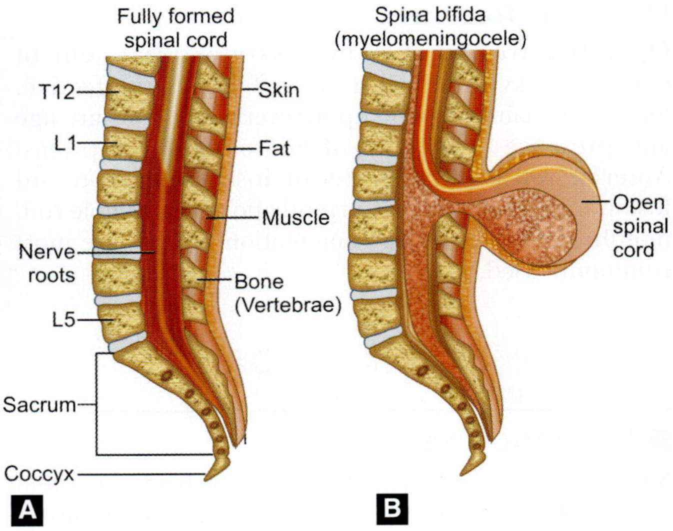

Figs 27.291A and B: Side views of spinal cord—(A) A fully formed spinal cord; (B) Myelomeningocele, with open neural tube, that may protrude in case of spina bifida

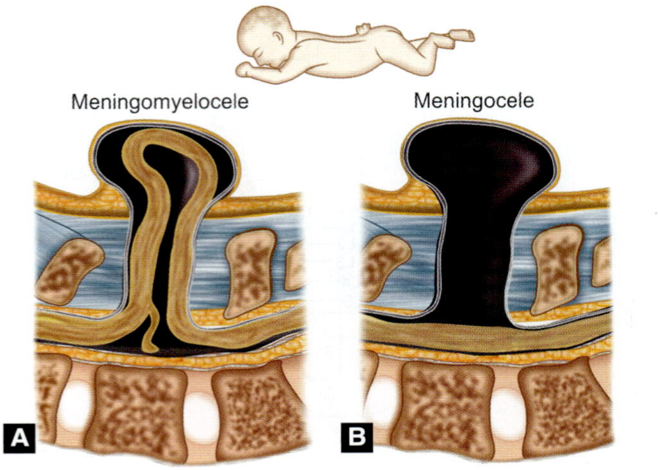

Figs 27.290A and B: (A) Presentation of meningomyelocele; (B) Meningocele (It is sacular protrusion of only the meninges)

Classification

Spina Bifida Cystica (Figs 27.290A and B)

Meningocele

- It is sacular protrusion of only the meninges.
- Spinal cord not involved.
- The sac contains only cerebrospinal fluid (CSF).
- This makes only 5 percent of spina bifida cystica.
- Surgical closure is required to avoid rupturing of the sac.

Myelomeningocele (Figs 27.291A and B)

- This is the most complex and severe form of spina bifida. Spina bifida cystica, usually involves neurological problems that can be very serious or even fatal. Ninety-five percent of cystica are of this type.
- Most infants with an open spine or myelomeningocele, undergo surgery within the first 48 hours of life, to close the defect. Antibiotics are given to prevent infection of the exposed spinal cord and nerves, until these structures can be protected by surgery.
- Before antibiotics were available, most children born with myelomeningocele died soon after birth. Those who survived, become severely disabled.
- With modern treatment, almost all children with myelomeningocele survive and most are able to live productive lives, with some degree of independence.

Syringomyelocele

In this spinal cord spreads out to form the lining of the sac and is thinned into cyst, by distension of central canal of the cord.

Myelocele

Presence of gross spinal cord deformity and elongated fissure, surrounded by telangiectasia or hair, which is in direct contact with central canal. Seen commonly in lumbosacral area.

Spina Bifida Occulta (Fig. 27.292)

- Occulta, means hidden, hence the defect is not visible.
- It is rarely linked with complications or symptoms.
- It is usually discovered accidentally, when the person has an X-ray or MRI for some other reason.
- The prevalence of occulta is not known, but it is probably the most common type of spina bifida. Prevalence rate from 5 percent to as high as 40 percent, has been proposed.

Causes

Both genetic factors (heredity) and environmental factors, such as nutrition and exposure to harmful substances, probably contribute to spina bifida. Spina bifida does seem to run in families, although with mixed patterns of

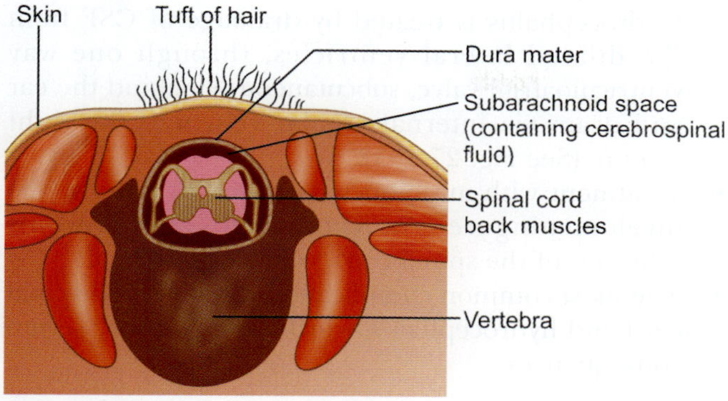

Fig. 27.292: Internal and external presentation of spina bifida occulta

inheritance. Having a child with spina bifida increases the chance that another child will also have spina bifida, to about eight times. Research has suggested that many cases of spina bifida can be prevented, by adequate intake of folic acid (folate) before and during early pregnancy. However, people with spina bifida, appear to have abnormal metabolism of folic acid. This suggests that the underlying problem in spina bifida may be an inborn defect in folic acid metabolism.

Clinical picture

- Spina bifida occulta, is rarely produces any symptoms. Occasionaly, local pigmented hairy patch.
- Patient with myelomeningocele has partial or total paraplegia, depending upon the level of the lesion.
- *Complete paralysis above L1:* No deformity of the legs develop, but patient is unlikely to walk independently.
- *Incomplete paralysis:* Deformity due to unbalanced paralysis, which progresses with growth.
- Dislocation of hip, with knee and foot deformities.
- Loss of sensation in the legs.
- Eighty percent of patient with hydrocephalus, secondary to Arnold-Chiari malformation (Figs 27.293 and 27.294).
- Urinary incontinence, urinary stasis and bladder dilatation, leads to hydronephrosis.
- Death can occur, due to back pressure and pylonephrosis.
- Many children with myelomeningocele, have or develop a tethered spinal cord.
- The cord is attached to the surrounding tissues and cannot move up and down freely, as it normally does. This can cause foot or leg deformities, hip dislocation or scoliosis. The problems can worsen as the child grows and the tethered cord is stretched.
- Obesity (due to inactivity).
- Pathologic bone fractures occur in as many as 25 percent of people with spina bifida.

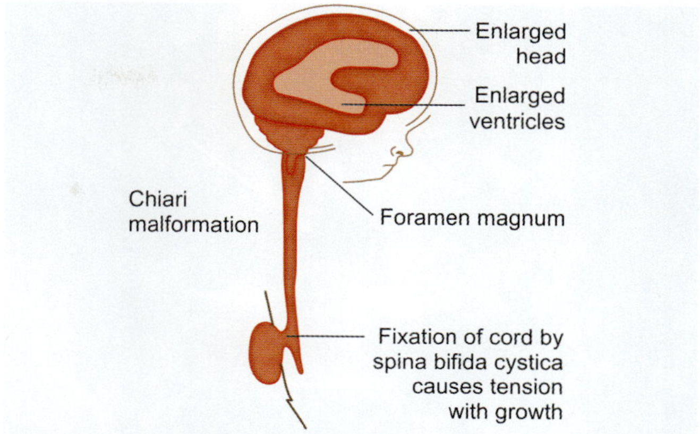

Fig. 27.293: Spina bifida with hydrocephalus, secondary to chiari malformation and secondary to fixation to cord by spina bifida cystic

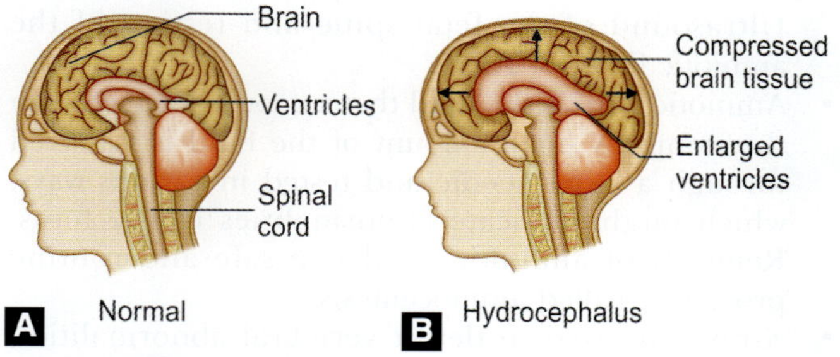

Figs 27.294A and B: Compression of brain tissues, due to hydrocephalus

- Psychological, social and sexual problems occur more often in people with spina bifida, than in the general population.
- Allergy to latex is very common in people with spina bifida. An allergic reaction to latex can be life threatening.

Subtle signs

- Have a dimple, darkening or small hairy patch on the skin, overlying the base of the spine.
- Others have a fatty growth called an epidural lipoma, which is formed within the spinal canal. This is usually harmless, but may result in tethering of the spinal cord.

Investigations

- A prenatal test measures the level of maternal serum alpha-fetoprotein (MSAFP or AFP), which is usually high in women carrying a fetus with spina bifida or other neural tube defect.
- Any pregnant woman, who has a high level of AFP, should undergo two additional tests that are very

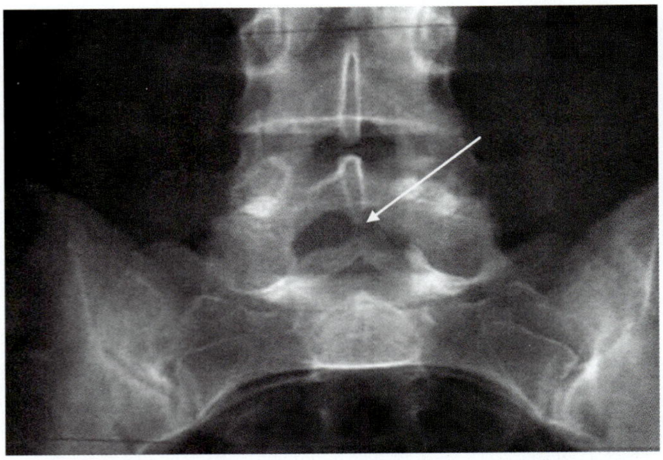

Fig. 27.295: X-ray of lower spine, showing spina bifida (arrow)

accurate in detecting severe spina bifida, these are: Ultrasound of the fetal spine and testing of the amniotic fluid for AFP.

- Amniotic fluid is the fluid that surrounds the fetus in the womb. A small amount of the fluid is removed through a large needle and tested in various ways, which might indicate abnormalities in the fetus. Removal of amniotic fluid is a safe and routine procedure called amniocentesis.
- X-rays are used to detect vertebral abnormalities, scoliosis, hip deformities, pathologic fractures and other bony abnormalities that are common and may or may not cause pain and other symptoms in spina bifida, as shown in Figure 27.295.
- Ultrasound may be used to assess an area of pain that suggests pathologic fracture. Sensitivity is 96 to 100 percent, specifity is 30 to 80 percent.
- CT scan of the head is used to evaluate for hydrocephalus.
- MRI provides the best detailed information on spinal cord abnormalities and the extent of cord and nerve root involvement.

Treatment

Combined management for following problems:

- – Myelomeningocele
- – Hydrocephalus
- – Urinary tract paralysis
- – Locomotor system
- – Education.

- Surgical closure of myelomeningocele within 48 hours after birth.
- Neural plaque, cord and nerve root are isolated and plaque is covered by suturing the dura over its surface.
- Skin closuring.
- After 2 to 3 weeks, air ventriculography is done, to assess presence and severity of hydrocephalus.
- Hydrocephalus is treated by drainage of CSF from the dilated lateral ventricles, through one way ventriculoatrial valve, subcutaneously behind the ear and drain via internal jugular vein into the right atrium, (See Fig. 27.293).
- Treatment with antibiotics is started as soon as the myelomeningocele is recognized. This prevents infection of the spinal cord, which can be fatal.
- The most common complications are tethered spinal cord and hydrocephalus, which can have very severe consequences.

Bowel bladder care

- Intermittent catheterization is helpful.
- Urinanalysis, intravenous pylography, estimation of plasma, urea and electrolytes is necessary.
- In males, urine retention with over flow is managed by fitting penile appliance.
- In females, bladder neck resection or urinary diversion.
- Orthopedic management of myelomeningocele.
- Unbalanced paralysis at different levels, leads to paralytic deformities in lower limb.
- Sharrard, classified the neurological defect in patients with myelomeningocele into six groups, according to the neurological level of paralysis. He also correlated the radiological state of the hip and the deformities of knees and feet, with lower limit of innervation.
- Three factors require for correction at hip.
  - – Adductor overactivity and contracture.
  - – Flexor overactivity.
  - – Valgus deformity of the femoral neck.

Neurological sequelae level

- T12 total flaccidity, postural deformity only
- L1 or L2 moderate hip flexor and adduct hip subluxation, occasional dislocation
- L3 or L4 hip flexors and adductor normal quadricep, hip extenxors and abductors paralysed dislocation of hip, recurvatum of knee
- L5 hip flexors, adductors and quadriceps normal hip exten paralysed, abductors moderate 50 percent hip have subluxation
- S1 or S2 hip exten weak other N. Hip stable normal no deformity.

Medical treatment

Children should be watched for signs of hydrocephalus, tethered spinal cord, seizure activity, obesity, bowel and/or bladder control problems, frequent urinary tract infections, learning disorders, emotional and psychosocial problems and other complications of spine. Despite, this assistance, some children with spina bifida will never be able to walk independently. These children will use a wheelchair for the rest of their lives. Parents should work with a physical therapist to learn how to exercise the baby's legs, to maximize strength and movement. They should begin these exercises soon after the first surgery. It will prevents osteoporosis due to disuse. Many children can become mobile, by wearing a brace or using crutches or an orthotic. These devices allow the child to function at the best possible level, by helping with balance, posture and control.

Other therapy

A child's emotional and social development can be deeply affected by physical disabilities, such as spina bifida. Children should be in the least restrictive environment. They should learn skills that help them to be as independent as possible. They should be encouraged to take on responsibility for their own care as much as possible. After childhood, group homes may be used to train patients with spina bifida to live independently.

Follow-up

- People with spina bifida should be seen frequently, for checking progressing deformities, disabilities or complications that may require intervention.
- The effectiveness of their physical therapy, including their braces, orthotics, crutches and wheelchair, should be checked often and changes made, if necessary.
- Development of hydrocephalus or worsening of deformities warrants the attention of the appropriate surgeon.
- Medical complications, such as obesity or urinary tract infection require appropriate treatment. The goal is to prevent secondary chronic complications, such as heart disease, diabetes and kidney problems.

Prevention

The only known way to prevent spina bifida and other neural tube defects is for the mother to have adequate folic acid levels, before and during early pregnancy. This does not work in all cases, but studies have shown that as many as 70 percent of cases of severe spina bifida could be prevented by adequate folic acid intake. Besides, fortified foods, other good sources of folic acid include dark green leafy vegetables (for example, broccoli, spinach, dark green lettuce, etc.) egg yolks, beans, whole grains, orange juice and citrus fruits.

TUBERCULOSIS OF THE SPINE

Introduction

- Tuberculosis disease of the spine is caused by *Mycobacterium tuberculosis.*
- "Tuber" in Latin means degenerative protuberances or tubercles.
- Phthisis is the Greek word for pulmonary disease.
- *Other names:* Include scrofula, tabes, hectic fever, gastric fever or great white plague (consumption).
- Tubercle bacilli are red bacilli seen in this microscopic specimen.

History

Mycobacterium tuberculosis has infected humans for thousands of years. Spinal column of Egyptian mummies from 2400 BCE, show signs of tubercular decay. In 460 BCE Hippocrates identified "phthisis" (Greek for consumption) as the most prevalent disease of the era, killing almost all who were infected and very contagious in the late stages. He warned physicians, not to visit their patients in the late stages.

Epidemiology

- The most common causative organism for spinal tuberculosis is *Mycobacterium tuberculosis.*
- The practice of boiling of milk before consumption has limited the disease caused by *Mycobacterium bovis. Mycobacterium africanum* is geographically limited to north-west Africa.
- Topographically, spinal tuberculosis constitutes about half the cases of skeletal tuberculosis.
- The dorsal spine is involved in half of the cases of spinal tuberculosis. The disease is always secondary to a primary visceral focus which may be in the lungs, lymph nodes or kidneys.
- Incidence of tuberculosis of the spine forms 50 to 60 percent of the total incidence of skeletal tuberculosis.
- It is a disease of childhood and adolescence, where 50 percent of the cases occur in the age group of 1 to 20 years. The most common level of the lesion is in the thoracolumbar level as shown in Figure 27.296
- This is because movement and the stress of weight bearing are maximum at this level. The proximity of the cysterna chyli may cause lymphatic spread of the infection from foci in the mesenteric lymph glands.
- Tuberculosis is still a major health problem in developing countries.
- In India nearly two million people develop active disease every year.
- In India—half a million die from this disease every year.
- It is predicted that in first decade of 21st century worldwide, greater than 15 million people and more than 4 million in India would die from tuberculosis.
- Spread of HIV has led to high prevalence of tuberculosis and *Mycobacterium avium* complex (MAC) infection among these patients as depicted in Tables 27.9 and 27.10.

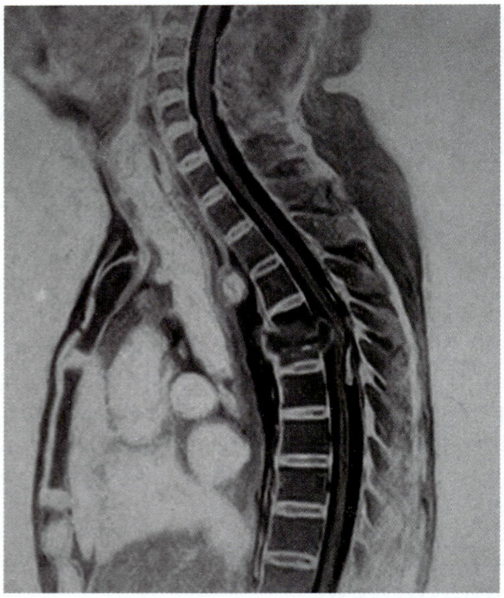

Fig. 27.296: Tuberculosis lesion in thoracolumbar area

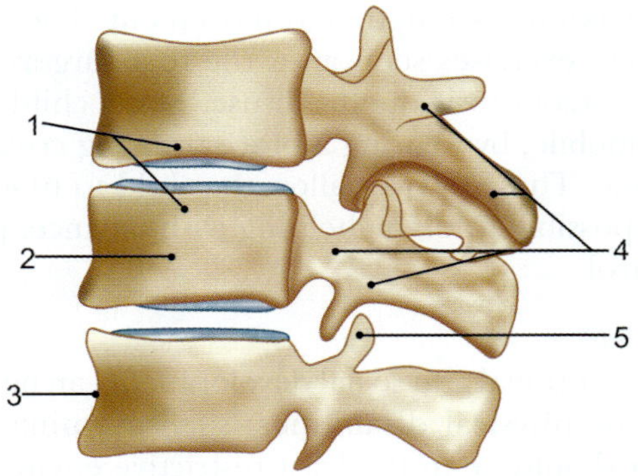

Fig. 27.297: Diagrammatic representation of the frequency of location of tuberculosis of the vertebral column—1. Paradiscal region; 2. Central body region; 3. Anterior vertebral region; 4. Appendicial lesion in the pedicle, lamina, transverse process and spinous process; 5. Articular lesion in the posterior intervertebral joint

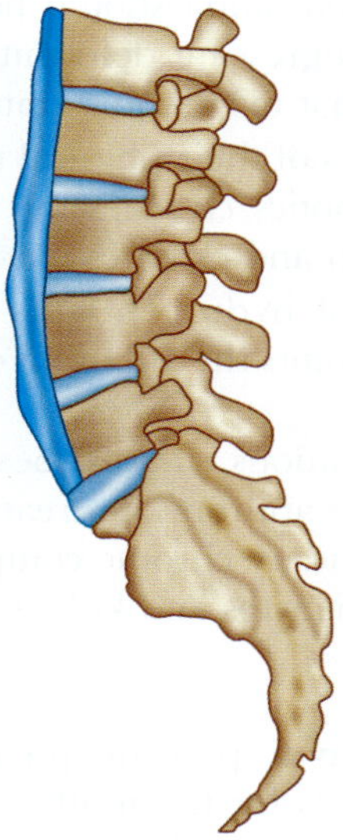

Fig. 27.298: Normal vertebrae (lateral view)

Table 27.9: Age distribution among male and female patients having vertebral tuberculosis

Age in years	*Percentage of patients*		
	Male	*Female*	*Total*
1 to 10	20	9	29
11 to 20	11	12	23
21 to 30	7	14	21
31 to 40	4	6	10
41 to 50	3	5	8
51 to 60	4	1	5
61 to 70	3	-	3
71 to 80	-	1	1
	52%	48%	

Table 27.10: Regional distribution of tuberculous lesions in vertebral column—expressed as percentage

Cervical (including atlanto-occipital)	12
Cervicodorsal	5
Dorsal	42
Dorsolumbar	12
Lumbar	26
Lumbosacral (including sacrum)	3

Pathology (Figs 27.297 to 27.301)

A minimum time lag of two to three years is present between the development of primary focus and manifestation of the disease in the spine. The bacteria may reach the spine through the arterial circulation or the Batson's plexus of veins. Initially, two contiguous vertebral bodies are involved due to a common vascular supply. Destruction of vertebral bodies compromises the nutrition of the intervertebral disk and leads to progressive disk destruction and vertebral collapse. The disease affects the spine secondarily from a primary focus in the lungs or mediastinal glands through the blood stream. The focus in the spine may be found in one of the following sites:

- Paradiscal lesion in the subchondral area of the vertebral body
- Central body lesion in the center of the vertebral body
- Anterior type in the anterior surface of the vertebral
- Appendicial lesion in the pedicle, lamina, transverse process and spinous process
- Articular lesion in the posterior intervertebral joint.

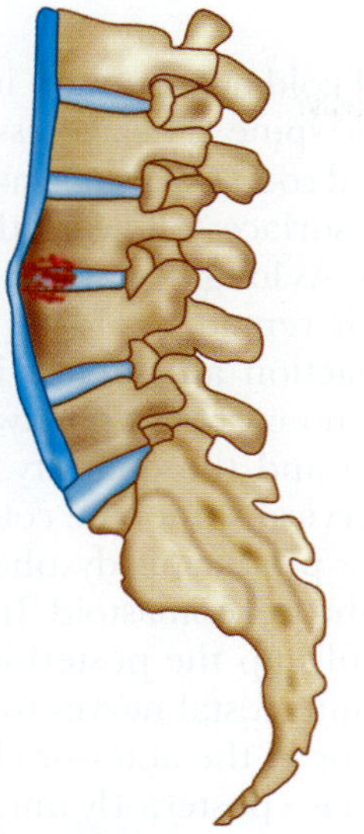

Fig. 27.299: Paradiscal tubercular lesion

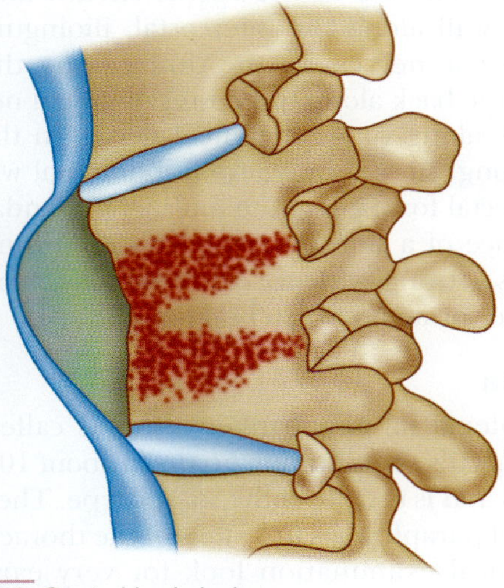

Fig. 27.300: Central body lesion

The lesion soon destroys the intervertebral disk and the adjacent surfaces of the vertebral bodies which slowly collapse and obliterate the intervertebral space. Destruction of the framework of the vertebral bodies results in their collapse and the development of an angular kyphosis called gibbus. The disease commonly involves two vertebrae, but in children it can rapidly destroy three or more vertebrae and cause gross deformities. The histological changes in the bone are typical of the tuberculous lesions elsewhere. Spreading caseation, results in osteolysis of the bony trabeculae, leading to the formation of cold abscess. Tuberculoma: compared to the total incidence of spinal tuberculosis, tuberculoma formation in the spinal cord is a rare phenomenon; it presents like an intramedullary spinal tumor causing cord compression and paraplegia.

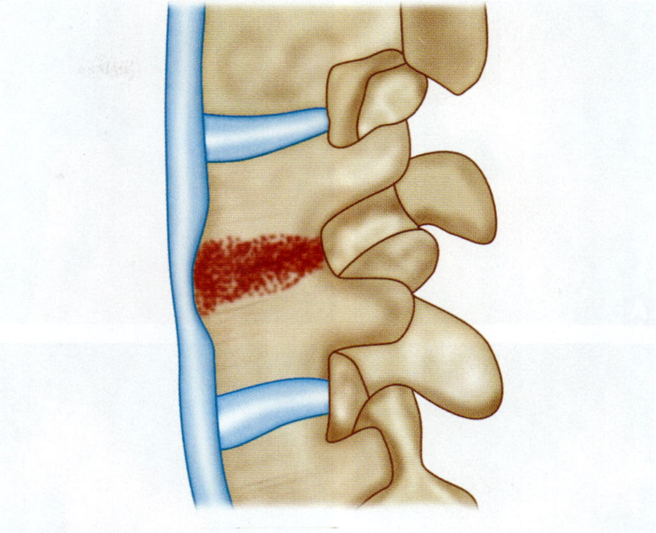

Fig. 27.301: Anterior vertebral region

Table 27.11: Clinical features of spinal tuberculosis (expressed as percentage)	
Clinical kyphosis	95
Palpable cold abscesses	20
Radiological perivertebral abscesses	21
Tuberculous sinuses (active/healed)	13
Associated extraspinal skeletal foci	12
Associated visceral or glandular foci	12
Neurological involvement	20
Lateral shift (radiological)	5
Skipped lesion in the spine	7

Clinical Features (Table 27.11)

The classical symptoms of tuberculosis of the spine as described by Percival Pott are as follows:

- Pain
- Rigidity
- Deformity
- Cold abscess
- Paraplegia.

Pain

It will be localized by the patient to one region of the spine. Localized tenderness over one vertebral spine is diagnostic of the level of the lesion. The disease can also present as referred pain. Disease in the cervical spine can present as pain in the ear or pain down the arm. Upper thoracic spine lesion can present as pain in the chest and as intercostal neuralgia. Lower thoracic

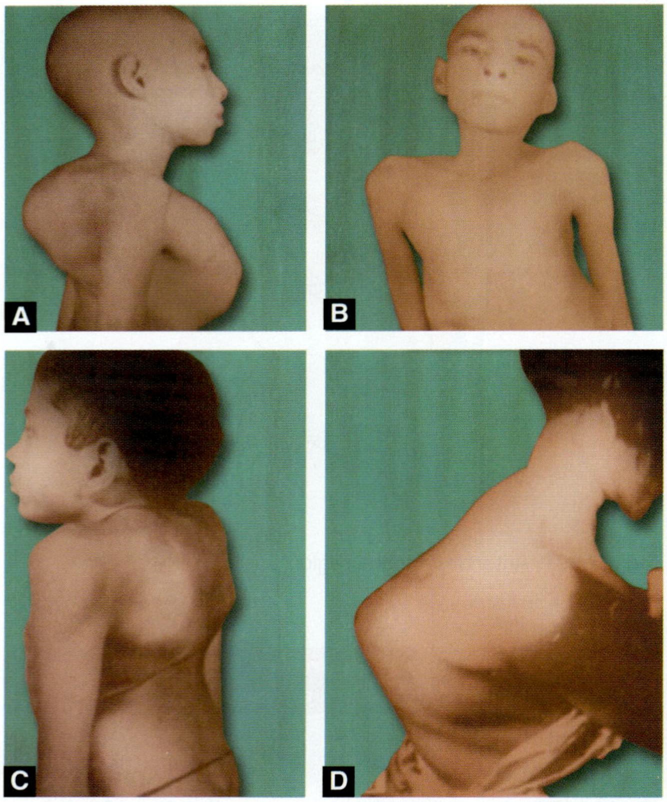

Figs 27.302A to D: Spinal deformities as outcome of tuberculosis lesions in spine

spine can cause referred pain in the abdomen. Whenever, a patient presents with pain in the back, examine the front by palpating the abdomen to detect a psoas abscess, aneurysm of the aorta or even a peptic ulcer.

Rigidity

It is caused by the spasm of the paraspinal muscles due to the disease in the spine. A cervical lesion causes rigidity of the neck which at times may be asymmetrical producing torticollis. In lumbar lesions, there is marked rigidity of the back and the spine moves in one piece when the patient attempts to bend forward. This is demonstrated by the coin test. The patient is asked to pick up a coin from the floor. He bends at the knee and hip and picks up the coin holding the spine rigid and straight all the time.

Deformity (Figs 27.302 and See Fig. 27.285)

In the cervical and lumbar spine the loss of the normal lordosis occurs first followed by the gibbus. In the thoracic spine angular kyphosis (gibbus) is characteristic. The prominence of gibbus depends on the number of the vertebrate involved. Gross kyphosis is seen in children when a number of dorsal vertebrae are destroyed.

Cold Abscess

The formation of cold abscess is an invariable feature of tuberculosis of the spine. The abscess forms in the paravertebral areas and soon tracks downwards due to gravity and towards the surface following the tracks of nerves and blood vessels. As long as the abscess remains deep to the deep fascia it remains cold to touch without any inflammatory reaction and hence it is called as cold abscess. There is no correlation between the size of the destructive lesion and the quantity of pus in the cold abscess. In the cervical spine, the cold abscess can point retropharyngeally producing dysphagia or show up in the neck behind the sternomastoid. In the thoracic spine, the cold abscess fills up the posterior mediastinum and tracks along the intercostal nerves to point either in the lateral chest wall or in the anterior chest wall. Abscesses also reach the surface posteriorly under the sacrospinalis muscles. The cold abscess sometimes enters the spinal canal causing pressure on the spinal cord, resulting in paraplegia. Involvement of the dorsolumbar spine may lead to cold abscess in the rectus sheath and lower abdominal wall along the intercostal, ilioinguinal and iliohypogastric nerves. In the thigh along the psoas sheath. In the back along the posterior spinal nerves. In the buttock along superior gluteal nerve. In the Petit's triangle along the flat muscles of abdominal wall or in the ischiorectal fossa along the internal pudendal nerve. The presence of a sinus in the back with a thin watery discharge is a strong evidence of tuberculous involvement of the posterior arch of vertebral bodies.

Paraplegia

The paraplegia in spinal tuberculosis is called 'Pott's paraplegia'. This complication occurs in about 10 percent of the cases and is usually of the spastic type. The highest incidence of paraplegia is in lesions of the thoracic spine. In the clinical examination look for very early signs pressure on the cord, like slight spasticity of the legs causing unsteady gait, exaggerated knee and ankle jerks and extensor plantar response. Depending on the severity of the paralysis, paraplegia is graded as grade I, II and III. 'grade I' being a partial paralysis (paresis) and 'grade III' being a total paraplegia.

Pott's Paraplegia

Pott's paraplegia is classified into two types.

1. Early onset paraplegia occurring during the active stage of the disease.
2. Late onset paraplegia occurring in patients whom lesion has reactivated after long years of quiescence.

The early onset paraplegia: The early onset paraplegia is due to the pressure on the cord by the following:

- Granulation tissue necrotic debris and sequestra from the bone or the intervertebral disk tissue

Table 27.12: Classification of tuberculous paraplegia/tetraplegia (predominantly based upon motor weakness) due to compression of cord and not cauda equina		
Stage		***Clinical features***
I	Negligible	Patient unaware of neural deficit, physician detects plantar extensor and/or ankle clonus
II	Mild	Patient aware of deficit but manages to walk with support
III	Moderate	Nonambulatory because of paralysis (in extension) sensory deficit less than 50%
IV	Severe	III+Flexor spasms/paralysis in flexion/flaccid/sensory deficit more than 50%/sphincters involved

Applicable to compression of cord and not cauda equina.

- Occasionally, a vascular thrombosis of the spinal arteries which produces a sudden total paraplegia.

■ Spinal Cord Tumor Syndrome

A rare type, is the gradual onset of paraplegia due to a granulomatous mass developing inside the spinal cord. Classification of tuberculous paraplegia/tetraplegia (Table 27.12).

Causes

Table 27.13 shows usual causeds of neurological complications in caries spine.

Table 27.13: Usual causes of neurological complications in caries spine	
Inflammatory	
• Inflammatory edema	Recovers by rest and drug therapy
• Tuberculous granulation tissue	Mostly recovers by rest and drug therapy
• Tuberculous abscess	Recovers by conservative therapy rarely requires evacuation and decompression
• Tuberculous caseous tissue	May subside by conservative therapy; sometimes requires evacuation and decompression
Mechanical	
• Tubercular debris	Solid debris requires operative removal and decompression
• Sequestra from vertebral body and disk	Require operative removal and decompression
• Constriction of cord due to stenosis of vertebral canal	Requires operative decompression
• Localized pressure due to salient (internal gibbus) along anterior wall of vertebral canal	Requires operative decompression
Intrinsic	
• Prolonged stretching of the cord over a sever deformity	• Stretched cord may be more vulnerable to other causes, them decompression, release or cord, and anterior transposition may lead to recovery
	• Rarely stretching leads to interstitial gliosis or atrophy of cord (may be visualized by myelo-CT and/or by MRI) which does not recover completely
• Infective thrombosis/endarteritis of spinal vessels	Difficult to prove/disprove, does not recover appreciably
• Pathological dislocation of spine	Rare complication, usually results from rough manipulation by masseur or indiscriminate laminectomy for caries spine; irreparable severance of cord
• Tuberculous meningomyelitis	Difficult to prove/disprove; myelitis does not recover completely
• Syringomyelic changes	Seen on MRI; poor recovery
Spinal tumor syndrome	
• Diffuse extradural granuloma or tuberculoma or peridural fibrosis	Present as spinal tumor syndrome, surgical approach is by laminectomy

Diagnosis

- No laboratory test is diagnostic.
- Antibody testing is unreliable as immunity is cell mediated.
- PCR test, it is not so specific as per recent reports.
- MR imaging cannot be diagnostic in most of the cases.

Laboratory Studies

- Tuberculin skin test (purified protein derivative (PPD) demonstrates a positive finding in 84 to 95 percent of patients who are non-HIV-positive.
- Erythrocyte sedimentation rate (ESR) may be markedly elevated (>100 mm/h).
- *Microbiology studies to confirm diagnosis:* Obtain bone tissue or abscess samples to stain for acid-fast bacilli (AFB) and isolate organisms for culture and susceptibility.
- CT-guided procedures can be used to guide percutaneous sampling of affected bone or soft tissue structures. These study findings may be positive in only about 50 percent of the cases.

Imaging Studies

Radiographic changes present relatively late. Plain radiography demonstrates the following characteristic changes of spinal tuberculosis:

- Lytic destruction of anterior portion of vertebral body
- Increased anterior wedging
- Collapse of vertebral body
- Reactive sclerosis on a progressive lytic process
- Enlarged psoas shadow with or without calcification.

Additional Findings

- Vertebral end-plates are osteoporotic
- Intervertebral disks may be shrunk or destroyed
- Vertebral bodies show variable degrees of destruction
- Fusiform paravertebral shadows suggest abscess formation
- Bone lesions may occur at more than one level.

Radiological Features

- The earliest radiological sign is the narrowing of the intervertebral disk space
- Later, there is erosion of the adjacent surfaces of the vertebral bodies
- Still later, there is destruction and collapse of the vertebral bodies with obliteration of the intervertebral space. Para or prevertebral soft tissue shadows of the abscess may also be present which may be calcified
- Sound healing usually ends in bony fusion of adjacent vertebrae. Neglected cases in children result in gross kyphotic deformities.

CT Scanning

- CT scanning provides much better bony detail of irregular lytic lesions, sclerosis, disk collapse and disruption of bone circumference
- Low-contrast resolution provides a better assessment of soft tissue, particularly in epidural and paraspinal areas
- It detects early lesions and is more effective for defining the shape and calcification of soft tissue abscesses
- In contrast to pyogenic disease, calcification is common in tuberculous lesions.

MRI

MRI is the criterion standard for evaluating disk space infection and osteomyelitis of the spine and is most effective for demonstrating the extension of disease into soft tissues and the spread of tuberculous debris under the anterior and posterior longitudinal ligaments. MRI is most effective for demonstrating neural compression.

Atypical presentations: They may be missed.

Early lesions: They are generally difficult to interpret. Recurrence and reactivation are difficult to diagnose on MRI after surgery, as shown in Figure 27.303 and Table 27.14.

Clinicoradiological classification of typical tubercular-spondylitis (Table 27.15).

Other Tests

- Radionuclide scanning is not useful
- Gallium and bone scans have a high false-negative rate of 70 percent and 35 percent, respectively.

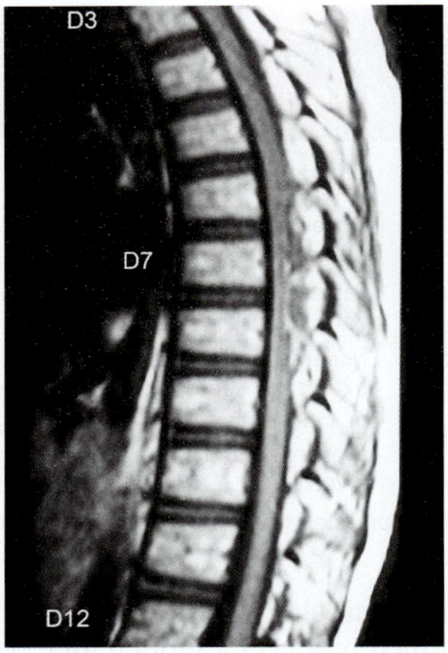

Fig. 27.303: MRI of spine (T2 image), showing early tubercular lesions

Table 27.14: Characteristics of different T_1 and T_2, MRI images

Tissue/fluids	*T_1 image*	*T_2 image*
Fat in marrow or cancellous bone or degenerated areas	White	Grayish-white
Muscles	Gray	Gray
CSF or clear fluid or water in tissues	Black	White
White matter brain/spine	Dark gray	Gray
Gray matter brain/spine	Blackish	Whitish gray
Granulation tissue	Gray	Whitish gray
Air	Black irregular	Black irregular
Bone	Black	Black
Flowing blood	Black	Black
Ligament or capsule (mature fibrous tissue)	Black line/band	Black line/band
Cord contusion or edema (myelitis)	Dark gray	Whitish
Prevertebral hematoma	White (Subacute stage)	Whitish
Ischemic/necrosed/ sequestrated bone	Gray dead bone surrounded by black zone	Gray dead bone surrounded by white zone
Syrinx	Black cavity in cord	White cavity in cord
Myelomalacia	Dark	White
Nucleus pulposus hydated	Black/gray	White
Nucleus pulposus desiccated	Black	Black

Procedures: Use a percutaneous CT-guided needle biopsy of bone lesions to obtain tissue samples. Percutaneous needle biopsy is not diagnostic. This is a safe procedure that also allows therapeutic drainage of large paraspinal abscesses. Obtain a tissue sample for microbiology and

Table 27.15: Clinicoradiological classification of typical tubercular-spondylitis

Stage	*Clinicoradiological features*	*Usual duration*
I. Predestructive	Straightening of curvatures, spasm of perivertebral muscles, scinit-scan would show hyperemia MRI shows marrow edema	<3 Months
II. Early-destructive	Diminished disk-space and Paradiscal erosion (Knuckle <10°) MRI-shows marrow edema and break of osseous margins, CT scan shows marginal erosions or cavitations	2-4 Months
III, IV, V all have vertebral-bodies destruction and collapse and appreciable kyphos:		
III. Mildangular kyphos	2-3 vertebrae involved (K:10-30°)	3-9 Months
IV. Moderate angular kyphos	>3 vertebrae involved (K:30-60°)	6-24 Months
V. Severe kyphos (Humpback)	*>3 vertebrae involved (K:>60°)*	*> 2 Years*

pathology studies to confirm diagnosis and to isolate organisms for culture and susceptibility.

Histologic Findings

- Since microbiologic studies may be nondiagnostic, anatomic pathology can be significant.
- Gross pathologic findings include exudative granulation tissue with interspersed abscesses.
- Coalescence of abscesses results in areas of caseating necrosis.

Bone Scan

- Technitium(Tc): Tc-99m bone scan showed increased uptake in 63 percent patients with active tuberculosis in the series reported by weaver and life so 21.
- The remaining patients showed a cold spot due to formation of avascular segments and abscesses.
- The Tc-99m scan is considered to be highly sensitive but nonspecific.
- It may only aid to localize the site of active disease and to detect multilevel involvement.

Treatment Algorithm

Flow chart 27.1 shows treatment algorithm (tuberculosis of spine).

Flow chart 27.1: Steps followed in treating tuberculosis of spine

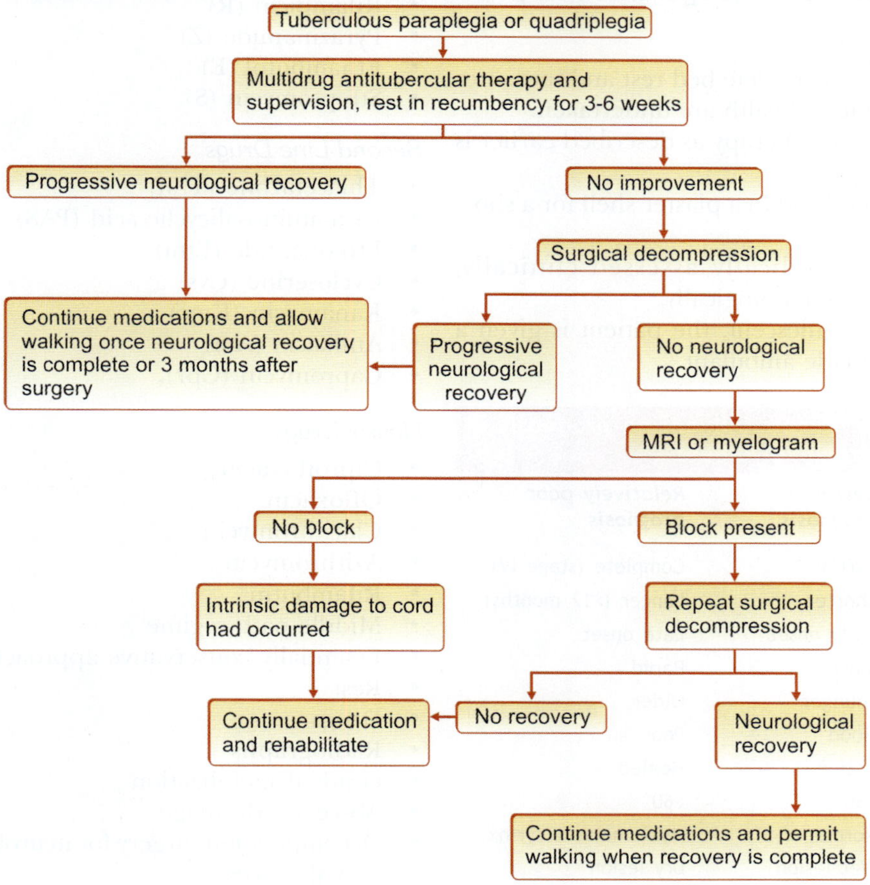

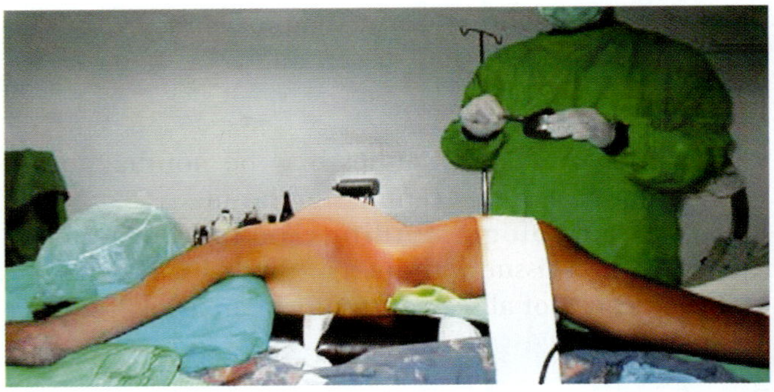

Fig. 27.304: Positioning, panting, drapping before spinal surgery

Problems in Management (Fig. 27.304)

Problems in management can be divided into:
- Diagnostic
- Medical
- Surgical
- Others.

Prognosis

Table 27.16 shows clinical factors influencing prognosis in cord involvement.

Treatment in Past (Fig. 27.305)

Conservative Treatment

- The patient is given complete bed rest and measures to improve his general health are undertaken.
- Antituberculous chemotherapy as described earlier is started.
- The spine is immobilized in a plaster shell for a short period.
- The patient is periodically assessed clinically, radiologically and hematologically.
- When the lesion is quiescent, the patient is given a spinal brace and made ambulant.

Table 27.16: Clinical factors influencing prognosis in cord involvement

Cord involvement	*Better prognosis*	*Relatively poor prognosis*
Degree	Partial	Complete (stage IV)
Duration	Shorter	Longer (>12 months)
Type	Early onset	Late onset
Speed of onset	Slow	Rapid
Age	Younger	Older
General condition	Good	Poor
Vertebral disease	Active	Healed
Kyphotic deformity	<60°	>60°
Cord on MRI	Normal	Myelomalacia/syrinx
Peroperative	Wet lesion	Dry lesion

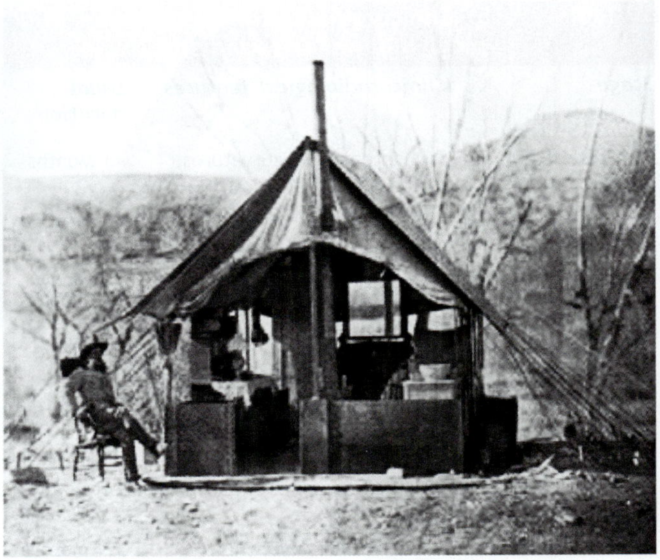

Fig. 27.305: Treatment of tubercular-spondylitis prevalent in past

- The chemotherapy is continued up to a total period of nine months.

First Line Drugs

- Isoniazid (H)
- Rifampicin (R)
- Pyrazinamide (Z)
- Ethambutol (E)
- Streptomycin (S).

Second Line Drugs

- Thiacetazone (TZn)
- Para-aminosalicyclic acid (PAS)
- Ethionamide (Etm)
- Cycloserine (Cys)
- Kanamycin (Kmc)
- Amikacin (Am)
- Capromycin (Cpr).

Newer Drugs

- Ciprofloxacin
- Ofloxacin
- Clarithromycin
- Azithromycin
- Rifambutin
- Middle path regime
- Essentially conservative approach
- Rest
- Drugs
- Radiographs
- Gradual mobilization
- Abscesses drainage
- Decompression surgery for neurological complications
- Spinal braces

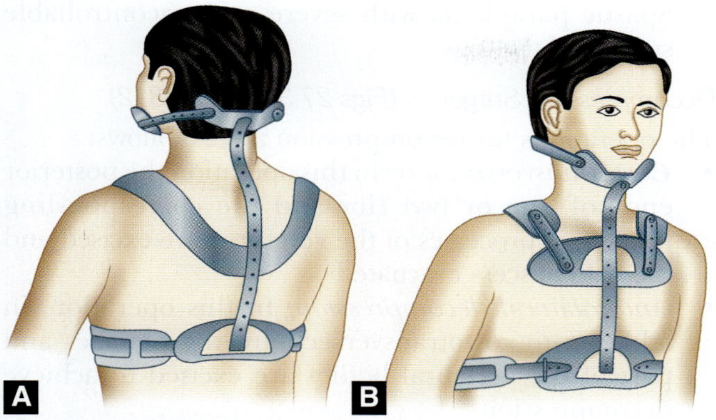

Figs 27.306A and B: Somi brace

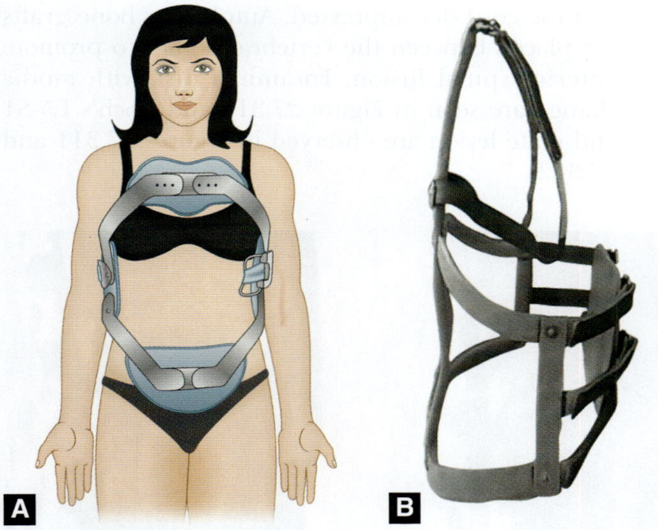

Figs 27.307A and B: (A) Jewett brace; (B) Taylor brace

- AKT
- *Intensive phase:* Five to six months of HRS/O
- *Continuation phase:* Seven to eight months
  - H and Z for three to four months
  - H and R for next four to five months
- *Prophylactic phase:* Four to five months of H and E.

Braces

Figures 27.306 to 27.308 show different types of braces.

Multidrug Resistant (MDR) Tuberculosis

- Most Common resistance to INH and rifampicin.
- Needs second-line drugs and new agents.
- Should be monitored by specialist as high chances of complications.
- Treatment expensive hence diagnosis needs to be certain.

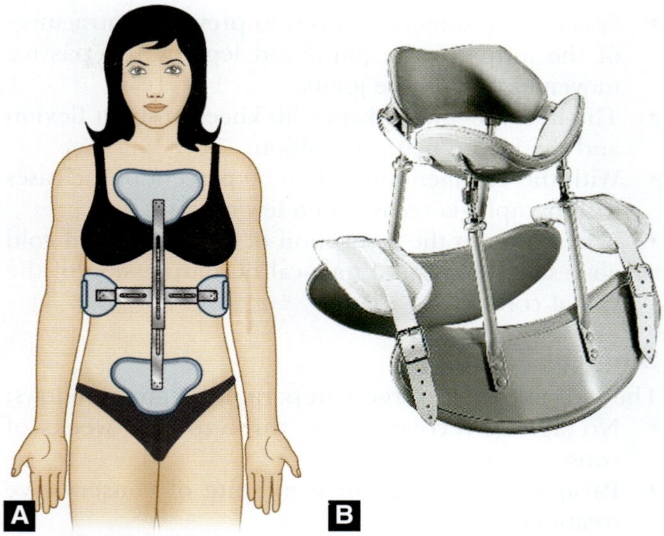

Figs 27.308A and B: (A) ASH brace; (B) Four-post collar

Table 27.17: Main indications for various operations for vertebral tuberculosis
- Decompression (± fusion) for neurological complications which failed to respond to conservative therapy/too advanced
- Debridement (± fusion) in failure of response after 3 to 6 months of nonoperative treatment
- Doubtful diagnosis
- Fusion for mechanical instability after healing
- Debridement ± decompression ± fusion in recurrence of disease or of neural complication
- Prevention of severe kyphosis by debridement + fusion by panvertebral operation in young children with extensive dorsal lesions
- Anterior transposition of cord through extrapleural antero-lateral approach for neural complications due to severe kyphosis

Note: Laminectomy has no place in tuberculosis of spine except for extradural granuloma/tuberculoma presenting as "spinal tumor syndrome", or a case of old healed disease (without much deformity) presenting with secondary "vertebral canal stenosis", or posterior spinal disease.

Surgical Management

- Indications need to be revised. These are illustrated in Table 27.17
- Decision based on merit of each case
- Imaging plays important role in decision making as seen in Figure 27.309.

Treatment of Pott's Paraplegia

- The initial treatment of the case is the same as before. The patient is immobilized in the plaster shell before the chemotherapy gets started.
- A neurological chart is maintained and the clinical status of the paraplegia recorded once a week.

- Special care should be taken to prevent contractures of the joints in the paralyzed legs by full passive movements of all the joints.
- The limbs should be kept with knees in slight flexion and the feet in neutral position.
- With this regimen more than 60 percent of the cases with paraplegia recover in a few months.
- This is due to the resorption of the intraspinal cold abscess resulting in a medical decompression of the spinal cord.

Surgical Treatment

The indications for surgery in paraplegia are as follows:

- No sign of recovery after three to four weeks of conservative treatment.
- Paraplegia getting worse in spite of conservative treatment.
- Spastic paraplegia with severe and uncontrollable spasms of the legs.

Decompression Surgeries (Figs 27.310 to 27.312)

The operations for decompression are as follows:

- *Costotransversectomy:* In this operation the posterior ends of one or two ribs and the corresponding transverse processes of the vertebrae are excised and the cold abscess evacuated
- *Anterolateral decompression:* In this operation, in addition to costotransversectomy, the pedicles and part of the vertebral bodies are excised to achieve decompression
- *Anterior decompression and spinal fusion:* (Hong Kong operation), through a standard thoracotomy; the abscess is evacuated and debridement is done. The diseased vertebral bodies are excised (vertebrectomy) and the cord decompressed. Autologous bone grafts are placed between the vertebral bodies to promote anterior spinal fusion. Foraminal disk with modic change are seen in Figure 27.310 and Koch's L5-S1 end plate lesion are observed in Figures 27.311 and 27.312.

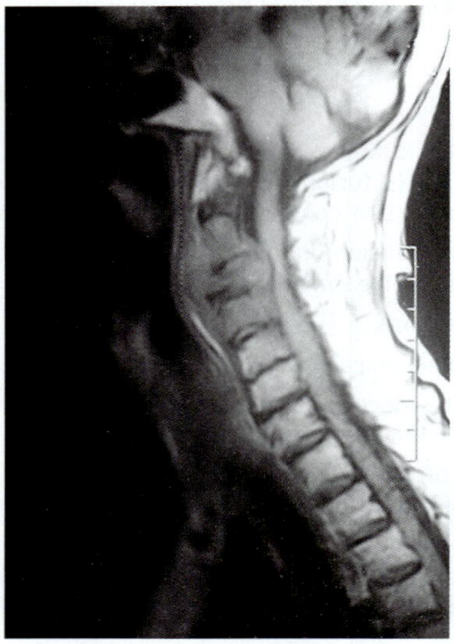

Fig. 27.309: MRI showing TB of spine

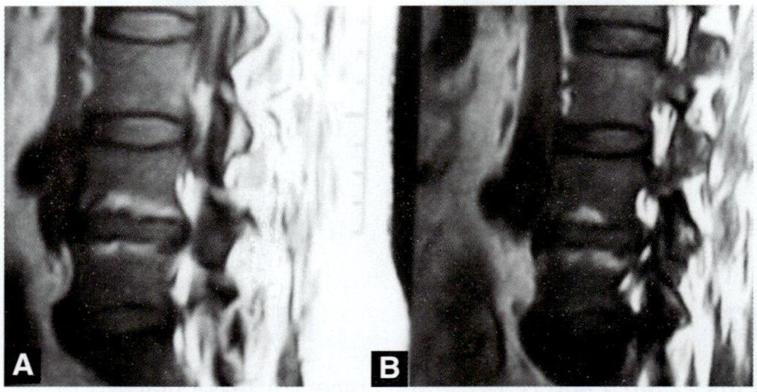

Figs 27.310A and B: Foraminal disk with modic changes

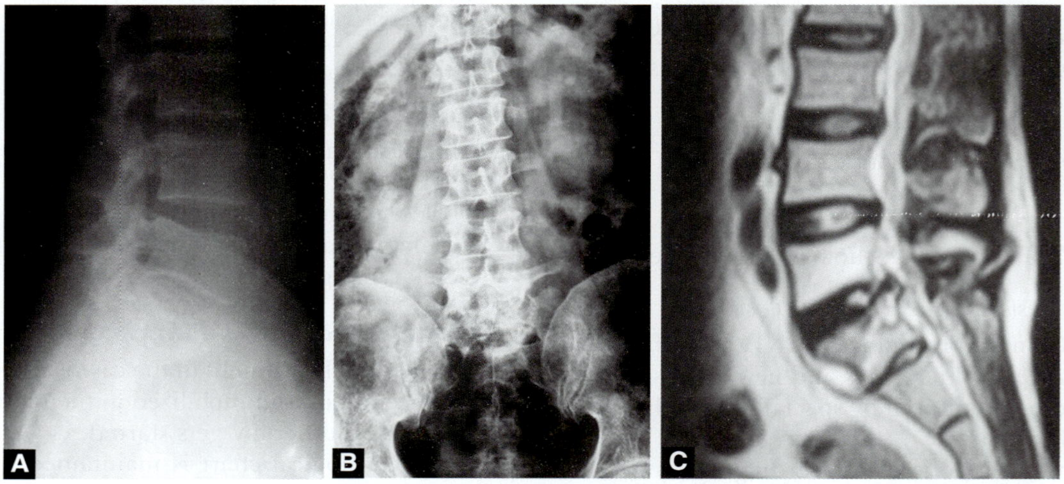

Figs 27.311A to C: Pott's spine, showing Koch's L5-S1 end-plate lesions—(A) and (B) X-ray images; (C) MRI of spine

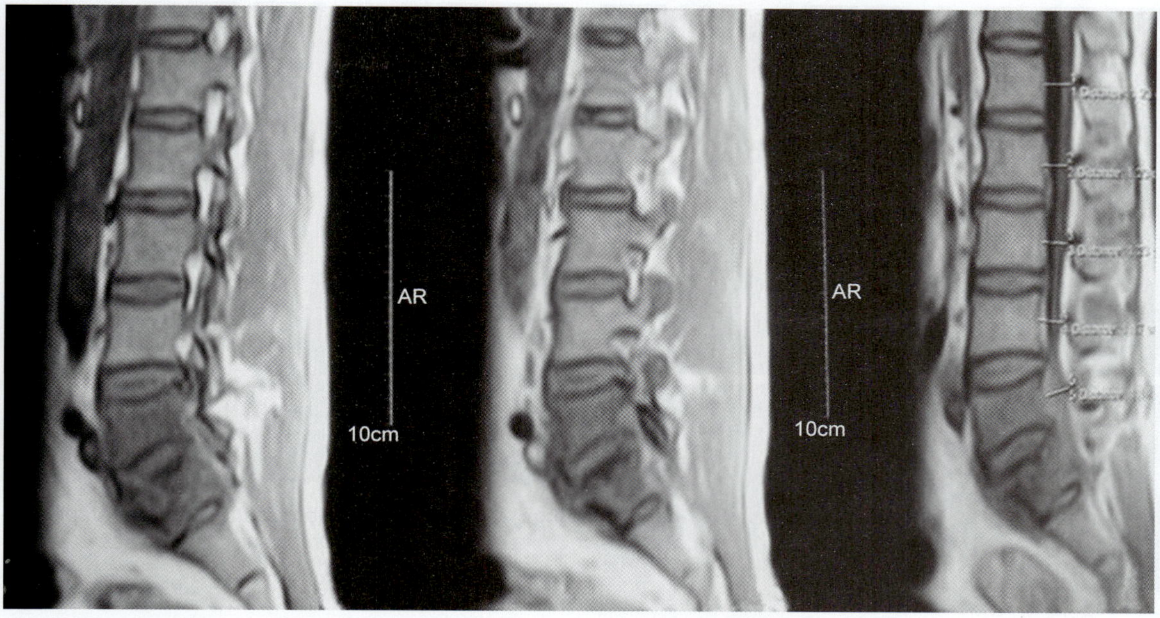

Fig. 27.312: Pott's spine—MRI showing Koch's spine L4-L5 with end-plate lesion

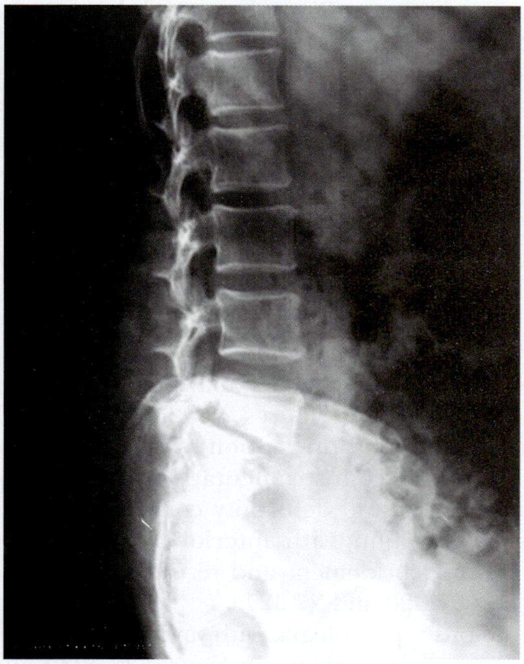

Fig. 27.313: Posterior involvement with pedicle destruction

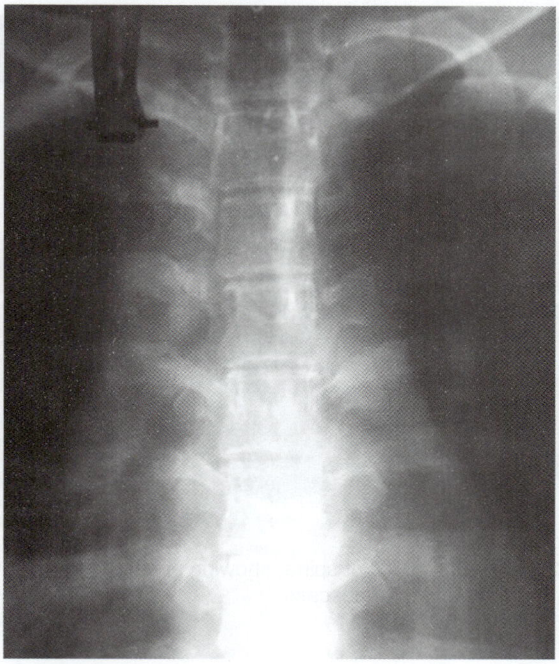

Fig. 27.314: Chest X-ray in posterior spine involvement and pedicle destruction

Posterior involvement with pedicle destruction are shown in Figures 27.313 to 27.315.

Acute onset paraplegia, with epidural abscess are shown in Figures 27.316A to C.

Tumors are likely to be mistaken for Koch's. Giant cell tumor with paraplegia, treated with ALD and anti-Koch's therapy for eight months, as depicted in Figures 27.317A and B.

D5 sarcoma with paraparesis, treated with AKT for 3 months as shown in Figures 27.318A to C.

Histopathological diagnosis is mandatory in many cases. Percutaneous biopsy procedures under image

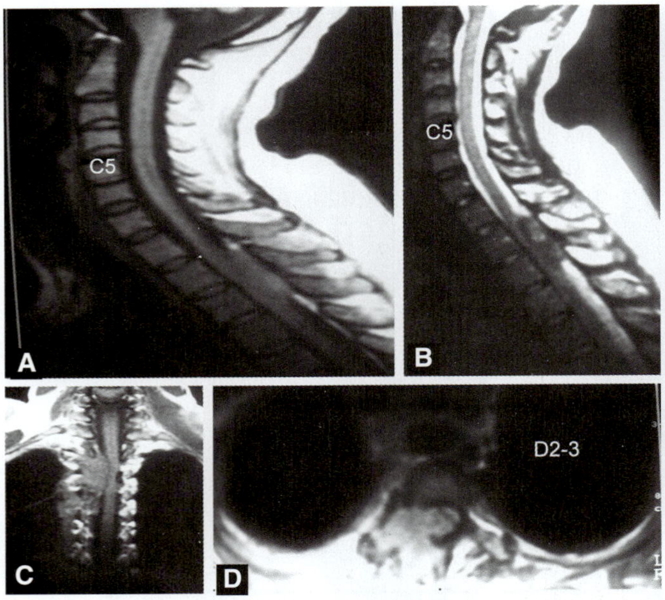

Figs 27.315A to D: MRI of spine, showing posterior spinal involvement with pedicle destruction

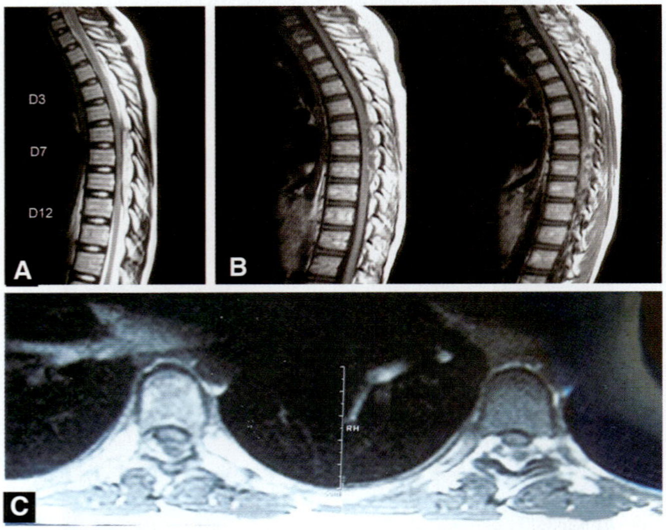

Figs 27.316A to C: MRI of spine, showing acute onset paraplegia with epidural abscess

guidance have a high success rate. Culture and sensitivity are very helpful but is time consuming. Bactec culture is faster, but a costly method. Tuberculosis is basically a medical disease and most important treatment is AKT. Since 1970, the efficacy of short course (six to nine months) and domiciliary regimens has been demonstrated. Fluoroquinolones, newer macrolides and some rifampicin congeners are the recent additions to the antimycobacterial drugs. Diagnosis is yet not clear.

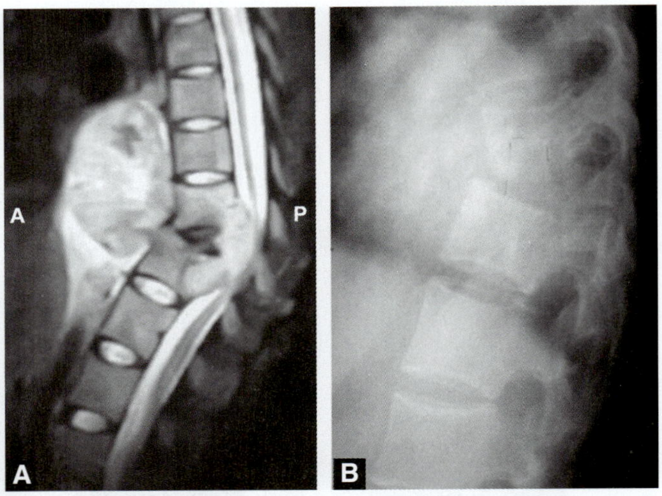

Figs 27.317A and B: Giant cell tumor with paraplegia—(A) MRI; (B) X-ray lateral spine

Extensive disease, which may leads to instability. Large abscesses or epidural granulation tissue, which can cause peridural fibrosis. Neurological deficit, where point has lost antigravity power. Retropharyngeal abscess are shown in Figures 27.319 and 27.320.

Costotransversectomy is useful only for abscess drainage and is rarely used. Anterolateral decompression or extrapleural approach reduces morbidity of thoracotomy. First preference for approach for anterior disease is anterior. Paradiscal Koch's with abscess as shown in Figures 27.321A to C.

TB spine L2-3 with paraparesis, as shown in Figures 27.322A to D.

Anterior decompression and bone grafting, as shown in Figures 27.323A to C.

Modification of approach may be required in many cases, as depicted in Figures 27.323 to 27.325. Deformity correction and prevention of kyphosis should be given importance. Instrumentation may be required for stabilization and deformity correction. No risk of persistent infection, with anterior implants are seen.

Anterior debridement and reconstruction observed in Figures 27.326 and 27.327.

Acute onset paraplegia, with multilevel Koch's spine and tuberculoma, as shown in Figures 27.328A and B.

Multiple level Koch's lesions with abscess formation with acute onset paraplegia treated with decompression, debridement and stabilization of spine by fusion with sublaminar wire fixation/Hartshill frame. Postoperative patients have been given ASHE brace as an external support for rehabilitation in addition to AKT (Figs 27.329 to 27.338)

Surgery in healed Koch's more demanding. Surgery for deformity in children may need global fusion. Surgery

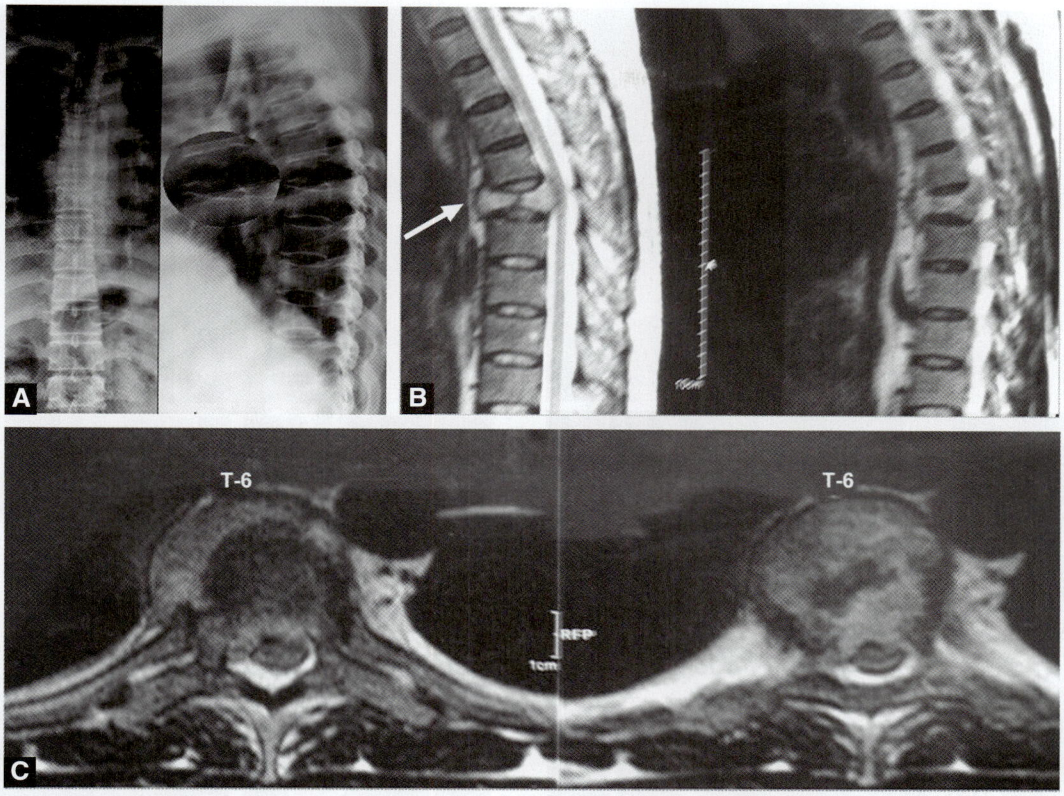

Figs 27.318A to C: D5 sarcoma with paraparesis, treated with AKT for 3 months

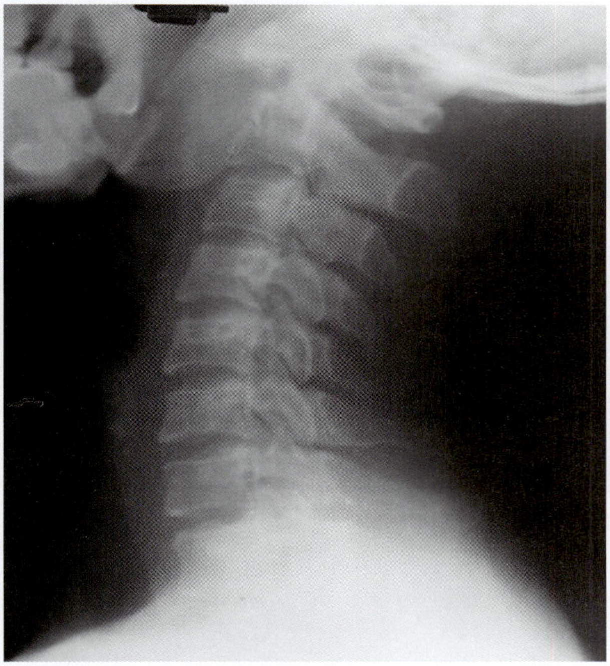

Fig. 27.319: Retropharyngeal abscess

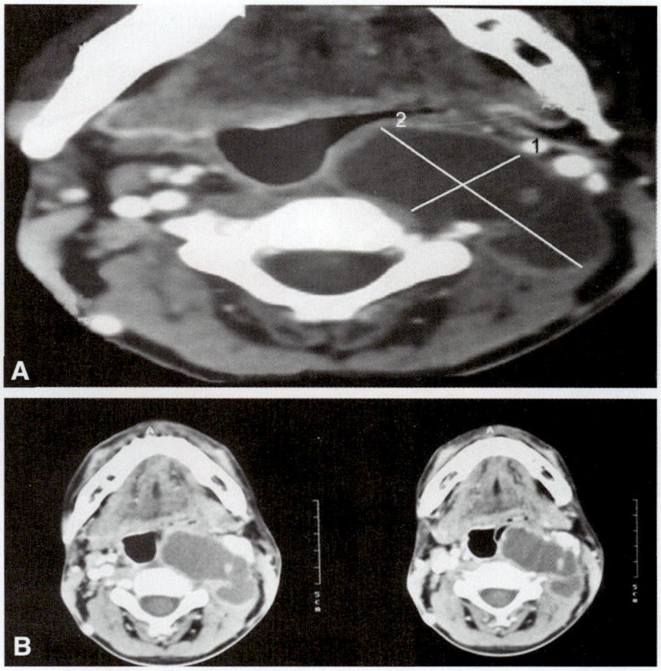

Figs 27.320A and B: PET scanning showing retropharyngeal abscess

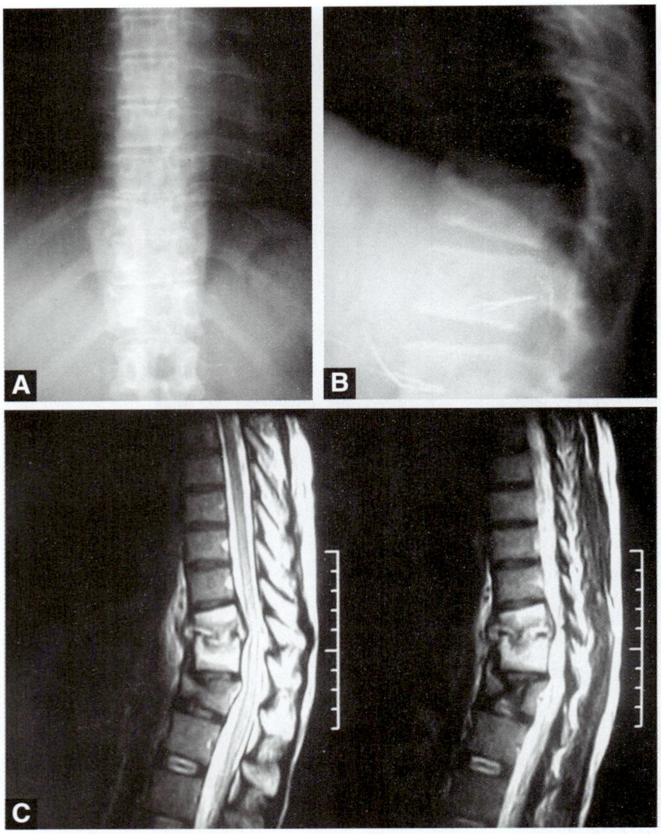

Figs 27.321A to C: Paradiscal Koch's with abscess. (A) and (B) X-rays; (C) MRI images

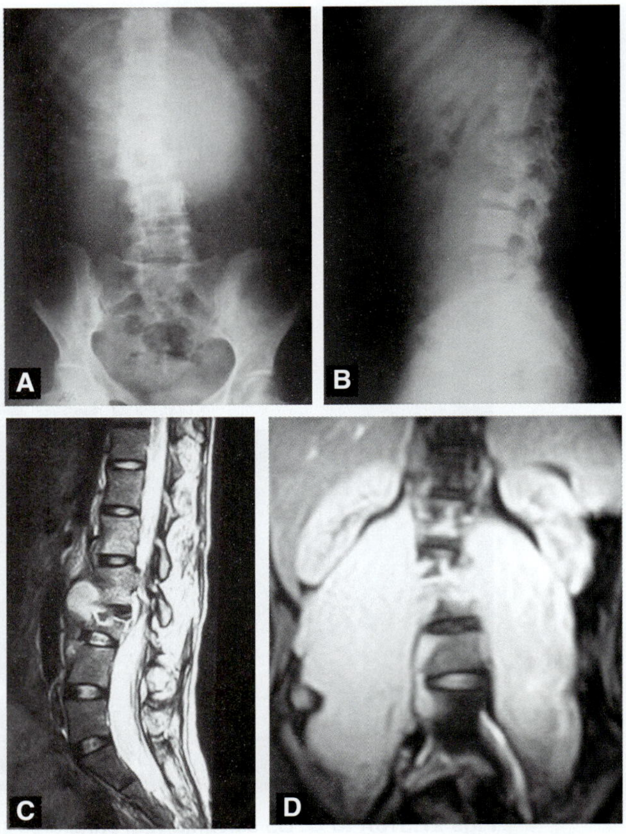

Figs 27.322A to D: TB spine L2-3 with paraparesis

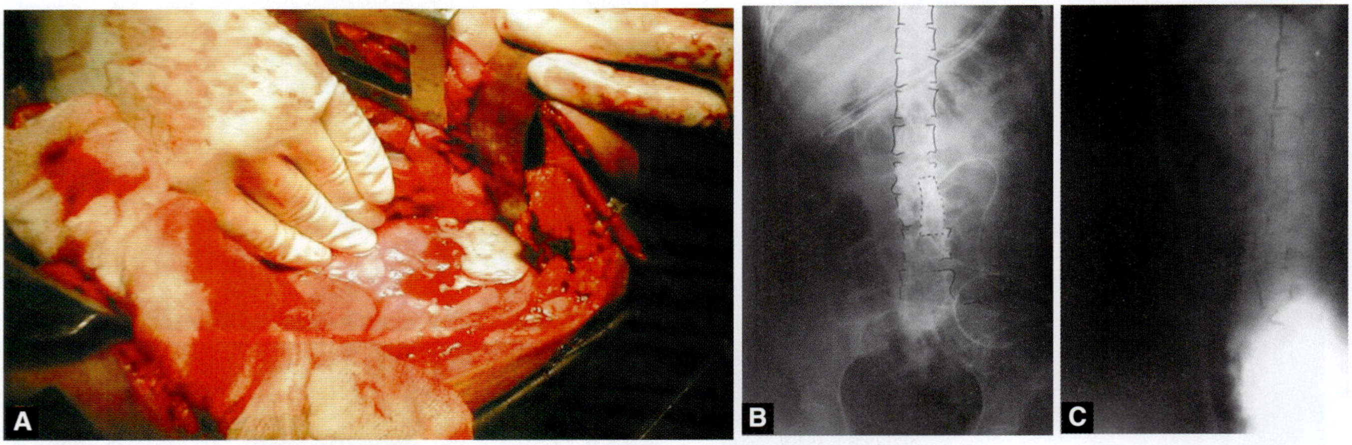

Figs 27.323A to C: Anterior decompression and bone grafting surgery being performed

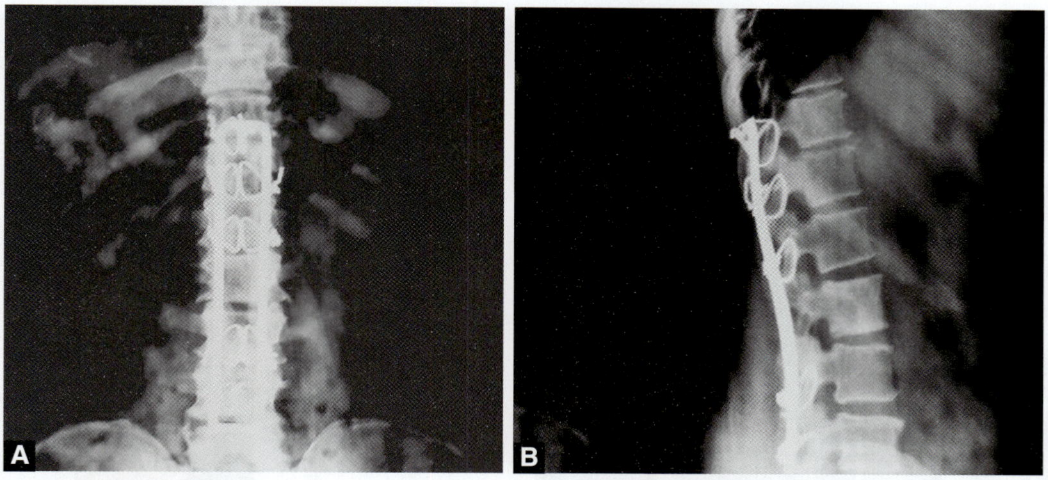

Figs 27.324A and B: Anterior implant used for anterior decompression and bone grafting surgery—(A) Anteroposterior view; (B) Lateral view

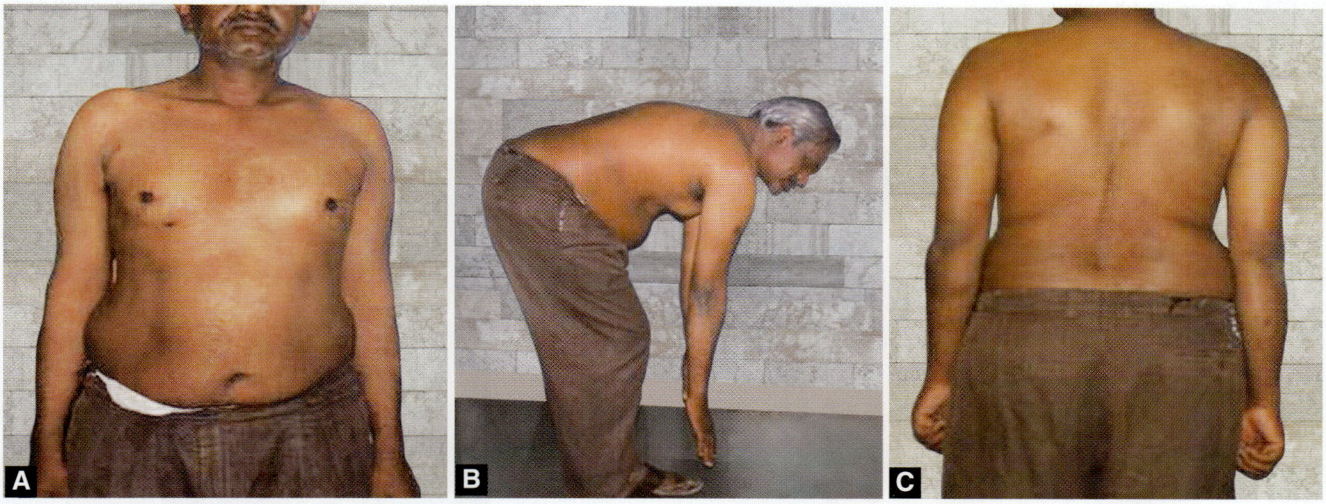

Figs 27.325A to C: Postsurgical inspection (after anterior decompression surgery)

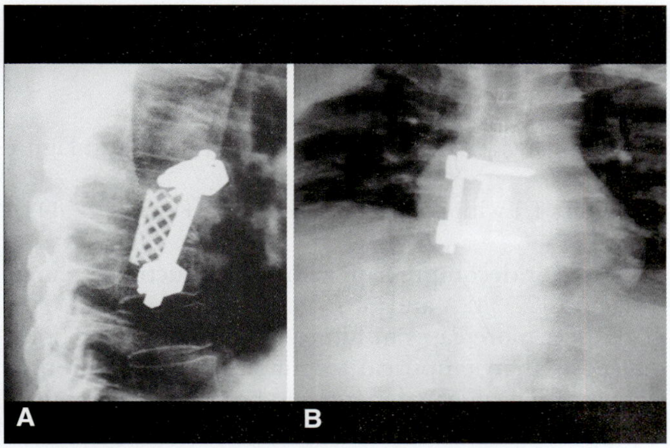

Figs 27.326A and B: Anterior debridement and reconstruction

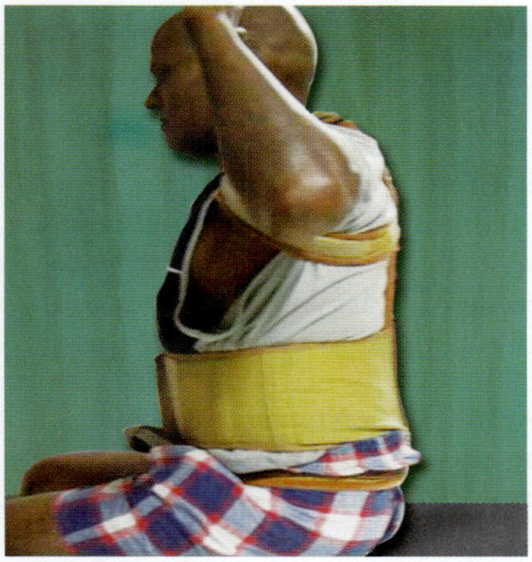

Fig. 27.327: Postsurgical inspection

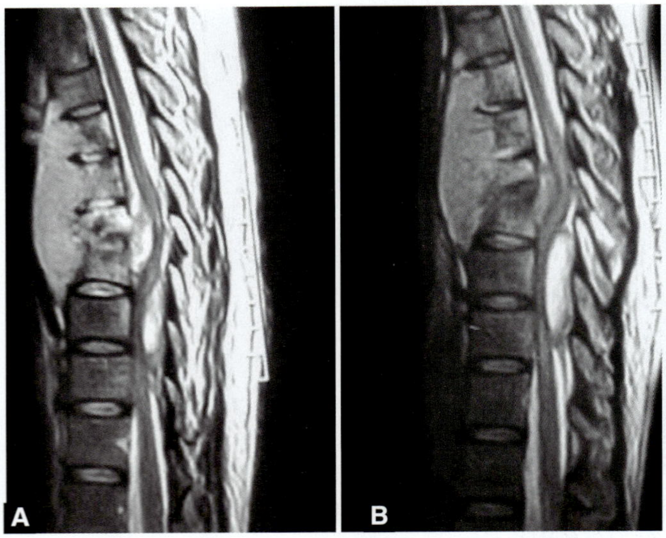

Figs 27.328A and B: Acute onset paraplegia with multilevel Koch's spine and tuberculoma

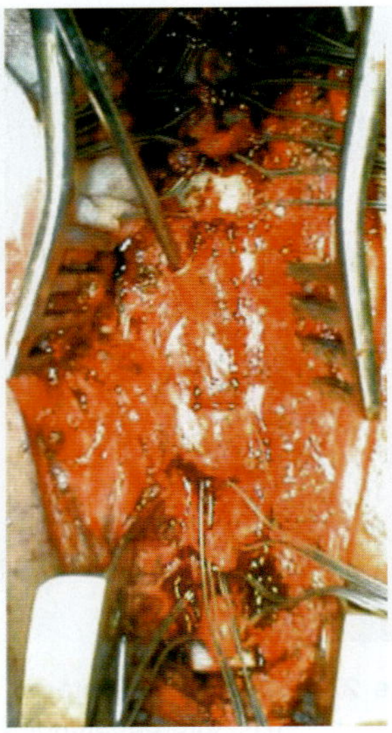

Fig. 27.330: L3-S1 Koch's lesion decompression, laminectomy, disectomy done and interspinous sublamilar wiring done

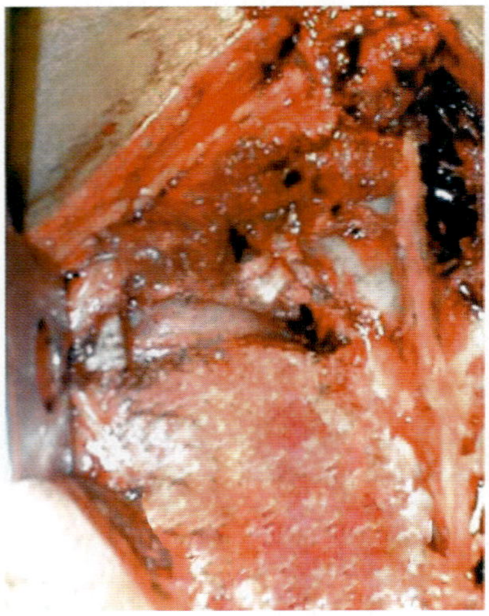

Fig. 27.329: L5–S1 Koch's lesion spinal fusion done

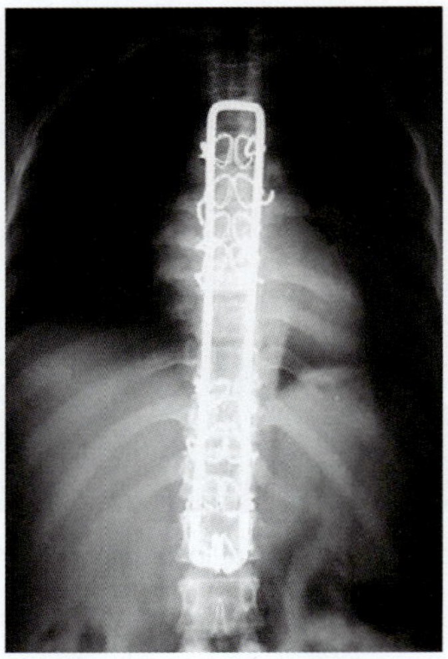

Fig. 27.331: X-ray AP view showing thoracolumbar spinal fusion with HAART shield after decompression

for reactivation is difficult to decide and execute. Instability following healed Koch's also poses challenge for the surgery. HIV is estimated to have infected 3.5 million people in India (WHO 1999) and these patients are specially vulnerable to severe forms of tubercular/MAC infection. Emergence of multidrug resistant (MDR) TB with overall 13 percent incidence in 35 countries is threatening the whole future of current antitubercular chemotherapy. For Pott's D4-5, periscapular approach is followed.

HIV positive point with Koch's D7-8 extrapleural approach, shown in Figures 27.339A and B.

Multidrug resistance in Pott's spine is shown in Figure 27.340.

Koch's L1 with paraparesis shown in Figures 27.341A to C.

Anterior decompression with reconstruction is shown in Figures 27.342A and B.

Expect more cases in future practices. Prompt tissue diagnosis than empirical treatment. Due attention to spinal stability and alignment must be given. Try to restore anatomy, whenever surgery is undertaken. Do not hesitate to use proper instrumentation when necessary, provided bone stock is good. No compromise done in AKT regimes.

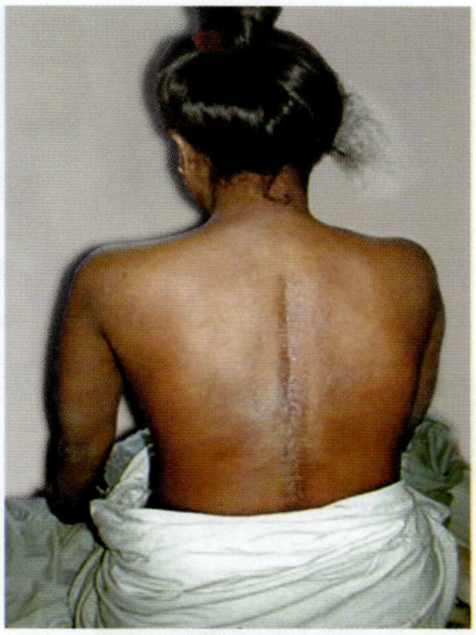

Fig. 27.332: Postoperative scar in a decompressed thoracolumbar Koch's spine

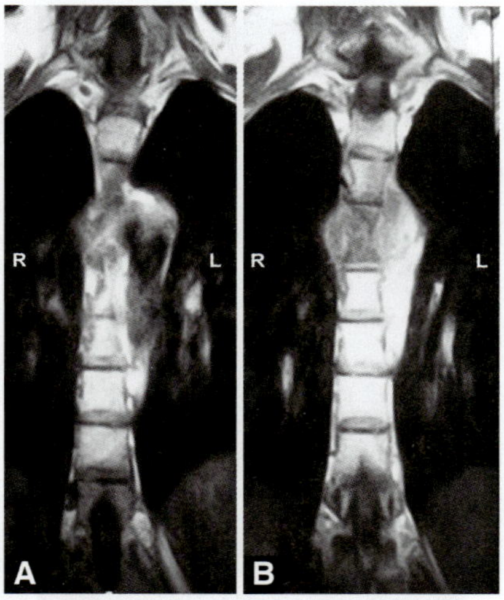

Figs 27.335A and B: MRI showing paraspinal collection in thoracic vertebrae region

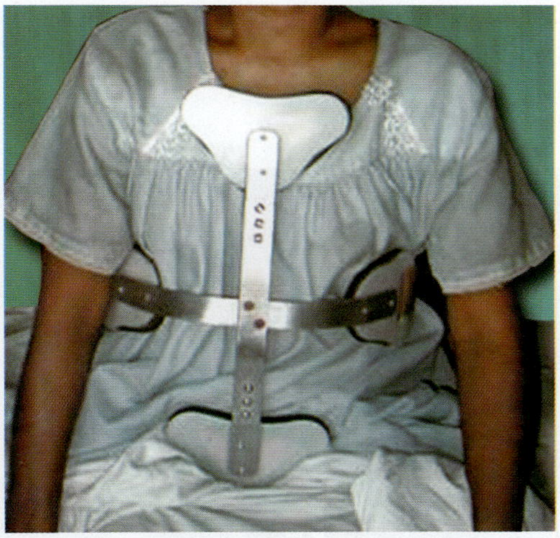

Fig. 27.333: Thoracolumbar immobilization after surgery with ASH brace

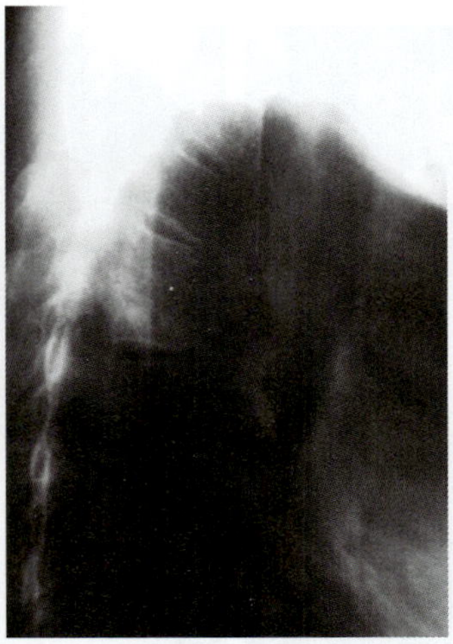

Fig. 27.336: X-ray lateral view Koch's spine showing upper thoracic vertebral lesion

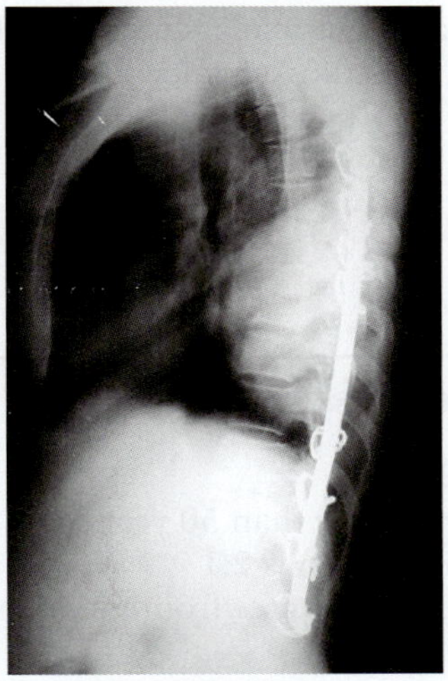

Fig. 27.334: X-ray lateral view showing thoracolumbar spinal fusion with Hartshill after decompression

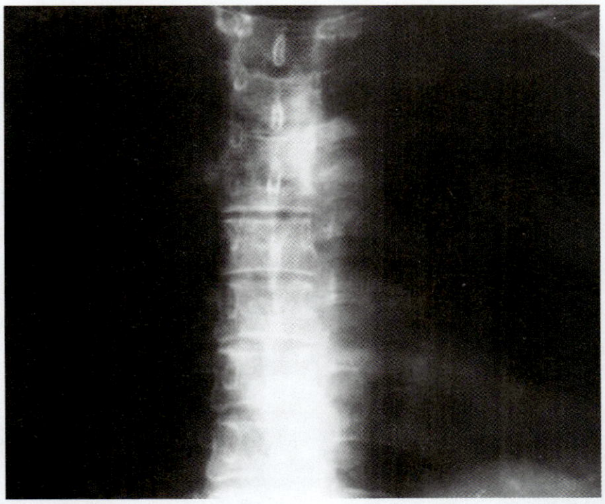

Fig. 27.337: X-ray AP view Koch's spine showing upper thoracic vertebral lesion

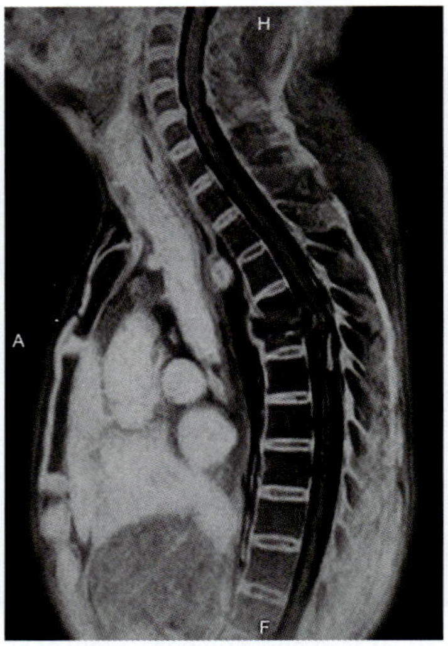

Fig. 27.338: MRI showing abscess anteriorly

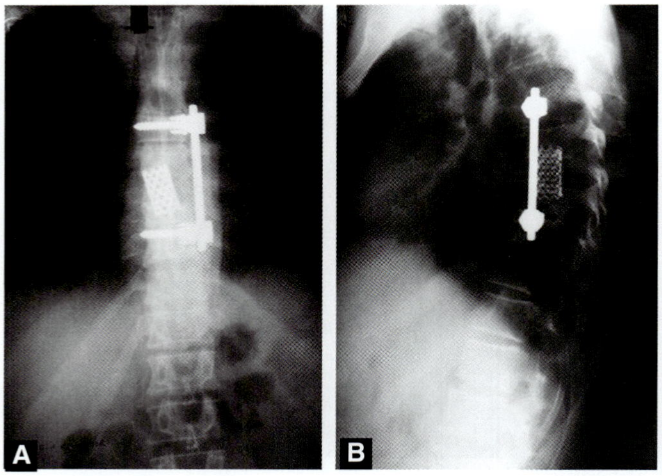

Figs 27.339A and B: Extrapleural approach for Koch's D7-8—(A) Anterior view; (B) Lateral view

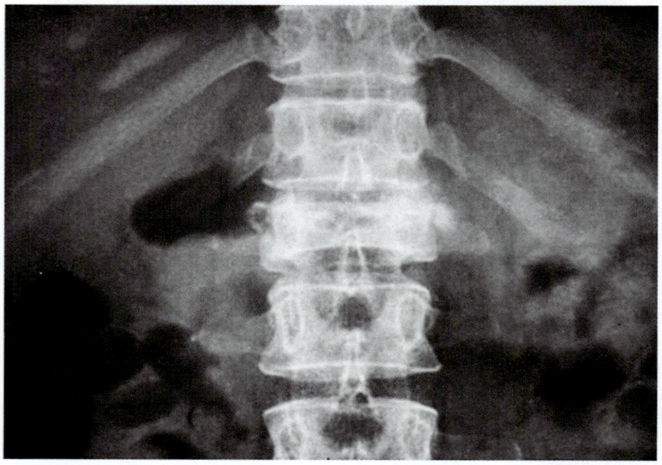

Fig. 27.340: X-ray showing TB of spine with MDR

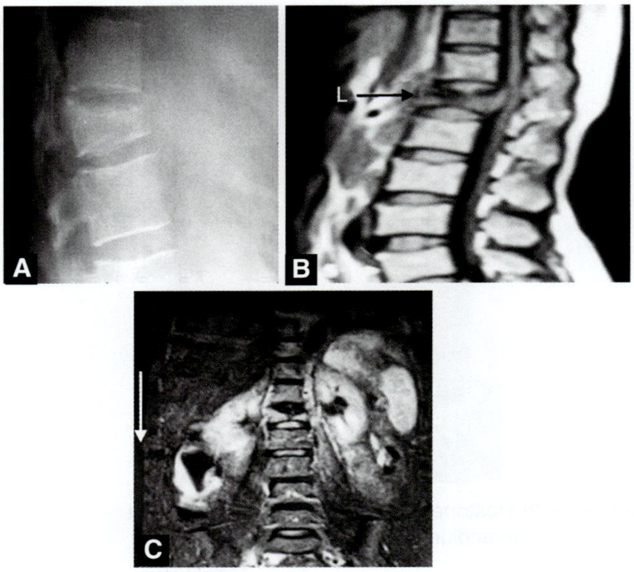

Figs 27.341A to C: Koch's L1 with paraparesis—(A) X-ray imaging; (B) and (C) MRI

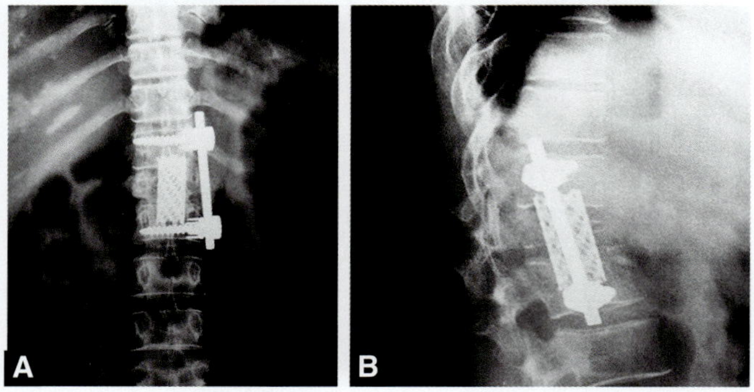

Figs 27.342A and B: Anterior decompression with reconstruction

For recent advances in management of TB spine please refer to TB of musculoskeletal system in general topics section.

NONTUBERCULAR INFECTIONS OF SPINE

Pyogenic Osteomyelitis

Epidemiology

- Age usually greater than 50 years old
- Male to female ratio is 2:1
- Steadily increasing rates from increasing:
  - Average age
  - Drug use
  - Increased instrumentation

Pathophysiology of Osteomyelitis

Common Sources

- Skin and soft tissue
- Respiratory tract
- Infected intravenous catheter sites
- Postoperative wound infection
- Endocarditis
- Dental infection.

Less Common Sources

- Infected native or prosthetic valvular infections.
- Direct spread from a ruptured esophagus diverticular or renal abscesses infected aortic lesions.

Rare: Lumbar puncture, myelography, translumbar aortography, chemonucleolysis or epidural catheter placement.

Hematogenous Spread

- Most common
- Marrow highly vascular
- Vessel change "corkscrew anatomy" with age may predispose to infection, usually causes bone destruction in two adjacent vertebral bodies and their intervertebral disk.
- Lumbar > thoracic >> cervical
- *Posterior extension:* Epidural and subdural abscesses, and meningitis anterior or lateral extension: paravertebral, retropharyngeal, mediastinal, subphrenic, retroperitoneal or psoas abscesses. In thoracic, empyema is possible.

Microbiology in Pyogenic Spinal Osteomyelitis

- *Staphylococcus aureus*: More than 50 percent of cases in most case series in developed western countries.
- Enteric gram-negative bacilli, particularly after urinary tract instrumentation
- *Pseudomonas aeruginosa* and *Candida*: Intravascular access sepsis or injection drug use
- Groups B and G hemolytic streptococci: Especially diabetes mellitus
- Tuberculous infection
- Geography: *Brucella melitensis* (Middle east)
  - *Burkholderia pseudomallei* (equatorial)
  - *Salmonella* and *Entamoeba histolytica* (Africa or South America).

Clinical Features

- Progressive LBP; local tenderness
- Pain often worse at night; relieved with rest initially
- Fever inconsistent (roughly ½)
- ESR and CRP elevated in more than 80 percent
- Blood cultures and more than 50 percent.

Diagnosis

- Mean duration symptoms ~2 months before diagnosis.
- High clinical suspicion, low back pain and elevated ESR.
- Imaging (plain films, CT, MRI).
- Aspiration of disk space/bone to confirm diagnosis and obtain organism.

Difference between pyogenic and tubercular osteomyelitis of vertebrae:

- Usually body and appendages
- Typical pyogenic infection (50)
- Sudden sometimes gradual
- Pyrexia marked
- Pain intense
- Leukocytosis may be marked
- Vertebral collapse none
- *X-ray:* Increased density
- New bone formation
- Spread through vertebrae
- *Cord invol:* Rare for acute onset
- *Course:* Short to bone fusion
- Invariably body
- Distant foci
- Gradual
- Seldom marked
- Dull aching
- Not a feature
- Usual
- *X-ray:* Decreased density
- No new bone formation
- Spread under ant common
- Ligament
- *Cord invol:* Common for gradual onset
- *Course:* Prolonged to recalcification? fibrous fusion?

Radiographs

Figures 27.343A to D show different radiographs of pyogenic spinal osteomyelitis.

■ Magnetic Resonance Imaging

- Magentic resonance imaging (MRI) is the most sensitive radiographic technique to detect vertebral osteomyelitis. MRI is also superior to CT scanning for detection of epidural abscesses.
- MRI showed either typical or suggestive changes of osteomyelitis in 91 percent of patients with symptoms of less than two weeks' duration and in 96 percent of those with symptoms of more than two weeks' duration (103 patients).
- *T1:* Decreased signal intensity in the vertebral body and disk and loss of end-plate definition.

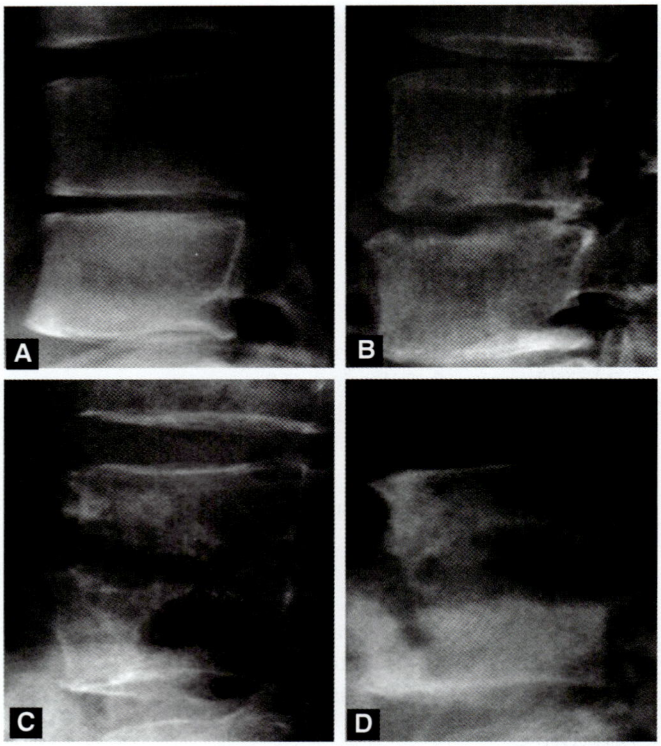

Figs 27.343A to D: Different radiographic images of pyogenic spinal osteomyelitis

- *T2-weighted images:* Increased disk and less often vertebral body signal intensity. Contrast enhancement of the vertebral body and disk. Ring enhancement of paraspinal and epidural processes can indicate abscess formation.
- *False-negative:* Meningitis.
- *False-positive results:* Bone fracture. Not useful in following disease progression; follow clinically and ESR often useful.

Controversies

- Duration of treatment?
- If cultures negative, treat medically?
- Late osteomyelitis of spine
- Hardware versus decompression?
- When to operate?
- Acute decline neurologically
- Location (e.g. often below conus).

■ Brucellosis of Spine

Introduction

- Uncommon generalized infectious disease.
- Undulant, Malta, Mediterranean or Gibraltar fever.
- Transmitted through the excretions and secretions of animals to humans.
- May be endemic in regions, where milk is unpasteurized, particularly in the Mediterranean countries.
- The spine is the most common pan of the musculoskeletal system affected and is involved in up to one-third of cases.
- Acute febrile stage lasting from a few days to several weeks.
- Followed by a protracted convalescent or chronic stage over several months to years .
- Characterized by recurring episodes of fever and a multiplicity of symptoms.
- A high index of suspicion is necessary to detect Brucellar vertebral osteomyelitis at an early stage.

Etiology

- Causative microorganisms:
  - *Brucella abortus* (cattle), most common type infecting humans.
  - *Brucella suis* (swine); suppurative osteomyelitis, usually in the vertebrae.
  - *Brucella melitensis* (sheep and goats), severe general symptoms, peripheral neuritis, cranial nerve palsies and meningoencephalitis.
  - *Brucella rangiferi* (caribou)
  - *Brucella canis* (dogs)
- The disease is prevalent in rural areas
- Farmers, veterinarians, and meat packers
- *41 to 60 years age group:* Susceptible.
- Undulant fever may affect children under 10 years of age.
- *Brucella* organisms occur in domestic animals and are transmitted through contact with secretions or excretions or handling of carcasses.

Pathology

- Tends to reside in the RES for prolonged periods: course of the disease tends to be protracted.
- Mononuclear infiltration, bone destruction, and abscess formation with tough fibrous capsules.
- Occasionally, sequestra are formed but early and extensive new bone formation is invariable and typical.
- Abscesses extend to the dura but do not penetrate it.
- Intervertebral disk is often destroyed and bony fusion between contiguous vertebrae may be seen.
- Collapse of the affected vertebrae is highly unusual.

Clinical Features

- *Incubation period:* 2 weeks (5 days to several months)
- *Acute stage:* 1 to 5 weeks
- Followed by recurring febrile episodes with highly variable symptoms and remissions lasting several days to 2 weeks.
- The chronic stage is protracted, lasting months to years.

Acute Stage

- Daily spiking fever, chills, headache, spelenomegaly, adenopathy, malaise, anemia and diarrhea occasionally.
- Vague arthralgias (neck, the shoulder, the lumbar region, the thigh, the knee) and evening rise of temperature may be seen.
- Meningoencephalitis, neuritis and severe backache may develop (earliest sign of vertebral affection).

Spine Involvement

- Lumbosacral region usually.
- Pain in the affected portion of the spine is the earliest manifestation of spondylitis
- Frequently, referred root pains to the abdomen or lower extremities may lead to erroneous diagnoses.
- Backache becomes progressively worse: Aggravated by activity and lessened by recumbency.
- May be referred in girdle-like fashion around to the front of the abdomen or to the lower extremities.
- Protective muscle spasm, and back motion becomes greatly restricted.
- Rarely, a peridural abscess may form and neurologic disturbances may result from irritation and compression of the spinal cord and cauda equina.
- Paraplegia is extremely rare.

Investigations

X-ray *(Fig. 27.344)*

- Changes are first detected after an interval of 1 to 6 months after the onset of local pain.

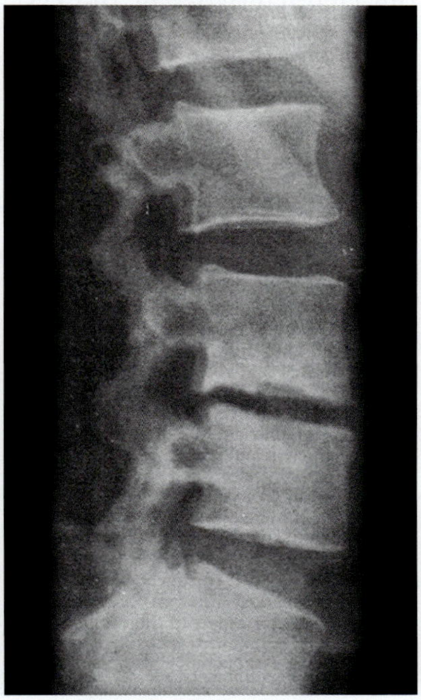

Fig. 27.344: Lateral X-ray showing brucellosis of spine

- Initially, only osteoporosis of contiguous vertebrae appears. Later, erosion of the cortical end plates develops and is followed by extensive ragged cavitation of those portions of the vertebrae that about on the intervening disk space.
- The disk interval gradually narrows.
- Bony proliferation about the destructive lesions is highly characteristic of this disease.
- At the margins of the vertebrae, large osteophytic outgrowths may appear to be within the substance of the anterior longitudinal ligament.
- As healing takes place, dense bone extends across and obliterates the vertebral cavitations and often bridges across the disk interval, creating a bony ankylosis between the vertebrae.

CT Scan/MRI Scan

Extent of vertebral involvement at an early stage but also for defining intraspinal extension and the formation of a compressive extradural mass.

Laboratory Findings

- Leukopenia is typical of the acute phase.
- Relative or actual lymphocytosis is common.
- Agglutinin antibodies to *Brucella.*
- Best isolated from specimens secured by needle biopsy.
- Rarely, a blood culture may be successful.

Treatment

- Chlortetracycline is very effective.
- Oxytetracycline, streptomycin and sulfa drugs are also effective.
- Combination of streptomycin and tetracycline is given during the first 3 weeks.
- Streptomycin, 1 g, intramuscularly twice daily and tetracycline orally 0.5 g, four times daily, are given for 3 weeks, then streptomycin is discontinued and tetracycline is continued until the erythrocyte sedimentation rate becomes normal and roentgenographic evidence of healing is achieved.
- Bed rest or continuous enforced recumbency on a Stryker frame is ordinarily sufficient, but immobilization in a body cast is more efficient and relieves pain quickly.
- Neurologic deficits usually clear up, and complete recovery takes place within 6 months to 2 years.
- Progressive neurologic impairment suggests peridural collection: surgical decompression is necessary.

■ Actinomycosis

Actinomycosis is a chronic granulomatous disease characterized by external sinuses. It is caused most commonly by *Actinomyces israelii. Actinomyces* actually are gram-positive anaerobic filamentous bacteria, not fungi.

Diagnosis usually is made by identifying sulfur granules or branching mycelia. Image-guided aspiration of infected regions is helpful in obtaining appropriate samples. With spinal involvement, there may be sclerotic changes; however, vertebral body height usually is preserved. Spinal involvement may resemble tuberculosis but usually does not affect the disk. Abscesses may extend to the skin and paravertebral abscesses may be present. Rib lesions have been described with sinus tract extension to the skin. Diagnosis is made by identification of the pathogen from an image-guided aspirant of infected tissue. Penicillin typically is used for treatment, although tetracycline, erythromycin and chloramphenicol can be used.

Fungal Infection

Fungal osteomyelitis generally develops slowly and therefore diagnosis and treatment may be delayed. As diagnosis depends on specific stains and cultures, the diagnosis must be suspected before it can be established. Treatment plans for these unusual infections should be made in collaboration with an infectious disease consultant.

Blastomycosis

- Infection usually occurs after inhalation of the spores of *Blastomyces dermatitidis*, a dimorphic soil-dwelling fungus.
- It is frequently found in immunocompromised patients.
- Osseous involvement is the third most frequent form of primary blastomycosis.
- Skeletal infection occurs by hematogenous spread from the lungs or by direct extension from a cutaneous infection.
- Osseous findings are not specific for blastomycosis and resemble other forms of osteomyelitis. Some asymptomatic regions may have osseous involvement with cortical erosions noted. The first sign of involvement may be a cutaneous sinus or abscess.
- Definitive diagnosis is made by demonstrating the characteristic broad-based budding yeast on microscopic examination of a joint or bone aspirate. Culture of the yeast or mold form establishes the diagnosis but may take 1 to 5 weeks to grow.
- Amphotericin B is the antibiotic of choice, with ketoconazole or itraconazole being an effective alternative drug.

Parasitic Infections of Spine

Echinococcosis

Echinococcosis is also called unilocular or human hydatid disease. It is caused by the larvae stage of *Echinococcus granulosus,* which is found most frequently in cattle and sheep-raising areas of the United States, similar diseases have been found in South America, Europe and Australia. Canidae (domestic dogs, fox, coyotes) serve as definitive hosts while sheep act as intermediate hosts. Bone involvement usually is seen in less than 1 percent of cases and is exhibited by cystic or lytic lesions in the trabecular bone that can extend into other subcortical areas. The most commonly affected areas in bone are the vertebrae, pelvis and the skull. Long bones also may be affected. Progressive changes may resemble tumor formation with an expansile cystic appearance. In rare cases, extension to the spinal cord has been described. Antigen or antibody titres are helpful in making the diagnosis and imaging studies (CT scan, ultrasonography Figs 27.345A to C) may delineate the characteristics of the cyst and guide treatment.

Treatment

The best treatment for a bone infection resulting from echinococcosis is to resect the involved bone or to amputate. However, curettage and instilling solutions,

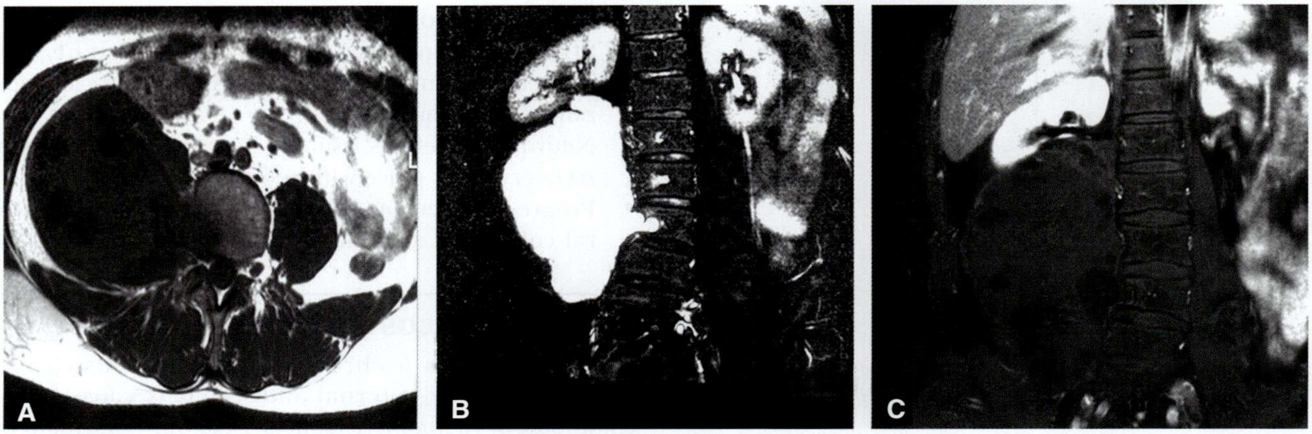

Figs 27.345A to C: CT scans—(A) Axial view; (B) and (C) Coronal views

such as hypertonic saline, 1 percent formalin or 0.5 percent silver nitrate have been tried. In suspected cases of echinococcosis, diagnostic biopsy or aspiration is contraindicated. Surgical management should include careful planning and meticulous technique to avoid spillage of the cyst contents, which may cause spread of the disease. If spillage occurs, application of cetyltrimethylammonium bromide (Cetrimide), 2-formalin or 1-iodine can reduce the danger of spreading. Albendazole or mebendazole also can be used chemotherapeutically, but resolution varies.

TRAUMATIC QUADRIPLEGIA AND PARAPLEGIA

Introduction

An acute pathologic insult to the spinal cord that completely or partially interrupts sensory and motor communications within the CNS and between the CNS and peripheral nervous system.

History

Spinal injury causing complete or incomplete paralysis has been recorded for thousands of years. The earliest mention is in Edwin Smith surgical papyrus in 1700, where the writer calls it an ailment not to be treated. Dr George Riddoch and Sir Ludwig Guttmann are the pioneers in the setting of spinal injury unit in second world war. The first spinal unit was set in India in military hospital in Pune by Col. Chahal in 1969. Annually 15,000 permanent spinal cord injuries are observed. Commonly seen in men in between 16 to 30 years old.

Mechanism of Injury

- *Vehicle crashes:* 48 percent
- *Falls:* 21 percent
- *Penetrating trauma:* 15 percent
- *Sports injury:* 14 percent

- Twenty-five percent of all the spinal cord injuries occur from improper handling of the spine and patient after injury.
  - Assumptions are based upon mechanism of injury (MOI) that patients have a spinal injury
  - Manage all spinal injuries with immediate and continued care.
- Lifelong care for spinal cord injury victim exceeds one million dollars.
- Best form of care is public safety and prevention programs.

Causes

- *Trauma is the most common cause:* Automobile or motorcycle accident
- Gunshot or knife wounds
- Falls
- Sports mishaps
- *Nontraumatic causes are as follows:*
  - Cervical spondylosis with myelopathy
  - Myelitis and osteoporosis
  - Syringomyelia
  - Tumors
  - Vascular disease.

Anatomy (Figs 27.346 and 27.347)

Anatomy of Spinal Cord (Figs 27.348A and B)

- Layers
  - Dura mater
  - Arachnoid
  - Pia mater.
- Cover entire spinal cord and peripheral nerve roots that exit
- Cerebrospinal fluid bathes spinal cord by filling the subarachnoid space
  - Exchange of nutrients and waste products
  - Absorbs shocks of sudden movement.

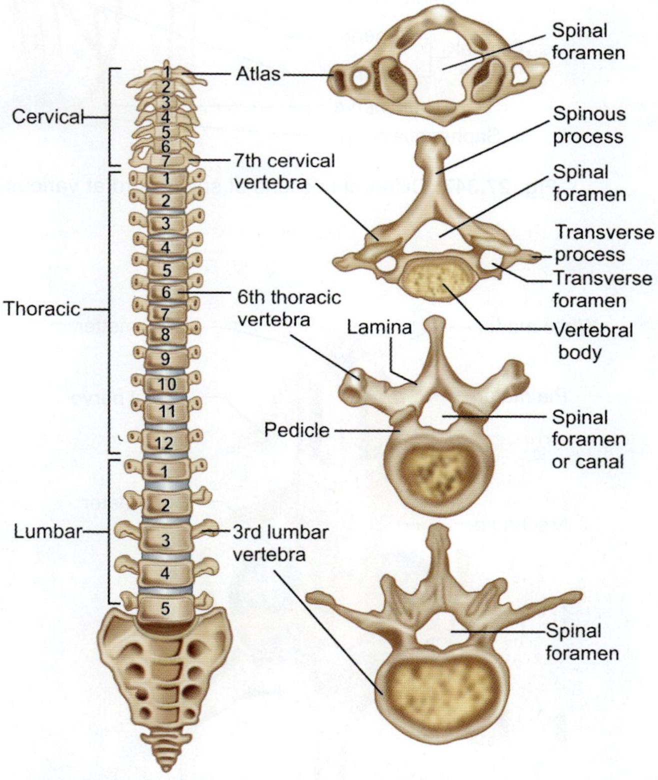

Fig. 27.346: Anatomy of spine showing structures of different types of vertebrae

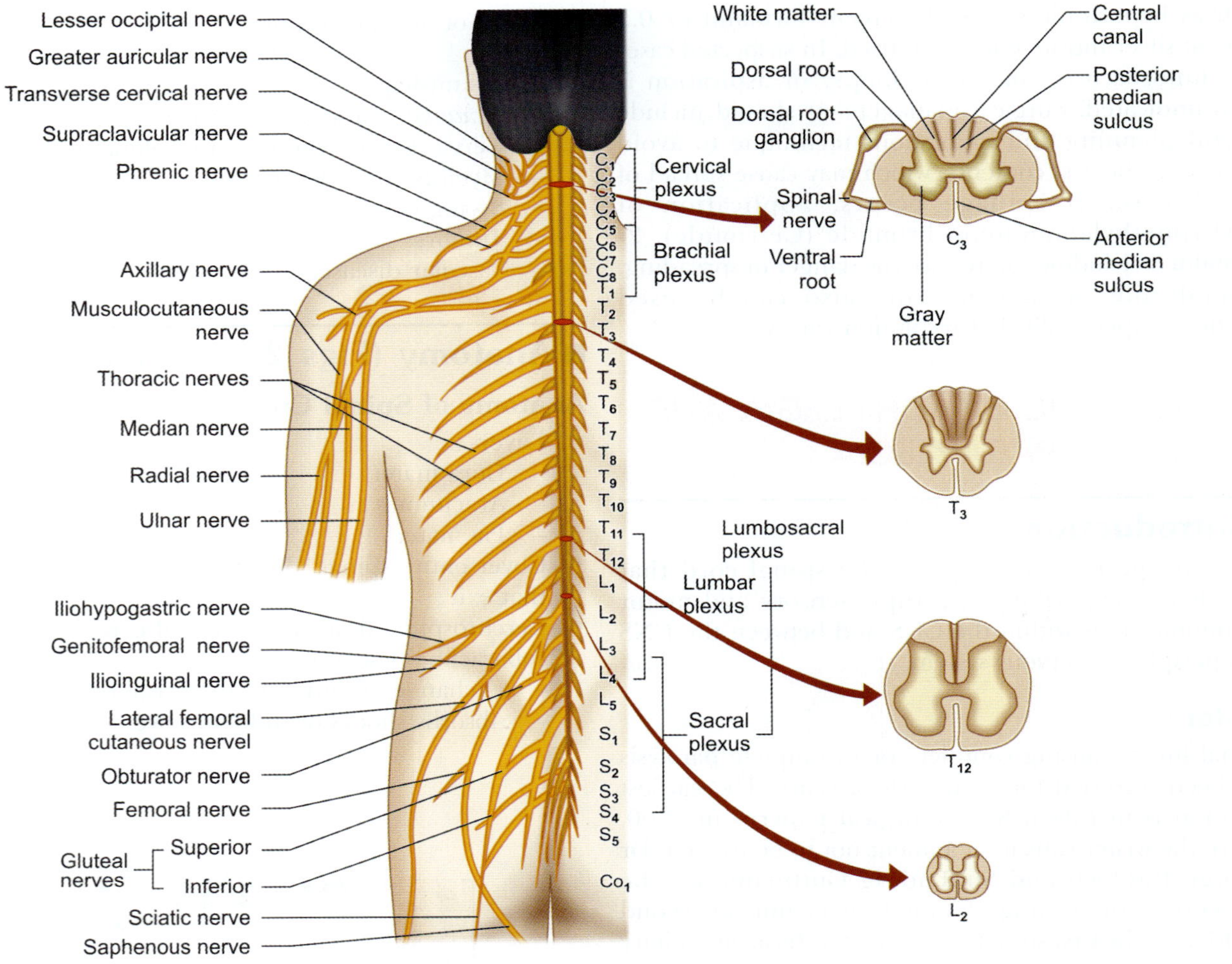

Fig. 27.347: Different sections of spinal cord at various spinal levels and spinal nerves arising from different regions

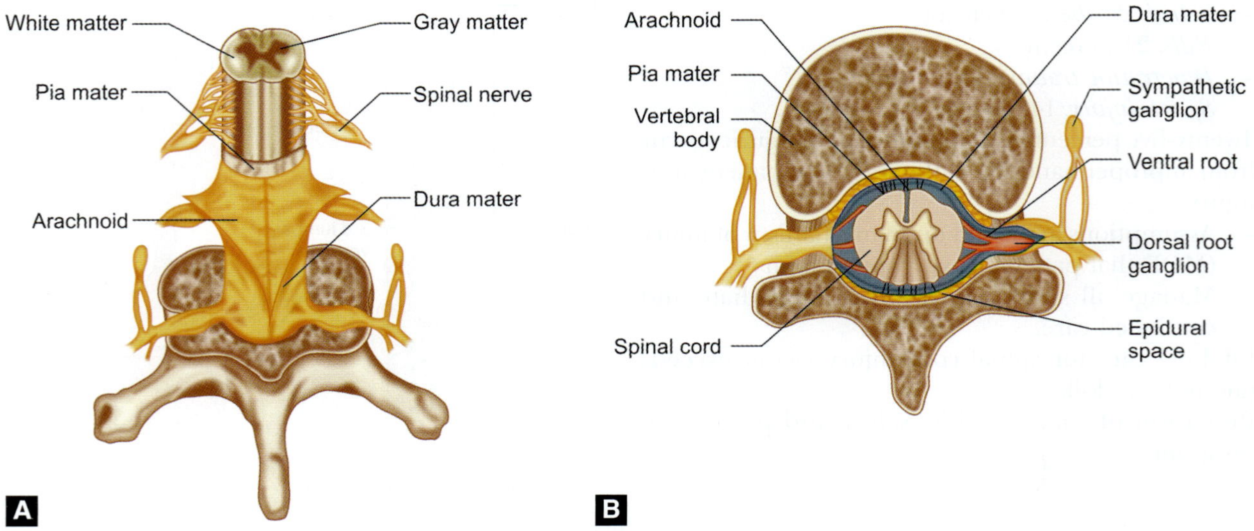

Figs 27.348A and B: Spinal cord anatomy with different meningeal layers

General Cord Anatomy

- *Anterior medial fissure*
  - Deep crease along the ventral surface of the spinal cord that divides cord into left and right halves.
- *Posterior medial fissure*
  - Shallow longitudinal groove along the dorsal surface.
- *Gray matter*
  - Area of the CNS dominated by nerve cell bodies
  - Central portion of the spinal cord.
- *White matter*
  - Surrounds gray matter
  - Comprised of axons.

Blood Supply

- *Paired spinal arteries*
  - Branch off the vertebral, cervical, thoracic and lumbar arteries
  - Travel through intervertebral foramina
  - Split into anterior and posterior arteries.

Physiology

- *Function*
  - Transmits sensory input from body to the brain
  - Conducts motor impulses from brain to muscles and organs
  - *Reflex center:* Intercepts sensory signals and initiates a reflex signal.
- *Growth*
  - *Fetus:* Entire cord fills entire spinal foramen
  - Adult
    - Base of brain to l-1 or l-2 level
    - Peripheral nerve roots pulled into spinal foramen at the distal end (cauda equina).
- *Axons*
  - Transmit signals upward to the brain and down to the body
  - Ascending tracts
    - Axons that transmit signals to the brain
    - These are called as 'sensory tracts'
  - Descending tracts
    - Axons that transmit signals to the body
    - These are called as 'motor tracts'
    - Voluntary and fine muscle movement.

Tracts of Spinal Cord

- *Ascending tracts (sensory tract):* Spinothalamic tract
- *Descending tract:* Corticol spinal tract, rubrospinal tract
- Corticospinal tracts (Fig. 27.349)
- Spinothalamic tract (Fig. 27.350)
- Spinocerebellar tract (Fig. 27.351)
- 31 pairs of nerves that originate along the spinal cord from anterior and posterior nerve roots
  - Sensory and motor functions
  - Travel through intervertebral foramina
- First pair exit between the skull and C-1
- Remainder of pairs exit below the vertebrae
- Each pair has two dorsal and two ventral roots
  - *Ventral roots:* Motor impulses from cord to body
  - *Dorsal roots:* Sensory impulses from body to cord
  - C-1 and CO-1 do not have dorsal roots.

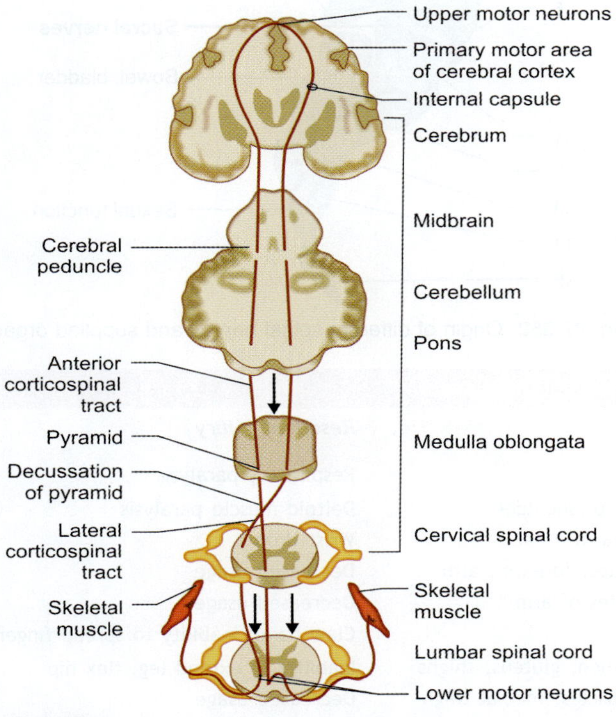

Fig. 27.349: Pyramidal lateral and anterior corticospinal tracts

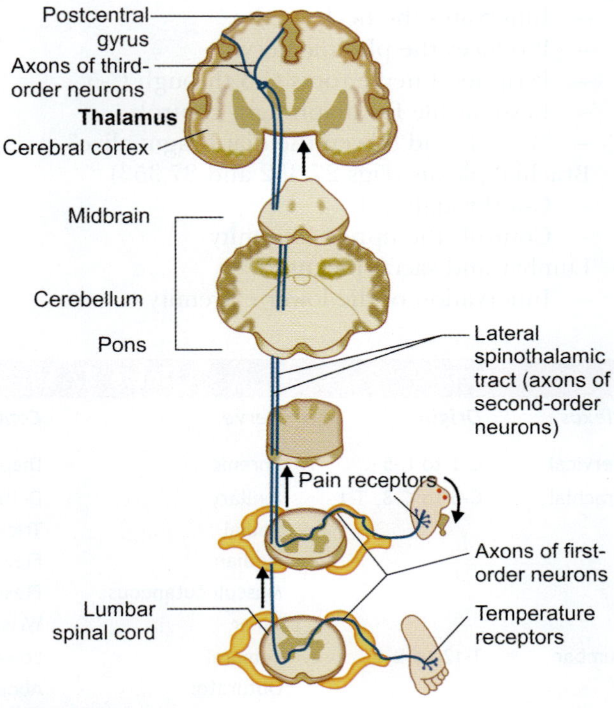

Fig. 27.350: Spinothalamic tract

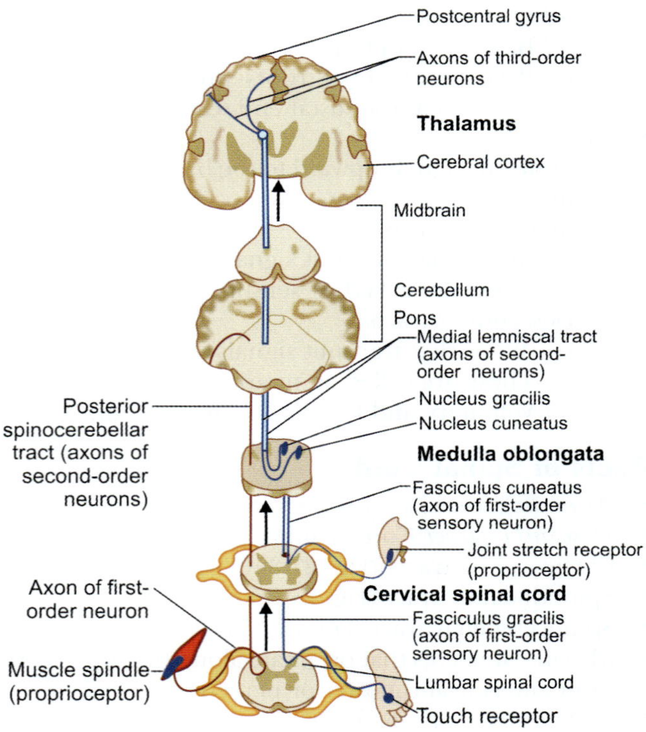

Fig. 27.351: Spinocerebellar tract

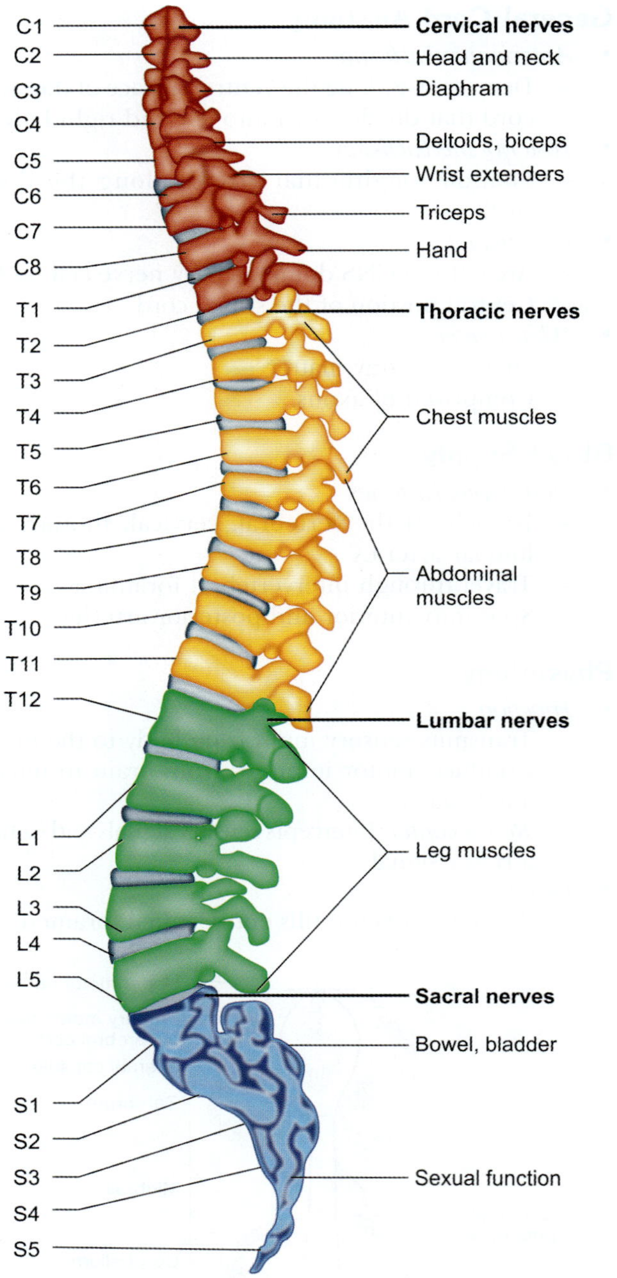

Fig. 27.352: Origin of different spinal nerves and supplied organs

Plexus

- Nerve roots that converge in a cluster of nerves
- Cervical plexus (Table 27.18)
  - Five cervical nerve roots
  - Innervates the neck
  - Produces the phrenic nerve
  - Peripheral nerve roots C-3 through C-5
  - Responsible for diaphragm control
  - "C-3, 4, and 5 keep the diaphragm alive"
- Brachial plexus (Figs 27.352 and 27.353)
  - C-5 through T-1
  - Controls the upper extremity
- Lumbar and sacral plexuses
  - Innervation of the lower extremity

Table 27.18: Spinal nerve plexuses

Plexus	*Origin*	*Nerve*	*Control*	*Result of injury*
Cervical	C-1 to C-5	Phrenic	Diaphragm	Respiratory paralysis
Brachial	C-5 to C-8, T-1	Axillary	Deltoid/skin of shoulder	Deltoid muscle paralysis
		Radial	Triceps/forearm	Wrist drop
		Median	Flexor muscles, forearm, arm	Decreased usage
		Musculocutaneous	Flexor muscles of arm	Decreased usage
		Ulnar	Wrist/hand	Claw hand; inability to spread fingers
Lumbar	T-12 to L-4	Femoral	Lower abdomen, gluteus, thighs	Inability to extend leg, flex hip
		Obturator	Abductor muscles, medial thigh	Decreased usage
Sacral	L-4 to S-3	Sciatic	Lower extremity	Decreased usage

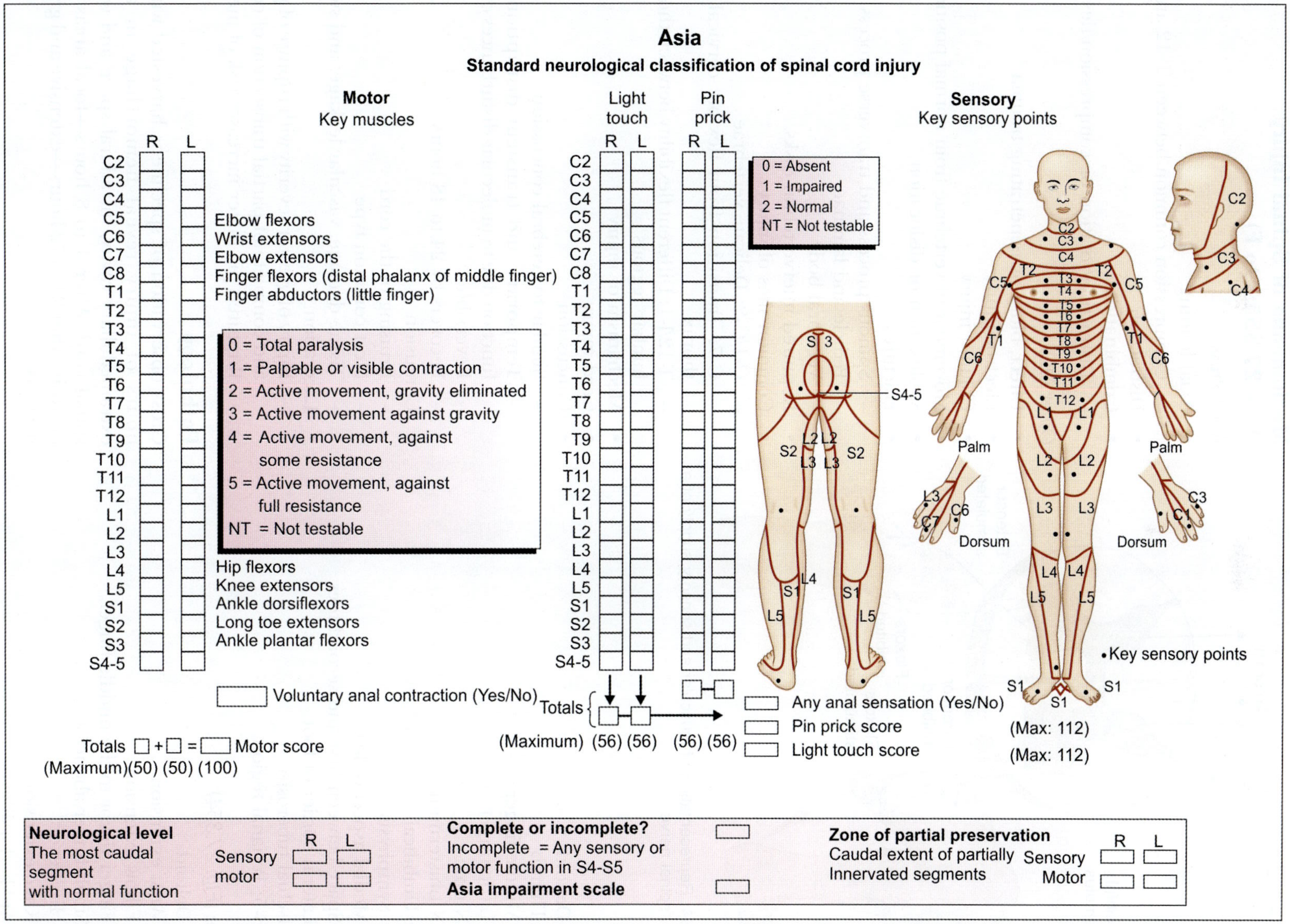

Fig. 27.353: Sensory distribution of spinal nerves

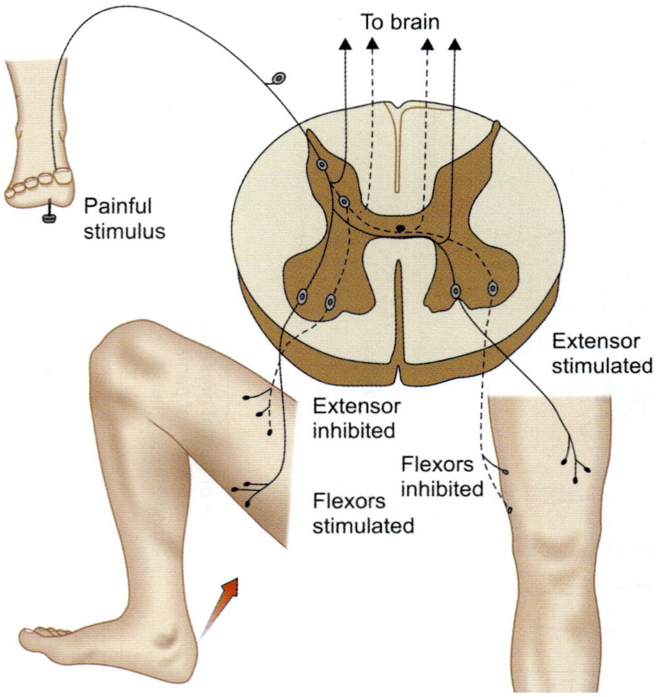

Fig. 27.354: Representation of muscular and sensory supply of a spinal nerve

- C-5: Deltoid
- C-6: Thumb
- C-7: Middle finger
- C-8: Little finger
- T-4: Nipple
- T-8: Xiphisternum
- T-10: Umbilical
- T-12: Symphysis
- L-4: Medial aspect of leg
- L-5: Space between first and second toes
- S-1: Lateral border of foot
- S-3: Ischial tuberosity
- S-4, S-5: Perianal region.

Myotome (Fig. 27.354)

- C-5: Deltoid
- C-6: Wrist extension
- C-7: Elbow extension
- C-8: Finger flexor to the middle finger
- T-1: Small finger abductor
- L-2: Hip flexor
- L-3: Knee extension
- L-4: Ankle dorsiflexor
- L-5: Long toe extensor
- S-1: Ankle plantar flexor
- Bilateral testing; digital exam (external anal sphincter).

Mechanisms of Spinal Injury (Figs 27.355A to F)

Axial stress

- Axial loading
  - Compression common between T-12 and l-2
- Distraction
- Combination
  - Distraction/rotation or compression/flexion.

Other MOI

- Direct, blunt or penetrating trauma
- Electrocution
- Column injury
- Movement of vertebrae from normal position
- Subluxation or dislocation
- Fractures
  - Spinous process and transverse process
  - Pedicle and laminae.
  - Vertebral body
- Ruptured intervertebral disks
- Common sites of injury
  - C-1/C-2: Delicate vertebrae
  - C-7: Transition from flexible cervical spine to thorax
  - T-12/l-1: Different flexibility between thoracic and lumbar regions
- Mechanism of injury
- Cord injury
- Concussion
  - Similar to cerebral concussion
  - Temporary and transient disruption of cord function due to molecular disturbances of neurons
  - Reversible
  - Recovers by 24 to 48 hours
- Contusion
  - Bruising of the cord
  - Most common type
  - Tissue damage, vascular leakage, and swelling.
- Laceration
  - Injury of greater severity with rupture of pia mater and complete of partial transection of cord
  - Ruptured pia mater increases risk of meningitis.

Pathology

Gross observation of specimens harvested within four hours of injury reveal hemorrhage in adjacent extramedullary cavity, intradural space and within the spinal cord. After 4 to 8 hours—focal areas of tissue necrosis. After 24 to 72 hours—extensive and gross tissue necrosis.

Microscopically

Hemorrhage is universally seen in intramedullary gray matter and in subdural space. Necrosis expands from the

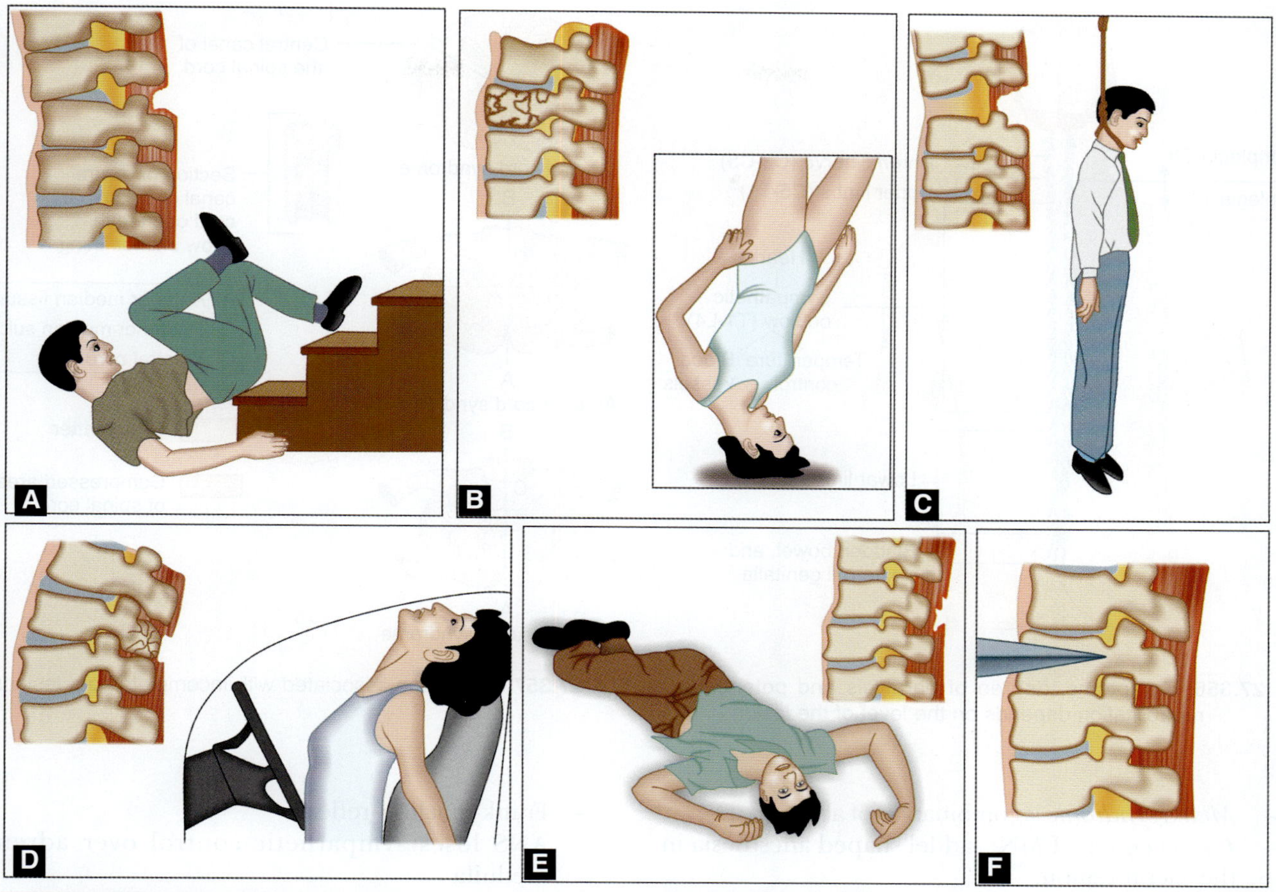

Figs 27.355A to F: Different mechanism of spinal injuries—(A) Flexion injury; (B) Compression injury; (C) Distraction injury; (D) Hyperextension injury; (E) Flexion-rotation injury; (F) Penetration injury

gray matter to engulf the progressive white matter. In mature form, cavities are filled with clear xanthochromic fluid and marginated with macrophages and astrocytes develop.

Transection Cord Injury

Injury that partially or completely severs the spinal cord

Complete

- Cervical spine
  - Quadriplegia
  - Incontinence
  - Respiratory paralysis
- Below T-1
- Incontinence
- Paraplegia.

Incomplete

Definition

- *Quadriplegia:* Paralysis of all the four limbs
- *Paraplegia:* Paralysis of the trunk and both lower limbs
- Depends on the level and degree of the injury
- Quadriplegia occurs with C-1 through C-8 injuries
- Paraplegia occurs with T-1 through L-4 (Fig. 27.356).

Incomplete Transection Cord Injury (Fig. 27.357)

- *Anterior cord syndrome*
  - Anterior vascular disruption
  - Loss of motor function and sensation of pain, light touch, and temperature below injury site
  - Retain motor, positional and vibration sensation
- *Central cord syndrome*
  - Hyperextension of cervical spine
  - Motor weakness affecting upper extremities
  - Bladder dysfunction
- *Brown-Sequard syndrome*
  - Penetrating injury that affects one side of the cord
  - Ipsilateral sensory and motor loss
  - Contralateral pain and temperature sensation loss
- *Posterior cord injury*
  - It is very rare
  - Only deep touch and loss of propioreception
  - *Conus medularis:* UMN and LMN sacral sparing present

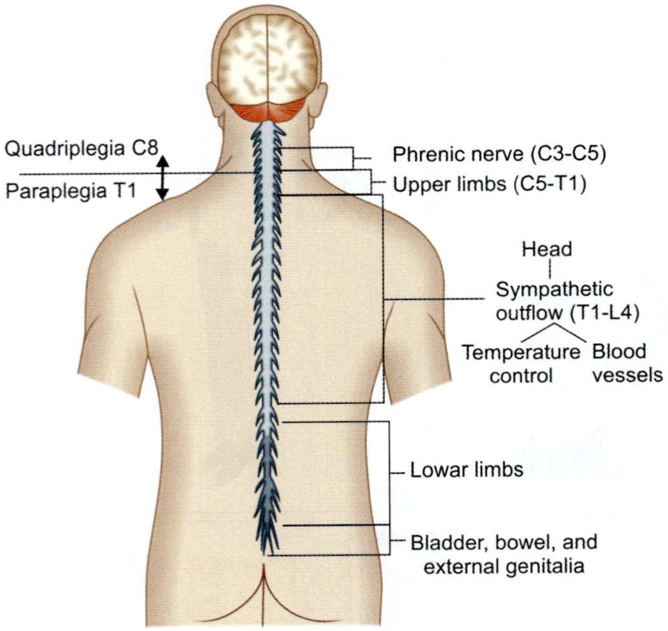

Fig. 27.356: Symptoms, degree of paralysis and potential for rehabilitation depends on the level of the lesion

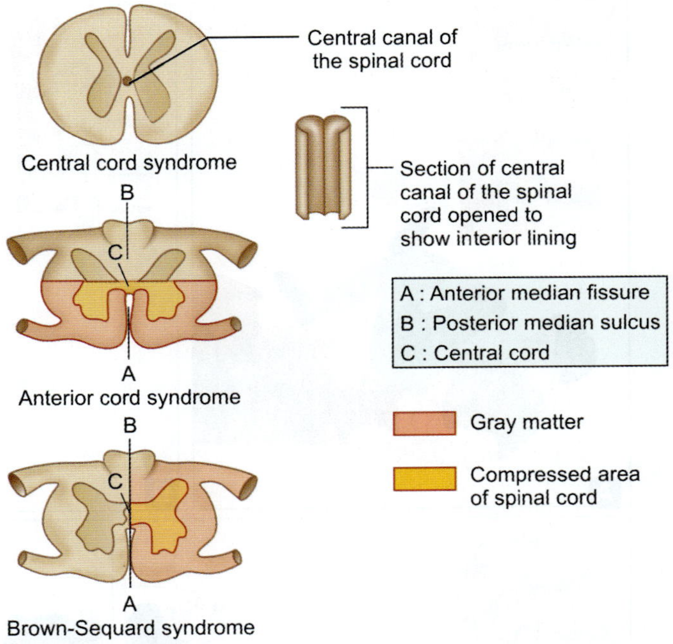

Fig. 27.357: Syndrome associated with incomplete cord lesions

- *Mixed syndrome* is combination of above
- *Cauda equina:* LMN; saddel shaped anesthesia in the sacral region.

General Signs and Symptoms

- Extremity paralysis
- Pain with and without movement
- Tenderness along spine
- Impaired breathing
- Spinal deformity
- Priapism
- Posturing
- Loss of bowel or bladder control
- Nerve impairment to extremities
- *Spinal shock:* It is a temporary insult to the cord. Affects body below the level of injury. Affected area is:
  - Flaccid
  - Without feeling
  - Loss of movement (flaccid paralysis)
  - Frequent loss of bowel and bladder control
  - Priapism
  - Hypotension secondary to vasodilation.
- *Spinal-vascular shock:* Occurs when injury to the spinal cord disrupts the brain's ability to control the body:
  - Loss of sympathetic tone
  - Dilation of arteries and veins
  - Expands vascular space
  - Results in relative hypotension
  - Reduced cardiac preload
  - Reduction of the strength of contraction
  - Frank-Starling reflex
  - ANS loses sympathetic control over adrenal medulla
  - Unable to control release of epinephrine and norepinephrine
  - Loss of positive inotropic and chronotropic effects.
- *Neurogenic shock:* Signs and symptoms include:
  - Bradycardia
  - Hypotension
  - Cool, moist and pale skin above the injury
  - Warm, dry and flushed skin below the injury
  - *Male:* Priapism.
- *Autonomic hyper-reflexia syndrome:* Associated with the body's resolution of the effects of spinal shock. Commonly associated with injuries at or above T-6. Typical presentation include:
  - Sudden hypertension
  - Bradycardia
  - Pounding headache
  - Blurred vision
  - Sweating and flushing of skin above the point of injury.
- *Specific signs*
  - *Injury at the level of C1 and C2:* Usually fatal, presence of quadriplegia, complete loss of sensory and motor control, artificial respiration mandatory for survival.
  - *Injury at the level of C3:* Usually fatal, presence of quadriplegia, complete loss of sensory and motor

control, artificial respiration mandatory for survival.

- *Injury at the level of C4:* Presence of quadriplegia. Slight breathing efforts present. Assisted ventilation injury at the level of C5—complete motor and sensory paralysis. Respiration present. Shrugging of shoulder present. Sensory at the deltoid region. Biceps reflex is absent.
- *C6 level:* Deltoid, biceps and wrist extensors are intact. Sensation laterally to thumb and index finger. Brachioradialis reflex is absent.
- *C7 level:* Only long flexors and intrinsic paralyzed. Sensation lost only on the ulnar side of the arm. Triceps reflex is absent.
- *C8 level:* Intrinsic muscles paralyzed with claw hand.
- *Level of T1:* Small muscles of the hand.
- *Level of T2 to T12:* Intercostal and rectus abdominis muscles to be tested. Upper limb have full power. Beevor's sign positive. Sensory T-4 nipple line, T-7 xiphoid process.
- *T12 to L3:* Iliopsoas, quadriceps and adductor group. No bowel and bladder control.
- *L4 level:* Tibialis anterior. Stepping gait. Patellar tendon reflex. No bowel and bladder voluntary control.
- *L5 level:* Extensor hallucis longus, extensor digitorum longus, gluteus medius. No bowel and bladder control.
- *S1 level:* Peroneus longus, gastrocnemius-soleus, gluteus maximus, achilles tendon reflex.
- *S2 to S4 level:* Superficial anal reflex.

Clinical Applications

- *Respiration:* Complete transection of the cord at C3 or higher is incompatible with life. Patient has to be permanently ventilated.
- *Wheel chair:* C6 level intact is the highest level for manipulation of wheel chair. However, independent transfer in and out of the wheel chair is still difficult due to lack of function of triceps.
- *Crutches:* Complete cord lesion above C8 is in compatible for the use of crutches since the intrinsic muscle of hand needs strong grip.
- *Complete or incomplete lesion:* Within first 24 hours, if returns is incomplete. Good prognosis.
- *Sacral sparing:* Prognostic indicator of cord return is sacral sparing as sacral nerves at the periphery. Check flexor muscle of the great toe, sensory testing of the perianal region and reflex testing of anal sphincter muscles.
- *T1 to T8:* Can use wheel chair independently. The person can not get up from floor on wheel chair.
- *T6:* Has full upper extremity and thoracic musculature and can stabilize himself against pectoral girdle.
- *T9 to T12:* Can walk independently with long leg braces and crutches.
- *Bowel and bladder:* If complete sacral sparing bowel and bladder recovers after few days. If only perianal sensation only partial recovery. If sacral sparing not there but anal wink and bulbocavernosus reflex present reflex bladder. Patient is trained to empty bladder.
- If all reflexes absent, atonic bladder has to be catheterized.

Investigations

- X-ray spine anteroposterior and lateral views, usually lateral oblique images are taken.
- CT scan
- MRI.

Management

- Emergency care at the scene of the accident and in the emergency room
- Definitive care of the patient
- Rehabilitation
- Emergency care
- At the scene of the accident:
  - Airway
  - Breathing
  - Circulation

Cervical Spine

Stabilize is a word commonly used to describe protecting the spinal cord from possible injury (or further injury), when vertebral column integrity is disrupted. Immobilize refers to the "splinting" of the head, neck and torso to limit any transmission of motion to the spine. Spinal motion restriction (SMR) is now suggested as a more accurate description of modern spinal injury care. However, this phrase could be misunderstood to indicate a more limited "immobilization" of the spine than is currently practiced.

Spinal Alignment (Figs 27.358A to C)

- Move patient to a neutral, in-line position
- Position of function
- Hips and knees should be slightly flexed for maximum comfort and minimum stress on muscles, joints and spine. Place a rolled blanket under the knees
- Always support the head and neck
- Contraindications to neutral position:
  - Movement causes a noticeable increase in pain
  - Noticeable resistance met during procedure
  - Increase in neurological deficits occurs during movement
  - Gross deformity of spine.
- Less movement is best

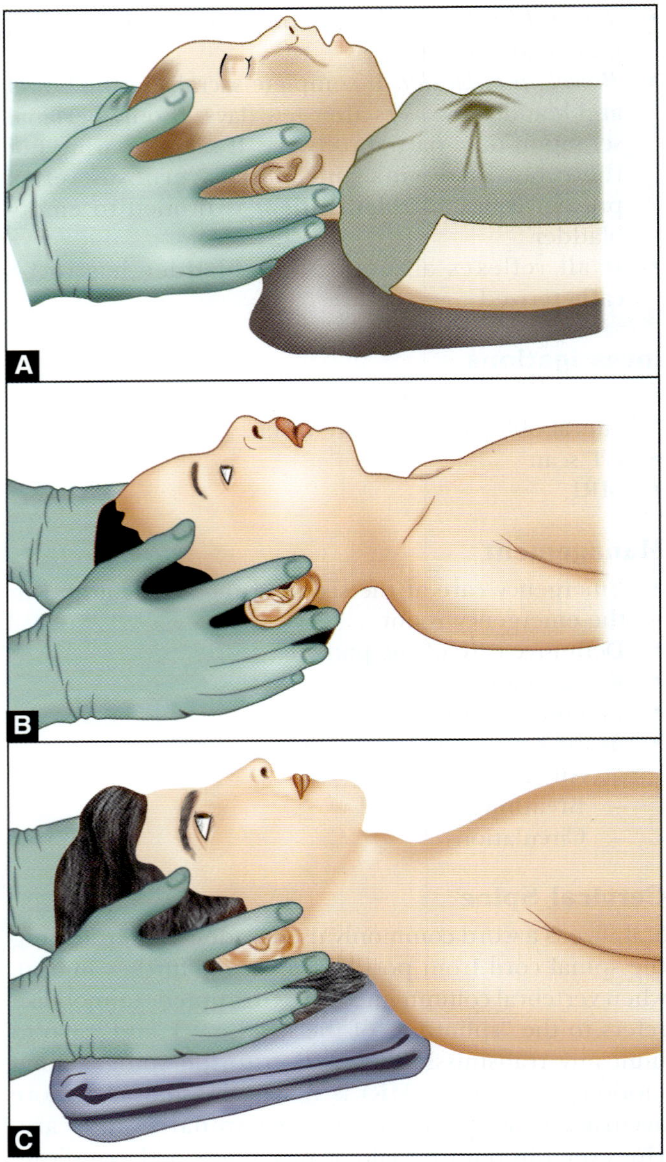

Figs 27.358A to C: Cervical spine positioning in different age groups—(A) Positioning in an infant; (B) In a child; (C) An adult

- In the emergency department rapid trauma assessment need to carried out. Focused versus rapid assessment.

Rapid Assessment

- Suspected or likely spinal cord/column injury
- Multisystem trauma patient
- Evaluate for
  - *Neck:* Deformity, pain, crepitus, warmth and tenderness
  - *Bilateral extremities:* Finger abduction/adduction. Push, pull, grip, etc.
  - Motor and sensory function
- Dermatome and myotome evaluation
- Babinski's sign test
- Hold-up position

Vital Signs

- Body temperature above and below the site of injury
- Pulse
- Blood pressure
- Respirations
- Stroke lateral aspect of the bottom of the foot
- Evaluate for movement of the toes
  - *Fanning and flexing (lifting):* Positive sign indicates injury along the pyramidal (descending spinal) tract.

Cervical Collar Application

- Apply the C-collar as soon as possible.
- Assess neck prior to placing.
- C-collar limits some movement and reduces axial loading.
- Does not completely prevent movement of the neck.
- Size and apply according to the manufacturer's recommendation.
  - Collar should fit snugly
  - Collar should not impede respirations
  - Head should continue to be in neutral position
  - Size it, size it, size it.
- Do not release manual control until the patient is fully secured in a spinal restriction device.

Definitive Care

- Clinical assessment of neurologic deficit
- GCS for level of consciousness
- Detailed neurological examination
- Radiological and special investigations: X-rays; CT-scan; MRI; Sciwora
- Conservative treatment
- Operative treatment

Medical Management

1. *Medications and spinal cord injury:* Steroids, if neurodeficit is identified, is given as IV 30 mg/kg for over 15 minutes. 5.4 mg/kg/hr for 23 hours given within 8 hours of the injury:
   - Reduce the body's response to injury
   - Reduce swelling and pressure on the cord
   - Administered within first 8 hours of injury
2. Me*dications and neurogenic shock*
   - Fluid challenge:
     - Isotonic solution: 20 ml/kg
     - 250 ml initially
     - Monitor response and repeat as needed
   - Dopamine: 2 to 20 mg/kg/min titrated to blood pressure
   - Atropine: 0.5-1.0 mg/3 to 5 min (maximum of 2.0 mg)

Operative Treatment

- *Cervical spine:* Facet wiring, orion anterior cervical plate and morscher plaing.
  - Decompression
  - Harrington distraction instrumentation
  - Harrington compression instrumentation
  - Edwards instrumentation
  - Luque instrumentation
  - Pedicle screw instrumentation
  - Conservative management
  - Care of the skin
  - Care of bladder
  - Care of bowel
  - Physiotherapy
  - Prevention of DVT
  - Rehabilitation
  - Physical rehabilitation
  - Social rehabilitation
  - Economic rehabilitation.

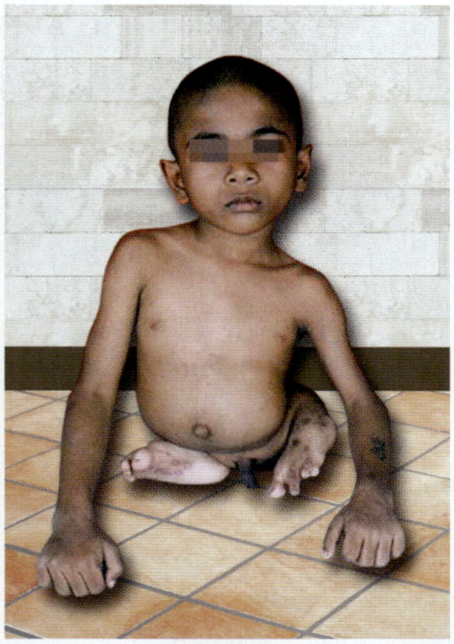

Fig. 27.359: Deformed limbs and accompanying spinal deformity can be corrected by using spinal orthosis

SPINAL ORTHOSIS

An externally applied device to assist the spine or spinal segment.

Nomenclature

- Cervical-thoracic-lumbar-sacral orthosis (CTLSO)
- Thoracic lumbosacral orthosis (TLSO)
- Lumbosacral orthosis (LSO)
- Sacral orthosis (SO)
- Lumbar orthosis (LO)
- Cervical orthosis (CO)
- Head CTLSO (HCTLSO).

Function (Fig. 27.359)

- To restore structure
- Musculoskeletal system
- Nervous system.

Restore Function

This is normally done by following:

- Stabilization
- Mobilization
- Corrective
- Protective
- Overlapping.

Stabilization

It generally supports the following:

- Largest group
- Controls an otherwise uncontrollable movements
- Prevention of deformities
- Architectural inadequacies
- Trauma
- Disease
- Congenital abnormalities.

Mobilization

- Prevents mobility
- Restricts mobility
- Resists.

Corrective

It corrects/resists/prevents the following:

- Traction
- Skeletal fixation
- Spinal orthosis with pads deformity must be correctable.

Protective

Protects the spine by following:

- Stabilization of spine
- Correction of deformity
- Correct alignment
- Postsurgical.

Biomechanics

- Movements of spine
- Alignment
- Mechanics of pain
- Materials used
- Trunk support
- Motion control
- Realignment
- Apply distraction force
- Pascal's law (Figs 27.360A and B)
- Spinal orthosis
- Materials used

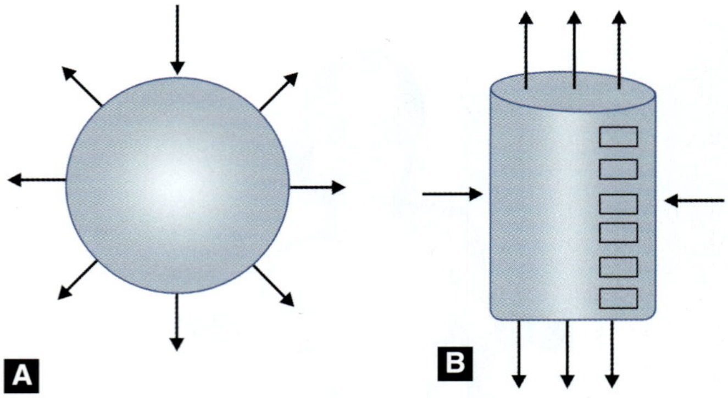

Figs 27.360A and B: Pascal's law

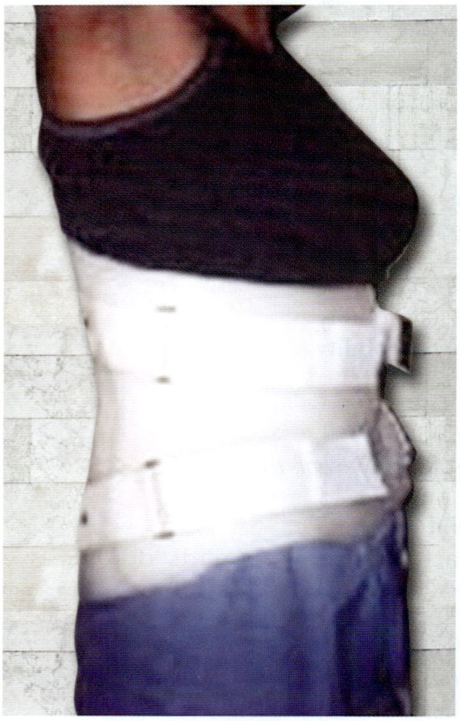

Fig. 27.361: Spinal braces for maintaining spinal biomechanics

- Plastics (thermoplastics)
  - Polyethylene (LD and HD)
  - Polypropylene (LD and HD)
  - Polyamide
  - Polyurethane
  - Polycarbolactine (low temp thermoplastics)
- Plastics (thermoplastics) (Fig. 27.361)
  - Epoxy
  - Polyester

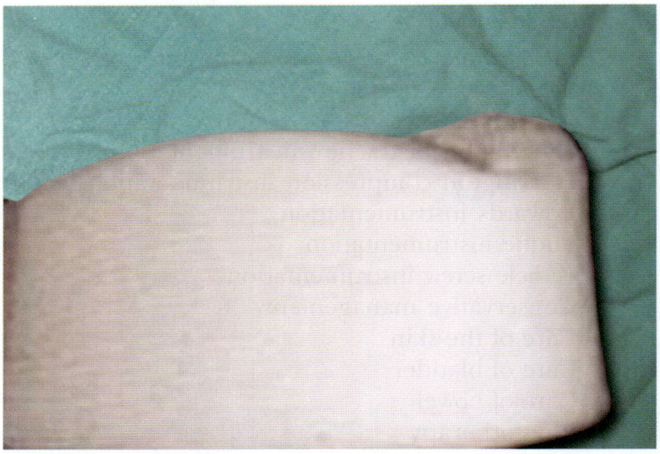

Fig. 27.362: Soft collar brace used for cervical spine

  - FRP
  - Carbon fiber reinforced plastics.

Spinal Orthosis

Types

- Soft
- Corset
- Belts
- Rigid orthosis.

Cervical Spinal Orthosis

- Supports weight of head
- Bypass the load from cervical spine
- Transportation of the patient
  - Soft collar (Fig. 27.362)
  - Moulded collar
  - Spinal orthosis
  - Soft modulated collar (Fig. 27.363)
  - Philadelphia collar
  - Somi brace (Fig. 27.364)
  - Four postcervical collar (Fig. 27.365).

Dorsolumbar Orthosis

- Chest/rib support
- Increased intracavity pressure
- Distraction force
- Restricted trunk motion
- Skeletal alignment

Lumbosacral Orthosis

- Increased intracavity pressure
- Restricted lumbosacral motion
- Skeletal alignment

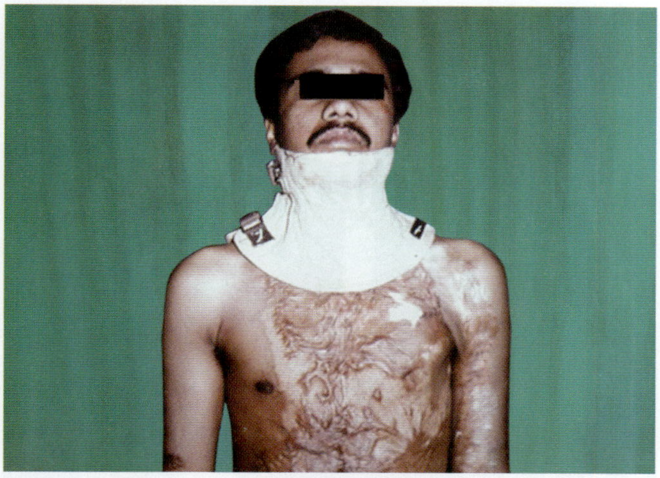

Fig. 27.363: Soft modulated cervical collar

- Abdominal brace
  - Taylor's brace (TLSO)

Taylor's Brace (Fig. 27.366)
Flexion-extension control.

Knight's Brace (Fig. 27.367)
Flexion-extension and lateral control.

Cow-Horn Brace
Flexion-extension, lateral and rotary control.

Boston's Brace (Figs 27.368A and B)

Cash/Ash Brace (Fig. 27.369)
Prevent flexion.

Jewett's Brace
Prevent flexion.

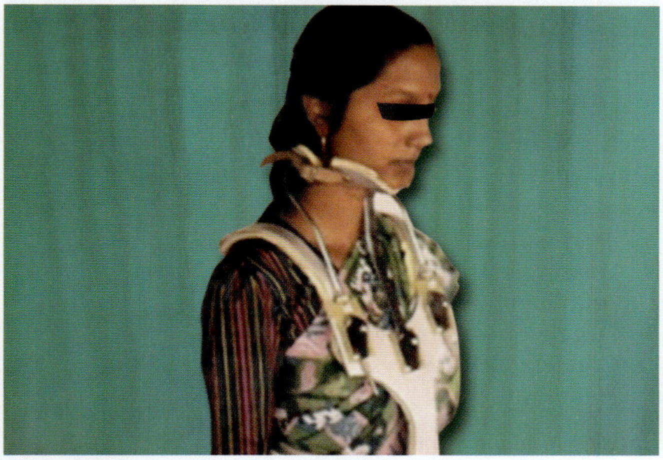

Fig. 27.364: A Somi brace

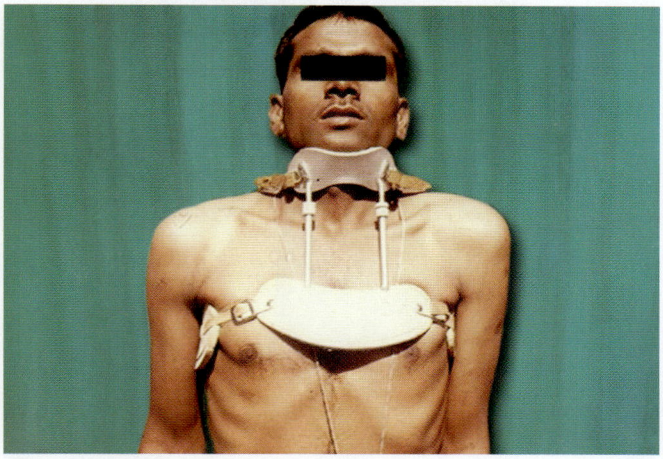

Fig. 27.365: Four-postcervical collar

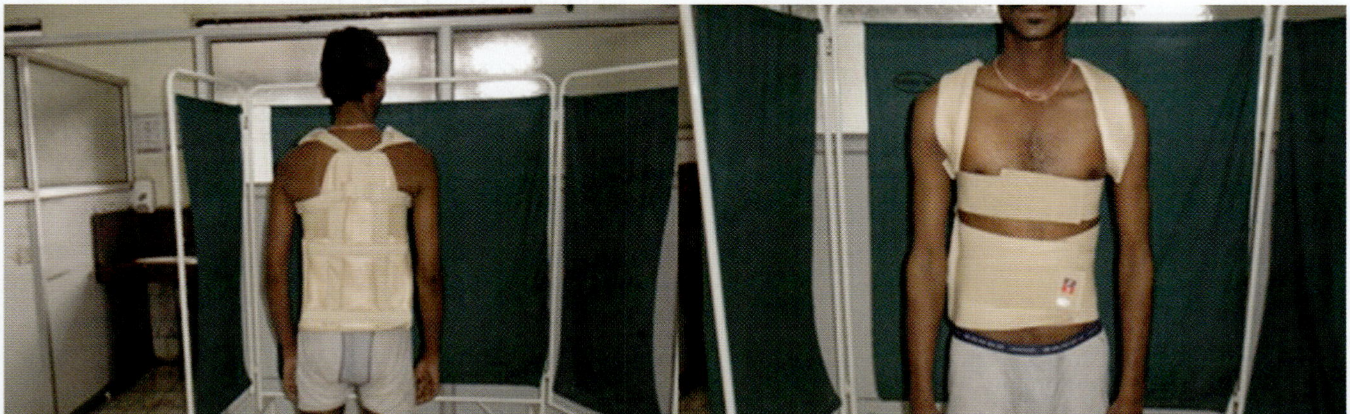

Fig. 27.366: A Taylor's brace seen from behind and front

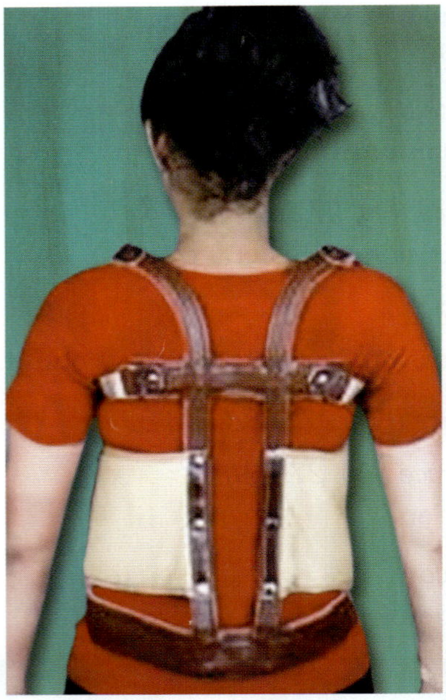

Fig. 27.367: Taylor-Knight's brace with lateral strips

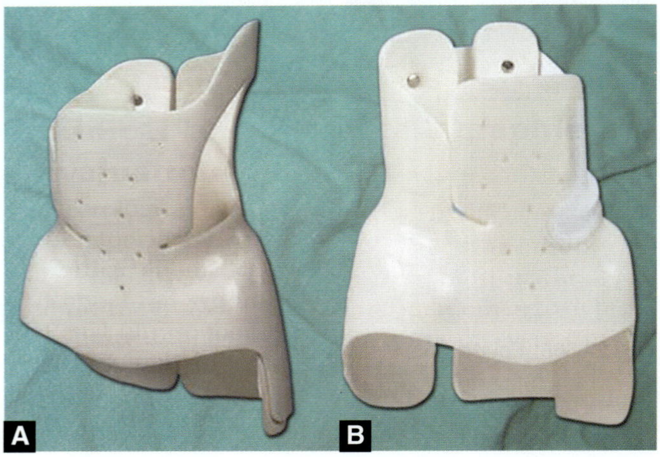

Fig. 27.368A and B: Boston's brace

Cervical Dorso-lumbosacral Orthosis

Milwaukee Brace (Figs 27.370A to C)

Head cervicodorsolumbar sacral orthosis (HCDLSO)

- Halo HCTO

Mechanism of Action

- Reduce trunk movements
- Improve skeletal alignment
- Increase intracavity pressure
- Thus restore structure
- Restore function
- Spinal orthosis.

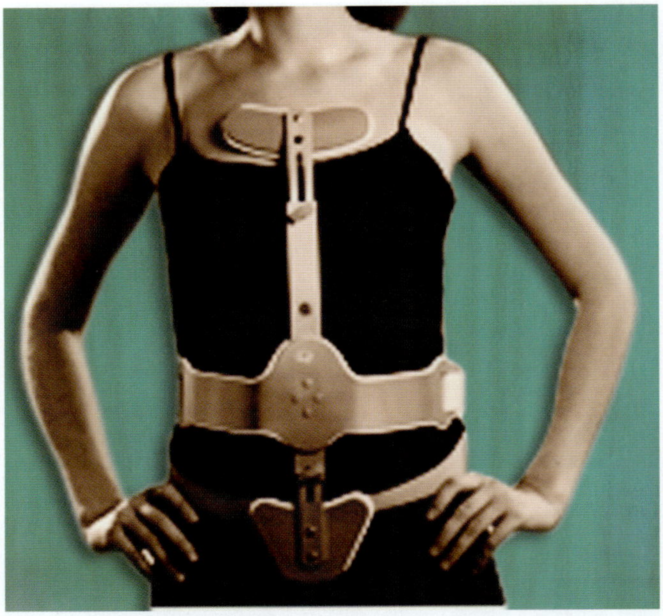

Fig. 27.369: Cash/Ash brace

Indications

- Pain
- Malignant
- Trauma
- Postsurgical
- Inflammation
- Degenerative disorders
- Congenital disorders
- Neoplasm.

Specific Management

- Low backache
  - Acute: Rigid orthosis
  - Mild: Soft orthosis.
- Deformities, e.g. scoliosis
  - TLO, LSO, TLSO (Taylor's brace)
  - CTLSO (Milwaukee orthosis)
  - With corrective pads.
- Kyphosis
  - TLO, LSO, TLSO (Taylor's brace)
  - Boston brace
  - CTLSO (Milwaukee orthosis)
  - With corrective pads.
- Lordosis
  - Abdominal corset
- Before spinal surgery
  - Preoperative orthosis
  - Pain relieved
  - Remove orthosis.
  - Pain reappear surgery
- Following disk surgery without fusion
  - Corset

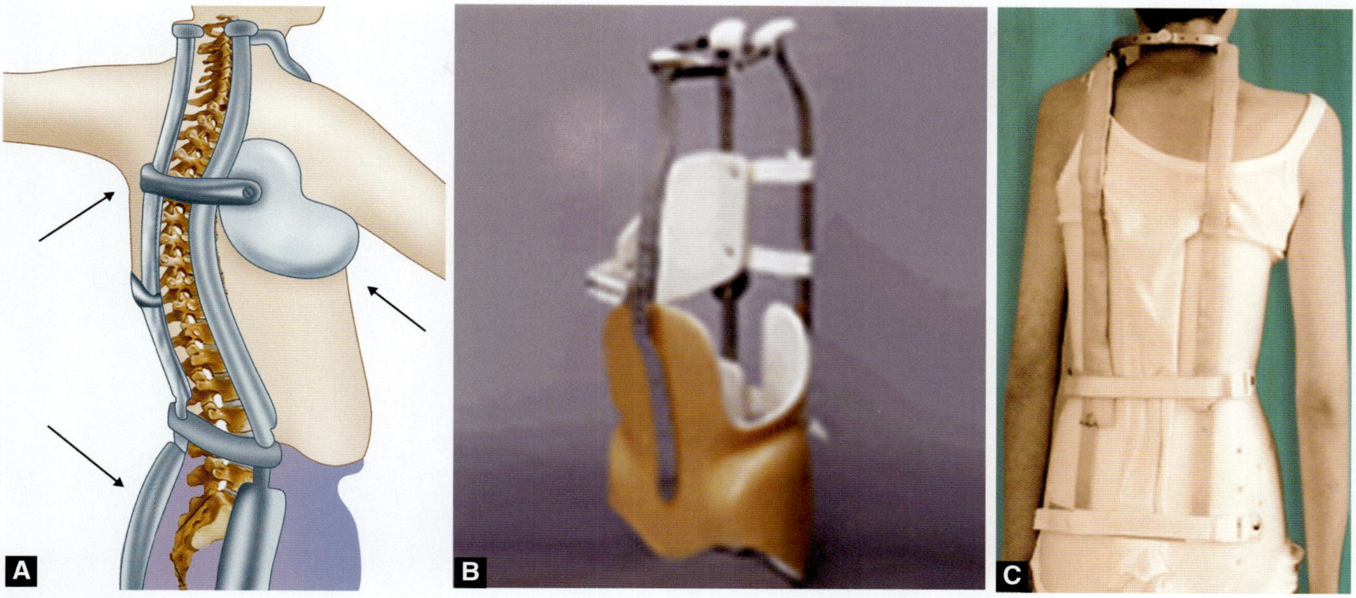

Figs 27.370A to C: Milwaukee brace—(A) Action of Milwaukee brace on body; (B) and (C) Brace applied to correct spinal alignment

- Following disk surgery with fusion: Rigid orthosis
- Other surgeries
  - Rigid orthosis
  - Bi-valve TLSO
- Fractures
  - Rigid orthosis in extension
  - As a substitute for surgery
  - Postoperatively
- Osteoporosis
  - Corset
- Inflammatory spinal arthritis
  - Orthosis to prevent flexion
- Infectious disorders like osteomyelitis and tuberculosis
  - TLSO with flexion, extension and lateral control orthosis
- Tumors of spine
  - TLSO with flexion, extension control orthosis
- Paralytic disorders
  - TLSO with corrective pads
  - Taylor's brace
  - Milwaukee's brace
  - Ash (Cash) brace
- Spondylolisthesis
  - Lumbosacral extension and lateral control orthosis
- Cervical conditions
  - Soft collar
  - Firm collar
  - Rigid collar
  - Halo traction

Positive Effects

- Trunk support
- Motion control
- Realignment.

Negative Effects

- Weakness and atrophy
- Psychological dependence.

Hazardous effects are due to the following:

- Wrong diagnosis
- Wrong prescription
- Wrong donning
- Prolonged use
- Wrongly manufactured
- Poor finish
- Hazards are:
  - Injury
  - Swelling
  - Ulceration
  - Bed sore
  - Increased symptoms.

Basic Principles of Orthotic Fitting

- Simplicity of design
- Easy donning and doffing
- Operational ease
- Comfortable
- Affordable.

Important Tips

- For prevention—early orthosis
- For correcting deformity—dynamic orthosis
- Orthosis to be given only for correctible deformity
- Proper selection of material.

Section 4

Recent Advancements in Orthopedics

28 Antibiotics in Orthopedics

- Penicillins
- Clavulanic Acid
- Sulbactam
- Cephalosporins
- Other Beta-lactam Antibiotics
- Macrolides
- Fluoroquinolones
- Antitubercular Drugs

■ History

History is divided into three phases—period of empirical use of "mouldy curd", by Chinese on boils, *chaulmoogra* oil by Hindus in leprosy, mercury by Paracelsus (16th century) for syphilis, cinchona bark (17th century) for fevers. Ehrlich's phase of dyes and organometallic compounds (1890–1935), with the discovery of microbes in later half of 19th century. Ehrich developed arsenicals, like arsphenamine in 1906 and neoarsphenamine in 1909 for syphilis.

Modern Era of Chemotherapy

- Phenomena of antibiotics was demonstrated by Pasteur in 1877
- Paul Gelmo discovered sulfonamide
- Fleming discovered penicillium in 1929, but could not purify penicillin out of it. It was eventually brought to clinical use, by Chain and Florey in 1941
- Genord Domagk, a bacteriologist and pathologist, who demonstrated therapeutic effect of prontosil, a sulfonamide dye in pyogenic infection. Sulfapyridine was first sulfonamide to be marketed in 1938
- Waksman and colleagues discovered streptomycin in 1944. Chloramphenicol was discovered in 1949 and erythromycin in 1952.

Definition

- Antibiotics are substances produced by microorganisms, which suppress the growth of or kill other organisms at very low concentration
- This definition excludes other natural substances, which also inhibit microorganisms, but are produced by higher forms, e.g. antibodies or even those produced by microbes, but are needed in high concentrations (ethanol, lactic acid, H_2O_2, etc.)
- Antimicrobial agents (AMAs) is term designated to synthetic, semisynthetic and naturally obtained drugs, which attenuate microorganisms.

Classification

Classified in many ways:

- Chemical structure
  - Sulfonamides, quinolones, aminoglycosides, macrolides, tetracyclines, etc.
- Mechanism of action
  - Inhibit cell wall synthesis (penicillins), inhibit protein synthesis (tetracyclines, macrolides), etc.
- Type of organism against which primarily active
  - Antibacterials, antivirals, antifungals and antiprotozoal
- Spectrum of activity
  - Narrow spectrum (penicillin G, streptomycin)
  - Intermediate spectrum (cephalosporins, fluoroquinolones, etc.)
  - Broadspectrum (tetracyclines, etc.)
- Type of action
  - Primarily bacteriostatic (ethambutol, erythromycin, etc.)
  - Primarily bactericidal (aminoglycosides, rifampicin, vancomycin, etc.).

Choosing an Antimicrobial Agent

It depends on following factors:

- Patient factors
- Infecting organism
- Drugs availability.

Patient Factors

- Age
- Renal and hepatic function
- Local factors, like presence of pus, hematomas, etc.

- Drug allergy
- Impaired host defence
- Pregnancy
- Genetic factors, e.g. primaquine is likely to produce hemolysis in glucose-6-phosphate dehydrogenase (G-6PD) deficient patients.

Organism Related Factors

- Clinical diagnosis
- Postbacteriological examination and culture sensitivity testing
- Virulence of the organism and coexisting diseases.

Drug Factors

- *Spectrum of activity:* Narrow or broadspectrum
- *Type of activity:* Bactericidal or bacteriostatic
- *Sensitivity of the organism:* On basis of minimum inhibitory concentration (MIC) values
- *Relative toxicity:* Beta-lactam over aminoglycoside
- *Pharmacokinetic profile:* Bioavailability, tissue penetration and elimination
- *Route of administration:* Oral/parenteral/topical
- *Evidence of clinical efficacy:* Based on clinical trials and US Food and Drug Administration (FDA) approval
- Cost.

Problems Arises with Antimicrobial Agents

- Toxicity, which can be local and systemic
- Hypersensitivity reactions
- Drug resistance
- Superinfection
- Nutritional deficiencies
- Masking of an infection, e.g. syphilis, masked by single dose of penicillin.

Mechanism of Action of AMA

Bacterial cell is different from eukaryotic cell in many ways, in its structure and organelles. For an AMA to do its desired action on a bacterial cells, their details are need to be understood, as shown in Figure 28.1. Bacterial cell are potential targets for attack of antibacterial drugs at some key biochemical reactions and formed structures, like cell wall, DNA, intracellular organelles, muscle fibers, etc.

Other mechanisms include:

- Inhibition of cell wall synthesis (most common mechanism)
- Inhibition of protein synthesis (translation) (second largest class)
- Alteration of cell membranes
- Inhibition of nucleic acid synthesis
- Antimetabolite activity.

Biochemical Reactions (Fig. 28.2)

Class I reactions: Using glucose and alternative carbon source for adenosine triphosphate (ATP) production. This is not very promising target, as both human and bacterial cell use Embden-Meyerhof pathway and tricarboxylic acid (TCA) cycle, for energy production and availibility of large variety of substrates, like lactate and amino acids by bacteria, if glucose pathways are blocked.

Class II reactions (Fig. 28.3): Utilizes energy and class I compounds, to make simple carbon compounds like

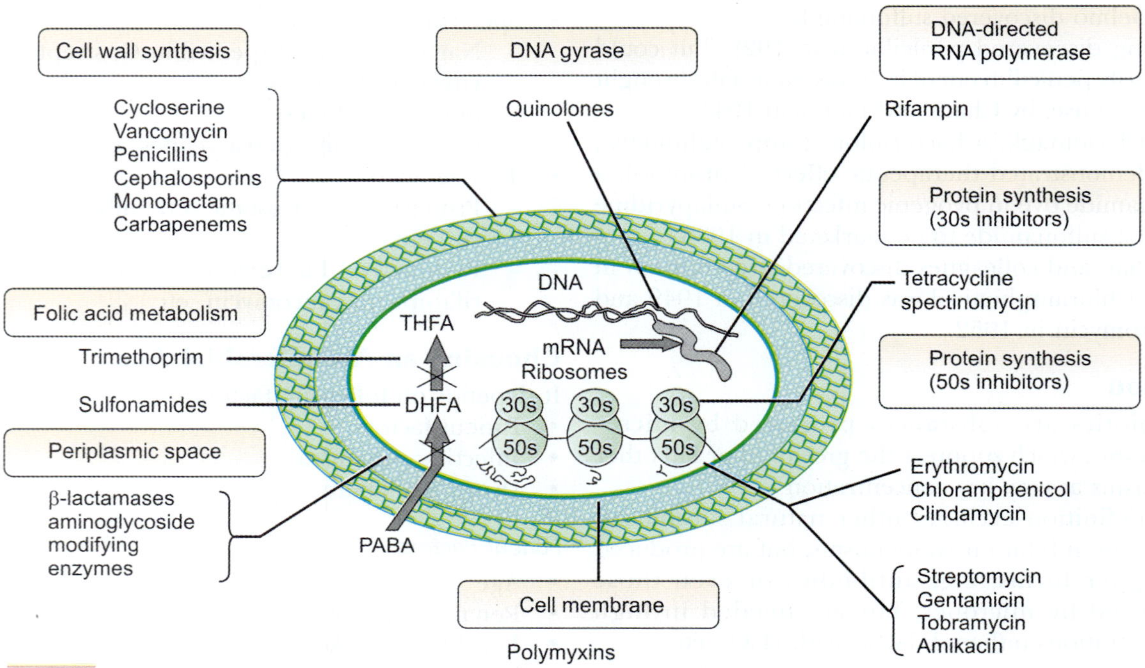

Fig. 28.1: Different types of AMA, for inhibiting different bacterial cell functions

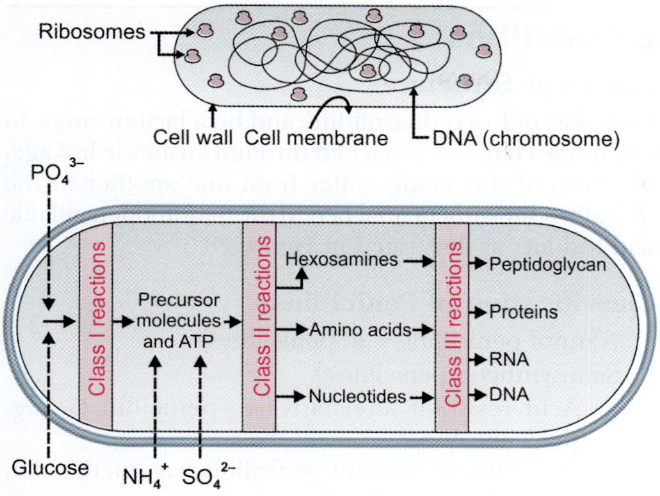

Fig. 28.2: Different types of biochemical reactions, occurring in a bacterial cell

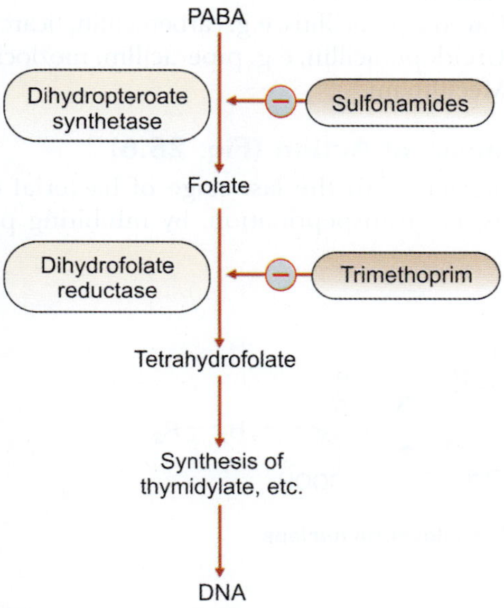

Fig. 28.3: Class II reaction, takes place in a bacterial cell—Sulfonamides compete with PABA for dihydropteroate synthetase, required for folate synthesis and is an important constituent for metabolic activities of the bacterial cell

amino acids, nucleotides and carbohydrates. They are better targets, since some of the pathways involved, exist in parasitic cells and not in human cells. For example, sulfonamides compete with para aminobenzoic acid (PABA), for dihydropteroate synthetase required for folate synthesis and thus the metabolism of bacteria.

Class III reactions (Figs 28.4A and B): Assembly of small molecules into macromolecules, e.g. proteins, ribonucleic

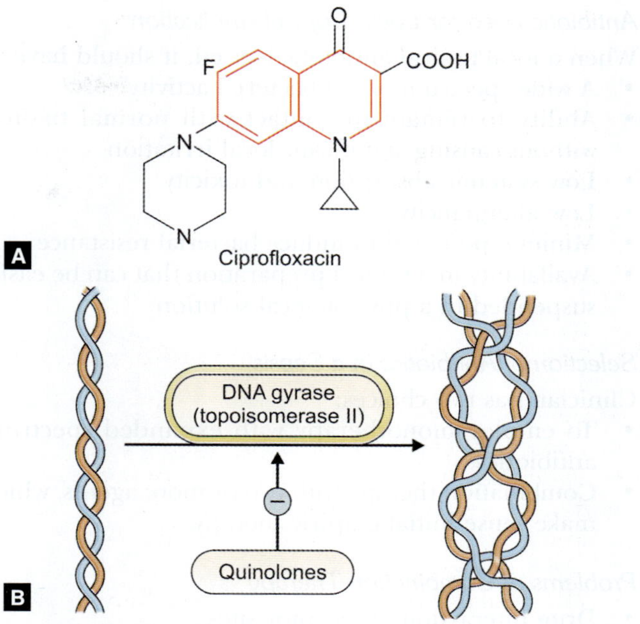

Figs 28.4A and B: Class III reaction of bacterial cell. (A) An example of a quinolone. (B) A simplified diagram of the mechanism of action of the fluoroquinolones

acid (RNA), deoxyribonucleic acid (DNA), polysaccharides and peptidoglycan. As shown in Figure 28.4, the mechanism of action of fluoroquinolones on DNA gyrase, preventing supercoiling of the DNA and hence replication and growth of bacteria is inhibited.

Antibiotic Prophylaxis

During the first 24 hours, the infection depends on the number of bacteria present. During the first 2 hours, the host defense mechanism works to decrease the overall number of bacteria, the 4 hours after that, the number of bacteria remains fairly constant. This first 6 hours is called 'golden period', after which the bacteria multiply exponentially. Administration of prophylactic antibiotics expands this golden period. Ideally the antibiotic therapy should begin immediately before the surgery (30–60 min. prior to skin incision). Maximal dosage of antibiotic can be repeated every 4 hours intraoperatively or whenever the blood loss exceeds 1000 ml. Commonly organisms of the skin cause operative infections, e.g. *Staphylococcus aureus*, *Staphylococcus epidermidis*, peptostreptococci, peptococci, *E.coli* and *Proteus*. More than 90 percent of infection after implant surgery is caused by *S. aureus* and *S. epidermidis*. First generation cephalosporins are the desirable choice, peak level are reached within 20 to 40 min. after a bolus intravenous (IV) infection. Most effective, when started within 3 hours of wound contamination.

Antibiotic Used for Local/Tropical Application

When a local/topical antibiotic is used, it should have:

- A wide spectrum of antibacterial activity
- Ability to remain in contact with normal tissues, without causing significant local irritation
- Low systemic absorption and toxicity
- Low allergenicity
- Minimal potential to induce bacterial resistance
- Availability in a topical preparation that can be easily suspended in a physiological solution.

Selection of Antibiotics in a Sepsis

Clinician has two choices:

- To employ monotherapy with expanded spectrum antibiotics
- Combination therapy with two or more agents, which make sense initial empiric therapy.

Problems of Combination Therapy

- Drug interaction at receptor sites
- Changes in elimination of drugs, by competition for elimination routes
- Potential for greater disruption of normal flora and risk of superinfections
- Adverse drug reactions
- Increased costs.

Penicillins

Chemical Structure

It consists of fused thiazolidine and beta lactum rings, to which side chains are attached through an amide linkage. Members of this family differ from one another in the "R" (alkyl) substituent attached to the 6-aminopenicillanic acid residue, as illustrated in Figure 28.5.

Classification of Penicillins

- Natural penicillins, e.g. penicillin G
- Semisynthetic penicillins
  - Acid resistant alternative to penicillin G, e.g. penicillin V
  - Penicillinase resistant penicillins, e.g. methicillin, cloxacillin, oxacillin, etc.
  - Extended spectrum penicillins
  - Aminopenicillins, e.g. ampicillin, bacampicillin, amoxicillin, etc.
  - Carboxypenicillins, e.g. carbenicillin, ticarcillin, etc.
  - Ureidopenicillin, e.g. piperacillin, mezlocillin, etc.
  - Mecillinam.

Mechanism of Action (Fig. 28.6)

They interfere with the last stage of bacterial cell wall synthesis, i.e. transpeptidation, by inhibiting penicillin

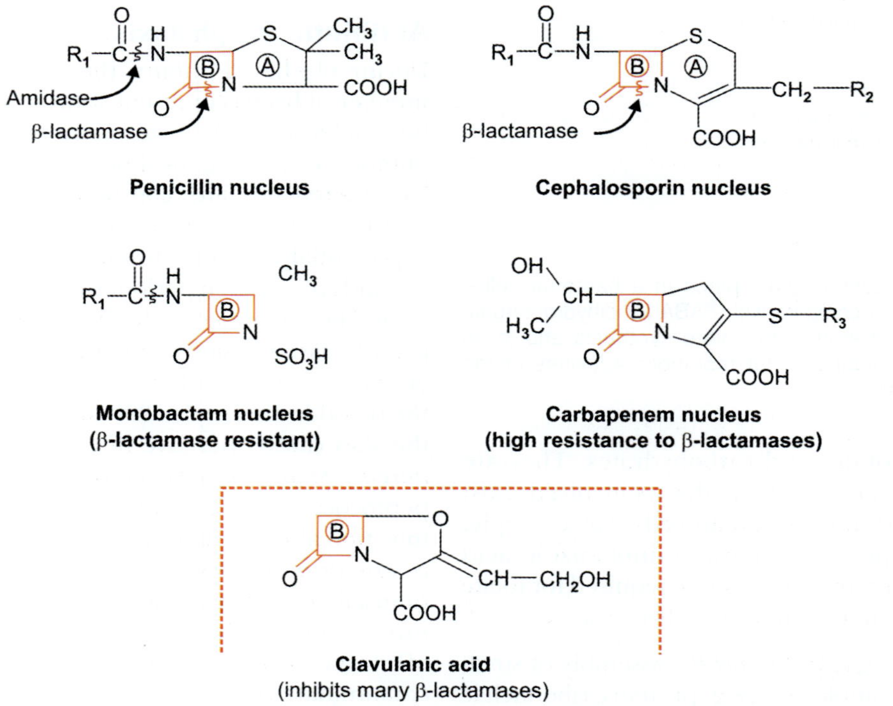

Fig. 28.5: Penicillin structure with other members of the same family, which differ from one another in the "R" substituent attached to the 6-aminopenicillanic acid residue

binding proteins (PBP) and activating autolysins resulting in an osmotically less stable membrane. They are hence, only active against organisms that synthesize a peptidoglycan cell wall. Antibacterial spectrum, shown in Figure 28.7.

Natural penicillins, e.g. penicillin G: A large number of gram-positive and gram-negative bacteria are now resistant to penicillins, due to development of penicillinase and lack of permeability through the porin channels.

Antistaphylococcal penicillins: Methicillin, oxacilllin, cloxacillin, dicloxacillin and naficillin are sensitive to penicillinase producing *Staphylococcus.*

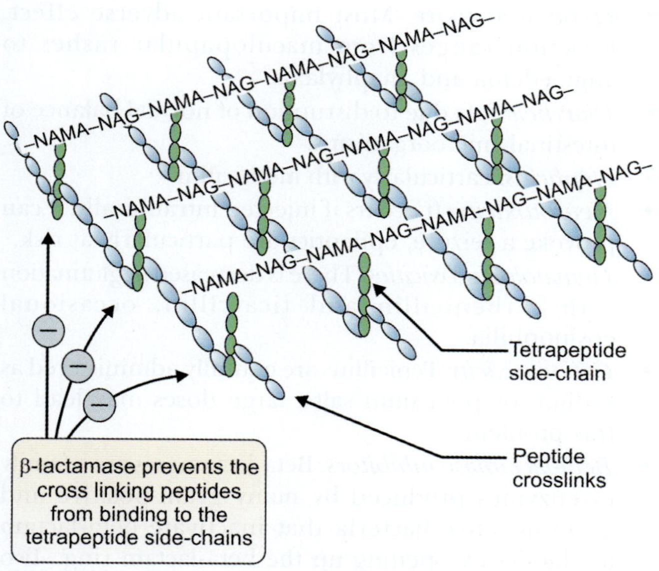

Fig. 28.6: Schematic representation of a single layer of peptidogycan, from a bacterial cell *(S. aureus)* showing the site of action of the β-lactam antibiotics

Extended spectrum penicillins: Ampicillin and amoxicillin have similar spectrum as that of penicillin G, but more effective to gram-negative bacilli. It is a drug of choice for listeria infection.

Antipseudomonal penicillins: Carbenicillin, ticarcillin and piperacillin.

Penicillins and aminoglycosides: Both are synergistic in action as penicillins inhibit cell wall synthesis, permitting entry for aminoglycosides, to their intracellular target sites.

Use of Penicillin

Penicillin G

It has limited use because of its relative lesser activity against penicillinase producing, *S. aureus* and most of the gram-negative pathogens. It is commonly used in the treatment of septic arthritis, caused by *Streptococcus* or Gonococci. As it is acid labile and only one-third of oral dose is absorbed, it is given parenterally. It acheives good concentration in synovium and bone, specially in inflammation.

Dosage and preparations

- Sodium penicillin G: 0.5 to 5 MU IM/IV, 6 to 12 hourly
- Repository penicillin G injections
- Procaine penicillin G: 0.5 to 1 MU IM, 12 to 24 hourly
- Fortified procaine penicillin G: 3 lakh U procaine penicillin and 1 lakh U Na penicillin G
- Benzathine penicillin G: 0.6 to 2.4 MU IM, 2 to 4 weekly.

Semisynthetic penicillin has enhanced gram-negative activity, used in infection caused by *Haemophilus influenzae* and susceptible strain of *E.coli* and *Proteus.*

Penicillin V

It is acid stable and get readily absorbed in gastrointestinal tract (GIT), eliminated mainly through kidney and have a serum half-life of 30 minutes.

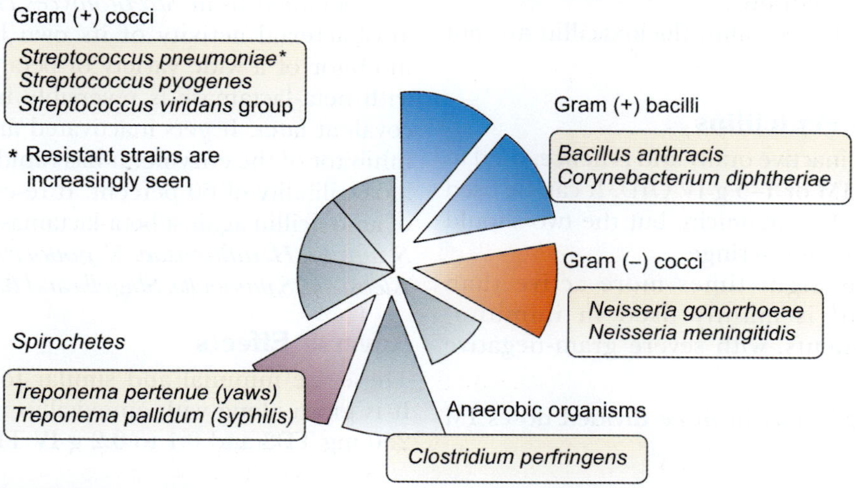

Fig. 28.7: Antibacterial spectrum for different pathogenic bacteria

Dose

- Adults: 500 to 1000 mg every 6 hours
- Children: 50 mg/kg/day in four divided doses.

Ampicillin

It is sensitive to all gram-positive and gram-negative organism. Food interferes with absorption, mostly excreted through kidney. Diarrhea is frequent after oral administration. Hydrocortisone inactivates ampicillin, if mixed in an IV solution:

Dose

- Adults: 0.5 to 2 g oral/IM/IV
- Children: 25 to 50 mg/kg/day in children.

Bacampicillin

It is an ester and a prodrug of ampicillin, attains higher plasma levels and is better tolerated as compared to ampicillin.

Dose: 400 to 800 mg, BD.

Amoxicillin

It is similar to ampicillin in all aspect except, food does not interfere with its absorption. Less chance of diarrhea. Less active against *Shigella and H. influenzae.*

Dose: 0.25 to 1g, TDS

Antistaphylococcal Penicillins

- *Methicillin:* It is active against penicillinase producing Staphylococci, but fails in *Methicillin resistant Staphylococcus aureus* (*MRSA*) infections. *Hematuria, albuminuria* and reversible interstitial nephritis are special adverse effects of this drug and is hence largely replaced by cloxacillin.
- *Cloxacillins:* It shows high penicillinase activity and is acid resistant, hence can be used in oral dose of 0.25 to 0.5 g, every 6 hour, as well as 0.25 to 1 g IM or IV in severe infections.
- *Nafcillin:* Used parenterally
- *Other:* Oxacillin, dicloxacillin, flucloxacillin are not marketed in india.

Antipseudomonal Penicillins

- *Carbenicillin:* It is inactive orally and is hence, used in dose of 1 to 2 gm IM or 1–5 g IV QID. It can be used in combination with gentamicin, but the two should not be used in the same syringe.
- *Piperacillin:* It is eight times more active than carbenicillin and is mainly used in immunocompromized patients, with severe gram-negative infection.

Dose: 100 to 150 mg/kg/day in three divided doses IM or IV.

Antibiotic Penetration in Different Tissues

- *Antibiotic penetration into synovial fluid:* It depends on following factors: Ability of drug to penetrate the semipermeable membrane of synovial membrane, depends upon its solute size. Permeability of membrane is inflammation dependent. In general 60 to 90 percent concentration is achieved in synovial fluid, as compared to serum.
- *Antibiotic penetration into bones:* Penicillin G does not penetrate into the bone. Oxacillin, an antipseudomonal penicillin, penetrates, less than 20 percent of simultaneous serum concentration.

Adverse Affects of Penicillins

- *Hypersensitivity:* Most important adverse effect. Reaction ranges from maculopapular rashes to angioedema and anaphylaxis.
- *Diarrhea:* It is due to disruption of normal balance of intestinal microorganisms.
- *Nephritis*: Particularly with methicillin
- *Neurotoxicity:* It occurs if injected intrathecally, it can provoke a seizure, epileptics are particularly at risk.
- *Hematologic toxicities:* There is decreased agglutination with carbenicillin and ticarcillin, occasional eosinophilia.
- *Cation toxicity:* Penicillins are genrally administered as sodium or potassium salts, large doses may lead to this problem.
- *Beta-lactamase inhibitors:* Beta-lactamases are a family of enzymes produced by many gram-positive and gram-negative bacteria that inactivate beta-lactam antibiotics by opening up the beta-lactam ring. Two inhibitors of this enzyme namely clavulanic acid and sulbactum are available.

■ Clavulanic Acid

It is obtained from *Streptomyces clavuligerus.* It has no antibacterial activity of its own but is a progressive inhibitor of a wide variety of beta lactamases. Its bond with beta-lactamase is reversible initially, but becomes covalent later. It gets inactivated and is hence a suicide inhibitor of the enzyme. It has rapid oral absorption with bioavailibility of 60 percent. It re-establishes the activity of amoxicillin against beta-lactamase producing resistant *S. aureus, H. influenzae, N. gonorrhoeae, E. coli, Proteus, Klebsiella, Salmonella, Shigella and Bacteroids fragilis.*

Adverse Effects

These are minimal and similar to that of amoxicillin. It is given along with amoxicillin in the dose of 125 to 250 mg TDS and 0.1 to 0.2 g IV TDS/QID.

■ Sulbactam

It is a semisynthetic progressive beta-lactamase inhibitor. It is two to three times less potent than clavulanic acid on weight basis, as compared to clavulanic acid. Its oral absorption is inconsistent and hence used parenterally. It is used in the dose of 0.5 g TDS/QID.

■ Cephalosporins (See Fig. 28.5)

Chemical Structure

They are group of semisynthetic antibiotics derived from cephalosporin-C obtained from a fungus cephalosprium. They consist of a beta-lactam ring fused to a dihydrothiazine ring.

Classification

This has been enumerated in the Table 28.1

- *First generation*
  - *Parenteral:* Cephalothin, cefazolin, etc.
  - *Oral:* Cephalexin, cephadrine, cefadroxil, etc.
- *Second generation*
  Parenteral: Cefuroxime, cefoxitin
  Oral: Cefaclor, cefuroxime axetil, etc.
- *Third generation*
  - *Parenteral:* Cefotaxime, ceftizoxime, ceftriaxone, ceftazidime, cefoperazone, etc.
  - *Oral:* Cefixime, cefpodoxime proxetil, cefdinir, ceftibuten, etc.
- *Fourth generation*
  - *Parenteral:* Cefepime, cefpirome, etc.

Mechanism of Action

Figure 28.9 shows mechanism of action of cephalosporin.

Spectrum of Action (Fig. 28.9)

As we precede from first generation to the third generation, the activity of cephalosporins shifts from gram-positive to gram-negative organisms. Fourth generation cephalosporins, like cefepime and cefpirome have further better range of action and are effective against resistant gram-negative organisms and hence are useful in hospital acquired infection, septicemia and bacteremia. First generation cephalosporins are active against bacteria, such as *S. aureus, Streptococcus pyogenes, Clostridia, Klebsiella, Proteus,* etc. Second generation cephalosporins have long serum half-life of 3 to 4 hours. Cefoxitin has arylsulfphatase A (ASA) activity same that of cephalaxin. They have more active against *H. influenzae.* Third generation cephalosporins shows more activity against *N. gonorrhoeae* and *H. influenzae.* Ceftazidime has nice activity against *Pseudomonas.* Serum binding protein ranges from 15 percent to 90 percent. All cephalosporins achieve good levels in interstitial, synovial and peritoneal fluids. All cephalosporins enter bone. The concentration

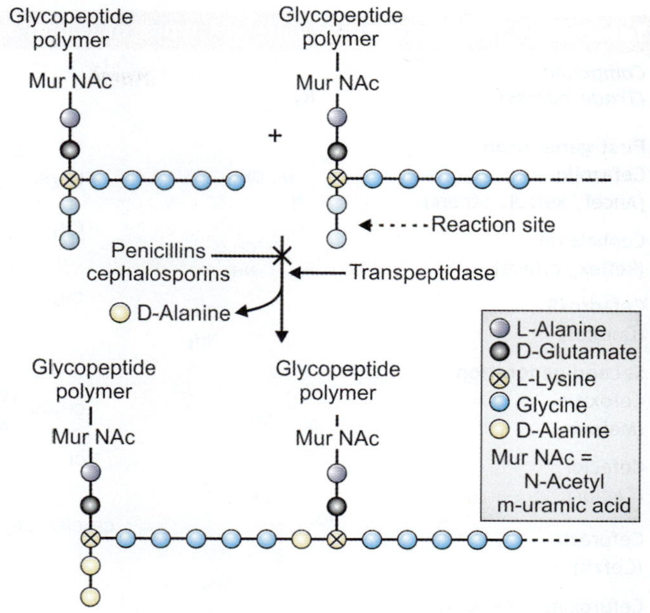

Fig. 28.8: Mechanism of action of cephalosporin, which is similar to that of penicillins, i.e. it blocks the last step of bacterial wall synthesis (transpeptidation or cross linkage)

of cefazolin are more than adequate for most of *Staphylococcus* to sensitive to *E. coli, Klebsiella* and *Pseudomonas aeruginosa.*

Side Effects

- Hypersensitivity reactions, rashes are most frequent, but anaphylaxis, angioderma, asthma and urticaria, has also been reported
- Nephrotoxicity is highest with cephaloridine
- Bleeding
- Neutropenia and thrombocytopenia
- Disulfiram like reaction.

Use of Cephalosporins

Infection caused by *Staphylococcus* treated by first generation cephalosporins. Anaerobic soft tissue and bone infection and infection caused by gram-positive organism. Gonococcal arthritis has been treated by cefoxitin and cefotaxim. Third generation cephalosporins are useful in septic arthritis and gram-negative osteomyelitis. Cefuroxime is heat stable and can be used in the treatment of osteomyelitis, with antibiotic impregnated bone cement.

■ Other Beta-lactam Antibiotics (Fig. 28.10)

Monobactams (Aztreonam) (Fig. 28.11)

Organisms inhibited are *Enterobacteriaceae* and *P. aeruginosa.* It is not effective against gram-positive and

Table 28.1: Classification of different types of cephalosporins, their trade names, chemical structure and dosages

Compound (Trade names)	*R_1*	*R_2*	*Dosage forms, adult dosage for severe infection, and $t_{½}$*
First-generation			
Cefazolin (Ancef, kefzol, others)	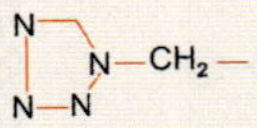	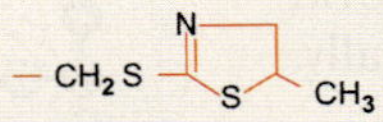	I: 1 to 1.5 g every 6 hours $t_{½}$ = about 2 hours
Cephalexin (keflex, others)	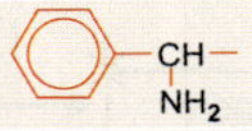	$-CH_3$	O: 1 g every 6 hours $t_{½}$ = 0.9 hours
Cefadroxil (Duricef)	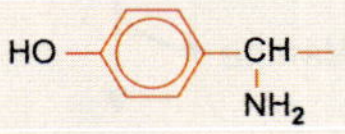	$-CH_3$	O: 1 g every 12 hours $t_{½}$ = 1.1 hours
Second-generation			
Cefoxitin (Mefoxin)	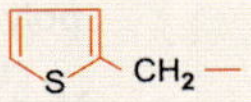	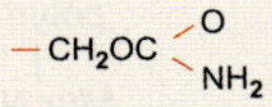	I:2 g every 4 hours or 3 g every 6 hours $t_{½}$ = 0.7 hours
Cefaclor (Ceclor)	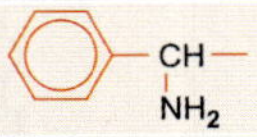	—Cl	O: 1 g every 8 hours $t_{½}$ = 0.7 hours
Cefprozil (Cefzil)	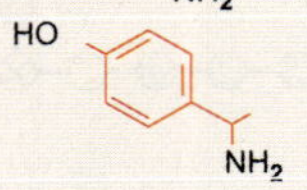	$CH=CH-CH_2$	O: 500 mg every 12 hours $t_{½}$ = 1.3 hours
Cefuroxime (Zinacef) Cefuroxime acetil (Ceptin)	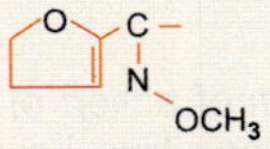	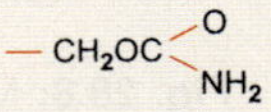	I: Up to 3 g every 8 hours $t_{½}$ = 1.7 hours T: 500 mg every 12 hours
Loracarbef (Lorabid)	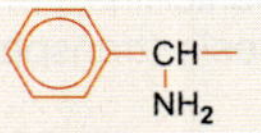	—Cl	O: 200 to 400 mg every 12 hours $t_{½}$ = 1.1 hours
Cefotetan (Cefotan)	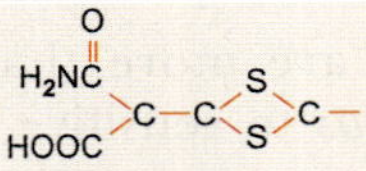	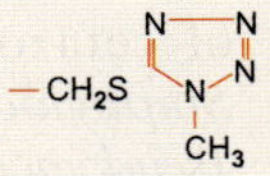	I: 2 to 3 g every 12 hours $t_{½}$ = 3.3 hours
Ceforanide (Precef)	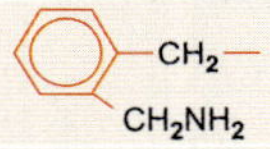		I: 1 g every 12 hours $t_{½}$ = 2.6 hours
Third-generation			
Cefotaxime (Claforan)	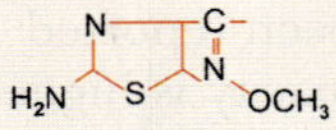	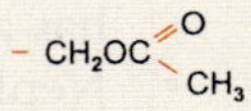	I: 2 g every 4 to 8 hours $t_{½}$ = 1.1 hours
Cefpodoxime proxetil (Vantin)	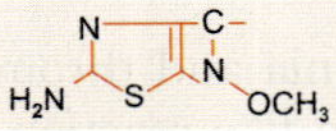	$-CH_2OCH_3$	O: 200 to 400 mg every 12 hours $t_{½}$ = 2.1 hours
Ceftibuten (Cedax)	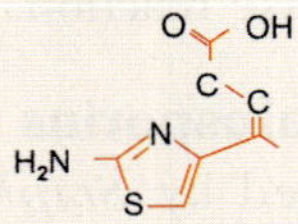	—H	O: 400 mg every 24 hours $t_{½}$ = 2.4 hours
Cefdinir (Omnicef)	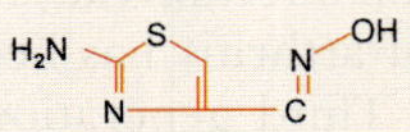	$CH=CH_2$	O: 300 mg every 12 hours or 600 mg every 24 hours $t_{½}$ = 1.7 hours
Cefditoren pivoxil (Spectracef)	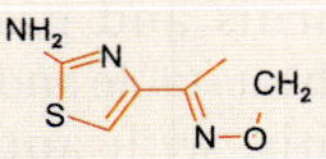	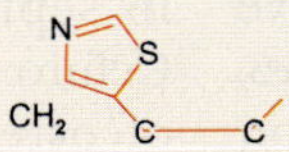	O: 400 mg every 12 hours $t_{½}$ = 1.6 hours
Ceftizoxime (Cefizox)	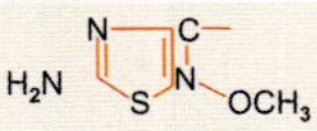	—H	I: 3 to 4 g every 8 hours $t_{½}$ = 1.8 hours
Ceftriaxone (Rochephin)	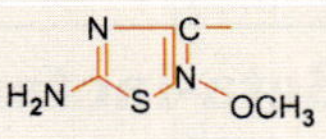	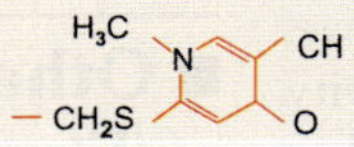	I: 2 g every 12 to 24 hours $t_{½}$ = 8 hours

Contd...

Contd...

Compound (Trade names)	**R_1**	**R_2**	**Dosage forms, adult dosage for severe infection, and $t_{½}$**
Cefoperazone (cefobid)	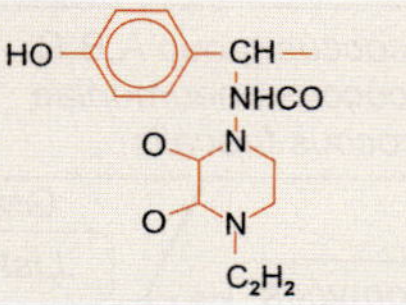	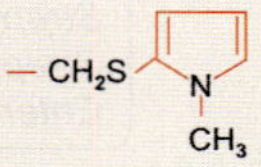	I: 1.5 to 4 g every 6 to 8 hours $t_{½}$ = 2.1 hours
Ceftazidime (Hortaz, others)	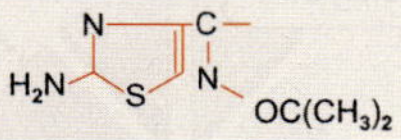	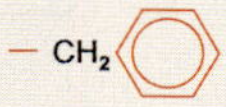	I: 2 g every 8 hours $t_{½}$ = 1.8 hours
Fourth-generation			
Cefepime (Maxipime)	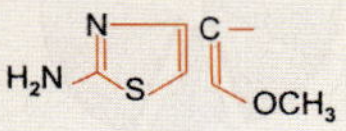	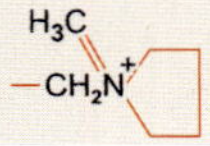	I: 2 g every 8 hours $t_{½}$ = 2 hours

R_1 and R_2—Side chains; $t_{½}$—Half line

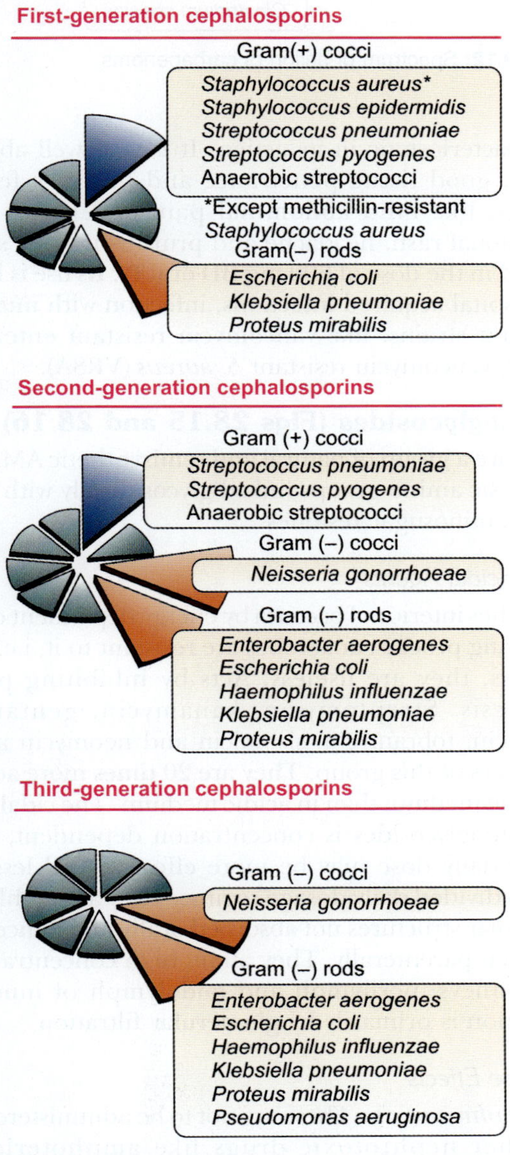

Fig. 28.9: Different spectrum of action of different generations of cephalosporins

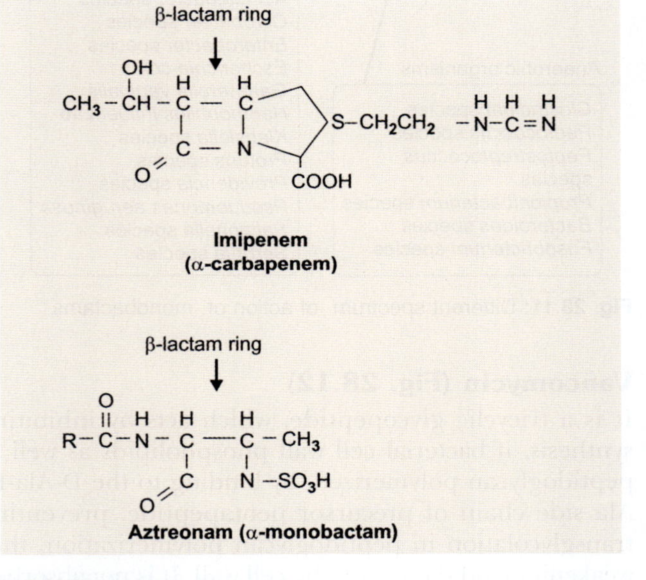

Fig. 28.10: Beta-lactum antibiotics

anaerobic organism. As it lacks cross sensitivity, it is useful in patients allergic to penicillins/cephalosporins and hospital acquired infections, originating from urinary, biliary and GIT.

Dose: 0.5 to 2g IM/IV 6 to 12 hourly.

Carbapenems

Imipenem and meropenem are extremely potent and very broad spectral antibiotics. Inhibit majority of gram-positive and negative organism. Rapidly hydrolyzed in the brush bordered renal tubular cells, It combines with cilastatin to overcome this problem.

Dose: 0.5 g IV 6 hourly.

Side effects: These include nausea, vomiting and diarrhea. High levels can provoke seizure.

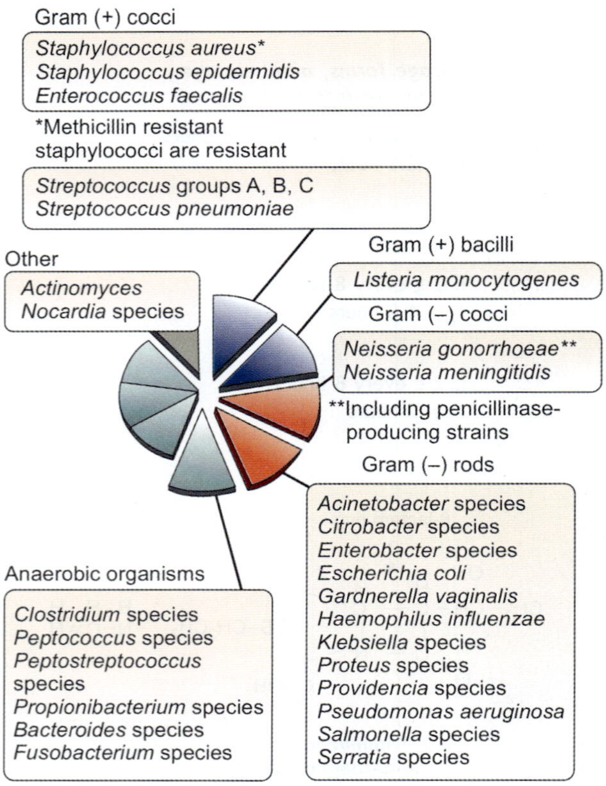

Fig. 28.11: Different spectrum of action of monobactams

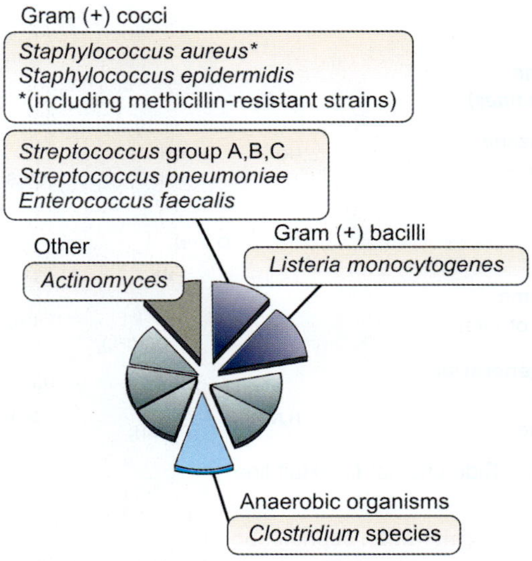

Fig. 28.12: Spectrum of action of carbapenems

Vancomycin (Fig. 28.12)

It is a tricyclic glycopeptide, which acts by inhibiting synthesis, if bacterial cell wall phospholipids as well as peptidoglycan polymerized, by binding to the D-Ala-D-Ala side chain of precursor pentapeptide, preventing transglycolation in peptidoglycan polymerization, thus weakening and damaging the cell wall. It is not absorbed orally and is hence used in the a dosage of 0.5 g, 6 hourly or 1 g, 12 hourly slow IV infusion over 1 hour. It is heat stable and hence used along with bone cement in case of osteomyelitis.

Adverse effects: Systemic toxicity is high. It can cause plasma concentration dependent nerve deafness, which may be permanent. Ototoxicity and nephrotoxicity is also noted. Skin allergy and fall in blood pressure during IV injection, due to histamine release. Rapid IV injection has caused chills, fever, urticaria and intense flushing called "red man syndrome."

Oxazolidinones (Figs 28.13 and 28.14)

Linezolid

Linezolid is a very newly discovered AMA.

Mechanism of action: It causes protein synthesis inhibition, by binding to the 23S fraction of 50S ribosome, interfering in the formation of 70S tRNA initiation complex. Hence, it is bacteriostatic in its action. It is very well absorbed orally, good tissue penetrance and has very few side effects, like mild abdominal pain and bowel upset. Occasional rash, headache and pruritus may be seen. It is used in the dose of 600 mg BD oral/IV. Its use is limited to hospital acquired infections, infection with multidrug resistant strains, like vancomycin resistant enterococci (VRE), vancomycin resistant *S. aureus* (VRSA).

Aminoglycosides (Figs 28.15 and 28.16)

They are a group of natural and semisynthetic AMA, with polybasic amino groups linked glycosidically with two or more aminosugar residues.

Bactericidal Agents

It reaches interior of bacteria by energy dependent oxygen requiring process, anaerobes are resistant to it, i.e. in big abscess, they are useless. Acts by inhibiting protein synthesis. Streptomycin, kanamycin, gentamicin, amikacin, tobramycin, sisomicin and neomycin are few members of this group. They are 20 times more active in alkaline medium than in acidic medium. The cidal action of aminoglycosides is concentration dependent, thus a single daily dose may be more effective and less toxic than a divided daily dosage regime. They are highly ionic and polar structures not absorbed orally and hence, must be given parenterally. They attain high concentration in the kidneys, perilymph and endolymph of inner ear. Excretion is primarily by glomerular filtration.

Adverse Effects

- *Nephrotoxicity:* These are not to be administered with other nephrotoxic drugs like amphotericin B, vancomycin, cephalothin, cyclosporine and cisplatin

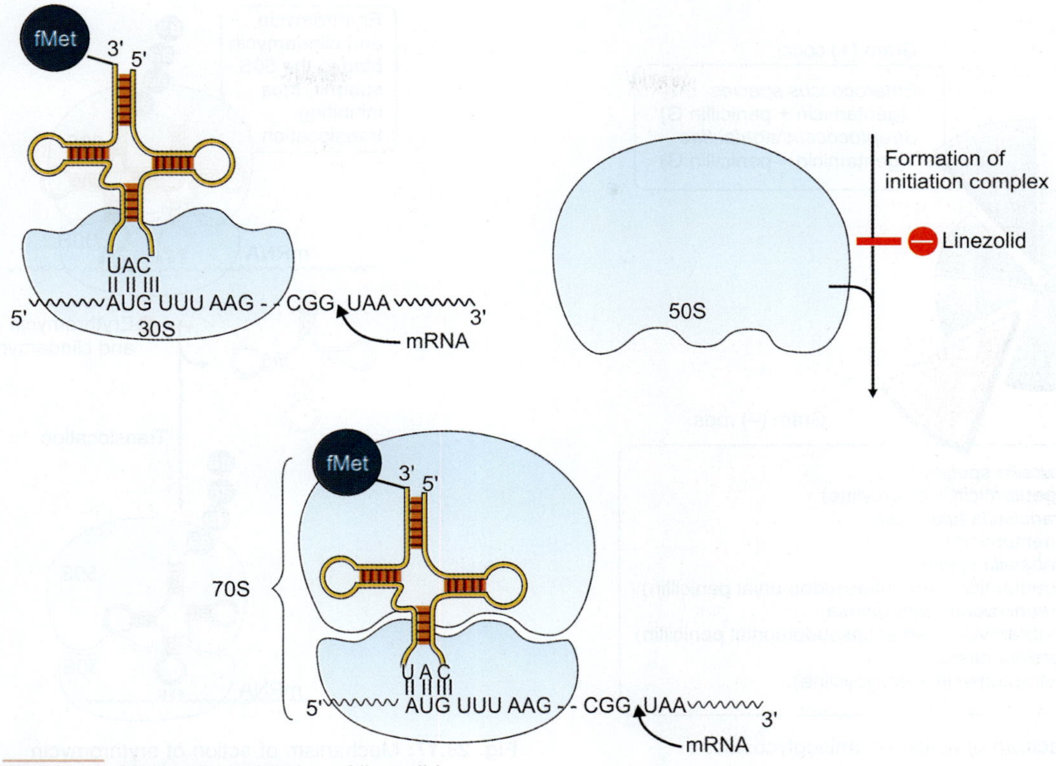

Fig. 28.13: Mechanism of action of linezolid

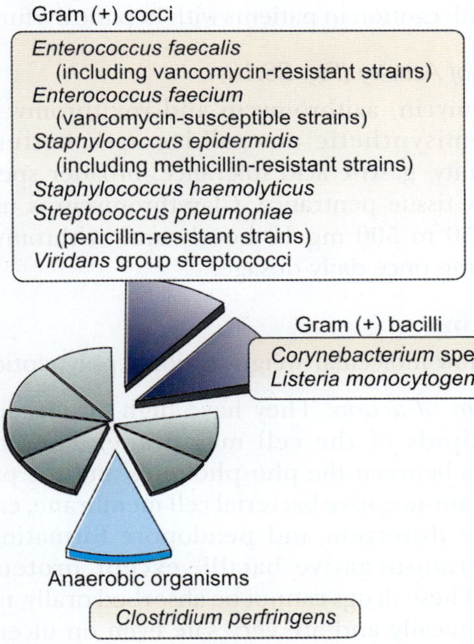

Fig. 28.14: Spectrum of action of linezolid

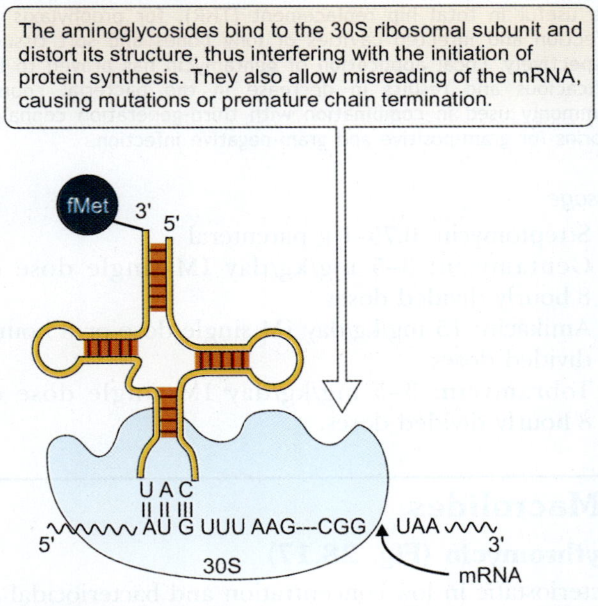

Fig. 28.15: Mechanism of action of aminoglycosides

- *Ototoxicity:* These drugs need to be avoided in pregnancy, to prevent fetal ototoxicity and concurrent use with other ototoxic drugs
- *Neurotoxicity:* Neomycin and streptomycin produce neuromuscular blockade.

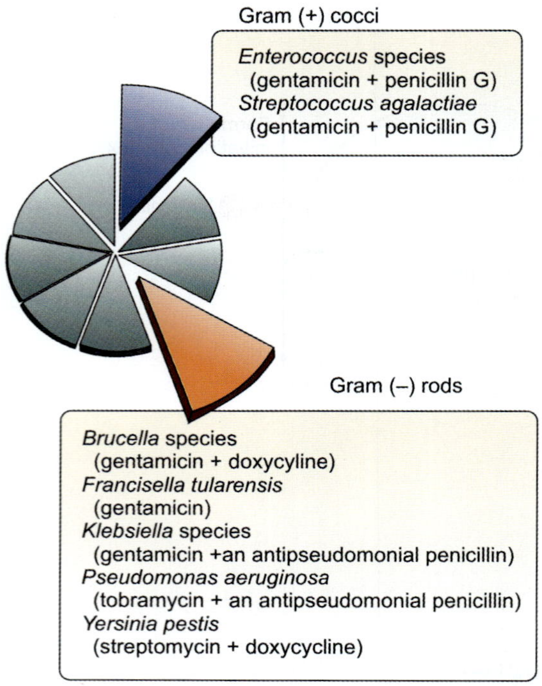

Fig. 28.16: Spectrum of action of aminoglycosides

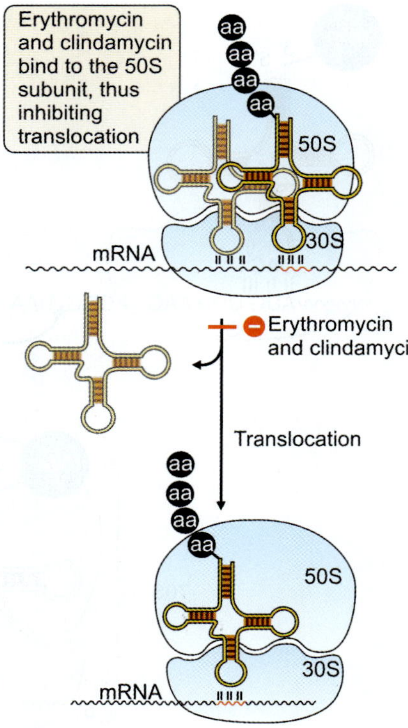

Fig. 28.17: Mechanism of action of erythromycin

Special orthopedic consideration

Incorporation of heat stable gentamycin and tobramycin into polymethyl methacrylate (PMMA) bone cement and beads, which are useful in total hip replacement (THR), for prophylaxis of infection and infected cavities of long bones and soft tissues respectively. Local application of gentamycin has proved to be efficacious and results in decrease in the bacterial count. Commonly used in combination with third-generation cephalosporins for gram-positive and gram-negative infection.

Dosage

- Streptomycin: 0.75–1 g parenteral
- Gentamycin: 3–5 mg/kg/day IM single dose or 8 hourly divided doses
- Amikacin: 15 mg/kg/day IM single dose or 8 hourly divided doses
- Tobramycin: 3–5 mg/kg/day IM single dose or 8 hourly divided doses.

■ Macrolides

Erythromycin (Fig. 28.17)

Bacteriostatic in low concentration and bacteriocidal in high concentration. It inhibits protein synthesis. It is acid labile, has short half-life (1.5–2 hours). Shows good bone penetration.

Dose: 250 mg to 1g 6 hourly.

Side effects: Comapatively very safe drug, mild-to-moderate epigastric pain, occasional diarrhea, hypersensitivity reaction, prolongation of QT interval. Hepatitis and cholestatic jaundice is also seen with this drug, so it should be used with caution in patients with hepatic dysfunction.

Spectrum of Activity (Fig. 28.18)

Clarythromycin, azithromycin and roxithromycin are newer semisynthetic macrolides with better oral bioavailibility, gastric acid tolerance, broader spectrum and better tissue pentrance. Clarythromycin is used in dose of 250 to 500 mg 12 hourly and azithromycin is used 500 mg once daily dosage.

Polymyxins

They are low molecular weight cationic polypeptides.

Mechanism of action: They have high affinity for the phospholipids of the cell membrane. They orient themselves between the phospholipids and the protein films in gram-negative bacterial cell membrane, causing membrane distortion and peudopore formation. All aerobic gram-negative bacilli, except proteus are sensitive. These drugs cannot be absorbed orally, usually applied topically and are very safe even on ulcers and denuded skin. Used as closed irrigation method for osteomyelitis.

Lincomycin and Clindamycin

Mechanism of action is similar to that of macrolides. Active against gram-positive and anaerobic infection, such as *Bacteriodes fragilis* and *S. aureus.*

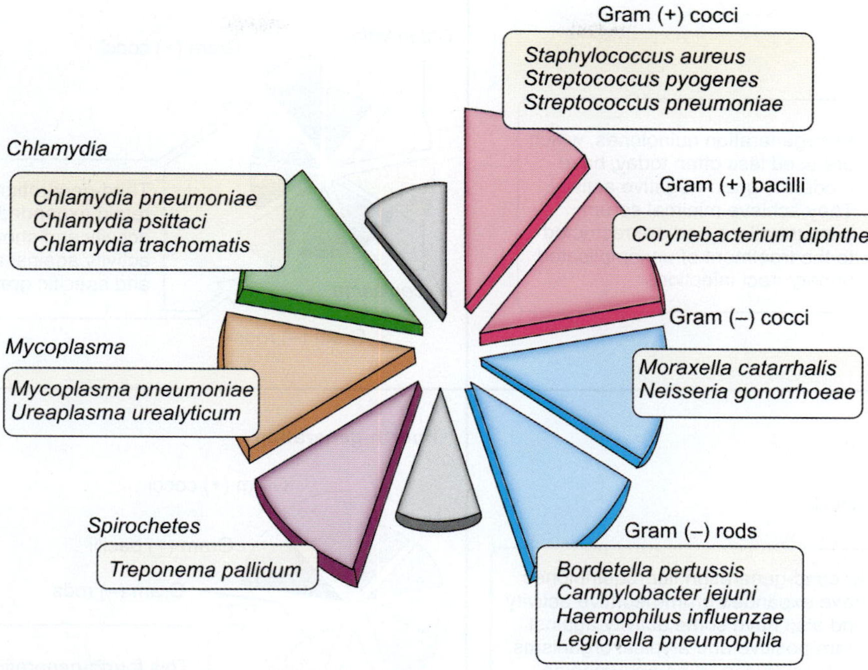

Fig. 28.18: Spectrum of action of macrolides

Doses: Clindamycin is used 150 to 300 g 6 to 8 hourly, lincomycin is used in dose of 500 mg 6–8 hourly and 600 mg IM/IV 6 to 12 hourly.

Adverse reaction: Pseudomembranous colitis and diarrhea.

■ Fluoroquinolones (Figs 28.19A to C)

Classification

- *First-generation:* Nalidixic acid
- *Second-generation:* Ciprofloxacin, norfloxacin, ofloxacin, etc.
- *Third-generation:* Gatifloxacin, levofloxacin, moxifloxacin, sparfloxacin, etc.
- *Fourth-generation:* Trovafloxacin, fluoroquinolones, etc.

Ciprofloxacin

It has a wide range of activity mainly against gram-negative and at higher concentration for gram-positive. Good penetration, including bone and synovium. Plasma half-life is 4 to 5 hours, with oral bioavailibilty up to 80 percent.

Spectrum of Action (Fig. 28.20)

Dosage

- *Ciprofloxacin:* 250 to 750 mg BD oral and 100 to 200 mg BD IV

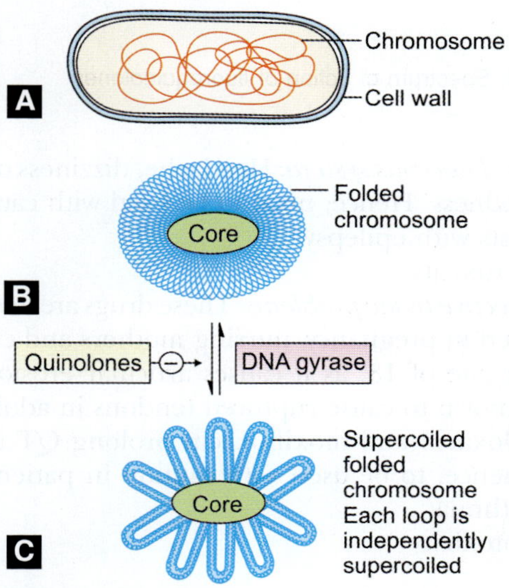

Figs 28.19A to C: Mode of action of quinolones, showing its negative affect on DNA gyrase enzyme

- *Ofloxacin:* 200 to 400 mg BD oral and 200 mg BD IV
- *Gatifloxacin:* 200 to 400 mg OD
- *Levofloxacin:* 500 mg OD oral and 500 mg IV OD
- *Sparfloxacin:* 200 to 400 mg OD oral.

Adverse Effects

- *Gastrointestinal:* Nausea, vomiting and diarrhea

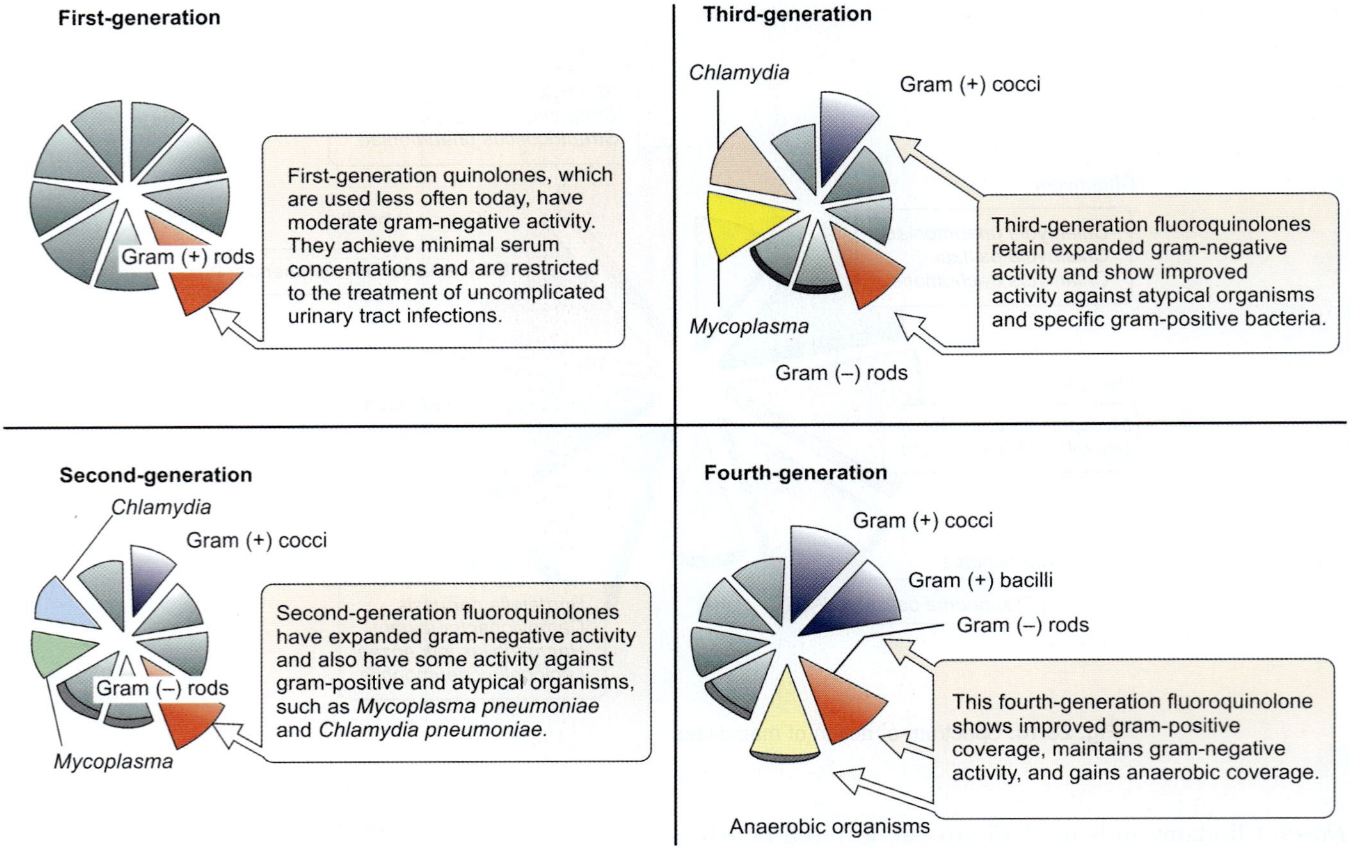

Fig. 28.20: Spectrum of action of fluoroquinolones

- *Central nervous system:* Headache, dizziness or light-headedness. Hence, need to be used with caution in patients with epilepsy.
- Liver toxicity
- *Connective tissue problems:* These drugs are need to be avoided in pregnancy, nursing mothers and children under age of 18, as it causes articular erosion. It is also known to cause ruptured tendons in adults.
- Sparfloxacin and moxifloxacin prolong QT interval and hence, to be used with caution in patients with arrhythmia.
- Phototoxicity

Tetracyclines

Mechanism of Action (Fig. 28.21)

Tetracyclines are active against gram-positive and negative bacteria, e.g. *Ricketisia, Mycoplasma, Brucella, etc.* Inhibit protein synthesis, by binding to 30S ribosome in susceptible organism.

Adverse Effects

1. They are known to cause epigastric pain, nausea, vomiting, diarrhea and intramuscular injections are very painful

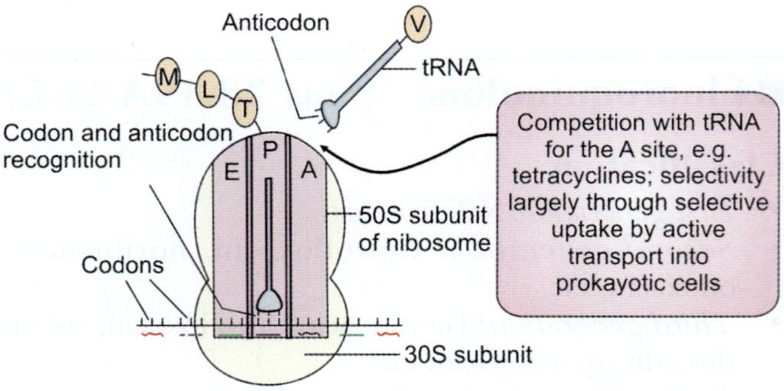

Fig. 28.21: Mechanism of action of tetracycline—The elements involved in protein synthesis are shown, a ribosome (with three binding sites for transfer RNA (tRNA)—the P, A and E sites, messenger RNA (mRNA) and (tRNA). The different mRNA codons (triplets of three nucleotides, which code for specific amino acids) are represented by dots, dashes and straight or wavy lines and are shown in different colors. A tRNA with the growing peptide chain (consisting so far of Met-Leu-Trp: MLT) is in the P-stes, bound by codon and anticodon recognition (i.e. by complementary base-pairing). The incoming tRNA carries valine (V), covalently linked

2. Dose related, liver and kidney damage is also seen
3. Phototoxicity

4. Brown discoloration of teeth and temporary suppression of bone growth
5. Hypersensitivity is also seen rarely.

Dosage: Tetracyclines are used in 250 to 500 mg oral TDS/ QID, doxycycline is used 100 to 200 mg OD and is more potent and better tolerated as compared to tetracyclin.

■ Antitubercular Drugs

Bactericidal Drugs

Rifampicin

It penetrates almost in all tissue membrane and is effective against intracellular and extracellular bacilli. It is also used for the treatment of brucellosis, along with doxcycline in dose of 600 mg/day for 6 weeks. Generally given on empty stomach.

Doses: 10 to 12 mg/kg body weight, 450 to 600 mg daily in divided doses and 900 mg for intermittent therapy.

Adverse effects: Hepatotoxicity, gastritis and purpura.

Isonicotinylhydrazine (INH) or Isoniazid

It is active against extracellular and intracellular bacilli.

Doses: 4 to 5 mg/kg/bodyweight. The INH should not be given in divided doses because peak level in serum is more important than sustained inhibitory level.

Adverse effect: Peripheral neuropathy and blood dyscrasia.

Streptomycin

It acts only on rapidly multiplying extracellular bacilli.

Dosage: 0.75 to 1 g parentral.

Adverse effects: Vestibular damage, nystagmus and renal damage.

Pyrazinamide

It is active against slow multiplying intracellular bacilli. It also increases sterilizing ability of rifampicin.

Doses: 1.5 to 2 g orally in two-three dicided doses.

Adverse effects: Hyperuricemia.

Bacteriostatic Drugs

Ethambutol

It is used in combination to prevent its resistance.

Doses: 15 mg/kg in two-three divided doses

Adverse effects: Retrobulbar neuritis.

Other Drugs

Thioacetazone, p-aminosalicylic acid (PAS), cycloserine, kanamycin and capreomycin.

Antifungal Drugs

Classification

- *Antibiotics:* Polyenes like amphotericin B, nystatin and heterocyclic benzofuran, like griseofulvin
- *Antimetabolite:* Flucytosine
- Azoles
  - Imidazoles: Clotrimazole, ketoconazole, etc.
  - Triazoles: Fluconazole, itraconazole, etc.

  Amphotericin B (AMB) and azoles are drugs of choice for *coccidioidomycosis, blastomycosis, histoplasmosis, cryptococcosis* and *sporotrichosis.* Amphotericin B is obtained from *Streptomyces nodosus,* it possess a macrocyclic ring with one end being hydrophilic and other lipophilic.
- *Antifungal spectrum*

  C. albicans, Cryptococcus, Histoplasma capsulatum, Coccidioides inmitis, Blastomyces dermatitidis, etc.

Dosage: 50 to 100 mg QID orally and 0.3 mg/kg infusion over 4 to 8 hours.

Adverse effects: Toxicity with AMB is high including chills, fever, aches, pain, nausea, vomiting and dypsnea, with each infusion, there is nephrotoxicity and bone marrow depression.

Ketoconazole: Broad spectrum antifungals, which work by inhibiting fungal cytochrome P450 enzyme lanosterol 14-demethylase and thus impair ergosterol synthesis. Dosage is 200 mg OD or BD. Adverse effects include nausea and vomiting, loss of appetite, headache, paresthesia, rashes, gynecomastia and hair loss. It is contraindicated in pregnant women and nursing mothers.

Antiparasitic Agents

Echinococcosis is the only parasitic infection, which is relevant orthopedically. It is treated with albendazole/ mebendazole. It is a congener of thiabendazole and acts by blocking glucose uptake in the parasite and depletion of its glycogen stores. It is well tolerated orally and is given in the dose of 400 mg BD for 4 weeks. Its use in pregnant women is contraindicated and should be used with caution in patients, with hepatic and renal disease.

Resistance to Antibiotics

Bacterial resistance to an antibiotic can be either:

- Intrinsic (inherent) or phenotypic
- Acquired via acquisition of foreign resistance genes
- Acquired via mutational events in the native genome.

Intrinsic Resistance

Organism is inherently not susceptible to the antibiotic, as in case of *M. tuberculosis*, which is insensitive to tetracyclines.

Phenotypic Resistance

Nongenetic, e.g. non-growing cells, gram-negative, outer cell membrane, etc.

Genotypic Resistance

Exchange of r-determinants (genes that confer resistance to specific antimicrobial agents). Transfer and recombination of resistant mutant genes is possible through normal bacterial genetic exchange mechanisms *(conjugation, transduction* or *transformation)*.

Plasmids

These are covalently closed and are circular extrachromosomal DNA. They may carry genes for drug resistance, metabolic enzymes and some virulence factors (e.g. exotoxins). Restricted or broad host range. Varies from small sized (nearly 5 Md), nonconjugal to large (20 to 200 Md), which can be conjugated. Plasmids can be transferred between cells—multidrug (multiple) resistance is possible. Can cross species barrier and closely related strains may acquire r-determinants.

Physiological and Biochemical Mechanisms of Drug Resistance

Bacteria may demonstrate any of the five general mechanisms of antibiotic resistance:

1. Lack of entry, e.g. decreased cell permeability
2. Greater exit, due to active efflux
3. Enzymatic inactivation of the antibiotic
4. Altered target, e.g. modification of drug receptor site
5. Synthesis of resistant metabolic pathway.

Beta-lactams

Mode of action: They inhibit peptidoglycan synthesis (bactericidal)

Resistance for these drugs:

- They fails to cross membrane (gram-negatives)
- Fails to bind to altered PBP
- Hydrolysis by beta-lactamases.

Vancomycin

Mode of action: Disrupts peptidoglycan cross-linkage

Resistance

- Fails to cross gram-negative outer membrane (too large)
- Some intrinsically resistant (pentapeptide terminus).

Bacitracin

Mode of action: Disrupts movement of peptidoglycan precursors (topical use).

Resistance: Fails to penetrate into cell.

Antimycobacterial Agents

Disrupt mycolic acid or arabinoglycan synthesis (bactericidal).

Resistance

- Reduced uptake
- Alteration of target sites.

29 Isotopes and Bone Scan in Orthopedics

- Atoms and Isotopes
- Bone Scan

Introduction

Greek Isos means equal, Topos means site or place. Isotopes of an element have nuclei with the same number of protons, but different numbers of neutrons. Isotopes can be any of the different types of atoms of the same chemical element, each having different atomic mass, as shown in Figure 29.1.

Atoms and Isotopes (Figs 29.2, 29.3 and Table 29.1)

What is Medical Isotope?

A medical isotope is a very small quantity of radioactive substance, used in safe, costeffective imaging and for the treatment of diseases. New technologies enable medical isotopes to be delivered directly to the site of diseased cells. This is different from external beam radiation treatment, where radiation is directed from outside of the body.

Uses in Orthopedics

Diagnostic

Therapeutic (still under trials)

Used in following conditions:

- Bone cancer pain
- Primary or metastatic bone carcinoma
- Rheumatoid arthritis
- Degenerative joint diseases.

Combined

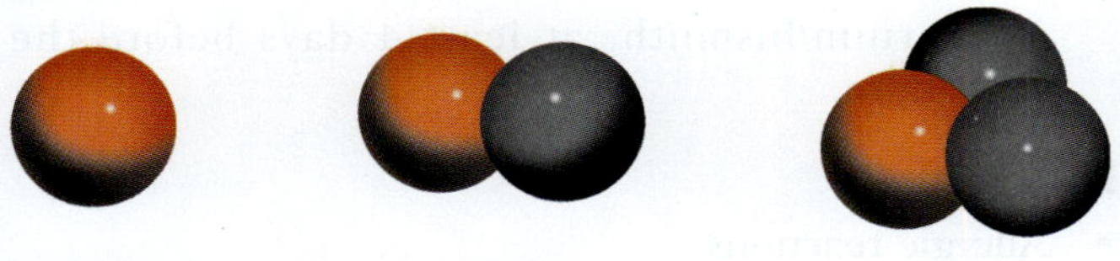

Fig. 29.1: Different isotopes of hydrogen element

Isotopes and Diagnosis

Radioisotopes give off energy, which can be detected by special equipment. When small quantities are introduced into the body, the imaging equipment tracks their location and movement. This enables the doctors to learn more about the diseased tissues than a diagnostic procedure, which just takes a picture from the outside. Medical isotope diagnostic procedures often facilitate an earlier and more complete disease diagnosis and therefore more rapid and effective treatment. Isotopes commonly used in orthopedics. The most commonly used isotopes are:

- Triphasic bone scan
- Gallium-67
- Indium-111, labeled leukocytes
- Technetium-99m
- Thallium-201
- Fluorine-18 fluorodeoxyglucose
- Samarium-153
- Gadolinium.

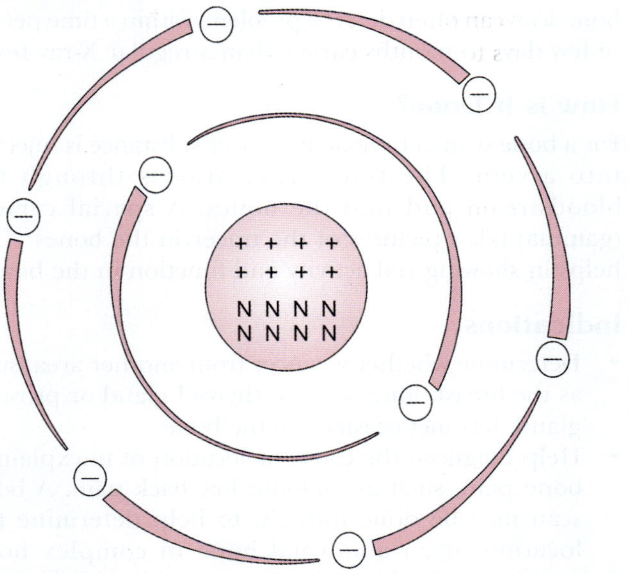

Fig. 29.2: Structure of an atom, with positive charged nucleus surrounded by negatively charged electrons

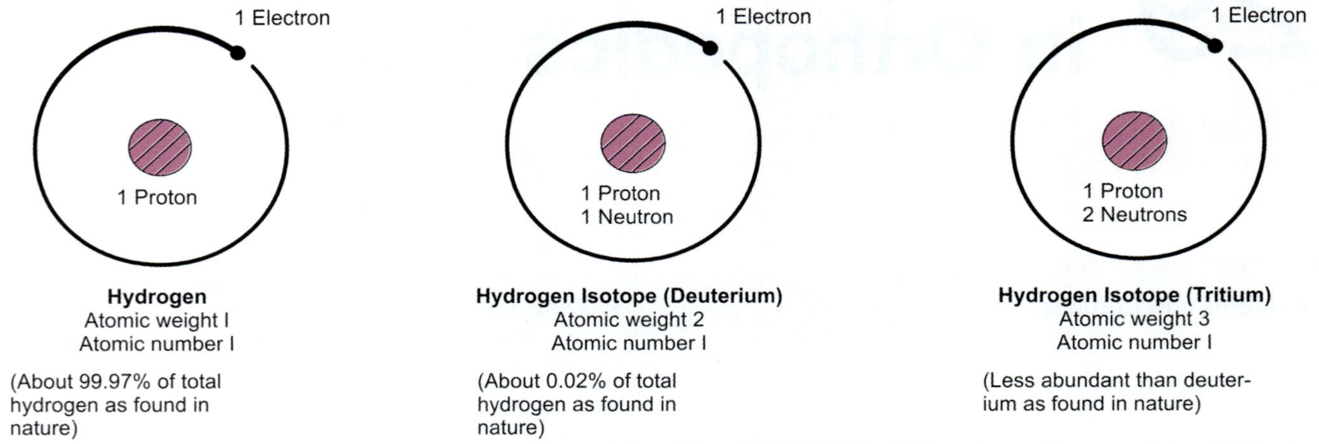

Fig. 29.3: A comparison between different hydrogen isotopes and their relative abundance

Table 29.1: Change in the number of any subatomic particles and its consequence

If you change the number of...	*It will affect the ...*	*And the result will be a...*
Protons	Identity of the atom	Completely different atom
Electrons	Charge	Ion
Neutrons	Mass	Isotope

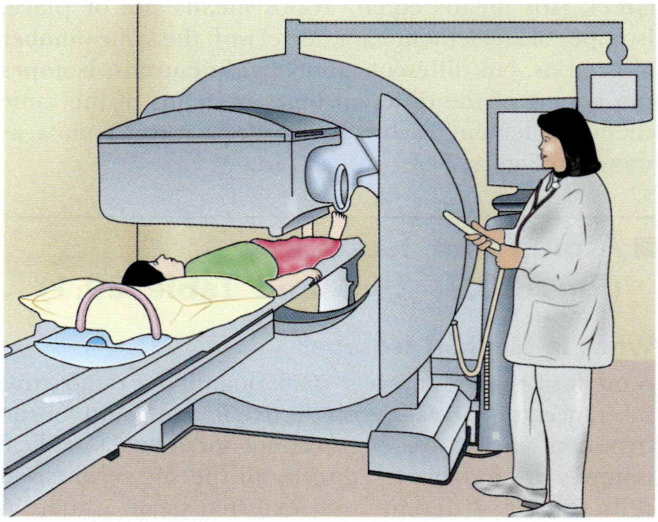

Fig. 29.4: Patient undergoing bone scan

Bone Scan (Figs 29.4 and 29.5)

A bone scan is a nuclear scanning test, which identifies new areas of bone growth or breakdown. It can be done to evaluate damage to the bones, detect cancer that has metastasized to the bones and monitor conditions that can affect the bones (including infection and trauma). A bone scan can often detect a problem, within a time period of few days to months earlier than a regular X-ray test.

How is it Done?

For a bone scan, a radioactive tracer substance is injected into a vein. The tracer then travels through the bloodstream and into the bones. A special camera (gamma) takes pictures of the tracer in the bones. This helps in showing cell activity and function in the bones.

Indications

- Determine whether a cancer from another area, such as the breast, lung, kidney, thyroid gland or prostate gland, has metastasized to the bone.
- Help diagnose the cause or location of unexplained bone pain, such as ongoing low back pain. A bone scan may be done initially, to help determine the location of an abnormal bone in complex bone structures, such as the foot or spine. Follow-up evaluation then may be done with a CT scan or MRI.
- Help diagnose broken bones, such as a hip fracture or a stress fracture, not clearly seen on X-ray.
- Detect damage to the bones, caused by infection or other conditions, such as Paget's disease.

Precautions or Contraindications

- Pregnancy
- Breastfeeding
- Any barium procedure (e.g. enema, swallow) within last 4 days
- Medicines containing bismuth. Barium and bismuth can interfere with test results. Patient should be taken off barium/bismuth, at least 4 days before the procedure.

Risks

- Allergic reactions
- Soreness at injection site
- Rarely, immune system depression.

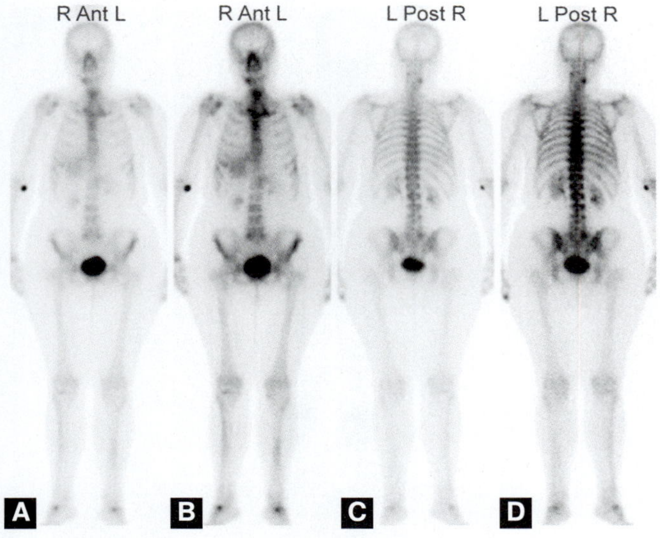

Figs 29.5A to D: Images showing bone scans of a patient—(A and B) Anterior view; (C and D) Posterior view. ("L" stands for left side and "R" stands for right side)

Table 29.2: Normal and abnormal findings of radioisotope bone scan

Normal:	The radioactive tracer is evenly distributed among the bones. No areas of too much or too little tracer are seen.
Abnormal:	The tracer may accumulate in certain area os the bone, indicating one or more hot spots. Hot spots may be caused by a fracture that is healing, bone cancer, a bone infection (osteomyelitis), arthritis, or a disease of abnormal bone metabolism (such as Paget's disease).
	Certain areas of the bone may lack the presence of tracer, indicating one or more cold spots. Cold spots may be caused by a certain type of cancer (such as multiple myeloma) or lack of blood supply to the bone (bone infarction).

Interpretation and Results

A bone scan does not distinguish between normal and abnormal bone growth by itself. Therefore, bone scan results must be interpreted along with symptoms and the results of X-ray tests. In addition, other tests, such as CT, MRI, blood tests or biopsies may also be needed to further evaluate abnormal bone scan results. This has been enumerated in Table 29.2.

Triphasic Bone Scan

Initial dynamic images are acquired over the area of concern and then followed immediately afterwards, by static images obtained over longer periods of time.

Phases of Triphasic Bone Scan

- *Flow phase:* It demonstrates perfusion to a lesion. Consists of serial 2 to 5 sec images of the area of suspected osteomyelitis, that are obtained during injection of the radiopharmaceutical. Classically, with cellulitis, diffuse increased uptake occurs in first two phases, but uptake is normal or diffusely increased in third phase. Osteomyelitis causes focally increased uptake in all three phases.
- *The blood pool image:* Obtained within 5 min after injection. In areas of inflammation, capillaries dilate, causing increased blood flow and blood pooling. First phase characterizes the blood flow to the area, while the second phase visualizes, the blood pool. These two early phases act to characterize, degree of inflammation and hyperemia that may be present. Diseases such as: degenerative disease, healing fractures, noninfected prosthesis with loosening and well treated osteomyelitis, may have little abnormal activity, on the early phases in spite of increase uptake on delayed images. It may be difficult to distinguish osteomyelitis from diabetic osteoarthropathy, which are also often abnormal on all three phases.
- *The bone image:* It demonstrates relative bone turnover associated with a lesion. In third phase, image is obtained about 3 hours later, when urinary excretion has decreased the amount of the radionuclide in soft tissues. If present, diffuse increased uptake in third phase is probably due to regional hyperemia, which is caused by cellulites. Osteomyelitis causes focally increased uptake in all three phases.

Triphasic Bone Scan and Neonates

In neonates, the sensitivity of the three phase bone scan decreases. Neonates with osteomyelitis, have falsely normal or cold defects, on three phase bone scans (22-68% of the time). Cold lesion on third phase may be caused by subperiosteal abscess. In children, large portion of blood supply to the bone comes from periosteal vessels and these are apparently disrupted by the subperiosteal abscess. When clinical findings strongly suggest osteomyelitis, but findings on three phase bone scan are normal, then consider gallium scan.

Osteomyelitis and Bone Scan (Figs 29.6A and B)

Differential diagnosis of osteomyelitis on bone scan:

- Soft tissue infection
- A neurotrophic lesion
- Gout
- Degenerative joint disease
- Postsurgical changes
- A healing fracture
- A noninfectious inflammatory reaction

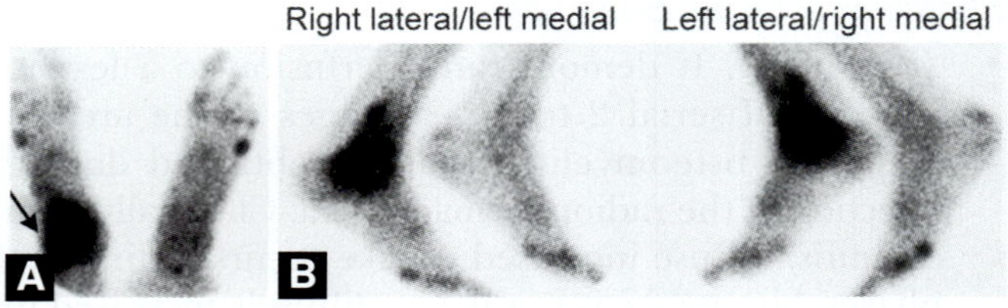

Figs 29.6A and B: Bone scanning in osteomyelitis

Table 29.3: Comparison of sensitivity and specificity of different types of diagnostic methods for osteomyelitis

	Sensitivity	*Specificity*
Radiography	67%	40%
3-Phase bone scan	85%	54%
Gallium scan	81%	69%
Technetium-99m	100%	70%
MRI	85%	

- A stress fracture
- Comparison of sensitivity and specificity of different types of diagnostic methods for osteomyelitis are shown in Table 29.3.

Gallium Bone Scan (Fig. 29.7)

Gallium works by localizing bacteria and inflammatory proteins. Borman et al. in 1986, reported an accuracy rate of 91 percent in 34 children, but cautioned that the radiation dose from gallium is higher than that from technetium or indium-111 and hence, recommended its use only in difficult cases. In a typical study, Ga-67 is intravenously injected and delayed images are acquired on next day. Early images are obtained, if urgent, but the target to background definition will be much better after 24 hours. Osteomyelitis is suggested, by focal uptake, however any reactive bone process, may also cause increased uptake. In cases of fractures, prosthesis and pre-existing complications, osteomyelitis cannot be confidently assessed with Ga.

Indium-111 (Fig. 29.8)

- If suspected osteomyelitis is superimposed on a disease, that causes increased bone remodeling.
- The combined indium-111-labeled leukocyte-Technetium-99m bone scan, is the procedure of choice in nonmarrow containing skeleton.
- The indium-111 labeled leukocyte scan is the procedures of choice in marrow containing skeleton.

Procedure: Indium WBC preparations, require withdrawing approximately 50 ml of autologous blood, with a leukocyte count of approximately 5,000 per ml. Leukocytes are collected by centerfuge, exposed to indium and reinjected IV.

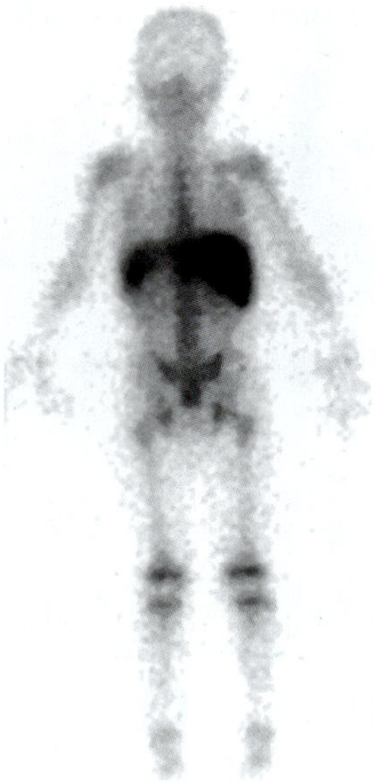

Fig. 29.7: Gallium bone scan imaging

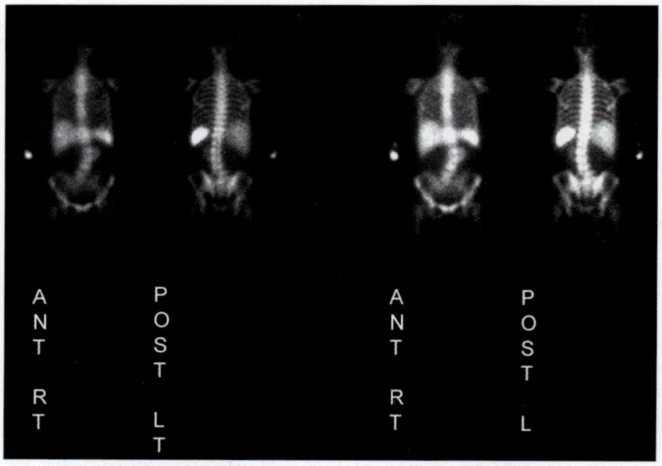

Fig. 29.8: Indium-111 imaging

Interpretation

- Images obtained after 24 hours, show activity only in the liver, spleen and bone marrow
- Most studies are taken at 24 hours
- Normal healing wounds and fully treated infections, with no significant degree of inflammation, show no discernable uptake.

Indium-111 False Positive

- IM injection sites
- Noninfected fracture
- Total joint prosthesis
- Rheumatoid arthritis
- Overlying soft tissue infection may also cause false positive.

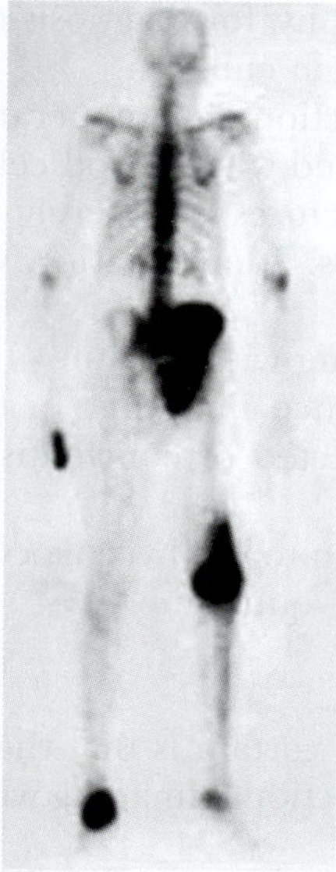

Fig. 29.9: Technetium-99m bone scan

Technetium-99m (Fig. 29.9)

- Half-life of technetium is 6 hours
- Over the course of several hours, half or more of the dose accumulates in bone and the remainder is excreted in urine.
- Images obtained over 2 to 4 hours
- Increased uptake in immature bone and metabolically active bone or where large numbers of osteoblasts are present.
- Intensity of the characteristic "hot lesion", reflects the degree of reactive new bone formation, as well as increased blood flow.
- In children the epiphyseal growth plates, display the most activity and nonossified bone is not visualized.
- In elderly, degenerative diseases are common and show typical distribution of increased, often focal, joint activity, at the sternocostal junction, shoulders, spine, knees, hips, hands and feet.
- Photopenic (cold) scans may indicate early osteomyelitis.

Bone Scan and THR (Fig. 29.10)

Normal THR

Normal study (minimal reactive bone formation), may be expected from months to a year after placement. Area of lesser trochanter to midshaft of prosthesis usually becomes normal in about 6 months. Area around acetabulum, greater trochanter and tip of prosthesis, may show increased activity for up to 2 years, but on an average, shows normal findings at about 1 year in majority of patients.

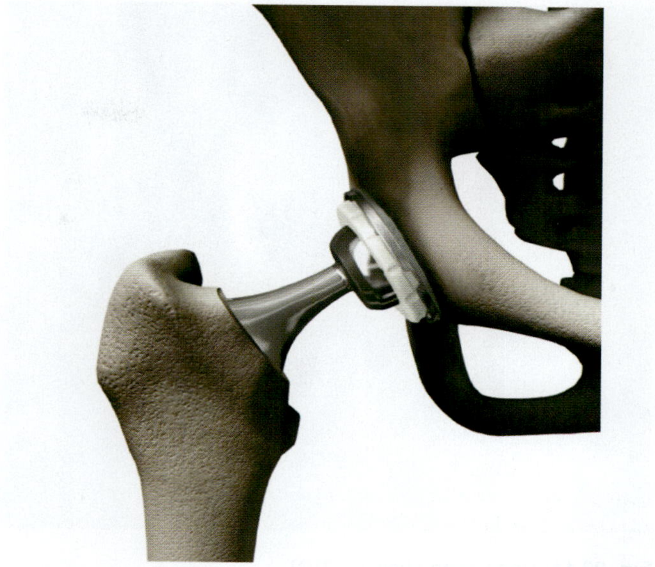

Fig. 29.10: Total hip replacement

Noncemented THR

Bone and fibrous tissue ingrowth into porous acetabular and intertrochanteric surfaces, may cause findings, unrelated to complications. With loosening, there is little inflammation and therefore, the first two phases of the bone scan are normal.

Bone Scan and Infected THR

Infection shows a more diffuse pattern of abnormality, occurring along prosthesis shaft and is usually positive on the early phases. Low grade infections, may consist of minimal hyperemia and may show a mild delayed uptake on bone scan, which is difficult to distinguish from loosening. False positive results may occur in up to 40 percent and false negatives in 5 to 10 percent. Indium-111 is more specific for making definitive diagnosis of infection, but may be less sensitive.

Bone Scan and Avascular Necrosis (AVN) (Fig. 29.11)

For detection of AVN, technetium-99 methylene-diphosphonate bone scanning, is a useful technique. Bone scanning may be less sensitive in the detection of AVN, at early stage of the disease or when both hips are involved symmetrically. Reactive bone at the edge of the infarcted segment, will show an increased uptake of the isotope on the delayed image. A photopenic area (cold area) located anterolaterally, which is surrounded by an area of increased activity is most consistent, with diagnosis of avascular necrosis.

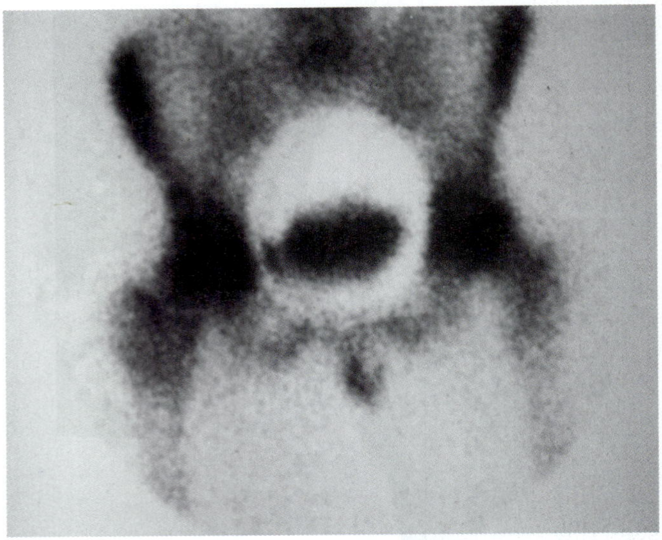

Fig. 29.11: Bone scan showing AVN

Some More Isotopes

- *Samarium-153:* Used in the treatment of pain, associated with bony metastases of primary tumors
- *Gadolinium:* Used in X-ray fluorescence.

Ongoing Studies

- The scintigraphic diagnosis of osteomyelitis.
- Comparison of indium-labeled leukocyte imaging, with sequential technetium-gallium scanning, in the diagnosis of low-grade musculoskeletal sepsis (a prospective study).
- Gallium scintigraphy, for diagnosis of septic arthritis and osteomyelitis in children.
- Diagnosis of infection by preoperative scintigraphy, with indium-labeled white blood cells.
- Undiagnosed fractures in severely injured children and young adults. Identification with technetium imaging.
- Leukocyte scanning with indium –111 is superior to magnetic resonance imaging, in the diagnosis of clinically unsuspected osteomyelitis in diabetic foot ulcer.
- Diagnosis and monitoring by leukocyte scanning, with indium in 111 oxyquinoline.

The Times to Come

- One thing that is certain is that the use of fusion of anatomic and functional imaging will become almost universal.
- More specialized radiopharmaceuticals will be developed, which will permit the distinction between malignant change and inflammatory process.
- This capability will have enormous value in the staging and follow-up of patients with malignant diseases.
- Radiopharmaceuticals will be "Made to Measure", with a particular molecular target in mind and the final product will be more specific, resulting in reduction in unnecessary radiation of nontarget tissues and maximization of specific target concentration.
- The future of nuclear medicine is bright on a worldwide scale.

30 New Bearing Materials in Orthopedics

• Bearing Material

Bearing Material

Bearing materials are materials that minimize implant wear and thus, reducing the effects of wear debris on the body and increasing the implant's life span, as shown in the Figure 30.1.

Introduction

Total joint replacement (also known as total joint arthroplasty), is regarded among the most valued developments in the history of orthopedics. It provides the surgeon, the ability to relieve pain and restore function to patients, whose joints have been destroyed by trauma or disease. An ongoing concern in joint replacement is, increased friction and wear of the joint, when utilizing man-made implants. It is important to recognize that the best bearing surface is human articular cartilage, but when the damage is too great to work on isolated smaller cartilage defects, we then look at man-made joint replacements. Compared to healthy organic cartilage surfaces, which have a surface friction of nearly negligible, the friction between these man-made bearing surfaces are hundreds times higher. This friction, subjects the implant to wear, which can limit the longevity of the joint replacement and induces inflammatory responses in the area surrounding the joint itself.

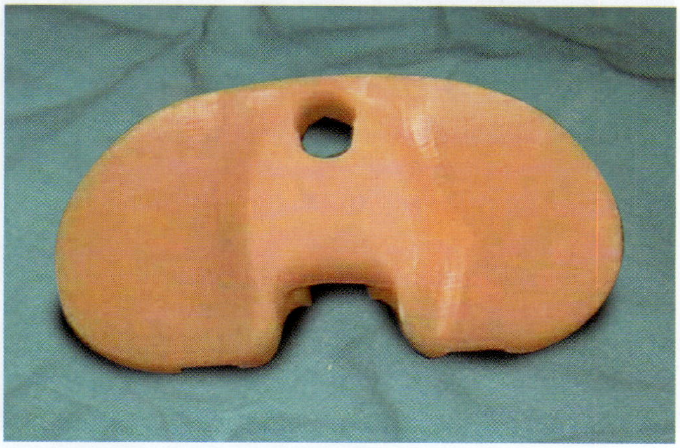

Fig. 30.1: A type of bearing materials, used with implants

Fundamental of Replacing Damaged Joint

- The requirement of producing
- A low friction bearing, to minimize surface wear
- Reducing inflammation, in surrounding tissues
- To delay possible eventual loosening of the implant, resulting in the need for an additional surgery.

What is Wear?

Wear is defined as the loss of material from the surface of the prosthesis, as a result of motion between those surfaces. It should be distinguished from plastic deformation or creep, which changes the shape of the implant, without causing loss of material or producing particulate debris.

Types of Wear

- Abrasive
- Adhesive
- Fatigue.

1. *Abrasive type:* In this the harder surfaces produces groove in the softer material.
2. *Adhesive type:* In this type the softer material is transferred, as a thin film onto the harder surface.
3. *Fatigue type:* In this repetitive loading produces subsurface cracks and particles or sheets of material, which subsequently delaminate and are lost from the surface.

Brief History of Joint Replacement Implant Materials

- In the 1960 and 1970, a number of materials were tried as bearing surfaces in joint arthroplasty.
- Including Teflon® and metallic alloys, such as stainless steel and cobalt-chromium alloy, but through the 1980s and much of the 1990s, the preferred bearing combination was ultra high molecular weight, polyethylene and cobalt-chromium.

- Polyethylene results in a low amount of friction, when bearing against a highly polished metallic surface. Today, metal-on-metal and ceramic-on-ceramic combinations are being considered as alternative bearing surfaces.
- *History and materials used:* The first successful wear couple was developed in 1962, involved a combination of hard and soft bearing materials in the form of a metal and in combination with ultra high molecular weight polyethylene (UHMWPE).

Types of Bearing Material

Several different bearing materials, used to minimize wear are:

- Ultra high molecular weight polyethylene (UHMWPE)
- Metallic alloys
- Ceramics
- Crosslinked polyethylene (XLPE)
- Polyetheretherketone (PEEK), there is a growing interest in this material because of its mechanical properties, biocompatibility and potentially low wear rates.

Why have so many Implant Bearing Combinations been Introduced?

It is the ongoing problem of wear, that has led to the reintroduction of a number of alternative bearing combinations, as shown in Figures 30.2 and 30.3. Clinically speaking, friction and wear result in very small wear particles (typically less than 4 per 100,000 of inches or about 200 times smaller than a grain of sand), that are released to the surrounding joint cavity, initiating an aggressive inflammatory response. The body mounts a cellular reaction, to try to deal with the wear debris, a reaction that unfortunately often leads to unwanted destruction of bone (called osteolysis), around the implant. When osteolysis becomes severe, it can cause pain and loosening of the implant and the need for revision surgery, to replace the components. One way to relieve the osteolysis problem and thus increase the longevity of joint replacements, is to improve the wear resistance of the bearing materials. Also facilitating this introduction of materials, is the shift toward younger and more active patients, seeking and receiving joint replacement.

Are Modern Implants Safe?

- All the materials are considered safe from a medical standpoint
- They are highly biocompatible
- Cause little, if any detrimental local or systemic problems due to immune response or an allergic reaction.
- Concern remains that adverse tissue responses could arise, as a result of the continual release of worn fragments of the prosthetic materials.
- This concern is most with the reintroduction of metal-on-metal bearing surfaces.

Concern in Development

- One of the main concerns in the development of implants is interaction of an implant bearing surfaces, with those materials that come in contact with each other, while in motion.
- This is an increasing concern, as progressively younger individuals, become candidates for joint replacement surgery.

Pathophysiology

- As the bearing couples rub against each other, tiny particles of debris are released into the body.
- As debris accumulates, the body activates macrophages, that stimulate the production of antibodies,

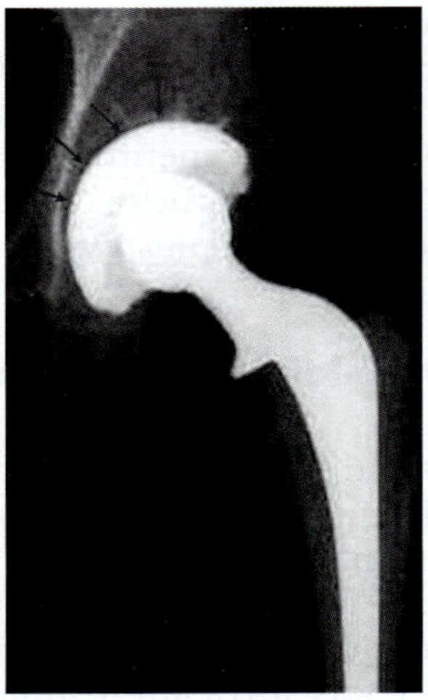

Fig. 30.2: One of the implants bearing combinations, with hip implant

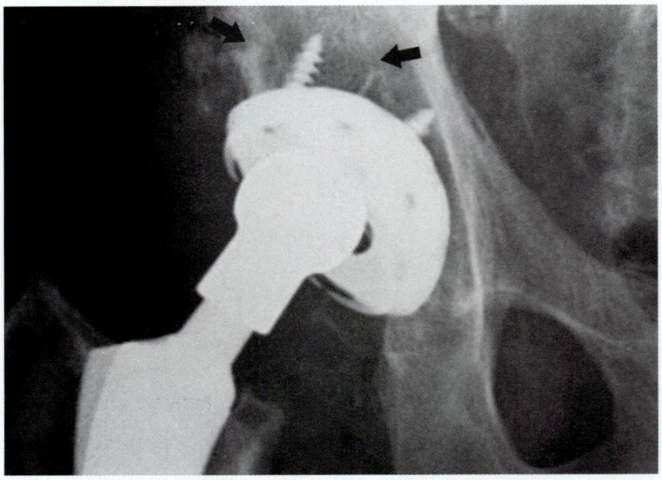

Fig. 30.3: Osteolysis around the implant

which attack the debris, the implant and the surrounding bone.
- The process can lead to osteolysis, possible implant loosening and subsequent failure of the implant.

Selection of Materials Used

Designers select materials based on following factors:
- Wear performance
- Biological response to wear debris
- Ease and reproducibility of manufacture
- Creep performance
- Fatigue resistance
- Impact strength
- Cost.

Wear Couple

Joints have bearing surfaces, which rub against each other, while in motion. It is extremely important in the hip, knee and shoulder for loading and range of motion. Wear performance is also a key, when selecting materials for ankle, finger and elbow joints in addition to new applications, such as motion preservation devices in spinal applications.

Importance of a Good Wear

In the hip, forces can reach six times a person's body weight and in the knee, forces can reach 17 times a person's body weight, when rising from a seated position. Therefore, the ability of a material to produce good wear performance must be assessed with respect to the relevant loads and motions.

Traditional Bearing Materials

The first successful wear couple was developed in 1962 and involved a combination of hard and soft bearing materials, in the form of metal, in combination with UHMWPE. This combination of bearing materials has proved extremely successful in terms of wear performance and cost. It remains the most commonly selected wear couple for total joint replacement in hips, knees and shoulders. Despite, the success of these restorative procedures, UHMWPE on metal or UHMWPE on ceramic prostheses have a limited implant life because of the wear and damage, that the metal component and to a lesser extent the ceramic, inflicts on the UHMWPE surface. This can lead to the production of small particles of UHMWPE debris, which can trigger osteolysis, as shown in Figure 30.4.

Wear must decrease to reduce bone resorption. One way of reducing wear volume is to incorporate hard bearing surfaces, such as metal-on-metal or ceramic-on-ceramic prostheses. Although, metal-on-metal bearings are associated with low wear rates, there are concerns that wear debris can trigger osteolysis. A further issue concerns

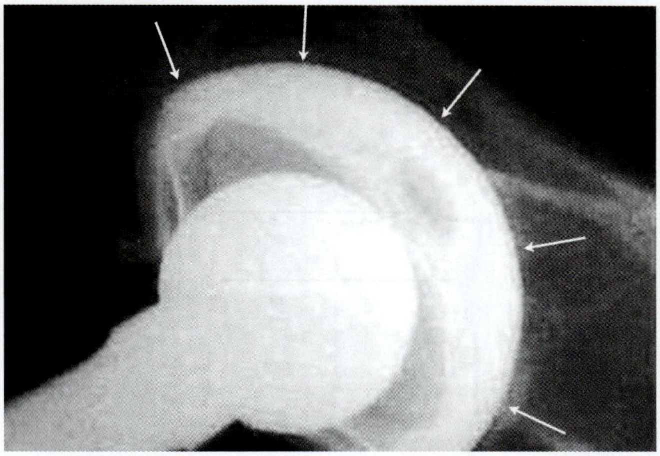

Fig. 30.4: Wear and damage, the metal component and the ceramic, inflicts on the UHMWPE surface

the release of chemically active metal ions into the surrounding tissues. Metal ions may also bind to protein moieties, which are transported into the bloodstream and lymphatics to remote organs. The use of ceramic-on-ceramic joints, avoids the issues of metal ions. The initial problems, concerning the brittle failure of ceramic implants, have largely been alleviated through improved fabrication techniques, with higher purity materials and finer grain sizes.

Metal-on-metal Bearings (Figs 30.5A and B)

Early Problems

Metal-on-metal bearings were among the first to be used in total hip arthroplasty and found clinical success in the 1960 and 1970. Metal-on-metal hip joints fell out of favor, by most orthopedic surgeons, as the clinical results with polyethylene-on-metal joints proved superior. However, failures during this earlier time period were due in part to poor metallurgy and implant design. The casting process used to make metallic implants suffered from poor quality control, sometimes leading to products, which had inferior wear resistance and were prone to fracture in the body. An early metal-on-metal designs often had small head to neck ratios, so that impingement between the neck of the femoral component and the rim of the acetabular components (joint socket), was a common occurrence. This impingement provides another source of wear and can knock the acetabular component (the joint socket), loose from the surrounding bone.

Benefits of Improved Modern Version

Improved metallurgy and manufacturing techniques, have led to resurgence in the use of metal-on-metal bearings for hip replacement. Cobalt-chromium alloys with

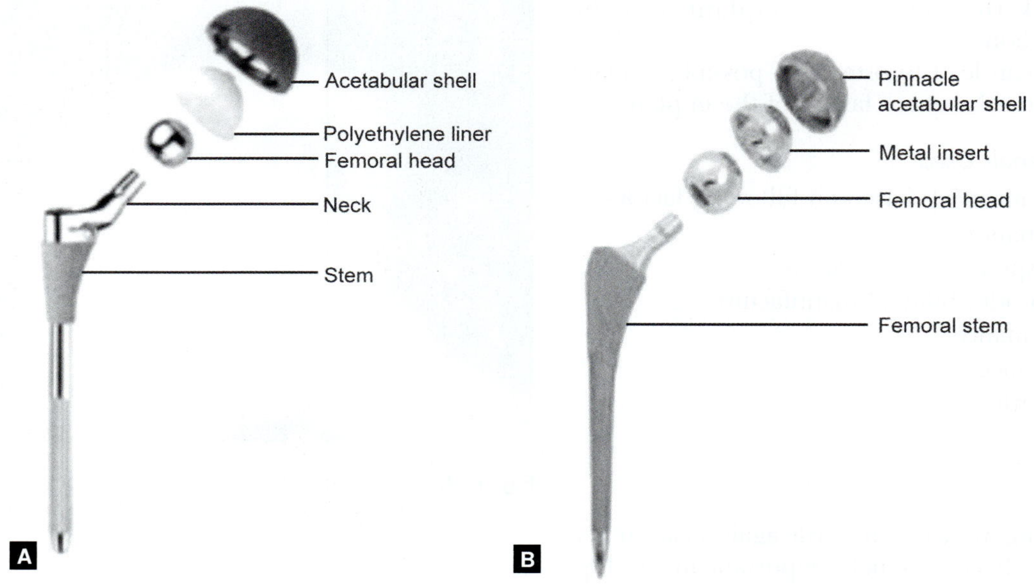

Figs 30.5A and B: (A) Metal on polyethylene bearings; (B) Metal-on-metal bearings

well-controlled grain sizes and finely distributed carbides provide superior hardness and wear resistance, compared to earlier versions of the alloy, to stainless steel and titanium alloy. Clearance and conformity between the bearing surfaces and a smooth surface, finish on the metallic bearings are now recognized as important factors that must be controlled as part of the design and manufacturing processes. The strength of cobalt-chromium alloys in comparison to polyethylene and their increased toughness over ceramics, provide additional benefits from the standpoint of hip implant design. Metal-on-metal bearings are not recommended for patients, with poorly functioning kidneys because metal ions excreted through the kidneys, can build up in the blood. Also, while being a pregnant woman or a woman of child-bearing age is not necessarily a contraindication for metal-on-metal bearings. Studies continue regarding metal ions crossing the placenta.

Metal on Polyethylene Bearings (Figs 30.5A and B)

It is one of the most commonly used bearing. Metal on polyethylene is a form of plastic that provides marked durability with an intended decrease in wear degradation. The goal of finding new means of reducing wear degradation in polyethylene has lead to some interesting developments in this material in the last two decades.

Ultra-high Molecular Weight Polyethylene Bearings

A substantial forward leap was made with the discovery in the late 1980, of the role of oxidation, in the wear performance of polyethylene, as shown in Figures 30.6.

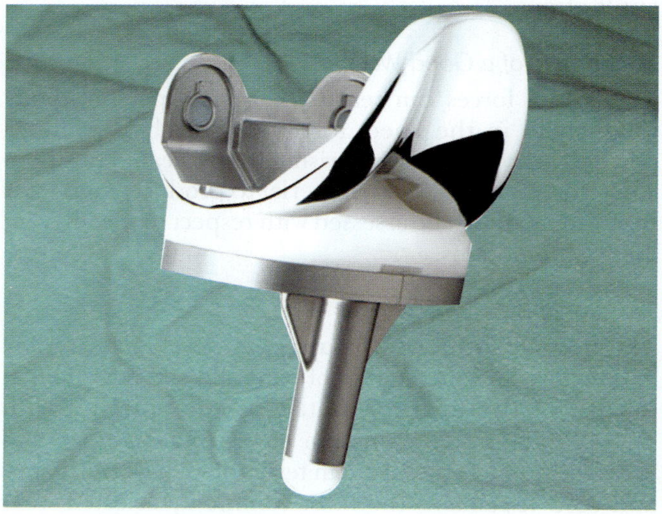

Fig. 30.6: Metal femoral component and tibial tray with polyspacer

Sterilization Options

There are two ways of sterilization, which are as follows:

- Placing polyethylene joint replacement components into sealed packages, which contain either vacuum or an inert gas, such as nitrogen or argon, instead of air.
- Replacing radiation altogether, instead exposing polyethylene components to ethylene oxide or gas plasma, neither of which imparts sufficient energy to cause oxidation, as shown in Figure 30.7.

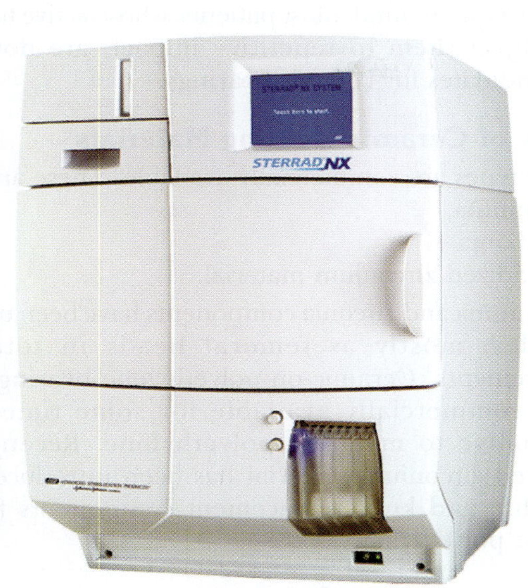

Fig. 30.7: Sterilization, by exposing polyethylene components to ethylene oxide or gas plasma

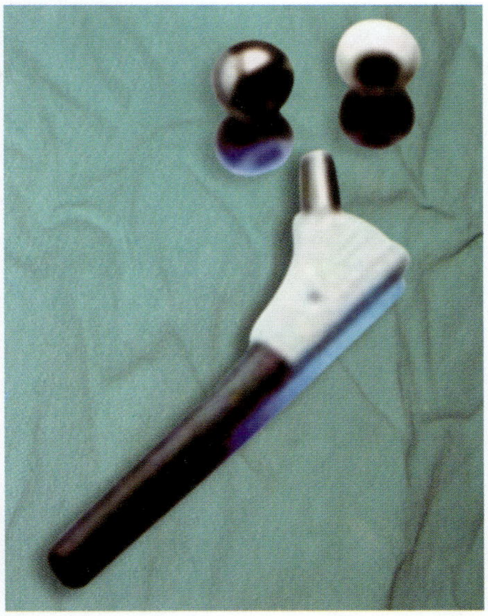

Fig. 30.8: A PEEK polymer

The Adverse Effects of Oxidation during Radiation Sterilization

- Polyethylene components, like most medical devices are sterilized by exposure to gamma radiation.
- Unfortunately, the radiation, while penetrating through the component has sufficient energy to break the chains that form the molecular backbone of the polymer.
- If the radiation exposure is performed, while the component is exposed to air, the broken ends can react with oxygen, causing harmful changes, which include:
  - Decrease in molecular weight
  - Dramatic loss of ductility
  - Decrease in strength
- The combined effect may make the polyethylene, markedly more susceptible to wear.

Development of Bearing Materials

Crossed-link polyethylene (XLPE), has been investigated, as a bearing material to address some of the limitations of UHMWPE. The process of cross-linking, has been shown to reduce wear, but the process can result in residual free radicals, which can lead to oxidative degradation and subsequent embrittlement within the material. Thermal treatments, following irradiation have been employed to reduce the concentration of free radicals. However, annealing or remelting treatments can reduce tensile and yield strength of XLPE as well as promote fatigue-crack propagation resistance. This is of particular importance in knees, where the articular surfaces are not completely congruent.

Polyether Ether Ketone (PEEK) Polymer (Fig. 30.8)

Due to its versatility, mechanical strength and biocompatibility, medical device manufacturers have routinely used, implantable-grade PEEK polymer in long run. One example of this potential is development of a carbon fiber reinforced PEEK (CF-PEEK) polymer, composite acetabular liner, which is used for articulation against a ceramic femoral head. Hip joint simulator testing up to 10 million cycles, showed that wear of the CF-PEEK polymer composite cups, was about 1 percent that of UHMWPE cups.

Ceramic Bearings (Fig. 30.9)

Advantages

Fully dense ceramics, alumina and zirconia are used in total joint replacements specifically for the purpose of providing, more wear resistant bearing surfaces, they have mechanical advantages over metallic alloys. Because of their hardness, ceramics can be polished to a very smooth finish and remain relatively scratch resistant, while in use as a bearing surface.

Disadvantages (Figs 30.10A and B)

- Their brittle nature, making them susceptible to fracture
- Strength and toughness remain issue, particularly in acetabular components of ceramic-on-ceramic hip replacements, where impingement of the femoral and acetabular components at extreme ranges of motion can lead to fracture

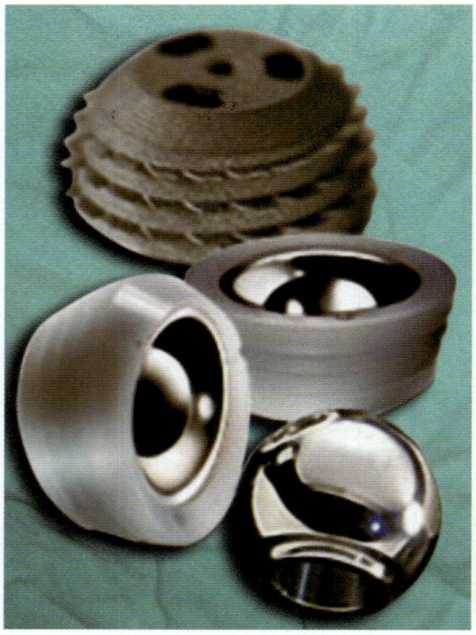

Fig. 30.9: Different ceramic bearings

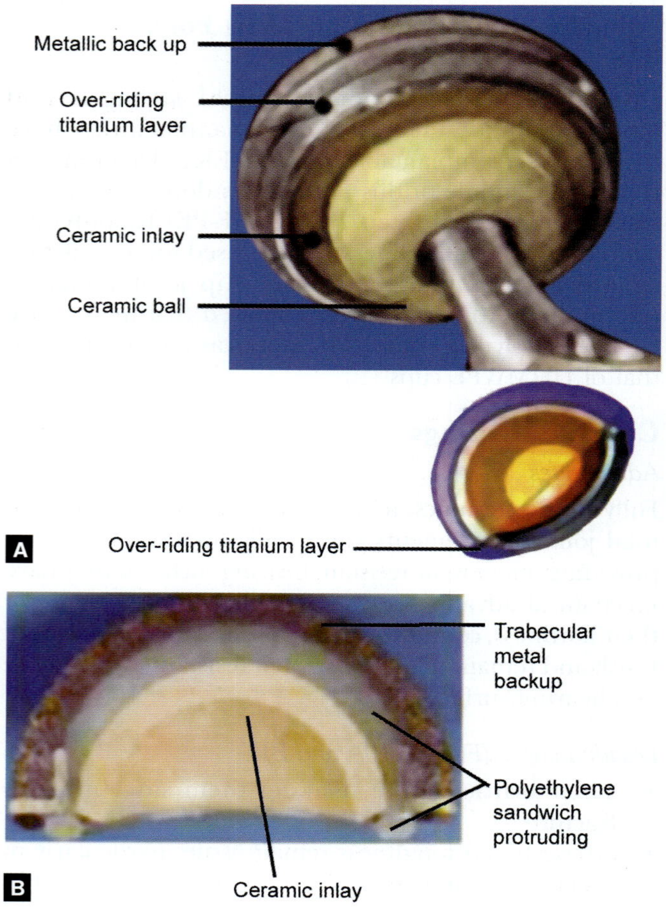

Figs 30.10A and B: Structure of a ceramic bearing and its different components

- With this in mind, most patients, whose active lifestyles subject them to repetitive impact, are not good candidates for ceramic bearings.

Types of Ceramic Bearing Materials

Three types are commercially available. These are:
- Alumina
- Zirconia
- Oxidized zirconium material.

Alumina and zirconia components have been used for decades, mostly as femoral heads in total hip replacements. Ceramic-on-polyethylene bearings have been commercially available for some time as an alternative to metal-on-polyethylene. Recently, an oxidized zirconium material has been introduced into both hip and knee replacement components for use against polyethylene.

Alumina-on-polyethylene

- Long-term experience
- Shows reduced wear rates over those typically seen, with metal-on-polyethylene bearings
- With an associated decrease in osteolysis
- Alumina-on-polyethylene bearings in knee replacements have found much more limited use.

Zirconia-on-polyethylene

- The use of zirconia, as a bearing surface against polyethylene has not proven as successful clinically, as alumina-on-polyethylene bearings.
- A direct comparison among alumina, zirconia and metal-on-conventional polyethylene bearings, in total hip patients, revealed the highest wear rate in the zirconia group.
- The tendency of zirconia, which is as wear resistant as alumina is to change its crystalline structure, to a form that is less tough, is one of the disadvantages of this material.
- The transformation is accompanied by a marked decrease in toughness, which makes the material more susceptible to roughening and increased wear.

Alumina-on-alumina

- In general, alumina-on-alumina joints have shown very low wear rates. Clinically, though the results are design dependent.
- Recent reports also show excellent wear resistance, in young patients, with no measurable wear and no evidence of osteolysis, even beyond a decade of follow-up.
- Furthermore, very few implant fractures have been observed, even in this high demand patient population, lending further credence, to the improved mechanical properties of alumina.

Oxinium (Oxidized Zirconium) on Polyethylene (Figs 30.11 to 30.16)

- Oxidized zirconium, popularly known as Oxinium (which is a brand name applied by orthopedic device manufacturer Smith and Nephew), is what is known as a hybrid technology
- Zirconium alloy is a metal, that is treated with high pressure and heat, which converts the surface of the implant to a ceramic
- This leads to an implant, which has surface properties of ceramic, which is harder, smoother and has less friction, as shown in the Figures 30.11 and 30.12.
- The advantage of this process is that the implant, made from oxidized zirconium do not share the brittle qualities of ceramics because the base material is metal.
- Oxinium is used for femoral heads in hip replacement and the femoral component in knee replacement.

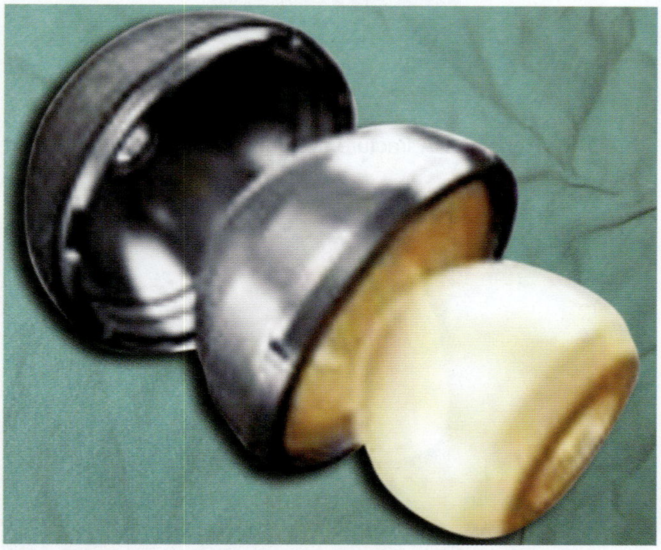

Fig. 30.11: Oxinium (oxidized zirconium) bearing on polyethylene

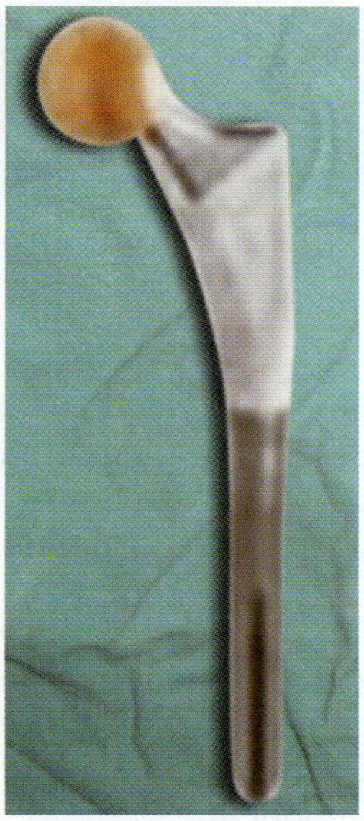

Fig. 30.12: Oxinium, applied on an implant

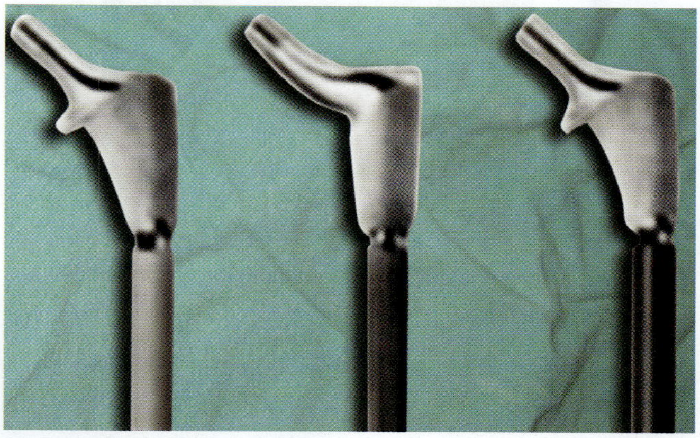

Fig. 30.13: Oxinium is used for femoral heads in hip replacement

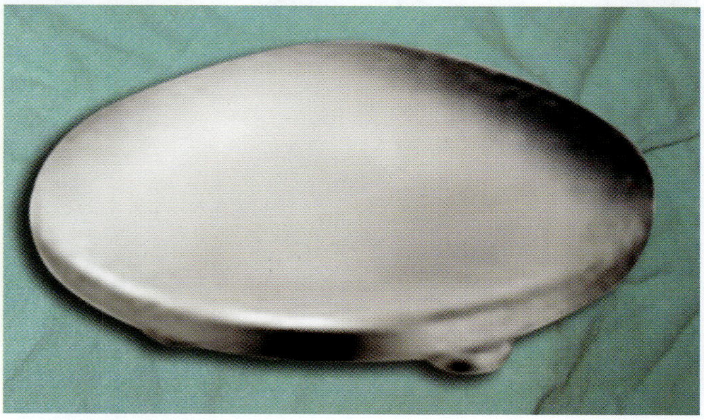

Fig. 30.14: A type of oxinium bearings

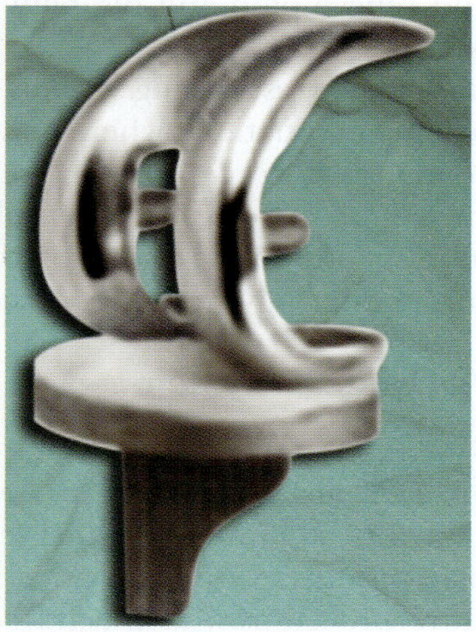

Fig. 30.15: Oxinium is used for the femoral component in knee replacement

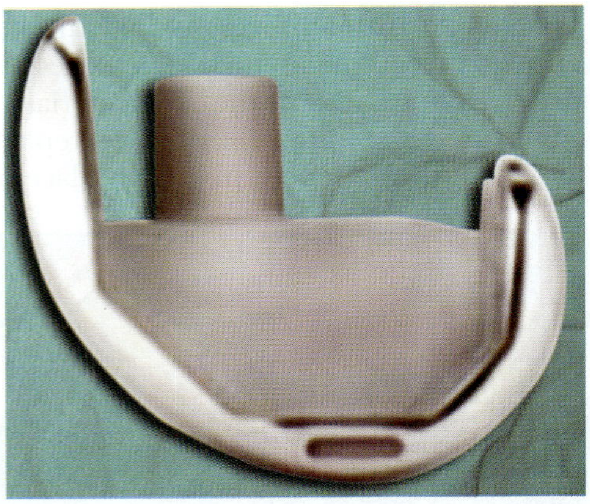

Fig. 30.16: Oxinium, used for different component of an implant

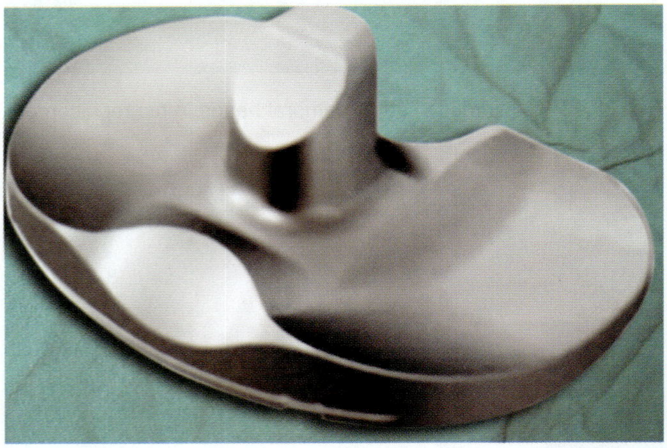

Fig. 30.17: Tibial tray for total knee replacement

Knee Replace System (Fig. 30.17)

- Total knee replacement systems, have helped restore function and relieve pain and disability for millions of patients
- Stryker's partial knee resurfacing systems are designed to conserve bone in situations, where only one portion of the knee joint is worn.
- Revision knee implants and instruments help prepare orthopedics surgeons, for any situation that may arise during complex oncology and knee revision surgeries.

Reunion HA Fracture System

Science of Success

The Reunion HA Fracture system consists of a revolutionary fracture stem design, which combines the heritage of solar products with innovative solutions for shoulder fracture procedures, as illustrated in Figures 30.18 and 30.19. Graft window and suture holes are

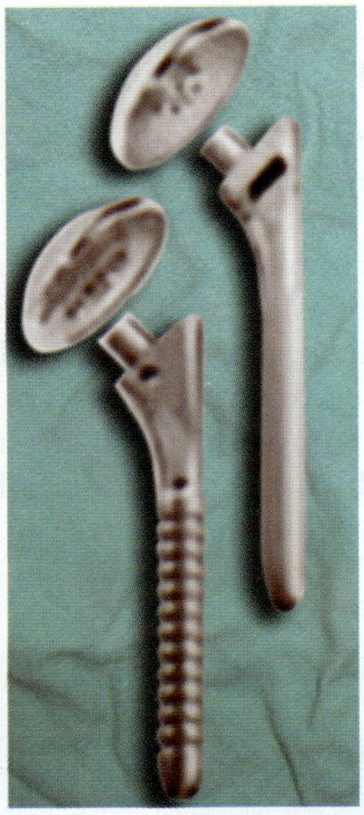

Fig. 30.18: Reunion HA fracture system

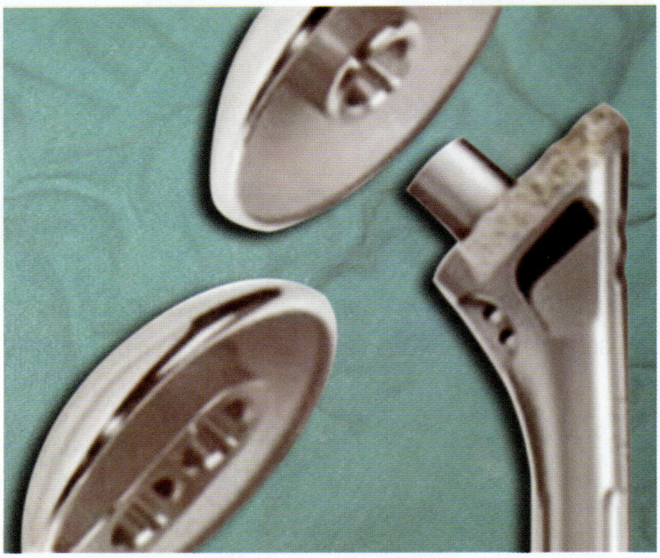

Fig. 30.19: Magnified view of HA fracture system, shown in Figure 30.18

positioned for technique preference, to help improve tuberosity attachment. Long-stem options are available for both difficult fractures and revision cases. A low profile design assists in tuberosity reduction for fractures.

Solar Shoulder (Figs 30.20 and 30.21)

The Solar total shoulder system is a completely modular system. All components are compatible, which allows any humeral component to be used with any humeral head on any glenoid component.

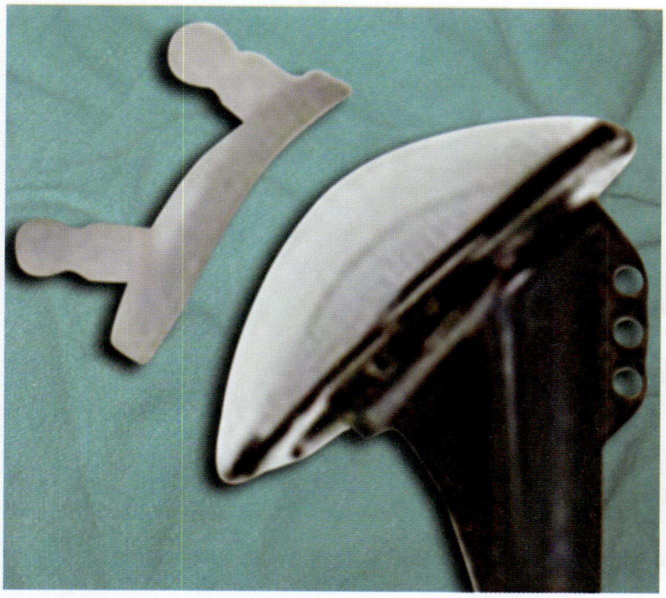

Fig. 30.20: A solar shoulder

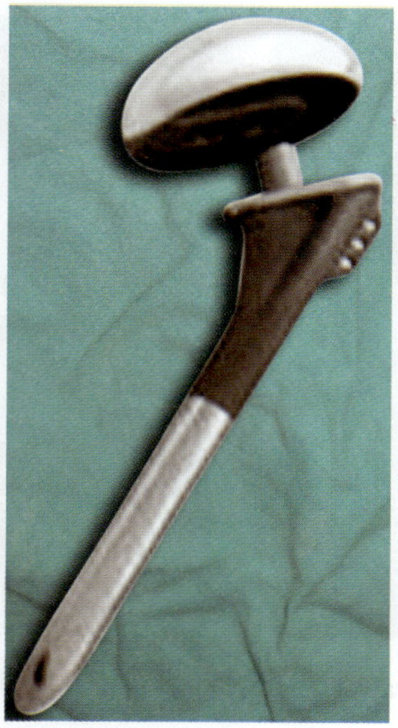

Fig. 30.21: A solar total shoulder system

Features and Benefits

- The system combines the most comprehensive selection of components, with the simplest instrumentation
- Unique dual offset humeral head
- Bipolar option design
- Modular dual radius humeral head
- Divergent peg glenoid components
- Solar stems.

Solar Elbow System (Figs 30.22 and 30.23)

Solar total elbow was designed, to recreate anatomy of the elbow and to optimize fixation. The prosthesis incorporates features that help restore the normal center of rotation of the elbow joint. Applications include rheumatoid, traumatic and degenerative arthritis. The solar elbow can achieve full extension and flexion up to 140° with approximately 7.5° of laxity in the varus/valgus plane during supination and pronation.

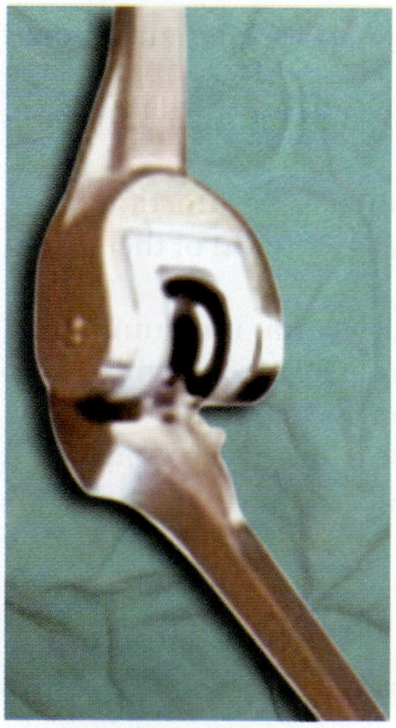

Fig. 30.22: A solar elbow system

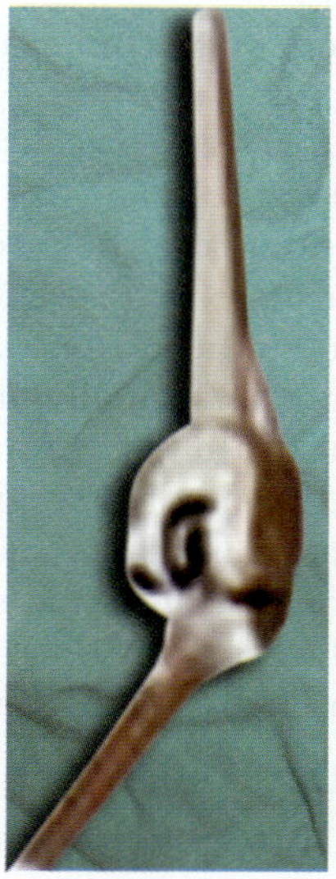

Fig. 30.23: A solar elbow system (extended view)

Features and Benefits

Humeral and ulnar components are anatomically designed to duplicate the functional motion of a normal elbow joint.

- Humeral component features:
  - Anatomic offset helps to recreate the natural anatomy of the elbow.
  - Lateral/medial fins help to resist rotational forces on humeral component.
  - Solar humeral component provides maximum contact in the epicondylar regions of the humerus, where the highest quality bone is present.
  - Designed to conserve the greatest possible amount of bone.
- Ulnar component features:
  - Helps to mimic the normal carrying angle of the elbow.
  - Anterior fin aids in mitigating rotational forces on ulnar component.

Solar Radial Head (Fig. 30.24)

For use in radial head arthroplasty, associated with comminuted fractures, rheumatoid disease and post-traumatic disease.

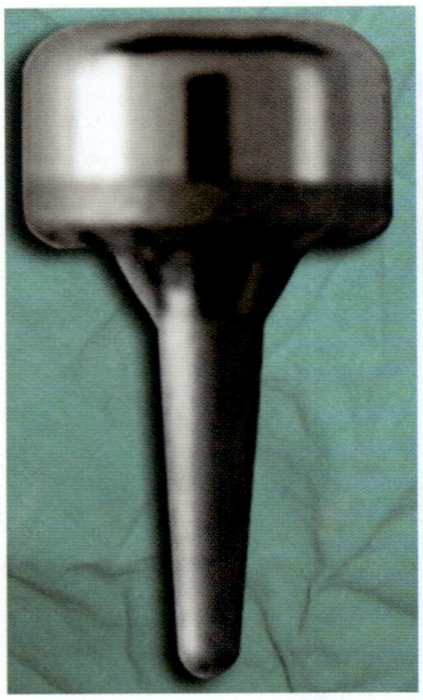

Fig. 30.24: A solar radial head

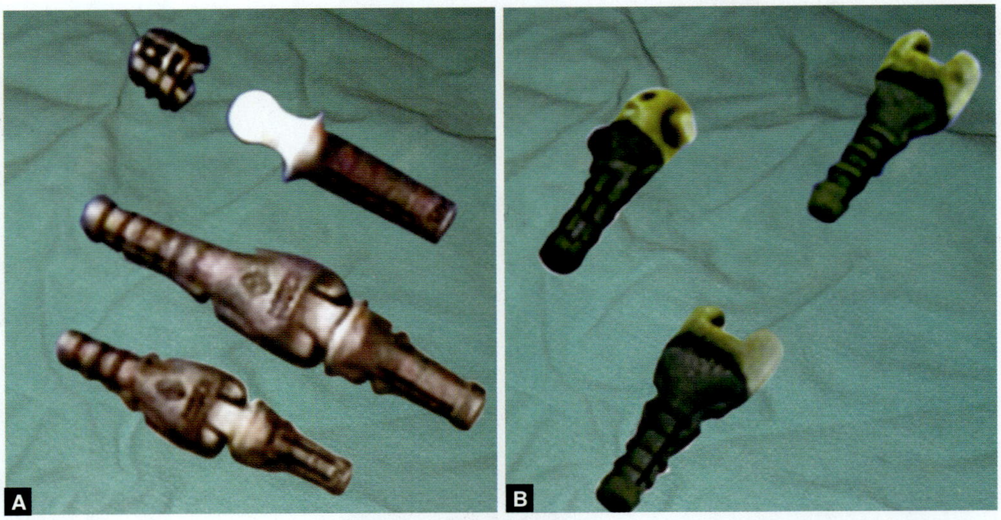

Figs 30.25A and B: Different solar finger implants, with PEEK-on-PEEK articulating surfaces

Features and Benefits

- Cemented component, designed for higher demand patients
- Superior wear characteristics, due to cobalt cromium material
- Designed to help restore proper joint function
- Designed to prevent proximal migration of the radius, due to head removal
- Five sizes (small 8 mm, small 11 mm, medium 9 mm, medium 12 mm and medium 15 mm), to accommodate surgical patient population.
- Finger implants, such as those feature PEEK-on-PEEK articulating surfaces. The material may reduce the risk of wear particles accumulating in the body, as shown in Figures 30.25A and B.

On the Horizon

The future of joint replacement may see the implementation of some very intriguing surface materials. Surfaces made of diamond have been produced recently, and there is much discussion of the promise of hardened titanium due to its smooth exterior.

Conclusion

- The final frontier (in man-made joint replacement), is the longevity of the implant, to prevent the problem of osteolysis.
- The alternate bearings are an attempt to bring it to the next level and get a further increase in longevity, by decreasing the wear degradation problems.
- At the end of the day, we have to customize, what we do for patients on an individual basis.
- The age of the patient, the patient's expected activity levels, the extent of the patient's joint problems are among a long list of factors that the surgeon must consider in choosing an implant.
- Despite the concern over wear and osteolysis, it must be remembered that joint replacement is a highly successful treatment with few complications.
- Perhaps one set of bearing materials will eventually emerge as the best for each joint in the body.
- For now, the decrease in wear afforded by the new bearing surfaces, represents an impressive milestone in the further improvement of total joint replacement.

31 Magnetic Resonance Imaging

- MRI of Spine
- MRI of Hip
- MRI of Knee
- MRI of Shoulder
- Recent Advances

Introduction

Magnetic resonance imaging (MRI) is the major medical imaging development of the century. It was developed by Purcell and Bloch independently in 1946, but its use for image production was started by Paul Lauterber in 1973. It provides a digital representation of tissue characteristics, related to spatial location and can be obtained in any tissue plane. The appearance of an MRI, is a function of the chemical composition of the tissue. Soft tissues are composed of around 70 percent water and 10 to 15 percent adipose, which generate the signal.

Fundamentals of MRI

Magnetic

There are two magnets essential to MRI:

1. *External magnet:* It is a part of the imaging machine and its strength is described in Tesla (T) units, like 0.5, 1.0 or 1.5 T
2. *Internal magnet:* These are the zillions of hydrogen atoms into the body.

Resonance: It is the matching of the frequency of the radiowaves, used for excitation, with the frequency of the spinning hydrogen atoms in the magnetic field. The hydrogen atoms have to be resonated with the correct frequency, which changes their magnetic vector.

Why Hydrogen Atom?

- Hydrogen is a simple element, with one proton in its nucleus
- It is everywhere in the body, i.e. water, lipids, proteins and nucleic acids
- The hydrogen ion in water contributes much to the signal, lipids to a lesser extent and proteins and nucleic acid, offer nothing to the signal
- The atom is positively charged and has a spinning or angular movement, which produces an internal magnetic field around the atom
- When these randomly oriented atoms are placed in an external magnetic field, some will align themselves parallel to the magnetic field, producing a net magnetic vector
- Other atoms, like sodium or potassium can also be used.

Common Terms Used in MRI

Pulse Sequence

These are of three types:

1. *Spin echo pulse sequence:* A combination of 90° and 180° Radiofrequency (RF) waves, result in hydrogen ion magnet, deflecting out of its position and spins like a top. The resulting signal is called the spin echo.
2. *Gradient echo pulse sequence:* These use less RF power, resulting in less anglular deflection of H^+ ion and these sequences require less time for recovery. This results in less time for the image gathering.
3. *Fast spin echo (FSE):* This delivers a faster image. Routine images take around 30-45 min for an image. FSE can get T2 SE images in less than 5 min.

Echo Time (TE)

It is the time between the initial RF pulse and the middle of the spin echo production, when the antenna detects the signal.

Repitition Time (TR)

It is the time between one RF pulse and the next. Varying TE and TR, different tissue relaxation times and different tissue contrasts, can be produced.

Relaxation Time

This is determined by the behavior of atoms in a magnetic field and can be used to produce images of varying tissue contrast. There are two types of relaxation:

- *T1 relaxation time (T1-weighted images):* It is the time required to restore 63 percent of the equilibrium population of atoms, to align with the magnetic field, following the excitation pulse. It is also known as spin lattice or longitudinal relaxation time.

- *T2 relaxation time (T2-weighted images):* It is the time required for 63 percent of the signal given, to disappear irreversibly. It occurs due to the interaction between adjacent nuclei. It is also known as spin-spin or transverse relaxation time.

Each tissue has a characteristic T1 and T2 relaxation times, which determine the signal intensity and thus the image produced. The set up of the machine, can be either of the combinations:

1. T1-TR: 600 ms
   TE: 30 ms
   Slice thickness: 4 to 5 mm
2. T2-TR: 2000 ms
   TE: 60/90 ms
   Slice thickness: 4 to 5 mm.

Technique

Place the patient in the magnetic coil. Broadcast a predetermined radiofrequency into the body and the series of the RF pulse is repeated in cycles. The hydrogen atoms absorb the energy from the RF and there is change in the net magnetic vector. During a gap in the pulse, the atoms try to reorient and release energy, they have absorbed. This energy is picked up by an antenna. It is recorded as digital data by the computer. Computer converts digital data into varying shades of gray to produce an image.

MRI Gray Scale

The varying shades of gray produced are based upon following factors:

- *Proton density:* The more number of free and mobile protons, brighter is the image and vice versa. Materials with high proton density are fat, CSF, blood and other fluids, these produce bright images. Materials with low proton density are calcium, air, cortical bone and fibrous tissue and these produce gray images.
- *T1 and T2 relaxation times:* Substances with the shortest T1, give off the brightest signal, e.g. fat, lipid containing molecules or proteinaceous fluid. Substances with the longest T1 give low signal and appear gray (edema, CSF, pure fluid and tumors). In T2 images, longer the T2 relaxation time, brighter the signal and vice versa.
- Motion or flow of materials, e.g. blood.

■ MRI of Spine

Sagittal T1 and T2 images of upper and lower spine is shown in Figures 31.1 and 31.2, respectively.

T1 Image

- Spinal cord—intermediate signal
- CSF—low (gray)
- Epidural fat—high
- Marrow intermediate to high
- Dorsal root ganglion—intermediate.

T2 Image

- Spinal cord—low
- CSF—high (white)
- Epidural fat—intermediate
- Marrow—intermediate to low
- Dorsal root ganglion—intermediate.

Axial T1 Images (Fig. 31.3)

- Spinal cord—intermediate
- CSF—low
- Marrow—high

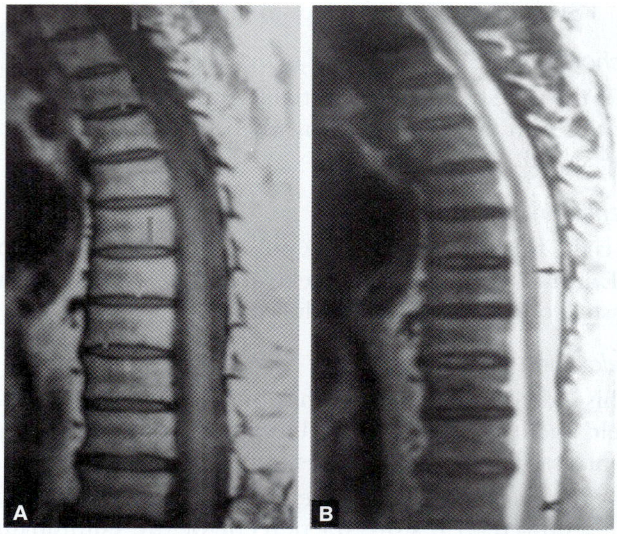

Figs 31.1A and B: MRI, sagittal T1 and T2 images of spine

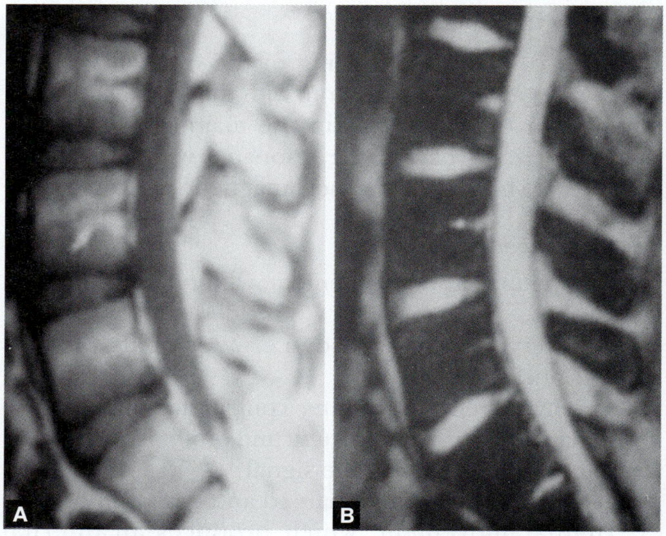

Figs 31.2A and B: MRI, sagittal T1 and T2 images of spine (magnified view)

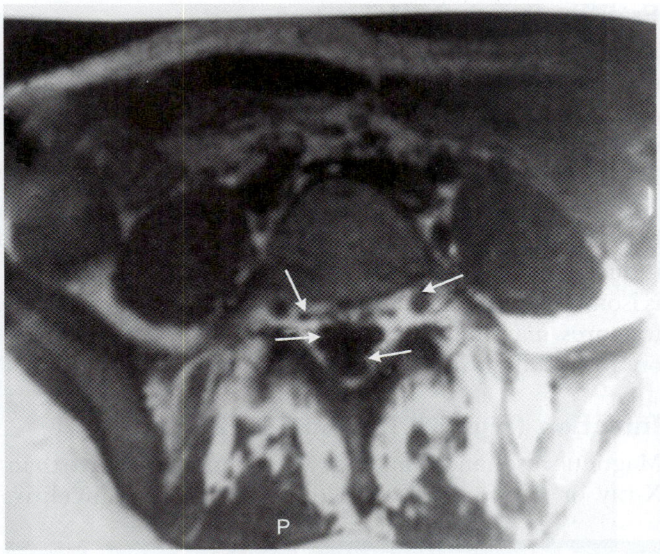

Fig. 31.3: Axial T1 MRI of spine

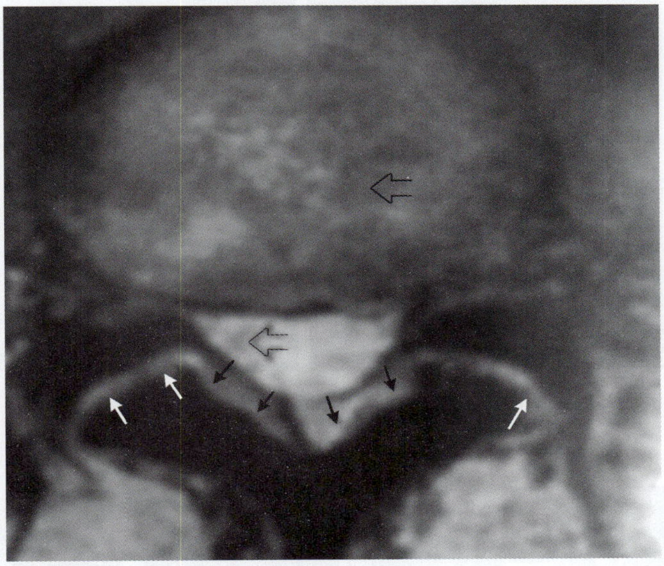

Fig. 31.4: Axial T2 MRI of spine

- Interforaminal vein—low
- Dorsal root ganglion—low, but well defined and surrounded by bright fat
- Ligamentum flavum—intermediate.

Axial T2 Images (Fig. 31.4)

- Spinal cord—low
- CSF—high
- Marrow—low
- Facet hyaline cartilage—intermediate
- Ligamentum flavum—high
- Intervertebral disk—high.

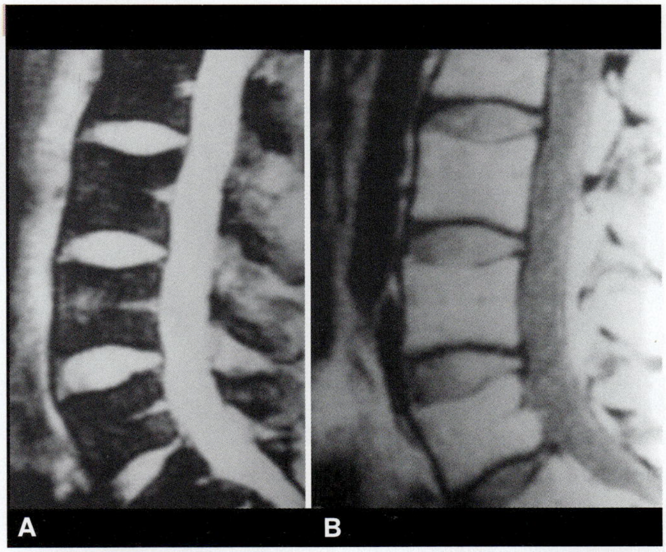

Figs 31.5A and B: T1 and T2 sagittal images of spine showing degenerative disk changes

Indications

- Degenerative disk disease
- Postoperative spine
- Infection
- Trauma
- Neoplasms of bone, soft tissue and cord
- Spondylolisthesis
- Marrow replacement disorders, e.g. leukemia, multiple myeloma and metastasis.
- Abnormalities of the pediatric spine.

Degenerative Disk Disease (Figs 31.5 to 31.7)

- Disk herniation is better seen in the T2 images, as there is white CSF as the background
- Lateral or posterolateral disk herniation are best seen in the axial images
- Schmorl's nodes and vacuum phenomenon can also be seen
- End-plate changes (modic), as illustrated in Figures 31.8 to 31.10.
- *Type I:* There is decreased signal intensity in T1 (Fig. 31.8A) and increased on T2 (Fig. 31.8B) and it represents subchondral vascularized fibrous tissue, associated with end-plate fissuring and disruption
- *Type II:* There is increased signal intensity on T1 (Fig. 31.9A) and isotense or hypotense signal on T2 (Fig. 31.9B). It represents fatty marrow end-plate conversion.
- *Type III:* There is low signal intensity on both T1 (Fig. 31.10A) and T2 (Fig. 31.10B) images. It represents sclerosis.

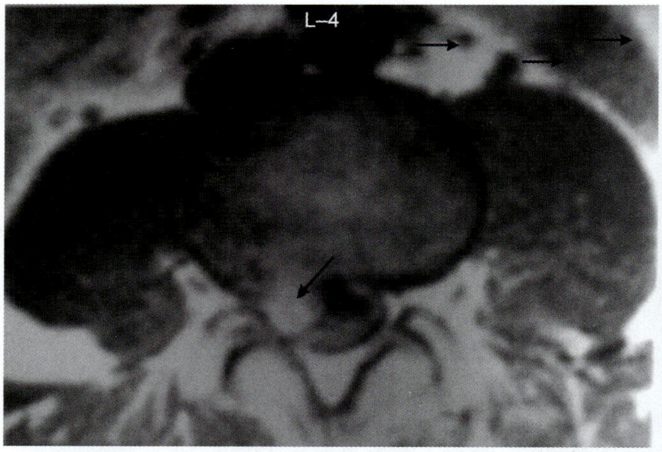

Fig. 31.6: Lateral or posterolateral disk herniation are best seen in the axial images

Fractures and Cord Trauma

Magnetic resonance imaging (MRI) has been used for traumatic and nontraumatic body fractures. In 28 percent of cases supraspinous ligament disruptions, associated with thoracolumbar burst fractures are identified on MRI. In post-traumatic myelopathy, there is low intensity on T1 and hyperintensity on T2. Syringomyelia shows hyperintensity on T2 images. Myelomalacia, i.e. gliosis induced microcystic degeneration of cord parenchyma, is isointense or hyperintense to cord on T1 images. Sacral fractures may mimic metastasis and show low intensity on T1 and high intensity on fat suppression images.

Infection (Figs 31.11 and 31.12)

Magnetic resonance imaging (MRI) is more sensitive than X-ray or CT for detection of vertebral osteomyelitis.

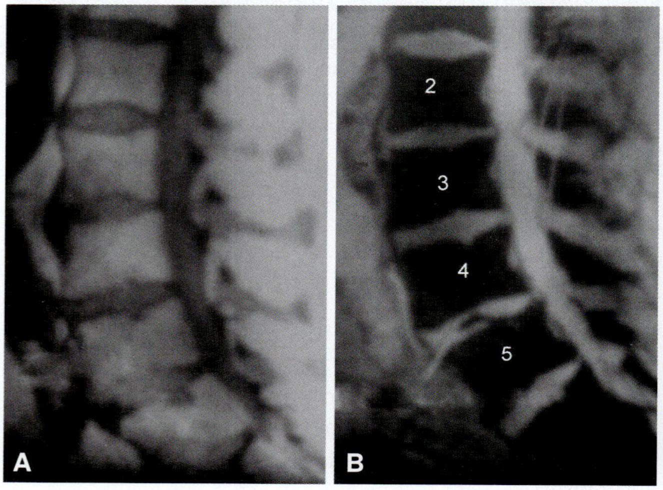

Fig. 31.7A and B: Degenerative disk changes and herniation in MRI imaging

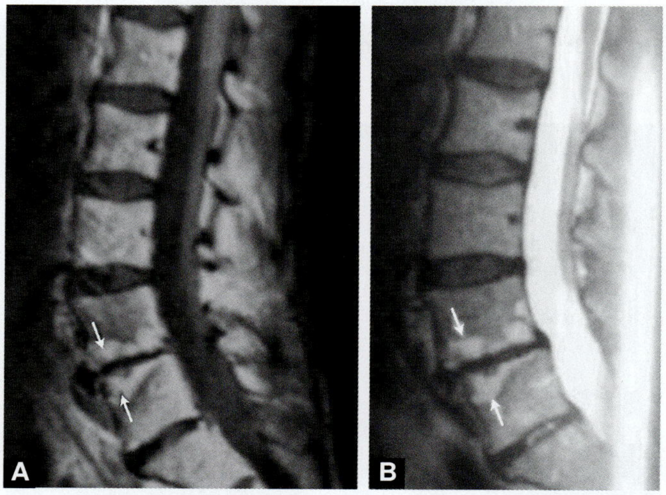

Figs 31.9A and B: Type II end-plate changes, seen in sagittal T1 (A) and T2 (B) MRIs

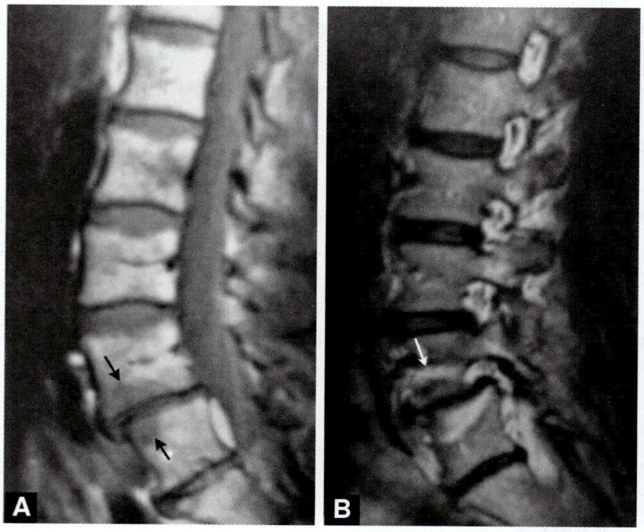

Figs 31.8A and B: Type I end-plate changes, seen in sagittal T1 (A) and T2 (B) MRIs

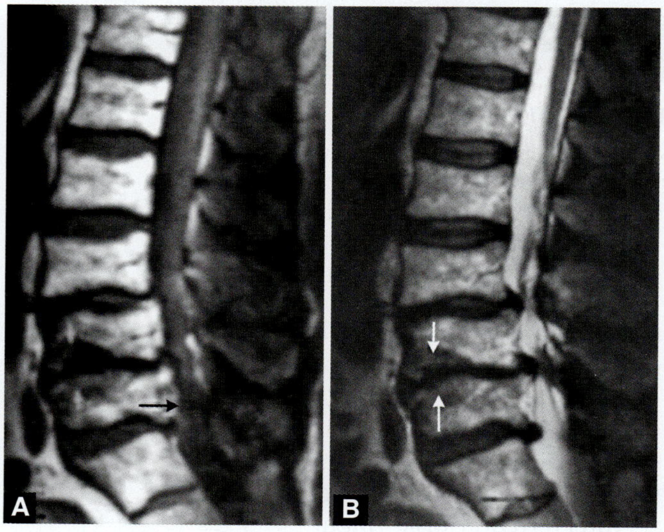

Figs 31.10A and B: Type III end-plate changes, seen in sagittal T1 (A) and T2 (B) MRIs

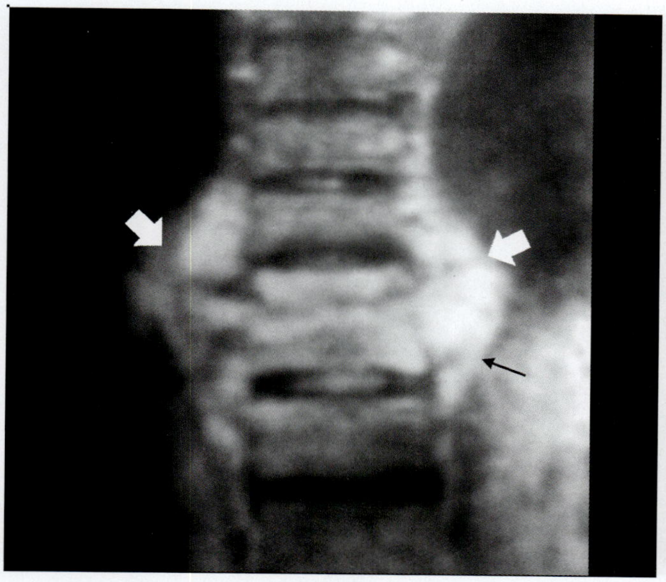

Fig. 31.11: Tubercular bone destruction with epidural and prevertebral abscess

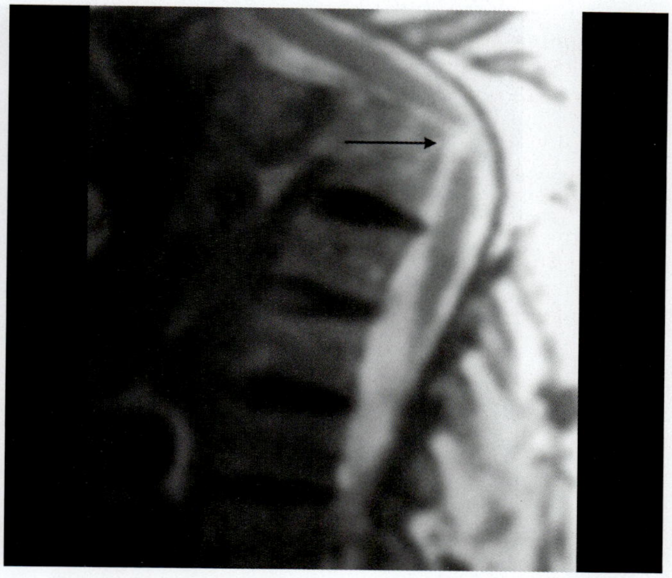

Fig. 31.12: Destruction and collapse of vertebral body with kyphotic deformity

Infection of vertebral body and the adjacent disk space is seen as low intensity on T1 images and high on T2 images. Tubercular (TB) spondylitis is characterized by intraosseous and paraspinal abscess formation, subligamentous extension of infection, destruction and collapse of the vertebral body and epidural space extension. Epidural abscesses are best demonstrated on T2 images.

Tumors and Marrow Disorders (Figs 31.13A to D)

Hemangiomas have increased signal intensity on T1 and T2 images. Aneurysmal bone cyst (ABC), demonstrates inhomogenous signal intensity on T1 and T2 images. Chordomas are hypointense on T1 and hyperintense on T2 images. Metastatic tumors having osteoclastic activity, have increased activity on T2 and osteoblastic have decreased activity on T2 images. Meningeal cysts may present with or without nerve root involvement (Tarlov cyst).

Spondylolisthesis (Figs 31.14A and B)

MR images are less sensitive than CT. The Anteroposterior (AP) diameter is increased in spondylolytic listhesis and narrowed in degenerative listhesis. Axial images demonstrate low signal intensity sclerosis, fragmentation or discontinuity in the region of the pars interarticularis. Reactive changes in the end plates can be seen (Modic Type II). The contours of the thecal sac may have an hourglass or constricted outline.

■ MRI of Hip

AVN of Hip

MRI Findings (Fig. 31.15)

- Bone marrow edema
- *Double line:* Head in head sign
- Crescent sign
- Collapse
- Joint effusion
- Involvement of acetabulum
- Status of other hip
- Marrow infiltrating disease
- Decreased signal from ischemic marrow
- Single band like area of low signal intensity
- Hundred percent sensitivity
- Ninety-eight percent specificity
- *Double line sign:* T2 image, as shown in Figure 31.16.
- A second high signal intensity seen within the line seen on T1 images, represents hypervascular granulation tissue.

Early Changes

See Figure 31.17.

Late Changes

See Figure 31.18.

■ MRI of Knee (Fig. 31.19)

MRI findings for lateral view of knee:

- Distal or lowest part of femur
- Patella (knee cap)

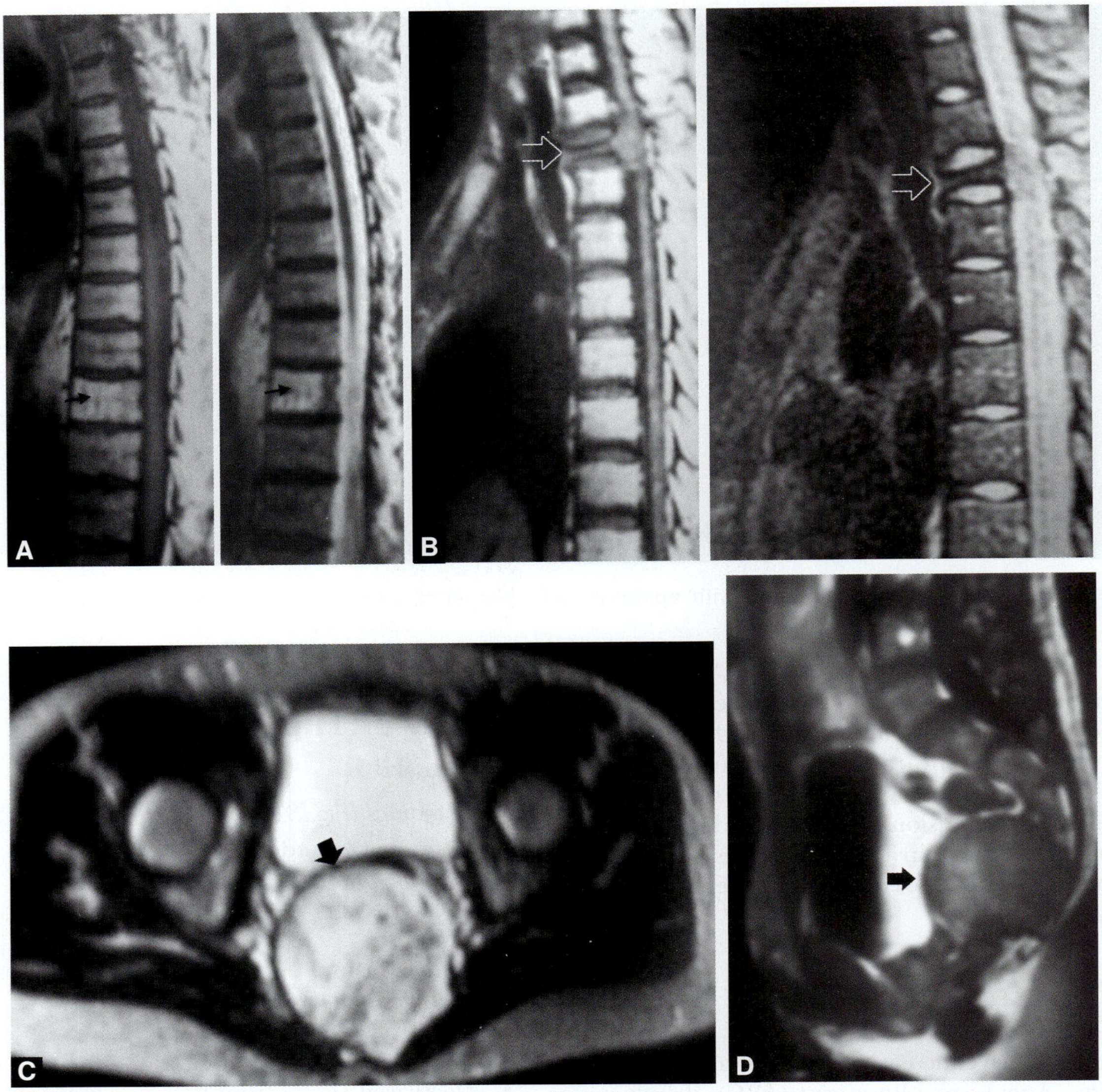

Figs 31.13A to D: (A) and (B) Sagittal MRI showing tumor and marrow changes; (C) and (D) Axial MRI showing tumor and marrow changes (arrows)

- Proximal (upper) tibia
- The lateral meniscus is seen as a dark bow tie like structure
- The patellar tendon is also clearly seen at the front of the knee, connecting the patella with the tibia.

■ MRI of Shoulder (Fig. 31.20)

Postoperative Spine

CT is important in assessing bony details, but MRI is useful in characterizing end-plate and associated marrow changes. Stable fusions show modic type II changes and increased intensity on T1 and isointense on T2 images. On T1, posterior scar has heterogenous intermediate intensity and isointense to hyperintense on T2 compared to the discectomy scar. Postoperative discitis, shows decreased intensity in the marrow on T1 images, hyperintensity on T2 images.

Arachnoiditis is classified as:

Group I: Central conglomeration of nerve roots within the thecal sac.

Group II: Nerve roots are clumped peripherally to the meninges, producing an apparent empty thecal sac.

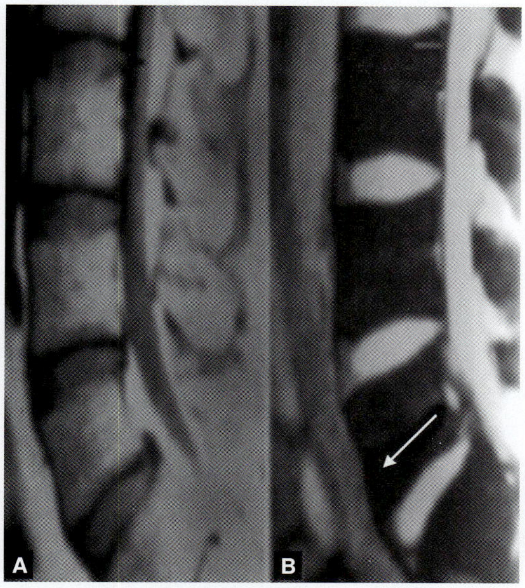

Figs 31.14A and B: MRI spine showing spondylolisthesis (arrow)

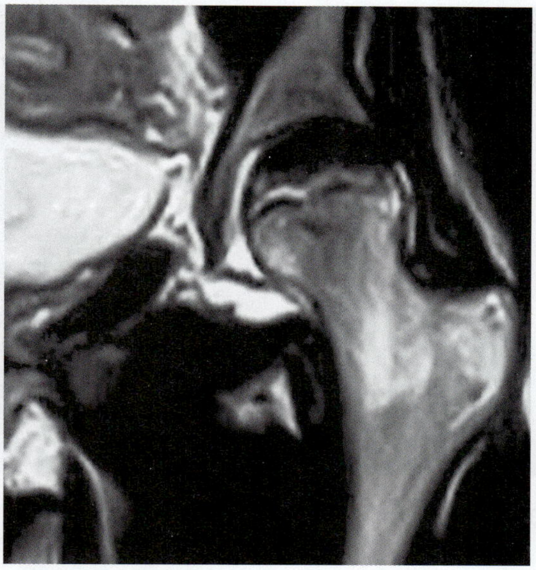

Fig. 31.16: Double line sign, seen in T2 image

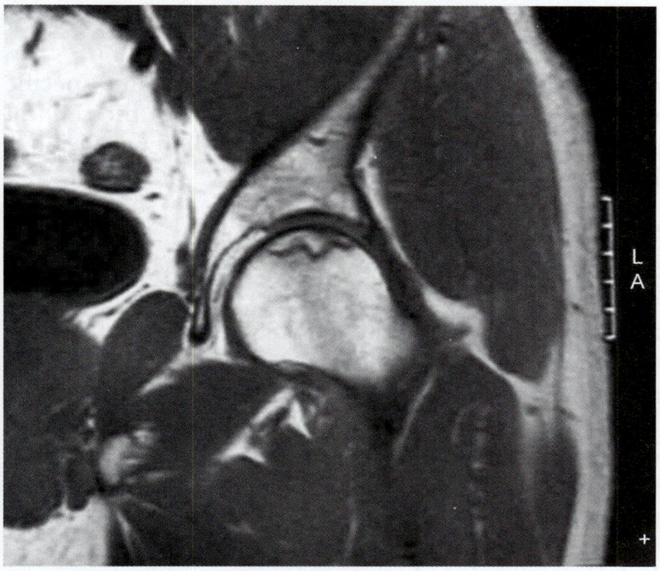

Fig. 31.15: MRI T1 image of hip

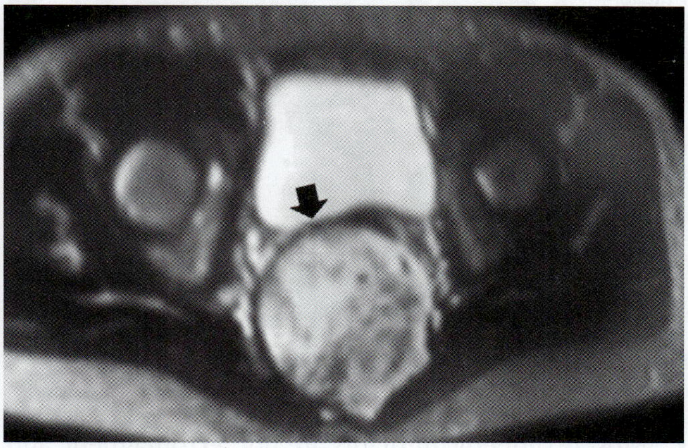

Fig. 31.17: Early tumor growth and marrow changes shown in MRI

Group III: Images show increased soft tissue signal, occupying the thecal sac with no discrimination of nerve roots.

Disadvantages

- The gantry is smaller and longer than CT and patient may have claustrophobia.
- The scan time is longer and the patient may find it difficult to be still for the time required.
- Patients with ferromagnetic materials in the body cannot be scanned. These include:
  - Cerebral aneurysmal clips
  - Pacemakers
  - Transcutaneous electrical nerve stimulation (TENS) units
  - Metallic cardiac valves
  - Life support devices.

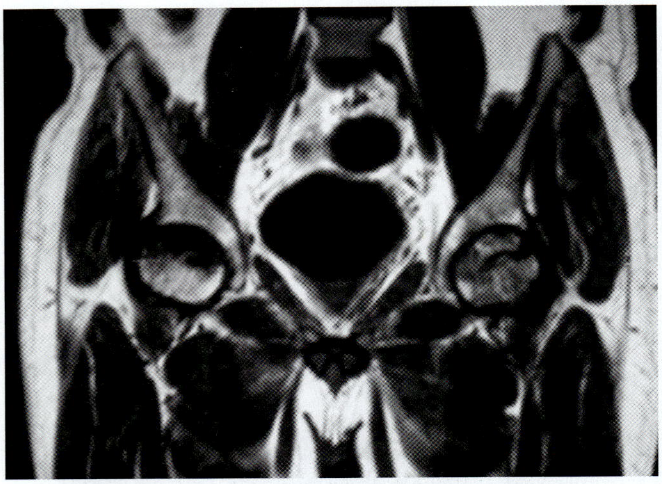

Fig. 31.18: Late tumor growth and marrow changes shown in MRI

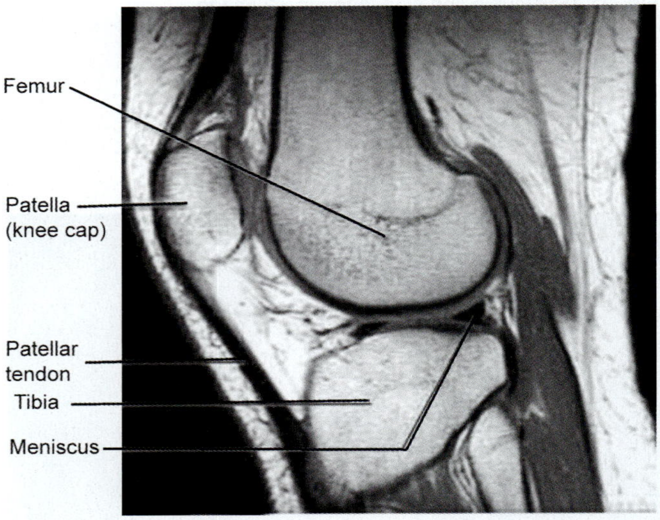

Fig. 31.19: MRI of the knee—side (lateral) view

- Most orthopedic implants are not ferromagnetic and do not affect image quality, unless are directly in the field, e.g. pedicle instrumentation.

Recent Advances

Kinematic MRI

It refers to the assessment of joint functions, with respect to various interactions of soft tissues, bony structures and relative alignment of these structures through a specific range of motion. It is used in evaluation of the cervical spine, temperomandibular joint, patellofemoral joint, knee, wrist, ankle and the shoulder.

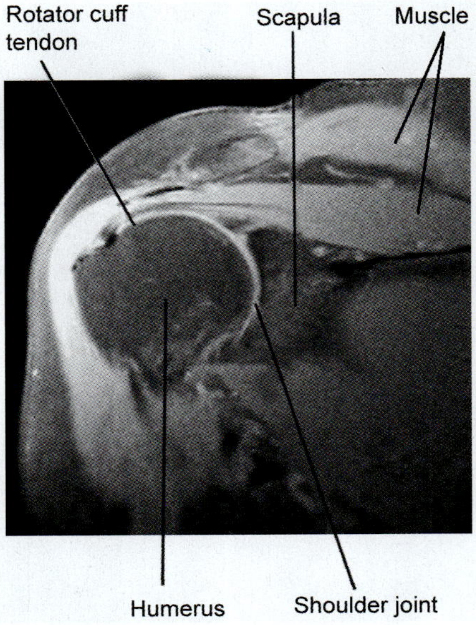

Fig. 31.20: MRI of the right shoulder, looking at rotator cuff and head of humerus as well as glenoid portion of scapula

STIR and GRASS

Short T1 inversion recovery (STIR), improves visualization of joint fluid. 3D gradient recalled acquisitions in steady state (GRASS) and spoiled GRASS (SPGR) images, optimize trabecular bone detail and the anatomy.

3D MRI Rendering Technique

Here, the 2D images obtained are converted into 3D by the computer. Finer structures can be visualized.

Fat Suppression Images

The adipose tissue gives a strong signal on the normal view and may hinder detection of pathology. Here, fat suppression offers improved visibility and sensitivity.

Contrast Enhanced MRI

Contrasts used are compounds known as gadolinium chelates. They are deposited in tissues with high water content and increase their signal intensity.

32 Introduction and Application of PET in Orthopedics

- Positron Emission Tomography
- Application of PET in Orthopedics

■ Positron Emission Tomography

Positron emission tomography (PET), shown in Figure 32.1, is a nuclear medicine imaging technique, which produces a three-dimensional image or map of functional processes in the body. It creates tomographic images, revealing certain biochemical properties of tissues by computer analysis of positrons emitted, when radioactively tagged substances are incorporated in the tissue. It is a new scanning technique in medical research.

Positron

- An antimatter equivalent of the electron
- The positron has an electric charge of +1, a spin of 1/2 and the same mass as an electron.
- Positrons are given off during the decay of the nuclei of specific radioisotopes, this is illustrated in Figure 32.2.
- When a low energy positron collides with a low energy electron, annihilation occurs, resulting in the production of two gamma ray photons, as depicted in Figure 32.3.

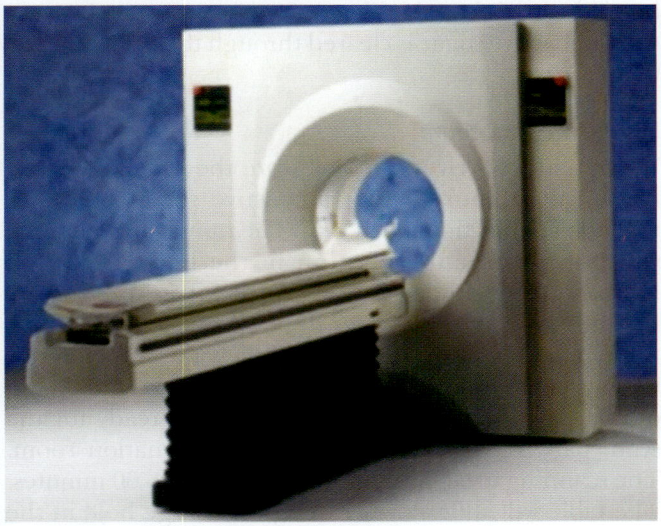

Fig. 32.1: A PET scanning table

- The first scientist deemed to have captured positrons through electron positron annihilation was Chung Yao Chao, a graduate student at Caltech in 1930, though he did not realize what they were at that time.

Radioisotopes

Radioisotopes are produced artificially by bombarding stable isotopes with a proton beam generated by a

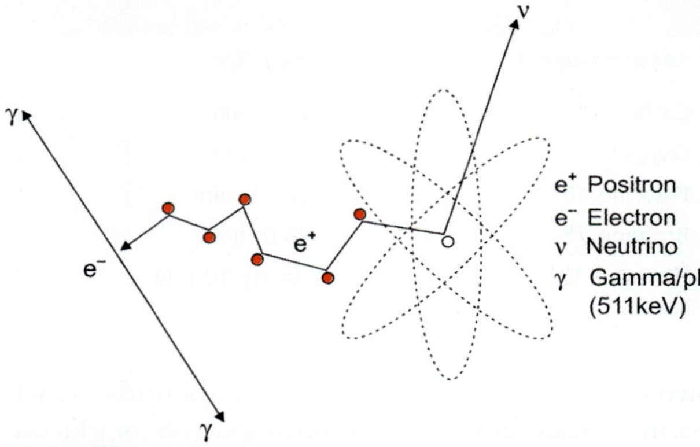

Fig. 32.2: Positron given away by a radioactive nuclei, is an antimatter equivalent of the electron

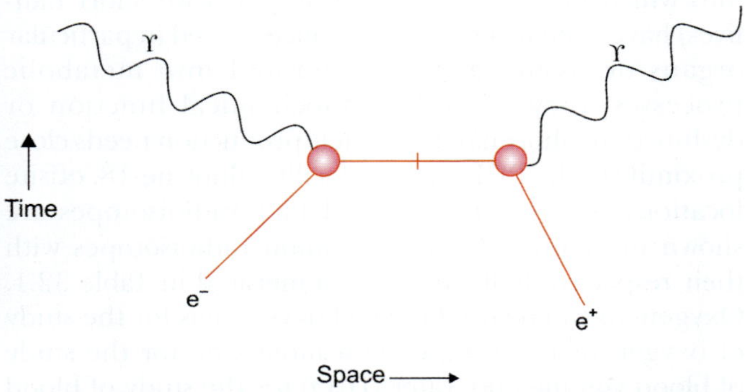

Fig. 32.3: A low energy positron collides with a low energy electron, causes annihilation, resulting in the production of two gamma ray photons

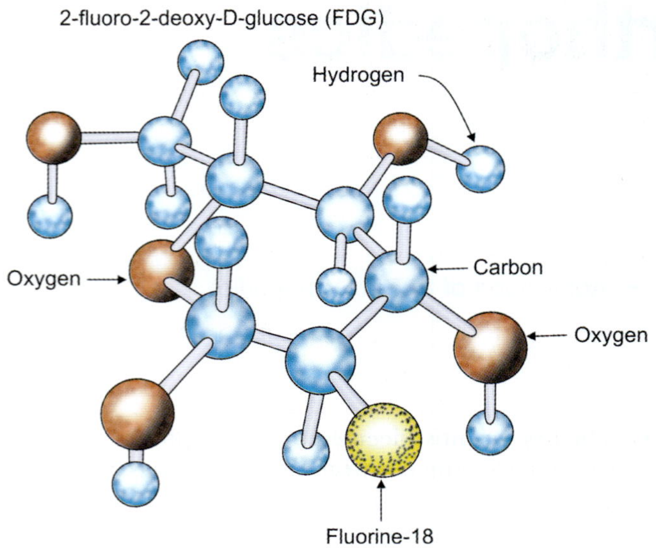

Fig. 32.4: Commonly used PET isotopes

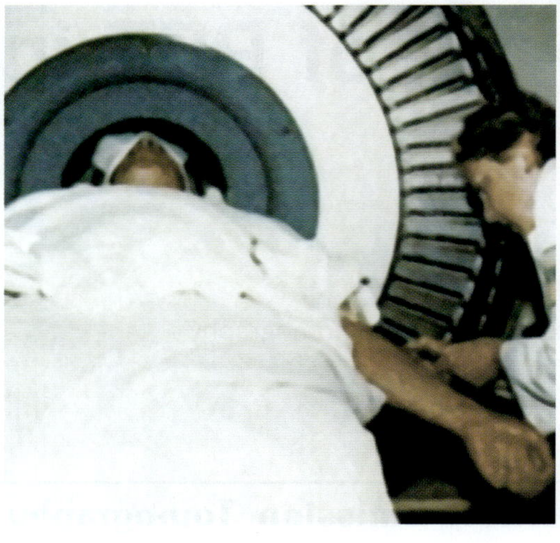

Fig. 32.5: Patient, undergoing PET scanning

Table 32.1: **Commonly used radioisotopes or labeling agents, with their half-life**

Labeling agent	*Half-life*
Carbon-11	20.3 min
Oxygen-15	2.03 min
Fluorine-18	109.8 min
Bromine-75	98.0 min
Nitrogen-13	Nearly 10 min

cyclotron. Incorporated either into compounds, which are normally used by the body, such as glucose (or glucose analogues), water or ammonia or into molecules that bind to receptors or other sites of drug action. Such labeled compounds are known as radiotracers. These radiotracers are analogues of physiologic or pharmaceutical agents, into which positron emitting isotopes (with short half-lives) have been incorporated. Concentrated in particular organs or tissues and incorporated into metabolic processes, they can reflect biochemical function or dysfunction. Short half lives: their production needs close proximity to the PET imaging facility (fluorine-18, offsite location). The commonly used PET radioisotopes are shown in Figure 32.4 and common radioisotopes with their respective half-lives are enumerated in Table 32.1. Oxygen-15 can be used to label oxygen gas for the study of oxygen metabolism, carbon monoxide for the study of blood volume and water (H_2O) for the study of blood flow in the brain. Fluorine-18 is attached to a glucose molecule to produce 2-fluoro-2-deoxy-D-glucose (FDG), for use in the observation of the brain's sugar metabolism.

How does It feel to have a PET Scan?

During a scan, as shown in Figure 32.5, the patient reclines on a comfortable couch with his or her head inside the large, doughnut shaped positron emission tomograph. While the patient's head must be kept very still, the only real discomfort involved, may be the pinprick of a hypodermic needle, as a minute amount of radiopharmaceutical is injected. The radiopharmaceutical could be administered as an intravenous injection or inhaled as a gas. How it is administered? It depends on the radiopharmaceutical. Which one is chosen? It depends on what function the researcher wants to study.

Preparing for the Procedure

Patient should be instructed to not eat or drink anything, except water for several hours prior to scan. Patient may be told to drink a significant amount of water because the radioactive sugar is cleared through the urine (if FDG used).

During the Procedure

When patient arrives for PET scan, the radiologist or a nurse will administer the radioactive sugar molecules through an injection into a vein. The radioactive material will not create any sensation in the body. After the injection, the radioactive substance will take 30 to 90 minutes to reach the tissues to be scanned. During that time, patient will need to lie quietly without moving or talking, as too much motion can disrupt the accumulation of the sugar molecules. When the body is ready for the scan, patient will be moved to the examination room. The scanning itself takes approximately 30 to 60 minutes. The table will slide slowly through the large hole in the center about six times during the test. Patient will need to lie still for the entire scan.

After the Procedure

Patient can expect to resume normal activities, immediately after PET scan. Advise the patient to drink several glasses of water to flush the radioactive material out of the body, though there are no side effects from the radiation.

How does PET Work?

A conventional X-ray is taken, by firing X-rays through a person and onto a film. This shadow image shows some structures in the body, such as cartilage and bone. A CT scanner uses fine streams of X-rays. By firing them through the body from several directions, the CT scanner is able to build up a composite picture of anatomical details within a slice, through the person. Magnetic resonance imaging (MRI) does much the same thing, but using magnetic and radiowave fields. In contrast, the PET scanner utilizes radiation, emitted from the patient to develop images. Each patient is given a minute amount of a radioactive pharmaceutical, which closely resembles a natural substance used by the body. A positron emitting radionuclide (tracer) is introduced into the body on a biologically active molecule. For example, 2-fluoro-2-deoxy-D-glucose (FDG), which is a glucose analogue and is widely used to locate zones of heightened energy metabolism. The radioisotope undergoes positron emission decay (also known as positive beta decay) and emits a positron. After travelling up to a few millimeters, the positron encounters and annihilates with an electron, the collision produces a pair of annihilation (gamma) photons having the same energy, but going in opposite directions (180°) (Fig. 32.6). The subject is positioned within a scanner, consisting of a ring of scintillation crystals, which convert gamma rays into flashes of visible light (Fig. 32.7). These flashes of light are detected by photomultiplier tubes or Silicon Avalanche Photodiodes (Si APD) and recorded electronically. A computer program assembles the data into a 3D and color coded image, to reflect the concentration density (Fig. 32.8). The technique depends on simultaneous or coincident detection of the pair of photons. Photons, which do not arrive in pairs (i.e. within a timing window of few nanoseconds) are ignored.

Localization of the Positron Annihilation Event

The most significant fraction of electron positron decays, result in two 511 keV gamma photons being emitted at almost 180° to each other, hence it is possible to localize their source along a straight line of coincidence (also called formally the Line of Response or LOR).

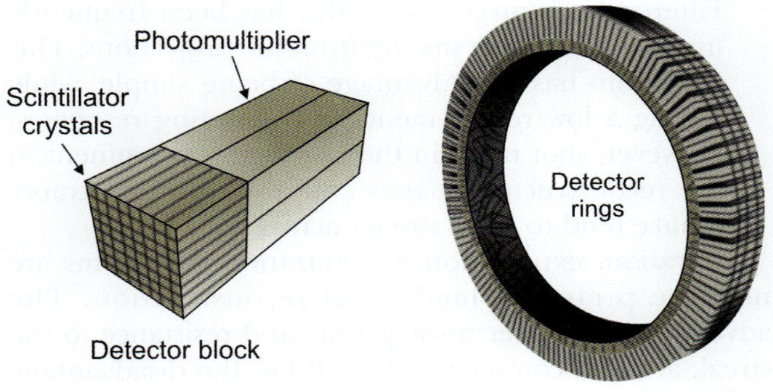

Fig. 32.7: Components of PET scanner—ring of scintillating crystals and photomultiplier tubes

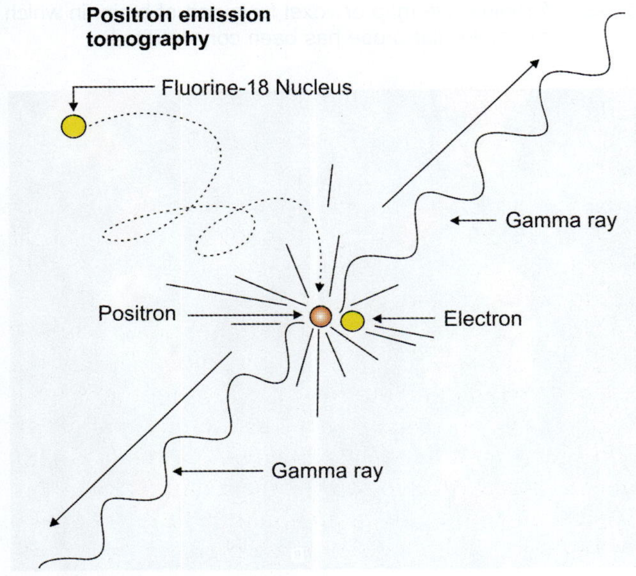

Fig. 32.6: Mechanism of working of PET scan

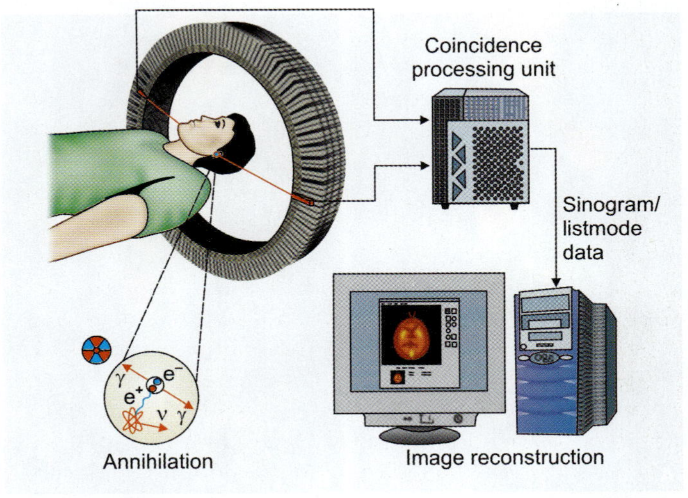

Fig. 32.8: Componets of PET scanner and their mechanism of working

Image Reconstruction

The raw data collected by a PET scanner, are a list of coincidence events, representing near simultaneous detection of annihilation photons by a pair of detectors. Each coincidence event, represents a line in space connecting the two detectors along which the positron emission occurred. Coincidence events can be grouped into projections images called sinograms. The sinograms are sorted by the angle of each view and tilt, the latter in 3D case images. The sinogram images are analogous to the projections captured by computed tomography (CT) scanners and can be reconstructed in a similar way.

In practice, considerable preprocessing of the data is required, for following:

- Correction for random coincidences
- Estimation and subtraction of scattered photons
- Detector dead time correction (after the detection of a photon, the detector must cool down again).
- Detector sensitivity correction, for both inherent detector sensitivity and changes in sensitivity due to angle of incidence.
- Filtered back projection (FBP) has been frequently used to reconstruct images from the projections. This algorithm has the advantage of being simple, while having a low requirement for computing resources. However, shot noise in the raw data is prominent in the reconstructed images and areas of high tracer uptake tend to form streaks across the image.

Iteration, expectation maximization algorithms are now the preferred method of reconstruction. The advantage is a better noise profile and resistance to the streak artifacts common with FBP, but the disadvantage is higher computer resource requirements. Using statistics collected from tens-of-thousands of coincidence events, a set of simultaneous equations for the total activity of each parcel of tissue along many LOR, can be solved by a number of techniques and thus a map of radioactivities, as a function of location for parcels or bits of tissue (also called voxels), may be constructed and plotted. The resulting map shows the tissues, in which the molecular probe has become concentrated and can be interpreted by a nuclear medicine physician or radiologist, in the context of the patient's diagnosis and treatment plan, as shown in Figures 32.9 and 32.10.

Attenuation Correction

As different LOR must traverse different thicknesses of tissue, the photons are attenuated differentially. The result is that structures deep in the body are reconstructed, as having falsely low tracer uptake. Contemporary scanners can estimate attenuation using integrated X-ray and CT

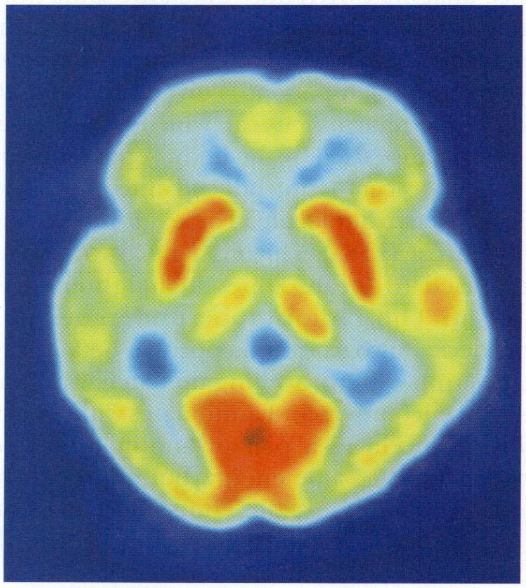

Fig. 32.9: A radioactive map or voxel for a part of brain, in which the molecular probe has been concentrated

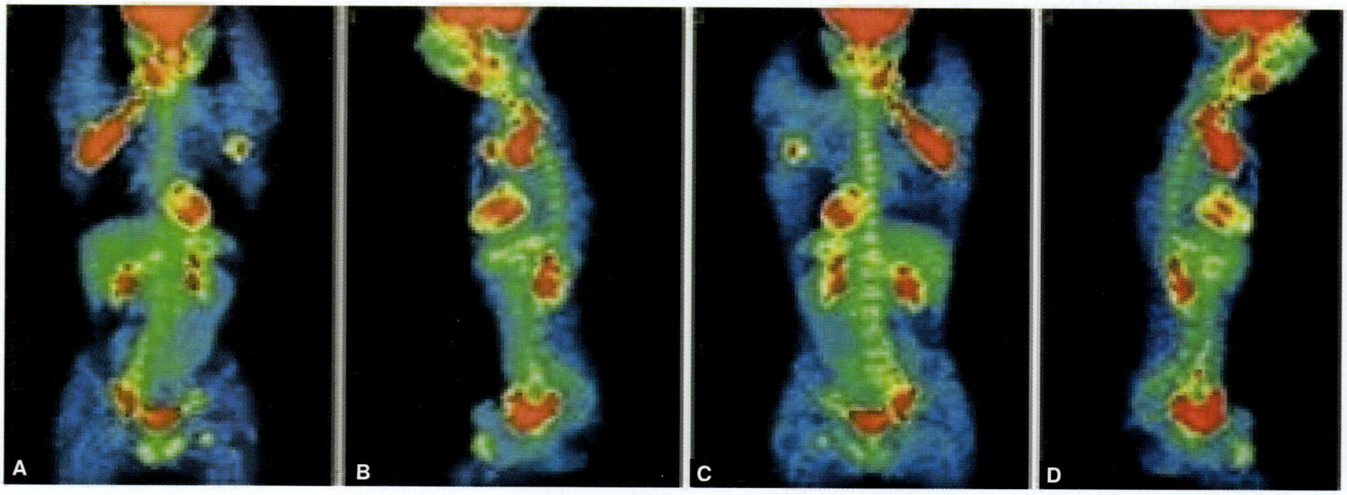

Figs 32.10A to D: Radioactive maps or voxels for different body parts (tissues), shown in different planes

equipment, however, earlier equipment offered a crude form of CT, using a gamma ray (positron emitting) source and the PET detectors. While attenuation corrected images are generally more faithful representations, the correction process is itself susceptible to significant artifacts. As a result, both corrected and uncorrected images are always reconstructed and read together.

2D and 3D Reconstruction (Fig. 32.11)

Early PET scanners had only a single ring of detectors. Hence, the acquisition of data and subsequent reconstruction was restricted to a single transverse plane. More modern scanners, now include multiple rings, essentially forming a cylinder of detectors. There are two approaches to reconstructing data from such a scanner, these are: (1) Treat each ring as a separate entity, so that only coincidences within a ring are detected, the image from each ring can then be reconstructed individually (2D reconstruction). (2) Allow coincidences to be detected between rings as well as within rings, then reconstruct the entire volume together (3D). 3D techniques have better sensitivity, because more coincidences are detected and used, therefore less noise, but are more sensitive to the effects of scatter and random coincidences as well as requiring correspondingly greater computer resources. The advent of subnanosecond timing resolution detectors, affords better random coincidence rejection, thus favoring 3D image reconstruction.

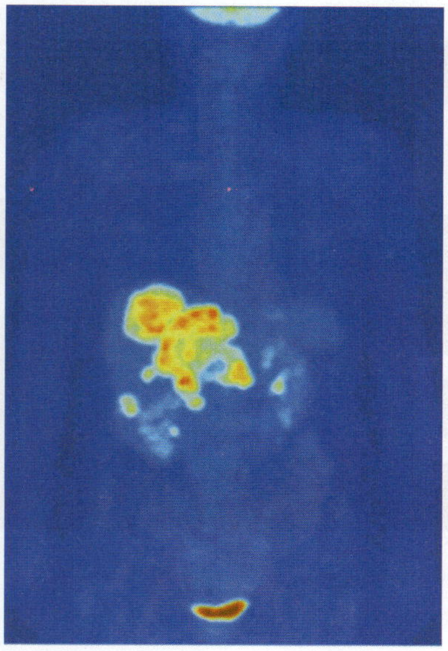

Fig. 32.11: 3D PET image

Combination of PET with CT and MRI (Figs 32.12 and 32.13)

PET scans are increasingly read alongside CT or MRI scans, the combination (coregistration), giving both anatomic and metabolic information (i.e. what the structure is and what it is doing biochemically?). As PET imaging is most useful in combination with anatomical imaging, such as CT, modern PET scanners are now available with integrated high end multidetector row CT scanners. The two scans can be performed in immediate sequence during the same session, with the patient not changing position between the two types of scans. Hence, the two sets of images are more precisely registered, so that areas of abnormality on the PET imaging can be more perfectly correlated with anatomy on the CT images. This is very useful in showing detailed views of moving organs or structures, with higher anatomical variation, which is more frequent outside of the brain.

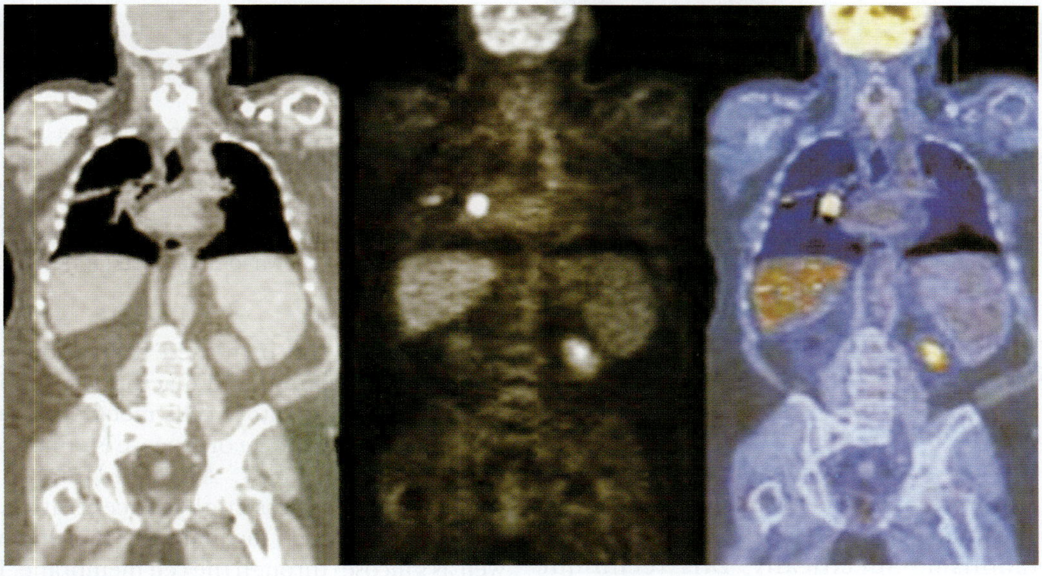

Fig. 32.12: Combination of PET with CT and MRI

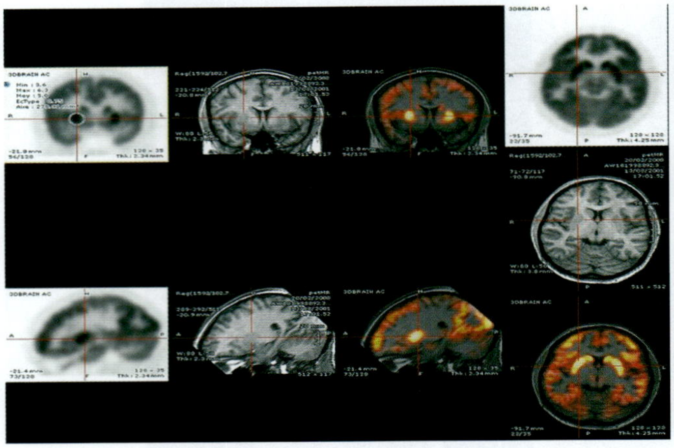

Fig. 32.13: Combination of PET with MRI of the brain

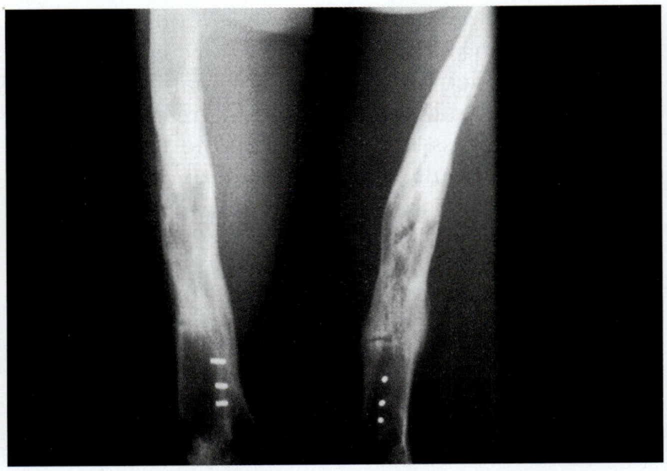

Fig. 32.15: Continued from Fig. 32.14, corresponding anteroposterior and lateral radiographs

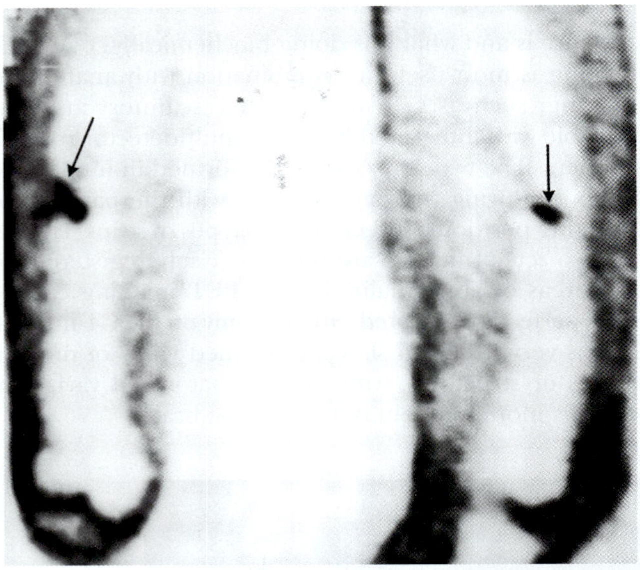

Fig. 32.14: Coronal and sagittal fluorodeoxyglucose positron emission tomography images showing intense uptake (arrows) in the anterolateral aspect of the middle third of the right femur after previous trauma. *Staphylococcus aureus* grew on culture of specimens taken from the site of increased uptake at the time of the operation

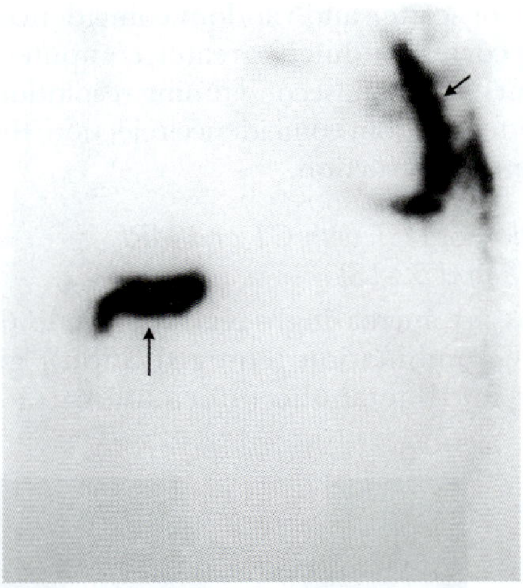

Fig. 32.16: Sagittal fluorodeoxyglucose positron emission tomography scan through the vertebral column of a patient, with microbiologically proven *S. aureus* spondylodiscitis of the eleventh and twelfth thoracic vertebrae (arrow). The myocardium of the left ventricle is also shown for reference (arrowhead)

Application of PET in Orthopedics

Diagnosis of Chronic Musculoskeletal Infections (Figs 32.14 to 32.18)

Fluorine-18 fluorodeoxyglucose positron emission tomography has made it possible to evaluate cellular glucose metabolism. Specifically, this technique demonstrates the increased utilization of glucose by activated neutrophils and macrophages in inflammatory reactions. Inflammatory cells metabolize predominantly glucose and the uptake of glucose is enhanced when such cells are stimulated. Activated macrophages and neutrophils express high concentrations of glucose transporters, which facilitate the movement of FDG (as well as glucose) through the cell membrane. Deoxyglucose

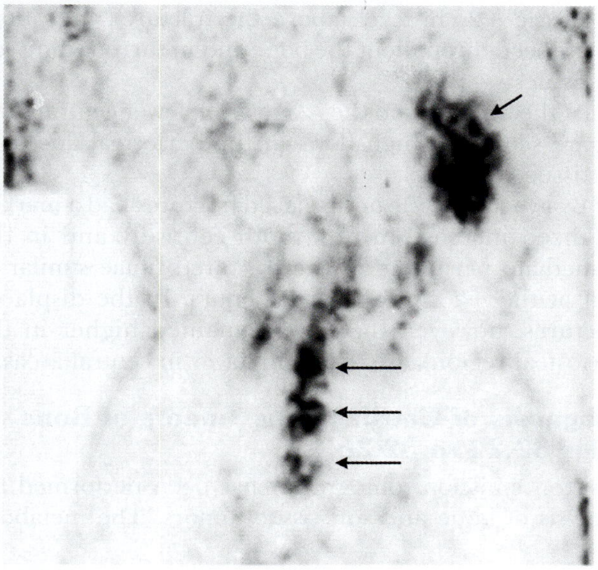

Fig. 32.17: Coronal, fluorodeoxyglucose positron emission tomography scans, through the lumbar vertebrae of a thirteen-year-old-girl, in whom extreme scoliosis had been treated with osteosynthesis nine months earlier. The fluorodeoxyglucose positron emission tomography scans, show increased uptake (arrows) in the bodies of the third, fourth, and fifth lumbar vertebrae, where uptake is normally very low, as well as increased splenic uptake (arrowhead). *S. aureus* grew on culture of specimens obtained at the time of the operation

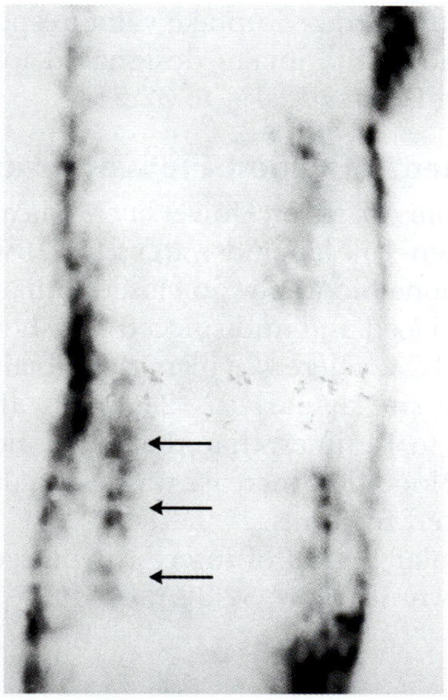

Fig. 32.18: Sagittal view for the above mention patient, fluorodeoxyglucose positron emission tomography scans showing increased uptake (arrows) in the bodies of the third, fourth, and fifth lumbar vertebrae, where uptake is normally very low

is phosphorylated to deoxyglucose-6-phosphate, which is not a substrate for glucose-6-phosphate dehydrogenase, so it becomes trapped in tissue long enough to allow PET imaging. Thus, FDG reflects glucose utilization and can indicate areas of inflammation. Sugawara et al. showed, in a rat model, that the uptake of fluorine-18 fluorodeoxyglucose at the site of infection is higher than the uptake of other tracers. Consequently, fluorine-18 fluorodeoxyglucose-positron emission tomography has been proposed as a promising technique for the evaluation of musculoskeletal infections.

Coronal and sagittal fluorodeoxyglucose positron emission tomography scans through the lumbar vertebrae of a thirteen-year-old girl, in whom extreme scoliosis had been treated with osteosynthesis nine months earlier. The fluorodeoxyglucose positron emission tomography scans show increased uptake (arrows) in the bodies of the third, fourth, and fifth lumbar vertebrae, where uptake is normally very low, as well as increased splenic uptake (arrowhead). *S. aureus* grew on culture of specimens obtained at the time of the operation, as shown in Figures 32.17 and 32.18.

Assessment of Chronic Osteomyelitis

In a study carried out at VU University Medical Center, Amsterdam, Netherlands (the accuracy of diagnostic imaging for the assessment of chronic osteomyelitis; a systematic review and meta-analysis). The meta-analysis showed that fluorodeoxyglucose positron emission tomography is the most sensitive technique for detecting chronic osteomyelitis and that it has a greater specificity than leukocyte scintigraphy, bone scintigraphy or magnetic resonance imaging. Fluorodeoxyglucose positron emission tomography was better than leukocyte scintigraphy for imaging chronic osteomyelitis in the axial skeleton.

Diagnosis of Periprosthetic Infection

The role of fluorodeoxyglucose positron emission tomography (FDG-PET) scans in the diagnosis of infections at the sites of arthroplasties has been evaluated at some centers. Studies have shown combined FDG-PET imaging to have variable sensitivity and specificity for diagnosing periprosthetic infection. One study, for example demonstrated approximately 91 percent sensitivity and 72 percent specificity for diagnosing infections around knee prosthesis and 90 percent sensitivity and 89 percent specificity for diagnosing infections around hip prostheses.

Imaging of Sarcomas with FDG-PET

Fluorine-18-fluorodeoxyglucose-positron emission tomography imaging provides a semiquantitative measure of tumor metabolism, which correlates to both tumor grade and necrosis. The corresponding semiquantitative analysis over multiple axial image planes yields the fluorine-18-fluorodeoxyglucose metabolic rate of the tissue or a standardized uptake value respectively, in an area of tissue in the image designated for analysis, as illustrated in Figures 32.19 to 32.21.

Measurement of Blood Flow at Fracture Sites

In a study from Aberdeen University Medical School, PET using Oxygen-15 labeled water (H_2O) was used, for measuring bone blood flow in closed unilateral fractures of tibia (displaced and undisplaced), as shown in Figures 32.22 and 32.23. There was increased tibial blood flow at the fracture site as early as 24 hours after fracture, reaching up to 14 times, than that in the normal limb at two weeks. Blood flow increase was less in displaced than in undisplaced fractures.

The circular region of interest is placed around the tibia, as shown in Figure 32.22A:

- At the +2 cm level (above the fracture), high flows are seen throughout the bone and in surrounding soft tissues
- At the fracture and the –2 cm level, lower central flows are seen with high flows in the periosteal and soft-tissue coverings.

By two weeks, the undisplaced fractures had a marked localized increase in flow, both centrally and in the immediate periphery of the fractured tibiae similar to that at the +2 cm level at 24 hours. In the displaced fractures, however, the flows remained higher in the periosteal region at +2 cm and lower in central areas.

Diagnosis of Cartilaginous Tumors of Bone (Figs 32.24 to 32.26)

Positron emission tomography has been performed for analysis of bone and soft tissue tumors. The metabolic

$$\text{Standardized uptake value} = \frac{\text{Tissue treacer activity (mCi/g)}}{\text{(injected dose [mCi] patient weight [kg])}}$$

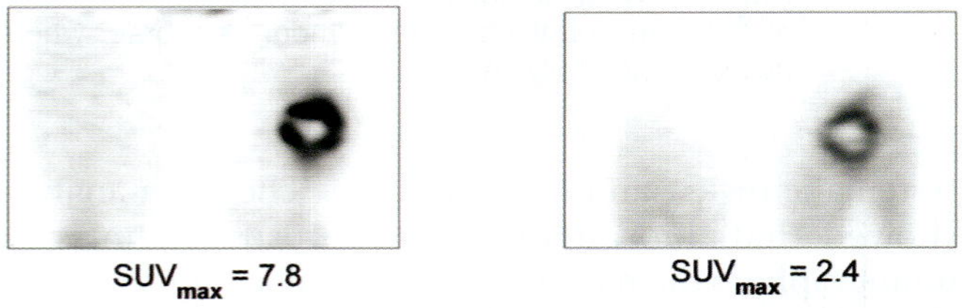

Fig. 32.19: A good response to treament of a soft tissue sarcoma of the thigh as seen by a substantial decrease in the maximum standardized uptake value (SUV) between baseline (left) and preresection (right) position emission tomography scans

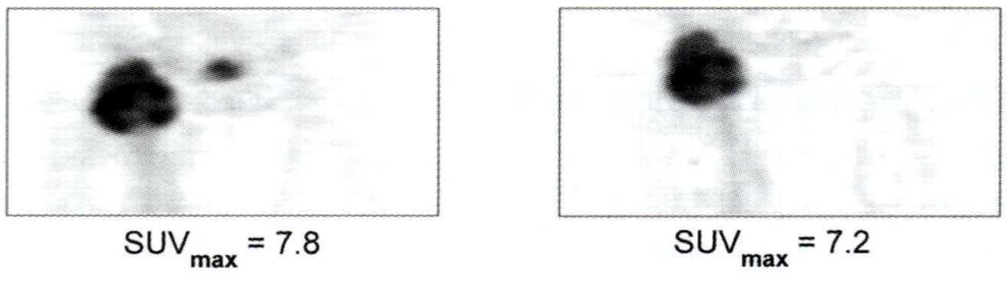

Fig 32.20: A poor response to treatment of a soft tissue sarcoma of the hip as evidenced by a minimal decrease in the maximum standardized uptake value (SUV) between baseline (left) and preresection (right) positron emission tomography scans

Fig 32.21: Disease progression as seen by an increase in the maximum standardized uptake value (SUV) over the interval between the baseline (left) and preresection (right) positron emission tomography scans

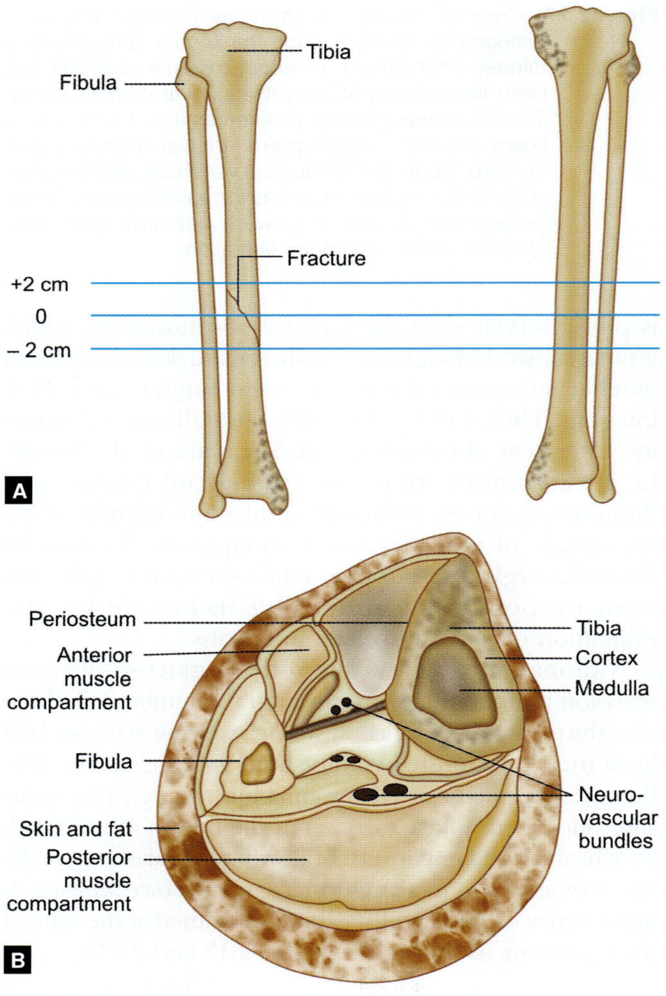

Figs 32.22A and B: (A) Diagram of both legs showing the levels of bone examined by PET; (B) The anatomy of a transaxial section of the right leg at midtibial level

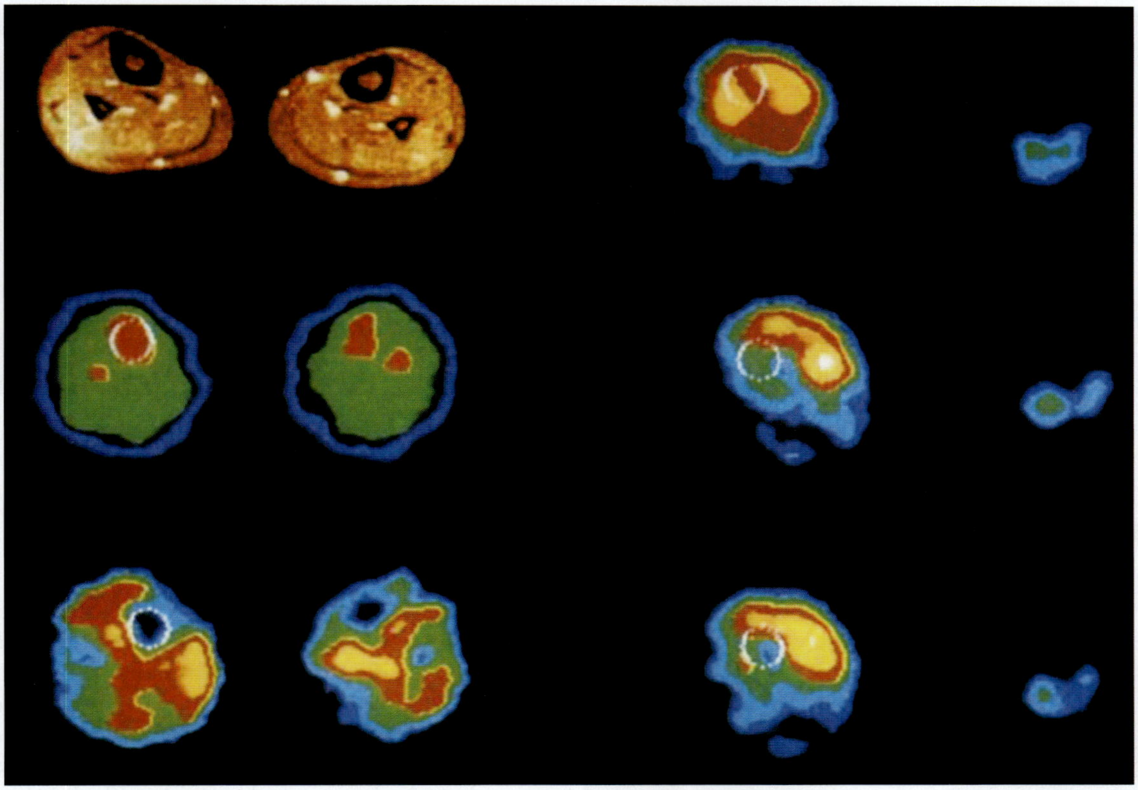

Fig. 32.23: (Top left) MRI scan of both legs of a volunteer for comparison with the PET images below. (Middle left) PET transmission image of the sections, used for attenuation correction and identifying regions of interest. The tibiae and fibulae are clearly seen, the right tibia is marked with a circular region of interest. (Bottom left) PET emission ($H_2^{15}O$) image, showing regional blood flow at rest in the normal volunteer. The region of interest has been transferred from the transmission image above, lying over the right tibia. The lowest flows are seen in the medullary areas with higher flows in the cortical bone. The highest flows are in the muscle compartments. (Right side) PET emission ($H_2^{15}O$) image at 24 hours after fracture. The three levels (+2 cm, 0, –2 cm) are shown from above down, with the region of interest over the fractured tibia marked in all scans. Distribution of flow (scans) showed large differences in the distribution of blood flow, as compared with the normal limb

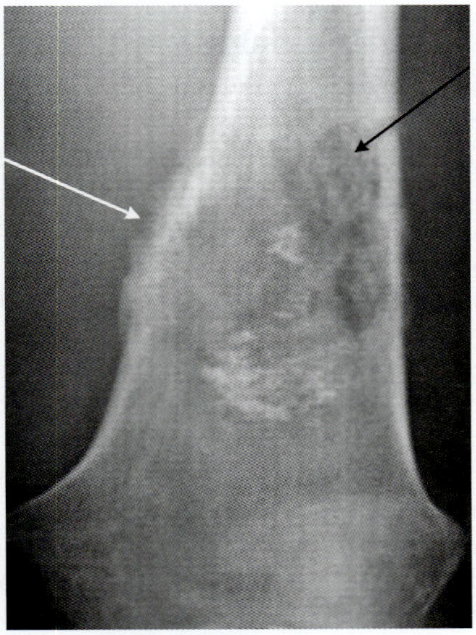

Fig. 32.24: Plain radiograph showing a mineralized lesion (chondrosarcoma), with radiolucency (black arrow) and cortical disruption (white arrow)

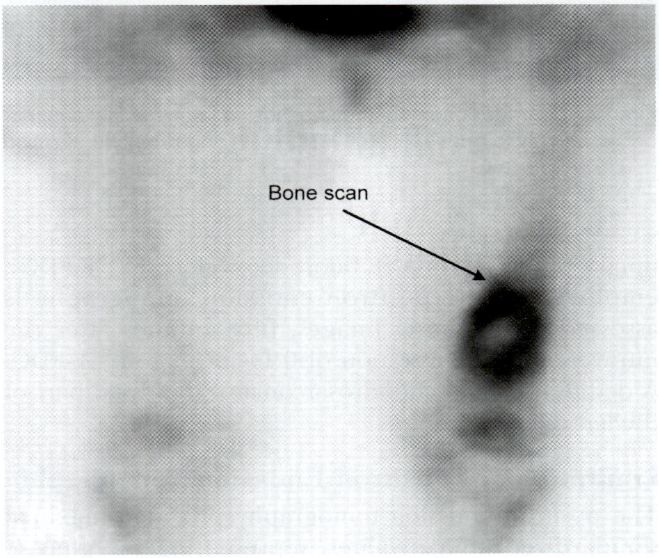

Fig. 32.25: Bone scan, showing increased uptake that is comparable with the plain radiograph

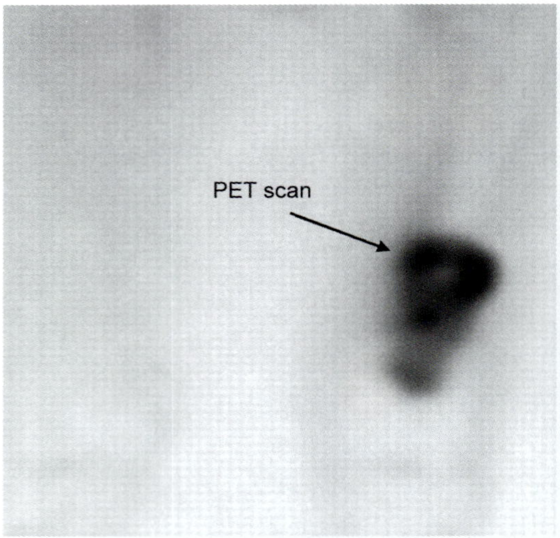

Fig. 32.26: PET scan showing a lesion with a high standardized uptake value

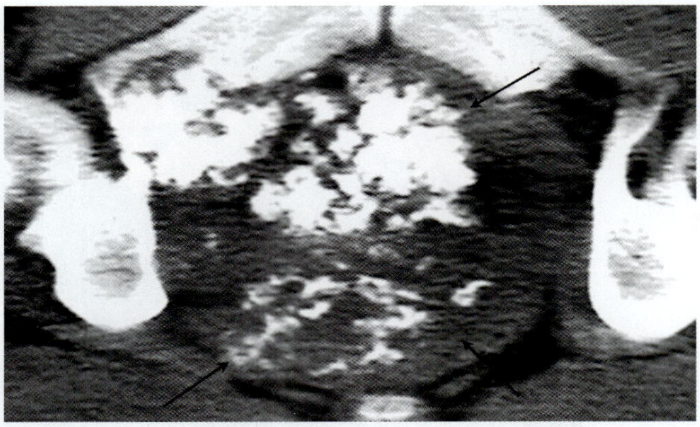

Fig. 32.28: An extremely large intrapelvic lesion displacing entire pelvic organs (arrows)

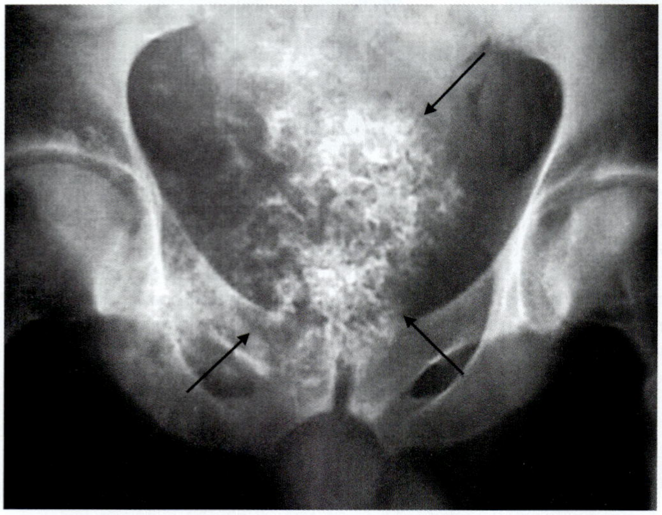

Fig. 32.27: Grade I chondrosarcoma, arising from the right superior pubic ramus. A large lesion with ring-like mineralization (arrows)

uptake of the fluorine 18 fluorodeoxyglucose (^{18}F-FDG), employed in the positron emission tomography is assessed by obtaining images, fifty minutes after the intravenous administration of 0.14 mCi/kg of ^{18}F-FDG. A dedifferentiated chondrosarcoma of the distal part of the left femur.

Limitations of Positron Emission Tomography

The positron emission tomography provided maximal standardized uptake values, representing the glucose metabolic profile of the lesion, in the regions of interest, that had been identified on plain radiographs, bone scans, computed tomography scans and magnetic resonance images, as shown in Figure 32.27. However, several large chondrosarcomas had low standardized uptake values, even though they caused considerable local morbidity, including one case of bowel obstruction and another case of obstruction of the inferior vena cava, due to their large size. When the tumor was located in the pelvis, adjacent structures such as the intestine, bladder and muscles could not be clearly distinguished from the peripheral borders of the large expansile lesion because of the limited resolution of the positron emission tomography (4.5-6.7 mm), this is illustrated in Figures 32.28.

Benefits of PET Scanning

- Very sensitive and specific test, may clarify the results of other tests
- Helps identify cancer that has spread, even if other tests (CT, MRI and ultrasound) cannot find it
- May allow patients to avoid unnecessary biopsies or surgery
- Can lead to more appropriate care and image guided therapy
- The benefits of a combined PET/CT scanner include:
  - Greater detail with a higher level of accuracy because both scans are performed at one time, without the patient having to change positions and there is less room for error.
  - Greater convenience for the patient, who undergoes two exams (CT and PET) at one sitting, rather than at two different times.

33 Stem Cells

• Bone Marrow

Introduction

A cell capable of unlimited cell cycles, with capacity to cease being a stem cell and become one of a wide variety of specialized cells, that can no longer divide. Stem cells are shown in Figure 33.1.

Properties of Stem Cells

- *Self-renewal:* The ability to go through numerous cell cycles of cell division, while maintaining the undifferentiated state
- Symmetric cell division
- *Potency:* The capacity to differentiate into specialized cells. This is illustrated in Figure 33.2.

Asymmetric replication in every cell division. One of the cells retains its self-renewing capacity, while the others enters a differentiation pathway and is converted into a mature nondividing population.

Cell Cycle (Fig. 33.3)

G1: Presynthetic phase
G2: Premitotic phase

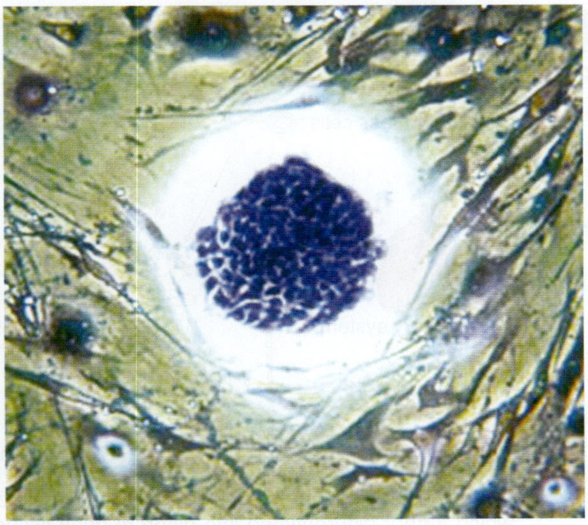

Fig. 33.1: Stem cells

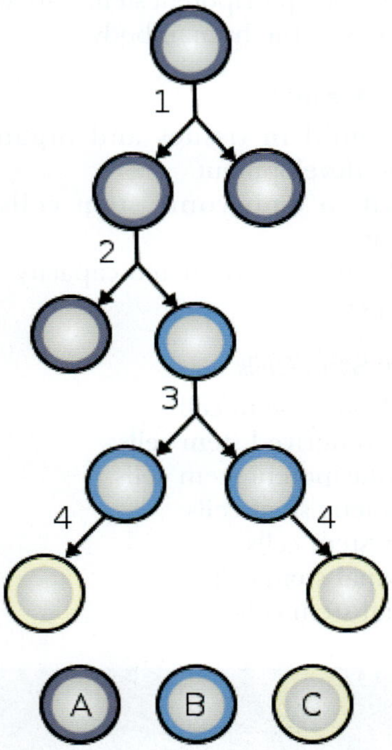

Fig. 33.2: Stem cell undergoing differentiated division into specialized cells

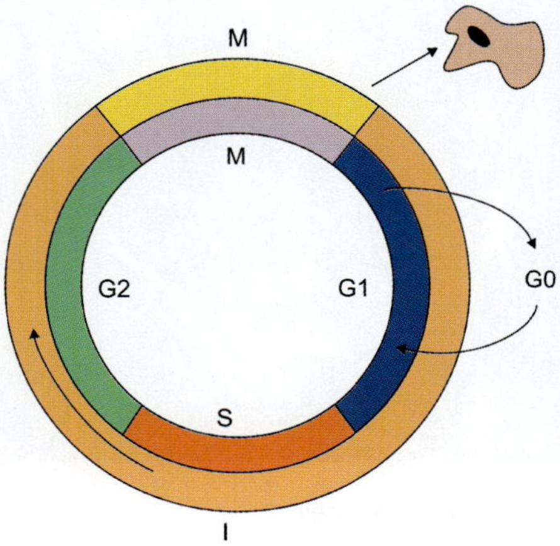

Fig. 33.3: Different phases of a cell cycle

G0: Quiescent stable phase
S: DNA synthesis
M: Mitotic phase.

Types of Stem Cells

- Adults stem cells
- Fetal tissue stem cells
- Embryonic stem cells
- Nuclear transplant stem cells.

Embryonic Stem Cells (Figs 33.4 and 33.5)

Source: Normal blastocysts (the structures formed at about 32 cell stage during embryonic development).

Properties: They are pluripotent stem cells, which can give rise to all tissues of the human body.

Adult Stem Cells

- *Source:* Found in tissues and organs, after the embryonic development
- Compared to embryonic stem cells, which are pluripotent
- More restricted differentiated capacity
- Lineage specific.

Types of Adult Stem Cells

- Adipose derived stem cells
- Dental pulp derived stem cells
- Induced pluripotent stem cells
- Hematopoietic stem cells
- Mammary stem cells
- Mesenchymal stem cells
- Endothelial stem cells
- Neural stem cell
- Olfactory adult stem cells
- Testicular stem cells.

Bone Marrow

- Bone marrow contains hemopoietic stem cells as well as mesenchymal or stromal cell
- Hemopoietic stem cells can generate all of the various blood cells and can reconstitute the bone marrow after depletion, caused by disease or irradiation.
- Bone marrow stromal cells or mesenchymal cells, depending on tissue environment, can generate:
  - Chondrocytes
  - Osteoblasts
  - Adipocytes
  - Myoblasts
  - Endothelial cell precursors
  - Hemopoietic stem cell (Fig. 33.6).

Mesenchymal Stem Cells (Figs 33.7 to 33.9)

- Mesenchymal cells can undergo following processes to get differentiated into different body tissues:
  - Osteogenesis
  - Chondrogenesis
  - Adipogenesis.

Multipotent Adult Progenitor Cells

- Adult bone marrow also harbors a heterogenous population of stem cells, which appear to have very broad developmental capabilities.
- These cells are called multipotent adult progenitor cells or MAPCs.

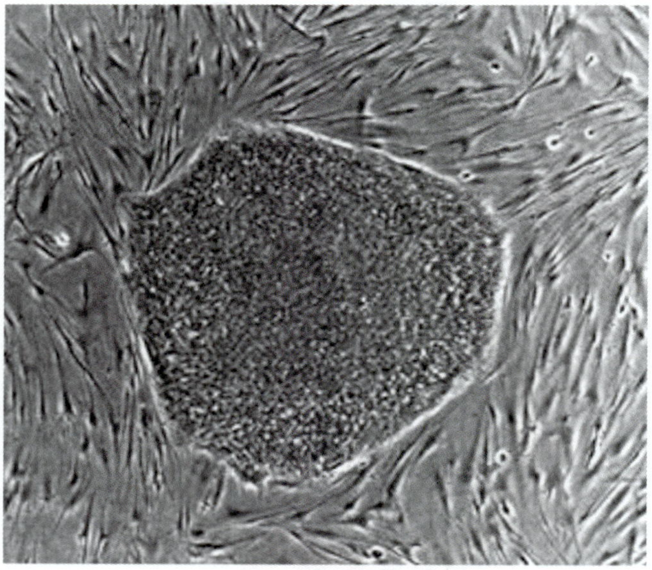

Fig. 33.4: Embryonic stem cells

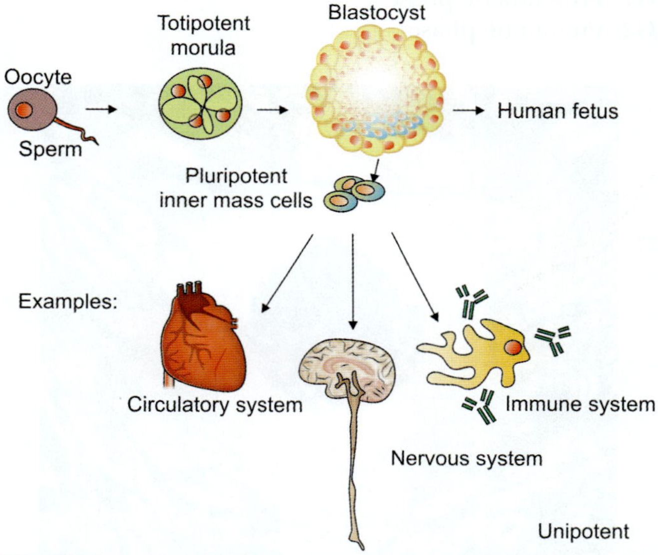

Fig. 33.5: Blastocytes, acting as a source for pluripotent stem cell, which further differentiated into different body tissues

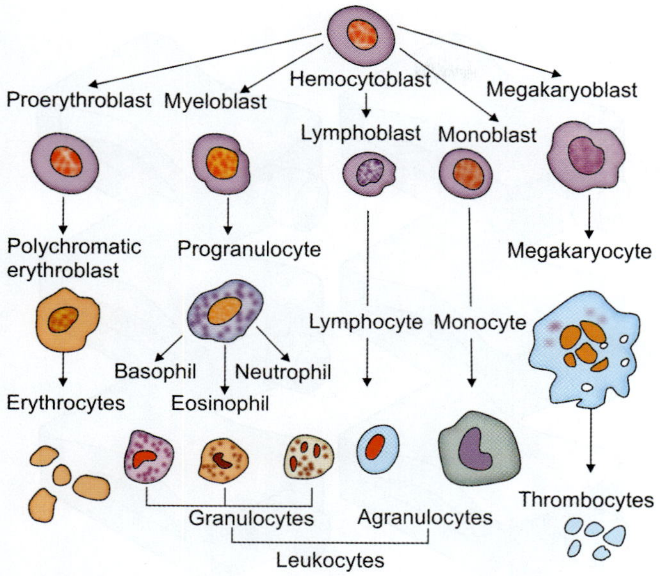

Fig. 33.6: Differentiation of hemocytoblast or hemopoietic stem cells into different blood cells

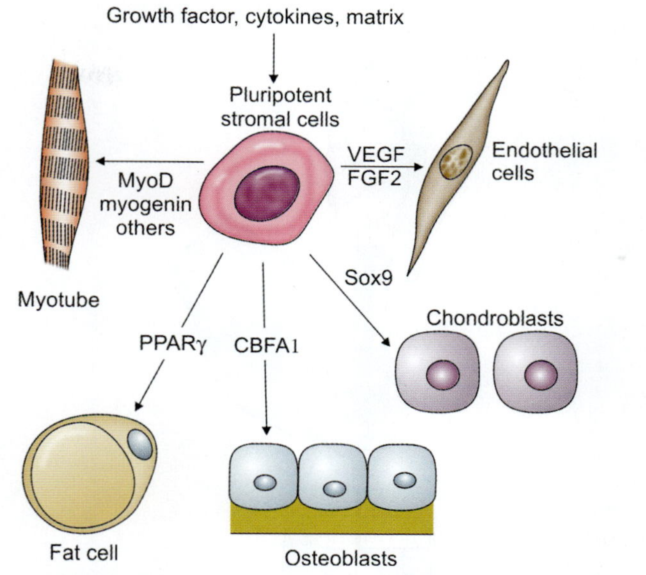

Fig. 33.8: Pluripotent stem cell differentiated into different body cells and tissues

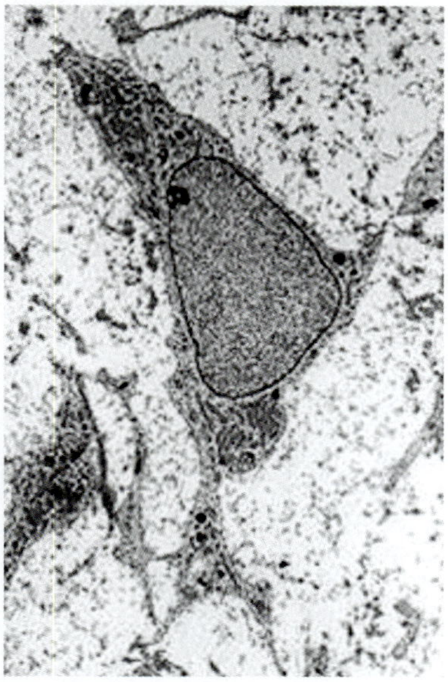

Fig. 33.7: Mesenchymal stem cell

- They can differentiate into mesodermal, endodermal and neuroectodermal cell types.
- They are not confined to bone marrow, they have been isolated from muscle, brain and skin.

Collection of Stem Cells (Figs 33.10 to 33.14)

- Bone marrow aspiration
- Mesenchymal stem cells (MSCs) are isolated and ready for culture
- Culture of MSC in flasks
- Easy handling because of their ability to adhere to the plastic container. After several passages, a sufficient number of MSC are collected. Trypsinization and collection of MSC from the flasks. MSC are then loaded in scaffold.

Role of Stem Cells in Orthopedics

- Nonunion (Fig. 33.15)
- Delayed union

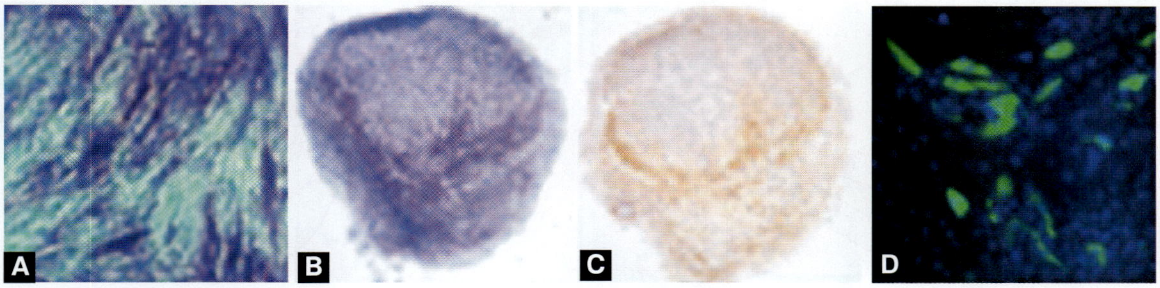

Figs 33.9A to D: Expansion and differentiation of bone marrow derived mesenchymal stem cell

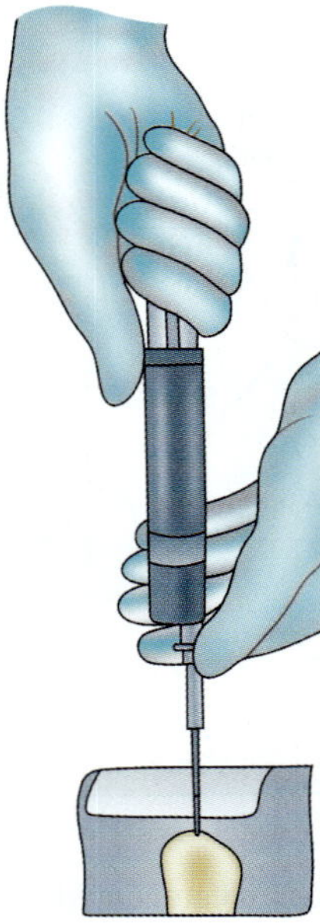

Fig. 33.10: Bone marrow aspiration

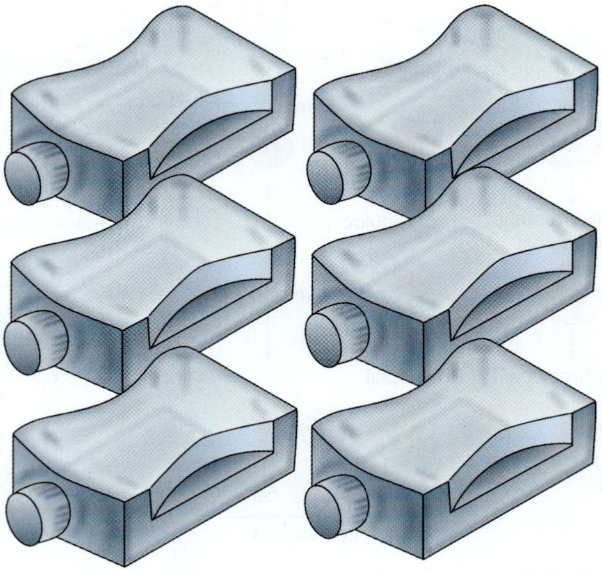

Fig. 33.13: After several passages, a sufficient number of MSC are collected

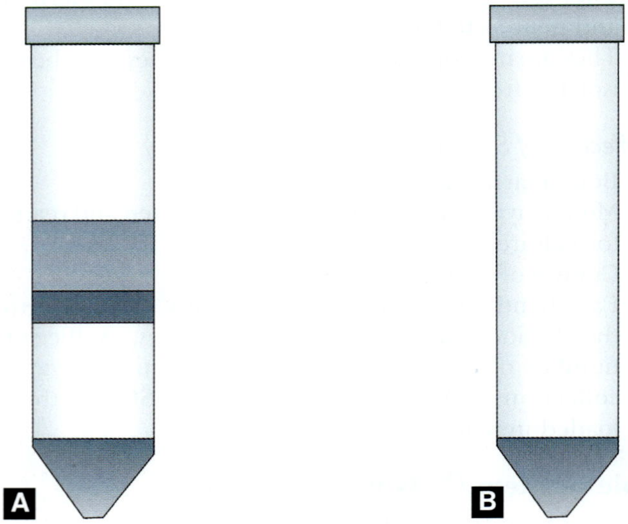

Figs 33.11A and B: Mesenchymal stem cells (MSCs) are isolated and ready for culture

Fig. 33.14: Trypsinization and collection of MSC from the flasks

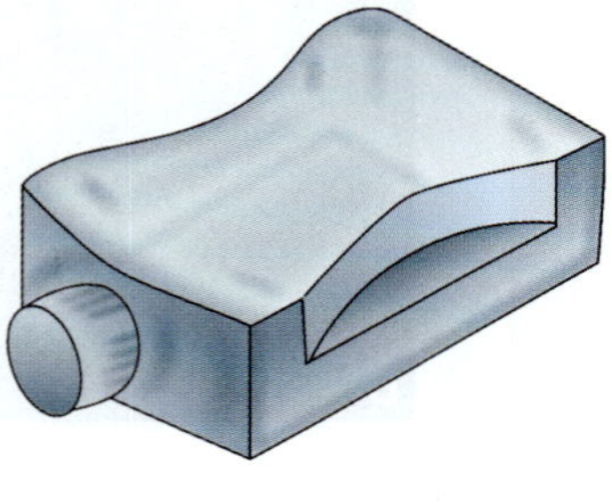

Fig. 33.12: Culture of MSC in flasks

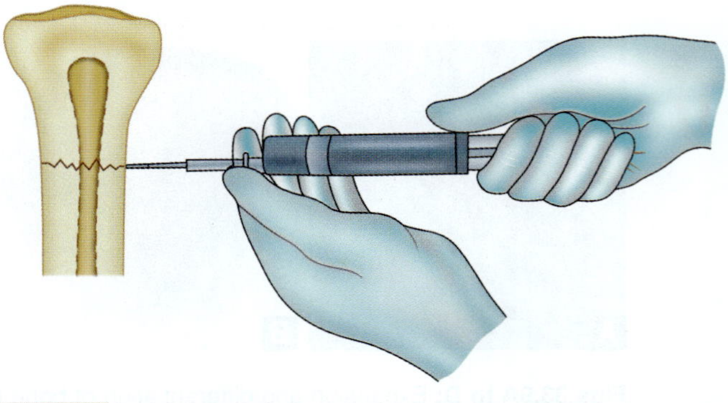

Fig. 33.15: Injection of MSC into the nonunion site

- Stabilization of fracture and scaffold implantation, as shown in Figure 33.16.
- Segmental bone defects
- Osteochondral defects
- Large bone defects
- Articular cartilage defects
- Articular defects
- Carriage defects repair, with chondrocyte implantation, as shown in Figure 33.17.
- Meniscal injury
- Femoral head osteonecrosis
- Spinal fusion in spinal cord injuries
- Physeal and bone cysts

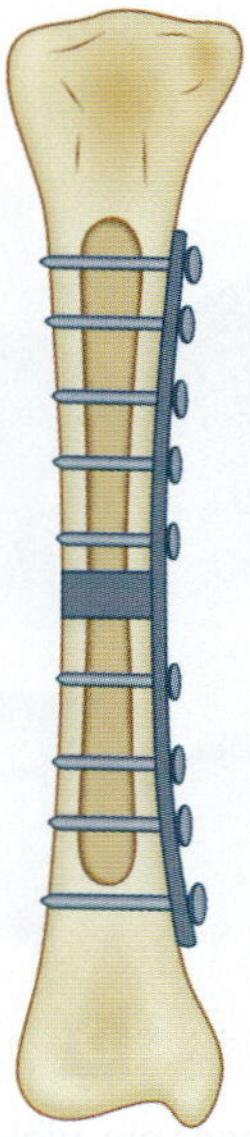

Fig. 33.16: Stabilization of fracture and scaffold implantation

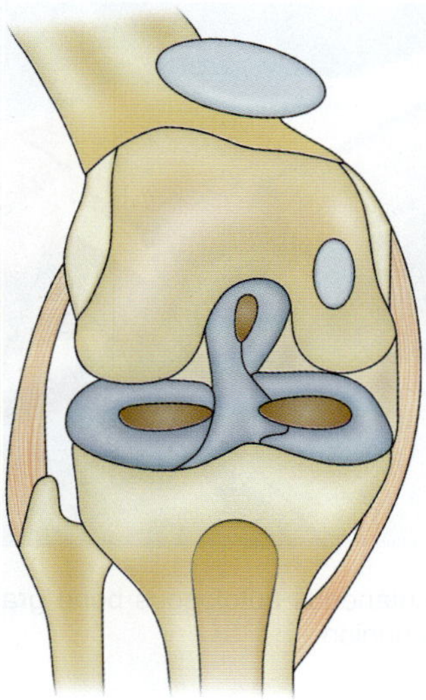

Fig. 33.17: Carriage defects repair, with chondrocyte implantation

- Spinal cord defects regeneration
- Criteria to achieve stable repair
- Generation of adequate number of cells and tissue, to fill the defect or complete the repair.
- Differentiation of cells towards correct phenotype and its maintenance.
- Ensuring the cells may adapt the appropriate three dimensional organization and produce extracellular matrix, this may require a structural support in the shape of resorbable scaffold.
- Production of tissues or cells, which are structurally and mechanically complaint with the normal demands of native tissues.
- Achievement of integration with local tissue, with vascularization, when required.
- Overcoming the risk of immunological repair.
- Articular cartilage repair, this is demonstrated in Figures 33.18A to F.

Mesenchymal Cell Implantation

See Figures 33.19 to 33.23 for mesenchymal cell implantation.

Nonunion (Figs 33.24 to 33.30)

Percutaneous Autologous Bone Grafting (Fig. 33.24)

- Mesenchymal stem cells are aspirated from bone marrow of iliac crest
- Centrifugation of the aspirate is done on cell separator

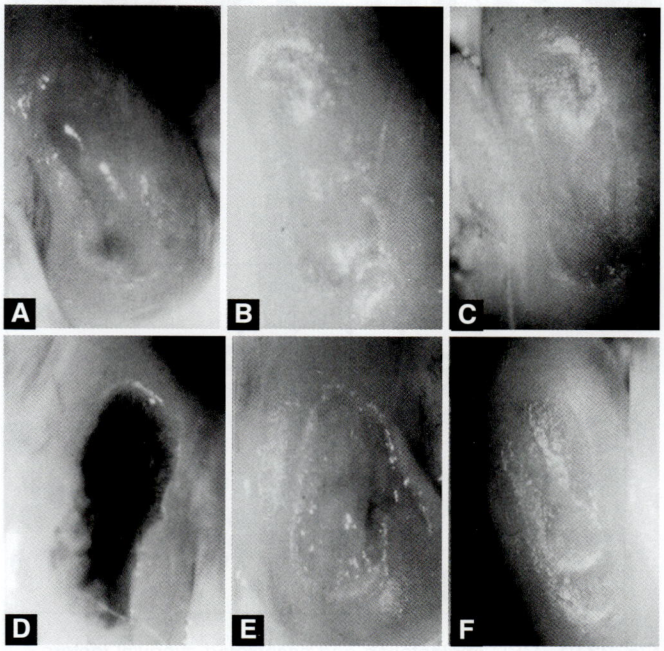

Figs 33.18A to F: (A) Two weeks after implantation; (B) 4 weeks after implantation; (C) 24 weeks after implantation; (D) Control defects, which left empty at 2 weeks; (E) 4 weeks; (F) 24 weeks

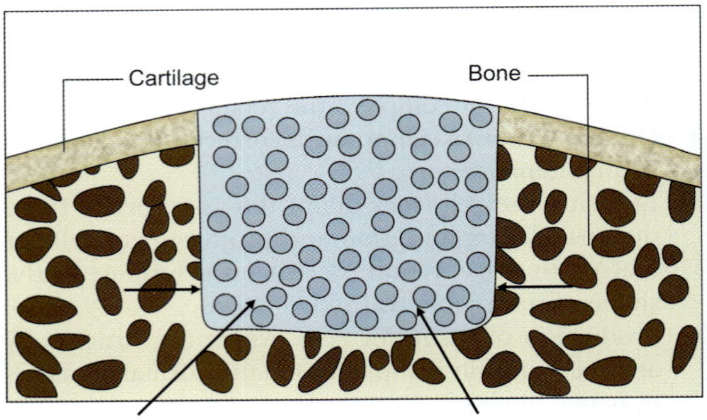

Fig. 33.19: MSC implantation

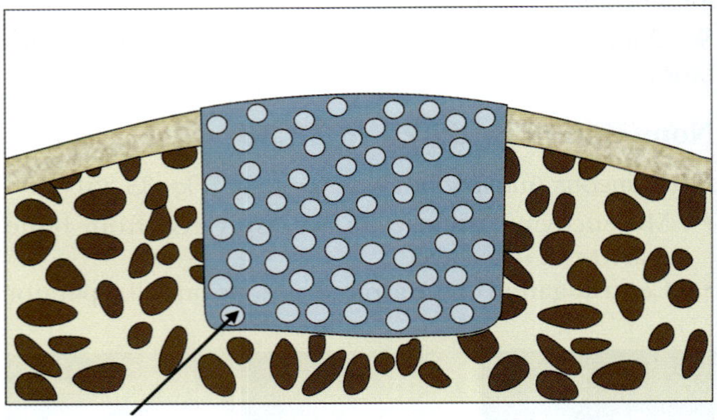

Fig. 33.20: Hypertrophic chondrocyte

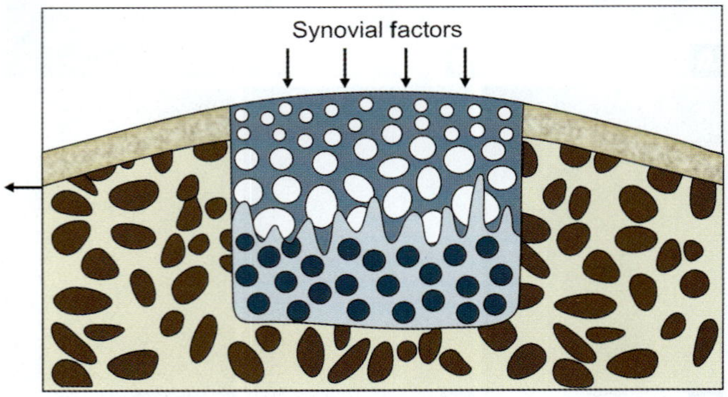

Fig. 33.21: MSC implantation and associated synovial factors

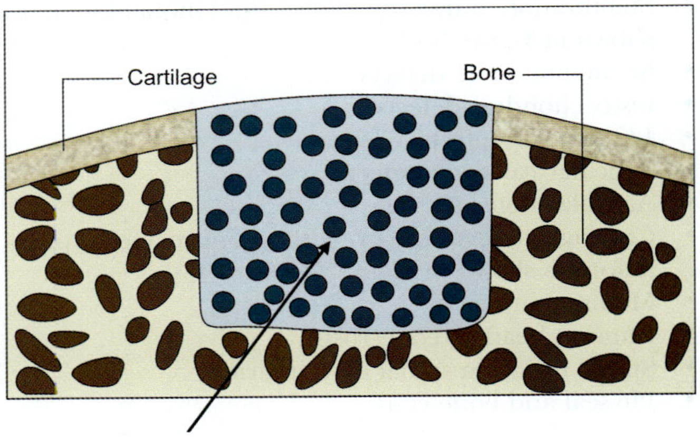

Fig. 33.22: New host bone develop

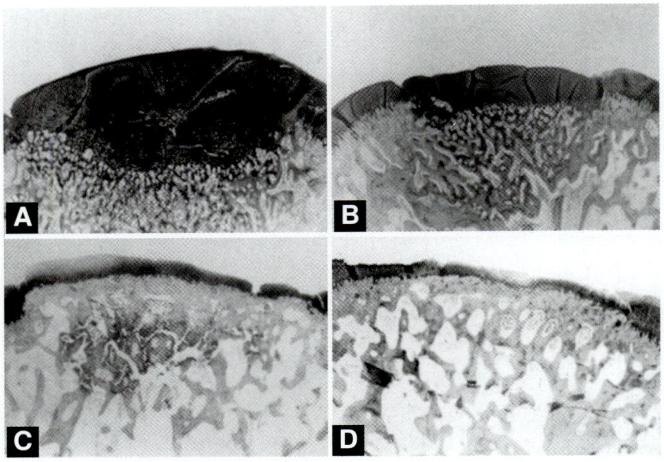

Figs 33.23A to D: Microscopic picture of mesenchymal cell implantation

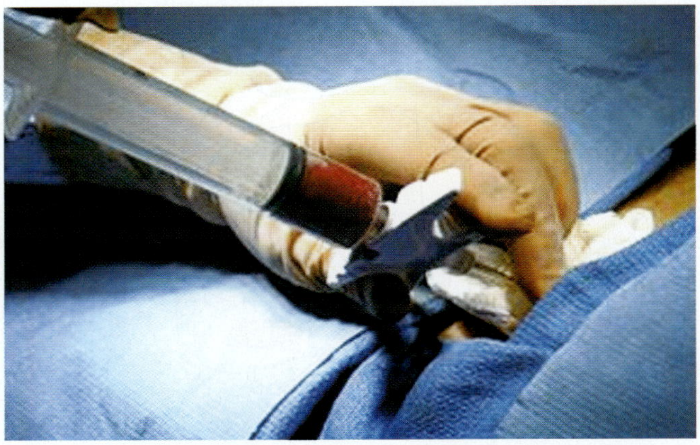

Fig. 33.24: Percutaneous autologous bone grafting is performed for nonunion

- The centrifugation method produces a buffy coat, that contains progenitor cells and other cells, which may be the source of angiogenic and osteogenic cytokines.
- The buffy coat is poured into a syringe for intraosseous injection.
- The trocar used to aspirate bone marrow, was placed both in nonunion gap and around the bone ends, as shown in Figure 33.25.
- The tip of the trocar was positioned with the use of image intensifier.

Osteonecrosis

Treatment of osteonecrosis of femoral head with implantation autologous bone marrow cells is illustrated in Figures 33.31 to 33.39.

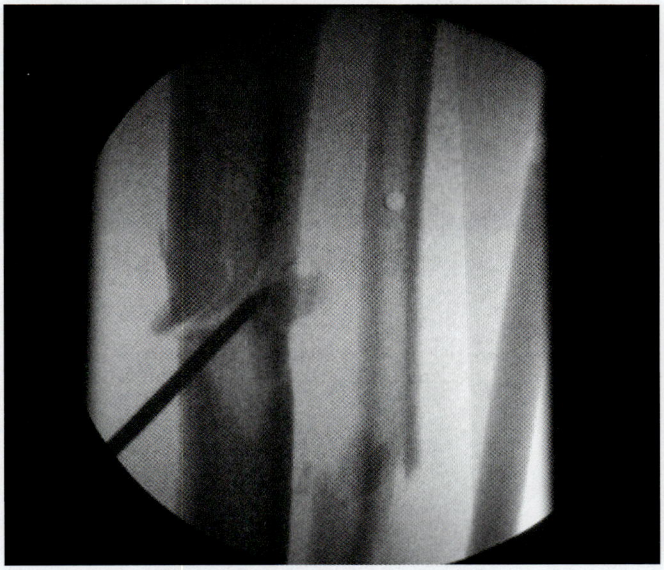

Fig. 33.25: The trocar placed in a nonunion gap

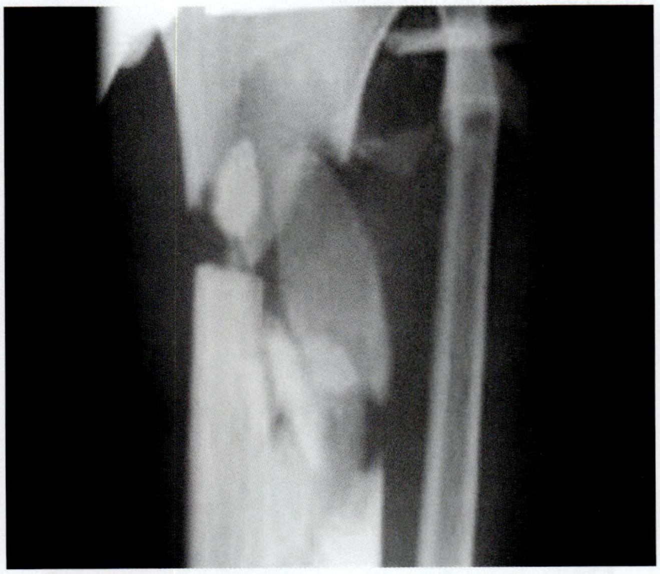

Fig. 33.26: Fracture at the time of nonunion

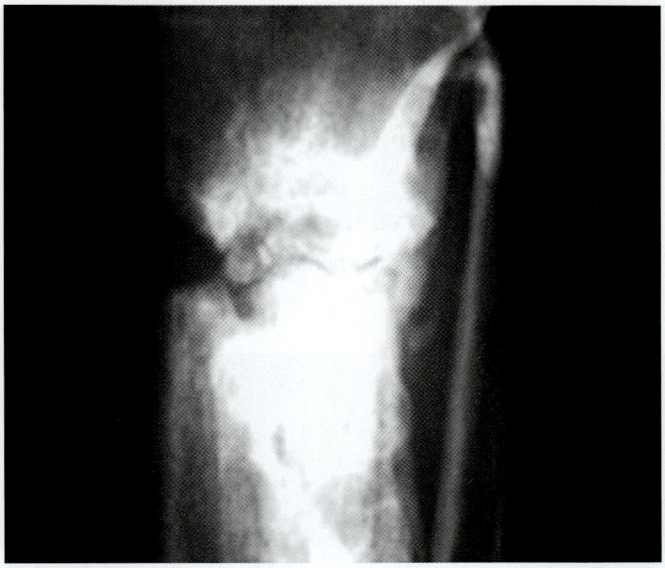

Fig. 33.27: Radiograph taken, one month after bone marrow injection

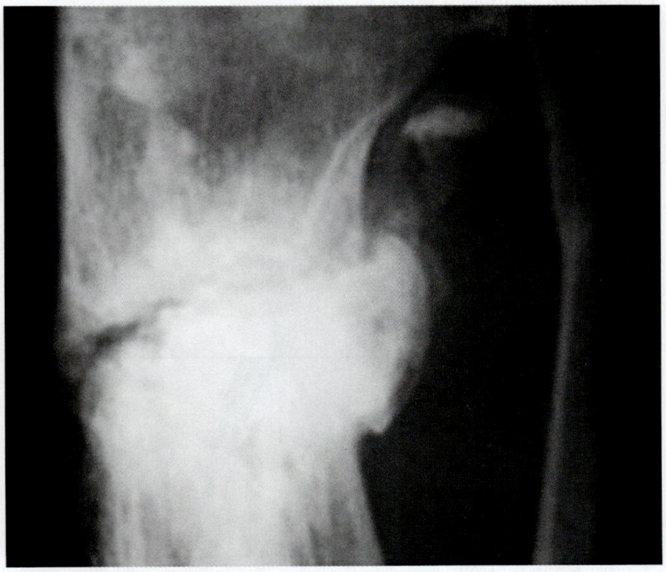

Fig. 33.28: Two months after bone marrow injection

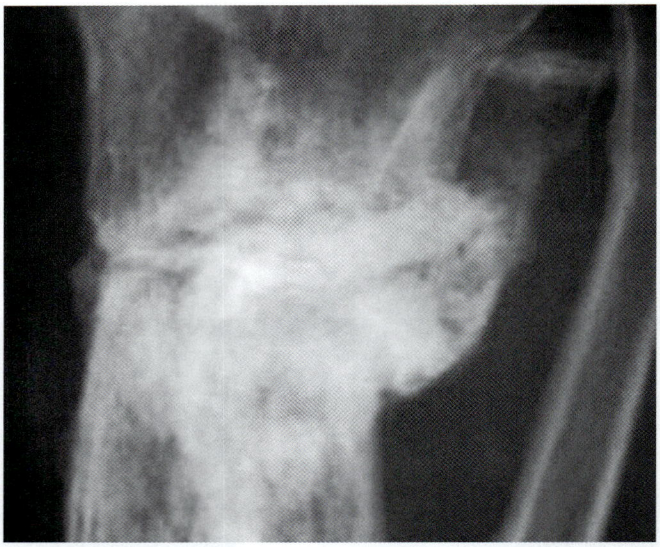

Fig. 33.29: Three months after bone marrow injection

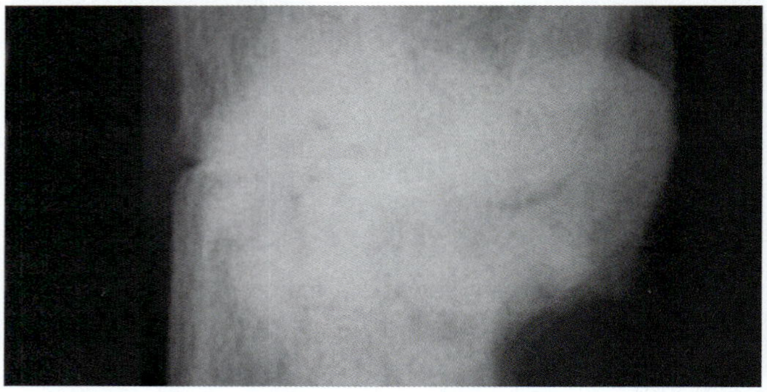

Fig. 33.30: Complete union of fracture site

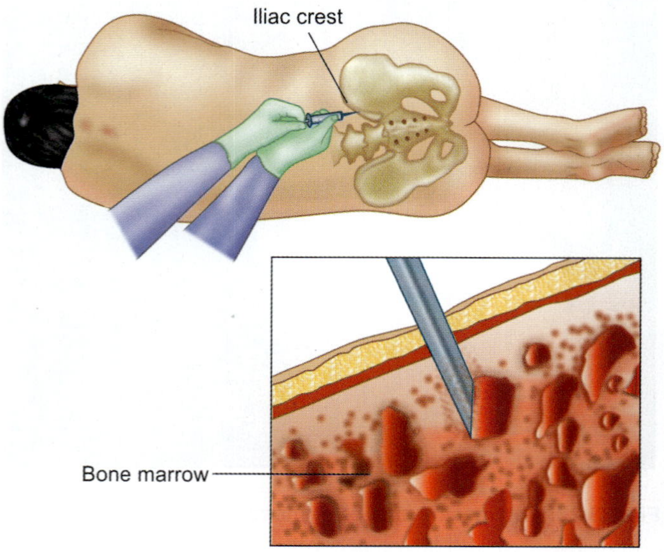

Fig. 33.31: Bone marrow aspiration

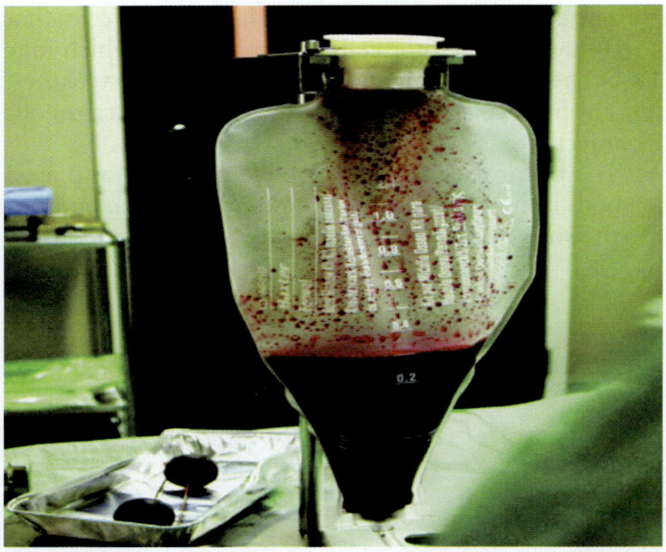

Fig. 33.32: Bone marrow collection unit (400 ml of bone marrow)

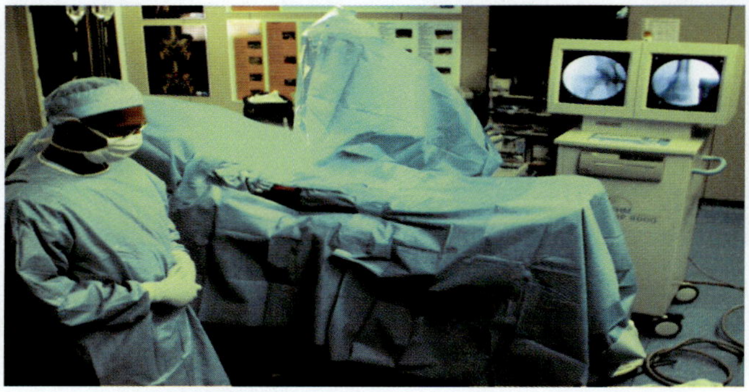

Fig. 33.33: Core decompression

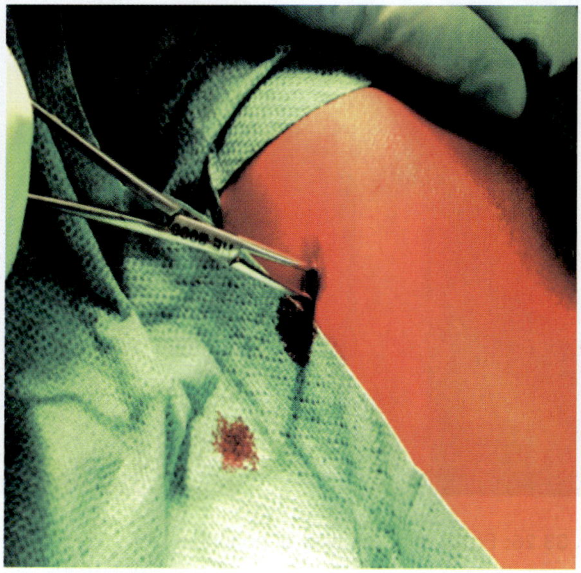

Fig. 33.34: Trephine is inserted, 3 mm from articular cartilage

Bone Marrow Aspiration Procedure (Figs 33.31 and 33.32)

Under aseptic condition and general anesthesia. Through 3 mm incision made at the level of anterior iliac crests on both sides, the needles of bone marrow aspiration are introduced by hands, deep into iliac crests. Bone marrow is aspirated with 10 ml syringes, rinsed with a buffer solution containing 400 ml of phosphate buffered saline solution, 25000 U of heparin and 100 ml of albumin, to avoid clotting. The contents of the syringes are transferred to bone marrow collection unit, to obtain a final volume of 400 ml of bone marrow.

Core Decompression (Figs 33.33 to 33.37)

A C-arm is draped and positioned at hip region. Using a 5 mm incision made laterally, a 3 mm trephine is then inserted under fluoroscopic control, through the trochanters, femoral neck and femoral head, to the necrotic lesion. The trephine is adjusted, 3 mm from articular cartilage.

- The 50 ml of mononuclear cells are injected through trephine, to be placed in necrotic lesion, as shown in Figure 33.38.

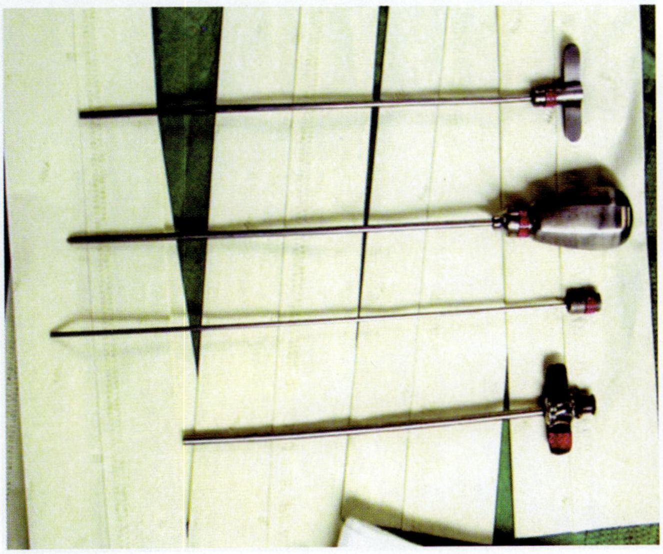

Fig. 33.35: Instrument for core decompression

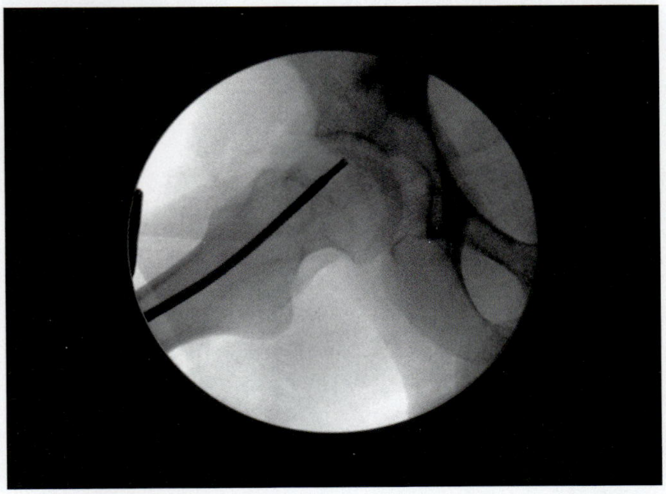

Fig. 33.37: Trephine in head of femur in lateral view

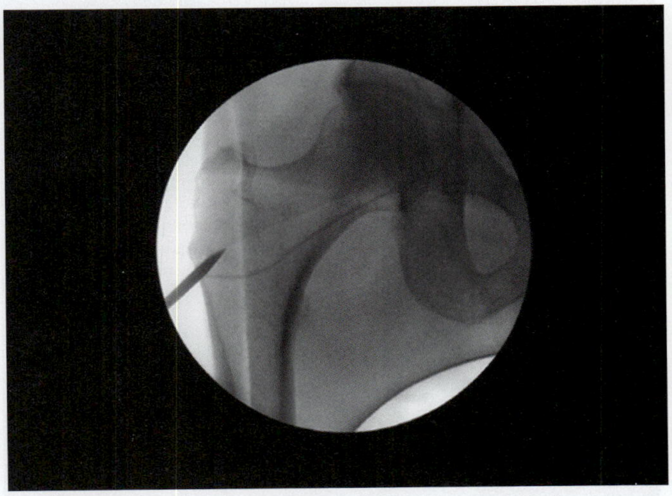

Fig. 33.36: Trephine introducing into femur in anteroposterior view

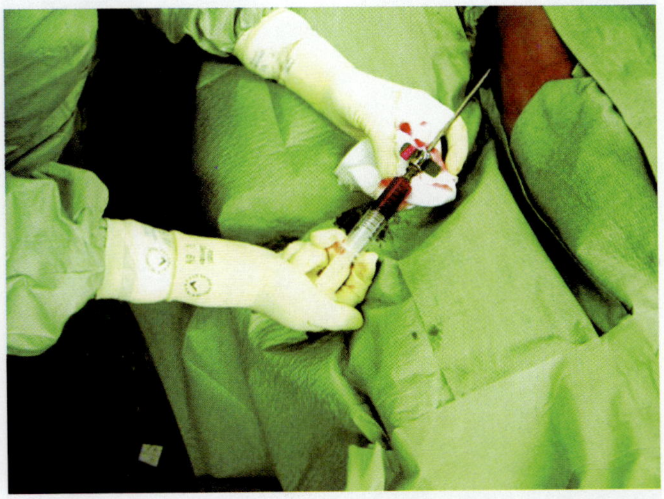

Fig. 33.38: The 50 ml of mononuclear cells are injected through trephine, to be placed in necrotic lesion

Radiographs (Figs 33.39 to 33.44)

Preoperative Radiographs

- Radiographs of segmental treated with ceramic cylinder, loaded with mesenchymal stem cell, shown in Figure 33.42.
- Use of stem cells in spinal fusion:
  - Before implantation 4 months (Fig. 33.43)
  - Postimplantation: Two years postimplantation (Fig. 33.44)

Spinal Cord Injury

See Figures 33.45A and B for spinal cord injury.

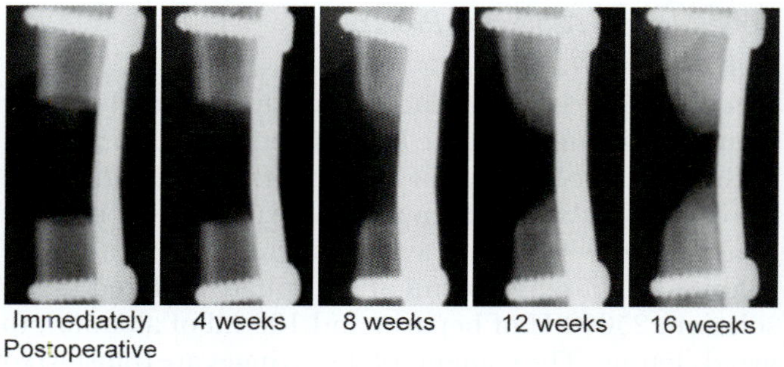

Fig. 33.41: The effect of implants, loaded with autologous MSC on healing of a segmental bone defect

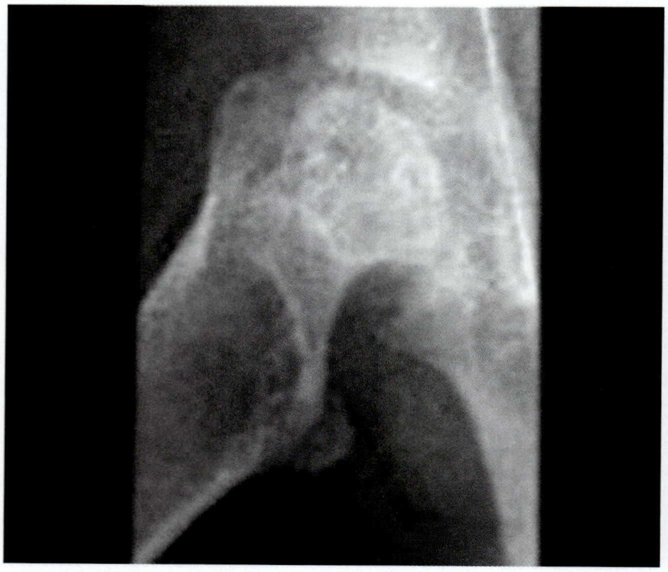

Fig. 33.39: Preoperative X-ray

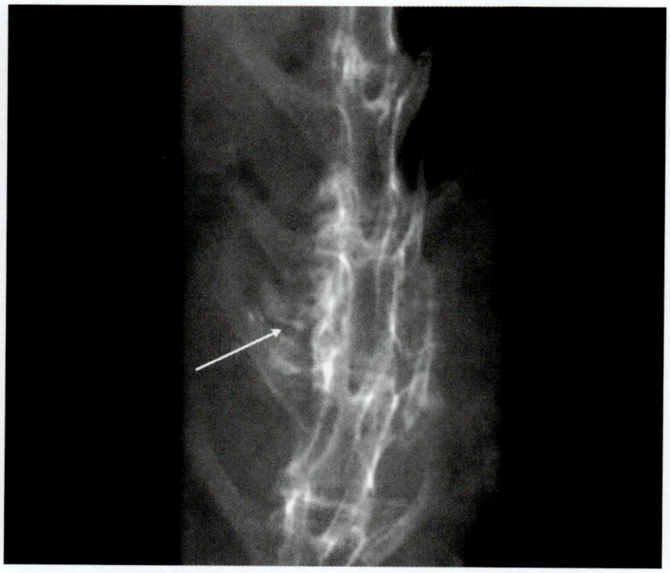

Fig. 33.42: Radiographs of segmental treated with ceramic cylinder, loaded with mesenchymal stem cell

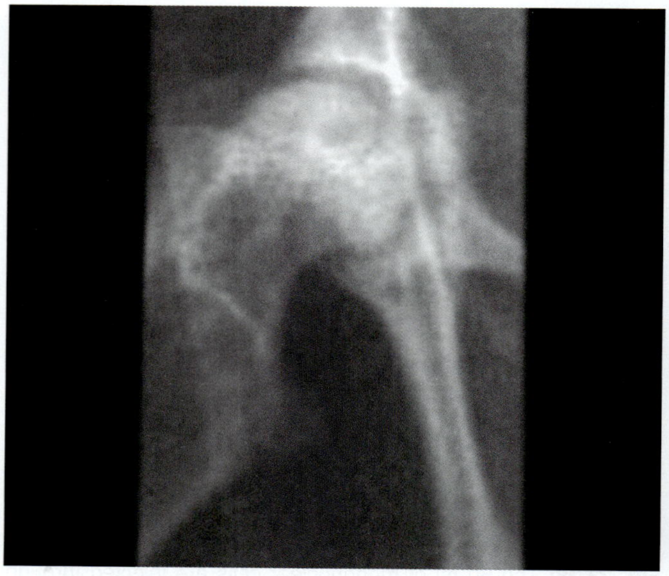

Fig. 33.40: Postoperative X-ray

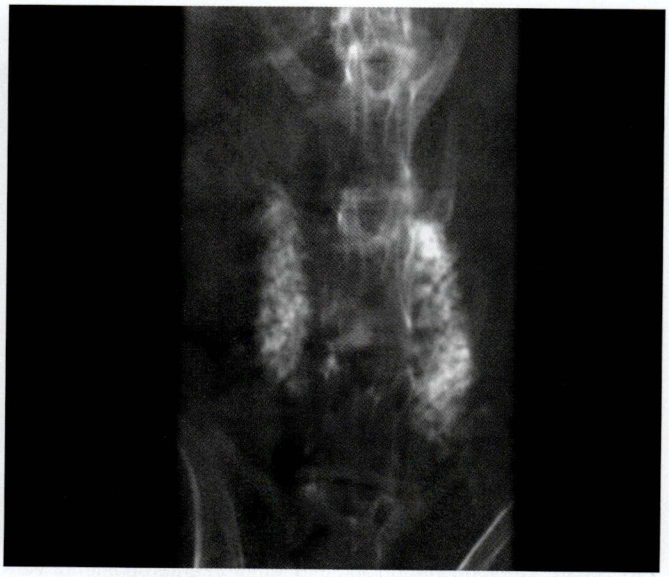

Fig. 33.43: Radiograph taken, before implantation 4 months

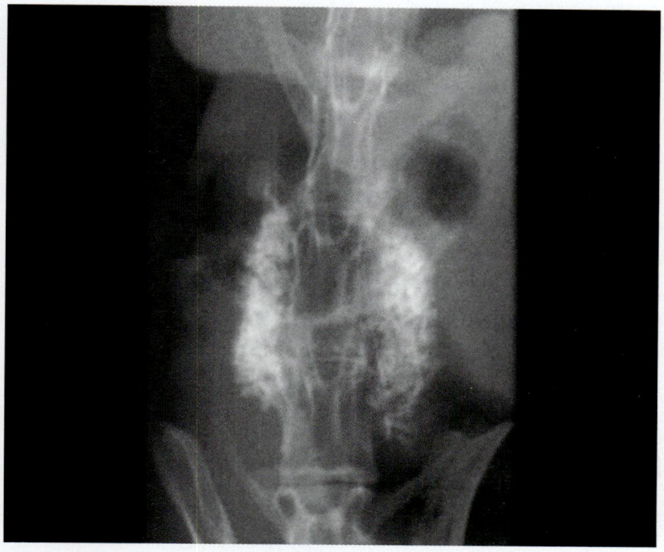

Fig. 33.44: Radiograph taken 2 years postimplantation

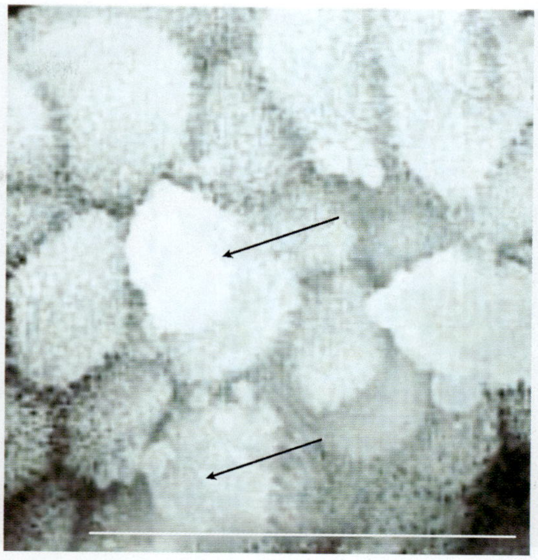

Fig. 33.47: Magnified image for Figure 33.48, arrows showing stem cells and membrane blebs

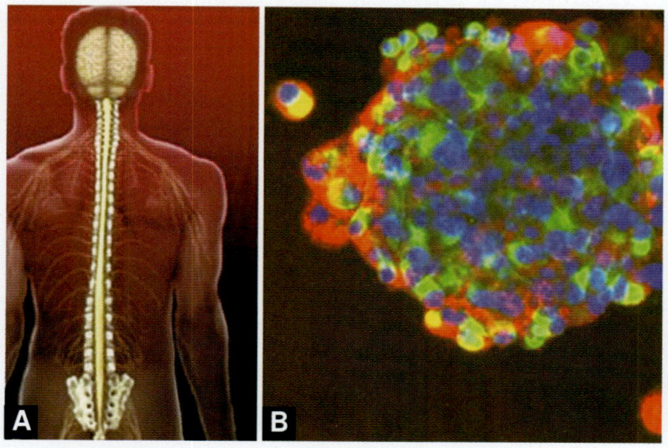

Figs 33.45A and B: Application of stem cells in spinal cord injuries

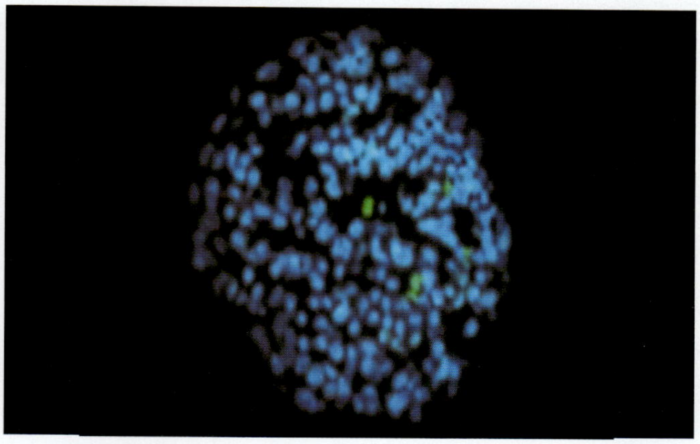

Fig. 33.48: Oligodendrocyte astrocyte

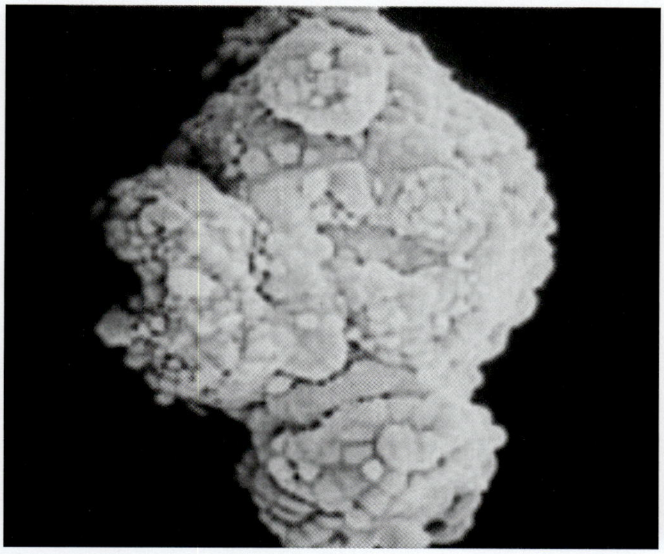

Fig. 33.46: Stem cells and membrane blebs

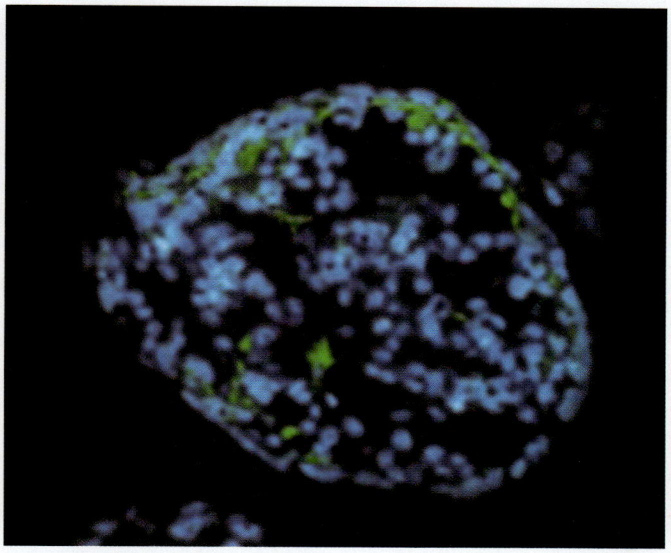

Fig. 33.49: Oligodendrocyte astrocyte (magnified)

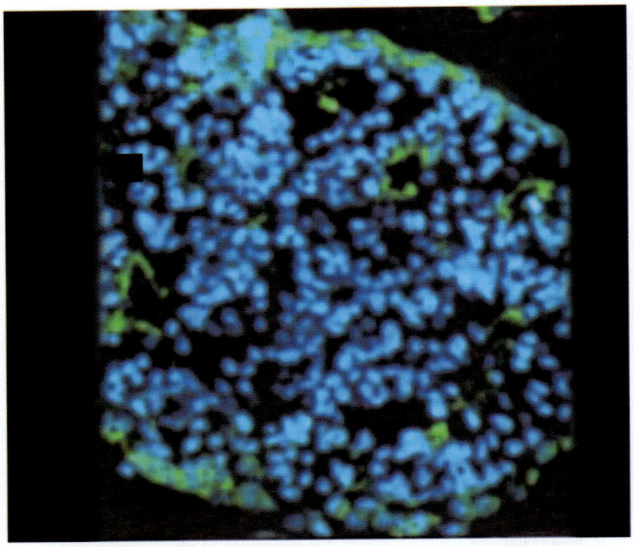

Fig. 33.50: Oligodendrocyte astrocyte (magnified with greater resolution)

Pathology

- Mechanical damage
- Neural tissue edema
- Axonal disruption.

Present researches on stem cells, promote regeneration of the gray tissues, for achieving axonal continuity in spinal cord injuries, using the adipose stem cells, neurotropic growth factors, embryonic stem cells and bone marrow stem cells. Undifferentiated multiple small processes markers being expressed. Stem cell and membrane blebs, developing consistent with neural cell, as shown in Figures 33.46 to 33.50.

Conclusion

An unlimited supply of cells capable of generating any tissue of the human body. A few years ago this could be the subject of science fiction, however today, they are called "stem cells".

34 Tumor Markers in Orthopedics

- Perfect Tumor Marker

Introduction

Tumor markers are biochemical indicators, of the presence of a tumor. They include cell surface antigens, cytoplasmic proteins, enzymes and hormones. In clinical practice, however, the term usually refers to a molecule, which can be detected in plasma or other body fluids. Tumor markers cannot be construed as primary modalities for the diagnosis of cancer. Their main utility has been as a laboratory test to support the diagnosis. Some tumor markers are also of value, in determining the response to therapy and in indicating relapse, during the follow-up period.

Perfect Tumor Marker

- Produced by the tumor cell alone
- Present in all patients, with a given malignancy
- Level in the blood, representative of the tumor mass
- Detectable in occult disease
- Absent in healthy person and benign disease
- No marker described till date meets all these criteria
- The ultimate application of tumor markers, is to target antibody bound cytogenic agents or the patient's own immune cells, to preferentially control or destroy malignant cells, by minimizing or excluding the damage to normal cells.

Some terms essential to understand the clinical use of tumor markers include:

- *Sensitivity:* The lowest amount of analyte that can be detected
- *Specificity:* The degree of interference, in the assay by extraneous substances, that may be present in the sample.
- *Predictive value:* Whether positive or negative, can give information, concerning clinical utility.

Clinical Classification of Tumor Markers

Classification of tumor markers, on the basis of chemical nature, i.e. hormones, enzymes and new molecular markers. This has been enumerated in Table 34.1 and the normal range or quantity used, for some commonly used markers, is given in Table 34.2. Further these tumor markers, can be classified as follows:

Clinically Useful Tumor Markers

- Carcinoembryonic antigen (CEA)
- Alphafetoprotein (AFP)
- Human chorionic gonadotropin (hCG)
- Calcitonin (CT)
- Prostate specific antigen (PSA)
- Estrogen receptor (ER) and progesterone receptor (PR).

Tumor Markers, with Clinical Promise

- CA 15-3
- CA 19-9
- CA 125
- Adrenocorticotropic hormone (ACTH)
- Neuron specific enolase (NSE)
- Lactate dehydrogenase (LDH)
- Squamous cell carcinoma antigen (SCC)
- Lipid bound sialic acid (LSA).

Markers Needing Further Evaluation

- Monoclonal antibodies, to specific tumors
- Oncogenes or tumor supressor gene.

Application and Interpretation

The hook effect (also known as high dose hook effect), is an artifact of tumor marker immunoassay kits, which causes the reported quantity of tumor marker to be incorrectly low when the quantity is high. An undetected hook effect may cause delayed recognition of a tumor. The hook effect can be detected by analyzing serial dilutions. Absent hook effect, reported quantities of tumor marker in a serial dilution, should be proportional to the dilution. If repeated measurements of tumor marker are needed, some clinical testing laboratories provide a special reporting mechanism, a serial monitor, which links

Table 34.1: Different tumor markers, their use in particular cancers and non-neoplastic conditions

Tumor markers	*Cancer*	*Non-neoplastic conditions*
hCG	Trophoblastic tumors, gonadal germ cell tumors	Pregnancy
Calcitonin	Medullary carcinoma of the thyroid	
Catecholamines	Pheochromocytoma	
Oncofetal antigens		
AFP	Hepatocellular carcinoma, gonadal germ cell tumor	Cirrhosis, hepatitis
CEA	Ca colon, pancreas, lung, stomach, breast, ovary	Pancreatitis, hepatitis, inflammatory bowel disease, smoking
Enzymes		
Prostatic acid phosphatase	Ca prostate	Prostatitis, BPH
Neuron specific enolase	Small cell Ca of lung, neuroblastoma	
LDH	Lymphoma, Ewing's sarcoma	Hepatitis, hemolytic anemia
Proteins		
PSA and PS membrane Ag	Ca prostate	Prostatitis, BPH
Immunoglobulins	Multiple myeloma	Infection
CA_{125}	Ca ovary, lymphomas	Menstruation, peritonitis, pregnancy
CA_{19-9}	Ca colon, pancreas, breast	Pancreatitis, ulcerative colitis
CA_{15-3}	Ca breast	
CD_{30}	Hodgkin's disease	
CD_{25}	Hairy cell leukemia	
New molecular markers		
P_{53}, APC, RAS mutations in stool and serum	Ca colon	
P_{53}, and RAS in stool and serum	Ca pancreas	
P_{53} and RAS mutations in sputum and serum	Ca lung	
P_{53} mutations in urine	Ca bladder	

test results and other data pertaining to the person being tested. This requires a unique identifier for the person. In the United States, a social security number is commonly used for this pupose. One important function of this mechanism is to ensure that each test is performed, using the same assay kit. For example for AFP, many different commercial assay kits, based on different technologies are available. AFP measurements obtained, using different assay kits are not comparable, unless special calculations are performed. Some of the primary tumors and their common sites of bony metastasis, are given in Table 34.3.

Table 34.2: Common tumor markers and their normal quantities used for the purpose of marking the tumors

Tumor markers	*Normal range*
CEA	Up to 5.0 ng/ml serum
AFP	Up to 15.0 ng/ml serum
B-hCG	<10.0 u/l serum
PSA	Up to 4.0 ng/ml serum
Calcitonin	6.0–30.0 pg/ml serum
CA_{125}	<35 u/ml serum
CA_{15-3}	<25 u/ml serum
NSE	Up to 12.5 µg/l serum
LDH	90–180 IU/ml serum
ER/PR	<10.0 fmol/mg cytosol protein

Table 34.3: Primary tumors and their common sites of bony metastasis

Primary tumors	*Common sites of bony metastasis*
Ca breast	Spine, pelvis, femur (upper 3rd), skull, ribs and humerus (at the junction of upper and middle 3rds)
Ca prostate	Vertebrae, femur, pelvis, skull, ribs, and sternum
Ca kidney	Humerus, spine, femur, pelvis, ribs, foot, skull and sternum
Ca thyroid	Skull, ribs, sternum, spine and humerus
Neuroblastomas	Skull (typical brush like appearance of skull vault)

Other cancers, which may metastasized to the bone are:
- Stomach
- Rectum
- Pancreas
- Lung
- Liver
- Urinary bladder
- Uterus
- Esophagus
- Large intestine
- Mouth or pharynx
- Seminoma of the testis
- Retinoblastoma
- Chorion epithelioma

- Melanotic tumors
- Ovary
- Retroperitoneal cancer
- Salivary mixed tumor
- Ureter
- Ewing's sarcoma
- Osteogenic sarcomas
- Lymphosarcomas
- Hodgkin's disease of lymphocytic depletion type.

Cancer of the bones, do not have any specific tumor marker, but from an orthopedician's point of view, metastasis to the bone can be ruled out, by ruling out any suspected cancer of any other organ, with the help of tumor markers.

35 Ultrasonography in Orthopedics

- Physics of Ultrasound
- Ultrasound in Physiotherapy

■ Physics of Ultrasound

Successful application of ultrasonography began shortly after World War II in late 1940 and early 1950. Ultrasound waves are produced by piezoelectric crystals. They pass through various interphases and are reflected back. That waves in form of electrical energy and is converted into mechanical energy.

Piezoelectric Effect (Figs 35.1A and B)

Described by, Pierre and Jacques Curie in 1880. It is defined as change in physical dimensions of certain materials, when subjected to an electric field. Such materials are made of innumerable dipoles arranged in a geometric pattern.

What is Dipole?

An electric dipole is a distorted molecule that has a positive charge on one end and a negative charge on other end. Positive and negative ends are so arranged that an electric field will cause them to realign, thus changing the dimension of crystal.

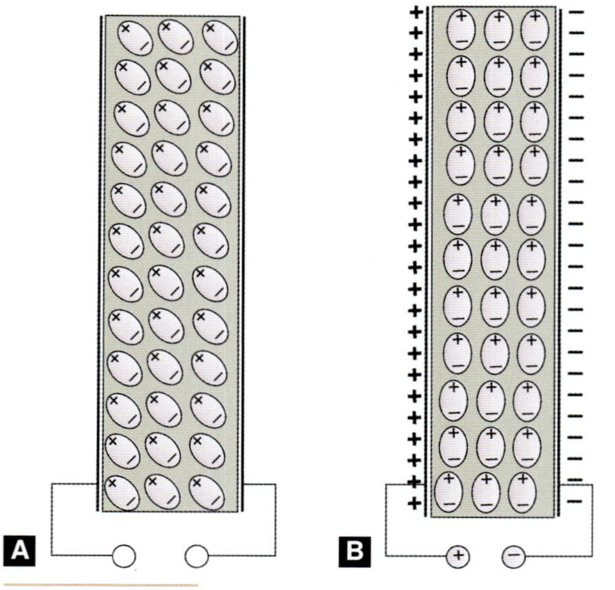

Figs 35.1A and B: An electric field realigns the dipoles in a piezoelectric crystal

Steps Involved in Generation of Ultrasonic Waves

Sudden burst or pulse of high frequency AC voltage causes crystal to vibrate and send ultrasound waves (as a beam in air and also back towards the damping block). Reflecting echoes from interphases carry energy, which causes physical compression of the crystal. This reorients the dipoles and induces voltage between electrodes and voltage amplification—ultrasonic signal for display. This compression force and associated voltage are responsible for the name piezoelectricity also called "pressure electricity".

Advantages of Ultrasonography

- Real time imaging capability allowing dynamic evaluation
- Low cost
- Easy accessibility
- Portability
- Noninvasiveness
- Multiplanar imaging.

Echogenicity of Tissues (Fig. 35.2)

- Hypoechoic (black)
- Hyperechoic (white).

Echogenicity of Different Tissues

Fat: Hypoechoic, but the echogenicity varies in different anatomy and pathology.

Muscle: Hyperechoic, separated by hypoechoic interfaces.

Fascia: Hyperechoic, thin well marginated soft tissue boundaries.

Tendon: Hyperechoic, consists of interdigitated parallel fibers running in long axis of tendon.

Paratenon: Some tendons do not have a true tendonsheath, instead they are surrounded by a hyperechoic boundary the paratenon, e.g. tendoachilles.

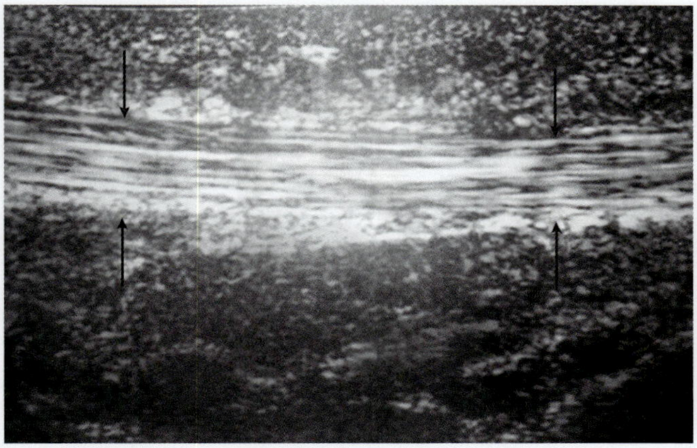

Fig. 35.2: USG of a normal patellar tendon, arrows showing fibrillar echotexture

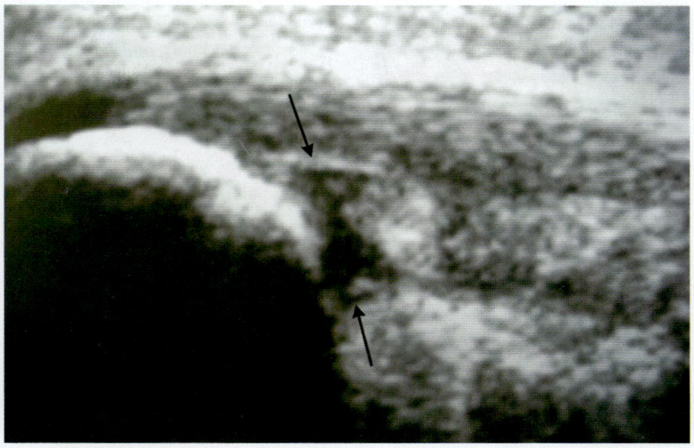

Fig. 35.3: USG showing partial detachment of patellar tendon from patella with arrows showing a small hematoma

Ligament: Hyperechoic, similar to tendons fibrillar pattern, may vary in multilayered ligaments.

Synovium/capsule: Both appear hypoechoic and similar to joint fluid.

Hyaline cartilage: Hypoechoic/transonic cartilage, seen against highly reflective cortical bone.

Bone/periosteum: Highly reflective hyperechoic/curvilinear line, with acoustic shadowing.

Nerve: Hypoechoic nerve bundles, separated by hyperechoic interfaces.

Air/gas: Highly reflective and creates characteristic comet tail artefacts.

Uses of USG

1. Diagnostic
2. Therapeutic.

Application of USG for different tissues and their associated conditions:

- Tendons
  - Tears
  - Tendinosis
  - Tendinitis
  - Peritendinitis
  - Tenosynovitis
- Enthesopathy
- Bursitis
- Postoperative patterns
- Cysts.

Tendon Tears USG (Figs 35.3 and 35.4)

- Discontinuity of muscle fibers (complete or incomplete)
- Focal thinning of tendon
- Hematoma of variable size, gap between the torn fragment is filled with hypoechoic hemorrhagic fluid.

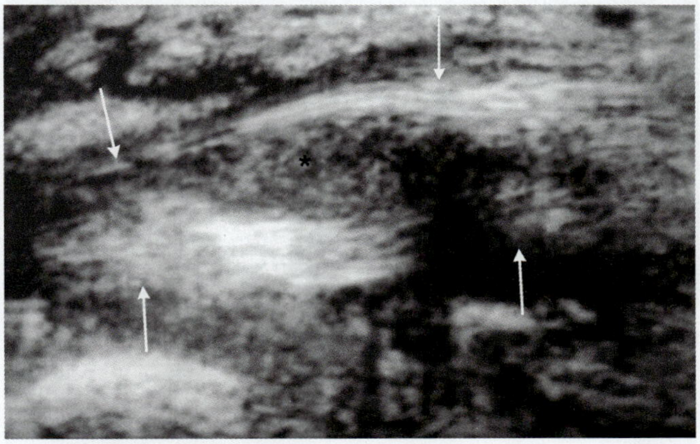

Fig. 35.4: Posterior tibial tendon split (central split)

- Bone fragment in case of bone avulsion, is seen as bright echogenic foci with acoustic shadowing.
- Partial tendon tears
- Nonvisualization of retracted tendon in case of complete tear, e.g. biceps brachii, rotator cuff and flexor tendons of finger (Figs 35.5 and 35.6).
- Except in achilles tendon rupture, hematoma develops around the whole tendon. Ruptures are associated with minimal focal hemorrhage.

Tendinosis

- Degenerative changes in a tendon, without clinical or histopathological signs of inflammation within the tendon or paratenon.
- Mostly associated with painful focal or diffuse nodular thickening of tendon
- Hypervascularity is seen on Doppler imaging, as shown in Figure 35.7.
- Mainly described with patellar tendon and achilles tendon (achillodynia).

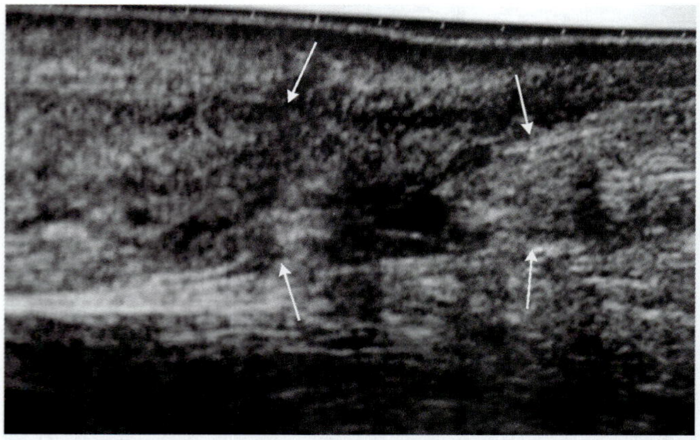

Fig. 35.5: Complete tear with nonvisualization of retracted tendon

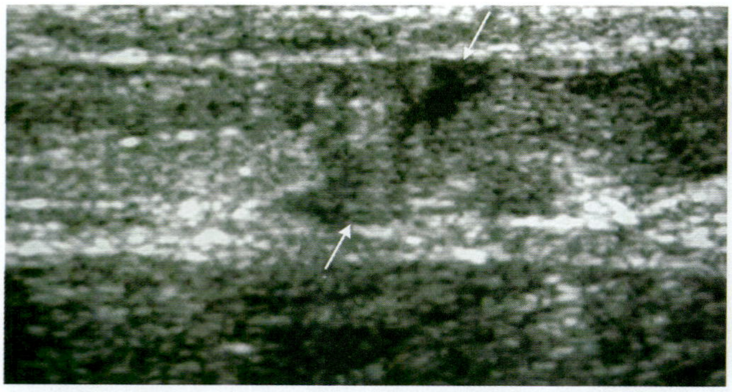

Fig. 35.6: Achilles tendon rupture with hematoma around the whole tendon

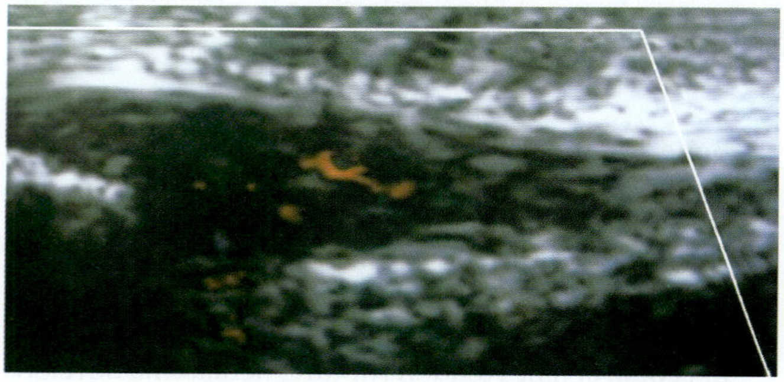

Fig. 35.7: Tendinosis with hypervascularity, seen on Doppler imaging

- Markedly decreased echogenicity and tendon enlargement
- Color Doppler imaging shows increased vascularity
- Early detection of occult tendinosis should prompt adequate treatment, to prevent chronic therapy resistant symptoms and subsequent tendon ruptures.

Tendinitis USG (Figs 35.8 and 35.9)

- Thickening of tendon
- Decreased echogenicity

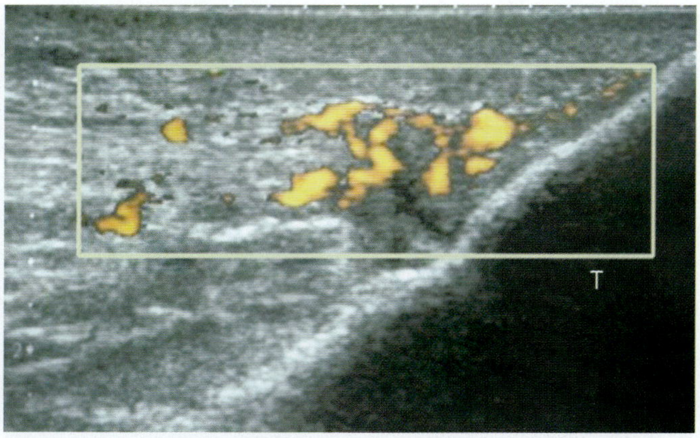

Fig. 35.8: Patellar tendinitis with decreased focal echogenicity and hypervascularity

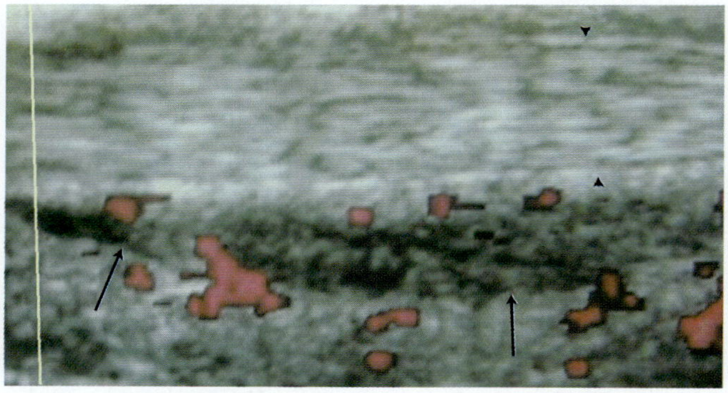

Fig. 35.9: Peritendinitis of achilles tendon with hypoechoic thickening of the paratenon, anterior to the tendon and associated increased vascularity

- Increased vascularity on Doppler imaging
- Calcification in chronic tendinitis
- Blurred margins.

Tenosynovitis USG (Figs 35.10 to 35.12)

- Acute tenosynovitis
  - Fluid, even of minimal quantity is seen in the sheath
- Suppurative tenosynovitis
  - Internal echoes representing debris, are seen
- Chronic tenosynovitis
  - Hypoechoic thickening of synovial sheath, with little or no fluid
- Rheumatoid tenosynovitis
  - Tendon sheath involved by a pannus is hypoechoic, with mild fluid may or may not be present
  - USG can be used to guide the injection of contrast medium into the sheath for tenography. A study that silhouttes the sheath wall of the tendon, guide for injecting steroid into the sheath for chronic inflammatory arthropathy.

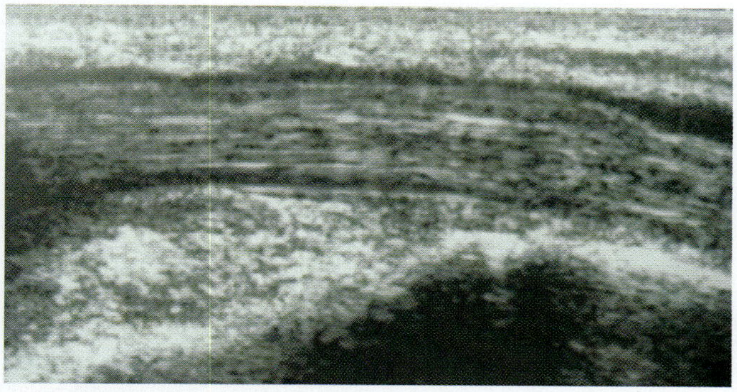

Fig. 35.10: Minimal amount of fluid collection, noted in posterior tibial tendon sheath

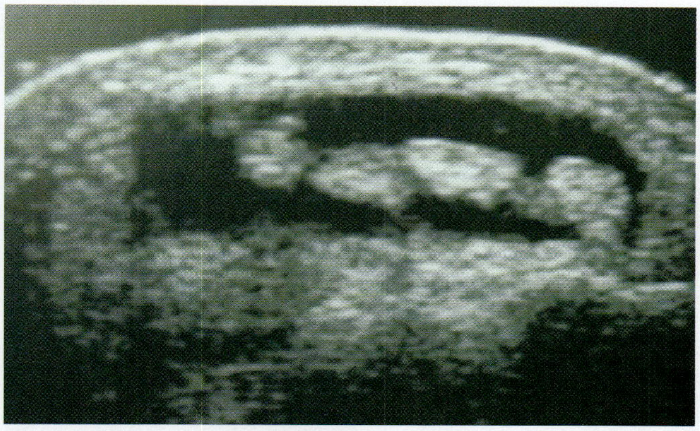

Fig. 35.11: Fluid around flexor tendons in wrist

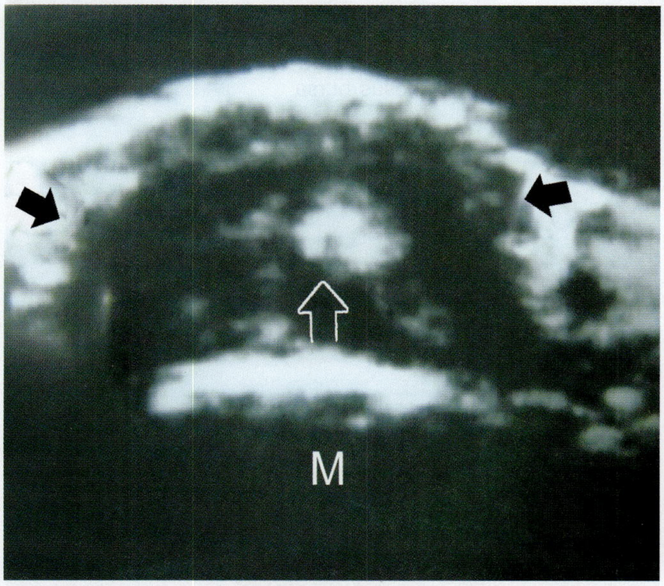

Fig. 35.12: Hypoechoic pannus (arrows) surrounding tendon (open arrow)

Bursitis (Fig. 35.13)

- Acute bursitis
  - There will be sonolucent and fluid filled collection, with ill-defined margins
- Chronic bursitis
  - Complex sonographic appearance with internal echogenic debris resulting from granulomatous tissue, precipitated fibrin and calcification.

Enthesopathy (Fig. 35.14)

It is defined as an inflammation of the tendons into the bones. Sonographically, the tendon appears swollen and hypoechoic, with calcification developing in chronic lesions.

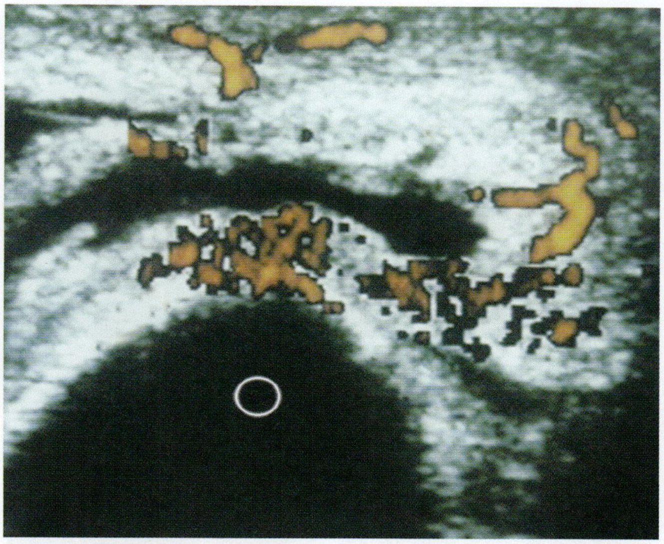

Fig. 35.13: Olecranon bursitis—posterior aspect of elbow shows thick walled fluid, containing olecranon bursa

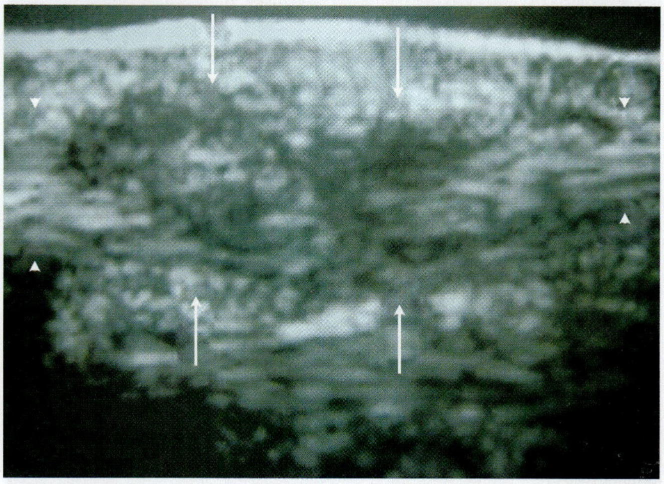

Fig. 35.14: Tendon of palmaris, after surgical repair, showing focal hypoechoic thickening

Postoperative Pattern

After surgical repair, tendons appear enlarged, hypoechoic and heterogenous, with blurred and irregular margins. Internal linear echo structure is shorter and thinner than in normal tendons. It may last from several months to years.

Ganglion Cysts (Figs 35.15 and 35.16)

USG demonstrates oval fluid collection adjacent to joint space or tendon. Chronic cysts may have internal echoes mimicing hypoechoic solid tumor.

Popliteal Cyst (Figs 35.17 to 35.20)

It is caused by an abnormal distension of the semimembranous bursa. On USG, present as hypoechoic fluid collection.

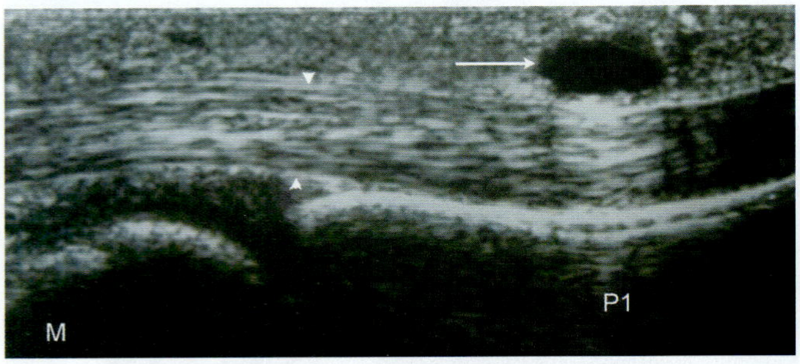

Fig. 35.15: Ganglion anterior to flexor tendon

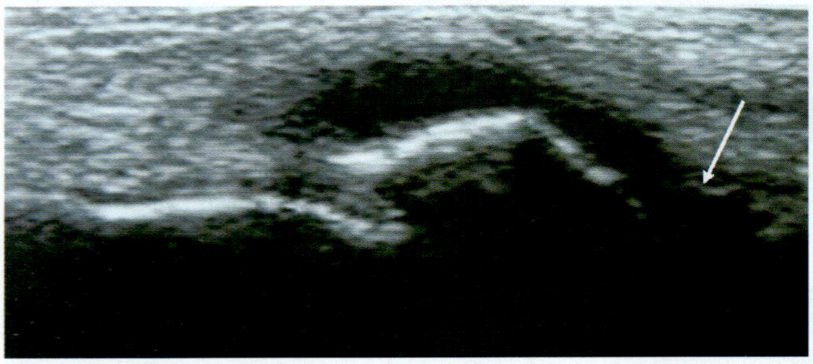

Fig. 35.16: Ganglion dorsal to wrist-connecting to joint

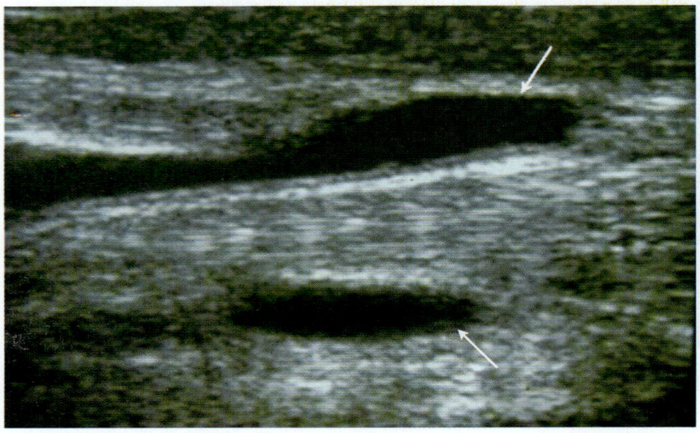

Fig. 35.17: Popliteal cyst, seen as hypoechoic fluid collection

Rotator Cuff Tear

Major criteria for diagnosis:
- Nonvisualization of the cuff
- Focal nonvisualization
- Discontinuity
- Abnormal echogenicity
- Wiener and Seitz classification, based on USG findings are enumerated in Table 35.1 and demonstrated in Figures 35.21A to E.

Minor Criteria for Diagnosis

- Intra- and extra-articular effusions
- Concave subdeltoid bursal contour
- Humeral head elevation
- Thickening of subdeltoid bursa.

Other Observations

- Cuff thickening
- Blood flow characteristic
- Developmental dysplasia of the hip (DDH).

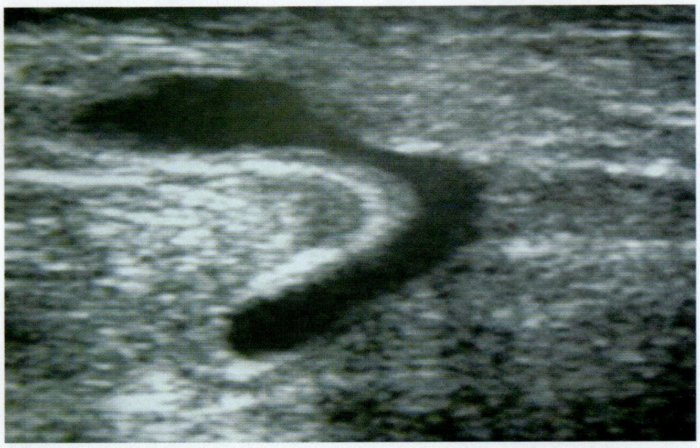

Fig. 35.18: Popliteal cyst caused by abnormal distension of semimembranosus bursa

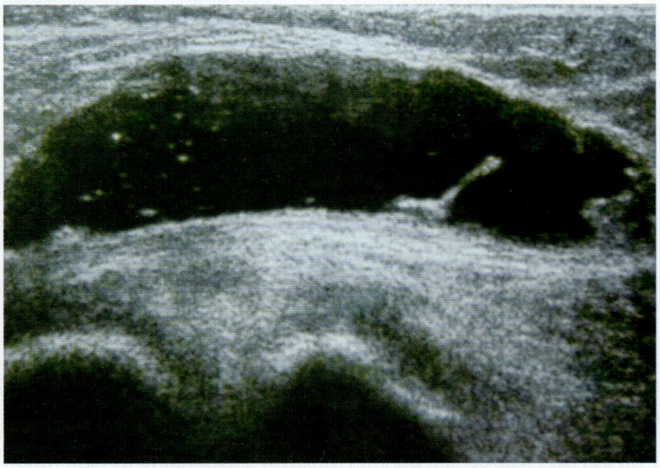

Fig. 35.19: Abnormal extension of semimembranosus bursa, in popliteal cyst, seen as hypoechoic fluid collection

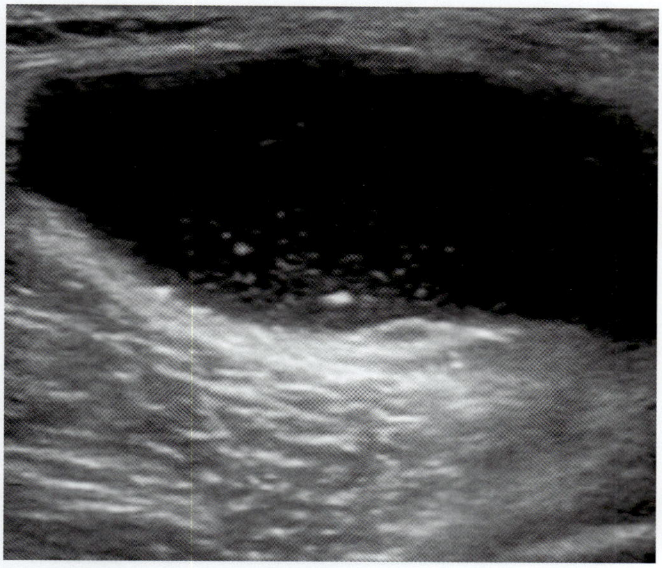

Fig. 35.20: Ruptured Baker's cysts

Table 35.1: Wiener and Seitz classification of rotator cuff tear visible in USG

Tear category	*Imaging features*
Normal	Normal
Partial thickness	Hypoechoic areas
Small full	
Thickness	<1 cm
Large full	
Thickness	1-3 cm
Massive	With or without cuff
	Arthropathy

Disadvantages of X-ray

- The exposure to ionizing radiation
- Lack of ossification of the femoral head in early infancy.

Methods of Screening DDH (Fig. 35.22)

- Morphologic evaluation of the location of the femoral head and the degree of acetabulum development
- Dynamic evaluation of the location of femoral head and degree of hip instability with stress
- A single coronal sonogram of each hip is done
- The image include lateral surface of iliac bone above acetabulum, deepest portion of acetabulum roof and proximal femoral metaphysis
- The depth of acetabulum and displacement of femoral head are measured by alpha and beta angles
- Draw three lines, one base line from lateral margin of ilium, second line from bony acetabular roof line and third line from lateral aspect of acetabular labrum

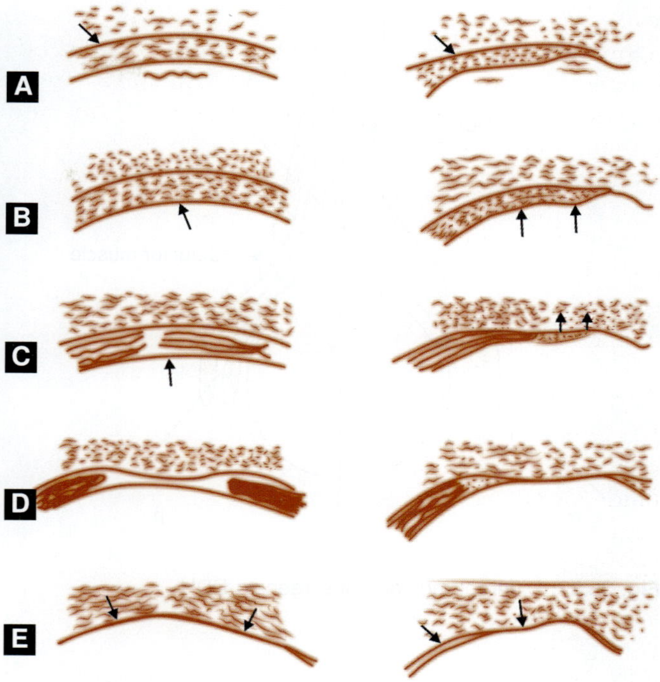

Figs 35.21A to E: Wiener and Seitz classification of rotator cuff tear visible in USG—(A) Normal; (B) Partial thickness tear, showing hypoechoic areas; (C) Small full thickness; (D) Large full thickness; (E) Massive rupture, showing region with or without cuff

- Alpha angle is between body weight base line and acetabular base line
- Beta angle is measured between body weight base line and acetabular labrum line, as shown in Figure 35.22.

Graf's Sonographic Classification of DDH (Table 35.2)

Table 35.2: Graf's sonographic classification of DDH

Type	*Alpha angle*	*Beta angle*	*Comment*
1	>=60°	<55°	Normal
2A	50-59°	55-77°	Physiologic immaturity, less than three months old
2B	50-59°	55-77°	Delayed ossification, greater than three months old
2C	43-49°	<77°	Labrum not everted
2D	43-49°	>77°	Subluxed, labrum everted
3	<43°	>77°	Dislocated
4	Unmeasurable	Unmeasurable	Dislocated with labrum interposing between femoral head and acetabulum

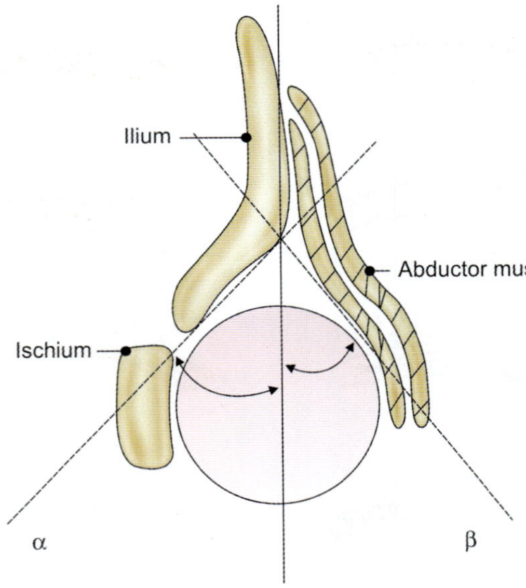

Fig. 35.22: Different methods of screening DDH

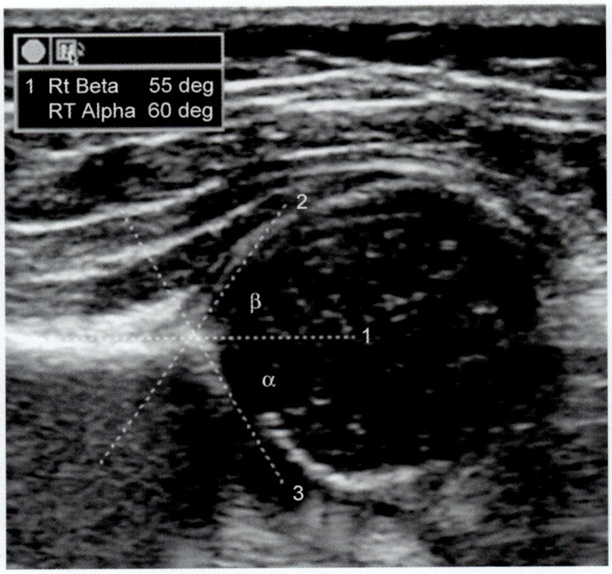

Fig. 35.23: USG hip showing alpha angle 60° and beta angle 55°

Simplified Graf's Classification (Table 35.3)

Table 35.3: Simplified Graf's classification of DDH

Type	*Alpha angle*	*Beta angle*	*Description*
1	>60°	<55°	Normal
2	43-60°	55-77°	Delayed ossification
3	<43°	>77°	Lateralization
4	Unmeasurable	Unmeasurable	Dislocated

Dynamic Stress Sonography by Harcke and Grissom (Figs 35.23 and 35.24)

In this sonographic evaluation, the hip is scanned in transverse and coronal planes in various position. While scanning the posterior lip of the acetabulum, a posterior push is performed to assess joint instability.

Disadvantages of X-ray

- The exposure to ionizing radiation
- Lack of ossification of the femoral head in early infancy.

Joint Effusions

Plane radiographic films are normal in the presence of small joint effusions, as shown in Figure 35.25. In such cases, USG can be used to determine, if effusion is present. USG can determine the nature of fluid collection, e.g. anechoic or hypoechoic fluid is seen in transient synovitis and more echogenic fluid in septic arthritis. To guide arthrocentesis, saline lavage can be used if fluid cannot be withdrawn.

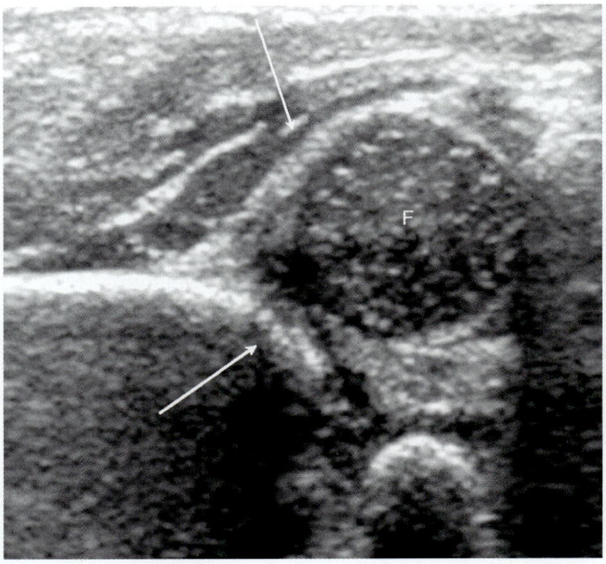

Fig. 35.24: USG hip showing dysplastic hip with reduced alpha angle

Infection

USG can be used to evaluate infection of soft tissues:

1. Cellulitis
2. Polymyositis
3. Abscess
4. In infection of osseous structure, it is used to supplement standard modalities.

Cellulitis USG

- Heterogeneous soft tissue thickening increase echogenesity in affected area, as shown in Figures 35.26A and B.

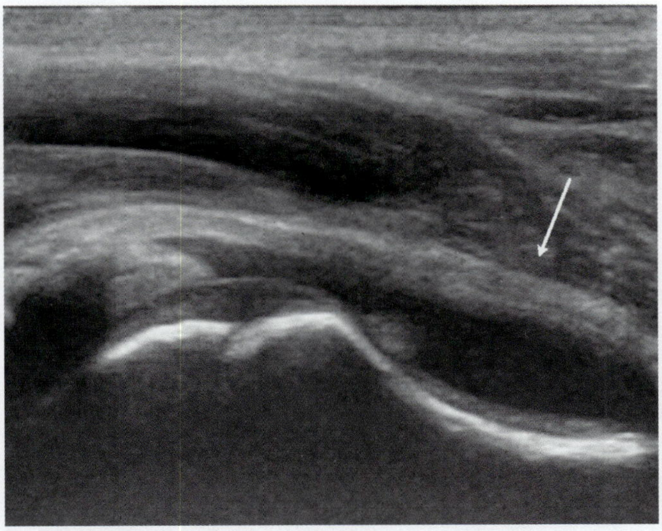

Fig. 35.25: Hip effusion with bulging joint capsule, with mixed echogenicity

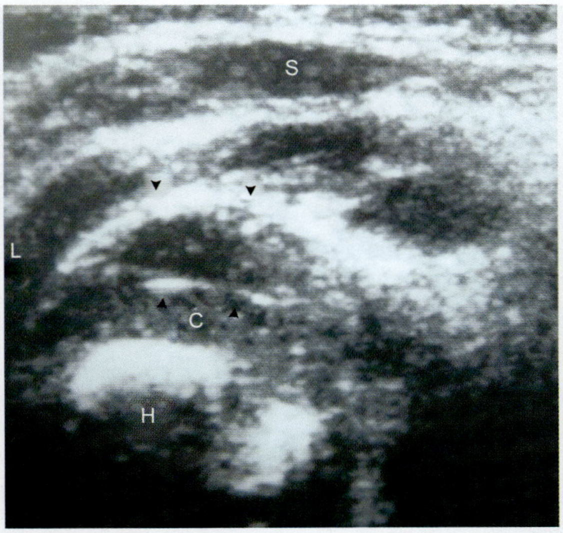

Fig. 35.27: Echogenic fluid, within the shoulder joint, superior to humeral head

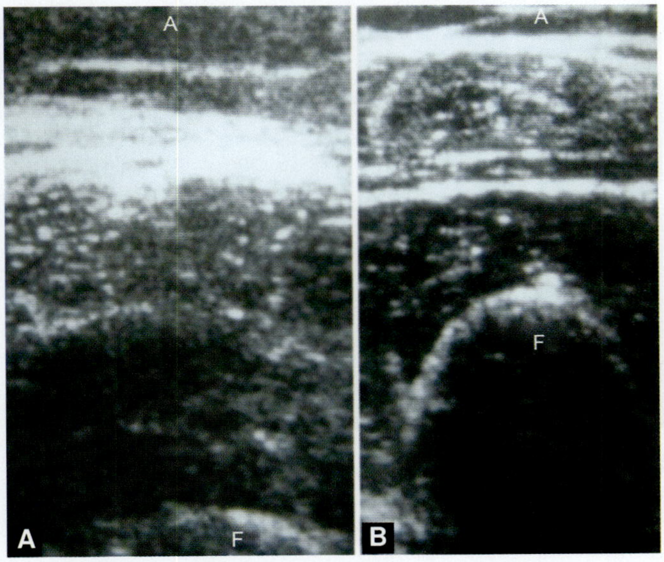

Figs 35.26A and B: Thickening and hyperechoic soft tissue in cellulitis

- Positive or negative adenopathy
- Foreign body can be identified if present
- Contralateral comparison aids diagnosis.

Abscess

- Inflammatory process can progress to abscess formation or necrosis
- USG appearance
  - Usually hypoechoic
  - Can be isoechoic/hyperechoic
- Moving internal echoes
- Doppler suggests increased flow at the rim and debris and is avascular within the cavity
- *Differential diagnosis:* Recent hematoma
  - Early myositis ossificans
  - Necrotic mass

Septic Arthritis (Figs 35.27)

- May be isolated abnormality or secondary to infection in adjacent soft tissue or bone.
- Fluid is seen as anechoic or hypoechoic areas
- *Differential diagnosis:* Articular cartilage, movement of the joint will show the cartilage fluid interface clearly.
- Doppler can demonstrate increased flow in capsule (infection causes hyperemia).
- Absence of hyperemia doesn't exclude septic arthritis.
- USG guided, joint fluid aspiration can be done.

Osteomyelitis (Figs 35.28)

Early sign: Deep soft tissue swelling.

Late sign

- Fluid along cortex of the bone or subperiosteally
- Fluid in adjacent joint (sterile or septic)
- Cortical disruption
- Doppler, increased flow at the margin of elevated periosteum in advanced infection.

Trauma (Figs 35.29 and 35.30)

- Radiographs are initial diagnostic modality
- USG helps, when symptoms are present and radiographs are unrevealing.

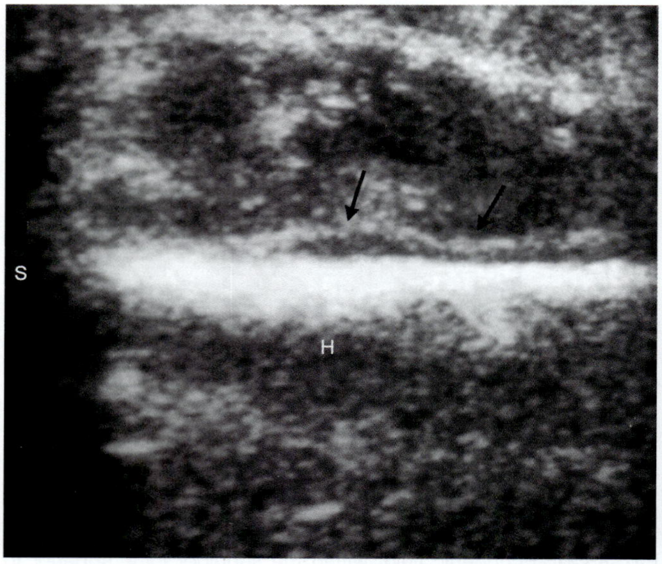

Fig. 35.28: Thickening and abnormal echogenisity of soft tissue with fluid along the bone

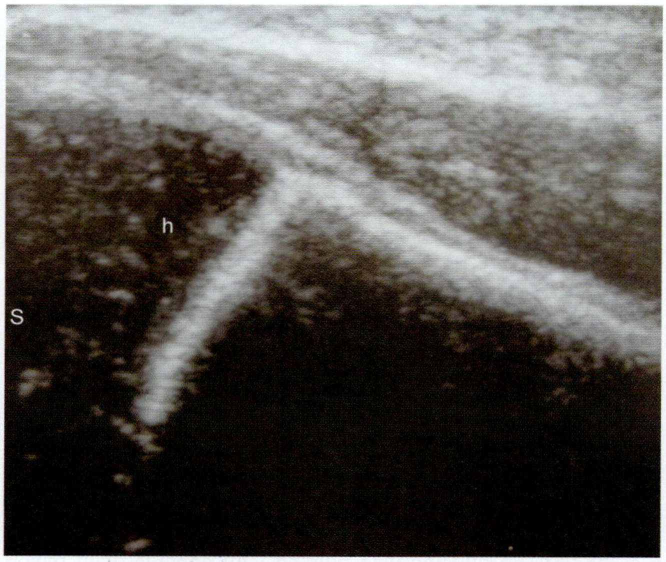

Fig. 35.30: Normal side for comparison

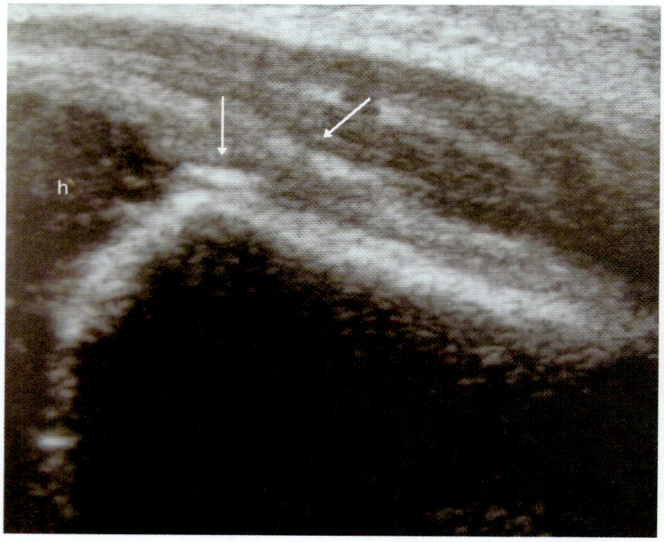

Fig. 35.29: Metaphyseal fracture fragment of infant, with non-accidental trauma

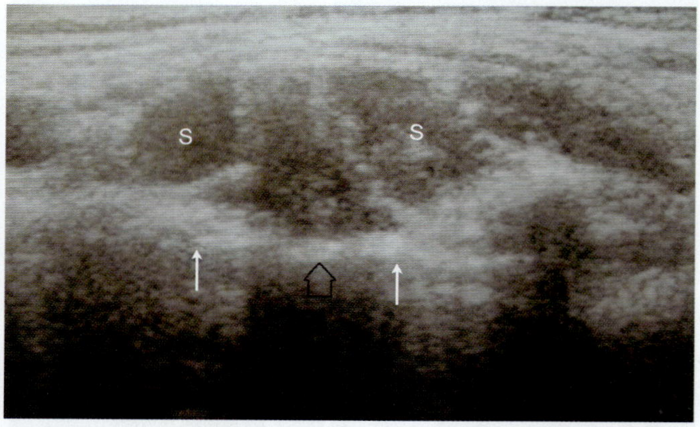

Fig. 35.31: Thickened and hyperechoic injured root

- Growth plate fractures, rib fractures and soft tissue injury, retained nonopaque foreign body.
- Brachial plexus injury from birth trauma can be identified.

Avulsed Nerve Roots (Figs 35.31 and 35.32)

- Meningocele and neurogenic tumors
- Congenital musculoskeletal abnormalities
- Proximal femoral focal deficiency

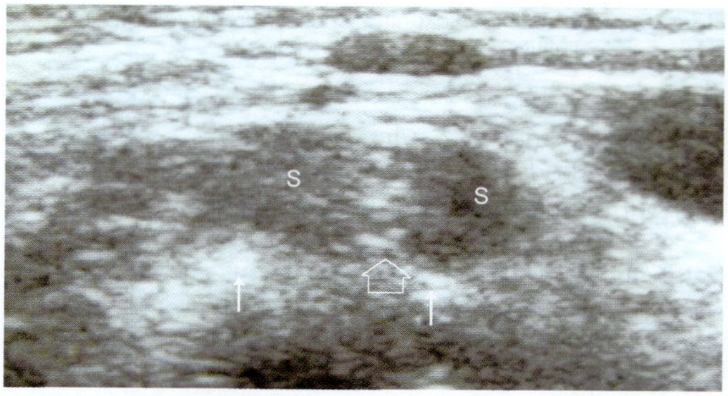

Fig. 35.32: Normal side for comparison

- Congenital joint dislocations
- Teratologic hip dislocation
- Skeletal dysplasia with 'atypical' hip
- Fibromatosis colli.

Therapeutic

- USG guided aspiration
- USG guided biopsy
- Aid in fracture healing in fresh fractures or non-unions. Act by upregulating the receptor activity of neurotransmitters at the fracture site
- Ultrasound in physiotherapy.

■ Ultrasound in Physiotherapy

Mechanism

- Thermal effect
  - Local rise in temperature
  - Increases extensibility of collagen
- Nonthermal effect
  - Increases the fragility of lysosome, thus enhances the release of their contained enzymes
  - Proliferative fibroblast and myofibroblast will drive Ca^{2+} ions towards the area of repair. Fibroblast will stimulate production of collagen tissue.

Uses of Ultrasound

- Recent injuries and inflammation
- Scar tissue
- Chronic indurated edema.

Adverse Effect

Burns

Contraindication

- Vascular conditions
- Acute sepsis
- Postradiotherapy
- Tumors.

36 Lasers in Orthopedics

- Characteristics of Laser

Introduction

The word 'laser' is an acronym for:
L: Light
A: Amplification by
S: Stimulated
E: Emission of
R: Radiation.

The atomic theories, leading to the discovery of lasers were established, by Einstein in 1917. The first practical ruby laser, was developed by Maiman in 1960 and the laser beam was visible red light with a wavelength of 694 nm.

Characteristics of Laser

1. Coherent
2. Monochromatic
3. Collimation (Rays travelling in a parallel beam).

Most of the lasers currently available for medical and operative applications are infrared, visible light and ultraviolet lasers (excimer lasers). The electromagnetic spectrum of various lasers include:

a. Ultraviolet (excimer) lasers: Wavelength ranging from 10 to 400 nm, e.g. xenon chloride laser
b. Visible light lasers (400 to 700 nm), e.g.:
  - Argon lasers
  - Potassium titanyl phosphate (KTP) laser.
c. Infrared lasers (700 nm to 300 micrometers), e.g. include:
  - Carbon dioxide lasers
  - Holmium: yttrium-aluminiumgarnet (Ho:YAG) lasers
  - Neodymium:YAG lasers
  - Erbium:YAG lasers.

Biological Effects of Lasers

Biological effects of laser can broadly be divided into following categories:

1. Electromechanical effect
2. Photoablation effect
3. Photothermal effect
4. Photochemical effect

Laser Physics

Current orthopedic lasers, function in the ultraviolet (excimer) or in the infrared portion of the electromagnetic spectrum. These lasers successfully combine the desired tissue effect and practical transmissibility for arthroscopic application. The optical properties of the material, determine the effectiveness of a given laser, by controlling the interaction between the laser light and the material. Mid-infrared and far-infrared lasers, such as the carbon dioxide laser and the holmium:YAG laser, are mostly absorbed by the water in tissues. The laser energy is absorbed by cellular water and is converted to heat. This vaporizes the tissue with little or no thermal damage to the adjacent tissues. Near infrared and visible light lasers, such as the neodymium:YAG laser, at 1.06 μm and the argon laser at 515 nm are absorbed relatively poorly, by water but are absorbed rapidly by pigments such as hemoglobin and melanin.

This optical property makes these lasers effective in the ablation of tissues rich in pigment, such as those in the retina, gastric mucosa and pigmented cutaneous lesions. However, the absence of pigment in cartilage, ligament and nucleus pulposus, makes these lasers less effective in most orthopedic applications. Ultraviolet light (excimer) lasers are absorbed by specific components of protein molecules, which vary with the wavelength of the laser. The absorption is due to a photochemical mechanism, in which the molecular bonds of tissue proteins are broken apart and the tissue is converted to gaseous plasma. The plasma is then expelled from the resultant tissue defect at supersonic speeds. This mode of operation contrasts with the photothermal mechanism of visible light and infrared lasers, which depend on the conversion of light to heat through the absorption of light by pigment on water.

Application in Orthopedics

- Laser arthroscopy
- Laser discectomy
- Removal of polymethylmethacrylate (bone cement)
- Tissue welding

- Biostimulation and treatment of tissue defects
- Photodynamic treatment of tumors with lasers.

Recent Applications of Laser

Laser Arthroscopy

To date, lasers have been used in orthopedics, primarily for arthroscopic procedures. Carbon dioxide laser was first used in arthroscopic procedures.

Demerits of carbon dioxide laser

– Because the carbon dioxide was well absorbed by water, gaseous insufflation of the joint was required, to prevent absorption of the laser, by the insufflating medium.
– There were reports of frequent postoperative effusions as well as problems with skin burns in the region of the laser hand piece.
– The characteristics and particulate organic material produced by the ablation of meniscal tissues caused a severe synovial reaction postoperatively.
– Subcutaneous emphysema with gaseous insufflation of the joint.
– Retroperitoneal and mediastinal emphysema have been reported in patients, in whom the knee joint had been distended with carbon dioxide.

The peaks of absorption, in human menisci, are at 280 nm and 340 nm wavelengths, which are in the ultraviolet range, and are attributed to the presence of tryptophan and hydroxypyridinoline, respectively. Thus, excimer lasers are used. Currently, 308 nm xenon chloride, excimer laser can be delivered fiberoptically and for this reason it is now used in arthroscopic procedures. There are also peaks of absorption in the mid infrared range and the far infrared range, corresponding to the water absorption peaks for infrared light. Lasers corresponding to these water absorption peaks are best suited to the cutting or ablation of tissue by photothermal vaporization.

The laser has been used successfully for:

– Partial meniscectomies and resections of the plica
– Lysis of adhesions
– Partial excision of a torn anterior-cruciate ligament
– Medial and lateral retinacular releases
– Tissue tightening (collagen shrinking)
– Ankle impingement decompression and debridement

Laser is also used in arthroscopy of the shoulder for:

– Subacromial decompression
– Acromioplasty
– Labral tear ablation
– Rotator cuff debridement
– Capsular releases

Advantages of laser in arthroscopy:

– Eliminate the need for the use of multiple instruments
– Less need for secondary trimming
– Better access to tight joint spaces with the narrow diameter hand pieces
– Improved properties of coagulation, compared with those obtained with mechanical devices.

308 nm xenon chloride, excimer laser can be delivered fiberoptically and for this reason, other ultraviolet wavelengths have not been used in arthroscopic procedures. The use of excimer lasers in arthroscopic procedures has been investigated by several authors and reported that the patients, who underwent laser surgery, had a significant reduction in pain and in reactive synovitis. The surgeons documented no complications, with use of the laser and cited the ease of operation of the flexible fiber light cable.

Laser Discectomy

At this time, laser discectomy has a limited role in the management of patients, who have low back pain and sciatica. The holmium:YAG and KPT (potassium titanyl phosphate) lasers have been approved for percutaneous discectomy. Application is currently restricted to patients, who have a prolapsed or extruded disk herniation and not a sequestered disk herniation. Reported rare complication is discitis. Excimer lasers, induce fluorescence to intervertebral disk tissue. The annulus fibrosus and nucleus pulposus become fluorescent at different wavelengths. The fluorescent spectroscopy can be developed into a valuable guidance system for percutaneous laser discectomy. This technology can lead to the development of so called 'smart lasers', that can be used to assess the fluorescence of the tissues; the fluorescence can either automatically deactivate the laser or warn the surgeon, that the nature of the tissue undergoing photoablation has changed.

Removal of Polymethylmethacrylate (Bone Cement)

The use of lasers in revision arthroplasty, is based on the optical property of polymethylmethacrylate, in which there is virtually complete absorption of light in the far infrared region. Hence, the carbon dioxide laser can ablate bone cement very efficiently, with little dissemination of the heat to the adjacent osseous tissue. Furthermore, bone absorbs light poorly at this wavelength and in the fluences, available in the carbon dioxide lasers that are currently on the market, there is little chance that bone would be thermally damaged by the laser. The products of vaporization are toxic and must be removed from the operating field with a high powered vacuum system, through a charcoal filter to prevent injury to individuals in the operating room. These products are also flammable, and a free beam carbon dioxide laser may generate enough heat to ignite the gases in the laser plume, during vaporization of polymethylmethacrylate.

The use of a laser wave guide with a jet of carbon dioxide or nitrogen gas can obviate the concern of igniting these gases, by diluting them and depriving them of enough oxygen to support combustion. Used in this way, lasers permit the removal of bone cement, without affecting the adjacent bone. This is an apparent advantage compared with the use of gouges, osteotomes and high speed burrs, which may produce fractures and perforations of the surrounding bone.

Tissue Welding

Use of lasers for joining tissues together, requires the uniform heating of the tissues to about 70 degrees Celsius. At that temperature, the collagen of the tissues changes its physical properties and the tissue becomes sticky. Milliwatt carbon dioxide lasers can achieve satisfactory tissue heating in thin walled structures, such as small arteries and veins and for this reason these lasers have been used successfully in sutureless anastomoses of small vessels and in thin walled hollow organs, such as the fallopian tube and the vas deferens. Tissue welding has the advantage of permitting healing without foreign body reaction to the suture material. It also produces a smoother intimal wall, which is less likely to clot. In addition, it allows unrestricted enlargement of growing vessels and preserves the mechanical properties at the site of the anastomosis. Small nerves can also be repaired with laser techniques.

Biostimulation and Treatment of Tissue Defects

Low powered helium neon laser light at 630 nm, penetrates several mm into tissues and several investigators have reported that it appears to decrease pain and swelling when used clinically in the treatment of tendinopathies and carpal tunnel syndrome. Lasers have also been used clinically, to hasten healing of skin ulcerations. Carbon dioxide lasers produce vaporization of the surface of infected skin wounds and ulcers. It also destroys surface bacteria. Sterilization of these lesions, with use of this technique has been found to promote granulation and healing. Whipple noted that treatment of decubitus ulcers, with a carbon dioxide laser before skin grafting appeared to permit rapid healing, without residual infection or loss of skin graft.

Photodynamic Treatment of Tumors with Lasers

This treatment modality depends on the selective absorption of laser light, by tumor cells that have been sensitized with a chromophore. It has been found that, after intravenous injection, hematoporpyrhin clears, from normal cells in twenty four to forty eight hours, but the compound is selectively retained by tumor cells for a maximum of twelve days. During that time, tumor cells labeled with a pigment actively absorb the light of specific wavelengths and in the presence of oxygen, produce free radicals, which destroy the labeled cells. Photodynamic therapy is particularly useful in the treatment of skin metastases and superficial gastrointestinal and urological lesions that are highly vascularized. In orthopedics, deeply seated, less vascular lesions may not be amenable to this form of treatment and very little clinical information is available on the use of lasers in musculoskeletal oncology.

Other Recent Applications

Muscles

Spasm, tension, myogelosis, hematoma, edema, neck/shoulder syndrome.

Bones

Fractures, periostitis.

Joints

Arthrosis/arthritis, bursitis, chondromalacia patellae and rheumatic inflammation.

Tendons

Tendovaginitis, tendinitis, Dupuytrens contracture, carpal tunnel syndrome and tennis elbow.

Nerves

Intercostal neuralgia, neuritis, lumbalgia and pain therapy.

Traumata

Distortions and hematoma.

Safety and Credentialing

A major concern with respect to the clinical use of lasers is the potential damage, to the eyes of all individuals in the operating room, including the patient. The lasers that are most completely absorbed by water (the carbon dioxide and erbium:YAG lasers), have the potential for producing corneal injury. Lasers that are less completely absorbed by water (the holmium:YAG and 1.44 micrometer neodymium:YAG lasers), can cause injury to the lens, while those that are absorbed by pigment only (argon lasers), pass through the cornea, lens and vitreum, to be absorbed by the retina. For this reason, goggles and protective glasses, tinted to absorb specific wavelengths, should be used, if there is any chance that the laser could be accidently deployed into the operating room.

If the laser is used endoscopically, protective eyewear may not be necessary. Other safety concerns are related to the contents of the laser plume that is produced by the vaporization of tissues and biomaterial, such as polymethylmethacrylate. The toxic gases, resulting from vaporization of the cement must be removed by a vacuum system. The products of vaporization of tissue should also be removed because of the possibility, that they may contain fragments of deoxyribonucleic acid (DNA). It has been speculated, that the papilloma virus might be transmitted to the respiratory tract of individuals, close to the working surfaces. A more serious threat is that fragments of the human immunodeficiency virus could be transmitted and spread by inhalation of the products of vaporization, from the tissues of a patient.

Concerns about the safety of lasers, also encompass the credentialing of surgeons, who are to use these devices. The American National Standards Institute has recommended that certification for the use of lasers, in a given hospital should be the function of a laser safety committee. Individuals, who are interested in employing lasers in the operating room, should be trained in their use and should present documentation of this instruction to the hospital.

■ Conclusion

Laser technology, is still developing and investigators are finding new applications for lasers. Use of lasers in arthroscopy and discectomy, appears to be reasonably well established and the experienced investigators have been fairly well identified. As new applications become available, it is important that a mechanism should be in place, so that they may be introduced in a way that will offer maximum benefit, with least risk to patients.

37 Computers in Orthopedics

- Role of Computers in Orthopedics
- Computed Tomography

Role of Computers in Orthopedics

Planning Surgeries

- Computer-assisted orthopedic surgery (CAOS)
- Computer guided joint replacements (Navigation)
- OPTOTRAK system
- Helix Izarov
- Computer-assisted oteotomy.

Investigations

- CT scans (CT guided biopsy)
- MRI (MRI guided biopsy)
- PET scans.

Other Latest Developments

- Learning aids (haptics)
- Simulating virtual surgeries.

Computer-assisted Orthopedic Surgery (Fig. 37.1)

Computer-assisted orthopedic surgery (CAOS) is a system, where a computer interacts with body parts via infrared lights and gate detectors. There are systems, that require C-arm images or CAT (Computed axial tomography) scans and the newest and most evolved systems are imageless systems, this means that no prescans of any kind are necessary. The imageless systems are far less complicated, of lower cost and more patient friendly, since the prescans are not necessary. The imageless systems will also bring down operation time.

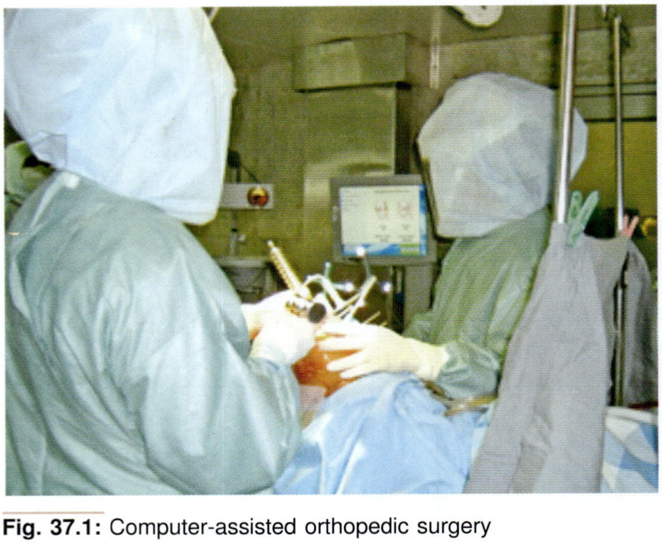

Fig. 37.1: Computer-assisted orthopedic surgery

Computer-assisted (Navigation) Joint Replacement

Over last decade, extensive research, has led to the development of a navigation system, for use in many surgical fields, including joint replacement surgery. Joint replacement surgery is a combination of mechanical engineering and surgical skills. Computer guided system is also called navigation, as it guides the surgeon in all the steps of surgery and even point out errors, before they are made.

Computer-assisted surgery is similar to a traditional surgery, except that the whole surgical process is carried out with the aid of the computer, in order to minimize the errors of the procedure and obtain optimum results. It includes a computer console, touch screen monitor and couple of infrared cameras, which track the position of the leg and the components. The computer has an infrared camera (sensor unit) and a screen. As the surgeon moves an instrument, within the patient's joint, the infrared camera calculates its position and then transfers that data to a computer in the operation theater. The computer then shows the direction and location of the instrument on the screen. The computer navigates the path of instruments, in such a way that the part will be fitted in the most optimum position. It also helps in adjusting the ligament tension, which is very vital to get a stable joint with good range of motion. During surgery, the anatomical landmarks are registered and data fed to the computer, using dedicated instruments, with reflective trackers. Computer generates a bone model, that guides the surgeon, in virtually all the steps of the surgery. The accuracy of the steps is improved to 0.5° and to 1 mm.

Apart from improving the precision of bone cuts, the computer also helps in restoring the soft tissue balancing, which is critical in getting the desired good results.

The computer also tells the surgeon what size of implant is correct. Since, the computer guides the accurate bony cuts, the surgical cut can remain limited with smaller incision and limited soft tissue dissection, i.e. minimally invasive surgery (MIS). In nonobese patients, knee and hip replacement is possible today through a 10 to 12 cm incision. The techniques have evolved, those minimizes or completely eliminate the damage to the muscles, thereby hastening the postsurgery recovery. Patients can stand and walk from third day onwards, after surgery and can be discharged from the hospital as early as fifth day after surgery. During conventional total knee replacement surgery, a rod is inserted in the cavity of the femur to set the alignment of the leg. In computer guided navigation surgery, the computer sets the alignment axis and therefore, rod does not require to be inserted in the femur. Any potential for the bone marrow and fat, reaching the lungs and cause fat embolism is thereby reduced.

The Advantages of Computer Guided Joint Replacement Surgery

- Restore accurate limb alignment.
- Increase the survival of the implanted joint.
- Reduce the risk of complications.
- No radiation during surgery.
- Constant guidance and monitoring during surgery.
- Range of motion analyses to achieve maximum function.
- Minimally invasive surgery, hence, less blood loss.
- Prevention of complications like fat embolism.
- Decreased hospital stay.
- Computer assisted surgery, is available for all total knee replacement surgeries, but is best used for difficult cases, like knock knee or bow leg deformities.
- There are similar softwares, for doing hip surgeries as well as spine surgeries.
- At the end of the surgery, the entire data can be stored on a CD and given to the patient for record keeping.

The OPTOTRAK System (Fig. 37.2)

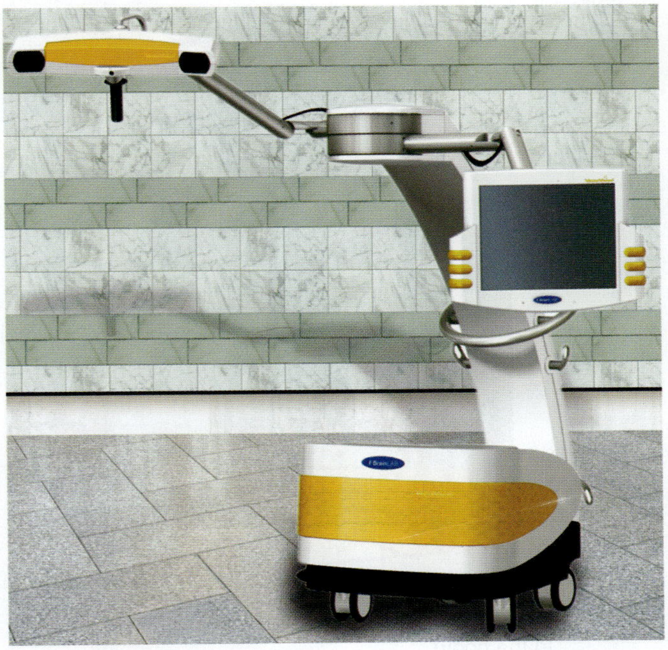

Fig. 37.2: An OPTOTRAK system

Developed at Northwestern University, Canada. The OPTOTRAK is a noncontact motion measurement system, which tracks small infrared (e.g. IRED) position sensors, which are attached to a subject, instead of reflective markers. Only one position sensor is required to determine the 3D position of each marker. The positions of the cameras, which track the sensors, are precalibrated. The position sensor must not be blocked at any time, since is it an optical system. If markers go out of view, they will be automatically identified by the system, when they return into view. Three position markers are needed to determine the 3D orientation of a body. However, more markers are preferred, since they can be blocked by the movement. The OPTOTRAK position sensor does not pick up interference from reflections and ambient lighting. The three-dimensional positions of markers are determined in realtime for viewing and processing. At the same time, data can be saved to file for postoperative analysis.

Uses

Most commonly used in osteotomy surgeries. Motion markers prior to joint replacements and osteotomy surgeries, as shown in Figure 37.3. The availability of high resolution, magnified and relatively noisefree endoscopic images, in a small workspace, 4 to 10 cm from the endoscope tip, opens up the possibility of using the endoscope as a tracking tool. They are developing a hybrid navigation system, in which image analysis based on 2D and 3D tracking is combined with optoelectronic tracking (OPTOTRAK) for computer assisted navigation, in laparoscopic ventral spine surgeries. Initial results are encouraging and confirm the ability of the endoscope, to serve as a tracking tool in surgical navigation, where sub-millimetric accuracy is mandatory.

Hex Ilizarov

The Hexapod, represents the kinematic mechanism, that realizes the three-dimensional movements by different lengths of the six distractors, connected to the two platforms. It is also used for imitation of flying and other machines. The Hexapod set for Ilizarov apparatus,

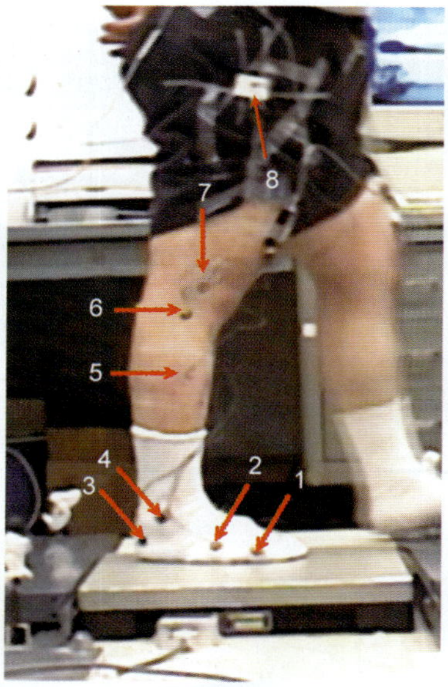

Fig. 37.3: Motion markers taken prior to surgeries, by using OPTOTRAK (1–8 represent motion markers attached to the body)

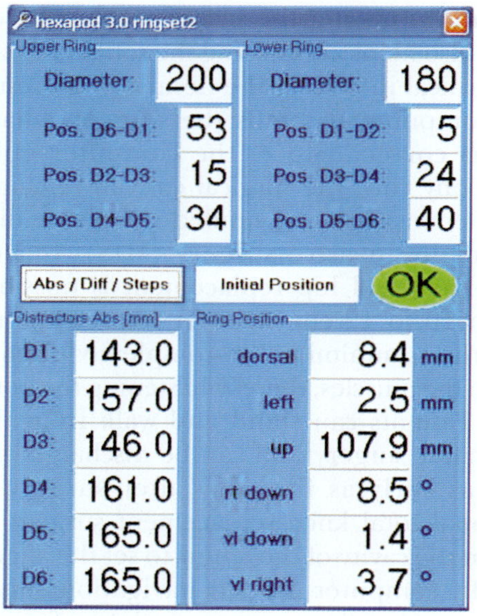

Fig. 37.5: An illustration of software model

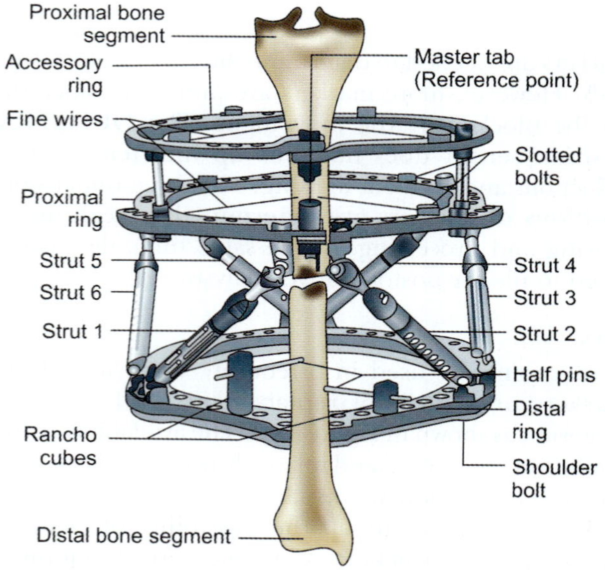

Fig. 37.4: Hex Ilizarov, fitted over a bone

consists of six telescopic distraction rods of varying length from 105 to 240 mm, 6 Y adaptors, a measuring stick and the software, as illustrated in Figures 37.4 and 37.5. The center of rotation and angulation (CORA) is entered in relation to the center of the distal ring and the desired correction, entered into the computer. The software then makes the appropriate adjustments for deformity correction, consistently for each plane according to the plan developed, on the basis of the malalignment test along three axes with six degrees of freedom.

The software is very simple to use. The base data needed, includes the diameter of the upper and lower rings, the positions of the Y adaptors on each ring and the length of the distraction rods. After the input of this data into the computer, the program shows the initial position of center of the upper ring, in relation to the lower. The software, displays a plan for correction, detailing the steps according to the surgeons input of the number of days and steps desired. All adjustments can be in three planes.

Uses

- Fracture treatment (especially compound fractures with bone loss)
- Correction of limb length disturbances
- Correction of rotational deformity, with limb length correction can be done in a single set-up.

Computer-assisted Osteotomy

A computer-assisted technique for correction osteotomy, of malunion of long bones. Outcome studies have shown that this procedure is accurate, reliable and safe. It has advantages over conventional technique, including less fluoroscopic radiation to the patient and surgical team, besides a quicker learning curve for nonexpert surgeons. This allows for full correction of the convergence, restoring the bow of the long bones. Improved fixation plate positioning and rotation (full forearm) post-operatively.

Haptics

Science of Haptics: An Artificial Touch Technology

Haptics, belongs to the category of virtual reality technologies, that create an artificial environment. Mostly such experiences are visual, either seen on a standard

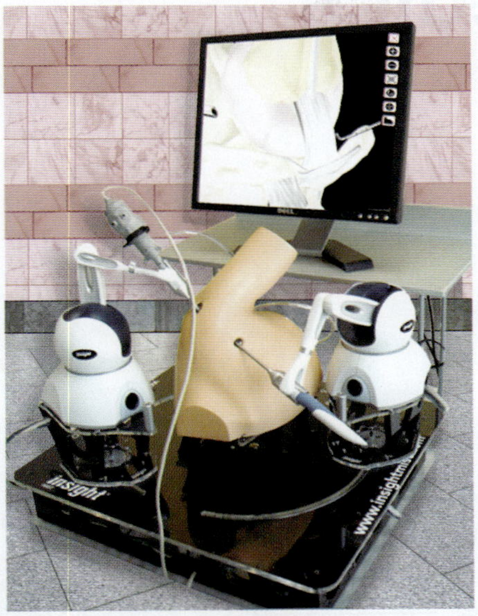

Fig. 37.6: Heptics, with the system consists of a base structure, a plastic model representing the anatomy of a shoulder joint and probe to perform the virtual surgery, a computer monitor, a computer that runs software, containing 3D anatomical models and learning modules

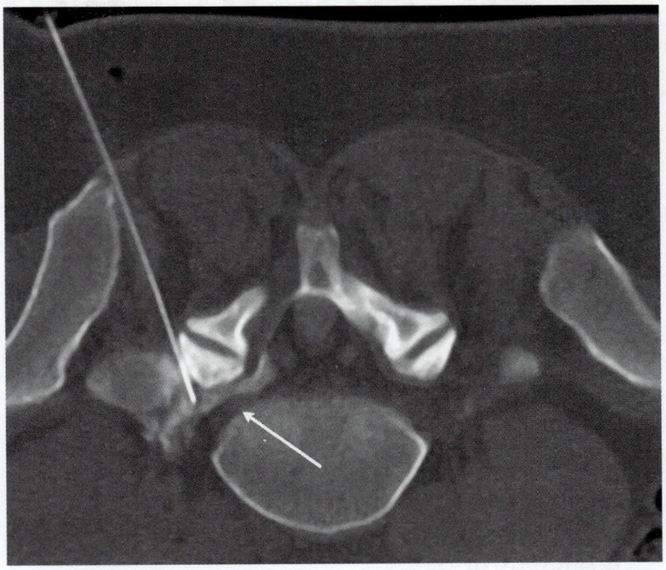

Fig. 37.7: CT guided transforaminal nerve root block for pain relief

computer screen or via stereoscopic displays worn by the user. The system consists of a base structure, a plastic model representing the anatomy of either the shoulder joint, knee joint or both arthroscope and probe to perform the virtual surgery, a computer monitor, a computer that runs software, containing 3D anatomical models and learning modules, as shown in Figure 37.6. In the case of knee arthroscopy, when the surgeon in training views a 3D image of the knee on screen and performs a simulated procedure, using the haptic stylus as his tool, the bone, cartilage, ligaments and meniscus, all feel different, depending on the virtually touched anatomic structure. The system also lets the surgeons, undergoing training, to differentiate between the feeling of healthy anatomy and pathological conditions.

Uses

- The touch component is a key for imparting accuracy and confidence to students, learning new procedures.
- Several specialty areas have seen a surge, in the availability of haptically enabled simulators, including arthroscopic surgery, spinal surgery and temporal bone drilling.

■ Computed Tomography

The word tomography, is derived from the Greek word, *tomos* (slice) and *graphein* (to write). Computed tomography (CT) is a medical imaging method, employing tomography. Digital geometry processing, is used to generate a three dimensional image, of the inside of an object from a large series of two-dimensional X-ray images, taken around a single axis of rotation. CT is often used to image complex fractures, especially around joints because of its ability to reconstruct the area of interest in multiple planes. Fractures, ligamentous injuries and dislocations, can easily be recognized with a 0.2 mm resolution.

Reconstruction of images, with the help of computer gives 3D images of individual bones and joints. For preoperative planning of following surgeries:

- Spine surgeries
- Joint replacements
- Corrective osteotomies
- Fracture fixation (trial and error of various implants, can be done on computer, even the biomechanics of fixation can be evaluated).

Fluoro CT imaging is now used to guide a number of minimally invasive, microtherapy procedures. Drainage of fluid collections such as cysts, abscesses (pus), lymphoceles (lymph fluid), hematomas (blood) or remove fluid from an infection or wound. Diagnostic biopsy, to remove a tissue sample, for pathologic or cytologic laboratory testing. Pain therapy, for example, the injection of therapeutic agents, into a spinal disk space to alleviate pain, as depicted in Figure 37.7. Minimally invasive operation, for example, cyst removal or ablation (cutting away) of tumors (such as brain/spinal tumors). Dynamic study of knee or elbow motion, swallowing or study of the larynx. CT arthrogram—injection of contrast into joint space, for easier diagnosis of injury. Guidance of embolization, to stop bleeding, for example, in liver and spleen trauma.

38 HIV in Orthopedics

- Statistics

Introduction

- AIDS first reported in 1981 in USA.
- Caused by HIV (human immunodeficiency virus).
- It is a retrovirus.
- Virus first isolated by Luc Montagnier in 1983, in Paris.
- Disability or life-threatening illness caused by HIV characterized by:
  - HIV encephalopathy
  - HIV wasting syndrome
  - Diseases due to immunodeficiency in a person with lab evidence of HIV infection or without other causes of immunodeficiency.

Statistics

- *Deaths annually:* 22,802 (2007)
- *Death rate:* 7.6 deaths per 100,000 population (2007).

Definition

As per Center for Disease Control (CDC):

Any HIV infected individual with a CD4+T cell count of less than 200/ml has AIDS regardless of the presence of symptoms or opportunistic disease.

Human Immunodeficiency Virus (Fig 38.1)

- Reverse transcriptase enzyme
- Infection life-long
- Asymptomatic for many years
- Virus is fragile—destroyed by boiling for one second
  - 1 percent bleach
  - 70 percent ethanol
  - 2 percent glutaraldehyde
  - 5 percent formaldehyde
  - 1 percent chlorine-sodium hypochlorite
  - 3 percent H_2O_2.

Modes of Transmission

- Sexual intercourse
- Transfusion
- Syringes and needles
- Prenatal and perinatal

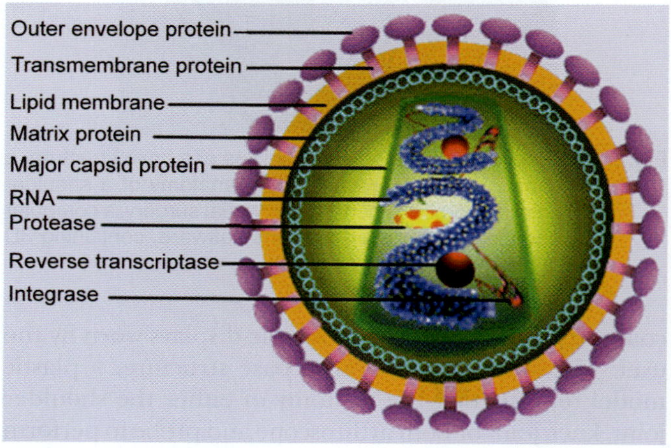

Fig. 38.1: Human immunodeficiency virus

- Organ transplants
- Dialysis.

Through bodily fluids:

- Blood products
- Semen
- Vaginal fluids
- Breast milk.

HIV is not Transmitted by Social Contacts.

Pathogenesis

- Primary HIV infection
- Initial viremia
- Dissemination of virus
- Establishment of chronic and persistent infection
- Advanced HIV disease.

Window Period

- It is the period before antibodies are produced in the blood stream.
- It is a seronegative infective stage.
- It is 2 to 12 weeks.
- During this period the person is infectious and he can infect others.

- Antibody test will be negative during this period.
- Infection can be detected by p24 antigen capture assay during this period.

Clinical Manifestations

- The acute HIV syndrome
- Asymptomatic stage
- Early symptomatic
- Opportunistic infection
- Orthopedic problem.

Four Stages of HIV

Stage 1: Primary

- Short, flu-like illness—occurs one to six weeks after infection
- No symptoms at all
- Infected person can infect other people.

Stage 2: Asymptomatic

- Lasts for an average of ten years
- This stage is free from symptoms
- There may be swollen glands
- The level of HIV in the blood drops to very low levels
- HIV antibodies are detectable in the blood.

Stage 3: Symptomatic

- The symptoms are mild
- The immune system deteriorates
- Emergence of opportunistic infections and cancers.

Stage 4: HIV—AIDS

- The immune system weakens
- The illnesses become more severe leading to an AIDS diagnosis.

Opportunistic Infections Associated with AIDS

- Bacterial
  - Tuberculosis (TB)
  - *Streptococcus pneumoniae*
- Viral
  - Kaposi sarcoma
  - Herpes
  - Influenza (flu)
- Parasitic
  - *Pneumocystis carinii*
- Fungal
  - *Candida*
  - *Cryptococcus*

Clinical Spectrum of HIV Infections

Two Major Signs Associated with atleast One Minor Sign

- Major signs
  - Weight loss of more than 10 percent of the body weight
  - Chronic diarrhea of more then 1 month
  - Prolonged fever of more than 1 month.
- Minor signs
  - Persistent cough of more than 1 month
  - Generalized pruritic dermatitis
  - Recurrent herpes zoster
  - Oropharyngeal candidiasis
  - Chronic disseminated and progressive herpes simplex infection
  - Generalized lymphadenopathy
  - Recurrent common infections
  - The presence of either Kaposi's sarcoma or cryptococcal meningitis alone is sufficient for the diagnosis.

Orthopedic Problems

- Rheumatoid arthritis
- Arthralgias
- Reactive arthritis
- AIDS associated arthropathy
- Fibromyalgia
- Septic arthritis.

HIV and Orthopedic Surgeon

Orthopedic surgery and HIV:

- Orthopedic and trauma surgeons are at a higher risk
- Power tools, screws and wires as well as bone spicules all contribute to the problem
- Routine testing is done for all undergoing surgery
- Patient should be convinced and consent taken
- His relationships should be fully informed
- It is unreliable after recent infection because serum conversion occurs 6 months or more after exposure
- Blood transfusion should be carefully done.

Trauma and the HIV Patient

The outcome of trauma in terms of union and complications has been greatly influenced by antiretroviral therapy.

Polytrauma

- Reported as a significant prognostic indicator for a worse outcome in acute injury and to the lung and adult respiratory distress syndrome intensive care
- Symptomatic HIV patient are more susceptible to secondary infection after polytrauma
- Impaired nutritional status will influence a negative outcome.

Closed Fracture

- Risk of wound infection after internal fixation, late sepsis around implants, union of the fracture and functional outcome
- Sepsis is the greatest fear, *Staphylococcus aureus* remains the most common

- Fungal and slow growing mycobacteria may occur
- Important determinants to infections are preoperative CD4 counts, wound healing and soft tissue handling
- Harrison—use of prophylactic antibiotics—first generation cephalosporins, a clean operating environment, strict operating theater discipline and careful soft tissue handling.

Compound Fractures

- Early debridement, prophylactic antibiotics and stabilization of the fracture with external fixator
- No risk of pin tract infection.

Fracture Union

- Increased risk of delayed union and nonunion
- Stable fixation can be achieved after stable internal fixation and autologus bone graft.

Implant Removal and Late Sepsis

- Risk of late sepsis around implants
- Some infections result in activation of latent bacteria.

Hemophiliacs and HIV

- Prone to bleeding around the joint
- Great risk of early degenerative arthropathy and require arthroplasty at an earlier age
- Bacteremia associated with their regular factor transfusions
- Increased rate of sepsis after arthroplasty.

Arthroplasty and HIV

- Degenerative arthropathy is uncommon
- They suffer from inflammatory arthropathy and avascular necrosis, sometime associated with antiretroviral therapy
- HIV patients are at a greater risk for late sepsis as well as aseptic loosening.

Cold Surgery

- Major surgery in HIV positive patients has increased risk of sepsis which rises steeply in those with physical signs
- Postoperative fevers and chest infection are also common.

Bone and Joint TB

- TB and HIV are synergistic and TB presents comparatively early in HIV
- Both are wasting disease with frequent night sweats
- Major surgery evokes serious postoperative complications
- Most respond to rest, food and drug therapy, prognosis is poor.

Other Musculoskeletal Infections

- Tropical pyomyositis, long bone hematogenous-osteomyelitis and late infections of orthopedic implants have become common presentations
- Signs—recent weight loss, skin and mouth signs of poor immune status and generalized lymphadenopathy
- They are usually anemic with high ESR and lymphopenia
- Postoperative complications are common.

Topical Pyomyositis

- Multiple abscesses and distal limb abscesses are particularly associated
- Adult long bone hematogenous osteomyelitis
- Common in African children
- Subacute onset and patients usually present with an abscess overlying the femoral or tibial metaphysis
- Bilateral infections are common and all four bones of the leg may be involved simultaneously.

Reactive Arthritis and Other Rheumatological Conditions

- Reactive arthritis is common Africa—related to outbreaks in rainy season
- Runs a more severe course with less chance of remission and poor response to therapy
- Knee and ankle joints are commonly affected.

Risks of Treating HIV—Positive Orthopedic Patients

- Risks at the operating table from patient to surgeon and vice versa is minimal
- HIV risks accumulate over a professional lifetime
- Most infective patient is one that is viremic from a newly acquired infection but still testing HIV negative
- In emergency situations there is no time to test the patients and most will carry no symptoms
- To be effective precautions must be universal
- Incisions are made larger and surgeons operate by sight rather than by feel
- No sharp instruments are handed directly between personnel
- Surgery may be more dangerous for an HIV positive patient, but there is little danger of the virus passing between the patients and surgeons as long as sensible precautions are universally applied.

Tuberculosis

- Dual epidemic
- HIV and TB are synergistic
- Wasting disease, night sweats
- Rest, food, drugs
- Prognosis poor.

Fractures

- Closed—heal normally with conservative treatment
- High infection rate with open reduction internal fixation.
- Open—infection and nonunion
- Surgery may promote clinical AIDS in seropositive patient.

Prevention

- Regular hand washing
- Cover wounds/skin lesions
- Protect eyes, mouth and nose
- Never transfer sharp objects directly
- Never recap a needle
- Proper disposal of sharp objects
- Consider every patient as a potential risk—stick to universal precautions.

Universal Precaution (Fig 38.2)

- Wear double gloves
- Plastic apron and water resistant shoe cover.
- Face shield and goggles
- Use no-touch technique
- Use a scalpel for skin incision then scissors and electrocautery
- Avoid simultaneous suture of same layer by two members of a team.

Precaution

- Put larger incision
- Operate by sight than feel
- No sharp instrument should be handed directly (Fig. 38.3)

Testing Options for HIV

Anonymous Testing

- No name is used
- Unique identifying number
- Results issued only to test recipient.

Confidential Testing

- Person's name is recorded along with HIV results
- Name and positive results are reported to the state department and the centers for disease control and prevention
- Results issued only to test recipient.

Administration

- Blood
- Urine
- Oral.

Blood Detection Tests

- Enzyme-linked immunosorbent assay/enzyme immunoassay (ELISA/EIA)
- Radio immunoprecipitation assay/indirect fluorescent antibody assay (RIP/IFA)
- Polymerase chain reaction (PCR)
- Western blot confirmatory test.

Urine Testing

- Urine western blot
- As sensitive as testing blood
- Safe way to screen for HIV
- Can cause false positives in certain people at high-risk for HIV.

Oral Testing

- Orasure
- The only FDA approved HIV antibody
- As accurate as blood testing
- Draws blood-derived fluids from the gum tissue.
- Not a saliva test!

Diagnosis

- Screening test—ELISA
- Confirmatory—Western blot
- Direct HIV detection:
  - P24 AG capture assay
  - HIV RNA by PCR.

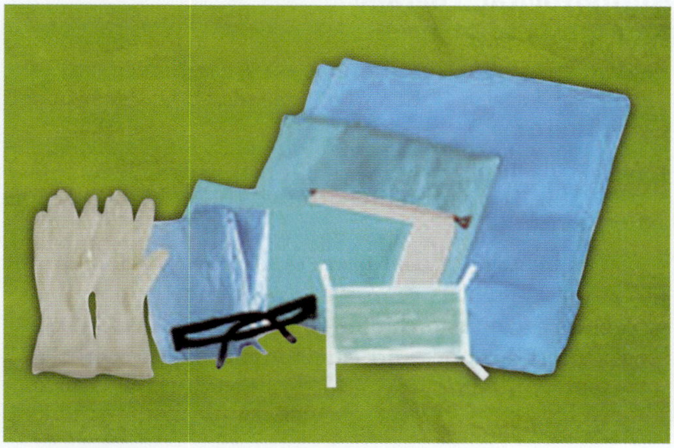

Fig 38.2: HIV surgery kit

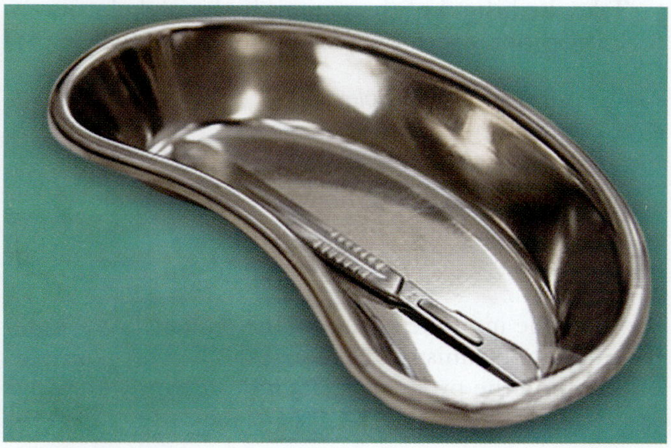

Fig. 38.3: Sharp instruments passed in kidney tray

Counseling

Pre-test counseling

- Transmission
- Prevention
- Risk factors
- Voluntary and confidential
- Reportability of positive test results.

Post-test counseling

- Clarifies test results
- Need for additional testing
- Promotion of safe behavior
- Release of results.

Needle Stick Injury

- Health care worker
- Risk of infection with a hollow bore needle prick – 0.3 percent
- Risk with suture needle is less.

Study Conducted by Center for Disease Control (CDC) on Needle Stick Injury

• Improper disposal of needle	27 percent
• During attempt to start IV line	23 percent
• During blood drawing	22 percent
• IM/SC injections	16 percent
• During giving IV infusion.	12 percent

Exposure

- Splash on the skin
- Wash thoroughly with soap and water
- Dip hands in undiluted savlon for 15 sec.
- Needle stick injury
- Let the wound bleed freely without pressing it
- Thoroughly wash
- Test the patient for HIV
- Test self at 3, 12 and 24 weeks.

Exposure

- If patient is negative follow-up at 3, 12, 24 weeks
- Take the history of the patient high-risk behavior
- Use condoms with the partner for 6 months.

Postexposure Drug Prophylaxis

- Azidothymidine
  - Within one hour of exposure
  - 200 mg q4h for 72 hours
  - 100 to 200 mg q4h for 25 days.

Strategies

- Boost the immune system of the patient
- Treat opportunistic infections
- Stopping the production of viral proteins with drugs
- Prevention of splicing
- Help the immune system.

Vaccine

Strategies

- Scientists have to make sure the vaccine itself does not make people ill
- HIV is constantly changing, so the defenses stimulated by a vaccine might not be effective in fighting the actual virus
- And if even a single virus escapes by hiding out inside a cell, it could go onto make thousands of copies of itself
- Artificial decoy CD4 units can be given
- HIV will attach to these instead of T cells
- Use of drugs that look like building blocks of DNA
- Prevent conversion of viral RNA into DNA
- HIV is constantly changing, and eventually it is no longer tricked by these faulty building blocks
- HIV becomes resistant to these drugs, and the life cycle continues the same as before
- Another problem is that these drugs can damage non-infected cells which also need to make DNA to reproduce
- Increased abdominal visceral fat is associated with reduced bone density in HIV-infected men with lipodystrophy
- Disrupted fat metabolism may account for HIV-related osteopenia
- Abnormal marrow or whole body fat metabolism may affect bone cell differentiation or the marrow cytokine environment in people with HIV-related lipodystrophy.

Antiretroviral Drugs

- Nucleoside analogues
- Protease inhibitors
- Non-nucleoside reverse transcriptase inhibitors.

Antiretroviral Therapy

- Triple therapy
- Two nucleosides and one protease inhibitor.

Conclusion

- Prevention of AIDS is our joint responsibility
- As there is no absolute curative therapy and vaccine for AIDS
- So education and awareness is only weapon in our hand
- Let us accept the challenge to fight against AIDS
- We must support and care for the people with HIV, AIDS with compassion and understanding.

Index

Page numbers followed by *'f'* refer to figure and *'t'* refer to table

B

D

E

G

H

M

N

O

P

Q

T